IMAGE-GUIDED INTERVENTIONS

OTHER VOLUMES IN THE EXPERT RADIOLOGY SERIES

IMAGE-GUIDED INTERVENTIONS

SECOND EDITION

MATTHEW A. MAURO, MD, FACR
The Ernest H. Wood Distinguished Professor of
Radiology and Surgery
Chairman, Department of Radiology
University of North Carolina School of Medicine
Chapel Hill, North Carolina

KIERAN P.J. MURPHY, MB, FRCPC, FSIR
Professor of Radiology
Joint Department of Medical Imaging
University Health Network
Mount Sinai Hospital
Women's College Hospital
Toronto, Ontario, Canada

KENNETH R. THOMSON, MD, FRANZCR
Professor of Radiology
Monash University Faculty of Medicine, Nursing, and
Health Sciences
Director, Radiology Department
Alfred Hospital
Melbourne, Victoria, Australia

ANTHONY C. VENBRUX, MD
Director, Cardiovascular and Interventional Radiology
George Washington University School of Medicine and
Health Sciences
Washington, DC

ROBERT A. MORGAN, MBChB, MRCP, FRCR, EBIR
Consultant, Vascular and Interventional Radiologist
Radiology Department
St. George's NHS Trust
London, United Kingdom

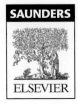

SAUNDERS

ELSEVIER

SAUNDERS

1600 John ~~F. Kennedy~~ Blvd.
Ste 1800
Philadelphia, PA 19103-2899

IMAGE-GUIDED INTERVENTIONS   ISBN: 978-1-4557-0596-2
(A Volume in the Expert Radiology Series)

Library of Congress Cataloging-in-Publication Data

Image-guided interventions / Matthew A. Mauro ... [et al.].—2nd ed.
       p. ; cm.—(Expert radiology series)
   Includes bibliographical references and index.
   ISBN 978-1-4557-0596-2 (hardcover : alk. paper)
   I. Mauro, Matthew A., 1951-   II. Series: Expert radiology series.
   [DNLM: 1. Radiography, Interventional–methods.   2. Diagnostic Techniques, Surgical.   3. Vascular Diseases–radiography.   4. Vascular Diseases–therapy.   5. Vascular Surgical Procedures–methods. WN 200]
   616.1′307572–dc23

                                                          2012046151

Content Strategist: Helene Caprari
Senior Content Development Specialist: Jennifer Shreiner
Publishing Services Manager: Anne Altepeter
Project Manager: Cindy Thoms
Design Direction: Steven Stave

Printed in China

Last digit is the print number: 9   8   7   6   5   4   3   2   1

To Pat, my wife, for her unwavering love and support and to our children, Lauren and David, my most precious accomplishments
Matt Mauro

To Rulan, my wife, Ronan and Anya, the three most interesting people I know in the world, thank you for allowing me the time and space to work on this book and all my other crazy ideas. To everyone who has taken the time to teach me, thank you for your patience
Kieran Murphy

To my wife, Barbara
Ken Thomson

To my family; to my patients, who have taught me so much; to my mentors; and to Michael Heinl
Tony Venbrux

To my family and friends for their forbearance, support, and good cheer over the years
Robert Morgan

Contributors

Hani H. Abujudeh, MD, MBA
Associate Professor of Radiology
Massachusetts General Hospital
Harvard Medical School
Boston, Massachusetts
Acute Lower Extremity Ischemia

Andreas Adam, PhD, FRCP, FRCS, FRCR
Professor
Department of Interventional Radiology
King's College
Consultant Radiologist
St. Thomas' Hospital
London, United Kingdom
*Esophageal Intervention in Malignant and Benign
    Esophageal Disease*

Allison S. Aguado, MD
Fellow
Department of Radiology
Memorial Sloan-Kettering Cancer Center
New York, New York
*Embolotherapy for the Management of Liver Malignancies
    Other Than Hepatocellular Carcinoma*

Muneeb Ahmed, MD
Assistant Professor of Radiology
Section of Interventional Radiology
Harvard Medical School
Beth Israel Deaconess Medical Center
Boston, Massachusets
*Image-Guided Thermal Tumor Ablation: Basic Science and
    Combination Therapies*

Kamran Ahrar, MD
Professor
Departments of Diagnostic Radiology and Thoracic and
    Cardivascular Surgery
University of Texas MD Anderson Cancer Center
Houston, Texas
Thermal Ablation of Renal Cell Carcinoma

Andrew Akman, MD
Assistant Professor of Radiology
Interventional Radiology
George Washington University School of Medicine and
    Health Sciences
Washington, DC
Management of Male Varicocele

Morvarid Alaghmand, MD
Internist
Riverside Primary Care Associates
District Heights, Maryland
Alimentary Tract Vasculature
Renal Vasculature

Ali Albayati, MBChB
Fellow
Division of Cardiovascular and Interventional Radiology
George Washington University Medical Center
Washington, DC
Principles of Intraprocedural Analgesics and Sedatives
Management of Male Varicocele

Agaicha Alfidja, MD
Faculty of Medicine
University Hospital
Clermont-Ferrand, France
Acute Mesenteric Ischemia

Ziyad Al-Otaibi, MD
Department of Anesthesiology and Critical Care Medicine
George Washington University Medical Canter
Washington, DC
Treatment of Medical Emergencies

John F. Angle, MD
Professor
Department of Radiology and Medical Imaging
Director
Division of Angiography and Interventional Radiology
University of Virgina Health System
Charlottesville, Virginia
Balloon Catheters
Closure Devices
Tracheobronchial Interventions

Gary M. Ansel, MD, FACC
Director, Center for Critical Limb Care
Riverside Methodist Hospital
Columbus, Ohio
Assistant Clinical Professor of Medicine
Medical University of Ohio
Toledo, Ohio
Chronic Upper Extremity Ischemia and Revascularization

Julien Auriol, MD
Praticien Hospitalier
Service de Radiologie
L'Hôpital Rangueil
Universitaire de Toulouse
Toulouse, France
Vascular Intervention in the Liver Transplant Patient

Chad Baarson, DO
Department of Radiology
National Capital Consortium
Walter Reed National Military Medical Canter
Bethesda, Maryland
Bipedal Lymphangiography

Juan Carlos Baez, MD
Resident
Department of Radiology
Brigham and Woman's Hospital
Boston, Massachusetts
Subarachnoid Hemorrhage
Image-Guided Intervention for Symptomatic Tarlov Cysts
Scalene Blocks and Their Role in Thoracic Outlet Syndrome

Curtis W. Bakal, MD, MPH
Chair, Radiology
Lahey Clinic
Burlington, Massachusetts
Professor of Radiology
Tufts University School of Medicine
Boston, Massachusetts
Diagnostic Catheters and Guidewires

Jörn O. Balzer, MD, PhD
Director
Department of Radiology and Nuclear Medicine
Catholic Clinic Mainz
Mainz, Germany
Endovascular Laser Therapy

Alex M. Barnacle, MRCP, FRCR
Consultant Interventional Radiologist
Department of Radiology
Great Ormond Street Hospital for Children
London, United Kingdom
Management of High-Flow Vascular Anomalies

Bradley P. Barnett, MD, PhD
Research Fellow
Department of Radiology
Johns Hopkins Medical Institutions
Baltimore, Maryland
Craniocervical Vascular Anatomy

Gamal Baroud, PhD
Professor
Department of Mechanical Engineering
Director, Biomechanics Laboratory
Canada Research Chair in Skeletal Reconstruction
University of Sherbrooke
Sherbrooke, Quebec, Canada
New Directions in Bone Materials

Carlo Bartolozzi, MD
Professor
Diagnostic and Interventional Radiology
University of Pisa
Pisa, Italy
Energy-Based Ablation of Hepatocellular Cancer

Jason R. Bauer, MD, RVT
Director of Interventional Oncology
Interventional and Vascular Consultants, PC
Portland, Oregon
Embolization Agents

Richard A. Baum, MD, MPA
Director, Interventional Radiology
The Herbert L. Abrams Director of Angiography and
   Interventional Radiology
Brigham and Women's Hospital
Associate Professor
Department of Radiology
Harvard Medical School
Boston, Massachusetts
Thoracic Duct Embolization for Postoperative Chylothorax

Kevin W. Bell, MBBS, FRANZCR
Clinical Associate Professor of Radiology
University of Melbourne Faculty of Medicine
Director
Department of Radiology
Western Health
Melbourne, Victoria, Australia
Vascular Anatomy of the Thorax, Including the Heart

Jacqueline A. Bello, MD
Professor
Departments of Radiology and Neurosurgery
Albert Einstein College of Medicine
Director of Neuroradiology
Department of Radiology
Montefiore Medical Center
Bronx, New York
Management of Head and Neck Tumors

Jennifer Berkeley, MD, PhD
Neurointensivist
Department of Neurology
Sinai Hospital of Baltimore
Baltimore, Maryland
Cervical Artery Dissection

Michael A. Bettmann, MD, FACR
Professor of Radiology Emeritus
Wake Forest University School of Medicine
Winston-Salem, North Carolina
Co-Chair
Task Force on Imaging Decision Support
American College of Radiology
Reston, Virginia
Contrast Agents

José I. Bilbao, MD, PhD
Professor of Radiology
Universidad de Navarra
Consultant Radiologist
Clínica Universitaria de Navarra
Pamplona, Spain
Portal-Mesenteric Venous Thrombosis

Deniz Bilecen, MD, PhD
Chief
Department of Radiology
Kantonsspital Laufen
Laufen, Switzerland
Transjugular Liver Biopsy

Tiago Bilhim, MD
Interventional Radiologist
Department of Radiology
St. Louis Hospital
Faculty of Medical Sciences
New University of Lisbon
Lisbon, Portugal
Treatment of High-Flow Priapism and Erectile Dysfunction

Christoph A. Binkert, MD, MBA
Chairman of Radiology
Institute of Radiology
Kantonsspital Winterthur
Winterthur, Switzerland
Inferior Vena Cava Filters
Caval Filtration

Haraldur Bjarnason, MD
Professor of Radiology
Division of Vascular and Interventional Radiology
Mayo Clinic
Rochester, Minnesota
Acute Lower Extremity Deep Venous Thrombosis

James H. Black, III, MD, FACS
Bertram M. Bernheim, MD Associate
Professor of Surgery
Johns Hopkins University School of Medicine
Baltimore, Maryland
Clinical Vascular Examination

Brian M. Block, MD, PhD
President
Baltimore Spine Center
Towson, Maryland
Instructor
Department of Anesthesiology and Critical Care Medicine
Johns Hopkins University School of Medicine
Baltimore, Maryland
Stellate Ganglion Block
Facet Joint Injection
Epidural Steroid Injection
Scalene Blocks and Their Role in Thoracic Outlet Syndrome

Marc Bohner, PhD
Material Science Engineer
Dr. Robert Mathys Foundation
Bettlach, Switzerland
New Directions in Bone Materials

Amman Bolia, MBChB, DMRD, FRCR
Consultant Vascular Radiologist
Departments of Imaging and Interventions
University Hospital of Leicester NHS Trust
Leicester, United Kingdom
Subintimal Angioplasty

Irene Boos, VMD
Clinical Research
Interventional Radiology
Woerth, Germany
Intraarterial Ports for Chemotherapy

Charles F. Botti, Jr., MD, FACC
Cardiac and Peripheral Vascular Interventionist
MidOhio Cardiology and Vascular Consultants
Riverside Methodist Hospital
Columbus, Ohio
Chronic Upper Extremity Ischemia and Revascularization

Nina M. Bowens, MD
General Surgery Resident
Department of Surgery
Hospital of the University of Pennsylvania
Philadelphia, Pennsylvania
Thoracic Aortic Stent-Grafting and Management of Traumatic Thoracic Aortic Lesions

Louis Boyer, MD, PhD
Professor of Radiology
Faculty of Medicine
ISIT, UMR CNRS 6284 University D'Auvergne
Head, Department of Radiology
University Hospital
Clermont-Ferrand, France
Acute Mesenteric Ischemia

Elena Bozzi, MD
Department of Diagnostic and Interventional Radiology
University of Pisa
Pisa, Italy
Energy-Based Ablation of Hepatocellular Cancer

Peter R. Bream, Jr., MD
Associate Professor
Departments of Radiology and Radiological Sciences and Medicine
Vanderbilt University School of Medicine
Director, PICC Service
Program Director, Interventional and Vascular Radiology
Vanderbilt University Medical Center
Nashville, Tennessee
Tunneled Central Venous Catheters

Rachel F. Brem, MD
Professor
Department of Radiology
George Washington University School of Medicine and
    Health Sciences
Director
Breast Imaging and Interventional Center
Vice Chair of Radiology
GW Medical Faculty Associates
Washington, DC
Minimally Invasive Image-Guided Breast Biopsy and Ablation

Mark F. Brodie, MD
Interventional Radiologist
Department of Radiology
Naval Medical Center
San Diego, California
Fallopian Tube Interventions

Allan L. Brook, MD
Associate Professor of Clinical Radiology and Neurosurgery
Departments of Radiology and Surgery
Albert Einstein College of Medicine
Bronx, New York
Director
Interventional Neuroradiology
Department of Radiology
Montefiore Medical Center
Brooklyn, New York
Management of Head and Neck Tumors

Benjamin S. Brooke, MD, PhD
Fellow
Vascular Surgery
Department of Surgery
Dartmouth-Hitchcock Medical Center
Lebanon, New Hampshire
Clinical Vascular Examination

Mark Duncan Brooks, MBBS, FRANZCR
Consultant Radiologist
Department of Radiology
Austin Hospital
Melbourne, Victoria, Australia
Transjugular Intrahepatic Portosystemic Shunts

Daniel B. Brown, MD
Director
Interventional Radiology
Department of Radiology
Thomas Jefferson University
Philadelphia, Pennsylvania
Management of Biliary Calculi

Karen T. Brown, MD, FSIR
Interventional Radiologist
Department of Medical Imaging
Memorial Sloan-Kettering Cancer Center
Professor of Clinical Radiology
Department of Radiology
Weill Cornell Medical College
New York, New York
Bland Embolization for Hepatic Malignancies

Jozef M. Brozyna, BS
West Virginia School of Osteopathic Medicine
Lewisburg, West Virginia
A Brief History of Image-Guided Therapy

Charles T. Burke, MD
Associate Professor
Department of Radiology
University of North Carolina School of Medicine
Chapel Hill, North Carolina
Management of Failing Hemodialysis Access
Hemodialysis Access: Catheters and Ports

James P. Burnes, MBBS, FRACR
Director
Body Intervention Unit
Department of Diagnostic Imaging
Monash Medical Centre Moorabbin
Southern Health
Clayton, Victoria, Australia
Endovascular Treatment of Peripheral Aneurysms

Patricia E. Burrows, MD
Professor of Radiology
Medical College of Wisconsin
Vascular Interventional Radiology
Children's Hospital of Wisconsin
Milwaukee, Wisconsin
Management of Low-Flow Vascular Malformations

Justin J. Campbell, MD
Staff Radiologist
Department of Radiology
South Shore Hospital
Weymouth, Massachusetts
Percutaneous Abscess Drainage Within the Abdomen and Pelvis
Renal and Perirenal Fluid Collection Drainage

**Colin P. Cantwell, MBBCh, BAO, Msc, MRCS,
FRCR, FFR(RCSI)**
Consultant Radiologist
Department of Radiology
St. Vincent's University Hospital
Dublin, Ireland
Peripherally Inserted Central Catheters and Nontunneled Central
    Venous Catheters

Thierry Carrères, MD
Cardio-vasculaire Radiologie
Hopital Européen Georges Pompidou
Paris, France
Infrapopliteal Revascularization

John A. Carrino, MD, MPH
Associate Professor of Radiology and Orthopedic Surgery
Section Chief, Musculoskeletal Radiology
The Russell H. Morgan Department of Radiology and
    Radiological Science
Johns Hopkins University
School of Medicine
Baltimore, Maryland
Image-Guided Percutaneous Biopsy of Musculoskeletal Lesions

Lucie Cassagnes, MD
Department of Radiology
University Hospital
Clemont-Ferrand, France
Acute Mesenteric Ischemia

Pascal Chabrot, MD, PhD
Faculty of Medicine
ISIT, UMR CNRS 6284 University D'Auvergne
Department of Radiology
University Hospital
Clermont-Ferrand, France
Acute Mesenteric Ischemia

Suma K. Chandra, MD
George Washington University Medical Center
Washington, DC
A Brief History of Image-Guided Therapy

Richard Chang, MD
Chief, Endocrine and Venous Services Section
Senior Clinician
Section of Interventional Radiology
National Institutes of Health
Bethesda, Maryland
*Arteriography and Arterial Stimulation with Venous Sampling
    for Localizing Pancreatic Endocrine Tumors*

Rishabh Chaudhari, BA
Medical Student
George Washington University School of Medicine and
    Health Sciences
Washington, DC
Renal Vasculature

Lakhmir S. Chawla, MD
Associate Professor
Department of Medicine
George Washington University Medical Center
Washington, DC
Treatment of Medical Emergencies

Hank K. Chen, MD
Section of Interventional Radiology
Department of Radiology
George Washington University Medical Center
Washington, DC
A Brief History of Image-Guided Therapy

Yung-Hsin Chen, MD
Assistant Clinical Professor of Radiology
Tufts University School of Medicine
Boston, Massachusetts
Image-Guided Percutaneous Biopsy of Musculoskeletal Lesions

Rush H. Chewning, MD
Chief Resident
Department of Radiology
University of Washington School of Medicine
Seattle, Washington
Endovascular Management of Epistaxis
Subarachnoid Hemorrhage

Albert K. Chun, MD
Assistant Professor of Radiology and Surgery
Division of Angiography and Interventional Radiology
George Washington University School of Medicine and
    Health Sciences
Washington, DC
Principles of Arterial Access

Joo-Young Chun, MMBS, BSc, MSc, MRCS, FBCR
Interventional Radiology Fellow
Department of Radiology
St. George's Hospital
London, United Kingdom
Aortic Endografting

Timothy W.I. Clark, MD, MSc, FRCP(C), FSIR
Associate Professor of Clinical Radiology
Department of Radiology
University of Pennsylvania School of Medicine
Philadelphia, Pennsylvania
Acute Upper Extremity Deep Venous Thrombosis
Management of Fluid Collections in Acute Pancreatitis
Chemical and Thermal Ablation of Desmoid Tumors

Wendy A. Cohen, MD
Professor of Radiology
University of Washington School of Medicine
Chief of Service
Department of Radiology
Harborview Medical Center
Seattle, Washington
Use of Skull Views in Visualization of Cerebral Vascular Anatomy

Bairbre Connolly, MB, FRCP(C)
Pediatric Interventional Radiologist
Department of Diagnostic Imaging
Hospital for Sick Children
Associate Professor
Medical Imaging Department
Earl Glenwood Coulson Chair
University of Toronto
Faculty of Medicine
Toronto, Ontario, Canada
Pediatric Gastrostomy and Gastrojejunostomy

Alison Corr, MBBCh, BSc
Faculty of Radiologists
Royal College of Surgeons
Dublin, Ireland
Percutaneous Biopsy of the Lung, Mediastinum, and Pleura

Anne M. Covey, MD, FSIR
Associate Professor of Radiology
Department of Diagnostic Radiology
Memorial Sloan-Kettering Cancer Center
New York, New York
Management of Malignant Biliary Tract Obstruction

Laura Crocetti, MD, PhD
Assistant Professor of Radiology
Department of Oncology, Transplants, and Advanced
    Technologies in Medicine
University of Pisa Faculty of Medicine
Pisa, Italy
Energy-Based Ablation of Hepatocellular Cancer

Charles D. Crum, MD
Neuroradiology Fellow
Department of Radiology
St. Joseph's Hospital and Medical Center
Phoenix, Arizona
Cryoablation of Liver Tumors

T. Andrew Currier, BSEE, LLB, P ENG
Barrister and Solicitor
Perry and Currier
Patent and Trademark Agents
Toronto, Ontario, Canada
Intellectual Property Management

Ferenc Czeyda-Pommersheim, MD
Resident in Radiology
Mallinckrodt Institute of Radiology
Washington University
Saint Louis, Missouri
Uterine Fibroid Embolization

Michael D. Dake, MD
Professor of Cardiothoracic Surgery
Stanford University School of Medicine
Director
Catheterization Angiography Laboratory
Stanford University Medical Center
Stanford, California
Balloon Catheters
*Endovascular Treatment of Dissection of the Aorta
    and Its Branches*

Michael D. Darcy, MD
Professor of Radiology
Washington University St. Louis
Chief of Intereventional Radiology
Mallinckrodt Institute of Radiology
Saint Louis, Missouri
Management of Lower Gastrointestinal Bleeding
Ambulatory Phlebectomy

Sean R. Dariushnia, MD
Assistant Professor of Radiology
Division of Interventional Radiology and
    Image-Guided Medicine
Emory School of Medicine
Atlanta, Georgia
Management of Extremity Vascular Trauma

**Robert S.M. Davies, MBChB, MRCS,
MMed, FRCS (England)**
Senior Clinical Fellow
British Society of Endovascular Therapy
Leicester, United Kingdom
Subintimal Angioplasty

Thierry de Baère, MD
Chief
Department of Interventional Radiology
Institut Gustave Roussy
Villejuif, France
Portal Vein Embolization
Intraarterial Ports for Chemotherapy

L. Mark Dean, MD
Interventional Radiologist
Riverside Methodist Hospital
Columbus, Ohio
Selective Nerve Root Block

Sudhen B. Desai, MD
Interventional Radiologist
Methodist Sugar Land Hospital
Houston, Texas
Percutaneous Biopsy
Treatment of Effusions and Abscesses

Massimiliano di Primio, MD
Division of Interventional Radiology
Hopital Européen Georges Pompidou
Paris, France
Infrapopliteal Revascularization

Robert G. Dixon, MD
Associate Professor
Department of Radiology
University of North Carolina School of Medicine
Chapel Hill, North Carolina
Subcutaneous Ports

Pablo D. Domínguez, MD
Department of Radiology
Clínica Universitaria de Navarra
Pamplona, Spain
Portal-Mesenteric Venous Thrombosis

Robert F. Dondelinger, MD, Hon FRCR
Professor and Chair
Department of Medical Imaging
University of Liège Faculty of Medicine
Liège, Belgium
Management of Trauma to the Liver and Spleen
Splenic Embolization in Nontraumatized Patients
Superior Vena Cava Occlusive Disease

Gregory J. Dubel, MD
Assistant Professor
Division of Vascular and Interventional Radiology
Warren Alpert Medical School
Brown University
Providence, Rhode Island
Stents

Damian E. Dupuy, MD, FACR
Professor
Department of Diagnostic Imaging
Warren Alpert Medical School
Brown University
Director of Tumor Ablation
Rhode Island Hospital
Providence, Rhode Island
Lung Ablation

Ghassan E. El-Haddad, MD
Assistant Member
Interventional Radiology
H. Lee Moffitt Cancer Center and Research Institute
Assistant Professor of Oncologic Sciences
University of South Florida
Tampa, Florida
Management of Renal Angiomyolipoma

Joseph P. Erinjeri, MD, PhD
Interventional Radiology Service
Memorial Sloan-Kettering Cancer Center
New York, New York
Chemical and Thermal Ablation of Desmoid Tumors

Clifford J. Eskey, MD
Assistant Professor
Department of Radiology
Dartmouth-Hitchcock Medical Center
Lebanon, New Hampshire
Vertebroplasty and Kyphoplasty

Thomas M. Fahrbach, MD
Radiology Fellow
Division of Interventional Radiology and
    Image-Guided Medicine
Emory School of Medicine
Atlanta, Georgia
Percutaneous Cholecystostomy

Ronald M. Fairman, MD
Clyde F. Barker-William Maul Measey Professor
Surgery
University of Pennsylvania School of Medicine
Chief of Vascular Surgery and Endovascular Therapy
University of Pennsylvania Health System
Philadelphia, Pennsylvania
*Thoracic Aortic Stent-Grafting and Management of Traumatic
    Thoracic Aortic Lesions*

Chieh-Min Fan, MD
Associate Director
Division of Angiography and Interventional Radiology
Brigham and Women's Hospital
Assistant Professor
Department of Radiology
Harvard Medical School
Boston, Massachusetts
Thoracic Duct Embolization for Postoperative Chylothorax

Mark A. Farber, MD
Associate Professor
Departments of Radiology and Surgery
Director
Heart and Vascular Center
University of North Carolina School of Medicine
Chapel Hill, North Carolina
Aortic Stent-Grafts
*Thoracic Aortic Stent-Grafting and Management of Traumatic
    Thoracic Aortic Lesions*

Laura M. Fayad, MD
Associate Professor of Radiology, Orthopedic Surgery, and
    Oncology
The Russell H. Morgan Department of Radiology and
    Radiological Science
Johns Hopkins University
School of Medicine
Baltimore, Maryland
Image-Guided Percutaneous Biopsy of Musculoskeletal Lesions

Dimitrios Filippiadis, MD, PhD
Consultant
Attikon University Hospital
Athens, Greece
Ablation and Combination Treatments of Bony Lesions
Sacroiliac Joint Injections

Kathleen R. Fink, MD
Assistant Professor of Neuroradiology
University of Washington School of Medicine
Seattle, Washington
*Use of Skull Views in Visualization of Cerebral
    Vascular Anatomy*

Sebastian Flacke, MD, PhD
Chief Interventional Radiology
Director of Non-Invasive Cardiovascular Imaging
Vice Chair, Department of Radiology
Lahey Clinic
Burlington, Massachusetts
Professor of Radiology
Tufts University Medical School
Boston, Massachusetts
Diagnostic Catheters and Guidewires

**Karen Flood, BMedSci, BMBS, MMedSciClinEd,
MRCS, FRCR**
Interventional Radiology Registrar
Department of Vascular Interventional Radiology
Leeds Teaching Hospitals NHS Trust
Leeds, United Kingdom
Principles of Venous Access

Matthew D. Forrester, MD
Resident
Department of Cardiothoracic Surgery
Stanford University School of Medicine
Stanford, California
*Endovascular Treatment of Dissection of the Aorta
and Its Branches*

Brian Funaki, MD
Professor
Department of Radiology
University of Chicago Pritzker School of Medicine
Section Chief
Division of Vascular and Interventional Radiology
University of Chicago Medical Center
Chicago, Illinois
Thombectomy Devices

Dimitri A. Gagarin, MD
Associate Professor of Medicine
Department of Internal Medicine
Virginia Commonwealth University
Richmond, Virginia
A Brief History of Image-Guided Therapy

Philippe Gailloud MD
Director
Division of Interventional Neuroradiology
Johns Hopkins Hospital
Baltimore, Maryland
*Craniocervical Vascular Anatomy
Arterial Anatomy of the Spine and Spinal Cord
Endovascular Management of Epistaxis*

Bhaskar Ganai, BSc(MedSci) Hons, MBChB, MRCS, FRCR
SpR in Radiology
Department of Interventional Radiology
Freeman Hospital
Newcastle upon Tyne, United Kingdom
Embolic Protection Devices

Debra A. Gervais, MD
Associate Professor
Department of Radiology
Harvard Medical School
Division Head
Abdominal Imaging and Intervention
Massachusetts General Hospital
Boston, Massachusetts
*Percutaneous Abscess Drainage Within the Abdomen and Pelvis
Renal and Perirenal Fluid Collection Drainage*

Jean-François H. Geschwind, MD
Professor
Departments of Radiology, Surgery, and Oncology
Johns Hopkins University School of Medicine
Director
Interventional Radiology Center
Director
Vascular and Interventional Radiology
Johns Hopkins Medical Institutions
Baltimore, Maryland
Radioembolization for Hepatocellular Carcinoma

Basavaraj V. Ghodke, MD
Associate Professor
Departments of Neuroradiology and Neurological Surgery
University of Washington School of Medicine
Director
Neuro-Interventional Radiology
Childrens Hospital and Research Center
Seattle, Washington
*Use of Skull Views in Visualization of Cerebral
Vascular Anatomy*

Brian B. Ghoshhajra, MD, MBA
Director
Clinical Cardiac Imaging
Department of Radiology
Massachusetts General Hospital
Boston, Massachusetts
Noninvasive Vascular Diagnosis

Mark F. Given, MD, BCh, BAO, AFRCSI, FFRCR
Consultant
Radiologist
Beaumont Hospital
Dublin, Ireland
*Anatomy of the Lower Limb
Acute Arterial Occlusive Disease of the Upper Extremity
Endovascular Treatment of Peripheral Aneurysms
Adrenal Venous Sampling
Parathyroid Venous Sampling
Percutaneous Biopsy of the Lung, Mediastinum, and Pleura*

Y. Pierre Gobin, MD, MS
Professor of Radiology
Neurosurgery Department
Weill Cornell Medical College
New York, New York
*Acute Stroke Management
Endovascular Management of Chronic Cerebral Ischemia*

S. Nahum Goldberg, MD
Professor
Department of Radiology
Harvard Medical School
Beth Israel Deaconess Medical Center
Boston, Massachusetts
Vice Chair
Research Department of Radiology
Hadassah Hebrew University Medical Center
Hadassah, Israel
*Image-Guided Thermal Tumor Ablation: Basic Science and
Combination Therapies*

Theodore S. Grabow, MD
Baltimore Spine Center and Maryland Pain Specialists
Adjunct Assistant Professor
Department of Anesthesiology and Critical Care Medicine
Johns Hopkins University School of Medicine
Baltimore, Maryland
*Facet Joint Injection
Epidural Steroid Injection*

Edward D. Greenberg, MD
Interventional Neuroradiology Fellow
Department of Radiology
Weill Cornell Medical College
New York-Presbyterian Hospital
New York, New York
Acute Stroke Management
Endovascular Management of Chronic Cerebral Ischemia

Bryan Grieme, MD
Medical Director
Interventional Radiology
St. Anthony Hospital
Oklahoma City, Oklahoma
Management of Male Varicocele

Gianluigi Guarnieri, MD
Neuroradiology Service
Cardarelli Hospital
Naples, Italy
Minimally Invasive Disk Interventions

Jeffrey P. Guenette, MD
Department of Diagnostic Imaging
Warren Alpert Medical School
Brown University
Providence, Rhode Island
Lung Ablation

Klaus D. Hagspiel, MD
Professor
Departments of Radiology, Medicine (Cardiology),
   and Pediatrics
Chief
Division of Noninvasive Cardiovascular Imaging
Department of Radiology and Medical Imaging
University of Virginia Health System
Charlottesville, Virginia
Balloon Catheters

Lee D. Hall, MD
Interventional Radiologist
Department of Radiology
Naval Medical Center
San Diego, California
Fallopian Tube Interventions

Danial K. Hallam, MD, MSc
Associate Professor
Departments of Radiology and Neurological Surgery
University of Washington School of Medicine
Seattle, Washington
*Use of Skull Views in Visualization of Cerebral
   Vascular Anatomy*

Mohomad Hamady, MBChB, FRCR
Consultant and Senior Lecturer
Department of Interventional Radiology
Imperial College
London, United Kingdom
Fenestrated Stent-Grafting of Juxtarenal Aortic Aneurysms

Stéphan Haulon, MD, PhD
Professor
Department of Vascular Surgery
Chief of Vascular Surgery
INSERM U1008, Université Lille Nord de France
Hôpital Cardiologique—CHRU
Lille, France
*Management of Thoracoabdominal Aneurysms by Branched
   Endograft Technology*

Klaus A. Hausegger, MD
Associate Professor and Head
Department of Radiology
Institute of Interventional and Diagnostic Radiology
Klagenfurt, Austria
Endoleaks: Classification, Diagnosis, and Treatment
Management of Biliary Leaks

Markus H. Heim, MD
Professor of Medicine
Department of Bioscience
University of Basel
Division of Gastroenterology and Hepatology
Department of Medicine
University Hospital Basel
Basel, Switzerland
Transjugular Liver Biopsy

Katharine Henderson, MS
Genetic Counselor
Yale School of Medicine
Co-Director
Yale HHT Center
New Haven, Connecticut
*Pulmonary Arteriovenous Malformations: Diagnosis
   and Management*

Robert C. Heng, MBBS, FRANZCR
Interventional Radiologist
Department of Radiology and Medical Imaging
Launceston General Hospital
Launceston, Tasmania, Australia
Vascular Anatomy of the Thorax, Including the Heart

Joshua A. Hirsch, MD
Associate Professor of Radiology
Harvard Medical School
Department of Radiology
Massachusetts General Hospital
Boston, Massachusetts
Vertebroplasty and Kyphoplasty

Andrew Hugh Holden, MBChB, FRANCZR
Associate Professor
Department of Radiology
Auckland University School of Medicine
Director
Body Imaging and Interventional Services
Auckland City Hospital
Auckland, New Zealand
Acute Renal Ischemia

Edward T. Horn, PharmD, BCPS
Clinical Pharmacy Specialist
Department of Pharmacy
Allegheny General Hospital
Pittsburgh, Pennsylvania
Vasoactive Agents

Joseph A. Hughes, MD
Fellow, Cardiovascular and Interventional Radiology
Department of Radiology
Pennsylvania State University College of Medicine
Penn State Hershey Medical Center
Hershey, Pennsylvania
Peripherally Inserted Central Catheters and Nontunneled Central Venous Catheters

Elizabeth A. Ignacio, MD
Associate Professor of Radiology
Division of Vascular and Interventional Radiology
George Washington University School of Medicine and Health Sciences
Washington, DC
Interventional Radiologist
Department of Radiology
Maui Memorial Medical Center
Wailuku, Hawaii
Vascular Anatomy of the Pelvis
Peripartum Hemorrhage

Zubin D. Irani, MD, MBBS
Instructor in Radiology
Harvard Medical School
Department of Medical Imaging
Massachusetts General Hospital
Boston, Massachusetts
Bronchial Artery Embolization

Roberto Izzo, MD
Neuroradiology Service
Carderelli Hospital
Naples, Italy

James E. Jackson, MBBS, FRCP, FRCR
Consultant Interventional Radiologist
Department of Imaging
Hammersmith Hospital
London, United Kingdom
Management of High-Flow Vascular Anomalies
Management of Visceral Aneurysms

Augustinus Ludwig Jacob, Prof MD
Professor
Department of Radiology
University of Basel
Head
Division of Interventional Radiology
Institute of Radiology
Basel, Switzerland
Transjugular Liver Biopsy

Abdel Aziz A. Jaffan, MD
Assistant Professor of Radiology
Division of Interventional Radiology and Image-Guided Medicine
Emory University School of Medicine
Atlanta, Georgia
Aortoiliac Revascularization

Priya Jagia, MD, DNB
Associate Professor
Department of Cardiac Radiology
All India Institute of Medical Sciences
New Delhi, India
Management of Vascular Arteritidies

Raagsudha Jhavar, MD
Special Volunteer
Urologic Oncology
National Cancer Institute
US National Institutes of Health
Bethesda, Maryland
Principles of Thrombolytic Agents

Francis Joffre, MD
Professeur
Service de Radiologie
L'Hôpital de Rangueil
Universitaire de Toulouse
Toulouse, France
Vascular Intervention in the Liver Transplant Patient

Matthew S. Johnson, MD
Professor
Departments of Radiology and Surgery
Indiana University School of Medicine
Indianapolis, Indiana
Restenosis

Amber Jones, CCRP
Senior Research Program Coordinator
Fellowship Program Coordinator
Endovascular Surgical Neuroradiology
Division of Interventional Neuroradiology
Johns Hopkins University School of Medicine
Baltimore, Maryland
Vascular Anatomy of the Upper Extremity
Abdominal Aorta and the Inferior Vena Cava

Verena Kahn, MD
Department of Diagnostic and Interventional Radiology
University of Frankfurt am Main
Frankfurt, am Main, Germany
Endovascular Laser Therapy

Özlem Tuğçe Kalayci, MD
Department of Radiology
Inonu University Medical Faculty
Malayta, Turkey
Congenital Vascular Anomalies: Classification and Terminology

Sanjeeva Prasad Kalva, MD
Assistant Radiologist
Department of Imaging
Massachusetts General Hospital
Assistant Professor
Department of Radiology
Harvard Medical School
Boston, Massachusetts
Noninvasive Vascular Diagnosis

Anthony W. Kam, MD, PhD
Assistant Professor
Department of Radiology
Johns Hopkins Medical Institutions
Baltimore, Maryland
*Arteriography and Arterial Stimulation with Venous Sampling
   for Localizing Pancreatic Endocrine Tumors*

Krishna Kandarpa, MD, PhD
Professor and Chair
Department of Radiology
University of Massachusetts School of Medicine
Adjunct Professor
Biomedical Engineering
Worcester Polytechnic Institute
Radiologist-in-Chief
Department of Radiology
University of Massachusetts Memorial Health Care
Worcester, Massachusetts
Acute Lower Extremity Ischemia

Zinvoy M. Katz, MD
Clinical Instructor
Division of Interventional Neuroradiology
Johns Hopkins University School of Medicine
Baltimore, Maryland
Carotid Revascularization

John A. Kaufman, MD, MS
Director
Dotter Interventional Institute
Oregon Health and Science University
Portland, Oregon
Invasive Vascular Diagnosis
Superior Vena Cava Occlusive Disease

Linda Kelahan, MD
Department of Radiology
Washington Hospital Center
Washington, DC
Bipedal Lymphangiography

Alexis D. Kelekis, MD, PhD, EBIR
Assistant Professor of Interventional Radiology
Second Radiology Department
Attikon University Hospital
University of Athens
Athens, Greece
Ablation and Combination Treatments of Bony Lesions
Sacroiliac Joint Injections

Frederick S. Keller, MD
Cook Professor
Dotter Interventional Institute
Oregon Health and Sciences University
Portland, Oregon
Bronchial Artery Embolization

Robert K. Kerlan, Jr., MD
Professor of Clinical Radiology and Surgery
Department of Radiology
University of California–San Francisco
San Francisco, California
Biliary Complications Associated with Liver Transplantation

David O. Kessel, MBBS, MA, MRCP, FRCR, EBIR
Consultant Radiologist
Department of Vascular Interventional Radiology
Leeds Teaching Hospitals NHS Trust
Leeds, United Kingdom
Principles of Venous Access

Ramy Khalil, MS
Department of Radiology
George Washington University School of Medicine and
   Health Sciences
Washington, DC
Renal Vasculature

Nadia J. Khati, MD
Associate Professor of Radiology
Abdominal Imaging Section
George Washington University Medical Center
Washington, DC
Alimentary Tract Vasculature
Renal Vasculature
Vascular Anatomy of the Pelvis

Neil M. Khilnani, MD
Associate Professor of Clinical Radiology
Division of Vascular and Interventional Radiology
Weill Cornell Medical College
Division of Cardiovascular and Interventional Radiology
New York-Presbyterian Hospital
New York, New York
Great Saphenous Vein Ablation
*Magnetic Resonance–Guided Focused Ultrasound Treatment of
   Uterine Leiomyomas*

Darren D. Kies, MD
Assistant Professor of Radiology
Department of Radiology and Imaging Sciences
Emory School of Medicine
Atlanta, Georgia
Management of Female Venous Congestion Syndrome

Hyun S. Kim, MD
Associate Professor of Radiology, Obstetrics and Gynecology,
   Hematology and Medical Oncology, and Surgery
Director
Interventional Radiology and Image-Guided Medicine
Department of Radiology and Imaging Sciences
Emory School of Medicine
Atlanta, Georgia
Management of Female Venous Congestion Syndrome
Percutaneous Cholecystostomy

Jin Hyoung Kim, MD, PhD
Assistant Professor
Department of Radiology
Asan Medical Center
University of Ulsan College of Medicine
Seoul, Republic of Korea
Intervention for Gastric Outlet and Duodenal Obstruction

Kyung Rae Kim, MD
Assistant Professor
Department of Radiology
University of North Carolina School of Medicine
Chapel Hill, North Carolina
Hemodialysis Access: Catheters and Ports

Hiro Kiyosue, MD
Associate Professor
Department of Radiology
Oita Medical University
Yufu, Oita, Japan
Retrograde Balloon Occlusion Variceal Ablation

Sebastian Kos, MD, EBIR
Chairman
Institute of Radiology and Nuclear Medicine
Lucerne, Switzerland
Transjugular Liver Biopsy

Jim Koukounaras, MBBS, FRANCZR
Interventional Radiologist
Department of Radiology
The Alfred Hospital
Melbourne, Victoria, Australia
Adrenal Venous Sampling

Andres Krauthamer, MD
Resident
Department of Diagnostic Radiology
George Washington University Medical Center
Washington, DC
Principles of Intraprocedural Analgesics and Sedatives
Vascular Anatomy of the Pelvis

Venkatesh Krishnasamy, MD
Interventional Radiology Fellow
Division of Vascular and Interventional Radiology
George Washington University School of Medicine and
    Health Sciences
Washington, DC
Vascular Anatomy of the Pelvis

William T. Kuo, MD
Associate Professor
Director, IR Fellowship Program
Division of Vascular and Interventional Radiology
Stanford University Medical Center
Stanford, California
Percutaneous Interventions for Acute Pulmonary Embolism

Max Kupershmidt, MBBS, FRANCZR, MMed (Radiology)
Director of Ultrasound
Barwon Medical Imaging
Geelong, Victoria, Australia
Treatment of High-Flow Priapism and Erectile Dysfunction

Vineel Kurli, MMBS
Vascular and Interventional Radiologist
Medical Diagnostic Imaging Group
Phoenix, Arizona
Acute Upper Extremity Deep Venous Thrombosis

Jeanne M. LaBerge, MD
Professor in Residence
Department of Radiology
University of California–San Francisco
San Francisco, California
Biliary Complications Associated with Liver Transplantation

Pierre-Yves Laffy, MD
Cardio-vasculaire Radiologie
Hopital Européen Georges Pompidou
Paris, France
Infrapopliteal Revascularization

Leo P. Lawler, MD, MBBS, BAO, FRCR
Assistant Professor of Radiology
The Russell H. Morgan Department of Radiology and
    Radiological Science
Johns Hopkins Medical Institutions
Baltimore, Maryland
Percutaneous Cholecystostomy

McKinley C. Lawson, MD, PhD
Resident
Diagnostic Radiology Department
University of Colorado–Denver
Anschutz Medical Center
Aurora, Colorado
Embolization Agents

Judy M. Lee, MD
Assistant Professor
Department of Obstetrics and Gynecology
Johns Hopkins University School of Medicine
Baltimore, Maryland
Management of Female Venous Congestion Syndrome

Michael J. Lee, M.Sc, FRCPI, FRCR, FFR(RCSI), FSIR, EBIR
Professor of Radiology
Consultant Interventional Radiologist
Beaumont Hospital
Professor of Radiology
Royal College of Surgeons in Ireland
Department of Radiology
Dublin, Ireland
Gastrostomy and Gastrojejunostomy

Thomas Lemettre, MD
Radiologue
Clinique Claude Bernard
Albi, France
Vascular Intervention in the Liver Transplant Patient

Riccardo Lencioni, MD, PhD
Associate Professor
Department of Radiology
University of Pisa Faculty of Medicine
Director
Division of Diagnostic Imaging and Intervention
Department of Hepatology and Liver Transplantation
Pisa University Hospital
Pisa, Italy
Energy-Based Ablation of Hepatocellular Cancer

Robert J. Lewandowski, MD
Associate Professor
Department of Radiology
Feinberg School of Medicine
Chicago, Illinois
Radioembolization of Liver Metastases
Percutaneous Biopsy
Treatment of Effusions and Abscesses

John J. Lewin, III, PharmD, MBA, BCPS
Division Director
Critical Care and Surgery
Department of Pharmacy
Johns Hopkins Hospital
Adjunct Assistant Professor
Department of Anesthesiology and Critical Care Medicine
Johns Hopkins University School of Medicine
Baltimore, Maryland
Vasoactive Agents

Curtis A. Lewis, MD, MBA, JD
Assistant Professor of Radiology
Division of Interventional Radiology and
   Image-Guided Medicine
Emory School of Medicine
Atlanta, Georgia
Management of Extremity Vascular Trauma

Changqing Li, MB
Interventional Radiologist
Department of Radiology
Beijing Ditan Hospital
Beijing, China
Transjugular Intrahepatic Portosystemic Shunts

Eleni A. Liapi, MD
Instructor
Interventional Radiology Department
Johns Hopkins Medical Institutions
Baltimore, Maryland
Radioembolization for Hepatocellular Carcinoma

Yean L. Lim, MD, PhD
Professorial Fellow
Department of Cardiology
University of Melbourne Faculty of Medicine
Professor and Director
Centre for Cardiovascular Therapeutics
Western Health
Melbourne, Victoria, Australia
Director
Raffles Heart Hospital
Changhi, Singapore
Permanent Secretary
Asian Pacific Society of Interventional Cardiology
Wanchai, Hong Kong
Vascular Anatomy of the Thorax, Including the Heart

Raymond W. Liu, MD
Assistant Radiologist
Division of Vascular Imaging and Intervention
Massachusetts General Hospital
Boston, Massachusetts
Acute Lower Extremity Ischemia

Rafael H. Llinas, MD
Associate Professor
Department of Neurology
Johns Hopkins University School of Medicine
Clinical Vice Chair of Neurology
Johns Hopkins Hospital
Baltimore, Maryland
Cerebral Functional Anatomy and Rapid Neurological Examination

Reinhard Loose, MD, PhD
Department of Diagnostic and Interventional Radiology
Klinikum Nürmberg-Nord
Nürmberg, Bavaria, Germany
Angioplasty

Stuart M. Lyon, MBBS, FRNZCR
Adjunct Clinical Associate Professor
Department of Surgery
Central Clinical School
Monash University
Director of Interventional Radiology
Alfred Hospital
Melbourne, Victoria, Australia
Acute Arterial Occlusive Disease of the Upper Extremity
Endovascular Treatment of Peripheral Aneurysms
Percutaneous Biopsy of the Lung, Mediastinum, and Pleura

Sumaira Macdonald, MBChB, FRCR, PhD, EBIR
Consultant
Vascular Radiologist
Department of Interventional Radiology
Freeman Hospital
Newcastle upon Tyne
United Kingdom
Embolic Protection Devices

Patrick C. Malloy, MD
Chairman
Department of Radiology
VA New York Harbor Healthcare System
New York, New York
Management of Pelvic Hemorrhage in Trauma

Mark D. Mamlouk, MD
Department of Radiological Sciences
University of California–Irvine
Orange, California
Cryoablation of Liver Tumors

Michael J. Manzano, MD
Radiologist
Private Practice
Pittsford, New York
Alimentary Tract Vasculature

Marie Agnès Marachet, MD
Praticien Hospitalier
Service de Radiologie
L'Hôpital de Rangueil
Universitaire de Toulouse
Toulouse, France
Vascular Intervention in the Liver Transplant Patient

Jean-Baptiste Martin, MD
Associate Radiologist
Radiology Department
Geneva University Hospital
Geneva, Switzerland
Ablation and Combination Treatments of Bony Lesions

Antonio Martínez-Cuesta, MD, MSc, FRCR
Department of Radiology
Hospital de Navarra
Pamplona, Spain
Portal-Mesenteric Venous Thrombosis

M. Victoria Marx, MD
Professor of Clinical Radiology
Radiology Keck School of Medicine
University of Southern California
Los Angeles, California
Radiation Safety and Protection in the Interventional Fluoroscopy Environment

Surena F. Matin, MD
Associate Professor
Department of Urology
University of Texas
MD Anderson Cancer Center
Houston, Texas
Thermal Ablation of Renal Cell Carcinoma

Alan H. Matsumoto, MD, FSIR, FACR, FAHA
Professor and Chair
Department of Radiology
University of Virginia School of Medicine
Division of Interventional Radiology, Angiography, and Special Procedures
Department of Radiology and Medical Imaging
University of Virginia Health System
Charlottesville, Virginia
Balloon Catheters
Closure Devices
Chronic Mesenetric Ischemia
Tracheobronchial Interventions

Matthew A. Mauro, MD, FACR
The Ernest H. Wood Distinguished Professor of Radiology and Surgery
Chairman, Department of Radiology
University of North Carolina School of Medicine
Chapel Hill, North Carolina
Percutaneous Management of Chronic Lower Extremity Venous Occlusive Disease

Gordon McLennan, MD, FISR
Department of Diagnostic Radiology
Cleveland Clinic Foundation
Cleveland, Ohio
Restenosis

Simon J. McPherson, MRCP, FRCR
Consultant
Vascular and Interventional Radiologist
Department of Radiology
Leeds General Infirmary
Leeds, United Kingdom
Management of Upper Gastrointestinal Hemorrhage

Khairuddin Memon, MD
Clinical Research Associate
Department of Radiology
Feinberg School of Medicine
Chicago, Illinois
Radioembolization of Liver Metastases

Steven G. Meranze, MD
Professor of Radiology and Surgery
Vice-Chair
Department of Radiology and Radiological Science
Vanderbilt University School of Medicine
Nashville, Tennessee
Percutaneous Nephrostomy, Cystostomy, and Nephroureteral Stenting

Todd S. Miller, MD
Faculty
Department of Interventional Neuroradiology
Montefiore Medical Center
Assistant Professor of Clinical Radiology
Department of Radiology
Albert Einstein College of Medicine
Bronx, New York
Management of Head and Neck Tumors

Robert J. Min, MD, MBA
Chairman of Radiology
Weill Cornell Medical College
Radiologist-in-Chief
New York-Presbyterian Hospital
New York, New York
Great Saphenous Vein Ablation

Sally E. Mitchell, MD, FISR, FCIRSE
Professor of Radiology, Surgery, and Pediatrics
Division of Interventional Radiology
Johns Hopkins Hospital
Baltimore, Maryland
Congenital Vascular Anomalies: Classification and Terminology
Urodynamics

Stephan Moll, MD
Associate Professor
Department of Medicine
Division of Hematology-Oncology
University of North Carolina School of Medicine
Chapel Hill, North Carolina
Antiplatelet Agents and Anticoagulants

Robert A. Morgan, MBChB, MRCP, FRCR, EBIR
Consultant, Vascular and Interventional Radiologist
Radiology Department
St George's NHS Trust
London, United Kingdom
Aortic Endografting

Hiromu Mori, MD
Professor and Chairperson
Department of Radiology
Oita Medical University
Yufu, Oita, Japan
Retrograde Balloon Occlusion Variceal Ablation

Paul R. Morrison, MS
Medical Physicist
Department of Radiology
Harvard Medical School
Brigham and Women's Hospital
Boston, Massachusetts
Cryoablation of Liver Tumors

Stefan Müller-Hülsbeck, MD, EBIR, FCIRSE, FICA
Professor of Radiology
Head
Department of Diagnostic and Interventional
    Radiology/Neuroradiology
Ev.-Luth. Diakonissenanstalt zu Flensburg
Flensburg, Germany
Atherectomy Devices

Kieran P.J. Murphy, MB, FRCPC, FSIR
Professor of Radiology
Joint Department of Medical Imaging
University Health Network
Mount Sinai Hospital
Women's College Hospital
Toronto, Ontario, Canada
Endovascular Management of Epistaxis
Subarachnoid Hemorrhage
Image-Guided Intervention for Symptomatic Tarlov Cysts
Scalene Blocks and Their Role in Thoracic Outlet Syndrome

Timothy P. Murphy, MD, FSIR, FAHA, FSVB, FACR
Professor
Department of Diagnostic Imaging
Warren Alpert Medical School
Brown University
Director
Vascular Disease Research Center
Department of Diagnostic Imaging
Rhode Island Hospital
Providence, Rhode Island
Stents
Aortoiliac Revascularization

Mario Muto, MD
Chair of Neuroradiology Service
Carderelli Hospital
Naples, Italy
Minimally Invasive Disk Interventions
Periradicular Therapy

Albert A. Nemcek, Jr., MD
Professor
Department of Radiology
Feinberg School of Medicine
Staff Interventional Radiologist
Northwestern Memorial Hospital
Chicago, Illinois
Percutaneous Biopsy
Treatment of Effusions and Abscesses

David B. Nicholson, C-RT
Radiologic Technologist
Department of Radiology
University of Virginia School of Medicine
Charlottesville, Virginia
Balloon Catheters

Ali Noor, MD
Department of Radiology
Mount Sinai Medical Center
New York, New York
Renal Vasculature
Bipedal Lymphangiography

Philippe Otal, MD
Professeur
Service de Radiologie
L'Hôpital Rangueil
Universitaire de Toulouse
Toulouse, France
Vascular Intervention in the Liver Transplant Patient

Randall P. Owen, MD
Department of Otolaryngology-Head and Neck Surgery
Mount Sinai Medical Center
New York, New York
Management of Head and Neck Tumors

Auh Whan Park, MD
Associate Professor
Department of Radiology
University of Virginia Medical Center
Charlottesville, Virginia
Closure Devices
Tracheobronchial Interventions

David A. Pastel, MD
Assistant Professor
Department of Radiology
Dartmouth-Hitchcock Medical Center
Lebanon, New Hampshire
Vertebroplasty and Kyphoplasty

Aalpen A. Patel, MD
Vice Chair
Clinical Operations
System Radiology
Geisinger Health System
Danville, Pennsylvania
Management of Clotted Hemodialysis Access Grafts

Rafiuddin Patel, MBChB (Honours), MRCS, FRCR
SpR in Interventional Radiology
Department of Vascular Radiology
Leeds General Infirmary
Leeds, United Kingdom
Management of Upper Gastrointestinal Hemorrhage

Monica Smith Pearl, MD
Assistant Professor of Radiology
Division of Interventional Neuroradiology
Johns Hopkins Hospital
Baltimore, Maryland
Director of Pediatric Neurointervention
Department of Radiology
Children's National Medical Center
Washington, DC
Vascular Anatomy of the Upper Extremity
Abdominal Aorta and the Inferior Vena Cava

Olivier Pellerin, MD, MSc
Faculté de Médecine
Université Paris Descartes
Sorbonne Paris-Cité
Paris, France
Infrapopliteal Revascularization

Daniel D. Picus, MD
Professor
Departments of Radiology and Surgery
Washington University School of Medicine
Chief
Division of Diagnostic Radiology
Interventional Radiology Section
Mallinckrodt Institute of Radiology
Barnes-Jewish Hospital
Saint Louis, Missouri
Management of Biliary Calculi

João M. Pisco, MD
Professor and Chair
Department of Radiology
Centro Hospitalar Lisboa Norte EPE Hospital
Pulido Valente, Lisbon, Portugal
Treatment of High-Flow Priapism and Erectile Dysfunction

Jeffrey S. Pollak, MD
Professor of Radiology
Co-Section Chief
Division of Vascular and Interventional Radiology
Department of Diagnostic Radiology
Yale School of Medicine
New Haven, Connecticut
Pulmonary Arteriovenous Malformations: Diagnosis and Management

Rupert H. Portugaller, MD
Associate Professor
Department of Vascular and Interventional Radiology
University Clinic of Radiology
Medical University Graz
Graz, Austria
Management of Biliary Leaks

Sarah Power, MD
Resident
Department of Radiology
Beaumont Hospital
Dublin, Ireland
Gastrostomy and Gastrojejunostomy

Denis Primakov, MD
Interventional Radiologist
Walter Reed National Military Medical Center
Assistant Professor of Radiology and Radiological Sciences
Uniformed Services University of the Health Sciences
Bethesda, Maryland
Bipedal Lymphangiography

David S. Pryluck, MD
Fellow
Vascular and Interventional Radiology
Department of Radiology
University of Pennsylvania School of Medicine
Philadelphia, Pennsylvania
Acute Upper Extremity Deep Venous Thrombosis
Management of Fluid Collections in Acute Pancreatitis
Chemical and Thermal Ablation of Desmoid Tumors

Martin G. Radvany, MD
Assistant Professor of Radiology,
    Neurological Surgery, and Neurology
Division of Interventional Neuroradiology
Johns Hopkins University School of Medicine
Baltimore, Maryland
Carotid Revascularization

Batya R. Radzik, MSN, CRNP, BC
Nurse Practitioner
Neurocritical Care
Department of Anesthesia and Critical Care Medicine
Johns Hopkins Hospital
Baltimore, Maryland
Cerebral Functional Anatomy and Rapid
    Neurological Examination

Suman Rathbun, MD, MS, RVT
Professor
Department of Medicine
University of Oklahoma Health Sciences Center
Oklahoma City, Oklahoma
Management of Risk Factors for Peripheral Artery Disease

Anne Ravel, MD
Faculty of Medicine
University Hospital
Clermont-Ferrand, France
Acute Mesenteric Ischemia

Charles E. Ray, Jr., MD, PhD
Professor and Vice-Chair of Research
Department of Radiology
Chief
Division of Interventional Radiology
University of Colorado–Denver
Anschutz Medical Center
Aurora, Colorado
Embolization Agents

Mahmood K. Razavi, MD
Director
Center for Clinical Trials and Research
Heart and Vascular Center
St. Joseph Hospital
Orange, California
Endovascular Management of Chronic Femoropopliteal Disease

Aaron Reposar
Medical Student
George Washington University School of Medicine and
    Health Sciences
Washington, DC
Renal Vasculature

Anne Roberts, MD
Professor
Department of Radiology
University of California–San Diego
Chief, Vascular and Interventional Radiology
UCSD Medical Center
Department of Radiology
VA Medical Center
San Diego, California
Surveillance of Hemodialysis Access

Alain Roche, MD
Professor and Chief
Department of Medical Imaging
Institut Gustave Roussy
Villejuif, France
Director
Laboratory UPRES EA 4040
Department of Interventional Radiology
University of Paris South
Paris, France
Portal Vein Embolization

Hervé Rousseau, MD
Professeur et Chef de service
Service de Radiologie L'Hôpital
Rangueil Universitaire de Toulouse
Toulouse, France
Vascular Intervention in the Liver Transplant Patient

Stefan G. Ruehm, MD, PhD
Professor
Department of Radiological Sciences
David Geffen School of Medicine at UCLA
University of California–Los Angeles
Director
Cardiovascular Imaging
Santa Monica-UCLA Medical Center and Orthopedic Hospital
Los Angeles, California
Clinical Manifestations of Lymphatic Disease

Diego San Millán Ruiz, MD
Neuroradiologist
Department of Diagnostic and Interventional Radiology
Hospital of Sion
Sion, Switzerland
Craniocervical Vascular Anatomy

John H. Rundback, MD, FAHA, FSVM, FSIR
Medical Director
Interventional Institute
Holy Name Medical Center
Teaneck, New Jersey
Renovascular Intervention
Chemical Ablation of Liver Lesions

Wael E.A. Saad, MD, FSIR
Associate Professor of Radiology
Division of Angiography and Interventional Radiology
University of Virginia School of Medicine
Charlottesville, Virginia
Balloon Catheters
Management of Postcatheterization Pseudoaneurysms
Management of Benign Biliary Strictures

Tarun Sabharwal, MBChB, FRCSI, FRCR
Consultant
Interventional Radiologist and Honorary Senior Lecturer
Department of Radiology
Guy's and St. Thomas' Hospital
London, United Kingdom
Esophageal Intervention in Malignant and Benign Esophageal Disease

Riad Salem, MD, MBA
Professor
Departments of Radiology, Medicine (Hematology-Oncology), and Surgery
Feinberg School of Medicine
Director
Interventional Oncology
Robert H. Lurie Comprehensive Cancer Center
Northwestern Memorial Hospital
Chicago, Illinois
Radioembolization of Liver Metastases

Marc Sapoval, MD, PhD
Head
Division of Interventional Radiology
Hopital Européen Georges Pompidou
Paris, France
Infrapopliteal Revascularization

Shawn N. Sarin, MD
Assistant Professor
Departments of Radiology and Surgery
Section of Vascular and Interventional Radiology
George Washington University Medical Center
Washington, DC
Balloon Catheters
Angioplasty

Matthew P. Schenker, MD
Associate Radiologist
Division of Angiography and Interventional Radiology
Brigham and Women's Hospital
Boston, Massachusetts
Thoracic Duct Embolization for Postoperative Chylothorax

Marc H. Schiffman, MD
Assistant Professor of Radiology
Division of Interventional Radiology
New York Hospital
Weill Cornell Medical College
New York, New York
Magnetic Resonance–Guided Focused Ultrasound Treatment of Uterine Leiomyomas

Sanjiv Sharma, MD
Professor
Department of Cardiac Radiology
All India Institute of Medical Sciences
New Delhi, India
Management of Vascular Arteritidies

Ji Hoon Shin, MD, PhD
Associate Professor
Department of Radiology
University of Ulsan College of Medicine
Research Institute of Radiology
Asan Medical Center
Seoul, Korea
Tracheobronchial Interventions

H. Omur Sildiroglu, MD
Department of Radiology and Medical Imaging
University of Virginia Health System
Charlottesville, Virginia
Chronic Mesenteric Ischemia

Naomi N. Silva, MD
Resident
Department of Radiology
Robert Wood Johnson
University Hospital
New Brunswick, New York
Vascular Anatomy of the Pelvis

Stuart G. Silverman, MD
Professor
Department of Radiology
Harvard Medical School
Director of Abdominal Imaging and Intervention
Brigham and Women's Hospital
Boston, Massachusetts
Cryoablation of Liver Tumors

Charan K. Singh, MMBS
Assistant Professor of Radiology
Department of Diagnostic Imaging and Therapeutics
University of Connecticut School of Medicine
Farmingham, Connecticut
Acute Upper Extremity Deep Venous Thrombosis
Management of Fluid Collections in Acute Pancreatitis

Tony P. Smith, MD
Professor
Department of Radiology
Duke University School of Medicine
Division Chief
Peripheral and Neurological Interventional Radiology
Department of Radiology
Duke University Medical Center
Durham, North Carolina
Antibiotic Prophylaxis in Interventional Radiology

Constantinos T. Sofocleous, MD, PhD, FSIR
Interventional Radiologist
Department of Radiology
Memorial Sloan-Kettering Cancer Center
New York, New York
Embolotherapy for the Management of Liver Malignancies Other Than Hepatocellular Carcinoma

Luigi Solbiati, MD
University of Milan
Postgraduate Medical School
Milan, Italy
Department of Radiology and Interventional Radiology
Busto Arsizio General Hospital
Busto Arsizio, Italy
Energy-Based Ablation of Other Liver Lesions

Stephen B. Solomon, MD
Chief
Interventional Radiology
Service Director
Center for Image-Guided Intervention
Memorial Sloan-Kettering Cancer Center
New York, New York
*Magnetic Resonance–Guided Focused Ultrasound Treatment of
Uterine Leiomyomas*

Ho-Young Song, MD, PhD
Professor
Department of Radiology
Asan Medical Center
University of Ulsan College of Medicine
Seoul, Republic of Korea
Intervention for Gastric Outlet and Duodenal Obstruction

Kean H. Soon, MMBS, PhD, FRACP, FCSANZ
Interventional Cardiologist
Centre for Cardiovascular Therapeutics
Western Hospital
Melbourne, Victoria, Australia
Vascular Anatomy of the Thorax, Including the Heart

David R. Sopko, MD
Associate
Department of Radiology
Duke University School of Medicine
Durham, North Carolina
Antibiotic Prophylaxis in Interventional Radiology

Thomas A. Sos, MD
Professor
Department of Radiology
Weill Cornell Medical College
New York-Presbyterian Hospital
New York, New York
Renal Vein Renin Sampling

Michael C. Soulen, MD, FSIR, FCIRSE
Professor of Radiology
Department of Interventional Radiology
University of Pennsylvania School of Medicine
Philadelphia, Pennsylvania
Chemoembolization for Hepatocellular Carcinoma

James B. Spies, MD, MPH
Professor and Chair
Department of Radiology
Georgetown University Hospital
Washington, DC
Uterine Fibroid Embolization

Stavros Spiliopoulos, MD, PhD, EBIR
Board Certified Interventional Radiologist
Department of Interventional Radiology
Patras University Hospital
Rion, Greece
*Esophageal Intervention in Malignant and Benign
Esophageal Disease*

M.J. Bernadette Stallmeyer, MD, PhD
Director
Division of Interventional Neuroradiology
Reading Hospital and Medical Center
West Reading, Pennsylvania
Management of Head and Neck Injuries

Joseph M. Stavas, MD
Professor
Department of Radiology
University of North Carolina School of Medicine
Chapel Hill, North Carolina
Biopsy Devices

LeAnn S. Stokes, MD
Assistant Professor
Department of Radiology and Radiological Sciences
Vanderbilt University Medical Center
Nashville, Tennessee
*Percutaneous Nephrostomy, Cystostomy, and
Nephroureteral Stenting*

Ernst-Peter Strecker, MD
Professor Emeritus
Consultant Physician
Department of Diagnostic and Interventional Radiology
Trudpert Klinikum Pforzheim
Pforzheim, Germany
Intraarterial Ports for Chemotherapy

Michael B. Streiff, MD
Associate Professor of Medicine
Department of Medicine (Hematology)
Johns Hopkins Medical Institutions
Baltimore, Maryland
Principles of Thrombolytic Agents

Deepak Sudheendra, MD
Assistant Professor of Clinical Radiology and Surgery
University of Pennsylvania School of Medicine
Division of Interventional Radiology
Hospital of the University of Pennsylvania
Philadelphia, Pennsylvania
Management of Renal Angiomyolipoma
Thermal Ablation of the Adrenal Gland

Paul V. Suhocki, MD
Associate Professor
Department of Radiology
Duke University Medical Center
Durham, North Carolina
Foreign Body Retrieval

Alfonso Tafur, MD, RPVI
Assistant Professor of Medicine
Department of Vascular Medicine
Oklahoma University Health and Science Center
Oklahoma City, Oklahoma
Management of Risk Factors for Peripheral Artery Disease

M. Reza Taheri, MD, PhD
Assistant Professor
Department of Radiology
George Washington University School of Medicine and
    Health Sciences
Washington, DC
Use of Skull Views in Visualization of Cerebral Vascular Anatomy

Jeff Dai-Chee Tam, MBBS, FRANCZR
Fellow
Interventional Radiology
Department of Radiology
Alfred Hospital
Melbourne, Victoria, Australia
Anatomy of the Lower Limb
Acute Arterial Occlusive Disease of the Upper Extremity
Parathyroid Venous Sampling

Elizabeth R. Tang, MD
Resident
Department of Radiology
Boston University
Boston, Massachusetts
Management of Head and Neck Tumors

Emily M. Tanski, PA-C
Physicians Assistant
Division of Vascular and Interventional Radiology
George Washington University School of Medicine
Washington, DC
Vascular Anatomy of the Pelvis
Management of Male Varicocele

Kiang Hiong Tay, MBBS, FRCR, FAMS, FSIR
Head and Senior Consultant
Department of Diagnostic Radiology
Singapore General Hospital
Associate Professor of Radiology
Duke NUS Graduate Medical School
Yong Loo Lin School of Medicine
National University of Singapore
Chairman
Cardiovascular and Interventional Radiology Subsection
Singapore Radiological Society
Honorary Secretary
College of Radiologists
Singapore
Peripartum Hemorrhage

Aylin Tekes, MD
Assistant Professor
Department of Radiology
Johns Hopkins University School of Medicine
Radiologist
Division of Pediatric Radiology
Johns Hopkins Hospital
Baltimore, Maryland
Congenital Vascular Anomalies: Classification and Terminology

Matthew M. Thompson, MD, FRCS
Professor of Vascular Surgery
St. George's Vascular Institute
St. George's Hospital
London, United Kingdom
Aortic Endografting

Kenneth R. Thomson, MD, FRANZCR
Adjunct Clinical Professor of Radiology
Department of Surgery
Central Clinical School
Monash University
Program Director
Department of Radiology and Nuclear Medicine
Alfred Hospital
Melbourne, Victoria, Australia
Anatomy of the Lower Limb
Acute Arterial Occlusive Disease of the Upper Extremity
Endovascular Treatment of Peripheral Aneurysms
Treatment of High-Flow Priapism and Erectile Dysfunction
Adrenal Venous Sampling
Parathyroid Venous Sampling
Percutaneous Biopsy of the Lung, Mediastinum, and Pleura

Raymond H. Thornton, MD
Vice Chair for Quality, Safety, and Performance Improvement
Department of Radiology
Division of Interventional Radiology
Memorial Sloan-Kettering Cancer Center
New York, New York
Management of Malignant Biliary Tract Obstruction

Emily J. Timmreck, RN, MSN, ACNP-BC
Nurse Practitioner
Division of Vascular and Interventional Radiology
George Washington University School of Medicine
Washington, DC
Vascular Anatomy of the Pelvis
Management of Male Varicocele

Jessica Torrente, MD
Assistant Professor of Radiology
Division of Breast Imaging and Intervention
George Washington University School of Medicine and
    Health Sciences
Washington, DC
Minimally Invasive Image-Guided Breast Biopsy and Ablation

Gina D. Tran, MD
Resident
Department of Family and Community Medicine
University of Nevada School of Medicine
Las Vegas, Nevada
A Brief History of Image-Guided Therapy

Scott Trerotola, MD
Associate Chair and Chief
Division of Interventional Radiology
University of Pennsylvania Medical Center
Philadelphia, Pennsylvania
Management of Clotted Hemodialysis Access Grafts

David W. Trost, MD
Associate Professor of Clinical Radiology
Division of Vascular and Interventional Radiology
Weill Medical College of Cornell University
Associate Attending Radiologist
Department of Radiology
New York-Presbyterian Hospital
New York, New York
Acute Lower Extremity Ischemia
Renal Vein Renin Sampling

Kemal Tuncali, MD
Instructor in Radiology
Harvard Medical School
Brigham and Women's Hospital
Boston, Massachusetts
Cryoablation of Liver Tumors

Ulku C. Turba, MD
Associate Professor of Radiology
Division of Interventional Radiology, Angiography, and
  Special Procedures
Rush University Medical Center
Chicago, Illinois
Balloon Catheters
Chronic Mesenteric Ischemia

Mark R. Tyrrell, PhD, FRCS
Consultant Vascular Surgeon
Department of Vascular Surgery
King's College Hospital
London, United Kingdom
*Management of Thoracoabdominal Aneurysms by Branched
  Endograft Technology*

Raghuveer Vallabhaneni, MD
Assistant Professor of Surgery
Division of Vascular Surgery
University of North Carolina School of Medicine
Chapel Hill, North Carolina
Aortic Stent-Grafts

Eric vanSonnenberg, MD
Visiting Professor of Medicine
David Geffen School of Medicine at UCLA
Chief Academic Officer
Chief of Interventional Radiology and Interventional
  Oncology
Kern/UCLA Medical Center
Bakersfield, California
Professor
Arizona State University
Tempe, Arizona
Cryoablation of Liver Tumors

Prasanna Vasudevan, MD
Chief Resident
Department of Diagnostic Radiology
George Washington University Medical Center
Washington, DC
Angioplasty

Anthony C. Venbrux, MD
Director, Cardiovascular and Interventional Radiology
George Washington University School of Medicine and
  Health Sciences
Washington, DC
A Brief History of Image-Guided Therapy
Angioplasty
Alimentary Tract Vasculature
Renal Vasculature
Management of Male Varicocele
Management of Female Venous Congestion Syndrome
Bipedal Lymphangiography

Bogdan Vierasu, MD
Praticien Hospitalier
Service Radiologie
L'Hôpital de Rangueil
Universitaire de Toulouse
Toulouse, France
Vascular Intervention in the Liver Transplant Patient

Isabel Vivas, MD
Professor of Radiology
Universidad de Navarra
Consultant Radiologist
Clínica Universitaria de Navarra
Pamplona, Spain
Portal-Mesenteric Venous Thrombosis

Dierk Vorwerk, MD
Professor and Director
Department of Radiology
Klinikum Ingolstadt
Ingolstadt, Germany
Renal Artery Embolization
*Percutaneous Management of Thrombosis in Native
  Hemodialysis Shunts*

David L. Waldman, MD, PhD
Professor and Chair
Department of Imaging Sciences
University of Rochester
Strong Memorial Hospital and Highland Hospital
Rochester, New York
FF Thompson Hospital
Canadaigua, New York
Management of Postcatheterization Pseudoaneurysms

Michael J. Wallace, MD
Professor
Department of Diagnostic Radiology
Section Chief
Interventional Radiology
University of Texas
MD Anderson Cancer Center
Houston, Texas
Thermal Ablation of Renal Cell Carcinoma

Eric M. Walser, MD
Professor and Interim Chair
Department of Radiology
University of Texas
Medical Branch
Galveston, Texas
Endovascular Management of Chronic Femoropopliteal Disease

Antony S. Walton, MD
Interventional Cardiologist
Alfred Hospital
Prahran, Victoria, Australia
Vascular Anatomy of the Thorax, Including the Heart

Thomas J. Ward, MD
Resident in Radiology
Department of Radiology
Mount Sinai School of Medicine
New York, New York
Chemical Ablation of Liver Lesions

Anthony F. Watkinson, BSc, MSc (Oxon), MMBS, FRCS, FRCR, EBIR
Honorary Professor of Radiology
Peninsula College of Medicine and Dentistry
Universities of Exeter and Plymouth
Consultant Radiologist
Royal Devon and Exeter Hospital
Exeter, United Kingdom
Transvenous Renal Biopsy

Peter N. Waybill, MD, FSIR
Professor of Radiology, Medicine, and Surgery
Chief, Division of Cardiovascular and Interventional Radiology
Department of Radiology
Pennsylvania State University College of Medicine
Penn State Hershey Medical Center
Hershey, Pennsylvania
Peripherally Inserted Central Catheters and Nontunneled Central Venous Catheters

Joshua L. Weintraub, MD, FSIR
Executive Vice Chairman
Department of Radiology
Professor of Radiology and Surgery
Columbia University College of Physicians and Surgeons
New York Presbyterian Hospital
New York, New York
Renovascular Interventions
Chemical Ablation of Liver Lesions

Robert I. White, Jr., MD
Professor Emeritus and Senior Research Scientist
Founder and Former Director
Yale HHT Center
Yale School of Medicine
New Haven, Connecticut
Pulmonary Arteriovenous Malformations: Diagnosis and Management

Mark H. Wholey, MD
Director of Peripheral Vascular Interventions
Chairman
Pittsburgh Vascular Institute
University of Pittsburgh Medical Center
Shadyside Hospital
Pittsburgh, Pennsylvania
Carotid Revascularization

C. Jason Wilkins, BMBCh, MRCP, FRCR
Consultant
Department of Radiology
King's College Hospital
London, United Kingdom
Management of Thoracoabdominal Aneurysms by Branched Endograft Technology

Bradford D. Winters, MD, PhD
Associate Professor
Departments of Anesthesiology and Critical Care Medicine, Neurology and Surgery
Johns Hopkins University School of Medicine
Baltimore, Maryland
Vasoactive Agents

Robert Wityk, MD
Associate Professor of Neurology
Johns Hopkins University School of Medicine
Baltimore, Maryland
Cervical Artery Dissection

Edward Y. Woo, MD
Associate Professor
Department of Surgery
University of Pennsylvania School of Medicine
Vice-Chief and Program Director
Division of Vascular Surgery and Endovascular Therapy
Director
Vascular Laboratory
University of Pennsylvania Health System
Philadelphia, Pennsylvania
Thoracic Aortic Stent-Grafting and Management of Traumatic Thoracic Aortic Lesions

Bradford J. Wood, MD
Director, Center for Interventional Oncology
Chief, Section of Interventional Radiology
Senior Investigator
National Institutes of Health
Bethesda, Maryland
*Arteriography and Arterial Stimulation with Venous Sampling
for Localizing Pancreatic Endocrine Tumors*
Thermal Ablation of the Adrenal Gland

Gerald M. Wyse, MBBCh, BAO, MRCPI, FFRCSI
Consultant Neuroradiologist
Department of Radiology
Cork University Hospital
Wilton, Cork, Ireland
Endovascular Management of Epistaxis
Subarachnoid Hemorrhage
Percutaneous Cholecystostomy
Image-Guided Intervention for Symptomatic Tarlov Cysts

Albert J. Yoo, MD
Assistant Professor of Radiology
Harvard Medical School
Department of Radiology
Massachusetts General Hospital
Boston, Massachusetts
Vertebroplasty and Kyphoplasty

Chang Jin Yoon, MD, PhD
Associate Professor
College of Medicine
Seoul National University
Seoul, Republic of Korea
Intervention for Gastric Outlet and Duodenal Obstruction

Hyeon Yu, MD
Assistant Professor
Department of Radiology
University of North Carolina School of Medicine
Chapel Hill, North Carolina
*Percutaneous Management of Chronic Lower Extremity Venous
Occlusive Disease*
Hemodialysis Access: Catheters and Ports

Steven Zangan, MD
Assistant Professor
Department of Radiology
University of Chicago Pritzker School of Medicine
Chicago, Illinois
Thombectomy Devices

Fabio Zeccolini, MD
Neuroradiology Service
Cardarelli Hospital
Naples, Italy
Minimally Invasive Disk Interventions

†Eberhard Zeitler, MD
Professor
Department of Diagnostic and Interventional Radiology
Friedrich-Alexander University
Erlangen-Nürmberg
Emeritus Director
Department of Diagnostic and Interventional Radiology
Klinikum Nürmberg-Nord
Nürmberg, Bavaria, Germany
Angioplasty

Dianbo Zhang, MD
Assistant Professor
Department of Radiology
State University of New York
SUNY Upstate Medical Center
Syracuse, New York
Restenosis

Christoph L. Zollikofer, MD
Professor
Department of Radiology
Kantonsspital Baden
Baden, Switzerland
Preoperative and Palliative Colonic Stenting

†Deceased

Preface

The second edition of *Image-Guided Interventions* builds on the success of the first as an international body of work that draws on the knowledge and experience of distinguished contributors from around the world. We believe the first edition fulfilled our intent of producing a practical, concise, well-illustrated textbook representative of the state of the art of interventional practice across the globe. Because modern-day textbooks are no longer needed for an exhaustive list of the current literature, only critical references were included. The second edition is a continuation of this goal. Its five principal editors were selected for their expertise and global representation. Four have returned for the second edition: Drs. Murphy, Venbrux, and Mauro from North America and Dr. Thomson from the Asia-Oceania region. We bid a fond farewell to Christoph Zollikofer (Europe), who has finally entered a well-deserved retirement, and welcome Robert Morgan as our European representative.

The second edition has been reduced to one volume. Several components of the text are offered only as an online resource; these include references and supplementary material. All of the core material with accompanying high-quality color illustrations are present in the traditional printed book form. The first edition received particular acclaim for its radiographic images, tables, charts, and color anatomic illustrations. These have been maintained and enhanced. We have also retained the basic organization of the text into two basic parts: vascular interventions and nonvascular Interventions. Part 1, Vascular Interventions, includes not only diagnosis and intervention of primary vascular disorders (arterial, venous, and lymphatic) but also diseases in other organ systems in which procedures are performed using the vascular system as a conduit for intervention. Part 2, Nonvascular Interventions, covers procedures performed via direct image-guided percutaneous access into the organ or site of interest. Part 1 again begins with core principles including vascular diagnosis, the instruments of intervention, patient care, and the principles of vascular intervention. The subsequent focus of Part 1 is on primary vascular disorders, including arterial, venous, and lymphatic diseases, followed by an anatomic-based discussion of a wide variety of entities in which the vascular tree is used as a conduit for intervention. Part 2 begins with an updated description of biopsy devices, followed by a similarly anatomic-based discussion of image-guided procedures utilizing direct access, including biopsy, drainages, stenting, ablation, injections, and augmentation. All chapters have been updated, and more than a third of the authors are newly appointed and offer specific expertise in the subject matter.

Image-Guided Interventions is designed to be read either primarily from cover to cover, or selectively in preparation for a specific procedure. We have maintained an organizational structure that highlights indications and contraindications for procedures at the outset. Materials required for procedures are clearly listed for easy reference, as are "Key Points" that sum up each chapter. High-quality illustrations and drawings are in abundance because they are typically worth the proverbial thousand words.

We have received tremendous positive feedback from seasoned interventionalists and trainees alike for the first edition of *Image-Guided Interventions*. The editors and Elsevier have strived in earnest to produce a sequel worthy of its namesake. Like its predecessor, *Image-Guided Interventions*, Second Edition, will maintain its relevance through constant Internet updating. It is a textbook created and designed not to gather dust on a bookshelf, but to be present in offices and procedural areas alike, well worn from constant use through reading and referral.

MATTHEW A. MAURO, MD, FACR
KIERAN P.J. MURPHY, MB, FRCPC, FSIR
KENNETH R. THOMSON, MD, FRANZCR
ANTHONY C. VENBRUX, MD
ROBERT A. MORGAN, MBChB, MRCP, FRCR, EBIR

Contents

CHAPTER **1**
A Brief History of Image-Guided Therapy
Anthony C. Venbrux, Jozef M. Brozyna, Suma Chandra, Hank K. Chen, Gina D. Tran, and Dmitri A. Gagarin

HISTORICAL HIGHLIGHTS OF ENDOVASCULAR THERAPY

- British dentist Charles Stent develops a plastic material for taking mouth impressions (i.e., creates a "scaffold") (1856).
- Image guidance was made possible by the discovery of x-rays by Wilhelm Conrad Röntgen, November 8, 1895 (Figs. 1-1 to 1-3).
- Sven Ivar Seldinger develops percutaneous vascular catheterization (1952) (Figs. 1-4 and 1-5).
- Percutaneous revascularization is accomplished by Charles Dotter with coaxial dilators (1964) (Figs. 1-6 and 1-7).
- Transcatheter embolotherapy is performed by Charles Dotter to control acute upper gastrointestinal bleeding (1970).
- Lazar Greenfield pioneers caval interruption with a vena cava filter (1973) (Fig. 1-8).
- Andreas Gruentzig performs percutaneous angioplasty (1977) (Figs. 1-9 and 1-10).
- Chemoembolization was performed by Cato (1981).
- Julio Palmaz develops the endovascular balloon-expandable stent (1985).
- Juan C. Parodi, Julio C. Palmaz, and H. D. Barone develop stent-grafts (1990).

ENDOVASCULAR MILESTONES

November 18, 1895, was a day of historical significance. In a physics laboratory in the southern part of Germany, Conrad Wilhelm von Roentgen accidentally discovered x-rays. The mysterious rays illuminated medical science, and radiology was born. From this serendipitous discovery, image-guided minimally invasive procedures evolved to provide patients with therapeutic options in the management of vascular and nonvascular diseases.

This chapter is neither comprehensive nor complete. Of the many potential technologic advances, arterial and venous endovascular therapy is the focus in this section. Later in the chapter, the history of nonvascular interventions is covered.

Arterial Endovascular Therapy: Revascularization and Vessel Reconstruction

An English dentist, Dr. Charles Stent, developed a thermoplastic material for taking impressions of toothless mouths in 1856. Thus the "stent" may be considered a "scaffold." For purposes of this discussion, a stent is used for reconstruction in the vascular (or nonvascular) systems.

Percutaneous vascular catheterization as a viable endovascular technique was described in June 1952, when Sven Ivar Seldinger presented his idea of replacing an arteriography needle with a catheter. Translumbar aortography and direct carotid puncture were effectively relegated to historical descriptions in textbooks.

The technique of percutaneous revascularization advanced rapidly in 1964, when Charles Dotter used coaxial "pencil-point" dilators to treat a superficial femoral artery stenosis. The era of image-guided revascularization of the lower extremities had begun.

Although Dotter was successful in dilating femoral arterial stenoses, the use of coaxial "pencil-point" dilators (Van Andel Catheters [Cook Inc., Bloomington, Ind.]) required progressive enlargement of the percutaneous puncture site. Development of the angioplasty balloon by Andreas Gruentzig in 1977 resulted in another major step forward that allowed the percutaneous arterial entry site to be kept to a minimum (see Figs. 1-9 and 1-10). Early balloon designs were hampered by uneven balloon dilation and frequent rupture. Such events often led to pseudoaneurysm formation or dissections and resulted in vessel thrombosis.

The arterial metallic stent was invented in the 1980s by Julio Palmaz at the University of Texas Health Science Center in San Antonio. Dr. Palmaz described his stent in 1985 and continued work on his device in 1986. Later developments included the use of a stent design consisting of a single stainless steel tube with parallel staggered slots in the wall. When the stainless steel tube was expanded, the slots formed diamond-shaped spaces that resisted arterial compression. This design became the first stent approved by the U.S. Food and Drug Administration (FDA) for vascular use.

Stanley Baum and Moreye Nusbaum pioneered catheter embolization in the mid-1960s for the purpose of treating

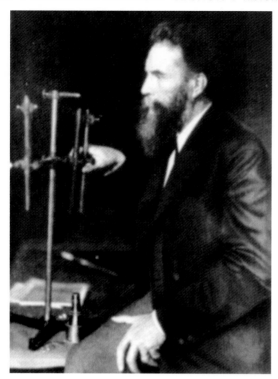

FIGURE 1-1. Photograph of Roentgen taken in 1906 while he was director of the Institute of Physics at the University of Munich. *(From Eisenberg RL. Radiology: an illustrated history. St Louis: Mosby–Year Book; 1992, p. 38.)*

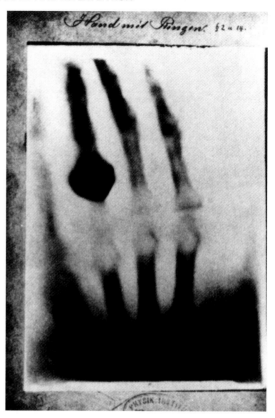

FIGURE 1-2. First roentgen photograph of Mrs. Roentgen's hand. *(From Glasser O. Wilhelm Conrad Röntgen and the early history of the roentgen rays. Springfield, Ill.: Charles C Thomas; 1933.)*

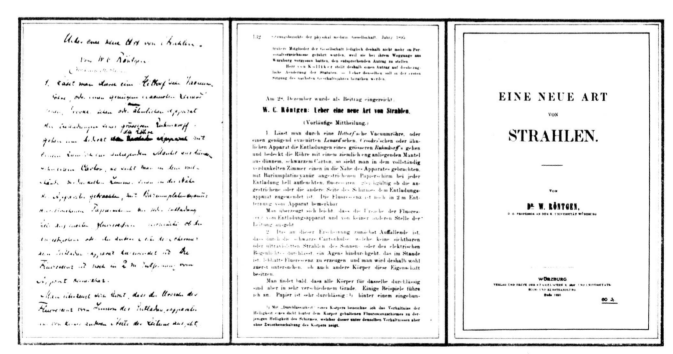

FIGURE 1-3. Roentgen's first communication. *Left,* First page of handwritten manuscript (1895). *Middle,* First page of published article on new type of ray. *Right,* Front cover of a reprint of initial paper. *(From Eisenberg RL. Radiology: an illustrated history. St Louis: Mosby–Year Book; 1992, p. 25.)*

acute gastrointestinal bleeding. In 1970, Charles Dotter reported utilizing an autologous clot as the embolic agent to control acute upper gastrointestinal bleeding by selective embolization of the right gastroepiploic artery in a patient who was a poor surgical candidate. Robert White used this technique in 1974 to control bleeding duodenal ulcers when the hemorrhage was unresponsive to intraarterial injections of vasopressin.

Chemoembolization was largely pioneered by the Japanese urologist Cato in 1981. Cato used particles about 200 μm in size to demonstrate that chemoembolization with microcapsules containing chemotherapeutic agents was superior to local intraarterial injection of antitumor agents.[1]

Stent-grafts, pioneered by Juan Parodi and Charles Dotter, became the major impetus for future endovascular reconstruction procedures used to exclude an aneurysm, close an arteriovenous fistula, and reconstruct the central lumen of a dissected vessel. Specifics of the history of endovascular grafts is worth mentioning. The technology has fundamentally changed the management of diseases of the abdominal and thoracic aorta.

The first abdominal aortic aneurysm (AAA) was described by Andreas Vesalius in the 16th century. By the 1800s, aortic ligation had become the surgical procedure of

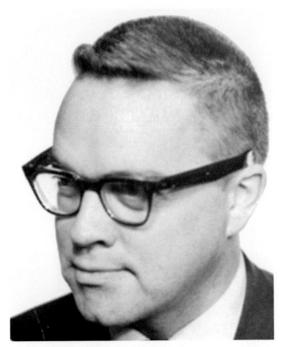

FIGURE 1-4. Sven Ivar Seldinger. *(From Eisenberg RL. Radiology: an illustrated history. St Louis: Mosby–Year Book; 1992, p. 442.)*

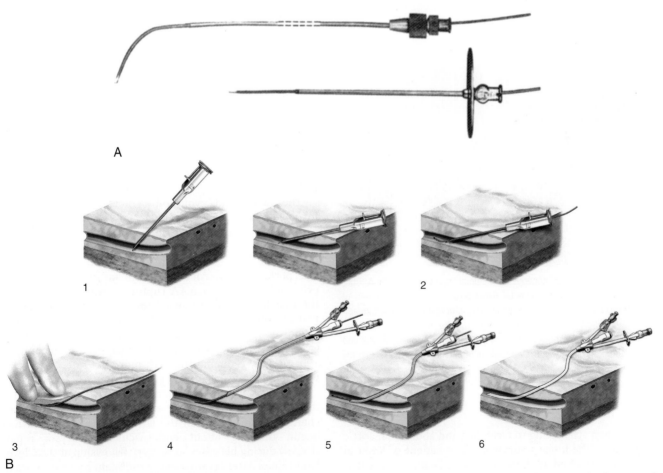

FIGURE 1-5. Seldinger technique (1953). **A,** Equipment. Stiletto is removed and leader inserted through needle and catheter. **B,** Diagram of technique used: *(1)* artery punctured and needle pushed upward, *(2)* leader inserted, *(3)* needle withdrawn and artery compressed, *(4)* catheter threaded onto leader, *(5)* catheter inserted into artery, *(6)* leader withdrawn. *(From Seldinger SI. Catheter replacement of the needle in the percutaneous arteriography: a new technique. Acta Radiol 1953;39:368–76.)*

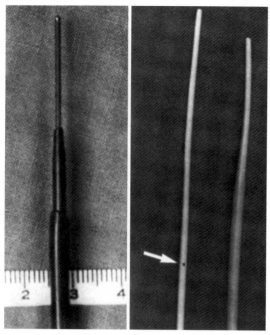

FIGURE 1-6. Dotter coaxial Teflon catheter system consisting of 12F catheter with tapered and beveled tip over inner 8F catheter with 0.044-inch guidewire. *(From Waltman AC, Greenfield AJ, Athanasoulis CA. Transluminal angioplasty: general rules and basic considerations. In Athanasoulis CA, Greene RE, Pfister RC, Roberson GH, editors. Interventional radiology. Philadelphia: WB Saunders; 1982.)*

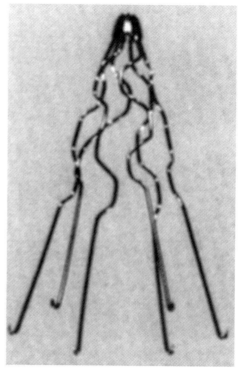

FIGURE 1-8. Kimray-Greenfield filter. *(From Dedrick CG, Novelline RA. Transvenous interruption of the inferior vena cava. In Athanasoulis CA, Greene RE, Pfister RC, Roberson GH, editors. Interventional radiology. Philadelphia: WB Saunders; 1982.)*

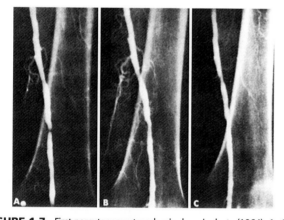

FIGURE 1-7. First percutaneous transluminal angioplasty (1964). **A,** Control arteriogram showing segmental narrowing, with threadlike lumen of left superficial femoral artery in region of adductor hiatus. **B,** Study immediately after dilation with catheter having an outer diameter of 3.2 mm. **C,** Three weeks after transluminal dilation, lumen remains open. Clinical and plethysmographic studies indicated continuing patency more than 6 months later. *(From Dotter CT, Judkins MP. Transluminal treatment of arteriosclerotic obstruction. Circulation 1964;30:654–70.)*

choice when attempting to treat iliac and abdominal aortic aneurysms. The longest survivor was a patient of Keen in 1899, who survived 48 days after aortic ligation at the diaphragm for a ruptured AAA. This was deemed a great success because previous aortic ligations for iliac aneurysms performed by Astley Cooper in 1817 and J.H. James in 1829 resulted in patient death within 48 hours. As the

years passed, many others attempted aortic ligations, and most were met with similar results; the most common mechanism of failure was ligature erosion into the aorta and massive hemorrhage. In April of 1923, over 100 years after Cooper's first attempts, Rudolph Matas performed the first successful aortic ligation on a patient with a syphilitic aortic and bilateral common iliac aneurysms, using cotton tape. The patient survived for 17 months before succumbing to tuberculosis.

The subsequent evolution of aortic aneurysm repair involved many varied techniques. Physicians experimented with different variations of aortic ligation, wires to induce thrombosis, and most notably, reactive polyethylene cellophane wrapping of aneurysms. This particular technique was performed on Albert Einstein in 1949; however, he eventually died of an AAA rupture 6 years later. In 1951, the first homograft was used for AAA repair by Charles DuBost, only to be superseded by nylon and then polytetrafluoroethylene (PTFE) grafts shortly thereafter. Javid and Creech first introduced surgical endoaneurysmorrhaphy in 1961, greatly reducing the high mortality rates associated with aneurysm excision and graft repair.

With the advent of minimally invasive techniques for the treatment of AAAs, the evolution of aneurysm repair changed dramatically. In the late 1970s, Juan Parodi had begun thinking about endovascular aneurysm repair (EVAR) during his vascular surgery fellowship at the Cleveland Clinic. After creating many rudimentary prototypes of varying designs, he became convinced that AAA repair was possible without laparotomy. However, he continuously ran into two problems: (1) the mechanics of delivering a minimally invasive system into the precise location needed,

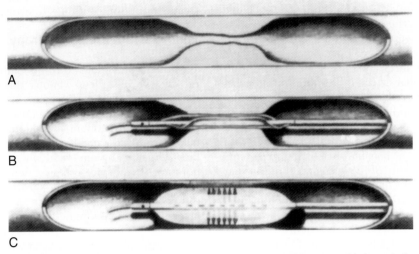

FIGURE 1-9. Percutaneous transluminal coronary angioplasty (1979). **A,** Stenosis of coronary artery. **B,** Double-lumen balloon catheter is introduced with guiding catheter positioned at orifice of left or right coronary artery. At tip of dilating catheter is a short soft wire to guide catheter through vessel. Proximal to wire is a side hole connected to main lumen of dilating catheter. This lumen is used for pressure recording and injection of contrast material. Dilating catheter is advanced through coronary artery with balloon deflated. **C,** Balloon is inflated across stenosis to its predetermined maximal outer diameter, thereby enlarging lumen. After balloon deflation, catheter is withdrawn. *(From Grüntzig AR, Senning A, Siegenthaler WE. Non-operative dilation of coronary artery stenosis. Percutaneous transluminal coronary angioplasty. N Engl J Med 1979;301:61–8. Copyright 1979 Massachusetts Medical Society. All rights reserved.)*

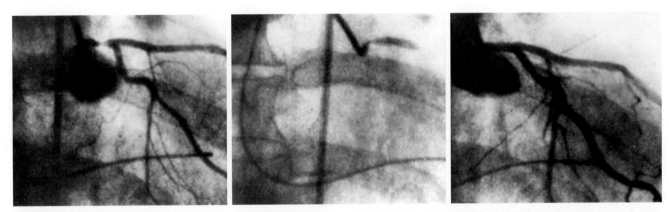

FIGURE 1-10. Transluminal dilation of coronary artery stenosis (1978). *Left,* Initial angiogram in 43-year-old man with severe angina pectoris reveals severe stenosis of main left coronary artery. *Middle,* After passage of dilation catheter, distensible balloon segment was inflated twice to a maximum outer diameter of 3.7 mm. *Right,* Postprocedure angiogram showing good result without complications. *(From Grüntzig AR. Transluminal dilation of coronary artery stenosis. Lancet 1978;1:263.)*

and (2) the absence of a fastening device that would take the place of surgical sutures in securing the graft in place and creating a seal between the intravascular graft and vessel wall.

The solution to these challenges came when Parodi met Julio Palmaz at the Transcatheter Cardiovascular Therapeutics meeting in Washington, DC, in 1988. Palmaz was attending to discuss a new stent design. Parodi was informed that Palmaz was presenting and thus was encouraged to attend. It became apparent to Parodi that the Palmaz design was precisely what he was looking for: a device with a high radial force (i.e., a balloon-expandable stent) that was deployed using endovascular techniques and would provide placement, precision, a secure anchor, and an aortic wall seal that his EVAR concept required. Palmaz was initially apprehensive about joining the project because of his many

professional commitments and perceived limitations of his device in the aorta. However, he later admitted that he envisioned his stent playing a role in aneurysm repair as early as 1986. Ultimately he decided to join efforts with Parodi. Work then began on the first EVAR in both Buenos Aires, where Parodi worked at the Instituto Cardiovascular de Buenos Aires (ICBA), and San Antonio, where Palmaz was Chief of Special Procedures at the University of Texas Health Science Center. During their efforts to perfect the device and the technique, Parodi was searching for an ideal candidate for the first EVAR.

On September 7, 1990, two patients were to undergo the new procedure, to be performed by both Parodi and Palmaz at the cardiac catheterization laboratory of ICBA. During the first procedure, the proximal portion of the stent was deployed just inferior to the renal arteries, and the distal portion placed just superior to the aortic bifurcation. The postprocedure angiogram displayed a completely excluded aneurysm, concluding the first EVAR procedure. The second patient was converted to traditional surgical AAA repair, because the proximal portion of the stent was deployed too low in the aorta, and the distal end of the graft ended in one common iliac artery. It was not until later that Parodi realized that the reflection of pressure waves from the aortic bifurcation and iliac arteries would cause an endoleak and failure of a single stent device.

This initial experience provided Parodi and Palmaz with clinical insight into patient benefits such as improvements in recovery time and quality of life, using an endovascular approach. The first patient quickly recovered and was discharged without complications, while the second remained intubated in the intensive care unit. Additionally, the second case provided the team with a possible mechanism of failure for their new procedure and delivery system. Over time, the procedure, delivery system, and methods of Parodi's team evolved. By December of 1992, 24 patients had undergone EVAR by one of three techniques that had evolved since the first case, the most common being an aorto-uni-iliac approach with contralateral common iliac embolization and femoral-femoral bypass. Prior to this, an interventional radiologist from Buenos Aires, Claudio Schonholz, had also joined the international team and played a significant role in the first EVAR performed in the United States.

In August of 1992, the vascular surgery department at Montefiore Medical Center in Bronx, New York, was consulted on a 76-year-old male patient with a 7.5-cm infrarenal AAA with several comorbidities that suggested he was not a candidate for open surgical repair. Frank Veith and Michael Marin quickly contacted Parodi and began discussing the logistics involved in traveling to South America, learning the procedure, and treating the aneurysm endovascularly. After several meetings, and convincing Johnson & Johnson (who was producing the Palmaz stent) executives to allow them to use a large Palmaz stent for the procedure (no FDA Investigational Device Exemption existed for it yet), they were ready to proceed. On November 23, 1992, Parodi, Schonholz, Veith, Marin, and Jacob Cynamon performed the first EVAR in the United States, using a 22-mm Dacron prosthesis sewn over a large Palmaz-like stent. The patient was discharged several days later and remained symptom free until his death 9 months later. Death was due to problems unrelated to the EVAR procedure.

Although Parodi is often credited with the first EVAR, it is important to mention that a Ukrainian surgeon, Nicholas Volodos, published an article in 1986 describing the endovascular repair of a traumatic thoracic aortic aneurysm with a homemade stent-graft. Also of note, Harrison Lazarus was awarded a U.S. patent in 1988 for an endovascular stent-graft that eventually served as the basis for the Guidant (Indianapolis, Ind.) Ancure device.

With advancements in technology and refinement of techniques, EVAR has become for selected patients the standard of care for treatment of AAAs. By the end of 2010, it was estimated that nearly three quarters of all abdominal aortic aneurysms in the United States were repaired endovascularly. There are an estimated 1.1 million Americans between the ages of 50 and 84 diagnosed with an AAA, and over 15,000 deaths annually due to abdominal aortic

aneurysms, so it is no surprise that this minimally invasive treatment option continues to evolve.

Venous Endovascular Therapy: Caval Interruption

Treatment of venous thromboembolic disease has also rapidly evolved. Deep venous thrombosis is one of the major causes of morbidity and mortality worldwide. "Caval interruption" with a filter was initially performed via surgical cutdown by Mobbin and Uddin. In 1973, Lazar Greenfield introduced a cone-shaped surgically placed vena cava filter. Greenfield pioneered his work with the Kimray Corporation. This device was first deployed percutaneously in 1984. The diameter of the sheath for the filter was 29F (outer diameter [OD]). Later developments reduced Greenfield's percutaneous puncture size from 29F (OD) to 16F (OD).

Because all permanent vena cava filters are associated with complications, including caval thrombosis (3%-40%), recent advances have provided patients at risk for venous thromboembolic disease with "optional devices," such as vena cava filters that may be permanent or removed, the latter when the patient's "window of vulnerability" has clinically passed. Removable devices were historically called *temporary filters* and were classified as either *tethered* or *retrievable*. A more accurate term in current clinical use is an *optional filter. Optional* implies that the device may either be a permanent implant or be used for a short interval. A *tethered* inferior vena cava (IVC) filter consists of a filter attached to a central venous catheter. A *retrievable* IVC filter is a device deployed in the IVC that attaches to the IVC wall with hooks but has no external tether. (The FDA approved use of the first tethered temporary vena cava filter in the United States in the early 1990s.) This tethered device (Tempofilter [B. Braun, Evanston, Ill.]), placed in a young trauma patient, remained in place for 13 days and trapped a large embolus, thereby preventing a potentially life-threatening pulmonary embolic event.

The FDA approved optional vena cava filters in the United States in 2003. The Recovery Filter (Bard Peripheral Vascular, Tempe, Ariz.), a permanent implant with the "option to remove" at any future date, was first deployed in the United States in July 2003. Since 2003, the Günther Tulip (Cook Medical, Bloomington, Ind.), the Opt Ease (Cordis Endovascular, Warren, N.J.), and other filters have also received FDA approval as optional vena cava filters. Thus, management of venous thromboembolic disease has further evolved with newer therapeutic options for patients who are at risk for pulmonary emboli but have a contraindication to or have had a complication of anticoagulant therapy.

SUMMARY

Arterial and venous endovascular procedures continue to progress rapidly. Future developments that might take place include continued use of mechanical devices in the vascular system, combination therapies to rapidly lyse and remove residual thrombi, further design modifications in endovascular devices to reduce the risk of metal fatigue/fracture, and the application of newer technologies to reduce intimal hyperplasia (e.g., drug-eluting stents). Such improvements will, one hopes, provide solutions for some of the limitations of our current technology.

HISTORICAL HIGHLIGHTS OF NONVASCULAR IMAGE-GUIDED THERAPY

- Wickbom, Weens, and Florence directly opacified the urinary tract with a needle (1954) (Fig. 1-11).
- Percutaneous urinary tract drainage is accomplished by Goodwin and colleagues (1955) (Figs. 1-12 and 1-13).
- Percutaneous biopsy of opacified lymph nodes is described by Sidney Wallace (1961).
- Percutaneous transhepatic cholangiography is described by Evans et al. (1962) (Fig. 1-14).
- Drainage of an abdominal viscus (e.g., gallbladder, stomach) with a retrievable anchoring device is described by Constantin Cope (1986).

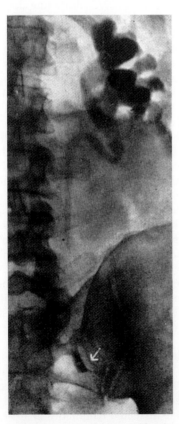

FIGURE 1-11. Antegrade pyelography (1954). After direct puncture of the left renal pelvis, contrast material demonstrates dilation of the pelvis and upper part of the ureter. There is complete obstruction of the ureter at the pelvic inlet *(arrow)*.

- Percutaneous image-guided drainage is extensively used and described by Eric Vansonnenberg, Peter R. Mueller, and Joseph T. Ferucci (1980s).

Urologic Interventions

In 1954, Wickbom opacified the renal pelvis directly by injecting contrast medium through a long needle. Thus, the antegrade pyeloureterogram (antegrade nephrostogram) as we know it was first performed. The following year, Goodwin et al. used a "catheter through a needle" for drainage. In

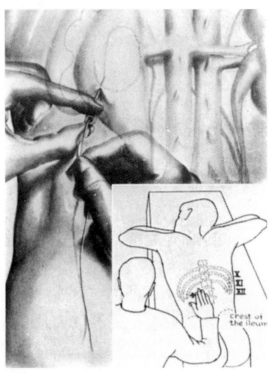

FIGURE 1-12. Percutaneous trocar nephrostomy (1955): method and landmarks. Optimum puncture site is usually about five fingerbreadths lateral to midline and at a level where a 13th rib would be. *(From Wickbom I. Pyelography after direct puncture of the renal pelvis. Acta Radiol 1954;41:505–12.)*

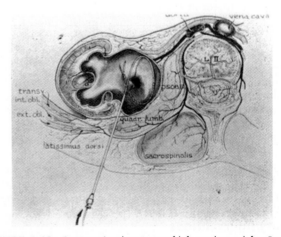

FIGURE 1-13. Cross-sectional anatomy of left renal area (after Brodel). About 2 inches of tubing is allowed to coil in hydronephrotic pelvis. *(From Wickbom I. Pyelography after direct puncture of the renal pelvis. Acta Radiol 1954;41:505–12.)*

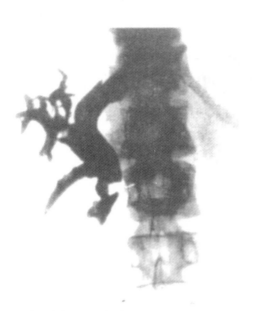 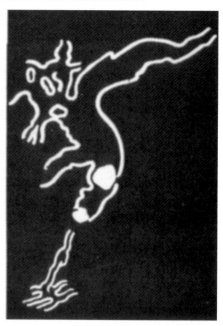

FIGURE 1-14. Operative cholangiography (1931). *Left,* Radiograph demonstrating biliary tract, with two sharply defined clear spaces in retroduodenal portion and at level of papilla of Vater. *Right,* Corresponding diagram with extracted calculi superimposed. Superior calculus is size of a hazelnut and inferior one size of a chickpea. *(From Mirizzi PL, Losada CQ. Exploration of the bile ducts during an operation. Paper presented at the Third Argentine Congress of Surgery, 1931, p. 694–703.)*

1965, Bartley used a guidewire technique for drainage of the urinary tract, and in 1976, Frenstrom and Johansson reported dilation of the nephrostomy tract for stone removal.[1]

By 1978, Stables reviewed the techniques used in the performance of 516 nephrostomies appearing in the medical literature. This series included 53 of his own patients. Thus, percutaneous techniques had received increasing attention in the published medical literature and were found to be a viable option for open surgical procedures.

Smith, in 1979, coined the term *endourology.* At that time he had begun work at the University of Minnesota, where the scientific/academic environment was conducive to new techniques. Smith and Amplatz together developed numerous endourologic techniques, including the Amplatz retention catheter in 1986.

In 1982, Castaneda-Zuniga and Amplatz published the technique for urinary stone removal. Once the percutaneous tract was dilated, they used fluoroscopic guidance to extract stones with a Randall forceps or a Dormia basket at the tip of the catheter. Coleman, in 1985, reported that the results of percutaneous removal of stones had improved since the early 1980s to a success rate of 99% in a study of 450 patients.

Thus, the technique of percutaneous drainage of the urinary tract with subsequent percutaneous removal of obstructing stones made significant advancements during the 1970s and 1980s. Today, percutaneous urinary tract interventions are an integral part of image-guided therapy.

Biliary Interventions

Percutaneous transhepatic cholangiography and percutaneous biliary drainage are based on needle/guidewire/catheter techniques developed simultaneously with endourology.

Nonsurgical management of biliary stones and strictures continues to be an essential part of the treatment of patients with biliary disease. In 1973, Burhenne described a technique for extraction of retained common duct stones through a T-tube tract.

The feasibility of percutaneous biliary duct dilation with balloon dilation catheters was reported by Berhenne in 1975.[2] Berhenne performed the technique through a mature T-tube tract. Molnar and Stockum described the dilation of biliary strictures via a transhepatic route in 1978.[3]

In 1980, Constantin Cope developed a simple drainage catheter to reduce the problem of nephrostomy tube dislodgement. Foley or Malecot nephrostomy drainage catheters were frequently pulled out or became dislodged. The Cope loop catheter was one of the most significant developments of nonvascular interventional procedures in the 1980s. A suture coursing through the lumen of the catheter allowed a locking mechanism, which today is the standard for most drainage catheters. Such catheters are used in the urinary tract and biliary system and for drainage of percutaneous abscesses.

Percutaneous application of biliary endoprostheses (plastic or metallic) to palliate patients with malignant biliary obstruction was described by Dotter, Gianturco, and Ring, among others.

Lymph Node Applications

As early as 1933, Hudack and McMaster used blue dye as a contrast agent to visualize the lymphatic system. The surgeon Servele dissected lymphatics in 1994 and inserted a needle, followed by the injection of Thorotrast.

Percutaneous biopsy of opacified lymph nodes (opacified with contrast material) was described by Sidney Wallace in 1961. The diagnostic and therapeutic potential of lymphangiography brought oncologic interventions to the forefront.

Other Nonvascular Interventions

The ability to nonsurgically access an abdominal viscus (percutaneous gastrostomy, etc.) was improved largely through the innovative efforts of Constantin Cope. Cope developed a suture-anchoring device. The retrievable anchoring device was reported by Cope in 1986 after he successfully drained the gallbladder and stomach without leakage. The technique of percutaneous abscess drainage was applied and described extensively by E. Vansonnenberg, P.R. Mueller, and J.T. Ferucci. Drainage of a percutaneous abscess or fluid collection is an integral part of image-guided nonvascular patient management.

KEY POINTS

- Nonvascular percutaneous interventions are an integral part of image-guided therapy.
- Significant advancements have allowed nonsurgical management of multiple medical conditions that previously required operative (open) procedures.
- Important percutaneous techniques in nonvascular interventions include those in the urinary tract, biliary system, lymphatic system, gastrointestinal tract, and drainage of abdominal fluid collections.

ACKNOWLEDGMENT

The authors would like to thank Shundra Dinkins, Toni Acfalle, and Dana Murphy for their expertise in preparation of this manuscript.

▶ SUGGESTED READINGS

Criado F. EVAR at 20: the unfolding of a revolutionary new technique that changed everything. J Endovasc Ther 2010;17:789–96.
Dotter CT, Frische LH, Judkins MP, Mueller R. Nonsurgical treatment of iliofemoral arteriosclerotic obstruction. Radiology 1966;86:871–5.
Dotter CT, Rosch J, Anderson JM, et al. Transluminal iliac artery dilation. JAMA 1974;230:117–24.

Friedman S. A history of vascular surgery. 2nd ed. Malden, MA: Blackwell Futura; 2005.
Gruentzig A, Senning A, Siegenthaler WE. Nonoperative dilation of coronary-artery stenosis. N Engl J Med 1979;301:61–8.
Grüntzig A, Hopf H. Perkutane recanalization chronisher arteriller verschüsse mit einen neuen dilatationskatheter: modification der Dottertechnik. Dtsch Med Wochenschr 1974;99:1502–51.
Hedin M. The origin of the word stent. Acta Radiol 1997;38:937–9.
Hurst JW. The first coronary angioplasty as described by Andreas Gruentzig. Am J Cardiol 1986;57:185–6.
Kent KC, Zwolak RM, Egorova NN, et al. Analysis of risk factors for abdominal aortic aneurysm in a cohort of more than 3 million individuals. J Vasc Surg 2010;52:539–48.
Lubarsky M, Ray CE, Funaki B. Embolization agents–which one should be used when? Part 1: large-vessel embolization. Semin Intervent Radiol 2009;26:352–7.
Margulis AR. Interventional diagnostic radiology; a new subspecialty [editorial]. AJR Am J Roentgenol 1967;99:761–2.
Palmaz JC, Parodi JC, Barone HD. Transluminal bypass of experimental abdominal aortic aneurysm. J Radiol 1990;11:177–202.
Palmaz JC, Sibbitt RR, Reuter SR, et al. Expandable intraluminal graft: a preliminary study. Work in progress. Radiology 1985;156:72–7.
Palmaz JC, Sibbitt RR, Tio FO, et al. Expandable intraluminal graft: a feasibility study. Surgery 1986;98:199–205.
Parodi JC, Ferreira M. Why endovascular abdominal aortic aneurysm repair? Semin Intervent Cardiol 2000;5:3–6.
Pearce W, Rowe VL. Abdominal aortic aneurysm. MedScape. Accessed September 4, 2011.
Ring ME. How a dentist's name became a synonym for a lifesaving device: the story of Dr. Charles Stent. J Hist Dent 2001;49:77–80.
Rosch J, Keller FS, Kaufman JA. The birth, early years, and future of interventional radiology. J Vasc Interv Radiol 2003;14:841–53.
Seldinger SI. Catheter replacement of needle in percutaneous arteriography: a new technique. Acta Radiol 1953;39:368–76.
Veith FJ, Marin MJ, Cynamon J, et al. 1992: Parodi, Montefiore, and the first abdominal aortic aneurysm stent graft in the United States. Ann Vasc Surg 2005;19(5):749–51.
Volodos NL, Shekhanin VE, Karpovich IP, et al. A self-fixing synthetic blood vessel endoprosthesis [in Russian]. Vestn Khir IM I I Grek 1986;137(11):123–5.
White RI, Giargian FA, Bell William. Bleeding duodenal ulcer control: selective arterial embolization with autologous blood clot. JAMA 1974;299:546–8.

The complete reference list is available onine at www.expertconsult.com.

CHAPTER **2**

Noninvasive Vascular Diagnosis

Brian B. Ghoshhajra and Sanjeeva Prasad Kalva

Most vascular diseases can be diagnosed with a combination of clinical history and examination, relevant laboratory tests, and appropriate noninvasive tests. Such tests include the ankle-brachial index, segmental pressure and pulse volume recording measurements, Doppler assessment of blood flow, ultrasound evaluation of vessels, computed tomographic angiography (CTA), and magnetic resonance angiography (MRA). Computed tomography (CT) and magnetic resonance imaging (MRI) are now the first-line tests or replacements for diagnostic catheter angiography in many cases. The imaging test should be chosen based on the clinical problem. Other factors that may affect the choice of a particular test include cost, availability, urgency, pretest probability, and underlying contraindications. As with any radiologic tests, radiation exposure should be kept as low as reasonably achievable. In this chapter we briefly discuss the principles of ultrasonography, CTA, and MRA and their clinical applications.

Ultrasonography is highly sensitive and specific for diagnosis of venous thrombosis in the extremities and superficial vessels. It remains the test of choice for evaluation of venous insufficiency, and is often useful in assessing hemodynamic significance of an arterial stenosis (sometimes in conjunction with pulse-volume recordings for peripheral arterial disease). Ultrasound is widely available, relatively inexpensive, and rapid, but is highly operator dependent and subject to technical challenges such as acoustic window limitations, especially in the obese patient. In peripheral vessels, ultrasound performs well and can obviate the need for further or invasive testing. In the abdominal vasculature, ultrasound can be reliably used when image quality allows.

CTA and MRA are comparable for evaluation of thoracoabdominal vessels and peripheral arteries. CTA is preferred in the acute setting, whereas MRA enjoys unique advantages when assessing inflammatory diseases affecting the large vessels. Both modalities are routinely useful in the neurovascular system, particularly in the setting of ischemic stroke workup.

MRA is preferable for evaluation of the vessel lumen in patients with extensive mural calcification. It is also operator dependent, often requiring expert physician oversight, and subject to numerous artifacts. Acquisition times can be long, particularly when imaging small vessels or using electrocardiogram (ECG) gating and respiratory gating or breath-hold techniques (especially in the cardiothoracic anatomy, where this is frequently necessary). However, MRA is less often limited by body habitus and generally allows unrestricted imaging planes. Recent advances in noncontrast MRA allow the technique to benefit those patients with contraindications to intravenous contrast.

CTA has also progressed dramatically in recent years as helical CT has moved to multidetector CT, and now wide-area-detector CT and dual-source CT. Recent advances now allow rapid and reliable angiographic imaging in nearly every circulatory bed. CT is less operator dependent than MRA but does require expert care. Although most acquisitions are axial, postprocessing of volumetric datasets allows near-unrestricted imaging planes. CT with cardiac gating is now widely available, allowing routine noninvasive ECG-synchronized imaging of the heart and great vessels. Coronary CTA is useful in assessing coronary artery anomalies, bypass grafts, and coronary artery disease. Although the capabilities of modern CTA are impressive, downsides include the need for rapid iodinated intravenous contrast administration and ionizing radiation. Numerous advances have decreased the radiation dose associated with CTA, particularly in the thorax. Limitations of the technique include poor assessment of small and peripherally calcified vessels, in which CTA can overestimate stenosis.

Noninvasive imaging now offers a large and diverse tool kit to the cardiovascular imager. Although ultrasound remains the first-line test in many vascular beds, MRI and CTA now offer reliable high-quality imaging of the vasculature in many settings. Choice of the appropriate test varies with the available technology, expertise, target vessel, and clinical question at hand.

The full discussion of noninvasive vascular diagnosis, as well as 10 illustrations, are available at www.expertconsult.com.

CHAPTER 3

Invasive Vascular Diagnosis

John A. Kaufman

Invasive vascular imaging is based on the technique described by Sven Ivar Seldinger in 1953 (Fig. 3-1).[1] This elegant innovation, now known by Seldinger's name, eliminated the need for surgical exposure of a blood vessel before catheterization, thus allowing the transfer of angiography from the operating room to the radiology department. Virtually all vascular invasive procedures and devices use this technique.

PREPROCEDURAL PATIENT EVALUATION AND MANAGEMENT

Every invasive procedure begins with a patient evaluation, determination of the appropriateness of the examination, and formulation of a procedural plan. In most cases the angiographer performing the procedure will have seen the patient previously in consultation and assumed primary responsibility for management of the disease to be diagnosed. A brief directed history should be obtained, with attention to the symptoms or signs that precipitated the study. Essential historical areas to cover include prior surgical procedures (especially vascular); evidence of atherosclerotic disease in "index" vascular beds, such as prior myocardial infarction or stroke; diabetes, with attention to medications; status of renal function; allergies; and known previous exposure to iodinated contrast agents. Office records or the patient's chart should be reviewed for similar information. Special attention should be applied to operative notes and reports from previous angiograms, because these provide valuable information that may alter the entire approach to the procedure. Most importantly, personal review of old angiograms or correlative imaging is essential before embarking on an invasive procedure.

The preprocedural physical examination is focused on the status of the vascular system and selection of a vascular access site. The person who will perform the procedure should conduct this examination. The quality of the pulses and the presence of an aneurysm (as suggested by a broad prominent pulse) should be recorded using a consistent system. Suspected integumentary infection, fresh surgical incisions, a large abdominal pannus, or a scar over the vessel all impact selection of an access site. Pulses distal to the anticipated access site must be evaluated because one of the potential complications of angiography is distal embolization. Furthermore, if an intervention is performed, this baseline information is important to help determine procedural endpoints. The physical examination should include both right and left sides of the patient so that a different access site can be used during the procedure if necessary. When an upper extremity approach is anticipated, the brachial blood pressure in both arms must be obtained.

Patients should be well hydrated before the procedure.[2,3] Outpatients should not be instructed to fast after midnight but encouraged to drink clear liquids until 2 hours before their scheduled appointment. In the preprocedural area, an intravenous infusion of 5% dextrose in 0.5% normal saline should be begun at 100 mL/h in normal patients. Fluid rates and characteristics should be adjusted in diabetics, patients on dialysis, and patients with congestive heart failure. Inpatients should have an established intravenous infusion in place before arriving in the angiographic suite. Most hospitals have established guidelines for oral intake before invasive procedures that must be followed, but remember that these are generally not designed for patients about to receive large doses of nephrotoxic contrast materials.

There are no laboratory studies that are absolutely necessary before starting an invasive vascular procedure; most problems that can be predicted from abnormal laboratory studies occur after the catheter is removed (e.g., bleeding, renal failure). A low platelet count is the single most important predictor of postprocedural bleeding complications.[4] The commonly acquired minimal laboratory studies are coagulation (international normalized ratio [INR], prothrombin time [PT], activated partial thromboplastin time [APTT], and platelet count) and serum creatinine value. Patients with renal failure undergoing central venous procedures that might entail intracardiac manipulation (e.g., central line placement) may require measurement of serum potassium concentration.

When the PT or INR is abnormal, fresh frozen plasma given the day or night before is useless or even dangerous because an INR drawn just after the plasma has been infused may be normal, but by the time the procedure is performed, the effect may dissipate. Fresh frozen plasma infused shortly before and during the procedure provides maximal correction when it is needed most. An abnormal APTT is usually due to administration of unfractionated heparin, which can be turned off when the patient arrives in the angiography suite. Because the half-life of unfractionated heparin is about 90 minutes, most patients will correct sufficiently for manual compression by the end of the procedure. Perhaps more importantly, platelet transfusion to restore a count to more than 50,000/µL is an empirical cutoff used in many departments for patients having an arterial access.

In the presence of an abnormal serum creatinine value, the risk of postprocedural renal failure should be weighed against the benefits of the procedure. Every hospital and practice should have guidelines for contrast administration to patients with abnormal renal function. Regardless of the renal protective strategy, the patient should be well hydrated before and after the examination. Renal protective strategies should be followed to maximize renal protection.

BASIC SAFETY CONSIDERATIONS

Operator precautions against exposure to body fluids should be applied to all situations, even for patients with no

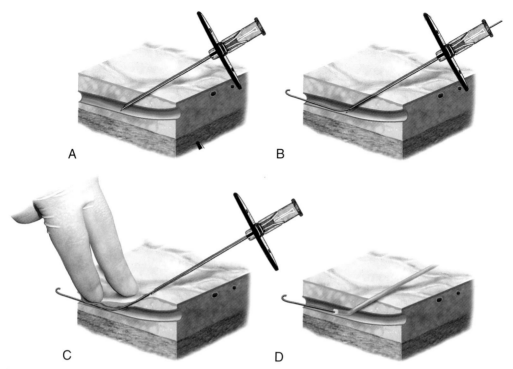

FIGURE 3-1. Seldinger technique. **A,** Percutaneous puncture of blood vessel with hollow needle. **B,** Introduction of atraumatic guidewire through needle into blood vessel lumen. **C,** Needle is removed while guidewire remains in place. Compression over puncture secures guidewire and prevents bleeding. **D,** Angiographic catheter is advanced into vessel over guidewire. *(From Kadir S. Diagnostic angiography. Philadelphia: WB Saunders; 1986.)*

known risk factors.[5] Masks, face shields or other protective eye wear, sterile gloves, and impermeable gowns are the minimal measures. Closed flush and contrast systems decrease the risk of splash exposures. All materials used during the case should be disposed of in waste containers designed and labeled for biological waste.

Sharp devices (e.g., needles, scalpels) should be carefully stored on the work surface in a red sharps container or removed immediately after use. Recapping needles is not advised owing to the puncture risk. The best sharps containers contain a foam block into which the point of the sharp device can be safely imbedded. At the end of the case, the angiographer can dispose of the sharps in one of the ubiquitous hard red plastic sharps receptacles. Puncture wounds from contaminated needles or scalpels are not only painful but also potentially life-altering events. If an accidental splash, puncture, or any other exposure occurs, immediate consultation with a physician experienced in management of exposure to occupational biohazards is essential.

Radiation exposure to the patient and staff should be kept to a minimum.[6] Use fluoroscopy only when needed to move catheters or guidewires. Prolonged fluoroscopy at high magnification with the x-ray tube in one position has been associated with radiation burns to the patient.[7] Exposure can be reduced during long cases by use of pulsed fluoroscopy modes. The typical pulse rate of 15 pulses per second can be decreased by 50% or more with only a minor degradation in image quality.

Accumulative radiation exposure to the angiographer can be substantial. Angiographers should wear wraparound lead, thyroid shields, leaded glasses, and radiation badges. Careful coning of the x-ray beam during the case can reduce

scatter. The operator's hands should never be seen on the fluoroscope during the case. When the angiographer must remain in the procedure room during filming, portable leaded shields should be positioned between the x-ray source and the physician.

Ergonomic considerations are important during invasive vascular imaging. Many angiographers develop degenerative spine disease in the neck and back.[8] Careful attention to the design of angiographic suites, especially the positioning of controls and monitors, can reduce twisting and bending. Similarly, patients should be positioned on the procedural table to minimize contortions on the part of the operator. The patient's comfort also requires careful consideration. For long procedures, careful padding of pressure points, especially when the patient is under general anesthesia, is important.

TOOLS

Access Needle

All angiographic procedures begin with a vascular access needle. There is great variety in vascular access needles, but all are designed to allow introduction of a guidewire through a central channel (Fig. 3-2). The simplest needle is a one-piece open needle with a sharp beveled tip. The guidewire is introduced directly through the needle once the tip is fully within the bleeding vessel lumen. This style of needle can be used for both arterial and venous punctures. Two-piece needles usually have a central sharp stylet that obturates the lumen and extends slightly beyond the needle tip. These needles have a blunted atraumatic beveled tip when the stylet is removed. The sharp stylet allows the needle to

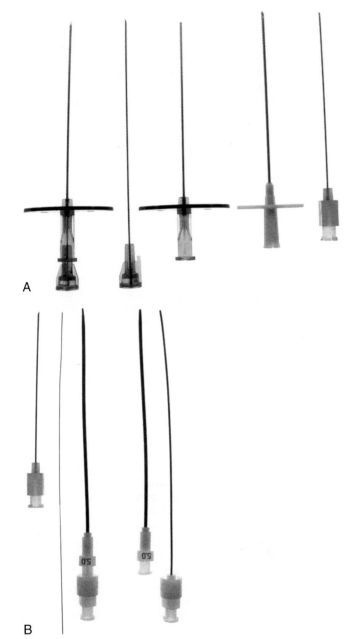

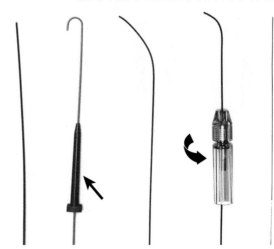

FIGURE 3-3. Common guidewires. *Left to right,* Straight 0.038-inch; J-tipped 0.038-inch with introducer device *(arrow)* to straighten guidewire during insertion into needle hub; angled high-torque 0.035-inch; angled hydrophilic-coated 0.038-inch nitinol wire with pinvise *(curved arrow)* for fine control; 0.018-inch platinum-tipped microwire. *(From Kaufman JA, Lee MJ, editors. Vascular and interventional radiology: the requisites. St. Louis: Mosby; 2004.)*

FIGURE 3-2. A, Typical access needles. *Left to right,* 18-gauge Seldinger needle with hollow, sharp, central stylet that extends beyond blunt tip of needle; stylet; Seldinger needle with stylet removed; 18-gauge sharp, hollow ("one-wall") needle; 21-gauge "microaccess" needle. **B,** Microaccess system. *Left to right,* 21-gauge needle; 0.018-inch guidewire for insertion through needle; 5F dilator with central 3F dilator tapered to 0.018-inch guidewire; 5F dilator with 3F dilator removed that accepts 0.038-inch guidewire; 3F dilator. *(From Kaufman JA, Lee MJ, editors. Vascular and interventional radiology: the requisites. St. Louis: Mosby; 2004.)*

puncture the vessel, but once it is removed the risk of vascular injury from the blunt needle tip is theoretically removed. The stylet can be solid or hollow. In the latter case, blood may be visualized on the stylet hub once the vessel lumen is entered. With all styleted needles, the stylet must be removed to insert the guidewire. Needles with stylets are generally used only for arterial punctures. The most common sizes for vascular access needles of the type

described above are 19 or 18 gauge in diameter and $2\frac{1}{4}$ to 5 inches in length.

Microaccess systems in which a very small-diameter access needle is used to enter the vessel and then converted to a larger short, plastic introducer with a larger lumen are very useful for both arterial and venous punctures. These systems usually employ a sharp, open, bevel-tipped 21-gauge needle for access. These needles are often modified to enhance visualization by ultrasound during the access procedure. After entering the blood vessel, a short, floppy-tipped 0.018-inch guidewire is inserted. The needle is removed over the guidewire and exchanged for a 4F or 5F dilator through which a 3F dilator has been coaxially inserted. Once the dilator assembly has been inserted, the 0.018-inch guidewire and the 3F dilator are removed, leaving the dilator with the larger lumen behind.

Guidewires

Guidewires are available in a number of thicknesses, lengths, tip configurations, stiffnesses, and materials of construction (Fig. 3-3). In general, the guidewire thickness (always referred to in hundredths of an inch—e.g., 0.038-inch) should be the same as or slightly smaller than the diameter of the lumen at the tip of the catheter or device that will slide over it. Guidewires that are too big will jam, usually at the tip of the catheter. However, if a guidewire is much smaller than the end hole of the catheter or device, there will be a gap between the guidewire and catheter that can cause vessel injury or prevent smooth movement over the guidewire.

The most commonly used style of guidewire has a central stiff core around which is tightly wrapped a smaller wire, just like a coiled spring (Fig. 3-4). The outer wire is often welded to the core at the back end but not the tip. The purpose of the coiled outer wrap is to decrease the area of contact between the surface of the guidewire and the

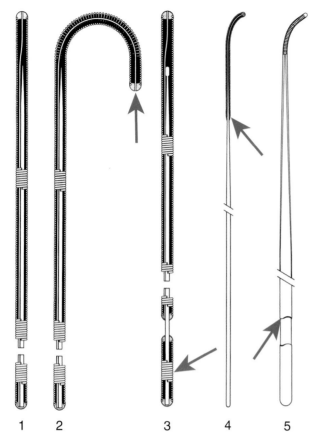

FIGURE 3-4. Basic construction of common guidewires. *1 and 2,* Curved and straight safety guidewires with outer coiled spring wrap, central stiffening mandril welded at back end only, and small safety wire *(arrow)* welded on inside at both ends. *3,* Movable-core guidewire in which mandril can be slid back and forth and even removed completely to change wire stiffness, using handle incorporated into guidewire *(arrow). 4,* Mandril guidewire in which soft spring wrap is limited to one end of guidewire *(arrow).* Remainder of guidewire is a plain mandril. *5,* Mandril guidewire coated with hydrophilic substance *(arrow). (Drawings reproduced with permission from Cook Group Inc., Bloomington, Ind.)*

tissues. A fine safety wire runs along the length of the inside of the guidewire between the inner core wire and outer wrap and is welded to the outer wrap at both ends. This safety wire prevents the outer wrap from unwinding should the weld break. This is where the term *safety guidewire* originated.

The composition and thickness of the inner core determine the degree of guidewire stiffness. Guidewires that are very flexible are important for negotiating tortuous or diseased vessels. Stiff guidewires provide the most support for introducing catheters and devices. A movable core guidewire is one in which the core is not welded to the tip but can be slid in and out of the spring wrap to adjust the guidewire stiffness as necessary. The mandril guidewire is an important design type in which the outer wrap is limited to the soft tip of guidewire. The majority of the guidewire is solid wire. This is a common construction for microguidewires (0.018 inch or smaller) or for extra-rigid large-diameter guidewires.

The features of the taper of the core at the leading end of the guidewire determine the softness or "floppiness" of the tip. The length and transition of the taper define the characteristics of the tip. The longer and more gradual the transition, the longer and floppier the tip. Bentson guidewires and movable core guidewires with the core retracted have the softest tips. With all guidewires, it is the soft end that goes in the patient.

A curved tip at the end of the guidewire provides an additional degree of safety in diseased vessels. As the guidewire is advanced, the rounded presenting part bounces over plaque rather than digging into it. A curve can be added to most straight guidewires by gently drawing the floppy tip across a firm edge (e.g., a fingernail, closed hemostat), much like curling a ribbon. A special type of wire is the tip-deflecting guidewire, which allows the operator to mechanically vary in the radius of the curve while in the patient. These guidewires have stiff tips and should never be advanced beyond the end of the catheter.

A wide range of special-purpose guidewires such as wires coated with slippery hydrophilic substances, highly torquable guidewires, kink-resistant nitinol-based wires, and microwires are available. These guidewires have been the difference between routine success and failure in the many challenging cases. The hydrophilic-coated guidewire is the most commonly used specialty guidewire; its central core is coated with an outer layer of hydrophilic material. This coating drastically reduces friction between the guidewire, blood vessel wall, and catheter. However, unless kept moist, hydrophilic guidewires actually become much stickier than a regular guidewire. When this happens, it is almost impossible to advance a catheter over the guidewire and easy to inadvertently pull the entire guidewire out of the body during an exchange. Of note, these guidewires should not be inserted through vascular access needles because the nonradiopaque coating can be easily sheared off by the metal edge of the needle if withdrawn.

The length of the average guidewire used in angiography is 145 to 160 cm. In circumstances in which a great deal of guidewire is needed inside the body, or the devices and catheters to be placed over the guidewire are very long, an "exchange-length" guidewire (260-300 cm long) is used. Extra-long guidewires are not used for routine cases because the excess length outside the body is cumbersome and easily contaminated.

Dilators

Vessel dilators are short, tapered, plastic catheters usually made of a stiffer material than diagnostic angiographic catheters (Fig. 3-5). The sole purpose of a dilator is to spread the soft tissues and the blood vessel wall to make introduction of a catheter or device easier. By inserting progressively larger dilators over a guidewire, a percutaneous puncture with an 18-gauge needle can be increased to almost any size. Sequential dilatation is important to minimize trauma to the vessel, since incremental steps in size (1F-2F) can be accomplished with much less resistance than one giant step. The initial dilator size after puncture with an 18-gauge access needle should be 5F. Larger dilators can follow as necessary. Dilatation of a puncture site beyond 50% of the expected diameter of the artery may obviate manual compression, because the muscular layer of the artery can no longer contract after removal of the catheter.

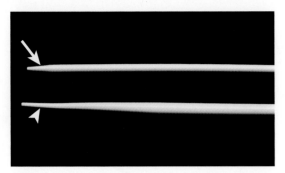

FIGURE 3-5. Vascular dilators. Standard taper *(arrow)* and longer taper *(arrowhead)* "Coons" tip, useful when more gradual dilation is required. *(From Kaufman JA, Lee MJ, editors. Vascular and interventional radiology: the requisites. St. Louis: Mosby; 2004.)*

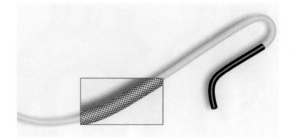

FIGURE 3-7. Drawing illustrating fine wire braid in shaft of a selective catheter. *(Reproduced with permission from Cook Group Inc., Bloomington, Ind.)*

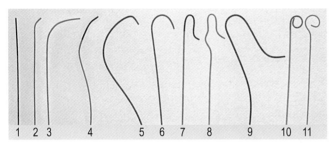

FIGURE 3-6. Common catheter shapes. *1,* Straight; *2,* Davis (short angled tip); *3,* multipurpose ("hockey-stick"); *4,* headhunter (H1); *5,* cobra-2 (cobra-1 has tighter curve, cobra-3 has larger and longer curve); *6,* Rösch celiac; *7,* visceral (very similar to Simmons 1); *8,* Mickelson; *9,* Simmons-2; *10,* pigtail; *11,* tennis racket. *(From Kaufman JA, Lee MJ, editors. Vascular and interventional radiology: the requisites. St. Louis: Mosby; 2004.)*

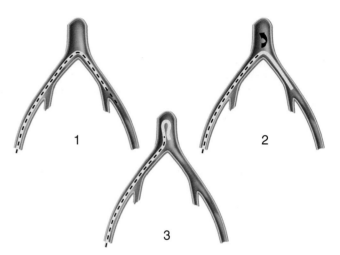

FIGURE 3-8. Branch technique for re-forming a Simmons catheter. *1,* Catheter is advanced into branch over guidewire *(dashed line).* Aortic bifurcation shown in this illustration. *2,* Guidewire withdrawn proximal to origin of branch but still in catheter. One may also remove guidewire and reinsert stiff end to same point. Catheter is then twisted and advanced at same time. *3,* Re-formed catheter. *(From Kaufman JA, Lee MJ, editors. Vascular and interventional radiology: the requisites. St. Louis: Mosby; 2004.)*

Catheters

Angiographic catheters are usually made of plastic (polyurethane, polyethylene, Teflon, or nylon). The exact catheter material, construction, coatings, inner diameter, outer diameter, length, tip shape, sidehole pattern, and endhole dimensions are determined by the intended use (Fig. 3-6). Catheters used for nonselective aortography are thick walled (to handle large-volume high-pressure injections) and often curled at the tip (the "pigtail," which keeps the end of the catheter away from the vessel wall) with multiple side holes proximal to the curl (so the majority of the contrast medium exits the catheter in a cloud). Conversely, selective catheters are generally thinner walled with a single end hole because injection rates are lower and directed into a small vessel. Precise control of the movement of a selective catheter, especially at the tip, is important. These catheters usually have fine metal or plastic strands incorporated into the wall ("braid") (Fig. 3-7). This results in a catheter tip that is responsive to gentle rotation of the shaft.

Catheter outer size is described in French gauge (3F = 1 mm), whereas the diameter of the end hole (and therefore the maximum size of the guidewire the catheter will accommodate) is described in hundredths of an inch. The length of the catheter is described in centimeters (usually between 65 and 100 cm). The shape of the tip is named for either something the catheter looks like ("pigtail," "cobra," "hockey

stick"), the person who designed it (Simmons, Berenstein, Rösch), or the intended use (celiac, left gastric, "headhunter") (see Fig. 3-6). There are so many different catheters that no one department can or should stock them all. The shape of some catheters (especially Teflon and polyethylene) can be modified by heating the catheter in steam while bending it into the desired configuration. Rapidly dunking the catheter into cool sterile water "sets" the shape.

Complex catheter shapes must be re-formed inside the body after insertion over a guidewire. Any catheter will resume its original shape, provided there is sufficient space within the vessel lumen and memory in the catheter material. Some catheter shapes cannot re-form spontaneously in a blood vessel, particularly the larger recurved designs like the Simmons. There are a number of strategies for re-forming these catheters (Figs. 3-8 to 3-12). These same techniques can be used to create a recurved catheter from a simple angled selective catheter by forming a Waltman loop (Fig. 3-13).[9]

Multiple side-hole straight or pigtail catheters are generally used for nonselective injections. Straight catheters should be advanced over a guidewire; otherwise the tip may

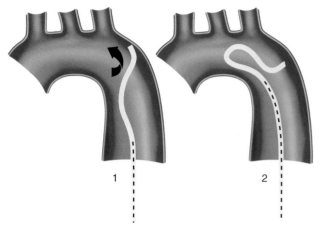

FIGURE 3-9. Aortic spin technique for re-forming a Simmons catheter (works best for Simmons 1). *1*, Catheter is simultaneously twisted and advanced in proximal descending thoracic aorta. Note wire is withdrawn below curved portion of catheter. *2*, Re-formed catheter. *(From Kaufman JA, Lee MJ, editors. Vascular and interventional radiology: the requisites. St. Louis: Mosby; 2004.)*

cause a dissection or perforation. Pigtail catheters can be safely advanced in normal vessels once the pigtail has re-formed, but should be advanced over a guidewire in abnormal blood vessels.

Selective catheters are chosen based on the particular vessel or anatomy that will be studied (Fig. 3-14). The technique used to catheterize a blood vessel with a selective catheter varies with the type of catheter (Figs. 3-15 and 3-16). The Waltman loop is particularly useful in the pelvis for selecting branches of the internal iliac artery on the same side as the arterial puncture.

Small catheters (3F or smaller outer diameter) that are specially designed to fit coaxially within the lumen of a standard angiographic catheter are termed *microcatheters*. These soft flexible catheters are typically 2F to 3F in diameter, with 0.010- to 0.027-inch inner lumens. They are designed to reach far beyond standard catheters in small or tortuous vessels. These catheters are technologically advanced and have a wide range of characteristics, such as stiffness, braiding, flow rates, and hydrophilic coatings. The ability to reliably catheterize small arteries without creating spasm, dissection, or thrombosis has allowed certain subspecialties (e.g., neurointerventional radiology) to flourish. When using a microcatheter, a standard angiographic catheter that accepts a 0.038- or 0.035-inch guidewire is first placed securely in a proximal position in the blood vessel. The microcatheter is then inserted through the outer catheter and advanced in conjunction with a specially designed 0.010- to 0.025-inch guidewire through the standard catheter lumen. Once a superselective position has been attained with the microcatheter, a variety of procedures can be performed, including embolization, sampling, or low-volume angiography. The small inner lumen and long length result in a high resistance to flow, so microcatheters are not used for routine angiography. Contrast and flush solutions are most easily injected through these catheters with 3-mL or smaller Luer-Lok syringes.

Guiding catheters are another class of catheters designed to make selective catheterization and interventions easier.

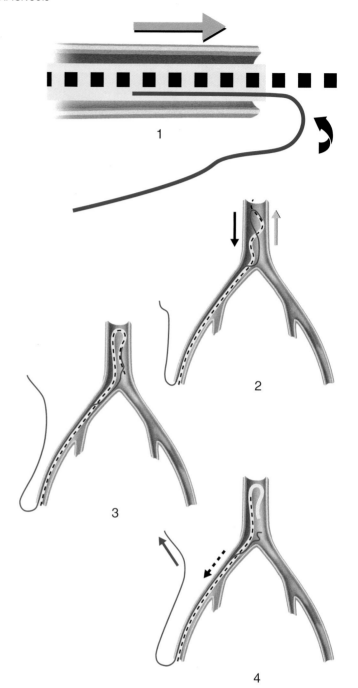

FIGURE 3-10. Cope string technique. Easily re-forms any size Simmons catheter. *1*, Three to 4 cm of 4-0 Tevdek II (Deknatel Inc., Fall River, Mass.) suture material *(curved arrow)* has been backloaded into catheter tip. Catheter is then advanced *(arrow)* onto floppy-tipped guidewire *(dashed line)*. *2*, Catheter has been advanced over guidewire into aorta, with suture material exiting groin adjacent to catheter. Floppy portion of guidewire still exits catheter, "locking" suture material in catheter tip. Suture material is pulled gently *(black arrow)* as slight forward force applied to catheter *(gray arrow)*. *3*, Simmons catheter has been re-formed. *4*, Suture removed by first retracting guidewire into catheter *(dashed arrow)*, "unlocking" suture material. Suture material can then gently be pulled out *(black arrow)*. *(From Kaufman JA, Lee MJ, editors. Vascular and interventional radiology: the requisites. St. Louis: Mosby; 2004.)*

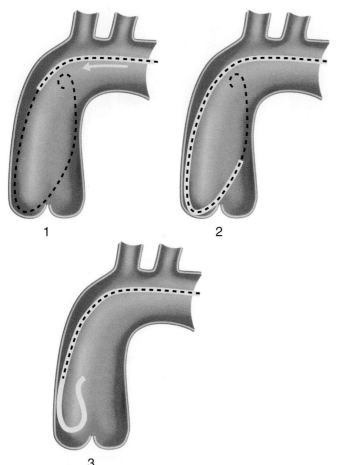

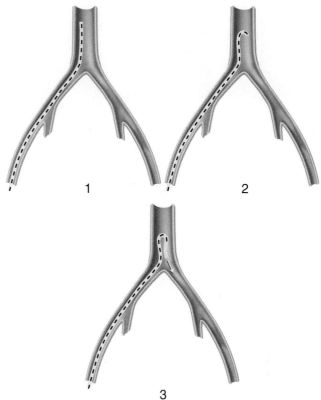

FIGURE 3-11. Ascending aorta technique for re-forming a Simmons catheter. *1,* Floppy-tipped 3-J guidewire reflected off of aortic valve. Catheter is advanced over guidewire. *2,* Catheter advanced around bend in guidewire. *3,* Retraction of guidewire completes re-formation. *(From Kaufman JA, Lee MJ, editors. Vascular and interventional radiology: the requisites. St. Louis: Mosby; 2004.)*

FIGURE 3-12. Deflecting wire technique (unsafe for use in small or diseased aortas). *1,* Deflecting wire is positioned near tip of catheter. *2,* Wire deflected, curving the catheter as well. *3,* With guidewire fixed, catheter is advanced *(arrow)* to re-form Simmons catheter. *(From Kaufman JA, Lee MJ, editors. Vascular and interventional radiology: the requisites. St. Louis: Mosby; 2004.)*

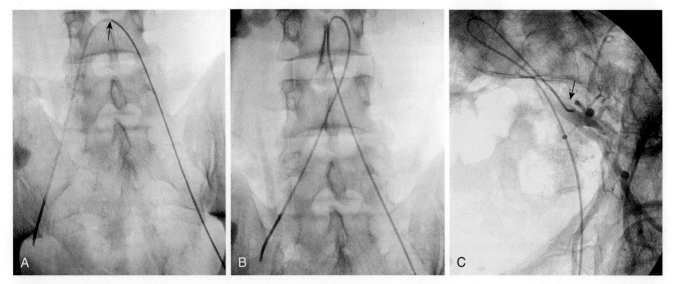

FIGURE 3-13. Waltman loop. This can be formed in any major aortic branch vessel with braided selective catheters. **A,** Angled catheter is positioned over aortic bifurcation. Note stiff end of guidewire at catheter apex *(arrow).* **B,** Catheter is advanced and twisted, forming loop. **C,** Looped catheter has been used to select ipsilateral internal iliac artery *(arrow).* *(From Kaufman JA, Lee MJ, editors. Vascular and interventional radiology: the requisites. St. Louis: Mosby; 2004.)*

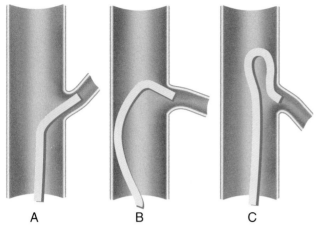

FIGURE 3-14. Choosing a selective catheter shape. **A,** Angled catheter when angle of axis of branch vessel from aortic axis is low. **B,** Curved catheter (e.g., cobra-2, celiac) when angle of axis of branch vessel is between 60 and 120 degrees. **C,** Recurved catheter (e.g., SOS, Simmons) when angle of axis of branch vessel from aorta is great. *(From Kaufman JA, Lee MJ, editors. Vascular and interventional radiology: the requisites. St. Louis: Mosby; 2004.)*

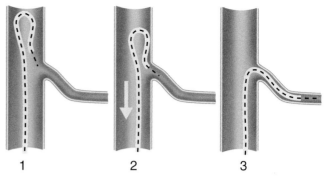

FIGURE 3-16. How to use a Simmons catheter. *1,* Catheter is positioned above branch vessel with at least 1 cm of floppy straight guidewire beyond catheter tip. *2,* Catheter is gently pulled down *(arrow)* until guidewire and tip engage orifice of branch. *3,* Continued gentle traction results in deeper placement of catheter tip. To deselect branch, push catheter back into aorta (reverse steps 1-3). To un-form a Simmons catheter, apply continued traction from this position. *(From Kaufman JA, Lee MJ, editors. Vascular and interventional radiology: the requisites. St. Louis: Mosby; 2004.)*

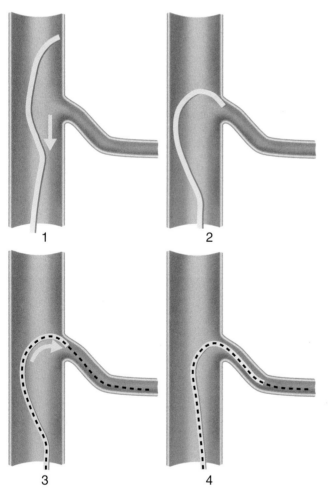

FIGURE 3-15. How to use a cobra catheter. *1,* Catheter advanced to position proximal to branch over guidewire, then pulled down *(arrow).* *2,* Catheter tip engages orifice of branch. Gentle injection of contrast agent to confirmed location. *3,* Soft-tipped selective guidewire has been advanced into branch. Guidewire is held firmly, and catheter is advanced *(arrow).* *4,* Catheter in selective position. *(From Kaufman JA, Lee MJ, editors. Vascular and interventional radiology: the requisites. St. Louis: Mosby; 2004.)*

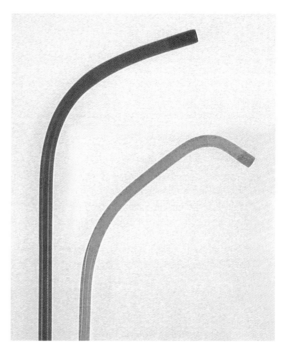

FIGURE 3-17. Two examples of nontapered large-diameter guide catheters that can accommodate standard 5F catheters. French size of guide catheters refers to outer diameter. *(From Kaufman JA, Lee MJ, editors. Vascular and interventional radiology: the requisites. St. Louis: Mosby; 2004.)*

These catheters can be used in some situations to help position and stabilize standard catheters. Guide catheters are nontapered catheters with extra-large lumens and a simple shape that accepts standard-sized catheters and devices (Fig. 3-17). They are used in circumstances in which standard catheters are difficult to position selectively. The larger outer catheter can provide direction and stability for the inner standard catheter. Guiding catheter size in French gauge refers to the *outer* diameter. This is the converse of the use of French sizes when describing standard catheters. The inner diameter of the guide catheter is usually described

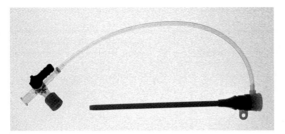

FIGURE 3-18. Typical hemostatic sheath. French size of sheaths refers to inner diameter. *(From Kaufman JA, Lee MJ, editors. Vascular and interventional radiology: the requisites. St. Louis: Mosby; 2004.)*

in hundredths of an inch, which must be converted to French gauge to determine which standard catheter will fit (1F = 0.012 inch = 0.333 mm).

Sheaths

Most vascular interventions and diagnostic procedures are performed through vascular access sheaths. These devices of varying thickness and construction are open at one end and capped with a hemostatic valve at the other (Fig. 3-18). The intravascular end is not tapered, although the edges are carefully beveled to create a smooth transition to the tapered dilator used to introduce the sheath over a guidewire. The valved end usually has a short, clear side-arm that can be connected to a constant flush (to prevent thrombus from forming in the sheath) or an arterial pressure monitor. The purpose of the sheath is to simplify multiple catheter exchanges through a single access site. When not using a sheath, it is unwise to downsize catheters during a procedure (i.e., place a small catheter through a big hole in the artery) because of the risk of bleeding. Devices that are irregular in contour or even nontapered can be introduced through a sheath without fear of trauma to the device or access vessel. In some cases, a long sheath can straighten a tortuous access artery.

Sheaths are described by the maximum-sized device (in French gauge) that will fit through the sheath. Because the walls of the sheath have some thickness, this means the actual hole in the blood vessel will be 1.5F to 2F *larger* than the sheath "size." Sheaths are available in a variety of lengths, depending on the requirements of the procedure. Short sheaths are more often used during diagnostic procedures, and long sheaths are used for interventions.

The peel-away sheath is a useful type of sheath (Fig. 3-19). The proximal end of this sheath terminates in two plastic wings, and there is no side port for flushing. Many of these sheaths have a break-away hemostatic valve. The sheath and dilator are introduced over a guidewire. Once they are in position, the dilator is removed. If there is no hemostatic valve, the only way to achieve hemostasis is to either block the open end of the sheath with a finger or clamp the sheath. After inserting a device or catheter through the sheath, the plastic wings are pulled in opposite directions parallel to the skin. This "peels" the sheath away in two long strips of plastic and allows complete disengagement from the catheter without having to slide off of the back end. The primary disadvantages of peel-away sheaths are that they kink easily, and those that are hemostatic are not designed for multiple catheter exchanges.[10]

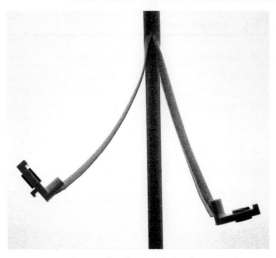

FIGURE 3-19. Peel-away sheath. To peel sheath away, wings are pulled in opposite directions at 90 degrees from catheter shaft. *(From Kaufman JA, Lee MJ, editors. Vascular and interventional radiology: the requisites. St. Louis: Mosby; 2004.)*

Contrast Agents

All the tools described previously are intended to facilitate delivery of a contrast agent into the vascular system. The development of safe and well-tolerated contrast agents was equally as important to angiography as the Seldinger technique.[11] The ideal contrast agent has excellent radiopacity, mixes well with blood, is easy to use, is inexpensive, and does not harm the patient. Iodinated contrast agents (which are based on benzene rings with three bound iodine atoms, termed *triiodinated contrast agents*) turn out to be as close to ideal as currently possible.

There are two major classes of triiodinated contrast agents: nonionic and ionic (Table 3-1). Ionic contrast agents use a nonradiopaque cation, usually sodium and meglumine (*N*-methylglucamine) but also sometimes magnesium and calcium. The result is a highly soluble, low-viscosity, but high-osmolar (two particles per iodinated ring) contrast agent. High osmolarity relative to human blood is believed to be a major contributing factor to adverse reactions to contrast agents. Nonionic contrast agents have no electric charge, so cations are not needed. This greatly reduces the osmolality of the contrast agent (one particle per iodinated ring), which improves the safety profile but increases viscosity. The two major classes of contrast agents are further subdivided into monomeric (one triiodinated benzene ring) or dimeric (two linked triiodinated benzene rings).

Adverse reactions to iodinated contrast agents are frequent, but the majority are minor, such as pain or nausea (Table 3-2).[12,13] Most minor complications are linked to the osmolality of the contrast agent, so the overall incidence is lower with nonionic contrast agents. Complications such as nausea and emesis are believed to be related to a central nervous system mechanism and are more frequent with venous than arterial injections. Late complications (occurring hours or days after the contrast exposure) are rare but include rash, urticaria, and parotitis.[14]

The two major adverse reactions to iodinated contrast agents are anaphylaxis and contrast-induced renal failure.[11] True anaphylaxis is distinguished from a vasovagal response

TABLE 3-1. Contrast Agents

Class of Contrast Agent	Contrast Agent	Commercial Names	Iodine Atoms per Molecule	Approximate Osmolality* (300 mg L/mL Concentration)
Ionic monomer	Diatrizoate Iothalamate	Hypaque, Renografin Conray	3	1500-1700
Nonionic monomer	Iopamidol Iohexol Ioversol Ioxilan Iopromide	Isovue Omnipaque Optiray Oxilan Optivist	3	600-700
Ionic dimer	Ioxaglate	Hexabrix	6	560
Nonionic dimer	Iodixanol	Visipaque	6	300

*mOsm/kg water.

TABLE 3-2. Contrast Reactions: Reported Incidence Rates

Reaction	Ionic Contrast	Nonionic Contrast
Nausea	4.6%	1%
Vomiting	1.8%	0.4%
Itching	3.0%	0.5%
Urticaria	3.2%	0.5%
Sneezing	1.7%	0.2%
Dyspnea	0.2%	0.04%
Hypotension	0.1%	0.01%
Sialadenitis	<0.1%	<0.1%
Death	1:40,000	1:170,000

TABLE 3-4. Preventive Measures for Contrast-Induced Acute Renal Failure

Agent	Protocol
Hydration	1 mL/kg D_5W for 12 hours before procedure; 0.5 mL/kg D_5W for 12 hours after procedure
Sodium bicarbonate	154 mmol/L at 3 mL/kg/h prior to procedure; 1 mL/kg/h for 6 hours after procedure
N-acetylcysteine	1200 mg orally every 12 hours beginning 24 hours before procedure, including one dose the morning of the angiogram and one dose the night after procedure. Total of four doses.

TABLE 3-3. Preparation of Patient with Contrast Allergy

Prednisone, 50 mg (oral), 13, 7, and 1 hour prior to the procedure
Cimetidine, 300 mg, intravenously on arrival in the angiography suite
Diphenhydramine (Benadryl), 50 mg, intravenously on arrival in the angiography suite
Use nonionic contrast

by tachycardia (in patients who are not on beta blockers) and respiratory distress. The incidence of life-threatening anaphylaxis due to iodinated contrast is roughly 1 in 40,000 to 170,000. Mild reactions (e.g., urticaria, nasal stuffiness) occur more commonly, especially with ionic contrast. Contrast reactions must be treated quickly and aggressively. The most common cause of death is airway obstruction.

A patient with a history of prior contrast allergy should receive pharmacologic prophylaxis beginning at least 12 hours before the procedure (unless a true emergency exists) (Table 3-3).[12] Patients may label many symptoms experienced during prior contrast studies as "allergy," such as nausea, vagal nerve-mediated bradycardia and hypotension, or ischemic cardiac events. Whenever the precise nature of the "allergic" reaction cannot be determined from the history, corticosteroid prophylaxis is wise. Nonionic contrast media should be used exclusively in any patient with a history of contrast allergy.

Renal failure after intravascular administration of iodinated contrast is more common in patients with diabetes, preexisting renal insufficiency (serum creatinine ≥ 1.5 mg/ dL), and multiple myeloma. The exact mechanism is not known, but the classic findings are a rise in creatinine concentration 24 to 48 hours after exposure to the contrast agent, peaking at 72 to 96 hours. Patients are usually oliguric but may be anuric. Management is usually expectant because the creatinine concentration will return to baseline in 7 to 14 days in most cases. However, in patients with severe preexisting renal insufficiency and diabetes, the risk of permanent dialysis may be as high as 15% despite protective measures (Table 3-4).

Contrast medium is administered during angiographic procedures by hand or mechanical injectors. Injection by hand is useful during the initial stages of the procedure, or for low-volume and low-pressure angiograms in small vessels, or through precariously situated catheters. The use of mechanical injectors is necessary for optimal contrast delivery, particularly when large volumes or high flow rates are needed. In addition, there is less radiation exposure to the angiographer if a mechanical injector is used. Catheters are rated for both contrast flow rates (mL/s) and maximum injection pressure in pounds per square inch (psi). Exceeding these limits may cause rupture of the catheter (usually at the hub) or premature termination of the injection by the injector software. Meticulous technique is necessary when connecting a catheter to a power injector to avoid air bubbles, contamination of the catheter, or disconnection during injection.

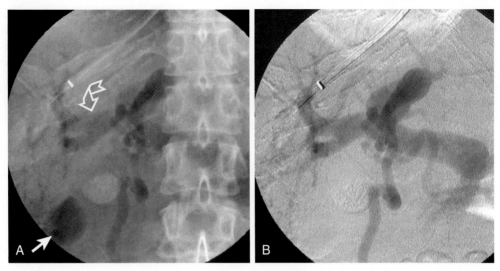

FIGURE 3-20. Carbon dioxide (CO_2) portal venogram. **A,** Unsubtracted image from wedged hepatic venogram shows CO_2 filling portal vein *(curved arrow)*. Density of CO_2 is same as gas in bowel *(straight arrow)*. **B,** Digital subtraction of same frame. Visualization of portal venous system is excellent. *(From Kaufman JA, Lee MJ, editors. Vascular and interventional radiology: the requisites. St. Louis: Mosby; 2004.)*

Alternative Contrast Agents

The low but real incidence of adverse reactions to iodinated contrast agents has led to the use of alternative contrast agents in selected circumstances. In particular, patients with past histories of true anaphylactic reactions to iodinated contrast or with precarious renal function may be considered for an alternative to iodinated contrast. Two alternative contrast agents have been described: carbon dioxide (CO_2) gas and gadolinium chelates.[15,16] Experience is most extensive with CO_2, which acts as a negative contrast agent. The gas temporarily displaces the blood in the lumen of the vessel, resulting in decreased attenuation of the x-ray beam. Digital subtraction technique is essential for diagnostic imaging with CO_2 (Fig. 3-20). The buoyant nature of CO_2 relative to blood results in preferential filling of anterior structures. The CO_2 gas is extremely soluble in blood and rapidly excreted from the lungs. The low viscosity of CO_2 is advantageous for demonstration of subtle bleeding or during wedged hepatic vein portography.[17] CO_2 can be used for abdominal aortography, selective visceral injections, lower extremity runoffs, and most venous studies. For abdomen studies it is helpful to administer intravenous glucagon to decrease bowel peristalsis. CO_2 is contraindicated in angiography of the thoracic aorta, cerebral arteries, or upper extremity arteries owing to potential neurologic complications. Rarely, CO_2 gas can cause a "vapor lock" in a small vessel, which obstructs blood flow and induces distal ischemia. An excessive volume of gas in the heart can obstruct the pulmonary outflow tract, with severe cardiac consequences.

Mechanical injectors that can be used for CO_2 are not available in the United States. Injections must therefore be performed by hand. Scrupulous handling of CO_2 is necessary to prevent contamination by less soluble room air. Explosive delivery of gas through the catheter can be avoided by first purging the ambient liquid in the catheter with a small volume of gas.

Gadolinium chelates were originally developed as contrast agents for magnetic resonance imaging (MRI). The acute safety profile of these contrast agents is superior to that of iodinated contrast, and there appears to be lower nephrotoxicity. There is no cross-sensitivity in patients with a history of anaphylaxis to iodinated contrast. However, patients with impaired renal function (creatinine clearance < 60 mg/dL) are at risk of developing a progressive systemic disorder—nephrogenic fibrosing sclerosis.[18] For this reason, this contrast agent may be most suited for patients with true anaphylaxis to iodinated contrast and normal or near-normal renal function.

The k-edge of gadolinium is 50 keV, slightly higher than iodine (33 keV). This allows visualization of gadolinium with current digital subtraction angiographic equipment. Although the approved doses of most gadolinium-based agents are 0.1 to 0.3 mL/kg, volumes of 40 to 60 mL have been used for many years. Special injection techniques or equipment are not required for gadolinium-based contrast agents. Digital subtraction angiography is necessary because the low gadolinium concentration in the available formulations results in weak opacification of deep vessels. Gadolinium-based contrast agents have been used safely in every vascular application, including carotid and coronary arteries. These contrast agents are very expensive compared to nonionic contrast agents and extremely expensive compared to CO_2.

ARTERIAL ACCESS

The patient should be positioned on the angiographic table in a manner that provides the easiest, most direct access to the puncture site. Patient comfort is extremely important, but the angiographer's ability to access the artery, manipulate the catheter, observe the puncture site, and use the table controls during the procedure are paramount. Also, all tools must be nearby before beginning so time is not wasted during the procedure looking for something needed routinely.

There are a few guidelines for selecting an arterial access for a procedure. The area of interest should be approachable from the access artery. The access artery must be large enough to accommodate devices needed for the procedure. There should be no critical or fragile organs between the skin and the artery to be accessed. The puncture should be over bone whenever possible so the vessel can be compressed against something stable at the end of the procedure. The pulse should be readily palpable to facilitate the puncture and, more important, the compression. The vessel to be punctured should be as normal as possible; bad arteries lead to bad complications. Lastly, the overlying skin should be free of infection and fresh surgical incisions.

Never underestimate the damage that can be caused by needles, guidewires, and catheters in the arterial system. Strict adherence to technique and respect for the delicacy of the arteries, especially when diseased, will maximize the safety of the procedure. Excellent guidelines for diagnostic angiography have been published by the Society of Interventional Radiology.[19,20]

Common Femoral Artery Access

The common femoral artery (CFA) is the most common access site for angiography. The CFA is usually near the skin (even in heavy individuals), large enough to accommodate standard angiographic tools, and easy to compress against the underlying femoral head. Furthermore, the CFA is contained within the femoral sheath, which helps control peripuncture bleeding.

The majority of CFA punctures are retrograde toward the abdomen (against arterial blood flow), as opposed to antegrade toward the leg (in the direction of arterial blood flow). For all approaches, the CFA should be accessed over the middle or lower third of the femoral head to facilitate compression at the termination of the procedure. The artery is localized by palpation or ultrasound. In large or elderly patients, the inguinal fold cannot be relied on to localize the CFA; it may hang down over the superficial femoral artery. A blunt metal instrument placed on the skin at the anticipated point of access can be fluoroscoped to determine its relationship to the femoral head. The entry site in the skin should be 1 to 2 cm lower than the intended entry site into the artery (for antegrade punctures, make the skin entry the same distance above) to allow a 45-degree angle of the needle relative to the artery during puncture. The skin and soft tissues are anesthetized with 1% to 2% lidocaine injection. Using the tip of a #11 scalpel blade, a 5-mm nick is made on the skin. The skin nick and a subcutaneous tract are then dilated gently with a straight surgical snap. This facilitates catheter insertion during the procedure and egress of blood in the event of postprocedural bleeding.

The access needle is held firmly by the hub in one hand while the skin nick is straddled by the tips of the second and third fingers (either one above and one below or one on each side) of the other hand (Fig. 3-21). The needle is advanced slowly through the nick at a 45-degree angle until arterial pulsation can be felt transmitted through the needle. The needle is then firmly thrust forward until the underlying bone is encountered. The periosteum can be anesthetized with an additional small amount of lidocaine injected directly through the needle (be sure that blood cannot be aspirated before injecting). The hub of the needle is slowly

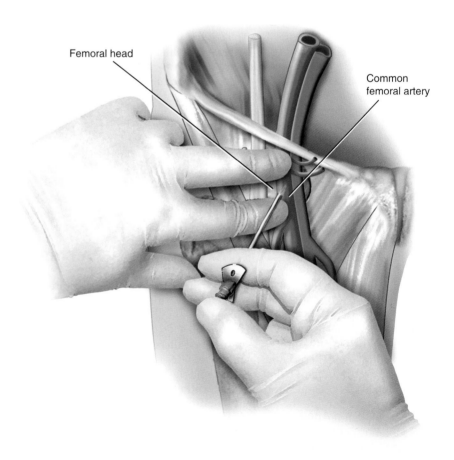

Femoral head

Common femoral artery

FIGURE 3-21. Technique for localization of arterial pulse during puncture. *(From Kadir S. Diagnostic angiography. Philadelphia: WB Saunders; 1986.)*

withdrawn until blood spurts out of the hub. A slight "pop" is frequently felt just as the needle tip enters the lumen of the artery. The flow of blood should be pulsatile and vigorous from an 18-gauge needle but may only drip from a 21-gauge needle. When the visible flow does not correlate with the quality of the pulse, the needle tip may be partially intramural ("side walled"), under a plaque, in a vein, or in the orifice of a small branch vessel.

Once satisfactory flow is obtained from the needle, an atraumatic guidewire (e.g., 3-J long taper or Bentson wire) is introduced through the hub. There should not be any resistance to advancement of the guidewire. If there is resistance, or the guidewire curls as it exits the needle, the tip may be only partially in the artery, or the guidewire may be being directed against the wall or under a plaque. When the guidewire will not advance freely, the tip should be inspected fluoroscopically. The angle of the needle can be changed slightly to align with the long axis of the artery. The guidewire is then gently readvanced while under continuous fluoroscopic monitoring. When adjusting the needle hub slightly does not correct the problem, remove the guidewire to check for good blood return through the needle. A small injection of contrast agent at this point may help resolve the problem, but this should only be done if there is good blood return. Otherwise, there is a risk of injection into the wall of the artery and creation of an obstructing dissection.

Antegrade access is different than retrograde access in that the direction is toward smaller peripheral rather than progressively larger central vessels. At the groin, the CFA bifurcates just below or at the inferior margin of the femoral head, so only a short length of artery may be available for access. Antegrade punctures can be difficult or impossible in obese patients, owing to excessive adipose tissue over the access site. On occasion, a large pannus can be sufficiently retracted with tape to allow an antegrade approach, but often this results in a very steep access. When performing an antegrade puncture, keep in mind that the superficial femoral artery (SFA) origin is medial and anterior to the profunda femoris artery (PFA) origin. A floppy-tipped 3-J guidewire should be used because the SFA is larger than the PFA.

Arterial punctures are characterized as double walled (as detailed above) or single walled. In a single-wall puncture, an open needle is advanced only a few millimeters after the tip touches the artery just through the anterior wall of the vessel. This creates one hole in the artery, which is plugged with the catheter during the procedure, thus theoretically decreasing the chance of a bleeding complication. Single-wall punctures are more difficult than double-wall punctures. If the open needle tip is only partially in the lumen, there may be good blood return, but the guidewire can enter into the subintimal layer as it exits the needle.

Accessing the nonpalpable artery can be challenging (either due to obstruction, low blood pressure, or patient obesity). Puncture under ultrasound guidance is an excellent approach in this situation, eliminating all guesswork. When ultrasound is not readily available, fluoroscopic evaluation of the groin may show calcification in the CFA. These calcified vessels can be punctured under direct fluoroscopic guidance. Another strategy is to opacify the vessel with contrast from a catheter placed through a different access site, but this is usually done only when two catheters

are needed, such as before an intervention. Blind puncture over the medial third of the femoral head may yield success but is the least productive strategy. However, if the femoral vein is entered during any of these attempts, a guidewire can be inserted. This can then be used as a guide to direct the needle lateral to the adjacent CFA during fluoroscopy.

Puncture of the postoperative groin requires knowledge of the type and age of the surgery, particularly if a vascular repair is present. Most angiographers prefer to wait 6 weeks before access through a recently operated groin, because the area can be very tender and there is a small concern about damaging the vascular repair. In reality, the artery and graft can be punctured immediately. Antibiotics are usually not necessary when puncturing a prosthetic graft. An important potential pitfall is present in the postoperative groin when an onlay graft is anastomosed to the CFA. This creates a wide "hood," with the native artery on the bottom and the graft on the top. During percutaneous access, it can be difficult to negotiate out of the native CFA into the more anterior graft, particularly if the external iliac artery is patent (Fig. 3-22). In addition, scarring in the groin may make it hard to introduce catheters. Overdilation of the tract by at least 1 French size and a stiff guidewire may be required to introduce even a 5F catheter.

Complications from CFA punctures are related primarily to vascular trauma during the procedure and lack of hemostasis afterward (Table 3-5). Attention to detail and a gentle touch help avoid most intraprocedural complications. Arterial dissections that occur during retrograde access are frequently subclinical because antegrade blood flow tends to compress the false lumen. Thrombosis is unusual unless a tight stenosis or very low flow is present; anticoagulation with heparin during the procedure is warranted in this situation.

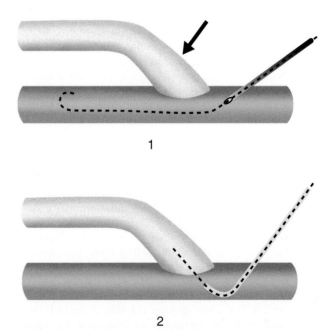

FIGURE 3-22. Puncture of groin after aortofemoral bypass. *1,* Guidewire is directed into native vessel by access needle. Note anterior relationship of graft *(arrow)* to native artery. *2,* Short, angled catheter is used to redirect guidewire into graft. *(From Kaufman JA, Lee MJ, editors. Vascular and interventional radiology: the requisites. St. Louis: Mosby; 2004.)*

TABLE 3-5. Complications of Common Femoral Artery Puncture

Complication	Acceptable Incidence
Hematoma (requiring transfusion, surgery, or delayed discharge)	<3%
Occlusion	<0.5%
Pseudoaneurysm	<0.5%
Arteriovenous fistula	<0.1%

The riskiest part of invasive vascular imaging is actually when the catheter has been removed, when arterial bleeding may occur. Patients who receive heparin during a procedure should have the activated coagulation time checked before removing the catheter or sheath. Protamine sulfate (10 mg/1000 units heparin still active) can be given slowly to correct a prolonged coagulation time. Patients with an abnormal INR (>1.5) can be given 2 units of fresh frozen plasma during the compression. The person performing manual compression must know the location of the catheter entry site in the artery relative to the skin nick and the quality of the pulse before the procedure. The pulse should be identified with certainty before the catheter is removed. Occlusive pressure is maintained for 1 to 2 minutes, after which it is reduced gradually to allow some prograde blood flow (usually this results in a palpable thrill or slight pulse under the finger tips). The occlusive pressure should be limited to 1 minute when compressing a graft, because the likelihood of thrombosis is higher than with a native vessel. After 15 minutes, only light pressure should be required. Should bleeding resume, pressure is reapplied and the 15-minute clock restarted. When a hematoma begins to form during compression, the pressure is either inadequate or being applied in the wrong place. Patients with heavily calcified vessels, with systolic blood pressure greater than 200 mmHg, or who are systemically anticoagulated are at greatest risk of bleeding and may require prolonged compressions. A sandbag should never be substituted for manual compression, because it is not only useless but also can hide development of a hematoma. Patients who undergo manual compression of the puncture should remain in bed with the head elevated to 30 degrees and with the leg immobilized for 6 hours.

There are several alternatives and adjuncts to manual compression of arteries, such as arterial closure devices, clamps, and hemostatic pads.[21] One major advantage of closure devices is that the patient may ambulate much sooner than after manual compression. The closure device strategies include remote suturing of the vessel, deposition of a hemostatic plug or procoagulant gel over the surface of the vessel, placement of an external clip on the surface of the artery, and applying a patch inside the lumen. A fibrotic reaction in the soft tissues may be associated with plug and patch devices. For some devices, the size of the hole in the artery wall must be increased to introduce the closure system. All these devices require training for proper use and are extremely useful in patients at risk for postcompression bleeding, such as those on anticoagulant therapy, with low platelets, or who cannot remain still for 6 hours. These devices fail to achieve hemostasis or require additional manual compression in 5% to 10% of patients.[21] Closure devices should not be used if there is any question of bacterial or fungal contamination of the access site. Infection of the soft tissues or arterial wall has been reported, as has pseudoaneurysm formation, bleeding, and arterial occlusion. An alternative strategy is to substitute an external clamp for manual compression. These patients must remain on bed rest for at least the same length of time as for manual compression.

Axillary/High Brachial Artery Access

The upper extremity approach to arterial access is an alternative to the CFA in patients with absent femoral pulses or groin conditions that preclude safe access or when an upper extremity intervention is anticipated (Fig. 3-23). This approach is a secondary access because of the small (0.5%) risk of stroke (related to the catheter crossing the origins of one or more great vessels) and peripheral upper extremity nerve injury (due to nerve compression by a hematoma in the medial brachial fascial compartment).[22] The upper extremity arteries tend to be smaller and more prone to spasm than the CFA, which limits the size of devices that can be introduced. In general, the axillary and high brachial arteries can accommodate up to a 7F sheath without difficulty. Patients with uncorrected coagulopathy, uncontrolled hypertension, and morbid obesity are contraindicated for axillary/brachial artery access.[23] In addition, because the arm must be placed over and behind the patient's head for the duration of the angiogram, individuals with severe arthritis or other shoulder pathology may not be able to tolerate an upper extremity access. The overall incidence of complications with axillary and high brachial artery punctures is higher than that of CFA puncture.

For procedures involving imaging of the abdominal aorta or the lower extremities, the left arm should be used so the catheter crosses only one cerebral artery (the left vertebral artery). For imaging the ascending thoracic aorta or selecting the cerebral vessels from the axillary approach, the right arm provides the best access. Before the procedure, upper extremity pulses should be palpated and blood pressures in both arms measured. A blood pressure differential of more than 10 to 20 mmHg suggests the presence of stenosis in the affected extremity, and access via the opposite arm should be considered.

The patient should be positioned on the angiographic table so the arm is abducted 90 degrees, with the elbow flexed and the hand placed under the back of the head. The arm should be supported with pillows or soft towels. A digital pulse oximeter on the side of the arterial access helps monitor perfusion of the extremity during the case. The axillary artery is located in the axilla and as it crosses the lateral edge of the pectoralis major muscle to become the brachial artery. Many angiographers prefer to access the high brachial artery where it lies against the humerus, rather than the axillary artery proper, because this site is easier to compress. The skin overlying the artery is anesthetized, but deep anesthesia should be avoided to prevent inadvertent nerve block (a confusing situation because nerve compression is a potential complication of the procedure). After making the skin nick and spreading the soft tissues, the arterial puncture is performed with the following modifications. The humerus is *superior* and posterior to

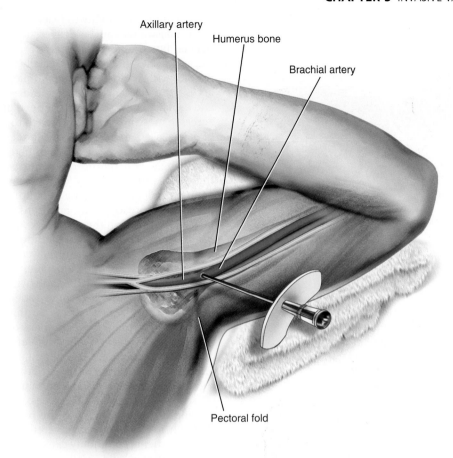

Axillary artery

Humerus bone

Brachial artery

Pectoral fold

FIGURE 3-23. High brachial artery puncture of left arm. Artery is entered lateral to pectoral fold. *(From Kadir S. Diagnostic angiography. Philadelphia: WB Saunders; 1986.)*

the high brachial artery (not directly posterior like the femoral head in relation to the CFA). The needle tip should be angled slightly toward the patient's head to hit the artery. A good initial guidewire for axillary or brachial artery puncture is a floppy 3-J to prevent accidental selection of the vertebral artery and other branch vessels. Many angiographers routinely use ultrasound guidance and microaccess needles for this access.

After the procedure, the arm should be immobilized in a sling for 6 hours, with the patient's back elevated in bed at least 30 degrees. Periodic pulse, access site, and neurologic examinations are mandatory during the 6-hour recovery period. Bleeding at the puncture site can result in compression of adjacent nerves, with ischemic damage. Development of a hematoma at the access site or weakness, paresthesias, or sensory changes in the hand require urgent evaluation for possible surgical decompression of the hematoma.

Additional techniques used in patients who have shoulder pathology or specific anatomic considerations (e.g., inability to bend the elbow) may have upper extremity arterial access from a low brachial artery or radial artery approach. These approaches also have risk and are mentioned here for completeness. In such instances, the patient may keep the arm straight and avoid the discomfort of the "hand behind the head" or elbow flexion (see "Unusual Arterial Access" later in this chapter).

Translumbar Aortic Access

The translumbar approach to the aorta (TLA) seems like a crude and dangerous approach to angiography but is actually an ancient (in angiographic terms), simple, and safe access.[24] The aorta is a large structure with a constant position, so it is usually easy to locate. The puncture is guided fluoroscopically using bony landmarks, allowing successful access in most cases. The main disadvantages of direct aortic puncture are that selective angiography (other than the cerebral vessels) is challenging, and the patient must remain in the prone position for the examination. This access is therefore usually restricted to aortic injections in patients who can lie on their stomachs for 1 to 2 hours. The chief complication of translumbar aortography is a symptomatic retroperitoneal hematoma. Virtually all patients have a small self-contained psoas hematoma (up to a half unit of blood), but fewer than 1% are symptomatic.[25] Very rarely, the pleural space may be entered, resulting in a hemopneumothorax. Visceral artery injury due to the needle has also been reported. Contraindications to TLA access include uncontrolled hypertension, coagulopathy, known supraceliac aortic aneurysm, severe lumbar scoliosis, and dense circumferential aortic calcification.

There are two types of TLA puncture: high (entry at the inferior end plate of the T12 vertebral body) and low (entry at the inferior end plate of L3) (Fig. 3-24). The high approach

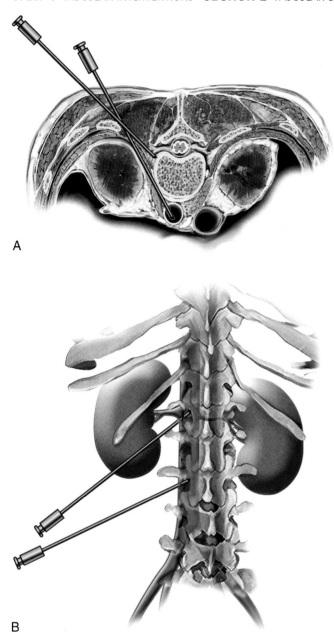

A

B

FIGURE 3-24. Translumbar puncture of abdominal aorta. **A,** Cross-sectional diagram demonstrates anterior redirection of needle away from vertebral body toward aorta. **B,** Two sites for puncture of aorta are at T12-L1 interspace (high) and L2-L3 interspace (low). *(From Kim D, Orron DE. Peripheral vascular imaging and intervention. St. Louis: Mosby; 1992.)*

is used most often because the low puncture is impossible in patients with infrarenal aortic occlusion (i.e., the typical TLA patient) and unwise in the presence of an infrarenal abdominal aortic aneurysm. With the patient prone, the T12 vertebral body and the left iliac crest are localized fluoroscopically. For a high access, the skin is anesthetized on the left at a point roughly midway between the lumbar spinous processes and the flank and several centimeters below the 12th rib. For a low access, the skin entry site is midway between the iliac crest and the 12th rib. If the skin nick is too medial, approach to the aorta will be blocked by the vertebral body. A lateral access may result in puncture

of the kidney or inability to reach the aorta with the needle. Deep anesthesia can be delivered with a 20-gauge spinal needle, but the aorta is rarely reached in normal adults. Access kits designed for TLA usually include a long 18-gauge needle, with preloaded coaxial Teflon dilators. For a high access, the needle is advanced under fluoroscopy medially and cephalad toward the inferior end plate of T12. For a low access, a more horizontal approach to the inferior end plate of L3 is used. If the vertebral body is encountered, the needle is withdrawn several centimeters, the angle adjusted accordingly, and the needle readvanced. Passing through the psoas muscle fascia can be uncomfortable for the patient. Deflection of aortic calcification by the needle may be visible fluoroscopically, or a transmitted aortic pulsation may be felt through the needle. At this point, the needle is firmly advanced forward a centimeter (but not across the midline). The stylet is removed, confirming blood return before introduction of a guidewire. In almost all instances, the natural direction of the guidewire will be cephalad. A 0.038-inch guidewire is recommended to minimize kinking in the retroperitoneal tissues during catheter exchanges. Insertion of a long 5F sheath allows catheter exchanges if necessary. Reversal of direction of the catheter can be accomplished if necessary by pulling a pigtail catheter or Simmons 1 catheter to the edge of the sheath, thus directing a guidewire into the distal abdominal aorta.

The best part of a TLA access is the compression: at the end of the procedure as the patient is rolled from the stomach to the back onto a stretcher, simply pull out the sheath. Patients commonly experience a mild backache due to accumulation of a small retroperitoneal hematoma, but otherwise should be asymptomatic. The blood pressure and vital signs should be checked frequently for several hours (and remain stable). Patients can ambulate after 4 to 6 hours of bed rest.

Unusual Arterial Access

Almost any artery in the body can be accessed percutaneously but not always safely. The radial artery can accommodate long catheters that can be advanced retrograde into the thoracic aorta.[26] The overall complication rate is low, and bed rest is not required after compression. Patients should have a normal Allen test before catheterization, because radial artery occlusion occurs in a small percentage of cases.

The popliteal artery can be accessed in the popliteal space using ultrasound guidance. The usual indication for this access is an intervention in the SFA and embolization of a distal limb lesion. Popliteal artery access is rare for diagnostic procedures. With the patient in the prone position, the popliteal artery is accessed with a microaccess needle and ultrasound guidance in a retrograde or antegrade direction as determined by the type of procedure. The popliteal vein, which lies superficial to the artery when the patient is in the prone position, can be avoided by using ultrasound guidance.[27]

VENOUS ACCESS

Percutaneous access of deep venous structures differs from arterial access in that the veins cannot be palpated. Superficial anatomy, anatomic relationships to palpable arterial

TABLE 3-6. Complications of Central Venous Punctures

Complication	Acceptable Incidence
Pneumothorax*	<2%
Hemothorax*	<2%
Air embolism*	<2%
Hematoma	<2%
Perforation of vein	<2%
Thrombosis of puncture site (symptomatic)	<4%
Arterial injury	<1%

*Jugular and thoracic veins only.

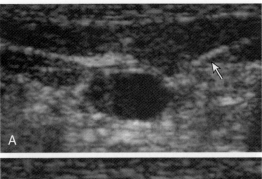
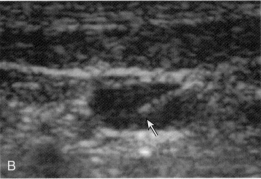

FIGURE 3-25. Ultrasound-guided puncture of internal jugular vein at base of neck. **A,** Axial view of vein shows microaccess needle *(arrow)* in sternocleidomastoid muscle. **B,** Needle tip *(arrow)* is in vein. *(From Kaufman JA, Lee MJ, editors. Vascular and interventional radiology: the requisites. St. Louis: Mosby; 2004.)*

or bony structures, or imaging with ultrasound or fluoroscopy are the major localization techniques. With the exception of femoral vein punctures, image guidance techniques are used for most venous punctures.[28,29]

Veins are forgiving structures with soft pliable walls and low or even negative ambient intraluminal pressures. Large catheters and devices are readily accommodated through most percutaneous central venous access sites, with satisfactory hemostasis at the end of the procedure. Compared to arterial punctures, primary complications associated with deep venous punctures are thrombosis, injury to adjacent structures (e.g., lung), and rarely, air embolism (Table 3-6).[30] Clinically important hematomas are rare but can occur in coagulopathic patients, especially in the presence of high central venous pressures.

Common Femoral Vein Access

The common femoral vein (CFV) is most often accessed over the femoral head, superior to the junction with the deep (profunda) femoral vein and saphenous vein. This segment of vein is similar to the CFA in that it is relatively large, constant in position, and contained within the fascia of the femoral sheath. The vein lies medial and deep to the palpable CFA pulse. To access the CFV, localize the CFA and then anesthetize the skin just medial to the pulse. The skin nick should be slightly lower than would be used for arterial puncture, because the goal is to enter the vein over the lower third of the femoral head. A sharp, open needle (without a stylet) is used, and suction is applied to the hub as the needle is advanced. Blood is aspirated when the needle enters the vessel. Continuous localization of the arterial pulse with fingers of the other hand while advancing the needle prevents inadvertent arterial puncture. If the underlying femoral head is reached without a blood return, slowly withdraw the needle while maintaining suction. Remove the fingers over the femoral pulse, because these can compress the adjacent vein. Vary the angle of the needle slightly with each pass if no blood return is obtained; the more lateral the trajectory, the higher the risk of arterial puncture. The femoral vein can be accessed in both an antegrade (toward the head) or retrograde (toward the foot) direction, depending on the needs of the procedure. Difficult punctures can be performed with continuous ultrasound guidance. Femoral venous punctures for diagnostic procedures require only 5 to 10 minutes of compression. Interventional procedures using large

sheaths in anticoagulated patients require longer compression times.

Internal Jugular Vein Access

The internal jugular vein (IJV) is a common access for many diagnostic and interventional procedures. The right IJV is the optimal access for insertion of tunneled catheters. The traditional approach to IJV access is based on anatomic landmarks, with a posterior, middle, or anterior approach. Access with ultrasound guidance is the preferred method by interventional radiologists. Puncture of the carotid artery and pneumothorax, the major complications of blind IJV access, can be almost eliminated by using ultrasound guidance.

The IJVs should be checked with ultrasound for location relative to the carotid arteries, compressibility, and change in size with respiration and cardiac cycle (indicating central patency) before final preparations.[28] The patient should be placed in Trendelenburg position or with the legs elevated on pillows to dilate the IJVs. Microaccess needles are optimal for ultrasound-guided IJV puncture.

The access site for an IJV access should be in the midportion of the neck for diagnostic and interventional procedures, and lower and posterior for tunneled venous catheters. The right IJV is the desirable vein for diagnostic or interventional venous procedures involving the thorax or abdomen, because it provides straight-line access to the superior and inferior venae cavae (SVC, IVC). The access needle is advanced under ultrasound guidance until it is seen to enter the vein or blood can be aspirated (Fig. 3-25). Aspiration of air may indicate transgression of the pleural cavity or (more often) that the syringe is not attached firmly to the needle. After achieving venous access, the guidewire should pass easily to the right atrium and often into the IVC. If accidental carotid puncture is suspected, either pull out everything or insert the 3F inner dilator from the microaccess kit over the 0.018-inch guidewire and inject a small amount of contrast agent to confirm the catheter location.

Percutaneous access via the IJV has a very low overall complication rate (see Table 3-6). Puncture-related thrombosis is less common in the IJV than most other venous access sites. However, a unique and potentially lethal risk of IJV (as well as subclavian vein) access is introduction of air (air embolism) through an open catheter, dilator, or sheath (particularly the peel-away type) into the central venous circulation if the patient takes a breath at the wrong moment. A small amount of air introduced into the central venous system is harmless, but a large amount (20-30 mL) can obstruct the pulmonary outflow tract. To minimize the risk, the patient should be instructed to perform a Valsalva maneuver or hum whenever a needle, catheter, or sheath is open to room air. Placing the patient in Trendelenburg position also helps decrease the chance of air embolism.

Should an air embolism occur during a procedure, first check the patient's vital signs for a drop in blood pressure or oxygen saturation. The patient may complain of chest pain or pressure. Stable patients can be observed for several minutes as air is absorbed. The air can sometimes be seen in pulmonary outflow tract with fluoroscopy. An unstable patient should be turned left side down to trap air in the capacious right atrium. In severe cases, a catheter can be introduced into the right atrium to aspirate the air.

After catheter removal, jugular veins can be compressed with the back of the patient's bed elevated. The patient should be instructed to perform a Valsalva maneuver during catheter removal, and occlusive pressure should be applied over the IJV as the catheter is removed. The duration of compression is usually 5 to 10 minutes. Keep in mind that air embolism through the subcutaneous tract can occur in thin patients.

Subclavian Vein Access

Percutaneous subclavian vein access has traditionally been based on superficial landmarks. With this approach, access is achieved in 90% to 95% of attempts, but pneumothorax and subclavian artery puncture also occur in 3% to 5%. With image-guided puncture, complications are reduced to less than 1%, with a 100% success rate.[29]

The safest place to access the subclavian vein is over the anterior aspect of the first rib, lateral to the clavicle. The vein should not be accessed under the clavicle, especially when placing long-term central venous catheters, because this may lead to compression and fracture of the catheter ("pinch-off syndrome") between the clavicle and first rib.[31] The subclavian vein is inferior and anterior to the subclavian artery over the first rib, so arterial puncture is less common in this location. The presence of underlying bone minimizes the risk of pneumothorax during puncture. At the lateral margin of the first rib, the vessel becomes the axillary vein, which is best accessed over the anterior portion of the second rib for the same reasons listed earlier.

Access of the subclavian vein can be guided with ultrasound or fluoroscopy. The disadvantage of ultrasonography is that the structures below the vein (rib and lung) may be difficult to visualize, and central venous patency cannot be assessed. The technique is virtually identical to that used for the jugular veins. The advantage of ultrasonography is that contrast medium is not necessary, so radiation exposure to the operator and patient is minimized. For fluoroscopic-guided puncture, an upper extremity venogram can be performed by injection of 10 to 20 mL of contrast material through a vein in the hand or forearm. This allows exact localization of the subclavian vein as it crosses the ribs and confirms patency of the central venous system. Puncture can then be performed with carefully coned-down fluoroscopy over the needle tip. A microaccess needle is advanced under direct visualization until blood is aspirated or the tip touches the anterior surface of the first rib.

Translumbar Inferior Vena Cava Access

Direct access to the IVC is used primarily for placement of long-term central venous access devices.[32] Diagnostic central venous procedures can almost always be performed from a peripheral approach. This access is similar in technique and materials to a low TLA, but the approach is from the right rather than the left.

Previous studies such as computed tomography (CT) scans and magnetic resonance imaging (MRI) should be reviewed before the procedure to determine IVC anatomy, particularly in a patient with an abdominal aortic aneurysm or retroperitoneal mass. When first performing this procedure, it may be helpful to place a 5F pigtail catheter into the IVC from a femoral approach to localize the IVC during puncture.

The patient is placed either prone or in left lateral decubitus position, with a small towel roll under the left flank to straighten the spine. A translumbar aortography needle/sheath system is inserted at a point approximately 10 cm to the right of the spinous process and just above the right iliac crest. The needle is advanced at a 45-degree angle cephalad toward the top of the L3 vertebral body until bone is encountered. The needle is then withdrawn, angled more anteriorly, and readvanced so it passes just anterior to the vertebral body. If a catheter has been placed in the IVC, it can be used as a target for puncture.

Puncture of an arterial structure is usually inconsequential unless the patient is coagulopathic; however, these patients should be observed with the same postprocedural protocol used for TLA punctures. Many patients have transient pain radiating to the right leg during the procedure. If pain is severe, the needle should be reinserted from a more lateral position to avoid the psoas muscle.

IMAGING

An essential element of angiography is the permanent recording of the contrast injection. Simple observation with fluoroscopy is not acceptable (no images = no diagnosis). Historically, there have been two basic modes of recording angiographic images: film-screen and digital angiography. The former is archaic. The latter is almost always displayed as a subtracted image (digital subtraction angiography

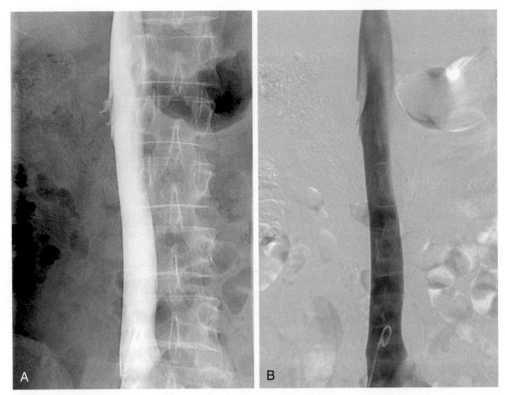

FIGURE 3-26. Digital subtraction angiography. **A,** Unsubtracted image of injection in inferior vena cava. Note that contrast in vein is dense (white), as are bones. Gas in bowel is black. **B,** Subtracted view of same image. Stationary bones and background tissues are now absent, greatly increasing visibility of contrast in vein. Because there is bowel peristalsis, gas artifact is seen in abdomen. *(From Kaufman JA, Lee MJ, editors. Vascular and interventional radiology: the requisites. St. Louis: Mosby; 2004.)*

[DSA]).[33] Cineradiography as used in cardiac catheterization has no role in noncardiac applications.

DSA is the most widely used angiographic technique in current practice (Fig. 3-26). The original clinical application of DSA was a large, rapid venous injection of contrast agent, with acquisition of digitally subtracted images timed to record arterial opacification by the bolus (IV-DSA).[34] This was an unsatisfactory application of a brilliant innovation because of unpredictable venous opacification due to variations in cardiac output, poor resolution of the weakly opacified arteries, inability to selectively inject arteries, and motion artifacts. Direct intraarterial injection of contrast medium, as used with film-screen angiography, rapidly replaced IV-DSA. Digital angiography still has lower resolution than film-screen, but the extremely rapid acquisition of images and processing (the subtraction is performed instantaneously and displayed on a monitor) as well as the ability to manipulate the image appearance online compensate for poor opacification, negating this disadvantage. The interchange between fluoroscopic and DSA modes is electronic and almost instantaneous rather than mechanical and slow. Images can be viewed in either subtracted or unsubtracted (raw) states. Filming can be as rapid as 30 frames per second with some angiographic equipment, with continuous acquisition while moving the angiographic table (bolus chase) or the tube (rotational angiography). Newer units can construct CT-like images and three-dimensional (3D) models from rotational angiographic data (cone-beam CT), a useful tool during complex diagnostic and interventional procedures (Fig 3-27). Lower-contrast concentrations can be used (30%-50% less iodine than the older film-screen angiography) without altering injection rates. The exquisite sensitivity of this technique allows use of negative contrast agents such as CO_2 for angiography. The limitations of DSA in addition to lower resolution include subtraction artifacts from involuntary motion such as bowel peristalsis, respiration, and cardiac pulsation and a tendency to "shoot first and ask questions later" (collect lots of images quickly, with only superficial review during the procedure).

Whether using film-screen or DSA, it is necessary to determine positioning and image acquisition rates for each injection. Patient positioning has been loosely standardized for most angiograms based on the anatomy under evaluation and the empiricism that two different views of the same vascular structure are necessary for evaluation of most pathologic processes (one view = no view) (Fig. 3-28). Similarly, contrast injection and image acquisition rates have been developed for different studies based on expected flow rates and pathologic processes. Individual variations in positioning, injection rates, and filming are frequently necessary because flow may be slower or faster than anticipated or the pathologic process may be visible only on delayed images. In general, images should be acquired faster during the arterial phase and then more slowly to follow the capillary and venous phases. Large vascular spaces such as aortic aneurysms require longer injections and large volumes of contrast (not faster injection rates) to be adequately opacified. Large vascular beds (e.g., lower extremities) require long injections at a lower rate to ensure complete

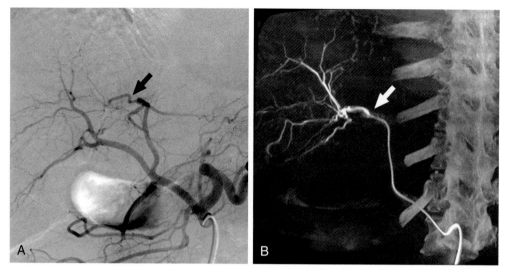

FIGURE 3-27. Postprocessed rotational digital subtraction angiogram (DSA) with a flat-panel image intensifier. **A,** Conventional DSA of celiac artery injection. Note medial branch of left hepatic artery *(arrow)* to segment 4 of liver. **B,** Maximum intensity projection (MIP) image from a rotational selective angiogram of segment 4 branch *(arrow)*. *(From Kaufman JA, Lee MJ editors. Vascular and interventional radiology: the requisites. 2nd ed. Philadelphia: Elsevier; 2013.)*

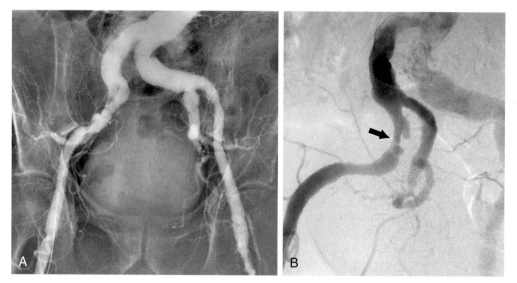

FIGURE 3-28. Evaluation of most vascular structures requires imaging in at least two views. **A,** Screen-film pelvic angiogram in anteroposterior projection. No obvious lesion present on right, but patient had slightly diminished right femoral pulse. **B,** Digital subtraction view of right external iliac artery in right posterior oblique projection. Eccentric stenosis *(arrow)* is now readily visible. Note that internal iliac artery origin is also clearly seen.

opacification, and rapidly flowing blood may require both high flow rates and large volumes (e.g., thoracic aortogram in a young hyperdynamic patient).

Intravascular Ultrasonography

Intravascular ultrasonography is an invasive technology that combines features of noninvasive imaging.[35] By placing a probe on the end of a catheter (usually 4F-9F), direct access to the vascular lumen can be obtained (Fig. 3-29). A hemostatic sheath is necessary to allow safe introduction of a probe. Rather than look from the outside in, intravascular ultrasonography is used to look from inside out (Fig. 3-30). This technique is a useful adjunct to conventional angiography when evaluating intraluminal processes such as dissections or vessel wall abnormalities such as eccentric stenoses that are difficult to visualize on an angiogram (Fig. 3-31). Precise luminal diameter measurements can be obtained, and stenoses can be localized. This may be particularly useful during complex interventions. The arterial wall can also be assessed for subtle changes of atherosclerosis, although the clinical utility of this information remains to be determined. The limitations of the technique are the expense of the additional equipment, the inability to look forward with the catheter (most designs are based on a rotating transducer that can image only in the axial plane), the small field of view when compared with external probes, and the limited penetration of smaller probes.

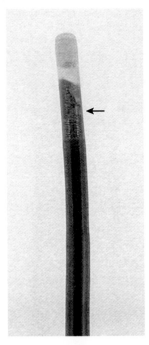

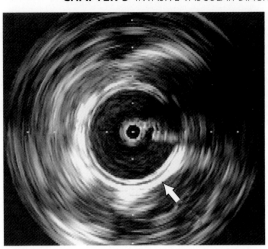

FIGURE 3-30. Normal intravascular ultrasound (IVUS) images of popliteal artery. A 6F probe (12.5 MHz) is visible in center of vessel. Echogenic intima, hypoechoic media, and echogenic media are clearly visualized *(arrow)*. *(From Kaufman JA, Lee MJ, editors. Vascular and interventional radiology: the requisites. St. Louis: Mosby; 2004.)*

FIGURE 3-29. Intravascular ultrasound probe (9F, 9 MHz). Transducer *(arrow)* is located proximal to tip of catheter. Smaller-diameter probes that can be inserted over a guidewire are readily available. *(From Kaufman JA, Lee MJ, editors. Vascular and interventional radiology: the requisites. St. Louis: Mosby; 2004.)*

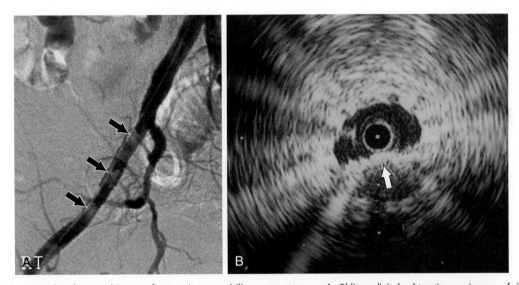

FIGURE 3-31. Intravascular ultrasound image of eccentric external iliac artery stenoses. **A,** Oblique digital subtraction angiogram of right external iliac artery shows several areas *(arrows)* of decreased contrast density consistent with bulky calcified plaque. **B,** Intravascular ultrasound image (7F, 12 MHz) of same vessel shows one of the calcified eccentric stenoses *(arrow)*. *(From Kaufman JA, Lee MJ, editors. Vascular and interventional radiology: the requisites. St. Louis: Mosby; 2004.)*

KEY POINTS

- Invasive vascular diagnosis remains an essential competency in image-guided intervention.
- Information is power; the more you have before the procedure, the better the outcomes.
- The interventionalist's responsibility includes providing preprocedural consultation and postprocedure care as well as performing the procedure.

- Vascular access selection requires consideration of the target vascular bed, devices that will be used, and the ability to obtain hemostasis at the end of the procedure.
- Imaging (the blood vessels injected and images collected) should match the vascular anatomy, physiology, and clinical scenario.

▸ **SUGGESTED READINGS**

Kandarpa K, Machan, L. Handbook of interventional radiologic procedures. 4th ed. Philadelphia: Wolters Kluwer/Lippincott Williams & Wilkins; 2011.

Kaufman JA, Lee MJ. Interventional radiology: the requisites, 2nd ed. Philadelphia: Elsevier; 2013.

Valji K. Vascular and interventional radiology, 2nd ed. Philadelphia: Saunders/Elsevier; 2006.

Waybill PN, Brown DB. Patient care in vascular and interventional radiology, 2nd ed. Fairfax: SIR Press; 2010.

The complete reference list is available onine at www.expertconsult.com.

CHAPTER 4

Diagnostic Catheters and Guidewires

Curtis W. Bakal and Sebastian Flacke

The basic principles of vascular access and catheter guidewire manipulation for selective and superselective angiography were described over a half century ago. Since the early days of direct puncture of the target vessel, continued refinement of puncture techniques and equipment facilitate the myriad of interventional procedures now considered current standard practice. Vascular access for diagnostic angiography requires a puncture needle, angiographic guidewires, sheath and dilator systems, and angiographic catheters. The basic principles of these materials and their manipulation are nearly universal, and an understanding of these fundamental concepts and techniques is crucial to successful contemporary interventional practice.

Single-wall puncture techniques using hollow nonstylet 18- or 19-gauge needles or a micropuncture system have now largely replaced the traditional double-wall puncture technique described by Seldinger. The single-wall puncture technique has many benefits if performed correctly, but the beveled tip of the needle may be error prone in inexperienced hands, since it can be both luminal and intraluminal and return pulsatile flow. Advancing the guidewire in this circumstance may initiate subintimal dissection. Other puncture needle designs are available and still have their niche for specific procedures.

Standard angiographic guidewires are composed of stainless steel springs tightly wound around a stiff mandrel core that is welded to the trailing end of the wire. A small-gauge internal safety wire is usually present to prevent the spring wire from uncoiling. Guidewires must interact with the needle, diagnostic catheter, and vessel wall in a manner that allows safe access, guidance along the vessel, and selective catheterization. The outer spring is usually coated with Teflon, which decreases its coefficient of friction. To date, hydrophilic copolymer–coated, nitinol-cored guidewires have largely replaced standard coil spring wires in most interventional suites. Characteristics that are independently incorporated into a specific guidewire design include mandrel tip tapering, mandrel stiffness, tip shape, length, and diameter. Mandrel shafts can be constructed with varying stiffness. Both straight and J-tipped standard guidewires are available. J tips are used for minimizing wall damage in atherosclerotic arteries during advancement, because the leading J edge is blunt. Knowledge of guidewire properties and appropriate sizes are keys to successful angiography; it is the interplay between the catheter and guidewire

characteristics, especially their relative leading stiffness, that determines how well a catheter can be advanced selectively.

Vascular dilators are stiff short catheters with tapered leading edges that are used to create a soft-tissue tract to facilitate passage of a diagnostic catheter. Vascular sheaths are thin-walled catheters inserted over tightly matched dilators. After removal of the inner dilator, the sheath is left in place to allow subsequent passage of a catheter. Sheaths are used during virtually all interventions. Sheaths of various length and tip design are available and can be used with angiographic catheters in coaxial fashion to facilitate and secure selective vascular access to aortic side branches.

Catheters are possibly the most varied products used by the typical interventional radiologist. It is useful to classify them functionally into two broad general categories: nonselective (flush) and selective.

Flush catheters must allow high-flow injections into the aorta or inferior vena cava, and uniform dispersal (with minimal recoil) of contrast media via multiple side holes. The tip of a flush catheter is usually designed to help center the shaft in the vessel and preclude engagement and injection into a branch vessel.

Selective catheters are designed with rotational stiffness to seek a vessel orifice, but with enough flexibility to pass the catheter far into the vessel. The shape of the catheter tip is perhaps its most essential or defining element, and a variety of more complex shapes are required because of the large size of the trunk vessel relative to the target vessel origin. Here, selection of the ostium, advancement down the vessel, and positional stability during subsequent manipulation and injection all depend on the wall-seeking behavior of the catheter; it must be in contact with the vessel wall opposite the target branch orifice. It is firm contact with the back wall that turns a catheter potentially flopping in midstream into an efficient device that will engage a branch origin and reorient the relatively vertical pushing force applied at the groin down the axis of the target vessel. Choice of the appropriate primary and secondary curve of a catheter is key to successful angiography.

This chapter, which can be viewed in its entirety at www.expertconsult.com, offers in-depth discussions of catheter, sheath, guidewire, and needle designs to help the clinician understand and choose the appropriate equipment for angiographic procedures.

CHAPTER 5

Balloon Catheters

Shawn N. Sarin, Wael E.A. Saad, David B. Nicholson, Ulku C. Turba, John F. Angle, Klaus D. Hagspiel, Michael D. Dake, and Alan H. Matsumoto

Although Dotter and Judkins first described percutaneous transluminal angioplasty (PTA) in 1964, use of the procedure did not gain momentum until 1976, when Gruentzig described his double-lumen balloon catheter. The Gruentzig balloon catheter incorporated balloon material that was relatively noncompliant and mounted on small catheters (7F-8F) that could be advanced coaxially over a guidewire. Since its introduction, the design of balloon catheters has improved as technology has evolved.

Two basic types of balloons are used by interventionalists: (1) *high-pressure*, relatively noncompliant, angioplasty-type balloons and (2) *low-pressure*, compliant balloons, typically made of latex, silicone, or polyurethane and used primarily for temporary vascular occlusion, embolectomy, or molding of stent-grafts. High-pressure balloons are made from relatively noncompliant polymers and are thin walled in design in order for them to be low profile (Table 5-1). These balloons exhibit high tensile strength with minimal expansion beyond their nominal diameter as inflation pressure is increased. Low-pressure balloons are typically molded into a tubular shape and then expanded beyond their original size during inflation. These balloons cannot be inflated to precise dimensions and enlarge with increasing inflation pressure. For angioplasty procedures, balloons must have a controllable or reproducible nominal diameter to ensure they will not continue to expand and damage or rupture the target vessel. For example, a low-compliance, high-pressure balloon might expand only 5% to 10% when inflated to its rated burst pressure. Conversely, low-pressure balloons—which are inflated by volume, not by pressure—can easily be enlarged by 600%.

Peripheral balloon dilation catheters can be divided into four broad categories:

- Standard balloons: 0.035-inch guidewire compatible
- Small vessel balloons: 0.014- to 0.018-inch guidewire compatible
- Large-diameter balloons: 12 mm or larger in diameter
- Other/specialty balloons: cutting, cryoplasty, occlusion, embolectomy, drug-eluting, and embolic capture balloons

These categories are very broad, so there may be some overlap between them. For example, a standard balloon product line might offer 12-mm sizes. Peripheral and noncompliant valvuloplasty balloons range from 12 to 33 mm in diameter and 1.5 to 12 cm in length. Catheter shaft lengths vary from product to product but generally range from 40 to 150 cm.

Balloon catheter technology has made remarkable strides over the past 3 decades. The goal of attaining low-profile systems with excellent trackability, rapid inflation/deflation times, noncompliance, and scratch resistance is quickly being met. There are now a large variety of balloons with higher burst pressures, smaller diameters, and low profiles that allow interventions in peripheral vessels as small as 2 mm. As it stands today, interventionalists have a wide assortment of balloon catheters to facilitate interventions (critical limb ischemia, intracranial procedures, esophageal intervention, etc.) not possible just a few years ago. Future advancements may see balloons combined with light therapy (lasers) and drug delivery systems or further integration with cutting blades, thermal energy, biodegradable stents, and other products.

For a full discussion of this topic, please visit the website www.expertconsult.com.

TABLE 5-1. Characteristics of Balloon Materials

Materials	Tensile Strength	Compliance (Relative)	Stiffness	Profile	Maximum Rated Pressure (atm)	Sterilization
PET	High	Low	High	Low	20	EtO or radiation
Nylon	Medium-high	Medium	Low	Low	16	EtO
PE	Medium	Medium	Low	Medium	10	EtO or radiation
PET/PE fibers and Pebax	Very high	Very low	High	Medium	30	EtO
PVC	Low	High	Medium	High	6-8	Radiation
NyBax	High	High	Low	Low	24	EtO or Radiation

EtO, Ethylene oxide gas; *PE,* polyethylene; *PET,* polyethylene terephthalate; *PVC,* polyvinyl chloride.

CHAPTER 6

Stents

Gregory J. Dubel and Timothy P. Murphy

Stents have revolutionized endovascular management of peripheral arterial disease and been responsible for the transition in revascularization from surgery to interventional means for many vascular territories, including coronary, subclavian, aortoiliac, carotid, renal, and visceral arteries. They may eventually be the preferred therapy for femoropopliteal obstruction. The impact of stents on clinical practice has been enormous. Many stents marketed in the United States are U.S. Food and Drug Administration (FDA) approved for treating biliary or tracheobronchial stenoses, although recently more have gained FDA approval for intravascular use. (Tables e6-1, e6-2, and e6-3 offer expansive lists.) Stents available today generally fall into two broad categories. The two fundamentally different classes of stent include self-expanding (SX) and balloon-expandable (BX) stents. BX stents require balloon dilation to increase their diameter from the compressed state. SX stents will attempt to regain diameter upon deployment. Many SX stents marketed today are made of nitinol.

Biological, mechanical, and technical factors influence stent design and placement considerations. Biological factors include resistance to corrosion and tissue biocompatibility. A basic understanding of the interplay between stent and vessel is useful because it has been speculated (but not proven) that host reaction and the biology of the stent may be the most important factors determining long-term patency. Important mechanical factors include properties such as radiopacity, flexibility, resistance to compression, and fatigue resistance. Fatigue resistance has proved to be problematic in the superficial femoral artery, and a great deal of research continues on this property. Important technical factors include things such as required delivery sheath, premounted versus unmounted stent, over-the-wire versus monorail delivery, available stent size, and delivery system. In the "real world" of daily patient care, technical and/or mechanical factors (e.g., flexibility, radiopacity, sizing, etc.) tend to dominate one's choice of stent. By understanding the basic biological, mechanical, and design properties of these devices, the practitioner is better able to select the appropriate device for individual applications.

For a comprehensive discussion of stents, including individual devices, please visit the accompanying website at www.expertconsult.com.

CHAPTER 7

Thrombectomy Devices
Steven Zangan and Brian Funaki

Catheter-directed thrombolysis (CDT) has advantages over surgical thrombectomy in the treatment of venous or arterial thrombosis. Thrombolytic therapy avoids the morbidity and mortality associated with conventional surgical techniques and general anesthesia. It is less traumatic and causes less intimal damage compared with surgical balloon thrombectomy. CDT has the distinct advantage of providing both diagnostic information about associated vascular disease that may have incited the occlusive event and the opportunity to treat coexistent lesions with angioplasty and stenting. However, CDT can be time consuming and expensive, and response to therapy may be nonuniform, especially in chronic occlusions. More importantly, some patients are excluded from treatment because of contraindications to anticoagulation. These shortcomings have driven the evolution of percutaneous mechanical thrombectomy (PMT). PMT is particularly well suited for the treatment of thrombosed hemodialysis access grafts, and most commercially available devices have been approved by the U.S. Food and Drug Administration (FDA) for this

TABLE 7-1. Mechanical Thrombectomy/Thrombolysis

Product	Company	Mode of Operation
Pronto Extraction Catheter	Vascular Solutions	Aspiration thrombectomy
Diver CE Clot Extraction Catheter Export AP Aspiration Catheter	Medtronic	Aspiration thrombectomy
Fetch Aspiration Catheter	Medrad	Aspiration thrombectomy
Helix ClotBuster Mechanical Thrombectomy Device	ev3	Rotational mechanical thrombectomy
Rinspirator Thrombus Removal System	ev3	Infusion and aspiration thrombectomy
Trellis Peripheral Infusion System	Covidien	Isolated pharmacomechanical thrombolysis via a dispersion wire between two occlusion balloons
AngioJet	Medrad/Possis	High-velocity water jets enclosed in the catheter capture, microfragment, and remove thrombus
ThromCat Thrombectomy Catheter System	Spectranetics	Internal helix produces a vacuum and macerates thrombus while simultaneous flushing and extraction facilitate thrombus removal
Arrow-Trerotola Percutaneous Thrombolytic Device	Arrow	Rotating wire fragmentation basket macerates thrombus
Cleaner Rotational Thrombectomy System	Argon Medical	Sinusoidal vortex wire rotates and macerates thrombus
D-Clot Thrombectomy Catheter System	Artegraft	Spiral conveyer shaft rotates and macerates thrombus while debris is aspirated through a sheath
Merci Retrievers	Concentric Medical	Mechanical thrombectomy with aspiration and proximal flow arrest via a balloon-guiding catheter (neurovasculature)
Penumbra System	Penumbra	Separator-assisted clot debulking and aspiration (neurovasculature)
Straub Rotarex Catheter	Straub Medical	Rotating spiral creates a vacuum and macerates thrombus, which is discharged into a collection bag
X-Sizer Thrombectomy Catheter System	ev3	Mechanical thrombectomy with a helical cutter
Fogarty Adherent Clot Catheter	Edwards Lifesciences	Mechanical thrombectomy via a corkscrew-shaped stainless steel cable
Fogarty Graft Thrombectomy Catheter	Edwards Lifesciences	Mechanical thrombectomy via a double helix ring
Xtraktor Thrombectomy Catheter	Xtrak Medical	Mechanical thrombectomy via a rotating spiral shaft
OmniWave Endovascular System	OmniSonics	Ultrasound-accelerated thrombolysis
EkoSonic Endovascular System	Ekos	Ultrasound-accelerated thrombolysis
Acolysis Ultrasound Thrombolysis System	Vascular Solutions	Ultrasound-accelerated thrombolysis

application. As device design continues to evolve, potential indications for PMT also expand. Literature documenting efficacy in native arterial and bypass graft occlusion, deep venous thrombosis, pulmonary embolism, and transjugular intrahepatic portocaval shunt (TIPS) and portal vein thrombosis is mounting.

All PMT devices engage thrombus, fragment it, and most dispose of the effluent. A variety of approaches have been developed to achieve these goals (Table 7-1). However, despite continued innovation, no single PMT device has emerged as superior. Each manufacturer claims benefits unique to their catheters owing to the specific mechanism of action, although these are often merely theoretical advantages and have not been sufficiently validated in clinical trials. Multiple studies have demonstrated that all PMT devices can achieve excellent technical success rates. As technology advances and more experience is gained, the safety and efficacy of these devices will continue to improve. It is expected that the scope of potential applications will also continue to expand.

For a full discussion of thrombectomy devices, please visit the website www.expertconsult.com.

CHAPTER 8

Embolic Protection Devices

Bhaskar Ganai and Sumaira Macdonald

Percutaneous endovascular procedures have transformed the management of arterial disease. It is known that peri-procedural thromboembolic events occur frequently as a result of manipulation of guidewires, balloons, and stents. The consequences and clinical manifestations of these emboli are dependent on size and number of emboli, as well as the target organ sensitivity to both emboli and ischemia. Efforts to make carotid artery stenting as safe as carotid endarterectomy have resulted in innovations with lower-profile devices and specifically designed stents. In addition, embolic protection devices (EPDs) were developed, aimed at preventing distal embolization of thrombus and plaque to the brain, and therefore reducing the adverse neurologic events associated with the procedure. Use of these EPDs is now regarded as mandatory for carotid intervention by the majority of interventionists.

There are a wide variety of EPDs available, but they all employ one or more of the following strategies:
- Vessel filtration
- Vessel occlusion (distal)
- Vessel occlusion (proximal) with:
  - Flow arrest
  - Flow reversal

Distal EPDs were the first to be developed. These devices originally employed a compliant balloon to occlude the distal internal carotid artery (ICA) during stent deployment. Filters were to follow and were initially constructed of perforated polyurethane membrane and later, nitinol mesh. These filters were placed in the distal ICA in an effort to capture emboli, which could then be retrieved along with the filter at the end of the procedure. Distal EPDs have continued to develop with new in-stent occlusion systems (TwinOne [Minvasys, Gennevilliers, France]) and Dacron mesh with flow stagnation (FiberNet [Lumen Biomedical Inc., Plymouth, Minn.]).

Proximal EPDs have the theoretical advantage of protecting the intracranial circulation throughout all phases of the procedure. These devices can result in flow reversal via the femoral approach (Gore Flow Reversal System [W.L. Gore & Associates, Flagstaff, Ariz.]) or via a direct common carotid artery approach (MICHI neuroprotection system [Silk Road Medical Inc., Sunnyvale, Calif.]). The Mo.Ma device (Medtronic Inc., Minneapolis, Minn.) results in relative flow arrest.

There have been numerous studies with regard to carotid stenting with EPDs, and we review the contemporary studies, including ARMOUR, DESERVE, EMPiRE, EPIC, and PROOF. These show improved outcomes compared to the more historical studies, namely the North American postmarketing surveillance registries employing specific manufacturers' filter and stent combinations, with proximal EPDs appearing more favorable.

Use of EPDs has been investigated outside the cerebral circulation. In the renal circulation, there is currently no strong evidence to support their routine use, and no specific EPD has been manufactured for the renal arterial territory. Although not supported by randomized trial data, filters are used in the peripheral circulation to capture debris liberated during the use of some atherectomy devices.

The full discussion of EPDs, as well as six illustrations and a table of comparisons, are available at www.expertconsult.com.

CHAPTER 9

Atherectomy Devices

Stefan Müller-Hülsbeck

Balloon angioplasty of femoropopliteal lesions is limited by a low primary patency rate of 30% to 61% after 3 years, depending on lesion length and clinical stage. Atherectomy physically removes plaque by cutting, pulverizing, or shaving it in atherosclerotic arteries, using a mechanical catheter-deliverable endarterectomy device. Four U.S. Food and Drug Administration (FDA)-approved atherectomy devices are currently available for treatment of peripheral arterial disease (PAD): SilverHawk Plaque Excision System (ev3/Covidien, Plymouth, Minn.) (Fig. 9-1), Orbital PAD System (Cardiovascular Systems Inc., St. Paul, Minn.), CVX-300 Excimer Laser (Spectranetics, Colorado Springs, Colo.), and Pathway PV Atherectomy System (Pathway Medical Technologies, Kirkland, Wash.). Theoretically,

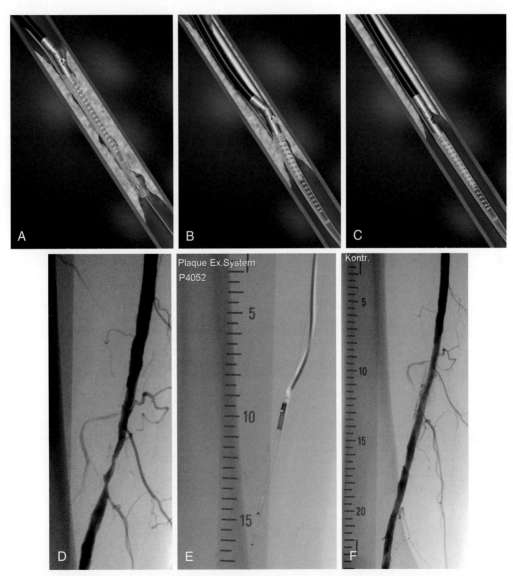

FIGURE 9-1. Three-step illustration of working principle of SilverHawk directional atherectomy catheter in a clinical case. **A,** Flexible shaft of device and rotating blade contained within tubular housing at proximal entrance of lesion. **B,** Device during activation, with rotating blade exposed and nosecone deflected in preparation for excision at distal part of lesion. **C,** Successful atherectomy procedure. **D,** Clinical case illustrates use of devices in treating a short, calcified superficial femoral artery lesion. **E,** SilverHawk was advanced over 0.014-inch guidewire. **F,** After four passes, no residual stenosis is present at completion angiography.

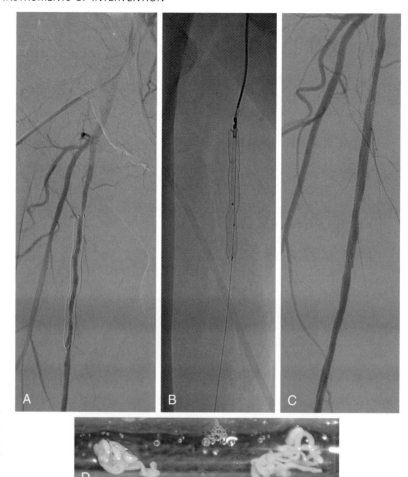

FIGURE 9-2. A, Angiography documenting intimal hyperplasia 6 months after placing self-expanding stent in proximal superficial femoral artery. **B,** Atherectomy of in-stent restenosis was performed with SilverHawk device. **C,** Final angiography after four passes shows no residual lumen loss. **D,** Intimal flaps collected.

atherectomy offers several advantages over percutaneous transluminal angioplasty (PTA). It shows a greater immediate success rate with less dissection and acute occlusion, treats complex lesions, and reduces the restenosis rate by minimizing barotrauma of the vessel wall.

At the moment, no specific recommendations are established for atherectomy devices for the treatment of lower limb artery disease. Current indications might be single, discrete, subtotal occlusion of a lower limb or lower limb artery bypass graft stenosis or restenosis, as well as post-PTA or in-stent restenosis (Fig. 9-2). Long-distance chronic total occlusions and acute occlusions seem contraindicated for current devices.

In this chapter, a balanced comprehensive overview of current devices will be given with respect to technical device-related details and outcomes, indicating that the immediate procedural success rate of atherectomy devices is high, but midterm restenosis rates are significant. Physicians have to ask themselves at the moment whether widespread use of these cost-intensive devices is justified. Complications due to atherectomy will also be discussed, as will postprocedure and follow-up care after atherectomy.

Please visit www.expertconsult.com for the complete discussion of current atherectomy devices, including their uses and pertinent procedural outcomes data.

CHAPTER 10

Embolization Agents

Charles E. Ray, Jr., McKinley C. Lawson, and Jason R. Bauer

The principle of catheter-directed embolization is to acutely stop flow in a blood vessel or vascular territory by way of mechanical occlusion using a temporary or permanent agent. Along with angioplasty, embolization has been a unique defining procedure in the history of interventional radiology. The elegance of the technique underscores the value of minimally invasive therapy. Since the first reported cases using autologous clot in the early 1970s, embolization techniques have evolved with the use of many agents and devices to yield truly impressive results. This technique has evolved to include nearly every vascular territory and has been used in such diverse clinical applications as treatment of tumors, vascular malformations, varicosities, aneurysms and pseudoaneurysms, fibroids, and gastrointestinal bleeding.

An understanding of the available agents and devices is key to using them appropriately (Table 10-1). Device selection is driven by the vascular territory to be embolized, the permanence of occlusion, and the degree of occlusion—proximal or distal—desired. In the past, choices were limited to a basic array of agents including polyvinyl alcohol (PVA) particles, Gelfoam, and coils. Now the armamentarium has expanded. Fundamentally, the techniques are unchanged, but the range of products available requires careful assessment in agent selection.

 Please visit www.expertconsult.com for a full discussion of the types of agents available and their applications resulting from both in vivo behavior and clinical results produced. Special attention will be paid to specific clinical scenarios that are historically challenging for the interventionalist. The discussion of biologically active embolic agents functioning as a vehicle for treatment, such as radioactive spheres and islet cell transplants, will be reviewed in other chapters.

TABLE 10-1. Commonly Used Embolization Materials

Permanent Large-Vessel Occlusions

Coils
Balloons
Amplatz Vascular Plug
Guidewires
Silk suture material
Porcine submucosa
Amplatz Vascular Obstruction Device

Permanent Small-Vessel Occlusions

Particles
Liquid sclerosants
Liquid adhesive
Ethiodol
Thrombin
Ethylene–vinyl alcohol copolymer

Temporary Large-Vessel Occlusions

Gelfoam sponge
Autologous clot

Temporary Small-Vessel Occlusions

Gelfoam powder
Starch microspheres
Fibrillated collagen

CHAPTER 11

Aortic Stent-Grafts

Raghuveer Vallabhaneni and Mark A. Farber

Over the past decade, stent-graft use for the treatment of aortic pathologies has steadily increased. Over 64% of infrarenal aortic aneurysms were treated with endovascular aneurysm repair (EVAR) in 2007.[1] Expanded indications have occurred as additional experience has been obtained using this technology and includes use of stent-grafts to treat aneurysms in the pararenal and visceral aorta, as well as emergent and nonaneurysmal pathologies.[2,3] This clinical application, however, has been associated with a rise in complication rates as devices are being implanted outside their intended "instructions for use" (IFU) guidelines.[4-6] To meet the demand for greater application of endovascular techniques, medical device manufacturers have made advancements in stent-graft design (Fig. 11-1) with new design modifications that are currently being evaluated in trials. Hopefully, this will enable the clinician to handle increasingly complex aortic pathologies that have traditionally been treated by open procedures.[7]

Successful EVAR is directly related to appropriate patient selection. Preprocedural computed tomographic angiography (CTA) with axial and multiplanar reformatted imaging can adequately identify and delineate anatomic characteristics. Axial imaging alone has some shortcomings with respect to accurately sizing tortuous anatomy.[14]

Absolute contraindications to infrarenal EVAR include those patients whose aortic neck is too short or too large to allow for exclusion of the aneurysm. EVAR would be contraindicated if repair requires occlusion of a critical branch vessel. This may include a patient with a patent inferior mesenteric artery when preexisting superior mesenteric artery and celiac artery stenosis or occlusion is present, accessory renal arteries supplying significant renal parenchymal mass (e.g., horseshoe kidney), and rarely a dominant lumbar artery providing critical blood supply to the spinal cord. Significant thrombus in the aortic landing zone may also be a relative contraindication for fear of embolization or lack of adequate seal. Additionally, alternative therapies or devices should be sought in patients with allergies to material components in a device's composition. Relative contraindications include patients whose anatomic criteria do not completely fit the IFU guidelines. This may include patients with small or diseased iliac arteries that require a conduit for device implantation.

In patients who have pararenal or type IV thoracoabdominal aneurysms and are not candidates for open repair, fenestrated endovascular aortic repair (FEVAR) or branched endovascular aortic repair (BEVAR) may be an option. However, clinical trials must be completed prior to these devices being commercially available. EVAR with physician-modified grafts may be considered in such patients, although this application would be outside the devices' IFU guidelines.

Early outcomes after EVAR have met with great success. Patients are discharged from the hospital and return to full activity much quicker than after open surgical repair. Using the latest-generation devices, technical success approaches 100%, with a mortality rate of less than 1% in experienced hands.[18] Morbidity rates have been reduced by over 50% compared to open surgery in most clinical trials, but this benefit may not be sustained beyond the first several years. Secondary procedures, although minimally invasive, add to the overall morbidity of the procedure. Recent reports demonstrated that at 2 to 4 years, the mortality between open and EVAR approach one another and are not statistically different.[19,20] This area is a major focus of research, and unless longer-term prospective studies are conducted, the answer remains unknown.

Compared to infrarenal devices, branched and fenestrated devices have had fewer studies to evaluate long-term follow-up. No randomized trials are available to compare fenestrated versus open repair of juxtarenal aneurysms. Fenestrated devices have allowed for the treatment of many patients with juxtarenal aneurysms who would not otherwise be surgical candidates with reasonable outcomes. These outcomes may improve as experience and technology advance.

The full discussion of aortic stent-grafts, as well as two detailed tables, are available at www.expertconsult.com.

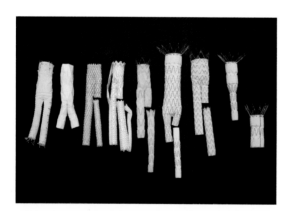

FIGURE 11-1. U.S. Food and Drug Administration (FDA)-approved infrarenal aortic aneurysm endovascular devices. *Left to right,* Ancure (Guidant, Menlo Park, Calif.), Endologix (Endologix, Irvine, Calif.), AneurX (Medtronic, Santa Rosa, Calif.), Gore Excluder (W.L. Gore & Associates, Flagstaff, Ariz.), Medtronic Talent, Cook Zenith (Cook Medical, Bloomington, Ind.), Medtronic Endurant, Cook Renu Converter, Cook Renu Cuff.

CHAPTER **12**

Inferior Vena Cava Filters

Christoph A. Binkert

Several different inferior vena cava (IVC) filter models are used to protect patients from pulmonary embolism. This chapter will provide descriptions of the IVC filters most commonly used in the United States, as well as filters that are unique from a device design or application perspective.

Before the individual IVC filters are described, some general comments about filter concepts and design are useful. In recent years there has been a trend toward the use of *optional filters*, which are permanent devices with the option to be removed if no longer clinically needed. There are two approaches: either the filter is entirely removed, or the filter is converted to a stent. Most optional filters are designed to be completely removed. Typically there is a hook at the cranial tip of the filter that can be grasped with a snare, then the filter can be pulled out. The access for these retrievals is typically the jugular vein. The OptEase filter from Cordis is one exception. The hook is placed at the caudal tip of the filter, allowing its retrieval from a femoral approach. The reason for a different retrieval mechanism is the design of the filter.

Most IVC filters have a conal shape, with the idea that the captured emboli are held in the center of the vein, allowing for dissolution of the trapped clot over time. Filtration can be done in one level (ALN, Option) or two (Eclipse, Celect). The OptEase filter has a two-level basket-shaped design with a hook at the bottom for retrieval. The reasons for retrieval from a femoral approach are the directional hooks at the upper portion of the filter that prevent cranial

migration. Prevention of migration is one of the major challenges of filter devices, and the mechanism most used is oversizing of a self-expanding design. Therefore it is important to be familiar with the maximum diameter of the IVC allowed for each filter. Most commonly, the filters are U.S. Food and Drug Administration (FDA) approved for 28 mm or 30 mm. In addition to this self-expansion, most filters have additional hooks to prevent migration. The hooks are located either at the legs of the filter (Celect, Eclipse, Greenfield), at the arms of the filter (ALN), or at the longitudinal struts (OptEase: hooks pointing up; TrapEase: hooks pointing both up and down; VenaTech LP: hooks pointing both up and down).

Over the last decade, the profile of IVC filters has decreased to about 6F to 8F, which allows a percutaneous placement. For profile comparison, it is important to distinguish between inner diameter (ID) and outer diameter (OD) of the introducer sheath. It is also important to select the right device for the access route chosen to avoid an upside-down filter placement. In today's difficult economic environment, the cost of each device must also be considered. When available, the list price in U.S. dollars is mentioned for each device.

The goal of this chapter, which can be viewed in its entirety at www.expertconsult.com, is to highlight the specific features of each device that should help the interventionist select the best possible filter for any given clinical situation. It is important to be familiar with the device chosen to use it safely and accurately.

CHAPTER 13

Endovascular Laser Therapy

Jörn O. Balzer and Verena Kahn

Chronic atherosclerotic obstructions are a leading cause of lifestyle-limiting intermittent claudication that occurs in 3% to 20% of the population older than 60 years of age.[1] Percutaneous transluminal angioplasty (PTA) is normally recommended as the primary treatment for short-segment femoropopliteal stenoses and occlusions,[1-3,9] but lengthy chronic occlusions are still mainly treated surgically.[1]

The pulsed excimer laser has been extensively evaluated for its ability to debulk atherosclerotic material in vitro and in vivo, demonstrating that the photoablative effect of laser light can recanalize even lesions not amenable to conventional PTA.[16-18] Thermal laser systems—the Nd:YAG and CO_2—were both found to be either dangerous or ineffective for laser-assisted angioplasty because of perforation or destruction of the vessel wall. In contrast, both the excimer and CO_2 lasers are "cold" laser systems that do not lead to heating at the treatment site, so the danger of vessel perforation from heating due to lasing is negligible.[21-27]

Most recanalizations are performed retrograde. The activated laser catheter is advanced for the first few millimeters into the occlusion without wire guidance. For further recanalization of the occluded vessel segment, the activated laser catheter is slowly advanced stepwise at a rate not exceeding 1 mm/s for a short (<5 mm) distance without wire guidance, followed by further crossing with the guidewire using a step-by-step technique. To enter the patent distal segment of the artery, it is recommended to cross the last 2 cm of the occlusion with the guidewire alone (angled or straight tip) before lasing. Particular attention should be paid to avoiding vessel wall dissections distal to the original occlusion. After initial passage, a repeat lasing during continuous saline flush increases the amount of ablation. In most cases, balloon angioplasty is then required. After contrast material application, thorough flushing of the vessel and laser catheter with saline is mandatory to remove remaining contrast medium, because the interaction of laser energy with contrast medium can produce shock waves that may result in disruption of the vessel wall.

Scientific data to demonstrate the benefits of laser therapy in occlusive disease are still lacking for many reasons. The LACI study[30] (Laser-Assisted Angioplasty for Critical Limb Ischemia) revealed a limb salvage rate of 93% in all treated limbs. In 89% of treated limbs, straight flow to the foot could be established. One of the major issues is that excimer laser–assisted angioplasty in long occlusions, if applied appropriately, is time consuming, expensive, and in a high proportion of cases requires adjunctive angioplasty.[31]

For a full discussion of excimer laser technology for treatment of atherosclerotic obstructions, please visit www.expertconsult.com.

CHAPTER **14**

Intellectual Property Management

T. Andrew Currier

OVERVIEW OF INTELLECTUAL PROPERTY

As the name suggests, the intellectual property (IP) regime can afford legal protection and ownership over intangible creations of the mind. The term *intellectual property* does not refer to one type of legal right but is a broad umbrella term encompassing different types of legal rights. Because IP is a creature of law, IP protection is provided on a country-by-country basis in accordance with the laws and registration systems of each country. The most common types of IP, which are found in virtually all countries of the world, are confidential information, patents, design patents, copyrights, and trademarks.

HOW TO USE THIS CHAPTER

As physicians and surgeons engage with hospitals, universities, corporations, and other entities, they are quite likely to be in the position of inventing new medical devices or treatments and such innovations may have significant commercial value. When considering the terms of these engagements, it is necessary to look carefully at the provisions that govern ownership of inventions and other intellectual property that may be created during that engagement. Use this chapter to familiarize yourself with the concepts of intellectual property law as you consider your compensation package associated with the engagement. Consider also whether your innovations could form the basis for a start-up company or sale to a large pharmaceutical company.

In your everyday work, recognize that you may be unaware you are inventing medical treatments and devices with significant commercial value. Keep careful written notes of what you conceive. Understand that you must maintain your inventions in confidence and that you should act quickly to secure legal protection for them. Students and academics, be wary of the desire to rush to publish your inventions before considering whether to legally protect them—publishing is akin to giving away your invention for free.

Intellectual property is an integral part of our modern capitalist economic system and plays a significant role in the economy of medical care. At the same time, medical practitioners often invent new devices, techniques, or drugs as part of their daily work. For the right inventions, there can be significant reward for inventors, provided they take active steps to protect their inventions and enforce those protections. Please visit www.expertconsult.com for the full version of this chapter. Readers will find basic guidelines to keep in mind when doing their daily work, and opportunities to consider whether those activities constitute protectable innovations.

CHAPTER 15

Clinical Vascular Examination

Benjamin S. Brooke and James H. Black, III

It is much more important to know what sort of patient has a disease than what sort of a disease a patient has.

—*William Osler 1849-1919*

Symptoms relating to vascular insufficiency are common complaints among patients presenting to emergency departments in westernized nations. Unfortunately, these symptoms are often misdiagnosed because of variability in presentation and overlap with other diseases. Vascular diseases may present and manifest in a number of different ways, but most can be evaluated after careful and thorough clinical examination. Although atherosclerosis will be asymptomatic in many patients, its natural progression may be identified by a patient's symptoms, which range from intermittent claudication to ischemic rest pain and gangrene. And although the majority of signs and symptoms result from chronic arterial insufficiency, it becomes essential to recognize acute symptoms that may be limb threatening and require immediate intervention. Moreover, there are many symptoms of nonvascular etiology that mimic vascular insufficiency. It is important to know how to recognize and differentiate symptoms attributed to these other organ systems and to make a differential diagnosis.

The goal of the clinical vascular examination is to identify the cause of the patient's symptoms while localizing the specific lesion and judging its relative severity. The astute clinician should be able to make a presumptive diagnosis after the examination, formulate a treatment strategy, and prevent the patient from undergoing unnecessary tests that are costly and may have additional risks. Although technology has greatly facilitated the ability to identify and localize vascular disease, it should not be relied on to make the diagnosis. The use of imaging modalities should merely confirm the clinician's diagnosis after the examination is complete. For some patients, in particular those with acute presentation, the decision to go to the operating room or angiography suite for intervention often has to be made by the end of the examination, without any adjuvant studies.

Detecting vascular disease is a comprehensive process that requires careful review of the medical history to reveal significant symptoms and risk factors, detection of relevant physical examination findings, and use of appropriate supplementary tests to confirm the diagnosis. A systematic head-to-toe approach should be undertaken with every patient, because many individuals will have multiple areas of vascular disease. In this chapter we review the important elements of the clinical vascular examination, including history and physical examination, risk factors, and bedside

procedures that can be used to confirm a diagnosis. Patterns of vascular disease are distinguished by anatomic and physiologic causes and differentiated from other conditions. In addition, relevant scientific studies that validate important findings of the history or physical examination are discussed.

HISTORY

Obtaining an accurate history of symptoms and their chronology is a critical initial component of a vascular examination. Often a presumptive diagnosis can be made after a detailed history even before the patient has been examined. Or conversely, a patient is referred with an established diagnosis that is determined to be inaccurate after a careful history and examination. Every patient must be queried as to the location of pain, duration of symptoms, whether the symptoms are intermittent or consistent, whether certain circumstances aggravate or alleviate symptoms, and the time relationship to other medical events. Knowing what questions to ask can help discriminate the severity and seriousness of disease as well as guide the diagnostic workup. It is imperative to discriminate symptoms in the history that indicate whether the disease is acute or due to chronic vascular insufficiency. Moreover, knowing a patient's history and risk factors can help distinguish whether symptoms are caused by an embolus or thrombosis. The presentation and patterns of symptoms for specific types of peripheral vascular diseases are discussed next in more detail.

Chronic Arterial Insufficiency

The natural history of arteriosclerosis in the lower extremity can be viewed as a progression of symptoms that reflect the degree of vessel occlusion and presence of collateral circulation. Symptoms classically begin with an intermittent and reproducible pain termed *claudication*, a derivation of the Latin word for "limp." Intermittent claudication is characteristically brought on by a given degree of exercise and relieved after a few minutes of rest. These symptoms reflect a demand for blood flow increases that cannot be met because of atherosclerotic narrowing in one or more arterial segments. Compression of stenotic arteries by exercising muscle and lack of compensatory vasodilation in

TABLE 15-1. Differential Diagnosis of Extremity Pain

Disorder	Location of Pain	Description of Pain	Onset of Symptoms	Effect of Rest	Positional Effects
Intermittent claudication	Buttock, thigh, or calf muscles	Cramping, aching, fatigue, or weakness	After same degree of exercise	Relieves pain quickly	None
Rest pain	Foot	Severe deep pain	At rest	None	Pain alleviated by elevation
Nerve root compression/ herniated disk	Radiates down posterior leg	Sharp pain	With exercise, but may also occur at rest	Not quickly relieved	Adjusting back position may help
Spinal stenosis (pseudoclaudication)	Follows dermatome distribution	Pain associated with motor weakness	After varying amounts of movement or exercise	Relief with changes in body position	Flexion of lumbar spine forward may help
Arthritis	Hip, knee, foot	Aching pain	After varying amounts of exercise	Not quickly relieved	Weight taken off joints may help
Symptomatic adventitial cysts (Baker)	Behind knee, down calf	Tenderness, swelling	Present at rest and with exercise	Does not help	None
Compartment/ entrapment syndromes	Usually calf muscles in muscular patient	Tight, bursting pain	After strenuous exercise	Subsides slowly	Helped by elevation
Venous claudication	Entire leg	Tight, bursting pain	After minimal exercise	Subsides slowly	Helped by elevation

Adapted from Dormandy JA, Rutherford RB. Management of peripheral arterial disease (PAD). TASC Working Group. TransAtlantic Inter-Society Consensus (TASC). J Vasc Surg 2000;31(Suppl):S1–S296.

diseased segments may also contribute to limited extremity perfusion. This pain is often described as aching, cramping, weakness, or fatigue and may present in the buttocks, thighs, calves, or feet. This diagnosis must be considered with any exertional limitation of the lower extremity muscles or any history of walking impairment that gets better shortly after rest. However, there are a number of other causes of extremity pain that must be considered and excluded from the diagnosis (Table 15-1). Among patients with claudication, 25% will experience worsening symptoms, 5% will eventually require revascularization, and only 1% to 2% will come to major amputation.[1]

A query of the specific distribution of claudication reported by the patient is an important focus of the history. Symptoms typically occur in the muscle groups immediately distal to the region of stenosis. The exact site(s) of discomfort or pain should be recorded, along with the relationship of this pain to rest or degree of exertion. Narrowing of the aortoiliac vessels classically presents as the constellation of buttock pain, impotence, and lower extremity muscle atrophy known as *Leriche syndrome.* Similarly, occlusion of the femoral, popliteal, or proximal tibial arteries will present as exertional calf pain. Multiple studies have found intermittent claudication to be a reliable symptom in the diagnosis of peripheral arterial disease. A recent meta-analysis found that the presence of claudication increased the likelihood of arterial disease being present by over threefold, whereas its absence lowers the likelihood by half that moderate to severe disease is present.[2]

Rest pain represents progression of ischemic disease in the lower extremity and is characterized by pain in the foot or calf that is made worse by elevation and is generally relieved by placing the extremity in a dependent position to allow gravity to assist in blood flow. This pain may start as a dull aching sensation in the toes that progresses to severe burning pain at night when the patient is lying supine. Patients may describe hanging a foot or limb over the bed or sleeping in a chair to obtain relief. The pain may intensify with cold exposure and be relieved somewhat with application of heat, although strong analgesics are usually needed to manage the discomfort. Skin ulceration and gangrene occur when the minimal nutritional and metabolic requirements of the extremity are not met by adequate blood flow. Usually, multiple levels of arterial disease (iliac, femoral, tibial) are present for this critical ischemia to occur. The pain associated with this process may intensify initially but then diminish or disappear as tissue necrosis involves peripheral sensory nerves.

Acute Arterial Insufficiency

The clinical presentation of acute arterial insufficiency and limb ischemia is characterized by new-onset extremity pain with concurrent changes in neurologic function. Pain is usually the first symptom to be described and is characteristically elicited by passive flexion or stretch of the extremity. This pain is not usually localized exclusively to the distal foot and not affected by limb position, which helps differentiate it from the rest pain of chronic arterial insufficiency. Sensory loss is the earliest neurologic sign; it may be very subtle at first but progresses quickly to frank paresthesias. When extremity perfusion continues to be compromised, muscle strength and motor control become diminished. This spectrum of clinical symptoms and findings are termed the *6 Ps: pain, pallor, poikilothermia, paresthesias, paralysis, and pulselessness* (Fig. 15-1).

The onset and pattern of these symptoms is an important clue to the cause of obstruction of blood flow. The diagnosis

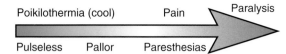

FIGURE 15-1. Stages of acute ischemia and clinical manifestations. Overlap of symptoms is common, especially early in clinical course. Patients with underlying chronic peripheral artery disease may experience slower progression than patients suffering acute limb ischemia without antecedent disease.

of arterial embolism is suggested by sudden onset of severe pain in an extremity not previously affected with claudication or other symptoms of obstructive arterial disease. This acute pain may be described as crippling and often may leave the distal extremity weakened. A careful review of the patient's history will usually reveal the source of emboli or associated risk factors. This includes ventricular thrombi generated weeks to months after a myocardial infarction, or during atrial fibrillation with or without adequate anticoagulation. Other origins of emboli include deep venous thrombus with a patent foramen ovale, mechanical heart valves, endocarditis, or aneurysms located in the aorta or infrainguinal arterial system.

Acute arterial thrombosis is the other main cause of acute insufficiency and is frequently superimposed on an already narrow atherosclerotic lesion. The pain associated with thrombosis is usually not as abrupt, typically following a crescendo course. Classically, a history of claudication or poor circulation is obtained in these patients. Severity and duration of symptoms often correlate with the presence of collateral circulation in the region of the narrowed vessel, helping restore distal perfusion. In the absence of collateral vessels, the pain of thrombosis may be similar to embolic disease. It is important to assess whether the patient has an antecedent coagulation disorder that may predispose to arterial thrombosis. In comparison, patients with deep vein thrombosis may have complaints related to swelling, erythema, and dull pain in the affected extremity. The presence of palpable pulses and/or signs of adequate perfusion in the affected extremity helps differentiate venous thrombosis from an arterial cause.

Cerebrovascular Disease

Patients presenting with carotid disease usually have had a recent transient ischemic attack, stroke in evolution, or completed stroke with persistent neurologic deficits. Transient ischemic attacks may include an account of transient monocular blindness or amaurosis fugax. These brief visual impairments are often described by patients as a "fog," "shade," or "curtain over the eye." When neurologic deficits are fixed, their distribution should be correlated with a point of occlusion in the cerebrovascular circulation. It is important to document the location and chronology of neurologic symptoms in all these patients. A great number of patients with carotid artery disease will be asymptomatic at presentation but may be identified by certain clues in the history. A recent report of nonspecific visual changes may be the first clue that a patient has significant carotid stenosis. Other sources of embolic disease must also be ruled out, including a patient history of cardiac arrhythmias or known patent foramen ovale.

Abdominal Aortic and Mesenteric Disease

The majority of abdominal aortic aneurysms (AAAs) remain asymptomatic until they dissect or rupture. As such, a ruptured AAA is the 13th leading cause of death in the United States.[3] Severe abdominal, back, or chest pain is the most common presenting symptom in the acute stage but must be differentiated from numerous other causes. The temporal pattern and location of pain can sometimes be used to help make the diagnosis. Large AAAs may occasionally cause specific symptoms that originate from compression of adjacent intraabdominal organs, including the stomach, duodenum, ureters, or inferior vena cava. Posterior compression into the adjacent vertebral column may lead to back pain. In many cases, this chronic pain is vague and ill defined until the aneurysm dissects or ruptures. The pain associated with these events is usually sudden and severe, with radiation from the point of injury. Dissections affecting the ascending aorta typically produce anterior chest pain, whereas descending aortic dissections typically cause back pain. The pain associated with aortic dissection is usually described as having a "tearing" quality and may radiate to the abdomen and extremities. Taking a family history of patients with symptoms of aortic disease may reveal first-degree relatives who died of a dissection or rupture. Alternatively, patients may have a history of sudden collapse that is often assumed to be a primary cardiac event.

Patients presenting with mesenteric ischemia can be differentiated by acute and chronic symptoms. Acute mesenteric ischemia produces sudden onset of severe periumbilical pain that is visceral in origin and poorly localized. This is usually accompanied by a history of gastrointestinal emptying (vomiting and diarrhea) and leukocytosis or bandemia (triad present in 10% to 20% of cases). All other causes of acute abdominal pain must be included in the differential diagnosis. In comparison, patients with chronic mesenteric disease usually describe periumbilical pain that has its onset shortly after meals and generally is dull in quality. This history of postprandial abdominal pain is consistently reproduced by eating food and is usually associated with avoidance of food and weight loss ("food fear").

RISK FACTOR IDENTIFICATION AND MODIFICATION

Many risk factors for vascular disease can be picked up by history or results of laboratory tests and help the clinician make a diagnosis. Identifying risk factors is an important part of the vascular examination because it can help stratify and predict the probability of vascular disease. These factors can be differentiated into hereditary, acquired, and modifiable risk factors (Table 15-2). Individuals with evidence of peripheral vascular disease by history and examination generally have evidence of atherosclerosis or other vessel disorders throughout their vascular tree, regardless of whether disease is in the preclinical state or symptomatic. There is considerable overlap between the pathogenesis of disease afflicting the aorta, carotid, coronary, and peripheral circulation, and most disease processes share common risk factors.

Identification of modifiable risk factors for arterial disease (e.g., smoking, hypertension, hyperlipidemia) during the physical examination is particularly important

TABLE 15-2. Risk Factors for Vascular Disease

Hereditary Risk Factors

Hypercoagulable states
Factor V Leiden mutation
Anticardiolipin antibodies
Antithrombin III deficiency
Protein(s) C and S deficiency
Homocystinuria
Diabetes mellitus
Familial hyperlipidemia
Hyperhomocysteinemia
Male sex

Acquired Risk Factors

Hypercoagulable states
Heparin-induced thrombosis (heparin antibodies)
Lupus anticoagulant and related antiphospholipid antibodies
Trousseau syndrome (cancer-associated thrombosis)
Pregnancy
Postoperative state
Oral contraceptives
Diabetes mellitus
Infection (cytomegalovirus, *Chlamydia*)
Age >60 years

Modifiable Risk Factors

Cigarette smoking
Hypertension
Hyperlipidemia
Physical inactivity

because it may allow an opportunity to initiate therapy, reduce symptoms, and prevent premature death. Among smokers, for instance, the progression of peripheral arterial disease from asymptomatic to claudication to ischemic rest pain has been shown to have a linear relationship with pack-years of exposure.[4,5] Formal smoking cessation efforts, which may include counseling, behavior modification, or pharmacotherapy, should be offered to all active smokers and may lead to rapid improvement in the incidence of intermittent claudication.[5] Similarly, the diagnosis of hypertension is associated with a two- to threefold increased risk for arterial disease and can be effectively managed with first-line agents such as thiazides and angiotensin-converting enzyme (ACE) inhibitors. In patients with hypertension and concomitant coronary arterial disease, initiation of β-blocker medications should be strongly considered for their established cardioprotective benefits. Finally, increased total cholesterol, triglycerides, and low-density lipoprotein levels are all independent risk factors for arterial disease that may be successfully treated with lipid-lowering agents such as statins, fibrates, and niacin. Statin use in particular has been consistently shown in randomized studies to reduce adverse cardiovascular events and improve symptoms of claudication in patients with arterial disease through a combination of cholesterol reduction and lipid-independent pleiotropic effects.[6,7]

PHYSICAL EXAMINATION

A thorough physical examination should be completed *from head to toe*, with concentration on anatomic areas that correlate with symptoms from the patient's history. Inspection of the skin and underlying tissue is an important step in the physical examination because skin coloration, temperature, and integrity are critical measures of vascular perfusion and associated tissue nutrition. Skin that has changed from its normal hue to shades of pale, red, blue, or black can indicate varying degrees of vascular insufficiency. Distal hair loss, trophic skin changes, and thickened nails should also be examined. Moreover, the presence of ulcers with their location and characteristics can be a critical finding in diagnosing the etiology of disease. Finally, assessment of blood flow should be made in all extremities. This includes measurement of blood pressure in both arms, with notation of symmetry and palpation of the brachial, radial, ulnar, femoral, popliteal, posterior tibial, and dorsalis pedis arterial pulses (Fig. 15-2). Pulses can be graded as absent, diminished, and normal on a scale from 0 to 2. Auscultation for bruits in the neck, abdomen, and groin should be routinely done and can help the clinician focus the examination. Combined examination findings can reveal patterns that may be useful in the characterization and diagnosis of specific vascular diseases and will be reviewed in greater detail from a head-to-toe approach.

The systematic vascular physical examination should begin at the head and neck and work its way down to the distal extremities to prevent missing any pertinent findings. The pupils should be inspected for symmetry, and an eye examination should be done to evaluate the visual fields for convergence and confrontation. Next, the facial musculature is inspected for tone and symmetry while the patient is asked to smile. Any drooping or inequality should be noted. Moving down to the neck, it is important to palpate both sides of the anterior triangle carefully and record the carotid upstrokes with amplitude. Bruits may be heard over an area beginning from just behind the upper end of the thyroid cartilage to just below the angle of the jaw. It may be useful to use the bell of the stethoscope and ask the patient to hold his or her breath momentarily to hear faint bruits. The presence of a carotid bruit in a symptomatic patient has been shown by several studies to increase the likelihood ratio of having high-grade stenosis (>70%) by up to fivefold.[8] However, the absence of a carotid bruit in a symptomatic patient may also indicate complete occlusion of the carotid artery. If a patient presents with a history of either transient or fixed neurologic deficits, occlusive disease of the cerebrovascular circulation may be present. A complete neurologic examination is required, including assessment of all cranial nerves as well as the peripheral nervous system. In addition, a more formal ocular examination may be required for patients having symptoms of amaurosis fugax or visual field deficits. The site of thromboembolic disease in the cerebrovascular circulation can often be deduced from neurologic deficits. In some cases, inspection of the patient's gait or movements may pick up abnormalities.

The circulation supplying the upper extremity should be examined and pulses palpated in the brachial, radial, and ulnar arteries. In addition, the brachial blood pressure should be taken in both upper extremities and compared for equality. Unequal blood pressures may be an important finding and correlate with symptoms of aortic dissection or occlusion in the great vessels, including coarctation. Complaints of pain, numbness, or weakness in the upper extremity may indicate thoracic outlet syndrome, which is most commonly due to compression of the brachial plexus but

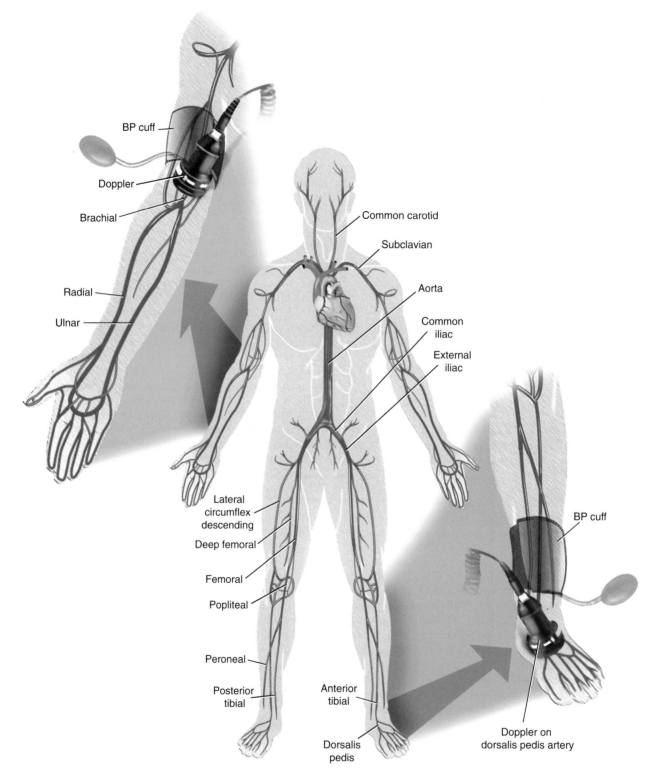

BP cuff

Doppler

Brachial

Radial

Ulnar

Common carotid

Subclavian

Aorta

Common iliac

External iliac

Lateral circumflex descending

Deep femoral

Femoral

Popliteal

Peroneal

Posterior tibial

Anterior tibial

Dorsalis pedis

BP cuff

Doppler on dorsalis pedis artery

FIGURE 15-2. Major arterial anatomy with positioning of Doppler probe for measurement of ankle-brachial index (ABI). Brachial artery is used for Doppler signal detection in upper extremity, and dorsalis pedis signal is detected in lower extremity for comparison. Ankle-brachial index is calculated by dividing ankle systolic pressure by brachial systolic pressure. *BP,* blood pressure.

may also involve compression of the subclavian vessels. Symptoms of thoracic outlet syndrome can usually be elicited by having the patient raise the afflicted arm, with pain dissipating when the extremity is lowered. If knowledge of hand perfusion is needed, the *Allen test* should be performed by holding the hand up, occluding both radial and ulnar arteries, and then lowering the hand while ulnar flow is allowed to resume. If collateral circulation through the palmar arch is adequate, the hand should be perfused when one of the two vessels is occluded.

Detecting vascular disease afflicting the thoracic aorta or great vessels in the chest by physical examination alone is difficult and must usually be correlated with the history, presence of associated symptoms, and results of imaging studies. The chest wall should be examined for symmetry and any irregularities. Auscultation of the heart for murmurs is important because murmurs may correlate with associated symptoms. Findings associated with the presence of a thoracic aortic dissection include an asymmetric pulse differential or deficit, a diastolic murmur, a pericardial rub, focal neurologic deficits, or electrocardiographic signs of myocardial ischemia. Presence of a widened aorta or mediastinum on chest radiography may also help narrow the differential diagnosis. When severe chest pain, asymmetric pulse or blood pressure differential, and mediastinal widening on a chest radiograph are combined, the likelihood of aortic dissection increases over 60-fold.[9] However, this classic triad is usually found in fewer than half of all patients with symptomatic disease. Aortic regurgitation is a common finding in patients with dissection of the aortic root. Other new murmurs such as mitral regurgitation may indicate a recent myocardial infarction and correlate with symptoms of embolic vascular disease.

Detecting vascular disease of the descending aorta and mesenteric circulation is similarly difficult, particularly with obese patients. Auscultation of the abdomen and flank for bruits should be performed but is generally not very sensitive or specific for detecting disease. AAAs may be detected during examination by palpation if sufficient in size and if the patient is not overly obese. The examination should be performed while the patient is supine with his or her knees raised and abdomen relaxed. Presence of an aortic pulsation is usually felt a few centimeters below the umbilicus and slightly to the left of midline. Aortic diameter can be estimated by placing an index finger on either side of a pulsatile area, with both hands on the abdomen. However, the absence of a palpable abdominal mass does not exclude the diagnosis. A meta-analysis showed that palpation alone was found to have a sensitivity ranging from 29% for AAAs of 3.0 to 3.9 cm, 50% for AAAs of 4.0 to 4.9 cm, and 76% for aneurysms 5.0 cm or larger in diameter.[10] The same analysis showed that the positive predictive value of detecting AAAs larger than 3.0 cm by palpation alone was only 43%. Moreover, the accuracy of physical examination in size estimation of an AAA is low. Thus, patients presenting with abdominal or back pain of new onset should have the diagnosis made or excluded by an imaging study, usually magnetic resonance angiography/imaging (MRA/MRI) or computed tomography (CT) with intravenous (IV) administration of contrast media.

The examination of a patient with acute mesenteric ischemia will generally be nonspecific. The pain of early disease is visceral and generalized. If compromised perfusion to the bowel continues, the patient may present with signs of peritoneal irritation, including rebound tenderness and involuntary guarding of the abdomen on examination. The tenderness is commonly described as pain out of proportion to physical findings. Frank peritonitis is generally a sign of severe bowel wall ischemia and necrosis, but the etiology cannot be differentiated from other causes of an acute abdomen. Similarly, examining a patient with chronic mesenteric ischemia does not typically yield a specific pattern of tenderness, and clinical diagnosis rests more

on history and exclusion of other possible causes. A rectal examination should always be completed, and the stool is usually found to be heme positive in mesenteric ischemia.

The lower extremity is the most common site for signs and symptoms of arterial insufficiency and must be examined carefully; a number of signs of chronic insufficiency may be elicited. Abnormalities in skin color may range from red to purple or black (necrotic skin). Skin overlying the dorsum of an extremity with decreased perfusion is typically characterized by lack of hair and a shiny, scaly, atrophic appearance. Underlying subcutaneous tissue and musculature may be atrophied, and nails are characteristically thickened. The extremity may transition from pallor when elevated to rubor when dependent. The clinician may test for this finding using the *Buerger test*: the patient lies supine, the affected leg is lowered from a 90-degree angle, and the level at which color transitions from pale to a red hue is determined. This test is considered positive if the angle is less than 0 degrees or the leg has to hang below the examining table for color to return.

Ulceration that develops from chronic ischemia in the lower extremities is generally located on the lateral malleolus or distally over pressure points such as the metatarsal heads, heel of the foot, or tips of the toes. These ulcers are painful, do not bleed a lot, and have an irregular "punched out" appearance with a pale base. The pain of these ulcers may be relieved somewhat by dependency of the limb. These ulcers tend to be dry unless they become infected and progress to wet gangrene. In comparison, the trophic ulcerations that may develop from long-standing diabetes are painless, usually with callused surrounding skin that has decreased sensation and associated neuropathy. Chronic arterial insufficiency is typically caused by stenoses at multiple levels of the periphery, and signs are generally appreciated in the tissue and muscle groups distal to these obstructions. Pulses distal to stenoses tend to be decreased. In many cases, collateral vessels will develop over time and ultimately supply the majority of blood flow to the extremity. An attempt to auscultate for bruits should also be made, particularly in the groin.

The physical examination during acute arterial insufficiency is unique and must be thorough so opportunities to restore flow are not lost. In the peripheral circulation, overlying skin distal to an obstruction may initially be red but becomes mottled with continued lack of blood flow. With sufficient time, the extremity becomes pale and cold to the touch. Capillary refill should be assessed by applying pressure to the lateral aspect of the great toe for at least 5 seconds. This will typically be abnormal (>5 seconds), and the skin will not blanch. Pulses should be examined at different levels of the extremities on both sides, including the radial and brachial in the upper extremity and the femoral, popliteal, posterotibial, and dorsalis pedis in the lower extremity. Presence of a weak pulse does *not* exclude the diagnosis; loss of palpable pulses is often the last physical sign to appear. However, absence of a pulse in one extremity but normal perfusion in the contralateral limb should raise suspicion. If unable to palpate a pulse with tactile sensation, detection with a handheld Doppler probe should also be attempted. The normal arterial pulse is triphasic, although patients with near occlusion may have only a biphasic or monophasic audible component. When ulceration and signs of chronic vascular insufficiency are present, these must be differentiated from the patient's acute symptoms.

Several studies have assessed the validity of clinical signs found during lower extremity examination. The presence of cool skin temperature and skin discoloration in symptomatic patients was found by one large study to increase the likelihood of arterial disease by almost sixfold and threefold, respectively.[11] Ulceration was also determined by this study to increase the likelihood of arterial disease by approximately sixfold, although absence of ulceration did not lessen the odds of arterial insufficiency. Another study conducted among diabetics found that traditional signs of arterial disease (e.g., skin changes, cool extremities) signaled only a limited increase in the likelihood (likelihood ratio [LR], 1.50; 95% confidence interval [CI], 1.2-1.7) of identifying severe arterial disease in this patient population.[12] A meta-analysis evaluated the presence of bruits at either the iliac, femoral, or popliteal artery during rest and found that this finding increased the likelihood of arterial disease approximately fivefold in both symptomatic and asymptomatic patients.[2] Likewise, the absence of bruits in all three positions among symptomatic patients was found to lower the likelihood of peripheral arterial disease by over half. Finally, the same analysis found that detection of absent or reduced pulses at any of the lower extremity arteries increases the likelihood of disease by close to fivefold in symptomatic patients and threefold in asymptomatic patients. The likelihood of arterial disease is reduced by over half in both symptomatic and asymptomatic patients found to have normal palpable pulses on examination.[2]

BEDSIDE PROCEDURES TO ASSIST WITH DIAGNOSIS

After a physical examination, several adjunctive procedures can be done at the bedside to confirm the diagnosis. These noninvasive diagnostics based on ultrasonography and plethysmography have become an integral part of the clinical examination. Test findings in conjunction with the patient's clinical presentation help the examiner decide whether further invasive tests or procedures are warranted.

Ankle-Brachial Index

The ankle-brachial systolic pressure index (ABI) is the most common and reliable bedside procedure to confirm the presence of arterial disease. It is a quick, noninvasive, cost-effective, and readily available means to establish or refute the diagnosis of peripheral arterial insufficiency and has been validated by numerous studies. This test is performed by placing an appropriately sized pneumatic cuff around the limb and inflating it to a level above the resting systolic blood pressure. While the cuff is being slowly deflated, a handheld Doppler probe positioned over the artery a few inches distal to the cuff is used to detect the systolic pressure at which Korotkoff sounds return (see Fig. 15-2). In the upper extremity, the brachial artery is used for Doppler signal detection, whereas either the dorsalis pedis or posterotibial signals can be detected at the ankle for comparison. The ABI is then calculated by dividing the higher ankle systolic pressure by the higher of two arm systolic pressures.

Interpretation of ABI values must always be made while taking the entire clinical scenario into consideration, but a standardized scale can be used to categorize the severity of vascular insufficiency. A value between 1.0 and 1.2 is expected in a normal individual, whereas a threshold value of 0.90 or less indicates abnormal vascular perfusion. Mild arterial occlusive disease is typically characterized by ABI values between 0.7 and 0.9, moderate disease by values between 0.4 and 0.7, and severe disease by values less than 0.4. Classic rest pain is normally associated with ABI values less than 0.4 to 0.5, whereas gangrene is usually found with values less than 0.2.

The accuracy of ABI has been validated by several studies comparing it to the gold standard of angiography for identifying occlusive disease. Sensitivity of ABI is approximately 95%, and specificity is close to 100%.[13] A false-negative ABI measurement may occur when peripheral arteries become heavily calcified and noncompressible, which occurs in approximately 10% of diabetics and older individuals with Mönckeberg-type calcification. Medial calcification prevents cuff occlusion from occurring with high systolic pressure readings, leading to ABI values above 1.3. These values are abnormal and may be associated with advanced vascular disease that requires further diagnostic workup. It may be necessary to test arterial flow with a Doppler probe at a vessel that is more distal, such as the radial artery or a toe vessel. A *toe-brachial index* may be measured in patients in whom lower extremity disease is suspected but noncompressible vessels render ABI unreliable. This technique may also be used to assess digital perfusion when small arterial occlusive disease is present. The limitation is that it requires a small cuff.

Pulse Volume Recordings

Pulse volume recordings (PVRs) are another noninvasive test to assess local tissue perfusion. This technique uses air plethysmography to provide waveform analysis of blood flow. PVRs may help establish the diagnosis as well as assess localization and severity of peripheral arterial disease. An air-filled cuff is applied around the extremity at segmental levels (i.e., thigh, calf, foot) and sequentially inflated to a standardized pressure. When the limb is normally perfused, there will be a characteristic change in volume that reflects the component of arterial flow. However, if the limb is not well perfused, there will be minimal or no change in cuff volume. Presence of an occlusive lesion can be determined by comparing the magnitude and contour of PVR readings between segments. The accuracy of PVRs is maintained in patients with noncompressible vessels. Previous studies show that PVR measurements have a sensitivity of approximately 85% when compared with angiography in detecting the presence of significant occlusive arterial lesions. The limitation of PVRs is that they do not give exact anatomic localization of vascular stenoses, nor do they characterize the degree of high-grade lesions. PVRs are not as precise in distal disease and may not be accurate in patients with congestive heart failure or low stroke volumes.

CORRELATING CLINICAL FINDINGS WITH PROBABILITY OF DISEASE

Knowing the probability of clinical findings found during the vascular examination helps the clinician determine the likelihood of disease and decide who may benefit from an interventional procedure. The significance of either positive or negative examination findings will impact a patient's pretest probability for disease. *Pretest probability* is estimated by combining a patient's risk factors (see Table 15-2) with a differential diagnosis (see Table 15-1) for their symptoms. Each risk factor for arterial insufficiency may be associated with a prevalence of disease ranging from 5% to 25%.[2] Patients with multiple coexistent risk factors will have an incrementally higher prevalence of disease. This is clinically relevant when evaluating patients with high numbers of risk factors for vascular disease because symptoms with even a low likelihood value may be significant. Similarly, the presence of a symptom with a high likelihood value may not guarantee the presence of vascular disease if that patient has no other risk factors.

The precision of detecting individual symptoms and signs of arterial disease is variable and depends on a clinician's experience.[14] When determining whether a pulse is present or absent by palpation alone, several studies have shown that interobserver agreement is only marginally reproducible.[15,16] The combination of several significant clinical findings augments the precision and accuracy of detecting vascular insufficiency. Several clinical decision scoring systems have been published that show increased accuracy in predicting arterial disease and necessity for additional testing by adding together important findings of the examination.[17,18] The combination of all normal findings likewise decreases the likelihood of having vascular disease.

SUMMARY

A thorough and comprehensive vascular examination is critical to making a diagnosis of vascular disease and preparing for potential interventions. This will require combining elements of the history, physical examination, risk factor profile, and ancillary studies to make an accurate diagnosis.

Knowing the association specific clinical findings have with arterial insufficiency can increase the likelihood of making the correct diagnosis. In an era of ever-increasing reliance on technology for diagnosis, an astute clinician can make sound clinical decisions that can significantly improve a patient's time to definitive therapy and reduce resource expenditure.

KEY POINTS

- The clinical vascular examination combines elements of the history, physical examination, risk factor profile, and ancillary studies to make an accurate diagnosis.
- Understanding the probability of positive and negative clinical findings found during the vascular examination helps the clinician determine the likelihood of disease and decide who will benefit from an interventional procedure.

▶ SUGGESTED READINGS

Boyco EJ, Ahroni JH, Davignon D, et al. Diagnostic utility of the history and physical examination for peripheral vascular disease among patients with diabetes mellitus. J Clin Epidemiol 1997;50:659–68.

Khan NA, Rahim SA, Anand SS, et al. Does the clinical examination predict lower extremity peripheral arterial disease? JAMA 2006; 295:536–46.

Stoffers HE, Kester AD, Saiser V, et al. Diagnostic value of signs and symptoms associated with peripheral arterial disease seen in general practice: a multivariate approach. Med Decis Making 1997;17:61–70.

The complete reference list is available online at www.expertconsult.com.

CHAPTER 16
Treatment of Medical Emergencies
Ziyad Al-Otaibi and Lakhmir S. Chawla

INTRODUCTION

The interventional suite plays host to a wide variety of patient types and procedures. Some of the patients who arrive into the suite are in good baseline health, while others are severely ill. In either case, patients can experience a life-threatening emergency during any interventional procedure. Unlike the operating room, where an anesthesiologist is routinely present to handle any non–procedure-related emergency, the level of support in the interventional suite is variable. When medical emergencies occur, it is not uncommon for interventionalists to have only their complement of nurses and technologists as support staff. In this brief chapter, we endeavor to provide a framework that will help mitigate the medical emergencies that can occur in patients undergoing interventional procedures.

The lion's share of medical emergencies can be placed into five categories: (1) oversedation, (2) airway compromise, (3) respiratory distress, (4) cardiac/hemodynamic emergencies, and (5) contrast reactions. The response to these medical emergencies often requires an anesthesiologist, an intensivist, and/or a surgeon. However, there are concrete steps and planning by the interventionalist and staff that can help lessen these emergencies and may prove life saving while appropriate personnel and resources are mobilized. This chapter will focus on these bridging and moderating techniques.

OVERSEDATION

Procedural sedation/analgesia is a common and important component of interventional procedures. Appropriate patient positioning and maintaining patient comfort are facilitated by proper sedation. However, reaching the perfect balance of sedation and comfort without oversedating the patient can be challenging. Striking the right balance can be particularly difficult in patients with underlying lung disease and in patients with unpredictable metabolism of common sedatives. In addition, patients with a marginal circulatory status may be prone to hemodynamic effects. The oversedated patient can experience hypercarbia, hypoxemia, and/or hypotension either related to the sedative itself or due to secondary effects. Prevention of oversedation and hypercarbia can be prevented with close patient monitoring and the use of pulse oximetry; the patient's response to verbal commands; observation of ventilation, blood pressure (BP), and heart rate every 5 minutes; electrocardiography for patients with significant cardiovascular disease; and use of exhaled capnography. When patients become oversedated, it is common for minute ventilation to decrease, which is often associated with a rise in end-tidal CO_2 (ETCO$_2$). This elevation typically precedes apnea and can alert the physician that the level of sedation is excessive. ETCO$_2$ above 50 mmHg, an absolute change of over 10 mmHg, or an absent waveform may detect subclinical respiratory depression not detected by pulse oximetry alone.[1] This is vitally important, since many patients have a variable response to hypnotic drugs. The choice of drugs that have minimal hemodynamic and respiratory depression may be considered (e.g., etomidate,[2] ketamine,[3] ketamine-propofol combination[4]).

In this section, we will focus on airway and respiratory management of the oversedated patient. Management of hypotension and arrhythmia is covered in the circulatory management section of the chapter. When patients become oversedated, their airway and respiratory centers can be compromised. The mechanisms by which this occurs are multiple:

- Use of narcotics can cause vomiting and aspiration.
- Narcotic and benzodiazepine use decreases respiratory drive and can cause central apnea.
- Muscle relaxation caused by sedatives can cause upper airway obstruction.

Typically the response to the oversedated patient is cessation of the sedative agent, increasing the inspired oxygen (e.g., placing a 100% FIO$_2$ face mask), and some form of stimulation (e.g., sternal rub) in an attempt to arouse the patient to stimulate breathing while the sedative wears off. This approach is often unsatisfactory owing to the half-life of the sedating agent. In addition, if the airway or respiratory center is compromised, subsequent hypercarbia may spiral toward complete respiratory arrest.

The approach to the oversedated patient should be managed in a more airway-centered manner. Once oversedation is recognized, a staff member in the interventional suite should be detailed to the head of the bed to manage the airway. Noninvasive airway management should be sufficient in most cases. If stimulation of the patient (e.g., calling the patient's name loudly, sternal rub) fails to immediately correct the compromise in oxygenation or respiratory effort, the airway should be assessed and optimized (Fig. 16-1; also see Airway Management and Optimization, later). At this point, if the sedative used has an antidote (e.g., flumazenil for benzodiazepines or, naloxone for narcotics), that antidote should be drawn up (Table 16-1).

Optimization of the airway often requires repositioning the patient's head and neck. A simple understanding of the anatomy allows anyone to place the patient's head in more favorable position for gas exchange. The tongue is the most common cause of upper airway obstruction. A head-tilt/chin-lift or jaw-thrust maneuver (Fig. 16-2) also called the *sniffing position* may establish an airway. If proper positioning fails to establish a viable airway, however, more invasive maneuvers such as using a nasopharyngeal/oropharyngeal airway or a laryngeal mask airway (LMA) may be necessary and will be discussed in a later section.[5]

Both benzodiazepines and narcotics have reversal agents that if used correctly could save an oversedated patient from having a respiratory arrest. Flumazenil antagonizes the action of benzodiazepines on the central nervous system and inhibits activity at γ-aminobutyric acid/benzodiazepine receptor sites. It is contraindicated in patients with serious tricyclic overdoses.[6] Available in injectable 0.1 mg/mL, flumazenil can be given undiluted or in D_5W, lactated Ringer's solution, or 0.9 normal saline. The initial intravenous (IV) dose is 0.2 to 0.4 mg over 15 seconds. If ineffective, a repeat dose can be given every 60 seconds. Maximum initial dose is 1 mg. If the patient becomes oversedated, a repeat dose can be given, and a drip may have to be started if the half-life of the offending benzodiazepine is longer than the half-life of flumazenil (41-79 minutes). Adverse effects include seizures, dizziness, headache, blurred vision, diplopia, visual field deficit, hyperventilation, nausea, and vomiting.[6]

Naloxone hydrochloride is a pure narcotic antagonist. It reverses the respiratory depression, sedation, and hypotensive effects of opioids. In the absence of narcotics, naloxone has no activity. Caution must be used in narcotic addiction, cardiac disease, and use of cardiotoxic drugs. Rapid reversal of narcotic depression may also cause nausea, vomiting, diaphoresis, and circulatory stress. The initial dose is 0.1 to 2 mg IV at 2- to 3-minute intervals until the desired effect of reversal is reached. It can be given undiluted as a bolus or as an IV infusion with D_5W or 0.9 normal saline. As with flumazenil, a drip may have to be started owing to a longer half-life of the offending agent. Naloxone has a half-life of 30 to 81 minutes. As an infusion, use 3.7 µg/kg/h. Adverse effects include seizures, ventricular tachycardia, ventricular fibrillation, acute narcotic abstinence syndrome, and return of pain.[7]

If stimulation, airway optimization, and reversal agents fail to rectify the situation, airway compromise may be the underlying problem, in which case the clinician should continue down the airway management algorithm (see Fig. 16-1).

Airway Management and Optimization

Airway management is a core skill for the medical specialties of anesthesiology, critical care medicine, and emergency medicine. A small section in a chapter will not be sufficient to cover all aspects of this topic. Our goal here is to arm the interventionalist with some basic noninvasive skills and maneuvers that can mitigate an impending airway calamity. As mentioned earlier, we recommend that some members of the interventional support staff should have some basic noninvasive airway management training. Advanced Cardiovascular Life Support (ACLS) training for all interventional nurses, technologists, and physicians is optimal and required in many institutions.[5]

A variety of noninvasive airway management maneuvers can dramatically improve ventilation and oxygenation pending a more durable intervention (e.g., endotracheal intubation). Suctioning, head positioning, and keeping a patent airway are the first and often highest-yield steps:

• The oropharynx should be suctioned under direct vision to remove any secretion accumulation. This can be diagnostic and therapeutic.

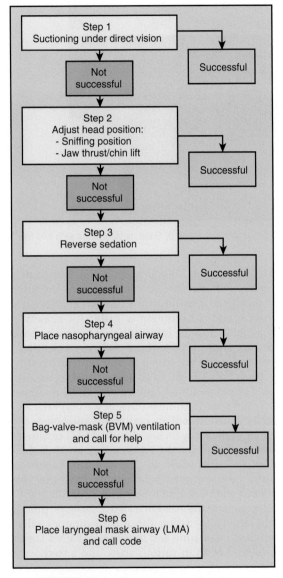

FIGURE 16-1. Airway management sequence.

TABLE 16-1. Sedative Antidote Administration

Antidote	Dosage and Comments	Side Effects
Naloxone	0.4-2 mg at a time; maximum dose 10 mg For typical doses used for conscious sedation, a dose of 0.2-0.4 mg should be sufficient Can be given as an infusion (2 mg/100 mL) 0.1 mg/min[7]	As narcotic reverses, elevated blood pressure, tachycardia, nausea, and vomiting can occur
Flumazenil	0.2-1 mg dose Each 0.2-mg increment should be given over 1 minute In clinical trials, 75% of patients responded to a dose of 1-3 mg	Frequent side effects (≈10%): nausea, vomiting, headache, blurred vision Major side effect (<1%): seizure[6]

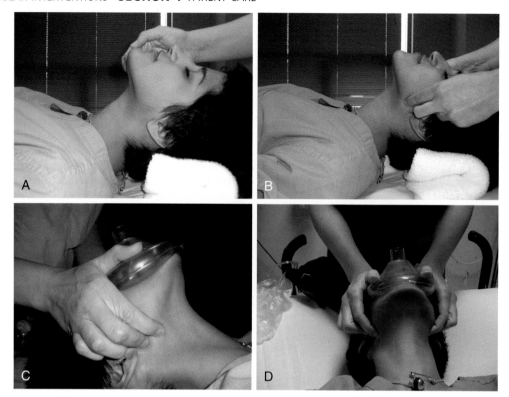

FIGURE 16-2. **A,** Chin lift into sniffing position. **B,** Jaw thrust. **C,** Good mask position with one hand. **D,** Good mask position with two hands.

+ The patient's head position should be adjusted to maximize airway patency. The sniffing position mentioned previously, with the head tilt/chin lift and/or jaw thrust should be performed to optimize the airway (see Fig. 16-2).

If these maneuvers do not rectify the situation:

+ A nasopharyngeal airway should be placed. This is a noxious stimulus, and the act of placing it may reestablish the airway. The nasopharyngeal airway must have lubricant applied at its end. It is placed in either naris until it is hubbed. Once applied, bag-valve-mask (BVM) ventilation should be reinstituted. The adequacy of BVM ventilation can be assessed by pulse oximetry and also by the rise of the thorax with each BVM-delivered breath.

+ If BVM ventilation with a nasopharyngeal airway in place fails to correct hypoxia and/or hypoventilation, an LMA should then be considered, and a code should be called.[5]

AIRWAY COMPROMISE

If the airway management steps fail to optimize the patient's airway, the next immediate step is using a BVM to breathe for the patient, with the understanding that a respiratory arrest may be imminent. Following a simple algorithm may prevent oversedation from becoming airway compromise and ultimately respiratory arrest. The interventionalist should feel comfortable with a certain sequence of events when a patient becomes unresponsive (see Fig. 16-1). Initial management should always be stimulation, airway optimization, use of reversal agents where appropriate, and finally use of a BVM. If BVM ventilation does not result in immediate resolution of hypoxemia, a code should be called,

and ACLS protocols should be initiated. Fortunately, this extreme level of intervention is uncommonly required. The simple skill set of breathing for a patient can prevent airway compromise from becoming a code. As already noted, having a member of the interventional team who has ACLS certification is important. If full ACLS certification is not possible, it takes an afternoon of time with an anesthesiologist to learn how to effectively use a BVM to breathe for a patient. Taking the time to train some of the interventional support staff to have some proficiency around the airway is an excellent investment in preventive medicine, even for those staff members who are already ACLS certified.

Table 16-2 outlines the contingency kit that should be immediately available for all interventional procedures. In short, the interventional suite should have the following materials at all times: a suction setup, accessibility to high-flow oxygen, oral and nasopharyngeal airways, pulse oximetry, the ability to assess BP and respiratory effort, the reversal drugs naloxone and flumazenil, BVMs (also called *Ambu bags*), LMAs in various sizes, and a stethoscope. In our experience of managing conscious sedation for a variety of different procedures, mask breathing for the patient while the sedative wears off to a more appropriate level is adequate therapy for the oversedated patient in the vast majority of cases.

RESPIRATORY DISTRESS

The next step is to assess for breathing. The simple acts of looking, listening, and feeling for breathing are essential. If the patient is not breathing, a code should be called and ACLS initiated. Breathing for the patient while optimizing their airway as described earlier should begin immediately while ACLS protocols are initiated.

There is one major caveat to respiratory distress in interventional procedures involving the thorax. When respiratory distress occurs during any procedure involving the thorax that may have resulted in violation of the pleural space, fluoroscopy should be used to assess for presumed tension pneumothorax. This should not be done at the expense of maintaining an airway or breathing for the patient. If fluoroscopy is not possible, auscultation for breath sounds is the next step. If pneumothorax or tension pneumothorax is suspected, insert a large-bore (14- or 16-gauge) needle with a catheter into the second intercostal space just superior to the third rib at the midclavicular line, 1 to 2 cm from the sternal edge (avoiding injury to the internal thoracic artery). A 3- to 6-cm-long needle should be used, holding it perpendicular to the chest wall when inserting. Some patients may have a chest wall thickness greater than 3 cm, and failure of symptom resolution may be inadequate needle length.

Once the needle is in the pleural space, there should be a hissing sound of air escaping. The needle may be removed while leaving the catheter in place. The next step is to call a surgeon for tube thoracostomy.

EMERGENCY CARDIAC/ HEMODYNAMIC EVENTS

When hypotension is identified in a patient, it should first be verified and not attributed to faulty equipment. An abbreviated differential diagnosis of the causes of hypotension should be conducted, and easily reversible causes should be corrected. The interventional suite is not the optimal venue for a diagnostic workup for a patient with significant hypotension, and this event would be a reason to cancel or abort a procedure. From a physiologic standpoint, BP = cardiac output × vascular resistance; if a patient's BP is low, either their vascular resistance or their cardiac output has decreased. A low BP that is new is often a result of sedative effects on vascular resistance. Processes that affect cardiac output and cause hypotension (e.g., myocardial infarction, pulmonary embolism) are not easily reversed and usually require rapid intervention. For the interventionalist, there are two key principles in the management of hypotension. *One, maintain blood pressure at all costs. Two, lead with volume, but do not fear short-term vasopressors.* All forms of shock are initially treated with volume, except left ventricular failure. Patients with acute left ventricular failure almost always require intubation, so if a patient becomes hypotensive, do not be afraid to give volume. Even if the patient ends up requiring intubation, that is much more reversible and benign than sustained hypotension.

The approach to the hypotensive patient (this assumes the patient does not have a dysrhythmia, and there is no obvious reason for the hypotension [e.g., obvious new hemorrhage]):

1. If the patient has just received sedation and BP drops, give a bolus of 500 mL of colloid (e.g., 5% albumin). If colloid is not immediately available, give 1 L of normal saline. Though there is no difference in crystalloid versus colloid in the long run, colloid has the advantage of having a greater effect with a smaller volume, which is helpful when the effect is needed quickly.
2. If BP does not improve within 5 minutes or continues to fall, administer 1 mL of phenylephrine (100 µg/mL; 10 mg in 100 mL NS)) from the contingency kit (see Table 16-2). If that fails to improve the BP, give up to 2 mL more of phenylephrine (100 µg/mL) (Table 16-3), and call for help. Another readily available drug in every code cart is epinephrine 1:10,000 (IV dose),

TABLE 16-2. Immediately Available Medications and Supplies

Item	Quantity
Flumazenil	(2) 1-mg vials
Naloxone	(2) 2-mg vials
Phenylephrine (Neo-Synephrine)	10 mg/100 mL
Diphenhydramine (Benadryl)	50 mg
Atropine	1-mg prefilled syringe
Epinephrine	1:1000 (SQ-IM concentration)
Epinephrine	1:10,000 (IV concentration)
Nasal airway and lubricant	
Oral airway	
Suctioning setup	
Bag valve mask	
Stethoscope	
Laryngeal mask airways	Various sizes
5% albumin or hetastarch (Hespan)	500 mL of either

IM, Intramuscular; *IV,* intravenous; *SQ,* subcutaneous.

TABLE 16-3. Vasoactive Medications Dose and Usage

Agent	Dosage	Use
Phenylephrine (Neo-Synephrine)	10 mg mixed in 100 mL normal saline	Can be given 1 mL IV q 1 minute for blood pressure support
Epinephrine	1:1000 (SQ-IM concentration)	Should be given in 0.3-mL increments (300 µg) For anaphylaxis or contrast reactions
Epinephrine	1:10,000 (IV concentration)	Should be given in 100- to 300-µg increments for severe anaphylaxis or contrast reactions Should be given as 10 µg every 3-5 min for blood pressure support
Atropine	1-mg vial	Should be given 0.5 mg at a time for bradycardia

IM, Intramuscular; *IV,* intravenous; *SQ,* subcutaneous.

which comes in 1 mg/10 mL. Mixing 1 mL with 9 mL normal saline will give a concentration of 10 µg/mL, which can be given at 1 mL (10 µg/mL) every 3 to 5 minutes, which is equivalent to an epinephrine drip. Next, call for help.

If these two maneuvers do not immediately achieve normotension, the low BP is unlikely to be due to sedative effects alone, and some other process is underway. In addition to calling for help, sustained hypotension will require large-bore IV access. Stat blood should be drawn for type and crossmatch for at least two units of packed red cells; a complete blood cell count and coagulation profile should be obtained as well.

A common cause of bradycardia is hypoxia, so an initial focus should be excluding and treating this disorder of oxygenation. Another cause may be vagal stimulation. The vagus nerve runs into the carotid sheath between the internal carotid artery and internal jugular vein down to the neck, chest, and abdomen, where it contributes to the innervation of the viscera. Any stimulation along its course can cause bradycardia, which should be treated with atropine 0.5 mg IV if the patient is symptomatic (i.e., chest pain, shortness of breath, altered level of consciousness).

An ACLS-trained person may aid evaluation of hemodynamic compromise, but the initial assessment can be done by anyone in the room. Large-bore IV access is essential because fluids must be given liberally and rapidly. Pulmonary edema is not an issue if the patient has no BP. ACLS protocols should be initiated immediately. In the event of a pulseless patient, ventilation and cardiac compressions should be started immediately, with an emphasis on compressions. Remember that the first drug in all pulseless algorithms is epinephrine, 1 mg IV every 3 to 5 minutes, until help arrives. See also Chapter 23.

CONTRAST REACTIONS

Reactions to contrast materials range from mild to life threatening. Recognizing a life-threatening contrast reaction is critical to initiating treatment and mitigating its effects. Severe allergic reactions to contrast are rare (<1:1000).[8,9] Nonetheless, these reactions represent a potentially preventable form of severe allergic injury. As always, a directed history and physical with a focus on allergic reactions should be conducted. Patients with a history of asthma are at a higher risk for contrast reactions than those patients without asthma.[10] Patients who have had a previous reaction to contrast have a 1 in 5 risk of having another reaction.[10] Pretreatment regimens for those patients known to be at risk have been published elsewhere.[11] The pretreatment cocktail usually includes corticosteroids and H_1 and H_2 antihistamines. However, available evidence suggests that pretreatment does not afford the clinician comfort

that a contrast reaction will actually be prevented.[11] The act of administering a prophylactic regimen should primarily serve to increase the clinician's vigilance.

If a contrast reaction is suspected, the first order of business is to stop the study and ascertain the severity of the reaction. If the reaction is a mild reaction, which would consist of urticaria, conjunctivitis, erythema/hives, and/or rhinitis, the treatment would consist of 25 to 50 mg of IV diphenhydramine. If the reaction involves angioedema, bronchospasm, laryngospasm, or hypotension, albuterol nebulizer treatments and intramuscular/subcutaneous epinephrine (0.3 mg of 1:1000 solution) or IV epinephrine (100-300 µg of 1:10,000) should be added to the regimen. The addition of airway symptoms should prompt the availability of more experienced help if the reaction fails to abate.

If the patient is having a major reaction, ACLS protocols should be initiated immediately, a code should be called, and epinephrine should be administered IV.[12] The ABCDs of ACLS should be initiated, and all attempts to restore oxygenation and circulation should commence without delay. The techniques described for airway optimization and BVM breathing can prove life saving while an airway (e.g., endotracheal intubation) is secured. At this point, the code cart, which should be immediately available, should be opened and used.

KEY POINTS

- Be prepared. Set up an emergency cart that is available immediately for common complications.
- In any emergency, detail an experienced member of the team to manage the airway.
- During an emergency, maintain blood pressure at all cost. "Bad memories are better than no memories."

▶ **SUGGESTED READINGS**

Tramer MR, von Elm E, Loubeyre P, Hauser C. Pharmacological prevention of serious anaphylactic reactions due to iodinated contrast media: systematic review. Br Med J 2006;333:675.

Vanden Hoek TL, Morrison LJ, Shuster M, et al. 2010 American Heart Association Guidelines for Cardiopulmonary Resuscitation and Emergency Cardiovascular Care Science, Part 12: Cardiac Arrest in Special Situations: 2010 American Heart Association Guidelines for Cardiopulmonary Resuscitation and Emergency Cardiovascular Care. Circulation 2010;122:S829–61, doi:10.1161/CIRCULATIONAHA.110.971069.

The complete reference list is available online at www.expertconsult.com.

CHAPTER 17

Radiation Safety and Protection in the Interventional Fluoroscopy Environment

M. Victoria Marx

Over the last 25 years, fluoroscopically guided interventional procedures have revolutionized medical care. Percutaneous stent placement has replaced surgical bypass for arterial revascularization. Surgical decompression of portal hypertension is rarely performed because of the efficacy of transjugular intrahepatic portosystemic shunt (TIPS) procedures. Hysterectomy for symptomatic fibroids is becoming less common as a result of the wide availability of uterine artery embolization. These developments have benefited thousands upon thousands of people because of less morbidity than in the surgical procedures they have replaced.

Fluoroscopy does, however, come with a price: exposure to ionizing radiation. It is the responsibility of each interventionalist to use fluoroscopy judiciously and in such a way that its immediate medical benefits outweigh its potential future risks. To do so, the practitioner must understand the bioeffects of ionizing radiation, provide meticulous preprocedural and postprocedural patient care, and develop optimal work habits in the fluoroscopic suite. A well-rounded radiation management program is important not only to minimize exposure to the patient but also to minimize occupational doses incurred by the interventional radiology team.

NEGATIVE EFFECTS OF IONIZING RADIATION

Ill effects of radiation can be divided into two basic categories: stochastic effects and deterministic effects.[1] *Stochastic effects* are those in which no clear relationship exists between the magnitude of the radiation dose and the severity of the effect. Stochastic effects include genetic mutation and induction of cancer. Estimations of the incidence of stochastic effects have been based on a no-threshold linear model assumption from the effects identified as a result of the atomic bomb detonations during World War II. These assumptions are not universally accepted. However, because of this uncertainty, the current approach is that stochastic effects have no threshold dose. Therefore, no radiation dose can be considered absolutely safe. It is imperative that fluoroscopically guided diagnostic and therapeutic procedures be performed under the safest conditions possible.

Deterministic effects are those in which the likelihood and severity of the effect are related to the magnitude of the radiation dose: the higher the dose, the more severe the effect. Deterministic effects have a minimum dose threshold below which no effect will occur. Examples of deterministic effects are radiation-induced skin injury (including epilation, acute burns, and delayed ulcers) and radiation-induced cataracts. The threshold dose for temporary epilation is about 3 Gy, whereas that for development of a cataract is about 2 Gy for a single exposure. Thresholds are higher for doses fractionated over time. Cataracts and epilation have occurred in patients as a consequence of complex intracranial neurointerventional procedures such as embolization of arteriovenous malformations (AVMs).

Since the mid-1980s, skin injuries have been reported in patients as a direct result of complex fluoroscopically guided interventional procedures, including arterial embolization, arterial revascularization, cardiac radiofrequency ablation, and TIPS.[2] The rise in reporting these adverse events resulted in U.S. Food and Drug Administration (FDA) action in 1994[3] and in U.S. federal regulations limiting the x-ray tube output of interventional fluoroscopic equipment. Similar actions have taken place throughout the world.

The threshold dose for acute skin erythema is about 2 Gy, and that for delayed deep skin ulcers is about 12 to 15 Gy. The risk for deterministic injury rises if multiple sequential procedures are performed at the same anatomic location (i.e., a TIPS procedure and TIPS revision 3 months apart). Other risk factors for skin injury include obesity, diabetes mellitus, and connective tissue disease.[4] Minimizing the risk of deterministic patient injury is a major focus of current radiation safety initiatives.

MANAGEMENT OF PATIENT EXPOSURE

Equipment Purchase and Maintenance

Optimal radiation exposure management begins with equipment purchase and room design. The interventionalist must be involved in both processes and must insist that radiation safety be a major factor in decision making. For an existing interventional radiology suite, adherence to a preventive maintenance schedule ensures that equipment will operate properly. Preventive maintenance also allows early replacement of parts before their deterioration contributes to unnecessarily high radiation exposure.

Preprocedural Patient Care

The interventional procedure must be medically necessary to justify exposure to ionizing radiation. This is particularly important for procedures known to be associated with high exposure: TIPS, visceral stent placement, visceral embolization, and neuroembolization.[5] For these interventions in particular, the risk for radiation-induced skin injury should be specifically discussed in the consent process. In addition, history taking should include questions about previous radiation exposure and factors that increase a person's susceptibility to radiation-related skin injury (e.g., diabetes). The physical examination should include inspection of the skin at previous x-ray beam entry sites.

Discussion of radiation-induced cancer risk is not typically included in the consent process because the immediate benefit of a medically necessary procedure far outweighs the risk for development of cancer in the distant future. However, the interventionalist should be prepared for patient questions regarding this issue. Discussion can include a review of the medical benefits of the planned procedure, a comparison between the relatively high overall risk for cancer in the general population and the small incremental risk engendered by medical radiation exposure, and mention of the long latent period between exposure and induction of cancer for most tumors.

Patient pregnancy is a contraindication to fluoroscopically guided procedures because of the risk of genetic mutation during early gestation and the risk of mental retardation and leukemia during late gestation. Because the life of the fetus depends on the life of the mother, however, occasional exceptions to this rule exist, particularly in the setting of acute trauma management. It is key for the interventionalist to collaborate closely with an obstetrician and a physicist during and after the procedure. In instances in which the woman and fetus survive the acute threat to life, formal fetal dose calculation may contribute to a recommendation that the pregnancy be terminated. The same collaboration should take place if it is found after the fact that a fetus was exposed unintentionally.

Intraprocedural Patient Care

Work habits of the interventionalist have a profound effect on patient radiation exposure.[6] Optimal work habits require knowledge of radiation physics, familiarity with tableside controls of the x-ray equipment, practice using these controls, and a commitment to radiation safety as a patient care priority.

For most interventional procedures, *fluoroscopy time* is the single most important determinant of patient radiation exposure that is under control of the operator. It correlates poorly with patient dose, however, because so many other variables, such as body habitus, affect the absorbed dose. It is possible to reach a skin dose of 2 Gy with a fluoroscopy time of 15 to 20 minutes in an obese abdomen. The operator should strive to keep the fluoroscopy time as brief as possible and should maintain awareness of the elapsed fluoroscopy time during the course of a procedure. New interventional rooms display the elapsed fluoroscopy time on an in-room monitor, whereas older equipment uses an audible signal at 5-minute intervals to note the elapsed fluoroscopy time.

Factors affecting fluoroscopy time include complexity of the procedure, operator experience, patient anatomy, image quality, inventory of disposables, and luck. One learned skill that can help lower fluoroscopy time is to make use of *last image hold*, a feature available on all digital interventional x-ray units. With last image hold, the operator can activate the fluoroscopy x-ray beam briefly by tapping the foot pedal. The resultant fluoroscopic image is saved on the monitor so the operator can review it rather than a live fluoroscopic image. Though not possible during deployment of an implantable device, it is a satisfactory way to review anatomy during decision-making times.

How much fluoroscopy time is too much? Although no standard or regulation has established a maximum fluoroscopy time, good patient care may require interruption of a procedure in instances in which prolonged fluoroscopy time puts the patient at risk for severe skin injury. One way to balance the risk-benefit ratio of prolonged fluoroscopy is to take stock of a procedure's progress at 30-minute intervals of elapsed fluoroscopy time. If 60 minutes of fluoroscopy time have passed and there has been no substantive progress toward achievement of the technical goal of the procedure over the previous 30 minutes, it may be in the best interests of the patient to stop and seek an alternative treatment path. On the other hand, if the goal is near, the patient's interests are best served by completing the procedure.

A patient's radiation dose for a fixed period of fluoroscopy time can vary by a factor of 5, depending on multiple technical factors, including x-ray tube output, beam geometry, imaging mode, and image sequence parameters.[6] *X-ray tube output* can be varied with modern digital interventional fluoroscopy equipment. Some types of equipment have modes of operation called "normal," "high dose," and "low dose." Others refer to fluoroscopic frame rates, such as "30 frames per second" (fps) (equivalent to analog fluoroscopy), 15 fps, and 7.5 fps. High-dose/fast-frame rate modes should be reserved for short periods when maximum resolution is necessary to guide treatment, such as positioning of a faintly visible stent. Low-dose/low-frame rate modes are most useful when the anatomy being imaged is very still (i.e., an extremity) and when precise visualization of an instrument is not needed. These latter modes may cause distracting image lag on the monitor if there is frequent or quick motion in the field of view (i.e., respiratory motion in the abdomen, cardiac pulsation in the chest). As a general rule, patient care is optimized during fluoroscopy by balancing image quality needs with as low a dose/frame rate as possible. With modern flat panel receptor technology, pulse rates as low as 3 to 4 pulses/s are commonly being used for low-intensity cases.

Radiation exposure can be limited by use of lead *collimators* to restrict the cross-sectional area of the beam exiting the x-ray tube. Although collimation does not decrease the peak skin dose to the patient, it does limit the volume of tissue being exposed. This serves to reduce the size of any potential skin injury and decrease the risk for stochastic effects. In addition, beam collimation can lead to improved image contrast by reducing Compton scatter within the field of view.

X-ray beam geometry includes three components: the distance between the x-ray source and the patient, the distance between the patient and the flat-panel receptor (or image intensifier), and the beam's angulation. Each component has an impact on patient dose. The patient should be positioned as far from the x-ray tube and as close to the image intensifier as possible for optimal image quality and minimal radiation dose. A vertical x-ray beam results in a lower dose to the patient than one at an oblique angle because more radiation is needed to penetrate the increased body-part thickness traversed by an angled beam, and the angulation of the C-arm results in a large air gap between the patient and the image receptor. Although the overall dose may be increased by beam angulation, the peak skin dose may be lowered by using this technique, because changes in beam angle cause changes in the entry point of the beam on the skin. Therefore, intraprocedural changes in tube angle may be a useful way to lower the risk for skin injury. When oblique fluoroscopy is used, doses to the operator are greater when the tube is rotated toward the operator.

All interventional fluoroscopic units provide multiple magnification settings for the image intensifier. Use of the image *magnification mode* has a complex effect on patient dose. Magnification of the image reduces the volume of tissue exposed but increases the dose to the remaining field of view. Therefore, use of the magnification mode may increase the risk for skin injury but leave the risk for stochastic effects unchanged. As a general rule, the magnification mode is best used sparingly and only when the technical demands of the procedure require a high level of fine detail. Use of the magnification mode throughout an entire procedure suggests there may be some other unmet imaging need; possibilities include a TV monitor positioned too far from the operator or an operator who needs new glasses!

Acquisition of digital subtraction angiography sequences (*DSA runs*) has an impact on patient dose, and DSA runs are the largest contributor to dose in neuroembolization procedures. Frame rates and the number of DSA runs should be tailored to each patient and kept as low as possible. For example, arterial flow through an AVM may be so fast, images have to be acquired at 7 fps, whereas an arterial tree in an ischemic extremity may be adequately imaged at 2 fps.

Postprocedural Patient Care

Information regarding the procedural radiation dose should be included in the patient's medical record.[7] The exact type of information depends on what dose metric is automatically recorded in the interventional equipment used to perform the procedure. Fluoroscopy time is always available. Also standard is a dose-area product (DAP) meter to provide a cumulative DAP (Gy/cm^2) for each procedure. DAP is a useful metric but correlates best with stochastic risk and has little relationship to peak skin dose. A brief procedure performed with a large field of view may result in the same DAP as a lengthy procedure performed at high magnification. The second procedure will have a much higher peak skin dose than the first. The newest generation of interventional fluoroscopy equipment incorporates sophisticated dose meters that can display real-time cumulative doses irrespective of the cross-sectional area of tissue exposed. As these rooms replace current equipment and become incorporated into clinical practice, it will be much easier to view dose information during a procedure and use that information to improve patient care. For example, decisions regarding whether to terminate a lengthy procedure can be made on the basis of real-time dose monitoring rather than fluoroscopy time, a poor substitute.

Dosimeters like those worn by radiation workers can be used to record a patient's dose. In clinical practice, however, these types of dosimeters are impractical for widespread use because they do not provide real-time information. They must be sent away for interpretation. This process takes time, requires employee time, and costs money not reimbursed by insurance payers.

Procedures with long fluoroscopy times (or high doses if a more precise metric is available) should be reviewed routinely as part of a quality assurance process to ensure the radiation exposure is medically justified and see whether practice trends emerge.

Standards for patient follow-up have not been established with respect to monitoring for potential fluoroscopy-induced skin injury. Multiple factors contribute to this lack. First, significant skin injury is rare, even in patients who have undergone long fluoroscopically guided procedures. Second, there is no clear evidence that early intervention changes outcomes when injury does occur. Finally, practitioners are reluctant to alarm patients when they have no clear recommendations for management of such an injury. In an ideal postprocedural setting, the patient should know that the procedure was medically necessary and performed in a way that optimizes the risk/benefit ratio, should be told that development of a rash in the region that was imaged could be due to radiation exposure, and should be instructed to call the interventionalist if a rash or irritation occurs. The interventionalist's responsibility is to then refer the patient to a dermatologist or plastic surgeon who is aware that radiation injury is a possibility and can incorporate that information into treatment planning. Biopsy of a radiation injury may not heal well.

MANAGEMENT OF OCCUPATIONAL EXPOSURE

Interventional radiologists work in close proximity to the x-ray tube and must use optimal radiation safety practices. The primary source of exposure to the operator is scatter from the patient at the beam entry point, which is typically at table level. Fortunately, for the most part, technical factors and work habits that minimize patient radiation dose also reduce occupational dose (see earlier). Shielding, distance, and dosimetry are the other protective tools available to the interventional team.

Shielding can be divided into three categories: shielding on the worker, shielding in the room, and shielding on the patient. These shields are commonly referred to as "leaded" barriers, although the metal alloys currently in use contain no lead and are lighter and more flexible than they would be if lead were used.

A *lead-equivalent apron* is mandatory for all workers in an interventional fluoroscopy environment. The lead apron covers almost all of the radiation-sensitive organs: gonads, lungs, gastrointestinal tract, and most of the bone marrow. The lead apron should fit well (custom-made is best) and be comfortable. For most people, a wraparound design provides the best protection and the least back strain. Dosimeters placed beneath a standard protective apron typically record radiation doses at or minimally above background during normal working circumstances.[8]

The thyroid gland is the most radiation-sensitive organ outside the lead apron and can be shielded by a small *thyroid shield* worn around the neck. The lens of the eye can acquire the threshold dose for cataracts over a long interventional radiology career and can be protected by *leaded goggles*. Again, these should be custom-made for optimal fit; if they do not fit, they will not be worn.

Additional *room-based lead shielding* can provide supplemental protection to the worker, especially to parts of the anatomy not covered by the apron, thyroid shield, and glasses. Commonly available shields include ceiling-mounted clear acrylic barriers on mobile booms, table-mounted flexible leaded strips, and mobile barriers on wheels. Boom-mounted shields can replace the need for leaded glasses and provide protection from body fluid splashes. Table-mounted shields provide protection to the legs. The main reason these ancillary shields are not used universally is that they can be cumbersome to position and move and can restrict access to the patient. Many interventionalists use them only in selected instances in which operator exposure may be high due to long fluoroscopy times, such as for TIPS and complex embolization procedures.

Relatively new are sterile *flexible leaded drapes* that can be placed on the patient in the sterile field.[9] These barriers are commercially available in a wide variety of designs and are disposable. They are much less cumbersome than boom-mounted shields. They can significantly reduce scatter to the operator's hands, arms, and head. It is important to note that these barriers should be kept out of the fluoroscopic image. When a leaded barrier is included in the fluoroscopic field of view, the automatic brightness control system in the imaging chain will cause x-ray tube output to increase in an attempt to penetrate the barrier.

Radiation-attenuating surgical gloves exist but may be ineffective in reducing hand exposure.[10] They provide no benefit if their use causes operators to put their hands in the visible x-ray beam.

Distance from the x-ray source is a powerful barrier to radiation exposure. According to the inverse square law, one's exposure diminishes by a factor of 4 when distance from the x-ray tube is doubled. Personnel not scrubbed in for a procedure should step into the control room when patient care does not require their presence in the procedure room with the patient. Scrubbed personnel can even step into the control room, or at least a few feet from the x-ray tube, during DSA acquisition.

Occupational Dose Monitoring

All medical radiation workers are required to participate in a facility-based radiation dosimetry monitoring program. Regulations regarding these programs vary from state to state. Typically workers are issued dosimeters to be worn outside the lead apron at neck level. These dosimeters record a dose that approximates that of the exposed head and neck. Some programs also include a second dosimeter to be worn under the lead at the waist level to serve as a proxy for the gonadal dose. Worker dosimeters are read at monthly intervals. Doses that exceed permissible levels are followed up by the facility's radiation safety office. Follow-up measures may include recommendations regarding a change in work habits or a change in shielding methods.

Some practitioners view compliance with dosimetry monitoring as pointless or an annoyance. They reason that a dosimeter left in the hallway will always record a low dose and thus allow the practitioner to avoid a visit from the radiation safety officer. In other facilities, the radiation safety office is woefully understaffed and simply cannot provide feedback in a timely or useful manner. The unfortunate outcome of these situations is that valuable feedback regarding occupational radiation exposure is lost.

SUMMARY

Optimal management of radiation exposure to patients and workers is an important aspect of interventional radiology. Together, a solid knowledge base, meticulous preprocedural and postprocedural patient care, and optimal work habits in the interventional fluoroscopy suite provide the best balance between the benefits and risks of radiation exposure in this environment.

KEY POINTS

- Exposure to ionizing radiation allows performance of lifesaving interventional procedures but has negative health implications, including stochastic and deterministic effects.
- Optimal management of patient radiation exposure requires the use of dedicated and well-maintained interventional fluoroscopy equipment, careful patient selection and preparation, adherence to work habits that can reduce patient exposure, and appropriate follow-up.
- Best-practice management of occupational exposure requires adherence to work habits that reduce worker exposure, use of appropriate shielding, and compliance with dosimetry regulations.

► **SUGGESTED READINGS**

Balter S. Interventional fluoroscopy: physics, technology, safety. New York: Wiley-Liss; 2001.

The complete reference list is available online at www.expertconsult.com.

CHAPTER **18**

Management of Risk Factors for Peripheral Artery Disease

Alfonso Tafur and Suman Rathbun

This chapter focuses on the management of *peripheral artery disease* (PAD), defined as atherosclerosis of the iliac and lower extremity arteries. PAD is a prevalent condition, with most patients in the community being asymptomatic. PAD confers risk for overall and cardiovascular mortality, especially among those with accelerated functional decline. A sensitive and inexpensive method to diagnose PAD is use of the *ankle-brachial index* (ABI), calculated by dividing the highest ankle pressure of each leg by the highest brachial pressure. Currently the PAD 2010 performance measures recommend measuring ABI in patients older than age 18 who have walking impairment or claudication, patients with lower extremity nonhealing wounds, patients aged 50 to 69 who have a history of smoking or diabetes, and all patients older than age 70.

The principal acquired risk factors for PAD are hypertension, chronic kidney disease, hyperlipidemia, diabetes mellitus, and a current or prior history of smoking. Nonmodifiable risk factors include advancing age, gender, and race. In addition, multiple biomarkers are emerging as potential indicators of disease progression. Prescribing lifestyle modifications such as regular exercise, maintaining ideal body weight, and moderate consumption of alcohol is the first step in treating vascular disease, but goal-directed management of the primary acquired risk factors will be essential for improving PAD-related outcomes.

For smoking cessation, bupropion, nicotine replacement therapy, and varenicline are well-tested medications that appear to be cost-effective. At the same time, the importance of intense counseling by the primary physician cannot be stressed enough. Current goals of therapy for hypertension control in patients with PAD are to achieve a target blood pressure less than 140/90 mmHg. β-Blockers and angiotensin-converting enzyme (ACE) inhibitors are valuable tools for achieving these goals among patients with PAD. Statin therapy to reduce LDL cholesterol to levels lower than 100 mg/dL is a well-accepted indication, and a target level of less than 70 mg/dL is advocated. For patients with PAD who require vascular surgery, perioperative initiation/continuation of statin therapy is necessary and proven to decrease postoperative rates of cardiovascular death and myocardial infarction. Finally, multiple recent trials have prompted a change in paradigms regarding diabetes treatment among patients with PAD. The American Diabetes Association recommends glycemic goals for nonpregnant adults of hemoglobin (Hb)A_{1c} of less than 7%, but personalization of care and less stringent treatment goals seem to be appropriate for adults with advanced PAD.

This chapter, which can be viewed in its entirety at www.expertconsult.com, will discuss in depth the management of PAD and its associated risk factors.

CHAPTER 19
Principles of Intraprocedural Analgesics and Sedatives

Ali Albayati and Andres Krauthamer

As the need for interventional radiologic procedures continues to grow, there is increased interest in better periprocedural pain control. Interventional radiology (IR) plays a significant role in pain management, both therapeutically (for chronic pain) and supplementally (for pain caused by intervention). Pain management is essential as IR practice becomes more invasive, readily available, and widely offered[1] to individuals at "high risk" for both operative procedures and anesthesia. One of the most noticeable changes in medical management is the migration toward more outpatient procedures, which has increased interest in providing sedation and analgesia modalities suitable to the outpatient setting, such as intraprocedural moderate sedation or monitored anesthesia care.[2] Some of the vascular surgical procedures for instance, can be performed with a combination of locoregional techniques and intravenous (IV) conscious sedation.[3] As a result, interventional radiologists and anesthesiologists face a variety of new challenges in ensuring the safety and comfort of their patients. Pain management is also important because it reduces patient discomfort and anxiety.

The interventionalist should obtain a proper history and physical examination and should discuss the procedure and pain management plan with all parties involved, including the patient and the nurse team member assigned to that particular procedure. Preprocedural consultation with an anesthesiologist is essential when there are ongoing or expected risk factors in terms of the patient's age, clinical status, unstable vital signs, complex intervention, or the potential for significant periprocedural pain. A point of caution is that during complex procedures, it is possible that numerous doses of intraprocedural analgesics and sedatives will be required to overcome stress and pain; this may result in deeper than intended postprocedure sedation after elimination of the procedure's painful stimuli. This can be avoided by adequate planning and communication with other disciplines. While a more active role for anesthesiologists in IR is being sought, the availability of anesthesia personnel to cover these procedures varies greatly among institutions.[4]

TECHNIQUES FOR PROVIDING ANALGESIA AND SEDATION

There is considerable overlap among the types of analgesia and/or sedation currently available. The determination of which is best is based on the type of procedure being performed, patient clinical status, patient preference, interventionalist preference, and availability of an anesthesiologist. The American Society of Anesthesiologists (ASA) Task Force on Sedation and Analgesia by Non-Anesthesiologists has developed practice guidelines[5] that define sedation and analgesia as a continuum that ranges from minimal sedation through general anesthesia (Table 19-1). Anesthesiologists recognize this continuum and thus are generally able to develop an anesthetic plan that meets the changing needs of the interventionalist. There are four main options of locoregional anesthesia and sedation available to the interventional patient:

1. *Local anesthesia* is indicated for minor procedures and includes infiltration of a local anesthetic to the region of planned procedure; there is no associated sedation. The patient will be fully awake. A subtype of this option is therapeutic (e.g., to eliminate a patient's chronic pain). A local anesthetic may be mixed with steroid and injected into a degenerative joint.

2. *Sedation* is indicated for most interventional radiology procedures and is coadministered with local anesthesia. There two main subtypes of sedation for this option:
   - *Moderate "conscious" sedation* will produce a state of decreased awareness with maintained protective reflexes. It is usually administered by the IR critical care nurse. The most frequently used combination of medications for moderate sedation is midazolam with fentanyl.
   - *Monitored anesthesia care (MAC)* is a deeper sedation administered by the anesthesiologist. Propofol is generally the first choice of anesthesiologists for MAC sedation.

   For more information on sedation, please visit www.expertconsult.com.

3. *Regional anesthesia* includes administration of local anesthetic to block main nerve trunks. There are two subtypes:
   - *Segmental anesthesia* (i.e., epidural anesthesia) is frequently provided by the anesthesiologist.
   - *Nerve block* can be an effective therapeutic technique. It is used to ameliorate chronic radicular pain when injected at the intervertebral foramina to block exiting spinal nerves.

4. *General anesthesia* is the deepest level of sedation and characterized by a state of unconsciousness, analgesia, anxiolysis, and amnesia. It is provided and maintained by the anesthesiologist and involves loss of response to painful stimuli and loss of the protective airway reflexes. The patient will not be able to recall procedural events.

INDICATIONS AND GOALS OF ANALGESIA AND SEDATION

Needs of Individual Patient

All patients vary in terms of their tolerance to discomfort and their ability to cooperate with the IR team. The main

TABLE 19-1. Continuum of Depth of Sedation: Definition of General Anesthesia and Levels of Sedation/Analgesia

	Minimal Sedation (Anxiolysis)	Moderate Sedation/Analgesia (Conscious Sedation)	Deep Sedation/ Analgesia	General Anesthesia
Responsiveness	Normal response to verbal stimulation	Purposeful response to verbal or tactile stimulation	Purposeful response after repeated or painful stimulation	Unarousable, even with painful stimulus
Airway	Unaffected	No intervention required	Intervention may be required	Intervention often required
Spontaneous ventilation	Unaffected	Adequate	May be inadequate	Frequently inadequate
Cardiovascular function	Unaffected	Usually maintained	Usually maintained	May be impaired

Adapted from American Society of Anesthesiologists Task Force on Sedation and Analgesia by Non-Anesthesiologists. Practice guidelines for sedation and analgesia by non-anesthesiologists. Anesthesiology 2002;96:1004–17.

indication is to decrease the pain that is experienced during a planned procedure. In nonemergent settings, the patient's needs can be addressed ahead of time at the consultation/informed consent visit, where the patient's anxiety can be reduced by a thorough explanation of the analgesia technique. This generally reduces the need for heavy preprocedural sedation. This also has a major impact on the type of analgesia and/or sedation offered; for example, such a discussion before a nontunneled central venous line placement can modify a patient's initial preference for moderate sedation to a more easily administered local anesthesia. In other instances, the discussion with the patient may result in a request for anesthesia support for a transjugular intrahepatic portosystemic shunt (TIPS) or endovascular aneurysm repair (EVAR). The final component in developing such a plan is how to make the patient most comfortable during the planned procedure.

Risks and Sequelae of Procedure

The ability to perform a rapid and accurate neurointerventional procedure, procedures involving a high risk of significant bleeding, postprocedure airway edema, or other potentially hemodynamic alterations are indicators for the interventionalist to consider moderate sedation or general anesthesia to have optimal control of the patient's movement, respiration, and other physiologic functions. The needs of an interventionalist may include the requirement of an absolutely still patient with controlled apnea and the expectation of avoiding a significant amount of patient pain or a prolonged procedure.

CONTRAINDICATIONS TO ANALGESIA AND SEDATION

Because of advances in monitoring and pharmaceutical agents, anesthesiologists rarely hear the statement "the patient is too sick for anesthesia." There are no defined contraindications for the patient to undergo some form of anesthesia. We are, however, occasionally presented with patients who are at such great risk for anesthetic morbidity and mortality that a careful discussion of the risk/benefit ratio of the proposed procedure should be undertaken before proceeding. Additionally, unless the procedure is emergent, all patients should be optimized medically before proceeding with elective procedures, including nothing-by-mouth status.[5]

EQUIPMENT

Please visit www.expertconsult.com for a full discussion of this topic.

PRECAUTIONS FOR PROVIDING ANALGESIA AND SEDATION

Please visit www.expertconsult.com for a full discussion of this topic.

PHARMACOLOGY OF ANALGESIC AND SEDATIVE AGENTS COMMONLY USED IN INTERVENTIONAL RADIOLOGY

Local Anesthetics

Subcutaneous or intradermal infiltration with a local anesthetic is frequently used in IR to achieve anesthesia of the skin. Local infiltration techniques typically involve extravascular injection of the drug at the procedure site. The discomfort due to the injection of a local anesthetic is often the worst aspect of commonly undertaken minor procedures; this is related to the acidic pH of the infiltrated solution.

Local anesthetics reversibly interrupt neural conduction by blocking sodium channels located on internal neuronal membranes. This results in inhibition of sodium permeability necessary for action potential propagation and pain signal formation.[11]

Adverse reactions associated with local anesthetics may arise from direct toxicity, reaction to an added vasoconstrictor or preservative, or allergic reaction. Toxicities result from high blood levels of local anesthetic, usually as a consequence of accidental intravascular injection, increased uptake from perivascular areas, or overdose. Common adverse reactions associated with local anesthetics include central nervous system toxicity, cardiovascular toxicity, neuronal toxicity, vasoconstrictor reactions, and allergic reactions.[13] Prevention of such reactions is contingent on both appropriate dosage administration, clinical vigilance for early detection of toxic reactions, and prevention methods such as syringe aspiration for blood prior to injection of the anesthetic.

The clinical action of a local anesthetic is often described by its potency, speed of onset, and duration of action. Lidocaine and bupivacaine are two of the most commonly used local anesthetics for skin infiltration in IR patients. Vasoconstrictors such as epinephrine are often added to local anesthetics to prolong the duration of action and improve the quality of the local anesthetic block.

For more information on the primary pharmacology of local anesthetics, please visit www.expertconsult.com.

Techniques for Delivering a Local Anesthetic

Efforts should be made to reduce pain during administration. These include warming the solution to be injected, use of topical anesthetics such as lidocaine gel prior to administration, using as small a needle as possible (e.g., 25-gauge needle for superficial infiltration) then changing to a longer and larger-caliber needle (e.g., 22-gauge) and slow injection of the agent along the expected tract or region of intervention. Mixing the injected solution with sodium bicarbonate and/or epinephrine can also be considered (see later discussion).

Lidocaine

Lidocaine (Lidocaine HCL [Hospira Inc., Lake Forest, Ill.]) was the first clinically used aminoamide local anesthetic, introduced into clinical practice by Nils Löfgren, a Swedish chemist. Lidocaine remains the most widely used agent because of its inherent potency, short latency, tissue penetration, and intermediate duration of action. Lidocaine concentration is expressed in percentage as grams per 100 mL (e.g., lidocaine 1% is 1 g/100 mL, which is 10 mg/mL). Available concentrations range from 0.5% to 5%. At concentrations of 0.5% to 1%, lidocaine provides local anesthesia with a duration of 1 to 2 hours. Lidocaine's versatility is demonstrated by clinical application for almost any regional anesthetic application. It is effective in infiltration, providing topical anesthesia, a peripheral nerve block, and both epidural and spinal blocks. There is a spectrum of toxicities directly related to the lidocaine serum concentration (Fig. 19-1).[1,14]

Bupivacaine

Bupivacaine (Marcaine [Hospira Inc.]) was the first long-acting amide agent to gain widespread use. Bupivacaine provides extended-duration anesthesia for infiltration, a peripheral nerve block, and epidural and spinal anesthesia.

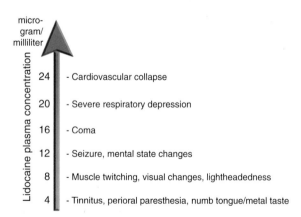

FIGURE 19-1. Spectrum of lidocaine's adverse effects relative to serum concentration levels. (*Adapted from Covino BG. Clinical pharmacology of local anesthetic agents. In: Cousin MJ, Bridenbaugh PO, editors. Neural blockade in clinical anesthesia and management of pain, 2nd ed. Philadelphia: Lippincott; 1988. p. 111–44.*)

Useful concentrations of the drug range from 0.125% to 0.75%. At concentrations of 0.25%, bupivacaine provides extended-duration anesthesia lasting 2 to 4 hours.[13] Bupivacaine has a unique property of both sensory and motor dissociation. By altering the concentration of bupivacaine, separation of sensory and motor blockade can be achieved. The main disadvantage of bupivacaine, in comparison to lidocaine, is its longer latency and increased potential for systemic toxicity.

Epinephrine

Please visit www.expertconsult.com for a full discussion of this topic.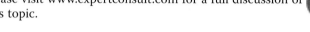

Sodium Bicarbonate

Please visit www.expertconsult.com for a full discussion of this topic.

Opioids

Fentanyl

Fentanyl (Sublimaze [Taylor Pharmaceuticals/Akorn Inc., Decatur, Ill.]) is a synthetic opioid that is structurally related to meperidine (Demerol [Hospira Inc.]) and binds to μ_1 and μ_2 receptors. The potency of most narcotics is described in relationship to morphine sulfate, and fentanyl is between 75 and 125 times as potent as morphine.[21] Fentanyl can more easily penetrate the central nervous system and thus has a rapid onset of action relative to morphine, owing to its high lipid solubility (lipophilic), a feature that facilitates rapid titration of the drug to patient effect. However, the maximal analgesic effect and potential respiratory depression may not be noted immediately. This lipophilicity also results in a longer elimination half-life for fentanyl (approximately 219 minutes) than morphine (approximately 120 minutes) because of its large volume of distribution,[21] but this effect is relevant only when fentanyl is administered in large doses over time. For a single dose of fentanyl, such as for an IR procedure, the effective half-life is shorter than for morphine and other intermediate-acting opiates such as meperidine or hydromorphone. Fentanyl has mild amnestic properties, so it is administered with other amnestics and anxiolytics such as midazolam.

For moderate sedation, fentanyl is generally given IV in the 1 to 3 µg/kg range in divided doses (increments of 25-50 µg). As a point of reference, doses as high as 50 to 100 µg/kg may be administered during an anesthetic for cardiac surgery.

Fentanyl and the other opiates have many side effects, most of which are well known to radiologists. Cardiovascular side effects of fentanyl include a centrally mediated bradycardia that may affect overall cardiac output, but the drug has surprisingly little effect on inotropy (preserving cardiac stability), leading to its widespread use by anesthesiologists for patients with poor cardiac function. Unlike morphine, fentanyl induces less nausea and urinary retention, as well as less histamine-mediated itching (particularly perinasal) or hypotension. The respiratory depressant effects of opiates are well recognized, and although anesthesiologists debate the relative potency of opioids for respiratory depression, these differences are generally not as significant.

Factors that may exaggerate respiratory depressant effects in individual patients include age, concurrent benzodiazepine or propofol administration, renal insufficiency, or reduced hepatic clearance.[22] Not only do opiates attenuate the normal ventilatory response to hypercapnia but they also reduce the patient's normal compensatory ventilatory response to hypoxia.[22] The combination of fentanyl with a benzodiazepine (e.g., midazolam) may result in respiratory depression and hypotension not seen with either drug alone. This is attributed to their synergistic action.[23]

For more information on fentanyl tolerance and side effects, please visit www.expertconsult.com.

Remifentanil

Recently developed synthetic opioids include sufentanil, alfentanil, and remifentanil. Although each has its unique qualities, as a group they are rarely used in IR, and for the purposes of this chapter they are similar to fentanyl, with the exception of remifentanil. Remifentanil (Ultiva [Bioniche Pharma USA LLC, Lake Forest, Ill.]) has been administered for pain control during a variety of interventional procedures.[25] It is similar in potency and structure to fentanyl and the other synthetic phenylpiperidine derivatives, except for a unique ester linkage which is hydrolyzed by nonspecific serum and tissue esterases and has a half-life in minutes. The half-life of the drug remains evanescent regardless of the duration of the infusion. It is routinely administered as an IV infusion in a 0.5 to 1 µg/kg/min dose rate, but it can be given as a bolus. There is some potential benefit of remifentanil over the conventional agents in patients with multiple organ failure because remifentanil's pharmacokinetics are not affected by hepatic or renal failure; routine use of remifentanil, however, is not recommended for critically ill adult patients.[26] It may be administered to nonintubated patients, but care must be taken because it has a narrow safety margin and a low total infused drug volume[27]; the intraluminal volume of the infusion tubing adds to the drug's clinical effect and may result in respiratory depression. Remifentanil is contraindicated for patients with known fentanyl hypersensitivity.

Naloxone

Naloxone (Narcan [Endo Pharmaceuticals, Chadds Ford, Pa.]) is a nonselective antagonist of all opiate receptors and has no agonist activity. It is generally used to reverse opiate-induced respiratory depression, but unfortunately also antagonizes other opiate effects such as analgesia. There are reports of extreme hypertension,[28] pulmonary edema,[29] and ventricular fibrillation[30] after naloxone administration, presumably due to the sudden and profound sympathetic stimulus as opiate-induced analgesia is reversed acutely. Standard teaching encourages IV administration of one ampule (400 µg) of naloxone to reverse opiate-induced respiratory depression. For the purposes of reversing respiratory depression produced in the course of moderate sedation, however, much smaller doses (e.g., 20-40 µg) should be titrated to effect while ventilatory support is provided as needed. In this way it may be possible to reverse respiratory depression while not eliminating all analgesic effects. The half-life of naloxone (60-90 minutes) is shorter than that of most opiates, so patients requiring naloxone administration should remain in a monitored setting for at least this period of time, and a continuous IV infusion of naloxone (e.g.,

5 µg/kg/h) may be required until serum levels of opiate have had time to decrease.

Benzodiazepines

Please visit www.expertconsult.com for a full discussion of this topic.

Midazolam

Midazolam (Midazolam HCL [Hospira Inc.]) is the most commonly used sedative agent for moderate sedation in IR procedures. It is two to three times more potent than diazepam, with a rapid onset, relatively short duration of action (elimination half-life, 1-4 hours[21]), and low toxicity level. Used primarily for anxiolysis, it is also a potent antegrade amnestic agent, this effect at least partially reversed by flumazenil.[31] These qualities make it an ideal agent for moderate sedation. Like the opiates, midazolam has little effect on cardiovascular function. It does produce a dose-dependent decrease in ventilation, and as stated previously, the respiratory depressant effects of midazolam are markedly accentuated when the drug is used in combination with other sedative agents. Typical dosage of midazolam for moderate sedation and anxiolysis ranges from 0.5 to 3 mg IV in divided (0.5 to 1 mg) doses. Enhanced effect of midazolam may be experienced in patients with significantly reduced hepatic or renal function secondary to accumulation of the drug or its active metabolites. Anesthesiologists occasionally use midazolam as an induction agent for general anesthesia, using an IV dose of 0.1 to 0.2 mg/kg.

As with other sedative agents, patients (particularly the elderly) may become disoriented or agitated when given midazolam and often will not recall the event, given the drug's amnestic properties. Whether this represents a "paradoxical" reaction is questionable. A frequent clinical response to this patient reaction is to administer more sedatives. Once factors such as hypoxia, hypotension, or other procedural causes of confusion are eliminated, the care team should consider actually reducing the level of sedation or alternatively, proceeding to a general anesthetic if the patient's medical condition and resources allow. In addition to having a more cooperative patient with a protected airway, elderly patients may awaken more rapidly from a carefully administered general anesthetic than from increasingly large doses of sedative agents.

Flumazenil

Flumazenil (Romazicon [Genentech/Roche, South San Francisco, Calif.]) is a highly specific competitive antagonist that has a high affinity for the benzodiazepine receptor. It is used for the reversal of benzodiazepine overdosage. Its elimination half-life is shorter than all clinically used benzodiazepines, including midazolam, implying that there exists the risk of re-sedation, and patients should continue to be monitored closely after its administration. The usual IV dosage for the reversal of benzodiazepines is 0.1 to 0.2 mg increments up to a total of 3 mg. Flumazenil should *never* be used for the routine reversal of benzodiazepine effects because of its possible weak agonist activity, resulting in re-sedation. Neave et al. showed that flumazenil administration to healthy volunteers causes hypotension and bradycardia and impairs patient awareness, attention, and long-term memory processing.[32]

Other Sedative Agents

Propofol

Propofol (Diprivan [APP Pharmaceuticals LLC, Schaumburg, Ill.]) is currently the most widely used IV anesthetic agent.[22] Propofol provides anxiolysis and sedation with variable amnestic effects. It has mild analgesic effects[33]; however, it is combined with fentanyl for better analgesic results. It is administered as an IV bolus (generally 1-2 mg/kg) for induction of general anesthesia or as a continuous IV infusion for moderate sedation (generally 10-50 µg/kg/min) or maintenance of general anesthesia (50-200 µg/kg/min IV). An alkylphenol, propofol is insoluble in water and is prepared as an emulsion, thus its milky white appearance. It can be quite painful on injection, and this effect may be attenuated by IV administration of lidocaine (0.5 to 1 mg/kg) immediately before propofol injection.

The pharmacokinetics of propofol are somewhat complicated, but the drug is rapidly metabolized by the liver as well as the lungs; inactive metabolites are excreted by the kidneys. A single bolus dose of drug is rapidly cleared by redistribution and elimination and has a distribution half-life of 2 to 8 minutes. The context-sensitive half-life (the period of time until plasma levels drop 50% after cessation of infusion) for propofol after infusions of up to 8 hours is less than 40 minutes, and thus it has a shorter recovery time than midazolam. Hemodynamic effects include systemic vasodilation and myocardial depression, which produce a fairly significant reduction in arterial blood pressure.[22] These effects are exaggerated in the elderly and in those with cardiovascular compromise. Propofol is also a profound depressant of ventilatory drive, and this effect is exaggerated in the presence of opiates.[22] It is important to recognize that there is potential for bacterial overgrowth in propofol, and current recommendations include discarding any drug not used within 6 hours of withdrawal from the original vial.

For more information on the benefits of propofol, please visit www.expertconsult.com.

Fospropofol

In 2008 the U.S. Food and Drug Administration (FDA) approved the use of a water-soluble prodrug of propofol, fospropofol (Lusedra [Eisai Inc., Woodcliff Lake, N.J.]), for MAC sedation in adult patients. Fospropofol is metabolized by endothelial and hepatic alkaline phosphatases to the active metabolite, propofol; therefore it has a longer onset time.

Propofol lipophilicity has known disadvantages, including pain on injection, narrow therapeutic window with the potential to cause deep sedation, high lipid intake during long-term sedation, and risk of infection resulting from bacterial contamination.[35] The hydrophilic fospropofol has slower pharmacokinetics with better predictable peak of the desired clinical effect and more gradual elimination. These features make fospropofol suitable for sedation for short diagnostic procedures such as colonoscopy or bronchoscopy and for other minor therapeutic surgical procedures. It is administered with other analgesics such as fentanyl.

Because fospropofol has a longer elimination half-life than propofol (44-57 minutes for fospropofol vs. 2-8 minutes for propofol), a deeper than intended sedation with fospropofol should be expected to last longer than deep sedation inadvertently induced with propofol.[1] The recommended dosage for fospropofol is 6.5 mg/kg as a bolus for induction, with 1.6 mg/kg as needed for maintenance to obtain the desired clinical effect.

In addition to cough, nausea, and vomiting, paresthesia and pruritus in the perineal region have been found to occur within 5 minutes of administration of the initial dose of fospropofol.[36]

Ketamine

Ketamine (Ketalar [JHP Pharmaceuticals, Rochester, Mich.]) is a curious drug, structurally related to phencyclidine. It produces what is called a "dissociative" anesthetic in which patients may appear to be awake, frequently with a slow nystagmus, but are uncommunicative. Potential advantages of ketamine include (1) it has profound analgesic effects, distinguishing it from all currently used induction agents, (2) it produces central sympathetic stimulation with resultant hypertension and tachycardia, (3) sympathetic stimulation also produces bronchial dilatation, and (4) it does not depress respiration as significantly as other induction agents.

It is the adverse effects of ketamine that limit its widespread use in adults. These include increased salivation, increased intracranial pressure in those with abnormal intracranial compliance, and most importantly, emergence delirium. Adult patients may have significant dysphoria and hallucinations after ketamine administration. This emergence delirium can be ameliorated with concurrent administration of benzodiazepines, particularly midazolam.[20] Dysphoric effects are much less frequent in children, and because of ketamine's beneficial effects—particularly its analgesic effects and lack of ventilatory depression—it is a commonly used sedative for painful procedures in young children. Ketamine is undergoing a "re-emergence" in anesthesia, and its preemptive use may reduce opioid tolerance and improve pain scores postsurgically.[38]

There is no absolutely fixed dose recommendation for ketamine because it varies with the desired clinical response, route of administration, and patient's age. However, the IV route is the easiest to titrate as 1 to 2 mg/kg over 1 minute for induction, then supplemented with 0.1 to 0.5 mg/kg for maintenance. Ketamine is also a common adjunct to total IV anesthesia (TIVA) for complex neurosurgical or neurointerventional procedures when electrophysiologic monitoring such as somatosensory or motor-evoked potentials is being done.

Dexmedetomidine

Dexmedetomidine (Precedex [Hospira, Inc.]) is a potent α_2-agonist that provides sympatholysis, sedation, anxiolysis, and analgesia.[39] It does not depress baseline ventilation when administered to adults within the recommended dose limits. It is easier to titrate and has a shorter recovery time (half-life 2 hours).

Dexmedetomidine is used in the intensive care unit (ICU) for sedation of mechanically ventilated patients during intubation/extubation. It has been used for moderate sedation in nonintubated patients prior to and/or during short interventional procedures.

Dexmedetomidine is metabolized extensively in the liver, and 95% is excreted in the urine. It should be given in small amounts to people who suffer from liver or kidney

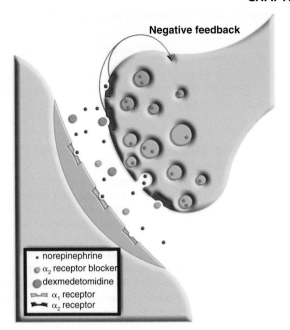

Negative feedback

- norepinephrine
- α_2 receptor blocker
- dexmedetomidine
- α_1 receptor
- α_2 receptor

FIGURE 19-2. Cross-section through a synapse in the brain with α-adrenergic receptor activity. Dexmedetomidine provides sympatholysis, sedation, anxiolysis, and analgesia via potent α_2-receptor agonist effect. Inadvertent prolonged sedation or cardiovascular adverse effects of dexmedetomidine can be potentially reversed by α_2-receptor blockers.

impairments. Some of dexmedetomidine's side effects are related to decreased sympathetic nervous system activity secondary to its α_2-agonist effect and may include hypotension, bradycardia, sinus arrest, atrial fibrillation, and dry mouth. Therefore dexmedetomidine is contraindicated in patients taking digoxin. Prolonged sedation or cardiovascular adverse effects of dexmedetomidine can be potentially reversed by α_2-receptor blockers (Fig. 19-2).

Adult dosage for moderate sedation is 1 µg/kg IV × 1, then supplemental as 0.6 µg/kg/h, which is titrated with a dose range of 0.2 to 0.7 µg/kg/h to achieve proper sedation. It should be administered with a controlled infusion device for less than 24 hours.

McCutcheon et al. found that dexmedetomidine produces mild analgesic effects that decrease analgesic requirements postoperatively.[40] Dexmedetomidine may be useful for selected IR procedures that require sedation with minimal analgesia; this could be more effective when coadminstered with an analgesic and/or local anesthetic. Dexmedetomidine has been used for sedation for endovascular repair of abdominal aortic aneurysms (AAAs)[41] and pediatric magnetic resonance imaging (MRI) studies.[42] Some patients receiving dexmedetomidine have been observed to be arousable and cooperative when stimulated; this is particularly useful for some interventional neuroradiologic procedures such as cerebral arteriovenous embolization. However, dexmedetomidine may impair the cognitive testing essential for proper neurologic monitoring.[43]

SUMMARY

Interventional radiology is one of the fastest-growing areas in medicine and is rapidly altering the way we approach traditional procedural medicine. Proper and safe sedation and analgesia of patients with multiple comorbidities is an essential component of high-quality medical care. The safe delivery of anesthesia and the pressure for rapid throughput of patients require trained personnel with a solid working knowledge of the pharmacology of currently used sedative/analgesic agents. A system that provides for safe and efficient preoperative evaluation, anesthesia delivery, and postprocedure recovery must be in place. Although a close relationship exists between interventional radiologists and anesthesiologists, a shortage of anesthesia personnel persists and may worsen in the near future[44] at a time when their services are increasingly needed in interventional suites. Other specialties, notably gastroenterology, have sought alternative approaches to providing deep sedation with propofol or fospropofol using a nonanesthesiologist provider. The ultimate safety of such a program remains undetermined.[45]

KEY POINTS

- Patient comfort and safety are priorities during a planned or emergent intervention. These can be achieved through coordination among different teams to come up with the sedation plan individualized for each patient and each procedure.

- Understanding the pharmacology of anesthetics, analgesics and sedatives is pertinent to provide safe and effective sedation and analgesia. This includes the fact that co-administration of analgesic and sedative results in synergistic effect with more pronounced cardiovascular and/or respiratory depression.

- Patients have variable responses to sedatives and analgesics, which depends primarily on the patients age, clinical status and intake of other analgesics. This variation affects the patient's post procedure recovery and pain control. Thus, it is very important to titrate the sedative and analgesic doses according to the patient needs.

▶ **SUGGESTED READINGS**

American Society of Anesthesiologists Task Force on Sedation and Analgesia by Non-Anesthesiologists. Practice guidelines for sedation and analgesia by non-anesthesiologists. Anesthesiology 2002;96:1004–17.

Ray CE. Pain management in interventional radiology. New York: Cambridge university press; 2008. ISBN-10 0521865921.

Stoelting RK, Hillier SC. Pharmacology and Physiology in Anesthetic Practice. 4th ed. Philadelphia: Lippincott Williams & Wilkins; 2006.

The complete reference list is available online at www.expertconsult.com.

CHAPTER 20

Contrast Agents

Michael A. Bettmann

There are probably no medications, with the possible exception of aspirin, that are more widely used than iodinated contrast agents. They are also among the safest of all medications. Their use is critical to the advancement of medical imaging, and to a certain extent the advances in contrast agents have paralleled the advances in x-ray technology. Although they have been widely used in various forms for over a century, and even though iodinated contrast agents have changed minimally over the past 20 years, some major questions remain regarding the mechanisms, significance, incidence, and prevention of adverse events. This chapter focuses on iodinated contrast agents. Other agents, such as barium and magnetic resonance imaging (MRI) contrast agents, have minimal roles at present in interventional radiology. This chapter addresses the nature of iodinated contrast agents, what is known about the adverse events associated with their use, prevention and treatment of such events, and alternatives to contrast agents.

HISTORY

The first reported use of a contrast agent, within a year of the description of x-rays by Roentgen, was for visualization of the vasculature in an amputated hand, highlighting the interest dating from the initial use of imaging in developing contrast agents to aid in defining arteries, veins, and other internal structures.[1] Over the next 30 years, the value of contrast agents was widely recognized and investigated. During this period, the major focus was on development of an intravenous (IV) agent for visualization of the urinary tract. Early on it was recognized that iodine was potentially a suitable agent because of its wide availability and its property of blocking x-rays. Organic iodine, however, was soon found to be too toxic to the endothelium to allow parenteral administration. A number of other agents were investigated. From the 1920s to 1950, perhaps the most promising and widely used was a colloidal suspension of thorium dioxide, Thorotrast. This compound was developed for clinical use by Egaz Moniz, a Portuguese scientist, neurosurgeon, and diplomat. He later received the Nobel Prize in Medicine for his development of the now-reviled procedure of prefrontal lobotomy for treatment of various forms of mental illness. Thorotrast was in many ways an ideal contrast agent. It was well tolerated when used for cerebral angiography and provided excellent vascular opacification. It was, however, an alpha emitter and was taken up and retained by the reticuloendothelial system after intravascular administration, thereby causing lifelong radiation exposure. It led to a high incidence of liver and hematologic malignancies as well as cirrhosis and was taken off the market.[2,3]

Biochemists in collaboration with physicians manufactured a series of compounds that used iodine in various combinations to achieve radiopacity with low levels of toxicity. During this period, toxicity was mainly pain on injection and sclerotic reaction in vessels. Among the investigators in the 1920s were Binz and his students and their collaborator Räth, who developed numerous compounds that were extensively investigated in vitro and in animal studies and even in humans. In the late 1920s, a young American urologist, Moses Swick, working in the laboratory of the eminent German physiologist and physician Professor von Lichtenberg, used several of these compounds. With trial and error, one of them, sodium-2-oxo-5-iodopyridine-N-acetate, was shown to achieve visualization of the urinary tract after IV administration, with limited acceptable endothelial and systemic toxicity. Swick was allowed to present his work, but as was the tradition in Germany at that time, the major credit and first authorship of the resultant paper went to von Lichtenberg.[4] Swick's substantial contributions were not fully recognized until 30 years later, when as an elderly urologist practicing in New York, his pivotal role in the development of intravascular contrast agents was finally publicly recognized and widely lauded.[5,6]

The compound Swick used consisted of an incompletely substituted four-carbon ring with a single iodine atom attached. Though a marked improvement over previously available agents, it was still somewhat toxic. From the late 1920s through 1954, a number of iodine-based agents were developed and tested in both animal models and the clinical setting. Swick and his collaborator Wallingford were the first to propose the use of a six-carbon (benzene) ring, but the toxicity of this compound, with a single iodine atom attached and not fully substituted, was too great.[6] In the early 1950s, three side chains were added to this six-carbon ring, and a second then a third iodine atom. This fully substituted six-carbon ring with three iodine molecules attached and various side chains at the other three positions had markedly decreased toxicity.[7] To achieve chemical stability in solution, this was manufactured as a salt. When placed into solution, one of the side chains dissociated into a positively charged cation (usually sodium) and the remaining iodine-containing anion. Consequently, in solution this compound had an osmolality that was twice what it needed to be: for each of the three iodine atoms, two osmotically active particles were present (Fig. 20-1).

The next major development came a little over a decade later.[8] Torsten Almen, at the time a young Swedish radiologist working as a research fellow in Philadelphia, noted that these high-osmolality ionic contrast agents (i.e., containing a positive and a negative charge) caused pain on intraarterial injection. He observed that if he swam in salt water with his eyes open, the water hurt his eyes. If he swam in fresh water, however, his eyes did not hurt. Almen then reasoned that the pain on injection was related to the high osmolality and to the property of the compound being a salt, with sodium as a dissociating side chain in most molecules. He

Available Iodine-based Contrast Agents

Molecular structure	Era	Examples	Comment
		Ionic monomer	
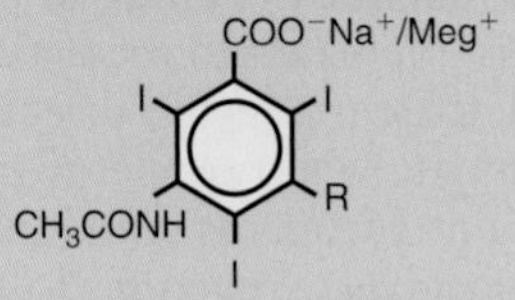	1950s	Diatrizoate Iothalamate	Hyperosmolar, 5–8× blood
		Non-ionic monomer	
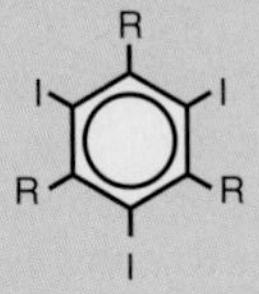	1980-present	Iopamidol Iohexol Ioversol Iopromide Oxilan	Lower osmolality, ~2× blood, improved hydrophilicity
		Ionic dimer	
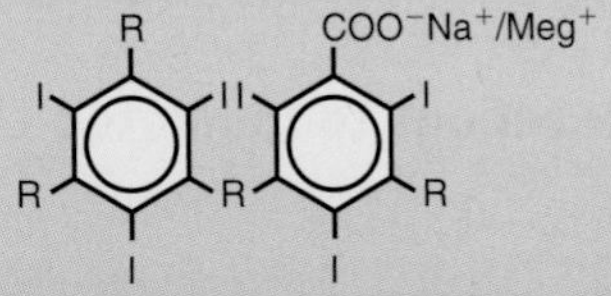	1980s	Ioxaglate	Osmolality, ~2× blood (300 mg I/mL)
		Non-ionic dimer	
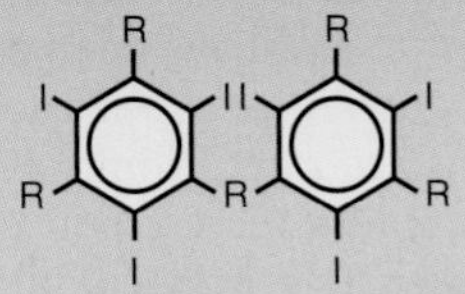	1990s–	Iodixanol Iotrolan	Osmolality = blood, increased viscosity, balanced Na^+/Ca^{2+}

FIGURE 20-1. Formulas and key characteristics of currently available iodinated contrast agents.

developed a nondissociating and nonionic (noncharged) compound, metrizamide (Amipaque). In creating this compound, he not only eliminated the charge but also decreased the osmolality of earlier compounds by half, at the same iodine concentration. Metrizamide, however, was not stable in solution. It was available as a lyophilized powder and had to be reconstituted before use. As Almen had predicted, the amount of discomfort encountered with intravascular injection of metrizamide was strikingly less than with previous agents. This was a major step forward, but because of the inconvenience of this formulation and the occurrence of some unexpected central nervous system complications, as well as the cost of producing the compound, extensive efforts were made to develop other more stable low-osmolality agents.

Numerous compounds resulted, many of which are still in use. There were two separate pathways, one of which is now essentially of only historical interest. With the aim of lowering the osmolality, two benzene rings were linked together, forming a dimeric compound. The resulting formulation still had a dissociating side chain in solution, but it now had six iodine atoms paired with two osmotically active particles and thus had an osmolality half that of the earlier contrast agents. This compound, ioxaglic acid (Hexabrix [Guerbet, Aulnay-sous-Bois, France]) was developed in France and widely used in the 1980s.[9] The other approach, which mimicked the development of metrizamide, was to create monomers of fully substituted benzene rings with three iodine atoms attached but without a dissociating side chain. This is the basic formulation of the vast majority of contrast agents currently in use.[10-12] These so-called low-osmolality agents, however, have an osmolality that is still twice that of blood (see Fig. 20-1). All the minor adverse events associated with the earlier higher-osmolality agents, including discomfort, pain, nausea, and vomiting, were markedly decreased with these low-osmolality agents, as were the direct cardiac effects[13-16]; but the very rare life-threatening reactions still occurred, perhaps at the same rate. It was theorized that both safety and comfort could be further improved if the osmolality could be decreased to that of blood. This was accomplished by creating a nondissociating nonionic dimer. Two such agents were developed in the 1980s. The first, iotrolan, was widely investigated and found to be generally safe and even more comfortable than the nonionic monomers.[17] After its release in much of Europe, to a limited extent in the United States, and in Japan, however, it was noted in Japan that there was a relatively high incidence of delayed cutaneous reactions, some of which were severe.[18] This led to removal of iotrolan from the market. The second nonionic monomer, iodixanol (Visipaque [GE Health Care, Princeton, N.J.]), was developed around the same time, was released widely in the mid- to late 1990s, and is now fairly widely used.[19] It is safe and causes minimal discomfort on injection, as expected, even less than the low-osmolality agents.

PHYSIOLOGY

As noted, all modern iodinated contrast agents consist of one or two fully substituted six-carbon rings (see Fig. 20-1). The conventional high-osmolality ionic contrast agents still exist, with a single benzene ring, three attached iodine atoms, and the property of dissociating into two charged particles in solution. They are very safe and inexpensive but are currently used to a limited extent, usually for injection in small volumes for opacification of collecting systems, as with placement or injection of biliary drains, nephrostomies, or abscess drains. Iothalamate (Conray) is perhaps the most widely used of this class of contrast agents. Various side chains unique to the commercially prepared individual nonionic molecules are attached at the three carbon sites not occupied by an iodine atom. All these so-called low-osmolality agents are nonionic, nondissociating, and stable in solution.

All iodinated contrast agents in current use are relatively small molecules with a molecular weight of less than 1 kD. They are therefore too small to act directly as antigens and induce an antigen-antibody (i.e., allergic) reaction. The degree of opacity achieved with contrast agents is a function of a number of variables. The iodine concentration is the most important. All contrast agents are prepared in a stable pH-balanced solution with various additives (e.g., calcium disodium EDTA) to maintain both the pH and stability during storage. In general, the higher the iodine concentration in a contrast agent, the higher the osmolality. For use in angiography, an iodine concentration of around 300 mg/mL is usually sufficient. It is important to keep in mind that an iodine concentration that is too low will not allow sufficient delineation of anatomic abnormalities such as vessel irregularities. On the other hand, if the iodine concentration is too high, there will be insufficient x-ray penetration to define certain structures such as plaque. Other obvious variables in visualization are viscosity of the contrast agent, rate and volume of injection, size of the vessel to be visualized, the patient's cardiac output, and blood flow in the specific region. Viscosity, which varies largely as a function of the side chains of the compound as well as the iodine concentration, has an effect on how well a bolus is maintained, in addition to how difficult it is to inject the contrast agent. The viscosity of most contrast agents is two to three times that of blood, and hand injection is not difficult. The single currently available nonionic dimer has a viscosity substantially greater than that of the monomers. On the one hand, this may allow the bolus of contrast to remain intact to a greater extent as it is injected into the bloodstream. Conversely, there may be a discernible difference when it is injected by hand through a small catheter. Various technical factors such as the contrast sensitivity of the imaging system and the use of subtraction techniques help define the optimal concentration plus volume of contrast agent that is necessary. If contrast material is injected into a small artery in a patient with low cardiac output and digital subtraction angiography (DSA) is performed, either a low concentration (e.g., 200 mg iodine per milliliter) or a very small volume can be used. On the other hand, if a large structure such as the aorta is to be visualized in a patient with high cardiac output, it is often necessary to use a higher iodine concentration (e.g., 320-360 mg of iodine per milliliter) and to use both a higher flow rate and a larger volume. With IV injection for visualization of vascular structures and organs, the quality of the images is similarly dependent on the aforementioned factors: imaging technology, patient's size and cardiac output, rate and volume of injection, and iodine concentration. With rapid multislice CT scanning, the iodine concentration, volume of injection, and timing of filming are crucial and still subject to wide debate.[20-22]

All iodinated contrast agents are essentially immediately distributed throughout the extravascular space. They are not metabolized and are excreted by glomerular filtration without tubular reabsorption. The half-life of contrast agents in general is about 60 minutes. Although there is still some debate, there is minimal if any free iodine in preparations of iodinated contrast agents. In general, therefore, there is no concern about the effect of contrast agents on the thyroid.[23,24] It is important to recognize that (1) organic iodine is relatively toxic if injected directly,[6] and (2) iodine is an essential element, so a true allergy to iodine is incompatible with life. Contrast agents bind minimally to protein. It is possible certain adverse reactions to contrast agents, as discussed later, are the result of complexes formed by binding to protein, with consequent antigenicity or activation of acute-phase reactants. It is important to reiterate, however, that iodinated contrast agents bind *minimally* to protein, and *no* antibodies to contrast agents have ever been found, despite varied extensive studies over decades.

Adverse Reactions to Iodinated Contrast Agents

General
Acute life-threatening and even fatal reactions to contrast agents clearly occur[25,26] and have been encountered with all contrast agents in current use, but there are two caveats. First, such reactions are rare. From large studies it is clear that the incidence is less than 1 per 100,000 patients.[27,28] Secondly, if appropriately treated, almost all reactions resolve. Third, most deaths that occur in association with the administration of a contrast agent are primarily due to underlying disease rather than the contrast agent itself. In large carefully controlled series, most or all fatalities have occurred in patients in whom the effects of the contrast agent were generally incidental or played a small additive role. For example, the vast majority of deaths in one large registry occurred in patients with severe multitrauma, advanced cancer, or end-stage congestive heart failure.[27]

It is clear, however, that severe acute reactions to contrast agents occur and can be rapidly fatal. It is therefore essential that before a contrast agent is administered, all patients be appropriately screened, and knowledge and expertise to treat severe life-threatening reactions be readily available. Multiple ways of screening patients have been recommended, and as in all clinical settings, it is important to adopt approaches based on the best available data. The basic requirements are that each patient has a targeted history taken (Table 20-1) and that vital signs and assessment of overall status be recorded. Because shellfish contain iodine, it was long believed that patients with shellfish or other seafood allergies would be more likely to experience reactions, particularly severe ones. This turns out to be completely false.[27] Although patients with a strong allergic diathesis do have a minor increased risk of having an adverse event associated with a contrast agent,[27,28] this relationship is a surprisingly weak one with no evidence that there is an increased incidence of severe reactions.[25] Again, it is crucial to remember that severe systemic reactions are not truly "allergic," although they may be "anaphylactoid"; that is, they appear to be immune-mediated. Similarly, it has been suggested that patients with asthma are at increased risk for systemic reactions to contrast agents. Although this is probably true, available studies suggest that the risk in such patients is mainly worsening bronchospasm, not an alternate severe systemic reaction. This bronchospasm almost invariably responds readily to β-agonist inhalers.

TABLE 20-1. Prescreening Questions for Patients Prior to Contrast Administration

1. Do you know why you have been scheduled for this procedure?
2. General risk factors:
   a. Do you have any heart or circulation problems? Do they affect how you live? Are you taking medicines for them?
   b. Do you have diabetes? Are you taking medicines for it? If you are, what are the medicines?
   c. Do you have kidney disease, bad kidney function, kidney stones, bladder problems?
   d. Do you have any allergies other than hay fever? What happens with your allergies?
   e. Do you have asthma? If so, are you taking medications for it?
3. Have you ever had an x-ray contrast agent or dye? If so, for what (a CT scan, a cardiac catheterization, an MRI)?
   a. Did you have any kind of reaction to the contrast agent? If so, what was the reaction and how was it treated?
   b. After the reaction, have you had any kind of contrast agent or dye again? If so, did you again have a reaction?
4. Do you have any questions about the procedure you are about to have?

These caveats notwithstanding, it is clear that the single best predictor of a reaction to an iodinated contrast agent is a previous reaction to such an agent. Again, if these reactions were truly manifestations of an allergy, readministration of a contrast agent would inevitability lead to another reaction, one at least as severe as the initial reaction. This is clearly not the case. From large studies, the incidence of recurrent reactions depends to some extent on the route of administration.[27] Another misconception, similar to the discredited belief that patients with shellfish allergies are at particular risk, is that the risk for a systemic reaction is higher with IV than with intraarterial injection. This also is clearly not true. Overall, far from approaching 100%, the risk of recurrent reactions in patients with a documented previous reaction is on the order of 7% with IV administration of contrast, 12% with intraarterial injection, and about 25% with intracoronary injection.[27] The reasons for these differences in risk are unclear. They may in fact be dependent in part on erroneously ascribing an adverse event to a contrast agent rather than to a procedure or underlying disease. For example, shortness of breath may be an anxiety response rather than bronchospasm, and hypotension more often occurs as a manifestation of a vasovagal reaction than as a sign of an anaphylactoid response to contrast administration. The important point is that the single best predictor of a reaction to a contrast agent (i.e., a prior contrast reaction) is not a very good predictor at all. Contrast agents are extremely safe. Serious life-threatening reactions, though very rare, occur unpredictably, so it is imperative that patients be appropriately screened and that the knowledge and expertise to treat reactions always be readily available.

Severe systemic reactions generally occur within 5 minutes of the administration of a contrast agent. It is very rare for true reactions, if they occur, to develop more than 15 minutes after the administration of a contrast agent. These acute life-threatening reactions may be present as loss of consciousness, confusion, severe shortness of breath or difficulty breathing, or diffuse erythema. As with any life-threatening clinical event, the first approach should be

the *ABCs* of basic life support: *assessment/airway*, *breathing*, and *circulation*. As soon as the radiologist becomes aware there is a problem, it is imperative to talk to the patient, auscultate the chest, assess for cyanosis, perfusion, and pulse, and obtain vital signs, particularly blood pressure and heart rate (immediately when the patient becomes symptomatic). As with all life-threatening events, the sooner the appropriate therapy is instituted, the higher the likelihood of a successful outcome.

There is a relatively narrow differential diagnosis in patients who appear to be having an acute life-threatening reaction to iodinated contrast agents. As already noted, many such patients have serious preexisting problems that may be life threatening; defining whether this is the case is a crucial part of screening *before* contrast agent injection. It is always possible for a patient to develop a life-threatening arrhythmia, myocardial infarction, or stroke, but such events more often than not occur in patients with risk factors for them. If patients are otherwise stable at baseline, the two major possibilities for what appears to be a major adverse event are an *anaphylactoid reaction* to the contrast agent and a *vasovagal response*. There can be substantial overlap between the symptoms of these two conditions, but the treatment is very different, so it is important to appropriately evaluate patients. With anaphylactoid reactions, patients are hypotensive and *tachycardic* and often rapidly progress to unconsciousness. A vasovagal reaction is characterized by hypotension and *bradycardia*, often presaged or accompanied by diaphoresis and feelings of anxiety. Again, screening of patients to determine vital signs at baseline is crucial. Patients taking β-blockers may be unable to mount a tachycardic response, thereby leading to the false conclusion that a vasovagal reaction is occurring. On the other hand, vagal reactions are far more frequent than life-threatening anaphylactoid reactions.

For a vasovagal reaction, treatment consists of leg elevation (more effectively increases intravascular volume than Trendelenburg position), administration of IV fluids at a high rate, and if necessary, administration of atropine, 0.5 to 1 mg IV. Vagal reactions, in general, are life threatening only if they do not resolve.[29] It is therefore crucial to monitor patients until their heart rate and blood pressure return to normal or to baseline levels. An acute anaphylactoid reaction, with hypotension and tachycardia, must be treated as is any cardiovascular collapse. Call a code, continuously assess and record vital signs, make sure there is good intravascular access, infuse fluids such as normal saline (depending on the patient's cardiac and diabetic status), and if necessary, administer epinephrine. As is rapidly apparent whenever it is administered, epinephrine is an extremely potent α- and β-adrenergic agonist and thus causes marked peripheral vasoconstriction and tachycardia. It should therefore be administered with great caution and only when really necessary, since it can be dangerous in patients with underlying coronary artery disease. Epinephrine is available on code carts in two preparations. Both contain 1 mg (1000 μg), but at a 10-fold difference in concentration: as a 1:10,000 mixture in a 10-mL syringe (100 μg/mL) or as a 1:1000 mixture in a 1-mL syringe (1000 μg/mL). A 1-mL vial of a 1:1000 mixture is also available. The 1:1000 preparation is recommended only for subcutaneous administration. In patients with existent or incipient cardiovascular collapse, subcutaneous administration is not appropriate;

cutaneous vasoconstriction occurs, and the drug will be slowly and unpredictably absorbed. Administration in an acute life-threatening setting should, if at all possible, be directly IV, using the 1 : 10,000 concentration. When needed, 1 to 2 mL (100-200 μg) should be administered IV as the initial dose. The same dose can be readministered at 2- to 5-minute intervals as needed while keeping in mind that although it should be administered as expeditiously as possible, the dose should also be limited so that as little as necessary is given.

There are medications that are often considered but are *not* appropriate for these rare acute life-threatening reactions. Administration of an antihistamine is often contemplated, but it has no efficacy or role in patients with cardiovascular collapse. Similarly, corticosteroids are often considered. The primary role of corticosteroids is to stabilize the basement membrane, a process that takes several hours. Acute administration of steroids is therefore an inappropriate treatment of cardiovascular collapse.

Bronchospasm and laryngospasm are other serious and potentially life-threatening adverse events. Bronchospasm presents as shortness of breath or difficulty breathing with *end-expiratory wheezing*, occurs primarily in patients with known asthma, and is best treated by the administration of a β-agonist inhaler. If the bronchospasm is severe, epinephrine may be necessary, but this should be handled by others more familiar with this treatment. Laryngospasm, conversely, is characterized by *inspiratory wheezing*, often with stridor, and it does not respond to inhaled bronchodilators. If true laryngospasm rather than an anxiety reaction is present, treatment consists of the use of a nonrebreather oxygen mask and administration of epinephrine. Although epinephrine can be injected subcutaneously, it is more effective if given IV as 1 mL of a 1 : 10,000 mixture. Clinical differentiation is obviously important. An anxiety reaction can mimic both laryngospasm and bronchospasm, but wheezing is not present and epinephrine is clearly not indicated. Rarely, prolonged hyperventilation can lead to bronchospasm.

Many additional adverse reactions to iodinated contrast agents have been documented, ranging from nausea and vomiting to pain, urticaria, and contrast medium–induced nephropathy (CIN).[30] Nausea, vomiting, and pain on injection are largely but not completely related to osmolality. As the osmolality of agents decreases from 1500 to 2000 mOsm/L (with the older high-osmolality ionic agents) to 500 to 700 mOsm/L, the incidence of nausea and vomiting decreases markedly. Both still occur, but infrequently. With isotonic agents, discomfort on injection is essentially absent. Although this is clearly an advantage, routine use of a nonionic dimer is largely obviated at this time due to the added cost.

Urticaria is a separate problem. Its occurrence in patients appears to increase the likelihood of recurrent urticaria, but NOT of a subsequent more severe contrast reaction. Urticaria occurs more often than it is diagnosed; if patients are thoroughly and carefully examined for hives, they are often seen in patients who are asymptomatic. If symptomatic, hives generally respond quickly to diphenhydramine (Benadryl, 25-50 mg orally or IV), but this medication can cause drowsiness, so it should only be used for symptomatic relief and only if the patient is not going to drive for the next 6 to 12 hours.[30]

Contrast Agents and the Kidneys

Contrast Medium–Induced Nephropathy

This complex, incompletely understood complication is clinically important. There has been awareness of CIN since the 1950s at least, but the incidence, etiology, and clinical relevance have been well defined only over the last 10 to 15 years, for various reasons, some of them commercial. CIN has been thought to be a major cause of in-hospital renal failure,[31] and this is probably true. As with all aspects of CIN, however, the problem lies in precise definition. Ultimately, *contrast-induced nephropathy* is defined as the worsening of renal function secondary to the administration of an iodinated contrast agent. The diagnosis has usually been based on serum creatinine, and a number of different specific definitions have been used, including an absolute increase (0.5 or 1.0 mg/dL) or percent of change (25% or 50% increase over baseline) in serum creatinine, or a decrease in estimated glomerular filtration rate (eGFR). There are problems with all these definitions. First, serum creatinine varies with age, muscle mass, diet, gender, and race. Thus, a serum creatinine level of 1.0 mg/dL may equate with totally normal renal function in some patients, such as young males, and may reflect a significant compromise of renal function in others, such as thin elderly women. The same concern holds for percent of change in serum creatinine because this is a logarithmic function: a 50% increase from 0.8 mg/dL in a young patient is almost certainly not associated with a serious decrease in renal function. A 50% increase from 1.4 mg/dL, however, is almost certainly indicative of renal dysfunction in any patient, but would reflect different degrees of alteration in GFR in different patients. These concerns make interpretation of the literature difficult because of varying methodologies. For example, demographics are not always matched, various definitions are used, and ultimately, serum creatinine is not necessarily an accurate reflection of GFR.[32,33]

There are numerous alternatives to the use of serum creatinine. In the past, absolute creatinine clearance has been used, but this requires a complete 12- or 24-hour urine collection and thus is impractical, expensive, and the urine collection is often not complete. Inulin clearance is also used and may be more accurate, but it is also impractical for routine use or large studies. The use of serum creatinine alone is simple and familiar, but there are limitations, as described. At present, calculated creatinine clearance is probably the best option both for defining patients at risk and for diagnosing CIN. Two formulas have been developed and validated, though not specifically in the patients of interest: the Cockroft-Gault[34] and MDRD (Modification of Diet in Renal Disease, or Levey) formulas.[35,36] Many clinical laboratories now routinely report not only serum creatinine but also GFR estimated with one of these formulas. Certainly for assessment of risk, this is better than a serum creatinine level alone, but the accuracy of these formulas is limited in the assessment of acute changes in renal function as occurs with CIN. An alternative that may be important in the future is cystatin C, a low-molecular-weight protein that is produced and circulates at a steady state, is excreted by glomerular filtration, and is then metabolized, resorbed, and excreted in an altered form. Circulating levels, then, accurately reflect the GFR. Furthermore, levels rise more rapidly than serum creatinine levels do.[37,38] Typically, cystatin C levels rise 4 to 12 hours after an insult, whereas serum creatinine may begin to rise by 24 hours but does not peak for 3 to 7 days. Several concerns have prevented widespread adoption of cystatin C, including lack of universal availability, increased cost compared to creatinine, and questions concerning its accuracy as a reflection of a renal insult alone.

The incidence of CIN clearly varies with the definition, parameter used, and timing of the assessments. It is apparent that CIN occurs only in patients with renal dysfunction at baseline.[39-42] As noted, this may not be reflected in serum creatinine. That is, normal GFR is defined as over 100 mL/min, and stage 1 chronic kidney disease (CKD) is defined as GFR = 60 to 99 mL/min. At this level, particularly in thin, debilitated, or elderly patients, serum creatinine is likely to be normal. In the presence of renal dysfunction, other risk factors are important, including primarily diabetes mellitus and increasing age. The coexistence of other nephrotoxic factors, such as surgery, aminoglycoside administration, and possibly nonsteroidal antiinflammatory drugs (NSAIDs), is also relevant. In patients with normal renal function, the volume of contrast material used is not a risk factor, except in neonates, infants, and patients with severely limited cardiac reserve, in whom volume of fluid and osmotic load are the concerns. In patients with renal dysfunction, on the other hand, the risk of CIN increases with increasing volume of contrast agent.[41,42]

The pathophysiology of CIN is not known. There are various theories, none of which can currently be fully substantiated because of the lack of a reliable animal model and the numerous clinical variables that exist.[43,44] It is likely, however, based on normal renal physiology, that CIN results from damage secondary to hypoxia in the region of the thick ascending limbs of the tubules in the outer medulla. In this area, tubular and vascular flow is normally slow and the adjacent renal parenchyma is normally borderline hypoxic. It is logical to assume that this region is tipped over into frank hypoxia, with resulting free radical formation and then cell damage and death, due perhaps to the osmotic or direct chemotoxic effects of contrast agents in the tubules. This hypothesized pathophysiology, logical but unproven, currently serves as a basis for prophylaxis for CIN.

The natural history of CIN is interesting. Most studies show that serum creatinine increases from days 1 to 7 after the insult and then gradually returns to baseline over the next 1 to 2 weeks. It is rare for patients to require dialysis after CIN, either chronically or acutely, even if renal function is very poor at baseline.[39,40] Because CIN does not usually cause end-stage renal disease, it is relevant to consider whether it is actually a clinically important event or merely a "creatinopathy" and not particularly important clinically. Natural history studies suggest that it *is* clinically important: overall morbidity and mortality are higher in patients in whom CIN develops than in those in whom it does not develop.[45-48] That is, CIN serves as a marker and perhaps a predictor of poor outcome. Why this is so is speculative at present, but it is known that CKD carries a poor prognosis.[49] CIN is important not because it leads acutely or eventually to dialysis, but rather because it increases the risk of death and major adverse cardiovascular events. In part this may be a reflection of the underlying risk factors in these patients, but that is not the only explanation, as careful case-control analysis has shown.

Ultimately, then, it is important to try to prevent CIN. Many regimens have been used and there are many high-quality studies, but it is still not possible to arrive at absolute conclusions or recommendations. In the 1990s and earlier it was thought that CIN was related to vasoconstriction involving glomeruli, so it was logical to assume that increasing renal blood flow, as with furosemide, would be beneficial. In a study comparing hydration alone with hydration plus either furosemide or mannitol, this was shown not to be true; the incidence of CIN was actually increased in the furosemide group.[50] It was assumed, however, that hydration was valuable, and this has been widely accepted, although it is somewhat problematic. First, to date no studies have directly compared hydration with *no* hydration. Second, there is no consensus on how to measure hydration, and most studies have not even tried. Nonetheless, a number of studies have evaluated various hydration regimens. They suggest that in general, oral hydration is not as effective as IV hydration.[51] This may simply be due to the fact that oral hydration is less reliable. Patients may forget to consume the prescribed volume or may be actively discouraged from oral intake, as they are often instructed to abstain from oral intake for 8 or more hours before the administration of contrast agents. Other studies have suggested that hydration with normal saline is more effective at preventing CIN than 0.45 saline, and that 12 hours of IV hydration is more effective than 4 hours.[52-54] The basic questions regarding the benefit of hydration and how to measure it remain incompletely answered, but it is widely accepted that hydration is of more benefit than either lack of hydration or, perhaps more importantly, dehydration, and that hydration is best achieved by the administration of IV fluids for more than 4 hours before and 6 hours after the administration of contrast.[52]

There have been many additional approaches to prophylaxis, with hundreds of published studies.[55] Many regimens have been either ineffective or impractical. For example, both hemodialysis and hemofiltration have been investigated. In several studies, hemodialysis has proved ineffective.[56-58] Hemofiltration, essentially slow hemodialysis during and immediately after the administration of contrast material, has been shown by one group to be effective.[59,60] It is, however, impractical and expensive and carries significant risks, so it is not a viable approach for most patients and institutions.

A number of studies have examined the use of theophylline, an adenosine antagonist, as prophylaxis for CIN. It has been hypothesized, though not proven, that vasoconstriction plays a role in inducing medullary hypoxia and that adenosine may mediate this effect, so the use of theophylline may be helpful. A meta-analysis suggests that this may be true, but the results to date are not conclusive.[61] Further, theophylline must be administered carefully and has a narrow toxic-to-therapeutic ratio. Another approach that has attracted interest is the use of various dopamine β_2-agonists, with the aim of inducing postglomerular vasodilation and thereby increased renal blood flow. This is largely based on an old theory, now discredited, that contrast agents cause a decrease in overall renal blood flow. Although some studies have been promising, a large prospective randomized trial showed no benefit with the specific agonist fenoldopam.[62] Several other approaches are promising, but there are insufficient studies to evaluate their real value.

Such approaches include the use of statins beginning immediately before administration of a contrast agent, with the rationale that they maintain endothelial function and increase nitric oxide production and reduce oxidative stress. One study showed a marginal protective effect when compared with hydration alone.[63] Another approach is the use of ascorbic acid, which is known to act as an antioxidant and free radical scavenger. It was shown to decrease the incidence of CIN in one study,[64] but further investigation is necessary. Prostaglandin E_1, a potent vasodilator, has been used in several studies, with promising but not yet replicated results in one.[65] Administration, however, was accompanied by a decrease in blood pressure that required careful monitoring. Prostaglandin E_1 deserves further evaluation, but its relatively narrow toxic-to-therapeutic ratio may limit its role.

The ideal approach to CIN prophylaxis should be safe, effective, inexpensive, and practical for use. In this light, two approaches merit more detailed consideration: N-acetylcysteine (NAC) and sodium bicarbonate (NaHCO₃). NaHCO₃ is essentially a form of hydration, but in theory it may be more effective because it is thought to alkalinize the at-risk outer medullary region of the kidney and thereby prevent or decrease oxidative stress, free radical formation, and resultant tissue damage. As first reported for this use, it was administered as an IV infusion. A total of 154 mEq of NaHCO₃ was mixed in 1 L of 5% dextrose in water and infused at a rate of 3 mL/kg/h for 1 hour before administration of the contrast agent and at a rate of 1 mL/kg/h over the subsequent 6 hours. This regimen led to a significant decrease in CIN, but the study was relatively small, the control regimen was a suboptimal infusion of normal saline (total infusion lasting 6 hours beginning 1 hour before the examination), and the study was stopped early.[66] Despite multiple subsequent studies, questions remain about the actual efficacy of NaHCO₃. Two high-quality studies evaluated it in combination with NAC. In one study involving patients undergoing percutaneous coronary interventions, when NAC and NaHCO₃ were administered together intravenously over 1 hour before the procedure, the incidence of CIN was lower than in the control group. The control group, however, received only postprocedural hydration, clearly suboptimal treatment.[67] In the other study,[68] three treatment regimens were compared in more than 300 patients undergoing coronary or peripheral interventions. This was a prospective randomized study, and all patients received NAC at a high dose. Patients were randomized to receive additional hydration with either normal saline, NaHCO₃, or saline plus ascorbic acid. The incidence of CIN was significantly decreased in the NaHCO₃ group. The conclusions, then, are that it is likely NaHCO₃ in combination with NAC decreases the risk for CIN, and that NaHCO₃ alone *may* decrease the risk. Further studies are clearly needed to determine the role of this potential prophylactic regimen.

The theoretical reasons why NAC should provide effective prophylaxis for CIN are that it is both a free radical scavenger and stimulates the production of endothelial nitric oxide synthase, an enzyme found in normal vascular endothelium that enhances vasodilation. It is available in both oral and parenteral preparations; the latter is currently indicated in the United States for the treatment of acetaminophen overdose to prevent the associated hepatic toxicity. It is generally easy to administer and safe, with rare anaphylactoid reactions being the only major complication. There are two drawbacks to NAC use. First, it tastes and smells bad, so patients are often reluctant to take it. In addition, in most studies it has been given in four oral doses of 600 mg each, two on the day before administration of the contrast agent and two on the day of the examination. This regimen presents a problem for many radiologic studies, particularly emergency or outpatient ones. As initially reported, NAC was the first medication to show a definite benefit in the prevention of CIN.[69] Many of the studies that have shown no benefit from NAC have used a different regimen, usually with elimination of the 24-hour preprocedure doses or with a limited IV dose. Two studies showed no benefit for NAC given IV 1 hour before the procedure, one at a dose of 500 mg immediately before the procedure[70] and the other at 1000 mg before and 4 hours after.[71] Conversely, when a higher dose of 150 mg/kg in 500 mL of normal saline was given over a 30-minute period before the administration of contrast material and 50 mg/kg in 500 mL of normal saline was given over a 30-minute period afterward, there was a significant reduction in the incidence of CIN.[72] Other studies have evaluated increased doses of NAC. Briguori et al. compared the standard oral four-dose regimen of 600 mg per dose to 1200 mg per dose and found additional benefit with the latter.[73] Multiple meta-analyses[73-77] have arrived at conflicting conclusions, not surprisingly since prospective studies have also had conflicting results. Almost all agree that there may be a benefit with NAC and that additional larger studies are necessary. There are several probable explanations for the lack of consistent findings and the need for further studies. First, definitions of CIN vary, as do levels of risk in different populations, as discussed earlier. Second, the type of examination, specific contrast agent, and volume of contrast agent used vary in the available studies. Some have controlled for these variables,[73] and some have not. Finally, most studies using the oral 600-mg, four-dose regimen have shown a benefit, and the negative studies have largely (although not exclusively) used a shorter or lower-dose approach. It is likely, then, that NAC *is* beneficial, probably more so at a higher oral dose of 1200 mg or a higher IV dose of 150 mg/kg. Because NAC is safe, available, inexpensive, and probably beneficial, its prophylactic use is generally indicated when relevant and practical.

NAC may, as one study suggests,[73] be even more effective when used in combination with NaHCO₃, although in this study NAC was given orally and NaHCO₃ parenterally. Whether this beneficial synergy exists when both are given orally (or IV) remains to be investigated. The advantage of combining NAC with theophylline has also been investigated, and this combination was found to be detrimental when compared with NAC alone.[75]

Another major consideration with CIN is whether there are differences between the various contrast agents. It is clear that there are some differences between high-osmolality and low-osmolality contrast agents, but predictably only in patients with renal dysfunction, and to a greater extent with renal dysfunction and diabetes mellitus.[39,40] These differences, however, are in the incidence of CIN, not in the incidence of the need for dialysis, since no such difference has been demonstrated. Moreover, it is not clear that these relatively minor differences translate into the major concern with CIN, which is an increase in mortality and morbidity among those who develop it versus those who do not. A related question, though one driven largely by commercial interests, is whether there are differences between nonionic monomers, or between the monomeric formulations and the single currently available nonionic dimer. The differences between these contrast agents chemically are relatively minor, since all are based on a single or two joined benzene rings, each with three iodine atoms on each 6-C ring and relatively small side chains attached to the remaining carbon atoms. There are differences in osmolality and viscosity, but it is not clear what the role of these two factors is in CIN. It has been hypothesized that increased viscosity may lead to alterations in capillary hemodynamics in the outer medulla and may precipitate oxidative stress.[76] Conversely, osmolality may play a role, so decreasing the osmolality of the contrast agent from 500 to 650 mOsm/kg to a level equal to that of blood, about 280 mOsm/kg, may be beneficial. Several studies and a number of opinions have addressed this question. The results are not conclusive, but the opinions are very strongly held. Two studies, for example, suggest that there is no advantage to the nonionic dimer,[77,78] although one is a relatively small multicenter study, and the other includes patients with renal function that ranges from very limited to normal, making a true direct comparison difficult. Two other studies, one a fairly small but carefully controlled multicenter one[79] and the other a single-center fairly large one,[80] both show that the incidence of CIN is lower with iodixanol. As is true with many aspects of CIN, no absolute conclusions can be drawn.

CIN remains an incompletely understood entity. To summarize, it is important not because of the transient decreases in renal function as reflected by a decrease in eGFR or a rise in serum creatinine, because these abnormalities rarely lead to signs or symptoms or to the need for either short- or long-term dialysis. Rather, it appears to be associated with an increased risk for mortality and major morbidity. The precise pathophysiology of CIN is unclear, but it is currently thought that CIN develops as a result of hypoxic stress in the region of the thick ascending limb of the tubules in the outer medulla. It occurs only in patients with some preexisting compromise in renal function, although this is not always reflected in serum creatinine values. It is essentially dogma that hydration to achieve and maintain normal intravascular volume is crucial to prevent CIN, and this should be an aim in all patients who are administered a contrast agent. It is likely that hydration is best achieved with a minimum of 12 hours of prehydration with IV normal saline, although this is clearly not always possible. There are several promising methods for preventing CIN, but none has an absolutely proven effect, nor are any always effective. The best current approach is to use NAC, either four oral doses of 1200 mg, two on the day before and two on the day of the examination, or intravenously starting 30 minutes before the examination at a dose of 150 mg/kg in 500 mL of normal saline, followed by 50 mg/kg over a 30-minute period after the examination, also in 500 mL normal saline. $NaHCO_3$ may likewise be effective, particularly in combination with NAC, but it must be started 1 hour before administration of the contrast agent and should be continued for 6 hours afterward. Most studies to date have included patients undergoing cardiac angiography or interventions, but although debated, limited studies suggest that the same concerns and approaches apply to other parenteral routes of administration.

Other Nephrotoxic Considerations
Another concern is the interaction of contrast agents and other medications. Specifically, there has been concern with the use of metformin, an effective and widely used medication for type 2 diabetes, marketed, among other names, as Glucophage and Glucovance. There is no real interaction between iodinated contrast agents and metformin, but in a small percentage of patients, primarily those with underlying renal dysfunction, poor renal perfusion, or poor hepatic function, severe lactic acidosis can develop.[81,82] Because contrast agents are known to depress renal function in those with underlying renal compromise, it has been hypothesized that the administration of contrast material and metformin together might increase the risk. Extensive data suggest that this is not true. The package insert for metformin preparations approved by the U.S. Food and Drug Administration (FDA) indicates that metformin should be stopped at the time an iodinated contrast agent is administered and not be restarted for 48 hours. Though this is a reasonable approach, mainly because it is mandated by the package insert, the crucial consideration is that metformin should not be used in patients with compromised renal function. This also is clearly stated in the FDA-mandated package insert. Unfortunately, it is not rare that patients on metformin are first identified as having compromised renal function not by their referring physicians but at the time of angiography or other contrast-enhanced examination. Conversely, a large recent study confirmed the safety of metformin, even in patients with CKD.[82]

A final question concerns the indications and timing for measuring parameters of renal function before administration of a contrast agent. As noted, the best practical approach is to use both serum creatinine and eGFR determined by one of the two widely used formulas. Not every patient needs to have renal function measured. In those known to have renal dysfunction or major risk factors (e.g., long-standing diabetes mellitus, bladder outlet obstruction, multiple recurrent renal calculi, current nephrotoxic medications [including aminoglycosides, some chemotherapeutic drugs, and perhaps high doses of NSAIDs], or other situations that might worsen renal function [recent major trauma or surgery, severe congestive heart failure, or hepatic failure]), serum creatinine should be measured within 24 hours of administration of the contrast agent. Advanced age by itself is probably an indication also, although this is hard to quantify. In all other patients it is wise to measure serum creatinine before repeated administration of contrast material, but a baseline measurement is unlikely to be particularly helpful or valuable.

Contrast agents have been thought to have detrimental effects in patients with other comorbid conditions such as paraproteinemia (e.g., multiple myeloma), myasthenia gravis, pheochromocytoma, or interferon therapy. Acute renal failure has developed after the administration of contrast material to patients with myeloma, but its etiology is clear. It is caused by precipitation of protein in the glomeruli, and this in turn is related to dehydration. If patients are well hydrated before administration of a contrast agent, there does not appear to be significant risk.[83] There have

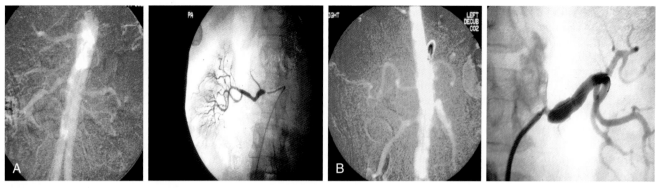

FIGURE 20-2. Selective renal arteriograms, each obtained with selective injection of 4 mL of nonionic dimeric contrast material, are compared with CO_2 aortograms in right anterior oblique **(A)** and left anterior oblique **(B)** projections. Both the CO_2- and contrast medium–enhanced angiograms show bilateral right renal artery stenosis.

been concerns in the past that administration of contrast agents may lead to release of catecholamines and an adrenergic hypertensive crisis in patients with metabolically active pheochromocytoma. Although incidents of this have been documented, particularly with selective injection of the artery feeding the tumor, it does not seem to be a real concern with nonionic contrast agents, even without the use of concurrent α-adrenergic blockers.[84] Myasthenic crises have been reported to occur (rarely) after the administration of contrast agents, but it is not clear that these incidents were specifically caused by the contrast agent.

ALTERNATIVES TO IODINATED CONTRAST AGENTS

Alternatives are most often considered in patients with renal dysfunction and in those with a history of a previous contrast agent–related adverse event. The most obvious approach is to use another imaging modality that does not require use of an iodinated contrast agent, such as ultrasound or a nuclear medicine study. In patients with a previous complication, as noted, it is important to carefully investigate exactly what that reaction was. Often it was unrelated or was not a complication at all. Steroids can be used for pretreatment, but if an imaging study is strongly indicated, it is appropriate to proceed, use a different contrast agent than the one that was associated with the complication, and be sure the equipment and expertise to treat a life-threatening reaction are immediately available.

In patients at risk for CIN, there are several additional options. One is to use a dilute iodinated contrast agent to limit the total volume of contrast. For example, it is often possible to perform selective arteriography and an intervention with less than 50 mL of contrast material, merely by using a high rate and a small volume for a limited aortogram (e.g., 8 mL of contrast medium at a rate of 20 mL/s) and then small injections of diluted contrast material for selective injections and intervention. Carbon dioxide (CO_2) is a useful adjunctive contrast agent, and there has been extensive experience with it. With care, it is safe and accurate[85] and produces images that, while aesthetically less pleasing than the usual DSA images, contain equivalent information. The concern with CO_2 is that it is a gas. It is invisible and compressible, so it is imperative that a closed

system be used to prevent contamination with air. In addition, because it is so compressible, it is easy to load 100 mL or more into a 20-mL syringe, and care must be taken to not inject so fast that the vessel becomes markedly distended. It is also important to not inject too slowly because CO_2 does not retain a bolus but rather rapidly fragments and is absorbed. The necessary injection volume and rate must be learned by experience. Furthermore, CO_2, unlike iodinated contrast agents, *decreases* density in comparison to surrounding structures. Obtaining adequate images, therefore, requires high-quality DSA and good patient cooperation (Fig. 20-2). This limits the utility of CO_2 in patients who cannot cooperate fully and in areas where there may be unpredictable motion, such as the bowel in the presence of bleeding. A final caution is that the safety of CO_2 in the central nervous system has not been proven, so care should be taken to avoid administration above the diaphragm.

Gadolinium chelates have been widely used in patients with renal dysfunction in the past and have been useful in eliminating or reducing the need for iodinated contrast agents. Unfortunately, over the last few years, it has become clear that gadolinium contrast agents, primarily certain formulations, lead to nephrogenic systemic fibrosis (NSF) in an unclear percentage of patients who have renal dysfunction.[86-92] This syndrome can be fatal. Its true incidence remains unknown, as does its pathophysiology, but deposition of gadolinium in the skin has been described.[86] The occurrence of NSF is related, at least to a large extent, to increasing severity of renal failure, and it has been described mainly in patients undergoing hemodialysis. It also seems to be related to increased doses of the gadolinium agent. The FDA has mandated a "black box" warning for all gadolinium contrast agents, and it is now widely accepted that an alternative be used in patients with marked renal dysfunction.[85] Some have suggested that dialysis be considered immediately after the administration of such agents in all at-risk patients, but this is probably neither a necessary nor a practical approach, and it is not clear that it is efficacious. At this time, as with iodinated contrast agents, gadolinium agents should be used in patients with renal dysfunction only when no viable alternatives exist, and they then should be used in as low a dose as possible. As with CIN, NSF is an entity that requires substantial further elucidation, but in distinction to CIN, it can be essentially eliminated by avoiding the use of gadolinium chelates in patients with severe renal dysfunction.[92]

KEY POINTS

- Iodinated contrast agents are among the most widely used and safest of all medications.
- Serious complications are rare but require rapid appropriate treatment.
- Prevention of systemic effects is not possible; steroid pretreatment is NOT effective prophylaxis.
- Contrast-induced nephropathy (CIN) is a risk in patients with diminished renal function, even when this is not reflected in serum creatinine levels.
- Hydration is important for all patients, particularly those with renal dysfunction. Intravenous normal saline is superior to all other hydration regimens.
- CIN is incompletely understood. The current best approach is to limit volume and pretreat with *N*-acetylcysteine, perhaps in combination with sodium bicarbonate, and to avoid iodinated contrast when possible.

▶ SUGGESTED READINGS

American College of Radiology Committee on Drugs and Contrast Media. Manual on contrast media. 7th ed. Reston, VA: American College of Radiology; 2010.

Bettmann MA, Heeren T, Greenfield A, Goudy C. Adverse events with radiographic contrast agents: results of the SCVIR registry. Radiology 1997;203:611–20.

Bolognese L, Falsini G, Schwenke C, et al. Impact of iso-osmolar versus low-osmolar contrast agents on contrast-induced nephropathy and tissue reperfusion in unselected patients with ST-segment elevation myocardial infarction undergoing primary percutaneous coronary intervention (from the Contrast Media and Nephrotoxicity Following Primary Angioplasty for Acute Myocardial Infarction [CONTRAST-AMI] Trial). Am J Cardiol 2012;109:67–74.

Maioli M, Toso A, Leoncini M, et al. Persistent renal damage after contrast-induced acute kidney injury: incidence, evolution, risk factors, and prognosis. Circulation 2012;125:3099–107.

Persson PB, Tepel M. Contrast medium-induced nephropathy: the pathophysiology. Kidney Int Suppl 2006;100:S8–S10.

The complete reference list is available online at www.expertconsult.com.

CHAPTER 21
Principles of Thrombolytic Agents
Michael B. Streiff and Raagsudha Jhavar

BIOLOGY OF THE FIBRINOLYTIC SYSTEM

Plasminogen/Plasmin

The fibrinolytic system is a critical regulatory network of proteins that provide balance to the hemostatic mechanism by ensuring maintenance of vascular patency by opposing the procoagulant forces of the coagulation cascade proteins. The key fibrinolytic enzyme in blood is *plasmin*, a serine protease that circulates as the inactive zymogen, *plasminogen*. Although plasminogen expression has been identified in a broad range of tissues, including the adrenal glands, brain, heart, intestine, kidney, lung, spleen, testis, thymus, and uterus, plasminogen is primarily synthesized in the liver. Plasminogen is a 92-kD, 791–amino acid glycoprotein whose plasma concentration in normal adults is 200 mg/L.[1-3] The concentration of plasminogen in premature infants and newborns, respectively, is 75% and 50% lower than in adults.[4] The half-life of plasminogen is 2.2 days, primarily because of catabolic degradation rather than consumption via conversion to plasmin. Although plasmin/plasminogen is primarily known for its function in the dissolution of fibrin thrombi, it also plays a key role in digestion of proteins critical for cellular migration, angiogenesis, and wound healing. Homozygous deficiency of plasminogen is associated with ligneous conjunctivitis, hydrocephalus, and abnormalities in wound healing, defects that can be corrected with plasminogen replacement therapy. Despite its role in thrombolysis, plasminogen deficiency or dysfunction has not been associated with an increased risk for thrombosis in affected patients.[1,5]

The plasminogen molecular structure consists of an N-terminal activation peptide followed by five disulfide-bonded kringle domains, an activation loop, and the serine protease active site domain at the C-terminus.

For more information on the molecular structure and function of plasminogen, including a structural diagram, please visit the website www.expertconsult.com.

α₂-Antiplasmin

In addition to plasminogen activators, which are discussed later in this chapter, the activity of the plasmin/plasminogen system is modulated by several negative regulatory proteins. The principal negative regulator of plasmin activity is α₂-antiplasmin.

More information on α₂-antiplasmin can be found at www.expertconsult.com.

The physiologic significance of α₂-antiplasmin is underscored by the clinical symptoms suffered by patients with homozygous α₂-antiplasmin deficiency. This rare bleeding disorder is inherited in an autosomal recessive fashion and is characterized by bleeding comparable in severity to that of hemophilia A. The bleeding typically occurs in delayed fashion after initial hemostasis, consistent with defective regulation of fibrinolysis. Laboratory testing demonstrates severely reduced levels of α₂-antiplasmin and a rapid euglobulin lysis time. Patients suffering from heterozygous deficiency of α₂-antiplasmin have also been rarely described, and some have suffered from a mild bleeding tendency. Symptomatic patients with α₂-antiplasmin can be successfully managed with antifibrinolytic agents such as ε-aminocaproic acid. Acquired causes of α₂-antiplasmin deficiency include disseminated intravascular coagulation, thrombolytic therapy, liver disease (secondary to impaired production), nephrotic syndrome (secondary to excretion), and systemic amyloidosis.[6]

α₂-Macroglobulin

α₂-Macroglobulin, a 725-kD glycoprotein synthesized by a variety of cells including hepatocytes and macrophages, plays a secondary role in the regulation of plasmin. α₂-Macroglobulin does not play a primary role in plasmin inhibition until α₂-antiplasmin is consumed. The plasma concentration of α₂-macroglobulin is 2 mg/mL. Unlike α₂-antiplasmin, α₂-macroglobulin does not inhibit plasmin by binding to its active site but rather by sequestering it. When the target protease cleaves a trigger peptide sequence in α₂-macroglobulin, a conformational change occurs that entraps the protease. The α₂-macroglobulin-protease complex is then rapidly cleared from the circulation by receptor-mediated endocytosis, primarily in the liver.[2,6,7]

Plasminogen Activator Inhibitors

The principal inhibitor of the endogenous plasminogen activators tPA and uPA is plasminogen activator inhibitor-1 (PAI-1).

More information on the molecular function of PAI-1 can be found at www.expertconsult.com.

Synthesis of PAI-1 is induced by a diverse group of substances including insulin, endotoxin, thrombin, and atherogenic lipoproteins and cytokines. Elevated levels of PAI-1 have been noted in association with sepsis, malignancy, pregnancy, the postoperative state, and acute thrombosis. These changes may contribute to the excess risk for thrombosis associated with these clinical states. The 4G/5G polymorphism in the PAI-1 promoter has been demonstrated to influence PAI-1 transcription rates, with individuals possessing the 4G/4G allele having higher PAI-1 levels. Some but not all studies have found an association between higher PAI-1 levels and venous thromboembolism. Conversely, rare individuals with PAI-1 deficiency have manifested a bleeding disorder.[2,3,6,7]

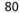

80

A second negative regulator of plasminogen activation, PAI-2, has also been identified. PAI-2 is generally found in detectable quantities only during pregnancy and appears to be synthesized by placental villous cells. The increase in plasma concentrations of PAI-2 probably contributes to the hypofibrinolytic state associated with pregnancy.[2,6,8] Other slower-acting inhibitors of tPA and uPA include α_1-antitrypsin, α_2-macroglobulin, α_2-antiplasmin, C1-inhibitor, and PAI-3.[8]

Thrombin-Activatable Fibrinolysis Inhibitor

The most recently identified negative regulator of the fibrinolytic system is thrombin activatable fibrinolysis inhibitor (TAFI). TAFI is a carboxypeptidase that removes C-terminal lysine or arginine residues that are exposed during digestion of fibrin by plasmin.

These residues are high-affinity binding sites for plasminogen and tPA that are generated with the initiation of fibrinolysis and explain the acceleration of fibrinolysis that occurs after initial lysis starts. Removal of these residues reduces plasminogen and tPA fibrin binding, and the conversion of Glu-plasminogen to Lys-plasminogen that prevents acceleration of fibrinolysis. TAFI is a 58-kD, 401–amino acid glycoprotein that is synthesized by the liver. TAFI is also released locally at the site of clot formation from platelet alpha granules during platelet activation. The mean plasma concentration of TAFI is 200 nM.[7,8]

TAFI as secreted is inactive until cleavage and release of an N-terminal activation peptide by serine proteases such as thrombin or plasmin. Activation of TAFI by free thrombin occurs slowly. This rate is accelerated 1250-fold by the thrombin-thrombomodulin complex, the same complex responsible for activating the endogenous anticoagulant protein C. Recognition that thrombin plays a key role in TAFI activation explains the previously noted observation that blood clots from hemophiliacs are much more susceptible to lysis than those from nonhemophiliacs.

The severely attenuated thrombin burst generated by hemophiliac plasma not only contributes to less fibrin generation but also activates less activated TAFI and factor XIII, such that the fibrin clot is more susceptible to

subsequent fibrinolysis. TAFI levels increase with age and in women taking hormonal therapy, although pregnancy has no effect on TAFI levels. Decreased TAFI levels have been noted in patients with severe liver disease and acute promyelocytic leukemia and may contribute to the bleeding diathesis seen in these conditions. Increased levels of TAFI have been associated with a moderate increase in the risk for venous thromboembolism.[7,8]

A MODEL OF REGULATED FIBRINOLYSIS

The fibrinolytic system plays a key role in balancing the procoagulant forces of the coagulation cascade to ensure that vascular patency is not sacrificed to maintain vascular continuity (Fig. 21-1). Vascular injury exposes tissue factor to initiate activation of the coagulation cascade through the extrinsic pathway of coagulation. Subsequent activation of the intrinsic pathway leads to amplification of the coagulation response and ultimately hemostatic plug formation. In addition to the negative regulatory response of endogenous anticoagulant proteins such as the protein C/protein S complex and antithrombin, the fibrinolytic system is also activated to dampen and focus clot formation strictly at the site of vascular injury. tPA is released from the surrounding undamaged endothelium in response to thrombin and venous stasis. tPA activates plasminogen poorly in solution but efficiently activates fibrin-bound plasminogen to form plasmin, which initiates clot dissolution. Circulating PAI-1 and α_2-antiplasmin efficiently inactivate tPA and plasmin, respectively, in solution, thereby ensuring that systemic activation of fibrinolysis does not occur. Conversely, covalent cross-linking of fibrin monomers and incorporation of α_2-antiplasmin into the substance of the clot ensure that clot lysis does not proceed too rapidly before vascular wall repair has progressed sufficiently to prevent delayed rebleeding. Inactivation of fibrin-bound plasmin is greatly slowed in comparison to plasmin free in solution.

This mechanism serves to concentrate activation of plasmin on the surface of the clot. Initial fibrinolysis exposes free lysine residues that serve as high-affinity binding sites for plasminogen and increase the sensitivity of plasminogen

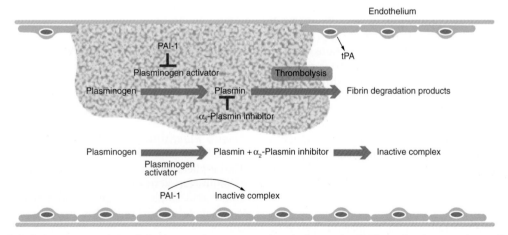

FIGURE 21-1. Fibrinolysis versus coagulation: balancing vascular patency against clotting needs. *tPA,* Tissue plasminogen activator. *(Adapted from Francis CW, Marder VJ. Mechanisms of fibrinolysis. In: Beutler E, Lichtman MA, Coller BS, Kipps TJ, editors. Williams hematology, 5th ed. New York: McGraw-Hill; 1995. p. 1255.)*

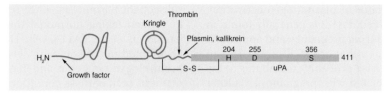

FIGURE 21-2. Urokinase. *uPA,* Urokinase plasminogen activator. *(Adapted from Dobrovolsky AB, Titaeva EV. The fibrinolysis system: regulation of activity and physiologic functions of its main components. Biochemistry [Mosc] 2002;67:99–108; and Francis CW, Marder VJ. Mechanisms of fibrinolysis. In: Beutler E, Lichtman MA, Coller BS, Kipps TJ, editors. Williams hematology, 5th ed. New York: McGraw-Hill; 1995. p. 1254.)*

to activation by tPA. This mechanism serves to accelerate fibrinolysis as it progresses and is negatively regulated by TAFI, which as a carboxypeptidase prunes away these free lysine residues. The interaction of these components ensures focused self-limited clot formation and remodeling that preserves vascular integrity and patency (see Fig. 21-1).

FIRST-GENERATION THROMBOLYTIC AGENTS

Streptokinase

Streptokinase (SK), the oldest known thrombolytic agent, is an extracellular protein of 415 amino acids (molecular weight 47,400 D) produced by β-hemolytic streptococci. It was first discovered by Tillett and Garner in 1933. Despite its name, SK is not a kinase. In contrast to most of the thrombolytic agents, SK indirectly activates plasminogen in a two-step process. In the initial step, SK forms an activator complex by binding to plasminogen. A conformational change occurs in plasminogen in which exposure of the active site allows it to convert free plasminogen molecules to plasmin. Because SK activates plasmin by fibrin-dependent and fibrin-independent mechanisms, fibrin as well as fibrinogen and other coagulation proteins are degraded, and a systemic "lytic state" is produced that is characterized by significant reductions in fibrinogen concentrations for 24 to 36 hours after the infusion of SK.[6,9,10]

SK has a biphasic pattern of elimination. Its initial half-life is 16 minutes, which corresponds to its inhibition by anti-SK antibodies formed as a result of previous streptococcal infections. The second half-life of 90 minutes corresponds to biological elimination of the SK-antibody complex by the liver. Because SK is a bacterial protein, its infusion can be associated with allergic reactions such as fever, hypotension, and (rarely) anaphylaxis. After exposure to SK, anti-SK antibody titers rise 100-fold within 5 to 10 days and last for up to 6 months after infusion. Consequently, SK cannot be effectively used within this window. These adverse effects and the nonfibrin selectivity of SK have curtailed its use within the United States, although it is still widely used elsewhere because it is less costly than other available agents.[6,9,10]

Urokinase

Urokinase (UK) is a naturally occurring plasminogen activator that was first isolated from human urine (hence its name). More recently, UK has been harvested from cultured human neonatal kidney cell lines. In the body, UK is

initially secreted as a 55-kD single-chain polypeptide zymogen (single-chain urokinase plasminogen activator [scuPA], or prourokinase) (Fig. 21-2) that is cleaved by plasmin at the Lys158-Ile 159 bond to generate two-chain uPA or UK.

Structurally, UK is a two-chain, 411–amino acid serine protease composed of one chain containing an amino-terminal epidermal growth factor domain and a kringle structure linked by a disulfide bond to the carboxy-terminal chain containing the protease active site.

The growth factor domain allows UK to bind to endogenous uPA receptors expressed on cell surfaces, whereas the kringle domain mediates inhibition of UK by PAI-1. Further proteolytic processing by plasmin and other serine proteases results in a lower-molecular-weight form of UK that lacks the growth factor and kringle domains. UK preparations derived from urinary sources contain primarily high-molecular-weight UK, whereas the low-molecular-weight forms predominate in UK derived from tissue culture lines.[3,5-7,10]

In contrast to SK, UK activates plasminogen directly. It also results in fewer allergic side effects given its human origin. Conversely, UK lacks significant fibrin selectivity and therefore results in extensive systemic fibrinolysis, similar to SK. The half-life of UK is approximately 15 minutes, with the liver primarily being responsible for its catabolism.[6] UK is approved by the U.S. Food and Drug Administration (FDA) for the treatment of pulmonary embolism. However, it has been used most often clinically for catheter-directed thrombolysis of venous or arterial thrombi or clearance of venous catheter occlusions. In recent years, production of UK has been disrupted by deficiencies in the manufacturing process.[9,10]

SECOND-GENERATION THROMBOLYTIC AGENTS

For a full discussion of the second-generation thrombolytic agents anistreplase and prourokinase, please visit the website www.expertconsult.com.

Tissue Plasminogen Activator

Tissue plasminogen activator is the principal endogenous plasminogen activator in humans. tPA is a 70-kD, 527–amino acid, single-chain glycoprotein that is synthesized by vascular endothelial cells. This single-chain molecule can be converted into a two-chain variety by plasmin-mediated hydrolysis of the Arg275-Ile276 bond. Unlike scuPA, both the single- and two-chain varieties of tPA are potent plasminogen activators.

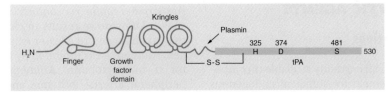

FIGURE 21-3. Tissue plasminogen activator (tPA). *(Adapted from Dobrovolsky AB, Titaeva EV: The fibrinolysis system: regulation of activity and physiologic functions of its main components. Biochemistry [Mosc] 2002;67:99–108; and Francis CW, Marder VJ. Mechanisms of fibrinolysis. In: Beutler E, Lichtman MA, Coller BS, Kipps TJ, editors. Williams hematology, 5th ed. New York: McGraw-Hill; 1995. p. 1254.)*

The molecular structure of tPA can be divided into four separate domains: an amino-terminal 47–amino acid finger domain (homologous to the finger domains of fibronectin), an epidermal growth factor domain, two kringle domains similar to the kringle domains of plasminogen, and a carboxy-terminal serine protease domain (Fig. 21-3). The finger domain and the second kringle domain mediate tPA's fibrin binding. Both kringle domains and the finger domain are responsible for accentuation of tPA's enzymatic activity when bound to fibrin. *In vivo* clearance of tPA is mediated by the finger and growth factor domains, whereas PAI-1, the physiologic inhibitor of tPA, binds to it through the active site and kringle 2 domains. The enzymatic activity of tPA resides in the serine protease domain, which has homology with other serine proteases, including trypsin, plasmin, and thrombin.[5,7,9,10,13]

Release of tPA from the endothelium is triggered by a variety of physiologic and biochemical stimuli, including venous stasis, exercise, mental stress, thrombin, hypoxia, acidosis, histamine, epinephrine, and bradykinin. Exogenous administration of desmopressin (DDAVP) can also induce endothelial secretion of tPA.[2,6] In solution, tPA is an inefficient plasminogen activator. Once bound to fibrin (through the finger and second kringle domains), tPA forms a ternary complex with plasminogen in which conformational changes are induced that increase tPA's catalytic efficiency by over 1000-fold. In addition to lysing fibrin, plasmin at the clot surface also leads to the conversion of single-chain tPA to two-chain tPA. The accentuation of tPA enzymatic activity by fibrin binding and the reduced susceptibility of fibrin-bound tPA and plasmin to inhibition by PAI-1 and α_2-antiplasmin, respectively, serve to focus fibrinolysis on the clot surface and limit the extent of systemic fibrinolysis. In response to a 100-mg dose of tPA, fibrinogen levels typically fall only 16% to 36% as opposed to 60% to 70% declines for comparable doses of UK and SK.[5,9,10]

Although two different forms of tPA are available commercially—the one-chain form of tPA, alteplase, and the two-chain form, duteplase—the one-chain form enjoys much wider use clinically. Alteplase is manufactured by recombinant DNA technology in Chinese hamster ovary (CHO) cells. It has a half-life of 4 minutes and is cleared by the liver. Because alteplase is an endogenous plasminogen activator, it does not appear to be significantly immunogenic, unlike SK and APSAC.[5,10] Alteplase has been approved by the FDA for the treatment of acute myocardial infarction, acute cerebrovascular accident, massive pulmonary embolism, and central venous catheter occlusion. It is also widely used for catheter-directed thrombolysis of venous and arterial thrombosis.

THIRD-GENERATION THROMBOLYTIC AGENTS

Reteplase

Reteplase is a 39-kD, 355–amino acid, recombinant nonglycosylated deletion mutant of wild-type tPA in which the finger, epidermal growth factor, and first kringle domains have been deleted. These changes result in a fourfold increase in the plasma half-life of the mutant (14-18 minutes) over wild-type tPA (4 minutes) because of elimination of the finger and epidermal growth factor domains, as well as carbohydrate side chains that mediate *in vivo* clearance of tPA. As a consequence, reteplase can be administered as a bolus rather than as a continuous infusion, a characteristic that facilitates prehospital initiation of thrombolysis for myocardial infarction. These structural changes also give rise to a fivefold reduction in fibrin binding as a result of loss of the fibrin-binding finger domain. PAI-1 inhibits reteplase and alteplase because the second kringle and active site domains remain intact in both molecules. Reteplase is synthesized through recombinant DNA technology by *E. coli* bacteria. It does not appear to be immunogenic.[5,10,13,16] Reteplase is approved by the FDA for the treatment of patients with acute myocardial infarction.[17] It has also been used for the treatment of patients with extensive deep venous thrombosis, peripheral arterial occlusion, and stroke.[18,19]

Tenecteplase

Tenecteplase is a tPA multiple point mutant in which Asp117, a glycosylation site in kringle 1, is replaced with glutamine, and Thr103 is replaced with asparagines to create a new glycosylation site in the first kringle domain. In addition, amino acids in the serine protease domain (Lys296, His297, Arg298, Arg299) are replaced with alanine. These changes result in an eightfold decrease in plasma clearance and a 200-fold reduction in PAI-1 inhibition in comparison to wild-type tPA. Tenecteplase's half-life is fourfold longer than that of tPA, and its fibrin specificity in plasma is greater than that of tPA. Its prolonged half-life and reduced inhibition by PAI-1 allow tenecteplase to be administered as a single bolus. Tenecteplase is produced by genetic engineering in CHO cells and has been approved by the FDA for use in acute myocardial infarction.[13,16,20]

For a full discussion of the third-generation thrombolytic agents lanoteplase, pamiteplase, staphylokinase, and desmoteplase (vampire bat plasminogen activator), please visit www.expertconsult.com.

DIRECT FIBRINOLYTIC AGENTS

Plasmin and Its Derivatives

A potential disadvantage of all currently available thrombolytic agents is their requirement for sufficient endogenous plasminogen to achieve clot lysis. Recognition of this limitation is not new. In the 1950s and 1960s, human (as well as bovine and porcine) plasmin was used as a thrombolytic agent; however, these early studies failed largely because of low purity and significant toxicity of the products.[23-25] Improvements in purification techniques over the last few decades have awakened new interest in the use of plasmin as a thrombolytic agent. Several *in vitro* and animal studies have demonstrated that purified plasmin can achieve equivalent or superior clot lysis with a lower incidence of bleeding than that seen with tPA.[26,27] Recombinant and transgenic forms of plasmin have been produced. A phase 2 trial investigating the efficacy of recombinant plasmin in peripheral arterial thrombosis is currently underway.[27]

For a discussion of microplasmin, miniplasmin, and deltaplasmin, please visit the website at www.expertconsult.com.

Alfimeprase (Recombinant Fibrolase)

Heterologous direct thrombolytic agents are also under development. Alfimeprase is a recombinant form of fibrolase, a fibrinolytic enzyme derived from the venom of

Agkistrodon contortrix contortrix, the southern copperhead snake. Alfimeprase results in clot lysis by directly cleaving the Aα chain and to a lesser extent the Bβ chain of fibrinogen. Alfimeprase is inhibited by the plasma protease inhibitor α$_2$-macroglobulin. Alfimeprase has been studied in peripheral arterial ischemia and central venous catheter occlusion. However, active clinical investigation has been suspended, perhaps due to hypotensive episodes in 18% of recipients and failure to demonstrate superiority over existing agents.[27,28]

SUMMARY

The fibrinolytic system is a network of proteins that modulate the procoagulant properties of the coagulation cascade and play a critical role in maintaining vascular patency.

Increasing knowledge of the fibrinolytic system and identification of naturally occurring plasminogen activators and fibrinolytic enzymes, as well as exploitation of genetically modified plasminogen activators and fibrinolytic enzymes, indicate that the therapeutic options available to clinicians will continue to expand (Table 21-1). Although the ideal fibrinolytic agent has yet to be identified, the increasing variety of available agents and mechanical thrombectomy devices ensures continued improvement in outcomes for patients with thrombotic disease.

TABLE 21-1. Selected Thrombolytic Agents

Agent	Type of Agent	Molecular Weight (D)	Plasma Half-Life (min)	Fibrin Selectivity	Antigenicity	Cost
First-Generation Plasminogen Activators						
Streptokinase	Bacterial proactivator	47,400	23	No	Yes	+
Urokinase	Direct PA	37,000 (LMW)-54,000 (HMW)	15	No	No	++
Second-Generation Plasminogen Activators						
Anistreplase	Bacterial proactivator	131,000	90	No	Yes	++
Prourokinase	Direct PA	55,000	8	++	No	?
Alteplase (tPA)	Direct PA	70,000	4	++	No	+++
Third-Generation Plasminogen Activators						
Reteplase	Direct PA*	39,000	14-18	+	No	++++
Tenecteplase	Direct PA*	70,000	18	+++	No	++++
Lanoteplase	Direct PA*	53,500	37	+	No	?
Pamiteplase	Direct PA*		30-47	++	No	?
Staphylokinase	Indirect bacterial proactivator	16,500	6	++++	Yes	?
Desmoteplase	Direct PA	52,000	168	++++	Yes	++++
Fibrinolytic Enzymes						
Plasmin	Fibrinolytic enzyme	85,000	0.02 sec		No	?
Microplasmin	Fibrinolytic enzyme	30,000	4 sec		No	?
Alfimeprase	Fibrinolytic enzyme	22,700	25		Yes	?

*PA deletion/point mutants.

- The fibrinolytic system is a network of proteins that (1) result in regulated dissolution of fibrin clots and (2) balance the procoagulant activity of coagulation proteins.

- Plasminogen, the key endogenous fibrinolytic enzyme, circulates in plasma as a zymogen until activated by plasminogen activators such as tPA to plasmin, the active form that digests fibrin clots.

- The profibrinolytic activity of the fibrinolytic system is negatively regulated by plasminogen activator inhibitors such as PAI-1 and plasmin inhibitors such as α_2-antiplasmin.

- First-generation plasminogen activators include the indirect bacterial plasminogen activator SK and the direct plasminogen activator UK.

- The second-generation plasminogen activator tPA is more fibrin specific than SK or UK but still results in significant fibrinogenolysis when administered in pharmacologic doses and thus is not associated with less bleeding than the less fibrin-specific plasminogen activators.

- Third-generation plasminogen activators such as reteplase and tenecteplase are tPA deletion mutants that have slower plasma clearance or greater fibrin selectivity, or both. However, these modifications have not resulted in clinically significant improvements in efficacy.

- Direct fibrinolytic enzymes such as plasmin, microplasmin, and deltaplasmin, which do not require plasminogen to function, are attractive agents theoretically but require additional testing to establish their clinical utility as thrombolytic agents.

► **SUGGESTED READINGS**

Baruah DB, Dash RN, Chaudhari MR, Kadam SS. Plasminogen activators: a comparison. Vasc Pharmacol 2006;44:1–9.

Castellino FJ, Ploplis VA. Structure and function of the plasminogen/plasmin system. Thromb Haemost 2005;93:647–54.

Dobrovolsky AB, Titaeva EV. The fibrinolysis system: regulation of activity and physiologic functions of its main components. Biochemistry (Mosc) 2002;67:99–108.

Khan IA, Gowda RM. Clinical perspectives and therapeutics of thrombolysis. Int J Cardiol 2003;91:115–27.

Lijnen HR. Elements of the fibrinolytic system. Ann N Y Acad Sci 2001;936:226–36.

Novokhatny VV, Jesmok GJ, Landskroner KA, et al. Locally delivered plasmin: why should it be superior to plasminogen activators for direct thrombolysis? Trends Pharmacol Sci 2004;25:72–5.

Rijken DC, Lijnen HR. New insights into the molecular mechanisms of the fibrinolytic system. J Thromb Haemost 2009;7(1):4–13.

Toombs CF. Alfimeprase: pharmacology of a novel fibrinolytic metalloproteinase for thrombolysis. Haemostasis 2001;31:141–7.

Ueshima S, Matsuo O. Development of new fibrinolytic agents. Curr Pharm Des 2006;12:849–57.

Verstraete M. Third-generation thrombolytic drugs. Am J Med 2000;109:52–8.

The complete reference list is available online at www.expertconsult.com.

CHAPTER 22

Antiplatelet Agents and Anticoagulants
Stephan Moll

PHYSIOLOGY OF BLOOD CLOTTING

Vascular injury leads to thrombus formation. As a first step, a platelet plug is formed, which is then surrounded and strengthened by a fibrin polymer meshwork. Several steps are involved in this process (Fig. 22-1):

1. *Platelet adhesion:* During the first step of hemostasis, von Willebrand factor multimers bind to exposed subendothelial collagen with one part of their structure and to the glycoprotein (GP)Ib receptor on the surface of platelets with another, thereby anchoring the platelet to the site of injury.

2. *Platelet aggregation:* Platelet adhesion leads to activation of the anchored platelet, which results in three major reactions:
   - *Release of platelet granules:* Platelet granules contain platelet agonists such as thromboxane A_2, adenosine diphosphate (ADP), and epinephrine. Thromboxane A_2 is synthesized with the help of the enzyme cyclooxygenase (COX)-1. Once released into the bloodstream, the agonists bind to receptors on the surface of platelets trying to float by, thus activating and recruiting them to the site of injury. The platelet receptors for ADP are termed $P2Y_1$ and $P2Y_{12}$, and it appears both must be activated for platelet aggregation to take place.
   - *Activation of platelet surface GPIIb/IIIa receptors:* Activation of the platelet leads to a change in shape of the GPIIb/IIIa receptor, enabling it to bind fibrinogen. One end of the fibrinogen molecule binds to the GPIIb/IIIa receptor of one activated platelet and the other to the receptor of another platelet, thus bridging platelets and creating a platelet plug.
   - *Flip-flop of phospholipids:* In nonactivated platelets, phospholipids are located on the inner side of the cell membrane. Platelet activation leads to a flip-flop of these phospholipids to the outside of the platelet membrane, where then they can bind coagulation factors and calcium and facilitate the various reactions of the coagulation cascade that lead to formation of fibrin.

3. *Plasmatic coagulation:* Vascular injury brings tissue factor on extracellular cells (fibroblasts, monocytes) into contact with circulating coagulation factor VIIa, thereby initiating the coagulation cascade that leads to thrombin and eventually fibrin formation. Coagulation factor activation reactions require phospholipids, which are provided by platelets during the flip-flop mechanism that occurs during platelet aggregation. A fibrin meshwork forms around the platelets anchored at the site of vascular injury. A thrombus is formed.

PATHOPHYSIOLOGY OF BLOOD CLOTTING

Venous thrombosis occurs mostly via the plasma coagulation system, with only minor platelet participation. In contrast, platelets play a major role in arterial thrombus formation, with additional participation of the plasma coagulation system. This paradigm helps explain why drugs that block the plasmatic coagulation reaction (i.e., anticoagulants) are very active in preventing venous thrombosis and also effective in preventing arterial thrombosis, whereas antiplatelet drugs, which successfully prevent arterial thrombosis, are less or not at all effective in venous disease. Table 22-1 lists the important antiplatelet agents and anticoagulants, discussed in further detail in the following sections.

ANTIPLATELET AGENTS

Aspirin

Aspirin (acetylsalicylic acid) inhibits the enzyme COX-1, which is needed to form thromboxane A_2 in platelets. Thromboxane A_2 is normally released from platelet granules upon platelet adhesion and during platelet aggregation (see Fig. 22-1, *B*) and serves as an agonist to activate and thereby recruit other platelets to the platelet plug. Because platelets do not synthesize new cyclooxygenase and aspirin binds irreversibly to the enzyme, aspirin's action lasts for the lifespan of a platelet (i.e., 7-10 days). Complete inactivation of platelet COX-1 is typically achieved with a daily aspirin dose of 160 mg. When used as an antithrombotic drug, aspirin is maximally effective at doses between 50 and 325 mg/day. Higher doses do not improve efficacy. However, there is considerable interindividual variability in aspirin's ability to inhibit COX-1. "Aspirin resistance" is a laboratory phenomenon in which there is an inability of aspirin to inhibit one or more in vitro tests of platelet function, such as platelet aggregometry, the Platelet Function Analyzer (PFA-100), the VerifyNow Aspirin rapid platelet function assay, or measurement of thromboxane generation in vitro or in vivo via serum levels of thromboxane B_2 or urinary levels of 11-dehydrothromboxane B_2. "Aspirin failure" is a clinical observation of treatment failure. Aspirin resistance does not necessarily lead to treatment failure, nor is clinical aspirin failure necessarily due to aspirin resistance.

Phosphodiesterase Inhibitors

Dipyridamole (Persantine)
Dipyridamole inhibits platelet aggregation by two mechanisms: (1) it inhibits cyclic nucleotide phosphodiesterase, and (2) it attenuates uptake of adenosine into platelets. Both these actions lead to an increase in intraplatelet cyclic adenosine monophosphate (cAMP), which inhibits platelet aggregation induced by several agonists. However, dipyridamole by itself has little or no effect as an antithrombotic drug. Its platelet aggregation inhibitory effect is reversible. The combination of aspirin (25 mg) and dipyridamole (200 mg) is available as Aggrenox. Dipyridamole also has

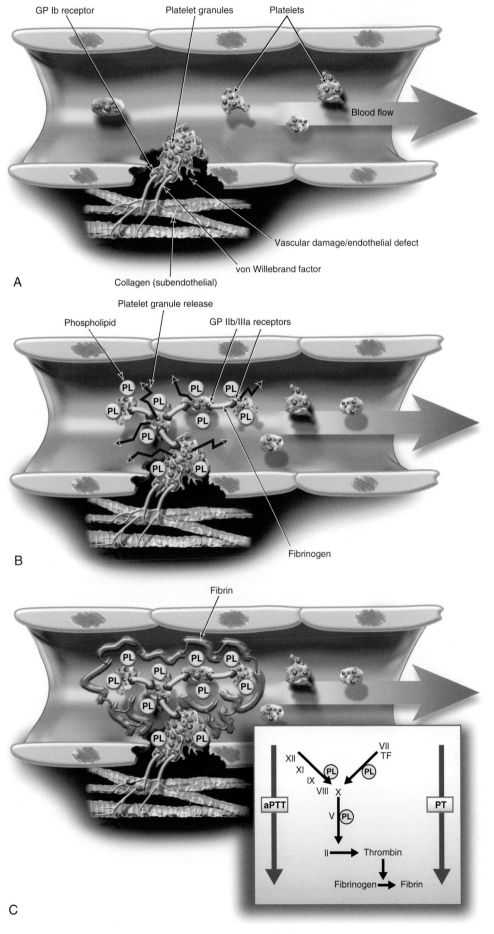

FIGURE 22-1. The three steps of thrombus formation. **A,** Platelet adhesion. **B,** Platelet aggregation: (1) granule release, (2) glycoprotein *(GP)* IIb/IIIa form shape and cross-linking, (3) flip-flop of phospholipids *(PL)*. **C,** Plasmatic coagulation (fibrin formation). *TF,* tissue factor.

TABLE 22-1. Antiplatelet Agents and Anticoagulants

Generic	Brand Name*	Dosing†
Platelet Aggregation Inhibitors		
Cyclooxygenase Inhibitor		
Aspirin		50-325 mg qd PO.
Phosphodiesterase Inhibitors		
Dipyridamole	Persantine	75-100 mg qid PO.
Dipyridamole + ASA	Aggrenox	1 tablet (200 mg/25 mg) q12h PO.
Cilostazol	Pletal	100 mg q12h PO.
ADP Receptor Blockers		
Clopidogrel	Plavix	Loading dose 300 mg PO; then 75 mg qd PO.
Ticlopidine	Ticlid	Loading dose 500 mg PO; then 250 mg q12h PO.
Prasugrel	Effient	Loading dose 60 mg PO; then 10 mg qd PO.
Ticagrelor	Brilinta	Loading dose 180 mg PO; then 90 mg q12h PO.
Cangrelor		In development.
Elinogrel		Development stopped.
Glycoprotein IIb/IIIa Receptor Blockers		
Abciximab	ReoPro	Bolus 0.25 mg/kg IV; then 0.125 µg/kg/min for 12 h IV.
Eptifibatide	Integrilin	Bolus 180 g/kg IV; then 0.5-2.0 µg/kg/min for up to 72 h IV.
Tirofiban	Aggrastat	0.4 µg/kg/min × 30 min IV; then 0.1 µg/kg/min × 12-24 h IV.

Oral agents‡
  Orbofiban
  Sibrafiban
  Xemilofiban
		Development stopped.

Others		
Pentoxifylline	Trental	400 mg tid PO.
Anticoagulants		
Heparins		
Unfractionated heparin	Various	Various nomograms—APTT or anti-Xa adjusted.
Enoxaparin	Lovenox Clexane	Prophylaxis: various doses Full-dose: 1 mg/kg q12h or 1.5 mg/kg qd SQ.
Dalteparin	Fragmin	Prophylaxis: various doses; full-dose: 100 units/kg q12h SQ or 200 units/kg qd SQ.
Tinzaparin	Innohep	Prophylaxis: various doses; full-dose: 175 units/kg qd SQ.
Certoparin	Monoembolex	Prophylaxis: various doses.
Reviparin	Clivarin	Not approved for full-dose anticoagulant treatment.
Nadroparin	Fraxiparin	
Anti-Xa Inhibitors		
Pentasaccharides: Fondaparinux	Arixtra	Prophylaxis: 2.5 mg qd SQ; full-dose: 7.5 mg qd SQ; 10 mg qd if body weight above 100 kg.
Idraparinux	None yet	In development.
Rivaroxaban	Xarelto	Atrial fibrillation with normal renal function: 20 mg qd PO. VTE prevention: 10 mg qd; Acute DVT or PE: 15 mg q12h for 3 weeks, then 20 mg qd PO with normal renal function.
Apixaban	Eliquis	2.5 mg q12h for VTE prevention. 5 mg bid for atrial fibrillation.
Edoxaban	Lixiana	30 mg PO once daily for VTE prevention after orthopedic surgery.
Thrombin Inhibitors		
Argatroban	Acova Novastan	No bolus. Continuous infusion: 2 µg/kg/min IV—APTT adjusted.
Lepirudin	Refludan	Bolus: 0.4 mg/kg IV. Continuous infusion: 0.15 mg/kg/h IV—APTT adjusted.

TABLE 22-1. Antiplatelet Agents and Anticoagulants—cont'd

Generic	Brand Name*	Dosing†
Desirudin	Iprivask Revasc	15 mg q12h SQ.
Bivalirudin	Angiomax	Bolus: 0.75 mg/kg IV. Continuous infusion: 1.75 mg/kg/h IV until 4 h after procedure; then 0.2 mg/kg/h for up to 20 h.
Danaparoid	Orgaran	Manufacturing discontinued.
Ximelagatran	Exanta	Withdrawn from market.
Dabigatran	Pradaxa	Atrial fibrillation with normal renal function: 150 mg q12h PO or 110 mg q12h.
Vitamin K Antagonists		
Coumarins		
Warfarin	Coumadin Jantoven	Interindividual variability; dosing is INR adjusted.
Phenprocoumon	Marcumar Falithrom Phenpro	
Acenocoumarol	Sinthrome	
Tioclomarol	Apegmone	
Indandiones		
Fluindione	Previscan	
Anisindione	Miradon	
Phenindione	Dindevan Pindione	

*Other products may exist.
†Drug approval and dosing regimens may vary depending on indication, country of use, presence or absence of renal or liver dysfunction, and concomitant use of antiplatelet drugs or anticoagulants.
‡Specific agents printed in italics are investigational.
ADP, Adenosine diphosphate; *APTT,* activated partial thromboplastin time; *h,* hour; *INR,* international normalized ratio; *IV,* intravenously; *q,* every; *qd,* once daily; *tid,* three times daily; *PO,* orally; *SQ,* subcutaneously; *VTE,* venous thromboembolism.

vasodilator effects and should therefore be used with caution in patients with severe coronary artery disease, in whom episodes of angina may increase as a result of the steal phenomenon. The most common side effects of Aggrenox are gastrointestinal complaints and headaches. The major indication for Aggrenox is secondary stroke prevention.

Cilostazol (Pletal)
A selective inhibitor of the phosphodiesterase 3 isoenzyme, cilostazol leads to inhibition of agonist-induced platelet aggregation, granule release, and thromboxane A₂ production. It also has vasodilator effects. The most common side effects are headache, palpitations, and diarrhea. It should not be used in patients with congestive heart failure. The major indication for cilostazol is disabling claudication, particularly when revascularization cannot be performed.

Pentoxifylline (Trental)
Pentoxifylline is a phosphodiesterase inhibitor that has been shown to have some beneficial effects in ischemic disease states. Its inhibitory effect on phosphodiesterase in erythrocytes leads to increased cAMP levels and improved erythrocyte flexibility, and its reduction of blood viscosity may be the result of decreased plasma fibrinogen concentrations and inhibition of red blood cell and platelet

aggregation. The most common side effects are gastrointestinal (dyspepsia, nausea, and vomiting) and neurologic (dizziness, headache). Its major indication is peripheral vascular disease with claudication.

Adenosine Diphosphate Receptor Antagonists

Clopidogrel, Ticlopidine, Prasugrel, Ticagrelor, and Others
Clopidogrel (Plavix), ticlopidine (Ticlid), and Prasugrel (Effient) inhibit the platelet ADP receptor P2Y₁₂ by irreversibly altering its structure. Clopidogrel and ticlopidine are closely related, but clopidogrel has a more favorable side-effect profile, with less frequent thrombocytopenia and leukopenia, and has largely replaced ticlopidine. Prasugrel is more rapid in onset and leads to less variable platelet response and more complete inhibition of platelet function than clopidogrel. Because maximal inhibition of platelet aggregation with all three drugs is not seen for a few days after starting therapy, loading doses of are often given to achieve a more rapid onset of action. Inhibition of platelet aggregation persists for the lifespan of the platelet. In all indications, clopidogrel appears to be equally effective as aspirin, except in peripheral arterial disease, where it has been shown to be slightly more effective than aspirin for prevention of ischemic events. Ticagrelor (Brilinta),

Cangrelor, and Elinogrel are also inhibitors of the platelet P2Y$_{12}$ ADP receptor, but their action is reversible. Prasugrel or ticagrelor given together with aspirin have been shown to be more efficacious than clopidogrel plus aspirin in certain acute coronary syndromes and percutaneous coronary interventions. Cangrelor is being studied in patients who require percutaneous coronary intervention. Development of Elinogrel was terminated in 2012.

Glycoprotein IIb/III Receptor Antagonists

The platelet GPIIb/IIIa receptors (also termed *integrin* $\alpha_{IIb}\beta_3$) are the sites where fibrinogen binds during platelet aggregation (see Fig. 22-1, *B*), leading to cross-linking of platelets and platelet plug formation. Several inhibitors of this receptor have been developed for clinical use.

Abciximab (ReoPro)
Abciximab is the Fab fragment of a chimeric human-murine monoclonal antibody against the IIb/IIIa receptor. The drug is given as a bolus followed by continuous infusion for 12 hours or longer. Unbound drug is cleared from the circulation with a half-life of about 30 minutes. Drug bound to the IIb/IIIa receptor inhibits platelet aggregation for 18 to 24 hours as measured in vitro, but bound drug is demonstrable in the circulation for up to 10 days. Ex vivo platelet clumping in ethylenediamine tetra-acetic acid (EDTA)-containing blood tubes can be seen in patients treated with the drug, and such clumping can lead to pseudothrombocytopenia when platelets are counted with an automatic blood cell counter. This phenomenon is clinically irrelevant and does not require discontinuation of the drug. However, true thrombocytopenia also occurs and, if severe enough, can require drug discontinuation.

Eptifibatide (Integrilin)
A synthetic peptide inhibitor of the so-called RGD binding site of the IIb/IIIa receptor, eptifibatide mimics the geometric and charge characteristics of the RGD sequence of fibrinogen, thus occupying the IIb/IIIa receptor and preventing binding of fibrinogen and hence platelet aggregation. It is given as a bolus followed by continuous infusion for up to 3 days. The platelet aggregation inhibitory effect lasts for 6 to 12 hours after cessation of infusion.

Tirofiban (Aggrastat)
Tirofiban is a nonpeptide (peptidomimetic) small-molecule inhibitor of the IIb/IIIa receptor that also binds to the RGD receptor site, similar to eptifibatide.

Oral Glycoprotein IIb/IIIa Antagonists
Antagonists such as orbofiban, sibrafiban, and xemilofiban have been associated with a surprising, not fully understood, excess in mortality. Development of these drugs has been stopped, and they are not clinically available.

ANTICOAGULANTS

Heparins

Mechanism of Action
Heparins are extracted from porcine intestine or bovine lung and consist of glycosaminoglycans of different lengths.

Unfractionated heparins have a mean length of 40 monosaccharide units. Low-molecular-weight heparins (LMWHs) are made from unfractionated heparin through chemical and physical processes and have a mean of 15 monosaccharide units. A pentasaccharide structure within these polysaccharide molecules binds to and enhances the action of antithrombin, which inactivates thrombin and factor Xa. Molecules with 18 monosaccharide units or more are required to bind thrombin and antithrombin simultaneously (i.e., to lead to heparin's antithrombin effect). The five sugars of the pentasaccharide structure, however, are sufficient to lead to a conformational change in antithrombin that can then inactivate factor Xa. LMWHs, therefore, inactivate mostly factor Xa, whereas unfractionated heparin acts primarily against thrombin. Fondaparinux (Arixtra) is a synthetic pentasaccharide based on the antithrombin binding region of heparin and has specific anti-Xa inhibitory action. Idraparinux is a new anticoagulant agent in development. It resembles fondaparinux, but modification of several side chains leads to a longer half-life, so it is dosed once weekly subcutaneously (SQ).

Management of Bleeding
If bleeding occurs in a patient taking unfractionated heparin, protamine can be given intravenously (IV), which binds to and neutralizes heparin. Protamine can impair platelet function and interact with coagulation factors and thereby cause an anticoagulant effect of its own. Therefore, the minimal amount of protamine needed to neutralize heparin should be given. LMWH is only partially reversed by protamine. However, in patients with significant bleeding while taking LMWH, protamine should be considered, and for major bleeding, recombinant factor VIIa (NovoSeven). Protamine is probably not successful in reversing the action of fondaparinux. Recombinant factor VIIa is the treatment of choice for major bleeding associated with fondaparinux. Fresh frozen plasma (FFP) probably has little if any effect on bleeding associated with heparin, LMWH, and fondaparinux and is not indicated.

Heparin-Induced Thrombocytopenia
Heparin-induced thrombocytopenia (HIT) is defined as the occurrence of thrombocytopenia and a positive test for heparin-associated antibodies in a patient treated with heparin. HIT associated with thrombosis, either arterial or venous, is referred to as *HITT*. Strict criteria for HIT require a decrease in platelet count to less than 100,000/μL or a count 50% lower than baseline. However, less strict definitions for HIT are a decrease in platelet count to less than 150,000/μL or a 30% decrease in the baseline value. HIT can occur in patients treated with heparin even with platelet counts remaining normal and unchanged. Confirmatory HIT antibody tests are (1) heparin-platelet factor 4 antibody enzyme-linked immunosorbent assay (HIT-PF4 ELISA), (2) heparin-induced platelet aggregation study, and (3) heparin-induced serotonin release assay. The HIT-PF4 ELISA is the most sensitive but the least specific. Heparin-PF4 antibodies develop in many patients exposed to high doses of heparin, such as after cardiopulmonary bypass surgery, but they often do not lead to thrombocytopenia or thrombosis and then appear to be clinically irrelevant. The HIT-PF4 ELISA is the test most widely used for the diagnosis of HIT. The heparin-induced platelet

aggregation test and the heparin-induced serotonin release assay are functional assays that are much more specific for the pathogenic antibodies that actually cause the clinical picture of HIT. However, they are more time consuming to perform, typically have a slower turnaround time, and are not widely available. HIT most commonly occurs in patients taking unfractionated heparin but can also develop in those taking LMWH. It more commonly occurs with IV heparin therapy but can also be seen with SQ dosing. In a patient with clinical suspicion of HIT, heparin should be discontinued and alternative anticoagulants started, such as:

- Hirudins (lepirudin or bivalirudin) IV
- Desirudin SQ
- Argatroban IV
- Orgaran IV or SQ
- Fondaparinux SQ

Vitamin K antagonists should not be used until platelet counts have substantially recovered, usually to at least 150×10^9/L. The alternative anticoagulant therapy should overlap with the vitamin K antagonist for a minimum of 5 days and until the international normalized ratio (INR) is within the target range. Because of cross-reactivity of the HIT-PF4 antibody between unfractionated heparin and LMWH, the latter is not a treatment alternative when HIT secondary to unfractionated heparin is diagnosed. HIT-PF4 antibodies do not appear to cross-react with fondaparinux in vivo to cause HIT, which has therefore led to SQ fondaparinux as an attractive treatment option in recent years. Detailed recommendations for monitoring the platelet count during heparin administration and for the diagnosis and treatment of HIT are available in the guidelines of the American College of Chest Physicians (ACCP).[1]

Heparin Resistance

Heparin resistance is a term used when patients require unusually high doses of unfractionated heparin, such as more than 40,000 units/day, to prolong their activated partial thromboplastin time (APTT) into the therapeutic range. Causes can be (1) very low baseline APTT, such as caused by elevations in factor VIII and fibrinogen; (2) increased heparin clearance; (3) increased nonspecific heparin-binding proteins; and (4) antithrombin deficiency. Because LMWH and fondaparinux also require the presence of antithrombin to be active as anticoagulants, antithrombin deficiency can cause LMWH and fondaparinux resistance, but this would not be noticeable by any routine laboratory tests, since routine laboratory monitoring of these drugs is not performed.

Unfractionated Heparin

Unfractionated heparin at therapeutic doses must typically be monitored with APTT. Therapeutic APTT range depends on the heparin sensitivity of the APTT reagent and the instrument used by the laboratory. A therapeutic APTT is considered to be one that corresponds to an anti-Xa plasma heparin level of 0.3 to 0.7 units/mL. Optimally, a coagulation laboratory should provide clinicians with the therapeutic APTT range for the reagent/instrument combination used in that laboratory, and clinicians should use a nomogram for heparin dosing. If the laboratory has not provided the clinician with the specific therapeutic APTT range used, an APTT ratio of 2.0 to 2.5 of the mean APTT of the normal range is often considered to be therapeutic. However, with some APTT reagents, this range is subtherapeutic, and underdosing of a patient may occur. Heparin is cleared mostly by the reticuloendothelial system and to a smaller degree by the kidney. Patients with renal failure may require less heparin to prolong their APTT into the therapeutic range. The half-life of heparin in plasma depends on the dose given. It is 60 minutes with a 100 units/kg bolus. A patient receiving a continuous IV infusion of unfractionated heparin at therapeutic doses will probably demonstrate a return to baseline APTT within 3 to 4 hours after discontinuation of heparin. In many patients at average risk for bleeding, a loading dose of heparin of 80 units/kg IV followed by a continuous infusion of 18 units/kg/h is appropriate. However, this dosing may have to be modified in a patient at higher risk for bleeding. The APTT should be determined 6 hours after initiation of heparin and each dose change, and once every 24 hours once the APTT is in the therapeutic range. In the occasional patient in whom the APTT is invalid, such as in a patient with a lupus anticoagulant or deficiency of coagulation factor XII, anti-Xa levels have to be used for heparin monitoring. Some laboratories routinely offer anti-Xa rather APTT testing for monitoring of heparin therapy, but it has not been shown to have an advantage (i.e., less bleeding and less thromboembolic complications).

Low-Molecular-Weight Heparin

The various LMWH drugs differ in their composition and degree of antithrombin and anti-Xa activity. Dosage recommendations for prophylaxis and treatment of venous thromboembolism (VTE) therefore vary for the LMWHs. Lack of significant binding of LMWH to plasma proteins gives them an anticoagulant effect that is more predictable than that of unfractionated heparin, so fixed or weight-adjusted dosing is possible without the need for routine anticoagulant laboratory monitoring. The peak plasma effect is reached 3 to 4 hours after SQ injection. The half-lives of the various agents differ, with ranges between 3 and 7 hours. Once- or twice-daily dosing regimens are available for the different drugs. Because the LMWHs are cleared by the kidney, dose reduction and anti-Xa monitoring are needed in patients with renal impairment. However, because the pharmacokinetic effect of impaired renal function may differ among LMWHs, there is not a single creatinine clearance cutoff value below which dose reduction is clearly needed. A value of less than 30 mL/min is a threshold in most patients and with most preparations below which dose adjustment is needed. In patients with severe renal impairment and those dependent on dialysis, choosing unfractionated heparin over LMWH is recommended. In obese patients, LMWH dosing should be based on absolute body weight, but above a body mass index of 40 kg/m^2 it may be reasonable to obtain anti-Xa levels to avoid overanticoagulation. A therapeutic anti-Xa level for once-daily dosing is on the order of 1 to 2 units/mL, and that for twice-daily dosing approximately 0.6 to 1.2 units/mL, obtained 3 to 4 hours after SQ injection. Anti-Xa levels should always be determined if a patient being treated with LMWH has recurrent thrombosis or significant bleeding; this will document whether the patient had subtherapeutic or supratherapeutic anti-Xa levels, possibly explaining the clotting or bleeding event.

Fondaparinux (Arixtra)

Fondaparinux is a synthetic antithrombin-dependent pentasaccharide that consists of the key five monosaccharides of heparin that bind to antithrombin, which then inhibits factor Xa. It is a specific anti-Xa agent without any activity against thrombin. It is given SQ, reaches its peak plasma level in 2 hours, and because of a half-life of 17 to 21 hours is dosed once daily. Because it does not bind significantly to plasma proteins, it can be given as a fixed dose, either in prophylactic or therapeutic doses. It is cleared by the kidney and should therefore not be used in patients with renal failure. It does not appear to cause the clinical syndrome of HIT and may be a good treatment option in patients with established HIT. There is no antidote for fondaparinux if major bleeding occurs. In case of life-threatening bleed, recombinant factor VIIa (NovoSeven) or hemodialysis may be considered.

Thrombin Inhibitors, Subcutaneous Drugs

Hirudins

Natural hirudin is a 65–amino acid direct thrombin inhibitor derived from saliva of the leech *Hirudo medicinalis.* It does not require the presence of antithrombin. Several derivatives and recombinant products have been developed. In case of major bleeding with any of the hirudins or with argatroban, recombinant factor VIIa (NovoSeven) should be considered; FFP may also have some limited effect, but probably very little. Lepirudin and argatroban are used mostly for treatment of HIT, bivalirudin is indicated for treatment of acute coronary syndrome, and desirudin for VTE prophylaxis.

- *Lepirudin* (Refludan) is a recombinant hirudin that consists of 65 amino acids; it is administered IV and monitored with the APTT. A therapeutic APTT range is considered to be 1.5 to 2.5 times the median of the laboratory's normal APTT range. The drug is cleared renally and has a half-life of about 80 minutes. It should not be used in patients with renal impairment. The indication for its use is HIT.
- *Desirudin* (Revasc, Iprivask) is also a 65–amino acid recombinant hirudin, administered SQ. Peak plasma levels are reached 1 to 3 hours after injection. It is primarily metabolized by the kidney, and dose reductions are needed in patients with moderate and severe renal impairment. It is indicated for deep vein thrombosis (DVT) prophylaxis. However, the manufacturer discontinued production in May 2012.
- *Bivalirudin* (Angiomax) is a synthetic 20–amino acid polypeptide that directly binds to and inhibits thrombin. It is given IV and has a half-life of 25 minutes. Dose adjustment for severe renal impairment is necessary. Bivalirudin is indicated in patients with acute coronary syndromes undergoing percutaneous transluminal coronary angioplasty.

Argatroban (Novastan)

Argatroban a small synthetic molecule that binds to and inhibits thrombin at its catalytic site. It is given IV. Because argatroban is metabolized in the liver, dosage reductions in patients with impaired liver function are necessary. Serum tests for liver function should always be performed before its use. Its half-life is 40 to 50 minutes. Argatroban can be started without the need for an initial bolus. The dosing is adjusted to an APTT of 1.5 to 3 times the initial baseline value (not to exceed 100 seconds). It is indicated for treatment of HIT.

Danaparoid (Orgaran)

Danaparoid is a mixture of non-heparin glycosaminoglycans isolated from porcine intestine. It has mostly anti-Xa activity, with a low degree of antithrombin activity; the anti-Xa/anti-IIa activity ratio is approximately 28. Danaparoid's anti-Xa activity has a half-life of 25 hours, whereas its antithrombin activity has a half-life of 7 hours. It can be given SQ for DVT prophylaxis but also IV, and is indicated for DVT prophylaxis and for management of HIT. Manufacturing in the United States was discontinued in 2002.

Vitamin K Antagonists

Mechanism of Action

All coagulation factors are synthesized primarily in the liver. Factors II, VII, IX, and X and proteins C and S have to be carboxylated in a final synthetic reaction to become biologically active. This step requires the presence of vitamin K. Vitamin K exists in two forms: vitamin K_1, produced in plants and termed *phylloquinone*, and vitamin K_2, synthesized by bacteria in our intestine and termed *menaquinone*. Half-lives of the vitamin K-dependent coagulation factors are 4 to 6 hours for factor VII, 24 hours for factor IX, 36 hours for factor X, 50 hours for factor II, 8 hours for protein C, and 30 hours for protein S. Because of the long half-lives of some of these factors, particularly factor II, the full antithrombotic effect of vitamin K antagonists is not reached for several days after starting these drugs. Since protein C has a relatively short half-life and levels decrease early, its lowering renders the patient hypercoagulable during the first few treatment days before factor II, with its long half-life, decreases and protects the patient from thrombosis. Thus, vitamin K antagonists create a prothrombotic state in the first 5 days before they have a full anticoagulant effect. This puts the patient at risk for warfarin-induced skin necrosis or progression of thrombosis unless a parenteral anticoagulant is given overlapping with the vitamin K antagonist. The former should be administered for at least 5 days and until the INR is above 2.0.

Monitoring, Dose Requirement

Vitamin K antagonists are monitored with the prothrombin time (PT). Because results of the PT depend on the sensitivity of the PT reagent used in the laboratory, PT measurements are converted to an INR by a calculation that includes a PT reagent's sensitivity (international sensitivity index). The coumarin vitamin K antagonists are metabolized by the cytochrome P450 enzyme complex, mostly the enzymes CYP2C9 and CYP1A2. Because of a high degree of interindividual variability in the activity of these enzymes, there is a high degree of variability in the daily drug dose that patients need to maintain their INR in the therapeutic range. Polymorphisms in the genes transcribing enzymes involved in the metabolism of vitamin K antagonists, such as *CYP2C9* (cytochrome P2C9 enzyme), and of vitamin K, such as *VKORC1* (vitamin K epoxide reductase complex 1), contribute to the variability in dose requirements. However, routine use of pharmacogenetic testing is not recommended at this time.

Management of Elevated International Normalized Ratios

Several options are available to manage elevated INRs and bleeding that occur during administration of vitamin K antagonists, and they depend on the degree of INR elevation and the presence or absence of risk factors for bleeding and active bleeding itself. These options have been published as recommendations from the ACCP[2] (Table 22-2) and consist of holding the next anticoagulant dose or doses and giving vitamin K. Administering too high a dose of vitamin K should be avoided if there is no major bleeding, because it will reverse the INR completely and might make re-anticoagulation more difficult. FFP can lower the INR some, but not completely or markedly, since the short half-life of coagulation factor VII (4-6 hours) would require the administration of huge doses of FFP for full reversal. If complete or immediate INR reversal is needed, such as when treating major bleeding while taking vitamin K antagonists, a prothrombin complex concentrate should be given or, if not available, recombinant factor VIIa (NovoSeven) considered.

Periprocedural Interruption of Oral Anticoagulant Therapy

Whether there is a need to stop oral anticoagulant therapy before a surgical or radiologic procedure depends on the bleeding risk associated with the procedure. How soon to stop the drug before the procedure depends on the patient's INR at the time administration of the drug is stopped as

well as the half-life of the drug used. In addition, whether bridging therapy with a SQ or IV anticoagulant should be given before and after the procedure depends on the patient's thromboembolic risk. Guidelines have been established by the ACCP[3] (Table 22-3).

Available Vitamin K Antagonists

Two classes of vitamin K antagonists exist: the most widely used coumarin derivatives (warfarin, phenprocoumon, acenocoumarol, tioclomarol) and the indandione derivatives (fluindione, anisindione, phenindione).

Coumarin derivatives differ in their half-lives and their onset and duration of action. It is possible that the difference in half-lives may influence the quality of anticoagulant management and thus efficacy and safety, but this issue has not been studied. For clinical purposes at this point, these drugs are classically viewed as equally effective and safe. The type of coumarin used is mostly a national preference primarily determined by marketing strategies and physician preferences. Warfarin is the most widely used coumarin in the United States, Canada, England, Italy, Australia, and Russia; acenocoumarol in the Netherlands and Spain; and phenprocoumon in Germany. Other regional preferences exist. *Warfarin* (Coumadin, Jantoven) has a half-life of 1 to 2.5 days, with a mean of about 40 hours. *Phenprocoumon* (Marcumar, Falithrom, Phenpro, etc.) has a longer half-life (5 days), a slower onset, and a longer duration of action than warfarin. *Acenocoumarol* (Sinthrome, etc.) has a shorter half-life (10-24 hours) than warfarin, a more rapid onset, and a shorter duration of action (2 days). The typical loading dose of warfarin in a hospitalized patient is 5 mg daily on days 1 and 2, with subsequent dosing based on the INR

TABLE 22-2. Recommendations for Management of Elevated International Normalized Ratios in Patients Taking Vitamin K Antagonists

INR	Bleeding?	Risk Factor for Bleeding?	Intervention
<5.0	No	No/yes	Omit next VKA dose and reduce dose
5.0-9.0	No	No	Omit next VKA dose and reduce dose
5.0-9.0	No	Yes	Vitamin K, 1-2.5 mg PO
>9.0	No		Vitamin K, 2.5-5 mg PO
Serious bleeding at any INR			Vitamin K, 10 mg IV, + FFP or PCCs
Life-threatening bleeding			Vitamin K, 10 mg IV, + PCCs; consider NovoSeven

FFP, Fresh frozen plasma; *PCCs,* prothrombin complex concentrates; *VKA,* vitamin K antagonist.
Modified after Ageno W, Gallus AS, Wittkowsky A, Crowther M, Hylek EM, Palareti G. Oral anticoagulant therapy: Antithrombotic therapy and prevention of thrombosis. 9th ed. American College of Chest Physicians evidence-based clinical practice guidelines. Chest 2012;141:e44S–88S.

TABLE 22-3. Recommendations When Interrupting Warfarin Therapy for Invasive Procedures*

Risk of Clot	Preoperatively	Postoperatively
Low	D/C warfarin ≈ 4 days preoperatively No LMWH/UFH	Prophylactic dose of LMWH/UFH (if intervention causes thrombotic risk) Restart warfarin
Intermediate	D/C warfarin ≈ 4 days preoperatively Prophylactic dose of LMWH/UFH	Prophylactic dose of LMWH/UFH Restart warfarin
High	D/C warfarin ≈ 4 days preoperatively Full-dose LMWH/UFH 2 days preoperatively	LMWH/UFH (no dose recommendation given) Restart warfarin

*These recommendations are all so-called grade C recommendations (i.e., very weak recommendations), and other alternatives may be equally reasonable.
D/C, Discontinue; *LMWH,* low-molecular-weight heparin; *UFH,* unfractionated heparin.
Modified after Ageno W, Gallus AS, Wittkowsky A, Crowther M, Hylek EM, Palareti G. Oral anticoagulant therapy: Antithrombotic therapy and prevention of thrombosis. 9th ed. American College of Chest Physicians evidence-based clinical practice guidelines. Chest 2012;141:e44S–88S.

after the first two doses. A frail or elderly patient or one who has been treated with prolonged antibiotics, has liver disease, or has undergone intestinal resection will need a lower dose in the first few days. Some clinicians prefer using higher loading doses of 7.5 to 10 mg, particularly in a well-nourished outpatient. For maintenance dosing, men younger than 50 years have the highest dose requirements to remain in the therapeutic range (median dose, 6.4 mg/day), and women older than 70 years have the lowest (median dose, 3.1 mg/day). Occasionally patients need doses as high as 20 or 30 mg/day.

Indandiones are a different class of drugs than coumarins. No head-to-head trials comparing these agents with coumarins have been published. *Fluindione* (Previscan), *anisindione* (Miradon), and *phenindione* (Dindevan, Pindione, etc.) are the drugs available. Fluindione is the most widely used oral anticoagulant in France. Its half-life is 30 hours. Phenindione is associated with hypersensitivity reactions in 1.5% to 3% of patients, which can be fatal, and its use is therefore not recommended.

NEW ORAL ANTICOAGULANTS

Advantages and Disadvantages

Several new oral anticoagulants have come onto the market in the last 2 years or are in the latter stages of clinical development. They all share a number of advantages compared to warfarin: (1) they do not require monitoring of their anticoagulant effect, because they have a wide therapeutic window and somewhat predictable dose-responses, (2) they are not influenced by vitamin K in the diet, since their mechanism of action is not through the vitamin K pathway, and (3) they have fewer interactions with other drugs than warfarin. The two disadvantages are that there is (1) no known effective reversal strategy in case of major bleeding and (2) limited knowledge on the performance of various coagulation tests in assessing the drugs' anticoagulant effects.

Management of Major Bleeding

Limited data exist on how to effectively manage major bleeding occurring in patients taking these drugs. Although in vitro data and studies in animals and healthy human volunteers indicate that some pharmacologic agents (e.g., prothrombin complex concentrates [PCCs], activated [a] PCCs, and recombinant factor VIIa) may have a reversal impact on the anticoagulant effects of some of these drugs, these agents have not been evaluated for management of bleeding events in patients on these drugs. Since the half-life of these drugs is relatively short (≈12 hours), for moderate and some more major bleeds, it may be sufficient to discontinue the drug and wait for it to clear from the circulation. If the drug was ingested in the preceding 2 hours, activated charcoal is indicated for any of these oral drugs. Depending on degree, location, and additional contributors to bleeding, the typical general measures should also be considered: symptomatic treatment, mechanical compression, surgical intervention, fluid replacement, hemodynamic support, and blood product transfusion. If hemostasis is not achieved with these strategies, PCCs, aPCCs, or

recombinant factor VIIa can be considered. FFP is unlikely to have any beneficial effect in this situation. A consensus statement on management of major bleeding on the various anticoagulants has been published.[4] Dabigatran is dialyzable; Rivaroxaban, Apixaban, and Edoxaban or not.

Measurement of Anticoagulant Effect

Limited data also exist on how various coagulation tests perform in patients treated with these drugs, and how coagulation test results correlate with plasma drug levels and clinical efficacy and safety of these drugs. Routine anticoagulation monitoring of patients on these new oral anticoagulants is not usually needed, but assessment of a patient's anticoagulation status may be desirable in certain clinical situations, such as assessing for sub- or supratherapeutic levels in patients with thromboembolic or hemorrhagic events during treatment, determining minimal residual drug anticoagulant effect prior to surgery and other interventions, or assessing the efficacy of reversal strategies when managing a patient who has a major bleed. Evaluation of coagulation tests in patients on these drugs is ongoing, and clinical trials are needed to determine the relationship of assay results with bleeding and thrombotic complications.

Dabigatran (Pradaxa)

Dabigatran etexilate is a synthetic small molecule, a prodrug that gets rapidly converted after oral ingestion to the active compound dabigatran. Dabigatran acts as an anticoagulant by directly inhibiting both free and clot-bound thrombin. Peak plasma level is reached approximately 1.5 hours after oral intake. Since the majority of dabigatran (up to 80%) is cleared by the kidney, its half-life depends on renal function. In individuals with normal renal function, the mean half-life is 13 hours (range 11-22 hours), increasing to a mean of 18 hours (range 13-23) in patients with a glomerular filtration rate (GFR) of 30 to 50 mL/min. It is dosed twice daily. The majority of dabigatran is renally cleared, so dose reduction is required in patients with impaired renal function, and the drug is not to be used in patients with severely impaired renal function with a GFR of less than 15 mL/min (Table 22-4). Dabigatran etexilate is approved in many countries (*not* including the United States) for prevention of VTE after orthopedic surgery, and in many countries (including the United States) for prevention of stroke and systemic arterial thromboembolism in patients with atrial fibrillation. A clinical practical guide is available, addressing issues of dabigatran dosing, interruption of therapy for surgeries and other interventions, and management options in case of major bleeding (Table 22-5). The PT and APTT are fairly insensitive to dabigatran and not useful in measuring its effect; they are often normal despite therapeutic dabigatran plasma levels. The *thrombin clot time* (TCT), also called *thrombin time* (TT), is quite sensitive to dabigatran; a normal TCT rules out significant residual presence of dabigatran. Other tests that appear to be useful for measuring dabigatran are presently being investigated, including the ecarin clotting time (ECT), ecarin chromogenic assay (ECA), dilute thrombin time (dTT), and prothrombin-induced clotting time (PiCT).

Rivaroxaban (Xarelto)

Rivaroxaban is a direct factor Xa inhibitor, a synthetic small molecule. Key pharmacokinetic data include a peak plasma drug level within 2 to 4 hours after oral administration and a half-life of 5 to 9 hours in patients with normal hepatic and renal function. Approximately 51% of rivaroxaban undergoes hepatic metabolism, and 66% is excreted in the urine (36% as unchanged parent drug). The oral bioavailability is more than 80%. It is dosed once daily. Dose reduction with decreasing renal function is necessary, and it is contraindicated below a GFR of 15 mL/min (Table 22-6). Rivaroxaban is approved in many countries, including the United States, for prevention of VTE after orthopedic surgery (with a lower dose [10 mg/day]) and in many countries, including the United States, for prevention of stroke and systemic arterial thromboembolism in patients with atrial fibrillation at a higher dose (20 mg/day if GFR is above 50 mL/min). It is also approved for the acute treatment and secondary prevention of deep vein thrombosis and pulmonary embolism. A clinical practical guide is available, addressing issues of rivaroxaban dosing, interruption of therapy for surgeries and other interventions, and management options in case of major bleeding (Table 22-7). A

TABLE 22-4. Dabigatran Dosing (FDA approval) in Atrial Fibrillation

Renal function* (CrCl mL/min)	>30	15-30	<15
Recommended starting dose†	150 mg bid	75 mg bid	Do not use

*For the purpose of dabigatran dosing, renal function should be estimated by the Cockcroft-Gault method. Cockcroft-Gault equation: CrCl = [(140 − age) × weight (kg)] / (SCr × 72) (× 0.85 if female).
†The median weight of patients treated with dabigatran in RE-LY1 was 82.5 ± 19.4 kg. No information is available on its safety and efficacy in overweight or obese patients, and anti-Xa levels are not useful for guiding drug dosing.
bid, Twice daily; *CrCl,* creatinine clearance.
Reed B, Miller A, Moll S. UNC guideline: management of dabigatran in adults. Available at http://professionalsblog.Clotconnect.Org/wp-content/uploads/2011/04/unc-pradaxa-5-2012.Pdf (last accessed December 28, 2012).

TABLE 22-5. Dabigatran Perioperative Management: Discontinuation Prior to Surgical Procedures

Renal Function (CrCl mL/min)	Half-life (hours) Mean (range)	Timing of Discontinuation Prior to Procedure (Minimum)	
		Standard Risk of Bleeding*	High Risk of Bleeding†
>80	13 (11-22)	24 hours	2-4 days
50-80	15 (12-34)	24 hours	2-4 days
30-50	18 (13-23)	≥48 hours	≥4 days
<30	27 (22-35)	48-120 hours	≥5 days

*Examples: electrophysiology procedures, cardiac catheterizations, no additional patient-specific risk factors.
†Examples: surgery involving major organs, procedures requiring complete hemostasis (e.g., spinal anesthesia), or when additional patient-specific risk factors are present.
Reed B, Miller A, Moll S. UNC guideline: management of dabigatran in adults. Available at http://professionalsblog.Clotconnect.Org/wp-content/uploads/2011/04/unc-pradaxa-5-2012.Pdf (last accessed December 28, 2012).

TABLE 22-6. Rivaroxaban Dosing

Indication	Renal Function (CrCl mL/min)*	Recommended Dose†
Atrial fibrillation‡,§	≥50 15-49 <15	20 mg once daily 15 mg once daily Do not use
Hip and knee replacement	≥30 <30	10 mg once daily Do not use
DVT and PE treatment	GFR ≥ 30	15 mg bid for 3 weeks after acute event, then 20 mg once daily <30 Do not use

*For the purpose of rivaroxaban dosing, renal function should be estimated by the Cockcroft-Gault method. Cockcroft-Gault equation: CrCl = [(140− age) × weight (kg)] / (SCr × 72) (× 0.85 if female).
†Co-administration with P-glycoprotein and strong CYP3A4 inducers (i.e., carbamazepine, phenytoin, rifampin) may warrant a dose increase. Doses > 10 mg should be taken with food.
‡The median body mass index of patients in ROCKET-AF1 was approximately 28 ± 3 kg/m². No information is available on its safety and efficacy in overweight or obese patients, and anti-Xa levels have not been evaluated for guiding drug dosing.
§In ROCKET-AF1, rivaroxaban was not studied in patients with CrCl < 30 mL/min, so recommendations in patients with CrCl 15-30 mL/min are based on the FDA-approved labeling.
Hunter M, Miller S, Reed B, Miller A, Moll S. UNC guideline: management of rivaroxaban in adults. Available at http://professionalsblog.Clotconnect.Org/wp-content/uploads/2012/05/unc-xarelto-2012.Pdf (last accessed December 28, 2012).

TABLE 22-7. Rivaroxaban Perioperative Management: Discontinuation Prior to Surgical Procedures

Renal Function (CrCl mL/min)	Half-life (hours)	Timing of Discontinuation Prior to Procedure* (Minimum)	
		Standard Risk of Bleeding†	High Risk of Bleeding‡
>50	5-9	18-24 hours	1-2 days
<50	>9	24-48 hours	>2 days
Hepatic Function (Child-Pugh Score)	**Half-life (hours)**	**Standard Risk of Bleeding†**	**High Risk of Bleeding‡**
Mild impairment (Child-Pugh A)	8	24 hours	1-2 days
Mild impairment (Child-Pugh B)	12-16	≥48 hours	≥4 days
Mild impairment (Child-Pugh C)	Unknown	72-120 hours	≥1 week

*No published data exist on optimal perioperative management of rivaroxaban, so the recommendations here have been extrapolated from the pharmacokinetics and pharmacodynamics of the drug.
†Examples: electrophysiology procedures, cardiac catheterizations, no additional patient-specific risk factors.
‡Examples: surgery involving major organs, procedures requiring complete hemostasis (e.g., spinal anesthesia), or when additional patient-specific risk factors are present.
Hunter M, Miller S, Reed B, Miller A, Moll S. UNC guideline: management of rivaroxaban in adults. Available at http://professionalsblog.Clotconnect.Org/wp-content/uploads/2012/05/unc-xarelto-2012.Pdf (last accessed December 28, 2012).

consensus statement on management of major bleeding has also been published.[4]

Given the available data, an anti-Xa assay appears preferable for monitoring rivaroxaban. Because anti-Xa assays may not be available in all clinical settings, there may be a role for PT/INR measurement in patients who are actively bleeding and suspected of having a high plasma drug concentration. A normal PT may rule out high rivaroxaban levels. However, caution should be taken in interpreting the PT, since there is significant interpatient variability as well as variation in results, depending on the specific PT reagent used by the laboratory. Further clinical data on other tests, such as PiCT, will have to determine whether such tests are worth their introduction into the routine clinical coagulation laboratory.

Apixaban

Apixaban is another synthetic small-molecule direct factor Xa inhibitor. After oral intake, it reaches peak plasma concentration in 1 to 3 hours. The half-life is 10 to 14 hours after repeated doses. Apixaban is metabolized in part by CYP3A4; it is partly eliminated by the kidneys (25%) and to some extent also processed via CYP-independent mechanisms in the liver. Apixaban does not induce or inhibit CYP enzymes and is expected to have a low likelihood of drug-drug interactions. It remains to be determined whether combined hepatic and renal elimination will allow apixaban to be safely given in patients with mild (or moderate) hepatic or renal impairment. As with rivaroxaban, reversal strategies for major bleeding on apixaban have not been studied, and it is not known whether PCCs, aPCCs, or factor VIIa have any beneficial effect.[4] Given the available data, an anti-Xa assay may be most suitable for measuring apixaban's anticoagulation effect. Less is known about the performance of other anticoagulation tests, and care must be taken to not assume a normal PT or APTT means no significant apixaban anticoagulant effect is present. Apixaban is approved in a number of countries (not in the United States) for the prevention of stroke and systemic arterial thromboembolism in atrial fibrillation.

PATIENT EDUCATION

Treatment with anticoagulants and antiplatelet agents is associated with a significant risk for bleeding, morbidity, and mortality. Therapy recommended and prescribed by healthcare providers may be optimized by having an educated patient. Patients can find information about antiplatelet and anticoagulant drugs, as well as the diseases treated with these drugs, at the following websites:

- www.clotconnect.org-nonprofit education website of the *Clot Connect* program of the University of North Carolina Hemostasis and Thrombosis Center.
- www.stoptheclot.org-website of the nonprofit patient organization National Blood Clot Alliance (NBCA)
- www.fvleiden.org-a nonprofit patient education website
- www.clotcare.com-an information website for patients and healthcare providers
- www.veinforum.org-website of the nonprofit organization American Venous Forum
- www.americanheart.org-website of the American Heart Association
- www.strokeassociation.org-website of the American Stroke Association
- www.vasculardisease.org-website of the nonprofit Venous Disease Coalition

---

KEY POINTS

- Arterial thrombosis is prevented and treated mostly with antiplatelet drugs.
- Venous thromboembolism is prevented and treated primarily with anticoagulant drugs.
- Guidelines and treatment recommendations exist for most clinical scenarios in which antiplatelet agents and anticoagulants are used.

► **SUGGESTED READINGS**

Ageno W, Gallus AS, Wittkowsky A, et al. Oral anticoagulant therapy: Antithrombotic therapy and prevention of thrombosis, 9th ed: American College of Chest Physicians evidence-based clinical practice guidelines. Chest 2012;141:e44S–88S.

Douketis JD, Spyropoulos AC, Spencer FA, et al. Perioperative management of antithrombotic therapy: Antithrombotic therapy and prevention of thrombosis, 9th ed: American College of Chest Physicians evidence-based clinical practice guidelines. Chest 2012;141: e326S–350S.

Kaatz S, Kouides PA, Garcia DA, et al. Guidance on the emergent reversal of oral thrombin and factor Xa inhibitors. Am J Hematol 2012;87(Suppl 1):S141–145.

Linkins LA, Dans AL, Moores LK, et al. Treatment and prevention of heparin-induced thrombocytopenia: Antithrombotic therapy and prevention of thrombosis, 9th ed: American College of Chest Physicians evidence-based clinical practice guidelines. Chest 2012;141: e495S–530S.

The complete reference list is available online at www.expertconsult.com.

CHAPTER 23

Vasoactive Agents

John J. Lewin, III, Edward T. Horn, and Bradford D. Winters

Vasoactive agents are commonly employed in a variety of settings in the hospitalized patient, including the interventional radiology suite. Safe and effective pharmacologic manipulation of an individual patient's hemodynamics for therapeutic or diagnostic purposes requires a thorough understanding of patient-specific factors and a firm comprehension of the pharmacology of the agents employed. In this chapter we review the pharmacology, hemodynamic impact, and intraarterial use (where indicated) of selected vasoactive agents that may be used in a variety of clinical settings in the interventional radiology suite. The reader is referred to Chapter 16 for more detail regarding the specific use of these agents in the setting of medical emergencies.

ADRENERGIC RECEPTOR PHARMACOLOGY

Vasopressors and inotropes act primarily through the adrenergic receptor class of transmembrane receptors. Additionally, the dopaminergic system plays a prominent role in the case of some agents. The overall physiologic response to many of the vasopressors and inotropes is determined in part by the pharmacology of their respective receptor interactions. The final clinical result of administering one of these agents is also influenced by other factors, including reflex mechanisms, the patient's volume status, overall cardiovascular state, and the complex balance between agonism and/or antagonism of the drugs at the receptors. Adrenergic receptors are a heterogeneous population of different subtypes whose response to various adrenergic agents varies with subtype. Distribution of receptors and their subtypes is heterogeneous across tissue beds, adding another layer of complexity. Adrenergic receptors historically were divided into two primary groups: the α receptors and the β receptors. More recent pharmacologic and molecular data have led to a reclassification into three main groups: α_1, α_2, and β. These groups are then further subdivided into three individual subtypes each, for a total of nine adrenergic receptor subtypes.

α_1-Adrenergic receptors are G protein–coupled transmembrane receptors whose intracellular signaling is through membrane phospholipids; they comprise three subtypes: 1a, 1b, and 1d. The subtypes have wide but variable distribution, with the highest expression for la being found in the liver and lower levels in the heart, cerebellum, and cerebral cortex. The lb subtype shows up greatest in the spleen, kidney, and cerebellum, whereas the 1d subtype has its greatest expression in the cerebral cortex and aorta.[1] Subtype-specific agonists and antagonists exist for these receptors but are for research purposes only. Clinically available agonists and antagonists are nonspecific in terms of subtype binding. Activation of these receptors by the clinically relevant agents leads to smooth muscle contraction that, in the vasculature, results in vasoconstriction.

α_2-Adrenergic receptors are transmembrane receptors whose intracellular signaling is mediated through G-protein inhibition of adenylate cyclase. The three subtypes—2a, 2b, and 2c—are widely distributed and each contribute uniquely though not completely for the various responses seen with α_2 agonists. The α_{2b} subtype has been demonstrated to be responsible for the short-term hypertensive response that may occur with α_2 agonists, whereas the α_{2a} subtype has been implicated in the sympatholytic response and elements of the anesthetic response to these agents. Currently there are no subtype selective α_2 agonists, and all α_2 agonists (clonidine and dexmedetomidine) are nonspecific in their action. Lower doses of these agents tend to produce hypotension through sympatholysis, whereas at higher doses the α_{2b} receptor present on the smooth muscle cells of resistance vessels predominates, leading to a hypertensive response.[2]

The β receptors are subdivided into β_1, β_2, and β_3 subtypes, and all generally use G protein–mediated activation of adenylyl cyclase as their intracellular signaling pathway. They have wide distribution and divergent clinical responses despite their biochemical relationship. β_1-Adrenoreceptors are predominantly found in the heart, whereas β_2 receptors are present in the smooth muscle beds of the lung, peripheral vasculature, and uterus. β_3-Adrenergic receptors are unique in that one of their roles appears to be in metabolic regulation.[3]

Activation of β_1 receptors is primarily responsible for increased inotropy and chronotropy in the heart. Other actions mediated by these receptors include release of renin from the kidneys and activation of lipolysis.[4] Their effect on cardiac contractility and heart rate results in increased cardiac output and sometimes blood pressure (BP), although this latter effect is often clinically blunted or even reversed by agonism at the β_2 receptor. Although β_1-specific antagonists (e.g., esmolol) are clinically available, there are no β_1-specific agonists (although there are some fairly β_2-specific agents, primarily used to treat bronchospasm). These improvements in cardiac output come at a price, however, because the increased contractility and heart rate significantly increase myocardial oxygen demand while reducing supply, putting the heart at ischemic risk. Long-term overstimulation of these receptors through humoral feedback mechanisms has been implicated in the molecular pathogenesis of chronic congestive heart failure (CHF), and strategies to interrupt these processes using β_1 antagonists (β-blockers) have led to some clinical success.[5]

The β_2 receptor is characterized by wide distribution throughout the respiratory tract and uterus as well as the vascular tree, where its primary effect is smooth muscle relaxation. In the respiratory tree, this results in bronchodilation; in the uterus, it affects tocolysis; and in the vascular tree, vasodilation. This vasodilatory effect is partly responsible for the often observed drop in BP when primary β agonists such as dobutamine are employed alone. Autonomic reflexes also play a role. Drugs such as epinephrine and norepinephrine have differential effects in that they stimulate not only β_1 and β_2 receptors but also α receptors. Thus, the end clinical hemodynamic result with these agents is determined by a complex interplay between increased cardiac contractility and possibly heart rate, peripheral vasoconstriction, and peripheral vasodilation. This interplay and other physiologic variables such as vagal reflexes are considered in the following discussions of the individual drugs.

β_3-Adrenergic receptors were originally thought to have little to no clinical relevance in terms of hemodynamics. Their primary role was believed to be in the metabolic regulation of energy metabolism via effects on adipose tissue. Although their ultimate place in terms of physiologic effects is still a matter of investigation, other mechanisms attributed to this subtype include gastric acid secretion, coupling to potassium channels in smooth muscle, and interactions with nitric oxide–dependent vasorelaxation.[6-8] Despite these possibilities, from a clinical point of view, the β_3 receptor does not yet have a defined role in the immediate clinical response to the commonly used vasopressors and inotropes.

A separate group of receptors involved in vasomotor tone are the dopamine receptors. Although they are not usually classified as adrenergic receptors, their primary agonist is the catecholamine dopamine. Like the adrenergic receptors, these are G protein–coupled transmembrane receptors. Dopamine receptors have two different nomenclature systems depending on whether they are in the central nervous system (CNS) or the peripheral vasculature. Those in the CNS were originally classified into two types, the D_1 and D_2 subtypes, based on their activation or inhibition of adenylate cyclase. Modern cloning techniques have further defined them into two superfamilies: the D_1-like group that includes the D_1 and D_5 subtypes and the D_2-like group that includes the D_2, D_3, and D_4 subtypes.[9]

Peripheral dopamine receptors are classified into two groups, the DA_1 and DA_2 subtypes. The DA_1 subtype is defined pharmacologically by its ability to mediate renal artery vasodilation and natriuresis. These receptors are widely distributed on vascular smooth muscle but are particularly dense in the renal and splanchnic beds. Agonism of these receptors leads to smooth muscle relaxation and vasodilation. The natriuretic effect is secondary to the receptor's impact on the sodium-hydrogen exchanger and sodium/potassium adenosine triphosphatase pumps in the proximal tubular cells and tubular cells of the thick ascending loop of Henle, as well as possible vascular effects on glomerular filtration rate (GFR) and renal blood flow. This subtype is thought to be similar to the D_1 receptor subtype in the CNS.

The DA_2 receptor subtype is similar to the CNS D_2-like receptors and is mostly found on the presynaptic adrenergic nerve terminals and in the sympathetic ganglia.[9] Agonism at these receptors leads indirectly to vasodilation by inhibiting the release of norepinephrine at the adrenergic nerve termini and by suppressing transmission at the sympathetic ganglia, leading to an overall drop in sympathetic activity.

AGENTS USED TO INCREASE BLOOD PRESSURE

Agents used to sustain BP in hypotensive patients can work through several mechanisms but usually exert their action via stimulation of adrenergic receptors. The medications discussed in this section can have very different pharmacologic actions based on their receptor-activity relationship. The BP elevation is due to either an increase in systemic vascular resistance or an increased cardiac contractility, resulting in increased cardiac output, or a combination of both. These differences are discussed individually within each drug section. These pharmacologic agents generally have the same adverse event profile, although there are nuances depending on the receptor-activity relationship. Agents that are potent α_1 agonists can produce excessive vasoconstriction and necrosis to poorly perfused tissues (especially in hypovolemic or under-resuscitated patients). Myocardial ischemia and dysrhythmias can occur due to β_1 stimulation. Other potential adverse effects that can occur are metabolic derangements (e.g., lactic acidosis) and soft-tissue damage from extravasation.[10-13] When the decision is being made to administer vasopressors, fluid status should always be assessed to truly determine the cause of the patient's hypotension.

Phenylephrine

Phenylephrine is a short-acting adrenergic agonist that is highly specific for the postsynaptic α_1 adrenoreceptor and has slight activity at the presynaptic α_2 adrenoreceptor.[14] This activity results in an overall increase in vascular tone, as demonstrated by an increase in systemic vascular resistance when a pulmonary artery catheter is in place. Owing to its lack of cardiac stimulation, phenylephrine has been used as a primary vasopressor in patients in septic shock who require hemodynamic support. It has been shown in multiple studies to have little effect on important cardiac indices, including cardiac index, in noncardiac patients. Adverse effects on cardiac performance have been shown in patients with cardiac dysfunction, resulting in decreased cardiac performance due to an increase in peripheral resistance.[15,16]

Phenylephrine can be dosed either as an intravenous (IV) bolus or a continuous infusion. For IV bolus administration, phenylephrine can be diluted to 100 μg/mL in a syringe, with 1 to 2 mL (100-200 μg) administered at a time, and doses given to achieve a goal mean arterial pressure (MAP) greater than 65 mmHg. This administration technique has been used in both obstetric patients and patients undergoing anesthetic induction during short procedures.[17,18] Phenylephrine IV infusions are more logical for patients who require hemodynamic support for prolonged periods. Doses for infusions are weight based and typically range from 0.1 to 4 μg/kg/min. Phenylephrine has been associated with decreased cardiac performance and increased splanchnic vasoconstriction (compared with norepinephrine), which limits its clinical usefulness.[19] For this reason, it is no longer considered first-line therapy for vasopressor-dependent septic shock.[20] Phenylephrine can be considered useful in the management of hypotension associated with anesthesia induction (including spinal), and

TABLE 23-1. Comparison of Relative Receptor Activity of Adrenergic Agonists

Agent	α_1	α_2	β_1	β_2	DA
Dobutamine	+	0	++++	++	0
Dopamine:					
0-3 µg/kg/min	0	0	+	0	++++
3-10 µg/kg/min	0/+	0	++++	++	++++
10-20 µg/kg/min	+++	0	++++	+	0
Epinephrine:					
<0.5 µg/kg/min	++	++	++++	+++	0
>0.5 µg/kg/min	++++	++++	+++	+	0
Norepinephrine	+++	+++	+++	+	0
Phenylephrine	++/+++	+	0	0	0
Isoproterenol	0	0	++++	++++	0

0, No activity; +, relative activity; DA, dopamine.

for the short-term management of hypotension not due to sepsis.

Ephedrine

Ephedrine is a mixed adrenoreceptor agonist. It has effects on both the α_1 and β_1 receptors in the cardiovascular system, resulting in vasoconstriction and tachycardia. It also has an indirect effect, causing postganglionic release of norepinephrine.[21-24] Ephedrine is effective with bolus dosing in preventing and treating epidural or spinal anesthesia–induced hypotension, with doses ranging from 10 to 50 mg intravenously or intramuscularly.[25-29] IV administration results in immediate effects that are short acting, whereas doses given intramuscularly may not take effect for 10 to 20 minutes, with a duration of 60 minutes. Continuous infusions of ephedrine have been thought to deplete norepinephrine stores, resulting in tachyphylaxis, but this is debatable.[23,24] Ephedrine is also known to possess stimulant, hallucinogenic, and euphoric properties that have resulted in its use being limited to short-term procedural use in obstetric and surgical/procedural settings.[30,31]

Norepinephrine

Norepinephrine is a potent α_1 and α_2 agonist and, to a lesser extent, a β_1 and β_2 agonist. Its primary effect is a profound increase in systemic vascular resistance through vasoconstriction of vascular beds. Whereas this is similar to phenylephrine, the β_1/β_2 stimulation supports cardiac function in the presence of increased resistance, so its effects on cardiac function range from no change to slight increase in cardiac output.[10,32] Recent published guidelines have promoted the use of norepinephrine or dopamine as the initial vasopressor in management of septic shock, which is a shift from previous clinical practice in which norepinephrine was only used in dopamine-resistant septic shock.[20,33] Norepinephrine may be preferable to dopamine in patients in whom β_1 stimulation would be deleterious, because norepinephrine possesses more potent α_1 and less potent β_1 activity. Excessive vasoconstriction due to the potent α_1 stimulation can occur, resulting in regional ischemia (skin, splanchnic perfusion).

Norepinephrine is dosed as a continuous IV infusion, with doses in clinical trials ranging from 0.1 to 2.2 µg/kg/min.[34] The hemodynamic effects one can expect are increases in systemic vascular resistance (and ultimately MAP), no to mild increase in cardiac output/cardiac index, and slight increases in heart rate. Norepinephrine should be used as a first-line vasopressor in patients with septic shock, who are at higher risk for adverse outcomes associated with arrhythmias. Norepinephrine should also be used in the presence of phenylephrine-resistant hypotension because it is a more potent α_1 agonist.

Dopamine

Dopamine is a vasoactive agent that has multiple receptor binding sites throughout the body, with varying dose-response activity at dopamine, β_1, β_2, and α_1 receptors (Table 23-1), although it has been shown that there is a degree of overlap in critically ill patients beginning at doses as low as 3 µg/kg/min.[35] The high doses of dopamine needed to maintain BP (15-20 µg/kg/min) can lead to tachyarrhythmias, limiting its usefulness as a first-line agent in managing shock. It can also cause disturbances in pulmonary function, including increases in pulmonary capillary wedge pressure, shunting, and decreased oxygen pressures.[36] Dopamine has also been shown to increase splanchnic and mesenteric ischemia.[11,37] Overall, norepinephrine has become the vasopressor of choice in the management of septic shock.[20,38] Low-dose dopamine (<3 µg/kg/min) had been thought to promote renal blood flow and increase renal function, especially in the critically ill, who are at increased risk for acute renal failure. Multiple studies have now shown that this management strategy has no effect on renal or survival outcomes and should be abandoned.[39,40]

AGENTS USED TO INCREASE CARDIAC OUTPUT

Dobutamine

Dobutamine is a synthetic catecholamine that possesses fairly selective β_1 and β_2 activity, with some slight α_1 stimulation, resulting in potent inotropy and relaxation of the vascular bed. Dobutamine has been shown to have an increased effect on cardiac output and may have less arrhythmogenic effects than dopamine at equal doses.[41,42]

Dobutamine will result in an increase in cardiac performance as measured by cardiac output/cardiac index and produce a slight decrease in systemic vascular resistance. These attributes make it a cornerstone of therapy in decompensated heart failure, together with other appropriate therapies such as vasodilators and diuretics. The dose range of dobutamine is 5 to 20 μg/kg/min, titrated to cardiac endpoints such as cardiac output or cardiac index. In most patients, BP is not affected significantly and remains stable. Dobutamine has been recommended as a first-line agent in the management of decreased cardiac performance associated with septic shock when used in conjunction with an agent that can provide BP support.[20,33] Overall, this drug is a useful agent to augment cardiac output in patients with septic or cardiogenic shock, but the patient must be monitored for tachyarrhythmias and hypotension.

Epinephrine

Epinephrine is a potent adrenergic agonist. Low-dose epinephrine infusions (<0.5 μg/kg/min) can produce effects similar to dobutamine, with increased cardiac indices. High-dose epinephrine infusions (doses > 0.5 μg/kg/min) are used to manage septic shock (typically after failure of norepinephrine) and are often employed after cardiac arrest. At this dose range, epinephrine produces profound peripheral vasoconstriction, resulting in increases in BP. This profound vasoconstriction produces regional ischemia, namely to the splanchnic and renal vasculature.[43,44] Epinephrine can also cause an increase in lactate production. Although the mechanism is not fully understood, it may be attributable to decreased oxygen delivery to the mesenteric bed or increases in calorigenesis and glycogen breakdown.[45] As with other agents that have β-adrenergic stimulation, epinephrine can cause arrhythmias and cardiac ischemia. Although it can produce significant increases in cardiac output, the potential for splanchnic and cardiac ischemia, metabolic disturbances, and arrhythmias typically limit epinephrine's use to a second- or third-line agent.

Isoproterenol

Isoproterenol is a potent β_1- and β_2-selective agent that is useful in the management of orthotopic cardiac transplant patients who have a denervated myocardium. This denervation can affect multiple pharmacologic agents, especially those that exert their effect through the atrioventricular node (e.g., atropine, digoxin), rendering them ineffective.[46] Isoproterenol is not affected by this mechanism. Other adrenergic agents, such as epinephrine and norepinephrine, have been demonstrated to produce an increased effect on contractility and chronotropy that is due to catecholamine hypersensitivity and may not be desirable.[47-49] Isoproterenol is dosed as a continuous infusion, with doses ranging from 0.05 to 0.2 μg/kg/min, titrated to an appropriate heart rate and/or cardiac output.

AGENTS USED TO LOWER BLOOD PRESSURE

Unlike the agents used to raise BP, which work almost exclusively through adrenergic pathways, agents used to lower BP can exert their effects through differing physiologic mechanisms related to regulation of vascular tone and BP control. Table 23-2 summarizes mechanisms of action, hemodynamic effects, and dosing of the antihypertensive agents discussed in this chapter.

Calcium Channel Blockers

Contraction of cardiac and smooth muscle cells requires an increase in intracellular calcium levels that occurs as the result of activation of calcium channels. This rise in intracellular calcium stimulates further release of intracellular calcium from its storage site in the sarcoplasmic reticulum. In turn, this causes the activation of calmodulin and myosin kinase, enabling myosin to interact with actin, resulting in excitation-contraction coupling and ultimately vasoconstriction. Calcium channel blockers exert their cardiovascular effects by inhibiting the influx of calcium through voltage-dependent L-type calcium channels located in the cell membrane. The net result is a reduction in intracellular calcium levels in the myocardial cells and smooth muscle cells in the peripheral vasculature, which results in dilation of arteries and arterioles. Calcium channel blockers can be divided into two classes based on their molecular structure and cardiovascular effects: dihydropyridines (DHPs) and non-dihydropyridines (non-DHPs).

Verapamil and Diltiazem

Verapamil and diltiazem are non-DHP calcium channel blockers. Both possess coronary and peripheral vasodilatory effects, resulting in a reduction in systemic vascular resistance and BP. In addition, unlike the DHP calcium channel blockers, these agents also suppress atrioventricular conduction and as such are used in the management of supraventricular arrhythmias. Both agents produce negative inotropic and chronotropic effects (especially verapamil). Because of their electrophysiologic and cardiodepressant effects, these agents should be avoided or used with extreme caution in patients with heart failure or second- or third-degree atrioventricular block. Both agents are available in oral and IV formulations. Intraarterial injection of verapamil has been used to help visualize the peripheral vascular system during hand angiography. Stoeckelhuber et al. studied the effects of verapamil, nitroglycerin, and tolazoline (an α_1-adrenergic antagonist) in 25 patients undergoing brachial artery angiography.[50] Injection of 100 μg of verapamil diluted in 10 mL of normal saline 30 seconds before contrast agent injection was more effective than nitroglycerin and as effective as tolazoline. All three agents were well tolerated with no reported cardiovascular adverse effects.

Intraarterial verapamil has also been used to manage cerebral vasospasm secondary to aneurysmal subarachnoid hemorrhage. In this setting, it has been employed to prevent catheter-induced vasospasm before balloon angioplasty and to treat vasospasm not amenable to balloon angioplasty because of vessel tortuosity or distal location. The average intraarterial dose in this setting is 3 mg, but doses as high as 8 mg have been reported.[51] Improvement is seen in some patients, but the duration of effect is unknown and is expected to be short-lived because of the drug's short

TABLE 23-2. Comparison of Agents Used to Lower Blood Pressure

Agent	Mechanism of Action	Hemodynamic Effects			Dosing
		HR	CO	SVR	
Verapamil	Non-DHP calcium channel blocker	↓	↓	↓	Tachyarrhythmias: 5-10 mg IV push over 2 minutes Hand angiography: 100 µg diluted in 10 mL of normal saline given _intraarterially_ 30 seconds before contrast agent injection Cerebral vasospasm in aneurysmal subarachnoid hemorrhage: 3-8 mg _intraarterially_ per vessel
Diltiazem	Non-DHP calcium channel blocker	↓	↓	↓	Tachyarrhythmias: 0.25 mg/kg IV push followed by a continuous infusion at 5 mg/h titrated to effect
Nicardipine	DHP calcium channel blocker	—/↑	—	↓	Hypertension: 5 mg/h continuous infusion and titrated every 5-15 minutes to a maximum of 15 mg/h Cerebral vasospasm in aneurysmal subarachnoid hemorrhage: 1-5 mg _intraarterially_ per vessel
Labetalol	α_1, β_1, and β_2 blocker	—/↓	—/↓	↓	Hypertension: IV bolus of 10-20 mg, repeated or doubled every 10 minutes (up to 300 mg) _or_ as a continuous infusion starting at 2 mg/min (after an initial bolus dose) and titrated to the desired effect
Esmolol	β_1 blocker	↓	↓	—/↓	Tachyarrhythmias/hypertension: 500 µg/kg loading dose (optional), followed by a continuous infusion at 25-50 µg/kg/min and titrated to desired effect
Nitroglycerin	↑ cGMP	—	—/↑	↓	Heart failure/unstable angina: continuous infusion of 25 to 200 µg/min
Nitroprusside	↑ cGMP	—/↑	↓/↑	↓	Heart failure/hypertension: 0.25-0.5 µg/kg/min, titrated every few minutes in 0.5 µg/kg/min increments to effect. Maximum dose 10 µg/kg/min
Enalaprilat	ACE inhibitor	—	↑	↓	Heart failure/hypertension: 0.625-1.25 mg IV q6h, titrated in 12-hour intervals to a maximum of 5 mg IV q6h
Hydralazine	Arteriolar vasodilator	↑	↑	↓	Hypertension: 10-20 mg IV q4-6h as needed
Papaverine	Phosphodiesterase inhibitor	—	—	↓	Cerebral vasospasm in aneurysmal subarachnoid hemorrhage: 300 mg of a 0.3% solution delivered to the affected vascular territory over 20-30 min

ACE, Angiotensin-converting enzyme; _cGMP,_ cyclic guanosine monophosphate; _CO,_ cardiac output; _DHP,_ dihydropyridine; _HR,_ heart rate; _IV,_ intravenous; _SVR,_ systemic vascular resistance.

half-life. Although effects on systemic hemodynamics are minimal, close monitoring is warranted.

Nicardipine

Nicardipine is a DHP calcium channel blocker available in an IV formulation. It has no effects on the sinoatrial or atrioventricular node and produces a dose-related decrease in systemic vascular resistance and small increases in cardiac output. Administration of nicardipine can produce a reflex tachycardia. Nicardipine has a rapid onset of action (5-15 minutes) and a half-life of 8.6 hours. It is given as a continuous infusion starting at 5 mg/h and titrated every 5 to 15 minutes to a maximum of 15 mg/h. Because nicardipine is metabolized in the liver, hepatic insufficiency can lead to accumulation and thus prolongation of its effects.

Intraarterial nicardipine, like verapamil, has been used for management of cerebral vasospasm in aneurysmal subarachnoid hemorrhage. It can be diluted to a concentration of 0.1 mg/mL with 0.9% NaCl and given in 1-mL aliquots up to a recommended maximum of 5 mg per vessel, with the total dose being determined by angiographic response. Badjatia et al. reported on 44 vessels in 18 patients with vasospasm receiving intraarterial nicardipine.[52] All vessels responded promptly, and mean peak systolic velocities as measured by transcranial Doppler imaging remained significantly reduced from baseline for 4 days after administration, suggesting a sustained effect. Hemodynamic changes were minimal, and 5 of the 14 patients experienced transient unsustained elevations in intracranial pressure. One patient experienced a sustained increase in intracranial pressure requiring discontinuation of therapy. Further study is warranted to determine safety and clinical outcomes.

Nifedipine

Nifedipine is a DHP calcium channel blocker available in immediate release (IR) and extended release (XL) oral formulations. Sublingual (SL) and IR nifedipine have been used in the management of hypertensive urgency and emergency. However, this method of BP management is strongly discouraged. Sublingual nifedipine has been associated with exacerbating myocardial ischemia and infarction in this setting, and its effects on BP are unpredictable and difficult to titrate.[53-55] Given the availability of safer and more titratable agents, use of SL or IR nifedipine should be completely abandoned.

ADRENERGIC ANTAGONISTS

Labetalol

Labetalol is an adrenergic antagonist available in both IV and oral formulations. It produces selective blockade of the α_1 receptor and nonselective blockade of the β_1 and β_2 receptors. The β-blockade effects predominate, the ratio of which is dependent on route of administration. Oral labetalol possesses a 3:1 β-to-α blockade ratio, whereas IV labetalol has a 7:1 ratio.[56] Hemodynamically, labetalol reduces systemic vascular resistance. In addition, the β_1 effects blunt any reflex tachycardia, maintaining or slightly reducing heart rate.

Labetalol can be administered as an IV bolus of 10 to 20 mg, which can be repeated or doubled every 10 minutes (up to a total of 300 mg), with peak effects occurring 5 to 10 minutes after a dose. Labetalol can also be administered as a continuous infusion starting at 2 mg/min (after an initial bolus dose) and titrated to the desired effect. The half-life of labetalol is 2 to 8 hours, with a single IV dose lasting 3 to 6 hours. It undergoes extensive metabolism in the liver, with 85% removed with a single pass; as such, patients with extensive hepatic disease may experience prolonged effects. Potential adverse effects are consistent with labetalol's pharmacodynamics and include bradycardia, second- or third-degree atrioventricular block, heart failure, and exacerbation of asthma or chronic obstructive pulmonary disease.

Esmolol

Esmolol is a "cardioselective" adrenergic antagonist producing selective β_1 blockade in usual doses. It is available in IV form only, and the effects are similar to those of other selective β-blockers and include reduction of heart rate, BP, and cardiac contractility. One advantage of esmolol over other β-blockers is its ultrashort half-life (9 minutes), making it easy to titrate and readily reversible in the event of hypotension. In addition, esmolol is metabolized by esterases in the cytosol of red blood cells, so its pharmacokinetics are unaltered in the setting of renal or hepatic dysfunction. Esmolol is given as a loading dose of 500 µg/kg, followed by a continuous infusion at 25 to 50 µg/kg/min titrated to effect. The bolus dose can be eliminated or reduced in patients with underlying cardiac pathology. Adverse effects are similar to those listed for labetalol. Although esmolol is highly selective for the β_1 receptor, caution should be exercised in patients with bronchospastic disease, particularly at higher doses.

NITRATES

Nitroglycerin

Nitroglycerin is an organic nitrate that is converted to nitric oxide. Nitric oxide then activates guanylate cyclase and produces vasodilatation of venous and arterial beds via the cyclic guanosine monophosphate pathway. In general, venous vasodilation predominates, producing a reduction in preload. In addition to effects on the systemic vasculature, nitroglycerin produces vasodilation of the coronary arteries and veins, resulting in increased coronary blood

flow. These effects, coupled with its ability to reduce preload, make this a useful agent in the management of heart failure and unstable angina. Usual doses of nitroglycerin range from 25 to 200 µg/min, but doses as high as 1000 µg/min have been used to treat pulmonary edema. It is important to note that tachyphylaxis to nitrates is not uncommon and typically presents as early as 24 hours after initiation, necessitating increasing doses to maintain the same hemodynamic effects. Tachyphylaxis can be overcome by providing a nitrate-free interval of 10 to 12 hours daily when clinically feasible.

Nitroprusside

Nitroprusside is a potent arterial and venous vasodilator, producing both preload and afterload reduction. On administration, nitroprusside is broken down to nitric oxide and cyanide, with the nitric oxide producing the vasodilatory effects. The cyanide produced from nitroprusside is converted in the liver to thiocyanate (this reaction requires adequate thiosulfate stores), which is less toxic than cyanide. Thiocyanate is then eliminated in the urine. Therefore, patients with hepatic and/or renal dysfunction are susceptible to the toxic effects of cyanide and thiocyanate, which are severe and potentially life threatening. The usual starting dose of nitroprusside is 0.25 to 0.5 µg/kg/min, titrated every few minutes in 0.5-µg/kg/min increments to effect. The maximal dose is 10 µg/kg/min, but cyanide toxicity has been manifested with doses as low as 3 to 5 µg/kg/min for a sustained period.[57] Nitroprusside is extremely fast acting (onset in seconds), is readily titratable with a half-life of 3 minutes, and has minimal effects on heart rate.

ANGIOTENSIN-CONVERTING ENZYME INHIBITORS

Inhibition of circulating angiotensin-converting enzyme (ACE) with ACE inhibitors (ACEIs) results in a reduction in angiotensin II and its vasoconstrictive effects, as well as an upregulation of bradykinin and its vasodilatory properties. This results in peripheral vasodilatation and a reduction in systemic vascular resistance, with no direct effects on heart rate or cardiac contractility. In addition, these agents exhibit a beneficial effect on renal hemodynamics through vasodilatation of the efferent arteriole, with resultant reduction in glomerular hydrostatic pressure. Although these properties produce a renoprotective effect in the long term, in the acute setting they could precipitate acute renal failure through a rapid reduction in glomerular filtration rate. These agents should be avoided in patients with underlying renal insufficiency or renal artery stenosis. In addition, ACEIs may make patients more susceptible to the nephrotoxic effects of IV contrast medium and should be discontinued before its use.

Enalaprilat is the only ACEI available in an IV formulation. Its onset of action is approximately 15 minutes, with peak response occurring 30 minutes after an IV dose. The usual IV dose is 1.25 mg every 6 hours, titrated in 12-hour intervals to a maximum of 5 mg every 6 hours. Of note, one adverse effect of ACE inhibition is angioedema, the cause of which is thought to be increased levels of bradykinin. Patients undergoing fibrinolysis with tissue plasminogen activator (tPA) in the presence of an ACEI may be at an increased risk of this adverse event, because tPA cleaves plasminogen to plasmin, which in turn cleaves high-molecular-weight kininogen, with resultant bradykinin production.[58]

OTHER VASODILATORS

Hydralazine

Hydralazine is a direct-acting arterial vasodilator available in IV and oral formulations. The usual IV dose of hydralazine is 10 to 20 mg (up to 40 mg) every 4 to 6 hours as needed. Its onset of action after an IV dose is 5 to 15 minutes. Hydralazine is eliminated via the liver and has a half-life of 3 to 5 hours. However, the duration of effect may last as long as 30 to 140 hours after a single dose, which may be related to binding of hydralazine to the arterial vasculature.[59,60] There are numerous adverse effects of hydralazine, including systemic lupus erythematosus with long-term use. Given the availability of alternative agents with more favorable side-effect profiles and more reliable dose-effect relationships, hydralazine is recommended only in patients with allergies or contraindications to alternative agents such as β-adrenergic blockers or ACEIs.

Papaverine

Papaverine is a nonspecific smooth muscle relaxant producing arterial and arteriolar vasodilation. Its mechanism of action is poorly understood but thought to be related to increased intracellular levels of cyclic adenosine monophosphate via inhibition of phosphodiesterase. Intraarterial papaverine has been used in the management of refractory vasospasm in the setting of aneurysmal subarachnoid hemorrhage. When administered for this purpose, the typical dose is 300 mg of a 0.3% solution (prepared by diluting 300 mg of papaverine in 100 mL of 0.9% NaCl) delivered to the affected vascular territory over 20 to 30 minutes.[61] Known side effects of intraarterial papaverine include mydriasis (particularly when infusion is proximal to the ophthalmic artery), seizure, hypotension, transient respiratory arrest and cardiac dysfunction (when infused into the posterior circulation), and papaverine precipitation and microcrystal deposition.[62] Because of these known side effects and the availability of intraarterial nicardipine and verapamil, intraarterial use of papaverine has fallen out of favor in many large interventional neuroradiology programs.

KEY POINTS

- Vasoactive agents may be employed for multiple therapeutic and diagnostic purposes.
- Safe and effective use of vasoactive agents requires:
  - An understanding of the pharmacology, hemodynamic effects, and adverse effects of the available agents.
  - Close observation and monitoring of predefined therapeutic and hemodynamic endpoints.

▸ SUGGESTED READINGS

Marik PE, Varon J. Hypertensive crises: challenges and management. Chest 2007;131:1949–62.
Dellinger RP, Levy MM, Carlet JM, et al. Surviving Sepsis Campaign: international guidelines for management of severe sepsis and septic shock: 2008. Crit Care Med 2008;36(1):296–327.

The complete reference list is available online at www.expertconsult.com.

CHAPTER 24
Antibiotic Prophylaxis in Interventional Radiology

David R. Sopko and Tony P. Smith

INTRODUCTION

Infection following any procedure that violates the skin's protective barrier is well known throughout all medical disciplines and contributes to significant morbidity, not to mention increased healthcare costs. Despite the universalization of aseptic technique and the expansive variety of antimicrobial drugs at our disposal, infection remains a frequent complication encountered by the interventional radiologist. In the recent past, numerous authors, including the Society of Interventional Radiology via their Practice Guidelines statement,[1] have performed comprehensive reviews of the current literature in an attempt to summarize and condense the body of data available. What these documents have revealed is that the practices currently in place at the majority of institutions have roots founded and supported primarily by the surgical literature.[2-5] Additionally noted is that despite the vastly prevailing opinion that antibiotic prophylaxis has become the standard of care, very little substantiation in the form of randomized controlled trials can be found.

The issue of appropriate periprocedural antibiotic prophylaxis will certainly continue to arise as the breadth of procedures provided by interventional radiology expands. For all procedures, patient-specific (age, weight, allergies, renal and hepatic function) and community-specific (formulary selection, local resistance) factors, in addition to weighting of the overall risks and benefits of antibiotic prophylaxis, must be considered. Consultation with appropriate specialists (e.g., pharmacy, infectious disease service) are highly encouraged when any questions or inconsistencies arise. It is important to note that the whole of medicine, not excluding the surgical or interventional radiology community, has in the recent past begun to reevaluate the role of periprocedural antibiotic prophylaxis as emerging issues such as resistance and cost-driven delivery of health care move to the forefront.[5-7] Ultimately, the responsibility lies with the interventional radiologist, who must conclude whether prophylactic antibiotic use is appropriate, identify the best antimicrobial agent, and oversee timely delivery.

ANTIBIOTIC PROPHYLAXIS

Many factors impact whether a patient is at elevated risk for periprocedural infection, and some aspects may not be resolved clinically (i.e., comorbidities, bacteremia) prior to the necessary performance of an intervention. However, preventive measures such as meticulous attention to sterile draping, handwashing, and sterile technique remain crucial to infection control in the interventional suite. Although universal application of these precautions should be independent of the decision for or against prophylactic antibiotic use, the National Academy of Sciences/National Research Council's surgical procedures classification system

can be applied in the interventional suite to guide use of prophylactic antimicrobial agents.[8] It is known that infection rates associated with interventional procedures differ from surgical counterparts,[9] but the characterization of a procedure as *clean, clean-contaminated, contaminated,* or *dirty* can predict infection risk associated with a given anatomic location. Importantly, these groupings take into consideration both the general health of tissues within the operative field and successful execution of aseptic technique for the duration of the procedure.

Clean procedures carry a 5% risk of infectious complication. These interventions maintain sterile technique in tissue with no obvious inflammation, and do not involve anatomic structures with potential bacterial colonization/infection (e.g., genitourinary [GU], gastrointestinal [GI], respiratory tract).[3,8] *Clean-contaminated procedures* convey a 10% risk of periprocedural infection. In this group, the GU, GI, or biliary tract may be entered, but inflammation is clearly absent at the time of the procedure, and aseptic techniques are maintained throughout.[3,8] Any major break in sterile technique results in a *contaminated procedure*, as does entry into obviously inflamed tissues,[3,8] save for those harboring purulent material. A contaminated intervention's risk of infection doubles that of clean-contaminated, at approximately 20%. Procedures with clearly infected material, including clinically infected GU or biliary systems or a GI perforation, make up the final conglomerate, *dirty procedures*. It is predicted that nearly 40% of dirty procedures result in infectious periprocedural complications.[3,8] Routine prophylactic antimicrobial agents are currently recommended for all procedures except those considered clean. Institution-specific formulary geographic bacterial resistance tendencies, as well as expense, should be considered prior to selection of an appropriate agent.[1,5,9]

Efficacious antibiotic prophylaxis has been shown to be a time- and dose-sensitive practice. A clearly defined window spanning from 1 hour prior to the procedure up to the time of initial incision has been validated by the surgical literature. A delay in administrating the prophylactic agent may increase the risk of periprocedural infectious complication by up to a factor of 5,[2,10,11] and several studies provide evidence that antimicrobial therapy initiated postoperatively is equivalent to no prophylaxis.[2,10] At our institution, we wait until the patient is in the interventional suite to initiate antibiotic prophylaxis. Providing prophylaxis via a reliable route (i.e., intravenously [IV]) and in adherence with temporal guidelines ensures that adequate serum antibiotic concentrations are achieved for maximal inhibitory effect.[12]

Several studies have disproved the previously held perception of superior efficacy of multidose prophylaxis regimens; a solitary dose achieves adequate prophylactic effect.[5,13,14] Important exceptions to single-dose prophylaxis include: (1) prolonged procedures lasting longer than 2 hours and (2) intervention on an obstructed structure such as the biliary tree, GU system, or other similar viscus. An auxiliary dose of the prophylactic agent should be administered under the direction of the interventionist for procedures exceeding 2 hours, taking into account the pharmacokinetics of the specific agent used.[5] In patients with a known obstructed system, the risk of bacterial translocation and inoculation of the lymphatic or vascular system, with resultant bacteremia or sepsis, is increased.[2,15] Therefore, therapeutic doses of antimicrobial agents should be continued for at least 48 hours following intervention or until adequate drainage has been achieved.[5] Particularly in the inpatient setting, it is not uncommon for the referring service to manage antibiotic administration in the immediate postprocedural period. Prompt communication of the necessity for continued treatment must be clearly provided by the interventionist and his/her team to ensure sustained therapy.

ANTIBIOTIC RESISTANCE

Similar to other procedural subspecialties, interventional radiology has realized a continuous increase in the overall volume of cases, particularly the placement of invasive devices. Concurrently, infectious periprocedural complications have followed a similar upward-sloping trend.[5] One would expect that, all other variables remaining constant, these tendencies would abide to a linear plot. It is striking then that the trends are not collinear, a finding that can be greatly attributed to the emergence of a variety of antibiotic-resistant microbial strains including methicillin-resistant *Staphylococcus aureus* (MRSA), vancomycin-resistant enterococci (VRE), and β-lactamase–producing gram-negative rods.[16] Resistance may be conferred between bacteria by horizontal gene transmission, known as *conjugation*, or by spontaneous mutation. These impressive microbial strategies are driven by the most clinically relevant contributor to the proliferation of resistant strains: inappropriate, nonspecific use of broad-spectrum antibiotics[17] in both healthy and immunocompromised patients.[5]

The latest generation of antibiotics for treatment of VRE species includes daptomycin, quinupristin-dalfopristin, and linezolid. These agents specifically attack the permeability of the bacterial membrane, or synthesis of protein/peptidoglycans integral to proper membrane function.[18] As the battle to develop newer antimicrobial agents continues, a refocusing of the medical community's efforts towards improved preventive techniques targeted at these dangerous strains and their mode of transmission is necessary. When a prophylactic antimicrobial agent is selected, special consideration of the most likely pathogen and source should guide the interventionist to not only prevent patient morbidity and mortality but also deter further contribution to antibiotic resistance. Complacency in the prevention of horizontal transmission and appropriate therapeutic selection today will inevitably result in a greater number of resistant organisms in the future.[19]

ANTIMICROBIAL HYPERSENSITIVITY

All too frequently, one is faced with the patient reporting an antibiotic allergy. It is known that many of these self-reported reactions do not represent a true immune-mediated reaction. Anaphylactic reactions are rare and include hives, bronchospasm, hypotension, and laryngospasm. An accurate detailed history should be obtained to determine the true nature of the complaint. The true incidence of hypersensitivity with the penicillins and other related β-lactams is near 2%. Cephalosporin cross-reactivity is a concern but occurs in only 15% of patients with previous adverse reaction to the penicillins. As a result, penicillins and cephalosporins should be withheld in patients with documentation of severe reaction. Instead, antimicrobials lacking the β-lactam fundamental structure, such as vancomycin, should be used,[5] with the monobactams and carbapenems other potential choices. Patients reporting minor reactions such as fever and/or a typical maculopapular rash can safely receive β-lactams without concern for anaphylactoid reaction.[20]

ANTIBIOTIC AGENTS

Antimicrobial agents achieve their desired toxicity by exploiting several mechanisms of bacterial homeostasis. Cell wall–specific agents include the penicillins, cephalosporins, and vancomycin (wall synthesis), in addition to amphotericin, polymyxin, and daptomycin (wall permeability). Protein synthesis is targeted by the aminoglycosides, macrolides, tetracycline, and linezolid, while nucleic acid synthesis is inhibited by the sulfonamides and quinolones. Even when correctly selected for the most likely bacteria, delivery of the agent must result in serum and tissue concentrations that exceed a minimum inhibitory concentration (MIC) of the organism so that effective interference with the desired process can occur.[12]

More information on the specific antibiotic agents commonly used in interventional procedures is available at www.expertconsult.com.

PROCEDURE-SPECIFIC ANTIBIOTIC PROPHYLAXIS

Generally, for clean procedures with associated periprocedural risk of infection near 5%, antibiotic prophylaxis is not indicated. However, the interventionist must appraise the clinical presentation, comorbidities, and anticipated microbes to decide whether prophylaxis is appropriate. In the setting of sparse level 1 data, the majority of what follows are guidelines. They are not intended to be restrictive, and considerable latitude with respect to selection and application is commonplace. Table e24-1 offers a brief overview of these recommendations.

Vascular Procedures

Venous Interventions
Central venous catheter (CVC) insertion is the most frequently performed procedure in the interventional suite, and has not been immune to controversy surrounding antibiotic prophylaxis. Because these are clean procedures, no prophylactic antibiotic use is recommended, even for tunneled catheter insertion, in the routine setting. Introduction of typical skin flora (coagulase-negative *S. aureus*) into the catheter tract is the predominant route of inoculation.[5] Aside from aseptic technique, several strategies can be used to minimize introduction of pathogens into the procedural

field. These include insertion of devices with the least number of lumens,[5] and placement of totally implantable devices for patients anticipating long-term use. The Centers for Disease Control and Prevention (CDC) issued guidelines further highlighting preventive strategies, including: (1) preferential use of 2% chlorhexidine cleansing solution, (2) minimizing catheter exchange to prevent infection, and (3) employment of antimicrobial-impregnated catheters in patients with previous infection.[21] Even though no unifying statement has been issued, patients with potentially depressed immune status, including initiation of chemotherapy, and those who possess an established history of frequent catheter-related infections may benefit from antimicrobial prophylaxis.[22] Oncology patients may also benefit from use of vancomycin/heparin flush following insertion.[22] Cefazolin 1 g IV is the preferred antimicrobial. Alternatively, vancomycin or clindamycin may be employed in the penicillin allergic when prophylaxis is desired.

Patients presenting with venous thromboembolism may possess contraindications to adequate anticoagulation, making them poor candidates for this therapeutic option. In these patients, placement of an inferior vena cava (IVC) filter may be indicated. There are little data describing significant morbidity associated with periprocedural infection related to IVC filter placement. To our knowledge, only one case report of infection following IVC filter placement exists.[23] In this patient, insertion was performed via a pre-existing CVC access site. Antibiotic prophylaxis is therefore not routine; it can be used at the interventionist's discretion for filter placement in patients with known bacteremia or outward signs of systemic infection.[3,23] In such patients, prophylaxis should be targeted to the known isolated organism or more generically to normal skin flora. It is unclear what role retrievable IVC filters may play in this particular patient population.

The armamentarium of procedures available to treat superficial venous insufficiency includes endovascular methods (i.e., thermal/laser ablation, sclerotherapy) or phlebectomy. Nerve injury, superficial phlebitis, and deep venous thrombosis (DVT) are more frequent complications in these patients. Infection is rare, so no recommendation for antimicrobial prophylaxis exists.

Arterial Interventions

When meticulous aseptic technique is observed, routine diagnostic angiography and associated simple percutaneous endovascular interventions such as angioplasty or thrombolysis are considered clean. Several authors have documented transient and inconsequential bacteremia in 4% to 8% of procedures requiring arterial puncture.[24,25] Similar to repeated surgical incision, recurrent arterial puncture at the same site may increase the risk of infection over that of primary access.[26] The pathogens encountered include typical skin flora (e. g., *Staphylococcus epidermidis*, *Streptococcus* spp., *Corynebacterium*), with inoculation most likely due to unintentional break in sterile technique during the preparation and handling of catheters and guidewires.[2,24] No antimicrobial prophylaxis is recommended for these procedures.

Infection related to percutaneous arterial stent placement is uncommon but potentially severe in consequence. Many patients are asymptomatic despite active infection and frequently present in a delayed fashion with fever, localized pain, and leukocytosis. Being a foreign body, a stent can contribute to both localized inflammation and arteritis.[27] It can also serve as a nidus for the adherence of bacteria, enabling subsequent translocation into the vascular/perivascular tissues. This may culminate in pseudoaneurysm formation[28] or acute vascular rupture. Known predictors of escalated risk for stent infection include use of a vascular sheath with over 24 hours of dwell time,[29] as well as secondary access in less than 1 week's time.[30] This is particularly true following use of percutaneous closure devices.[31] Current recommendations for stent placement parallel those of routine angiography, though in patients with known risk factors, their use is not uncommon. Standard regimens include cefazolin 1 g IV in appropriately selected patients. For penicillin-allergic individuals, either vancomycin 1 g or clindamycin 600 to 900 mg are acceptable substitutes.

Infection related to synthetic graft material is associated with high morbidity and mortality.[5,32] Routine antibiotic prophylaxis for endovascular aneurysm repair (EVAR) is administered at many institutions, but its use is certainly a point of contention. Reintervention is frequent following EVAR,[33] as are repeat interventions in dialysis accesses that may also necessitate stent-graft use. Protocols for stent-graft placement prophylaxis are similar to those for high-risk angiographic procedures.

Nonvascular Procedures: Hepatobiliary Interventions

Biliary Interventions

The unaltered native biliary tree should be free from bacterial colonization. In contradistinction, intervention in the setting of biliary obstruction (either benign or malignant) and/or the presence of hepatolithiasis must be approached carefully, and the target system assumed contaminated.[34,35] Antimicrobial prophylaxis is nearly universal in most practices[4] because infectious complications can approach 50% in its absence.[34] One can account for the greater risk of infectious complications with percutaneous biliary drain (PBD) placement when compared to simple percutaneous cholangiography (PTC) by noting more prolonged procedure time and greater intraprocedural manipulation necessary for the former.[36] Microbes of particular virulence with a higher potential for mortality include *Clostridium* spp. and *Escherichia coli*,[5] with regimens targeting these groups in addition to other gram-negative aerobes. Predictors of colonization and subsequent infectious complication include febrile illness, cholangitis, hepatolithiasis/choledocholithiasis, coagulopathy, proximal or malignant obstruction, bilioenteric anastomosis, and prior biliary intervention.[37,38] Indeed, extended administration of antimicrobial agents beyond the periprocedural period is frequent following biliary interventions. Biliary cultures, though rarely acquired, can help one formulate appropriately targeted therapeutic continuation of antibiotics until relief of obstruction is successfully attained.[5,34,37]

Ceftriaxone (1 g IV) is the drug most frequently used at our and other institutions, owing to its simple dosage, biliary excretion, and long biological half-life. Ampicillin/sulbactam (1.5-3 g IV) is an excellent alternative, with potent activity against most *Enterococcus* spp., as are ampicillin (2 g IV) with gentamicin (1.5 mg/kg IV).[5] In the patient with penicillin allergy and previous cephalosporin cross-reactivity, vancomycin or clindamycin may be employed.

Transjugular Intrahepatic Portosystemic Shunt

With the advent of a covered stent platform and its resultant superior patency profile, creation of a transjugular intrahepatic portosystemic shunt (TIPS) is now widely advocated in patients with clinical manifestations of portal hypertension. When considering TIPS-related infection, there are those with and (more commonly) those without stent infection.[5,34] In patients referred for TIPS, multiple comorbidities are the rule and likely contribute to decreased ability to mount an appropriate immune response to infection. For this reason, the majority of interventionists use antibiotic prophylaxis despite the data being far from convincing.[39] Target microbes are skin flora, in addition to *E. coli, Enterobacter/Enterococcus* spp., and other gram-negatives including anaerobes.[34] Typical regimens include ceftriaxone 1 g IV or ampicillin/sulbactam 1.5 to 3 g IV, with vancomycin or clindamycin reserved for the penicillin allergic.

Stent infection does demand discussion, typically occurring approximately 3 months following TIPS creation. This must be considered in the patient with fever and bacteremia of unknown cause[40] or other clinical manifestations such as tender hepatomegaly, septic pulmonary emboli, or sepsis.[5,41] Appropriate investigation of the TIPS for thrombosis or stent-associated vegetation should be undertaken. Most patients respond to IV antimicrobial therapy with resolution of bacteremia.

Nonvascular Procedures: Genitourinary Interventions

Percutaneous Nephrostomy Tubes and Nephroureteral Stents

Fortunately, septic shock, even in the setting of pyonephrosis, is uncommon.[42-44] However, bacteremia is frequent following even simple GU interventions such as percutaneous nephrostomy (PCN) tube exchange.[43] In the absence of obstruction, infection, and/or previous intervention, common GU procedures are classified as clean-contaminated. On the opposite end of the spectrum, a clinically infected collecting system must be considered dirty,[3] with gram-negative bacilli (i.e., *E. coli, Proteus/Klebsiella/Enterococcus* species) the most likely culprits. All other conditions may therefore collectively be considered contaminated. Risk factors such as diabetes mellitus, indwelling catheters, previous GU intervention, ureteroenteric anastomosis, detrusor dysfunction, and nephrolithiasis all predispose the patient to periprocedural infection.[3,5] Accurate identification of such comorbidities assists in triage of patients requiring antimicrobial prophylaxis, resulting in up to a fivefold reduction in serious periprocedural infections.[45]

Most agree antibiotic prophylaxis is generally indicated for GU interventions. The cephalosporins cefazolin/ceftriaxone (1 g IV) are most commonly used, especially in patients with no known risk factors. Ampicillin/sulbactam (1.5-3 g IV) or ampicillin (2 g IV) combined with gentamicin (1.5 mg/kg IV) may be alternatively used, particularly for those patients with documented risk factors for infection related to GU procedures. For the penicillin allergic, either vancomycin or clindamycin may be substituted. Similar to the biliary tree, antimicrobial therapy should ideally be guided by urinary cultures and continued in the setting of obstruction until adequate diversion or restoration of native flow is achieved. If no signs or symptoms of sepsis arise following intervention, antimicrobial agents need not be continued further. No clear benefit of antibiotic prophylaxis during routine tube exchanges has been shown,[43] so its use is at the discretion of the operator.

Uterine Artery Embolization

Infection following uterine artery embolization (UAE) is exceedingly rare (<1%) and often delayed in presentation. Trends in antibiotic prophylaxis are mainly guided by case reports of fatal sepsis.[46-50] No specific risk factors have as of yet been clearly identified to accurately predict periprocedural infection.[51,52] Nonetheless, many interventionists do give prophylactic antibiotics to patients with hydrosalpinx or intrauterine devices.[1]

The typical pathogens are skin flora, and the usual antimicrobial agent is cefazolin 1 g IV. Ampicillin/sulbactam 1.5 to 3 g IV may also be used, and either clindamycin 900 mg IV with gentamicin 1.5 mg/kg IV or vancomycin reserved for the penicillin allergic. A prolonged prophylactic course of doxycycline 100 mg twice daily for 1 week prior to UAE may be considered for hydrosalpinx.[1]

Interventional Oncology Procedures

Hepatic Embolization and Chemoembolization

Bacteremia following angiography paired with either particle or chemoembolization is known to be more frequent than with angiography alone.[25] Hepatic abscess following embolization, while less common than bacteremia, may be more frequent in the setting of prior biliary surgery or in those lacking an intact sphincter of Oddi.[53] The suspected mechanism is bile duct ischemia with potential infarct of colonized biliary radicals. Portal vein occlusion and biliary obstruction also result in an increased risk of periprocedural infection/abscess formation.[54] Skin flora are the most commonly encountered pathogens, with gram-negative intestinal isolates following in prevalence. The latter are found in greater frequency in patients with biliary obstruction or prior biliary surgery.

Similar to other solid organ/tumor embolizations, to avoid bacterial translocation, abscess, and possible sepsis, antibiotic prophylaxis is recommended for hepatic embolization.[5,9,25] Ceftriaxone 1 g IV may be effectively used for either. Patients undergoing chemoembolization may receive ampicillin/sulbactam 1.5 to 3 g IV, ampicillin 2 g IV with gentamicin 1.5 mg/kg IV, or cefazolin 1 g IV with metronidazole 500 mg IV.[5,9] Following bilioenteric anastomoses, patients should undergo bowel preparation on the day prior to chemoembolization, in addition to antimicrobial prophylaxis with piperacillin/tazobactam or other agent.[53,55] No specialized recommendation currently exists for radio-embolization with yttrium-90.

Percutaneous Tumor Ablation

Percutaneous ablative techniques once confined to the liver are now used throughout the body, including the lung, bone, and GU tract. Cholangitis and liver abscess following percutaneous hepatic radiofrequency ablation (RFA) are uncommon (<1.5%) but possibly fatal.[56] Abscess formation may be delayed for several weeks and may be identified early with careful postoperative clinical evaluation and follow-up. Similar to hepatic embolization, altered sphincter of Oddi function (e.g., sphincterotomy, bilioenteric anastomosis, stent placement) is thought to portend a greater risk for periprocedural infection with hepatic ablation,[34] whereas in the GU system, nephrolithiasis and hydronephrosis are thought to increase the risk of periprocedural infection. In contradistinction to embolization, where bacterial translocation is thought to be the mechanism, infection following thermal therapy occurs via direct inoculation of the ablation zone,[57] most frequently by typical skin flora but potentially from enteric sources.

Administration of prophylactic antimicrobial agents is variable and controversial, with no unified recommendation. The most frequent agent is ampicillin/sulbactam 1.5 to 3 g IV, followed by third-generation cephalosporins with gram-negative coverage.

VALVULAR HEART DISEASE

The most recent (2007) American Heart Association (AHA) recommendations for infective endocarditis (IE) prophylaxis brought significant changes.[58] Patients at greatest risk for unexpected and untoward outcomes should receive appropriate prophylactic regimens and include: previous IE, prosthetic valves, unrepaired cyanotic congenital heart disease (CHD), CHD with conduits or shunts, CHD partially repaired with prosthetic material and persistent defects, and cardiac transplant recipients with valvular dysfunction.[58,59] Special consideration is given to CHD completely repaired with prosthetic material, where antimicrobial prophylaxis is recommended regardless of approach—surgical or percutaneous—for a period of 6 months postoperatively. Revised from previous recommendations, mitral valve prolapse and hypertrophic cardiomyopathy no longer need prophylaxis. Percutaneous valves are emerging as a therapeutic option in patients with valvular disease and relative poor health contributing to poor surgical candidacy. It is likely antibiotic prophylaxis will be indicated for these procedures, but to date this has not been defined.

The prophylactic agent chosen depends upon the anatomic location of the intended intervention and suspected pathogens. For respiratory interventions, the regimen should target *Streptococcus viridans*, so ampicillin or amoxicillin (2 g IV) or cephalosporins (cefazolin or ceftriaxone 1 g IV) are preferred. Clindamycin 600 mg or vancomycin 1 g IV for penicillin-reactive patients may be used. Prophylaxis is no longer recommended for routine GI and GU procedures if the sole purpose is to prevent infective endocarditis. However, *Enterococcus* spp. draw the greatest attention in this anatomic distribution, especially given rapidly developing resistance.[60] Treatment and elimination of known enterococcal colonization prior to even routine exchange would be ideal, but if not achievable, amoxicillin

or ampicillin 2 g IV, vancomycin 1 g IV, or clindamycin 600 to 900 mg IV are the most favorable prophylactic agents.

SUMMARY

Optimal, accurate, and efficacious use of antibiotic prophylaxis in the interventional radiology suite demands a wide breadth of knowledge spanning pharmacology and infectious disease, in addition to anatomy and physiology.[61] Current practice tendencies and guidelines continue to lack level 1 support. Prior to selecting an appropriate agent, the prudent operator must take into account the risk of the procedure, anatomic distribution, and likely microbes to be encountered, as well as factors unique to the individual patient (e.g., comorbidities, allergic history, culture and sensitivity data). Specifically targeted therapy is preferred when possible. When challenging cases arise, one must not be afraid to request expert consultation from infectious disease and pharmacy specialists to guide and optimize antibiotic prophylaxis.

KEY POINTS

- The variety of interventional procedures continues to expand, yet the body of literature regarding the use of antibiotic prophylaxis remains sparse.

- Procedure and patient-specific factors, as well as evolving antibiotic resistance and institution-specific considerations, must be accounted for when selecting appropriate prophylactic regimens.

- Specialist consultation should be sought should questions arise, or for particularly challenging cases.

► **SUGGESTED READINGS**

Brown DB, Cardella JF, Sacks D, et al. Quality improvement guidelines for transhepatic arterial chemoembolization, embolization, and chemotherapeutic infusion for hepatic malignancy. J Vasc Interv Radiol 2009;20(7 Suppl):S219–S226.

Miller DL, O'Grady NP. Guidelines for the prevention of intravascular catheter-related infections: recommendations relevant to interventional radiology. J Vasc Interv Radiol 2003;14(2 part 1):133–6.

Venkatesan, AM, Kundu S, Sacks D, et al. Practice guideline for adult antibiotic prophylaxis during vascular and interventional radiology procedures. J Vasc Interv Radiol 2010;121:1611–30.

Wilson W, Taubert KA, Gewitz M, et al. Prevention of infective endocarditis: guidelines from the American Heart Association. A guideline from the American Heart Association Rheumatic Fever, Endocarditis, and Kawasaki Disease Committee, Council on Cardiovascular Disease in the Young, and the Council on Clinical Cardiology, Council on Cardiovascular Surgery and Anesthesia, and the Quality of Care and Outcomes Research Interdisciplinary Working Group. Circulation 2007;116(15):1736–54.

The complete reference list is available online at www.expertconsult.com.

CHAPTER 25

Angioplasty

Shawn N. Sarin, Eberhard Zeitler*, Reinhard Loose, Prasanna Vasudevan, and Anthony C. Venbrux

Percutaneous transluminal angioplasty (PTA) is based on the diagnostic percutaneous catheter techniques introduced by Sven Seldinger in 1953. PTA was first introduced by Charles Dotter and Melvin Judkins in Portland, Oregon, in 1964 as a method to treat arteriosclerotic occlusion in arteries.

The year 1974 marked the beginning of a new era of PTA, with introduction of the double-lumen balloon catheter by Andreas Gruentzig. Remarkable technical and clinical results were achieved. Because of the smaller outer diameter of the balloon catheter in the deflated state, local complications at the puncture site could be reduced, and the dilation force on stenotic lesions in the vessel could be adapted to the diameter of each artery by using different balloon diameters. Balloons were inflated to maximal force with solutions of contrast material. Such inflation enabled the operator to achieve excellent control during fluoroscopy.

Since its introduction, PTA (with and without stenting) has become standard practice in all arteries of the extremities, as well as in other areas of the body, including the coronary[1,2] and carotid[3] circulations. The increasing success of angioplasty of the coronary arteries led to general clinical acceptance of angioplasty as an alternative to open surgery. Subsequent technical developments and the introduction of additional antiplatelet aggregation drugs helped improve clinical results.

STENTING

Intravascular stents are mechanical devices used to solve problems arising during or after recanalization and balloon angioplasty. Stents are inserted for the management of intimal dissection or elastic recoil and have been found to improve long-term patency.

Stents can also be used as a primary technique for vascular recanalization. They are used in highly stenotic arteries, followed by PTA to optimize vessel diameter and the inner surface of the arteriosclerotic artery and to reduce intimal hyperplasia.

There are basically two types of stent configurations: balloon-expandable (BX) and self-expandable (SX) stents. They are constructed of different materials and have different designs (Table 25-1). To reduce the problem of in-stent restenosis, drug-eluting stents and bioabsorbable stents are now being evaluated in clinical trials. At present, PTA without stents is less costly than PTA with stents, so stent use requires specific clinical indications derived from results of randomized trials. Use of drug-eluting stents is

safe for acute complications, but for elective applications, results from randomized prospective trials are necessary.

CLINICAL RELEVANCE

Global Prevalence of Peripheral Occlusive Vascular Disease

The incidence of peripheral occlusive vascular disease (POVD) varies between 2.7% and 4.0%, without regard to differences in age and sex. Between the ages of 70 and 79 years, the prevalence of POVD is 9.8% in men and 7.7% in women. Coronary artery disease (CAD) is 2.5 times more frequent in patients with POVD than in individuals with healthy peripheral arteries. In contrast, POVD develops 2.3 times more often in patients with CAD than in persons without coronary symptoms; a strong correlation exists between CAD and POVD.[4,5]

The prognosis for POVD if untreated is poor, with about 25% of patients dying within 5 years and 17% requiring leg amputation. Follow-up studies of patients with intermittent claudication (Rutherford classification 2 and 3) show that 50% die within 10 years, 20% do not change, and 20% experience symptom deterioration. Clinically, only 10% improve spontaneously.[6]

In such circumstances, any treatment modality that helps improve the overall clinical situation and prognosis is important. Thus, the basis of therapy is modification of risk factors, including control of hypertension, diabetes mellitus, smoking, hyperlipidemia, and infection. The last 30 years' experience in angioplasty of the extremities has shown that in addition to conservative management (e.g., exercise, different types of open vascular surgery), image-guided endovascular treatment plays an important role.

Most patients with claudication, pain at rest, and gangrene with Trans-Atlantic Inter-Society Consensus (TASC) type A or B arterial occlusion can be successfully treated with either balloon angioplasty or stent-assisted angioplasty (stenting). The results of endovascular techniques vary depending on the clinical stage (Rutherford grading), extent of arterial occlusion (length and diameter; TASC classification), and experience of the interventionalist.

Results can be optimized with the combination of open surgery and endovascular treatment. The original TASC classification gives recommendations for the management of POVD secondary to atherosclerosis affecting the lower limbs and seeks to aid physicians in selecting a suitable treatment. TASC II (2007),[7] more recently released, reflects the evolution of the preferred options for treating femoropopliteal lesions.

*The authors dedicate this chapter to the memory of Eberhard Zeitler, MD.

TABLE 25-1. Stents

Self-Expandable

Wallstent (Boston Scientific, Natick, Mass.)
Easy Wallstent (Boston Scientific)
Nitinol stents (various manufacturers)
Cragg, Symphony (Boston Scientific)
Memotherm (Bard Peripheral Technologies, Covington, Ga.)
Instent
AVE Stent (Medtronic AVE, Santa Rosa, Calif.)
Perflex Stent (Cordis Corp., Warren, N.J.)

Balloon-Expandable

Palmaz (Cordis Corp.)
Palmaz Long-Medium Stent (Cordis Corp.)
Strecker (Boston Scientific)

Stent-Grafts

Cragg, Passager (Boston Scientific)
Corvita (Boston Scientific)
Hemobahn (W.L. Gore & Associates, Flagstaff, Ariz.)

Angioplasty is generally the preferred minimally invasive technique. In most cases, it requires shorter hospitalization time, no general anesthesia, and less intensive postprocedural monitoring. In 20% of patients, mainly with TASC A and B lesions, angioplasty can be performed on an outpatient basis.

EQUIPMENT

Today a wide range of equipment for diagnostic and interventional procedures is commercially available. For optimal function, a dedicated interventional room has to be large and versatile enough to allow different types of sophisticated interventional procedures to be performed. Additional modalities that should be available to the interventionalist include electrocardiography, Doppler ultrasound, or other studies that do not require moving the patient to different examination rooms.

The suite should be equipped much like an operating room: equipment for monitoring, life support, and resuscitation of critically ill patients. Illumination should be bright and shadowless, and operation of room lights should be controllable with an on/off foot switch.

Commonly used diagnostic and interventional materials such as catheters, guidewires, stents, drugs, and contrast material should be stored in the interventional suite for quick access. In situations involving critically ill patients, immediate access to the staff of the intensive care unit, critical care unit, and anesthesia department should be available through a paging system.

Most diagnostic and interventional angiography systems are designed as a "C-arm" or a "U-arm" so the equipment can be moved around the patient easily to acquire multidirectional imaging projections during dynamic fluoroscopic imaging without subtraction or during digital subtraction angiography. If possible, the systems should be designed with the x-ray tube under the table to reduce occupational exposure. If horizontal or oblique projections are necessary, the physician should always stand at the detector side of the patient and not at the tube side. Additional and mandatory options for reduction of patient and occupational exposure

include last image hold, a second monitor for reference images, pulsed fluoroscopy, and virtual collimation without radiation.[8]

In 2002, the first dynamic flat-panel detectors were introduced, replacing the image intensifier. These detectors are now available with dimensions up to 40×40 cm. When compared with image intensifier systems, they provide higher spatial resolution (up to 3.25 line pairs per millimeter), homogeneous signal intensity over the entire image, no geometric distortion, and a better signal-to-noise ratio with a smaller dose of radiation.[9] In 2004 the first flat-panel detector computed tomography (CT) systems were introduced for clinical use. With a single rotation for unsubtracted images or two rotations (forward/backward) for subtracted images, up to 2000 thin CT slices can be reconstructed. The time needed for a 240-degree rotation ranges from 5 to 20 seconds, and the dose to the patient does not exceed that of a conventional multislice CT.[10]

TECHNIQUE

Anatomy and Approach

Descriptions of normal arterial anatomy of the abdominal aorta, pelvic arteries, and upper and lower extremities are derived from several standard texts and included elsewhere in this book. Knowledge of vascular variations and sites for percutaneous introduction of catheters into the arterial system is important for performing interventional techniques.[11,12]

The common femoral artery, which is the continuation of the external iliac artery distal to the inguinal ligament, and the superficial femoral artery (SFA) are most often the sites of percutaneous puncture for access to the arterial system. In specific clinical circumstances and with availability of smaller-diameter catheters, the brachial artery can also be punctured retrograde for catheterization of the aorta and aortic side branches, as well as the lower extremity arteries.

The SFA is a unique vessel in its anatomy, function, and interventional requirements. It is not comparable to any other arterial vascular bed. The SFA is a long vessel with high resistance to flow in varied hemodynamic conditions. In the past, the unique characteristics of the SFA have resulted in suboptimal outcomes for specific endovascular procedures. Although some endovascular techniques used in the SFA have been studied in prospective randomized trials, the results have been disappointing. Five-year long-term patency rates ranging between 50% and 60% have been reported. This is lower than rates reported in other arterial vascular beds.[13]

The interventional procedure starts with local anesthesia and percutaneous puncture of the artery in a retrograde or antegrade direction. For most diagnostic procedures, including cardiac and cerebrovascular angiography, retrograde puncture of the femoral artery below the inguinal ligament is most desirable. The Seldinger technique is used. To reduce local groin complications, use of a catheter introducer sheath is important. Such sheaths are of value in several specific clinical situations, such as introduction of closed-tip catheters; delivery of interventional devices such as balloon catheters, stents, atherectomy devices, intravascular duplex ultrasound catheters, intravascular radiation devices; and for removal of clots, embolic material, or intravascular foreign bodies.

Angioplasty of the iliac arteries, renal arteries, aortic branches, and the aorta itself most often requires the retrograde puncture technique followed by introduction of sheaths of different sizes.

Angioplasty of lower extremity arteries, especially the SFA, can be performed after antegrade puncture of the CFA or retrograde puncture from the contralateral CFA and manipulation of the catheter at the aortic bifurcation (the so-called up-and-over approach). This technique requires special catheters with preshaped tips and a stabilizing guidewire. This combination is generally more rigid to facilitate downstream manipulation of angioplasty catheters, stents, balloons, and other endovascular devices.

Technical Aspects

Angioplasty for treating arterial stenosis or obstruction may be divided into steps:

1. Pretreatment angiography with localization of the arterial obstruction
2. Crossing the lesion with a guidewire or catheter with a flexible tip
3. Advancement of the treating catheter or instrument over the guidewire and confirming patency of runoff arteries
4. Exchange of the diagnostic catheter for the balloon catheter or stent
5. Dilation of the stenosis with the angioplasty balloon, followed by deflation
6. Completion angiography followed by treatment of runoff vessels with different balloon catheters or stents
7. Exchange of catheter materials and occlusion of the arterial puncture site by manual compression or a closure device
8. Placement of a compression bandage above the puncture site, followed by patient monitoring for a minimum of 2 hours
9. Depending on the patient's clinical situation and condition and the outcome of the angioplasty procedure, monitoring the patient for several more hours
10. After discharge, if there is no contraindication, patients may be treated for 2 more days with medications such as anticoagulant or antiplatelet drugs. Modification of risk factors is also important.

In summary, the pathomorphologic mechanism of angioplasty can be described as a "controlled traumatic injury" that leads to dilation, with a free arterial lumen. This effect can be verified by histologic and angiographic examination and is summarized in Table 25-2.

TABLE 25-2. Mechanisms of Percutaneous Transluminal Angioplasty*

Rupture of fibers in the intima and media
Compression of thrombus
Compression of medial layers
Distribution of thrombus at inner surface of artery
Overstretching of artery

*There is a risk of distal embolization and vessel rupture (infrequent).

Angioplasty for Occlusion of the Iliac Artery

Angioplasty with balloon catheters as originally described by Gruentzig is successful in treating single stenoses of the common and external iliac arteries (Figs. 25-1 to 25-3) via a retrograde transfemoral approach. To treat stenoses in the groin region, the CFA of the contralateral side is punctured, and treatment is accomplished as described earlier (i.e., "up and over" the iliac bifurcation).

In patients with stenosis of the infrarenal aorta or occlusion of the iliac arteries on both sides (see Fig. 25-2), bilateral retrograde femoral artery puncture is required. To dilate stenoses close to the aortic bifurcation or in the aorta itself, simultaneous dilation with two balloons (i.e., the kissing balloon technique) or a balloon with a large diameter is necessary. Dilation with three balloons has been reported in the literature (i.e., balloon catheters inserted from the groin puncture sites and one from the brachial artery directed downstream [i.e., caudally]).

In some situations, atherosclerotic changes are so severe that balloon dilation results in rupture of the inner layers, followed by dissection, incomplete dilation, and reduced blood flow. This can be visualized immediately with a completion angiogram. In addition to angiography, this problem can be further evaluated with duplex or intravascular ultrasound guidance. At the time of angioplasty, intraarterial blood pressure readings confirm the presence of a significant gradient (i.e., suboptimal angioplasty). In this circumstance, an optimal outcome can be achieved by stenting the lesion, which results in a patent lumen and good blood flow.

After angioplasty or stenting, a completion angiogram of the treated lesion and runoff vessel is necessary. Ankle and arm pressures should be obtained to calculate the ankle-brachial index (ABI) using a Doppler technique.

Indications for the different types of treatment of POVD in the aortoiliac segment are summarized in the TASC 2007[7] document, which states that treatment of type C lesions can be endovascular or surgical. If endovascular techniques and conventional surgery have comparable short- and long-term results, the technique associated with the least morbidity and mortality is preferred.

Regarding type D lesions, treatment is generally surgical, although endovascular repair may be considered in special clinical and local situations.

Angioplasty of the Superficial Femoral and Popliteal and Tibioperoneal Arteries

In most patients, angioplasty of the superficial femoral, popliteal, and tibioperoneal arteries generally starts with an antegrade puncture in the groin under local anesthesia. A sheath is placed, and a guidewire with a soft, flexible tip for crossing the stenosis is advanced. A more rigid guidewire may be used if necessary to recanalize a total occlusion. The combined diagnostic and therapeutic procedure is monitored with image guidance. In most patients, this is accomplished fluoroscopically, but occasionally ultrasound and magnetic resonance imaging (MRI) may be used. In some patients with complete vascular occlusion, laser technology or a rotating device (Rotablator [Boston Scientific, Natick, Mass.]) can be used.

In patients with claudication, more often single (Figs. 25-4 and 25-5) or multiple stenoses can be crossed safely with the guidewire and catheter. In some patients, the diagnostic catheter is exchanged for the balloon catheter. In

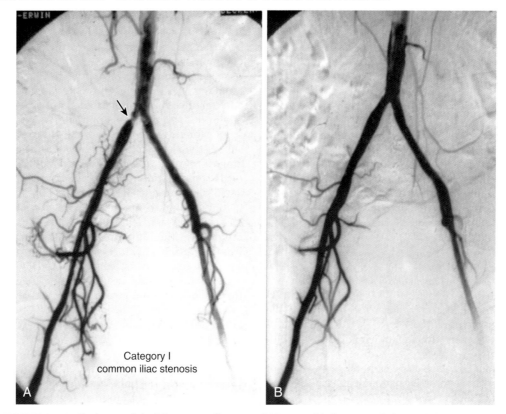

FIGURE 25-1. Single stenosis in right common iliac artery (TASC type A) before **(A)** and after **(B)** balloon angioplasty.

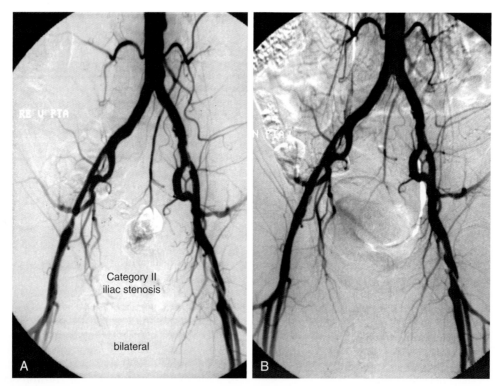

FIGURE 25-2. Bilateral iliac artery stenoses before **(A)** and after **(B)** balloon angioplasty performed from left groin, with downstream catheterization across aortic bifurcation to right iliac artery.

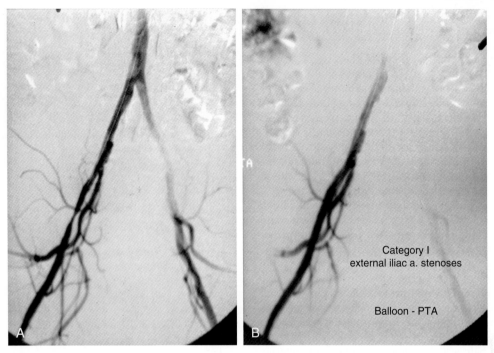

Category I
external iliac a. stenoses

Balloon - PTA

FIGURE 25-3. External iliac artery stenosis (TASC 2000 type B) before **(A)** and after **(B)** balloon angioplasty. *PTA,* Percutaneous transluminal angioplasty.

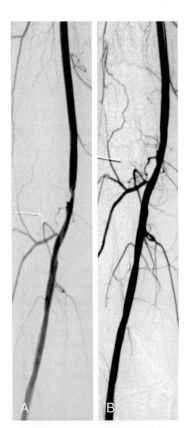

FIGURE 25-4. Single stenosis in superior femoral artery (TASC 2000 type A) before **(A)** and after **(B)** balloon angioplasty.

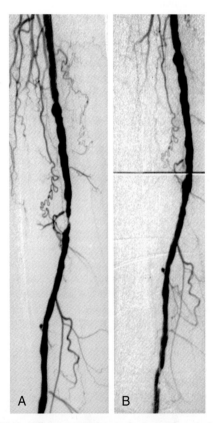

FIGURE 25-5. Diffuse arteriosclerotic disease with a single stenosis in superior femoral artery (TASC 2000 type B) before **(A)** and after **(B)** balloon angioplasty.

others, after carefully advancing the guidewire, the balloon catheter can be introduced directly over the guidewire in situ.

Before angioplasty, the diameter of the arterial lumen is measured so an appropriate-diameter balloon can be selected. In leg arteries, measuring the diameter of the inner arterial lumen in one projection is adequate, but in the iliac or other arteries (i.e., renal, carotid), biplane measurements are recommended to prevent underinflation and overdilation. Significant overdilation can disrupt the artery. In the event of arterial rupture at the site of balloon dilation, the best technique to control bleeding is to inflate the balloon at the perforation site. If accidental rupture of the SFA occurs and the catheter and sheath have already been removed, a blood pressure cuff is placed at this site and inflated while carefully monitoring the patient and immediately consulting with a vascular surgeon to discuss treatment options for the complication.

In the majority of cases, especially those involving the SFA, a simple 10-mL syringe provides adequate dilating force. In cases where precise incremental pressure increases are required, special inflation syringes with a manometer may be used.

Patients with pain at rest or gangrene may have arteries with multiple arteriosclerotic lesions, both in the SFA and tibioperoneal arteries. Femoral artery occlusions may also be present (Figs. 25-6 to 25-8). Recanalization can be successfully performed with standard guidewires, hydrophilic coated guidewires, and lasers.

Additional stenotic lesions in the lower leg require catheters with smaller balloon diameters (see Fig. 25-8). In

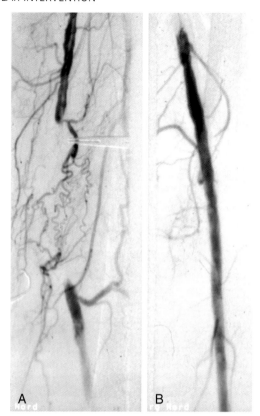

FIGURE 25-7. An 8-cm occlusion of superficial femoral artery (TASC type C) before (**A**) and after (**B**) percutaneous transluminal angioplasty and local intraarterial thrombolysis.

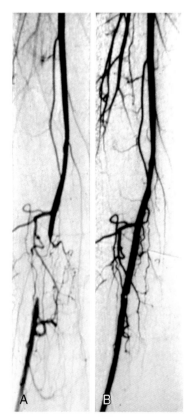

FIGURE 25-6. A 3-cm occlusion of superficial femoral artery (TASC type B) before (**A**) and after (**B**) percutaneous transluminal angioplasty.

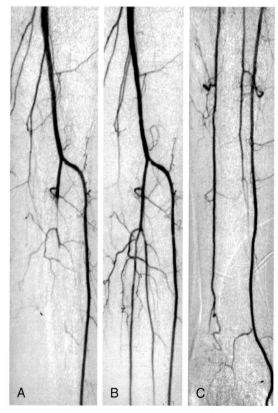

FIGURE 25-8. Tibioperoneal occlusions (**A**) before (**B**) and after (**C**) treatment (same patient as in Fig. 25-7).

special circumstances, such as scarring in the groin or extreme obesity, puncture and catheter advancement can be accomplished retrograde from the popliteal artery. The patient is placed in the prone position for this approach. Puncture is facilitated with ultrasound imaging. Retrograde transpopliteal catheterization can also be of assistance in dissections occurring after an antegrade intervention by allowing successful entry into the true arterial lumen.

In special situations with stenoses at arterial bifurcations (e.g., common femoral artery, SFA, or deep femoral artery junctions or at bifurcations of the common iliac artery and external and internal iliac arteries), use of two kissing balloons can be important (Fig. 25-9). This technique generally necessitates placement of a larger-diameter sheath or requires multiple arterial puncture sites (e.g., contralateral femoral artery, brachial artery).

It is very important before angioplasty to review the different treatment options; discuss the treatment plan with the primary care physician, vascular surgeon, and interventionalist to reduce the chance of complications; and agree that angioplasty plus stenting is an appropriate minimally invasive therapeutic option.

The TASC 2007 classification of occlusion of the femoropopliteal arteries is shown in Figure 25-10. The majority of lower extremity interventions are performed under fluoroscopic guidance; duplex ultrasound imaging may also be useful. In many institutions, MR or CT angiography (MRA, CTA) is becoming the diagnostic screening examination for vascular disease. MR fluoroscopic imaging during an interventional procedure is still problematic. CTA requires use of iodinated contrast and is associated with a considerable total radiation dose.

Type A lesions
- Unilateral or bilateral stenoses of CIA
- Unilateral or bilateral single short (≤3 cm) stenosis of EIA

Type B lesions
- Short (≤3 cm) stenosis of infrarenal aorta
- Unilateral CIA occlusion
- Single or multiple stenosis totaling 3–10 cm involving the EIA not extending into the CFA
- Unilateral EIA occlusion not involving the origins of internal iliac or CFA

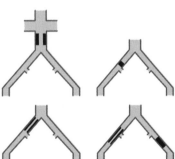

Type C lesions
- Bilateral CIA occlusions
- Bilateral EIA stenoses 3–10 cm long not extending into the CFA
- Unilateral EIA stenosis extending into the CFA
- Unilateral EIA occlusion that involves the origins of internal iliac and/or CFA
- Heavily calcified unilateral EIA occlusion with or without involvement of origins of internal iliac and/or CFA

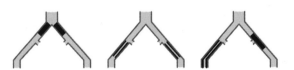

Type D lesions
- Infra-renal aortoiliac occlusion
- Diffuse disease involving the aorta and both iliac arteries requiring treatment
- Diffuse multiple stenoses involving the unilateral CIA, EIA, and CFA
- Unilateral occlusions of both CIA and EIA
- Bilateral occlusions of EIA
- Iliac stenoses in patients with AAA requiring treatment and not amenable to endograft placement or other lesions requiring open aortic or iliac surgery

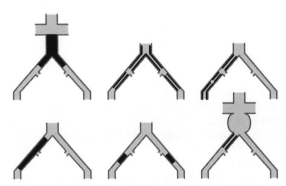

FIGURE 25-9. TASC II morphologic stratification of aortoiliac lesions. *AAA,* Abdominal aortic aneurysm; *CFA,* common femoral artery; *CIA,* common iliac artery, *EIA,* external iliac artery. (Redrawn from Norgren L, Hiatt WR, Dormandy JA, et al.; TASC II Working Group. Inter-Society Consensus for the Management of Peripheral Arterial Disease [TASC II]. J Vasc Surg 2007;45 Suppl S:S5–S67.)

Type A lesions
• Single stenosis ≤10 cm in length
• Single occlusion ≤5 cm in length

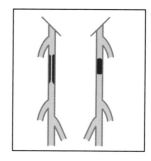

Type B lesions
• Multiple lesions (stenoses or occlusions), each ≤5 cm
• Single stenosis or occlusion ≤15 cm not involving the infrageniculate popliteal artery
• Single or multiple lesions in the absence of continuous tibial vessels to improve inflow for a distal bypass
• Heavily calcified occlusion ≤5 cm in length
• Single popliteal stenosis

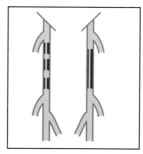 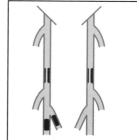

Type C lesions
• Multiple stenoses or occlusions totaling >15 cm, with or without heavy calcification
• Recurrent stenoses or occlusions that need treatment after two endovascular interventions

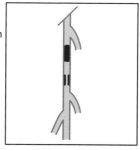

Type D lesions
• Chronic total occlusions of CFA or SFA (>20 cm, involving the popliteal artery)
• Chronic total occlusion of popliteal artery and proximal trifurcation vessels

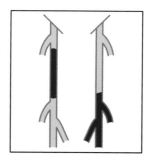

FIGURE 25-10. Classification of femoropopliteal occlusions with modified TASC 2007 recommendations. *CFA,* Common femoral artery; *SFA,* superficial femoral artery. *(Redrawn from Norgren L, Hiatt WR, Dormandy JA, et al.; TASC II Working Group. Inter-Society Consensus for the Management of Peripheral Arterial Disease [TASC II]. J Vasc Surg 2007;45 Suppl S:S5–S67.)*

CONTROVERSIES

Over the years, several techniques have been developed besides simple balloon angioplasty. With the wide range of newer guidewires, balloon catheters, and stents now available, mechanical and laser atherectomy has played a reduced role.

Indications for vascular stent placement remain controversial; for example, it is debatable whether there should be a general indication for stenting or whether stenting should be used only as an adjunct to balloon angioplasty. After recanalization of occlusions in the iliac arteries, stenting has often become the standard of practice. Stents are generally required after balloon angioplasty of iliac artery stenoses in about 40% to 50% of patients. In some published series, stent placement is required only about 5% to 20% of the time after angioplasty of the SFA, as demonstrated in a 2-year study from the Nürnberg Clinic South,[14] as well as in other publications by Mahler (Table 25-3).[15]

In the SFA, several studies have shown long-term outcomes to be no better after stenting. However, in SFA occlusions longer than 8 cm, early results with drug-eluting stents have given some hope that better long-term results will be achieved.[16,42] In general, covered stents in the SFA and popliteal artery are indicated only for treating aneurysmal disease. In the tibial arteries, use of newer technologies

TABLE 25-3. Stent-Assisted Angioplasty—Comparison of Use in Superficial Femoral and Iliac Arteries

Year	Total Number	SFA (n) + Stent		Iliac Artery (n) + Stent	
1997	705	284	34 (12%)	183	72 (40%)
1998	919	301	22 (7%)	144	68 (47%)

SFA, Superficial femoral artery.
Data from Ritter W, Bar I. Stent implantation in femoral and iliac arteries. Personal communication, 2000.

such as absorbable stents may give better results (e.g., in diabetic patients with limb-threatening ischemia, so amputations can be prevented or reduced in level or degree).

Another controversy is widespread use of the TASC recommendations (Figs. 25-11 and 25-12; also see Figs. 25-9 and 25-10). New technologies and the publication of a number of randomized double-blinded studies may change the indications and treatment algorithms. Cooperation between vascular surgeons and interventionalists in

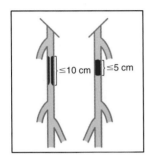

TASC TYPE A
• Single stenosis ≤10 cm in length
• Single occlusion ≤5 cm in length

Endovascular therapy is the treatment of choice.

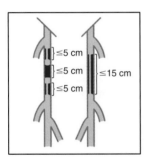

TASC TYPE B
• Multiple lesions each ≤5 cm (stenoses or occlusions)
• Single stenosis or occlusion ≤15 cm not involving the infrageniculate popliteal artery
• Single or multiple lesions in the absence of a continuous tibial vessel to improve inflow for a distal bypass
• Heavily calcified occlusion ≤5 cm long
• Single popliteal stenosis

Endovascular therapy is the preferred treatment.
Patient's comorbidities, fully informed patient preference, and the local operator long-term success rates must be considered when making treatment recommendations.

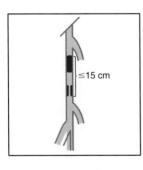

TASC TYPE C
• Multiple stenoses or occlusions totaling >15 cm in length, with or without heavy calcification
• Recurrent stenoses or occlusions that need treatment after two endovascular interventions

Surgery is the preferred treatment for good risk patients.
Patient's comorbidities, fully informed patient preference, and the local operator long-term success rates must be considered when making treatment recommendations.

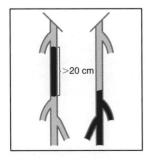

TASC TYPE D
• Chronic total occlusion of the common femoral artery or SFA >20 cm in length involving the popliteal artery
• Chronic total occlusion of popliteal artery and proximal trifurcation vessels

Surgery is the treatment of choice.

FIGURE 25-11. TASC II 2007 preferred options for treating femoropopliteal occlusions. *(From Norgren L, Hiatt WR, Dormandy JA, et al.; TASC II Working Group. Inter-Society Consensus for the Management of Peripheral Arterial Disease [TASC II]. Eur J Vasc Endovasc Surg 2007;33 Suppl 1:S1–S75.)*

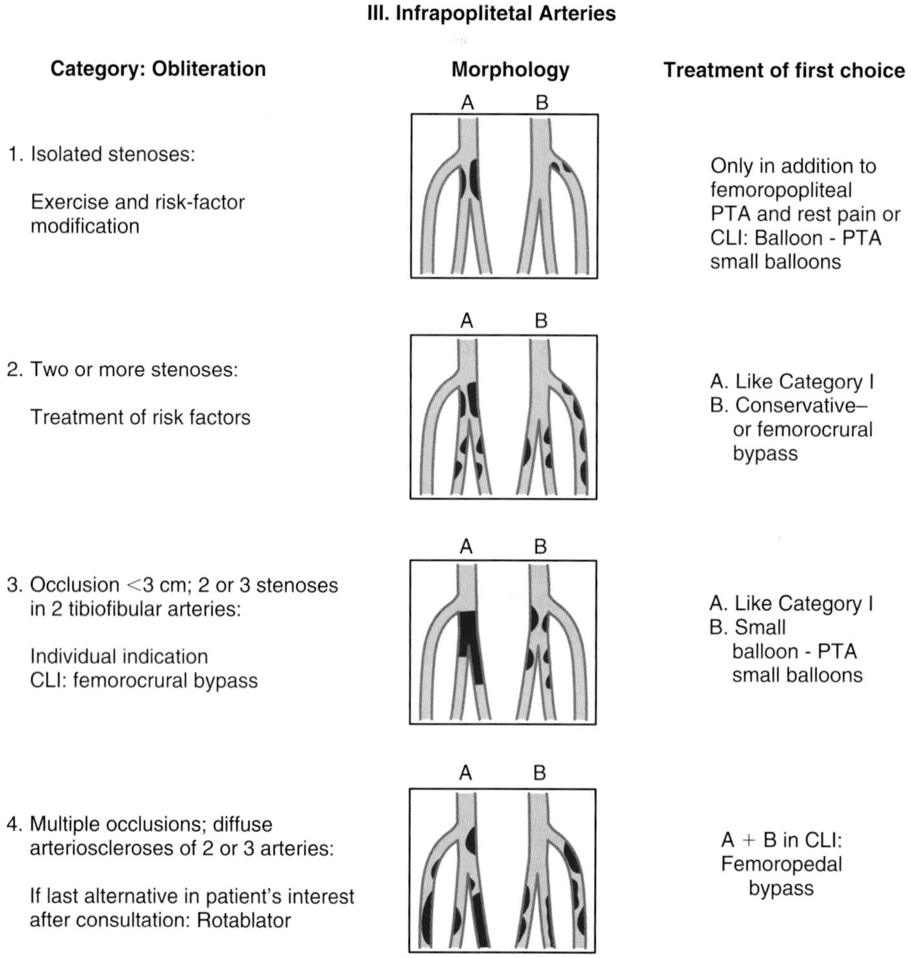

III. Infrapoplitetal Arteries

Category: Obliteration	Morphology	Treatment of first choice
1. Isolated stenoses: Exercise and risk-factor modification	A B	Only in addition to femoropopliteal PTA and rest pain or CLI: Balloon - PTA small balloons
2. Two or more stenoses: Treatment of risk factors	A B	A. Like Category I B. Conservative– or femorocrural bypass
3. Occlusion <3 cm; 2 or 3 stenoses in 2 tibiofibular arteries: Individual indication CLI: femorocrural bypass	A B	A. Like Category I B. Small balloon - PTA small balloons
4. Multiple occlusions; diffuse arterioscleroses of 2 or 3 arteries: If last alternative in patient's interest after consultation: Rotablator	A B	A + B in CLI: Femoropedal bypass

FIGURE 25-12. Classification of infrapopliteal occlusions with modified TASC 2000 recommendations. *CLI*, Critical limb ischemia; *PTA*, percutaneous transluminal angioplasty.

vascular centers has also changed the clinical approach to therapy.[17,18]

Still another long-standing controversy is use of the subintimal angioplasty technique.[19] It is technically successful in most patients, with few complications.[20] Data show short-term clinical success followed by wound healing and temporary relief of pain at rest.[21] However, long-term arterial patency is poor, with a high rate of symptom recurrence. The 2-year patency rate is reported to be 40%, but the limb salvage rate can be as high as 90%. Therefore, we view this technique as a valid alternative therapy in patients with pain at rest and gangrene if open surgery is contraindicated.[22,23]

OUTCOMES

In the majority of stenoses and short atherosclerotic occlusions in the iliac and femoropopliteal arteries, PTA with or without adjunctive stent placement has become the gold standard. Compared to the more invasive treatment option of open surgery, the percutaneous endovascular procedure is associated with reduced morbidity, mortality, and expense and has a low procedure-related complication rate. There are significant differences in long-term patency rates of the iliac and femoropopliteal arteries after angioplasty.

Primary success and long-term patency rates of angioplasty vary with the following conditions: (1) clinical stage of disease (Fontaine classification I, IIA, IIB, III, IV; Rutherford classification 1-6), (2) presence of disease in the iliac, femoral, popliteal, and tibioperoneal arteries, and (3) extent of atherosclerotic disease (i.e., stenosis, occlusion). Outcomes also differ depending on integrity of runoff arteries and whether the patient is diabetic. In reviewing published results, it is necessary to study the specifics of the patient population being treated.

The TASC 2000 and TASC II 2007 classifications[23] are the results of review and analysis of many published series involving management of POVD. Their definition of clinical success includes:

- A 75% reduction in stenosis as demonstrated by imaging such as angiography, ultrasound, CTA, or MRA
- Improvement in pulse status and ankle blood pressure
- Change in the stenotic bruit by auscultation
- Change in clinical symptoms such as pain at rest, improvement in walking distance, reduction in claudication, tissue healing

Improvement can vary between scores of 1 and 3 (Table 25-4).

The *primary success rate* is the percentage of technically successful procedures. The *primary patency rate* defines the

TABLE 25-4. Definitions of Success After Angioplasty

Score	Degree of Improvement	Symptomatic Changes
+3	Markedly improved	Symptoms gone/markedly improved; ABI increased to > 0.90
+2	Moderately improved	Symptomatic but at least single-category improvement (Rutherford or Fontaine classification)
+1	Minimally improved	ABI increased by > 0.1
0		No improvement in category

ABI, Ankle-brachial index.
From Rutherford RB, Baker JD, Ernst C, et al. Recommended standards for dealing with lower extremity ischemia: revised version. J Vasc Surg 1997;26:517–38.

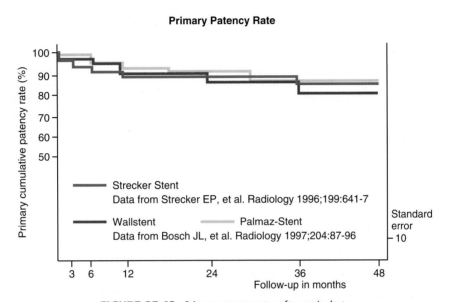

FIGURE 25-13. Primary patency rates after angioplasty.

clinical and imaging results after technically successful angioplasty. A different analysis of long-term success is provided by the life-table method[24] or by nonparametric estimation from incomplete observation.[25]

The 1- to 3-month primary patency rate after angioplasty of iliac artery stenoses (TASC 2000 A and B) varies in the literature between 93% and 96%. In the femoropopliteal arteries with stenoses and occlusions up to 3 cm (TASC 2000 A and B), the 1- to 3-month primary patency rate is between 82% and 87%. After PTA of multiple stenoses or occlusions up to 10 cm in length (TASC 2000 C), primary patency rate varies widely between 38% and 75%, depending on the degree of calcification and arteriosclerotic disease in the tibioperoneal arteries. Figure 25-13 gives an overview of primary patency rates.

Ankle blood pressure cannot be measured reliably when arterial calcification (i.e., diabetics) is present, because these vessels are not compressible, so such measurements lead to falsely elevated pressure. In this situation, angiographic and clinical results combined with duplex ultrasound are far more reliable than ankle pressure measurement.

There is little doubt that long-term patency rates correlate with the length of the arterial occlusion, particularly in the femoropopliteal arteries. This has been documented in the past[26] and is repeatedly confirmed by more recent findings. It has substantially influenced the TASC 2000 classification. The evolution and improvement of endovascular devices and techniques reflect changing recommendations

for endovascular management in TASC 2007. Differences found in patients younger or older than 65 years[27] concentrated on complication rates (2% vs. 9%) rather than varying patency rates (79% vs. 74%). Numerous reports of patency rates at 3 and 5 years after PTA for iliac artery stenoses without additional stenting vary between 81% and 92%. In the femoropopliteal system, PTA of stenoses and occlusions up to 10 cm in length has resulted in patency rates of 53% and 88% at 3 and 5 years, respectively.

Long or total SFA occlusions in the TASC 2007 D category were preferably managed with bypass surgery. As shown in a recent randomized study by van der Zaag et al.,[28] the 1-year patency rate after PTA was only 43%, whereas after above-knee bypass surgery it was 82%. However, of 18 centers, only 52 patients could be randomized to PTA or bypass surgery. The relative lack of data in this subset of patients continues to fuel controversy between vascular surgeons and interventionalists. With continued use and evolution of metallic stents in this vascular territory, patency rates and long-term results could be improved.[29] It should be noted, however, that in TASC 2007, TASC D category lesions were longer and more complex than TASC D lesions in the TASC 2000 document.

Stenting of iliac arteries with TASC 2007 A or B lesions is an accepted option if the angiographic and hemodynamic results are not optimal. For TASC 2007 C and D lesions, primary stenting may be the first step in treatment. In the treatment of TASC 2000 type A and B femoropopliteal artery lesions, it has been suggested that stenting is indicated only for patients with residual stenosis and dissection after balloon angioplasty or during reintervention.[15,27,29] In all other patients, simple balloon angioplasty had similar primary and long-term results without stenting.

Recent series have shown that after PTA for iliac artery occlusions (TASC 2000 C and D lesions), stenting increases the ABI of patients from 0.45 to 0.83 and is associated with a 3-year primary patency rate of 76% and a secondary patency rate of 90%.[30] The limb salvage rate after 3 years was 97%. The primary patency rate in diabetic patients in this population was only 57%, whereas the rate in nondiabetic patients was 83%.

In another publication, significant clinical improvement in TASC 2000 C and D lesions was noted in patients with iliac artery occlusions treated by stent-assisted angioplasty; 97.3% of patients with TASC 2000 C and 88.5% with TASC 2000 D lesions reported clinical improvement. The primary patency rate after 3 years was 89.9%, and the secondary patency rate was 95.5%. With an overall complication rate of 5.6%, the authors recommend endovascular treatment of TASC 2000 C and D iliac lesions rather than open aortoiliac surgical reconstruction.[31]

This leads to the conclusion that complex long-segmental and even bilateral iliac occlusions can be treated safely with endovascular techniques, with high rates of clinical improvement. The initial technical success, morbidity, and midterm durability (3 years) are comparable to that after surgical reconstruction.

In a randomized prospective study,[32] stenoses and occlusions of the SFA with a mean length of 13.2 cm were treated by either PTA or stent insertion. At 1 year, duplex ultrasound was performed and showed a 37% restenosis rate in lesions that underwent stenting and a 63% restenosis rate in the PTA-alone group. From these data, the authors suggest that SFA occlusions up to 7 cm in length should be treated with PTA alone, and stents used only for technical failure. Primary stenting was recommended for SFA occlusions longer than 7 cm.

The differing results seen in the literature led to TASC 2000 recommendations (see Figs. 25-9 to 25-12) that modifications be individualized for each patient.

A combination of PTA for iliac artery occlusions (TASC 2000 C and D) and surgical crossover bypass (femorofemoral bypass) for bilateral pelvic artery occlusions has also resulted in a 10-year primary patency rate of 60.6% and a secondary patency rate of 86.4%, with a limb salvage rate of 91.3%. The combined endovascular-surgical approach is a favorable alternative to conventional aortoiliac reconstruction[33] or angioplasty alone in some cases. This combined procedure for treating aortoiliac disease has 5-year primary patency rates of 81% and a secondary patency rate of 85%, with lower morbidity and mortality than seen with traditional aortoiliac reconstruction.[34]

In patients with critical limb ischemia and unfavorable surgical options, percutaneous subintimal/extraluminal recanalization can be an alternative, even if the initial technical success rate is just 72%.[20] The 3-year patency rate varies between 50% and 60%, with a complication rate of 1% to 3%. This technique is not widely accepted but may be the only available option for selected patients.

In femoropopliteal and popliteotibial occlusions, Haider et al.[35] demonstrated excellent results with infrainguinal

PTA or use of subintimal angioplasty (or both; Bolia technique) in patients with pain at rest and tissue loss. In 198 limbs, the technical success rate was 92%. Cumulative primary (and secondary) patency rates for TASC 2000 lesions at 2 years were TASC A, 73% (84%); TASC B, 62% (74%); TASC C, 65% (72%); and TASC D, 55% (72%).

Limb salvage rates at 1, 2, and 3 years were 94.9%, 89%, and 87%, respectively. The authors concluded this series by stating that angioplasty combined with subintimal techniques, when used preferentially for critical limb ischemia, provides very acceptable limb salvage and survival rates despite a relatively high restenosis rate. Therefore, some authors recommend subintimal angioplasty and stenting for femoropopliteal and tibial artery obstructions in patients with critical limb ischemia.[19,21,23,36]

Most patients experience short-term clinical success followed by wound healing and temporary relief of pain. However, patency rates after 2 years are poor in comparison to limb salvage rates, which range from 80% to 90%. Reintervention can be performed if symptoms or tissue loss recurs. This technique is indicated in patients who are poor surgical candidates.

Vascular Stents

As noted earlier, there are two broad categories of vascular stents: BX and SX (see Table 25-1). Examples of the BX variety include the Palmaz, Strecker, Iostent Peripheral, and Saxx Medium, among others. Examples of SX stents include the Wallstent and Easy Wallstent, Luminexx, Iostent, Sinus SuperFlex, SMART, and others.

Self-expandable stents maintain their shape with a spring mechanism or the memory of the metal of which the stent is made. The MAAS prosthesis is spiraled, whereas the Wright prosthesis consists of a zigzag wire component on the longitudinal axis of the prosthesis. The Wallstent is composed of woven mesh made of filaments of stainless steel alloy.

Balloon-expandable stents include the Palmaz and Strecker. The Palmaz stent is made of wire mesh, the different branches of which are joined together. The Strecker stent consists of a tubular wire netting that is knitted from a single metallic filament of tantalum.

Experimental studies have shown that SX stents have considerably less radial force.[37] Because of their deployment mechanism, these stents may offer less precision than BX stents.

Clinical results with the different types of stents were similar, although different complications were observed with BX and SX nitinol stents. Nitinol stents were noted to have a higher incidence of fracturing.

A prospective controlled study of SFA stenoses treated by stent-assisted angioplasty (with the Wallstent)[15] revealed that length of stenosis or SFA occlusion influences patency rates of endovascular intervention. The 2-year primary (and secondary) patency rate for occlusions longer than 90 mm was 22% (46%); the rate for occlusions shorter than 90 mm was 59% (79%).

Covered stents and, to a lesser extent, drug-eluting stents have broadened the horizons of endovascular therapy. Covered stents can be used for treatment of aneurysms, trauma, and vascular injury. Research into the use of drug-eluting stents in the peripheral vessels is ongoing.

COMPLICATIONS

Complications of angioplasty/stenting include those of diagnostic arteriography and consist of puncture site hematoma, vascular injury, and contrast nephropathy, among others. Additionally, angioplasty carries the risk of vessel dissection, thrombosis, and possible distal embolization. The incidence of distal embolization is reported to vary from 2% to 8%.[38]

It is important to recognize which complications can be managed conservatively and which require acute surgical management.[27] The incidence of complications that can be controlled conservatively or in the interventional radiology room varies between 1% and 8%, and the incidence of complications that require surgical correction varies between 2% and 3%. Possible complications include early thrombosis (2%-10%) and restenosis (20%-40%). It is important that the interventionalist be prepared to manage potential complications, including use of percutaneous aspiration thromboembolectomy[39,40] and catheter-directed intraarterial thrombolysis.[41]

POSTPROCEDURE AND FOLLOW-UP CARE

Patients with POVD often have other manifestations of arteriosclerotic disease, such as coronary heart disease or cerebrovascular arteriosclerotic disease. In these patients, evaluation plus management of comorbid conditions such as hypertension and diabetes is essential. Before the procedure, for both inpatients and outpatients, it is recommended that the patient be without oral intake if conscious sedation is to be administered.

If the patient has no contraindication and is not taking aspirin, intravenous injection of Aspisol or a loading dose of clopidogrel bisulfate will reduce platelet aggregation at the time of the procedure. Diuretics and laxatives should *not* be administered.

Adjunctive treatment with medications before, during, or after PTA has the following goals:

1. Avoid platelet aggregation leading to early thrombosis.
2. Avoid acute thrombosis during the procedure when flow is reduced or sluggish.
3. Avoid mechanically induced spasm.
4. Maintain peripheral perfusion during catheter manipulation and subsequent manual compression at the arterial puncture site after removal of the catheter to prevent adjacent venous thrombosis.

These objectives can be achieved by administering the following suggested medications. Of course, their use depends on the patient's clinical status:

- Premedication: oral acetylsalicylic acid, 100 to 330 mg
- To prevent early thrombosis after successful arterial puncture of the artery: heparin, 5000 units
- To prevent arterial spasm: oral calcium antagonists, nifedipine or nitroglycerin spray, 1% lidocaine (3 mL), or intraarterial nitroglycerin
- After successful PTA: anticoagulation with heparin or warfarin (coumarin) or only inhibitors of aggregation: aspirin 100 mg, two to three times daily, plus clopidogrel for 3 to 6 weeks

Smoking cessation, diet, and exercise are important adjuncts to preventing progression of arteriosclerosis and restenosis.

After hemostasis at the puncture site is achieved, a sterile dressing and bandage are applied. Bed rest and leg extension are essential after the procedure to maintain hemostasis, especially if a closure device is not used. Documentation of pedal pulses after the procedure is necessary. Calculation of the ABI at follow-up can define the technical success and clinical outcome. Repeated ABI measurements at 3-month intervals in the first year and every 6 months over the following 5 years are recommended. In hemodynamic situations suggesting restenosis, duplex ultrasonography or angiography may be indicated. Some interventionalists recommend lifelong administration of platelet aggregation inhibitors if there is no contraindication.

KEY POINTS

- Patients with peripheral occlusive vascular disease (POVD) need to undergo evaluation for coronary heart disease.
- Risk factors such as diabetes and arterial hypertension must be controlled in patients with POVD.
- An ankle-brachial index (ABI) in the nondiabetic patient is an inexpensive screening tool for POVD and useful at postintervention follow up visits. Deterioration of ABI may indicate restenosis or progression of disease. Defining the percentage of arterial stenosis and the length of an occlusion are important for understanding outcomes after interventions.
- Measurement of the pressure gradient within a lesion assists in determining whether there is a clear indication for intervention.
- It is important that follow-up be carried out at 1, 3, and 12 months and ABI and duplex ultrasound be performed before redo procedures.
- The interventionalist must be qualified, and interdisciplinary cooperation is a necessity.

▶ SUGGESTED READINGS

Abahji TN, Tató F, Rieger J, et al. Stenting of the superficial femoral artery after suboptimal balloon angioplasty. Int Angiol 2006;25:184–9.

Akopian G, Katz SG. Peripheral angioplasty with same-day discharge in patients with intermittent claudication. J Vasc Surg 2006;43:41–7.

Ascher E, Markus NA, Schutzer RW, et al. Duplex-guided balloon angioplasty and stenting for femoropopliteal arterial occlusive disease: an alternative in patients with renal insufficiency. J Vasc Surg 2005;42:1108–13.

Athanasoulis CHA. Interventional radiology. Philadelphia: WB Saunders; 1982.

Becker G, Katzen B, Dake MD, et al. Noncoronary angioplasty. Radiology 1989;170:921–40.

Bosch JL, van der Graf Y, Hunick MGM. Health-related quality of life after angioplasty and stent placement in patients with iliac artery occlusive disease; results of a randomised controlled trial. Circulation 1999;99:3150–60.

Capek D, McLean GK, Berkowitz HD. Femoropopliteal angioplasty: factors influencing long-term success. Circulation 1991;83(Suppl I):70–80.

Cope C, Burke DR, Meranze S. Interventional radiology. Philadelphia: JB Lippincott; 1990.

Dondelinger RF, Rossi P, Kurdziel JC, Wallace S. Interventional radiology. New York: Thieme; 1999.

Dotter CT, Grüntzig AR, Schoop W, Zeitler E. Percutaneous transluminal angioplasty. Berlin: Springer-Verlag; 1984.

Günther R, Thelen M. Interventionelle radiologie. Stuttgart, Germany: Thieme; 1988.

Janka R, Wenkel E, Fellner C, et al. Magnetic resonance angiography of the peripheral arterial occlusive disease: when is an additional conventional angiography required? Cardiovasc Intervent Radiol 2006;29: 220–9.

Johnston KW. Femoral and popliteal arteries: reanalysis of results of balloon angioplasty. Radiology 1992;183:767–71.

Kadir S. Current practice of interventional radiology. Philadelphia: BC Decker; 1991.

Kreitner KF, Kalden P, Neufang A, et al. Diabetes and peripheral arterial disease: prospective comparison of contrast-enhanced three-dimensional MR angiography with conventional digital subtraction angiography. AJR Am J Roentgenol 2000;174:171–9.

Lammer J, Schreyer H. Praxis der interventionellen radiology. Stuttgart, Germany: Hippokrates-Verlag; 1991.

Mahler F. Katheterinterventionen in der angiology. Stuttgart, Germany: Thieme; 1990.

Olbert F, Muzika N, Schlegl A. Transluminale dilatation und rekanalisation im Gefäßbereich. Nürnberg, Germany: DE Wachholz; 1985.

Palmaz J, Laborde J, Rivera FJ, et al. Stenting of iliac arteries with the Palmaz stent: experience of a multicentre trial. Cardiovasc Intervent Radiol 1992;15:291–7.

Reekers JA. Short-term results of femoropopliteal subintimal angioplasty. Br J Surg 2000;87:1361–5.

Reekers JA, Vorwerk D, Rousseau H, et al. Results of European multicentre iliac stent trial with a flexible balloon expandable stent. Eur J Vasc Endovasc Surg 2002;24:511–5.

Sigwart U, Bertrand M, Serruys PW. Cardiovascular interventions—handbook. New York: Churchill Livingstone; 1996.

Silber S. When are drug-eluting stents effective? A critical analysis of the presently available data. Z Kardiol 2004;93:649–63.

Strecker E, Hagen B, Liermann D, et al. Iliac and femoropopliteal vascular obstruction disease treated with flexible tantalum stents. Cardiovasc Intervent Radiol 1993;16:158–64.

Tettero E, van der Graaf Y, Bosch JL. Randomised comparison of primary stent placement versus primary angioplasty followed by selective stent placement in patients with iliac artery obstructive disease. Lancet 1998;351:1153–9.

Wilkins RA, Viamonte M Jr. Interventional radiology. Boston: Blackwell Scientific; 1982.

Zeitler E. Radiology of peripheral vascular diseases. New York: Springer-Verlag; 2000.

Zeitler E, Grüntzig A, Schoop W. Percutaneous vascular recanalization; technique, application; clinical results. New York: Springer-Verlag; 1978.

Zeitler E, Seyferth W. Pros and cons in PTA and auxiliary methods. New York: Springer-Verlag; 1989.

The complete reference list is available online at www.expertconsult.com.

CHAPTER 26

Restenosis

Dianbo Zhang, Matthew S. Johnson, and Gordon McLennan

BACKGROUND

When a vessel is dilated by percutaneous transluminal angioplasty (PTA) or stenting, there is an "initial gain" in lumen size. *Restenosis*, an iatrogenic "disease," is defined as a reduction in luminal size due to a "loss of gain." Restenosis has been defined in several ways. Greater than 50% stenosis at follow-up angiography or duplex ultrasonography has become the most frequently used definition in recent trials. In-stent restenosis (ISR) is usually defined as 50% stenosis at the stented site or at a proximal or distal site adjacent to a segment without stenosis. *Clinical patency* and *clinical restenosis* are other terms used to describe the clinical outcome of vascular intervention. The clinical patency rate is the percentage of patients who have undergone an initially successful procedure, with the symptomatic improvements being uninterrupted in any specified period. Clinical patency is ended when symptoms recur to the same degree as present before the intervention. Clinical restenosis is defined as the need for target lesion revascularization (TLR), which is any clinically driven repeat percutaneous intervention of the target lesion or bypass surgery of the target vessel performed for a clinical indication. *Clinical indications* refer to ischemic symptoms or greater than 50% in-lesion stenosis, or both, by quantitative angiography or ultrasound. The period from primary percutaneous intervention to repeat intervention is defined as "freedom from TLR."

Restenosis is a multifactorial process involving three major mechanisms: remodeling, neointimal hyperplasia, and thrombosis. In vascular remodeling, arteries structurally adapt in size and composition. Using serial intravascular ultrasound imaging to observe the coronary artery after percutaneous transluminal coronary angioplasty (PTCA), Mintz et al.[1] demonstrated that remodeling was a bidirectional phenomenon. Of 212 native coronary lesions in 209 patients after PTCA, 22% of the lesions showed positive remodeling (adaptive or expansive remodeling), and 78% of the lesions exhibited negative remodeling (constrictive or restrictive remodeling) with a decrease in lumen area (from $6.6 \pm 2.5 \text{ mm}^2$ to $4.0 \pm 3.7 \text{ mm}^2$; $P < 0.0001$). The SURE (Serial Ultrasound Restenosis) study[2] examined the time course of this phenomenon by performing serial intravascular ultrasonography and revealed that the decrease in lumen and external elastic membrane volume occurred between 1 and 6 months after PTCA. The remodeling event was related to the adventitial fibrosis. Preliminary animal studies have demonstrated that arterial injury triggers the differentiation of adventitial fibroblasts into activated myofibroblasts by day 3 after injury.[3] Myofibroblasts have both synthetic capability (type I collagen) and the ability to translocate to the vessel intima.[4] They contribute to restenosis by proliferating, forming a fibrotic scar around the injury

site, and migrating into the neointima.[5] The source of the early proliferating cells causing stenosis formation is likely to be derived from the adventitia and media.[6]

Neointimal hyperplasia has been extensively investigated and described. First, the interventional damage to the endothelium and the subsequent exposure of subintimal collagen and tissue factors lead to loss of nitric oxide,[7] prostacyclin,[8] tissue plasminogen activator,[9] heparan sulfate proteoglycans,[10] and endothelial-derived hyperpolarizing factor.[11] This process results in thrombosis, vasoconstriction, inflammation, and cellular activation and growth. Second, dysfunctional endothelial cells overexpress plasminogen activator inhibitor (PAI)-1, fibronectin, thrombospondin, integrins, selectins, angiotensinogen, angiotensin-converting enzyme, endothelin, and several growth factors, thereby leading to smooth muscle cell activation and growth.[12] Proliferation plus migration of smooth muscle cells from the adventitial and medial layers of the vessel wall to the intima is a universal phenomenon in animal models of restenosis. However, the bulk of neointimal tissue is composed not primarily of smooth muscle cells themselves but of the fibrocollagenous extracellular matrix they secreted after activation. In human neointima, only 11% of the neointimal tissue mass is composed of cellular elements.[13] The cytokines and growth factors released have the ability to promote proto-oncogene expression (e.g., c-myc, c-myb, c-fos), believed to regulate transformation of smooth muscle cells from a contractile phenotype to a secretory phenotype.[14] The secretory phenotype of smooth muscle cells produces a loose extracellular matrix that represents the major portion of neointimal hyperplasia. Meanwhile, the whole process leads not only to tissue growth but also to fibrotic constriction of the adventitia, also responsible for constrictive remodeling.[15]

Mural thrombosis is a fundamental participant in the restenosis process. Immediately after vascular injury, circulating platelets adhere to exposed subintimal elements such as collagen, von Willebrand factor, fibronectin, and laminin via a number of glycoprotein membrane receptors. Platelet adhesion in turn promotes release of cytokines and growth factors, including platelet-derived growth factor, transforming growth factor (TGF)-β, and basic fibroblast growth factor, which can result in smooth muscle cell proliferation and, ultimately, neointima formation.[16,17] Thrombus formation also acts as a scaffold for vascular smooth muscle cell migration, proliferation, and synthesis of matrix. The role of thrombosis in the restenosis process is supported by a clinical study by Bauters et al.[18] In 117 consecutive patients who underwent successful PTCA and coronary angioscopy before/immediately after the procedure and at 6 months' follow-up, they found that an angioscopically protruding thrombus at the PTCA site was associated with significantly greater loss of luminal diameter.

Elastic recoil is a direct result of the elastic properties of the vessel wall, and it occurs immediately at the site of PTA. Ardissino et al.[19] demonstrated that mean elastic recoil averaged 17.7% ± 16% in a study involving 98 consecutive patients and was correlated to the degree of residual stenosis immediately after coronary angioplasty ($r = 0.64$; $P < 0.001$). During 8 to 12 months of follow-up, no correlation was observed between the degree of elastic recoil and changes in minimal lesion diameter, but a positive correlation between the amount of elastic recoil and the incidence of restenosis was documented ($r = 0.84$; $P < 0.05$). Stenting virtually eliminates vessel elastic recoil and negative remodeling, the mechanical component of restenosis, but it also stimulates the cellular mechanisms that result in neointimal hyperplasia and subsequent ISR.[20]

CLINICAL RELEVANCE

Restenosis remains the major limitation of many endovascular interventions, despite new technologies and devices. In noncoronary vessels, restenosis is seen mainly in small and medium-sized arteries.

Peripheral Arteries

In peripheral artery interventions, the iliac, femoropopliteal, and infrapopliteal arteries are distinguished by differences in interventional approaches and results.[21] Primary patency of interventions is directly related to TransAtlantic Inter-Society Consensus (TASC) classification.[22,23]

In the iliac arteries, an endovascular approach is usually considered for TASC A and B lesions. Restenosis is not a principal limiting factor. The 2-year primary patency rate of iliac artery PTA/stenting was 81% to 83%.[24,25]

In the femoropopliteal region, restenosis is a major limitation. In a regression analysis of 330 consecutive patients undergoing femoropopliteal PTA or stenting, 6- and 12-month patency rates were 55% and 39% after PTA and 70% and 41% after stenting, respectively ($P = 0.19$).[26] An analysis of 11 publications indicated that 1- and 3-year primary patency rates were 67% and 58% after femoropopliteal stenting.[27] Recent studies showed that self-expandable nitinol stents appeared to perform better than PTA in the superficial femoral artery. The RESILIENT (Randomized Study Comparing the Edwards Self-Expanding LifeStent versus Angioplasty Alone in Lesions Involving the SFA and/or Proximal Popliteal Artery) trial showed 12-month freedom from target lesion revascularization was 87.3% for the stent group compared with 45.1% for the angioplasty group ($P < 0.0001$), and duplex ultrasound–derived primary patency at 12 months was better for the stent group (81.3% vs. 36.7%; $P < 0.0001$).[28] It is reported that the 3-year patency rate of nitinol stents was as high as 76%.[29]

Infrapopliteal angioplasty has proved to be a reasonable primary treatment for critical limb ischemia (CLI) patients with TASC A, B, or C lesions. Freedom from restenosis, reintervention, or amputation was reported to be 39% at 1 year and 36% at 2 years.[30,31] Higher patency rates can be expected with infrapopliteal stenting. In a randomized prospective study, 95 infrapopliteal lesions in 51 patients were treated by PTA or Carbofilm-coated stents. The 6-month primary patency rate of stenting was higher than that of PTA (45.6% vs. 79.7%; $P < 0.05$).[32]

Renal Artery

Percutaneous transluminal renal angioplasty, alone or in conjunction with stenting, is a treatment strategy for atherosclerotic or fibromuscular dysplastic renal artery stenosis. In a prospective study of 31 fibromuscular dysplastic renal artery lesions in 27 patients, there was a cumulative 23% restenosis rate 12 months after PTA.[33]

Stenting has proved a better technique than PTA to achieve vessel patency in ostial atherosclerotic renal artery stenosis. In a nonrandomized prospective study of 163 patients with 200 atherosclerotic renal arterial lesions after PTA or stenting, there was a significant difference after PTA in 12-month patency rates of ostial, proximal, and truncal renal arterial stenoses (34% vs. 65% vs. 83%; $P < 0.001$), which essentially was based on a higher rate of restenoses in ostial lesions ($P < 0.001$). There was no statistically significant difference after stenting in patency rates of ostial, proximal, and truncal stenoses (80% vs. 72% vs. 66%). The stent-related reduction in relative risk of developing restenosis in 12 months was 70% in ostial stenoses ($P = 0.002$).[34] In a randomized prospective study comparing PTA with stenting in 84 patients with ostial atherosclerotic renal artery stenosis, 6-month patency rates of PTA and stenting were 29% and 75%, respectively. Restenosis occurred in 48% of PTA and 14% of stenting procedures.[35] The restenosis rate of renal artery stenting ranges from 15% to 20%.[36]

Mesenteric Arteries

Stenoses of mesenteric arteries are usually focal and located at the ostium. Percutaneous endovascular PTA/stenting is becoming an alternative to surgery in patients with chronic mesenteric ischemia. The primary 1-year patency rates were 65% to 86%.[37,38] In a retrospective analysis of 33 consecutive patients from a single institution who underwent PTA, stenting, or both for the treatment of chronic mesenteric ischemia, the primary long-term (mean, 38 months) clinical success rate was 83.3%, and the restenosis rate was 17.7%.[39]

Subclavian and Carotid Arteries

Atherosclerosis of the brachiocephalic and subclavian arteries is not as common as that of the extracranial carotid arteries. The primary success rate was almost 100% for stenoses and 82% to 87% for total occlusions in the brachiocephalic and subclavian arteries. The 1-year primary patency rate was as high as 88% to 97.9%.[40,41] In a study of 110 patients with symptomatic stenosis or occlusion of the proximal subclavian artery, PTA and stenting were technically and clinically successful in 102 patients. The 5-year primary clinical patency rate was 89%, with a median recurrent obstruction-free period of 23 months. The 5-year binary restenosis rate was as low as 13.7%.[42]

Carotid artery stenting has been proposed as an alternative to surgery for carotid artery obstruction in patients at high risk. In a meta-analysis of 34 studies on a total of 4185 patients with a follow-up of 3814 arteries over a median of 13 months, the cumulative restenosis rates after 1 and 2 years were approximately 6% and 7.5%.[43]

Hemodialysis Access

The patency of hemodialysis prosthetic grafts and arteriovenous fistulas is limited primarily by venous obstruction due to intimal hyperplasia and thrombosis. Stenosis can be treated by PTA, stenting, and in selected instances, atherectomy. Restenosis is still a principal factor in the low patency rate. PTA is the standard of care for treatment of vascular access stenosis and occlusions, providing a primary patency rate of 31% to 75% at 6 months.[44] Life-table analysis revealed a 6-month patency rate of 63% and a 1-year patency rate of 41% for the first angioplasty in a given graft, and a 6-month patency rate of 44% and a 1-year patency rate of 22% for the second angioplasty.[45]

PREVENTION OF RESTENOSIS

Physician knowledge of appropriate endovascular interventions is crucial. Appropriate indications and accurate balloon or stent placement and expansion may help prevent restenosis. Various pharmacologic strategies have been shown to modulate the restenotic processes in vitro and have been efficient in reducing restenosis in animal models. Still, in clinical trials most of these attempts did not successfully limit neointima formation.

Systemic pharmacotherapies have targeted different mechanisms that have been identified as potential participants in the development of restenosis. Antithrombotic agents were associated with improved outcomes, especially cilostazol. In a study of 141 consecutive patients scheduled for PTA in the femoropopliteal artery, the incidence of TLR was significantly lower in the cilostazol-treated than in the non–cilostazol-treated patients (12% vs. 32%; $P < 0.01$).[46] Antiinflammatory agents such as steroids did not reduce restenosis in a multicenter double-blind placebo-controlled trial involving 915 PTCA patients. A restenosis rate of 40% was noted after intravenous steroid treatment, and 39% after placebo.[47] The clinical restenosis benefit of treatment with statins (3-hydroxy-3-methylglutaryl coenzyme A [HMG CoA] reductase inhibitors) is still in doubt. Calcium channel blockers and angiotensin-converting enzyme inhibitors have been considered for preventing restenosis because of their ability to reduce elastic recoil and smooth muscle cell vasoconstriction, but several clinical trials have failed to demonstrate a decrease in restenosis rates. Large numbers of antiproliferative agents administered orally or by infusion have been investigated for prevention of restenosis. Conflicting results on the efficacy of reducing the frequency of restenosis have been reported for most of these agents in clinical trials.[48] Pemirolast[49] and systemic rapamycin[50] have shown promising results in several clinical trials, but large-scale long-term trials are still needed to confirm the benefit.

Local therapy provides the opportunity to deliver drugs exactly where they are needed and to use the smallest effective dose required to achieve a drug concentration at the vessel wall sufficient to prevent restenosis. Stent devices have been coupled with local delivery of drugs and are classified into two groups: simple coated stents and drug-eluting stents. Simple coated stents are covered either with a polymer (e.g., phosphorylcholine, silicon carbide) or a drug applied directly to the metal (e.g., heparin, gold, turbostratic carbon), used mainly to decrease the metal's thrombogenicity. In contrast, drug-eluting stents have both a polymer and a drug spread over the metal, enabling slow release of a drug (e.g., steroids, AVI-4126, rapamycin and its analogs, paclitaxel and its analogs, actinomycin D, batimastat, tyrphostin) that usually targets the process of neointimal proliferation. Recent clinical studies demonstrated that drug-eluting stents containing sirolimus and paclitaxel have been the most encouraging. In a hierarchic bayesian meta-analysis of 11 randomized trials involving 5103 patients in which bare metal stents were compared with stents eluting sirolimus or paclitaxel, sirolimus- and paclitaxel-eluting stents were more effective in decreasing rates of angiographic restenosis than bare metal stents (8.9% vs. 29.3%).[51] However, the results of limited peripheral trials of drug-eluting stents were not as exciting as those of coronary trials. In the SIROCCO II study (Sirolimus-Coated Cordis S.M.A.R.T. Nitinol Self-Expandable Stent for Treatment of Obstructive Superficial Femoral Artery Disease) involving 57 patients, the diameter of the target lesion tended to be larger, and percentage of stenosis tended to be lower with the sirolimus-eluting stent, but there were no statistically significant differences between treatments in terms of any of the variables. Binary restenosis rates at 6 months were zero in the sirolimus-eluting stent group and 7.7% in the bare stent group ($P = 0.49$).[52]

Perivascular local drug delivery is under investigation. Drug-loaded polymer formulations, polymer cuffs, and gelatin or pluronic (fluorine-127) gels have shown the feasibility of perivascular delivery.[53] Several antiproliferative agents, including dexamethasone, paclitaxel, and rapamycin, have demonstrated positive results with perivascular delivery in animal peripheral arteries or vein graft models.[54]

Restenosis has become a target for local intravascular gene therapy. Genes are directly introduced and transferred to the desired location, most commonly via adenovirus vectors or plasmid DNA. Several strategies have been used that have targeted the various roles of cellular proliferation and migration of vascular smooth muscle cells, matrix, fibroblasts, and endothelial cells, as well as antithrombotic genes. Animal studies have shown a dramatic improvement in inhibition of neointimal proliferation after PTA, but limited small clinical trials, in which vascular endothelial growth factor was the target gene, have shown conflicting results.[55,56]

ENDOVASCULAR TREATMENT OF RESTENOSIS

Repeat Balloon Angioplasty

Conventional PTA is a basic therapy for managing restenosis in peripheral vessels, especially in noncalcified nondiffuse lesions and for treatment of focal ISR. Despite a favorable acute procedural outcome, restenosis after repeat angioplasty develops in 32% to 37% of treated patients.[57,58] Angiographic dissection is the main complication of PTA, especially in superior femoral artery lesions, which are associated with some degree of dissection in as many as 69% of patients.[59] PTA is also a basic therapy for ISR, with excellent immediate results. The mechanism of improvement in lumen diameter by PTA is primarily due to compression or extrusion of hyperplastic tissue through the stent struts, rather than further stent expansion. However, the restenosis rate is remarkable despite successful repeat PTA. Patients with diffuse, severe, or body-location ISR were at higher risk for recurrent restenosis.[58]

Cutting Balloon Angioplasty

Cutting balloon catheters have three or four microsurgical blades mounted longitudinally on the balloon that cut directly into the stenotic lesion during initial balloon inflation. Cutting balloon angioplasty (CBA) is increasingly being used for tight stenoses as an alternative to conventional angioplasty, particularly in the coronary arteries and arteriovenous dialysis fistulas. Successful results have also been reported for other applications such as in-stent, renal, and popliteal restenosis. Several studies have revealed that CBA is effective in reducing residual stenosis in lesions unresponsive to conventional PTA.[60,61,62] Potential complications of CBA are vessel dissection, perforation, and pseudoaneurysm.[63]

Cryoplasty and Atherectomy

In cryoplasty (cryoballoon angioplasty), a balloon is filled with liquid nitrous oxide, which evaporates into a gas on entering the balloon and causes it to dilate and cool to −10°C. Preliminary clinical studies showed a good success rate and short-term efficacy, especially at noncalcified lesions.[64,65] The freedom-from-restenosis rate at 1 year was 55% to 57%, an improvement over standard PTA.[66,67] There is a case report of successful cryoplasty for treatment of renal artery ISR.[68]

Atherectomy is a debulking method used primarily to modify heavily calcified plaque. Atherectomy has been reported to effectively treat restenotic lesions resulting from the crushing of stents in severely calcified lesions.[69]

Brachytherapy

Ionizing radiation inhibits cellular proliferation. In endovascular brachytherapy, gamma and beta emitters are delivered by catheter-based systems. Brachytherapy has shown potential in controlling the neointimal hyperplasia process in animal models of restenosis.[70] In a clinical trial of 100 patients with postangioplasty femoropopliteal restenosis, the patients receiving brachytherapy had a restenosis rate of 23% at 1-year follow-up, which differed significantly ($P < 0.028$) from the 42% rate in controls undergoing angioplasty.[71] Pokrajac et al. reported a clinical study of brachytherapy with a strontium-90 beta source in 11 superficial femoral artery restenoses and 17 ISR. The cumulative restenosis rates at 1, 2, and 3 years were 9%, 28%, and 40%, respectively.[72]

Stent

Stents decrease the relative risk of restenosis by reducing vessel recoil and vascular remodeling and providing a large postprocedural luminal diameter. Stenting is recommended for unsuccessful PTA, postangioplasty vessel dissection, or perforation. Repeat stent placement for ISR with a resulting "stent sandwich" has the conceptual disadvantage of overexpansion of the arterial wall, which acts as a stimulus for neointimal proliferation in patients known to be prone to neointimal hyperplasia.

Drug-eluting stents have been introduced successfully to prevent or treat restenosis in coronary interventions. Recent study on below-the-knee drug-eluting stents is very promising. In the PARADISE (Preventing Amputations Using Drug-Eluting Stents) trial, 228 drug-eluting stents (83% Cypher [Cordis Corp., Miami Lakes, Fla.], 17% Taxus [Boston Scientific, Natick, Mass.]) were implanted in 118 limbs of 106 patients. The 3-year cumulative incidence of amputation was 6%, survival was 71%, and amputation-free survival was 68%.[73]

Stent-grafts have the potential to reduce restenosis by impeding intimal hyperplasia and reducing tissue ingrowth. In a randomized prospective study of 100 limbs in 86 patients comparing the treatment of superficial femoral artery occlusive disease with an expanded polytetrafluoroethylene (ePTFE)/nitinol self-expanding stent-graft versus surgical femoral-to–above knee popliteal artery bypass with synthetic graft material, the stent-graft group demonstrated comparative results with surgery in primary patency (72% vs. 76%, 63% vs. 63%, 63% vs. 63%, and 59% vs. 58%; $P = 0.807$) and secondary patency (83% vs. 86%, 74% vs. 76%, 74% vs. 76%, and 74% vs. 71%; $P = 0.891$) at 12, 24, 36, and 48 months, respectively.[74] In a randomized prospective multicenter trial of 190 patients with venous anastomotic stenosis of dialysis access grafts, who underwent either balloon angioplasty alone or balloon angioplasty plus placement of a stent-graft, reduction in the incidence of binary restenosis at 6 months was significantly better in the stent-graft group than the balloon angioplasty group (28% vs. 78%; $P < 0.001$).[75] However, the problem of edge restenosis has not been eliminated.

A preliminary clinical trial of a bioabsorbable everolimus-eluting coronary stent system (ABSORB) has demonstrated excellent clinical safety, with the hope of a normal healed vessel that could be without the risk of late stent thrombosis or ISR.[76]

KEY POINTS

- Restenosis remains the major limitation of many endovascular interventions. In noncoronary vessels, restenosis is seen mainly in small and medium-sized arteries.

- Stenting virtually eliminates vessel elastic recoil and constrictive remodeling, the mechanical component of restenosis, but it also stimulates the cellular mechanisms for neointimal hyperplasia and results in in-stent restenosis (ISR).

- Various pharmacologic strategies have been shown to modulate the restenotic processes in vitro and in animal models. Drug-eluting stents containing sirolimus or paclitaxel were the most encouraging therapy clinically; the results of limited peripheral vessel trials of drug-eluting stents were not as exciting as those of coronary trials.

- Conventional percutaneous transluminal angioplasty is a basic therapy for the management of restenosis in peripheral vessels, especially in noncalcified nondiffuse lesions and for the treatment of focal ISR. Stenting, cutting balloon angioplasty, cryoplasty, and brachytherapy have demonstrated potential in reducing restenosis in some specific situations.

► **SUGGESTED READINGS**

Bauters C, Meurice T, Hamon M, et al. Mechanisms and prevention of restenosis: from experimental models to clinical practice. Cardiovasc Res 1996;31:835–46.

Dzau VJ, Gibbons GH, Cooke JP, Omoigui N. Vascular biology and medicine in the 1990s: scope, concepts, potentials, and perspectives. Circulation 1993;87:705–19.

Giles KA, Pomposelli FB, Hamdan AD, et al. Infrapopliteal angioplasty for critical limb ischemia: relation of TransAtlantic Inter-Society Consensus class to outcome in 176 limbs. J Vasc Surg 2008;48:128–36

The complete reference list is available online at www.expertconsult.com.

CHAPTER 27
Principles of Arterial Access
Albert K. Chun

TECHNIQUE

Before any arterial access, the operator should assess and document pulses distal to the puncture site. The technique for percutaneous arterial access was first described by Seldinger in 1953.[1] In short, the arterial pulse was palpated, local anesthesia was applied, and a needle with stylet was advanced into the artery. After removal of the stylet, a wire was advanced into the artery, and the needle was withdrawn. A catheter was then placed into the artery over the wire.

Because of its relative size and superficial location, the common femoral artery is the most frequent access point for arterial interventions. The point of maximal impulse is palpated, and a radiopaque marker (e.g., clamp) is placed at the site. Care is taken to enter the artery over the inferior and medial quadrant of the femoral head (Figs. 27-1 and 27-2). This location allows adequate compression of the artery between bone and the operator's fingers. In addition, entry at this site is generally below the inguinal ligament,[2] which ensures that the external iliac is not punctured, allows manual control of the puncture site, and prevents retroperitoneal bleeding. It should be noted that the operator cannot rely on the inguinal fold because the location of the skin "crease" is variable and frequently inferior to the femoral head in obese patients. Care should be taken to retract or displace an overlying pannus before groin puncture to reduce the depth of the artery from the skin (Fig. 27-3).

On occasion, the arterial pulse cannot be palpated. In these instances, the artery may be punctured under fluoroscopic control alone (if the artery is calcified) or with ultrasound guidance[3] (Fig. 27-4).

After the puncture site is identified, local anesthesia is administered subcutaneously (typically 1% lidocaine without epinephrine). A very small and superficial incision is made, and an 18-gauge bevel-tipped needle is advanced through the incision at a 45-degree angle. The needle may be directed in retrograde or antegrade fashion. The antegrade approach allows a shorter working distance when ipsilateral interventions are planned. However, there is the potential for symptomatic dissection as a result of normal antegrade blood flow.

The needle is advanced while palpating the arterial pulse or under direct visualization. If immediate return of pulsatile blood (single-wall technique, in which only the anterior vessel wall is punctured) is not seen, the needle is advanced to the periosteum and then slowly withdrawn (double-wall technique). Once the needle tip is in the artery, a 0.035-inch wire with a floppy straight or J-shaped tip is gently advanced into the artery. The wire should be advanced under direct fluoroscopic visualization to ensure proper position without any kinking of the wire. In addition, the operator should feel little or no resistance.

If resistance is encountered or the wire is deformed, the operator should withdraw the wire and confirm the needle's position. If pulsatile blood flow is no longer present, distal pulses should be reconfirmed and the needle then carefully repositioned. If blood return is satisfactory but the wire still cannot be advanced, the operator may choose a different access site, a smaller access set (e.g., 0.018-inch wire and 21-gauge needle), or injection of contrast material to assess for the presence of dissection, stenosis, or spasm.

Selection of a straight, angled, or J-tipped wire is largely operator dependent but should be adjusted to the clinical situation. If, for instance, atherosclerotic plaque is present at the origin of the right external iliac artery (Fig. 27-5, A), there is a short excursion from a right common femoral access to the point of stenosis. Thus, the risk of intimal dissection or disruption of the plaque with distal embolization is increased when an angled-tip wire is used as opposed to a J-wire (Fig. 27-5, B).

In Figure 27-5, C there is stenosis at the right common iliac artery—slightly farther from the point of access than the previous example. The degree of stenosis in this example is unfavorable for passage of a J-wire, but there is room for passage of an angled glide or floppy-tipped straight wire (Fig. 27-5, D).

Once the wire is in position, the needle is removed, and a catheter or vascular sheath may be advanced safely over the wire. For diagnostic arteriography, a 4F or 5F sheath is most commonly placed, through which a diagnostic catheter may then be advanced. The presence of a sheath allows multiple wire and catheter exchanges with minimal or no trauma at the arteriotomy site. The sheath may be exchanged for larger-diameter sheaths to accommodate larger catheters or other instruments required for intervention.

Occasionally it is necessary or advantageous to access the arterial system from a site other than the common femoral artery. The brachial artery approach is often used in the setting of iliac artery occlusion, groin infection or hematoma (particularly if bilateral), recent surgery involving the groin (as with graft placement), or some upper extremity interventions. Brachial artery access may also offer a more advantageous approach in certain renal or mesenteric interventions and may additionally serve as secondary or tertiary access (as with planned fenestration of an aortic dissection flap).

As with other arterial punctures, contraindications include uncorrected coagulopathy and uncontrolled hypertension. Contraindications specific to brachial arterial access include proximal arterial stenosis (e.g., subclavian stenosis suggested by decreased systolic pressure in the affected arm) or decreased shoulder mobility.

When intervention within the descending aorta or its branches is anticipated, the left brachial artery is favored because it offers a more advantageous angle of approach and minimizes the risk of dissection of the brachiocephalic

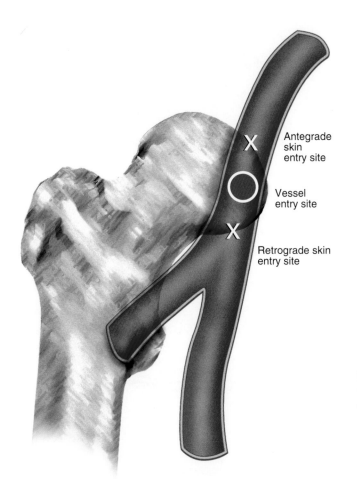

FIGURE 27-1. Schematic of puncture sites for right common femoral arterial puncture. Note that actual vessel entry site is the same for both antegrade and retrograde puncture. *(Courtesy Chieh-Min Fan, M.D.)*

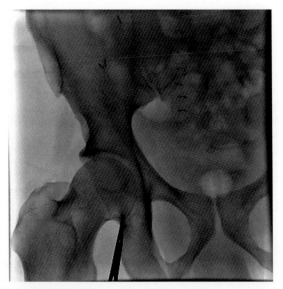

FIGURE 27-2. Fluoroscopic image showing metallic clamp marking skin entry site for retrograde puncture of right common femoral artery.

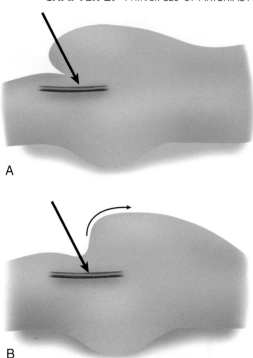

FIGURE 27-3. A, Path of access needle *(straight arrows)* traversing overhanging pannus. **B,** Femoral artery becomes much more superficial with cephalad retraction of pannus. *(Courtesy Chieh-Min Fan, M.D.)*

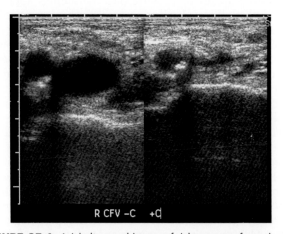

FIGURE 27-4. Axial ultrasound images of right common femoral artery and vein. Note larger and more medial vein *(left)*, which is completely compressible (not visualized in image on right).

and left carotid arteries or inadvertent embolization to these vessels.[4] Radial and ulnar pulses should be documented and the patient's arm placed in abduction, with the hand behind the head or on an armboard.

The axillary artery, a continuation of the subclavian artery, becomes the brachial artery at the lateral edge of the pectoralis major. A direct axillary artery approach is not favored because of the proximity of the brachial plexus. The brachial artery is localized by palpation or with ultrasound guidance. Lidocaine is administered superficially (to avoid a nerve block of the median nerve, which runs along the

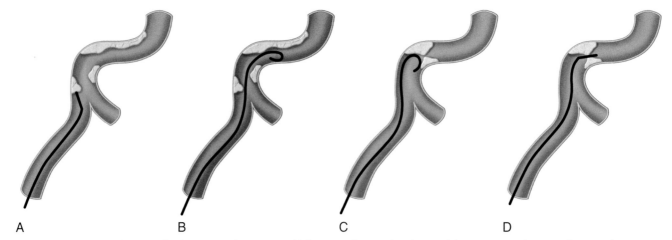

FIGURE 27-5. A-D, Schematic of right common iliac artery and bifurcation of external and internal iliac arteries, with retrograde access from common femoral artery. *(Courtesy Chieh-Min Fan, M.D.)*

superolateral aspect of the brachial artery). The artery should be stabilized above and below the puncture site with two fingers, and a single-wall puncture is made. A sheath is then advanced, which should be no larger than 7F.

Risks associated with the procedure include thrombosis, pseudoaneurysm, and hematoma. In addition, there is a risk of compartment syndrome and neuropathy as a result of either direct nerve injury or a mass effect from an expanding hematoma.

Direct puncture of the aorta via a translumbar approach was historically used when aortography was required in patients with severe bilateral iliac occlusion (thereby precluding femoral access). With the advent of computed tomographic angiography (CTA) and magnetic resonance angiography (MRA), this has become less common, although the translumbar approach may still be useful in selected instances (e.g., embolization of an aneurysm sac in the setting of an endoleak).

First described by Amplatz in 1963,[5] a translumbar aortic puncture begins with the patient in the prone position and demarcation of the spine, iliac crest, and lower edge of the left 12th rib (costal margin). An entry site a few centimeters lateral to the midline is chosen at the lower end plate of either T12 or L3. Selection of a T12 or L3 ("high" or "low") approach is determined by the underlying pathology and expected intervention. Entry at these levels from a posterior approach minimizes the chance of crossing a visceral arterial branch.

A long 18-gauge needle is advanced toward T12 or L3. Care is taken to avoid transgressing the descending colon, left kidney, and spinous processes. When the needle strikes the vertebral body, it is withdrawn slightly and redirected laterally with a short, decisive puncture. Entry is confirmed by pulsatile blood return.

Contraindications to translumbar aortic puncture include inability of the patient to lie prone, dense calcification of the aorta (rendering the aorta impervious to puncture), and severe scoliosis (preventing use of bony landmarks for guidance), in addition to uncontrolled hypertension or coagulopathy. As with other arterial access, intimal dissection and thrombosis are risks associated with the translumbar approach. In addition, there is a risk of pneumothorax

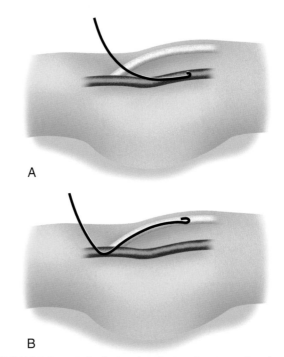

FIGURE 27-6. A, Path of J-tipped guidewire traversing graft and passing retrograde into native common femoral artery. **B,** Path of J-tipped guidewire is redirected anteriorly and passes retrograde into graft. *(Courtesy Chieh-Min Fan, M.D.)*

with the "high" translumbar access because the pleura extends to the level of the 12th rib posteriorly.

Finally, when attempting retrograde access in a patient who has undergone aortofemoral bypass, it should be noted that the anastomosis of the graft is generally at the anterior wall of the femoral artery (formation of a "hood") (Fig. 27-6). Direct puncture of a graft, even if recently placed, is generally safe, despite concern for suture disruption, infection, thrombosis, or pseudoaneurysm formation.[6] However, with puncture of the native artery just caudal to the anastomosis, it may be difficult to prevent the guidewire from

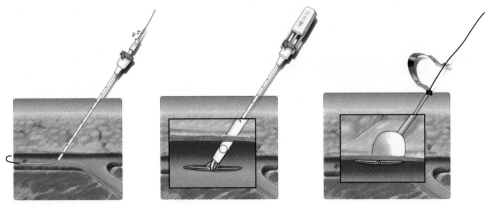

FIGURE 27-7. Collagen-type closure device (Angioseal [St. Jude Medical, St. Paul, Minn.]). *(From Hoffer EK, Bloch RD. Percutaneous arterial closure devices. J Vasc Interv Radiol 2003;14:865–86.)*

traveling retrograde into the native artery. Therefore, an angled- or curved-tip catheter with the tip directed anteriorly may be necessary to direct the wire into the graft.

POSTPROCEDURAL AND FOLLOW-UP CARE

At the conclusion of any percutaneous arterial intervention, hemostasis at the access site is typically achieved by manual compression. Most commonly, compression is applied for 15 minutes, followed by 6 hours of bed rest with the hip in extension (for common femoral artery access). The pulse should be palpable above and below the arterial entry point, and direct pressure applied at these points with the fingers of one hand as the sheath or catheter is removed with the other hand.

The access site should be inspected after the procedure for hematoma or pseudoaneurysm formation. In addition, the arterial pulses distal to the arteriotomy should be reexamined after the procedure. With diagnostic catheterization, there is about a 1% risk of hematoma or pseudoaneurysm formation.

A number of external compression devices are available, which may free a staff member from the duty of holding pressure. These devices do not, however, reduce the duration or amount of discomfort to the patient.

Alternatively, arteriotomy closure devices that use sutures, collagen plugs, or nitinol clips have been developed (Figs. 27-7 and 27-8; also see Chapter 28, Closure Devices). These closure devices are useful in patients who are unable to keep the hip in extension for several hours, are incapable of tolerating prolonged compression, or have an uncorrectable bleeding disorder. In certain situations, such as percutaneous endograft placement, closure devices may be partially deployed before the intervention in preparation for closure of the larger arteriotomy required for deployment of the endograft.

Techniques for deployment of these devices vary, but all require initial verification of the arterial entry site. For common femoral artery access, this is done by performing an arteriogram in a 15-degree ipsilateral oblique projection. The vessel to be closed should not be densely calcified. Closure of an arteriotomy at a bifurcation point (e.g., superficial femoral artery and profunda femoris artery) should also be avoided.

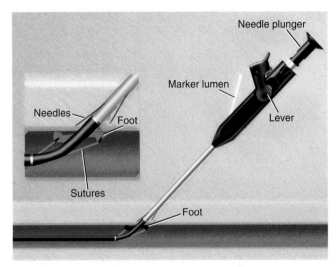

FIGURE 27-8. Suture-type closure device (Perclose [Abbott Laboratories, Abbott Park, Ill.]). *(From Hoffer EK, Bloch RD. Percutaneous arterial closure devices. J Vasc Interv Radiol 2003;14:865–86.)*

Closure devices have a technical success rate of 92% to 97% and have been shown to reduce time to hemostasis and time to ambulation when compared with manual compression. However, these devices are also associated with an increased rate of hematoma, pseudoaneurysm formation, occlusion, distal embolization, and other complications requiring transfusion or surgery.[7] Therefore, as with other aspects of the procedure, the risks and benefits of using a particular closure device must be considered carefully.

Manual compression is generally preferred after brachial artery catheterization because the brachial artery is relatively small and prone to vasospasm. Radial and ulnar pulses should be documented, and hourly neurologic examination (with assessment of upper extremity sensation and grip strength) is recommended. Any change from the preprocedure examination should prompt immediate surgical exploration for possible nerve sheath hematoma and compartment syndrome.[8]

By contrast, direct compression of the aorta is not possible because of the depth of the aorta and its location below the psoas muscle. Therefore, a small retroperitoneal hematoma may be expected, but this should be self-limited in patients lying supine after the procedure and who have their blood pressure under control and normal coagulation.

- Pulses distal to the access site should be documented before and after any arterial puncture.

- Access to the common femoral artery should be over the inferior and medial quadrant of the femoral head. This ensures entry below the inguinal ligament (preventing retroperitoneal bleeding) and above the bifurcation of the smaller superficial and deep femoral arteries.

- Risks associated with arterial puncture include hematoma, pseudoaneurysm, dissection, thrombosis, distal embolism, infection, and damage to surrounding structures (e.g., median nerve neuropathy secondary to brachial artery puncture).

- Arterial puncture is contraindicated in patients with pre-existing pseudoaneurysm, hematoma, or infection of the puncture site. Relative contraindications include recent surgery, dense calcification of the artery, and uncontrolled hypertension or coagulopathy.

- Hemostasis may be achieved with manual compression or various closure devices. In general, closure devices provide more rapid hemostasis but are associated with higher complication rates than manual compression.

▶ **SUGGESTED READINGS**

Hoffer EK, Bloch RD. Percutaneous arterial closure devices. J Vasc Interv Radiol 2003;14:865–86.

Spies JB, Bakal CW, Burke DR, et al. Standard for diagnostic arteriography in adults. Standards of practice committee of the Society of Cardiovascular and Interventional Radiology. J Vasc Interv Radiol 1993;4: 385–95.

The complete reference list is available onine at www.expertconsult.com.

CHAPTER 28

Closure Devices

John F. Angle, Auh Whan Park, and Alan H. Matsumoto

Manual compression (MC) after femoral arterial access removal has a high success rate with a relatively short compression time (5-15 minutes). The biggest drawback to MC is that 1 to 6 hours of postprocedure bedrest are required. In patients with orthopnea, musculoskeletal disorders, or other conditions that make lying supine difficult or painful, it can be challenging or nearly impossible to manage the puncture site with MC. Anticoagulation and antiplatelet drugs can prolong the time to hemostasis, increase the time to safely pull the sheath, and increase the risk of delayed complications. Roughly 2% of MC leads to a major complication. The origins of the current interest in vascular closure devices is unclear but likely was the result of an effort to decrease the need for MC, speed the time to ambulation, and potentially reduce hematoma rates. Since the first edition of this chapter, their use has skyrocketed: in 2007 approximately 30% of the 10 million endovascular procedures performed in the United States employed a closure device.

There are several classes of devices that can aid MC or provide artery closure. The most mature class of devices is the group of compression devices that includes bedside C clamps and pneumatic compression straps. These do little to minimize groin complications or shorten bedrest time, but they do free up the operator and his/her assistants from compression. The second class is the topical agents; all the products in this class are procoagulants applied to the puncture site at the time of the MC. They are generally very safe, but their utility remains unproven because of the lack of appropriate clinical testing. It makes intuitive sense that these devices are most useful when the puncture is superficial, such as with radial artery punctures or dialysis graft access. The third class is invasive devices where no foreign body is left behind. The final class of devices are the invasive device where the arteriotomy is mechanically or pharmacologically closed. This group includes all the devices that instantly seal the arteriotomy, but they are invasive in that they require the operator to deposit either a procoagulant (e.g., piece of bovine collagen) next to the artery or deliver a suture or clip into the arteriotomy. One important point to consider at this step is whether not vessel access is given up in the case of device failure. For example, the Perclose and ProStar devices (Abbott Vascular, Redwood City, Calif.), or the Quick Seal (Sub-Q Inc., San Clemente, Calif.) allow a guidewire to be left in the vessel until hemostasis is obtained. With most of the remaining devices, a leap of faith is made that the device is going to work, and if it does not seal the artery, immediate MC or open femoral artery repair must be performed.

All these aids to hemostasis and closure devices add a cost to procedures, but the cost of these devices may be offset by a shortened stay and fewer admissions for complications. One randomized study of 193 patients looked at costs. Patients received either the Perclose device (Abbott

Vascular) with 4-hour ambulation or MC with next-day ambulation, and it did show a cost savings. A similar study demonstrated that the Duett device did not increase overall costs and improved patient quality of life in the short term (7 days). On the other hand, invasive devices may not shorten the stay, which negates the cost savings. A study of transarterial chemoembolization demonstrated earlier ambulation but no change in length of stay.

Topical patches appear to shorten the compression time required to achieve hemostasis, but questions remain about their use in anticoagulated patients and their effect on time to ambulation. In addition, although studies show a statistically significant reduction in time to hemostasis, the shortening may not be of clinical significance (MC was shortened 2, 3, and 6 minutes in three randomized trials). Probably the most practical observation is that use of a procoagulant patch or pad during MC can shorten the time to ambulation, if only because it allows the sheath to be removed earlier after an intervention where anticoagulation was employed.

Compression device outcomes are well published, with several trials comparing these devices to MC. In experienced hands, technical success can approach 100%, and complications are similar or lower than those of MC. When compression devices are compared to some of the invasive devices, hemostasis rates are similar at several hours, but the invasive devices provide hemostasis earlier.

There are two invasive devices that do not involve deposition of foreign material. Such devices have the theoretical advantage of fewer thromboembolic or infectious complications compared to other invasive devices. The first device of this class consists of an umbrella temporarily inserted into the artery and pulled back against the arteriotomy to provide temporary hemostasis. The second is a device that directs the arterial puncture to aid with hemostasis. The Boomerang (Cardiva Medical, Mountain View, Calif.) has been shown to have a shorter time to hemostasis than MC. Very recently, a device that creates an intramural track during the initial femoral artery puncture, Axera (Arstasis, Redwood City, Calif.), is being evaluated in a single-arm study to determine whether there is a shorter time to hemostasis compared to MC.

The results of the invasive devices that actively seal the artery for patients on anticoagulation or antiplatelet therapy are even more encouraging, providing hemostasis and early ambulation where MC would not be possible until anticoagulation was discontinued. There are some data comparing one vascular closure device to another, but few studies predict a marked difference between devices, which makes choosing a device difficult. In addition, the reported differences in success may or may not be clinically significant. Although all the available devices appear to speed the time to ambulation, the minimum times required, particularly in the presence of anticoagulation, remain unclear.

In most cases, any of the invasive devices can achieve immediate hemostasis, but these vascular closure devices do not appear to markedly reduce the number or severity of vascular complications compared to MC alone in any of the multiple meta-analyses of the literature. Even in experienced hands, early or late hematomas can occur. Just like with MC, bleeding is more common when patients are ambulated early or when they are on anticoagulation. In addition, there are immediate device failures that must be managed with MC, or in some cases emergent arterial cutdown. In one study, 2% of invasive device applications resulted in emergent femoral cutdown. One large analysis of 5093 patients demonstrated a drop in hematocrit of at least 15% in 5.2% of the invasive closure device group compared to 2.5% in the MC group. A meta-analysis by Koreny of 30 studies using six different devices demonstrated the relative risk (RR) of pseudoaneurysm is higher in patients receiving an invasive device application compared to MC (RR, 5.40; 95% confidence interval [CI], 1.21-24.5). Yet most of the comparison trials and four different meta-analyses of the literature show bleeding complication rates are similar or slightly lower than with MC.

After assessing the risks and benefits of the three classes of devices, each practice will have to decide when to use which device. When considering use of the invasive devices, the three broad practice pattern options are to use them in all cases, to never use them, or to use them in selected cases. Criteria for the third option might include patients with difficulty lying flat (e.g., congestive heart failure or lumbar spine disease), difficulty holding still, large sheaths, need for continuous antiplatelet or anticoagulation therapy, or patients with coagulation disorders. As experience with these devices grows and more comparative studies are undertaken, these choices may become easier to make. In the meantime, when to use these devices is unclear.

There are fortunately a large number of devices offering a range of closure options. These devices also range in cost, effectiveness, and risk, but success rates are encouraging. Although complications are very rare, they can be devastating. In summary, the application of these devices to previously challenging clinical situations has greatly enhanced our ability to safely perform arteriography in a wider range of patients. Yet questions remain on the utility and safety of using these devices in every case. There are important differences among the wide array of devices, and careful case and device selection are essential.

The full discussion of closure devices is available at www.expertconsult.com.

CHAPTER 29

Principles of Venous Access

David O. Kessel and Karen Flood

CLINICAL RELEVANCE

The National Institute of Clinical Excellence has recommended that ultrasound guidance should be used when inserting elective central venous lines.[1] There is clear evidence that using imaging guidance increases success rates and reduces complications associated with jugular and subclavian vein puncture. Most of these routine procedures do not require interventional radiologic input, but interventional radiologists become indispensable in cases where central venous access is difficult, as is often the case in hemodialysis and cancer patients.[2]

INDICATIONS

Venous access is the starting point for a large number of diagnostic and therapeutic interventions in the systemic and portal venous circulations. Table 29-1 lists typical indications.

CONTRAINDICATIONS

There are few absolute contraindications to obtaining venous access. Reversal of coagulopathy should be considered if clotting is severely deranged. This is particularly important if solid organ puncture is required or large-bore catheters are being used.

Venous thrombosis, stenosis, and occlusion are frequently encountered but are not contraindications to access. Rather, these are the reasons an interventional radiologist (i.e., an individual with skill in thrombolysis and recanalization of vessels, etc.) is required. With regard to venous thrombosis and risk of causing emboli, care should be taken to avoid puncturing into iliofemoral deep venous thromboses (DVT) when placing an inferior vena cava (IVC) filter. This is one reason for considering the jugular route as a standard approach for IVC filter placement.

EQUIPMENT

Ultrasound

The key item of equipment is an ultrasound machine with a suitable-frequency probe (typically 4-9 MHz for jugular vein puncture and 3-5 MHz for transhepatic, transrenal, or transsplenic puncture) and color Doppler. Poor-quality ultrasound is the most common cause of failure to obtain venous access. Certain compact ultrasound systems such as those used in wards for venous puncture are often of insufficient quality for this purpose.

Needles

For uncomplicated femoral or jugular access, 18-gauge needles are suitable, but smaller 21-gauge "mini-access systems" are recommended in difficult situations. These minimize venous trauma and spasm, which may herald the end of a procedure before it even begins. Note that some proprietary line insertion kits use 0.038-inch guidewires, so it is essential that the interventionist use a needle that will accommodate this. Traditionally, a syringe is attached to the needle to allow aspiration of venous blood, confirming the intraluminal position of the needle tip.

Guidewires

Many line insertion kits include a J-tip guidewire. This is sufficient for simple access but of little use in more difficult or complex situations. In these circumstances, it is wise to ensure that the full range of wires are available for the procedure, particularly steerable hydrophilic wires, highly supportive wires such as the Cook Lunderquist wire, and also 0.018-inch wires, which allow use of low-profile angioplasty balloons.

Sheaths and Catheters

The choice between sheaths and catheters depends largely on the planned procedure, but it is worth noting that the jugular vein is a very forgiving vessel, especially if large-bore catheters are being used. When inserting tunneled central venous catheters, peel-away sheaths are required. These are normally included in the line kits, but on occasion a longer peel-away sheath is needed to negotiate around tortuous vessels.

Angioplasty Balloons and Stents

It is sometimes necessary to predilate a stenosed or occluded vein prior to passage of a line (Fig. 29-1). Stents are generally unnecessary, however, if access rather than patency is the desired outcome.

TECHNIQUE

Veins are typically thin walled and perfused at low pressure. These characteristics increase the challenge of puncture. To improve the odds, it helps to increase the venous pressure. A tourniquet is fine in the periphery but is of little use in the jugular vein. The Valsalva maneuver will distend a vein if the patient is able to follow the instruction to "strain

TABLE 29-1. Interventional Procedures Requiring Venous Access

Procedure	Typical Approach
Diagnostic	
Venography	Appropriate peripheral vein
Venous sampling	Femoral vein
Pulmonary angiography	Femoral vein
Therapeutic—Systemic	
Venous angioplasty, stenting, and thrombolysis	Appropriate peripheral vein
IVC filter placement	Jugular vein
Tunneled central line insertion	Jugular vein
Repositioning/stripping of lines	Femoral vein
Management of SVCO/IVCO	Jugular vein
Transjugular liver biopsy	Jugular vein
Varicocele and ovarian vein embolization	Femoral vein
Varicose vein ablation	Appropriate peripheral vein
Therapeutic—Portal	
TIPS	Jugular vein
Portal vein embolization	Transhepatic
Post transplant portal vein intervention	Transhepatic

IVC, Inferior vena cava; *IVCO,* inferior vena cava occlusion; *SVCO,* superior vena cava occlusion; *TIPS,* transjugular intrahepatic portosystemic shunt.

gently down." It is often helpful to ask the patient to hum to achieve this desired effect. Ensuring the patient is adequately hydrated can also help, and if necessary, administering a liter of intravenous saline will also work to increase the venous pressure. An alternative is to use the head-down (Trendelenburg) position or temporarily elevate the patient's legs to increase venous return. Unfortunately, few interventional radiology suites are equipped with tilting tables, so Trendelenburg is often not an option. Interventionists will also typically be referred all patients who cannot lie flat for one reason or another, so it is important that he or she be familiar with the different means of increasing venous pressure in these patients.

Whatever technique is adopted, one should be sure that the final positioning allows scanning the vein while performing the puncture. It is best to choose an approach that allows the needle to pass along the scan plane so it can be seen throughout its passage, but this is often impossible when using a standard linear array probe to guide jugular puncture because there is insufficient space in the neck. In these circumstances, it is necessary to scan transversely and "triangulate" the needle position as it approaches the vein. It is worth remembering that thin-walled veins will often be compressed by pressure transmission from the needle in soft tissues superficial to or even adjacent to the vein. This is no substitute for observing the needle tip come into contact with the anterior vein wall. When the needle actually abuts the vein, the wall will be indented by the needle, and the anterior wall may even come into contact with the posterior wall. Further needle advancement in this

circumstance leads to transfixing the vein. To puncture the anterior wall and enter the lumen, it is best to advance the needle with a short stab as soon as it abuts the anterior wall. If a syringe was attached at the start of the procedure, blood should be aspirated to confirm intraluminal position. If aspiration is not possible, it is likely the needle has been advanced through the posterior vein wall. In this case, the needle should be pulled back slowly, aspirating as it goes, until flow is restored. If this does not succeed, one should start again, ensuring the needle is flushed before beginning.

Anatomy and Approach

Several considerations may be relevant when planning the optimal approach for venous access. The general adage that the shortest, straightest route is best often applies, but this should be weighed against possible disadvantages of choosing a particular site. Typical approaches are outlined in Table 29-1, but there are also some esoteric routes typically reserved for cases wherein all other options have failed. These include utilizing collateral veins, transhepatic, translumbar, or transrenal access to the systemic veins and transsplenic or transmesenteric access to the portal venous system. There are occasions when dual access is helpful, especially when the most direct route is through a small vessel or via an artery.

Virtually any vein can be used, but the most common sites depend on the indication. The following section will outline a rational approach for the most common procedures.

Central Venous Access
Central venous access is the starting point for many procedures (see Table 29-1). The most common points of access are the internal jugular and subclavian veins. The jugular vein is superior to the subclavian vein because it is less prone to symptomatic thrombosis.[3] The right internal jugular vein also provides the shortest, straightest route and is the first-choice point of access. The left jugular approach is often possible, but it is important to be aware of any sharp bends in the mediastinum that may result in kinking of sheaths (Fig. 29-2). It is prudent to check the manufacturer's instructions for use; there are sometimes caveats to using the left jugular approach for this reason.

Ultrasound-guided jugular puncture is a simple procedure and provides an excellent opportunity to learn basic ultrasound guidance. A preliminary scan before starting is always advisable, especially if access is known to be problematic. Particular attention should be paid to any signs that may indicate a potential venous obstruction, especially venous distension, loss of normal jugular vein pulsatility, and spontaneous contrast within the vein due to slow flow. The presence of visible jugular vein tributaries (Fig. 29-3) is strongly suggestive of a central occlusion, and any vein seen to course across the neck should raise suspicions. Alternative approaches in these circumstances are through the external/anterior jugular veins or the thyroid veins[4] (Fig. 29-4). These may allow the line to be tunneled close to the conventional position for an internal jugular line. Whenever using these veins, it is prudent to perform a venogram to establish whether there is in fact a direct route into the central veins rather than an impenetrable network of

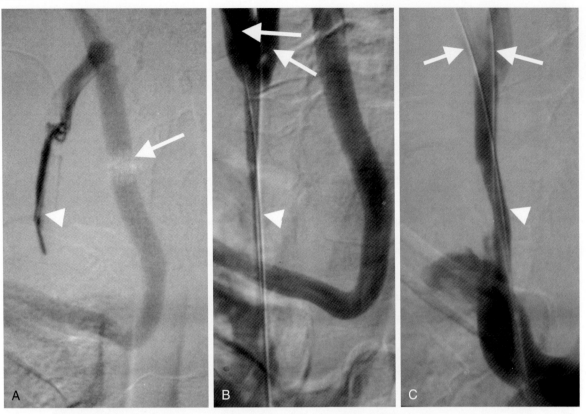

FIGURE 29-1. Insertion of Tesio lines (Medcomp, Harleysville, Pa.) through an occluded jugular vein (same patient as Fig. 29-3). **A,** Remnant of jugular vein *(arrowhead)* and collateral vein passing into subclavian vein *(arrow).* **B,** Occluded internal jugular vein has been recanalized and a guidewire passed from each of two veins *(arrows)* cranial to occlusion. **C,** Following balloon angioplasty, jugular vein is now patent, and collateral vein seen in **A** no longer fills. Lines were inserted uneventfully.

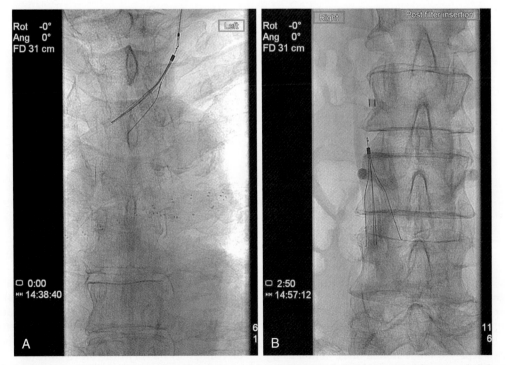

FIGURE 29-2. During insertion of inferior vena cava (IVC) filter through left internal jugular vein (right internal jugular was occluded, and iliofemoral deep venous thrombosis was present), filter strut perforated through side wall of sheath **(A).** Fortunately, left brachiocephalic vein was not perforated. Filter was withdrawn back into sheath. Both were removed and replaced with a new sheath, and successful placement of filter in infrarenal IVC was achieved **(B).**

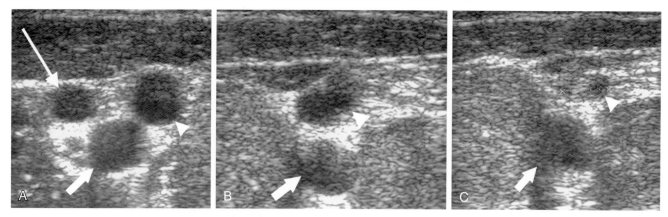

FIGURE 29-3. Abnormal ultrasound indicating jugular vein occlusion. **A,** In most cranial image, jugular vein *(arrowhead)* and a collateral vein *(long thin arrow)* are seen anterior to common carotid artery *(short thick arrow)*. **B,** Note that 1 cm caudal to this, jugular vein and collateral have merged to form a single vein *(arrowhead)*. **C,** Occluded jugular vein remnant is seen 1 cm caudal *(arrowhead)*.

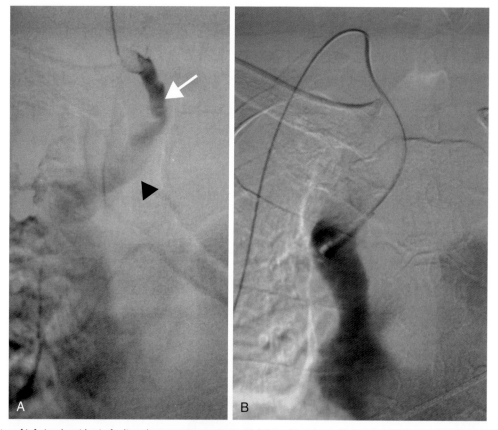

FIGURE 29-4. Use of inferior thyroid vein for line placement in a patient with bilateral jugular occlusion. **A,** Initial venogram demonstrates inferior thyroid vein *(white arrow)* draining into left brachiocephalic vein *(black arrowhead)*. **B,** Tunneled line has been uneventfully inserted. Note that position of neck puncture and tunnel are not dissimilar to conventional jugular vein placement.

collaterals (Fig. 29-5). In difficult cases, it is often necessary to employ angiographic techniques to recanalize venous stenosis and occlusion[5] (see Fig. 29-1).

When attempting "last-ditch" line placement for hemodialysis access, it is often better to use a single dual-lumen catheter than two separate single-lumen lines. When using a peel-away sheath, it is usually possible to "persuade" a single line through even the most tortuous vein, but virtually impossible to pass two separate lines down the same

vessel. If using two separate lines, it is sometimes tempting to convert a single puncture into a double puncture by passing two guidewires down a single sheath. This should be generally avoided, though, because placement of the two peel-away sheaths tends to tear the vein, and the resultant bleeding may be very difficult to control.

The techniques just described will generally suffice for the vast majority of cases, but occasionally it will be necessary to consider more obscure venous access approaches for

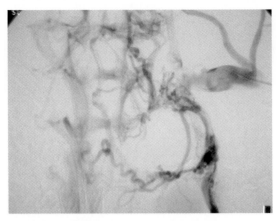

FIGURE 29-5. Occlusion of distal left subclavian and brachiocephalic veins. There are multiple collateral veins draining across root of neck, which communicate via small vessels, giving a moyamoya-like ("puff of smoke") appearance. These vessels are not suitable for passage of a line.

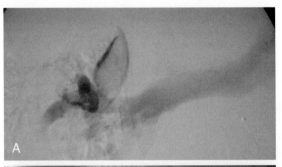

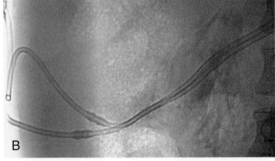

FIGURE 29-6. Transrenal placement of hemodialysis catheter in a patient with no other site of access. **A,** Initial venogram. **B,** Post line insertion.

dialysis access. These include transhepatic, transrenal, and translumbar routes.[6] The transhepatic route involves ultrasound-guided hepatic vein puncture, but is generally unsatisfactory because the catheter position tends toward instability due to the large respiratory excursion of the liver. The kidneys move rather less, and a transrenal approach through a nonfunctioning native kidney can be used for hemodialysis access (Fig. 29-6). The translumbar route is exactly analogous to translumbar aortic puncture, but using the right rather than left paravertebral approach. This can be achieved under fluoroscopic or computed tomography (CT) guidance.

Upper Limb Veins
Venous interventions in the upper limb are most often performed for problems associated with hemodialysis or

thoracic inlet syndrome. Dialysis access intervention is covered elsewhere (see Chapters 114-117), but it is worth mentioning here that there are often branch veins that can be used to access the fistula without the need to directly puncture the fistula, which frequently causes significant spasm. When dealing with peripheral stenoses via a transvenous approach, it is essential to decide how to position the patient's arm and where to stand. It is often simplest to abduct the arm and work from the contralateral side of the patient, since this allows the operator and assistant adequate space to maneuver. Whichever approach is chosen, care should be taken to ensure that the interventionist will be able to view the ultrasound screen and fluoroscopy monitors without undue contortion.

The ipsilateral basilic vein is the most direct approach to central venous stenoses. The cephalic vein is more tortuous, and the junction with the axillary vein must be negotiated. When the basilic vein is the principal efferent vein from a fistula, placement of a 4F sheath and an approach from this route to traverse an occlusive lesion should be considered. Subsequently, if a large sheath is required for angioplasty or stenting, it can either be placed in the basilic vein or, alternatively, a rendezvous maneuver can be performed from the femoral vein, thus minimizing the risk of damage to the fistula.

Lower Limb Veins
The femoral vein is a common point of access for many endovenous procedures. Many operators will puncture it blind, relying on its position medial to the femoral artery. As always, ultrasound guidance should be considered in case of any difficulty. Alternative approaches may be considered for venous thrombolysis; these include the posterior tibial vein posterior to the medial malleolus and the popliteal vein. Both of these require ultrasound guidance. The paired posterior tibial veins are readily identified adjacent to the posterior tibial artery and should be punctured with a mini-access set.

Varicose vein intervention may require direct catheterization of the varicosity or the more proximal or distal long or short saphenous vein.

Portal and Hepatic Vein Approaches
The hepatic veins course cranially up through the liver to join the IVC just caudal to the right atrium. Their angulation permits approach from the right internal jugular vein, and this is easily the most practical approach for transjugular liver biopsy. It is sometimes impossible to access the hepatic veins in patients with Budd-Chiari syndrome and large vein occlusion. In this circumstance, ultrasound will demonstrate whether the peripheral hepatic veins are patent; if they are, it is usually relatively straightforward to puncture them transhepatically (Fig. 29-7). This allows direct access to the point of occlusion and simplifies crossing the lesion. The liver is a vascular organ, and when diseased is typically associated with coagulopathy. This condition should be reversed whenever possible. To further minimize the risk of hemorrhage, use of a 3F or 4F system for the transhepatic puncture should be considered; the tract should then be plugged with Gelfoam upon completion. If angioplasty or stenting are performed, a rendezvous can be achieved by snaring the guidewire from the jugular or femoral approach.

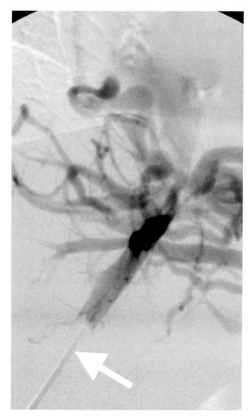

FIGURE 29-7. Transhepatic hepatic vein puncture in a patient with Budd-Chiari syndrome. A 4F sheath *(white arrow)* has been inserted into a peripheral hepatic vein branch. Typical leash of intrahepatic collateral veins is clearly seen. Central hepatic vein was completely occluded and subsequently traversed via transhepatic route. Guidewire was then snared and a stent placed from right internal jugular vein.

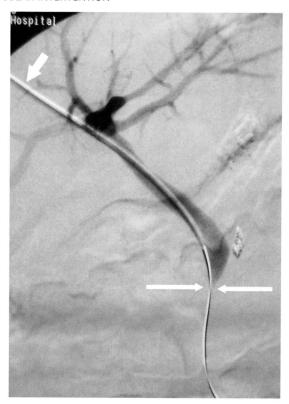

FIGURE 29-8. Stenosis of a surgical portal vein shunt (Rex Shunt [Rex Medical, Conshohocken, Pa.]) in a child with congenital portal vein atresia. Peripheral branch of right portal vein has been entered *(short white arrow)* and a 4F sheath placed. Venogram delineates portal vein and stenosis *(long thin arrows)* in distal shunt. Note that portal vein radical that has been catheterized does not opacify because 4F sheath completely fills its lumen. Stenosis was uneventfully dilated to 6 mm.

To perform procedures on the portal vein such as embolization, angioplasty, and stenting, it is necessary to negotiate a passage into the portal system. This can either be via direct entry into the portal system (Fig. 29-8) using ultrasound-guided puncture of the liver or spleen,[7] or surgical exposure of a peripheral portal vein tributary in the mesentery. The alternative is to enter the portal system from the systemic venous circulation using a transjugular intrahepatic portosystemic shunt (TIPS) set to puncture from the hepatic vein or IVC into the portal vein. Obviously these procedures involve considerably more risk than conventional systemic venous access.

COMPLICATIONS

On the whole, even large-bore devices can be readily inserted via the jugular vein. This has the advantage that hemostasis is readily achieved. For jugular vein punctures, hemostasis is actually helped by allowing the patient to sit up immediately after the device is removed, since this lowers venous pressure. This allows most transvenous procedures to be performed on an outpatient basis.

Fortunately, complications of venous access should be low, but some are significant and even life threatening and merit further consideration. There is clear evidence from

TABLE 29-2. Effect of Ultrasound Guidance on Complications of Central Venous Access*

Complication	Blind Puncture	Guided Puncture
Failure to access	5%-13%	0%-1%
Malposition	1%-8%	0%-12%
Pneumothorax	0%-12%	0%-1.4%
Hemothorax	0%-2.5%	0%
Arterial puncture	Up to 3%	0%-1%

*Data from References 9-22.

trials that complications of central venous catheterization are reduced by using ultrasound guidance (Table 29-2).[8]

Air Embolism

Air embolism is a potentially fatal complication of central venous access in which the negative intrathoracic pressure during inspiration results in air being aspirated into the superior vena cava. From here it passes through the right heart and into the pulmonary trunk. A large volume of air can obstruct the pulmonary trunk or prevent the ventricle from pumping effectively. This is a medical emergency. The patient should be turned onto the left side and placed head down if possible. Traditionally, the carotid arteries are also compressed in the case of a right-to-left shunt, which may result in a cerebrovascular accident. In practice, this first aid should never be necessary; *prevention* of air embolism is key.

Prevention is achieved by the simple expedient of never leaving the hub of any needle or catheter open to air. A syringe is attached during vein puncture, and a finger is placed over the hub while waiting for a guidewire. In reality, significant air embolization only occurs in one circumstance: when using a peel-away sheath to introduce a large catheter. Not all of these sheaths have a hemostatic valve, so there is always a moment between removal of the dilator and introduction of the catheter when air can enter. The best strategy to avoid this is to instruct the patient to hum whenever the catheter might be open to air (e.g., when removing a dilator or wire). This should be rehearsed to ensure the patient understands what is required. An alternative is to ask the patient to breathe in, then breathe out, then stop still. Humming or stopping at end expiration raises the intrathoracic pressure above atmospheric pressure, so if there are any problems, they will result in bleeding rather than aspiration. In practice, the patient can usually start breathing again a few seconds after the catheter is placed within the sheath. This strategy will only succeed in a compliant patient. In other patients, if the Trendelenburg position is not possible, the best strategy is to carefully observe their respiration over a few cycles and then time catheter insertion to expiration. A finger can always be placed over the hub again until the sheath has been split.

Pneumothorax

Pneumothorax is another complication better prevented than cured. In our local practice, there has not been a single pneumothorax case in 10 years of performing ultrasound-guided venous access. The same cannot be said for "blind puncture" techniques[9-22] (see Table 29-2).

Arterial Puncture and Catheterization

Arterial puncture is extremely rare with ultrasound guidance. A large meta-analysis showed that arterial puncture was more frequent with jugular than subclavian puncture, but the majority of procedures were performed without ultrasound guidance.[23,24] Following inadvertent carotid artery puncture, the puncture alone is unlikely to have serious sequelae, but incidences of stroke have been reported. If the artery is punctured, compression hemostasis should be obtained immediately, as for femoral arterial puncture. Periarterial hematoma is inevitable and may compromise subsequent access of the adjacent vein.

More serious is arterial catheterization, normally a complication of "blind" puncture or failure to visualize the puncture properly during ultrasound guidance. Unfortunately this is often associated with placement of a large hemodialysis catheter. This presents a serious problem. It is essential that the referring team remains calm and leaves the catheter in situ, allowing the interventional radiologist to arrange a rescue. Solutions include using a balloon to tamponade the hole during surgical or compression hemostasis, use of a percutaneous closure device, or an endoluminal stent-graft (Fig. 29-9).[25] Less can be done in the case of mediastinal hematoma or cardiac tamponade due to perforation of a central vessel.

Venous Thrombosis

All venous catheterization is associated with a risk of causing venous thrombosis. The risk is low but is of practical importance when using large devices. In one study, placement of an IVC filter was associated with an increased rate of recurrent DVT.[26] Although the devices in this study have largely been superseded by lower-profile systems, it is important to consider the morbidity from femoral vein puncture. This is less of an issue if the jugular vein is used as the point of access.

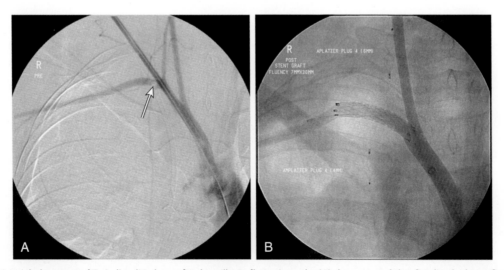

FIGURE 29-9. Arterial placement of Tesio line (Medcomp [Harleysville, Pa.]). Angiography **(A)** demonstrated that first line had transfixed right subclavian artery *(arrow)* and was sitting within pleural cavity. Second line had been placed directly into proximal right subclavian artery. Amplatzer plugs were placed in right vertebral and internal mammary arteries. **B,** Both lines were then sequentially removed while a stent-graft was successfully deployed to seal arterial defects.

▶ **SUGGESTED READINGS**

Chapman GA, Johnson D, Bodenham AR. Visualisation of needle position using ultrasonography. Anaesthesia 2006;61(2):148–58.

Flood SM, Bodenham AR. Central venous cannulation: ultrasound techniques. Anaesth Intensive Care Med 2010;11(1):16–8.

Funaki B. Diagnostic and interventional radiology in central venous access. Semin Roentgenol 2002;37:343–53.

Galloway S, Bodenham A. Long-term central venous access. Br J Anaesth 2004;92(5):722–34.

Hind D, Calvert N, McWilliams R, et al. Ultrasonic locating devices for central venous cannulation: meta-analysis. Br Med J 2003;327:361.

Keenan SP. Use of ultrasound to place central lines. J Crit Care 2002; 17(2):126–37.

Kumar A, Chuan A. Ultrasound guided vascular access: efficacy and safety. Best Pract Res Clin Anaesthesiol 2009;23(3):299–311.

Maecken T, Grau T. Ultrasound imaging in vascular access. Crit Care Med 2007;35(5):S178–S185.

Magee DC, Gould MK. Preventing complications of central venous catheterisation. N Engl J Med 2003;348:1123–33.

Ruesch S, Walder B, Tramer MR. Complications of central venous catheters: internal jugular versus subclavian access–a systematic review. Crit Care Med 2002;30:454–60.

Weeks SM. Unconventional venous access. Tech Vasc Interv Radiol 2002; 5:114–20.

The complete reference list is available onine at www.expertconsult.com.

CHAPTER **30**

Vascular Anatomy of the Upper Extremity

Amber Jones and Monica Smith Pearl

In this chapter, the classic arterial and venous anatomy of the upper extremity will be presented. Congenital variants will be discussed, as well as clinical correlates. It should be noted that fuller descriptions can be found in standard anatomy texts.

VASCULAR IMAGING OF THE UPPER EXTREMITY

Imaging of the arterial and venous systems is an important component of the evaluation in many vascular disorders involving the upper extremity. In combination with clinical and laboratory observations, imaging provides crucial information for both diagnosis and management of these complex processes. This section will provide a brief overview of vascular imaging, including ultrasonography (US), computed tomographic angiography (CTA), magnetic resonance angiography (MRA), and conventional angiography. For a complete discussion of vascular imaging techniques, please see Chapters 2 and 3.

Real-time grayscale and color Doppler US is a useful, rapid, and portable imaging modality used to evaluate both the arterial and venous systems of the upper extremity. Arterial interrogation may be performed to assess for suspected limb ischemia, arterial stenosis, or patency of a hemodialysis arteriovenous fistula or graft. Assessment of the integrity of the venous side of the dialysis graft or fistula is also important, as is evaluation of thrombosis or compression of upper extremity veins. US can investigate flow hemodynamics along with vessel lumen and wall morphology. It is, however, operator dependent, does not fully evaluate upper extremity arterial inflow and central thoracic venous anatomy, and is limited in spatial display.[1]

CTA is a widely available technique that may be performed on all existing multidetector CT (MDCT) scanners (4 through 320 channels) to assess upper extremity vasculature. An excellent review on state-of-the-art techniques and clinical applications of CTA in the upper extremity by Hellinger et al. proposes four upper extremity CTA protocols: Aortic Arch with Upper Extremity Runoff, Upper Extremity Runoff, Upper Extremity Indirect CT Venography (CTV), and Upper Extremity Direct CTV based upon different clinical indications.[1] This review highlights the various clinical scenarios in which CTA is useful and provides the technical parameters for acquisition, which are beyond the scope of this chapter.

Contrast-enhanced MRA is a rapid noninvasive imaging technique that aids in treatment planning and preoperative mapping of various vascular disorders of the upper extremity.[2] It evaluates vascular integrity and patency, which may be compromised in cases of trauma, atherosclerosis, vasculitis, and malignancy. MRA not only defines the site, degree, and extent of stenosis or occlusion but also demonstrates collateral pathways in these processes. Advantages of contrast-enhanced MRA in the upper extremity include its noninvasive nature, lack of flow artifact, multiangular projection capability, and ability to delineate the small vessels of the hand. Limitations of this imaging technique in the upper extremity include limited coverage of 40 to 50 cm, variable circulation time among individuals, and overlapping of the arteries and veins in the hand.[2] Other considerations include the effects of partial volume averaging and susceptibility artifacts, which may lead to an overestimation of stenosis in small blood vessels.

Conventional angiography is the gold standard for vascular imaging of the upper extremity, but it is an invasive procedure and is currently reserved for situations in which clinical questions remain despite information provided by the above-described noninvasive imaging modalities. It may also be used as the primary diagnostic modality when direct hemodynamic analysis is required for treatment planning or when there is intent to perform endovascular intervention in one combined procedure.[1]

ARTERIAL ANATOMY OF THE UPPER EXTREMITY

Subclavian Artery

The arterial blood supply of the upper extremity originates with the subclavian artery, whose typical diameter is 8 to 10 mm. The right subclavian artery arises from the brachiocephalic trunk, whereas the left subclavian artery is a direct branch from the aortic arch (Fig. 30-1). From its origin to the lateral border of the first rib, the subclavian artery supplies blood to the upper part of the chest, arms, and central nervous system (via the vertebral artery). The subclavian artery is divided into three segments based on its medial, posterior, or lateral relationship to the anterior scalene muscle. The first segments of the right and left subclavian arteries differ, whereas the second and third are nearly identical bilaterally. The first segment of the right subclavian artery begins at its origin from the brachiocephalic (innominate) trunk posterior to the upper border of the right sternoclavicular joint. It arches superolaterally, passes anterior to the extension of the pleural cavity in the root of the neck, and extends to the medial margin of the right anterior scalene muscle. It ascends variably 2 to 4 cm above the clavicle. The first segment of the left subclavian artery begins as a direct branch of the aortic arch after the origin

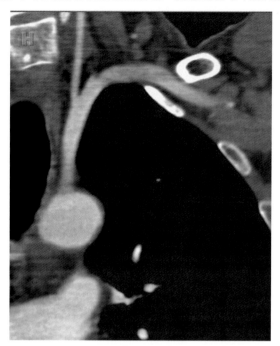

FIGURE 30-1. Coned-in computed tomographic angiography (CTA) of chest demonstrates left subclavian artery originating from aortic arch and axillary artery, which begins at lateral border of first rib.

subclavian artery in the neck, whereas more distal regions of the plexus surround the axillary artery (Fig. 30-2).

Variations in subclavian arterial anatomy are related to its origin and pathway. The right subclavian artery may arise above or below the sternoclavicular level as a distinct aortic arch branch, either the first or the last. When it arises as the first branch, it is in the position of a brachiocephalic trunk, as in the "classic" anatomy. If it arises as the last branch off the aortic arch, it ascends obliquely to the right and courses behind the trachea, esophagus, and right common carotid artery; alternatively in this scenario, it may pass between the trachea and esophagus. Occasionally, the left subclavian artery is combined at its origin with the left common carotid artery. Other variations in the pathway of the subclavian artery have also been described in relation to the anterior scalene muscle: perforating the muscle or, very rarely, passing anterior to it. Most of the branches of the subclavian artery arise from the artery's first segment. Its branches include the vertebral artery, thyrocervical trunk, internal thoracic artery, and costocervical trunk (Fig. 30-3). These branches all arise from the first segment of the subclavian artery on the left. On the right, the costocervical trunk usually originates from the second segment of the subclavian artery. Additionally, on either side the dorsal scapular artery may arise from the third or, less often, the second segment of the subclavian artery or continue as the deep branch of the transverse cervical artery, a branch of the thyrocervical trunk.

Vertebral Artery

In more than 80% of cases, the vertebral artery originates from the superoposterior aspect of the first segment of the subclavian artery as its most proximal and largest branch. The vertebral artery ascends and enters the transverse foramen of the sixth cervical vertebra and continues superiorly through the foramina of the fifth through first cervical vertebrae. At the superior border of the first cervical vertebra, the artery curves medially, crosses the posterior arch of the first cervical vertebra, and passes through the foramen magnum to enter the posterior cranial fossa. Size of the vertebral arteries is variable, but a left-dominant artery is more common.

Variations involving the vertebral artery are related to its origin, usually a more proximal one. The left vertebral artery originates from the aortic arch between the left common carotid and the left subclavian artery in up to 5.8% of cases (Fig. 30-4). Its entrance into the cervical transverse foramen is also variable, but it most commonly enters at the level of the fifth cervical vertebra. Other rare variations involving the left vertebral artery that have been described include an origin from the aortic arch distal to the left subclavian artery, an origin from the left common carotid artery, or an origin from the external carotid artery. In less than 1% of cases, the right vertebral artery originates from the right common carotid artery or the aortic arch.

Thyrocervical Trunk

The thyrocervical trunk is the second branch of the subclavian artery, and it arises just distal to the vertebral artery from the superior surface of the first segment of the subclavian artery. Near the medial border of the anterior scalene

of the left common carotid artery at the level of the third and fourth thoracic intervertebral disk spaces. It also ascends into the neck and arches laterally to the medial border of the left anterior scalene muscle. The second segment of the subclavian artery is posterior to the anterior scalene muscle. It is short and the most superior part of the vessel. The third segment descends from the lateral margin of the anterior scalene muscle and extends to the lateral border of the first rib, where it becomes the axillary artery. This portion is the most superficial part of the artery and lies partly in the supraclavicular triangle, the lower and smaller subdivision of the posterior cervical triangle.

The posterior cervical triangle of the neck is located in the lateral aspect of the neck in direct continuity with the upper limb. It is bordered anteriorly by the posterior edge of the sternocleidomastoid muscle, posteriorly by the anterior edge of the trapezius muscle, and inferiorly by the middle third of the clavicle. Its apex is the occipital bone, just posterior to the mastoid process where attachments of the trapezius and sternocleidomastoid converge. About 2.5 cm above the clavicle, it is crossed by the inferior belly of the omohyoid muscle, which divides the posterior triangle into the occipital and supraclavicular triangles.

All major nerves that innervate the upper limb originate from the brachial plexus, a somatic plexus that begins in the neck and passes laterally and inferiorly over the first rib into the axilla. Medially to laterally, it is composed of roots, trunks, divisions, and cords. The roots are formed by the anterior rami of C5 to C8 and most of T1. The roots and trunks enter the posterior triangle of the neck by passing between the anterior and middle scalene muscles and lie superior and posterior to the subclavian artery. The proximal parts of the brachial plexus are posterior to the

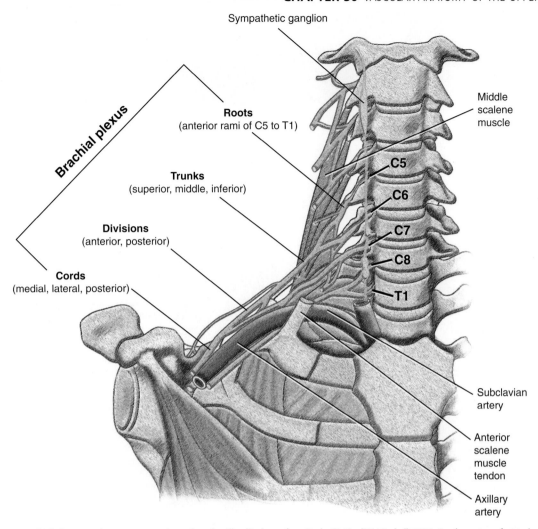

FIGURE 30-2. Brachial plexus: major components in neck and axilla. *(Redrawn from Drake RL, Vogl W, Mitchell AWM. Gray's anatomy for students. Philadelphia: Elsevier/Churchill Livingstone; 2005.)*

muscle, the thyrocervical trunk classically divides into the inferior thyroid, transverse cervical, and suprascapular arteries. Only slightly more than 50% of individuals have this classic anatomy. Independent origins of one or more of these vessels from the subclavian artery are common.

The inferior thyroid artery is the superior continuation of the thyrocervical trunk. It ascends anterior to the anterior scalene muscle and turns medially just below the sixth cervical transverse process. Here it passes anterior to the vertebral vessels and posterior to the carotid sheath and its contents. It finally descends on the longus colli muscle to the inferior pole of the lateral lobe of the thyroid gland.

Branches of the inferior thyroid artery include muscular branches supplying the infrahyoid muscles, longus colli muscle, anterior scalene muscle, and the inferior pharyngeal constrictor, as well as pharyngeal branches supplying the lower pharynx, thyroid, and parathyroid glands. An important muscular branch is the ascending cervical artery, which arises as the inferior thyroid artery turns medially behind the carotid sheath; it ascends on the anterior surface of the prevertebral muscles, which it supplies, and sends branches to the spinal cord.

The middle branch of the thyrocervical trunk is the transverse cervical artery. This branch passes laterally and

slightly posteriorly, anterior to the brachial plexus and the anterior scalene muscle, and enters and crosses the base of the posterior triangle. As it reaches the deep surface of the trapezius muscle, it divides into superficial and deep branches. The superficial branch continues on the deep surface of the trapezius muscle, and the deep branch continues on the deep surface of the rhomboid muscles near the medial border of the scapula. Alternatively, these branches may not arise in common as a transverse cervical artery. The superficial branch frequently arises directly from the thyrocervical trunk as a superficial cervical artery, and the deep branch may arise from the third or, less commonly, from the second part of the subclavian artery as the dorsal scapular artery.

The most inferior branch of the thyrocervical trunk is the suprascapular artery. It descends laterally and crosses anterior to the anterior scalene muscle, phrenic nerve, third part of the subclavian artery, and trunks of the brachial plexus. It reaches the superior scapular border, passes above the superior transverse scapular ligament, which separates it from the suprascapular nerve, and enters the suprascapular fossa. In addition to supplying the supraspinatus and infraspinatus muscles, the suprascapular artery contributes branches to numerous structures along its course. Other

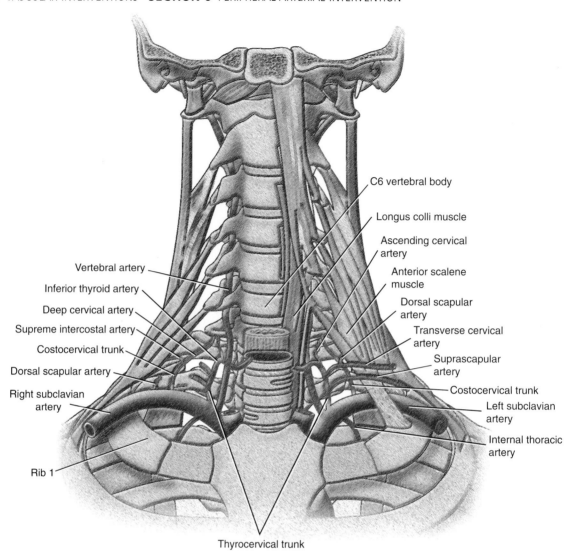

FIGURE 30-3. Subclavian artery and branches in root of neck. *(Redrawn from Drake RL, Vogl W, Mitchell AWM. Gray's anatomy for students. Philadelphia: Elsevier/Churchill Livingstone; 2005.)*

alternative origins of the suprascapular artery include a direct origin from the third part of the subclavian artery or as a branch of the internal thoracic artery.

Internal Thoracic Artery

The internal thoracic artery arises from the anteroinferior aspect of the first part of the subclavian artery, directly below the origin of the thyrocervical trunk. It courses anteromedially behind the clavicle and the internal jugular and brachiocephalic veins. It descends behind the first six costal cartilages about 1 cm from the lateral sternal border, divides into numerous intermediate branches, and terminates in the musculophrenic and superior epigastric arteries at the level of the sixth intercostal space.

In the event of thoracic or abdominal aortic obstruction, the internal thoracic arteries are important potential sources of collateral blood supply via anterior anastomoses with the intercostal arteries and inferior epigastric arteries, respectively. Additionally, the internal thoracic arteries may provide collateral blood supply to the bronchial arteries.

Costocervical Trunk

The final branch of the subclavian artery in the root of the neck is the costocervical trunk. Depending on the side, it arises in a slightly different position. On the left it arises from the first segment of the subclavian artery, whereas on the right it arises from the second segment. On both sides it arches back above the cervical pleura to the neck of the first rib, where it divides into the deep cervical and supreme intercostal branches. The deep cervical artery anastomoses with the descending branch of the occipital artery and branches of the vertebral artery. In most cases the deep cervical artery arises from the costocervical trunk, but on occasion it may be a separate branch of the subclavian artery. The supreme intercostal artery descends anterior to the first rib and divides to form the posterior intercostal arteries for the first two intercostal spaces.

Clinically relevant scenarios related to stenosis or occlusion of the origin of the subclavian artery involve the potential collateral blood supply, including all the branches of the subclavian and axillary arteries. Subclavian steal, which

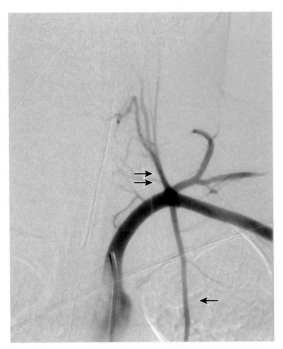

FIGURE 30-4. Left subclavian artery angiogram. Note absence of left vertebral artery, which arises from aortic arch. Thyrocervical trunk *(double arrow)* is first branch of left subclavian artery. Single arrow points to internal thoracic artery.

may be associated with arm pain or central neurologic symptoms, is caused by retrograde flow in the ipsilateral vertebral artery. Additionally, steal physiology may affect other vessels in the upper extremity. For example, reversal of flow can occur in smaller subclavian artery branches such as the thyrocervical trunk and the internal mammary artery. In patients who undergo cardiac bypass surgery based on an internal mammary artery, proximal subclavian stenosis can cause a steal phenomenon involving the internal mammary artery that results in angina.

The axilla is the transition zone between the neck and arm, through which all major structures pass into and out of the upper limb. It is formed by the clavicle, scapula, upper thoracic wall, humerus, and related muscles.

Axillary Artery

The axillary artery, as a continuation of the subclavian artery, begins at the lateral margin of the first rib and ends normally at the inferior border of the teres major, where it becomes the brachial artery. The axillary artery supplies the walls of the axilla and related regions and continues as the major blood supply to more distal parts of the upper limb. Similar to the division of the subclavian artery based on its relationship to the anterior scalene muscle, the axillary artery is also divided into three segments based on its relationship to the pectoralis minor muscle: proximal, posterior, and distal.

As mentioned previously, the more distal regions of the brachial plexus surround the axillary artery. The brachial plexus trunks divide into anterior and posterior divisions, which ultimately give rise to peripheral nerves associated with the anterior and posterior compartments of the arm and forearm, respectively. The divisions give rise to lateral,

medial, and posterior cords that are lateral, medial, and posterior to the second part of the axillary artery, respectively. In general, nerves associated with the anterior compartments of the upper limb arise from the medial and lateral cords, and nerves associated with the posterior compartments originate from the posterior cord.

Branches of the axillary artery are highly variable in origin, but six branches are generally present (Fig. 30-5). One branch, the superior thoracic artery, originates from the first segment. Two branches, the thoracoacromial and lateral thoracic arteries, originate from the second segment. Three branches, the subscapular, anterior circumflex humeral, and posterior circumflex humeral arteries, originate from the third segment. With the exception of the vertebral artery, all the axillary and subclavian artery branches have potential anastomoses with each other that become apparent in the presence of occlusive disease or vascular tumors.

The superior thoracic artery is small and originates from the anterior surface of the first part of the axillary artery near the inferior border of the subclavius muscle. It runs anteromedially above the medial border of the pectoralis minor muscle and then passes between it and the pectoralis major muscle to the thoracic wall. It supplies these muscles and the thoracic wall and anastomoses with the internal thoracic and upper intercostal arteries.

The second segment of the axillary artery gives off two branches, the thoracoacromial and lateral thoracic arteries. The thoracoacromial artery is short and curves around the superior margin of the pectoralis minor muscle. It penetrates the clavipectoral fascia and divides into four branches, the pectoral, deltoid, clavicular, and acromial, that supply the anterior axillary wall and related regions. The pectoral branch contributes vascular supply to the breast as it descends between the pectoral muscles and anastomoses with the intercostal branches of the internal thoracic and lateral thoracic arteries. The deltoid branch often arises with the acromial and crosses the pectoralis minor to accompany the cephalic vein between the pectoralis major and deltoid, both of which it supplies.

The lateral thoracic artery also arises from the anterior surface of the second segment of the axillary artery posterior to the inferolateral margin of the pectoralis minor. It follows the lateral margin of the muscle to the thoracic wall and supplies the serratus anterior and pectoral muscles, axillary lymph nodes, and subscapularis. It anastomoses with the internal thoracic, subscapular, and intercostal arteries and the pectoral branch of the thoracoacromial artery. In women, it is large and has lateral mammary branches that curve around the lateral border of the pectoralis major and contribute to the vascular supply of the breast.

Branches of the third segment of the axillary artery include the subscapular and anterior and posterior circumflex humeral arteries. The subscapular artery, the largest branch of the axillary artery, is the major blood supply to the posterior wall of the axilla and contributes to the blood supply of the posterior scapular region. It originates from the posterior surface of the third part of the axillary artery, follows the inferior margin of the subscapularis muscle, and then divides into its two terminal branches, the circumflex scapular and thoracodorsal arteries. The circumflex scapular artery passes through the triangular space between the

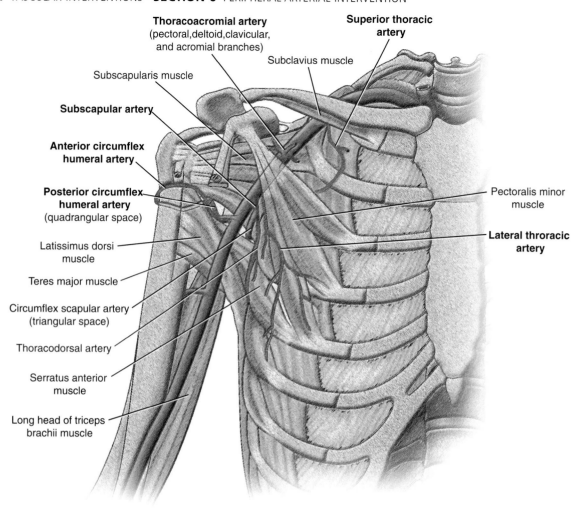

FIGURE 30-5. Branches of axillary artery. *(Redrawn from Drake RL, Vogl W, Mitchell AWM. Gray's anatomy for students. Philadelphia: Elsevier/Churchill Livingstone; 2005.)*

subscapularis, teres major, and long head of the triceps muscles. It contributes to an anastomotic network of vessels around the scapula and anastomoses with the suprascapular artery and the deep branch (dorsal scapular artery) of the transverse cervical artery (Fig. 30-6). The thoracodorsal artery, which follows the lateral border of the scapula to the inferior angle, contributes to the vascular supply of the posterior and medial walls of the axilla.

The anterior and posterior circumflex humeral arteries both originate from the lateral side of the third segment of the axillary artery. The anterior circumflex humeral artery is small in comparison to the posterior circumflex humeral artery. It passes anterior to the surgical neck of the humerus and anastomoses with the posterior circumflex humeral artery while supplying branches to surrounding tissues, including the glenohumeral joint and the humeral head. A variation described is a common origin of this artery with the posterior circumflex humeral artery.

The posterior circumflex humeral artery originates from the axillary artery immediately posterior to the origin of the anterior circumflex humeral artery. With the axillary nerve it leaves the axilla by passing through the quadrangular space between the teres major, teres minor, and the long head of the triceps brachii muscle and the surgical neck of

the humerus. The posterior circumflex humeral artery also curves around the surgical neck of the humerus and supplies the surrounding muscles and the glenohumeral joint. It anastomoses with the anterior circumflex humeral artery and with branches from the profunda brachii, suprascapular, and thoracoacromial arteries.

Clinically relevant scenarios involving the axillary artery are related to axillary puncture and trauma. The radial, ulnar, and median nerves are in close proximity to the axillary artery. Contained in a sheath of connective tissue along with the artery, these neural structures are at risk for compression by hematomas after puncture of the axillary artery. In traumatic settings, the axillary artery is more frequently lacerated than any other except for the popliteal artery. It has been ruptured in attempts to reduce old dislocations, especially when the artery is adherent to the articular capsule. Additionally, fractures of the first rib may compromise the distal part of the subclavian artery or the first part of the axillary artery.

The axilla, antecubital fossa, and carpal tunnel are significant areas of transition between the different parts of the limb. As stated previously, all major structures that pass between the neck and arm pass through the axilla. The next major transition zone is the antecubital fossa, a triangular

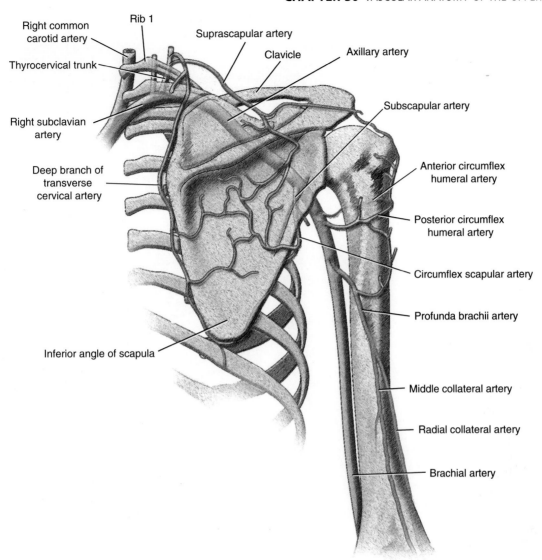

FIGURE 30-6. Arterial anastomoses around shoulder. *(Redrawn from Drake RL, Vogl W, Mitchell AWM. Gray's anatomy for students. Philadelphia: Elsevier/ Churchill Livingstone; 2005.)*

depression anterior to the elbow joint that is formed by the brachioradialis muscle laterally, the pronator teres muscle medially, and an imaginary line drawn between the medial and lateral epicondyles superiorly. The brachial artery, which passes from the arm to the forearm, travels through this fossa, as does the median nerve.

Brachial Artery

The brachial artery, the major artery of the arm, is a continuation of the axillary artery and is found in the anterior compartment. Proximally, the brachial artery begins at the lower border of the teres major muscle and lies on the medial side of the arm. Distally, it moves laterally and lies between the medial and lateral epicondyles of the humerus. It crosses anterior to the elbow joint, where it lies immediately medial to the biceps brachii muscle tendon. The brachial artery gives off numerous branches along its path, the largest of which is the profunda brachii artery, before it divides into the radial and ulnar arteries. Other named

branches of the brachial artery include the humeral nutrient artery, muscular branches, and the superior and inferior ulnar collateral arteries (Fig. 30-7).

The profunda brachii artery is the largest branch of the brachial artery; it arises from its posteromedial aspect and passes into and supplies the posterior compartment of the arm. It enters the posterior compartment with the radial nerve, and together they pass through the triangular interval, which is formed by the shaft of the humerus, the inferior margin of the teres major muscle, and the lateral margin of the long head of the triceps muscle. They continue along the radial groove on the posterior humeral surface deep to the lateral head of the triceps brachii muscle. Branches of the profunda brachii artery supply adjacent muscles and anastomose with the posterior circumflex humeral artery. The artery terminates as two collateral vessels, the middle collateral and radial collateral arteries, which contribute to an anastomotic network of arteries around the elbow joint.

Variations in anatomy involving the axillary and brachial arteries and their branches include common trunks for a

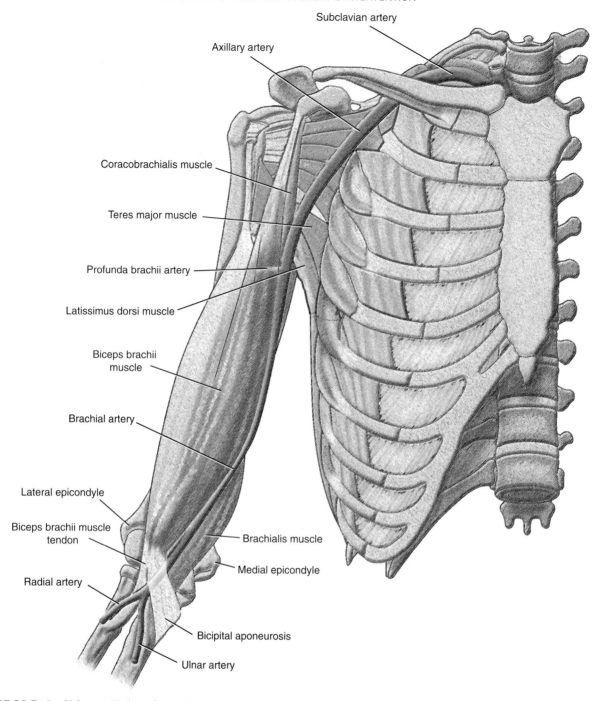

FIGURE 30-7. Brachial artery. *(Redrawn from Drake RL, Vogl W, Mitchell AWM. Gray's anatomy for students. Philadelphia: Elsevier/Churchill Livingstone; 2005.)*

number of branches and more proximal divisions or high origins. Occasionally, the subscapular, circumflex humeral, and profunda brachii arteries arise from a common trunk from the axillary artery. Additionally, the axillary artery may be the source of the profunda brachii artery, radial artery, or anterior interosseous artery of the forearm, or it may divide into the radial and ulnar arteries. Anomalous high origins of the radial or ulnar artery from the brachial or axillary artery are present in 15% and 3% of patients, respectively. These variants are important to consider during upper extremity angiography, especially if the catheter is unknowingly placed distal to an anomalous high origin.

Variants of the brachial artery itself are uncommon but include a small accessory branch to the radial artery called the *persistent superficial brachial artery*, which exists in 1% to 2%, and duplication in 0.1%. More common variations involve more proximal divisions of the brachial artery as described earlier. Occasionally it divides more proximally into two trunks that reunite. Frequently it divides more proximally than usual into the radial, ulnar, and common interosseous arteries. Most often it is the radial branch that arises proximally, leaving a common trunk for the ulnar and common interosseous arteries. However, either the ulnar or common interosseous artery may alternatively arise

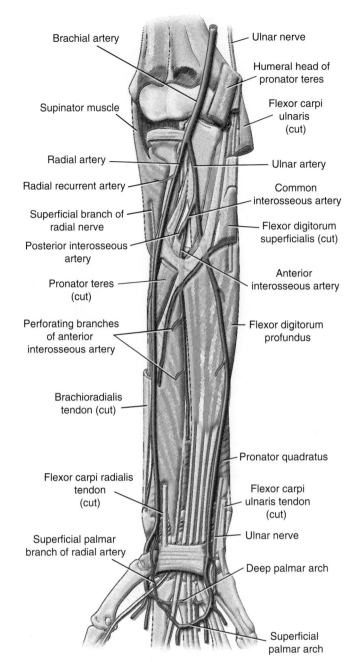

Brachial artery

Supinator muscle

Radial artery

Radial recurrent artery

Superficial branch of radial nerve

Posterior interosseous artery

Pronator teres (cut)

Perforating branches of anterior interosseous artery

Brachioradialis tendon (cut)

Flexor carpi radialis tendon (cut)

Superficial palmar branch of radial artery

Ulnar nerve

Humeral head of pronator teres

Flexor carpi ulnaris (cut)

Ulnar artery

Common interosseous artery

Flexor digitorum superficialis (cut)

Anterior interosseous artery

Flexor digitorum profundus

Pronator quadratus

Flexor carpi ulnaris tendon (cut)

Ulnar nerve

Deep palmar arch

Superficial palmar arch

FIGURE 30-8. Arteries of anterior compartment of forearm. *(Redrawn from Drake RL, Vogl W, Mitchell AWM. Gray's anatomy for students. Philadelphia: Elsevier/Churchill Livingstone; 2005.)*

proximally and leave the other branches to form the other division.

Radial Artery

The terminal branches of the brachial artery are the radial, ulnar, and interosseus arteries (Fig. 30-8). The forearm arteries supply the adjacent muscles, whereas the radial and ulnar arteries continue into the hand and form anastomoses at the wrist with the palmar and dorsal carpal arches, and in the hand with the superficial and deep palmar arches between their digital and metacarpal branches (Fig. 30-9). Considerable variation exists in the distribution of the

arteries of the hand. In most cases the radial and ulnar arteries both supply the hand, although one vessel may dominate. In less than 2% of individuals, the interosseus artery may continue into the hand as the median artery.

The radial artery, though smaller than the ulnar artery, is the more direct continuation of the brachial artery. There are three main segments of the radial artery: one in the forearm, one at the wrist, and one in the hand. In the proximal portion of the forearm, the radial artery begins from the medial aspect of the radial neck and is just deep to the brachioradialis muscle. In the middle third, it descends along the lateral aspect of the forearm and is medial to the superficial branch of the radial nerve. In the distal part of the forearm, the radial artery is medial to the brachioradialis muscle tendon and is covered only by the skin and superficial and deep fasciae. Other distal landmarks include its lateral relationship to the flexor carpi radialis muscle tendon and its position anterior to the pronator quadratus muscle and the distal end of the radius. In the distal end of the forearm, the flexor carpi radialis muscle may be used as a landmark to locate the radial artery.

Branches of the radial artery that originate in the forearm include the radial recurrent artery, muscular branches, and more distally, the palmar carpal and superficial palmar branches. The radial recurrent artery arises just distal to the elbow and ascends; it contributes to an anastomotic network around the elbow joint and to numerous vessels that supply muscles on the lateral side of the forearm. The muscular branches are distributed to the extensor muscles on the radial side of the forearm. The palmar carpal branch is a small vessel that arises near the distal border of the pronator quadratus muscle and contributes to an anastomotic network of vessels supplying the carpal bones and joints. The superficial palmar branch arises from the radial artery just before it curves around the carpus. It passes through and occasionally over the thenar muscles and anastomoses with the end of the ulnar artery to complete a superficial palmar arch (Fig. 30-10).

As the radial artery leaves the forearm, it curves laterally around the wrist and passes over the floor of the anatomic snuffbox, a triangular depression formed on the posterolateral side of the wrist and the first metacarpal by the extensor tendons passing into the thumb (Fig. 30-11). Before penetrating the back of the hand, the radial artery gives rise to two vessels: a dorsal carpal branch and the first dorsal metacarpal artery. The dorsal carpal branch arises deep to the extensor pollicis tendons, passes medially across the wrist, and anastomoses with the ulnar dorsal carpal branch and with the anterior and posterior interosseous arteries to form a dorsal carpal arch. From the dorsal arch, three dorsal metacarpal arteries arise and subsequently bifurcate into the small dorsal digital arteries, which enter the fingers and anastomose with the palmar digital branches of the superficial palmar arch. Just before it passes between the heads of the first dorsal interosseous, the radial artery gives off the first dorsal metacarpal artery, which supplies adjacent sides of the index finger and thumb. The radial side of the thumb receives a branch directly from the radial artery itself.

The radial artery continues and penetrates the dorsolateral aspect of the hand between the bases of the first and second metacarpals to provide the major blood supply to the thumb and lateral side of the index finger. It passes between the two heads of the first dorsal interosseus muscle

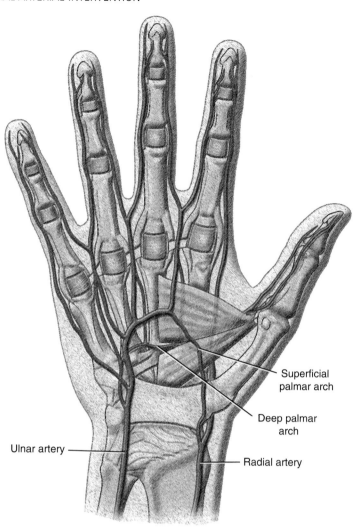

Superficial
palmar arch

Deep palmar
arch

Ulnar artery

Radial artery

FIGURE 30-9. Arterial supply to hand. *(Redrawn from Drake RL, Vogl W, Mitchell AWM. Gray's anatomy for students. Philadelphia: Elsevier/Churchill Livingstone; 2005.)*

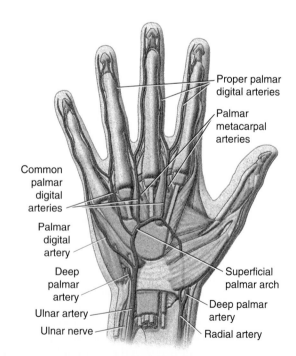

Proper palmar
digital arteries

Palmar
metacarpal
arteries

Common
palmar
digital
arteries

Palmar
digital
artery

Deep
palmar
artery

Superficial
palmar arch

Ulnar artery

Deep palmar
artery

Ulnar nerve

Radial artery

FIGURE 30-10. Superficial palmar arch. *(Redrawn from Drake RL, Vogl W, Mitchell AWM. Gray's anatomy for students. Philadelphia: Elsevier/Churchill Livingstone; 2005.)*

and then between the two heads of the adductor pollicis to access the deep plane of the palm and form the deep palmar arch (Fig. 30-12).

The deep palmar arch passes medially through the palm between the metacarpal bones and the long flexor tendons of the digits. On the medial side of the palm, it anastomoses with the deep palmar branch of the ulnar artery. Branches of the deep palmar arch include the three palmar metacarpal arteries, three perforating branches, and the recurrent branches. The palmar metacarpal arteries run distally from the convexity of the arch on the interosseous muscles of the second to fourth spaces and join the common palmar digital arteries from the superficial palmar arch. The perforating branches traverse the second to fourth interosseous spaces between the heads of the corresponding dorsal interossei to anastomose with the dorsal metacarpal arteries from the dorsal carpal arch. The recurrent branches ascend proximally from the deep palmar arch anterior to the carpus to supply the carpal bones and end in the palmar carpal arch.

Two vessels, the princeps pollicis artery and the radialis indicis artery, arise from the radial artery in the plane between the first dorsal interosseous and adductor pollicis. The princeps pollicis artery is the major blood supply to the thumb and arises from the radial artery as it turns medially into the palm of the hand. At the base of the proximal muscular branches arise directly from the main vessel and distribute to muscles in the ulnar region.

The common interosseous artery is a short branch of the ulnar artery just distal to the radial tuberosity. It passes back to the proximal border of the interosseous membrane and divides into the anterior and posterior interosseous arteries.

The anterior interosseous artery descends along the anterior aspect of the interosseous membrane and gives off muscular branches as well as nutrient arteries to the radius and ulna. Additionally, numerous perforating branches pass through the interosseous membrane to supply deep muscles of the posterior compartment. It also has a small branch that contributes to the vascular network around the carpal bones and joints. In the distal end of the forearm, it perforates the interosseous membrane and terminates by anastomosing with the posterior interosseous artery.

The posterior interosseous artery is usually smaller than the anterior and also originates from the common interosseous artery in the anterior compartment of the forearm. It passes dorsally over the proximal border of the interosseous membrane into the posterior compartment. It contributes the recurrent interosseous artery to the vascular network around the elbow joint and then passes between the supinator and abductor pollicis longus muscles to supply the superficial extensors. Distally, it anastomoses with the end of the anterior interosseous artery and dorsal carpal arch of the wrist.

The dorsal carpal branch arises just proximal to the pisiform bone and anastomoses with the radial dorsal carpal branch to complete the dorsal carpal arch. The palmar carpal branch is a small vessel that anastomoses with the radial palmar carpal branch; it receives branches from the anterior interosseous artery and forms the palmar carpal arch at the wrist and carpus.

The ulnar artery reaches the wrist, enters the hand on the medial side of the wrist, and crosses lateral to the pisiform bone and ulnar nerve. It is anterior to the flexor retinaculum, a thick band of connective tissue that forms the anterior wall of the carpal tunnel, the gateway to the palm of the hand. The posterior, lateral, and medial walls of the carpal tunnel are made of small proximal carpal bones that form an arch through which the median nerve and long flexor tendons pass from the forearm to the digits of the hand. The ulnar artery is often the major blood supply to the medial three and one-half digits. Distally, the ulnar artery is medial to the hook of the hamate bone and swings laterally across the palm to form the superficial palmar arch, which is superficial to the long flexor tendons of the digits and just deep to the palmar aponeurosis. On the lateral side of the palm, the arch communicates with a palmar branch of the radial artery.

Branches from the superficial palmar arch include a palmar digital artery to the medial side of the fifth digit and three common palmar digital arteries. The three large common palmar digital arteries provide the principal blood supply to the lateral side of the fifth digit, both sides of the fourth and third digits, and the medial side of the second digit. The common palmar digital arteries are joined by the corresponding palmar metacarpal arteries from the deep palmar arch before bifurcating into the proper palmar digital arteries, which enter the fingers.

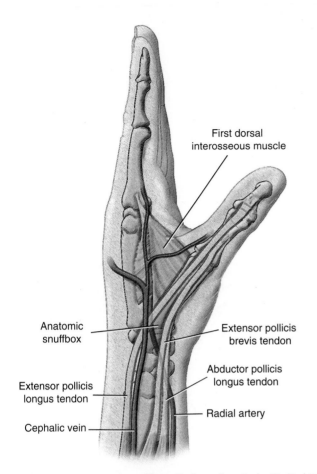

FIGURE 30-11. Anatomic snuffbox. *(Redrawn from Drake RL, Vogl W, Mitchell AWM. Gray's anatomy for students. Philadelphia: Elsevier/Churchill Livingstone; 2005.)*

Labels on figure: First dorsal interosseous muscle; Anatomic snuffbox; Extensor pollicis longus tendon; Cephalic vein; Extensor pollicis brevis tendon; Abductor pollicis longus tendon; Radial artery

phalanx, it divides into two branches that run along the sides of the thumb and supply the skin and subcutaneous tissue. The radialis indicis artery arises from the deep palmar arch and frequently from the princeps pollicis artery and supplies the lateral side of the index finger.

Ulnar Artery

The ulnar artery is the larger terminal branch of the brachial artery; it begins at the level of the radial neck and passes downward and medially to reach the ulnar side of the forearm. As it leaves the cubital fossa, the ulnar artery passes deep to the pronator teres muscle and through the forearm in the fascial plane between the flexor carpi ulnaris and flexor digitorum profundus muscles. In the distal part of the forearm, the ulnar artery is lateral to the ulnar nerve and is not easily palpable because it often remains positioned under the anterolateral lip of the flexor carpi ulnaris tendon.

Branches arising in the forearm include the ulnar recurrent artery, muscular branches, the common interosseous artery, and two small carpal arteries, the dorsal carpal branch and the palmar carpal branch, that supply the wrist.

The ulnar recurrent artery is composed of anterior and posterior branches that contribute to an anastomotic network of vessels around the elbow joint. Numerous

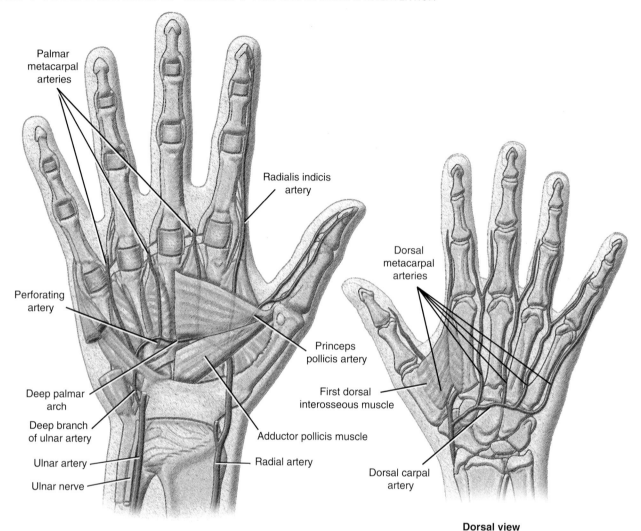

FIGURE 30-12. Deep palmar arch. *(Redrawn from Drake RL, Vogl W, Mitchell AWM. Gray's anatomy for students. Philadelphia: Elsevier/Churchill Livingstone; 2005.)*

The deep palmar branch of the ulnar artery arises from the medial aspect of the ulnar artery just distal to the pisiform and penetrates the origin of the hypothenar muscles. It curves medially around the hook of the hamate to anastomose with the deep palmar arch derived from the radial artery.

In general, the classic arterial anatomy of the hand includes two complete palmar arches, each of which receives blood supply from both the radial and ulnar arteries. The deep palmar arch is the more proximal arcade and is supplied primarily by the radial artery. The superficial palmar arch is the more distal arcade and is ulnar artery dominant. Numerous variations are commonly present, with less than 50% of patients having both complete classic arcades. In patients with an incomplete arch system, ischemic symptoms may develop after trauma because of deficient collateral blood supply.

A clinically relevant scenario involving ischemia of the hand and fingers is the hypothenar hammer syndrome. It has been classically described in men of working age with industrial occupations who use the hypothenar side of the palm as a hammer, but it has also been reported in mountain bikers, tennis players, and other athletes. Blunt repetitive trauma to the ulnar artery and superficial palmar arch against the hook of the hamate bone results in damage to the arterial wall that may lead to pseudoaneurysm formation, with or without vessel thrombosis, microemboli, and compression of the sensory branch of the ulnar nerve. Treatment options include conservative management with thrombolytics and smoking cessation or surgery.

VENOUS SYSTEM

The veins of the upper extremities are divided into superficial and deep systems, with free anastomoses between them. The superficial veins are subcutaneous in the superficial fascia; deep veins accompany arteries between the muscles of the limb. Both groups have valves, but they are more numerous in the deep veins. From the hand to the shoulder, the superficial veins are the major drainage pathway. At the shoulder, the deep veins become the primary drainage route. This is different from the anatomy of the lower extremities, where the deep veins are dominant throughout.

The superficial veins of the upper extremity are large veins embedded in the superficial fascia of the upper limb

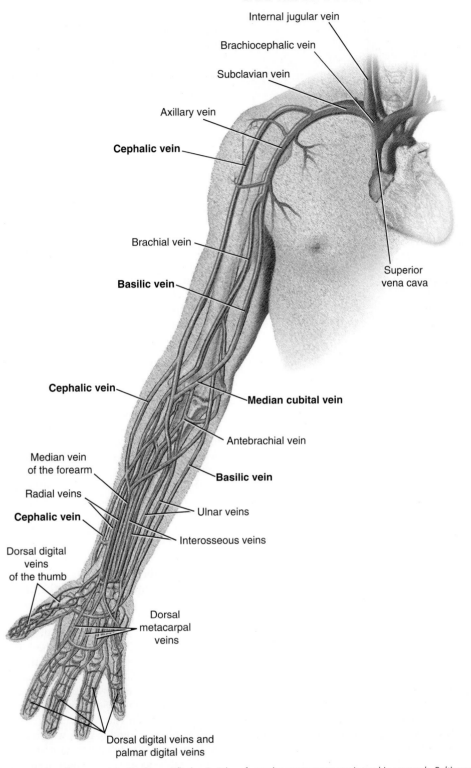

Internal jugular vein

Brachiocephalic vein

Subclavian vein

Axillary vein

Cephalic vein

Brachial vein

Basilic vein

Superior
vena cava

Cephalic vein

Median cubital vein

Antebrachial vein

Median vein
of the forearm

Basilic vein

Radial veins

Ulnar veins

Cephalic vein

Interosseous veins

Dorsal digital
veins
of the thumb

Dorsal
metacarpal
veins

Dorsal digital veins and
palmar digital veins

FIGURE 30-13. Venous anatomy of upper extremity. *(From Uflacker R. Atlas of vascular anatomy: an angiographic approach. Baltimore: Lippincott Williams & Wilkins; 1997, p. 339–403.)*

and are often used to access a patient's vascular system and withdraw blood. The most significant of these veins are the cephalic along the anterior radial edge, the basilic along the posterior ulnar edge, and the median cubital along the anterior aspect in the midline (Fig. 30-13).

As generally found in the upper limb, the hand contains interconnected networks of deep and superficial veins. The

deep veins follow the arteries, whereas the superficial veins drain into a dorsal venous network. Dorsal digital veins pass along the sides of the fingers and unite into three dorsal metacarpal veins that form the dorsal venous network on the back of the hand over the metacarpal bones (Fig. 30-14). The cephalic vein originates from the lateral side of the dorsal venous network, and the basilic vein originates from

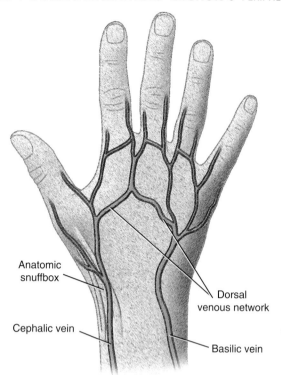

FIGURE 30-14. Dorsal venous arch of hand. *(Redrawn from Drake RL, Vogl W, Mitchell AWM. Gray's anatomy for students. Philadelphia: Elsevier/Churchill Livingstone; 2005.)*

its medial side. Additionally, palmar digital veins connect to the dorsal system and drain into the superficial palmar venous plexus. This superficial plexus drains into the median vein, which ascends anteriorly in the forearm to join the basilic or median cubital vein.

The cephalic vein is a superficial vein that drains the lateral and posterior parts of the hand, forearm, and arm. As a lateral continuation of the dorsal venous network, the cephalic vein passes over the anatomic snuffbox at the base of the thumb and continues superiorly along the anterolateral aspect of the arm. It ascends anterior to the elbow, superficial to a groove between the biceps and brachialis muscles, and ascends lateral to the biceps. In the area of the shoulder, it passes into the clavipectoral triangle, a triangular depression between the pectoralis major muscle, deltoid muscle, and clavicle. In the superior part of the clavipectoral triangle, the cephalic vein passes deep to the clavicular head of the pectoralis major muscle and pierces the clavipectoral fascia to join the axillary vein. There are no critical arterial or neural structures near the cephalic vein.

The basilic vein is the medial continuation of the hand's dorsal venous network and passes proximally up the posteromedial surface of the forearm. It passes onto the anterior surface of the forearm just inferior to the elbow and ascends along the medial border of the biceps muscle, accompanied by only a few small superficial nerves. At the junction of the distal and middle thirds of the upper part of the arm, the basilic vein penetrates the deep fascia and continues medial to the brachial artery to the lower border of the teres major muscle, where it becomes the axillary

vein. The basilic vein is easily identified in the upper part of the arm as the largest single, most superficial medial draining vein.

At the antecubital fossa just below the elbow joint, the cephalic vein sends a branch, the median cubital vein, obliquely across to join the basilic vein.

The deep veins of the arm are small paired structures that parallel their associated namesake arteries. The deep veins of the forearm are the ulnar, interosseous, and radial veins. These vessels drain into the paired brachial veins at the level of the antecubital fossa. In the upper part of the arm, the brachial veins are closely related to the median and radial nerves and the brachial artery. The brachial veins pass along the medial and lateral sides of the brachial artery and receive tributaries that accompany branches of the artery. The brachial veins have a variable relationship with the basilic vein; they may join either the basilic or the axillary vein near the inferior margin of the teres major muscle. Of the paired brachial veins, the medial one often joins the basilic vein before it becomes the axillary vein. Up until this point, the deep veins are smaller than the superficial veins. However, from the axillary vein centrally, the deep veins assume dominance.

The axillary vein, which begins at the lower margin of the teres major muscle as a continuation of the basilic vein, continues to the lateral border of the first rib, where it becomes the subclavian vein. As the axillary vein passes through the axilla, it is medial and anterior to the axillary artery. Tributaries of the axillary vein generally follow branches of the axillary artery and include the brachial veins, which follow the brachial artery, and the cephalic vein.

The subclavian vein is a continuation of the axillary vein that begins at the lateral border of the first rib. It crosses the base of the posterior triangle, passes between the first rib and clavicle, and extends to the medial border of the anterior scalene muscle, where it joins the internal jugular vein to form the brachiocephalic vein. In the posterior triangle, the subclavian vein is anterior to the anterior scalene muscle and anterior and slightly inferior to the subclavian artery.

The external jugular vein is a large vein that forms near the angle of the mandible and descends through the neck in the superficial fascia. It pierces the investing layer of cervical fascia in the lower part of the posterior triangle and ends in the subclavian vein. Transverse cervical and suprascapular veins travel with their corresponding arteries and may become tributaries of either the external jugular vein or the subclavian vein.

The internal jugular vein, which collects blood from the skull, brain, superficial aspect of the face, and parts of the neck, begins as a continuation of the sigmoid sinus, a dural venous sinus. The internal jugular vein traverses the neck within the carotid sheath, initially posterior to the internal carotid artery and becoming more lateral inferiorly. It joins with the subclavian vein to form the brachiocephalic (innominate) vein.

Blood from the upper extremities and head returns to the heart via the brachiocephalic veins and the superior vena cava. The right and left brachiocephalic veins, located immediately posterior to the thymus, form on each side at the junction between the internal jugular and subclavian veins.

The right brachiocephalic vein is about 2.5 cm long, begins posterior to the sternal end of the right clavicle, and descends vertically to join the left brachiocephalic vein and form the superior vena cava. It is anterolateral to the brachiocephalic artery and right vagus nerve. The right pleura, phrenic nerve, and internal thoracic artery are posterior to it above but are located laterally to it inferiorly. Its tributaries are the right vertebral, first right posterior intercostal, internal thoracic, and sometimes the inferior thyroid and thymic veins.

The left brachiocephalic vein is approximately 6 cm long and begins posterior to the sternal end of the left clavicle. It crosses the midline obliquely in a slightly inferior direction and joins with the right brachiocephalic vein to form the superior vena cava posterior to the lower edge of the right first costal cartilage near the right sternal border. It crosses anterior to the left internal thoracic, subclavian, and common carotid arteries, the left phrenic and vagus nerves, the trachea, and the brachiocephalic artery. The aortic arch is inferior to it. Its venous tributaries are the left vertebral, left superior intercostal, inferior thyroid, internal thoracic, and sometimes the thymic and pericardial veins.

Variations involving the brachiocephalic veins are related to return pathways to the heart. The brachiocephalic veins may enter the right atrium separately, with the right vein taking the course of a normal superior vena cava. The left vein acts like a left-sided superior vena cava, which may communicate via a small branch with the right superior vena cava and then cross the aortic arch to pass anterior to the left pulmonary hilum before turning to enter the right atrium.

The superior vena cava, generally 6 to 8 cm in length and up to 2 cm in diameter, is vertically oriented and begins posterior to the lower edge of the right first costal cartilage where the right and left brachiocephalic veins unite. It continues inferiorly and terminates at the lower edge of the right third costal cartilage in the upper right atrium. The inferior half of the superior vena cava is within the pericardial sac and forms part of the right superolateral border on a chest radiograph. The other main tributary of the superior vena cava is the azygos vein.

The azygos vein arises opposite the L1 or L2 vertebral body level at the junction between the right ascending lumbar and the right subcostal veins. Alternatively, it may arise as a direct branch of the inferior vena cava and be joined by a common trunk from the junction of the right ascending lumbar and right subcostal veins. It enters the thorax and ascends through the posterior mediastinum to about the T4 level, where it arches anteriorly over the root of the right hilum to join the superior vena cava before the superior vena cava enters the pericardial sac.

The hemiazygos vein usually arises at the junction between the left ascending lumbar and left subcostal veins. Alternatively, it may arise from either of these veins alone and often has a connection to the left renal vein. The hemiazygos vein enters the thorax and ascends through the posterior mediastinum on the left side to about the T8 level, where it crosses the vertebral column posterior to the thoracic aorta, esophagus, and thoracic duct to enter the azygos vein.

The accessory hemiazygos is a small vein that descends on the left side from the superior portion of the posterior mediastinum to about the T8 level. At this point it crosses the vertebral column and joins either the azygos vein, the hemiazygos vein, or both. Usually it also has a connection superiorly to the left superior intercostal vein. Occasionally, this vein will empty anteriorly and superiorly into the left brachiocephalic vein, in which case it can be visualized along the lateral border of the proximal descending thoracic aorta.

A number of collateral pathways exist between the superficial and deep venous systems of the upper extremity and become important when occlusion is present. Occlusion of a brachiocephalic vein results in obstruction of flow from both the ipsilateral arm and neck. However, as long as the contralateral internal jugular vein is patent, facial swelling on the side of the occlusion is rare. Venous blood from the arm may drain across the back, chest, and neck via deep and superficial collaterals to the opposite jugular, subclavian, and brachiocephalic veins. Superficial chest wall veins, such as the internal mammary and intercostal veins, may also serve as collateral drainage pathways. These veins drain into the azygos vein on the right and the hemiazygos vein on the left, or they may continue down the abdominal wall to the inferior epigastric veins. Additionally, pericardial and phrenic veins may also be recruited as collateral drainage pathways.

With occlusion involving the superior vena cava, the level of occlusion determines which collateral pathway will be dominant. When the occlusion is above the azygos vein, collateral drainage involves primarily the chest wall and intercostal veins, which empty into the azygos system, with the normal direction of flow being toward the superior vena cava. Additionally, some drainage through the pericardial and abdominal wall veins may be present. When the occlusion is below the azygos vein, flow reverses in the vein, with drainage into the inferior vena cava and chest wall; pericardial collaterals may develop.

KEY POINTS

- Knowledge of normal and variant upper extremity vascular anatomy is essential for upper extremity angiography and intervention.
- Multiple potential collateral pathways in both the arterial and venous systems of the upper extremity exist and become significant in the setting of occlusion or stenosis.

▶ **SUGGESTED READINGS**

Drake RL, Vogl W, Mitchell AWM. Gray's anatomy for students. Philadelphia: Elsevier/Churchill Livingstone; 2005. p. 607–1033.

Kaufman JA, Lee MJ. Vascular & interventional radiology: the requisites. St Louis: Mosby; 2004. p. 142–93.

Uflacker R. Atlas of vascular anatomy: an angiographic approach. Baltimore: Lippincott Williams & Wilkins; 1997. p. 339–403.

The complete reference list is available online at www.expertconsult.com.

CHAPTER 31

Anatomy of the Lower Limb

Kenneth R. Thomson, Mark F. Given, and Jeff Dai-Chee Tam

This chapter is not intended to replace standard anatomy texts. For the purposes of this chapter, the lower limb is considered to extend from the thigh to the foot. The thigh extends from the base of the femoral triangle at the inguinal ligament anteriorly and the gluteal fold posteriorly to the level of the knee joint. The femoral triangle provides the portal for most angiography and vascular interventional procedures. Additionally, knowledge of the anatomy of the venous system of the lower limb is critical for the treatment of venous disorders, including thrombosis and varicose veins. Deep and cutaneous nerves may be injured by needle puncture for the treatment of varicose veins or vascular malformations.

COMPARTMENTS OF THE LOWER LIMB

The lower limb is encased in a dense layer of connective tissue—the deep fascia—that acts to contain the leg muscles and improve venous flow as the muscles contract. In the lateral aspect of the thigh, the fascia is thickened and forms the iliotibial tract. This tract is a conjoint aponeurosis of the gluteus maximus and tensor fasciae latae. The distal portion of the iliotibial tract is attached to the lateral condyle of the tibia.

Septae from the deep fascia separate the thigh muscles into three compartments. The lateral intermuscular septum between the anterior and posterior groups is thicker and stronger than the other two septa. At the knee, the subcutaneous fascia and deep fascia merge, but in the thigh and calf there is fatty connective tissue between the superficial and deep fascia. The superficial veins, cutaneous nerves, and lymphatics lie in this subcutaneous tissue.

In the calf, the fascia is called the *crural fascia*, and it also separates the deep and superficial posterior muscles. The interosseous membrane and the crural intermuscular septa separate the anterior, extensor, and posterior muscle groups. In the lower portion of the calf, the crural fascia forms the extensor retinaculum. Accumulation of excess fluid in a compartment may compromise both nerve and vascular supply to muscles within the compartment.

The *saphenous opening* is a deficiency in the fascia lata inferior to the medial part of the inguinal ligament over the upper portion of the femoral triangle. The opening has a well-defined crescentic margin, except on its medial aspect. A thin connective tissue—the cribriform fascia—covers the opening. The long saphenous vein and lymphatics pass through the fascia and enter the femoral triangle.

The *femoral triangle* is a space in the upper part of the thigh that is bounded above by the inguinal ligament, medially by the adductor longus, and laterally by the sartorius muscles (Fig. 31-1). The floor of the triangle is formed by the iliopsoas laterally and the pectineus medially. The roof of the triangle is composed of the cribriform fascia and fascia lata, subcutaneous tissue, and skin. The contents of the triangle are, from lateral to medial, the femoral nerve and its branches, the femoral artery and its branches, the femoral vein and its proximal tributaries, including the long saphenous vein and the deep inguinal lymph node, and associated lymphatics.

The femoral vein and artery and the lymphatics, but not the femoral nerve, are enclosed in the *femoral sheath*, which is an extension of the extraperitoneal fascia overlying the iliopsoas and transversalis abdominis. The femoral sheath is further divided into compartments for the femoral artery, femoral vein, and lymphatics. At the inferior extent of the femoral triangle the sheath becomes continuous with the adventitia of the vessels. The medial compartment is called the *femoral canal*, and its proximal extent under the inguinal ligament is termed the *femoral ring*. This opening is usually closed by fibrofatty tissue and is the site of a femoral hernia should one develop (Fig. 31-2).

The *femoral nerve* is the largest branch of the lumbar plexus and is composed of sensory and motor fibers from L2 to L4. It is formed within the psoas and enters the femoral triangle at about the midpoint of the inguinal ligament. Within the triangle, the femoral nerve divides into multiple branches to the quadriceps, sartorius, and the hip and knee joints. Its cutaneous branches supply the skin on the anterior and medial aspect of the thigh. Its largest cutaneous branch—the *saphenous nerve*—runs obliquely downward in the femoral triangle to lie adjacent to the femoral artery and vein. The saphenous nerve then passes into the adductor canal and exits proximal to the adductor hiatus by passing superficially between the gracilis and sartorius. The saphenous nerve passes along the anteromedial aspect of the calf close to the long saphenous nerve to supply skin on the anteromedial aspect of the calf and foot. At the medial malleolus, it may be damaged by a cutdown for access to the long saphenous vein.

The *femoral artery* arises as a continuation of the external iliac artery beneath the inguinal ligament. In the femoral triangle, it lies centrally between the femoral nerve and vein. It enters the adductor canal and continues as the popliteal artery once it passes through the adductor hiatus to the popliteal fossa. The femoral artery gives off the superficial epigastric artery, superficial circumflex iliac artery, and superficial and deep external pudendal arteries in the upper portion of the triangle before it gives off the deep artery of the thigh (profunda femoris) and continues as the (superficial) femoral artery in the adductor canal (Fig. 31-3). Within the canal, the femoral artery gives off several muscular branches and the descending genicular artery. The proximal superficial branches of the femoral artery are important collateral pathways in the event of arterial occlusion.

Branching variations at the origin of the deep artery of the thigh are common, and the length of the (common) femoral artery before the origin of the deep artery of the thigh is variable. Occasionally, the deep artery of the thigh

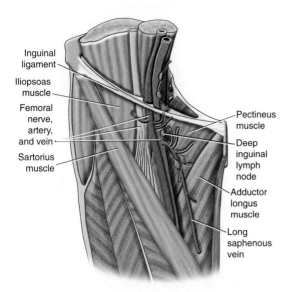

Inguinal ligament

Iliopsoas muscle

Femoral nerve, artery, and vein

Sartorius muscle

Pectineus muscle

Deep inguinal lymph node

Adductor longus muscle

Long saphenous vein

FIGURE 31-1. The femoral triangle is a space in the upper part of the thigh that is bounded above by the inguinal ligament, medially by the adductor longus, and laterally by the sartorius.

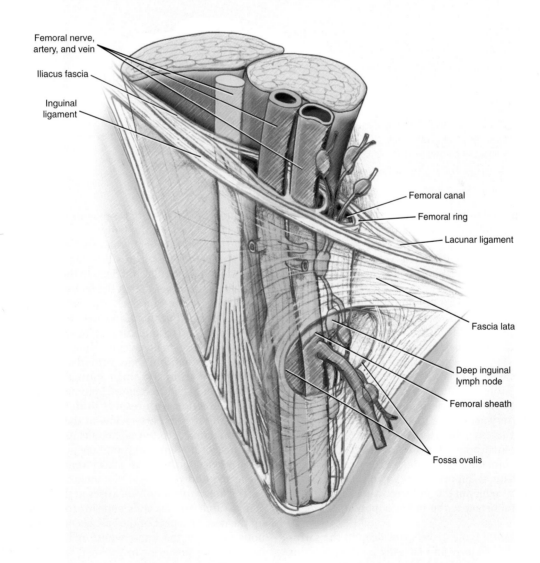

Femoral nerve, artery, and vein

Iliacus fascia

Inguinal ligament

Femoral canal

Femoral ring

Lacunar ligament

Fascia lata

Deep inguinal lymph node

Femoral sheath

Fossa ovalis

FIGURE 31-2. The femoral sheath is further divided into compartments for the femoral artery, femoral vein, and lymphatics. At the inferior extent of the femoral triangle, the sheath becomes continuous with the adventitia of the vessels.

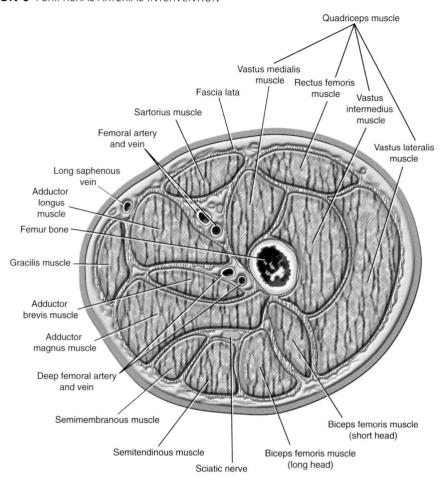

FIGURE 31-3. Cross-section of thigh. Femoral artery lies deep to sartorius and is separated from deep femoral vessels by adductor muscles.

is absent and replaced by direct branches from the femoral artery. Rarely, the anterior division of the internal iliac artery may continue from the pelvis as the sciatic artery, which terminates as the popliteal artery. In such cases, the femoral artery is small and supplies only the upper part of the thigh.

The *deep artery of the thigh* lies posterior to the femoral artery and passes deeply between the pectineus and adductor longus. Proximally, the deep artery of the thigh gives off medial and lateral circumflex femoral branches that form the cruciate anastomosis with obturator branches of the inferior gluteal and superficial circumflex femoral arteries. The cruciate anastomosis often supplies a branch to the sciatic nerve. Sometimes the obturator artery or an accessory obturator artery arises as a branch of the inferior epigastric artery. In this case, the artery lies on the femoral ring and may become incorporated in a femoral hernia.

The muscular branches of the deep artery of the thigh provide large collateral opportunities when there is occlusion of the femoral artery in the adductor canal. The medial circumflex femoral artery is the major supply to the head of the femur.

The *adductor canal* is a narrow space deep to the sartorius and bounded anteriorly and laterally by the posterior aspect of the vastus medialis and posteriorly by the adductor longus and adductor magnus. It contains the saphenous nerve, the (superficial) femoral artery, and the femoral vein. The adductor hiatus is an opening between the distal

attachments of the adductor magnus immediately above the adductor tubercle of the femur.

The *femoral vein* begins as a continuation of the popliteal vein at the adductor hiatus and runs superiorly within the adductor canal medial and deep to the femoral artery. There are numerous valves within the femoral vein that aid venous flow up the limb. The deep femoral vein accompanies the deep artery of the thigh and may be multiple. Unlike the arteries, there is significant variation in the number and position of the smaller veins. Numerous perforating veins connect the femoral vein with the superficial veins and drain blood from the thigh muscles. At the apex of the femoral triangle, the femoral vein passes in a posterior-to-medial direction with respect to the femoral artery. Puncture of the femoral artery low in the femoral triangle may result in damage to the saphenous nerve and unintentional puncture of the femoral vein. Low punctures are also more often associated with an arteriovenous fistula when both the artery and vein are simultaneously punctured.

The *long saphenous vein* arises in the foot from the dorsal venous arch and ascends anterior to the medial malleolus up the medial aspect of the calf, accompanied by the saphenous nerve to the knee, where it lies approximately one handbreadth posterior to the medial femoral condyle. The saphenous nerve separates from the vein above the knee joint, and it is at this point that the long saphenous vein is usually punctured for thermal ablation. Several perforating veins connect the long saphenous vein to the deep femoral

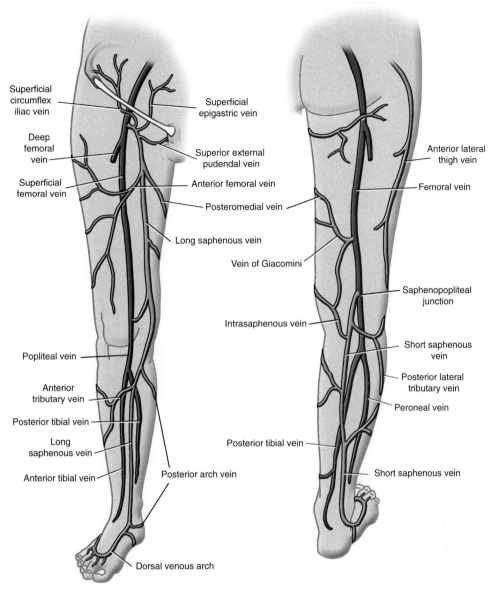

FIGURE 31-4. Diagram of venous system of lower limb.

veins. They are grouped above the ankle, below and just above the knee, and along the lower half of the adductor canal. These perforating veins also contain valves that direct flow to the deep system through the fascia lata. The oblique course of these veins through the fascia causes mechanical compression during muscle contraction. Several of the perforating veins have eponymous names (Fig. 31-4). The long saphenous vein also receives large cutaneous veins from the lateral and anterior aspect of the thigh just before it passes through the cribriform fascia. Within the femoral opening, the long saphenous vein receives the superficial circumflex iliac, superficial epigastric, and external pudendal veins. These veins provide connection between the saphenous vein and the deep pelvic veins. Ovarian vein reflux may cause an increase in pressure in these tributaries of the long saphenous vein at the femoral opening.

The *short saphenous vein* is formed from the lateral end of the dorsal venous arch and passes upward on the posterior aspect of the calf to enter the popliteal vein at the lower border of the popliteal fossa. Throughout its course, it is in close proximity to the sural nerve.

The deep veins of the foot follow the arteries, and contrast material injected into the superficial veins can be directed into the deep veins by obstructing the saphenous veins at the ankle with a tourniquet.

Lymphatic drainage is supplied by the deep and superficial lymphatic vessels that accompany the veins of the thigh. Superficial lymphatics drain to the superficial inguinal lymph nodes and then to the external iliac lymph nodes. Lymph may also pass directly to the deep inguinal lymph nodes, particularly if it originated below the knee. These nodes lie in the medial aspect of the femoral sheath within the femoral triangle. In the popliteal fossa, the lymph nodes are arranged in superficial and deep groups. They are usually small. There is a superficial lymph node at the termination of the short saphenous vein and a group of deep nodes draining the knee joint. Lymphatic channels ascend in the leg with the femoral vessels and join the deep inguinal

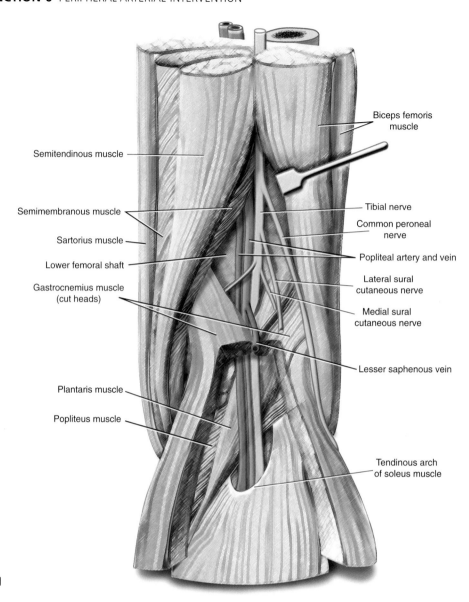

FIGURE 31-5. Popliteal fossa with popliteal vessels and sciatic nerve.

lymph nodes. The easiest place to access the lymphatic system of the leg is on the dorsum of the foot. Patent blue dye injected into the interdigital web spaces will outline the lymphatic channels, and they can easily be cannulated with a 25-gauge needle.

The *sciatic nerve* is the largest nerve in the body and is formed from the ventral rami of L4 to S3. It consists of two nerves connected by a common connective tissue sheath. It receives direct arterial supply from the inferior gluteal artery—a fact that makes embolization of this artery with small particles or liquids dangerous. The sciatic nerve enters the gluteal region through the greater sciatic foramen, usually inferior to the piriformis. In about 12% of people, the common fibular (peroneal) division passes through the piriformis and may be compressed. Below the piriformis, the sciatic nerve lies at the midpoint of a line drawn from the superior border of the greater trochanter to the posterior-superior iliac spine. An injection of local anesthetic at this point will block the function of the sciatic

nerve. Any deep intramuscular injections should be made above this line in the superolateral aspect of the buttock or in the anterior aspect of the thigh to avoid injury to the sciatic nerve.

In the thigh, the sciatic nerve lies on the posterior surface of the adductor brevis in the space between the biceps femoris and the adductor magnus. It usually enters the popliteal fossa as two separate nerves, the common peroneal (fibular) and the tibial nerves (Fig. 31-5). This separation may occur anywhere from the pelvis to the popliteal fossa. Through its two major branches, the sciatic nerve supplies the skin of the foot, most of the calf, and the muscles of the foot and calf.

The *popliteal fossa* is a space bounded by the hamstrings above and the two heads of the gastrocnemius below (see Fig. 31-5). The anterior border (floor) is the lower femoral shaft and the knee joint, with the popliteus muscle forming the lower extent of the fossa. The popliteal artery and vein and the tibial and peroneal nerves lie from deep to superficial in the central portion of the fossa. The popliteal artery and vein share a common fibrous sheath, and a hematoma in the sheath may cause venous or arterial compression.

Frequently, the popliteal vein lies directly superficial to the popliteal artery, and a slightly oblique approach from the medial side under ultrasound guidance is preferred for direct needle access. The tibial and peroneal nerves are situated slightly lateral to the artery. Lying in the superficial portion (roof) are the lateral cutaneous nerve of the thigh and the short saphenous vein.

From an angiographer's standpoint, the major interest is the geniculate anastomosis between the branches of the femoral and tibial arteries because these vessels form a major collateral blood supply in case of major artery occlusion (Fig. 31-6). This anastomosis is formed by a double ring of vessels, one at the level of the supracondylar ridge of the

lower part of the femur, and one at the level of the tibial plateau.

When the knee is flexed, the popliteal artery flexes several centimeters above the knee joint close to the adductor hiatus (Fig. 31-7). Recognition of this point of flexure is important because arterial stents placed at the point of flexure are more likely to fracture or occlude.

The *popliteal artery* begins at the adductor hiatus and extends through the popliteal fossa to divide into a posterior tibial trunk and an anterior tibial artery (Fig. 31-8). The anterior tibial artery passes through a hiatus in the upper border of the interosseous membrane; it joins the tibia and fibula, runs inferiorly in the anterior compartment, and ends as the dorsalis pedis artery of the foot. This artery runs over the navicular and intermediate cuneiform bones and lies in the space between the heads of the first and second metatarsals, where it can easily be palpated below the extensor retinaculum between the tendons of the extensor hallucis longus and extensor digitorum longus to the second toe.

The *posterior tibial artery* divides a variable distance from the popliteal artery into a larger posterior tibial branch and a smaller peroneal branch. The peroneal branch passes inferiorly on the lateral side of the deep compartment and

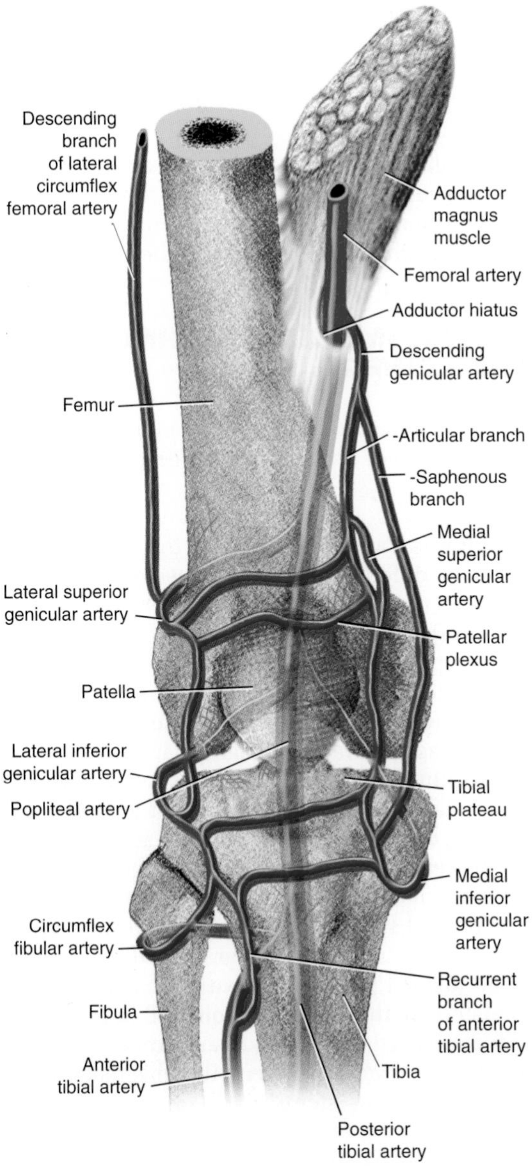

FIGURE 31-6. Geniculate anastomosis. Note that there are two rings of anastomoses.

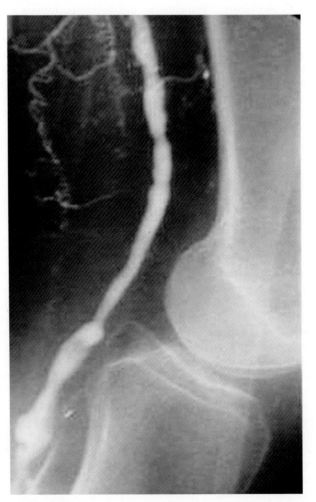

FIGURE 31-7. Lateral angiogram at level of popliteal fossa. Note that the arterial flexion point is above the level of the knee joint. This has implications for stent placement in this region.

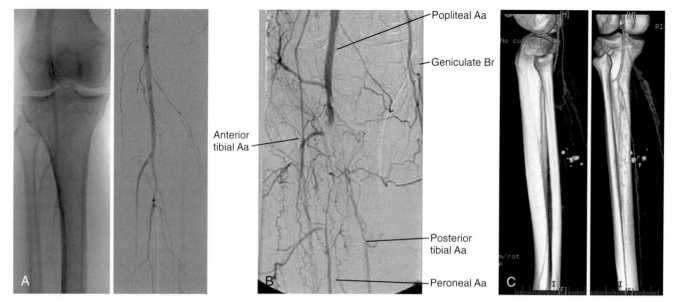

FIGURE 31-8. A, Termination of popliteal artery. Artery usually divides below knee joint, but one tibial artery may arise high in popliteal fossa. **B,** As a result of geniculate anastomosis, tibial vessels may fill even when popliteal artery is occluded, as in this case. **C,** Computed tomographic angiogram (CTA) shows anterior tibial artery passing to anterior compartment near neck of fibula.

sends perforating branches to the peroneus longus and brevis muscles in the lateral compartment. More distally it crosses below the lower portion of the interosseous membrane to anastomose with the anterior tibial artery. The posterior tibial artery continues to the ankle with the tibial nerve and deep tibial vein; it passes posterior to the medial malleolus and enters the sole of the foot, where it divides into a smaller medial and larger lateral plantar artery (Fig. 31-9).

There are anastomotic connections between the deep plantar arch and the arcuate branch of the dorsalis pedis artery at the level of the metatarsal heads (Fig. 31-10). As the posterior tibial artery rounds the medial malleolus, it is superficial and easily palpable. Palpation of the plantar artery is difficult because it lies deep to the flexor digitorum brevis muscles and the plantar aponeurosis.

The *tibial nerve* passes between the femoral and tibial heads of the soleus muscle to lie on the tibialis posterior, usually just lateral to the posterior tibial artery and vein. The tibial nerve supplies all the muscles of the posterior compartment of the calf and two cutaneous branches, the sural nerve and the medial calcaneal nerve. The sural nerve arises in the popliteal fossa and joins the lateral sural branch from the peroneal nerve. This conjoined nerve lies deep to the fascia over the gastrocnemius as far as the midcalf, where it penetrates the deep fascia to become subcutaneous.

The tibial nerve and its sural branch may be damaged by percutaneous puncture of the popliteal fossa while seeking the artery or vein. Generally, the nerves lie lateral to the vein and artery, with the artery situated most deeply. Injury to the tibial nerve causes numbness of the sole of the foot and paralysis of the flexor muscles in the leg and intrinsic muscles of the foot.

The *peroneal (common fibular) nerve* is the smaller branch of the sciatic nerve. It leaves the popliteal fossa above the sural nerve, crosses laterally across the lateral

head of the gastrocnemius, and winds around the head of the fibula, where it is prone to injury. The peroneal nerve supplies the muscles of the lateral compartment with its superficial branch and the muscles of the anterior compartment with its deep branch.

VASCULAR IMAGING TECHNIQUES IN THE LOWER LIMB

Various techniques are available in imaging the vascular system of the lower limb, each with its own strengths and limitations.

Angiography is the gold standard vascular imaging modality. It was traditionally used as the sole imaging technique, but as different modalities developed, angiography has now been reserved for those patients who require intervention, or prior to intervention as a planning investigation. It involves a puncture with a needle into an artery or vein, which provides access for injection of iodinated contrast material, allowing visualization using subtracted or unsubtracted imaging. Subtracted imaging has allowed for greater contrast within the images, requiring less contrast material and less radiation. One disadvantage of angiography is its invasiveness, but this is also its greatest advantage in that it allows intervention. Advantages include greater sensitivity, smaller doses of contrast compared with computed tomography (CT), and functional assessment of flow. Angiography can also be used for venography of the lower limb, usually performed prior to intervention. A superficial vein is cannulated in the foot and contrast injected IV (IV). Tourniquets placed at the ankle and knee force blood to flow into the deep venous system, thereby imaging both the superficial and deep systems.

Computed tomographic angiography (CTA) is a noninvasive alternative to conventional angiography as a diagnostic tool in the lower limbs (Fig. 31-11). It requires injection of IV iodinated contrast from a peripheral vein, usually in

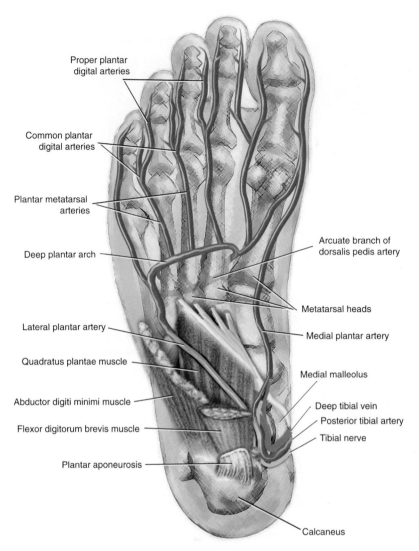

Proper plantar
digital arteries

Common plantar
digital arteries

Plantar metatarsal
arteries

Deep plantar arch

Lateral plantar artery

Quadratus plantae muscle

Abductor digiti minimi muscle

Flexor digitorum brevis muscle

Plantar aponeurosis

Arcuate branch of
dorsalis pedis artery

Metatarsal heads

Medial plantar artery

Medial malleolus

Deep tibial vein

Posterior tibial artery

Tibial nerve

Calcaneus

FIGURE 31-9. Diagram of tarsal arterial arches between plantar and dorsalis pedis arteries.

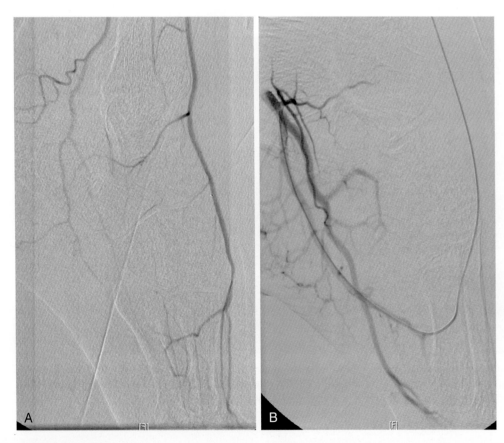

FIGURE 31-10. A, Angiogram of foot, showing tarsal arches and dorsalis pedis and plantar arteries. **B,** Arch can be catheterized in either direction with a microcatheter. In this example in a different patient, plantar arteries have been accessed from dorsalis pedis.

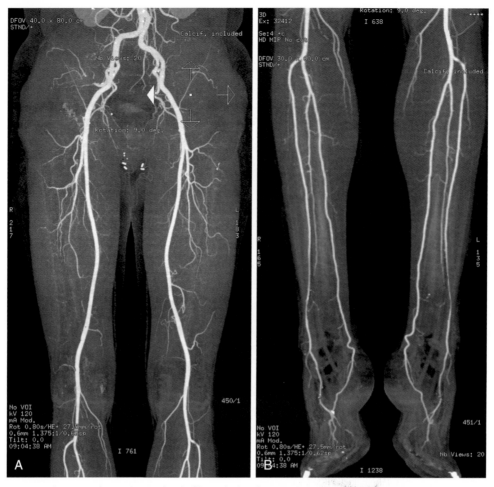

FIGURE 31-11. **A,** Computed tomographic angiogram (CTA) of lower limb to knee. **B,** CTA of lower limb from knee to foot. In this example, two separate injections were made because of low cardiac output. It can be difficult to obtain adequate maximum-intensity projection (MIP) images from low-contrast objects.

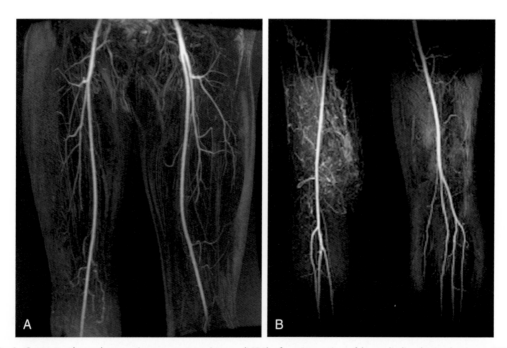

FIGURE 31-12. **A,** Contrast-enhanced magnetic resonance angiogram (MRA) of upper portion of lower limbs obtained using a TRICKS sequence (GE Healthcare [TRICKS is Time Resolved Imaging of Contrast KineticS]). **B,** Contrast-enhanced MRA of popliteal region using a TRICKS sequence. Note anomalous origin of anterior tibial artery on left side. This example used a small field of view to increase image resolution.

the upper limb. More accurate assessment can be made of structures that do not enhance, such as the size of the thrombosed false lumen in an aneurysm, which angiography will not be able to image. In addition, multidetector CT enables volume rendering of the vascular system. Limitations include the inability to assess rates of flow, and higher doses of radiation and contrast. In addition, CT venography (CTV) of the lower limb has been described, particularly in combination with CT pulmonary angiography, to look for deep venous thrombosis (DVT) in patients with pulmonary embolism. However, the extra dose of radiation to look for DVT when ultrasound can give identical information *without* use of radiation has resulted in limited use of this technique. It is also more difficult to derive maximum-intensity projection (MIP) images of venous phase CT because of the dilution of contrast.

Ultrasound is an accurate noninvasive modality that can be used to assess both arterial and venous systems in the lower limb. It has no ionizing radiation and requires no contrast or IV cannulation. Doppler studies are able to assess flow within a vessel, and this is a major advantage over CTA. However, ultrasound is user dependent and unable to display anatomic information as well as CT.

Magnetic resonance imaging (MRI) has many advantages over the other imaging modalities in vascular anatomy investigation. There is no ionizing radiation, and contrast material may or may not be used, depending on the specific indication. In the lower limbs, MRI can be useful in the investigation of runoff vessels in planning for bypass surgery. The major advantage of MRI is its high soft tissue contrast resolution, making it ideal to investigate arteriovenous malformations (AVMs). Its magnetic resonance venography (MRV) capability is also a major strength, and investigation of low-flow vessels, such as veins or lymphatics, is best performed using MRV. Injection of contrast does improve sensitivity, particularly when a subtraction technique is used (Fig. 31-12), but not all indications require IV contrast. Limitations of MRI include its inability to visualize metallic stents, which is particularly important in patients with possible in-stent stenosis or occlusion. Widespread use of MRI to investigate DVT has been limited by the ease and availability of ultrasound.

KEY POINTS

- Arterial access is through the femoral triangle.
- Venous access requires awareness of the position of the cutaneous nerves.

CHAPTER 32
Acute Arterial Occlusive Disease of the Upper Extremity

Jeff Dai-Chee Tam, Mark F. Given, Stuart M. Lyon, and Kenneth R. Thomson

In the absence of trauma, acute upper limb arterial disease is relatively uncommon, particularly in comparison with lower limb disease. Some authors suggest that it is one sixth as common as that in the leg.[1] The majority of patients will have small vessel disease.[2] Blunt trauma and repetitive use of the arm—for example, in athletes or associated with certain occupations—are the usual causes in the proximal upper extremity.[3,4] More distal upper limb ischemia is usually the result of emboli from a proximal stenosis or a cardiac origin. Occlusive disease of the upper extremity is as important as lower limb occlusive disease, not least because it may reflect an underlying systemic illness.[5,6]

Atherosclerotic disease is the most common cause of large vessel stenosis or occlusion, but it may also present as small vessel occlusion via thromboembolism. Aneurysmal disease, including cystic adventitial disease, may also be a source of emboli.[7]

Other primary causes include thoracic outlet compression syndrome, drug-induced occlusion, post-radiotherapy stenoses, and iatrogenic catheter injury.[5,8,9]

INDICATIONS

Upper limb evaluation, including clinical examination, serologic analysis, noninvasive vascular studies, duplex Doppler ultrasound, and digital subtraction angiography, is indicated in any patient who presents with arm claudication, rest pain, ulceration, gangrene, or Raynaud syndrome. Acute total ischemia of an upper limb is unusual except in cases of trauma, where a subintimal dissection may occur. These injuries are more common in the axilla and proximal portion of the upper limb, and in most cases are still treated surgically. Where there is no external compression of the vessel, a case can be made for stenting as an alternative. Acute arterial occlusion in the distal portion of the upper limb is more likely to be treated by endovascular means.

CONTRAINDICATIONS

The only absolute contraindication to angiographic intervention, particularly if considering administering thrombolytics, is uncontrollable coagulopathy. Other relative contraindications include renal failure and infection at the puncture site. In cases of renal failure, duplex Doppler ultrasound can be used for most mapping of vessels, and diluted nonionic dimer contrast used for any catheter angiography.

EQUIPMENT

- 5F to 6F vascular sheath
- J and hydrophilic angled guidewires
- Pigtail, Hinck, Davis-T, Simmons catheters
- Progreat microcatheter system (Terumo, Somerset, N.J.)
- Angioplasty balloons (4- to 10-mm diameter)
- Self- or balloon-expandable stents
- Mechanical thrombectomy device or balloon thrombectomy catheter
- Drugs: anticoagulants, thrombolytics, antispasmodics
- Nonionic dimer contrast medium: iodine, 300 mg/mL

TECHNIQUE

Anatomy and Approaches

The arterial supply to the upper limb originates from the subclavian arteries. The left subclavian artery arises directly from the aortic arch in the majority of cases, whereas the right subclavian originates from the brachiocephalic artery. The subclavian vessels first pass between the scalene muscles and then between the clavicle and first rib. At the lateral border of the clavicle they become the axillary arteries.

The branches of the subclavian artery include the vertebral, internal mammary, thyrocervical trunk, costocervical trunk, and supreme intercostal arteries.

The axillary artery extends to the lateral margin of teres minor, where it becomes the brachial artery. Its branches include the superior and lateral thoracic arteries and the thoracoacromial, subscapular, scapular circumflex, and circumflex humeral arteries. The radial, ulnar, and median nerves are contained in a connective tissue sheath along with this vessel and are at risk of damage if one is considering puncture of an axillary artery. Also of importance is that there are multiple potential collateral pathways involving the branches of both the subclavian and axillary arteries in the presence of stenosis or occlusion.

Lateral to the teres minor, the axillary artery becomes the brachial artery, which has the profunda brachialis as its first branch in the upper arm. This branch travels posterolaterally around the humerus, giving off multiple muscular branches and providing collateral branches around the elbow.

At the elbow joint, the brachial artery then terminates into the radial, ulnar, and interosseus arteries. The interosseus artery then divides into an anterior and posterior branch. The radial and ulnar arteries continue down the forearm to form the superficial and deep palmar arches and supply the hand. The deep palmar arch is more proximal and is mainly supplied by the radial artery, whereas the superficial arch is more distal and has the ulnar artery as its main supply. These classic palmar arcades occur in fewer than 50% of patients, but there are multiple variations. The classic anatomic description of the more proximal upper limb arteries noted earlier is also subject to variation, particularly in the origin of their branches, and this can be a potential source of confusion on angiography.

Within the hand, paired common palmar metacarpal and common palmar digital arteries originate from the arches and join at the web spaces to form the proper palmar digital arteries, which supply the fingers. As a rule, the radial artery supplies the thumb (princeps pollicis artery) and second digit, and the ulnar artery supplies the fourth and fifth digits. The third digit has a variable arterial supply. Provided that one or both of these arches are complete, occlusion of either the radial or ulnar arteries may be well tolerated. However, if they are incomplete or absent, severe hand/digital ischemia may develop. The Allen test may be performed prior to intervention to assess the dominance of the radial and ulna artery. This test requires elevation and exercise of the hand until pallor occurs while both radial and ulnar arteries are compressed. Sequential removal of compression allows one to define the degree of contribution of the radial and ulnar arteries to the arterial supply to the hand.

Technical Aspects

Before performing angiography of the upper limb vessels, the presence of the axillary, brachial, radial, and ulnar pulses should be confirmed. Bilateral brachial artery blood pressure measurements should also be taken.

It is important to ensure overlap of images to confirm that the vessels are seen in their entirety. For an arch aortogram, a 5F pigtail catheter should be placed just proximal to the takeoff of the brachiocephalic artery. A right anterior oblique projection will show the bifurcation of the brachiocephalic artery; a left anterior oblique projection is required to adequately demonstrate the left common carotid and subclavian origins. A powered injection of approximately 20 mL at 20 mL/s should be adequate to visualize these vessels.

For selective catheterization of the subclavian arteries, a 5F angled catheter such as a Hinck or Davis should be used in conjunction with a long J or angled hydrophilic guidewire. In young patients, it is easy to catheterize the left vertebral artery because it lies in a straight line from the aortic arch. If the great vessels arise at an acute angle from the arch, use of a "formed" catheter such as a Simmons-1 or Simmons-2 may be required. To image the subclavian and axillary vessels, the catheter tip should be positioned distal to the origin of the vertebral artery, using meticulous technique to avoid cerebral emboli.

An angled guidewire can then be employed to advance the catheter into the proximal axillary artery, where an angiogram is performed to assess the brachial artery. The catheter should not be placed in the brachial artery before this, or one may miss a high takeoff of either the ulnar or radial arteries and also a proximal plaque that may be the source of distal emboli. Six to 8 mL of nonionic dimer contrast at 3 mL/s with overlapping angiograms is adequate to look at the vessels of the upper limb.

Angiography of the forearm vessels and hand is performed with the catheter in the mid-brachial artery and with the hand in the anatomic position. Vasodilation with warm towels or a vasodilator may be necessary to obtain optimal views of the digital vessels. Selective catheterization of the forearm vessels can be achieved using

microcatheters and wires to lessen the risk of spasm. Vasospasm may also be treated with intraarterial glyceryl trinitrate in 50-μg aliquots. Patient discomfort and spasm is much less likely when nonionic dimer contrast is used.

CONTROVERSIES

The investigation of patients with upper limb ischemia is widely accepted to include a variety of invasive and noninvasive tests. Of these, the most dominant is duplex Doppler ultrasound. However, very detailed imaging of the upper limbs can be achieved with computed tomography (CT) or magnetic resonance imaging (MRI), and diagnostic angiography is not usually performed unless a therapeutic interventional procedure—whether that be angioplasty, stenting, or thrombolysis—is planned.

Although the majority of stenoses may be successfully treated with angioplasty or the placement of stents, certain lesions, in particular those secondary to radiation therapy, may respond better to surgical reconstruction techniques.[9]

OUTCOMES

Acute upper limb ischemia is often secondary to an embolus from a cardiac origin. If the hand is viable, catheter-directed thrombolysis using a standard 5F catheter or microcatheter may be performed from either a brachial or femoral approach, with excellent results. Mechanical thrombectomy devices may also be deployed cautiously in the more proximal vessels. Aspiration thrombectomy via a transbrachial approach has also been successful in treatment of acute upper limb ischemia.[10]

If the source of embolization is from a proximal atherosclerotic plaque, the proximal lesion should be definitively treated with either angioplasty or stent placement. Angioplasty balloon diameters range from 3 to 10 mm.

Balloon-expandable stents should be used for stenoses involving the origins of these vessels because they can be deployed more accurately. Self-expandable stents may be used more peripherally in these vessels. Stents should not be placed within the subclavian artery as it passes behind the clavicle and first rib because they may fracture. The technical success rate of angioplasty and stenting in this region is over 90%, with a complication rate of less than 1% (Figs. 32-1 to 32-4).[11]

COMPLICATIONS

Potential complications include those associated with angiography in general, such as puncture site hematoma, pseudoaneurysm formation, dissection, arteriovenous fistula, and so on. The accepted rate of these adverse occurrences for a common femoral arterial puncture ranges from 0.2% to 0.5%.[12]

Specific complications, particularly those associated with a brachial approach, include vasospasm, nerve injury, and the risk of stroke because the catheter may cross the origin of the great vessels. The overall incidence of complications, including hemorrhagic, neurologic, and occlusive complications, tends to be higher with brachial artery punctures than with femoral artery punctures. If a brachial puncture site occludes, it is a simple procedure to repair the

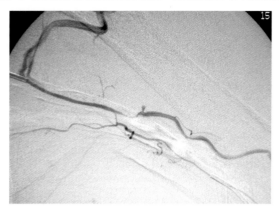

FIGURE 32-1. Angiography of left upper arm performed from a left subclavian catheter shows diffuse disease in profunda brachii and occlusion of deep brachial artery itself. No veins were available for bypass. Access has also been obtained via the brachial artery at the elbow with a second catheter.

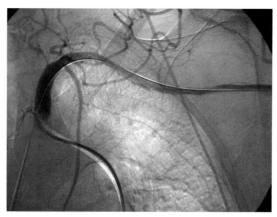

FIGURE 32-4. Final result after angioplasty with a 10-cm-long, 5-mm-diameter balloon shows a widely patent lumen, but there was poor perfusion of the hand (see Fig. 32-5).

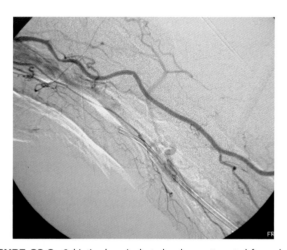

FIGURE 32-2. Subintimal angioplasty has been attempted from above, but this has not been successful. A new attempt was made from the elbow.

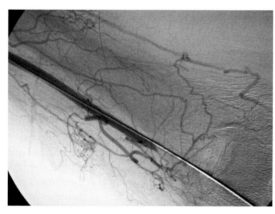

FIGURE 32-5. View of elbow shows occlusion of brachial artery by an embolus. It is advisable to not remove the guidewire before runoff has been established to be normal. This occlusion was treated by a simple open arteriotomy; outcome was excellent.

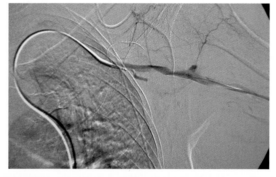

FIGURE 32-3. Subintimal angioplasty from the elbow has resulted in an irregular but patent lumen and good flow.

artery and extract the thrombus, provided this is done soon after the procedure (Fig. 32-5).

POSTPROCEDURAL AND FOLLOW-UP CARE

Routine postprocedural care for a femoral or brachial angiogram is employed. The radial pulses must be recorded before removal of the access. Records should include regular neurovascular observations and, for femoral punctures, semi-supine bed rest for 4 hours.

If the patient is conscious, it is useful to ask him or her to report immediately any change in color, temperature, or pain. Pain out of proportion to the apparent abnormality may indicate development of a compartment syndrome and is usually associated with poor perfusion.

The patient may ambulate earlier if a closure device has been used or if only a brachial puncture has been performed. To limit use of the punctured arm, a triangular bandage sling is recommended if the patient is ambulatory.

- Acute upper limb arterial disease is uncommon.
- Small vessels are most affected.
- There may be an underlying systemic illness or remote emboli.
- Techniques that work for the lower limb also work in the arm.
- Spasm is more likely in the upper limb than the lower limb.

The majority of patients may be discharged home the same day. Some may require postprocedural anticoagulation, depending on angiographic findings and treatment.

▶ **SUGGESTED READINGS**

Kaufman JA, Lee MJ. Vascular and interventional radiology: the requisites. St. Louis: Mosby; 2003.

The complete reference list is available online at www.expertconsult.com.

CHAPTER 33

Acute Lower Extremity Ischemia

Raymond W. Liu, Hani H. Abujudeh, David W. Trost, and Krishna Kandarpa

Acute lower extremity ischemia (ALEI) is a serious condition with substantial morbidity and mortality. ALEI refers to recent onset of lower extremity pain; long-standing lower extremity ischemia is dealt with elsewhere in this book. If ALEI is severe and prolonged, the patient may develop progressive paresthesia, motor dysfunction, and eventually tissue infarction in the lower extremity. The rapidity plus severity of the onset of symptoms is dependent on the location, extent, and degree of collateral pathways around the obstruction. The estimated incidence of ALEI is approximately 1.5 cases per million each year. The two principal causes of ALEI are (1) embolic, in which an artery may become occluded when an embolus becomes dislodged from a proximal source, and (2) thrombotic, in which occlusion of a native artery occurs in the setting of severe atherosclerotic disease. Patients who have an embolic etiology to their presentation often present early (within hours of the embolic event) owing to lack of collateral flow, whereas patients with a thrombotic etiology may present more slowly over a day or so. The clinical presentation of ALEI has classically been stated as the six Ps: pain, pallor, pulselessness, paresthesia, paralysis, and poikilothermia (inability to regulate body temperature).

An acute profoundly ischemic limb is a surgical emergency. Cell death begins within 4 hours of total ischemia and is irreversible after 6 hours. Revascularization in this setting may result in sudden tissue reperfusion and lead to a systemic acid-base disorder and impaired cardiopulmonary function.[1] In the late 1970s, Blaisdell et al. documented mortality rates in excess of 25% after open surgical repair of ALEI.[2] Operative mortality remains high despite advances in surgical technique and management.[3] Amputation rates can vary from 10% to 30%.[4]

Treatment generally begins with early anticoagulation with heparin to limit propagation of the thrombus. This has traditionally been followed by surgical thromboembolectomy and correction (patch angioplasty or bypass graft) of the culprit lesion to restore arterial flow.[5]

Thrombolytic therapy provides an attractive alternative to open surgery because it offers several advantages. It is a less invasive procedure, since it not only dissolves the primary arterial thrombus but also helps clear the microcirculation, thereby resulting in gradual reperfusion and averting the release of anaerobic metabolites and thus helping reduce the potential for sudden reperfusion and compartment syndrome.[1]

In the 1970s, intravenous thrombolytic agents (e.g., streptokinase) were shown to restore patency in acutely occluded arteries in 75% of cases.[6] However, systemic infusion of thrombolytic agents carries a high risk of remote bleeding complications and has largely been abandoned in favor of catheter-directed local thrombolytic therapy. Local intraarterial thrombolytic therapy has gained popularity over the past 20 years and in many cases, barring contraindications, is the initial intervention of choice. Thrombolytic agents are infused directly into the occluding thrombus in a concentrated fashion so systemic drug concentration and the total dose required for the procedure are reduced. As flow is restored, the underlying culprit lesion is usually unmasked and managed by interventional or surgical techniques.

INDICATIONS

A classification system was devised by the Society for Vascular Surgery (SVS, United States) and updated by The TransAtlantic Inter-Society Consensus (TASC) II guidelines in 2007 for describing the degree of acute limb ischemia (Table 33-1). The main objective of this categorization is to stratify the acuity of limb ischemia into defined groups for decision-making purposes. The TASC II guidelines also suggest an algorithm for the diagnosis and treatment of acute limb ischemia (Fig. 33-1).[7]

Percutaneous intraarterial thrombolysis (PIAT) is indicated in patients who have acute-onset claudication (SVS I, the limb is generally viable) or limb-threatening ischemia (generally SVS II-a, but also SVS II-b) due to thrombotic or embolic arterial occlusion.[5,8] McNamara et al. described occlusion patterns and found that all patients with a single occluded segment but normal inflow and patent collaterals (generally SVS I) successfully underwent PIAT, with no deaths or amputations.[5] In patients with normal inflow and patent collaterals but tandem occluded segments, PIAT was successful in 90% and had a mortality of 0.7% and a limb loss rate of 8.2%. In patients with irreversible limb ischemia (SVS III), PIAT has unacceptably high morbidity and mortality and is therefore not indicated (see Fig. 33-1). Patients who are considered to have viable or marginally threatened limbs may have imaging performed prior to angiography and thrombolytic therapy. Available modalities include duplex ultrasonography, computed tomographic angiography (CTA), and magnetic resonance angiography (MRA).

Previously thrombolysis was used to clear the acute thrombosis of a popliteal aneurysm to visualize a suitable distal runoff vessel for surgical bypass when the initial diagnostic arteriogram failed to do so.[9] These days, with the availability of MRA, which has high sensitivity for demonstrating these distal vessels, this practice has been abandoned for the most part.

Indications for salvage of a graft require consideration of the individual case.[10] There are twin goals of removing the clot and correcting the underlying lesion. If the underlying lesion is secondary to diseased inflow or outflow, progression of atherosclerotic disease is usually the primary etiology. In this scenario, treatment with angioplasty/stent or bypass grafting has demonstrated success. If the underlying

TABLE 33-1. Society for Vascular Surgery Clinical Categories of Acute Limb Ischemia

			Physical Examination		Doppler Signals	
Category	Definition	Prognosis	Sensory Loss	Muscle Weakness	Arterial	Venous
I	Viable	Not immediately threatened	None	None	+	+
II	Threatened					
II-a	Marginally	Salvageable with prompt treatment	Minimal (toes)	None	Occasional +, frequently −	+
II-b	Immediately	Salvageable with immediate treatment	More than toes, pain at rest	Mild to moderate	Rare +, usually −	+
III	Irreversible	Major permanent tissue loss	Anesthetic	Paralysis	−	−

Modified from Rutherford RB, Baker JD, Ernst C, et al. Recommended standards for reports dealing with lower extremity ischemia: revised version. J Vasc Surg 1997;26:517–38. ©The Society for Vascular Surgery and the North American Chapter of the International Society for Cardiovascular Surgery.

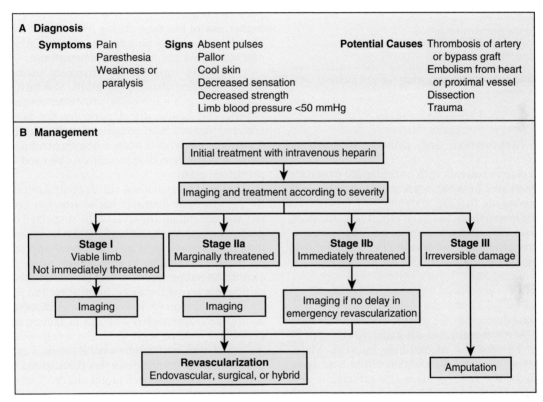

FIGURE 33-1. Clinical algorithm for management of acute lower extremity ischemia. *(From Creager MA, Kaufman JA, Conte MS. Acute limb ischemia. N Engl J Med 2012;366:2198–206.)*

lesion is secondary to intrinsic graft disease, either intimal hyperplasia or graft stenosis is usually the primary etiology. The type of conduit can guide treatment, since prosthetic grafts will develop intimal hyperplasia, while venous bypass grafts often develop stenosis at the site of a valve. Prosthetic grafts may not have successful long-term results with angioplasty and require surgical graft thrombectomy and patch angioplasty. Venous bypass grafts can be treated successfully by angioplasty and/or stenting.

CONTRAINDICATIONS

Relative and absolute contraindications are listed in Table 33-2. Absolute contraindications include active internal bleeding, cerebrovascular events such as a recent (within

6-12 months) cerebrovascular accident or a transient ischemic attack (within 2 months), known intracranial neoplasm, or craniotomy within 2 months.

Irreversible ischemia (SVS III) accompanied by severe sensory loss, along with the onset of muscle rigor and absent arterial and venous signals on Doppler interrogation, puts the patient at high risk for the consequences of acute reperfusion. In this setting, PIAT is associated with a high rate of amputation (25%) and mortality (13%).[10] A surgical approach is advised in this clinical setting.

Most relative contraindications to PIAT are aimed at minimizing the risk of bleeding. The benefits of PIAT should be weighed against this risk. Relative contraindications include recent major surgery, organ biopsy, trauma, gastrointestinal bleeding, pregnancy, postpartum status,

TABLE 33-2. Contraindications to Local Catheter-Directed Thrombolytic Therapy

Absolute
Active internal bleeding
Irreversible limb ischemia (severe sensory deficits, muscle rigor)
Recent stroke (arbitrary guidelines: TIA within 2 months or CVA within 6-12 months)
Intracranial neoplasm or recent (2 months) craniotomy
Protruding mobile left heart thrombus

Relative
History of gastrointestinal bleeding
Recent (10-14 days) major surgery, including biopsy
Recent trauma
Recent CPR
Severe uncontrolled high blood pressure
Emboli from a cardiac source
Subacute bacterial endocarditis
Coagulopathy
Pregnancy and the postpartum period
Severe cerebrovascular disease
Diabetic retinopathy

CPR, Cardiopulmonary resuscitation; *CVA,* cerebrovascular accident; *TIA,* transient ischemic attack.

uncontrolled hypertension, and diabetic hemorrhagic retinopathy.

Of note, in elderly patients with uncontrolled hypertension who were treated for acute myocardial infarction with systemic thrombolytic therapy, a significantly greater risk for intracranial hemorrhage has been reported.[11] The presence of a mobile intracardiac thrombus on echocardiography is predictive of a higher risk of embolization and should therefore be considered a relative risk for lytic therapy.[12]

EQUIPMENT

There are several devices on the market that facilitate infusion of thrombolytic therapy, but any standard catheter, 5F or under, can be used for an end-hole infusion. Multisidehole catheters allow for distribution of the lytic agent along the axis of the catheter once the catheter is well embedded within the thrombus. These catheters come with different effective infusion lengths (segment of distribution of the sideholes) to match the length of the thrombus, and most can be used for both slow continuous and pulsed-spray infusion. One such catheter has pressure-responsive side slits through which jets of fluid lace the thrombus during pulse spray infusion, in addition to allowing slow continuous infusion (Uni-Fuse, SpeedLyser, and Pulse-Spray Infusion Systems [AngioDynamics Inc., Queensbury, N.Y.]). An approach increasingly used is the EkoSonic Endovascular System (Ekos Corporation, Bothell, Wash.). The system consists of a multiple-sidehole catheter through which a wire is placed that emits high-frequency, low-power microsonic energy. By exposing the thrombus to an energy source while infusing a thrombolytic, the interventionalist can achieve improved efficacy in a shorter period of time.[13]

Although there is a large choice of potential delivery catheters, there is no compelling evidence that any of the more complex catheters offer any advantage over a single end-hole catheter for the delivery of lytic agent.

TECHNIQUE

Anatomy and Approach

All previous imaging (angiograms and noninvasive studies) should be reviewed before the procedure, and the choice of puncture site should provide the most direct route possible to the thrombus. Previous ultrasound and CT scans are particularly helpful to decide the approach for the initial puncture. The cohort of patients who have critical limb ischemia often have difficult arterial access secondary to extensive atherosclerotic disease and possibly previous arterial surgery. Real-time ultrasound during the puncture can facilitate access and ensure a minimal number of attempts to gain access. Anterior wall puncture alone of the femoral artery should be performed, since posterior wall puncture is more difficult to control manually and carries a higher risk of bleeding during lysis. Use of an intraarterial sheath is mandatory because it facilitates catheter exchange and minimizes trauma to the puncture site.

Ultrasound can also be extremely useful in directly accessing occluded prosthetic grafts. This technique is often applied for extra-anatomic prosthetic bypass grafts. In experienced hands, direct puncture has been associated with low rates of local complication. Prophylactic antibiotics are recommended when using this technique. Alternatively, a contralateral approach can be used to access the prosthetic graft.

Choice of an ipsilateral versus contralateral approach to the puncture site for either native artery or prosthetic graft remains debatable. The level of the suspected occlusion will guide the approach, as will operator preference. Many interventionalists favor a contralateral approach, allowing for pelvic angiography to evaluate for inflow disease. After a contralateral puncture, a long crossover sheath is used to gain access across the aortic bifurcation and provide stability for all subsequent interventions. A disadvantage of the contralateral approach is difficulty in gaining access for very peripheral lesions, such as in the infrapopliteal area. An ipsilateral approach can be used if physical exam and noninvasive studies demonstrate that the majority of the disease is distal to the common femoral artery.

Technical Aspects

A baseline arteriogram should be obtained to document the extent of thrombus. Once the occluded artery is catheterized, attempts should be made to cross the entirety of the thrombus with a wire. Failure to cross the thrombus with a guidewire ("guidewire traversal test") indicates that the thrombus may be chronic and more difficult to lyse. In such cases, an initial short trial of infusion into the proximal clot may facilitate traversal at a later time.

After successful guidewire traversal, the infusion catheter is used to bathe the entire thrombus with the lytic agent. There are several techniques and devices for delivering thrombolytic agents locally. Table 33-3 summarizes the nomenclature and descriptions of these techniques.

To accelerate thrombolysis, an initial high-dose "trans-thrombus bolus" has been advocated.[14] The authors prefer pulse-spray boluses via catheters with multiple side orifices.[15] After transthrombus lacing, a continuous slow infusion is started, and the lytic therapy is administered via the

TABLE 33-3. Description and Nomenclature of Infusion Techniques

Stepwise infusion	The tip of the catheter is placed in the proximal aspect of the thrombus, and a fixed amount of lyric agent is infused. As the thrombus dissolves, the catheter is advanced and the process is repeated.
Continuous infusion	Refers to steady infusion of the lytic agent, with or without lacing the thrombus.
Graded infusion	Refers to periodic tapering of infusion rates, with the highest rates given initially.
Accelerated thrombolysis	Involves lacing of the thrombus with a high-dose lytic agent initially to bathe the thrombus.
Pulse-spray infusion	This technique forcefully injects the lytic agent into the thrombus to fragment it and increases the surface area exposed to the lytic enzyme.
Pulse-spray pharmacomechanical thrombolysis	Refers to mechanical thrombus disruption and infusion of lytic agents. The mechanical effect can be achieved with the use of pulse-spray catheters, microporous infusion balloons, or mechanical thrombectomy devices.
Enclosed thrombolysis	Refers to infusion of a lytic agent between two balloons spaced across the length of the thrombus.

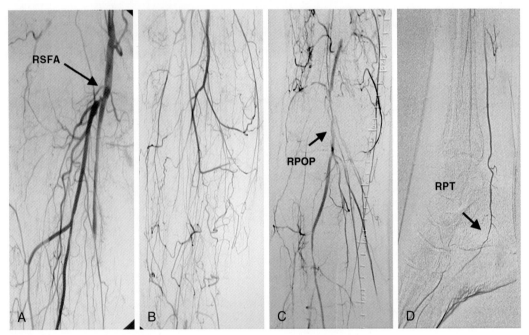

FIGURE 33-2. Elderly man with acutely worsening claudication in right calf and foot. Baseline angiogram shows proximal occlusion of right superficial femoral artery *(RSFA)* **(A)**, extensive thigh collaterals **(B)**, distal reconstitution of a popliteal segment **(C)**, and filling of right posterior tibial *(RPT)* artery at foot **(D)**. Access was via left common femoral artery.

coaxial catheter technique as just described. To minimize concurrent rethrombosis during therapy, intravenous anticoagulation with heparin is recommended, and on occasion, antiplatelet agents are administered. Figures 33-2 through 33-5 illustrate a case in which such a regimen has been successfully used.

Once therapy is initiated, the patient should be transferred to an intensive care or high-dependency unit for frequent monitoring of clinical status and vital signs. Pulses on the treated extremity should be checked every 4 hours or more often if needed. The puncture site should be frequently examined for bleeding, particularly initially.

Laboratory evaluation is important to ensure adequate anticoagulation and detect occult hemorrhage. Partial thromboplastin time (PTT) should be 2 to 2.5 times the control level, and activated clotting time (ACT) should be around 300 seconds. PTT and ACT should be checked

often initially (every 2 hours) to adjust heparin infusion rates, and less frequently thereafter as adequate anticoagulation is attained. Decreasing hematocrit or fibrinogen levels (especially values < 100 mg/dL) are useful signs of potential or occult bleeding.

A repeat angiogram should be obtained 4 to 12 hours after initiating therapy to monitor progress. During therapy, it is not unusual for symptoms to sometimes get worse as a result of distal embolization. The patient and referring physician should be made aware of this possibility. The embolized clot is likely to lyse without change in therapy; however, if symptoms fail to abate, the catheter occasionally has to be advanced to the embolized clot. Alternatively, a persistent embolus can be removed by suction thrombectomy.

After documentation of successful recanalization, the lytic agent and heparin are discontinued simultaneously.

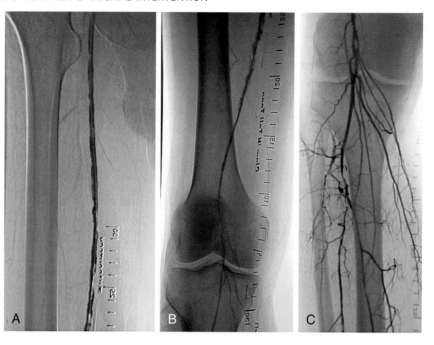

FIGURE 33-3. A-C, After performing a diagnostic angiogram, a multi-sidehole pulse-spray catheter was placed to bridge entire thrombus, and it was laced with 10 mg of tissue plasminogen activator (tPA); an intra-arterial infusion was started at 1 mg/h. Patient also received a 3000-unit bolus of heparin and infusion at 500 units/h, along with a 15-mg intravenous bolus of abciximab and infusion at 10 μg/min (maximum, 12 hours). At 6-hour check, superior femoral artery is patent with residual thrombus, and diseased popliteal and calf vessels are patent. Considerable resolution of thrombus allowed tPA infusion to be lowered to 0.5 mg/h.

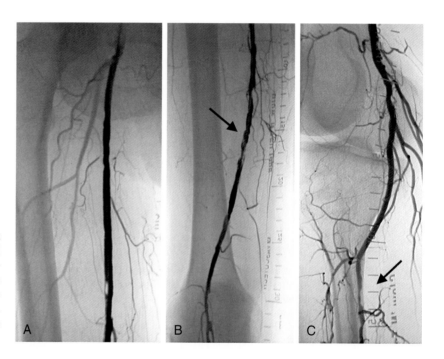

FIGURE 33-4. For logistical reasons, next check angiogram was performed at 18 hours. **A,** Superficial femoral artery *(SFA)* thrombus is almost completely dissolved, and there are stenoses **(B)** in distal SFA and **(C)** tibioperoneal segments *(arrows).* Brisk flow was reestablished, and patient and his leg were doing well clinically. Patient had received a total dose of 22 mg of tissue plasminogen activator.

The catheters are removed, but the arterial sheath is left in place and is infused with heparinized saline to keep it patent until it can be removed when the lytic and coagulation status has normalized. Successful thrombolysis often reveals an underlying culprit lesion that should be treated by endovascular (e.g., focal stenosis) or surgical (e.g., long-segment disease, failed graft) techniques.

Thrombolytic Agents

In the 1990s, urokinase (UK) and recombinant tissue plasminogen activator (rtPA) largely replaced streptokinase in the United States because of their better efficacy and safety records. UK (Abbokinase [Abbott Laboratories, Abbott Park, Ill.) has since been withdrawn from the U.S. market.

The plasma half-life of rtPA is 5 minutes, compared to 20 minutes for UK, but prolonged use can extend the duration of the systemic lytic and hypocoagulation status. A popular scheme for the delivery of UK was (and where available, is) 240,000 international units (IU)/h for 2 hours or until restoration of antegrade flow, reduced to 120,000 IU/h for another 2 hours, and then to 60,000 IU/h until treatment is complete.[16] The PURPOSE trial in part validated these previously empirical dose ranges.[17]

Based on its established efficacy in the intravenous treatment of myocardial infarction, pulmonary embolism, and stroke, rtPA has also been used for the treatment of peripheral arterial occlusion. In addition, prospective controlled trials, such as the STILE trial, have shown that UK and rtPA

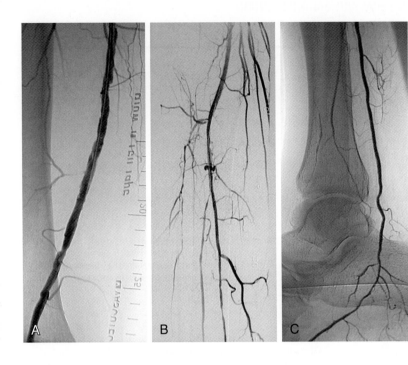

FIGURE 33-5. A, Superficial femoral artery stenosis was successfully dilated with a 6 mm × 4 cm angioplasty balloon. **B,** Tibioperoneal trunk was successfully dilated with a 3.5 mm × 2 cm percutaneous angioplasty balloon. **C,** Brisk antegrade flow to posterior tibial artery has been reestablished. Access at left common femoral artery was closed with a percutaneous suture device, and effects of the lytic, anticoagulation, and antiplatelet agents were allowed to resolve spontaneously.

are equivalent in efficacy and safety, but rtPA and UK do not have U.S. Food and Drug Administration (FDA) approval for direct intraarterial infusion to treat peripheral arterial occlusion. The dosage of rtPA for use in peripheral arterial occlusion is 0.5 to 1 mg/h intraarterially after a thrombus-lacing dose (if used) of 5 to 10 mg. Studies comparing different dosages of rtPA have not revealed significant benefit with higher doses.[18] Studies evaluating more recent agents such as reteplase[19] and tenecteplase[20] report thrombus dissolution and bleeding rates that appear comparable to those of older thrombolytic agents. Direct-acting fibrinolytic agents such as alfimeprase (Nuvelo, Sunnyvale, Calif.) that do not have to convert plasminogen to plasmin to achieve fibrinolysis have shown promising initial results and may potentially reduce the risk of remote bleeding.[21]

CONTROVERSIES

Although contrary opinions exist regarding the appropriate use of thrombolytic therapy or surgery (or both), it is important to realize that these treatment options are complementary rather than exclusive of each other. Proper treatment should be tailored to the individual patient, his or her ability to tolerate further ischemia, and treatment options and skills most immediately available at any given center.

OUTCOMES

The Rochester, STILE, and TOPAS trials are three prospective controlled randomized studies in which thrombolytic therapy was compared to surgery for the treatment of acute peripheral arterial occlusion (Table 33-4).

The Rochester trial included 114 patients at a single center and compared UK therapy with primary surgery in patients with "hyperacute ischemia."[16] The limb salvage rate was the same between the two arms of the study (80%). However, the mortality rate at 1 year was 16% in patients treated with UK and 42% in patients treated surgically. This

difference in survival was thought to be due to increased in-hospital complications in the surgical group.

The STILE trial (Surgery or Thrombolysis for the Ischemic Lower Extremity) was a multicenter study of 393 patients. There were three treatment arms; patients were randomized to rtPA (Activase [Genentech, San Francisco]), UK (Abbokinase), or primary surgery. Because the outcomes for the two thrombolytic agents were comparable, their results were combined and compared with the operative arm. The results of thrombolysis versus surgery were as follows: 30-day mortality rate, 4% versus 5%; amputation rate, 5% versus 6%; and major morbidity, 21% versus 16%, respectively. At 1 year, the amputation rate in patients with native artery occlusions was higher in the thrombolysis group (10% vs. 0%; P = .0024).[22] By contrast, in patients with acute graft occlusion, the amputation rate was lower in those who received thrombolysis (P = .026).[23] Subsequent subgroup analysis suggested there may also be a temporal difference, with patients having limb ischemia for more than 14 days having a better clinical outcome with surgery.

The TOPAS (Thrombolysis or Peripheral Arterial Surgery) multicenter trial included 544 patients. Patients were randomized to recombinant UK or a primary operative intervention. The findings in this study confirmed that acute limb ischemia can be managed by catheter-directed thrombolysis, which achieved amputation and mortality rates similar to those of surgery while minimizing the need for and degree of open surgical procedures in a significant number of patients.[24]

A meta-analysis of five randomized controlled trials with a total of 1283 participants was updated in 2009 and suggests that either thrombolysis or surgery can be considered as first-line treatment for patients presenting with acute limb ischemia. Because of the heterogeneity of the studies, subgroup analysis of patients with different classifications of acute limb ischemia was not possible. This review does demonstrate that there was no significant difference in limb salvage or death at 30 days, 6 months, or 1 year in patients

TABLE 33-4. Comparison of Thrombolysis Outcomes

Trial	Methods	Outcomes
Rochester (1994)[16] Comparison of thrombolytic therapy to operative revascularization in initial treatment of acute peripheral arterial ischemia	114 patients in single center comparing UK therapy with primary surgery	Similar limb salvage rate (80%) with decreased mortality at 1 year (16% vs. 42%) for UK patients.
STILE (1994)[22] Surgery or Thrombolysis for the Ischemic Lower Extremity	Multicenter study of 393 patients randomized to rtPA, UK, or primary surgery	Thrombolysis vs. surgery demonstrates similar clinical outcomes at 30 days, despite greater reduction in ongoing/recurring ischemia in the surgical group.
TOPAS (1996)[24] Thrombolysis or Peripheral Arterial Surgery	Prospective, multicenter study of 213 patients randomized to UK or surgery	Thrombolysis had similar amputation and mortality rates.
Cochrane Systematic Review (2002)[27]	Meta-analysis of five randomized trials with a total of 1283 patients	Similar rates of limb salvage and death at 30 days, 6 months, and 1 year between thrombolysis or surgery. Increased rate of stroke, hemorrhage, and distal embolization in thrombolysis.

rtPA, Recombinant tissue plasminogen activator; *UK,* urokinase.

undergoing either procedure. However, within 30 days, there was an increase in the number of strokes (1.3% vs. 0%), major hemorrhage (8.8% vs. 3.3%), and distal embolization (12.4% vs. 0%) in patients undergoing thrombolysis. The authors concluded that the higher risk of complications for patients undergoing thrombolysis should be weighed against the risks of surgery for the individual patient.

COMPLICATIONS

Although the reported total complication rates associated with local thrombolytic therapy are as high as 50%, the vast majority do not have significant clinical consequences.[13] The most dreaded complication of thrombolytic therapy is intracranial bleeding or severe intraabdominal bleeding. Bleeding is theorized to occur as a result of dissolution of a preexisting remote hemostatic plug during therapy. The reported rate of intracranial bleeding was 2.1% in TOPAS-I, 1.6% in TOPAS-II,[25] and 1.6% in STILE.[26] In the STILE study, there was no difference in bleeding complications between UK and rtPA, and this is generally corroborated by other experience.

Retroperitoneal bleeding occurs in about 0.3% of patients[11] and is more likely to occur with a high puncture above the inguinal ligament. It often goes undetected until hypotension develops, so any complaints such as nausea or back pain should be diligently evaluated and monitored.

When bleeding occurs during thrombolytic therapy, both the thrombolytic agent and heparin infusions should be stopped immediately. If bleeding continues, administration of fresh frozen plasma should be considered. The site of bleeding should be determined immediately, and appropriate interventions should be taken. Pericatheter bleeding at the arterial puncture site is very common, may be delayed in onset, and can typically be controlled by applying local pressure. If severe, thrombolysis may have to be stopped.

Distal embolization of partially lysed fragments after cleavage of thrombus can develop in 10% to 15% of cases. These are usually of minor clinical significance and can be treated by continuing the therapy, adjusting the region of therapy, or performing aspiration thrombectomy.

Allergic reactions are rare with UK and rtPA, but they have been reported more frequently with streptokinase. They can be managed by oral prophylaxis with antihistamines or histamine H_2 blockers such as cimetidine or ranitidine.

POSTPROCEDURAL AND FOLLOW-UP CARE

In the immediate postprocedure time frame, the patient should be monitored for reperfusion injury and possible compartment syndrome. Patients will present with pain out of proportion to physical exam, paresthesia, and edema. Compartment pressures above 20 mmHg are an indication for a fasciotomy. Fasciotomy has been required in up to 5.3% of cases in the United States following successful revascularization.

After successful treatment by either endovascular or surgical means, patients should be placed on a long-term regimen of anticoagulant and antiplatelet therapy (aspirin or clopidogrel, or both) in the appropriate setting. Adequate levels of anticoagulation should be monitored in an ambulatory setting. Patients should generally be observed for possible worsening of native disease, and patients with vascular grafts should be entered into a surveillance program.

SUMMARY

Thrombolytic therapy is a viable treatment option, barring known contraindications to the use of lytic agents and so long as the limb is not irreversibly threatened (SVS III). Intraarterial catheter-directed thrombolytic therapy provides an attractive alternative to open surgery for patients with ALEI (SVS I and II-a). Depending on local expertise, patients with SVS II-b limb ischemia may be treated by either lytic therapy or surgery. There are several techniques that use different drugs and dosing regimens aimed at achieving thrombus dissolution. An underlying lesion is usually revealed for immediate endovascular or operative management.

KEY POINTS

- Acute ischemia of the lower extremity is a serious condition with substantial morbidity and mortality.

- Classification helps with decision making.

- Treatment generally begins with early anticoagulation with heparin. Various forms of thrombolysis or surgery (or both) may follow. Catheter-directed local thrombolytic therapy has largely replaced systemic infusion.

- Contraindications share the common themes of bleeding risk, previous cerebrovascular events, reperfusion injury risk, and certain embolization risks.

- Baseline imaging and a guidewire traversal test inform the process. Many catheter designs can be used for thrombolysis. A direct route to the thrombus and an intraarterial sheath should be used.

- Close patient monitoring is necessary. Laboratory evaluation is important to ensure adequate anticoagulation and detect occult hemorrhage.

- Complications include bleeding (especially intracranial or severe intraabdominal bleeding), distal embolization, and (less frequently) allergic reactions to the lytic agent.

- Although contrary opinions exist regarding the appropriate use of thrombolytic therapy or surgery (or both), it is important to realize these treatment options are complementary rather than exclusive of each other.

- Successful thrombolysis often reveals an underlying culprit lesion that may have to be treated by endovascular or surgical techniques.

▸ **SUGGESTED READINGS**

Camerota AJ, Weaver FA, Hosking JD, et al. Results of a prospective randomized trial of surgery versus thrombolysis for occluded lower extremity bypass grafts. Am J Surg 1996;172:105–12.

Dormandy J, Heek L, Vig S. Acute limb ischemia. Semin Vasc Surg 1999;12:148–53.

Ouriel K, Shortell CK, De Weese JA, et al. A comparison of thrombolytic therapy with operative vascularization in the initial treatment of acute peripheral arterial ischemia. J Vasc Surg 1994;19:1021–30.

Ouriel K, Veith FJ, Sasahara AA, for the Thrombolysis of Peripheral Arterial Surgery (TOPAS) Investigators. A comparison of recombinant urokinase with vascular surgery as initial treatment for acute arterial occlusion of the legs. N Engl J Med 1998;338:1105–11.

STILE Investigators. Results of a prospective randomized trial evaluating surgery versus thrombolysis for ischemia of the lower extremity. The STILE Trial. Ann Surg 1994;220:251–68.

Weaver FA, Camerota AJ, Youngblood M, et al. Surgical revascularization versus thrombolysis for nonembolic lower extremity native artery occlusions: results of a prospective randomized trial. The STILE Investigators. Surgery versus thrombolysis for ischemia of the lower extremity. J Vasc Surg 1996;24:513–21.

The complete reference list is available online at www.expertconsult.com.

CHAPTER 34
Chronic Upper Extremity Ischemia and Revascularization

Gary M. Ansel and Charles F. Botti, Jr.

The majority of this chapter is dedicated to a discussion of the management of occlusive disease of the subclavian and brachiocephalic arteries. Treatment of various conditions such as thoracic outlet syndrome and more distal lesions will also be covered.

SUBCLAVIAN AND BRACHIOCEPHALIC DISEASE

Symptomatic chronic ischemia of the upper extremity is commonly encountered in clinical vascular practice, comprising about 17% of symptomatic extracranial cerebrovascular disease[1]; 80% occurs in males. In contradistinction to chronic lower extremity ischemia, presenting symptoms in the upper extremity are often due to remote ischemia in the bed supplying collateral flow—namely, vertebral-subclavian and coronary-subclavian steal.[2-8] This intimate association between the vascular territories of the arm, hindbrain, and heart (in post left internal mammary artery [LIMA] coronary artery bypass graft [CABG] patients) is unique and may present technical challenges and potential complications not typically encountered in other vascular beds. With modern techniques and equipment, however, operators treating underlying stenotic or occlusive lesions of the proximal upper extremity arteries by interventional techniques can expect high degrees of success with low complication rates.[2,4,7,9-13]

INDICATIONS

- Symptomatic chronic upper extremity ischemia
- Symptomatic vertebral-subclavian steal syndrome
- Symptomatic coronary-subclavian steal syndrome
- Asymptomatic subclavian stenosis or occlusion in a patient about to undergo CABG with LIMA engraftment
- Preservation of dialysis or other vascular access

CONTRAINDICATIONS

- Asymptomatic disease (in general, except as noted earlier)
- Renal insufficiency, severe aortic arch atherosclerosis (relative)

EQUIPMENT

- 6F to 9F sheaths, 45 and 90 cm, long enough to extend through the area of intervention from the access site
- Straight and angled hydrophilic wires
- Diagnostic catheters of various shapes, such as Judkins right (JR)4, multipurpose, headhunter, LIMA, VTK, Amplatz, and Simmons
- Straight or angled tip glide catheter

- 0.035-inch exchange wire, atraumatic, straight, or J tipped
- Balloons 4- to 10-mm diameter, 2 to 4 cm in length, with a long shaft length (110 cm long), if the site of access is from the femoral artery
- Balloon-expandable stents capable of achieving these diameters, and lengths from 20 to 40 mm
- Covered stents in similar sizes for treatment of restenosis or for emergency use in vessel perforations
- Coronary stents in 3.0, 3.5, and 4.0 mm for vertebral or LIMA salvage (with compatible 0.014-inch wire)

TECHNIQUE

Anatomy and Approaches

Symptomatic disease of the left subclavian artery is roughly eight to ten times more frequent than in the brachiocephalic trunk or right subclavian artery.[9,10] This can be considered fortunate because intervention in the brachiocephalic or right subclavian artery naturally involves working in close proximity to the right common carotid artery, subjecting it to potential embolization, dissection, ostial compression, or stent coverage.

Proper technique, as always, begins with case planning and selection of vascular access. The strength of the indications must be weighed against the relative contraindications (severe generalized arch disease, renal insufficiency, long occlusions) and operator experience for good case selection. Most complications will happen early in an operator's experience in more difficult cases.

Aorto-ostial flush occlusions, long occlusions, and lesions in close approximation with the vertebral, right common carotid, or internal mammary artery (IMA) are all "yellow flags," to be given thoughtful consideration.

The operator should select the vascular access point that yields the highest chance of success with the lowest risk of complication at both the access and intervention site. In general, this is femoral access. Brachial access should be considered first in cases with heavily diseased or tortuous iliofemoral vessels and in severely tortuous aortic arches, particularly those with flush occlusions. Brachial access is also often used when guidewire access cannot be gained in antegrade fashion from a first femoral approach. In such cases, retrograde passage of the guidewire is often surprisingly easy.

Technical Aspects

Once vascular access has been selected and gained, a diagnostic catheter is selected based on the angulation involved and the need for coaxial support.

From a femoral or brachial access, a simple JR4 or IMA catheter may suffice for guiding a wire through a stenotic lesion; an occlusion, especially approached from the arch, may need the additional backup support offered by a VTK, Amplatz, or Simmons shaped catheter. Great care must be used with such aggressive catheter shapes to avoid disrupting aortic plaque. When tempted to use them, brachial access should at least be considered as an alternate approach. Appropriate wire selection may include an 0.018- to 0.035-inch transition wire, a Wholey wire, or other similar metallic wire for stenosis, but a hydrophilic straight or angled wire will be necessary to cross most occlusions. Careful fluoroscopic guidance with road map support (if available) is necessary to ensure wire passage safely into the lumen beyond the occlusion. Care must be taken, especially with hydrophilic wires, to avoid propagating a dissection plane, either toward the vertebral artery or into the aorta retrogradely. Although helpful in infrainguinal revascularization, a subintimal approach in brachiocephalic disease is best avoided.

In occlusive disease, once the hydrophilic wire is free in the distal lumen, it is advisable to pass a diagnostic catheter (hydrophilic if necessary) through the occlusion, then remove the wire and confirm luminal placement by blood aspiration and gentle injection of contrast medium. A stiff exchange-length guidewire is then advanced through the catheter for completion of the procedure.

Although there is no conclusive evidence in favor of primary stenting for subclavian and brachiocephalic artery lesions, most operators treat these lesions by stenting in preference to angioplasty alone.

Once guidewire access across the lesion has been achieved, one has the choice of whether or not to predilate before stent placement. Predilation has several advantages, including better visualization of the lesion length, especially of the distal stent landing point, proof of distensibility (especially in calcific lesions), and the ability to visually confirm correct balloon size. The main disadvantages are the possibility of propagating a dissection and, in theory, relieving the subclavian gradient enough to restore antegrade vertebral flow and lose the inherent protection against vertebral embolization retrograde flow provides. There is controversial evidence from a small study done over 20 years ago that restoration of antegrade flow may take several minutes,[14] perhaps owing to chronic ischemic vasodilation in the arm. In our experience, however, restoration of antegrade flow in the vertebral artery occurs immediately on relief of the pressure gradient across the lesion, either with aggressive predilation or stenting. There is some evidence that direct stenting (i.e., without predilation) may be associated with a lower restenosis rate as well.[10] In general, we gently predilate occlusions with undersized balloons to allow some antegrade flow for better visualization, and primary stent most stenoses that are not heavily calcified.

As is the case with most aortic branch vessel disease, most subclavian disease is ostial or near ostial. This includes the right subclavian artery, where typically the lesion is at the brachiocephalic bifurcation. In general, these lesions have a high degree of resistance to dilation and subsequent recoil; accordingly, balloon-expandable stents are generally preferred to self-expanding stents or angioplasty alone.[9,10]

When positioning the stent, it is important to fully cover the lesion, but every attempt should be made to leave the ostium of the common carotid, internal mammary, and/or vertebral artery uncovered. One should be mindful,

especially if predilation was not performed, that the vertebral or IMA may not be visible owing to reversed blood flow. If any of these ostia become compromised, rescue angioplasty with or without coronary-sized stent placement should be considered. In the case of the ostial right subclavian artery, consideration may be given to placing an additional guidewire in the proximal right common carotid artery in the event the ostium is severely compromised when the stent is deployed.

Many cases of stent migration before deployment in the lesion have been reported.[7,12] This usually arises from either the stent edge catching in the lesion during attempted passage through the lesion, or the rear of the stent catching on the guiding catheter during attempted stent withdrawal if the stent cannot be passed across the lesion. In both instances, the stent may be loosened ("skimmed") off the balloon and left free on the wire. Although there are several methods available to rescue this event, including safely deploying the stent in a more proximal vessel,[7] this situation is best avoided. Stents that are factory rather than hand mounted may be more resistant to skimming, and the risk can be eliminated entirely by readvancing the dilator and sheath through the lesion before the stent is advanced. In this way, the stent can be positioned while it is still protected inside the sheath, which can subsequently be withdrawn, and the exposed stent deployed. Especially when using 6F guiding sheaths, the potential for distal embolization is minimized.

Finally, after stent deployment, repeat angiography to assess optimal sizing should be undertaken, and postdilation can be performed if necessary, aiming for no more than a 1:1 balloon size–to–vessel ratio.

Figures 34-1 to 34-6 illustrate various aspects of the interventions discussed.

CONTROVERSIES

Much of the controversy originally surrounding endovascular treatment of the brachiocephalic and subclavian vessels has subsided because of the reproducibility and good clinical outcome of stenting compared with the perioperative complication rate of carotid subclavian bypass.[7,12] It can now be stated that with the exception of chronic occlusions that cannot be crossed with a guidewire, carotid subclavian bypass should no longer be performed as primary therapy.

The major controversies still discussed are whether to predilate (as addressed earlier) and whether prophylactic stenting of the subclavian artery can safely allow for the use of the IMA for subsequent coronary bypass. In this second concern, the protean reports of good long-term results in subclavian stents suggest that in the absence of small vessels or diffuse disease, the IMA can indeed be counted on to be a reliable conduit in subsequent bypass. Several studies report prospectively on this very issue.[4,9,16] With the recent advent of balloon-expandable polytetrafluoroethylene (PTFE) stent-grafts for the biliary circulation, improved patency of total occlusions is an important question. The COBEST (Covered vs. Balloon Expandable Stent) Trial demonstrated improved patency of PTFE-covered stents when compared with bare metal stents in this randomized trial. In view of the relatively small patient population with subclavian stenosis, a randomized trial comparing covered with bare stents in this anatomic territory may not be

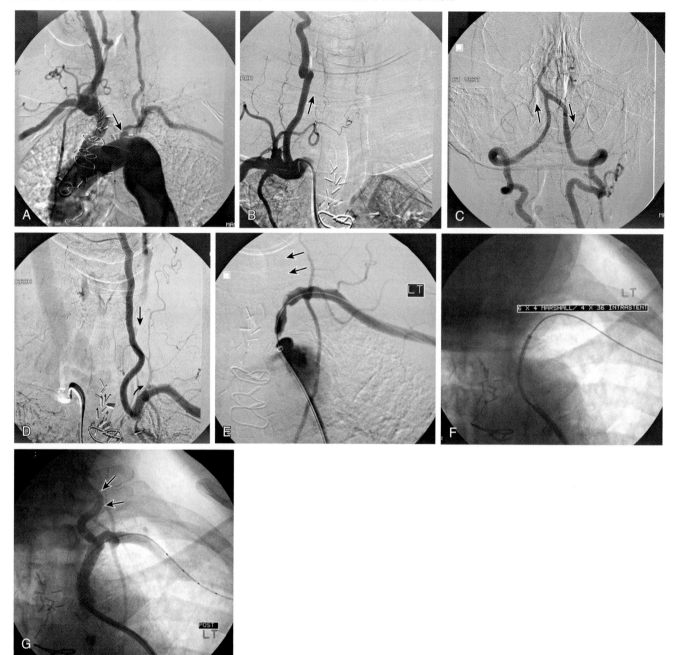

FIGURE 34-1. Subclavian steal. **A,** Arch aortogram shows a diffusely diseased arch with critical left subclavian stenosis *(arrow)*. Right subclavian arterial injection **(B)** shows antegrade right vertebral flow, crossover flow *(arrows)* into left vertebral artery **(C)** at level of basilar artery, and retrograde flow down left vertebral artery to reconstitute left subclavian artery **(D). E,** Injection of left subclavian artery directly demonstrates critical stenosis. Note apparent absence of vertebral artery owing to unopacified retrograde flow. After stenting **(F),** stenosis is relieved **(G)** and antegrade flow returns to vertebral artery *(arrows)*.

feasible, and physician discretion should be used. Certainly this appears to be a promising technology, especially for treatment of restenosis.[17]

Even more controversial is the approach to severe asymptomatic but technically low-risk stenoses. Close questioning may actually reveal that the patient has insidious symptoms that have been circumvented. There are no data to guide therapy in truly asymptomatic patients, and decisions regarding intervention in such situations should be made on a case-by-case basis, with a bias toward conservative therapy.

OUTCOMES

Initial clinical success is generally seen in nearly 100% of stenotic lesions and 60% to 100% of occlusions.[2,4,7,9-13,15] No doubt some of these results are time dependent, with increased success as technology has advanced, particularly with the advent of hydrophilic wires. Among contemporary studies, differences in success likely reflect differences in operator experience and patient selection as well.

Long-term outcomes have been reported in multiple studies.[2,9-13,18] At 1 year, primary patency is seen in 91% to

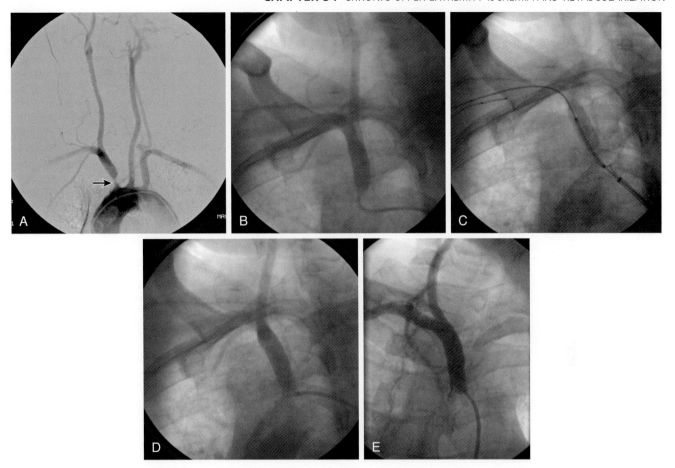

FIGURE 34-2. Brachiocephalic stenosis. **A,** Arch aortogram shows severe brachiocephalic stenosis *(arrow)* in a mildly diseased arch. **B,** Selective angiogram obtained with a JR4 catheter confirms critical stenosis with damping. A 0.035-inch wire is advanced, and a long sheath is placed. **C,** A short balloon-expandable stent is placed, with care to cover the ostium, but not compress left carotid proximally (left anterior oblique view) or brachiocephalic division distally (right anterior oblique view). **D-E,** Final result in both views is satisfactory.

100%, falling to 82% to 86% at 3 years and 77% at 5 years. Other studies reported restenosis rates at variable intervals of 1 year or greater range from 6% to 15%. In 110 patients followed by duplex ultrasonography for patency up to 10 years (mean, 3 years), De Vries and colleagues reported a 93% success rate, one major complication, and 8% symptomatic restenosis; an additional 6% of patients had asymptomatic 50% to 70% restenosis.[9]

Few studies have directly compared stent-supported angioplasty with carotid subclavian bypass. In 1999, Hadjipetrou and associates eloquently summarized all published series of both endovascular and surgical treatment of brachiocephalic arch vessels.[12] In 52 series encompassing 2184 patients, surgical approaches included endarterectomy, axilloaxillary, intrathoracic, and carotid-subclavian bypass. The overall rate of stroke was 3% (range, 0%-9%), and that of death was 2% (range, 0%-11%). Of course, intrathoracic procedures would be expected to have higher risks. However, when trials reporting only carotid subclavian bypass are considered, the stroke rate in 267 patients is 2%, with a death rate of 1.5%; complications including transient ischemic attack, myocardial infarction, and Horner syndrome were seen in 12%. In that same series, 126 patients treated with stenting had 0% stroke and death rates and a

6% complication rate, mostly consisting of minor complications related to vascular access.

COMPLICATIONS

Major complication rates for endovascular non–carotid arch vessel intervention have been uniformly low, running from 0% to 1%.[2,4,7,9-13] The majority are neurologic events that likely arise as often from arch embolization as from the site of intervention. Other infrequent complications include transient ischemic attacks, distal embolization to the arm, major bleeding, and vessel perforation,[19] all seen in less than 1%. There are no good data on the treatment of embolic events. Large emboli in accessible arteries may be treated with catheter aspiration. Smaller emboli may be treated by thrombolysis, and intravenous (IV) antiplatelet therapy may be helpful in either circumstance.

Operators should also be familiar with techniques used in the event of balloon rupture early during stent deployment.[20] This has become less common with current higher-pressure balloons. Initial management may include attempting rapid inflation with a large syringe. If this is unsuccessful, care must be taken to get another balloon in place without causing stent migration. The access sheath

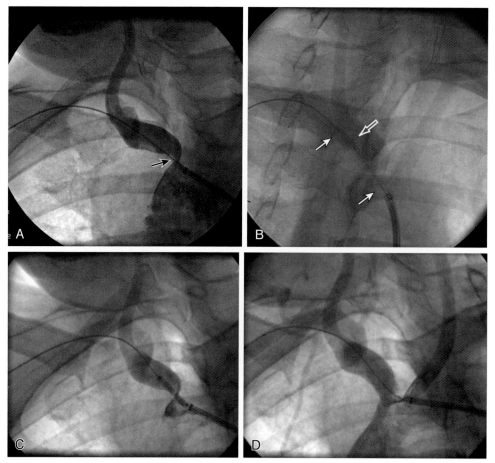

FIGURE 34-3. Brachiocephalic stenosis, incorrect stent choice. **A,** Selective angiography demonstrates critical brachiocephalic stenosis *(arrow)*. **B,** Initial 29-mm stent selection proves too long, impinging on right carotid/subclavian division. **C,** Shorter 18-mm stent is placed and distally postdilated with 12-mm balloon. **D,** Final result conforms to the vessel without overly stretching the ostium.

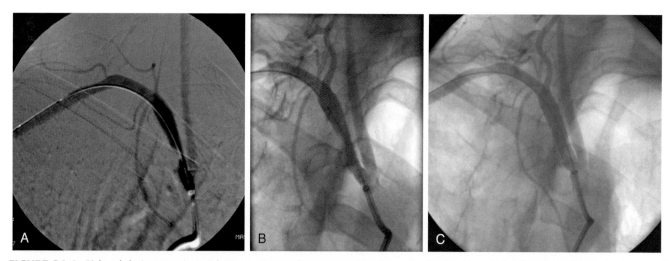

FIGURE 34-4. Right subclavian stenosis. **A,** Selective angiogram shows severe stenosis just distal to brachiocephalic bifurcation, with nonvisualization of reversed right vertebral artery. **B,** After predilation, vertebral artery appears and a 29-mm stent is carefully positioned so as not to cover right carotid proximally or vertebral artery distally. **C,** Final angiogram shows antegrade vertebral flow.

can be used to buttress the stent in place during exchange. If the ruptured balloon is entrapped or if a portion of the stent is not yet deployed at all, it may be best to first replace the 0.035-inch wire with a 0.014-inch wire so that once the balloon is withdrawn, a coronary balloon can be used to open the stent enough to allow passage of a new peripheral balloon without pushing the partially deployed stent distally.

Management of vessel rupture may be handled conservatively by prolonged balloon inflation combined with

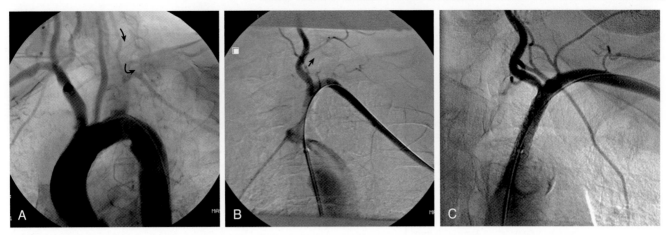

FIGURE 34-5. Left subclavian occlusion. **A,** Arch aortogram demonstrates complete occlusion of left subclavian artery, with retrograde vertebral reconstitution. **B,** After predilation, flow in vertebral artery is immediately reversed. **C,** After stent placement, there is no residual stenosis.

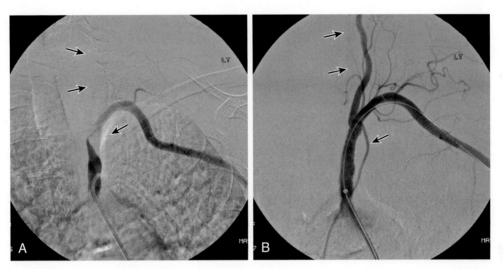

FIGURE 34-6. Left subclavian occlusion. **A,** Arch aortogram demonstrates complete occlusion of left subclavian artery *(arrows)*, with retrograde vertebral reconstitution. **B,** After predilation, flow in vertebral artery is immediately reversed *(arrows)*. After stent placement, there is no residual stenosis.

reversal of anticoagulation in the majority of cases.[16] Larger perforations should generally be handled with balloon tamponade and stent-graft placement. If necessary, this may have to be performed from a second access site to allow the tamponading balloon to remain *in situ* during graft preparation and insertion.

Minor complications common to all endovascular procedures include access site bleeding, infection, reactions to contrast media, and cholesterol embolization.

POSTPROCEDURAL AND FOLLOW-UP CARE

Postprocedural care after brachiocephalic and subclavian stenting should include long-term antiplatelet therapy with aspirin and/or clopidogrel. Aggressive risk factor modification with smoking cessation and statin therapy should be given to all patients to achieve National Cholesterol Education Program guidelines.[21]

Given that arch vessel disease is a marker for advanced atherosclerosis, strong consideration should be given to coronary and carotid artery evaluation, because the vast majority of patients will ultimately succumb to cardiovascular death.

Noninvasive ultrasound follow-up of stents in the brachiocephalic circulation is recommended for at least 2 years,[4] after which progression of disease rather than restenosis would be the main concern.

OTHER DISORDERS OF UPPER EXTREMITY ARTERIES

Thoracic Outlet Syndrome

The neurovascular structures that exit the thorax may be compressed, leading to manifestations of both vascular and neurologic symptoms. Thoracic outlet syndrome may be divided into neurologic (brachial plexus), venous

Thoracic Outlet Syndrome

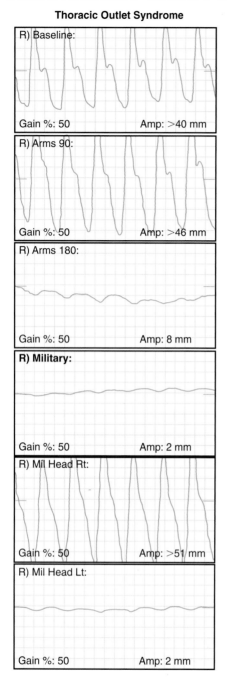

FIGURE 34-7. Pulse volume recording (PVR) of patient with thoracic outlet syndrome of right upper extremity, Note that with appropriate maneuvers, arterial waveform flattens due to arterial compression.

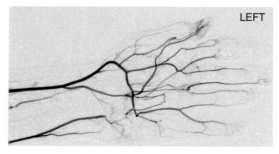

FIGURE 34-8. Angiography of lower arm of a minor league pitcher with thoracic outlet syndrome, who developed a subclavian artery aneurysm. Note embolization of distal ulnar artery and digits.

(subclavian vein), and arterial (subclavian artery) categories. The arterial form (the least common type) occurs as external compression of the subclavian artery from a cervical rib or callus of a previously broken clavicle, leading to turbulent flow. This may lead to a stenosis or aneurysm formation and platelet thrombi that may embolize and cause digital ischemia (Fig. 34-7). Noninvasive imaging typically demonstrates compression with maneuvers that lead to narrowing of the outlet (Fig. 34-8).

Thoracic outlet syndrome is typically treated by open surgical treatment of the offending stimulus (e.g., cervical rib). Angioplasty may be employed as a temporizing treatment to maintain patency until definitive surgical repair is completed. Stenting should be avoided owing to continued external trauma that can lead to stent fracture. Local thrombolysis may be useful to restore patency prior to surgery.

Distal Upper Extremity Arterial Disease

Chronic ischemia of the upper extremities due to arterial lesions distal to the subclavian arteries is much less common than more proximal disease. The axillary, brachial, radial, and ulnar arteries all may be affected by typically nonatherosclerotic disease that may manifest in various patterns.

Axillary Artery Disease
Atherosclerosis rarely affects arteries distal to the subclavian artery. The typically reported etiologies of axillary artery stenosis are Takayasu aortoarteritis,[22] giant cell arteritis,[23] and radiation-induced arteritis.[24] Less commonly, neurofibromatosis and collagen vascular diseases may affect the axillary artery. Repetitive trauma to any artery may lead to arterial stenosis. The axillary artery may be affected by prolonged use of crutches, and more rarely by repetitive injury in gymnasts.[25,26]

Brachial, Ulnar, and Radial Artery Disease
The brachial and more rarely the ulnar and radial arteries may be involved by fibromuscular dysplasia (FMD). FMD mainly affects young girls and women younger than 40 years of age. The FMD process is a noninflammatory, nonatherosclerotic process that affects the arterial vascular system. FMD can affect the arterial intima, media, or adventitia. Although the intima is typically intact, dysplasia in these layers decreases lumen size and increases turbulence, leading to diminished flow through the involved segment. Embolization and ischemia may occur, but overt thrombosis is rarely seen.[27] Management of FMD is surgical and/or interventional. As in the renal vasculature, it appears that angioplasty is typically sufficient for a successful clinical result.

Chronic hand ischemia may occur in patients who use the palms of their hands for manual labor or use vibrating power equipment. The repetitive trauma may cause irreversible damage to primarily the distal radial or ulnar arteries. In this process, there is often damage to the intima lining that may lead to arterial thrombosis.[28] If the trauma primarily leads to damage of the media, it may cause aneurysm formation. These aneurysms may lead to embolization of the digital arteries, causing symptoms of ischemia. These patients may have symptoms of Raynaud syndrome, or they may have ischemic ulceration of their fingers.

Hypothenar hammer syndrome with involvement of the ulnar artery is much more frequently encountered than thenar hammer syndrome, which is caused by damage to the radial artery. Both conservative and surgical treatments have been used successfully. In long segment occlusions, thrombolysis may play a role in treatment and may uncover an aneurysm.[29] Avoidance of the precipitating activities is important in long-term management of these patients.

FMD typically responds to simple balloon angioplasty. Thrombolysis may restore patency to occluded digital arteries and uncover underlying lesions in arterial occlusions.[29] The aneurysm formation of hypothenar hammer syndrome is typically treated by microsurgical bypass.

IMAGING OF UPPER EXTREMITY ARTERIES

The ability to evaluate and image the upper extremity arterial system continues to evolve. Pulse volume recording (PVR), although still used, has been largely superseded by modern noninvasive imaging modalities. Duplex ultrasound is effective for assessment of the peripheral upper extremity arteries and is inexpensive.[30] However, the refinement of magnetic resonance imaging (MRI), especially with contrast agents, has enabled much improved demonstration of the upper extremity arteries, especially the central vessels (Fig. 34-9). The lack of radiation exposure makes this the current procedure of choice for those patients without a contraindication to magnetic resonance angiography (MRA). Similarly, computed tomographic angiography (CTA) is highly effective for imaging this arterial territory, especially the central arteries that cannot be readily imaged by duplex ultrasound (Fig. 34-10). Imaging plays an important role in planning for both endovascular and surgical treatment of appropriately selected patients.

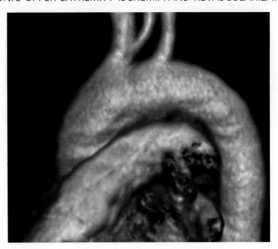

FIGURE 34-9. Magnetic resonance angiogram (MRA) of a patient with subclavian artery disease.

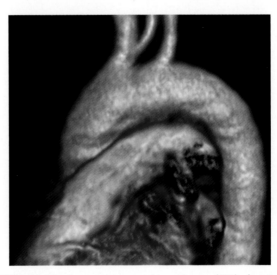

FIGURE 34-10. Computed tomographic angiogram (CTA) of aortic arch and brachiocephalic vessels.

KEY POINTS

- Upper extremity arterial insufficiency is common in vascular practice.
- Symptoms may result from cerebral, coronary, or upper extremity ischemia.
- The overwhelming majority of cases are atherosclerotic in nature. Other causes include inflammatory arteritis, spontaneous dissection, and thoracic outlet syndrome.
- Endovascular intervention is the revascularization method of choice.
- Key differences exist between right and left subclavian intervention, owing to involvement of the right common carotid in the brachiocephalic trunk.
- High success and low complication rates can be expected if case selection is commensurate with experience level.
- Distal upper extremity blockage is rarely atherosclerotic in etiology and is generally due to uncommon conditions. Thrombolysis is useful to treat digital embolization and help define the underlying process.

▶ SUGGESTED READINGS

Amann-Vesti BR, Koppensteiner R, Rainoni L, et al. Immediate and long-term outcome of upper extremity balloon angioplasty in giant cell arteritis. J Endovasc Ther 2003;10:371–5.

De Vries JP, Jager LC, Van den Berg JC, et al. Durability of percutaneous transluminal angioplasty for obstructive lesions of proximal subclavian artery: long-term results. J Vasc Surg 2005;41:19–23.

Fields WS, Lemak NA. Joint Study of extracranial arterial occlusion: VII. Subclavian steal—a review of 168 cases. JAMA 1972;222:1139–43.

Gray BH. Endovascular treatment of peripheral arterial disease. J Am Osteopath Assoc 2000;100(20 Suppl pt 2):S15–20.

Hadjipetrou P, Cox S, Piemonte T, Eisenhauer A. Percutaneous revascularization of atherosclerotic obstruction of aortic arch vessels. Comment in: J Am Coll Cardiol 1999;33:1246–7.

Keshava SN, Falk A. Revascularization of aortic arch branches and visceral arteries using minimally invasive endovascular techniques. Mt Sinai J Med 2003;70:401–9.

Olsen CO, Dunton RF, Maggs PR, Lahey SJ. Review of coronary-subclavian steal following internal mammary artery-coronary artery bypass surgery. Comment in: Ann Thorac Surg 1989;46:675–8.

Phatouros CC, Higashida RT, Malek AM, et al. Endovascular treatment of noncarotid extracranial cerebrovascular disease. Neurosurg Clin North Am 2000;11:331–50.

Westerband A, Rodriguez JA, Ramaiah VG, Diethrich EB. Endovascular therapy in prevention and management of coronary-subclavian steal. J Vasc Surg 2003;38:699–703; discussion 704.

The complete reference list is available online at www.expertconsult.com.

CHAPTER 35

Aortoiliac Revascularization

Abdel Aziz A. Jaffan and Timothy P. Murphy

EPIDEMIOLOGY

Peripheral arterial disease (PAD) is a common medical condition that is underdiagnosed, undertreated, poorly understood, and much more common than previously thought.[1] According to the Framingham (Massachusetts) Heart Study results, annual incidence of symptomatic PAD is 26:10,000 in men and 12:10,000 in women; PAD is at least as frequent as angina in the U.S. population.[2] Historical prevalence data vary with the method of detection. Questionnaires designed to elicit symptoms, such as the Rose Questionnaire, typically underestimate the prevalence of PAD. Relying on the presence of intermittent claudication (IC) alone to make a diagnosis or screen for PAD would miss the majority of patients. In community cohort studies like the Rotterdam Study and the Edinburgh Artery Study, classic symptoms of IC occurred only in a minority (6%-9%) of patients.[1,3-5] Population studies using noninvasive tests such as the ankle-brachial index (ABI) are more likely to yield a truer estimation because asymptomatic occurrences would also be included. ABI is currently accepted as a diagnostic reference standard for PAD, with a high sensitivity and specificity. It is noninvasive, inexpensive, and readily available.[6] Criqui et al., using segmental blood pressures, flow velocity on Doppler ultrasound, postocclusive reactive hyperemia, and pulse return half-times, reported a prevalence of large vessel PAD of 11.7% in a population with an average age of 66 years.[7] The prevalence of PAD is also related to age, as shown by Kannel in the Framingham Study, who found 2.5%, 8.3%, and 18.8% of Americans aged 60 years or younger, 61 to 70 years, and older than 70 years, respectively, to have PAD.[8] In 2005, the Centers for Disease Control and Prevention (CDC) estimated that PAD affected 5% of the U.S. population older than 40 years of age.[9] Higher prevalence is anticipated in the future as the average age of the U.S. population rises. Among those with advanced age (>70 years), history of smoking, and presence of diabetes mellitus, prevalence of PAD can be as high as 50%.[3] In general, prevalence of PAD is estimated at 3% in middle-aged patients when noninvasive testing is used, increasing to 20% in patients older than 70. The aortoiliac territory is affected in one third of theses cases.[10]

HISTORY

In 1964, radiologists Dotter and Judkins published a seminal paper describing the first cases of percutaneous transluminal revascularization.[11] What followed was a revolutionary change in management of PAD, best exemplified by aortoiliac interventions. The first iliac artery angioplasty was done using a "caged" compliant Fogarty balloon in 1965 by Dr. Charles Dotter[12,13] shortly after he devised the method of serial dilation of the femoropopliteal arteries.[11] Consistently good outcomes were achieved with conventional angioplasty and stent techniques in the aorta and iliac arteries. In an analysis of treatment patterns of aortoiliac occlusive disease in the United States, Upchurch et al. reported more than an eight fold increase in angioplasty and stenting, 15.5% decrease in aortobifemoral bypass surgery, and 34% increase in total number of interventions from 1996 to 2000.[14] Endovascular therapy is generally accepted as the primary mode of revascularization therapy for most patients with aortoiliac disease.

INDICATIONS

Although thigh and/or buttock claudication can help localize PAD symptoms to the proximal segment, the most common symptom of aortoiliac insufficiency is calf claudication. Patients can present with critical limb ischemia and tissue loss, but usually these patients have multisegmental disease involving infrainguinal arteries in addition to the aortoiliac segment. Erectile dysfunction in males can also be seen. Rarely, ulcerated plaques can result in cholesterol or thrombotic embolization and result in blue toe syndrome.[1,3]

Claudication is managed conservatively or by percutaneous or surgical revascularization. A previous report of relatively benign natural history of claudication,[2] which may have fostered a conservative attitude, is contradicted by more recent studies.[15,16] Of those who present with typical IC, after 5 years, 70% to 80% will have stable claudication, 10% to 20% will have worsening claudication, and 5% to 10% will develop critical limb ischemia. Less than 2% will undergo a major amputation.[17] In a review of over 2307 patients in six studies, 30% of patients with IC eventually required surgery for critical limb ischemia, and 6% required amputations.[16] Exercise programs have shown improvements in quality of life and walking distance, but benefits gained in an unsupervised setting are poor.[18] Surgery, in combination with an exercise program, has proven superior to both exercise or surgery alone, albeit with higher complications.[19] Despite excellent long-term outcome, surgical revascularization is associated with up to 4.6% perioperative mortality and a 13.1% major early complication rate.[20] With the significant improvement in endovascular techniques and materials, endovascular therapy can be now considered the initial safe and effective therapeutic option for aorto-occlusive disease, with a high rate of technical success and excellent long-term patency rates.[21]

The TransAtlantic Inter-Society Consensus (TASC) document classified aortoiliac disease by angiographic appearance and pattern (see Chap. 25, Fig. 25-9). Initially published in 2000 and intended to provide recommendations regarding percutaneous vs. surgical revascularization based on severity of anatomic obstruction, it has been revised twice, each time broadening the indications for percutaneous revascularization. Briefly, TASC categorizes lesions of increasing severity, with TASC A lesions being focal and singular, and advancing categories describing longer, multiple, or occlusive lesions, through category D. It is the authors' opinion that TASC is useful as a descriptive description of anatomy but does not impact clinical decision making in the aortoiliac segment because nearly all disease types are amenable to percutaneous revascularization, and except in cases of total aortoiliac occlusion from the renal arteries to the inguinal ligaments, where the patient has a good surgical risk profile, surgery should be reserved for those who fail percutaneous revascularization.[22-26]

CONTRAINDICATIONS

Contraindications to arteriography generally apply also to aortoiliac interventions. Patients with uncorrectable coagulopathy, inability to lie supine, severe non–dialysis dependent renal insufficiency, or current systemic infections have relative contraindications to elective percutaneous revascularization, and alternate management should be considered until the risk profile is more suitable. Limited procedures can be performed with alternative contrast agents (namely, carbon dioxide) in patients with renal insufficiency, depending on the clinical situation. No absolute contraindications exist for endovascular treatment of aortoiliac disease per se. Relative contraindications are mainly anatomic and include juxtarenal aortic occlusion, circumferential heavy calcification (>1 mm in thickness), hypoplastic aortic syndrome, and juxtaposition to aneurysmal disease.[27]

EQUIPMENT

- Directional catheter
- Hydrophilic guidewire
- Exchange wires
- Angioplasty balloon
- Self-expanding stent
- Balloon-expandable stent (mounted or unmounted)
- Covered stent
- Reentry catheter
- Vascular sheath
- Hemodynamic pressure monitor

A standard room for angiography equipped with single projection fluoroscopy, movable table, and power contrast injection pump are necessary. Most modern rooms for angiography have digital subtraction capability with features such as live road mapping and bolus-chasing capability. A sterile table should contain heparinized flush saline, hand-injectable contrast media, room for catheters and wires, lidocaine for dermal anesthesia, and a sharps container. The diagnostic portion of the examination can be performed using a multipurpose flush catheter. Femoral access can be challenging in patients with aortoiliac disease. Although most attempts at access can be attained using landmarks, ultrasound guidance may be useful. Alternatives to femoral access are brachial or even radial access.[28] Continuous patient monitoring is essential and requires cooperation among the patient, nurse, technologist, and interventionalist. A cardiac monitor, pulse oximeter, and automated sphygmomanometer are mandatory. Emergent patient resuscitation equipment including a code cart should be readily available, and all providers should be Advanced Cardiac Life Support (ACLS) certified. Working familiarity with conscious sedation medications including reversal agents is required.

Many varieties of catheters and guidewires are now available to facilitate the treatment of aortoiliac disease. The following recommendations are based on our experience and review of published reports. Simple stenosis may only require a straight tapered spring-coil guidewire. These wires are also very useful at traversing chronic arterial occlusions. A combination of hydrophilic guidewires (e.g., Glidewire [Terumo Medical Corp., Somerset, N.J.]) and directional catheters (e.g., Kumpe [Cook Inc., Bloomington, Ind.]) can be used for complex stenosis and occlusions, especially if in the latter case a spring coil fails to cross the lesion. Exchange length guidewires with greater stiffness (e.g., Rosen or Amplatz [Cook Medical]) are needed to pass subsequent sheaths, balloons, and stents. Although larger-diameter angioplasty balloons up to 15 mm may be necessary for distal aortic purposes, many patients will experience symptomatic relief with 10- or 12-mm-diameter stents, even in the aorta. Dilation to larger diameters increases the risk of aortic rupture. For iliac arteries, balloon diameters between 6 and 10 mm suffice, usually 7 to 9 mm in the common iliac arteries and 6 to 8 mm in the external iliac arteries. Inflation devices with an atmospheric pressure gauge offer greater control over manual balloon inflation with a syringe and are useful for large arteries in the chest, abdomen, and pelvis. Pressurized bags of saline for continuous flushing of catheters, and transducers for simultaneous pressure-gradient measurements between the access sheath and the angioplasty catheter should be readily available.

Many types of stents are now available for use in the aortoiliac system. Stents can vary in their metallic composition, construction, radiopacity, trackability, flexibility, radial force, hoop strength, and foreshortening. For aortoiliac purposes, the vast majority of available stents can be divided into self-expanding types such as the Wallstent RP (Boston Scientific Corp., Natick, Mass.) or balloon-expandable types such as the Palmaz Genesis (Cordis Corp., Miami Lakes, Fla.). Self-expanding stents tend to have greater flexibility, trackability, and vessel wall apposition and are more likely to be crush resistant. Most balloon-expandable stents are made of stainless steel and possess greater hoop strength and radial force. The major advantage of balloon-mounted stents is the greater ability for precise placement—required, for example, for common iliac origin lesions or lesions extending to the iliac artery bifurcation (Fig. 35-1). Covered stents are increasingly used primarily in aortoiliac intervention, but definitely needed in case of vascular perforation; they can be self-expanding (e.g., Viahbahn [Gore Medical, Flagstaff, Ariz.]) or balloon-expandable (e.g., ICast [Atrium Medical, Hudson, N.H.]). With diffusion of technology, however, distinctions between stents are now becoming blurred. As a result, the authors stock a tailored list of stents, acquired over time with personal experience. Vascular sheaths, preferably with a radiopaque tip (e.g., Brite Tip [Cordis, Bridgewater, N.J.]), sizes between 5F and 10F and lengths up to 90 cm may be necessary to deliver appropriate-diameter balloons and stents, depending on the route of access.

For chronic long-segment occlusions, subintimal recanalization is increasingly performed, and in many times is unavoidable. Once in the subintimal tract, reentry into the

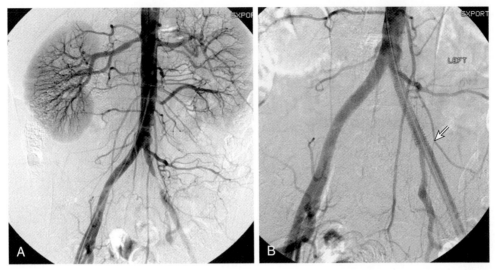

FIGURE 35-1. **A,** Digital subtraction angiogram demonstrates high-grade left common iliac artery (CIA) stenosis extending to bifurcation. **B,** Completion angiogram after placement of balloon-mounted stent with preservation of left internal iliac artery (IIA) patency. Use of balloon-mounted stent allowed precise placement to level of CIA bifurcation *(arrow)* without covering left IIA origin.

true lumen can pose a challenge. Reentry can be achieved using low-technology off-the-shelf devices like the back end of guidewires, stainless steel stiffening cannulas in combination with needle-tip guidewires,[29] or with dedicated chronic total occlusion (CTO) reentry catheters (discussed later) like the Outback catheter (Cordis) and the Pioneer catheter (Medtronic, Minneapolis, Minn.), shown to increase technical success of crossing complete arterial occlusions. A reentry catheter should be available in case needed.

TECHNIQUE

Preprocedure Patient Evaluation

Patients should be evaluated by the interventionalist before any procedure. A directed history and physical examination should be performed to determine the presence and severity of PAD. Physical examination may reveal diminished or absent femoral artery pulses and decreased ABI. Other vascular systems should be examined (e.g., for carotid artery bruit or abdominal aortic aneurysm (AAA)). At the time of consultation, all available previous test results should be reviewed, including pulse volume recording (PVR), segmental pressures (Fig. 35-2), computed tomographic and magnetic resonance angiography (CTA, MRA), and records of prior interventions and surgeries. Necessary tests should be ordered. Pertinent laboratory values include platelet count, prothrombin time, and serum creatinine and blood urea nitrogen (BUN) levels. Presence of severe renal insufficiency may preclude use of iodinated contrast agents. There is a lack of consensus regarding appropriate contrast nephropathy prophylaxis, but most authors recommend (1) hydration with 0.9% saline at 1 mL/kg/h for 24 hours beginning at 2 to 12 hours before the procedure and (2) use of the least amount possible of low-osmolar iodinated contrast agent.[30] Use of *N*-acetylcysteine and sodium bicarbonate infusion may be helpful, but results of clinical trials have been equivocal or limited. If a non–life threatening contrast allergy (e.g., urticaria) is present, a prophylaxis regimen such as 32 mg of oral methylprednisolone 12 and 2 hours before contrast agent administration has been recommended. A history of life-threatening allergic reaction (e.g., cardiopulmonary collapse, laryngeal edema, bronchospasm) should prompt an investigation of an alternative to contrast (e.g., carbon dioxide possibly supplemented with intraarterial (IA) pressure measurements during intervention). Insulin-dependent diabetics should take half their dose of insulin the morning of their procedure. Warfarin compounds and metformin should be held when appropriate. An assessment of cardiovascular risk in conjunction with their cardiologist should be done, and if anticoagulation cannot be stopped, they may need to be converted to subcutaneous low-molecular-weight heparin while the warfarin is held. It is not routine to evaluate patients for myocardial ischemia before percutaneous interventions. All patients with PAD also should be assumed to have significant coronary artery disease,[31] but percutaneous revascularization is not contraindicated for such patients.

A clear liquid diet is recommended for at least 6 hours before the procedure. On the morning of the procedure, conscious sedation evaluation should be performed, and peripheral intravenous (IV) access is required. Aspirin is administered to any patient not already taking the medication. A bladder catheter is routinely placed in patients in whom intervention is anticipated.

Noninvasive Imaging

With the advances and widespread availability of noninvasive imaging modalities, performing catheter arteriography for a purely diagnostic purpose is now rarely indicated. For aortoiliac evaluation, duplex arterial mapping, CTA, and MRA can provide very accurate anatomic details in terms of location and extent of disease and eligibility for endovascular intervention, without the need for the relatively invasive catheter angiography, its substantial costs, and small risk of complications.[32]

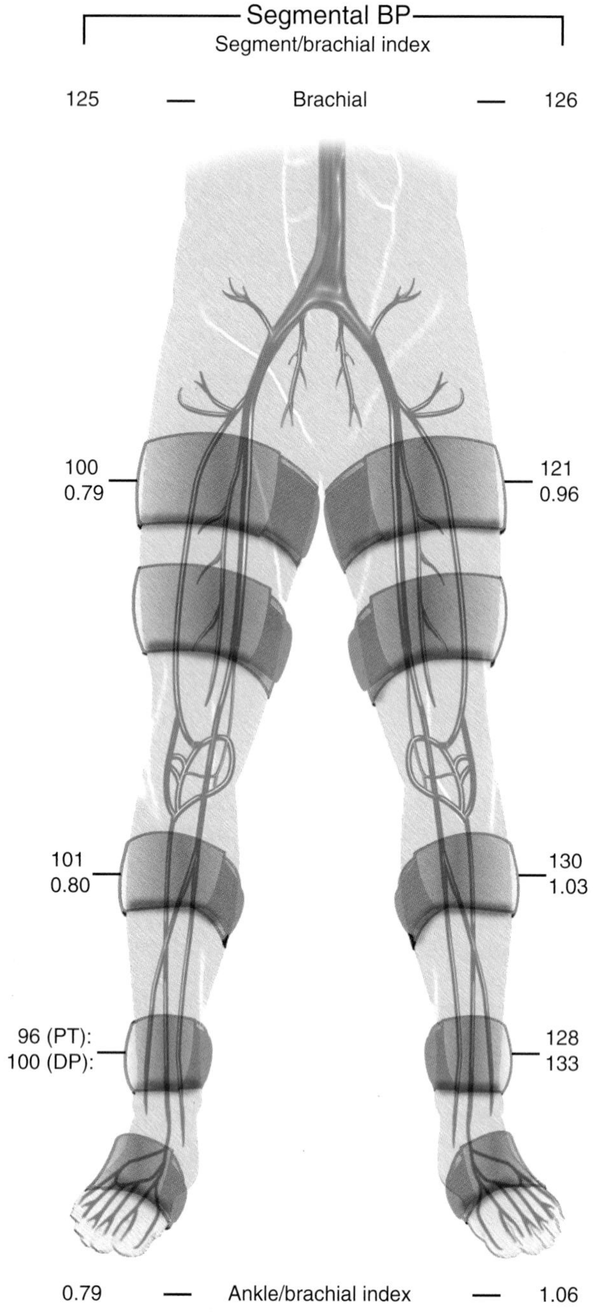

```
┌─────────── Segmental BP ───────────┐
        Segment/brachial index

  125  ──      Brachial      ──  126

  100                              121
  0.79                            0.96

  101                              130
  0.80                            1.03

  96 (PT):                         128
 100 (DP):                         133

  0.79  ──  Ankle/brachial index  ──  1.06
```

FIGURE 35-2. Segmental blood pressures with measurements at high thigh, calf, and ankle levels in a patient with right thigh claudication. Note significant decrease in right thigh brachial index (0.79), demonstrating a likely right iliac–common femoral occlusive disease. Also note smaller but still abnormal decrease in the left thigh brachial index (asymptomatic side). No significant dropoff in level below thigh is noted. Segmental pressures are useful to delineate level(s) of occlusive disease.

Duplex Arterial Mapping

Duplex arterial mapping can provide a safe and inexpensive means of assessing the location and extent of hemodynamically significant stenosis in the aortoiliac territory. Limitations to this technique, including the presence of significant arterial calcifications, overlying bowel gas, large body habitus, and dependence on highly trained vascular technologists, made it fall out of favor as a primary tool for preprocedure noninvasive imaging.[27]

Computed Tomographic Angiography

Developed shortly after the introduction of spiral (helical) computed tomography, CTA made it possible to cover body regions so rapidly, that transient enhancement of the vascular system following IV contrast injection would be captured in one scan (Fig. 35-3).[33] With the introduction of multidetector (MD) row technology, spatial and temporal resolutions improved significantly, and CTA became an easy-to-perform standard technique for vascular imaging, taking over most diagnostic vascular procedures. Compared to intraarterial digital subtraction angiography (IA-DSA), CTA is noninvasive, permits three-dimensional (3D) visualization of vessels from any angle, has lower cost and shorter examination times, lowers overall effective radiation dose, and lowers the volume of intravascular contrast.[34] Sensitivity and specificity of MD-CTA compared to conventional IA-DSA are reported to be between 93% and 100%. In a meta-analysis including 436 patients and 9541 arterial segments, Heijenbrok-Kal et al. found that MD-CTA has a sensitivity of 92% and a specificity of 93% for detection of hemodynamically significant (>50%) stenosis in patients with claudication or critical limb ischemia, with a diagnostic performance almost as good as IA-DSA.[32] CTA is an accurate tool for assessment of all treatment-relevant morphologic information of PAD: gradation, length, and number of stenoses.[35] Various 3D postprocessing techniques now available, such as maximum intensity projection (MIP), volume rendering (VR), and multiplanar reformatting (MPR), can improve diagnostic performance. Oto et al. found that curved MPR resulted in higher sensitivity (97% vs. 89%) and specificity (100% vs. 96%) than use of transverse images.[36] A major drawback of MD-CTA is hampered vessel assessment due to arterial wall calcifications, which may cause overestimation of stenosis.[33] Detection of calcification, however, has significant implications for treatment planning. Circumferential calcifications thicker than 1 mm are considered a relative contraindication to aortoiliac angioplasty and stenting because of the potential risk of fracture and rupture. A covered stent should be considered in this case to minimize the impact of a clinically significant arterial perforation.[27]

Magnetic Resonance Angiography

MRA is a noninvasive technique that does not employ ionizing radiation or iodinated contrast material (Fig. 35-4). Very fast 3D sequences in contrast-enhanced MRA (CE-MRA) allow study of the arteries from the abdominal aorta to the feet with a single injection of contrast material. With CE-MRA, the limitations of the older non-contrast MRA (NC-MRA) techniques (e.g., time of flight [TOF], phase contrast), such as long acquisition time and flow and movement artifacts, have been overcome.[37] NC-MRA relies on inflow phenomena prone to saturation effects, which can lead to overestimation of the degree of stenosis in areas where the vessels run in a more horizontal course, such as the pelvis.[38] CE-MRA is not susceptible to in-plane saturation. Other advantages include reduced imaging acquisition time and higher spatial resolution. In a multicenter controlled trial comparing NC-MRA, CE-MRA, and IA-DSA

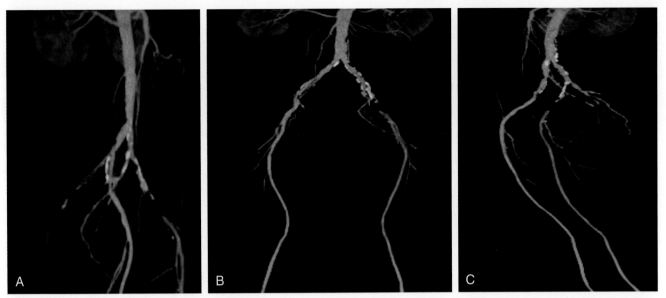

FIGURE 35-3. A-C, Volume rendering from computed tomographic angiography of distal aorta to bilateral superficial femoral arteries demonstrated occlusion of left external iliac artery, with reconstitution at level of left common femoral artery. Mild stenosis was noted at origin of right external iliac artery.

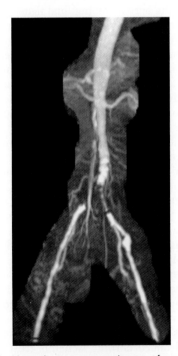

FIGURE 35-4. Magnetic resonance angiogram of aortoiliac arteries in patient with buttock claudication. Bilateral common iliac artery occlusions are shown.

in 407 patients referred to investigate PAD in the aortoiliac region, Bui et al.[38] showed that CE-MRA was superior to and more consistent than NC-MRA for detecting hemodynamically significant stenosis in patients with a suspected or proven PAD, and compared favorably with IA-DSA as a reference standard. A fundamental limitation to this modality is lack of visualization of vascular calcifications, important for surgical planning. Venous contamination is another limitation to this technique.[37,38]

Diagnostic Arteriography

Catheter arteriography is rarely performed nowadays for a purely diagnostic purpose, except in rare cases where noninvasive imaging is inconclusive. In patients undergoing catheter arteriography, a treatment plan has already been formulated and a decision for an endovascular therapy made. Common femoral artery (CFA) access is most desirable. Prior to the advent of CTA and MRA, puncture of the CFA was performed on the side with the better palpable pulse, and angiogram was performed to assess disease and decide whether a lesion should be treated from an ipsilateral or contralateral approach. Nowadays, preprocedural CTA/MRA should have determined the puncture site with the safest and most direct route to the target lesion. In general, common iliac artery (CIA) lesions are best treated ipsilaterally, and external iliac artery (EIA) lesions best approached from the contralateral access.[39] If the lesion is close to the aortic bifurcation, bilateral CFA access for a kissing technique may be required; however, if the plaque is limited to the proximal CIA and does not involve stenosis of the distal aorta, our practice is to not deploy stents bilaterally but rather to use a balloon-expandable stent placed accurately to cover only the lesion in the CIA.

If a femoral pulse is absent on the puncture side, fluoroscopically guided femoral access can be done using palpation in individuals whose body habitus permits because atherosclerotic arteries are often hard and can be palpated even if pulseless. If that is not the case, calcification is often present and permits access using fluoroscopy. Of course, ultrasound guidance can be used to gain access if these methods fail, and it is highly successful. Presence of calcifications in the wall of the vessel and the lateral location of the artery in the groin will help differentiate the CFA from the common femoral vein by ultrasound. Alternatively, brachial access can be obtained, especially in patients with complete aortoiliac occlusion. Once access is gained, a short 5F sheath is placed and set to a flush. A diagnostic

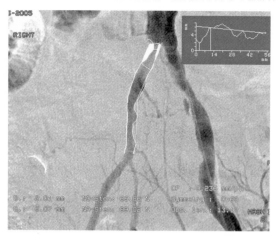

FIGURE 35-5. Quantification of right common iliac artery stenosis using commercially available software.

arteriogram of the abdominal aorta and pelvis is obtained via a multisidehole flush catheter. Oblique projections may be helpful in the pelvis. Greater than 50% reduction of diameter is generally considered to represent hemodynamic significance. Commercially available software can be used to facilitate accurate measurements (Fig. 35-5). However, IA pressure measurements above and below the lesion are preferred because pressure gradients have been shown to be more accurate in detecting hemodynamically significant stenosis.[40] Pressure gradients can be obtained simultaneously with single or double access, with the former requiring a 2F size difference between the coaxial catheter and the sheath. Pull-back measurement is less favored because blood pressure varies over time, and nonsimultaneous measurements may artifactually introduce a substantial difference (10-15 mmHg systolic) where none really exists, especially after pharmacologic augmentation. A systolic difference of 10 to 15 mmHg or a mean difference of 5 mmHg is considered significant. To mimic the increased flow situation that exists with exercise, patients with IC may require pharmacologic augmentation (e.g., IA nitroglycerin administered to the affected extremity) to unmask a hemodynamic significance when a lesion does not yield a pressure difference at rest. With pharmacologic augmentation, a difference of 20 mmHg systolic or 10 mmHg mean is necessary to be a significant gradient.[40] For patients with critical limb ischemia, many clinicians use a gradient of 5 mmHg mean to indicate the need for revascularization.[40,41] Pressure measurements are not routinely done for occlusions because it is self-evident that arterial occlusions are hemodynamically important. In the presence of occlusion, delayed images or ipsilateral access below the occlusion may be required to determine the exact length of the occluded vessel segment and the appropriateness of the artery to receive the distal portion of the stent. For example, if the occlusion extends below the inguinal ligament, an endovascular approach may not be beneficial.

Intervention

Usually, systemic anticoagulation is accomplished with intravenous (IV) heparin as soon as the determination for endovascular treatment course is made, but this is not universal, and simple procedures can be safely accomplished without anticoagulation if they can be done within a few minutes. Once the stenosis is traversed with a guidewire, a stent is properly positioned to cover the entire lesion and deployed. Negotiation of complex stenoses and occlusions can be challenging but facilitated with directable catheters and hydrophilic guidewires. Chronic occlusions are addressed later. Most patients will experience some level of discomfort due to adventitial stretching during inflation of the angioplasty balloon. Typically, 6 to 8 atmospheres of pressure is applied. Although arterial perforation can occur at lower pressures,[42] the patient's discomfort level should guide the degree of inflation. In cases of severe pain, aggressive dilation should be avoided. An appropriate level of conscious sedation is crucial to obtain real-time patient feedback. Self-expanding stents often require dilation to desired diameter with an angioplasty balloon and will usually recoil about 1 mm from the inflation diameter after the balloon is deflated.

When placing a stent in the aortoiliac system, three areas merit special consideration. Stent extension below the inguinal ligament should be avoided, usually because it can interfere with future femoral endarterectomy or planned femoral distal bypass surgery. In circumstances in which stenting across the inguinal ligament is required, a self-expanding stent is recommended, given its resistance to being irreversibly crushed. Internal iliac artery insufficiency may lead to problems with impotence, and patency should be maintained. However, stenting across the internal iliac artery origin is often required and is usually not associated with adverse outcomes (Fig. 35-6). The internal iliac artery has been shown to remain patent despite stent coverage in 89% to 100% in prior reports.[43,44] Internal iliac artery occlusions immediately after stenting are usually the result of overlapping stents in the area of the origin of the internal iliac artery. A recent study showed no new cases of impotence with aortoiliac stenting, unlike in the bypass cohort (where the reported rate of impotence was 28%).[45] Nevertheless, if technical success can be achieved with sparing of the origin of the internal iliac artery, the origin should be spared. CIA ostial lesions will be discussed later.

Sizing of angioplasty balloons and stents is dictated by the lesion's characteristics. Typically, CIAs are 7 to 10 mm in diameter, and EIAs are 6 to 9 mm in diameter. A minimal diameter of 6 mm is desired for most people so that significant gradients are not present at rest. Paradoxically, those with more advanced chronic ischemia (rest pain or ischemic tissue loss) will often require *less* aggressive dilation of their obstructions than those with IC because any improvement in blood flow at rest will usually be sufficient to reverse their symptoms. Those complaining of IC will require a larger-diameter vessel to accommodate the high flow volumes on demand for symptom relief to be satisfactory.

As mentioned earlier, numerous stents are available for iliac revascularization, although most qualify as off-label use.[46] Given similarities between current stents, few factors besides personal preference dictate stent selection. Self-expanding stents come in longer lengths, allowing use of a single stent for diffuse disease even for very long lesions. Conversely, focal, ostial, and lesions with high elastic recoil, such as eccentric and calcific stenoses, may predicate use

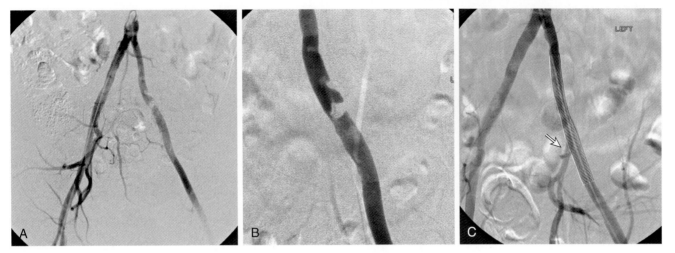

FIGURE 35-6. A, Digital subtraction angiogram demonstrates multifocal eccentric nodular plaque in left common iliac artery (CIA). **B,** Magnified view of left CIA stenosis. **C,** Completion angiogram shows complete alleviation of stenosis. Note maintenance of left internal iliac artery perfusion despite stent coverage of ostium.

of a balloon-mounted stent for precise placement and greater hoop strength. Contralateral delivery of stents is now no longer limited to self-expanding stents. Improved trackability allows contralateral placement of newer-generation balloon-mounted stents, unlike the first-generation Palmaz stent that could be problematic if delivered over the bifurcation because of its rigidity. Choice of an appropriate stent depends on the lesion morphology and location. In tortuous vessels, self-expending stents assure good flexibility and vessel conformability. Nitinol stents are appropriate for treating vascular segments with abrupt transition in size. Covered stents are usually reserved for treatment of isolated iliac aneurysms, iatrogenic perforation, ruptures, and arteriovenous fistulas. More studies are needed on their primary use in aortoiliac occlusive disease.[10]

After angioplasty or stent placement, a completion angiogram is mandatory. As in any case of endovascular interventions, a guidewire should be kept across the treated vessel until a satisfactory completion angiogram is obtained. Presence of residual stenosis, flow-limiting dissection, or arterial rupture should be swiftly managed. If balloon angioplasty is done, a low threshold of stent placement after angioplasty should exist, and most residual stenosis and dissections can be effectively alleviated with stents.

Successful revascularization is predicated on reduction of the mean pressure gradient below 5 mmHg. As such, completion pressure gradients should accompany a post-procedural angiogram. In cases of initial percutaneous transluminal angioplasty (PTA), subsequent stent placement should reduce the gradient to acceptable levels. Finally, distal embolization should be excluded angiographically. If a procedure has been long and a large amount of contrast agent has been used, an abbreviated runoff can be done to check for distal emboli at bifurcation points. Alternatively, in a patient with intact infrainguinal runoff, an on-the-table pulse examination may be sufficient to exclude distal atheroembolization and be in the patient's best interest, depending on contrast total, procedure duration, and patient comorbid conditions.

Aortic Bifurcation

Kissing stents (Fig. 35-7) are usually done when atherosclerotic plaque involves one or both CIA ostia and extends proximally to involve the terminal aorta.[47-49] It is our practice however to not reconstruct the aortic bifurcation more than a few millimeters proximally. Aortic stenosis often involves the segment caudal to the inferior mesenteric artery (IMA), and it is usually our practice to place a balloon-expandable stent in that segment, then treat the CIAs separately, if possible, even if a small gap (1-2 mm) is left unstented between the aorta and CIAs.

When ostial CIA stenosis is unilateral and does not involve the terminal aorta, usually a single balloon-expandable stent can achieve the desired result without the need to stent the nonstenotic CIA. Smith et al. reviewed a series of 175 patients with unilateral ostial CIA lesions who were treated with PTA or stenting unilaterally and without contralateral protection. On follow-up, mild non–hemodynamically significant stenosis in the unprotected contralateral CIA was reported in 2 of the 175 treated patients. The authors concluded that protection of the contralateral CIA during PTA or stenting of a proximal CIA lesion is not mandatory.[50]

There is controversy about outcomes after kissing stent placement. Siskin et al. found that younger age is not a significant risk factor for iliac artery stent failure.[51] In a review of 68 patients who underwent kissing iliac stents, however, Yilmaz et al. found that age younger than 50 years was a predictor of lower patency.[49] In a retrospective review of 66 patients who underwent endovascular aortoiliac reconstruction, Sharafuddin et al. found that female gender, presence of occlusions, and residual stenosis were predictors of restenosis.[48] A few studies showed worse outcomes when treating extensive aortoiliac disease (TASC C/D lesions) with kissing stents compared to less extensive disease. In a retrospective review of 173 patients treated with kissing stents, Björsens et al. found no difference in outcome in patients with TASC C/D compared to TASC A/B lesions, however.[52]

A few studies found geometric mismatch to be a significant predictor of decreased patency.[47-49,52] *Geometric*

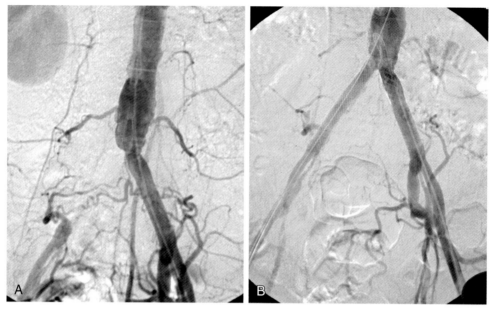

FIGURE 35-7. Kissing stents for right common iliac artery (CIA) occlusion. **A,** Digital subtraction angiogram demonstrates a proximal chronic right CIA occlusion. **B,** After placement of balloon-mounted kissing stents. Contralateral stent was placed in left CIA for protection. *(From Murphy TP, Vorwerk D. Advanced aortoiliac interventions. Tech Vasc Interv Radiol 2000;3:195–207.)*

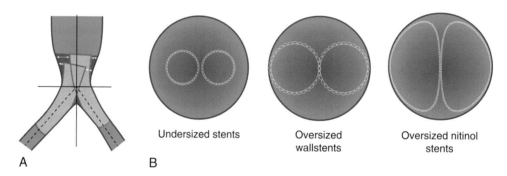

FIGURE 35-8. A, Determinants of anatomic matching of iliac stents to distal aortic lumen depends on aortic shape (straight vs. tapered), radial mismatch (radial or transverse dead space), and protrusion mismatch. **B,** Effect of stent sizing and material on geometric matching of the stent pair with native aortic lumen. Dead space between stent pair and native aortic wall can be minimized by using oversized nitinol stents. *(From Sharafuddin MJ, Hoballah JJ, Kresowik TF, et al. Long-term outcome following stent reconstruction of the aortic bifurcation and the role of geometric determinants. Ann Vasc Surg 2008;22:346–57).*

mismatch is defined by nonconformities between the native aortic lumen and the final configuration of the stents following aortoiliac reconstruction. Determinants of mismatch include aortic anatomy and configuration (straight vs. tapered shaped) and the stenting geometry itself, which is a reflection of stent material and sizing and stenting configuration.[48] If "double-barrel" stents are extended into the distal aorta, a configuration that is not favored in our practice, the dead space between the stent pair and the aortic wall can be reduced by using oversized nitinol self-expanding stents, which can allow a mirror-D configuration and reduce dead space (Fig. 35-8).[48] Greiner et al. found a primary patency rate (PPR) and assisted primary patency rate (APR) at 2 years significantly higher for the iliac stenting group without stent extension into the distal aorta (94.1% and 100%, respectively) than those in the group with a double-barrel stent configuration (33.2% and 45.3%).[53]

It is generally recommended that the proximal end of a stent should not extend more than 0.5 cm over the aortic bifurcation.[49] The results are particularly poor when stents extend into the aorta far enough to overlap at least half the width of a stent.[54] In the aortoiliac region, like elsewhere in the body, stent type is usually chosen based on lesion characteristics, location, vessel tortuosity, and stent profile. Other factors, however, such as ease of deployment, familiarity of the physician, cost, and availability, are also considerations.[49] Self-expanding stents are typically used in longer tortuous lesions. Balloon-expandable stents are commonly used in shorter, more calcified lesions and unilateral or bilateral CIA ostial lesions.[48,52]

In very calcified lesions with predicted high risk of rupture, primary use of a covered stent can be considered. It has been hypothesized that reconstruction of the aortic bifurcation with covered stents may provide better laminar flow, decreased thrombogenicity, less chance of prolapse of plaque through the covered stent, and less ingrowth of hyperplastic tissue compared to bare metal stents.[54] In a retrospective review of 54 patients with aortoiliac disease who received reconstruction with kissing stents (26 with covered stents and 28 with bare metal stents) Sabri et al. found higher primary patency in the covered stent group (92% at 1 and 2 years) compared to the bare metal stent (78% and 62% at 1 and 2 years, respectively).[54] Several studies demonstrated the efficacy of using stent-grafts for aortoiliac disease, with overall primary patency ranging from 70% to 85% at 1 year. Limitations to stent-grafting include larger introducer sheaths, costs, and lack of U.S. Food and Drug Administration (FDA) approval.[54]

Chronic Occlusions

Chronic occlusions can represent a technically challenging subset of aortoiliac disease (Fig. 35-9). Long-term outcome of stents for chronic iliac artery occlusions rivals those of bypass surgery, with less morbidity and mortality.[41,55-57] When faced with a chronic arterial occlusion, identification of the true lumen may be challenging if not impossible. Injection of contrast medium directed at the occlusion may reveal a sliver of occluded true lumen. Probing with a spring-coil guidewire initially is often successful. If occlusion traversal is not readily achieved, hydrophilic guidewires are often used. In a long-length occlusion, partial traversal from either direction only may be possible. In such cases, a snare introduced into the occluded segment often can be used to pull the other guidewire across from the opposite direction.[58] Once the occlusion is traversed, stents are deployed to restore a patent lumen to a desired diameter.

Role of Thrombolysis

Thrombolysis may theoretically facilitate successful revascularization by facilitating traversal, reducing potential distal embolization, and improving stent apposition to the arterial wall. This may hold true for fresh thrombus superimposed on a stenosis or short occlusion. Unfortunately, chronic occlusions are often resistant to thrombolysis, in which case, thrombolysis only adds to procedural time, prolongs hospitalization, and exposes the patient to potential bleeding complications. In a retrospective review of 25

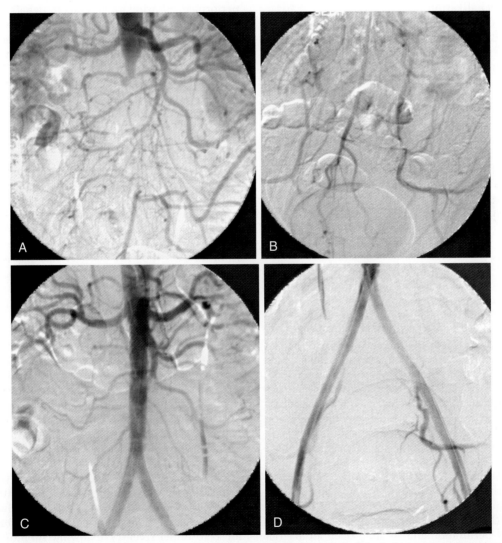

FIGURE 35-9. Total infrarenal aortoiliac artery occlusion reconstructed with aortoiliac stents. **A-B,** Abdominal aortogram demonstrates occlusion of infrarenal aorta and iliac arteries. **C-D,** After overnight thrombolysis, two Palmaz stents in the aorta and Wallstents in the bilateral iliac arteries were placed. *(From Murphy TP, Vorwerk D. Advanced aortoiliac interventions. Tech Vasc Interv Radiol 2000;3:195–207.)*

patients with iliac disease with subacute (1 week to 3 months) and chronic (>3 months) symptoms of claudication who underwent thrombolysis prior to intervention, treatment was completed in 21 patients with complete recanalization of the iliac axis, and the underlying lesion was clearly identified in 20 out of 21 patients (95%), and occlusions were transformed into stenosis.[59] The complication rate was 8% and consisted of peripheral embolization. Thrombolysis can turn a long occlusion into a shorter and more treatable stenotic lesion, allowing less extensive stenting.[59] Martinez and Diethrich reported 100% technical success with a preliminary thrombolysis before PTA and stenting in 6 and 7 patients, respectively. Some authors recently recommended primary stenting without thrombolysis. Their argument was that thrombolysis may increase cost, time, and complications such as distal embolization. Distal embolization, however, can still occur even in the absence of thrombolytic use. The exact role of thrombolysis in chronic aortoiliac disease is still unclear.[60] It may be useful in reducing the length of stented segments in those with long occlusions, such as those involving the entire infrarenal aortic segment.

Subintimal Recanalization

Subintimal angioplasty (SIA) was first described by Bolia in 1989. Usually this technique is used for infrainguinal occluded arteries. Often when crossing iliac artery CTO, an intramural path is used; the "true" lumen has long been obliterated. This is often addressed by stenting after lesion traversal. Although early descriptions of angioplasty for chronically occluded iliac arteries were not positive,[61] subintimal angioplasty alone has been described as a definitive treatment for chronic occlusions in the iliac arteries. Meta-analysis of SIA analyzing 37 studies of SIA found a technical success rate of 86%, 1-year PPR of 56%, and limb salvage rate of 89%.[62] Only two of these studies included iliac artery interventions, for a total of 79 patients. Technical success rates, limb salvage rates, and primary and secondary patency rates are high, as shown by the recent series of stent-supported SIA in the treatment of CTO of the iliac arteries.[62,63]

Intraluminal reentry can be challenging. It is critical to reenter the true lumen beyond the occlusion but below the aortic bifurcation. Often this may be a challenging task and may require additional maneuvers. Steerable catheters can redirect the wire into the true lumen. Alternatively, using an occlusion balloon as a target, the stiff end of a guidewire can be used to poke into the true lumen. Use of a needle aimed toward an occlusion balloon also has been successful but is rarely required.[29] Although sharp recanalization can be successfully accomplished, steps should be taken to ensure safe passage. Distance between the needle and the occlusion balloon should be minimized. Indentation of the occlusion balloon should be noted before an attempt at needle advancement. The occlusion balloon should be sufficiently inflated to avoid collapse of the intimal flap. This is confirmed by conformity of the occlusion balloon to the luminal shape owing to its compliance. Lastly, contrast medium should be injected along the tract once passage has been created to exclude arterial perforation and stenting open an arterial rent (Fig. 35-10). Initial reports of SIA recommended against anticoagulation until after the occlusion was crossed to reduce the risk of bleeding in case of perforation. The risk of thrombus formation in the subintimal space is higher, with subsequent risk of embolization, so anticoagulation is recommended prior to recanalization.[64]

During subintimal recanalization, it is very important to monitor the behavior of the hydrophilic wire under fluoroscopy. After initial penetration into the subintimal plane, the wire may initially spiral; this is not the preferred path of the wire. Rather than intentionally dissecting where the hydrophilic guidewire assumes a spiral or serpentine configuration, it is usually best to keep the tip free and rapidly rotate the guidewire, probing for the best path. Once the wire is near the end of the occlusion, the catheter is used to straighten the wire which is then advanced freely into the distal lumen in case of true lumen reentry. Another method of penetrating into an occlusion is to use the back end of a standard Glidewire.[64] This technique can be used in locations where the direction of the wire exiting the catheter is in the direction of the axis of the occluded vessel. The wire is advanced only a short distance, the catheter is advanced to that point, and the soft end of the wire is again used to cross a remaining occlusion.[64] If reentry into the true lumen is not possible distally, centering the wire in the distal portion of the occlusion using an angioplasty balloon can be performed, allowing for support to penetrate back into the true lumen. Inflating a balloon can also cause disruption of the distal cap of the occlusion and allows reentry. If reentry is still not possible, extending the dissection beyond the end of the occlusion may allow reentry, but this may affect branch points and collaterals in areas not otherwise involved and is usually discouraged, especially in the distal aorta, where creation of a dissection that propagates proximally is possible. To avoid this, reentry catheters can be used.[64]

Reentry Catheters

Reentry catheters are devices designed to allow true lumen reentry. Two devices are currently available: Outback and Pioneer.

OUTBACK The Outback LTD catheter (Cordis, Miami Lakes, FL) is a 6F compatible single-lumen system guided over a 0.014-inch guidewire. Initially the wire emanates from its distal tip. The catheter has also a hollow nitinol curved needle that can be advanced through a side hole at the tip. When the device is in the subintimal space, the needle is retracted inside the catheter, and the wire is withdrawn back inside the catheter proximal to the needle tip. The nosecone at the catheter tip has an L-shaped radiopaque marker that indicates needle direction, with the tip of the horizontal limb of the L indicating the direction of entry into the vessel. The marker becomes a T when the fluoroscope is rotated 90 degrees, and the horizontal position of the T should be overlying the artery. The needle is deployed once the catheter is in line with the vessel (T marker on top of the vessel and L marker toward the artery) through the intima and into the lumen. Usually multiple attempts are required. The 0.014-inch wire is advanced into the true lumen and the Outback catheter removed (Fig. 35-11).

In a retrospective review of 51 patients with CTO (inflow, outflow, and runoff disease), Aslam et al. showed a technical success rate of 96.1% when using the Outback catheter for true lumen reentry following subintimal recanalization.[65] Small series that focused on aortoiliac occlusions showed a technical success of 91% to 100%.[66-68] Very few reports of long-term patency following recanalization with

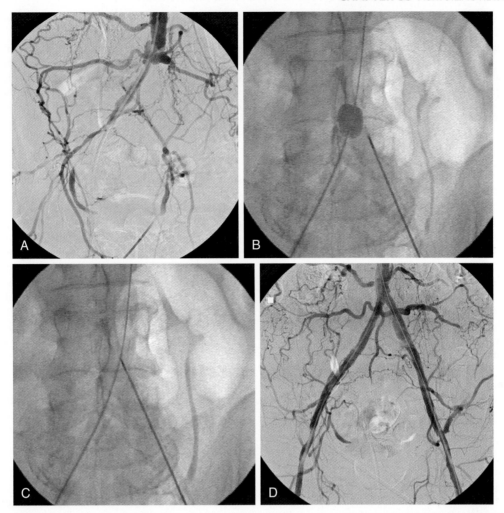

FIGURE 35-10. Sharp recanalization technique for chronic occlusions. **A,** Digital subtraction angiogram revealed right external artery and left common iliac and external iliac artery occlusions. **B,** Occlusion balloon is placed as a target for needle recanalization of the left occlusion. **C,** Spot radiograph after the occlusion is crossed with the needle. **D,** Completion angiogram after right external iliac artery and left common and external iliac artery reconstruction with stents.

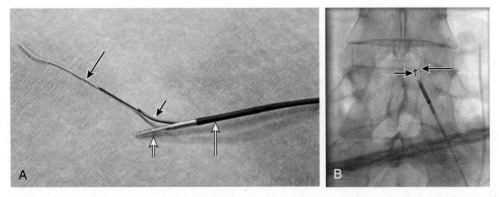

FIGURE 35-11. Reentry catheters. **A,** Outback LTD catheter. Hollow curved nitinol needle *(large black arrow)* is deployed, allowing side passage of 0.014-inch guidewire *(small black arrow)*. Nosecone *(large white arrow)* has radiopaque "LT" orientation marker. Catheter shaft is indicated by small white arrow. **B,** Outback catheter. Needle is deployed *(large arrow)* with free passage of guidewire into true aortic lumen. Note "L" configuration *(small arrow)*. *(Powell RJ, Rzucildo EM. Aorto-iliac disease: endovascular treatment. In: Cronenwett JL, Johnston W, editors. Rutherford's Vascular Surgery. 7th ed. Philadelphia: Saunders; 2010.)*

Outback exist. Abisi et al. reported a patency rate of 89% at a mean follow-up of 13 (±11 months) in 48 patients with aortoiliac disease where the Outback was used.[69] A disadvantage of this device is that it usually requires multiple needle passes, which is relatively innocuous in the superficial femoral artery (SFA) but carries a potential risk of clinically important hemorrhage in the aortoiliac territory.[64,69]

PIONEER The Pioneer catheter (Medtronic, Santa Rosa, Calif.) is a 7F compatible dual-lumen monorail catheter that tracks over a 0.014-inch guidewire. It has a 64-element phased-array 20 MHz intravascular ultrasound (IVUS) transducer that works in combination with the Volcano In-Vision Gold IVUS console (Volcano, San Diego, Calif.). This helps identify the blood flow in the true vessel lumen via a color flow mode (Chroma Flo feature). The second lumen of the catheter contains a curved needle that can be deployed and retracted through the side port just proximal to the IVUS transducer. The side port is fixed at the 12 o'clock position on the IVUS image. Once the catheter is in the subintimal space at the level of the presumed reentry site, the device is rotated to place the true lumen at 12 o'clock, and the needle is then deployed across the intimal membrane separating the false and the true lumen. Another 0.014-inch guidewire is then passed into the true lumen.[64,70]

The technical success rate using the Pioneer catheter is reported to be between 95% and 100%.[71,72] In a retrospective review of 11 patients with CTO of the iliac arteries where a Pioneer device was used, the success rate was 100%. At a mean follow-up of 10.5 months, all patients had palpable femoral pulses, with improvement of their ABIs and their symptoms; amputation-free survival was 100%.[72] An advantage of the Pioneer catheter is its ability to show the true lumen, limiting the number of needle passes and potentially the risk of perforation. Presence of calcifications can limit the IVUS imaging. The catheter requires a 7F sheath at minimum and will not track in sharply angulated bifurcation owing to the 0.014-inch monorail delivery system and size and rigidity of the transducer at the end of the catheter. Other drawbacks are catheter cost and requirement for an available IVUS machine.[64,73]

Evaluation for Common Femoral Artery Disease

Classically, the presence of significant (>50% stenosis) concomitant disease of the CFA determined whether to proceed with percutaneous endovascular therapy or an open surgical approach. Nowadays, hybrid repair has become an acceptable alternative to total open surgical repair for patients with iliofemoral occlusive disease; aortoiliac disease is treated endovascularly and femoral disease is treated with an open approach such as endarterectomy and patch angioplasty. In a retrospective review comparing hybrid repair with open repair in patients with severe iliofemoral occlusive disease, Piazza et al. showed that hybrid repair has similar early and long-term efficacy when compared to open repair, with shorter hospitalization, and should be considered in all patients with iliofemoral occlusive disease. Long-term patency was similar between the two groups regardless of lesion severity. Recently, treating CFA disease with an endovascular approach (angioplasty, atherectomy, etc.) is gaining acceptance in certain situations. It is often useful to angioplasty the CFA if needed, which usually responds well in our experience.[27,74]

Infrarenal Aortic Steno-occlusive Disease

Two patterns of atherosclerotic disease can affect the infrarenal aorta: (1) lesions of the aortic bifurcation involving the lower part of the abdominal aorta and CIAs, and (2) isolated lesions of the infrarenal aorta without involvement of the aortic bifurcation. The most common presentation of aortic disease is focal stenosis of the distal aorta caudal to the IMA. Fortunately, total infrarenal aortic occlusion is rare but this anatomy can be often seen with bilateral CIA occlusion and distal aortic occlusion may be caused by it. We have not seen total occlusion of the infrarenal aortic segment without bilateral CIA occlusion.

Isolated disease of the infrarenal aorta is rare compared to the other patterns of PAD. It affects mainly younger patients with less extensive atherosclerotic disease. The most important risk factors include female sex, heavy smoking, dyslipidemia, and hypoplastic aortic syndrome.[75,76] Although at higher risk of cardiovascular events than those with isolated infrainguinal atherosclerotic disease, because of their younger age at presentation, these patients have a longer life expectancy than the average patient with claudication.[77] Total occlusion of the aorta has a prevalence of 0.15% and is identified in 3% to 8.5% of patients with aortoiliac occlusive disease.[78] Historically, management of aortic steno-occlusive disease involves endarterectomy for focal lesions or surgical bypass for more extensive disease.[70] Surgery has an established and favorable long-term outcome, with a patency of 90% at 5 years and 75% at 10 years.[76,79] The complication rate is non-negligible, however, and varies between 5% and 10%.[77] In a meta-analysis of 25 series, the perioperative mortality rate was 4.4%, and the major complication rate was 12.2%.[79]

PTA was introduced in 1980 by Grollmann et al., Velasquez et al., and Tegtmeyer at al. as an alternative to open surgery for localized stenosis of the infrarenal aorta[76] as well as the aortic bifurcation. Aortic PTA has an initial technical success rate of 95% to 100%, with a primary patency around 70% and secondary patency over 85%. Since then, multiple series have been published in favor of the successful results in PTA in focal infrarenal aortic stenosis.[76] Although the initial technical success rate is high, mid- and long-term efficacy is frequently compromised by restenosis; elastic recoil is increased by the extensive presence of elastic fibers in the aortic wall.[76] Theoretical disadvantages of PTA alone include distal embolization—mainly in complex, eccentric, irregular, ulcerated, or calcified lesions—and risk of aortic rupture during dilatation due to large aortic diameter (according to Laplace law).[75]

Primary or direct stenting has been proposed because of favorable outcomes obtained in iliac arteries, including higher patency rates compared to PTA, and has been used selectively in complex ulcerated, eccentric, irregular, and/or calcified plaques as well as total occlusions.[80] In 1990, Diethrich et al. began to offer stent therapy to patients with abdominal aortic lesions that were considered to be high risk for conventional surgery. Cumulative primary patency at 5 years was 100% in 24 patients. Since then, a limited number of series have studied the efficacy of stent placement in the infrarenal aorta. Technical success rates were 82% to 100%, and PPRs were 83% to 100% during the short and midterm follow-up. The secondary patency rate was around 100%.[76]

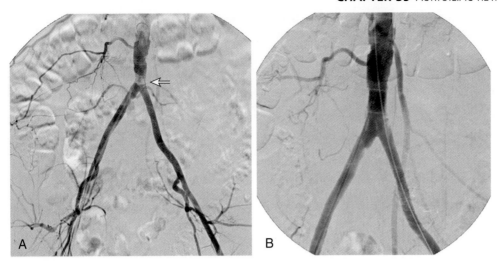

FIGURE 35-12. Stent treatment of distal aortic stenosis. **A,** Digital subtraction angiogram demonstrates a high-grade distal aortic stenosis. **B,** Appearance after placement of short distal aortic stent.

A review by Yilmaz et al. of previously published data revealed 586 patients in 24 series with 75% of lesions located in the distal aorta treated with angioplasty alone, angioplasty with selective stenting, or primary stenting. Technical success, major complication, minor complication, and PPRs were 66% to 94% (100% in three fourths of series), 3%, 4.7%, and 89.2%, respectively.[81] No published study comparing PTA alone to primary stent placement in the distal infrarenal aorta exists.[77] The more uniform distribution of radial forces during stenting should decrease the risk of aortic rupture in comparison to PTA (Fig. 35-12).[76,79,80]

In many cases, the disease involves or is near the origin of the IMA. One could argue that implantation of a stent across the IMA could cause occlusion of the ostium, but this does not appear to carry a major risk. Indeed, in surgical bypass, the IMA is almost always sacrificed, with a 2% risk of bowel ischemia.[80,82] In a series of 12 patients with infrarenal aortic steno-occlusive disease treated with primary stenting, Klonaris et al. found no symptoms of mesenteric ischemia in any patients on follow-up. In another series of 19 patients, Laganà et al. found one case of transient angina abdominis that completely resolved. In general, covering the origin of IMA is safe to do if needed; however, careful preprocedural evaluation to assess the patency of all relevant splanchnic vessels is crucial (celiac trunk, superior mesenteric, and hypogastric arteries).[76,80]

Chronic obstruction of the aortic bifurcation involving to a varying degree both the infrarenal aortic and CIAs can result in a triad of symptoms in men, consisting of IC, absent or diminished peripheral pulses, and impotence. The clinical condition was first described in 1814 by Sir Gilbert Blane. The underlying mechanism and pathology, however, was defined later by French surgeon René Leriche. Although classically found in males, the anatomic pattern of obstruction is equally common in males and females.[83] Onset is mainly between 40 and 60 years of age and can lead to severe impairment of walking capacity, rest pain, and wheelchair dependence.[74,83] Multiple case reports described a purely endovascular approach for treatment of Leriche disease. In a small series of 11 patients with total aortobiiliac occlusion treated with endovascular reconstruction,

Krakenberg et al. described a technical success rate of 73%, with unilateral success in the other 27%. There was one intraprocedural complication (complete thrombotic occlusion successfully managed with thrombolysis). At the median follow-up of 14 months, all patients were alive and reported marked relief of symptoms, with improvement in clinical status by at least one Rutherford category. Pending long-term outcomes and experience with a greater number of patients, the endovascular approach holds promise to replace surgery as the first line of treatment in patients with extensive aortoiliac disease.[83]

Internal Iliac Artery Disease

Atherosclerotic disease involving the IIA is a common finding on angiography. The occurrence of symptomatic internal IIA disease is uncommon, however. When it occurs it presents with isolated buttock or proximal thigh claudication and/or vasculogenic erectile dysfunction. Pelvic claudication has become more prevalent with the increase in the practice of unilateral embolization of the IIA as an adjunct during endovascular aortic aneurysm repair (EVAR). Afflicted individuals can experience signs and symptoms of pelvic ischemia that resolve with time with development of collateral flow from the patient's contralateral IIA. Unilateral embolization of the hypogastric artery is well tolerated, and the extensive network of collateral circulation in the pelvis makes severe buttock and proximal thigh ischemia a rare event. Patients who undergo bilateral IIA embolization, however, can have significant symptoms of pelvic ischemia.[84]

ABI is nonspecific for the detection of IIA disease. Duplex scanning has high sensitivity but is technically demanding, requires experienced physicians, and is impossible in obese patients. Transcutaneous oxygen pressure measurement ($TcPO_2$) on the buttock during exercise is 83% sensitive and 82% specific in detecting gluteal ischemia secondary to hemodynamically significant occlusive IIA disease; the criterion used is a drop of $TcPO_2$ greater than 15 mmHg during stress testing.[85]

Contemporary experience with IIA disease has centered around revascularization in the face of bilateral ischemia.

Direct open reconstruction via endarterectomy or bypass of the IIA has for years been the gold standard treatment of occlusive IIA disease.[84] Open reconstruction has a high technical success rate but increased morbidity and mortality. In a retrospective review of a series of 40 patients with symptomatic occlusive IIA disease who underwent 44 open IIA revascularizations concomitant to aorto- or iliofemoral bypass, the PPR was 89% at 1 year and 72.5% at 5 years. Symptomatic relief was seen in 85% of cases.[86] Endovascular experience with IIA stenosis or occlusion and coexisting severe buttock claudication is still limited.[87] In a series of nine patients (15 IIAs treated) who underwent angioplasty and/or stenting of unilateral or bilateral IIA, Thompson et al. had a 100% technical success rate; 7/9 patients (78%) had symptomatic relief, and the mean follow-up was 1 month. No intraoperative or postoperative complications were found.[84] Donas et al. reviewed 21 consecutive patients with 22 cases of buttock claudication (one patient with bilateral symptoms); 14 cases underwent PTA, and 8 cases underwent secondary stenting for suboptimal results. The success rate was 100%. All patients had relief of buttock claudication. There was significant increase in maximum walking distance from 85 to 225 meters, sustained nonsignificant improvement of ipsilateral ABI was seen, and the cumulative PPR was 95.5% over a mean follow-up of 14.7 ± 5.7 months.[79] Stent placement should be reserved for suboptimal PTA, owing to the risk of compression at the level of the gluteal canal.[87]

Persistent Sciatic Artery

Persistent sciatic artery is a rare congenital abnormality that is due to lack of regression of the axial artery during embryologic development. The axial artery persists and continues as the main blood supply to the lower limb, while the iliofemoral system remains hypoplastic and underdeveloped. The incidence is 0.025% to 0.04% in the general population. It is associated with increased incidence of aneurysmal disease, early atherosclerotic changes, thrombosis, and distal embolization. Originating from the IIA as a continuation of the inferior gluteal artery, the sciatic artery accompanies the sciatic nerve and continues as the popliteal artery and then the runoff vessels. The EIA and CFA are hypoplastic and continue as the femoral profunda. There are two types of persistent sciatic artery: (1) complete, where the sciatic artery forms the popliteal artery (in this case, the SFA is hypoplastic/absent), and (2) incomplete, where the persistent sciatic artery is hypoplastic and the SFA is the major blood supply to the lower limb. The most common presentation is aneurysmal disease with distal embolization; more rare presentations include atypical sciatica and IC. Knowledge of aberrant anatomy is crucial because it is essential to preserve the IIA in this case. The persistent sciatic artery can be diseased itself. Contralateral femoral or axillary access is mandatory, if needed. Ipsilateral CFA access is not an option in this case.[88]

OUTCOMES

Primary Stenting vs. PTA with Selective Stenting

With an acceptable associated risk for patients with aortoiliac disease and IC, PTA can be considered an acceptable option for focal, concentric, noncalcified, nonstial lesions. Becker et al. analyzed 2697 angioplasty procedures and reported a technical success rate of 92%, a 2-year patency rate of 81%, and a 5-year patency rate of 72%.[89] In two of the largest series published, 4-year patency rates (including technical failures) were between 60% and 80%.[90] In their review of iliac angioplasty for focal stenosis, Pentecost et al. reported a mean technical success rate of 95% and a 5-year patency rate of 80% to 90%. These results closely approximate a meta-analysis of aortoiliac bypass surgery with an 88% to 91% patency at 5 years. This is also reflected in the only randomized controlled trial comparing angioplasty with surgery, which showed the same 3-year patency rate between the two study arms of 73%.[91] The success of iliac PTA is reduced, however, by initial residual stenosis and late restenosis.[86] In 1990, Palmaz et al. published results of the first 171 iliac stent interventions.[92] Subsequent studies followed that reported long-term results. It is still unclear whether a stent should be inserted primarily or selectively (i.e., for primary PTA failure).[93] PTA in irregular, eccentric, long, ulcerated stenosis and occlusions demonstrated unsatisfactory long-term patency rates.[94] Selective stenting should be performed in PTA failure, defined as residual stenosis greater than 30%, trans-stenotic mean pressure gradient over 5 mmHg or systolic pressure gradient over 10 mmHg, or flow-limiting dissection (Fig. 35-13).[89,93,95,96] One area of continued debate is the role of primary stenting. Although stenting clearly has increased the applicability of endovascular revascularization, proponents of PTA question the benefits of primary stenting. The Dutch Iliac Stent Trial (DIST) is the only prospective randomized controlled trial published to date comparing PTA with selective stenting to primary stenting in iliac lesions. It randomized 279 patients to PTA and selective stenting (136 patients) or primary stenting (143 patients) and followed them for 5 to 8 years. Consensus was that PTA and selective stenting in the iliac artery has better symptomatic success than primary stent placement. Patency, ABI, and quality of life were similar in both groups. However, 43% of those in the provisional stent group ended up needing stents, even with the liberal pressure gradient threshold used, and complications were nearly twice as frequent in the provisional stent group.[97] The study included only patients with a stenosis less than 10 cm in length or occlusion less than 5 cm in length, excluding the more complex patients,[89] so the results are of dubitable value in contemporary clinical practice.

In most reviews of iliac stenting, both technical success (88%-100%) and clinical success (93%-95%) are excellent. Many series advocate routine primary stent placement. Arguments are that with their mechanism of fixing the plaque against the arterial wall, stenting in the short term would prevent immediate recoil and obstructive plaque dissection, with decreased risk of distal embolization. Long term, however, there is a tendency to develop intrastent myointimal hyperplasia and subsequent stent restenosis, a phenomenon responsible for most late failures.[93] Many authorities advocate the use of routine primary iliac stenting in extensive lesions (TASC C and TASC D). In their retrospective review of 110 patients who underwent primary stenting and 41 patients who underwent PTA plus selective stenting for aortoiliac occlusive disease, AbuRahma et al. found perioperative complications lower in the first group (2.7% vs. 24%). The early clinical success rate was higher in

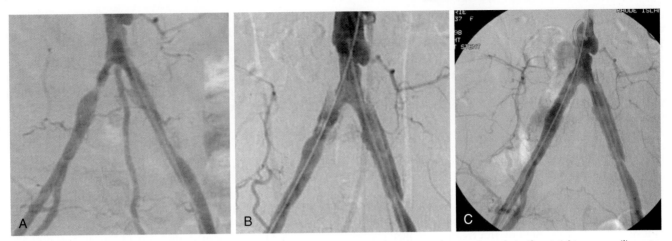

FIGURE 35-13. Suboptimal result after angioplasty followed by stent. **A,** Digital subtraction angiogram showed significant right common iliac artery stenosis. **B,** After angioplasty, there is suboptimal technical success, with significant residual stenosis and dissection. **C,** After stent placement, there is complete resolution of stenosis and dissection.

the primary stenting group (97% vs. 83%). Success rate was equal in both groups (100%) for short lesions (TASC A and B). Success was significantly higher for complex lesions (TASC C and D) in the primary stenting group (93% vs. 46%). This difference was maintained on follow-up (84% vs. 46%). Primary patency at 1, 2, 3, and 5 years was 98%, 94%, 87%, and 77% in the primary stenting group, and 83%, 78%, 69%, and 69% for the PTA and selective stenting group. Rates were comparable in both groups for shorter lesions but were superior in the primary stent group for longer lesions.[95] Other series reported similar results in patients with advanced iliac disease with primary stenting.[94,98,99] Although no strong scientific evidence is available to support this claim, simple lesions can be managed with PTA or primary stenting, whereas advanced complex lesions should be managed with primary stenting.

Bare Metal Stent vs. Stent-Graft

Restenosis after PTA is a common problem. It is caused by residual obstructive plaque, constrictive remodeling, or intimal hyperplasia. Stent placement improved midterm patency by improving technical success rate and reducing delayed remodeling. The 1-year primary patency of iliac stenting is 78% to 97% (mean 90%). Stenting improves technical success rates by fixing obstructive flaps and dissection, preventing elastic recoil, and by permanently compressing the plaque. Covered stents may theoretically prevent remodeling in the long-term, and the fabric tube may prevent tissue infiltration and intimal hyperplasia by excluding the diseased segment from the circulation. Experimental data, however, showed that stent-grafts may in fact induce more new intimal overgrowth at the end of the stent-graft than a bare metal stent.[27,100] In a prospective nonrandomized multicenter trial where a self-expanding nitinol stent covered with e-polytetrafluoroethylene (ePTFE) (Hemobahn [Gore, Flagstaff, Ariz.]) was implanted in 127 patients with symptomatic PAD (iliac disease, 61 limbs; femoral disease, 80 limbs), Lammer et al. found a 100% technical success rate, with a PPR of 98% and 91% at 6 and 12 months, respectively. Secondary patency rate was 95% at 12 months for iliac arteries.[101] Chang et al. reported

a series of 171 patients with advanced iliac disease who underwent a hybrid procedure where 193 CFA endarterectomy and patch angioplasty procedures were performed with primary iliac stenting (bare metal or stent-graft); 39% had EIA disease exclusively, and 61% had EIA and CIA lesions. The technical success rate was 98%. Primary patency was significantly higher at 5 years in patients who underwent stent-graft (87% ± 5% vs. 53% ± 7% in patients who had bare metal stents placed). There was no difference in primary assisted patency and secondary patency.[102] Rzucidlo et al. reported a series of 134 patients with advanced aortoiliac disease (TASC C and D lesions) who underwent endovascular iliac recanalization using covered stents (Wallgraft [Boston Scientific, Natick, Mass.] or Viabahn [Gore]); 53% of patients underwent concomitant CFA endarterectomy. At 6 and 12 months after intervention, PPR for aortoiliac segments was 87% and 70%, respectively, and secondary patency rates were 88% and 88%, respectively. Although not statistically significant (owing to small sample size), improvement in PPR was noted in patients who underwent concomitant CFA endarterectomy. At 6 and 12 months, the PPR in patients who underwent CFA endarterectomy was 94% and 94%, compared with 79% and 53% in patients who did not have CFA endarterectomy.[103]

Use of the bifurcated aortoiliac stent-graft has been described in the treatment of aortoiliac disease. Maynar et al. used the Excluder bifurcated endograft (Gore) to treat five patients with aortoiliac disease. The technical success rate was 100%. After a 17-month follow-up (3-36 months), 100% patency rate was noted.[104] In a series of 60 patients where the balloon-expandable covered stent iCast (Atrium) was used to treat 40 iliac lesions, PPR was 97% at 6 months, 84% at 12 months, and 77% at 18 months. The primary assisted patency was 100% at 18 months.[100] Despite the encouraging results, there is still no solid scientific evidence to support primary use of stent-grafts in aortoiliac occlusive disease.

Long-Term Outcomes

Despite recommended reporting standards,[105] published reports lack uniformity of severity of treated lesions, definition of patency, indication for treatment, and follow-up time period and methods. In iliac arteries, the reported 1-year PPR is 78% (67%-92%) after PTA and 90% (78%-97%) after stenting.[39] In long diffuse lesions involving the EIA, the 1-year primary patency after PTA is lower (67%-74%). Technical and clinical success of PTA in iliac artery stenosis was better than 90% in most series. The 5-year patency rate varies between 54% and 93%. Becker et al. in an analysis of 2697 cases of iliac PTA found a 5-year patency rate of 72%, better in claudicants (79%) and less favorable with long stenosis, EIA stenosis, and tandem lesions. In iliac artery occlusions, the technical success rate of PTA is 78% to 98%, with a 3-year patency rate of 48% to 85%. For iliac artery stenting, the 3-year patency rate is 41% to 92% for stenosis and 64% to 85% for occlusions.[106] Murphy et al. reported a PPR of 74% at 8 years. Schurmann treated 126 iliac lesions (66 stenosis and 60 occlusions) and reported 10-year primary patency of 46%. A meta-analysis by Bosch and Hunink comparing results of aortoiliac occlusive disease PTA to stenting in 2116 patients showed that with respect to long-term patency, stenting contributed to relative risk reductions of long term failures of 39% compared to PTA. The primary technical success rate for PTA of iliac artery stenosis is 95% (88%-99%); in occlusion, 83% (78%-98%). The technical success rate for stents in iliac artery stenosis is 99% (91%-100%); in occlusion, 82% (80%-92%).[107]

Gandini et al. reviewed 138 patients with iliac artery occlusion (150 occlusions) who underwent recanalization and stenting. Mean follow-up was 108 months, and technical success was 99%. PPRs were 90%, 85%, 80%, and 68% at 3, 5, 7, and 10 years, respectively. The cumulative secondary patency rate was 93%, 90%, 88%, and 78%, respectively. Occlusion hazard was 24%, higher in patients with EIA disease than in patients with CIA disease. In patients with CIA and EIA lesions, occlusion hazard was 9% higher than in patients with CIA-only lesions. Stents with diameters over 10 mm showed a 9% higher occlusion hazard rate than stents with a diameter less than 10 mm. Vowerk et al. reported 4-year patency rates of 78% and 82% for primary and secondary stenting procedures, respectively, in 100 patients.[108] Cikrit et al. reported a 5-year patency rate of 63% in 38 limbs that were treated by Palmaz stent placement, where as Palmaz et al. reported a 92% patency rate at 9 months. Primary 4-year patency as high as 86% has been reported.[108] In a retrospective review of 118 patients with endovascular treatment of 127 chronic iliac artery occlusions, all treated with stent placement with or without preballoon dilatation, Ozkan et al. found an initial technical success of 92%. Primary patency at 5 years was 63%, and secondary patency was 93%[109] (Table 35-1).

Predictors of Outcome

Predictors of outcome in endovascular aortoiliac revascularization have not been consistently substantiated. Murphy et al. in their long-term follow-up of 505 treated arterial segments in 365 patients, including 88 occlusions and 193 patients with critical limb ischemia, found stent length over 7.5 cm to be the only statistically significant risk factor for loss of primary patency. Placement of an EIA stent only, compared with one in the CIA only or CIA with EIA or aorta, lowered risk of loss of primary patency. Interestingly, older age and presence of critical limb ischemia contributed

to maintenance of primary patency.[110] Other predictors of failure mentioned in the literature include female sex, small vessel diameter, renal failure, critical limb ischemia, poor runoffs, extensive vascular calcifications, long lesion, residual postprocedure stenosis, disease of the superficial femoral artery, perioperative vascular complications, and hypercholesterolemia.[100,111-113]

External Iliac Lesions

External iliac artery lesions have been the subject of much controversy. Park et al. found a higher occlusion hazard rate in EIA lesions than in CIA lesions in a series of 249 limbs treated with stents.[114] In a study of 69 males treated with iliac stents (EIA, 49 limbs; CIA, 31 limbs), a nonstatistically significant trend favoring PPR in the EIA group was noted.[115] Powell et al. studied iliac patency after PTA and selective stenting and found that lesions located in the EIA were significantly predictive of bad results, with 47% and 18% PPR at 12 and 36 months. In another study, they defined a score according to the extent of EIA lesions and found a statistically significant difference in primary patency with EIA lesions longer than 5.0 cm. Timaran et al. retrospectively reviewed 67 patients with IC or critical limb ischemia who had EIA stents placed. Global PPRs of 76% and 56% were found, and in women only 61% and 47% at 1 and 3 years, respectively. They concluded that EIA treatment gives significantly worse results in women.[116,117]

In a more recent review, Maurel et al. reviewed the results of primary stenting of 90 EIAs in 81 patients with IC. The PPR was 97% at 1 year, 90% at 2 years, and 84% at 3 years. Secondary patency rate was 98% at 1 year, 93% at 2 years, and 93% at 3 years. Their conclusion was that in a population of patients with IC, endovascular therapy of EIA lesions yields better results after a systematic stenting than after selective stenting. Long lesions are usually treated with self-expanding nitinol stents because of their flexibility in the anteroposterior curved anatomy of the EIA. Rigid stainless steel or balloon-expandable stents are used for short lesions.[117]

Outcomes and TASC Classification

Higher lesion complexity and higher TASC category have been implicated as increased risk factors for patency loss. As shown by Bosch and Hunink, in general, stenoses have higher long-term patency compared to occlusion, regardless of PTA or stenting.[107] A fairly limited number of studies directly compared results in occlusions and stenosis. Most studies in fact categorize and analyze patients by TASC classification, which often include in the same class a wide range of different lesions, both occlusions and stenosis. In a retrospective review of 223 interventions performed for aortoiliac occlusive disease in 212 patients, Pulli et al. found that primary, primary assisted, and secondary patency were 82.4%, 90.6%, and 93% in the occlusion group and 77.7%, 85.5%, and 92.8% in the stenosis group, respectively, with no significant difference between the groups.[21] In another retrospective cohort of 375 patients with aortoiliac disease who underwent endovascular intervention for 438 lesions (stenosis or occlusion), Sixt et al. found a PPR similar for all TASC groups: 89%, 86%, 86%, and 85% for TASC A, B, C, and D, respectively. The secondary patency rate was also

TABLE 35-1. Literature Review of Endovascularly Treated Iliac Occlusive Disease

Study	Year	Study Design	No. of Iliac Lesions	Type of Treatment (No. of Lesions Treated)	Primary Patency (%)						Long Term (yr)	Secondary Patency % (yr)
					1 yr	2 yr	3 yr	4 yr	5 yr	7 yr		
Ichihashi[23]	2011	Retrospective	334 (TASC A/B)	Stenting (334)	95		91		88			97 (10)
			199 (TASC C/D)	Stenting (199)	90		88		83			98 (10)
Chen[62]	2011	Retrospective	121	Stenting (82)	86		68					80 (3)
Pulli[21]	2011	Prospective	109 (occlusions)	Stenting (97)					82			93 (5)
			114 (stenosis)	Stenting (101)					78			93 (5)
Jaff[137]	2010	Prospective	177	Stenting (177)	94	90						
Stockx[138]	2010	Prospective	163	Stenting (163)	92*	88						
Ozkan[109]	2010	Retrospective	127	Stenting (127)					63			93 (5)
Koizumi[111]	2009	Retrospective	487	Stenting (296)			88		82		75 (10)	
				PTA (177)			67		54		50 (10)	
Gandini[108]	2008	Retrospective	150	Stenting (150)	95	93	90	88	85	80	68 (10)	78 (10)
Sixt[139]	2008	Retrospective	438	All (438)	86							98 (1)
				PTA (84)	71							99 (1)
				Stenting (354)	90							97 (1)
Hans[121]	2008	Retrospective	68	Stenting (68)				69				89 (4)
Carreira[140]	2008	Prospective	31	Stenting (31)	97	87	83	79	75	67	67 (8)	86 (8)
Kashyap[25]	2008	Retrospective	127	Stenting (127)	90		74					96 (3)
Kondo[98]	2008	Retrospective	24 (occlusions)	Stenting (24)		91						96 (2)†
			90 (stenosis)	Stenting (24)		89						100 (2)†
AbuRahma[95]	2007	Retrospective	190	Primary stent (149)	98	94	87		77			
				Selective stent (41)	83	78	69		69			
De Roeck[99]	2006	Retrospective	38	Stenting (38)	94		89		77			94 (3)
Leville[141]	2006	Retrospective	92	Stenting (92)			76					90 (3)
Park[94]	2005	Retrospective	249	Stenting (249)			87		83	61	49 (10)	
Kudo[142]	2005	Retrospective	151	Stenting (34)	76		59		45			99 (7)
Picquet[143]	2005	Retrospective	34	Stenting (34)	95		84					89 (3)
Onal[144]	2005	Retrospective	32	Stenting (32)	97	90						
Galaria[145]	2005	Retrospective	394	Stenting (201)							72 (10)	87 (10)
Reyes[146]	2004	Retrospective	303	Stenting (259)					70	65		87 (9)
Ponec[147]	2004	Prospective	203	Stenting (203)	93							
Timaran[148]	2003	Retrospective	68	Stenting (68)	76		66		55			
Rzucidlo[103]	2003	Retrospective	34	Stenting (34)	88							
Timaran[149]	2003	Retrospective	136	Stenting (136)	85		72		64			
Reekers[150]	2002	Prospective	126	Stenting (126)	89							
Schurmann[151]	2002	Retrospective	110	Stenting (110)					66		46 (10)	55 (10)
Siskin[152]	2002	Retrospective	59	Stenting (59)	86		65					88 (3)
Uher[55]	2002	Retrospective	76	Stenting (76)	79		69					81 (3)
Scheinert[56]	2001	Retrospective	53	Stenting (53)	100		98		95			
Powell[153]	2000	Retrospective	210	Stenting (115)	87		72					
Uher[154]	1999	Retrospective	81	Stenting (81)	75		61					75 (3)
Nawaz[155]	1999	Retrospective	140	Stenting (140)	90		84					87 (3)
Becquemin[156]	1999	Retrospective	281	Stenting (67)	87		81		79		76 (6)	
Parsons[157]	1998	Retrospective	307	PTA (307)	87							

Continued

TABLE 35-1. Literature Review of Endovascularly Treated Iliac Occlusive Disease—cont'd

Study	Year	Study Design	No. of Iliac Lesions	Type of Treatment (No. of Lesions Treated)	Primary Patency (%)						Long Term (yr)	Secondary Patency % (yr)
					1 yr	2 yr	3 yr	4 yr	5 yr	7 yr		
Tettero[158]	1998	Prospective	279	Stenting (143)		71						
Toogood[159]	1998	Prospective	50	Stenting (40)		65						
Sullivan[160]	1997	Retrospective	501	Stenting (510)	75	57						
Murphy[41]	1996	Retrospective	94	Stenting (94)	78		53					82 (3)

*Six months primary patency was reported.
†Primary assisted patency was reported.
NOTE: Secondary patency was not reported in all studies.

similar in all groups, reported at 98% to 100%. The 1-year PPR following stenting was significantly better than balloon angioplasty alone (90% vs. 71%) and was comparable between stenosis and occlusions (88% and 83%, respectively).[118] In a recent meta-analysis of 958 patients with aortoiliac disease classified as TASC C and D lesions treated endovascularly, technical success rate and PPR at 12 months were higher in the TASC C than the TASC D group, although this difference was not statistically significant. Primary stenting showed a higher patency rate than selective stenting at 24 and 36 months; however, at 5 years, both groups showed comparable patency (67.1% vs. 63%).[22] In summary, outcome of endovascular therapy for complex aortoiliac disease has significantly improved over the years, and these lesions can be managed effectively through an endovascular approach. Although some debate about the EIA exists, there is no compelling reason to take a "surgery first" approach for this artery, since restenosis, if it occurs, can almost always be managed percutaneously; if it cannot, surgery is usually not impeded.

Endovascular vs. Open Surgical Treatment

To date, there is one randomized controlled trial comparing PTA and open surgical therapy for aortoiliac disease,[91,119] but none published comparing iliac stenting and open surgical therapy. In the multicenter prospective controlled trial, Wolf et al. randomized 263 patients with PAD to undergo either bypass surgery (133 patients) or PTA (130 patients). The study defined four disease categories: (1) iliac disease with claudication, (2) iliac disease with rest pain, (3) femoropopliteal disease with claudication, and (4) femoropopliteal disease with rest pain. The median follow-up was 4.1 years (2-6 years). The operative mortality in the surgical group was less than 1%, with no mortality in the PTA group. The surgical cohort had more late death and better PPR at 4 years, and PTA had better limb salvage rate, however all differences between the two treatment arms were not statistically significant. Claudicants had better outcome than patient with rest pain, and patients with iliac disease had better outcome with either intervention than did patients with femoropopliteal disease. Improvement of functional status was seen equally in all groups with no statistically significant difference. The conclusion was that both bypass surgery and PTA are equally effective. Moise and Kashyap et al. in a retrospective review compared open reconstructions in 96 patients (161 limbs) to 83 patients (127 limbs) undergoing PTA/stenting. The lesions were all occlusions (TASC B, C and D).[18,120] Limb-based PPR at 3 years was significantly higher for aortobifemoral bypass than for PTA/stenting. Secondary patency rate (97% vs. 95%), limb salvage (98% vs. 98%), and long-term survival (80% vs. 80%) were similar in both groups.[25] Similar results were reported by Hans et al. where at a follow-up of 48 months, primary patency in the endovascular group was 69%, significantly lower than that of aortobifemoral bypass which is 93%. The secondary patency rate was statistically similar in both groups: 89% in the endovascular group and 100% in the aortobifemoral.[121] In a recent retrospective study comparing 118 aortobifemoral bypass and 174 PTA/stenting procedure in patients with aortoiliac disease, with a follow-up of 10 years, Burke et al. showed no difference in 30-day mortality rate, myocardial infarction rate, and stroke rate between the two groups. The aortobifemoral had more perioperative complications including additional emergency surgery, infection/sepsis, transfusion, and lymph leak. The aortobifemoral group had a greater improvement in ABI; freedom from amputation and revision rates were similar in both groups however.[122] Moreover, given that percutaneous re-interventions can usually be performed without much difficulty and with minimal morbidity, secondary patency rates may be more appropriate when comparing endovascular and surgical outcome data.

Endovascular vs. Medical Therapy

Patients with mild to moderate symptoms of IC can be managed conservatively. Two medications approved by the FDA for symptomatic relief of IC are available. Pentoxifylline was the first drug approved and was shown to only mildly improve symptoms of IC; for this reason, it has fallen out of favor. The other medication, cilostazol (Pletal [Otsuka Pharmaceuticals]), has been shown to increase maximum walking distance and pain-free walking distance 22% to 51% and 21% to 67% above baseline, respectively. The drug is contraindicated in patients with congestive heart failure. Although minor, the side effects (e.g., headaches, diarrhea, dizziness, palpitations) of cilostazol affect one third of patients taking the medication, reducing compliance and limiting its widespread use.

A supervised walking program for at least 30 minutes three times a week significantly improved pain-free walking distance and absolute walking distance in some series by 100%. The benefits of exercise in an unsupervised setting are controversial. In a study comparing the cost-effectiveness of a supervised exercise program to PTA of the iliac arteries, Treesak et al. found that at 3 months, PTA was more effective with regard to absolute walking distance but more costly; at 6 months, exercise was found to be more effective and less costly. Reimbursement for these programs is low to nonexistent, and Medicare does not cover costs. The adjuvant benefit of angioplasty in patients with mild to moderate IC (MIMIC) was studied in two simultaneous multicenter prospective, randomized, controlled trials that randomized patients with mild to moderate femoropopliteal and aortoiliac occlusive disease to receive supervised exercise therapy and best medical therapy with and without PTA. Participants were followed for 24 months. The study suggested that PTA significantly improves symptoms compared to best medical therapy and supervised exercise, and that the benefit of PTA persisted up to 24 months in both the aortoiliac and femoropopliteal groups. The study was limited by small sample size.[121,123] CLEVER (Claudication: Exercise vs. Endoluminal Revascularization) is an ongoing prospective multicenter randomized controlled trial designed to compare the relative clinical benefit and cost-effectiveness of revascularization with stents to supervised exercise rehabilitation in a cohort with moderate to severe claudication due to aortoiliac insufficiency.[124,125] The preliminary 6 month results showed that patients treated with supervised exercise walked better on the treadmill than those treated with stent revascularization. Those with stent revascularization, however, reported better quality of life. The final 18-month results are still pending.[126]

COMPLICATIONS

The Society of Interventional Radiology defines *minor complications* as those requiring no or nominal therapy, including observation admission. *Major complications* include those that (1) require therapy or minor hospitalization (<48 hr); (2) require major therapy, unexpected increase in level of care, or prolonged hospitalization; (3) result in permanent adverse sequelae; or (4) result in death.[127] Unfortunately, published papers lack uniformity in reporting complications.

In a meta-analysis of 1300 iliac PTA patients (six series) and 816 iliac stent patients (eight series), Bosch and Hunink demonstrated low complication rates for both procedures. Procedural-related complications or deaths during the same hospital stay for PTA and stent groups occurred at rates of 0.14% and 0.3%, respectively. The 30-day all-inclusive mortality rates were 1.0% and 0.8% for PTA and stent groups, respectively.[107] The rates of major complications requiring therapy for PTA and stent studies were 4.3% and 5.2%, respectively. The list of complications included access hematomas, pseudoaneurysms, dissections, emboli, arterial ruptures, thromboses, postdilation dissections, upper gastrointestinal tract bleeding, septicemia, acute pulmonary edema, renal failure, and myocardial infarction.[107] These rates compare favorably with those of aortofemoral bypass surgery. In a meta-analysis of 23 series of aortic bifurcation grafts for aortoiliac occlusive disease, de Vries and Hunink reported mean rates of 4.1% and 4.8% for procedural related deaths and 30-day mortality, respectively.[128]

Combined local and systemic complications, which excluded minor complications and early graft failures, occurred in 19.7%.[128]

Stent infection represents one of the most serious potential complications of aortoiliac revascularization and may result in devastating outcomes, including amputation or death,[129] especially when complicated by delayed diagnosis. Fortunately, stent infections are extremely rare. However, with increased use of iliac stents, several single case reports have been published.[130,131] Darcy reported a total of eight published cases of iliac stent infections as of the year 2000 but also intimated that the true incidence is likely higher due to underreporting.[129] Proposed risk factors include repeated accesses to the same segment of the CFA, use of prolonged indwelling arterial sheaths or catheters for repeat procedures,[132] increased procedural time, and presence of hematomas.[133] Complications with chronically implanted iliac stents can also occur, as in the case of an infected pseudoaneurysm that developed 22 months after stent placement.[130]

A high level of clinical suspicion may aid timely diagnosis. Fever, pain, and positive blood cultures are likely present, and progression to pseudoaneurysm formation and sepsis may ensue.[134] If a stent infection is suspected, aggressive treatment including immediate administration of appropriate antibiotics is warranted. Moreover, when the infecting organism is *Staphylococcus aureus*, consideration for surgical resection of the infected artery and explantation of the stent is recommended to avoid frequent amputation and death. Infection with less virulent organisms, such as *Streptococcus*, have been successfully treated with antibiotics without surgery.[130,134] Prophylactic antibiotics, however, are not routinely recommended for iliac artery stent placement. Patients with high-risk factors mentioned previously may be pretreated with 1 g of cefazolin 2 hours before the procedure.[135]

Aortoiliac angioplasty may rarely be complicated by arterial ruptures. A prospective analysis of over 657 aortoiliac PTA procedures performed over a 20-year period resulted in 0.8% of iliac artery rupture or delayed pseudoaneurysm formation.[136] Eleven years earlier, Palmaz et al. reported almost the exact same rate: 0.9%.[94] Ruptures are typically diagnosed during the procedure. The patient may complain of persistent pain after deflation of the angioplasty balloon. Postintervention arteriography may show extravasation of contrast agent. In cases of free intraabdominal rupture, hemodynamic embarrassment may quickly follow. Patient resuscitation with IV fluids and chronotropic medications (e.g., atropine for bradycardia) should be done as needed, and blood sent for cross-matching. Reversal of anticoagulation with protamine sulfate and immediate reinflation of the balloon to a low pressure should be performed in an attempt to temporarily tamponade the bleeding. Effective hemostasis can usually be confirmed by injecting contrast agent above and below the occluding balloon (often through the lumen of the balloon catheter and through a sheath) and imaging. It is possible to maintain balloon tamponade for 10 to 15 minutes; once the balloon is deflated, the hemorrhage has often stopped, and patients can be observed overnight in intensive care settings. Follow-up imaging can be done (e.g., CT, MRA, contrast arteriography) to evaluate for development of a pseudoaneurysm (Fig. 35-14). In the current era, placement

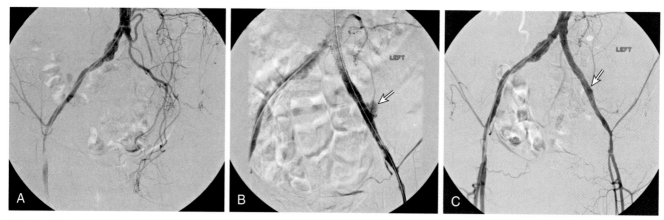

FIGURE 35-14. External iliac artery (EIA) rupture after stenting, treated with balloon tamponade. **A,** Digital subtraction angiogram demonstrates left common iliac artery and EIA chronic occlusion. **B,** Contained left EIA rupture *(arrow)* after stent placement. **C,** After balloon tamponade and anticoagulation reversal, extravasation was no longer evident. A small pseudoaneurysm is present *(arrow)*. Patient did well after procedure, and 1-month computed tomography scan (not shown) revealed no persistent pseudoaneurysm. Currently, this type of lesion would be managed by placement of a stent-graft.

of a covered stent is often performed. Emergent surgical management should be considered if hemostasis cannot be achieved promptly by any means. However, measures must be taken in the angiography suite to tamponade hemorrhage.

POSTPROCEDURAL AND FOLLOW-UP CARE

On completion of the procedure, catheters and sheaths should be removed after sufficient time has been allowed to reduce the effects of heparin, usually 1 to 2 hours. Although not necessarily routine, an activated clotting time of less than 160 seconds or a partial thromboplastin time less than 1.5 times the control is usually acceptable for sheath removal. Once hemostasis is obtained, the ABI should be checked. During the next 6 hours, patients should remain on bed rest. Access site, femoral pulses, and distal pulses should be serially monitored. Diet can be reinitiated starting with clear liquids and advanced as tolerated once effects of conscious sedation are resolved. Urine outputs are recorded. Routine postprocedure serum creatinine levels are not necessary. Depending on the amount of contrast medium administration during the procedure and the presence of preexisting renal insufficiency, continued hydration and/or bicarbonate drip infusion are recommended. Limited ambulation is suggested after 6 hours and for the first 24 hours. Typically, patients are admitted for 23-hour observation. Discharge is contingent on the ability to tolerate solid food intake, ambulate, and void. Before discharge, a 1- to 2-week follow-up appointment is made. Discharge instructions including emergency contact number are provided.

On discharge, strenuous activity is to be avoided within the first week. At follow-up visitation, potential access site complications, femoral pulses, and distal pulses should be documented. Clinical improvement status and ABI should be evaluated. Additional follow-up routines vary; in our practice we see people at 6 months and 18 months. If symptoms recur or worsen, noninvasive tests (i.e., ABI, PVR) should be performed to identify patients with recurrent

disease. If restenosis is suspected, repeat angiography should be scheduled to promptly address recurrence of disease.

All patients with atherosclerotic aortoiliac occlusive disease have a coronary artery disease equivalent, and long-term management should include aggressive risk factor modification to reduce their risk of cardiovascular events. This includes lowering the low-density lipoprotein value to below 100 mg/dL (perhaps to below 70 mg/dL), increasing the high-density lipoprotein number, reducing triglycerides, controlling blood pressure, increasing activity, ingesting a low-fat ("DASH") diet, and smoking cessation. Whether or not a patient's primary care physician has included such measures in the long-term care plan, it behooves the vascular specialist to check that these efforts are underway and coordinate or institute them if they are lacking.

KEY POINTS

- Percutaneous revascularization is generally accepted as the primary mode of treatment for most patients with aortoiliac disease.

- Aortoiliac occlusive disease, including complex stenoses and chronic occlusions, can be safely and effectively treated with stents, with long-term patency rates similar to those of bypass surgery and less morbidity and mortality.

- Preprocedural consultation and postprocedural follow-up by the interventionalist are essential for optimal patient care.

▶ **SUGGESTED READINGS**

Bosch JL, Hunink MG. Meta-analysis of the results of percutaneous transluminal angioplasty and stent placement for aortoiliac occlusive disease. Radiology 1997;204:87–96.

de Vries SO, Hunink MG. Results of aortic bifurcation grafts for aortoiliac occlusive disease: a meta-analysis. J Vasc Surg 1997;26:558–69.

Leung DA, Spinosa DJ, Hagspiel KD, et al. Selection of stents for treating iliac arterial occlusive disease. J Vasc Interv Radiol 2003;14(2 pt 1):137–52.

Pentecost MJ, Criqui MH, Dorros G, et al. Guidelines for peripheral percutaneous transluminal angioplasty of the abdominal aorta and lower extremity vessels. A statement for health professionals from a Special Writing Group of the Councils on Cardiovascular Radiology, Arteriosclerosis, Cardio-Thoracic and Vascular Surgery, Clinical Cardiology, and Epidemiology and Prevention, the American Heart Association. J Vasc Interv Radiol 2003;14(9 pt 2):S495–S515.

Rutherford RB, Baker JD, Ernst C, et al. Recommended standards for reports dealing with lower extremity ischemia: revised version. J Vasc Surg 1997;26:517–38.

Tetteroo E, Van Der Graaf Y, Bosch JL, et al. Randomised comparison of primary stent placement versus primary angioplasty followed by selective stent placement in patients with iliac-artery occlusive disease. Dutch Iliac Stent Trial Study Group. Lancet 1998;351:1153–9.

Yilmaz S, Sindel T, Yegin A, et al. Primary stenting of focal atherosclerotic infrarenal aortic stenoses: long-term results in 13 patients and a literature review. Cardiovasc Interv Radiol 2004;27:121–8.

The complete reference list is available online at www.expertconsult.com.

CHAPTER 36

Endovascular Management of Chronic Femoropopliteal Disease

Eric M. Walser and Mahmood K. Razavi

Femoropopliteal occlusive disease is present in a significant proportion of older patients, with about 20% of men and 17% of women older than 55 living with ankle-brachial indices (ABI) under 0.9. A smaller percentage (3%-7%) present with symptoms of intermittent claudication (IC) between the ages of 60 and 70.[1-5] After the age of 70, however, 25% of patients with IC clinically deteriorate, with 1% to 3.3% progressing to critical limb ischemia (CLI) and eventual amputation.[6,7] Although only some patients experience worsening claudication or gangrene, many more adjust to this reduction in circulation by becoming progressively more sedentary. As such, the femoropopliteal arteries deserve respect as critical determinants in the health and mobility of our older citizens. To be sure, significant lower extremity occlusive arterial disease has ominous associations with generalized vascular disease, and the estimated 5-, 10-, and 15-year morbidity and mortality of these patients is 30%, 50%, and 70%, respectively, with 70% to 80% of deaths related to cardiovascular events (myocardial infarction, cerebrovascular accidents, and ruptured aneurysms). These figures are 2.5 times higher than that of nonclaudicants.[2]

The anatomy and physiology of the femoropopliteal artery is unique and poses specific challenges for both percutaneous and surgical treatments. The femoral artery is the longest artery in our body, with the fewest branches. It has thick muscular walls so that it can tolerate the variety of longitudinal and lateral compressive forces delivered to it by virtue of its fixation at the highly mobile hip and knee joints. In this milieu, catheter-based intervention often falters because this powerful artery scars, proliferates, and thromboses under the injuries inflicted by angioplasty, and it fractures and deforms metallic stents placed within its lumen.[8] No wonder that multiple devices have tried and failed to tame occlusive disease in the femoropopliteal arteries.

In this chapter, the discussion of femoropopliteal occlusive disease begins with its clinical and noninvasive diagnosis. Then we describe established medical and surgical therapies. Finally, we will focus on endovascular methods, including the multitude of past failures and their evolution to more modern devices and treatments available today and in the near future.

With almost 2000 articles pertaining to femoral artery stents available in the recent medical literature,[8] the importance of critical manuscript review in this subject area cannot be understated. Therefore, the reader must consider important comparative data when evaluating the various treatments for femoropopliteal arterial disease—including, but not limited to, the status of the runoff and inflow vessels, the length and degree of calcification of lesions treated, clinical versus imaging follow-up, and the presence of concomitant disease states such as diabetes, continued smoking, or renal failure.

CLINICAL PRESENTATION

Peripheral arterial disease (PAD) involving the lower extremities is defined as the presence of disease causing hemodynamic compromise resulting in a resting ABI of less than 0.9. The clinical presentation of PAD can range from no symptoms to gangrene and tissue loss. PAD is a strong marker for the presence of systemic atherosclerotic disease and is therefore associated with an increased risk of major cardiovascular events (5%-7% annually).[2] The most common cause of occlusive disease in the femoropopliteal segment (FPS) is atherosclerosis, with the major risk factors presented in Table 36-1 along with targets for reduction and the means for reaching those targets.

Intermittent claudication is the most common symptom related to PAD. Typical symptoms consist of muscle fatigue, ache, or cramps induced by exertion and relieved by rest (Rutherford-Becker classification II). Involvement of calves, thighs, or buttocks indicates the level of anatomic disease.

Critical limb ischemia is the most severe manifestation of PAD and refers to chronic ischemic rest pain and/or ulceration and gangrene (Rutherford-Becker classifications III and IV). This group carries the worst prognosis of all PAD patients, with an amputation-free survival of only 50% at 1 year. Approximately 25% of patients with CLI die, and another 25% require a major amputation at 1 year. The main manifestation of CLI is ischemic rest pain in the foot, which is worse at night or when the foot is in a nondependent position. Edema is another common manifestation due to prolonged dependency of the foot and/or inflammation. Ulceration and gangrene are other clinical manifestations of CLI. Gangrene typically involves the digits or the heel and may progress to affect the distal forefoot. Although ulcers above the foot can be of arterial etiology, the majority are caused by venous disease.

DIAGNOSIS

Patients with IC give a history of leg muscle pain that is relieved by rest. The differential diagnosis of IC includes arthritis of the hip, knee, and ankle joints; spinal stenosis; nerve root compression; Baker cyst; and venous claudication. The clinical features of IC that differentiate it from other conditions include quick relief of symptoms by rest and lack of dependence on patient or extremity position. Frequently, musculoskeletal pain or pain due to spinal stenosis is worse in the morning before any significant muscular exertion, whereas claudication virtually never affects patients before they get out of bed.

Key components of the physical examination in patients with PAD include palpation of extremity pulses and evaluation of the extremities for color, temperature, chronic hair loss, nail changes, and skin ulcerations. Those patients with

TABLE 36-1. Risk Factors for Peripheral Vascular Disease

Risk Factor	Risk of Developing Peripheral Vascular Disease	Threshold Value	Means of Risk Reduction	Target
Race	7.8% vs. 4.4% non-Hispanic blacks over whites	NA	NA	NA
Sex	2 or 3:1 males over females	NA	NA	NA
Age	2.5% age 40-59, increasing to almost 20% over age 70[65]	NA	NA	NA
Smoking	Odds ratio 2.6 for men and 4.6 for women[66,67]	Any smoking	Combination of physician encouragement, bupropion, and nicotine replacement therapy[68]	Cessation of smoking has twofold increase in 5-year survival rate and 3 times decreased risk of amputation compared to continued smoking[69]
Hypertension	Odds ratio 2.2 for men and 2.8 for women[66,67]	Over 140 systolic and 90 diastolic	Aggressive medical management	Below 140/90 mmHg generally, but below 130/80 mmHg in diabetics or renal failure
Diabetes	Odds ratio 6.1 for men and 3.6 for women[66,67]	Persistently elevated glucose	Insulin if not controlled with antihyperglycemic agents	Hemoglobin A_{1c} under 7%
Hyperlipidemia	Odds ratio 1.02 for each 1 mg/dL increase in serum LDL in men or women[66,67]	Normal range	Diet before statins, niacin, or fibrates	Keep LDL below 100 mg/dL (2.59 mmol/L)[70]

Other risk factors: Hyperhomocysteinemia, hypothyroidism, increased inflammatory markers (C-reactive protein), increased blood viscosity, chronic renal failure.
LDL, Low-density lipoprotein.

a history and/or physical findings suggestive of PAD should proceed to objective testing, including the ABI.

As mentioned earlier, an ABI of less than 0.9 is a highly sensitive measure for the presence of obstructive lesions in the arterial supply to the leg. Thus, measurement of the ABI is a good screening tool for the presence of PAD. A formal noninvasive test of the lower extremity should also include segmental limb systolic pressure measurement and segmental plethysmography or pulse-volume recordings. Measurement of toe pressures and toe-brachial index would be desirable in the presence of CLI and noncompressible arteries that may occur with conditions such as diabetes and renal failure. The toe pressure is usually 30 mmHg below the ankle pressure, and hence an abnormal toe-brachial index is defined as less than 0.7. Doppler velocity waveform analysis is also a useful tool that is frequently done as part of a formal noninvasive vascular study. Triphasic arterial waveforms become biphasic, then flat (monophasic) as arterial flow diminishes.

Computed tomographic angiography (CTA) and magnetic resonance angiography (MRA) are moderately sensitive and specific for arterial occlusive disease in the large and medium-sized vessels. Most practitioners reserve costly cross-sectional imaging for those patients with symptoms warranting intervention and segmental limb pressures indicative of potentially correctable arterial disease. A more detailed discussion of CTA and MRA is presented elsewhere in this book.

The diagnosis of CLI cannot be made based on clinical presentation alone and should be confirmed by ABI, toe systolic pressure, or transcutaneous oxygen tension. Patients with CLI typically have ankle and toe systolic pressures of less than 50 mmHg and 30 mmHg, respectively. The presence of ulceration or rest pain alone does not confirm the diagnosis of CLI. The differential diagnosis of ischemic ulceration includes traumatic, neuropathic, or venous ulcerations. A combination of these causes is not uncommon, especially in diabetic patients. The differential diagnosis of ischemic rest pain includes diabetic neuropathy, nerve root compression, complex regional pain syndrome (previously known as *reflex sympathetic dystrophy*), and miscellaneous conditions such as various inflammatory conditions affecting the foot or digits and peripheral neuropathy caused by vitamin B_{12} deficiency or some chemotherapeutic agents.

TREATMENT

Treatment planning for patients with femoropopliteal disease should consider the epidemiology and natural history of the disease, as well as the risks and benefits of the proposed therapy. The treatment of patients with IC and CLI will hence be considered separately owing to their disparate natural histories and risk/benefit ratio of therapy. The overall goals of therapy for both groups, however, remain the relief of symptoms, limb preservation, and reduction of cardiovascular morbidity and mortality. As such, risk factor modification should be an integral part of therapy in any patient with PAD.

Medical Management

As discussed earlier, many factors contribute to the development and progression of atherosclerosis (see Table 36-1). Attempts should be made to address all modifiable risk factors. Surprisingly, medical therapies have not been instituted or optimized in a large proportion of patients referred for lower extremity revascularization. This represents an opportunity and an obligation for the interventionalist to evaluate and institute appropriate therapies for various risk factors.

Along with efforts to modify a patient's risk factors, a program of structured exercise is the recommended initial step in the treatment of IC. Patients with CLI, however, bypass this step and generally proceed directly to revascularization owing to their advanced occlusive disease and walking impairment. Supervised exercise conducted for 3 months or longer increases treadmill performance and lessens the severity of claudication,[9] but there are three major limitations to exercise programs. First, unfortunately, exercise is contraindicated in 9% to 34% of PAD patients, such as those with severe coronary artery disease or neurologic and musculoskeletal impairment. Second, PAD patients are usually poorly compliant with exercise programs, which are furthermore not widely available. Finally, and even worse, these exercise programs are not reimbursed by most insurance companies even though they are proven to be cost-effective compared to surgical or endovascular vascular procedures.[10,11] Structured exercise programs are therefore not widely prescribed.

Many pharmacologic agents have been studied for the relief of symptoms of IC. Only a few, however, have shown any evidence of clinical utility, and they do not provide the same level of symptom relief as a successful revascularization.[12] The first U.S. Food and Drug Administration (FDA) agent approved for claudication was pentoxifylline, a methylxanthine derivative thought to increase red blood cell membrane deformability and decrease fibrinogen activity and platelet adhesion, with the overall effect of reduced blood viscosity. Multiple trials have failed to show other than mild clinical benefit, so this drug is probably beneficial only to those who cannot tolerate cilostazol,[13] a better claudication drug. Cilostazol is a phosphodiesterase-III inhibitor with some antiplatelet and vasodilatation activity. As such it should not be prescribed to patients with congestive heart failure (CHF), owing to decreased survival compared to placebo in patients with class III-IV CHF. Cilostazol increases maximal and pain-free walking distances by half and two thirds, respectively, after 3 to 6 months of therapy,[14] but its side effects of diarrhea, headaches, and dizziness present a compliance issue, with up to 60% of patients stopping the drug within 3 years.[15]

Use of antiplatelet agents, specifically aspirin, is an important topic and deserves more attention. Aspirin use has been associated with a 25% odds reduction in subsequent cardiovascular events in patients with cardiovascular disease.[16] Although an initial meta-analysis by the Antithrombotic Trialists' Collaboration concluded aspirin use in patients without any evidence of vascular disease does not statistically reduce cardiovascular events,[17] more recent studies combining data from trials using not only aspirin but also other antiplatelet agents showed a significant reduction in ischemic events in patients with PAD. The American College of Cardiology and American Heart Association (ACC/AHA) recommend aspirin or clopidogrel daily for cardiovascular risk reduction in patients with PAD, and studies do indicate a relative risk reduction in all cardiovascular events for patients receiving such agents, especially clopidogrel.[18] Other agents such as naftidrofuryl, propionyl-L-carnitine, and some lipid-lowering agents have also shown promise in improving walking distance in patients with IC.

Other critical elements of treatment include adequate pain control and treatment of infections if present. Care of ulcerations will require specialized treatment and should be done in conjunction with specialists in foot and wound care. Primary major amputation may become necessary if anatomic or comorbid medical conditions do not allow for a successful revascularization. Frequently, minor amputations are done after a revascularization procedure for limb salvage.

Surgical Revascularization Procedures

Bypass surgery has been the traditional treatment modality in the majority of patients in need of lower extremity revascularization, but the less invasive nature of endovascular approaches and better outcomes data are shifting this paradigm. The change was reflected in the 2007 TransAtlantic Inter-Society Consensus (TASC II) document that expanded recommendations for endovascular therapies.[2] TASC II classification of diseases of the FPS is shown in Table 36-2. Although TASC class A and B lesions in symptomatic patients are best treated endovascularly, the recommended treatment for class D patients is surgical bypass in suitable candidates. Class C patients represent the "gray area" where endovascular techniques are applicable in selected patients not suitable or agreeable to surgical bypass. These recommendations are based on the consensus of a panel of experts after reviewing the current literature. For comparison purposes, the surgical gold standard for treating the diseased FPS is femoral-to–above knee popliteal venous bypass with 6-month, 1-, 2-, 3-, and 4-year primary patency rates of 87%, 81%, 77%, 71%, and 70%, respectively, with these numbers slightly decreasing when prosthetic material is used as the bypass conduit (85%, 77%, 66%, 59%, and 51% at the same time intervals).[19]

The remainder of this chapter describes current endovascular approaches to femoropopliteal occlusive disease. Table 36-3 lists patency rates, complications, and the lesion types and locations suitable for various techniques as described in the recent literature. These data are best compared and contrasted with the results from best medical therapy, surgical bypass, and balloon angioplasty (also included, where possible, in Table 36-3). Even the most modern endovascular devices marketed for the FPS (and there have been many) struggle to achieve results comparable to balloon angioplasty, and most remain woefully inferior to surgical bypass. We will briefly describe those devices falling short of expectations, then conclude with a discussion of the best currently available techniques to reliably open diseased femoropopliteal arteries—namely nitinol stents and stent-grafts.

Endovascular Procedures

This section concentrates mainly on various endovascular procedures for treating occlusive lesions of the FPS. This is a very active area of research and development marked by rapid change. The information contained herein, especially in the area of outcome, is hence likely to change over time, and the reader is encouraged to seek updates from the current literature.

The main determinants of outcome in all endovascular procedures in the limb include the anatomic location of the

TABLE 36-2. TASC II Classification of Femoropopliteal Segment Disease

TASC II Group	Stenosis	Occlusion	Involvement of Infrageniculate Popliteal Artery	Heavily Calcified	Continuous Tibial Artery Runoff
A	Single <10 cm	Single <5 cm	Ok	No	Yes
B	Multiple <5 cm	Multiple <5 cm	Ok	No	Yes
	Single <15 cm		No	No	Yes
	Single popliteal stenosis		Ok	No	Yes
	Single or multiple lesions		Ok	No	No
	Single lesion <5 cm		Ok	Yes	Yes
C	Multiple stenoses or occlusions >15 cm		Ok	Yes or No	Yes
	Recurrent stenoses or occlusions requiring more than two endovascular treatments		Ok	Yes or No	Yes or No
D	Chronic total occlusions of common and superficial femoral artery >20 cm		Yes	Yes or No	Yes or no
	Chronic total occlusion of popliteal artery and proximal trifurcation vessels		Yes	Yes or no	No

Adapted from Norgren L, Hiatt WR, Dormandy JA, et al. Inter-Society Consensus for the management of peripheral arterial disease (TASC II). J Vasc Surg 2007;45:1S–68S.

TABLE 36-3. Comparison of Current Treatment Methods for Superficial Femoral Artery Occlusive Disease

Treatment	Initial Success (%)	Primary Patency (%) 6 mo	1 yr	Longer (time)	Secondary Patency (%) 6 mo	1 yr	Longer (time)	Adjunct Use of Stents or Angioplasty (%)	Restenosis on Ultrasound (%)
Venous above-knee femoropopliteal bypass		87	81	77 (3 yr)					
Prosthetic above-knee femoropopliteal bypass		85	77	66 (3 yr)					
Balloon angioplasty	95	63	58	55-68 (3 yr)					
Atherectomy (SilverHawk)		62	52 (18 mo)		80.3	75 (18 mo)		35	
Atherectomy (Pathway)	99	73						50	30 (6 mo) 40 (1 yr)
Laser (Spectranetics)	90.5		59	54		75		88	41 (6 mo) 46 (1 yr)
Cryoplasty	94	63	55		91	91			30 (9 mo)
Bare stents (non-nitinol)	98	81	65	55 (3 yr)					
Nitinol stents (newer devices)	98		81-90	69 (4 yr)		93-96	90 (4 yr)		
Stent-grafts (Viabahn)	95	82	74	63 (2 yr)		84			

disease, extent of the diseased and treated segments, quality of the inflow and outflow vessels, occlusion versus stenosis, clinical stage of the disease (IC vs. CLI), the presence of diabetes or renal failure, and the nature of the therapeutic technology. Undoubtedly, certain pathophysiologic conditions affecting the vascular wall, such as inflammation, will also impact outcome. Schillinger et al. observed a correlation between C-reactive protein levels and 6-month patency of percutaneous transluminal angioplasty (PTA) in the superficial femoral artery (SFA).[20] Although not yet proven, certain pharmacologic adjuncts such as prolonged antiplatelet therapy are also likely to change the outcome of an endovascular procedure.

In addition to these general factors affecting outcome, certain device-specific technical considerations have also been noted to improve long-term performance. For example, when employing bare stents, stent-grafts, or cryoplasty, it is recommended that the treatment segment extend beyond the focal lesion per se and include the entire diseased segment between two adjacent normal areas. Whereas one may choose not to overdilate using simple angioplasty, a certain degree of oversizing is necessary when applying cryoplasty or stenting. Complete knowledge of and careful attention to performance characteristics of devices is thus important to their optimal use.

Balloon angioplasty is an established approach to patients with IC and CLI and has been the mainstay of endovascular therapy for lesions of the SFA and tibial arteries. Angioplasty catheters are inexpensive, widely available, easy to use, and require no costly generators or other supplemental supplies. The technical success of PTA in stenoses of the SFA exceeds 95% in all reported series.[13] Patency rates, however, are limited; this is probably due to the large amount of calcification and long-segment disease in the FPS. These characteristics lead to extensive recoil and angioplasty failure in up to 30% of cases.[21] In fact, a meta-analysis by Muradin et al. found a 3-year patency rate ranging from 55% to 68%. Patency rates strongly correlated with lesion morphology and fell to 52% to 62% in patients with chronic occlusions and long-segment disease of the SFA.[22]

Comparison of angioplasty to bypass surgery is difficult owing to the relative paucity of prospective randomized trials. Up until recently, PTA was done for short-segment disease and in patients with IC. Bypass was frequently reserved for patients with more advanced disease and those with CLI. Wolf et al. reported a multicenter prospective randomized trial in 263 men with diseases of iliac and femoropopliteal lesions, comparing PTA to bypass surgery.[23] They observed no statistically significant difference in outcome measures of patency, survival, and limb salvage between the two groups. Subgroup analysis of patients with long-segment SFA disease, however, showed a better 1-year cumulative patency for surgery.

In another multicenter prospective randomized study of patients with CLI, angioplasty alone (no stenting) was compared with bypass surgery.[24] There was no difference in the clinical outcome, with 1-year amputation-free survival of 56% and 50% in surgical and angioplasty groups, respectively. The health-related quality of life was also similar between the two groups. The 1-year cost of care, however, was significantly lower in the angioplasty group.

For short-segment stenoses of the FPS, angioplasty was and remains the treatment of choice. However, it soon became clear that we needed new approaches and innovative technology to tackle the longer and more complex lesions so characteristic of the FPS. From the early bare-metal stenting bailout of angioplasty failures exploded a great controversial experiment into femoropopliteal "gadgetry" that still exists today. The following is a discussion of the milestones (and headstones) of the ongoing FPS treatment evolution and where it has taken us today.

Early Stent Placement in the Femoropopliteal Segment
Metallic stent implantation in the FPS arose initially as a logical response to failed angioplasty (residual stenosis, recoil, or flow-limiting dissection). Although the high technical success and immediate results were greeted enthusiastically, several clinical trials conclusively showed no superiority of balloon-expandable stents over angioplasty[25-29]—a disappointing result that repeated when

Elgiloy-based self-expanding Wallstents failed to provide superior results to angioplasty,[30,31] and yet again when early stent-graft implantations failed to improve patency over angioplasty.[32,33] Common to all these early devices were rigid stent design and abrupt edge construction that led to stent fractures, thromboses, and early restenosis at the ends of the devices. As the search for a better device continued, indications for stent placement seemed forever confined to angioplasty failures only.

Atherectomy
In recent years there have been improvements in percutaneous atherectomy technology, including plaque excision and laser plaque ablation. These techniques purport to improve recanalization rates of chronic total occlusion, reduce the length of the artery stented, and improve results in diseased vessels that cannot be stented by virtue of their small caliber or hostile location. Although these devices were intended to replace angioplasty and stents, experience dictates that they are best used as adjunctive procedures. Occasionally, atherectomy can be used as a stand-alone technique without the use of stents (Fig. 36-1).

Atherectomy Methods: Devices and Their Advantages and Limitations
Plaque excision techniques include the directional atherectomy device, SilverHawk (ev3, Minneapolis, Minn.), orbital atherectomy devices (e.g., CSI Diamond-Back 360 [CSI, Minneapolis, Minn.]), the rotational atherectomy device (e.g., Pathway Jetstream [Pathway Medical Technologies Inc., Kirkland, Wash.]) or the Rotablator device (Boston Scientific, Natick, Mass.), and finally, the laser atherectomy devices, including the Spectranetics Excimer Laser (Spectranetics, Colorado Springs, Colo.).

Of late, the device most commonly used for this purpose is the SilverHawk. This device is a revision of earlier atherectomy devices in that the blade is placed against the target plaque by angulation of the catheter tip, rather than being crushed into the plaque by an eccentric balloon (the method used by the now discredited Simpson atherectomy device). The theoretical advantage of this approach is that there is potentially no barotrauma to the vessel wall. The other major advantage of plaque excision is in avoiding or limiting placement of stents in undesirable locations across joints, as in the common femoral and popliteal arteries (Fig. 36-2).

As with other treatment modalities of FPS, there are limitations to this device. The delivery device is larger and procedure time is longer compared to stent placement. The SilverHawk has a limited ability to clear large densely calcified intraluminal plaques. Although dissection can occur with this device, the dissection flap can be cut and removed. Care must be taken not to cut plaque too aggressively because vessel perforation is a known complication of this device. Another complication associated with excisional atherectomy is distal embolization, particularly when treating long lesions with repeated passes of the device.

Although robust data on restenosis rate of this device are not yet available, several studies have reported clinical outcome in patients with both CLI and claudication. In a prospective registry of 69 patients with CLI, Kandzari et al. used the SilverHawk device for lower extremity

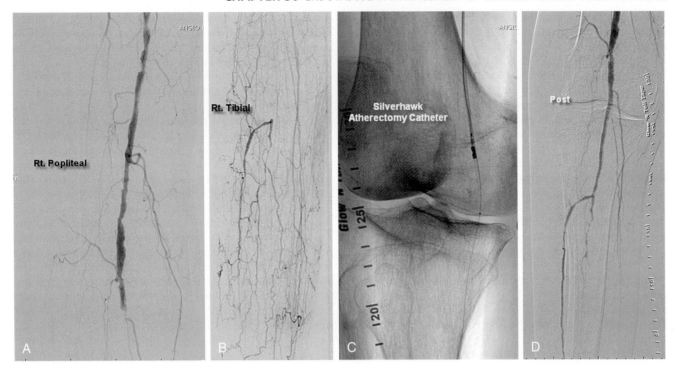

FIGURE 36-1. **A-B,** Arteriograms of right lower extremity of 87-year-old man with rest pain and nonhealing ulceration involving heel and three toes. Note diffuse superficial femoral artery disease with occlusion of popliteal and mid–anterior tibial arteries. **C-D,** After popliteal artery recanalization, vessel was treated by atherectomy alone using SilverHawk MS device, with resumption of flow as shown. Superficial femoral artery and mid–anterior tibial artery were balloon dilated. Patient's rest pain resolved, and ulceration healed; he remained asymptomatic at last follow-up 18 months later.

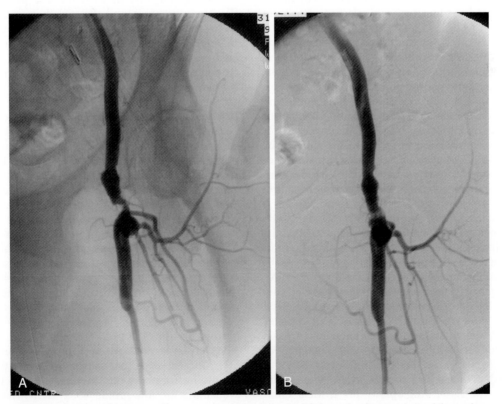

FIGURE 36-2. **A,** Angiogram of 67-year-old woman with recurrent symptoms following left femoral endarterectomy and three subsequent revisions including a femoral/superficial femoral artery bypass. Stenosis of left common femoral artery was resistant to balloon angioplasty, requiring excisional atherectomy using SilverHawk device. **B,** After atherectomy, angiogram shows improved luminal diameter.

revascularization. Procedural success occurred in 99% of cases with a limb salvage rate of 82% at 6 months.[34] Amputation was less extensive than initially planned or avoided altogether in 92% of patients at 30 days and 82% at 6 months. Some physicians remained skeptical of efficacy claims based on registry data, however, and this skepticism increased when the *Wall Street Journal* reported that some physician contributors to the data registry received consultancy fees and stock options from the parent company, FoxHollow Technologies Inc.[35] With time, however, more data have accumulated, and one of the largest series consists of 579 lesions in 275 patients treated by physicians at Columbia University. Primary patency for all lesions at 12 and 18 months was 62.2% and 52.7%, respectively. Secondary patency at 12 and 18 months for all lesions was 80.3% and 75.0%, respectively. Limb salvage was 93.1% at 12 months and 92.4% at 18 months. Interestingly, only 65% of patients had atherectomy only, with the remainder requiring adjunctive angioplasty (75%) or stent placement (25%), again indicating that atherectomy is often not a "stand-alone" procedure. Additionally, there was a significant drop in patency rates after SilverHawk treatment of restenotic versus *de novo* lesions and for long versus short lesions.[36] For those "unstentable" complex lesions in unfavorable locations (long, heavily calcified lesions across joints), one series reported 88% technical success and 69% 1-year primary patency using the SilverHawk.[37]

The newer rotational atherectomy device (Pathway PV system) passes through lesions while cutting a channel with rotating blades. Small series report good technical success even in calcified or otherwise challenging lesions. At 6 and 12 months, 30% and 40% restenosis rates, respectively, were noted by surveillance ultrasound; about half of the reported cases needed adjunctive angioplasty and/or stent placement.[38,39]

Laser Plaque Ablation: Advantages and Limitations

Similar to excisional atherectomy, initial clinical results with laser angioplasty were disappointing. The current generation of "cool tip" lasers uses a different wavelength and delivery method, overcoming the limitations of prior devices. The most common laser system in use today for lower extremity revascularization is manufactured by Spectranetics Inc. (Colorado Springs, Colo.). This excimer laser primarily works through contact photoablation, converting plaque and thrombus to water vapor and carbon dioxide.

Advantages of the current excimer laser catheters include the ability for ablation of clot and plaque (debulking) and a tool for recanalization of chronic total occlusions. Preliminary unconfirmed observations suggest that after recanalization of a chronic total occlusion by hydrophilic wire/catheter technique, passage of the laser appears to clear any clot or unstable plaque, thereby reducing the risk of distal embolization. In its current form, the excimer laser catheter can create only a limited luminal diameter and hence needs adjunctive angioplasty and/or stenting in the majority of FPS cases (Fig. 36-3).

Laser photoablation has been rigorously evaluated in the setting of CLI. The Laser Angioplasty for Critical Limb Ischemia (LACI) phase 2 registry was a prospective multicenter study of 145 patients with CLI (155 limbs with Rutherford category 4 to 6) who were deemed poor surgical

candidates. Poor surgical status was based on an absent target vessel for bypass, absence of a venous conduit, or significant cardiac comorbidity. Straight-line flow to the foot was established in 89% of the limbs. After a follow-up of 6 months, only 9 of the 127 patients who were alive had required major amputation, for a limb salvage rate of 93% among survivors.[40]

Newer versions of the excimer laser catheter are available for wider applications. Data from the CELLO trial (ClirPath Excimer Laser System to Enlarge Luminal Openings) followed 65 claudicants after laser recanalization and adjunctive therapy of 13 occlusions and 52 stenoses (>70%) of the femoral artery ranging from 1 to 15 cm in length. As expected, about 88% of patients required angioplasty and/or stent placement after laser treatment. Ultrasound surveillance showed 59% and 54% patency rates at 6 and 12 months post procedure, respectively. No major adverse events occurred, and all patients experienced relief of claudication symptoms.[41] Time-tested angioplasty and bailout stent placement is, however, certainly less expensive and time-consuming while producing essentially equivalent results (see Table 36-3).

Cryoplasty

The observations of cold-induced apoptosis of endothelial and smooth muscle cells led to the development of cryoplasty in an effort to reduce the restenosis rate after vascular interventions. Cryoplasty achieves apoptosis by producing a hypertonic intracellular environment that triggers programmed cell death. The resultant reduction in the number of smooth muscle cells theoretically reduces restenosis.[42]

The current system used for this purpose (PolarCath [Boston Scientific]) is a balloon catheter capable of cooling the interface between the delivery balloon and arterial wall to −10°C by the delivery of nitrous oxide into the dilation balloon. Balloon inflation and delivery of nitrous oxide is automated and regulated by an inflation unit supplied with the catheters.

The only prospective clinical evaluation of cryoplasty in FPS to date has been a single-arm, multicenter registry of 102 patients.[43] In this study, the mean lesion length was 4.7 ± 2.6 cm, and technical success was achieved in 94% of patients. After a 9-month follow-up, 18% of patients required target lesion revascularization, for a clinical patency of 82%. By ultrasound criteria, a restenosis rate of 30% was observed. Compared to angioplasty alone, some recent reports confirm the reduced rate of dissection with cryoplasty, with one group reporting dissections in only 12% of patients, none of whom required additional intervention.[44] However, these same reports also report disappointing long-term results of cryoplasty, with reintervention required in 42% of patients and 63% and 55% primary patency rates at 6 and 12 months, respectively.[44,45]

Nitinol Stents

A variety of stents have been used to treat lesions of the FPS. Current experience strongly favors the use of self-expanding nitinol stents in this vascular territory.[46] The availability of low-profile long stents has substantially improved the immediate technical outcome of FPS interventions (Fig. 36-4). In early studies of nitinol stents, Mewissen reported an initial success rate of 98% in complex FPS

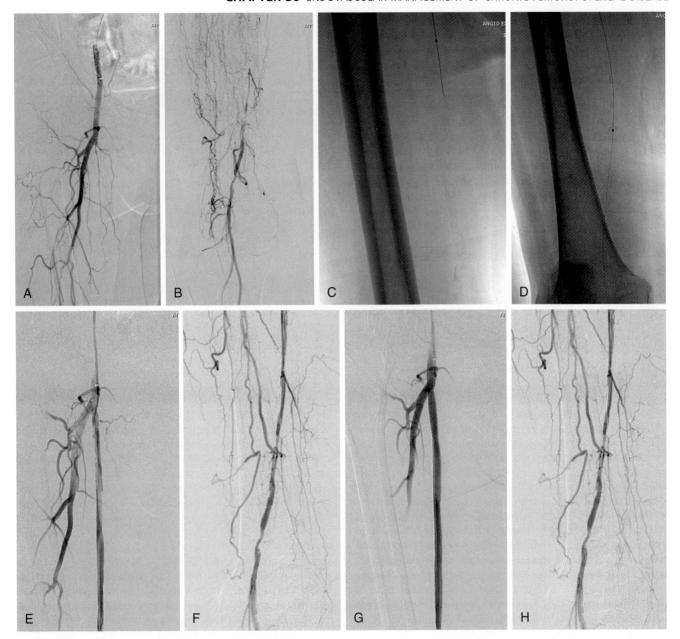

FIGURE 36-3. A, Chronic total occlusion of right superficial femoral artery in 71-year-old man with lifestyle-limiting claudication. **B,** Reconstitution of popliteal artery at level of adductor canal is noted, as is focal stenosis in popliteal artery just above knee. Anterior tibial artery has a high origin from popliteal artery. **C-D,** A cool-tip excimer laser catheter was used as an adjunct to a hydrophilic wire to recanalize occluded artery. Once wire was passed through occlusion, laser was used again as a debulking tool. **E-F,** Flow channel has been established by laser catheter alone. **G-H,** Reestablished lumen was augmented by nitinol self-expanding stents, including stenotic lesion in popliteal artery.

lesions with a mean length of 12.2 cm.[46] Reported patency rates were 76% and 60% at 12 and 24 months, respectively, using the standard duplex velocity criteria.

Despite publication of many single-center studies reporting improved patency of stents in comparison to historical data of angioplasty alone, controversy over the best method of therapy continues. This is mostly fueled by economic considerations of stent costs. A prospective randomized study of 104 patients with relatively long FPS lesions addressed this controversy. Trial subjects were randomized to either angioplasty or primary stenting using nitinol stents. Mean lengths of treated segments were 132 ± 71 mm in the stent group and 127 ± 55 mm in the angioplasty group. At 6 months, the angiographic rate of restenosis was 24% in the stent group and 43% in the angioplasty group (P = .05). At 12 months, duplex restenosis rates were 37% and 63%, respectively (P = .01). This study confirmed the clinical experience of many operators that primary stent placement has a better outcome than angioplasty alone.[47] The RESILIENT I and II trials comparing PTA with optional stenting and primary nitinol stenting alone provided further confirmation of the superiority of stents for FPS disease, with 80% primary patency by duplex ultrasound compared to 38% in the PTA group.[48] Primary nitinol stenting also provided

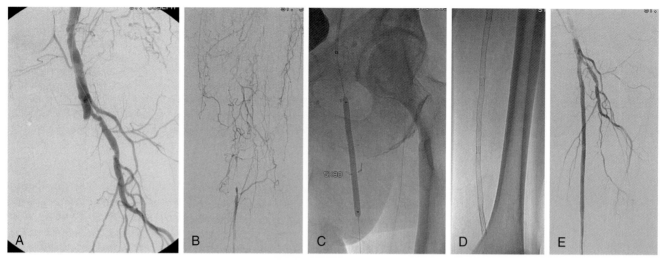

FIGURE 36-4. A-B, Digital subtraction arteriograms of left lower extremity of 76-year-old man with lifestyle-limiting claudication reveal chronic total occlusion of left superficial femoral artery, with reconstitution of suprageniculate popliteal artery. **C-D,** After recanalization, occluded segment was initially balloon dilated and stented using nitinol self-expanding stents. **E,** Angiogram 6 months after recanalization and stenting shows widely patent vessel with continued relief of symptoms.

larger increases in ABI and treadmill walking capacity over the PTA group.[47]

An important consideration in the use of stents in the FPS is the issue of stent fracture, possibly contributing to earlier treatment failure. Scheinert et al. observed that fracture rates and their deleterious consequences vary from one type of stent to another, suggesting that stent properties such as design and surface characteristics play an important role in structural integrity.[49] The anatomic conditions and metal characteristics predisposing to such fractures are currently the subject of intense investigations. It is established that stent fractures increase significantly with length of lesion treated and number of overlapping stents, with fractures noted in 13% of stents positioned in lesions less than 8 cm, compared to over 50% of stents covering lesions exceeding 16 cm.[49] Additionally, stent fractures occur with lower frequency in newer-generation nitinol stent designs as manufacturers adapt these devices to the unique environment of the femoropopliteal artery.

Stent-Grafts

In an effort to improve long-term patency of angioplasty and stents, interest in stent-grafts has been intensified. Early results of covered stents using the Wallgraft and Cragg Endopro systems to treat FPS were disappointing. Improved graft materials, such as expanded polytetrafluoroethylene (ePTFE), which has a lower inflammatory response and thrombogenicity compared to earlier devices, have emerged as suitable alternatives.

The largest experience in the FPS is with the Viabahn endoprosthesis (W.L. Gore & Associates Inc., Flagstaff, Ariz.). A multicenter prospective registry using the earlier version of this device, Hemobahn, included 80 patients with occlusive FPS lesions and was associated with 79% primary patency at 1 year.[50] More recent single-center studies using the Viabahn have reported similar 1- and 2-year patency of 82% and 77%, respectively.[51,52] In a 6-year study of this device in 57 patients, Fischer et al. reported primary and

secondary patencies of 57% and 80%, respectively, after 3 years and 45% and 69% after 5 years.[53]

Although no studies directly comparing bare stents to stent-grafts exist, Viabahn has been compared with prosthetic bypass grafts in a prospective randomized study.[54] In this report, percutaneous angioplasty plus stent-graft placement was prospectively compared with femoral-to–above knee popliteal artery bypass in 100 limbs (86 patients). After a median of 18 months, no difference in either primary or secondary patency was observed between the two groups. Primary patency at 3, 6, 9, and 12 months of follow-up was 84%, 82%, 75.6%, and 73.5% for the stent-graft group and 90%, 81.8%, 79.7%, and 74.2% for the femoral-popliteal surgical group. Secondary patencies of 83.9% and 83.7% in the stent-graft and bypass groups, respectively, were almost identical. The same authors recently released data on 2-year patency rates for these patients, with equivalent primary patency rates of 63% and 64% for the Viabahn and surgical group, respectively.[55] Early occlusions of stent-grafts in FPS are usually due to technical failures. Ansel et al. describes lack of sufficient anticoagulation, incomplete stent-graft dilation, excessive oversizing leading to graft redundancy, and unrecognized proximal or distal dissections as causes of early failure.[56]

Factors associated with good outcome are similar to angioplasty and bare stenting and include good inflow and outflow vessels, lack of severe calcifications allowing optimal vessel dilation, and adequate antiplatelet therapy. Viabahn stent-graft diameters of 6 or 7 mm also fared better than 5-mm devices, and as expected, patency rates improved for TASC II A or B lesions compared with C or D lesions.[55] To easily pass the delivery catheters of stent-grafts through occlusion or stenoses of the FPS, predilation is highly desirable. In cases of chronic total occlusion of any segment of the vessel, predilation is indeed mandatory. If more than one device is necessary, an overlap of approximately 1 cm is recommended.

In treating patients with FPS disease using stent-grafts, the risk/benefit ratio of covering collateral vessels must be

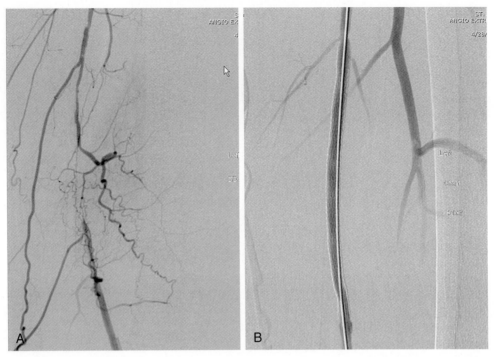

FIGURE 36-5. A, Left lower extremity arteriogram of 38-year-old man with long history of coronary and peripheral vascular disease reveals chronic occlusion of mid–superficial femoral artery. Multiple collateral vessels are noted around occluded segment. **B,** Occluded segment was recanalized and treated with Viabahn stent-graft. Device was placed over inflow collaterals distally. Repeat arteriogram shows decompression of proximal collaterals and coverage of distal one.

carefully weighed. Deploying these devices over long segments, especially more distally, may compromise the reentry point of some important collateral vessels (Fig. 36-5). Whether this loss of potential collateral circulation has a significant deleterious effect is not yet known.

The major advantage of Viabahn over the current generation of metallic stents is its flexibility and relative resistance to fracture. This makes it particularly suitable for placement in the distal FPS and behind-the-knee popliteal artery (Fig. 36-6). Its main disadvantages include the large delivery catheter and blockage of any potential collateral circulation, as described. An ongoing trial, VIBRANT, will compare bare nitinol stents to stent-grafts for long-segment femoropopliteal occlusive disease. Preliminary 6-month data in 148 patients indicate equivalent safety profiles between the devices and no differences in primary patency or freedom from target limb revascularization.[57] A new trial (VIPER) is designed to evaluate whether the redesigned Viabahn stent-graft with heparin coating and smoother edges can outperform uncovered nitinol stents in FPS occlusive disease.

Drug-Eluting Stents

Drug-eluting stents have been successful in reducing restenosis rates in the coronary circulation, so their application may also improve patency rates in the peripheral circulation in general and in FPS in particular. The first study to address this issue in FPS disease was the SIROCCO I trial, in which 57 patients with obstructive disease of the SFA were randomized to either a bare metal stent or a drug-eluting self-expanding nitinol stent.[58] Mean lesion length was 81.5 ± 41.2 mm, with 66.7% of patients having total

occlusion of the lesion. After a 6-month follow-up, the binary restenosis rates were 0% and 7.7%, respectively, in the drug-eluting and bare metal stent groups ($P = .49$). There were no statistically significant differences in late lumen loss and in-stent mean lumen diameter at 6 months. In a follow-up study, Duda et al. followed the 93 patients enrolled in both the SIROCCO I and II trials and reported similar restenosis rates of 22.9% (drug-eluting stent) and 21.1% (bare metal stent) after 24 months.[59] The restenosis rate in the bare metal stent group was unexpectedly low, and hence no difference was observed between the two treatment groups.

Although the results of the SIROCCO trial cooled initial enthusiasm about the use of drug-eluting stents in lower extremity arteries, subsequent studies have been undertaken using different drug and stent platforms. Results of these studies are pending. Newer directions include use of an everolimus-coated stent (STRIDES trial) or a paclitaxel-coated stent (ZILVER trial).

PHARMACOTHERAPY DURING AND AFTER INTERVENTION

Antithrombotic and antiplatelet agents prevent acute thrombosis and adverse ischemic events,[16] and use of heparin during vascular interventions is a well-established practice. The efficacy of anticoagulation is assessed by measurement of activated coagulation time. In most procedures in which anticoagulation is necessary, an activated coagulation time of 250 seconds or more is the optimal target. Heparin is an indirect thrombin inhibitor with nonspecific binding to serine proteases in plasma and

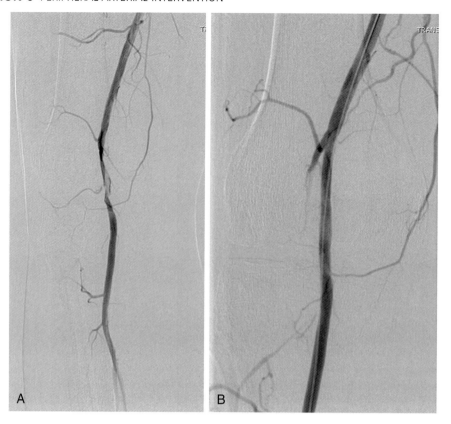

FIGURE 36-6. A, Angiogram of 65-year-old man who underwent iliofemoropopliteal embolectomy for acute limb ischemia 1 day earlier. Flow-limiting dissection is noted in popliteal artery, likely caused by embolectomy catheter. **B,** Because of its flexibility, a Viabahn stent-graft was used to treat dissected popliteal artery, with resumption of unobstructed flow.

endothelial cells. This and other factors may lead to nonlinear pharmacokinetics of heparin (nonuniform response to heparin). For this reason, many practitioners have switched to the use of the direct thrombin inhibitor bivalirudin. In our practice, we use bivalirudin instead of heparin in complex interventions and during carotid stenting. Bivalirudin has been shown to be safer than heparin in terms of hemorrhagic complications and just as effective as heparin plus antiplatelet therapy during coronary interventions.[60] Its safety and efficacy have also been established in peripheral interventions.[61]

Platelets play an important role in the development and propagation of clot. Antiplatelet agents include aspirin, thienopyridines (clopidogrel and ticlopidine), and glycoprotein (GP) IIb/IIIa receptor inhibitors. If it is not contraindicated, aspirin should be routinely used before and after the procedure in all patients undergoing FPS interventions. Evidence in favor of aspirin administration for prevention of myocardial infarction, stroke, and thromboembolic peripheral vascular ischemic events in at-risk patients is extensive.[62]

Thienopyridine derivatives, such as clopidogrel and ticlopidine, in combination with aspirin have been shown to be highly effective in reducing coronary stent thrombosis.[63] Clopidogrel is preferred to ticlopidine, owing to its better safety profile. A loading dose of 300 mg can be administered before the procedure, with a daily maintenance dose of 75 mg. More rapid platelet inhibition can be achieved by giving a loading dose of 600 mg of clopidogrel, reducing the effective inhibition time from 6 to 2 hours. Dual therapy with aspirin and clopidogrel has been shown to reduce the risk of future cardiovascular events over aspirin monotherapy alone.[64] For this reason, most practitioners prescribe dual antiplatelet therapy after peripheral interventions as well. It should be noted that dual therapy increases the incidence of non–life-threatening bleeding from 1.3% (monotherapy) to 2.1% ($P < .001$).

GP IIb/IIIa receptor inhibitors are effective platelet inhibitors with proven efficacy in the coronary circulation. Their use in peripheral vascular disease, however, has not been well studied, so there are no clear indications for their use. In our laboratory, we use this class of antiplatelet agents if acute intraprocedural thrombus is noted at the site of intervention. Their use can also be justified in patients with aspirin and clopidogrel resistance who are undergoing complex interventions for CLI.

Summary

Treatment of FPS disease must include institution of therapies for the causes of disease as well as correction of anatomic obstruction to flow. Reduction of long-term risk of cardiovascular morbidity and mortality is an integral part of the overall treatment strategy for patients with peripheral vascular disease.

Given the abundance of available treatment modalities for these patients, the need for revascularization and method of therapy have to be strictly based on available evidence. In considering such evidence, however, it should be noted that conduit patency should not be the sole measure of outcome. Other important factors in making such determinations must include the morbidity, mortality, and impact on a patient's quality of life.

KEY POINTS

- Peripheral arterial disease (PAD) is a common condition occurring in 15% to 20% of individuals older than 70 years of age, with manifestations ranging from asymptomatic disease to gangrene.

- Appropriate conservative treatment for less symptomatic intermittent claudication (IC) includes reduction of risk factors, exercise therapy, and oral cilostazol therapy.

- Surgical or endovascular treatment is reserved for patients with lifestyle-limiting IC not responding to conservative measures, or for patients with critical limb ischemia (CLI).

- TASC II classification dictates appropriate interventions, with endovascular treatment reserved for class A and B disease and class C patients deemed poor surgical candidates. Most class C or D disease requires surgical bypass.

- The highly muscular FPS is subject to considerable torque and external forces that challenge the capabilities of many available devices. Treatments such as cryoplasty, atherectomy, and bare metal stenting offer few advantages over inexpensive balloon angioplasty and fall far short of the surgical gold standard of the above-knee femoropopliteal bypass graft and its associated 70% to 80% primary patency rate at 3 years.

- Current endovascular care for the FPS includes balloon angioplasty with "bailout" nitinol stent placement, although ongoing trials may shift this treatment to primary stent or stent-graft placement. Atherectomy devices have utility in treating lesions where stents perform poorly (small arteries or across joints). Long or complex lesions respond best to stents or stent-grafts.

- Drug-eluting stents, which confer excellent long-term patency in the coronary arteries, provide no similar benefits in the FPS when compared with nitinol stents.

▶ SUGGESTED READINGS

Lin PH, Weakly SM, Kougias P. How to interpret data from the superficial femoral artery stenting trials and registries. Semin Vasc Surg 2010; 23:138–47.

Schillinger M, Sabeti S, Loewe C. Balloon angioplasty versus implantation of nitinol stents in the superficial femoral artery. N Engl J Med 2006;354:1879–88.

The complete reference list is available online at www.expertconsult.com.

CHAPTER 37

Infrapopliteal Revascularization

Marc Sapoval, Massimiliano di Primio, Olivier Pellerin, Thierry Carrères, and Pierre-Yves Laffy

In most countries, critical limb ischemia (CLI) has an incidence estimated to be 50 to 100 per 100,000 every year. CLI has a high mortality and morbidity rate and consumes important health and social care resources.[1,2] Aging of the population, increasing incidence of diabetes and renal failure, and limitations in the ability to reduce tobacco consumption explain the high likelihood of increased incidence in the near future. Treatment options include amputation, surgical or endovascular revascularization, and novel techniques of arteriogenesis or angiogenesis using stem cell or gene transfer. Amputation should be avoided as much as possible because it carries its own risk of complications and increased mortality.

Bypass surgery requires good-quality saphenous veins (not always present) and routine ultrasound-guided graft surveillance.[3] The optimal approach should be selected according to multidisciplinary consensus and is generally based on local and general clinical factors, high-quality anatomic workup, and experience. As stated in the TransAtlantic Inter-Society Consensus (TASC) document in 2000[1] and confirmed by the recent results of the BASIL trial,[4] the endovascular approach is generally regarded as the initial treatment of choice.

INDICATIONS

Based on current evidence, the indication for below-the-knee (BTK) angioplasty is limited to patients presenting with chronic CLI as defined in the TASC consensus document.[1] Indications for BTK angioplasty are based on clinical assessment of the patient and evaluation of the extent of arterial disease. Revascularization is the only method that will prevent amputation and prolong life. These patients are at high risk for limb loss and other vascular events like stroke and myocardial infarction (MI). Studies have shown that 25% of patients who cannot be revascularized will die within 1 year after the initial diagnosis of CLI.[5,6]

Clinical examination should follow a sequential approach: (1) documentation of the quality of lower limb pulses, (2) assessment of the skin surface and ankle pressures (should include toe pressure in diabetic patients [critical level < 50 mmHg], and (3) overall evaluation of the patient's general status (renal function, cardiac and carotid evaluation). Also important is the patient's social environment because chronic care will be needed in all cases. An appropriate link to a postoperative care network to ensure appropriate global management and nursing is key to optimal clinical management.

Next is appropriate imaging, which should be performed by well-trained radiologic personnel in a hospital environment.

With the endovascular approach, many patients can have successful reestablishment of improved flow down to the foot and healing of any ulcers. Stents may improve the results of angioplasty, but an important breakthrough has been the use of subintimal recanalization, which dramatically increases the number of patients who can be helped by the endovascular approach.

CONTRAINDICATIONS

Contraindications to revascularization are rare. This is because endovascular techniques are less invasive and can be undertaken in patients who cannot undergo open repair. However, a patent distal vessel (whether in the lower leg or foot) is an essential prerequisite before an attempt at revascularization should be considered. In patients with CLI who have no patent distal target vessel to justify an attempt at recanalization, work is ongoing looking at the potential for other methods to improve distal arterial perfusion, such as angiogenesis using stem cell therapy or gene transfer. However, beneficial results from clinical evaluation in patients are awaited.

In patients with distal limb infection, urgent amputation should be performed to avoid septicemia and other systemic complications.

EQUIPMENT

Imaging

Both noninvasive and invasive imaging techniques are of utmost importance before considering an endovascular or surgical approach.

The initial workup should be by color duplex ultrasound imaging, which can provide (in expert hands) essential anatomic and hemodynamic information. However, the results of duplex ultrasound are variable at the BTK level, so for evaluation of the BTK circulation, many centers use computed tomographic angiography (CTA) or magnetic resonance angiography (MRA).

MRA has several advantages that are well recognized, but it is limited by the possibility of claustrophobia and other well-known contraindications. MRA for the demonstration of BTK lesions has a sensitivity of about 93%, and with recent technical refinements (venous occlusion cuff, parallel imaging), the results should further improve.[7,8]

Multidetector CTA (MDCTA) is now rivaling digital subtraction angiography (DSA) in the quality of imaging sensitivity and specificity.[9] MDCTA requires iodinated contrast medium, but careful hydration can overcome most of the problems related to nephrotoxicity. A significant limitation is analysis of small and calcified vessels. The results of high-quality MRA and CTA for the diagnosis of BTK disease are broadly comparable.

The gold standard for imaging BTK circulation is DSA, which has become easier to perform thanks to the development of smaller-caliber diagnostic catheters and less toxic iodinated contrast media. A unifemoral approach, where only the ipsilateral femoral artery is punctured and subsequent angiography limited to the symptomatic leg, requires substantially less contrast medium than required for classic bilateral angiography. Patients taking metformin or other biguanides should undergo interruption of these medications for at least 48 hours after DSA, with reintroduction only after verification of unimpaired creatinine clearance (European Society of Urological Radiology guidelines).[10] In practice, puncture of the ipsilateral common femoral artery (CFA) with a Teflon needle and injection of less than 60 mL of a contrast agent can provide adequate images of the lower limb arterial supply. Delayed images with selective injections, appropriate pixel shifting, and masking are also key elements to allow high-quality images.

Endovascular Revascularization

Equipment needed for endovascular revascularization includes:

1. Arterial puncture needle:
   a. Metallic 18-gauge needle.
   b. Teflon 18-gauge needle.
   c. 21-gauge micropuncture needle.
2. Catheters:
   a. To assist in the crossover technique: pigtail or Cobra, sometimes internal mammary catheter.
   b. To assist in catheterizing the origin of the superficial femoral artery (SFA): any catheter with an angulated tip (e.g., Bolia Minicath [Terumo Medical Corp., Somerset, N.J.], Vanshi 2 or 3 [Cook Medical, Bloomington, Ind.] Van Andel catheter for subintimal use [Cook Medical]).
3. Sheath:
   a. Antegrade approach: 4F or 6F (Terumo): 10, 25, or 40 cm long.
   b. Crossover: first choice is KSAW-5.0 (Cook Medical) with a removable Y-connector that can be replaced with a hemostatic valve. The Shuttle-SL flexor sheath (up to 80 cm) (Cook Medical) is also useful, as is the Destination sheath 5F to 6F (Terumo).
4. Guidewires:
   a. Intraluminal recanalization: first choice is the Pilot 200 (Abbott Vascular, Santa Clara, Calif.). Other dedicated 0.014-inch wires such as the guide approach CTO (chronic total occlusion) (Cook Medical), Winn (Abbott Vascular), and V14 (Boston Scientific, Natick, Mass.). Coronary CTO 0.014-inch wires such as PT Graphix (Boston Scientific) and Choice PT (Boston Scientific) can be helpful in selected cases.
   b. Subintimal recanalization: hydrophilic 0.035-inch J and straight (stiff in some cases) (Terumo) and previously mentioned 0.014-inch wires advanced in a loop shape.
   c. 0.014-inch wires for calcified occlusions (Cross-it [Abbott Laboratories, Abbott Park, Ill.]; Pilot intermediate [Guidant, Santa Ana, Calif.]).
5. Contrast media (low-osmolar contrast media preferred because of frequent renal failure in these patients): Xenetix 320 (Roissy, France) or Visipaque 320 (GE Healthcare Inc, Princeton, N.J.).
6. Balloons:
   a. Size 0.014- or 0.018-inch coaxial balloons are preferable because they allow better crossability of calcified lesions (lower profile). Small (1.25 or 2 mm) balloons can be used to predilate difficult lesions. Short coronary balloons have better lesion crossability (Ryujin [Terumo]).
   b. Size 0.035-inch balloons are preferred in subintimal angioplasty because they provide better pushability and allow progressive dilation by very short iterative inflation/deflation.
   c. High-pressure (up to 30 atm) balloons (Dorado [Bard Peripheral Vascular, Tempe, Ariz.]) are useful to overcome recoil in subintimal recanalization.
   d. 0.035-inch ReKross Catheter (Bard PV) is useful in a very tight subintimal space.
7. Stents:
   a. Self-expandable dedicated stents: Xpert (Abbott Vascular) self-expandable thin-strut nitinol stent, Maris Deep (Medtronic Inc., Minneapolis, Minn.) thin-strut nitinol stent, Astron Pulsar (Biotronik, Bulack, Switzerland).
   b. Coronary balloon expandable stents: PRO-Kinetic explorer (Biotronik, Berlin, Germany), cobalt chromium (CoCr) and passive coating (silicon carbide), diameter 2.0-5.0 mm, length 8-40 mm.
   c. Dedicated balloon-expandable stents: Chromis Deep (Medtronic Inc.) CoCr stent up to 8 cm in length, Inperia (Maquet, Orleans, France) (Not available in the U.S.).

TECHNIQUE

Anatomy and Approaches

In general, when performing BTK interventions, the ipsilateral antegrade approach should be used to enable direct access to the BTK circulation. According to the level of bifurcation of the CFA, antegrade puncture may be easy or very difficult. When the CFA is short or the patient is obese, antegrade puncture may be technically challenging. Ultrasound-guided puncture is very useful to enable successful and rapid antegrade femoral artery puncture. In obese patients or if the common femoral bifurcation is high, the SFA can be punctured directly. A contralateral technique is rarely required.

When popliteal puncture is considered, ultrasound guidance is mandatory, and one should remember the relationship of the artery to the nerves in the popliteal fossa.

Technical Aspects

Heparin should be administered (70 units/kg) intraarterially after arterial puncture. A vasodilator should also be administered to prevent spasm in the BTK arteries (e.g., tolazoline in 5-mg doses intraarterially, up to 10 to 15 mg, glyceryl trinitrate in 100-μg bolus injections).

After the intervention, all patients should be treated with aspirin (75-125 mg/day) and clopidogrel (300-mg loading dose and 75 mg/day thereafter until healing of the ulcer or until the relief of rest pain).

Analgesia should be administered during the procedure for patient comfort, to reduce limb movement, and therefore to enhance the chance of technical success. General anesthesia is seldom required but may be used for noncompliant patients.

The usual technique can be summarized in the following steps: arterial puncture, sheath insertion, crossing the lesion with a hydrophilic guidewire, percutaneous transluminal angioplasty (PTA), withdrawal of the balloon (while leaving the guidewire in place), and control angiography. In certain cases, prolonged balloon inflation (3 minutes at 3 atm) can overcome severe dissection without stent placement (Fig. 37-1).

For intraluminal recanalization of the SFA, we usually start with a 0.035-inch metallic straight wire and an angled-tip catheter (Terumo 4/5F Glide or Mallinckrodt), but for BTK complete occlusion, the first choice is a Pilot 200 mounted on a 3-mm balloon for progressive advancement (Fig. 37-2).

For subintimal arterial revascularization, if the lesion is at the origin of the SFA, we perform an ultrasound-guided puncture of the upper part of the CFA, enter the stump of

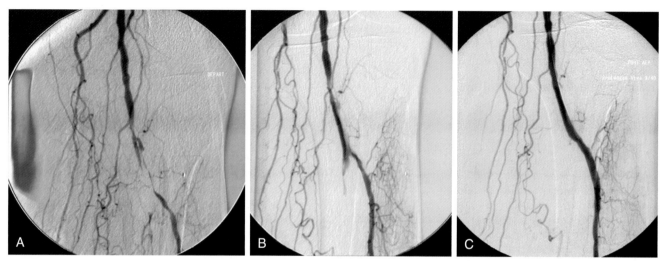

FIGURE 37-1. Images from 74-year-old insulin-dependent diabetic patient with renal failure and ulcer on left foot. **A,** Long stenosis of lower popliteal artery extended down to anterior tibial artery, the only distal vessel. **B,** After percutaneous transluminal angioplasty (0.014-inch wire, 4-mm balloon), there was a severe dissection. **C,** After prolonged low-pressure inflation (3 minutes at 3 atm).

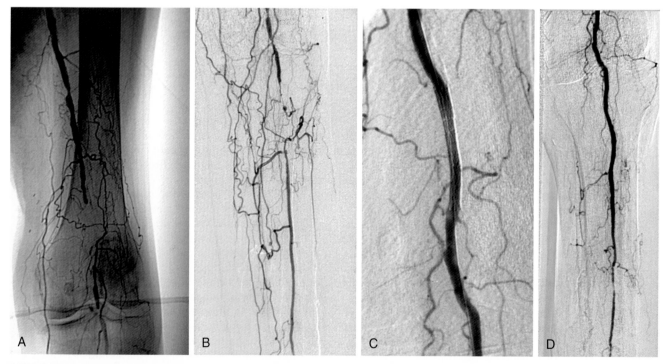

FIGURE 37-2. Images from 82-year-old woman with insulin-dependent diabetes and left foot ulcer. **A,** Diagnostic angiogram shows occlusion of proximal popliteal artery. **B,** Occlusion of distal popliteal artery and tibioperoneal trunk. **C-D,** Result after recanalization, angioplasty with 4-mm balloon, and stent placement for recoil in upper popliteal artery.

the SFA occlusion (in the case of a flush occlusion) or catch (dissect) a plaque above the occlusion, enter the subintimal space with the tip of the catheter, create a loop with the hydrophilic 0.035-inch J-type wire, push the loop, reenter the lumen distal to the occlusion, and perform PTA. Reentry into the true lumen can be difficult and is associated with an approximate failure rate of 20% using the wire-catheter technique (Fig. 37-3).

In case of failure to reenter the lumen, reentry assistive devices such as the Outback device (Cordis Corp., Warren, N.J.) can be used (6F sheath). Alternatively, we favor the double approach (SAFARI [subintimal arterial flossing with antegrade-retrograde intervention] technique) that consists of performing retrograde puncture of a distal vessel (popliteal or tibial vessel) followed by snaring the distal guidewire into a proximal catheter in the subintimal lumen. To minimize the risk of thrombosis, the distal puncture site should not be manually compressed, but we routinely perform a prolonged gentle angioplasty (5 minutes) at the distal vascular access.

Whatever the technique used, the goal is to restore direct flow to the foot if possible using the angiosome-based target vessel revascularization. For this purpose, one should choose the best vessel according to its global aspect and its chance of success of recanalization. Even in cases where this cannot be achieved, reopening a stenosis above a large collateral vessel can be sufficient to achieve clinical success.

Stenting is recommended if PTA fails because of severe dissection or recoil (Fig. 37-4).

The cutting balloon may be used to treat short calcified lesions, although evidence of benefit is limited (Fig. 37-5).

CONTROVERSIES

It is generally recognized that the endovascular approach is the first method to be used in CLI patients. A small subset of patients probably benefit from amputation first (those with severe wound infections and septicemia).

The current controversies are the role of bare metal stents, drug-eluting stents, and drug-eluting balloons. There is accumulating evidence in support of the use of drug-eluting devices in cases of short lesions. For longer lesions, we should know in the next few years whether the initial gain in patency is reflected in clinical benefit in terms of limb salvage and is worthwhile in terms of cost-effectiveness.

There is some controversy regarding the initial imaging strategy for CLI patients.[11] In general, duplex ultrasound is the usual initial study, but in some centers, MRA and/or CTA are used as first imaging methods. Whichever modality is chosen generally reflects local preference and is usually guided by availability of expertise and equipment.

OUTCOMES

Survival and Limb Salvage

The most frequent causes of death in patients with CLI are myocardial infarction, stroke, and cancer. If amputation is required, mortality is increased, as demonstrated by Kalra et al., who recorded a 5-year survival of 60% in the case of limb salvage as compared with 26% in the case of amputation.[5] At the end of the follow-up period in the BASIL trial,

amputation-free survival was 71% and 52% at 1 year and 3 years, respectively, in the angioplasty arm of the trial, with no significant difference between the two arms.

In nonrandomized trials, Wagner and Rager did a 1998 meta-analysis of studies published between 1984 and 1997 and found a limb salvage rate of 86% at 2 years in 1284 limbs.[12] Recent experience reported a 6-month limb salvage rate of 89%[13]; it was 88% at 1 year,[14] 87% at 2 years,[15] and 49% to 65% at 3 years.[16] The CIRSE Foundation Registry reported a 77% limb salvage rate at 6 months for 390 patients.[17]

Stents

Stenting is still a work in progress at this level, but encouraging results have been presented recently. Four different kinds of stents are available: regular coronary stents, carbon-coated stents, drug-eluting stents, and biodegradable stents. Biodegradable stents could be a breakthrough: the stent remains in place for 5 to 6 weeks and then disappears. Peeters et al. reported a clinical patency of 89% and limb salvage of 100% of the limbs treated in a group of 20 patients.[18] Sirolimus-eluting stents have been investigated by Bosiers et al., who report an overall 6-month survival and limb salvage rate of 94.4% and 94%, respectively, in 18 consecutive patients.[19] Carbon-coated stents have also been studied in 51 patients (95 lesions) randomized between provisional stenting and direct stenting. Six-month patency in patients treated with direct stenting was 84%, versus 61% in the PTA group ($P < 05$).[20]

With short lesions, there seems to be increasing evidence that drug-eluting metal stents prolong vessel patency and enable sustained patient improvement, including a reduced number of repeat procedures and a trend toward improved wound healing.[21]

Drug-Eluting Balloons

The rationale of these devices is to reduce neointimal hyperplasia post angioplasty. Schmidt et al. reported restenosis in 27.4% of patients at 3 months using a drug-eluting balloon, which compares favorably with a restenosis rate of 69% at 3 months after standard balloon angioplasty. Moreover, at 1 year, clinical improvement was present in 91.2% of patients treated with the drug-eluting balloon. Randomized trials are required to show whether this difference will lead to prolonged improvement in clinical outcomes.[22]

Quality of Life

There is no health-related quality-of-life questionnaire dedicated to patients with CLI. According to the TASC study, the most acceptable is the SF36 (Short Form Health Survey) document. The Nottingham Health Profile score was used for evaluation at 4 years, and the authors found a clear improvement in energy, emotion, pain, sleep, and mobility in 62 patients.[23] In the Basil trial, quality of life after angioplasty and surgery improved significantly according to results from the SF36 and EQD5D questionnaires. Physical improvement was more important than mental status, but the latter was also improved. Interestingly, the patients' overwhelming concern was to have their pain relieved and

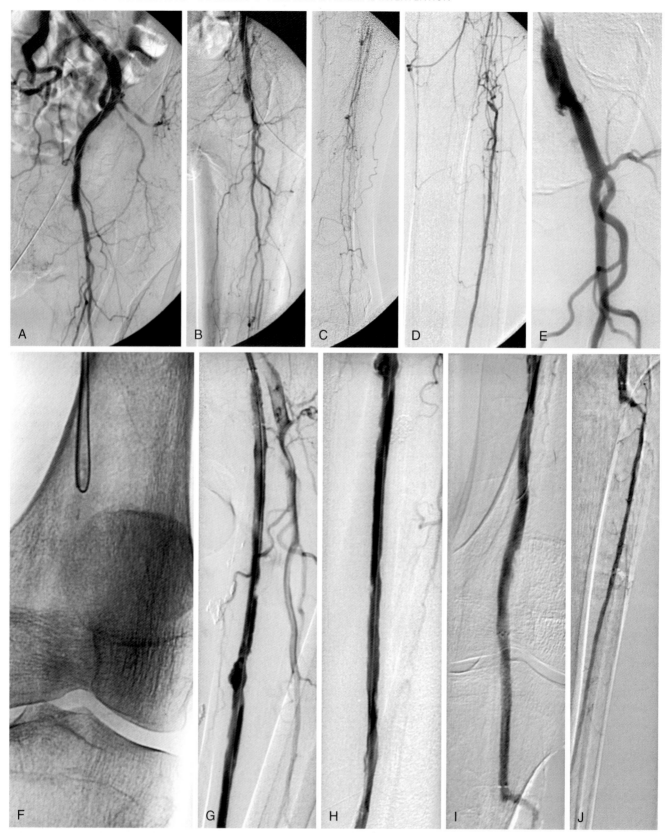

FIGURE 37-3. Images from 62-year-old man who presented with large foot ulcer. **A-D,** Diagnostic angiography shows a flush occlusion of superficial femoral and popliteal arteries, with a small stump and reconstitution of a good anterior tibial artery patent to ankle. **E,** Antegrade femoral puncture was performed, and subintimal space was entered using the Bolia Minicath (Terumo Europe N.V., Leuven, Belgium). **F,** Progression of a J wire down the subintimal space (note small loop). **G-J,** After subintimal angioplasty, there was rapid flow and a regular lumen (a short stent was implanted at ostium of the superficial femoral artery to cover a recoiling plaque).

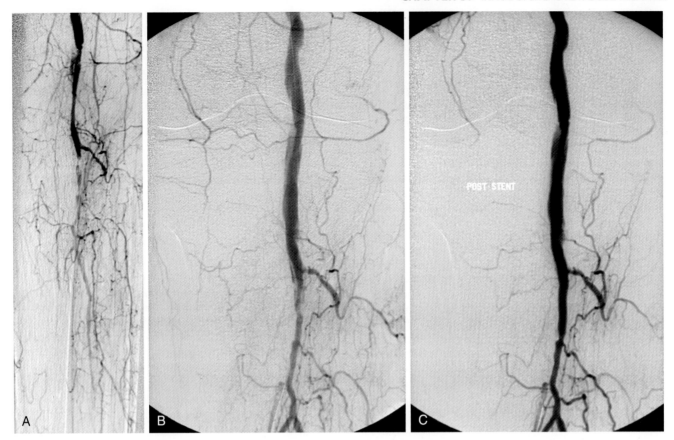

FIGURE 37-4. Short occlusion of tibioperoneal trunk, with angioplasty and stenting for severe dissection. **A,** Occlusion of tibioperoneal trunk. **B,** Recanalization and percutaneous transluminal angioplasty; severe dissection of tibioperoneal trunk. **C,** Appearance after stenting (Inperia 4 × 18 mm Datascope).

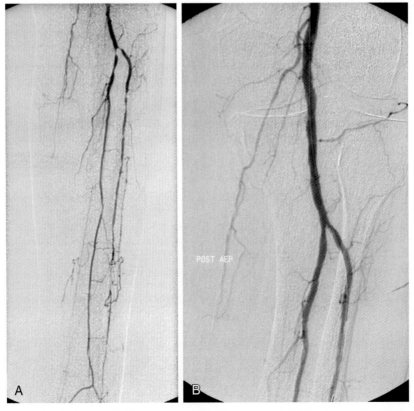

FIGURE 37-5. **A,** Stenosis of anterior tibial artery. **B,** After treatment with 3.5-mm (upper lesion) and 3-mm (lower lesion) cutting balloons, result was very good.

amputation avoided, with less concern in terms of health-related quality of life.

Cost

Cost evaluation and comparison shows that angioplasty is less expensive in the short to midterm than bypass surgery. In 1994, Hunink et al. reported an in-hospital cost of $11,353 ± $7658 for PTA versus $15,059 ± $7313 for bypass.[24] In 2000, Laurilla et al. found a relative cost of PTA over surgery of 41% in 772 patients.[25] In the Basil trial, for the first year the hospital costs associated with a surgery-first strategy were about one third higher than those with an angioplasty-first strategy (£17,419 UK for an angioplasty-first strategy versus £23,322 UK for a bypass-first strategy).[4] This is related to a higher need for high-dependency unit care (23% during the first year vs. 7% in the PTA-first group). When comparing the cost of different strategies, Yost found a dramatic decrease in costs after successful revascularization compared to after amputation ($600/yr vs. $49,000/yr).[26] In the same study, it was estimated that the cost savings if only 25% of amputation could be avoided would be $3 billion per annum in the United States.[26]

The financial implications of using drug-eluting stents in the infrapopliteal arteries has been recently studied by Katsanos et al., who found that use of these devices could be cost-effective.[27]

COMPLICATIONS

These patients have significant cardiorespiratory and renal comorbidity, so any intervention carries its own risk. Most studies show that compared to distal bypass, an endovascular approach is associated with reduced mortality and morbidity. Mortality rates after endovascular treatment are generally 2% to 3% (2.3% in the CIRSE Foundation Registry).[17] In the Basil randomized trial, the 30-day mortality was 5% after bypass and 3% after angioplasty.[4] In the same trial, 56% of patients developed a complication after surgery and 41% after angioplasty, but in reality, among these patients, 20 had no complication after angioplasty but did so after secondary surgery due to a failure of angioplasty. Therefore, the complication rate after angioplasty itself was in reality 32%. The most frequent immediate complications are myocardial infarction and wound infection, followed by urinary and pulmonary infection. Immediate failure of angioplasty (20% in the angioplasty arm of the Basil trial) is usually related to the morphology of the lesions, although the technical expertise of the operator plays a significant role in deciding whether the procedure will succeed or not. It is notable that an initial failure of angioplasty does not compromise the possibility of secondary surgery.

POSTPROCEDURAL AND FOLLOW-UP CARE

All patients should be considered high-risk cardiovascular patients. In the short term, the principal goal is to maintain patency of the treated site and prevent acute complications. In the mid- to long term, the goal is to provide the longest possible period for limb salvage and prevent secondary cardiovascular events.

Immediate monitoring, in addition to puncture site surveillance, should comprise hourly blood pressure measurements, continuous pulse oximetry, and continuous electrocardiography.

Specific wound care to ensure protection of the foot is very important. This will consist of débridement of dead tissue and local amputation of gangrenous toe(s).

All these patients should be aggressively treated with double antiplatelet treatment, lipid-lowering drugs, and angiotensin-converting enzyme inhibitors. There is no evidence for the need of follow-up imaging if clinical success is maintained.

KEY POINTS

- All patients should undergo diagnostic imaging to assess the possibility of revascularization. The reference method remains digital angiography; duplex ultrasonography is not sufficient to rule out the possibility of performing endovascular intervention.

- All diabetic patients with a foot ulcer should undergo vascular imaging screening to detect any arterial lesion that could be treated.

- To date, revascularization is the only method that prevents amputation and therefore the extension of life.

- Optimal medical treatment is of crucial importance and includes lipid-lowering drugs, antiplatelet therapy, and smoking cessation.

- Gene and stem cell therapy to stimulate angiogenesis are being studied.

▶ **SUGGESTED READINGS**

Adam DJ, Beard JD, Cleveland T, et al. Bypass versus angioplasty in severe ischaemia of the leg (BASIL): multicentre, randomised controlled trial. Lancet 2005;366:1925–34.

Dormandy JA, Rutherford RB. Management of peripheral arterial disease (PAD). TASC Working Group. TransAtlantic Inter-Society Consensus (TASC). J Vasc Surg 2000;31:S1–S296.

Katsanos K, Spiliopoulos S, Krokidis M, et al. Does below-the-knee placement of drug-eluting stents improve clinical outcomes? J Cardiovasc Surg (Torino) 2012;53(2):195–203.

Norgren L, Hiatt WR, Dormandy JA. Inter-Society Consensus for the Management of Peripheral Arterial Disease (TASC II). J Vasc Surg 2007;43(Suppl A):1A–116A, S:S5-S67.

The complete reference list is available onine at www.expertconsult.com.

CHAPTER 38
Subintimal Angioplasty

Amman Bolia and Robert S.M. Davies

CLINICAL RELEVANCE

Subintimal angioplasty (SIA) was first introduced in 1987 as a minimally invasive percutaneous technique for the treatment of femoropopliteal occlusive disease in patients with intermittent claudication (IC).[1] Early positive results led to use of the technique for the popliteal artery and trifurcation vessels as well, where it has proved to be invaluable as an alternative to surgical bypass for treating critical limb ischemia (CLI).

Recent results indicate that SIA treatment of femoropopliteal occlusive disease for IC is durable,[2-20] and in chronic CLI it has proved so useful that it has become the first-line treatment in many patients with this condition.[21-35] The treatment has application in long superficial femoral artery (SFA), popliteal, and tibial occlusions and has the ability to reconstitute bifurcations and trifurcations[36] that would otherwise not be possible. Long tibial occlusions extending down to the ankle and below have been treated in cases in which surgery would not be applicable. The technique has made its biggest impact in the treatment of CLI, where reported limb salvage rates are between 80% and 90%.[25,28,29] In patients with IC, secondary patency rates of up to 64% at 5 years have been reported, close to those achieved by surgical bypass.[2]

INDICATIONS

1. Chronic femoropopliteal and tibial occlusions that have become hard, possibly calcified, thus making it impossible for the guidewire to be negotiated through an "intraluminal" approach. A subintimal dissection plane is relatively easy to create in these situations.
2. Long occlusions of the femoropopliteal and tibial arteries can be recanalized through a subintimal channel in cases where it would be difficult to maintain an intraluminal position of the guidewire.
3. An occlusion in an underlying diffusely diseased vessel would make it difficult for the guidewire to traverse the occlusion intraluminally, and hence is an indication for SIA.
4. Previously failed intraluminal attempts at angioplasty may be suitable for a subintimal approach.
5. Flush SFA occlusions in which there may be a very small stump or none at all. An intraluminal approach in these situations is difficult if not impossible.
6. Moderately calcified vessels, which are often difficult to treat by conventional angioplasty but are relatively easily managed with SIA because the wire follows the path of least resistance along the subintimal plane.
7. The presence of a large collateral vessel proximal to an occlusion that lacks a stump, which is necessary to engage the guidewire for transluminal angioplasty. This situation can be dealt with by creating a subintimal dissection above the collateral, thus avoiding persistent wire entry into the collateral.
8. When an arterial perforation occurs during attempted intraluminal crossing of an occlusion, subintimal dissection helps avoid the site of the perforation by negotiating the plane of dissection away from the site of the perforation.[37,38]
9. A common femoral occlusion that extends into the profunda and SFA. Recanalization of both these vessels may be achieved by the subintimal approach, thus reconstituting the bifurcation.
10. A popliteal occlusion that extends into the trifurcation vessels can be treated with SIA whereby the recanalization can be extended into all three runoff vessels, achieving a three-vessel runoff.
11. SIA has a role in recanalization of native SFA occlusions in patients who have undergone femoropopliteal bypass grafting that has subsequently occluded.[39,40] Similarly, tibial occlusions can be recanalized after failure of a femorodistal bypass graft.[41]

CONTRAINDICATIONS

When an occlusion is fresh (<3 months old), subintimal and intraluminal angioplasties are unlikely to be successful because of the softness of the thrombus, which fails to be displaced when the lumen is being reestablished with a balloon. In fact, attempting angioplasty for such lesions increases the risk for embolism because a fresh thrombus is more likely to be disrupted and released downstream.

For more information on imaging for fresh thrombi, please visit the website at www.expertconsult.com.

Although heavy calcification is not a contraindication, it is sometimes difficult to pass through a heavily calcified length of SFA because of failure of forward progression of the catheter or the occurrence of perforation. The presence of fine cylindrical calcification, as seen in renal failure patients, can make SIA a difficult undertaking. It is usually not difficult to initiate a dissection, but this form of calcification can make it very difficult to reenter the true lumen distally. Even when reentry has been achieved, chances of recoil due to the calcification are fairly high, and this may result in an unfavorable outcome.

Finally, calcified common femoral artery (CFA) occlusions are difficult to cross because such occlusions have to be approached from the contralateral side. The contralateral approach does not allow sufficient push to cross the occlusion, and in any case, the bulk of the calcification present does not permit a satisfactory and durable channel to be created.

EQUIPMENT

Angiography equipment with high-quality digital subtraction and roadmap facilities using a 40-cm image intensifier is desirable.

The technique requires minimal materials. A standard Teflon-coated 0.035-inch, 180-cm long guidewire is used for entry into the artery through the needle. Once entry has been achieved and a catheter introduced, the wire is substituted for a hydrophilic wire (Terumo) in either standard or stiff format, depending on the nature of the lesion. Once again, these wires are 0.035 inch in diameter and 180 cm long, with a curved tip and a 3-cm floppy end.

The most widely used catheter, particularly for flush occlusions where there is no available stump or only a small stump, is the 4F short-angled catheter (Bolia Mini-cath [Terumo Medical Corp., Tokyo, Japan]), which comes in a 20-cm length with a 30- or 60-degree curved tip. Similar shaped catheters (e.g., Bernstein [Boston Scientific, Natick, Mass.]), vertebral, or even a cobra-shaped Glidecath (Terumo Medical Corp., Somerset, N.J.) may be used for this purpose. However, the advantage of the Bolia Mini-cath is twofold: (1) being 4F and short in length, it facilitates entry into the CFA when there is only a short length of wire engaged within the vessel; (2) it is easier to handle and manipulate than longer catheters, particularly important when entering the origin of the SFA or initiating a dissection at this level through an ipsilateral antegrade CFA puncture.

The two most useful balloon catheters for use in the infrainguinal segment are 5 mm × 4 cm with a length of 80 cm for the femoropopliteal segment, and 3 mm × 2 cm with a length of 120 cm for infrapopliteal disease. Both these balloon catheters are used in a 5F format, necessary to overcome resistance offered by long length occlusions in the infrainguinal and infrapopliteal segments. A simple inflation device consisting of a 10-mL high-pressure syringe with a flow switch is used for quick inflations and deflations.

Most patients who undergo these procedures are pretreated with aspirin, 75 to 150 mg/day. Heparin, 3000 to 5000 units, is used during the procedure. The vasodilator tolazoline (a nonselective competitive α-adrenergic receptor antagonist) is given intraarterially in a dose of 5 mg before crossing a lesion, and usually 5 mg at the conclusion of the procedure to prevent vasospasm. When vasospasm does occur, glyceryl trinitrate (GTN) is used in 100 μg increments up to a total dose of 500 μg. A GTN patch is also applied to the treated leg to deliver 5 mg of GTN over a 24-hour period to sustain vasodilation in the immediate postprocedure situation, particularly when the subintimal procedure involves infrapopliteal vessels. A closure device is most useful in patients in whom a high puncture has been made. The authors currently prefer Angioseal (St. Jude Medical, Minneapolis, Minn.) unless contraindicated.

TECHNIQUE

Anatomy and Approach

SIA has its main application in the femoropopliteal and tibial arteries. Therefore, the approach to these vessels is via an ipsilateral antegrade puncture unless there is a specific reason to the contrary. If a groin site puncture is not possible because of scarring from previous surgery, infection, a high CFA bifurcation, or because of severe obesity in which an antegrade puncture may be difficult, a crossover or popliteal approach is more appropriate.

For more information on the anatomy and approach to these vessels, please visit the website at www.expertconsult.com.

Technical Aspects

Femoropopliteal Artery Occlusions

After a correct high puncture, a standard Teflon-coated guidewire is advanced into the profunda artery into which the angled 4F short catheter (Bolia Mini-cath) is positioned. An introducer sheath is not recommended for flush occlusions. A diagnostic angiogram is carried out through this catheter position to outline the full length of the occlusion and all the vessels down to the foot. It is important to obtain a detailed diagnostic study so that should a complication occur, such as embolism, one has an exact idea of which vessels were patent preintervention and which vessels have occluded postintervention. Heparin, 3000 to 5000 units, is injected IA as soon as the decision for angioplasty of the artery is made. At the same time, 5 mg of tolazoline is injected to prevent spasm in the distal vessels.

With an appropriate oblique projection (right anterior oblique for a right SFA occlusion) and small puffs of contrast material, the catheter tip is slowly withdrawn from the profunda artery into the CFA. The tip of the catheter is directed away from the profunda to the occluded SFA origin. Then, with the use of a roadmap facility, a curved hydrophilic guidewire is advanced into the origin of the SFA when a small stump is available. If no stump is available, one will usually have an idea of where the origin of the SFA should be, at the level where the profunda artery dips downward away from the line of the CFA as seen on the appropriate oblique projection. A curved hydrophilic guidewire is then run along the junction of the common femoral and profunda arteries. Usually the wire will be seen to engage at the origin of the SFA. Once engagement is achieved, the wire is advanced into the occlusion, and if necessary, the Mini-cath is positioned at the entry point of the SFA to provide support so that the wire can enter the occlusion rather than being pushed away from it. After the wire has entered the occlusion, the Mini-cath is advanced into the occlusion, and the wire is then manipulated into a loop. The loop is advanced 5 to 10 cm further, and when this position is achieved, the purpose of the Mini-cath is over, and it is replaced by a balloon catheter that is usually 5 mm in diameter × 4 cm in length on an 80-cm shaft. The loop is then advanced further, with the balloon catheter following immediately behind it. When the loop stops advancing, the balloon catheter is advanced toward the leading edge of the loop for support, which will allow the loop to be advanced further. The length of the loop is shortened every so often, and when the end of the occlusion is reached, the length of the loop must be 5 cm or less. A little twisting and forward action allows reentry to be achieved in the distal part of the artery, and in most cases this takes place without effort. Should the loop fail to reenter the artery, it is usually due to diffuse disease beyond the end of the occlusion. In such situations, the dissection can be extended further until the disease-free part of the artery is reached, where the loop has its most favorable situation for reentry. There is a natural tendency for the loop to reenter at the junction between the diseased and nondiseased segment of the artery (the line of "demarcation"). It is important at the time of the baseline angiogram to mentally mark the level beyond which one does not want a subintimal channel to extend. For femoropopliteal occlusion, extension of the subintimal tract into the below-knee popliteal artery puts runoff vessel patency at risk unless they are also occluded, and should be avoided. The authors recommend withdrawing the guidewire and reattempting to reenter the true lumen proximally should this occur. Failure to reenter using standard techniques may result in a reentry device being employed (see later discussion).

Once the entire length of the occlusion has been crossed, the balloon is inflated from the distal part to the proximal part of the occlusion. High-pressure (10-12 atm) but short inflations are carried out throughout the length of the occlusion. The balloon is usually inflated twice, once from the distal to proximal part of the occlusion, and then from proximal to distal. The balloon catheter is then positioned beyond the occlusion before the guidewire is taken out. Injection of contrast material through the catheter will confirm rapid flow in the distal vessels beyond the recanalized segment, which is a measure of a successful outcome. The catheter is gradually withdrawn to a level proximal to the recanalized segment, and during withdrawal, small puffs of contrast material are used to ensure the channel is open and flowing. A final angiogram of the newly recanalized segment is carried out. Although the recanalized segment almost invariably appears smooth and disease free, the measure of a successful outcome is usually determined by the speed of flow rather than cosmetic appearances. A completion angiogram of the distal vessels ensures that if any emboli have been released, they will be detected and dealt with appropriately.

At the conclusion of the procedure, a further dose of tolazoline (5 mg) is given to facilitate peripheral vasodilation and reduce peripheral resistance, helping enhance flow through the recanalized segment. Aspirin, if not contraindicated, is prescribed for patients who have undergone successful recanalization, the usual dose being 150 mg daily for 3 months tailored to 75 mg/day thereafter indefinitely. Some authors opt for dual antiplatelet therapy with the addition of clopidogrel (75 mg/day) or ticlopidine (500 mg/day) for 1 month post procedure. This regimen may be of benefit, particularly in those patients with known aspirin resistance.

Tibial Occlusions

Tibial occlusions can also be treated by SIA. Short occlusions are usually easily crossed intraluminally, but SIA is applicable for longer occlusions (>3 cm). The technique for crossing a tibial occlusion is similar to that used in the femoropopliteal segment. Unlike the treatment of tibial stenotic disease, in which a small wire and balloon system is used (0.018 inch and 3.5F), in the case of tibial occlusive disease it is important to use a 0.035-inch guidewire and a balloon catheter with a 5F shaft. The larger guidewire and catheter are needed because when a long tibial occlusion must be crossed (e.g., 30 cm), resistance to the wire-catheter

combination is quite substantial; a larger device ensures enough strength in the system to allow progression of the catheter-wire combination throughout the length of the occlusion. The system can be further strengthened with the use of a stiff hydrophilic guidewire if necessary. The most popular catheter for this procedure is one with a 3-mm diameter, 2-cm long balloon on a 120-cm-long 5F shaft.

Once again, the aim is to form a loop in the hydrophilic guidewire that allows one to cross the entire length of the lesion with minimal risk of perforation. This loop is desirable for achieving dissection throughout the length of the tibial artery as well as reentry into the true lumen distally. Because the intima becomes thinner as the distal arterial tree is approached, it is usually not difficult to reenter the true lumen in the distal tibial artery. However, it is important to keep the length of the loop short so that the softer part (floppy tip) of the guidewire forms the leading edge of the loop and therefore reduces the chance of perforation in these small, delicate vessels. Having crossed the lesion, balloon dilation is performed in a similar manner as for the femoropopliteal segment.

In the case of a long femoropopliteal occlusion with concomitant trifurcation disease and a single vessel runoff, it is of vital importance for true-lumen reentry to occur in the patent crural vessel. This does not necessarily occur using the standard aforementioned technique, since the guidewire will have a natural tendency to take the path of least resistance—which does not always equate to the least-diseased crural vessel. In an attempt to address this potential complication, Spinosa et al. described *subintimal arterial flossing with antegrade-retrograde intervention* (SAFARI).[42] This technique is described in depth elsewhere in the book.

Reentry Devices

Percutaneous subintimal revascularization of chronically occluded femoropopliteal or crural vessels is associated with a reported failure rate of 10% to 20% (Table 38-1). The primary limitation is the failure to reenter the distal true lumen after crossing the occlusion subintimally. Furthermore, true-lumen reentry may be significantly remote from the level of patency, thereby unnecessarily extending the length of subintimal dissection beyond that of the occluded segment. Inadvertent lengthening of the lesion may itself cause complications including loss of patent branches and collaterals distal to the treated occlusion.

These limitations have been addressed in recent years with the use of reentry devices that facilitate true-lumen reentry. The two most commonly used reentry devices are the Outback LTD Reentry Catheter (Cordis Corp., Bridgewater, N.J.) and the Pioneer catheter (Medtronic Inc., Minneapolis, Minn.), recently updated to the Pioneer Plus Catheter PPlus 120.

To date within the English literature, Bausback et al.[12] report the largest experience of using the Outback catheter. They report 118 limbs with femoropopliteal occlusion in which the Outback catheter system was used because of failure to reenter the true lumen using standard techniques. Success was achieved in 108 (91.5%) limbs, with minor bleeding of the target vessel in 5 limbs (5.2%) (Table 38-2).

TABLE 38-1. Summary Data for All Studies with Over 100 Limbs Treated with Subintimal Angioplasty

Study	Study Type	No. of Patients	No. of SIAs	Disease Severity	Lesion Location	Technical Success	Stents Used	Primary Patency (Months)	Primary Assisted Patency (Months)	Secondary Patency (Months)	Limb Salvage (Months)	Survival (Months)
Bausback et al.[12]	Case note review	113	118	Claudication & CLI	Femoropopliteal	107 (91%)	Y	57% (12)	83% (12)	89% (12)	NA	NA
Siablis et al.[11]	Cohort	98	105	Claudication & CLI	Femoropopliteal	96 (91%)	Y	42% (24)	NA	NA	89% (36)	84% (36)
Sidhu et al.[14]	Case note review	120	128	Claudication & CLI	Femoropopliteal	117 (91%)	Y	NA	73% (12)	85% (12)	98% (12)	NA
Setacci et al.[34]	Cohort	145	145	CLI	Femoropopliteal	121 (83%)	Y	70% (12), 34% (36)	NA	77% (12), 43% (36)	88% (12), 49% (36)	NA
Sultan et al.[35]	Cohort	190	206	CLI	Infrainguinal	NA	Y	73% (60)	NA	NA	73% (60) amputation-free survival	79% (60)
Köcher et al.[54]	Case note review	123	133	Claudication & CLI	Femoropopliteal	115 (86%)	Y	58% (12), 50% (24)	NA	NA	81% (12) for CLI	NA
Marks et al.[55]	Cohort	108	116	NA	Femoropopliteal	99 (85%)	Y	59% (12) for technically successful procedures	NA	NA	NA	NA
Scott et al.[15]	Case note review	472	506	Claudication & CLI	Infrainguinal	439 (87%)	Y	45% (12)	NA	76% (12)	75% (36) for CLI	55% (36) for CLI; 84% (36) for claudication
Akesson et al.[33]	Case note review	181	193	>95% CLI	Infrainguinal	148 (77%)	Y	45% (12)	NA	NA	NA	62% patients died at a median of 17 (IQR 3-31) months after SIA
Scott et al.[16]	Case note review	104	105	Claudication & CLI	Femoropopliteal	91 (87%)	Y	31% (36)	NA	44% (36)	78% (36) for CLI	17 patients died at a mean of 23.4 (range 0-46) months after SIA

Study	Study type												
Tartari et al.[56]	Case note review	105	117	CLI	Infrainguinal	92 (84%)	Y	NA	NA	NA	NA	87% (12)	88% (12)
Hynes et al.[32]	Case note review/database review	158	158	CLI	All	158 (100%)	N	>95% (12)	NA	NA	NA	>95% (12)	NA
Trocciola et al.[17]	Registry review	115	121	Claudication & CLI	Femoropopliteal	121 (100%)	Y	72% (12) for CLI; 85% for claudication	NA	NA	NA	91% (12) for CLI	NA
Desgranges et al.[18]	Case note review	96	100	Claudication & CLI	Infrainguinal	88 (88%)	N	61% (24)	69% (24)	NA	NA	78% (24)	85% (24)
Florenes et al.[19]	Cohort	104	116	Claudication	Infrainguinal	101 (87%)	N	NA	64% (60) for technically successful procedures	NA	NA	NA	14 patients died at a median of 41 (range 1-79) months after successful SIA
Laxdal et al.[20]	Registry review	186	88 (43%)	Claudication & CLI	Femoropopliteal	72 (82%)	N	31% (12)	NA	NA	NA	63% (12) for CLI	NA
Lazaris et al.[26]	Case note review	99	112	CLI	Infrainguinal	100 (89%)	N	69% (24)	NA	NA	NA	88% (36)	60% (36)
Laxdal et al.[8]	Case note review	109	124	Claudication & CLI	Femoropopliteal	112 (90%)	N	NA	37% (12)	NA	NA	NA	NA
Tisi et al.[23]	Case note review	148	158	Claudication & CLI	Infrainguinal	135 (85%)	N	27% (12)	NA	33% (12)	NA	84% (24) for CLI	60% (24) for CLI, 97% (24) for claudication
London et al.[5]	Case note review	NA	200	Claudication & CLI	All	159 (80%)	N	58% (36) for technically successful procedures	NA	NA	NA	NA	NA

CLI, Critical limb ischemia; *IQR*, interquartile range; *NA*, not available; *SIA*, subintimal angioplasty.

TABLE 38-2. Summary Data of Studies Reporting Use of Reentry Catheters

Study	Study Type	No. of Limbs	Reentry System (Manufacturer)	Reason for Using Reentry Device	Occlusion Location	Reentry Level	Reentry Success
Airoldi, et al.[57]	Case note review	6	SPOT System (S.I. Therapies, Israel)	Failure of standard technique	SFA	SFA	83%
Bausback, et al.[12]	Case note review	118	Outback LTD (Cordis Corp., Hialeah, Fla.)	Failure of standard technique	Femoropopliteal	SFA/popliteal	91.5%
Shin, et al.[58]	Case note review	52	Outback LTD (Cordis)	Failure of standard technique	Femoropopliteal	Adductor canal (62.5%), AK popliteal (27.1%)	64.5%
Smith et al.[59]	Case note review	51	Outback LTD (Cordis)	Failure of standard technique	SFA	Femoropopliteal	87%
		8	Pioneer (Medtronic Inc., Minneapolis, Minn.)	Failure of standard technique	SFA	Femoropopliteal	100%
Aslam et al.[60]	Case note review	51	Outback LTD (Cordis)	Failure of standard technique	All	NA	96.1%
Al-Ameri et al.[61]	Case note review	13	Pioneer (Medtronic)	Failure of standard technique	CFA/SFA	Femoropopliteal	92%
Beschorner et al.[62]	Case note review	65	Outback LTD (Cordis)	Failure of standard technique	Femoropopliteal	SFA/popliteal	88%
Husmann et al.[63]	Cohort	20	Outback LTD (Cordis)	Failure of standard technique	SFA	SFA/popliteal	95%
Setacci et al.[34]	Cohort	24	Outback LTD (Cordis)	Failure of standard technique	Femoropopliteal	NA	79%
Jacobs et al.[64]	Case note review		Pioneer (Medtronic)	Failure of standard technique	Iliac/femoral	Within 2 cm of lesion	100%
			Outback LTD (Cordis)	Failure of standard technique	Iliac/femoral	Within 2 cm of lesion	100%
Scheinert et al.[65]	Cohort	25	Pioneer (Medtronic)	Failure of standard technique	SFA	NA	100%
Wiesinger et al.[66]	Cohort	10	Outback LTD (Cordis)	Proof-of-concept	Iliac/femoral	Femoropopliteal	50%
Hausegger et al.[67]	Case note review	10	Outback LTD (Cordis)	Failure of standard technique	Femoropopliteal	Femoropopliteal	80%
Saket et al.[68]	Cohort	3	CrossPoint TransAccess catheter (Medtronic Inc., Menlo Park, Calif.)	Failure of standard technique	Femoropopliteal	Femoropopliteal	100%

AK, Above the knee; *CFA,* common femoral artery; *NA,* not available; *SFA,* superficial femoral artery.

For more information on reentry devices, please visit the website at www.expertconsult.com.

CONTROVERSIES

The preferred approach for SIA is an ipsilateral common femoral puncture to treat flush occlusions and all occlusions below this level. However, some advocate a crossover or a popliteal approach. The crossover approach is applicable when either the ipsilateral groin is unavailable (scarring or infection) or the patient is grossly obese and the antegrade approach would be difficult. The crossover approach has its disadvantages. For example, during manipulations, the feel imparted by the guidewire to the operator is reduced, and therefore one's ability to perform delicate manipulations is reduced, as is the ability to push from the contralateral approach, which could be a significant

hindrance with very long and calcified occlusions. Moreover, if an embolic complication occurs, it becomes difficult to perform percutaneous embolectomy, and a contralateral puncture also puts the "good side" at risk from the embolus if it happens to be released on this side during retrieval.

The popliteal approach makes it easier to treat either flush occlusions[7] or occlusions with a large proximal collateral and no entry point (equivalent to a flush occlusion). However, there are some disadvantages. For example, tibial vessel disease cannot be treated at the same time as the SFA lesion without having to make an additional puncture. This is particularly important in patients with CLI, who often have tandem lesions in the femoropopliteal and tibial arteries. Without management of the latter, treatment would be deemed incomplete. Additionally, any embolic complication in which the embolus is located in the midportion of the popliteal artery or below would be impossible to aspirate percutaneously without having to make an additional puncture.

Use of an introducer sheath is the norm for percutaneous interventions. Flush SFA occlusions and disease in the proximal SFA cannot be treated with a sheath in place, because the sheath occupies space in the CFA and makes manipulations difficult. The majority of flush SFA occlusions can be treated successfully without the need to use an introducer sheath.

There is continuing uncertainty regarding the use of selective or routine stenting following subintimal recanalization of femoropopliteal occlusions.

In the authors' view, stenting improves the angiographic appearance and hemodynamics of a suboptimal SIA where flow is seen to be compromised. In these patients, selective stenting would appear to be a reasonable undertaking.

For more information on controversies surrounding SIA, please visit the website at www.expertconsult.com.

OUTCOMES

SIA has a definite learning curve. Our first 200 procedures had a technical success rate of 80%,[5] which increased to 90% in the subsequent 200 cases. Yilmaz et al. reported an initial technical success rate of 83% for the first 30 patients and 100% for the last 30.[6] This learning curve should be borne in mind when assessing the results of SIA from centers with little experience that are reporting results of initial attempts with this technique. London et al. provided the first major report of the technique of SIA in 200 consecutive femoropopliteal artery occlusions with a mean length of 11 cm.[5] The technical success rate was 80%. The actuarial hemodynamic patency rate of technically successful procedures at 12 and 36 months was 71% and 58%, respectively, with the symptomatic patency rate being 73% and 61%, respectively. The majority of reports on the results of SIA quote a primary success rate of between 80% and 90%,[2,6-11,14-16,34] with the latter rate being more likely as experience increases (see Table 38-1).

In terms of patency, the best results thus far have been reported by Flørenes et al. in Oslo and Sultan and Hynes. in Ireland.[2,35] Both these studies report patency rates in excess of 60% at 60 months follow-up. One of the keys to this success has been a comprehensive duplex surveillance program whereby patients have been prospectively assessed not only to determine patency but also to detect any treatable lesions that could be dealt with to improve the secondary patency rate.

SIA has made its biggest impact in CLI because it has a very effective role to play in recanalization of long tibial artery occlusions, the predominant disease in patients with CLI.[21-30] Ingle et al. reported limb salvage rates of 94% at 36 months in patients who had CLI and tibial vessel disease.[29] The study was specifically designed to assess the durability of SIA in tibial vessel recanalization. It is important to stress that occlusion following successful subintimal recanalization does not necessarily correspond with clinical status deterioration. This is particularly advantageous in cases of CLI for which SIA may allow minor limb amputation of wounds or ulcers to heal and provide time for improved collateralization of the diseased arterial segment, thereby eliminating symptom recurrence if the recanalized segment should occlude.

Figures 38-1 through 38-8 show some case examples in which successful outcomes were achieved.

COMPLICATIONS

SIA appears to have a slightly higher incidence of some complications, mainly perforation and embolism. Fortunately, both these situations can be managed percutaneously at the same setting and are very rarely of serious consequence. The overall incidence of patients requiring surgery for a complication is 1% or less.[37,51] Only four main complications of SIA are of any significance: vessel perforation, peripheral embolism, retroperitoneal bleeding after a high puncture, and elastic recoil.

Perforation

Perforation of an occluded segment during SIA appears to be more common than with conventional percutaneous transluminal angioplasty (PTA) and occurs in about 5% of cases. A recent large study showed that perforation was twice as likely to occur during SIA as during PTA.[37] After arterial perforation, an alternative dissection tract is formed and the procedure carried out as usual.[38] This treats the perforation in two ways. First, it diverts the flow of blood along the path of least resistance away from the perforation and more distally into the leg. Second, the atheroma is shifted to the damaged side of the vessel, where it compresses the site of perforation.

If the perforation is large, as assessed by substantial leakage of contrast material into the tissues, particularly in a hypertensive patient, it may be difficult to find an alternative dissection tract. In such situations, an embolization coil is placed immediately above the site of the perforation to recreate the occlusion and stop the flow of blood into the perforation. The majority of these patients are then recalled for a repeat attempt, usually in a few weeks. Experience indicates that most of these patients achieve a successful outcome, and the presence of the embolization coil does not hinder the procedure or affect the outcome.

Perforation may also occur during balloon dilation. In this situation, the perforation is normally large, and therefore a covered stent may have a role in management.

Embolism

An embolic complication occurs in about 5% of patients. The majority of emboli can be removed by percutaneous embolectomy with a large (8F) nontapered catheter and a 50-mL suction syringe. If the embolus is large and fails to attach itself to the embolectomy catheter despite adequate suction, an alternative way of dealing with it is to "push and park."[9] This concept, first described by Higginson,[52,53] becomes very useful when more than one runoff vessel is present. The embolus can be pushed with either the already available nontapered embolectomy catheter or a balloon catheter to advance it into one of the runoff vessels. Because the embolus is likely to advance down a straight line, it usually ends up in the peroneal artery, thus relieving one of the other vessels and allowing flow to continue down to the foot. It is very rare for surgical embolectomy to be required after SIA.

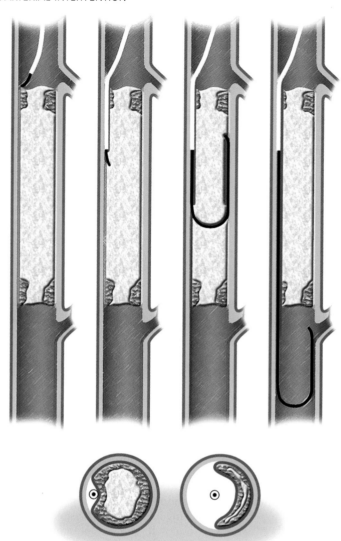

FIGURE 38-1. Dissection is initiated at origin of occlusion, away from any important collaterals, with use of a guidewire protruding from a Van Andel catheter. Forward push of this combination usually results in dissection. Once in the dissection, hydrophilic wire is manipulated into a loop, which is then advanced through length of occlusion, and once again, with help of loop, reentry into lumen is achieved.

Retroperitoneal Hematoma

A flush occlusion of the SFA requires a high antegrade puncture of the CFA. In these situations, the puncture should be high enough to allow manipulations so one can enter the SFA occlusion, but not so high that the risk of retroperitoneal hematoma is increased. The nursing staff caring for the patient should be warned to exercise particular vigilance because of the increased risk of retroperitoneal hemorrhage in high-puncture situations. We are increasingly using closure devices for high punctures. Closure devices also prove useful for patients taking multiple antiplatelet agents, restless patients, and those still receiving therapeutic doses of warfarin or heparin.

Elastic Recoil

The phenomenon of elastic recoil is unfortunately unpredictable. An occlusion in the SFA or femoropopliteal segment may be dissected and crossed with a hydrophilic wire and catheter to achieve reentry in the artery distally. During the dissection maneuver, it is conceivable that damage to collateral vessels can occur. If this happens to the most important distal collateral beyond the occlusion, and subsequently the occluded segment fails to remain open because of elastic recoil despite multiple balloon dilations, the distal limb will receive no blood flow from either the recanalized segment or the collateral. In other words, the flow in the artery beyond the occluded segment becomes static, and an emergency situation has been created. In the past, an emergency bypass would have been required to establish flow in the leg. The operation is usually difficult because by the time the patient undergoes surgery, blood flow to the limb would have been absent for quite some time, and thrombosis of the distal vessels would have resulted. Thus, the operative procedure requires embolectomy in the first instance, followed by thrombolysis and then a bypass graft, all of which usually takes several hours.

More recently, the majority of these situations have been treated successfully by placement of a long self-expanding stent at the site of the occlusion where the recoil is supposed to have been maximal. The incidence of this complication is 1% or less.

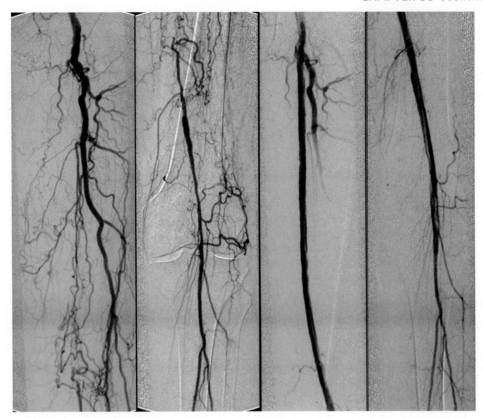

FIGURE 38-2. Long occlusion in the left superficial femoral artery. After successful recanalization, smooth disease-free vessel is noted. Collaterals do not fill, mainly because of preferential flow through recanalized segment.

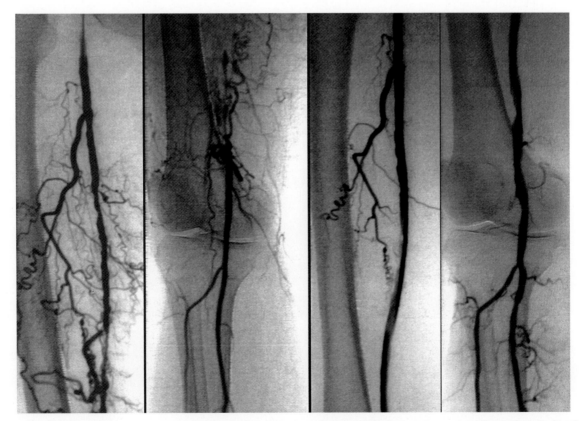

FIGURE 38-3. Long diffuse segment of disease in middle and distal thirds of superficial femoral artery, terminating in occlusion of proximal popliteal artery. Dissection was initiated at origin of diffuse disease then extended throughout diseased and occluded segments. Successful recanalization was achieved.

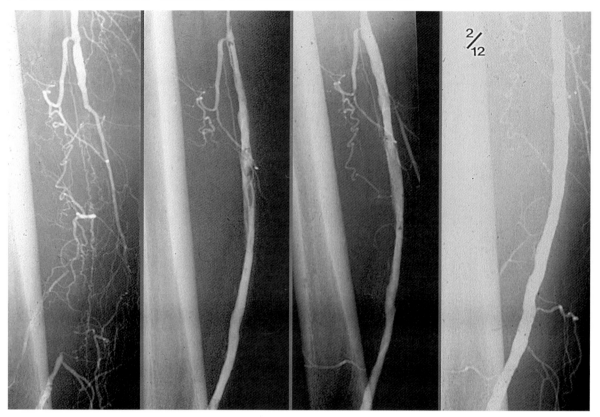

FIGURE 38-4. Long right superficial femoral artery (SFA) occlusion was successfully recanalized, but thrombus was noted in recanalized segment and aspirated percutaneously. At 2 months, recanalized segment has remodeled and shows an excellent and wider lumen throughout SFA. In addition, branch vessels have developed from recanalized segment.

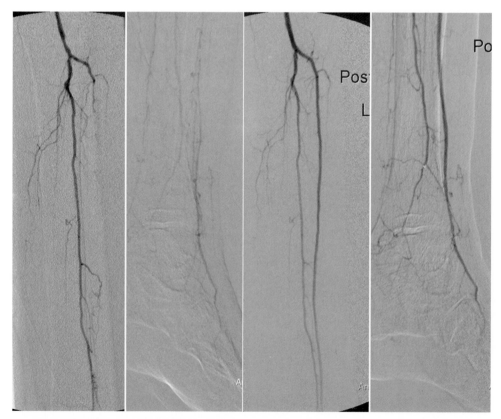

FIGURE 38-5. Disease of popliteal artery trifurcation, with occlusion of left anterior tibial artery and posterior tibial artery. Diseased segments and anterior tibial artery occlusions were successfully treated with angioplasty.

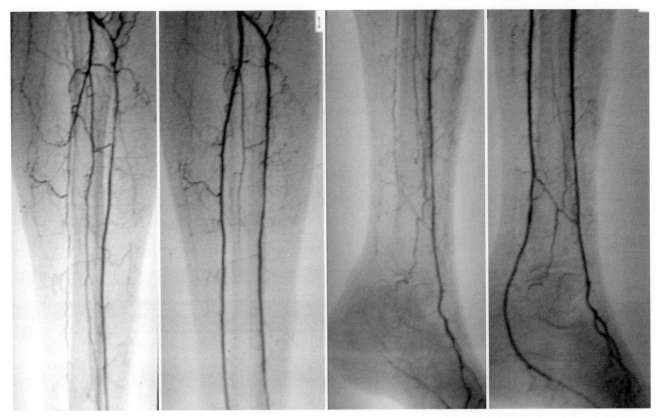

FIGURE 38-6. Some disease is present in proximal anterior tibial artery. Long occlusion of posterior tibial artery extends into lateral plantar arch. Diseased segments and occlusions were successfully treated with angioplasty.

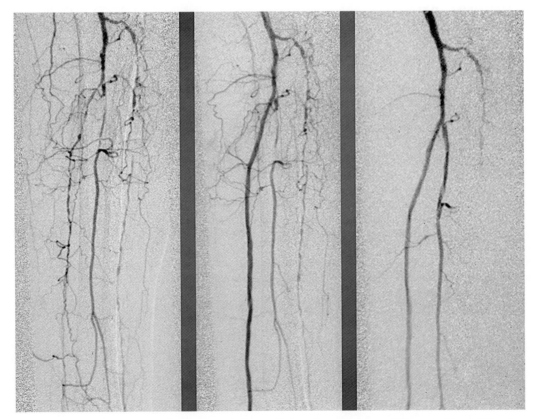

FIGURE 38-7. Long occlusion of left posterior tibial artery and short occlusion of peroneal artery. Tibioperoneal trunk bifurcation was successfully reconstituted.

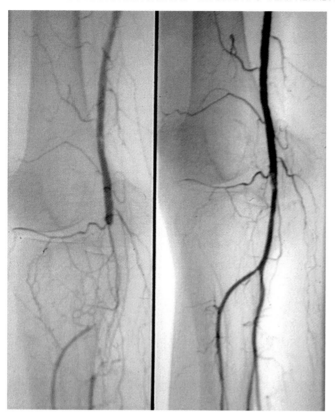

FIGURE 38-8. Occlusion of midportion of popliteal artery extending into anterior tibial and tibioperoneal trunk arteries. Trifurcation was successfully reconstituted.

POSTPROCEDURAL AND FOLLOW-UP CARE

After successful SIA, patients need no special attention beyond that for conventional angioplasty. Most patients are taking aspirin at the start of the procedure, but if not and there are no contraindications, they receive 150 mg/day for at least 3 months. During angioplasty, patients receive 3000 to 5000 units of heparin, but no anticoagulants after the procedure. If the subintimal procedure has involved the tibial vessels, a patch containing 5 mg of GTN released gradually over a period of 24 hours should be given. The patch is normally applied to the treated foot; its aim is to produce sustained vasodilation of the distal vessels, encouraging enhanced flow through any proximal segments that have undergone angioplasty, helping ensure patency in the early postprocedural phase.

If a high puncture has been made, the Angioseal closure device (St. Jude Medical, Minneapolis, Minn.) is preferred.

Close monitoring of the patient's blood pressure and pulse should be ordered. Should blood pressure fall or the pulse rise (or both), retroperitoneal bleeding may be a possibility. In straightforward situations in which a high puncture has not been made, patients may start mobilization after 4 to 6 hours of bed rest.

Patients are monitored at the outpatient clinic for determination of their clinical status. The history will usually reveal any improvement in claudication or CLI. A history and clinical examination are performed as a matter of routine 3 weeks and 3 months following the procedure, after which patients are discharged if all is well. Duplex examination follow-up is the most useful tool for surveillance to detect any stenoses that may be treatable, which would then improve the secondary patency rate. Duplex scanning is recommended at 1, 3, 6, and 12 months after the procedure and then at yearly intervals.

KEY POINTS

- Subintimal angioplasty produces durable results in the femoropopliteal segment for intermittent claudication.
- Subintimal angioplasty is most useful in the treatment of tibial vessels for chronic critical limb ischemia.
- Limb salvage rates of around 90% at 1 year can be expected with subintimal angioplasty.
- Primary success rates of 80% to 90% are achievable, and complications requiring surgery occur in less than 1% of patients.
- Subintimal angioplasty has an extended role in situations in which intraluminal angioplasty would fail.
- Reentry devices may play a roll in improving primary success rates.
- Stents are not used as a matter of routine but are very useful to combat flow-limiting elastic recoil.

▶ SUGGESTED READINGS

Bolia A. Percutaneous intentional extraluminal (subintimal) recanalisation of crural arteries. Eur J Radiol 1998;28:199–204.

Bolia A, Bell PRF. Femoropopliteal and crural artery recanalisation using subintimal angioplasty. Semin Vasc Surg 1995;3:253–64.

Reekers JA, Bolia A. Percutaneous intentional extraluminal (subintimal) recanalisation: how to do it yourself. Eur J Radiol 1998;28:192–8.

The complete reference list is available online at www.expertconsult.com

CHAPTER 39
Management of Extremity Vascular Trauma
Sean R. Dariushnia and Curtis A. Lewis

Vascular injury has two main consequences—hemorrhage and ischemia. Or, in the words of an anonymous Czech surgeon, "Bloody vascular trauma—it's either bleeding too much or it's not bleeding enough."[1] Unrecognized and uncontrolled hemorrhage can rapidly lead to a trauma patient's demise. Unrecognized and untreated ischemia can lead to limb loss, stroke, bowel necrosis, and multiple organ failure. The aim of this chapter is to highlight the fundamentals of peripheral vascular trauma and provide an approach to the diagnosis and management of vascular injury.

Arterial and venous structures are most commonly injured by penetrating trauma, with a much higher incidence in gunshot wounds than for stab injury. Blunt trauma also carries a significant vascular injury rate, and iatrogenic vascular injuries are increasing as radiologic and minimal-access procedures become more commonplace.

Hemorrhage is the prime consequence of vascular injury. Bleeding may be obvious, with visible arterial hemorrhage, or it may be concealed. Classically, concealed arterial hemorrhage may be in the chest, abdomen, and pelvis. Hemorrhage may also be concealed in the soft tissues of the buttock and thigh, and blood from facial fractures may be swallowed and go unnoticed.

Ischemia results from acute interruption of blood flow to a limb or organ. When oxygen supply is inadequate to meet demand, anaerobic metabolism takes over, producing lactic acidosis and activating cellular and humoral inflammatory pathways. If the arterial supply is not reestablished in time, cell death occurs. Skeletal muscle can be rendered ischemic for 3 to 6 hours and still recover function. Peripheral nerves are more sensitive to ischemia, and prolonged neurologic deficit may result from relatively short periods of tissue ischemia.

If arterial supply is restored to ischemic tissue, the sudden release of inflammatory mediators, lactic acid, potassium, and other intracellular material into the circulation can cause profound myocardial depression and generalized vasodilatation and may initiate a systemic inflammatory response.

Vascular trauma can result in serious and potentially fatal consequences. Percutaneous intervention can provide immediate control of hemorrhage and in many cases can be lifesaving.

INDICATIONS

Patterns of Vascular Injury

Laceration with either complete or incomplete vessel transection is the most common form of vascular injury. Hemorrhage tends to be more severe in partially transected vessels because complete transection results in retraction and vasoconstriction of the vessel, limiting or even preventing arterial hemorrhage.

Blunt trauma injures vessels by crushing, distraction, or shearing. This results in contusion to the vessel, which may extend for some distance along its length. An intimal flap may be formed that will lead to thrombosis or dissection and subsequent rupture. Thrombosis may propagate for some distance down the vessel, or there may be embolization to produce effects more distally.

Arterial hemorrhage may continue within a contained hematoma, leading to a pulsatile mass, a pseudoaneurysm. Commonly, distal flow is preserved with false aneurysm formation, and diagnosis may be difficult. Aneurysms are at risk of rupture if undiagnosed, and often present late after the initial injury is forgotten.

If there is injury to an adjacent vein as well as to the artery, an arteriovenous fistula (AVF) can form, which may subsequently lead to rupture or cardiovascular compromise. AVFs may present some time after the initial injury.

Spasm as a unique entity is never the result of trauma and should not be assumed to be the cause of limb ischemia.

Hard Signs of Vascular Injury

- Pulsatile bleeding
- Expanding hematoma
- Absent distal pulses
- Cold, pale limb
- Palpable thrill
- Audible bruit

Soft Signs of Vascular Injury

- Peripheral nerve deficit
- History of moderate hemorrhage at the scene
- Reduced but palpable pulse or an injury in proximity to a major artery
- Unexplained hypotension
- Mechanism and location of injury

EQUIPMENT

For the diagnosis of arterial injury, no special equipment is required other than what is usually found in the radiology department, such as angiography, ultrasound, computed tomography (CT), and the simple sphygmomanometer.

In the operating room, the surgeon is usually able to provide direct access to the artery, but it is easier and safer to use the Seldinger technique to insert a catheter than via an arteriotomy.

TECHNIQUE

The diagnosis of significant vascular injury rests almost entirely on the physical examination. An absence of hard signs of vascular injury does not exclude the presence of vascular trauma. In contrast, the presence of hard signs mandates immediate action.

Diagnostic Tests

Computed Tomographic Angiography

CT scanners are present in nearly every hospital. In trauma centers, 16- and 64-MDCT technology is commonplace and allows for fast image acquisition of the entire body (seconds). Routinely, if the patient presents with polytrauma and is hemodynamically stable, a head, chest, and abdomen/pelvis CT (PAN-SCAN) can be obtained. With multidetector scanners, an extremity computed tomographic angiography (CTA) examination can easily be added to the PAN-SCAN with the same contrast injection, without significantly adding to image acquisition time.[3] Axial images can be viewed immediately after image acquisition and most injuries identified. Postprocessing three-dimensional (3D) reconstructions can provide an easily understandable format obtainable within minutes of the scan and can be of benefit to both the radiologist and nonradiologist clinician, especially the vascular or trauma surgeon (Fig. 39-1).

Arterial findings on CT correspond closely with those findings on conventional angiography. Vascular lacerations with active bleeding on CT are seen as an irregular collection of contrast medium adjacent to the vessel. A pseudoaneurysm may be seen as a rounded collection of contrast contiguous with the vessel. Opacification of a vein adjacent to an artery (when CT images are acquired in the arterial phase) could be related to a traumatic AVF. A short- or long-segment narrowing of the artery on CT could represent dissection, external compression (e.g., perivascular hematoma), or spasm. An intraluminal filling defect in the artery may represent thrombus or dissection.[4]

In some trauma centers, patients with hard signs of vascular injury immediately go to surgery. Hemodynamically stable patients with soft signs of vascular injury and an ankle-brachial index (ABI) below 0.9 are stratified to CTA, the results of which may be used to plan for surgical or interventional radiology intervention.[5] CTA has high accuracy in assessing arterial injury. In the original series comparing CTA with conventional angiography, Foster et al.

stated that CTA demonstrated a 90% sensitivity and 100% specificity for large artery and proximal extremity injury.[3]

Angiography

Angiography remains the gold standard for further investigation and delineation of vascular injury and may be used to treat selected injuries where expertise and technical facilities are available. Proximal control may be possible with an angioplasty catheter before transfer to the operating room. Overall diagnostic accuracy for angiography has been reported as high as 98%.[6]

Arteriography is also cost-effective for vascular injury in asymptomatic penetrating extremity trauma.[7]

Please visit the website at www.expertconsult.com for a full discussion of diagnostic tests.

Categories of Injury

Although traditionally, vascular injuries have been classified as contusion, intimal disruption, puncture, lateral disruption, transection, AVFs, and pseudoaneurysm,[7-9] for the sake of our discussion, a narrower classification will be used:

- Vascular laceration with active bleeding. Typically, these are arterial injuries, because peripheral venous laceration rarely poses a clinical concern.
- Traumatic pseudoaneurysm formation.
- Traumatic AVF formation.
- Vascular occlusion, which can be due to arterial dissection and thrombosis. Venous thrombosis involving large veins (femoral, iliac, axillary, subclavian) may become a concern.
- Foreign body embolization.

Anatomy and Approaches

Vascular Laceration with Active Bleeding, Traumatic Pseudoaneurysm, and Arteriovenous Fistula

In patients with rapidly expanding hematoma, surgical intervention remains the mainstay of therapy. The specific injury is identified and repaired at the time of surgical exploration. This allows management of the injury well within the critical ischemic time. Arteriography is usually unnecessary for the diagnosis.

Endovascular management of hemodynamically stable patients with traumatic vascular lesions has evolved into the standard of care in many trauma centers; many injuries

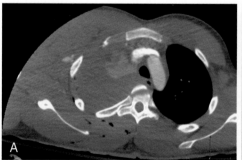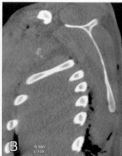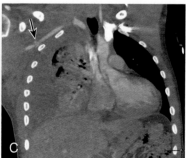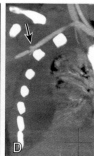

FIGURE 39-1. Traumatic pseudoaneurysm. Patient with history of gunshot wound to right upper extremity. Computed tomographic angiogram was initially obtained. Axial (**A**), sagittal (**B**), and coronal (**C**) thin-slice images demonstrate luminal irregularity and extraluminal contrast involving right axillary artery, consistent with pseudoaneurysm. **D,** Coronal maximum intensity projection (MIP) shows pseudoaneurysm to better advantage.

detected at the time of diagnostic angiography can be treated in the same setting. Even among more surgically accessible vascular injuries, endovascular management may be the better treatment option. A hematoma or pseudoaneurysm may obliterate natural tissue planes, and an AVF with associated regional venous hypertension may complicate surgical dissection.[10] An endovascular approach can allow easier access to the target lesion, limit the morbidity often associated with surgical exploration, and reduce transfusion requirements.

Percutaneous transcatheter embolization is routinely successfully performed for active hemorrhage from traumatic injuries of retroperitoneal vessels associated with pelvic fractures, iatrogenic and posttraumatic hepatic pseudoaneurysms, splenic pseudoaneurysms, and peripheral arterial trauma[11] (Fig. 39-2).

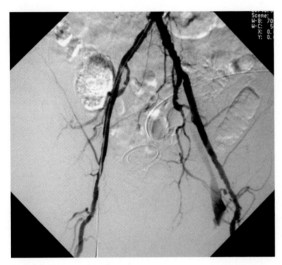

FIGURE 39-2. Penetrating trauma to left groin, with formation of arteriovenous fistula. Note early filling of left common femoral vein.

Endovascular repair of peripheral arterial injuries such as pseudoaneurysms or AVFs is widely used as an alternative treatment to surgery, with good results.[12] The fundamental principle of endovascular repair is exclusion of the lesion (pseudoaneurysm, AVF) from the lumen of the artery by placement of stent-grafts[13] (Figs. 39-3 and 39-4). A disadvantage of this technique is that in addition to sealing the lesion, the stent-graft also excludes any arterial branches covered by the stent-graft. An alternative treatment method for arterial pseudoaneurysms, though in general less satisfactory, involves deployment of an uncovered stent across the lesion, followed by occlusion of the pseudoaneurysm by placement of coils though the mesh of the stent. The coils eventually thrombose the pseudoaneurysm, and the uncovered stent prevents the coils from reentering the arterial lumen.[14]

Pseudoaneurysms of the common femoral artery (CFA) are an infrequent complication after cardiac/interventional catheterization, and are generally treated by ultrasound-guided compression therapy, or more usually by ultrasound-guided percutaneous injection of thrombin.[15-17] Traumatic pseudoaneurysms in other locations can also be treated by thrombin injection.[18]

For illustrations of traumatic pseudoaneurysms and their management see Figures e39-1 and e39-2.

Pseudoaneurysms or AVFs involving peripheral and nonessential small arteries may be treated by coil embolization.[13] This may be performed from the arterial or venous side (Fig. 39-5). In nonessential small peripheral vessels, traumatic AVFs or pseudoaneurysms may be treated by exclusion of the area of injury ("jailing") by embolizing the distal and proximal ends of the injured artery (Fig. 39-6).[19]

Vascular Occlusion

Traumatic arterial occlusion, especially when associated with orthopedic trauma, is associated with an especially poor prognosis. Clearly the important variable is ischemic time since injury. Although not yet proven, the most rapid restoration of flow distally may best be achieved by

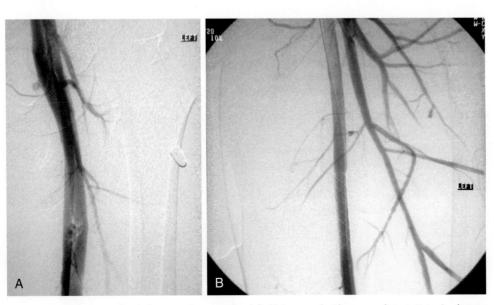

FIGURE 39-3. A-B, Traumatic arteriovenous fistula from gunshot wound to left thigh, treated with a covered stent. Note simultaneous filling of superficial femoral artery and corresponding femoral vein.

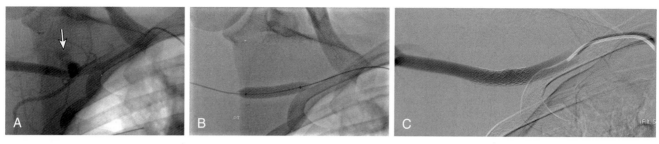

FIGURE 39-4. A, Traumatic pseudoaneurysm (same patient as Fig. 39-1). Patient underwent right upper extremity arteriography that showed a contained rounded collection of contrast adjacent to right axillary artery, consistent with pseudoaneurysm. Covered stent was placed across lesion **(B)** and balloon-expanded, with expected covering of lateral thoracic artery and resultant exclusion of pseudoaneurysm **(C).** Patient did well and required no further intervention.

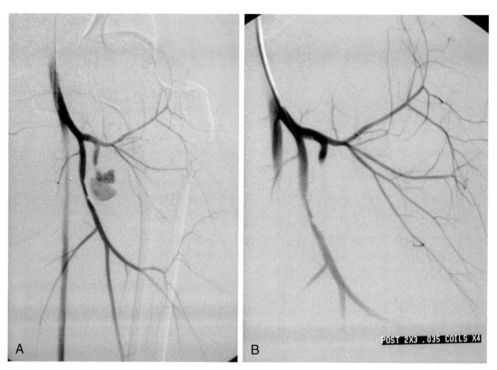

FIGURE 39-5. Coil embolization of a bleeding branch of left profunda femoris artery **(A)**, with immediate hemostasis **(B).**

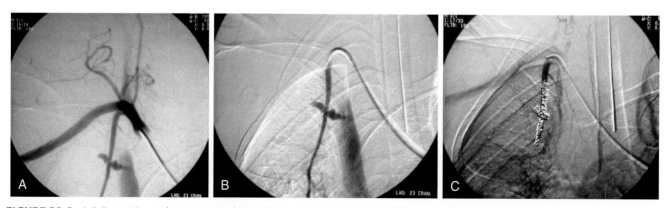

FIGURE 39-6. A-B, Traumatic pseudoaneurysm involving right internal mammary artery, with formation of arteriovenous fistula to adjacent right innominate vein. **C,** After embolization and "jailing" of the pseudoaneurysm, no residual contrast extravasation or flow to venous lumen is seen.

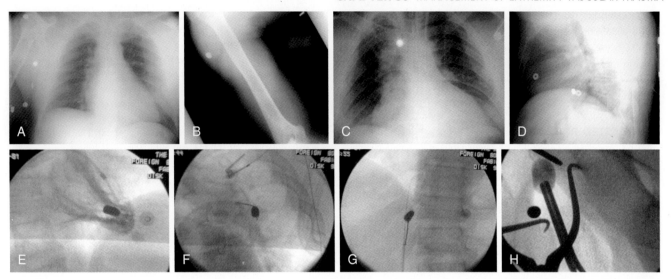

FIGURE 39-7. Bullet embolization to heart. **A,** Initial chest radiograph of gunshot wound injury to right arm reveals a bullet in right arm soft tissue. **B,** Six hours later, a radiograph of right arm did not show bullet. Bullet was seen in right ventricle on posteroanterior **(C)** and lateral **(D)** chest radiographs. Bullet embolized to right pulmonary artery during an attempt at retrieval and was eventually snared. **E-H,** A cutdown was made on right groin to remove bullet.

catheter/guidewire techniques followed by placement of stents or stent-grafts.

Foreign Body Embolization

Foreign body embolism can be traumatic or iatrogenic. Traumatic foreign body emboli are almost always induced by gunshot wounds. Central vessels with a large lumen are the most frequent site of entry. Foreign bodies are transported to the periphery or heart and lungs. Clinical manifestations depend on foreign body size and location. Treatment depends on the patient's clinical signs and size, shape, and location of the foreign body. Symptomatic foreign body embolism and large irregularly shaped foreign bodies should be extracted. When only a small foreign body with no clinical symptoms is present, conservative management is most appropriate (Fig. 39-7).

CONTROVERSIES

Thrombin injection treatment of false aneurysms, particularly after arterial access procedures, remains controversial because in many countries the use of intravascular thrombin is not approved.

OUTCOMES

In most cases of acute trauma, the outcome is determined by factors other than radiologic interventions. However, excellent long-term outcomes are possible after percutaneous interventions, particularly embolization of remote bleeding vessels, coiling of aneurysms, and stent-graft occlusion of false aneurysms and AVFs.[19-22]

Outcomes of thrombin injection involving false aneurysms are discussed elsewhere in this text.

COMPLICATIONS

The most common complications after endovascular interventions for ischemic vascular injuries are compartment syndromes and systemic trauma responses due to lactic acidosis and late reperfusion of severely ischemic tissue. In some cases, there may be significant nerve injury even though other tissues have been preserved by the intervention.

POSTPROCEDURAL AND FOLLOW-UP CARE

Postprocedural and follow-up care is usually dictated by the other injuries the patient has sustained, rather than angiography or percutaneous interventions.

It is important to consider the possibility of late false aneurysm formation when follow-up imaging is performed.

Stent-grafts are not immune from restenosis or occlusion, and these patients should be observed to ensure that late complications do not develop.

KEY POINTS

- Diagnosis of significant vascular injury rests almost entirely on the physical examination. Computed tomographic angiography and conventional angiography can help localize vascular injury when the physical examination is equivocal.

- Hard signs of vascular injury include pulsatile bleeding, expanding hematoma, absent distal pulses, a cold pale limb, palpable thrill, and audible bruit. Hemodynamically unstable patients who present with these signs should proceed to surgery. Patients who are hemodynamically stable and demonstrate hard or soft signs of vascular injury may be candidates for angiography and intervention.

- Laceration with either complete or incomplete vessel transection is the most common form of vascular injury. Hemorrhage tends to be more severe in partially transected vessels.

- Categories of injury include vascular laceration with active bleeding, traumatic pseudoaneurysm, traumatic arteriovenous fistula, vascular occlusion, and foreign body embolization.

- Endovascular techniques—stents, stent-grafts, and coils—are being increasingly used to treat vascular injuries.

▸ SUGGESTED READINGS

Foster BR, Anderson SW, Soto JA. CT angiography of extremity trauma. Tech Vasc Interv Radiol 2006;9(4):156–66.

Hanks S, Pentecost MJ. Angiography and transcatheter treatment of extremity trauma. Semin Intervent Radiol 1992;9:20–5.

Hilfiker PR, Razavi MK, Kee ST, et al. Stent-graft therapy for subclavian artery aneurysms and fistulas: single-center mid-term results. J Vasc Interv Radiol 2000;11(5):578–84.

Krueger K, Zaehringer M, Strohe D, et al. Postcatheterization pseudoaneurysm: results of US-guided percutaneous thrombin injection in 240 patients. Radiology 2005;236(3):1104–10.

Parodi JC, Schönholz C, Ferreira LM, et al. Endovascular stent-graft treatment of traumatic arterial lesions. Ann Vasc Surg 1999;13(2):121–9.

Peng PD, Spain DA, Tataria M, et al. CT angiography effectively evaluates extremity vascular trauma. Am Surg 2008;74(2):103–7.

The complete reference list is available online at www.expertconsult.com

CHAPTER 40

Management of Postcatheterization Pseudoaneurysms
Wael E.A. Saad and David L. Waldman

Arterial pseudoaneurysms are the most common complication (61%) of interventions requiring femoral artery catheterization (Table 40-1).[1-3] The overall incidence of postcatheterization pseudoaneurysms ranges from 0.11% to 1.52%.[4-10] In six studies involving 107,052 femoral catheterizations, 757 patients (0.71%) exhibited postcatheterization pseudoaneurysms.[4-10] The incidence of access pseudoaneurysms increases with transcatheter therapeutic interventions (3.5%-5.5%) as compared with studies confined to diagnostic arterial catheterization (0.1%-1.1%).[1,4,11] Because of the ongoing paradigm shift in transcatheter endoluminal interventions as opposed to traditional open surgical interventions, the incidence of postcatheterization pseudoaneurysms is on the rise, with approximately 15,000 femoral pseudoaneurysms diagnosed in the United States annually as of the year 2000.[1,4,5,9,11-17]

Postcatheterization pseudoaneurysms are associated with increased morbidity (Table 40-2).[1,4,11] Numerous methods, including variants within each method, have been described for the management of postcatheterization pseudoaneurysms (Table 40-3; also see Table e40-1). For the purposes of this chapter, the two most commonly described approaches—pseudoaneurysm compression and direct percutaneous thrombin injection and their variant techniques—will be discussed. The limited role of stent-grafts will also be mentioned.

INDICATIONS

Pseudoaneurysm Compression

Pseudoaneurysms that are most amenable to compression are small pseudoaneurysms less than 2 weeks old with long accessible necks, in a patient not taking anticoagulants who has intact overlying skin. Some authors report that large pseudoaneurysms are associated with a lower success rate or require longer compression times.[18-20] In addition, patients receiving anticoagulation therapy represent 64% to 100% of reported failures in studies of patients undergoing compression therapy.[10,18-24] In eight reports describing a total of 684 cases with detailed analysis of failures (133 failures), 100 failures (75%) were associated with anticoagulation therapy.[10,18-24]

Direct Percutaneous Thrombin Injection

With its high success and low complication rates (see later discussion), and the risk/benefit ratio largely in favor of treatment, the indication for treatment of access pseudoaneurysms by direct percutaneous thrombin injection is broad and involves almost all patients except those with uncommon contraindications.

Stent-Graft Placement

Stent-grafts are preferred as first-line therapy by some clinicians, although there is no evidence for their preferential use over compression or thrombin injection. They may occasionally be useful as a temporizing measure until definitive surgery is performed.

CONTRAINDICATIONS

Pseudoaneurysm Compression

Poor patient/lesion candidates for compression therapy include (1) pain intolerance/painful pseudoaneurysms (25%-34% of failures), (2) morbid obesity (13% of failures), (3) large pseudoaneurysms obliterating adjacent vascular structures (19% of failures), (4) associated arteriovenous fistulous component (1%-2% of pseudoaneurysms), (5) superadded infection or overlying skin breakdown, and (6) unstable patients (2% of failures).[18,22,25,26] Poor candidates for compression represent approximately 10% of all patients and 50% of intent-to-treat technical failures.[7,18,27-31]

Direct Percutaneous Thrombin Injection

Contraindications to direct percutaneous thrombin injection therapy include (1) infected pseudoaneurysms or overlying skin erosion/breakdown, (2) ruptured pseudoaneurysms, (3) associated arteriovenous fistulous component, (4) associated ipsilateral deep venous thrombosis (DVT), and (5) previous treatment/exposure to bovine thrombin because of concern for allergic reactions (relative contraindication).[32]

Stent-Graft Placement

The main relative contraindication to stent-graft use is the location of the femoral artery, which predisposes stent-grafts to fracture and occlusion. Therefore, most authors avoid using these devices for this indication.

EQUIPMENT

Pseudoaneurysm Compression

Little equipment is required other than the ultrasound transducer for real-time ultrasound compression. Institutions that adopt ultrasound-guided compression may use stationary (vice-like) mechanical compression devices such as the FemoStop (Femoral Compression System, RADI Medical Systems AB, Uppsala, Sweden, distributed by Radi Medical Systems, Inc., Reading, Mass.).[29,33-35]

TABLE 40-1. Type of Arterial Catheterization Complications Requiring Intervention

Access Complication	Incidence (%)
Pseudoaneurysm	61.2
Hematoma	11.2
Arteriovenous fistula	10.2
External bleeding	6.1
Retroperitoneal hematoma	5.1
Arterial thrombosis	3.1
Groin abscess	2.0
Mycotic aneurysm	1.0

Data from Lumsden AB, Peden EK, Bush RL, Lin PH. Complications of endovascular procedures at the target site. In: Ouriel K, Katzen BT, Rosenfield K, editors. Complications in endovascular therapy. New York: Taylor & Francis; 2006. p. 29–53.

TABLE 40-2. Type of Complications Caused by Postcatheterization Pseudoaneurysms

Complication	Descriptive Incidence
Large, painful thigh/groin hematoma limiting patient ambulation	Common
Overlying skin erosion/breakdown	Not common (large PsAs)
Associated/superadded infection	Not uncommon (most subclinical)
Venous stasis/leg edema/DVT	Not common
Sensory-motor femoral neuralgia	Not uncommon with large PsAs
Anterior abdominal wall hematoma	Uncommon
PsA rupture and bleeding	Rare

DVT, Deep venous thrombosis; *PsA*, pseudoaneurysm. Data from references 1, 4, 11and .

TABLE 40-3. General Approaches to Management of Postcatheterization Pseudoaneurysms and Their Variant Techniques

Management Approach	Indications	Problems/Disadvantages
Observation	Asymptomatic patients Small PsA (<1.8-2 cm in diameter, <6 cm in volume) No anticoagulation therapy	Requires frequent Doppler examination Reduced patient activity (increased morbidity) Not inexpensive in view of above 2 points Limited indications
Surgery	Historically: standard management Currently: when minimally invasive methods fail Associated overt infection Complex (associated) vascular injuries (AVF component)	High complication rate (11%-32%) Most are wound infection/dehiscence, bleeding, and femoral neuralgia
Endoluminal coiling	PFA branches Circumflex branches	More involved and probably more expensive than other minimally invasive approaches Aesthetic problems (nest of coils subcutaneously)
Temporary endoluminal balloon exclusion of PsA	Wide and short PsA necks; 15% of PsAs thrombose within minutes	More involved and probably more expensive than other minimally invasive approaches Requires heparinized saline infusion through balloon shaft to maintain distal patency
Endoluminal stent-graft exclusion of PsA	PsA originating above inguinal ligament No infection	More involved and more expensive than other minimally invasive approaches Limited application/indications
Direct percutaneous coil or glue into PsA	Potentially all patients Preferably (if ever resorted to) small PsAs (aesthetics)	More expensive than thrombin injection Aesthetic problems (nest of coils/lump of glue subcutaneously)

AVF, Arteriovenous fistula; *PFA*, profunda femoris artery; *PsA*, pseudoaneurysm.

Direct Percutaneous Thrombin Injection

Thrombin and Tissue Adhesives

Varying preparations of thrombin, fibrinogen, and fibrin have been used.[36-43] The following are some of the more commonly used products.

Lyophilized, sterilized, and virus-inactivated powdered bovine thrombin reconstituted with saline (1000 U/mL and can be diluted to 100 to 500 U/mL):

- Gentrac Inc., for Johnson & Johnson Medical Inc., Middleton, Wis.
- Jones Medical Industries, St. Louis, Mo.
- Vascular Solutions, Bochum, Germany.

- Thrombostat, Parke-Davis, Scarborough, Ontario, Canada.

Sterilized and virus-inactivated human thrombin, tissue sealant to be defrosted (500 U/mL):

- Tissuecol Duo S 500, Immuno AG, Vienna, Austria.
- Tisseal, Baxter Healthcare Corp., Glendale, Calif.

Autologous centrifuged and suspended human thrombin:

- Laboratory preparation details have been published by Quarmby and colleagues.[40]

Fibrinogen, aprotinin, thrombin, and factor XIII composite tissue adhesive (three doses available: 0.5, 1, and 3.9 mL):

• Beriplast P Combiset, Centeon Pharmaceuticals Ltd., Marburg, Germany.

Ultrasound Transducer

Most authors use a linear array transducer ranging in frequency between 5 and 7.5 MHz, and use a lower-frequency transducer (3.5-4.0 MHz) for morbidly obese patients or those who have excessively large overlying hematomas.[32,36] Some authors use higher-frequency transducers (7.5 to 12 MHz).[32,44]

Needle

Most authors use a needle ranging between 20 and 22 gauge in diameter.[5,27,30,32,33,36,37,42,44,53] However, the use of 19-gauge and 23- to 25-gauge needles has been described.[33,38,43,53,54]

Stent-Graft Placement

Self-expanding stent-grafts are the devices of choice. Balloon-expandable stents are not used because they will be distorted or crushed owing to continuous flexion and extension at the hip joint or external compression.

TECHNIQUE

Pseudoaneurysm Compression

Numerous variations of the compression management of access pseudoaneurysms have been described. One variable is the guidance method, which includes blind compression (by palpation and without image guidance),[6,35,55] ultrasound examination to determine the ideal site for subsequent compression,[6,29,33,35,56,58] and real-time ultrasound-guided compression.[17,18,20,26,56,57,59] A second variable is the means with which the pseudoaneurysm neck is compressed, including manual/digital compression,[43,56,58,60] use of stationary (vice-like) contraptions such as a FemoStop device,[29,33,35] and finally, use of the ultrasound transducer itself to compress the pseudoaneurysm neck.[18,20,51,52,59,61,63]

Largely Adopted Real-Time Ultrasound-Guided Pseudoaneurysm Neck Compression Technique

Before pseudoaneurysm neck compression is applied, baseline distal arterial pulses are determined. Ankle-brachial indices (ABIs) may even be calculated. Via color-flow Doppler sonography, the pseudoaneurysm is carefully evaluated for overall size, pseudoaneurysm neck location, dimensions, and hemodynamics. The relationship of the pseudoaneurysm with the supplying femoral artery is also evaluated, in addition to associated arterial injuries such as arteriovenous fistulous components. The overlying skin is likewise evaluated for necrosis and infection. Assessment is also made of the direction required to apply pressure to occlude flow into the pseudoaneurysm sac. The ideal trajectory for applying pressure is one that avoids gross compression of the pseudoaneurysm sac itself, as well as the adjacent normal vasculature (femoral vein and artery) (Fig. 40-1).

Some authors routinely use moderate sedation in patients undergoing pseudoaneurysm neck compression. For those who do not routinely sedate patients, 25% to 34% of their patients eventually require moderate sedation to tolerate

the pseudoaneurysm compression.[18,27,64] The ultrasound probe is positioned directly over the pseudoaneurysm neck, and downward pressure is applied until flow into the pseudoaneurysm ceases (see Fig. 40-1, B and C). The ideal degree of pressure will abolish flow into the pseudoaneurysm and, if avoidable, not compress the adjacent femoral artery. In some patients, temporary occlusion of the femoral artery is unavoidable, but there are usually no untoward sequelae.[65] Compression of the femoral vein is unavoidable when the pseudoaneurysm swings medially and overlies the femoral vein. If the pseudoaneurysm neck is not clearly identified by color-flow Doppler examination, ultrasound-guided compression directed at the pseudoaneurysm sac itself can be performed until cessation of flow in the pseudoaneurysm is achieved.[65] The pseudoaneurysm neck is compressed intermittently for intervals extending between 6 and 20 minutes.[7,23,25,34,66-68] It is not uncommon during ultrasound-guided compression to lose the ideal position over the pseudoaneurysm neck, thus necessitating adjustment of the ultrasound transducer's position. Between pressure applications, the pseudoaneurysm is evaluated for flow by color-flow Doppler ultrasound. If the pseudoaneurysm has thrombosed, the procedure is deemed technically successful (see Fig. 40-1, D). If there is still residual flow, a repeat compression interval is performed. Most operators will not exceed three or four such intervals. In addition, it is not uncommon for patients to not tolerate repeat compression intervals/sessions.

Direct Percutaneous Thrombin Injection

The technique of direct percutaneous intrapseudoaneurysm injection of thrombin or tissue fibrin sealant varied considerably in earlier reports. The two main variants were the site of needle application (see Fig. e40-1) and whether to occlude the neck. Over the past decade, the technique has been refined, and numerous authors have recently described a more uniform and simplified method to obliterate postcatheterization pseudoaneurysms with direct thrombin injection[5,32,36,41,45,47,49,73-77] (see later discussion).

Insertion of the needle tip into the pseudoaneurysm neck for injection of thrombin has been performed in an attempt to rid the thrombin clot formed around the needle tip by flow carrying it away from the needle tip and neck into the pseudoaneurysm sac (see Fig. e40-1, A). However, this location has largely been abandoned because of concern for an increased risk of femoral artery thrombin embolization. A second needle tip insertion site is at the juncture of the pseudoaneurysm neck and the pseudoaneurysm sac (see Fig. e40-1, B). The hypothetical advantage of this site is that blood flow at this juncture carries the thrombin clot that forms around the needle tip into the pseudoaneurysm neck, without the risk of femoral artery embolization.[74] However, this precise site for needle tip placement can be clearly identified in only 42% of patients with the use of ultrasound contrast agents.[74] The added expense of ultrasound contrast agents, the increased time needed to perform an ultrasound contrast–enhanced evaluation, and the increased technical challenge to place the needle tip at that precise location make this needle tip placement site unpopular. Furthermore, the safety (low risk of femoral embolization; Tables 40-4 and 40-5) achieved by placing the needle tip at the fundus (*authors' definition*) of the

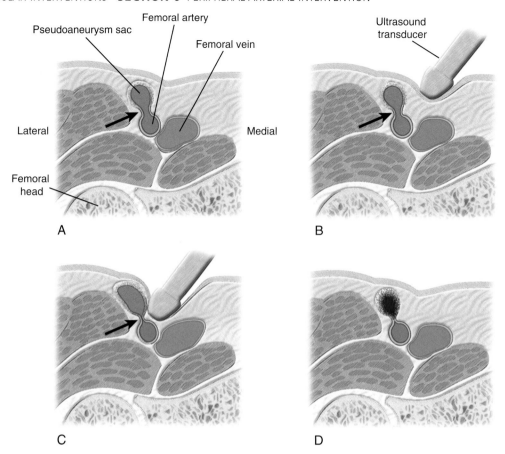

FIGURE 40-1. Cross-sectional (axial) anatomic depiction of right thigh at level of femoral head, along with schematic depiction of stages of Doppler ultrasound evaluation and compression therapy for a postcatheterization pseudoaneurysm. **A,** Cross-sectional (axial) anatomic depiction of right thigh at level of femoral head. Larger striated structures are muscle groups (quadriceps femoris, adductor femoris groups), and arrow points to pseudoaneurysm neck. **B,** Ultrasound transducer overlying femoral vessels. It is tilted laterally to be orthogonal to pseudoaneurysm neck *(arrow).* **C,** Pressure is held with the ultrasound transducer at the same orthogonal plane decided on in **B** so pseudoaneurysm neck *(arrow)* is compressed and flow within the pseudoaneurysm sac is obliterated. Pressure is maintained for 5- to 20-minute intervals, with Doppler evaluation of femoral vasculature performed between compression intervals. **D,** No further compression is applied when pseudoaneurysm is thrombosed *(shaded pseudoaneurysm).*

TABLE 40-4. Comparison of Outcomes Between Compression and Direct Thrombin Injection Therapies for Treating Postcatheterization Pseudoaneurysms

Criteria		Compression	Thrombin Injection
Rate of unsuitable candidates		10%	<2%
Success rate*	Ultimate success	80%	97%
	First-attempt success	73%	89%
	Proportion of ultimate successes requiring >1 session	13%	8%
Procedure time (including setup)[†]		37-75 minutes (61 minutes)	15-25 minutes (21 minutes)
Complications[‡]	Overall	1.3%	1.4%
	Major	0.5%	0.4%
	Minor	0.8%	1.0%
	Most common complication	Pain related: 0.7%[§] (17% are major)	Distal arterial embolization: 1% (29% are major)

*Overall references for analysis of success rates: 5-10, 17-40, 43-49, 51-63, 66-76, 79, 81-90, 92.
[†]Procedure time (including setup time for the procedure) is calculated from studies with intrainstitutional comparisons between compression and thrombin injection therapies.[30,51,52,86] The majority of authors report that the actual time for thrombosis of the pseudoaneurysm with direct thrombin injection is within seconds (setup time for the entire procedure not included).
[‡]Complication rates are calculated from studies that have a sample size that exceeds 90 patients.[6,18,20,24,27,28,31,32,36,45,52,73,74,83,88]
[§]Pain-related complications include vasovagal episodes, pain intolerance, and cardiovascular responses possibly secondary to pain, such as hypertension, atrial fibrillation, and even angina/myocardial infarction.

TABLE 40-5. Complications Encountered with Compression Management of Postcatheterization Pseudoaneurysms in Studies with a Sample Size Greater than 90 Pseudoaneurysms (Total of 1637 Cases)

Complications*		Range within Individual Studies	Overall Case-Weighted Rate
All complications	Overall	0.0%-5.5%	1.3% ($n = 21/1637$)
	Major		0.5% ($n = 8/1637$)
	Minor		0.8% ($n = 15/1657$)
Pain-associated complications	Overall	0.0%-4.1%	0.7% ($n = 12/1637$)
	Major (angina/atrial fibrillation)		0.2% ($n = 3/1637$)
	Minor (vasovagal/hypertension)		0.5% ($n = 9/1637$)
Pseudoaneurysm rupture		0.0%-0.9%	0.2% ($n = 4/1637$)
Distal arterial embolization		0.0%-0.8%	0.1% ($n = 1/1637$)
DVT		0.0%-0.3%	0.1% ($n = 1/1637$)
Pulmonary embolism†		Rarely reported	0.0% ($n = 0/1637$)

*Complication rates are calculated from studies that have a sample size exceeding 90 patients.[6,18,20,24,28,31,52,83]
†Not reported in studies with more than 90 cases.
DVT, Deep venous thrombosis.

pseudoaneurysm sac reduces the validity of ultrasound contrast–aided needle insertion at the pseudoaneurysm neck. The third needle tip insertion site, most popular and preferred by the current authors, is in the pseudoaneurysm sac itself at a point as far away from the pseudoaneurysm neck as possible (see Fig. e40-1, *C*). There is, however, controversy regarding which pseudoaneurysm lobe to insert the needle tip in cases where the pseudoaneurysm has more than one lobe (complex postcatheterization pseudoaneurysm). Some authors prefer to place the needle tip at the most proximal lobe (closest to the femoral artery/pseudoaneurysm neck), whereas others prefer the most distal lobe to maximize the distance between the thrombin injection site and the pseudoaneurysm neck (see Fig. e40-2).[32,36,48,49]

Exclusion of the pseudoaneurysm by occluding the pseudoaneurysm neck (endoluminally with a balloon or by external manual compression) was originally described in earlier reports from 1998 to 2001.[75-77] In fact, mere occlusion of the neck by placing a coaxial balloon across the neck from a contralateral femoral approach has been described solely in the treatment of postcatheterization pseudoaneurysms[78] (see Fig. e40-3). Furthermore, balloon exclusion of the pseudoaneurysm with the intention of subsequent thrombin injection leads to thrombosis of 15% of pseudoaneurysms before commencement of the thrombin injection.[79] Recent reports (2001-2005), however, have described a simple technique without pseudoaneurysm neck occlusion.[5,32,36,41,45,47,49,69-73]

Simplified and Largely Adopted Direct Pseudoaneurysm Thrombin Injection Technique

A baseline assessment of the distal arterial vasculature is performed (palpation, Doppler imaging, or even ABIs). In addition, and with the use of color-flow Doppler sonography, the pseudoaneurysm is carefully evaluated for overall size and complexity (number of lobes), pseudoaneurysm neck dimensions, and hemodynamics. The relationship of the pseudoaneurysm to the supplying femoral artery is also evaluated, along with associated arterial injuries such as arteriovenous fistulous components. In addition, the overlying skin is evaluated for necrosis and infection. Whether to proceed with treatment and identification of the ideal

needle access site and approach are determined on the basis of these findings.

Subsequently, the overlying skin is sterilely cleansed and draped in the standard surgical manner. The ultrasound transducer probe is sterilely draped. Real-time grayscale ultrasound is used to image the needle tip longitudinally along the needle shaft. Once the needle tip is in adequate position in the pseudoaneurysm sac, ultrasound is switched to color-flow Doppler imaging with a low pulse repetition frequency (Fig. 40-2, *A*). Hemodynamic flow within the pseudoaneurysm does not alter needle tip position.[36] Slow and steady thrombin injection ensues under real-time color-flow Doppler ultrasound visualization. The rate of injection is slow enough to gradually form an isoechoic to hyperechoic thrombus that fills the pseudoaneurysm gradually, but fast enough to not allow it to encase the needle tip (Fig. 40-2, *B*). A quoted injection rate is 0.1 to 0.3 mL of thrombin injected per second.[32] If the needle tip becomes encased by a thrombus ball/mound, further injection of thrombin into the thrombin ball/mound can be ineffective. To alleviate this problem, the needle tip can be gently manipulated to rid the thrombus ball within the pseudoaneurysm lobe and free the needle tip to resume thrombin injection (Fig. 40-2, *C*). It is not uncommon (23%) for patients to experience a local heat sensation.[47]

Complete or nearly complete thrombosis of the entire pseudoaneurysm is usually achieved within seconds (Fig. 40-2, *D*). Figure 40-3 demonstrates an actual postcatheterization pseudoaneurysm before, during, and after thrombin injection. Residual pockets free of thrombus are left to thrombose spontaneously as long as there are no high rates of flow through them (usually requiring communication with the original pseudoaneurysm neck). Such high-flow pockets communicating with the pseudoaneurysm neck are uncommon but, if identified, may require additional needle punctures with subsequent thrombin injection. Some authors apply gentle pressure to obliterate these pockets.[37]

The technique of thrombin obliteration of the pseudoaneurysm is physiologic; a temporary hematoma forms, which is then degraded in normal fashion by fibrinolysis and phagocytosis. Any remaining cavities fill with granulation tissue.[79,80]

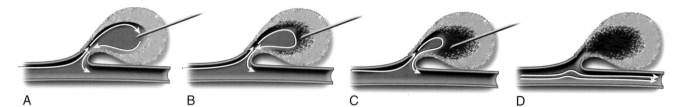

FIGURE 40-2. Schematic illustration of simple (one-lobe) postcatheterization pseudoaneurysm along long axis of femoral artery and pseudoaneurysm neck and sac during direct percutaneous thrombin injection. **A,** Localization of needle tip in pseudoaneurysm sac, ideally positioned to commence thrombin injection. **B,** Needle tip located in pseudoaneurysm sac, with commencement of thrombin injection. Thrombin/clot formation is starting to accumulate around needle tip. **C,** Needle tip pushed in/manipulated in pseudoaneurysm sac to maximize amount of thrombin injected and achieve complete obliteration of pseudoaneurysm sac. **D,** Needle removed from pseudoaneurysm sac after complete thrombosis/obliteration of postcatheterization pseudoaneurysm. In essence, residual (thrombosed pseudoaneurysm) is a temporary hematoma, which is then degraded in normal fashion by fibrinolysis and phagocytosis. Any remaining cavities fill with granulation tissue. Femoral artery laceration heals with granulation and fibrosis and endoluminal intimal proliferation.[77,86]

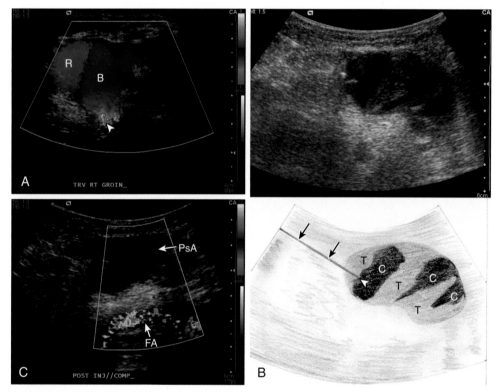

FIGURE 40-3. Actual color Doppler ultrasound images of a postcatheterization pseudoaneurysm before, during (with supplementary schematic illustration), and after successful obliteration by direct percutaneous injection of thrombin. **A,** Color Doppler evaluation of a postcatheterization femoral pseudoaneurysm, demonstrating typical to-and-fro (red [R] toward transducer, blue [B] away from transducer) blood flow (bidirectional flow, "yin-yang" sign) within pseudoaneurysm sac. Aliasing at origin of pseudoaneurysm neck *(arrowhead)* is seen. Note that flow within pseudoaneurysm neck at any moment in time is in one direction (into sac during systole and out of sac during diastole), and schematic depiction of flow *(curved arrows)* in Figures 40-2 and 40-5 is misleading with respect to a given moment in time. **B,** Real-time grayscale ultrasound image and schematic illustration of it during direct percutaneous thrombin injection along long axis of needle shaft *(arrows).* Arrowhead points to needle tip. *C,* Residual cavity; *T,* thrombus. **C,** Color Doppler evaluation of a postcatheterization femoral pseudoaneurysm after thrombin injection. Typical bidirectional flow (yin-yang sign) in pseudoaneurysm is lost, as is any color Doppler–perceptible flow within thrombosed pseudoaneurysm sac *(PsA).* Flow is maintained in adjacent femoral artery *(FA).* (Courtesy Dr. Christine Mentas, Mallinckrodt Institute of Radiology, Washington University, St. Louis, Mo.)

Stent-Graft Placement

The technique of self-expanding stent-graft placement is no different from stent placement in the iliac or femoral arteries, and will not be discussed further. An example is presented in Figure 40-4.

OUTCOMES

Pseudoaneurysm Compression

Ultimate success (multiple compression sessions if needed) is achieved in 33% to 100% of patients. In 47 studies describing compression management of 2480 cases of

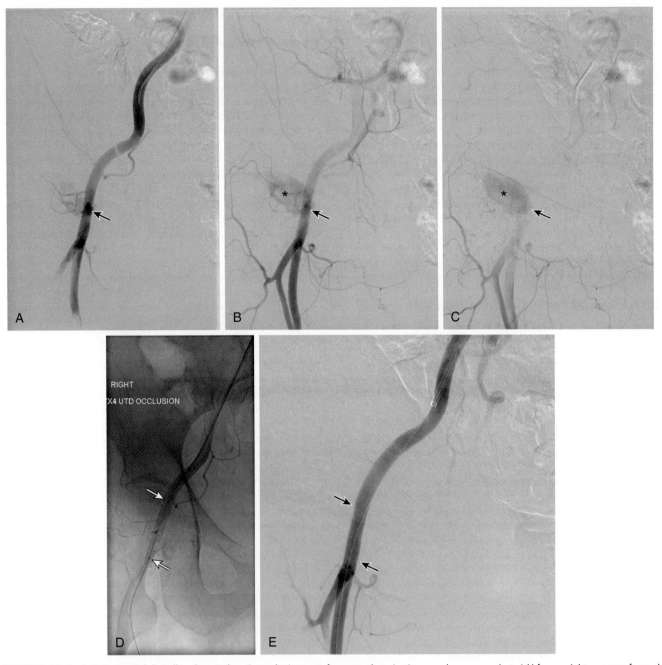

FIGURE 40-4. **A-C,** Sequential digitally subtracted angiography images of a postcatheterization pseudoaneurysm *(asterisk)* from a right common femoral artery injury *(arrow)*. **D,** Fluoroscopic image with contrast being injected through sheath as a 7-mm balloon is used to tamponade bleeding and temporize hemodynamically unstable patient. No bleeding is seen. **E,** A 7-mm self-expanding stent-graft has been deployed across common femoral artery/inguinal ligament, sparing common femoral artery bifurcation. There is no bleeding (filling of pseudoaneurysm) seen on angiogram. Patient hemodynamically stabilized and did well.

access pseudoaneurysms, 1991 (80.3%) were ultimately treated successfully.[6-10,17-31,33-35,43,51,52,54-63,71-77,79,81-83] The first-attempt success rate for studies (14 studies) clearly identifying success per session ranged from 13% to 93%, with an average of 73.3% (*n* = 773/1054). In the same group of studies, 12.9% (range, 3.3%-73%) of ultimately successful cases required more than one compression session.[6,18,21,24,68,5-35,43,51,55,64,82,85] The three most common causes of failure (based on an intent-to-treat analysis) are, in order, anticoagulation therapy (representing 75% of actual failed attempts), poor candidates (10% of all patients),

and pain intolerance without sedation (25%-34% of failures).[18,27] In addition, it should be noted that anticoagulation therapy is more likely than antiplatelet regimens to be associated with compression failure.[55]

Higher success rates can be achieved with experience because compression therapy for access pseudoaneurysms is closely associated with a learning curve.[7] As seen in an analysis of the literature, institutions reporting less than 80 pseudoaneurysm compression cases have an inconsistent and broad success rate ranging from 33% to 100%, with an average success rate of 76% (*n* = 659/868); whereas institutions reporting more than 80 cases have a more consistent and higher success rate of 74% to 98%, with an average success rate of 83% (n = 1332/1612).

When comparing the results of compression management of access pseudoaneurysms with the results of direct percutaneous thrombin injection (see later discussion), the former shows relatively variable rates (wide range of success) in comparison to the latter. This is most likely because compression management is subject to numerous population, technical, and methodological variables, including differing populations (varying percentages of obese patients and those receiving anticoagulation therapy), varying thresholds and indications for patient/lesion selection, varying technical factors such as the percentage of patients undergoing sedation and the degree of sedation/analgesia, length of compression times, presence of image guidance (non–image guided real-time ultrasound guidance, site-localized ultrasound guidance, etc.), and the associated learning curve.[7]

Direct Percutaneous Thrombin Injection

Ultimate success (multiple thrombin injection sessions if needed) is achieved in 86% to 100% of patients. In 36 studies describing direct percutaneous thrombin injection management of 1722 cases of access pseudoaneurysm, 1668 (96.9%) were ultimately successfully treated. The overall first-attempt success rate for these 36 studies ranged from 57% to 100%, with an average of 89.0% (n = 1507/1693). In the same group of studies, 8.0% (range, 0%-39%) of ultimately successful cases required more than one thrombin injection session.[5,27,29,30,32,33,37-40,43-49,51-53,60,69-76,79,84,86-90]

In 12 studies with intra-institutional comparisons (n = 802) between compression and direct thrombin injection (n = 388), varying from randomized prospective evaluations to intra-institutional historical comparisons, success rates for compression and thrombin injection were 74.3% (n = 596/802; range, 33%-100%) and 96.6% (n = 375/388; range, 92%-100%), respectively. One reason for the improved success of thrombin injection over compression management is its wide clinical application, including its limited contraindications and higher patient candidacy rate (10% of patients are not candidates for compression vs. probably <1% for thrombin injection). The second and possibly most important reason is that direct thrombin injection is not hindered by anticoagulation or antiplatelet therapy.[79] A third reason is that direct thrombin injection is tolerated by most patients and does not generally require sedation, whereas 25% to 34% of patients undergoing compression therapy fail because of pain associated with intolerance to the procedure.[27,29,30,33,43,51,52,54,60,83,84,86]

Stent-Graft Placement

There are no large case series addressing expanded polytetrafluoroethylene (ePTFE) self-expanding stent-grafts for the management of access pseudoaneurysms. Anecdotally, the authors believe these devices are very effective in selected cases. When the injury is very high above the inguinal ligament (well within the external iliac artery) and in the absence of infection, stent-grafts are effective from a definitive treatment standpoint (see Fig. 40-4).

COMPLICATIONS

Pseudoaneurysm Compression

Complication rates and specifics are displayed in Tables 40-4 and 40-5. The most common complications resulting from compression therapy are pain-associated complications such as vasovagal reactions, pain itself, and possibly cardiovascular responses to pain such as hypertension, atrial fibrillation, and chest angina (see Tables 40-4 and 40-5). Seventeen percent of these pain-associated complications are considered major complications by the current authors (see Table 40-4), and the majority may be avoided by sedation, which is required in up to 34% of patients undergoing compression therapy but not usually required in those undergoing direct percutaneous thrombin injection.

An interesting finding during compression, and defined as a complication requiring premature termination of a compression session (failed treatment) by one study, is acute and rapid expansion of a pseudoaneurysm proper or its neck (impending rupture) during compression. This complication was encountered in 1% of 297 cases.[24]

Direct Percutaneous Thrombin Injection

Complication rates and specifics are displayed in Table 40-6 (also see Table 40-4). The most common and concerning complication resulting from direct percutaneous thrombin injection therapy is distal arterial embolic events (see Tables 40-4 and 40-6). Some 29% of these arterial embolic complications are considered major, requiring surgical or endoluminal intervention; the remainder (71%) are clinically transient without sequelae and do not require further management (see Table 40-6).

Distal arterial embolization is thought to be due to leakage of thrombin from the pseudoaneurysm into the femoral artery. Leakage of thrombin into the circulation is probably more common than generally believed and clinically realized.[36,91] However, thromboembolic events are rare, probably because thrombin is rapidly diluted and deactivated by natural inherent thrombolytic mechanisms.[36] The incidence of this clinical complication can be reduced by diluting the thrombin, especially in the case of small pseudoaneurysms, which theoretically have a higher risk of systemic circulatory escape of thrombin during direct percutaneous thrombin injection.[36]

Stent-Graft Placement

Occlusion and infection are the main potential complications of stent-graft placement.

POSTPROCEDURAL AND FOLLOW-UP CARE

There is no clear consensus on clinical and imaging follow-up intervals for patients who have successfully undergone minimally invasive postcatheterization pseudoaneurysm treatment. All authors keep patients on bed rest for 1 to 24 hours, with the majority recommending 2 to 12 hours.[30,33,36,38,43,48,49,51,52,60] The vast majority of authors perform a follow-up Doppler evaluation within 24 hours of

TABLE 40-6. Complications Encountered with Direct Percutaneous Management of Postcatheterization Pseudoaneurysms in Studies with a Sample Size Greater than 90 Pseudoaneurysms (Total of 719 Cases)

Complications*		Range within Individual Studies	Overall Case-Weighted Rate
All complications	Overall	0.0%-3.5%	1.4% (*n* = 10/719)
	Major		0.4% (*n* = 3/719)
	Minor		1.0% (*n* = 7/719)
Distal arterial embolization	Overall	0.0%-2.6%	1.0% (*n* = 7/719)
	Major (requiring intervention)	0.0%-1.5%	0.3% (*n* = 2/719)
	Minor (transient/self-limited)	0.0%-2.6%	0.7% (*n* = 5/719)
Allergic reaction		0.0%-0.4%	0.1% (*n* = 1/719)
Infection		0.05-0.9%	0.1% (*n* = 1/719)
Pseudoaneurysm rupture		0.0%-0.8%	0.1% (*n* = 1/719)
Pain with or without vasovagal reaction		0.0%-0.4%	0.1% (*n* = 1/719)
Hypotension and bradycardia[†]		Rarely reported	0.0% (*n* = 0/719)
Deep venous thrombosis[†]		Rarely reported	0.0% (*n* = 0/719)

*Complication rates are calculated from studies that have a sample size exceeding 90 patients.[27,32,36,45,73,74,88]
[†]Not reported in studies with more than 90 cases.

the initial treatment.[27,32,36,38,43,46,49,51,52,74,75] This evaluation is usually performed in conjunction with clinical evaluation of the distal pulses, which may include calculation of the ABI. Some authors perform a follow-up Doppler ultrasound evaluation at 24 hours for inpatients, and not earlier than 1 week for patients treated on an outpatient basis in whom there is no clinical concern for persistent or recurrent pseudoaneurysms subsequent to successful obliteration.[5] Authors who mention subsequent short- to midterm follow-up perform a Doppler evaluation at 3 to 10 days and occasionally later Doppler evaluations, varying widely from 3 weeks to 6 months.[5,27,32,36-38,42,46-50,74,75]

- Pseudoaneurysm compression and direct percutaneous thrombin injection are the two main types of treatment technique; each has variants in technique.
- The use of stent-grafts is limited to noninfected pseudoaneurysms of the external iliac artery that are a distance from the inguinal ligament, or as a temporizing measure, stabilizing patients until definitive treatment is performed.

▶ SUGGESTED READINGS

Kronzon I. Diagnosis and treatment of iatrogenic femoral artery pseudoaneurysm: a review. J Am Soc Echocardiogr 1997;10:236–45.

Middleton WD, Dasyam A, Teefey SA. Diagnosis and treatment of iatrogenic femoral artery pseudoaneurysms. Ultrasound Q 2005;21:3–17.

Morgan R, Belli A-M. Current treatment methods for postcatheterization pseudoaneurysms. J Vasc Interv Radiol 2003;14:697–710.

Saad NEA, Saad WEA, Davies MG, et al. Pseudoaneurysms and the role of minimally invasive techniques in their management. Radiographics 2005;25:S173–S189.

Saad NEA, Saad WEA, Rubens DJ, Fultz P. Ultrasound diagnosis of arterial injuries and the role of minimally invasive techniques in their management. Ultrasound Clin N Am Vasc Ultrasound 2006;1:183–200.

The complete reference list is available online at www.expertconsult.com.

KEY POINTS

- Arterial pseudoaneurysms are the most common complication (61%) of interventions requiring femoral artery catheterization.
- Because of the ongoing paradigm shift in transcatheter endoluminal interventions as opposed to traditional open surgical interventions, the incidence of postcatheterization pseudoaneurysms is on the rise.
- Postcatheterization pseudoaneurysms are associated with increased morbidity.

CHAPTER 41

Endovascular Treatment of Peripheral Aneurysms

Kenneth R. Thomson, Stuart M. Lyon, Mark F. Given, and James P. Burnes

Peripheral aneurysms are classified as true or false depending on the composition of the aneurysm wall. The type of treatment depends on the shape (saccular or fusiform), location, and cause.

Vascular surgery has been the preferred method of treatment, especially if the aneurysm is superficial,[1] but more recently, computed tomography (CT) has shown that endoleaks occur in peripheral aneurysms post surgery, just as they do after aortic endovascular repair.[2] Recent advances in endovascular methods of treatment and development of new endovascular tools for peripheral aneurysms have made this method a reasonable alternative to conventional surgery.

False aneurysms are most common after trauma (including angiographic access). The cause of an aneurysm may be obvious (trauma or iatrogenic) or more obscure (due to atheromatous change, increased flow, or infection), and it may be impossible to determine which type of aneurysm is present based on angiography alone. Multidetector-row CT and Doppler ultrasonography have increased detection of asymptomatic peripheral aneurysms. Aneurysms related to thoracic outlet compression are commonly symptomatic owing to peripheral embolization.[3]

Permanent occlusion of an aneurysm requires more than just proximal occlusion of the supplying artery. If arterial occlusion is performed, the vessel should be occluded both proximal and distal to the site of the aneurysm to prevent retrograde filling of it via collateral vessels. In the case of an abdominal pseudoaneurysm (e.g., splenic artery pseudoaneurysm) in an unstable patient, proximal arterial occlusion may provide equivalent results to the more conventional segmental occlusion.[4]

INDICATIONS

Aneurysms will eventually enlarge and rupture once the tension on the wall is greater than the intrinsic wall strength. Tension on the wall is a function of the pressure multiplied by the radius divided by the wall thickness (Laplace law).

Rupture is more common in false aneurysms, probably related to wall thickness. In the absence of trauma, peripheral aneurysms are less prone to spontaneous rupture than intracranial aneurysms. Larger aneurysms are believed to be at greater risk of rupture than smaller ones, and this is particularly so in the case of splenic aneurysms, whether they are true or false.

In addition, aneurysms may extrinsically compress surrounding structures like nerves or arteries and lead to symptoms.

In general, false aneurysms, particularly those caused by an arterial puncture, are more likely to be associated with pain than true aneurysms. Early treatment of false aneurysms is important to reduce the risk of rupture. Factors that influence rupture of cerebral aneurysms are disturbed flow patterns, small impingement regions, and narrow jets.[5] The same factors probably apply in peripheral aneurysms.

CONTRAINDICATIONS

Major contraindications to endovascular treatment of peripheral aneurysms are active/uncontrolled infection or arteritis, and an aneurysm that is unlikely to enlarge further or rupture (e.g., circumferentially calcified aneurysms). If an aneurysm is to be left untreated, careful follow-up is mandatory.

In the case of infection, aggressive treatment with high doses of intravenous antibiotics is required if endovascular treatment is contemplated. Most vascular surgeons prefer to perform an extra-anatomic bypass for infected aneurysms. However, if the risk of surgery and rupture is unacceptable, infected aneurysms can be treated by endovascular methods.

Patients with aneurysms related to arteritis should ideally be treated until the erythrocyte sedimentation rate and other inflammatory markers are within normal range and the etiologic disease is under control, if this is possible. However, aneurysms related to Behçet disease are more likely to arise suddenly and are prone to early rupture.[6]

Patients who know they have an aneurysm are usually very anxious about it and will request treatment, even when the aneurysm is small and asymptomatic.

EQUIPMENT

- Micropuncture access kit (Cook Inc., Bloomington, Ind.; AngioDynamics Inc., Queensbury, N.Y.)
- 0.035-inch guidewire (1.5-mm J or Terumo guidewire [Cook Inc.; Terumo Corp., Somerset, N.J.])
- 5F access sheath (Cook Inc.)
- 4F or 5F diagnostic catheter (Cobra 2) (Cook Inc., Angio-Dynamics Inc., Terumo Corp.)
- Guide catheters (Cordis Corp., Hialeah, Fla.; Abbott Vascular, Santa Clara, Calif.)
- Microcatheter (Terumo Progreat or equivalent)
- Ultravist 370 or equivalent nonionic contrast media
- Arterial stent (balloon-expandable or self-expanding), provided the interstices of the stent allow passage of a catheter
- Peripheral endograft (Symbiot [Boston Scientific, Natick, Mass.], Atrium [Atrium Medical, Hudson, N.H.], Jo-Graft [Abbott Vascular, Abbott Park, Ill.])
- Balloon angioplasty catheter for use with vinyl alcohol copolymer (Onyx [ev3/Covidien, Irvine, Calif.])
- Occlusion coils (fiber coils are preferred in 0.018- or 0.035-inch wire diameters [Cook Inc., Boston Scientific])
- Detachable coils (Micro Therapeutics Inc. [Irvine, Calif.], Cook Inc., Boston Scientific)
- Vinyl alcohol copolymer (Onyx)

- *N*-butyl cyanoacrylate (NBCA) adhesive and iodized oil (Cordis Corp.)
- Thrombin (USP), 1000 IU/mL or 5000 IU/5 mL (Thrombin-JMI [GenTrac Inc., Middleton, Wis.])

TECHNIQUE

Anatomy and Approaches

Approach to the aneurysm will be determined by its site. If the aneurysm cannot be accessed angiographically, it may be possible to directly puncture it using a 22-gauge needle. Of the visceral aneurysms, splenic artery aneurysms are the most common.[7]

Because of the short gastric supply to the spleen, it is usually possible to occlude the main splenic artery without causing splenic infarction. However, preservation of pancreatic blood supply is critical to avoid pancreatitis. If possible, distal splenic artery embolization should be avoided to reduce the risk of splenic infarction. Provided it will adequately treat the aneurysm, proximal splenic artery embolization is preferred.

In the limbs, it is essential to maintain blood supply to the distal limb and avoid embolization of the distal vessels.

Technical Aspects

There are several methods of treating peripheral aneurysms.

Thrombin Injection Into a False Aneurysm

The concept of this procedure is that introducing a small amount of thrombin into the aneurysmal sac will induce a rapid and localized coagulation cascade that will be confined to the aneurysm and not lead to any thrombosis or distal embolization within the native vessel (Fig. 41-1).

Under Doppler ultrasound visualization, a 22-gauge needle is inserted into the false aneurysm, and thrombin injection is commenced. Injection must be slow and sufficient time allowed for thrombus to form. Thrombus can be seen to develop at the tip of the needle by ultrasound.

Care should be taken not to compress the developing thrombus during this process because thrombus may be squeezed from the false aneurysm into the parent artery,

with extensive thrombosis of the distal arteries beyond the false aneurysm.[8] In addition, great care must be taken to ensure that thrombin is not inadvertently injected into the venous side of the circulation; this can induce a systemic venous thrombosis.

Because the average amount of thrombin required is in the range of 100 to 500 IU, and thrombin is supplied in ampules of 1000 IU/mL or 5000 IU/5 mL,[4] thrombin should be injected very slowly using a 1-mL hypodermic syringe. On occasion, it may be necessary to inject larger doses. This is particularly so in the setting of complex multilobulated pseudoaneurysms.

The manufacturer's recommendations indicate that thrombin is not suited for intravascular use. For this reason, it is extremely important that thrombin only be injected into the false aneurysm.

Once ultrasound demonstrates the beginning of thrombus formation within the aneurysm, complete thrombosis of the false aneurysm is surprisingly quick and will occur with little or no further thrombin. The most common error in this procedure is to use more thrombin than required. It is unnecessary to compress the aneurysm sac after thrombin injection, even in the setting of a wide-necked aneurysm.

If it is decided to treat an infected aneurysm by endovascular methods, injection of thrombin is worth considering. This is the only method that will not leave a foreign body at the site of the aneurysm.

Placement of Peripheral Endograft Across Neck of Aneurysm

Where the anatomy permits, this is the quickest and probably the most reliable method of exclusion of an aneurysm (Fig. 41-2). However, in many situations, tortuosity of the proximal feeding artery precludes endograft placement, or the position of the aneurysm neck is at a vessel bifurcation. This method is particularly suited to cervical carotid arteries. Theoretically, the endograft should be self-expanding in areas where the vessel is subject to compression, but we have successfully placed balloon-expanded endografts in the cervical portion of the carotid artery, with excellent long-term results.

If the endograft is self-expanding, it should be slightly oversized to prevent development of a type I endoleak. Where there are branch arteries arising from the area of the

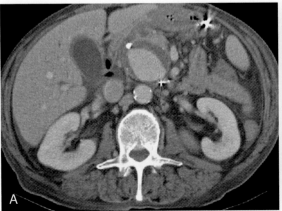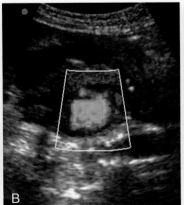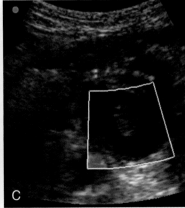

FIGURE 41-1. A-C, Thrombin injection into false aneurysm (see text for description).

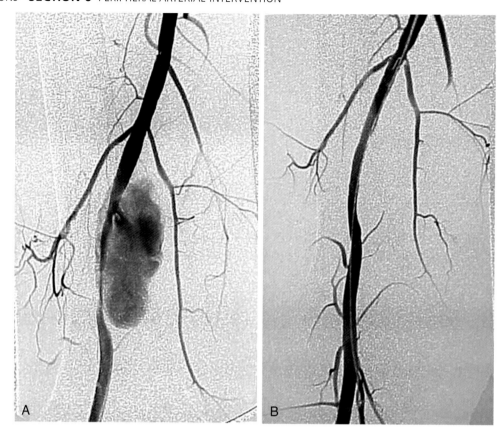

FIGURE 41-2. A-B, Placement of peripheral endograft across aneurysm neck.

aneurysm, there is also risk of a type II endoleak if the aneurysm is not completely thrombosed.

Coiling of a Narrow-Necked Aneurysm

Peripheral aneurysms rarely have a narrow neck, but in these situations it can be relatively easy to completely pack the aneurysm with coils in exactly the same way as an intracranial aneurysm. When possible, the microcatheter should be inserted into the aneurysmal sac and a three-dimensional coil inserted first to form a structure upon which to deposit further coils. Fiber coils are preferred because they will promote thrombosis in the event of interstices between coils. Placement of coils in the aneurysm is continued until it is completely packed or until complete aneurysm thrombosis has been demonstrated angiographically. It is unnecessary to place a coil in the aneurysm neck if it is very short. In very large peripheral aneurysms, movable-core guidewires may be used as a less expensive alternative to embolization coils (Fig. 41-3). For this process, the removable guidewire core is taken out, the guidewire's external spring component is curved over the back edge of a scalpel, then the core is replaced. During insertion of the wire into the aneurysm sac, the movable core is progressively removed, and the final portion of the wire is pushed into place using a new guidewire. Movable guidewires are available in 65-cm and 145-cm lengths.

Coiling an Aneurysm Through a Stent Placed Across Aneurysm Neck

When an aneurysm's neck is wide and there is a risk of coils extruding from the aneurysm, a bare arterial stent may be placed across the neck to keep the coils in place within the

aneurysm (Fig. 41-4). This technique requires that the interstices of the stent are of sufficient width to allow either a 4F catheter or a microcatheter to be safely passed and retrieved. The tip of the catheter is positioned at the most distal point of the aneurysm, and coils are inserted until the aneurysm is completely filled. This method provides a very secure and complete occlusion of the aneurysm. The only limitation is the ability to place a stent across the aneurysm neck. Self-expanding stents are less suitable than balloon-expanded stents because they tend to have narrower interstices.

Balloon-Protected Occlusion of an Aneurysm with Onyx

A newer method of treating aneurysms is to fill them with Onyx, a nonadhesive liquid embolic compound, while a balloon is in place in the adjacent portion of the artery to prevent reflux of the agent. The most viscous Onyx is required, and the aneurysm is catheterized with a microcatheter before instillation of the balloon in the parent artery. Onyx should be injected very slowly so that the surface exposed to the balloon sets slightly. Further injections of Onyx will expand the collection and fill the aneurysm. Once the Onyx has "cured," the balloon is deflated and removed.

Coiling of a Wide-Necked Aneurysm

In situations where vascular anatomy precludes placement of a peripheral endograft or covered stent, and stent placement across the aneurysm neck to hold the coils in place within the aneurysm is impossible, it may be necessary to use a three-dimensional coil on which to deposit further coils (Fig. 41-5). When there is doubt that the coils will stay

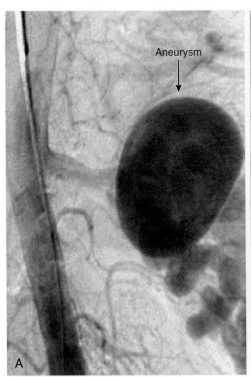
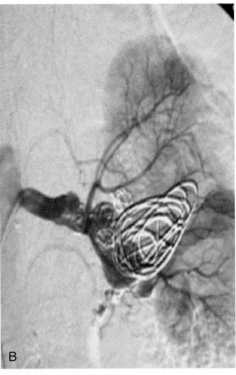

FIGURE 41-3. A-B, In very large peripheral aneurysms, movable core guidewires may be used as a less expensive alternative to embolization coils.

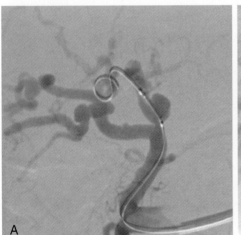
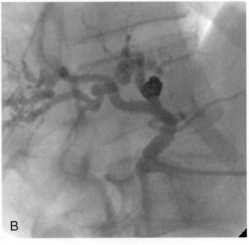

FIGURE 41-4. A-B, Coiling an aneurysm through stent placed across aneurysm neck.

within the aneurysm, use of a detachable coil system is recommended. By using this technique, the final coil will often prolapse slightly into the parent vessel. Follow-up of the aneurysm with multidetector-row CT or digital subtraction angiography at 3 months is suggested; if necessary, further coils can be placed within the aneurysm if the previous coils have contracted and there is recurrent filling of the aneurysm. Incomplete coiling of an aneurysm may result in increased size owing to pressure effects of the coils on the aneurysm wall.

Embolization of Arteries Supplying Aneurysm

When an aneurysm cannot be treated directly, equivalent results can be obtained by occluding the artery proximal and distal to the aneurysm with coils or NBCA "glue" (Fig. 41-6). As noted earlier, it is important to perform embolization in the artery both proximal and distal to the aneurysm to prevent retrograde filling via a collateral vessel supplying distal arterial branches. This is referred to as "shutting the front and back doors." In the emergency situation of a ruptured aneurysm or hemodynamically unstable patient, occlusion of just the proximal artery may be sufficient. Although we have seen evidence of continued aneurysm filling by distal branches after occlusion of the proximal artery, others have found no difference between proximal or proximal and distal embolization.

Treatment of Flow-Related Aneurysms in Conjunction with a High-Flow Vascular Malformation

Unless aneurysms are extremely large and there is a risk of rupture, it is preferable to reduce flow in the malformation by embolizing it before attempting to treat the aneurysm directly. An aneurysm may disappear spontaneously once the high-flow situation has been reversed (Fig. 41-7).

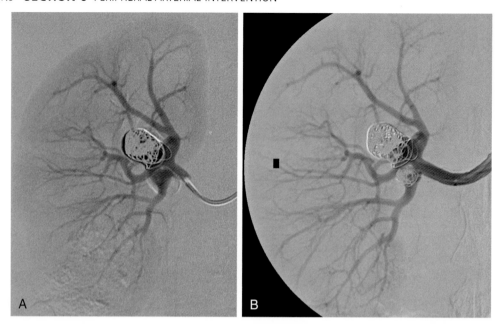

FIGURE 41-5. A-B, Using three-dimensional coil upon which to deposit further coils.

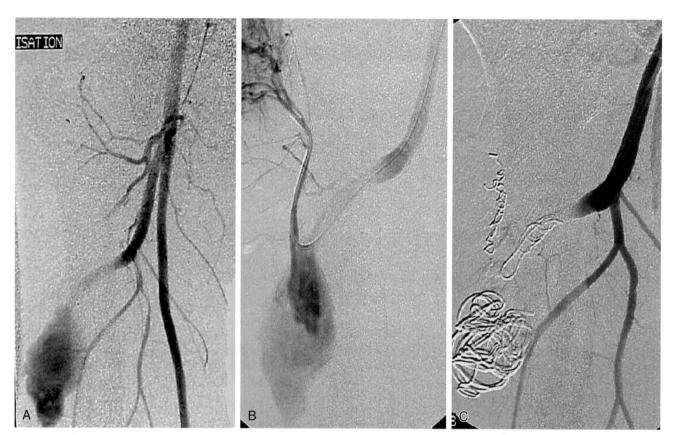

FIGURE 41-6. A-C, When aneurysm cannot be treated directly, equivalent results can be obtained by occluding the artery proximal and distal to aneurysm with coils or *N*-butyl cyanoacrylate "glue."

CONTROVERSIES

Many surgeons believe aneurysms are best treated surgically, but with newer techniques and improved and refined hardware, including coils and other embolic materials, there are very few aneurysms that cannot be treated easily and just as effectively by endovascular means. These techniques are, however, dependent on significant familiarity, training, and expertise with a variety of catheters, guidewires, and coils, which requires considerable experience to achieve.

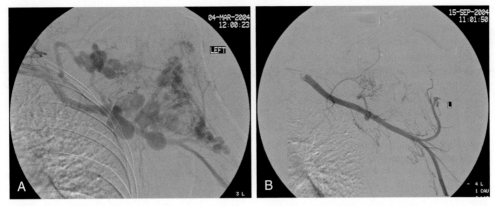

FIGURE 41-7. **A-B,** Flow-related aneurysms may disappear spontaneously once high-flow situation has been reversed.

Because the manufacturer of thrombin states that it is not intended for intravascular use, using thrombin for the treatment of false aneurysms requires off-label notification, and approval by the patient and probably the institution where the procedure is performed.

OUTCOMES

The only existing randomized data comparing endovascular techniques to open surgery in aneurysm treatment are for intracranial aneurysms, where surgical approach is much more difficult. Once vascular surgeons begin to adopt an endovascular approach to treating peripheral aneurysms, these methods will become much more widely accepted.

COMPLICATIONS

Rupture of peripheral aneurysms during treatment is rare. The most likely complication is ectopic embolization of thrombus or embolic material from the aneurysm during or after the procedure. Metallic coils can usually be retrieved relatively easily, but if thrombin or blood clot escapes into a critical vessel, thrombolysis or thrombectomy may be urgently required. In a series of 240 cases of thrombin injection of false aneurysms, there were two embolic complications and six late reperfusions.[9]

Coil treatment of aneurysms is durable, but follow-up is required to exclude reperfusion or vessel thrombosis.

Regarding use of endografts to exclude peripheral aneurysms, follow-up is essential, particularly after treatment of popliteal artery aneurysms because knee flexion can cause endografts to thrombose or fracture.[10] Long-term results in a small number of cases showed a primary patency of only 55% and several acute occlusions of the endograft.

POSTPROCEDURAL AND FOLLOW-UP CARE

Once an aneurysm has completely thrombosed, it will usually reduce in size. Degree of size reduction will be limited by the coils within it or any calcified shell around it. Follow-up is most easily and effectively done by multidetector-row computed tomographic angiography (MD-CTA) because this method alone demonstrates the entire aneurysm. If the artifact produced by metallic coils precludes CTA review, peripheral aneurysms may be reviewed by Doppler ultrasonography. Most coils, although magnetic resonance imaging (MRI) compatible, produce a susceptibility artifact that degrades imaging of the aneurysm.

Normally, unless the aneurysm is very large or in an anatomically critical location, the patient will be unaware of symptoms related to embolization. In large aneurysms, pain and some fever may occur, similar to the syndrome seen after endovascular treatment of aortic aneurysms. Where there is a risk of contamination of the area—for example, after gunshot wounds or penetrating injury—periprocedural and postprocedural antibiotics are recommended.

In very superficial areas, the patient may become aware of the presence of the coils under the skin and need reassurance that this is normal.

KEY POINTS

- The term *peripheral* excludes intracranial and aortic aneurysms.
- There is more than one way to occlude an aneurysm.
- Exclude the possibility of infection and arteritides.
- Maintain arterial flow where possible.
- In emergencies, proximal arterial occlusion may be sufficient.

▶ **SUGGESTED READINGS**

Sueyoshi E, Sakamoto I, Nakashima K, et al. Visceral and peripheral arterial pseudoaneurysms. AJR Am J Roentgenol 2005;185:741–9.

Tisi PV, Callum MJ. Surgery versus non-surgical treatment for femoral pseudoaneurysms. Cochrane Database Syst Rev 2006;CD004981.

The complete reference list is available online at www.expertconsult.com.

CHAPTER **42**
Management of Vascular Arteritides
Sanjiv Sharma and Priya Jagia

Nonspecific aortoarteritis is characterized by an initial phase marked by nonspecific constitutional symptoms and signs. Presence of active vascular inflammation may include aggravation of symptoms and signs of active disease, aggravation or appearance of new angiographic lesions, or abnormal results of serologic tests showing increased levels of acute-phase reactants, such as erythrocyte sedimentation rate (ESR), C-reactive protein, or antistreptolysin-O titers.

IMAGING

Noninvasive imaging, including duplex sonography, computed tomography (CT) and magnetic resonance imaging (MRI), are used for diagnosis and detection of disease activity. High-resolution B-mode ultrasound can detect intima media thickness (IMT) with or without obstructive stenosis. Increased IMT may suggest presence of active disease.[1] Maeda et al. reported circumferential arterial wall thickening of the common carotid arteries, which may or may not be bilateral.[2] MRI and CT have both been used to demonstrate arterial wall thickness. Noncontrast CT scans may show a high-density wall of variable thickness in the aorta or its branches, along with calcification if present. CT post contrast may show enhancement of the thickened aortic wall in patients with active inflammation.[3] MRI shows subtle wall thickening, and T2-weighted images may show bright signal due to edema in the inflamed vessel. During the acute phase, enhancement of the aortic wall and periadventitial soft tissues can also be observed.[4] It has been suggested that contrast-enhanced MRI may be more sensitive than serologic markers of clinical activity in this disease. Overall, these MR criteria are not highly sensitive but are highly specific for disease activity. We have observed that the sensitivity of T2-weighted imaging in detecting active disease seems inferior to contrast-enhanced T1-weighted imaging. Aortic wall thickness by itself may also reflect disease activity.[5] Most of our patients with inactive disease had a wall thickness of less than 4 mm, and most of them with acute or chronic active disease had a wall thickness greater than 5 mm.

The differential diagnosis includes a variety of conditions that can cause vasculitis. These are summarized in Table 42-1.

INDICATIONS

Therapeutic goals include control of clinical activity by pharmacologic treatment with corticosteroids and/or immunosuppressive therapy, restoration of blood flow to the obstructed vessel by surgical or endovascular techniques, pharmacologic control of blood pressure, and supportive management.

Renovascular hypertension (RVH) is the most common form of treatable clinical presentation of this disease. It is usually due to obstructing lesions involving the aorta and renal arteries.[6,7] Takayasu disease is a common cause of RVH in India. Chugh et al.[8] studied the causes of RVH in India and reported that nonspecific aortoarteritis was responsible for 61%, fibromuscular dysplasia (FMD) for 28%, and atherosclerosis for 8% of cases. Some form of revascularization is necessary to relieve ischemia secondary to a hemodynamically significant stenosis. The complexity of pathologic changes in the wall of the aorta and the widespread nature of involvement make surgical revascularization difficult. There is also a high prevalence of graft occlusion or aneurysm formation at the treatment site.[9-11] Because of this, nonsurgical revascularization techniques have been increasingly used to treat this disease.[6,7,12-22]

Percutaneous transluminal angioplasty (PTA) for treatment of aortic stenosis in the presence of nonspecific aortitis has been infrequently reported.[7,17,23] In these patients, the angiographic morphology of 140 stenoses has been correlated with the outcome of balloon angioplasty. Patients with short-segment (<4 cm) stenosis show better overall results than those with long-segment (>4 cm) stenosis. The angiographic features, including eccentricity of the stenosis and presence of diffuse adjacent disease, location of the stenosis in the juxtadiaphragmatic segment of the aorta, and presence of calcification adversely affect the outcome of PTA, with most patients developing large intimal flaps. Such patients should be electively treated by stent placement. Stents have also been used as a "bailout" measure in salvaging an obstructive dissection.[22,23] Our results show that stents provide immediate relief of symptomatic obstructive dissection and are also useful to treat recurrent stenosis after successful angioplasty. Except for the situations just mentioned, we do not advocate elective use of stents because of the young age of patients, cost involved, and lack of knowledge about the long-term behavior of stents in the aorta at a growing age.

CONTRAINDICATIONS

Presence of active disease has important therapeutic implications and adversely affects outcomes of various revascularization techniques. It is important to identify clinical remission before advocating endovascular or surgical revascularization to treat the complications of vascular inflammation.

Various methods have been used to identify active disease. Constitutional signs and symptoms include fever, anorexia, arthralgia, limb ischemia, hypertension, and raised ESR. These acute-phase features may be present in 50% of patients. The other 50% of patients present with advanced obstructive changes with no acute-phase symptoms. Surgical biopsy specimens from patients with clinically inactive disease showed histologically active disease in as many as 44%.[24] From a study in 1998, researchers

TABLE 42-1. Potential Underlying Systemic Illnesses in Upper Limb Arterial Disease

Connective Tissue Disorders
Systemic lupus erythematosus
Scleroderma
Polyarteritis nodosa
Arthritides
Rheumatoid arthritis
Takayasu arteritis
Giant cell arteritis
Myeloproliferative Disorder
Polycythemia rubra vera
Immunoglobulin Abnormalities
Cryoglobulinemia
Multiple myeloma

concluded that no known serologic test could supplant vascular histopathologic examination in determining disease activity. Similarly, 61% of patients with remitting disease showed new lesions on angiography, emphasizing the need for more reliable and accurate markers for disease activity.

The National Institutes of Health describes "active" disease as fresh onset or progression of at least two of the following features[25]:

- Signs and symptoms of vasculitis or ischemia (claudication, feeble or absent pulses, differential blood pressure in extremities, bruits, or carotidynia)
- Raised ESR
- Angiographic abnormalities
- Systemic symptoms such as fever, polyarthralgia, or polymyalgia

A study by the International Network for the Study of Systemic Vasculitides (INSSYS) enlisted 29 patients with Takayasu arteritis and 26 healthy controls. Activity was assessed based on Birmingham vasculitis activity scores.[26] Serologic tests including ESR, C-reactive protein, tissue factor, von Willebrand factor, thrombomodulin, tissue plasminogen activator (tPA), intercellular adhesion molecule-1, vascular cell adhesion molecule-1, E-selectin, and platelet endothelial cell adhesion molecule-1 were performed on all patients but could not reliably differentiate between healthy volunteers and patients with Takayasu arteritis. Clinical and biochemical markers remain poor predictors of clinical activity, but patients with an elevated ESR and/or positive C-reactive protein test are considered to have active arteritis and are not accepted for this treatment.

EQUIPMENT

Standard angioplasty techniques are employed.

- Arterial sheath: for placement in both femoral arteries
- Pigtail catheter: to be placed in the abdominal aorta above the origin of the renal arteries for continuous pressure measurement and diagnostic digital subtraction angiography
- Selective angiographic catheter: for transstenotic gradient measurement
- Appropriate-sized balloon catheter (not oversized)

Alternatively, a coaxial technique with a preshaped guiding catheter and an over-the-wire or monorail technique can be used. When a branch vessel originates or is involved in the stenosis, a kissing balloon technique is employed using a coaxial approach.

TECHNIQUE

Anatomy and Approaches

It has been traditionally reported that nonspecific aortoarteritis involves all layers of the vessel wall.[27,28] Histopathologic findings are characterized by inflammatory changes, with marked tissue destruction and connective tissue proliferation initiated at the junction of the media and adventitia or the outer layer of the media. There is an endarteritis obliterans or onion skin–type fibrosis in the vasa vasorum. Thickening of the intima results from an increase in ground substance and proliferation of connective tissue.[27-30] Underlying chronic inflammation, extensive periarterial fibrosis, thickening, and adhesions combine to produce tough, noncompliant, rigid vessel walls.

The femoral route is preferred for access to renal and aortic lesions. In difficult situations, such as an acute downward angulation of the involved artery, or unavailability of the femoral route due to concomitant obstructive disease, a brachial approach is used.

Technical Aspects

Use of an angled hydrophilic guidewire reduces the risk of complications related to vessel spasm and perforation. Predilation by a Teflon catheter is required in most patients before the balloon catheter can be positioned across the stenosis. Stenotic lesions often resist prolonged repeated mechanical distention before responding to balloon dilation. In addition, the risk of arterial tear or rupture is significant if the vessel is overdistended during angioplasty. Multiple prolonged balloon inflations are usually necessary to obtain a substantial decrease in stenosis.

Most patients experience an intense transient backache during balloon inflation, often accompanied by a transient fall in blood pressure. This subsides soon after balloon deflation. If pain persists, an obstructive dissection should be suspected.

Angiographic features including eccentricity of the stenosis and presence of diffuse adjacent disease, location of the stenosis in a juxtadiaphragmatic segment of the aorta, and presence of calcification adversely affect the outcome of PTA, with an increased risk of large intimal flaps.

Elective use of stents is not recommended, owing to the young age of patients and lack of knowledge about the long-term behavior of stents in the aorta at a growing age, except as "bailout" for dissection or restenosis.

CONTROVERSIES

The morphologic pattern of involvement in Takayasu disease shows racial and geographic differences.[31] In Japan, thoracic aortic involvement is more common, and neck vessels are most often involved.[28] In most other Asian countries, the abdominal aorta is most frequently affected, with the renal and subclavian arteries being the most commonly involved branches.[32] Although pulmonary artery involvement is common in most studies, among Indian patients it is less frequent. In a prospective study, we found pulmonary arterial involvement in 14.9% of patients.[33]

Reports of familial incidence of Takayasu arteritis may point to a genetic origin. In Japan, 16 families with familial Takayasu arteritis have been reported.[34] In India, Mehra et al.[35] studied 104 patients and suggested an association of this disease with human immune response genes, namely HLA-B5 and its serologic subtypes B51 and B52. In HLA B52–positive patients, aortic regurgitation, ischemic heart disease, and pulmonary infarction are more common. Renal artery stenosis is reported more frequently in HLA B39–positive patients. The human leukocyte antigen association is thought by some to strengthen the argument in favor of an autoimmune pathogenesis. However, no specific autoantigens have been identified, and for any adaptive immune response to occur, whether against exogenous or endogenous antigen, presentation of antigen to T cells in the context of the major histocompatibility complex is central.

The predominant involvement of females has prompted investigators to study the role of sex hormones. In one study, urinary estrogens were elevated in 80% (16 of 20) of patients, compared with healthy controls.[36] In most studies that have evaluated the angiographic morphology, obstructive lesions predominate.[27,28,32,37] When present, aneurysmal lesions also show distinct geographic predilections. There is a disproportionately high incidence of these lesions in the Philippines, Thailand, Israel, Japan, and Western India.[38,39] Fusiform aneurysms probably have a genetic predilection because they are seen in a distinct racial subset. In this regard, it is worth mentioning that the phenotype frequencies of various loci of HLA-A and HLA-B antigens show significant differences between patients from Japan and India. Such differences may also account for different angiographic morphologies of the disease in different locations.[37]

OUTCOMES

Using interventional radiologic techniques over a 14-year period, the authors have treated a total of 276 patients with renovascular hypertension caused by this disease (Figs. 42-1 to 42-14). These included 264 renal arteries in 193 patients and 88 aortas in 83 patients. Among the renal arteries, stenosis decreased from 87% ± 6% to 11% ± 11%, and the pressure gradient fell from 95 ± 22 to 9 ± 8 mmHg ($P < .01$). The drug requirement for control of hypertension decreased from 3.9 ± 0.5 to 1.1 ± 0.9, systolic blood pressure improved from 181 ± 16 to 136 ± 25 mmHg, and diastolic blood pressure fell from 115 ± 10 to 86 ±16 mmHg ($P < .01$). An obstructive dissection was seen in two patients, both of whom were successfully treated by stent placement. The follow-up period ranged from 3 to 104 (49 ± 22) months. Remodeling at the percutaneous transluminal renal artery angioplasty (PTRA) site, with further angiographic improvement, was seen in most patients who underwent repeat angiography. Cumulative 5-year patency rate was 67%. Results are summarized in Table 42-2.

Results of PTRA have been reported by many authors.[6,7,13-22] Most of them concern a single case or a small group of patients. Dong et al.[16] reported 30 patients. Of these, the lesion was associated with nonspecific arteritis in 22. The procedure was successful in treating hypertension in 86% of patients. Complications were encountered in seven (excessive bleeding in three, pseudoaneurysm requiring surgery in one, occlusion of the renal artery in two, and dissection of the renal artery in one). Kumar et al.[17] reported results in nine patients, with clinical success in 55%. Procedure-related complications occurred in 33% of cases. Tyagi et al.[22] performed renal angioplasty in 35 patients. Nonspecific arteritis was the cause in 31 of the cases. Clinical benefit was seen in 92% of cases. Complications were not reported.

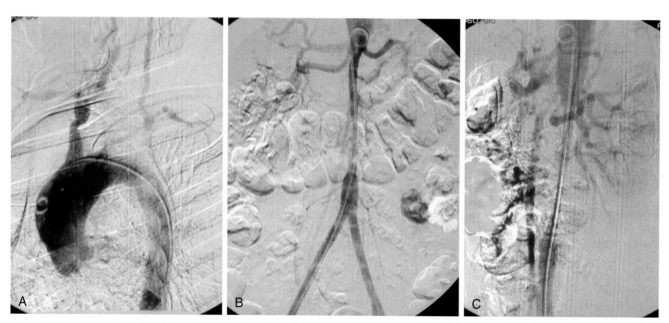

FIGURE 42-1. This 17-year-old girl presented with bilateral limb claudication and underwent intraarterial digital subtraction angiography. **A,** Left common carotid artery occlusion and significant proximal disease of left subclavian artery. **B,** Tight infrarenal aortic stenosis with normal renal arteries and aortic bifurcation. **C,** Lateral view showing ostial stenosis of celiac and superior mesenteric arteries.

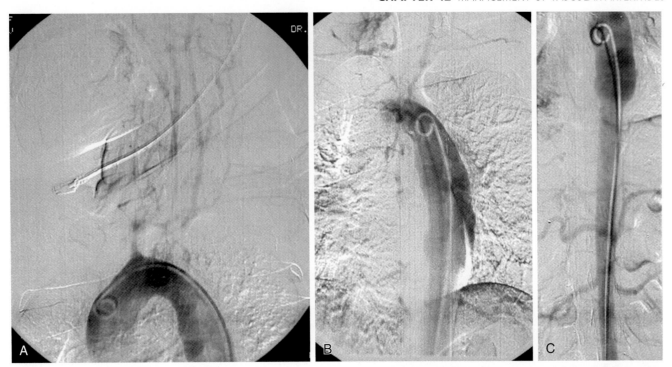

FIGURE 42-2. Intraarterial digital subtraction arteriography in a 20-year-old woman with absent upper limb pulses. **A,** Steno-occlusive lesions involving all the arch vessels. **B-C,** Dilative lesion in proximal descending thoracic aorta.

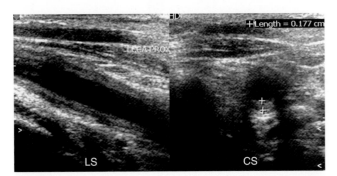

FIGURE 42-3. Patient with Takayasu arteritis has increased common carotid artery intima media thickness on B-mode ultrasonography.

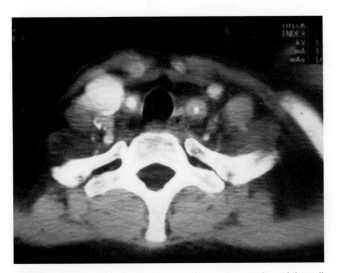

FIGURE 42-4. Axial computed tomographic angiogram shows bilaterally thickened common carotid artery walls with mural contrast enhancement.

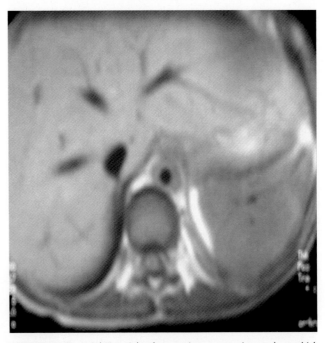

FIGURE 42-5. Axial T2-weighted magnetic resonance image shows thickened abdominal aortic wall with bright mural signals, suggestive of active disease.

Among the aortic lesions, stenosis decreased from 81% ± 7% to 19% ± 18%, pressure gradient fell from 76 ± 19 to 26 ± 11 mmHg, blood pressure fell from 185 ± 20/112 ± 12 to l46 ± 12/90 ± 7 mmHg, and the drug requirement fell from 4 ± 1 to 1 ± 1 (P < .001 for all). Results are summarized in Table 42-2. Localized nonobstructing flaps at the PTA site were seen in approximately half of patients (see Fig. 42-7). The follow-up period ranged from 3 to 97 (37 ± 17) months. Remodeling at the angioplasty site with further angiographic improvement was seen in most patients. Some patients showed a delayed clinical benefit despite a poor technical result, probably due to late remodeling. One patient had recurrent stenosis despite three successful angioplasties within a period of 14 months and was treated by stent placement. Cumulative 5-year patency rate was 71%.

Outcomes of endovascular interventions in the supra-aortic branches are less rewarding. Because of the presence

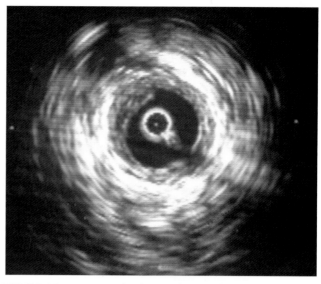

FIGURE 42-7. Intravascular ultrasound image of thoracic aorta shows a normal intimal shadow and thickened media and adventitia with altered echogenicity.

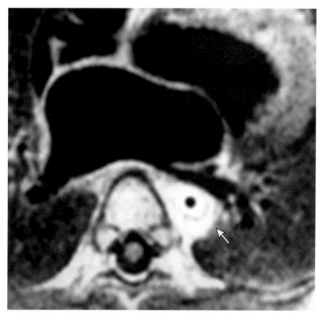

FIGURE 42-6. Axial magnetic resonance image shows enhancement of the thick aortic wall (arrow) after administration of gadolinium.

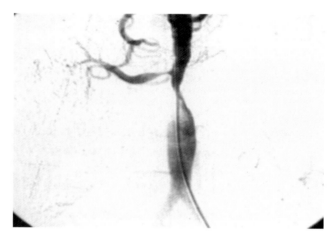

FIGURE 42-8. This 22-year-old woman presented with hypertension and claudication. Digital subtraction angiogram shows right renal artery stenosis and juxtarenal aortic stenosis.

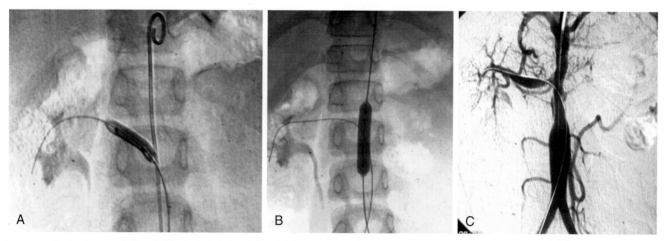

FIGURE 42-9. Same patient as in Figure 42-8. Angioplasty of right renal artery (A) and aorta (B) was performed. C, Follow-up angiogram shows good opening of right renal artery; nondestructive flap was noted in aorta.

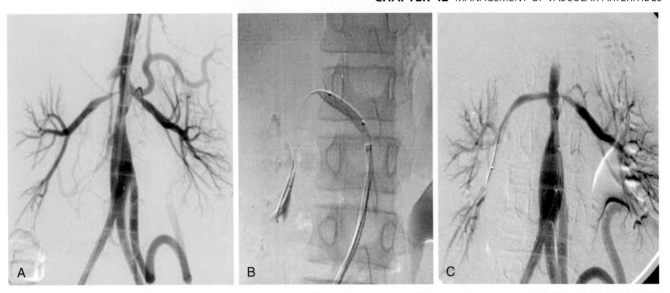

FIGURE 42-10. This 14-year-old girl presented with hypertension. Right renal artery stenosis **(A)** at the ostium was treated with a coaxial technique **(B)**. **C,** Postangioplasty angiogram shows good end result.

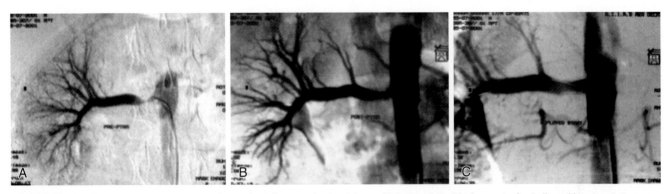

FIGURE 42-11. Right renal stenosis in a young hypertensive boy. **A,** Selective right renal injection. **B,** Residual stenosis after balloon dilatation. **C,** Aortogram after renal stenting.

TABLE 42-2. Outcomes After Percutaneous Transluminal Angioplasty in Takayasu Arteritis

	No. of Patients	Technical Success	Clinical Success	Complications	Restenosis Rate
Renal artery stenosis	193 (264 vessels)	96%	91% Cure: 32% Improvement: 68%	15 patients Groin hematoma: 8 Transient renal artery spasm: 7 Renal vein injury: 1	17%
Aortic stenosis	83 (88 aortas) Descending thoracic: 56% Abdominal aortic: 44%	84%	89%	Pseudoaneurysm at PTA site: 2 Obstructive dissection: 11 Stent: 8 Surgery: 2	5%

PTA, Percutaneous transluminal angioplasty.

of diffuse lesions and increased wall thickening, stenosis in the carotid and subclavian arteries responds less well to balloon angioplasty. We treat these lesions less often because even though they are commonly present, they are largely asymptomatic. When symptomatic, most lesions are very long and not well suited for endovascular management. Among patients with suitable angiographic morphology, luminal stenosis and trans-stenotic pressure gradients are difficult to abolish because stenosis often does not respond to multiple high-pressure balloon dilatations. Even after initial successful angioplasty, the restenosis rate is high.

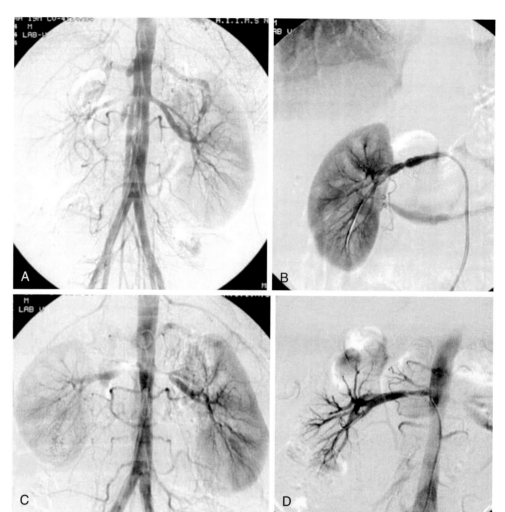

FIGURE 42-12. This 19-year-old man presented with hypertension. **A,** Percutaneous transluminal renal artery angioplasty (PTRA) was performed for a tight ostial right renal artery stenosis. **B,** Post-PTRA angiogram shows mild residual disease. **C,** Follow-up angiogram after 15 months shows restenosis of right renal artery ostium. Left renal artery also shows tight ostial disease. **D,** Right PTRA was again performed, with good opening of lesion with mild residual disease.

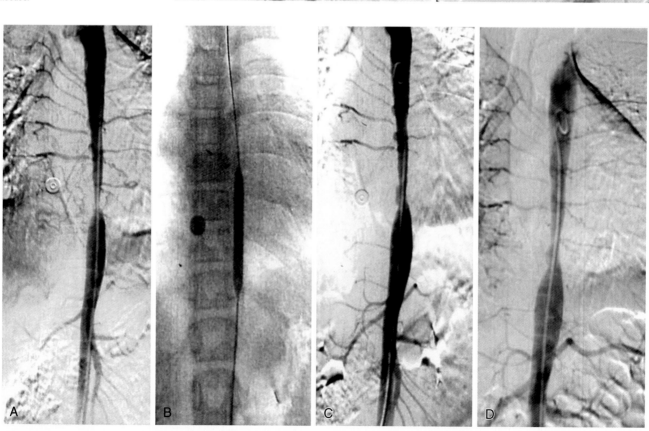

FIGURE 42-13. This 11-year-old girl presented with hypertension. **A,** Intraarterial digital subtraction angiogram shows a tight lower-thoracic aortic stenosis. **B,** Balloon inflated across stenosis during angioplasty. **C,** Postangioplasty intraarterial digital subtraction angiogram shows a nonobstructive dissection at angioplasty site. **D,** At 2-month follow-up, there is remodeling at angioplasty site, with no gradient across residual stenosis.

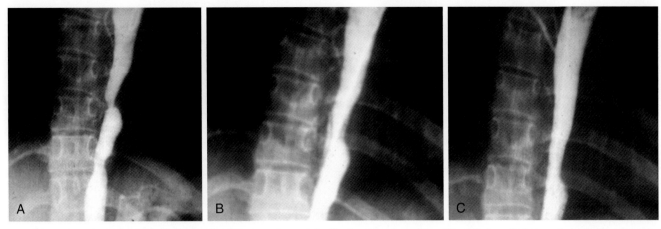

FIGURE 42-14. This 16-year-old girl presented with hypertension and claudication. Aortogram shows **(A)** a tight juxtadiaphragmatic aortic stenosis, treated by balloon angioplasty, and an obstructive dissection flap at the angioplasty site **(B)** that was treated by placing a self-expanding stent, with immediate hemodynamic and angiographic improvement **(C)**.

COMPLICATIONS

Complications common to angiography and angioplasty may be expected. Major complications associated with nonspecific aortoarteritis are obstructive intimal dissection from guidewires and vessel rupture due to overdistention with a too-large balloon. Use of hydrophilic wires and careful balloon sizing will minimize these complications. Prolonged and high-pressure inflations may be required to achieve a satisfactory result. Restenosis (17%) is less likely than might be expected because remodeling of the lesion after angioplasty is common.

POSTPROCEDURAL AND FOLLOW-UP CARE

Standard postangiography/angioplasty observations are performed. Antihypertensive medication is stopped 24 hours before angioplasty, except for use of short-acting drugs such as sublingual administration of 5 to 10 mg nifedipine if blood pressure is over 170/110 mmHg.

Patients are treated with aspirin (175-330 mg) daily for 3 days before angioplasty, and this treatment is continued for 6 months after treatment. Heparin (100 IU/kg) is given intravenously during the procedure and not reversed afterward.

Blood pressure medication is withheld for 24 hours after the procedure, except for use of short-acting drugs if blood pressure is over 160/100 mmHg.

If stent placement is considered, additional pretreatment with clopidogrel (75 mg once daily) is desirable, beginning 3 days before the angioplasty procedure. Alternatively, a single 300-mg dose of clopidogrel is given to patients in whom bailout stenting is performed. Subsequently, oral clopidogrel (75 mg daily) is continued for 6 weeks after the procedure.

Angioplasty is considered technically successful if [40,41]:

* The aortic or renal artery lumen after angioplasty has less than 30% residual stenosis.
* The arterial lumen is at least 50% larger than its pre-treatment diameter.

* The pressure gradient is less than 20 mmHg and has decreased at least 15 mmHg from the pretreatment gradient.

Clinical results of renal angioplasty are judged as follows:

* Cure (normal blood pressure after the procedure, without antihypertensive drug therapy).
* Improved (at least 15% reduction in diastolic pressure or diastolic pressure < 90 mmHg, with the patient taking less antihypertensive medication than before the procedure).
* Failed (no change in blood pressure after the procedure).

All patients cured or improved are considered to have benefited from angioplasty. Follow-up is performed by blood pressure and medication evaluation 1 day, 1 week, and 4 to 6 weeks after treatment and then at 6-month intervals. Follow-up angiograms are performed in patients with recurrence of hypertension and in whom contralateral nephrectomy of a poorly or nonfunctioning kidney for residual hypertension is planned.

Angioplasty is repeated if restenosis is detected.

KEY POINTS

* Nonspecific aortoarteritis (Takayasu disease) is a chronic and progressive disease of unknown cause that affects the aorta, its major branches, and the pulmonary arteries, most commonly in the second and third decades of life.

* Even though the disease is more common in parts of Japan, Korea, China, Thailand, Philippines, and India, it has a worldwide distribution.

* It is possible that this disease probably starts in a genetically predisposed individual with a specific hormonal milieu, who on later exposure to specific unidentified antigens (e.g., *Mycobacterium tuberculosis*) develops an immune response affecting the vessels.

* The outcome of various revascularization techniques is adversely affected by the presence of active disease.

* Underlying chronic inflammation, extensive periarterial fibrosis, thickening, and adhesions combine to produce tough,

noncompliant, and rigid vessel walls. In view of these features, stenotic lesions resist prolonged repeated mechanical distention before responding to balloon dilatation.

- Standard angioplasty techniques with particular care not to overdilate lesions produces a cumulative patency rate of 67% to 71%.
- Results of cross-sectional imaging suggest that there are extensive wall changes even in angiographically normal areas that may have a profound effect on outcome of localized therapy.

► **SUGGESTED READINGS**

Aggarwal A, Chag M, Sinha N, Naik S. Takayasu's arteritis: role of *Mycobacterium tuberculosis* and its 65 kDa heat shock protein. Int J Cardiol 1996;55:49–55.

Bahl VK, Seth S. Takayasu's arteritis revisited. Indian Heart J 2002; 54:147–51.

Baltazares M, Mendoza F, Dabague J, Reyes PA. Antiaorta antibodies and Takayasu arteritis. Int J Cardiol 1998;66(Suppl 1):S183–S187, discussion S189.

Chopra P, Datta RK, Dasgupta A, Bhargava S. Nonspecific aortoarteritis (Takayasu's disease): an immunologic and autopsy study. Jpn Heart J 1983;24:549–56.

Inada K, Swashima Y, Okada A, Shimizu Y. Aortitis syndrome: the diagnostic criteria. Gendai-Iryo 1976;8:1183–8.

Ishikawa K. Diagnostic approach and proposed criteria for the clinical diagnosis of Takayasu's arteriopathy. J Am Coll Cardiol 1988;12: 964–72.

Johnston SL, Lock RJ, Gompels MM. Takayasu arteritis: a review. J Clin Pathol 2002;55:481–6.

Judge DR. Takayasu's arteritis and aortic arch syndrome. Am J Med 1962;32:379–83.

Liu YQ. Radiology of aorto-arteritis. Radiol Clin North Am 1985;23: 671–88.

Lupi-Herrera E, Sanchez-Torres G, Marcushamer J, et al. Takayasu's arteritis: clinical study of 107 cases. Am Heart J 1977;93:94–103.

Pantell RH, Goodman BW Jr. Takayasu's arteritis: the relationship with tuberculosis. Pediatrics 1981;67:84–8.

Sagar S, Ganguly NK, Koicha M, Sharma BK. Immunopathogenesis of Takayasu arteritis. Heart Vessels Suppl 1992;7:85–90.

Sen PK, Kinare SG, Kelkar MD, Nanivadekar SA. Nonspecific stenosing arteritis of the aorta and its branches: a study of possible etiology. Mt Sinai J Med 1972;39:221–42.

Sharma S, Kamalakar T, Rajani M, et al. The incidence and patterns of pulmonary artery involvement in Takayasu's arteritis. Clin Radiol 1990;42:177–81.

Sharma S, Rajani M, Shrivastava S, et al. Nonspecific aortoarteritis (Takayasu's disease) in children. Br J Radiol 1991;64:690–8.

Sharma S, Rajani M, Talwar KK. Angiographic morphology in nonspecific aortoarteritis (Takayasu's arteritis): a study of 126 patients from North India. Cardiovasc Intervent Radiol 1992;15:160–5.

Sharma S, Sharma S, Taneja K, et al. Morphologic mural changes in the aorta in nonspecific aortoarteritis (Takayasu's arteritis): assessment by intravascular ultrasound. Clin Radiol 1998;53:37–43.

Talwar KK, Chopra P, Narula J, et al. Myocardial involvement and its response to immunosuppressive therapy in nonspecific aortoarteritis (Takayasu's disease)—a study by endomyocardial biopsy. Int J Cardiol 1988;21:323–34.

Webb M, Chambers A, Al-Nahhas A, et al. The role of 18F-FDG PET in characterizing disease activity in Takayasu arteritis. Eur J Nucl Med Mol Imaging 2004;31:627–34.

Yamato M, Lecky JW, Hiramatsu K, Kohda E. Takayasu's arteritis: radiographic and angiographic findings in 59 patients. Radiology 1986; 161:329–34.

The complete reference list is available online at www.expertconsult.com.

CHAPTER **43**

Congenital Vascular Anomalies: Classification and Terminology

Aylin Tekes, Özlem Tuğçe Kalayci, and Sally E. Mitchell

BIOLOGICAL CLASSIFICATION OF CONGENITAL SOFT-TISSUE VASCULAR ANOMALIES

The classification of vascular anomalies is confusing to most physicians. Overlapping clinical and imaging findings, the rarity of the vascular anomalies, lack of physician experience with the entity, and lack of a multidisciplinary approach in many centers contribute to the chaos in diagnosis and management of vascular anomalies.

To clarify this situation, the correct terminology for each entity should be consistently used. Even as recently as 2009, Hassanein and Mulliken found that the term *hemangioma* was used incorrectly in 71.3% of publications that year.[1] This emphasizes the importance of understanding the current classification system that was approved by the International Society for the Study of Vascular Anomalies (ISSVA) in 1996 (Table 43-1), which stems from the biological behavior–based classification system introduced by Drs. Mulliken and Glowacki in 1982.[2]

Congenital soft-tissue vascular anomalies can present anywhere in the body from head to toe, with variable size and infiltration, so a multidisciplinary approach is crucial in the management/treatment of these patients. Consistent use of correct terminology will improve communication between different specialists and avoid misunderstandings.

Given the rarity of some of the vascular anomalies, as well as overlapping clinical and imaging features, the experience of the team taking care of the patient is extremely important. Accurate classification and treatment of vascular anomalies is best performed by groups who see a large volume of patients and can begin to see the patterns of vascular anomalies in coordinated clinical and imaging appearances. This is why development of multidisciplinary vascular anomalies centers is essential for accurate diagnosis and management of these patients. In our clinical practice, we often see patients who say that their doctor had never seen anything like that before and had no idea what it was, let alone how to treat it.

Vascular anomalies can be imaged by ultrasonography (US), computed tomography (CT), computed tomographic angiography (CTA), digital subtraction angiography (DSA), magnetic resonance imaging (MRI), and MR angiography/venography (MRA/MRV). US is often used as first-line imaging, given its lack of ionizing radiation, no need for sedation/general anesthesia, and bedside imaging capabilities. Structural imaging data can be combined with flow dynamics of the vascular anomaly, which is very valuable for classification. However, operator dependence and small field of view are limiting factors in diagnosis and follow-up. MRI sets the gold standard in most cases, given its high soft-tissue resolution, different sequences, and fat-suppression capabilities, enabling clear differentiation/demarcation of the vascular anomaly from surrounding soft tissues, along with dynamic contrast-enhanced (CE) imaging information. The full anatomic extent of the anomaly can be evaluated in relation to adjacent nerves, and MRA/MRV can identify the feeding artery and draining vein. Response to treatment can be reliably evaluated over time by changes in size and flow characteristics.

In this chapter, we will review the ISSVA classification system, which will include both common vascular anomalies and the more complex syndromes. We will describe the clinical presentation and imaging findings of each group/subgroup of vascular anomalies, using a practical approach to correlate clinical presentation with imaging findings (Fig. 43-1 and Table 43-2).

Vascular anomalies are divided into two main groups: vascular tumors and vascular malformations.[3] The morbidity and treatment for vascular tumors differ dramatically from vascular malformations, and also differ dramatically for each type of vascular tumor and each type of vascular malformation, which is the overriding impetus for clear, standardized classification in the first place.

Vascular Tumors

Vascular tumors include infantile hemangiomas (IHs); congenital hemangiomas, including noninvoluting congenital hemangiomas (NICHs) and rapidly involuting congenital hemangiomas (RICHs); and kaposiform hemangioendotheliomas (KHEs). Age at presentation (prenatal, at birth, early childhood/adult), presence or absence of overlying telangiectatic vessels, a lighter peripheral ring, presence of fast-flow, and temporal evolution of the mass (involution vs. no involution) are important clinical criteria to approach the diagnosis of vascular tumors.

Infantile Hemangiomas

IHs comprise approximately 90% of all vascular tumors. They are the most common vascular tumors of infancy, with a higher incidence in white infants. The highest incidence is noted in preterm infants weighing less than 1000 g.[4] Head and neck regions are involved most frequently (60% of cases), followed by the trunk (25% of cases), and extremities (15% of cases).[5]

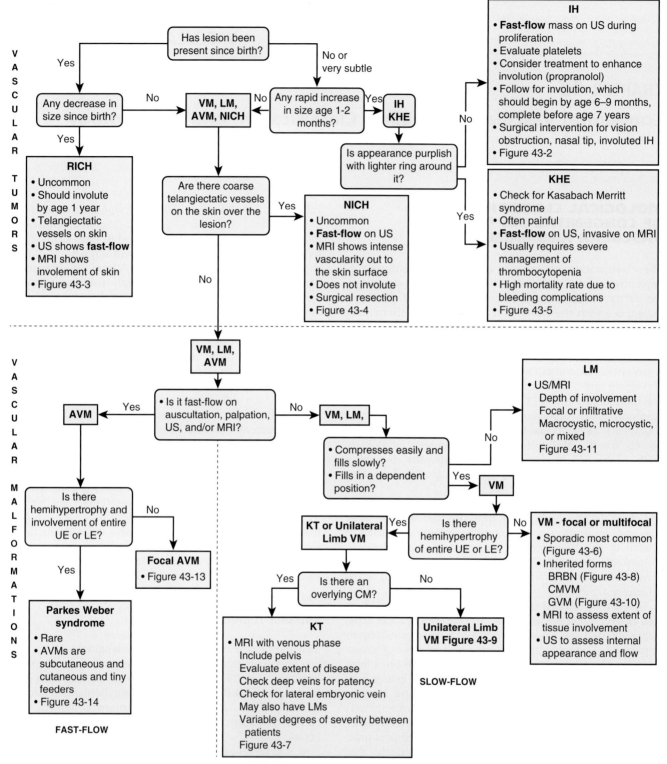

FIGURE 43-1. Vascular anomalies flowchart.

IHs are often not apparent at birth but most appear within the first 6 weeks of life as a soft, noncompressible mass with a typical triphasic evolution: proliferation, plateau, and involution. Superficial hemangiomas are generally cherry red macules and papules; deep hemangiomas are firm, rubbery subcutaneous masses, sometimes with a bluish skin hue. Compound hemangiomas combine aspects of both types. Most IHs double in size in the first 2 months of life, and approximately 80% reach their maximum size by 6 months of age.[6]

Spontaneous regression in early childhood (≈7 years of age) is typical,[7,8] but up to 40% of IHs may have residual skin changes and fibrofatty residuum, especially if they involve the head and neck. Patients with large IHs in the head and neck region—where there may be a concern for airway compromise, ulceration, or bleeding—can be medically treated, and propranolol is the leading drug of choice (Fig. 43-2; also see Fig 43-1).

The immunohistochemical marker glucose transporter protein isoform 1 (GLUT1) has become a major tool in diagnosing infantile hemangioma, with endothelial cells staining strongly.[21] The overwhelming majority of other vascular lesions, including congenital hemangiomas and vascular tumors, do not stain positive for GLUT1.[9,10]

Imaging is not required for the majority of IHs but can be useful to confirm the suspected diagnosis in atypical lesions, to determine the extent of deep lesions, and to exclude other vascular tumors (such as KHE) or soft-tissue malignancies. US demonstrates a solid mass with increased color flow within the mass.[11] The arterial inflow and venous drainage can be visualized by Doppler US.[12]

MRI reveals a T2 bright, T1 isointense mass with homogenous avid contrast enhancement.[13] Internal serpiginous flow voids within the IH noted in T2-weighted imaging represents the arterial inflow, an important diagnostic clue. Dynamic contrast-enhanced MRA (DCE-MRA) demonstrates early arterial enhancement in a soft-tissue mass with a draining vein. Typically, no perilesional edema is observed, which facilitates differentiation from other soft-tissue malignancies. Fibrofatty infiltration can be observed during the involuting phase.

TABLE 43-1. Vascular Anomalies

Vascular Tumors
Infantile hemangiomas
Congenital hemangiomas
• Rapidly involuting congenital hemangiomas
• Noninvoluting congenital hemangiomas
Kaposiform hemangioendothelioma
Others

Vascular Malformations
Slow-flow vascular malformations
• Venous malformations
• Lymphatic malformations
• Capillary malformations
Fast-flow vascular malformation
• Arteriovenous malformations/fistulas
Combined complex vascular malformations
• Capillary-venous
• Capillary-arteriovenous
• Lymphovenous

Simplified and adapted from the International Society for the Study of Vascular Anomalies (ISSVA) classification, 1996.

Congenital Hemangiomas

Unlike IH, congenital hemangiomas are fully formed at birth, with nearly no growth after birth, and lack positive staining with GLUT1.

Clinically, RICH (Fig. 43-3) and NICH (Fig. 43-4; also see Fig. 43-1) appear similar, often presenting as violaceous gray tumors with prominent overlying veins or telangiectases that extend beyond the periphery of the lesion. Many have a lighter or bluish halo on the surrounding skin. In practice, RICH and NICH are distinguished in retrospect, since the former involutes by 12 months of age, and the latter involutes either partially or not at all and requires surgical excision. In addition, RICH can leave significant textural change necessitating reconstructive surgery after involution.[14]

Early and accurate diagnosis is critical to avoid unnecessary biopsy/surgical intervention.[15] Similar histologic and clinical features of RICH and NICH raise the possibility that the latter may undergo involutional arrest to become a noninvoluting tumor.[16]

Kaposiform Hemangioendothelioma

KHE is a rare, distinct vascular tumor.[17] It may present at birth or within the first few months of life as an ill-defined purpuric mass, often painful, with an encircling pale ring; however, presentation may be later in childhood.[18] The destructive/infiltrative nature and very rapid growth of this vascular tumor facilitates differentiation from IH. *Kasabach-Merritt phenomenon* (KMP, a rare life-threatening condition in which a vascular tumor traps and destroys platelets) can be seen up to 50% of patients. KHE has a high mortality rate (24%) related to coagulopathy or complications from local tumor infiltration.

The firm, indurated lesion of KHE has a more invasive appearance and a purplish coloration (Fig. 43-5; also see Fig. 43-1). These cells form slitlike lumina containing erythrocytes that resemble Kaposi sarcoma, thus the name *kaposiform hemangioendothelioma*.[19] KHE appears as a solid mass with ill-defined borders and variable echogenicity on US imaging.[20] MRI demonstrates an infiltrative pattern, with crossing of multiple soft-tissue planes and involvement of overlying skin and subcutaneous fat. These more aggressive imaging features distinguish KHE from IH, as do the atypical clinical features.

Syndromic Associations with Hemangiomas

Although the clinical course of the vast majority of hemangiomas is benign, there are some associated abnormalities that should be noted and that may require further diagnostic evaluation. Patients with large segmental facial

TABLE 43-2. Key Magnetic Resonance Imaging Features of Vascular Anomalies

	IH	VM	LM	AVM
Solid mass	Yes	No	No	No
Phlebolith	No	Yes	No	No
Enhancement	Avid homogenous	Variable	None (cysts' periphery)	Avid serpiginous
DCE-MRA	Arterial	Venous	None	Arterial with early venous drainage

AVM, Arteriovenous malformation; *DCE-MRA*, dynamic contrast-enhanced magnetic resonance angiography; *IH*, infantile hemangioma; *LM*, lymphatic malformation; *VM*, venous malformation.

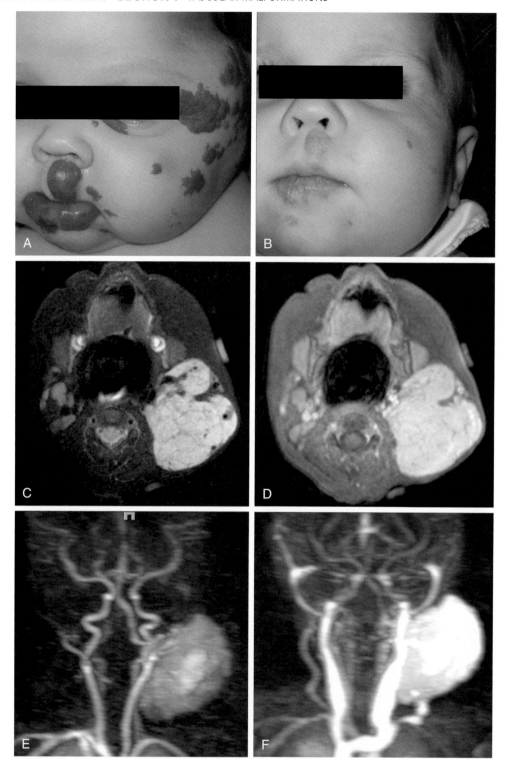

FIGURE 43-2. **A,** This 10-week-old infant girl had multiple segmental facial red hemangiomas, ulceration on bottom lip, and subcutaneous hemangioma of left upper medial eyelid that caused swelling and partial obscuring of left eye. **B,** Same patient after 9 months on propranolol. Note degree of involution of lesions shown in **A.** **C,** Magnetic resonance imaging of 6-month-old girl with palpable soft mass in left lateral neck, an infantile hemangioma (IH). Axial T2-weighted image with fat saturation demonstrates well-defined hyperintense soft-tissue mass in left neck, with few internal serpiginous flow voids. **D,** Same patient as in **C;** postcontrast T1-weighted image with fat saturation demonstrates avid homogenous internal contrast enhancement of the solid vascular mass. **E,** Same patient as in **C;** time-resolved dynamic contrast-enhanced magnetic resonance angiography (DCE-MRA) in arterial phase demonstrates that avid homogenous enhancement of IH starts in arterial phase (note that only arteries are enhanced, no veins visualized) from a feeding artery taking off from left external carotid artery. Serpiginous flow voids noted in **C** were demonstrated to represent feeding arteries and draining veins of the IH. Note draining vein into left subclavian/internal jugular junction **(F).**

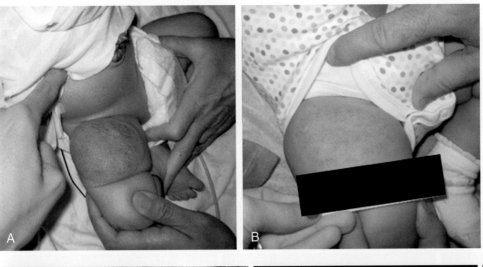

FIGURE 43-3. A, Newborn with round purple mass on right thigh. Note coarse telangiectasia of skin and peripheral pallor typical of congenital hemangiomas. **B,** Same patient at 5 months of age. Note that lesion has spontaneously involuted very rapidly, confirming this is a rapidly involuting congenital hemangioma (RICH).

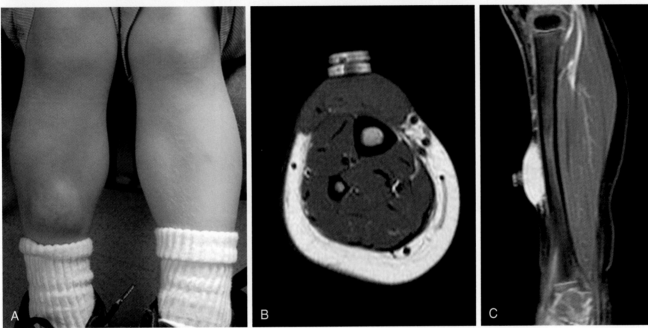

FIGURE 43-4. A, This 4-year-old boy had a raised round lesion on right shin since birth, without regression. Note coarse purple telangiectasia on skin. **B,** Axial T1-weighted image without fat saturation clearly demonstrates infiltration of skin typical of congenital hemangiomas. **C,** Axial postcontrast T1-weighted image with fat saturation demonstrates avidly enhancing solid vascular mass with skin infiltration. This constellation of imaging findings together with patient's age and absence of regression since presentation at birth confirms diagnosis of noninvoluting congenital hemangioma (NICH).

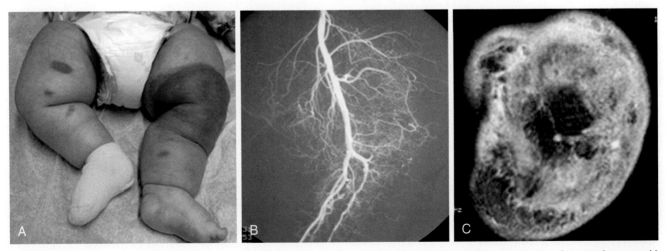

FIGURE 43-5. A, This 11-month-old girl was born with an ill-defined purple, firm, indurated lesion overlying left knee region. Vascular anomaly was notable for being extremely painful and limiting movement of left lower extremity. **B,** Lateral view of arteriogram of left knee, demonstrating enlarged feeders off lower superficial femoral and popliteal arteries filling the hypervascular mass. **C,** Axial postcontrast T1-weighted image with fat saturation demonstrates infiltration of skin, subcutaneous fat, muscle groups, and cortex of bone by this enhancing infiltrative vascular anomaly. Infiltrative and aggressive nature of this painful solid mass in a young child confirms diagnosis of kaposiform hemangioendothelioma.

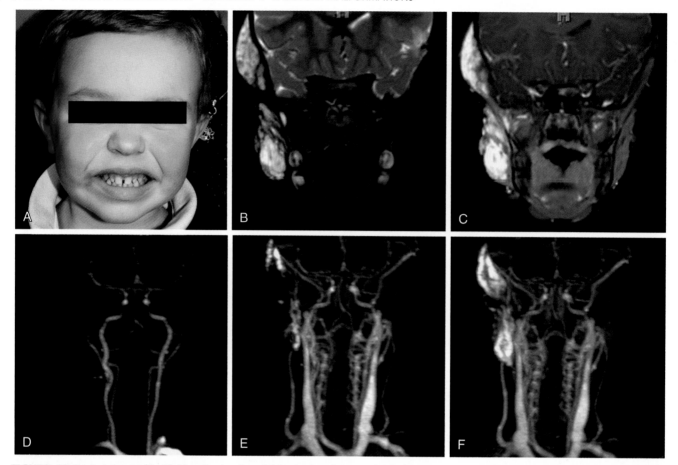

FIGURE 43-6. **A,** A 4-year-old with blue discoloration of right cheek and corner of right lip, noted to be present since birth and stable; note that right cheek is fuller than left. Lesions were soft and compressible. Coronal images show infiltration of right temporalis muscle and right masticator space by a T2 bright (**B**) and enhancing (**C**) mass. Note T2 dark round foci in **B**, representing phleboliths. Dynamic contrast-enhanced magnetic resonance angiography (MRA) demonstrates no enhancement in arterial phase (**D**). Enhancement starts in venous phase (**E**) and progressively increases in delayed venous phase (**F**), typical for venous malformation.

hemangiomas should be evaluated for signs and symptoms of PHACES syndrome. *PHACES syndrome* refers to a constellation of Posterior fossa brain malformations, Hemangiomas, Arterial anomalies, Coarctation of the aorta and cardiac defects, Eye abnormalities, and Sternal defects.[21]

Patients with hemangiomas overlying the lumbosacral spine can have associated abnormalities, the most common of which is a tethered spinal cord. MRI should be performed to exclude this abnormality.[22] Genitourinary anomalies are possible, although less common.

Airway hemangiomas should be investigated in patients who have cutaneous cervicofacial hemangiomas distributed in the chin, anterior neck, lower lip, and preauricular areas (a "beard" distribution).[23]

Vascular Malformations

Vascular anomalies that are present at birth, grow slowly proportionally to the patient, and do not demonstrate spontaneous regression are consistent with vascular malformations—that is, congenital errors in vascular development. Although present at birth, they may remain dormant and present in later childhood or adult life. Histologic evaluation of these lesions supports this classification,

with types of malformations delineated by the basic type of constituent vessel and presence or absence of arteriovenous shunting. They demonstrate vascular spaces lined with flat, mature epithelium that is mitotically quiescent. Vascular malformations are subclassified based on flow dynamics as slow-flow and fast-flow vascular malformations.[24]

Slow-Flow Vascular Malformations
Venous Malformations

Venous malformations (VMs) are the most common vascular malformation. They present as soft, compressible lesions that typically infiltrate multiple tissue planes. Physical examination generally reveals bluish lesions (Fig. 43-6; also see Fig. 43-1) that may enlarge with the Valsalva maneuver or gravity. There may be overlying skin involvement. They usually present during mid- to late childhood and become more symptomatic as time passes.

Ultrasound examination of VMs demonstrates a sponge-like network of tubular structures with low velocity or no venous flow. The vessels are easily compressible by the US probe. MRI typically demonstrates increased T2 signal with a variable degree of contrast enhancement. Phleboliths are often observed (round/oval-shaped T2 dark foci), representing calcification within the veins. DCE-MRA

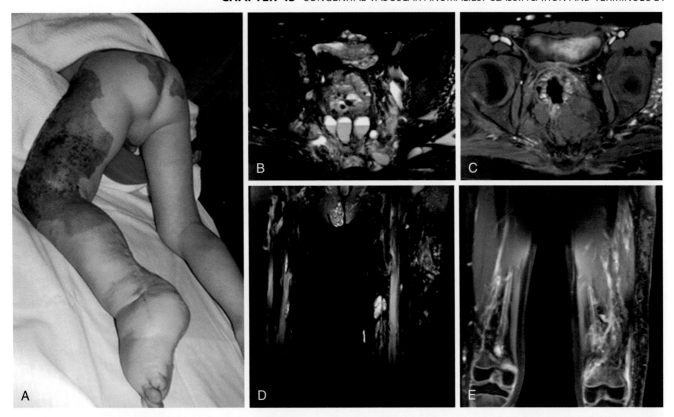

FIGURE 43-7. A, A 4-year-old with hemihypertrophy of left lower extremity and capillary, venous, and lymphatic malformations in left lower extremity; status post surgical resection of a lower leg microcystic lymphatic malformation. Note pelvic involvement, with perineal swelling. **B,** Axial T2-weighted image with fat saturation shows multiple cysts, with fluid-fluid levels noted deep in pelvis. **C,** Axial postcontrast T1-weighted image demonstrates lack of contrast enhancement in cysts, confirming that these represent lymphatic malformations. **D,** Coronal T2-weighted image with fat saturation shows increased thickness of subcutaneous fat in left thigh. Note infiltration of subcutaneous fat and muscle groups by the venous malformation, which shows heterogenous enhancement **(E).** Also note enlarged/patulous deep venous system.

demonstrates enhancement in the venous phase that may be progressive in nature.[25]

Syndromes Associated with Venous Malformations

KLIPPEL-TRÉNAUNAY SYNDROME Klippel-Trénaunay syndrome (KT) is characterized by hypertrophy of the affected limb, with underlying extensive VM and/or lymphatic malformation (LM) (Fig. 43-7; also see Fig. 43-1). Dysplastic/anomalous veins or persistent embryonic veins can be observed. The deep venous system may be atretic, hypoplastic, or abnormal in approximately 50% of patients with KT, and must be confirmed patent prior to ablation of the superficial abnormal veins. These patients can vary from a mild form of KT to a more severe form with extensive involvement of the pelvis and viscera as well as the legs. Some may have more LMs, others may have more VMs, and some may have enlarged ectatic pelvic and leg veins. KT patients may also be at higher risk for pulmonary embolism[26] and need to be evaluated for potential long-term anticoagulation.

BLUE RUBBER BLEB NEVUS SYNDROME Blue rubber bleb nevus syndrome (BRBNS) is characterized by multiple cutaneous VMs as well as internal VMs, typically involving subcutaneous tissues and muscles in numerous locations (Fig. 43-8; also see Fig. 43-1). These patients must be followed owing to multiple small-bowel lesions that frequently bleed, presenting in early adulthood as slow, chronic gastrointestinal (GI) bleeding and chronic iron-deficiency anemia. Removal of these small-bowel lesions without bowel resection has been pioneered by Fishman et al.[27]

UNILATERAL LIMB VENOUS MALFORMATIONS Some patients with diffuse VMs in an extremity do not have KT (no hypertrophy, no LM, no port-wine stain) and are classified as having a unilateral limb venous malformation[28] (Fig. 43-9; also see Fig. 43-1). Venous malformation in the subcutaneous region may cause the skin to appear bluish. They typically have numerous deeper VMs within muscles from the pelvis to the feet.

MUCOCUTANEOUS VENOUS MALFORMATIONS This is an autosomal dominant inherited venous malformation with multiple bluish spots that are usually small and punctuate and painful to touch, but may be larger in size.[29]

GLOMUVENOUS MALFORMATIONS This is also an autosomal dominant inherited VM in which there are multiple small bluish to purple skin lesions[29] (Fig. 43-10; also see Fig. 43-1).

Lymphatic Malformations

Lymphatic malformations are soft compressible lesions of lymphatic origin (Fig. 43-11; also see Fig. 43-1). These have also been referred to as "cystic hygromas" or "lymphangiomas," but this terminology is confusing and should be

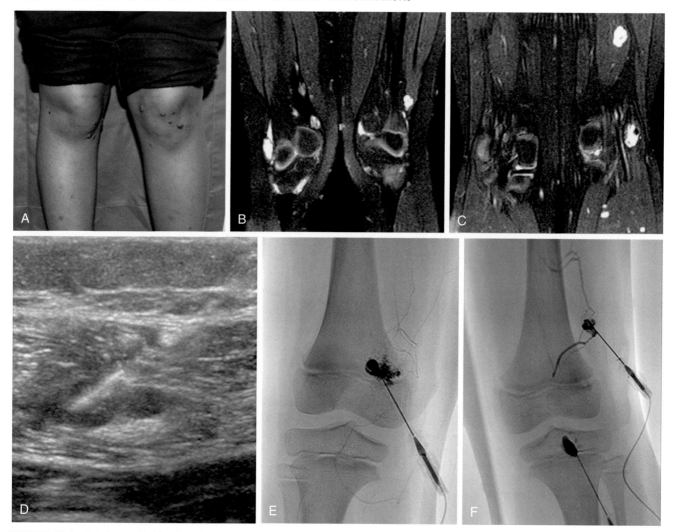

FIGURE 43-8. **A,** A 7-year-old girl with multiple dark, slightly raised, firm skin lesions on both knees and over the entire body as well, characteristic of blue rubber bleb nevus syndrome. Multiple deep venous malformations (VMs) on shoulder and right arm were previously percutaneously sclerosed. Recent onset of severe pain around both knees and thighs prompted magnetic resonance imaging. **B-C,** Coronal T2-weighted images demonstrate multiple small lobular T2 bright lesions in muscle groups and medulla of bones, representing venous malformations. **D,** Ultrasound images show an intramuscular VM, with needle accessing it for percutaneous sclerotherapy. **E,** Percutaneous venogram of right leg intramuscular VM, demonstrating type II drainage into normal veins. **F,** Percutaneous venogram of left leg intramuscular VM and infrapatellar venous malformation. Note again the drainage into normal veins, confirming this is a VM.

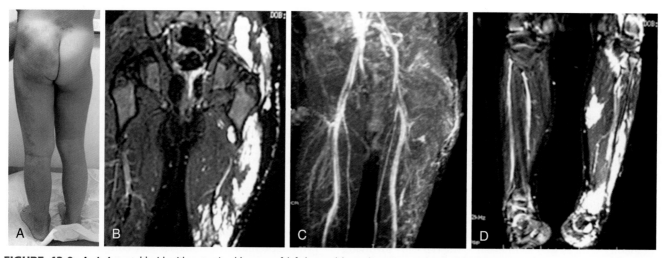

FIGURE 43-9. **A,** A 4-year-old girl with extensive blueness of left leg and buttock region; no leg length discrepancy on measurement. **B-C,** Coronal T2-weighted image shows intensive venous malformation (VM) infiltrating muscle groups in left lower extremity and buttock. Note skin infiltration. **D,** Dynamic contrast-enhanced magnetic resonance angiography shows enhancement of VM in venous phase.

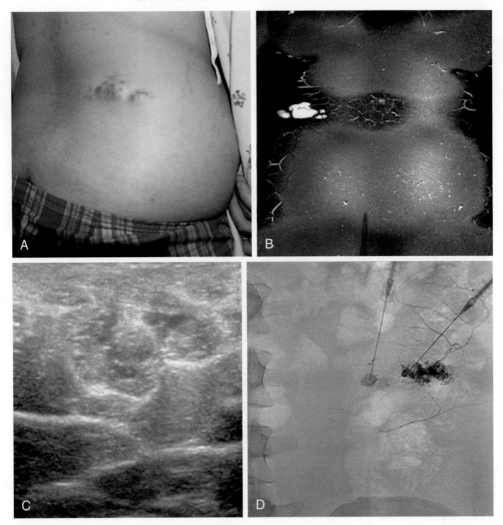

FIGURE 43-10. A, This 20-year-old man had a bluish lesion on right lower flank. Similar lesions were also noted on buttocks, right and left thighs, left wrist, and right forearm (not shown). His father had a similar lesion on left forearm. Pressure elicited pain. Lesions were cutaneous and subcutaneous, raised, with some firmness, yet compressible. **B,** Coronal T2-weighted image shows lobular T2 bright lesion in subcutaneous fat. **C,** Ultrasound during needle access for sclerotherapy. Lesion had firm borders but extensive venous spaces. No flow seen on power Doppler (not shown). **D,** Percutaneous venogram of lesion during sclerotherapy treatment. Based on magnetic resonance imaging only, diagnosis of glomuvenous malformation is very difficult, since imaging features overlap with those of venous malformation. Presence of similar lesions in patient's father, along with superficial location and painful nature, are very helpful in establishing diagnosis of glomuvenous malformation.

avoided. LMs are collections of cystic spaces filled with chylous material.[30] These cystic spaces may be macrocystic, microcystic, or mixed. Microcystic LMs are not as compressible as macrocystic LMs. The microcysts may be so small as to be indistinguishable on cross-sectional imaging.

US evaluation shows no flow within the major spaces, although small arteries and veins can traverse interstitial spaces. MRI appearances can be variable on T1-weighted imaging, depending on internal hemorrhage and inflammation, but the lesions are usually high signal on T2 weighting and show no internal enhancement with gadolinium.

Capillary Malformations

Capillary malformations (CMs) are commonly known as *port-wine stains* as well as *nevus flammeus* and can be confused with IH. They are typically red or pink in infancy and may darken with age. They grow in proportion with the patient and do not resolve spontaneously. CMs in certain locations can be associated with other abnormalities. For example, midline posterior CMs may be associated with a tethered spinal cord. Facial CMs may be associated with Sturge-Weber syndrome, particularly in the V1 distribution (Fig. 43-12; also see Fig. 43-1). Patients with V1-distribution CMs should undergo early neurologic and ophthalmologic evaluation. Patients with V2 and V3 involvement are generally not at risk. Other conditions associated with CMs include KT and Parkes Weber syndrome. CMs may be associated with underlying arteriovenous malformations (AVMs) as part of the RASA1 mutation.[14]

CMs associated with Sturge-Weber syndrome have a tendency to become thickened and lobulated with age. These are very difficult to treat and may require difficult and repeated plastic surgical procedures to keep the growth under control. Angiography rarely demonstrates enough visible hypervascularity to suggest a role for embolization

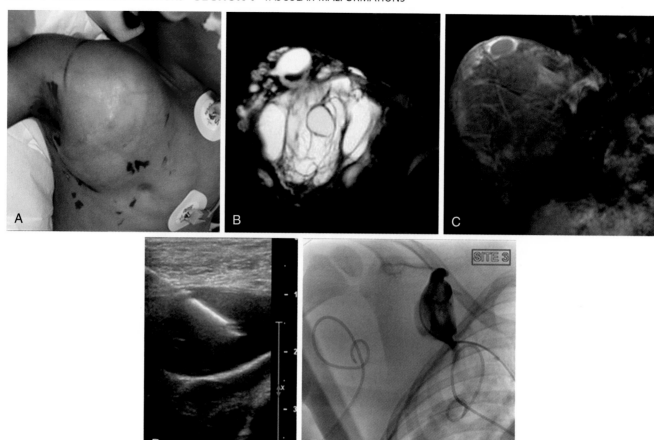

FIGURE 43-11. **A,** A 4-year-old boy with large firm mass on right shoulder/chest wall, first noted soon after birth; he underwent surgical debulking at that time. Diagnosis was lymphatic malformation (LM). Patient had noticed recent enlargement of residual malformation. **B,** Coronal T2-weighted image with fat saturation shows a T2 bright multicystic/septated large mass that only shows enhancement of cyst walls and septa **(C),** typical of LM. Relatively large size of each cyst qualifies for macrocystic LM. **D,** Ultrasound during percutaneous access demonstrates a macrocystic LM. **E,** Contrast injection into one of three macrocysts being treated with doxycycline sclerotherapy.

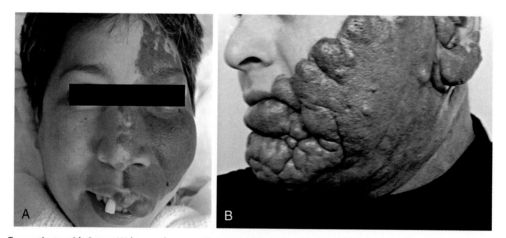

FIGURE 43-12. Two patients with Sturge-Weber syndrome: a 23-year-old **(A)** and a 35-year-old **(B),** both with extensive facial capillary malformations (CMs). Note thickening of CM, especially in **B,** which can be seen in CMs over time.

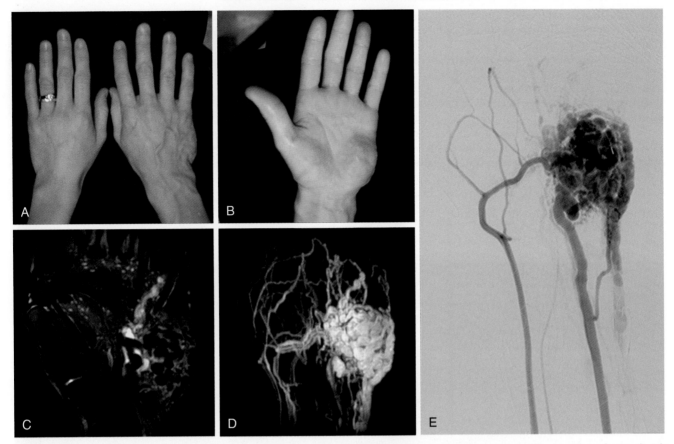

FIGURE 43-13. A, A 30-year-old woman with a swollen pulsatile mass on hypothenar eminence of right hand. View of dorsal surface of patient's right hand compared to left. Note enlarged draining veins and relatively bigger size of right hand. **B,** Note hypothenar eminence mass on palmar surface of right hand. **C,** Coronal T2-weighted image with fat saturation demonstrates a serpiginous tangle of flow voids, indicating fast-flow, and infiltration of hypothenar eminence and subcutaneous fat. Note absence of an associated soft-tissue mass. **D,** Magnetic resonance angiogram demonstrates strong enhancement of arteriovenous malformation (AVM), with arterial supply from ulnar artery and venous drainage into basilic vein. **E,** Angiogram demonstrating predominant arterial supply from ulnar artery to AVM. Note early venous drainage.

as an alternative to controlling these lesions. In addition, there may be bony overgrowth that cannot be controlled. MRI demonstrates the superficial thickening.[31]

Fast-Flow Vascular Malformations
Arteriovenous Malformations/Fistulas
AVMs and arteriovenous fistulas (AVFs) are pulsatile lesions without a mass and without the capillary transition between artery and vein, typically with an associated bruit or murmur (Fig. 43-13; also see Fig. 43-1). They can present in early childhood and may grow with the child. They may also present in adulthood. AVMs can undergo periods of more rapid growth associated with growth spurts and puberty. Rapid growth may also occur after trauma, pregnancy, or surgery. They can be complicated by arterial steal in affected extremities. Venous congestion from AVMs can lead to pain, bleeding, and skin breakdown. In some cases, they can cause high-output cardiac failure. Diagnosis can be made by MRI or CTA. Biopsy should be avoided because of the high risk of bleeding. Treatment typically involves transcatheter embolization, with or without additional modalities.[32,33]

AVMs are clinically classified by the Schobinger scale of AVM severity (Table 43-3).[34] Grayscale evaluation of

TABLE 43-3. Schobinger Scale of Severity of Arteriovenous Malformations

Stage	Stage Name	Description
I	Quiescence	Only pink-bluish stain and warmth
II	Expansion	Enlarged swelling with pulsation, thrill, and bruit; veins are tense and tortuous
III	Destruction	Same as stage II with ulceration, bleeding, pain, and tissue necrosis
IV	Decompensation	Same as stage III with cardiac failure

Modified from Kohout MP, Hansen M, Pribaz JJ, Mulliken JB. Arteriovenous malformation of head and neck: natural history and management. Plast Reconstr Surg 1998;102:643–54.

AVMs demonstrates a tangle of vessels with no associated mass. Doppler evaluation shows arterial flow within the vessels, with prominent draining veins that also exhibit fast-flow. Magnetic resonance imaging reflects this high-flow state by prominent flow-related signal voids, as well as

# #

# # #

easier visualization of feeding and draining vessels. MRA/MRV is frequently helpful in the preprocedural planning for treatment of these lesions.

Pathologic examination demonstrates beds of venules and arterioles intermixed with numerous larger-caliber arteries and thick-walled veins.

SYNDROMES ASSOCIATED WITH ARTERIOVENOUS MALFORMATIONS

Parkes Weber Syndrome Parkes Weber syndrome (previously called *Klippel-Trénaunay-Weber syndrome*) is not a venous malformation syndrome but is characterized by hemihypertrophy, CM, and diffuse multiple tiny superficial arteriovenous shunts[35] (Fig. 43-14; also see Fig. 43-1).

Combined Complex Vascular Malformations
Capillary Malformation–Arteriovenous Malformation
These lesions are a RASA1 mutation in which there are multiple CMs with an encircling pale halo, with an underlying AVM.[36]

Lymphaticovenous Malformation
Lymphaticovenous malformations (LVMs) are slow-flow lesions that contain both lymphatic and venous elements.[37] In the authors' experience, these lesions are rare and often seen in the setting of syndromes such as KT. Even in patients with KT, lymphatic and venous malformations are seen

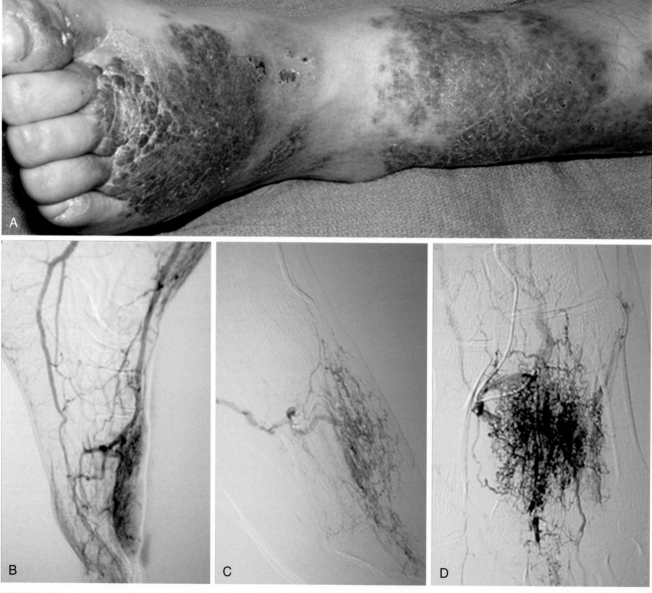

FIGURE 43-14. A, Foot and lower leg of 24-year-old man with Parkes Weber syndrome. Note thickened skin lesions on anterior lower shin and dorsum of foot. **B,** Lateral arteriogram of foot from a popliteal artery injection. Note hypervascularity of skin lesions in same location as thickened skin lesions on photograph. **C,** Selective angiogram on dorsum of foot, lateral view. **D,** Selective angiogram on dorsum of foot, anteroposterior view.

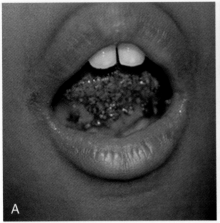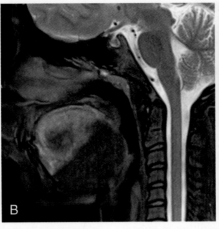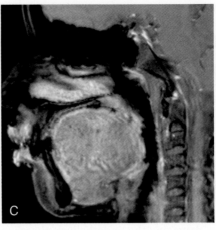

FIGURE 43-15. **A,** An 11-year-old girl with a lymphovenous malformation of the tongue, status post tongue reduction surgery and prior laser treatment. Note recurrent blue-black small numerous tiny cystic lesions on tongue. They weep both clear lymphatic and bloody fluid. **B,** Sagittal T2-weighted image of tongue shows increased T2 signal in intrinsic tongue muscles, which show mild enhancement on postcontrast T1-weighted sagittal image **(C).** Magnetic resonance imaging is helpful in identifying that this lesion is not only superficial but also infiltrates intrinsic muscles of tongue.

separately (see Fig. 43-7). Mixed LVMs are generally found as superficial lesions infiltrating the skin or tongue (Fig. 43-15; also see Fig. 43-1).

KEY POINTS

- *Vascular anomalies* are divided into two major groups: *vascular tumors* and *vascular malformations*. It is of critical importance to first make the differentiation between the two groups, since morbidity and treatment options are very different, and then subclassify these lesions. This process involves combining patient history, physical exam, and imaging to determine the correct diagnosis.

- The term *vascular tumor* refers generically to any solid lesion of predominantly endothelial etiology, but that is not neoplastic. Within this group of vascular anomalies, treatment differs widely, making further subclassification necessary.

- *Vascular malformations* clinically present as soft masses or lesions, frequently with red or bluish coloration. A wide assortment of haphazard names creates confusion that can lead to inappropriate patient management by well-intentioned but poorly informed healthcare providers. Correct classification and proper use of appropriate terminology may result in earlier diagnosis and facilitate referral and treatment of patients who would benefit from early intervention.

- All centers/practitioners involved in the care of vascular anomalies should adhere to the classification system approved by the International Society for the Study of Vascular Anomalies (ISSVA).

► **SUGGESTED READINGS**

Dubois J, Alison M. Vascular anomalies: what a radiologist needs to know. Pediatr Radiol 2010;40(6):895–905.

Dubois J, Garel L, David M, Powell J. Vascular soft-tissue tumors in infancy: distinguishing features on Doppler sonography. AJR Am J Roentgenol 2002;178(6):1541–5.

Finn M, Glowacki J, Mulliken J. Congenital vascular lesions: clinical application of a new classification. J Pediatr Surg 1983;18(6):894–900.

Hassanein AH, Mulliken JB, Fishman SJ, et al. Evaluation of terminology for vascular anomalies in current literature. Plast Reconstr Surg 2011;127(1):347–51.

Siegel MJ. Magnetic resonance imaging of musculoskeletal soft tissue masses. Radiol Clin North Am 2001;39(4):701–20.

The complete reference list is available online at www.expertconsult.com.

CHAPTER 44

Management of Low-Flow Vascular Malformations

Patricia E. Burrows

CLINICAL RELEVANCE

The goal of sclerotherapy is to obliterate abnormal channels by damaging the endothelium, thereby resulting in subsequent inflammation and fibrosis. Venous malformations (VMs) are caused by abnormal development of the vein wall, with thinning and asymmetric disruption of the smooth muscle layer of the vein in association with endothelial cell abnormalities. This results in progressive, often asymmetric, dilation of the affected channels. Associated absence or insufficiency of valves in the conducting veins contributes to swelling. Affected channels become progressively enlarged, and the resulting stagnation of blood causes thrombosis, swelling, and pain. Most VMs undergo a continuous cycle of spontaneous thrombosis and thrombolysis.[1] Calcification of thrombi results in formation of phleboliths. Symptoms and signs include blue or purple cutaneous lesions, swelling with dependency or effort, pain, deformity, and consumption coagulopathy. Pulmonary embolism can occur, especially when the conducting venous channels are malformed.

The angioarchitecture of VMs includes focal (Fig. 44-1), multifocal (Fig. 44-2; also see Fig. e44-1), and diffuse forms (Fig. 44-3; also see Fig. e44-2). The degree to which the lesion communicates with adjacent conducting veins is the key factor in planning treatment.[2,3] VMs with minimal communication can be considered "sequestered," whereas those with free drainage are confluent or "nonsequestered" (see Fig. 44-3 and Fig. e44-2). Focal lesions may be intramuscular, cutaneous, or mucosal and usually consist of collections of abnormal interconnecting channels or spaces that are sequestered or drain through fairly small channels to normal adjacent conducting veins. This type of lesion is characterized by focal pain or a sensation of fullness with dependency, after exercise, or on arising in the morning (due to stasis). These lesions are easily and effectively treated by injection of sclerosant.

Diffuse VMs involve multiple tissue layers, usually including muscle, subcutaneous fat, skin, and sometimes bone. In diffuse lesions, the malformed veins are nonsequestered and communicate directly with the main conducting veins, which are frequently also abnormal.[4] Diffuse VMs are difficult to treat effectively because injected sclerosant can directly enter the circulation and potentially cause deep venous thrombosis, pulmonary embolism, or systemic effects of ethanol. Recanalization is also more likely than after sclerotherapy for nonsequestered lesions.[5] Some patients with diffuse VMs have focal eccentric varices that can exert a considerable mass effect on adjacent structures. These varices can be obliterated by endovascular treatment.

Multifocal lesions are most commonly seen in familial forms of VM, including blue rubber bleb nevus syndrome (see Fig. 44-2 and Fig. e44-2), mucocutaneous familial VMs, glomuvenous malformation, and Maffucci syndrome.

Lymphatic malformations (LMs) result from regional maldevelopment of lymphatic channels and include cystic and channel-type anomalies. Cystic LMs are generally classified into three groups: microcystic (cystic components <1 to 2 cm diameter), macrocystic, and combined forms. Macrocystic lesions are most common in the neck, axilla, and pelvis (Fig. 44-4). LMs are frequently combined with cutaneous capillary malformations (capillary-lymphatic malformations [CLMs]) and anomalies of conducting venous channels (LM with venous dilation, lymphatic-venous malformations [LVMs], or capillary-lymphatic-venous malformations [CLVMs]). Generally, LMs manifest either as focal mass lesions (macrocystic) or as diffuse tissue swelling or overgrowth.[6] Unlike VMs, they do not expand with the Valsalva maneuver but rather expand or swell intermittently, especially in association with systemic viral illness. Swelling can occur acutely as a result of infection or bleeding into the lesion. Bleeding is presumably due to either adjacent abnormal venous channels or rupture of small arteries, frequently seen in the septa. Sepsis is most frequently a problem with lesions close to the alimentary tract (e.g., face, pelvis). Cutaneous extensions of LMs are manifested as vesicles that may leak clear, bloody, or chylous fluid. Diffuse and multifocal LMs (generalized lymphatic anomaly) are composed of incompetent lymphatic channels, often associated with chylous reflux and leaks. Life-threatening chylothorax or chylous ascites may develop in patients with generalized lymphatic anomaly. Gorham syndrome (vanishing bone disease) is a type of CLM associated with increased osteoclastic activity and progressive osteolysis of affected bone, most often in the shoulder and pelvis.

Magnetic resonance imaging (MRI) is the best technique to confirm the diagnosis and extent of low-flow vascular malformations.[7,8] VMs and LMs are hyperintense on fluid-sensitive sequences and do not have fast-flow components on gradient-recalled echo sequences. VMs enhance inhomogeneously, whereas LMs typically show minimal or rim enhancement. Arteriography is not routinely necessary.

INDICATIONS

Endovascular or percutaneous treatment is warranted in patients with significant symptomatology not well controlled by conservative treatment. For VMs, standard nonoperative treatment includes use of graded elastic compression garments (for limbs) and aspirin or

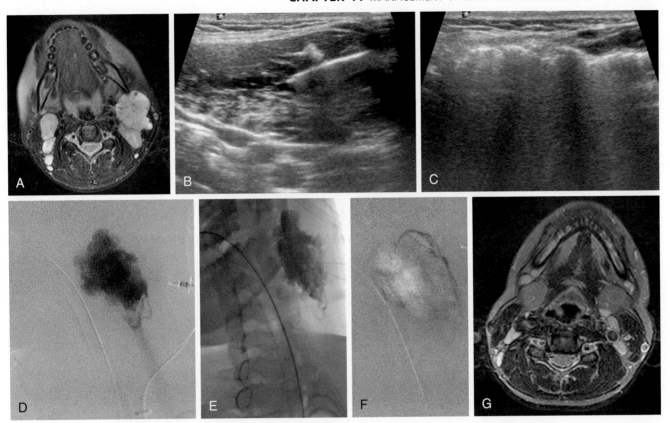

FIGURE 44-1. Sclerotherapy of focal venous malformation (VM) of left neck using sodium tetradecyl sulfate (STS) foam and bleomycin. **A,** Axial STIR image of the next shows a focal T-2 hyperintense lesion containing thrombi or phleboliths in left retromandibular space. Patient also has adenopathy related to a viral illness. **B,** Sonographic image demonstrating needle placement within center of focal VM. **C,** Sonographic image demonstrates foam within VM. **D,** Roadmap image of contrast injection into VM demonstrates a focal lobulated lesion with late opacification of internal jugular vein. **E,** Unsubtracted fluoroscopic image shows collection of opacified venous spaces within malformation. **F,** Roadmap image during injection of STS foam, using double needle technique; 15 units of bleomycin were injected through same cannula 5 minutes after foam injection. **G,** Axial T2-weighted image 2 months following sclerotherapy demonstrates dramatic decrease in size. Small residual lesion enlarged over next 6 months and was treated with a second session.

anticoagulation. Indications for invasive treatment include pain secondary to swelling, a mass effect resulting in functional impairment (e.g., interference with ambulation, breathing, swallowing, speech), and disfigurement. For macrocystic LMs, sclerotherapy is now the preferred treatment over resection. Indications include pain, recurrent infection or bleeding, and a significant mass effect in the presence of macrocysts on imaging.

CONTRAINDICATIONS

Pulmonary hypertension and atrial septal defects are contraindications to sclerotherapy for VMs unless the malformation is completely sequestered from the venous circulation.[9,10] Relative contraindications include diffuse involvement of a closed space, such as the orbit or a muscle compartment (because of the risk of compartment syndrome), confluent or nonsequestered VMs, and severe consumption coagulopathy. The latter can often be corrected or improved with use of anticoagulants for 2 weeks before treatment. In patients with vascular malformations involving or adjacent to the airway, precautions for airway protection must be taken. Patients who have had cardiovascular complications from ethanol should not receive this agent

again. Those with lesion-related neuropathy may be made worse by sclerotherapy.

EQUIPMENT

Low-flow vascular malformations are best treated in an angiography suite with road-mapping capability and anesthesia support. Ultrasound equipment with high-frequency probes and sterile probe covers and gel is useful. An automated tourniquet system with sterile cuffs is important for control of flow in some VMs of the limbs. Sclerosants include 95% to 98% ethanol, 3% sodium tetradecyl sulfate (STS), sodium morrhuate, ethanolamine, and bleomycin for VMs, and doxycycline, OK-432, bleomycin, or ethanol for LMs. Ethiodol or Lipiodol can be used to opacify sclerosants with minimal dilution. An agent that combines ethanol and ethyl cellulose for greater viscosity has been developed but is not yet clinically available.[11] Useful needles include angiocatheters, 21-gauge single-wall needles, and 25- and 27-gauge butterfly needles. Plastic connecting tubes and three-way stopcocks are useful for hand-injected imaging. If oily contrast medium is used, plastic stopcocks must be checked for compatibility (see Fig e44-2).

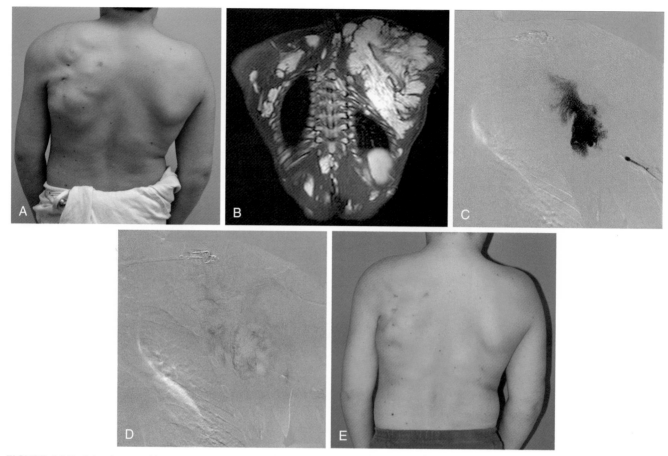

FIGURE 44-2. Sclerotherapy of large venous malformation (VM) in a patient with blue rubber bleb nevus syndrome using 3% sodium tetradecyl sulfate (STS) foam followed by bleomycin. **A,** Photograph demonstrates extensive soft-tissue masses around posterior left shoulder and back. Note numerous cutaneous lesions typical of this syndrome. **B,** Coronal STIR image demonstrates multiple focal VMs and extensive confluent lesion around left scapula. **C,** Percutaneous contrast injection (roadmap technique) shows an intramuscular compartment of VM without drainage. **D,** Roadmap image after injection of foamed STS (visible as negative opacity). **E,** Photograph taken 8 months after **A,** showing dramatic response of VMs to sclerotherapy. Patient's range of movement and pain were vastly improved.

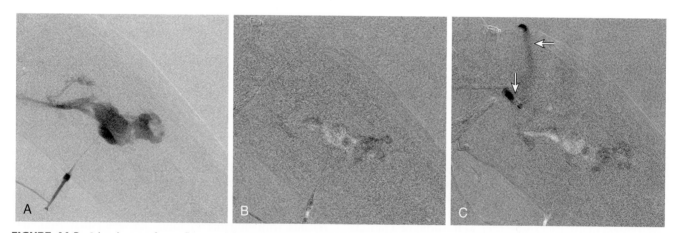

FIGURE 44-3. Sclerotherapy of a confluent multifocal intramuscular venous malformation (VM) of forearm, using double-needle technique. **A,** Contrast injection into intramuscular varix demonstrates direct drainage into antecubital vein. **B,** Injection of 3% sodium tetradecyl sulfate (STS) foam (roadmap image), with tourniquet occluding venous outflow. Second cannula was placed in proximal part of venous sac. **C,** Contrast medium is seen exiting second cannula *(arrows).* Sclerosant is gradually backfilling more of malformation.

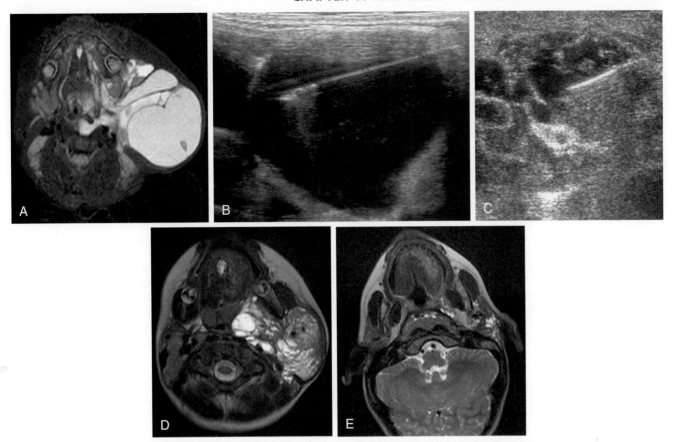

FIGURE 44-4. Sclerotherapy of a complex left cervical facial lymphatic malformation (LM) with OK-432 followed by bleomycin. **A,** Axial STIR image of lower face demonstrates LM involving multiple tissue layers, extending into parapharyngeal space. Lesion consists of macrocystic and microcystic components and involves parotid gland. **B,** Sonographic image demonstrating needle placement within large macrocyst prior to fluid aspiration. **C,** Sonographic image after aspirating fluid and injecting sclerosant. **D,** Axial T2-weighted image after three injections of OK-432. Note solid mass-like appearance of residual lesion in left parotid gland. This is commonly seen early after OK-432 sclerotherapy and usually resolves. **E,** Axial STIR image after further sclerotherapy using bleomycin shows nearly complete resolution of LM, resulting in symmetrical contour.

TECHNIQUE

Vascular Malformations

Anatomy and Approach
Sclerotherapy is performed by direct percutaneous cannulation of vascular channels, usually with a simple needle.[3,12-16] Previously obtained MRIs are used to determine the location and extent of the lesion and are available in the procedure room to help plan the percutaneous access. Sonographic guidance of needle placement is useful (see Fig. 44-1, *B*). MRI guidance is feasible and may be advantageous for deep lesions not easily seen with sonography. Small localized lesions can be injected with detergent sclerosants under regional anesthesia. Patients with extensive VMs and those undergoing ethanol sclerotherapy are anesthetized, pretreated with corticosteroids, and have a Foley catheter placed. Patients undergoing sclerotherapy for VMs must be kept well hydrated to compensate for the hemolysis caused by the sclerosant.

Technical Aspects
Affected limbs are widely prepared to permit observation of the skin and placement of a peripheral intravenous cannula and tourniquet or other occlusion device.

Compression of proximal veins is useful to distend the malformation before cannulation. The abnormal channels or spaces are cannulated with a needle after localization by either palpation or sonography. After obtaining blood return, contrast medium is injected into the lesion, followed by sclerosant. The process is repeated until the selected components of the malformation are all injected.

Contrast medium is injected, usually with imaging by digital subtraction radiography, to exclude arterial cannulation or extravasation, assess the nature of the lesion and its drainage, determine how much of the lesion is accessed, and calculate how much liquid is necessary to displace the blood into the draining vein. If possible, blood is displaced from the malformation. The appropriate sclerosant drug is then injected. The initial volume injected is less than the amount of contrast medium required to opacify the draining vein. Ethanol should not be used in lesions adjacent to major nerves or cutaneous lesions or in confluent or non-sequestered venous channels without some form of outflow control. The total volume of ethanol injected in one session should be less than 0.5 mL/kg or 40 mL. The volume of 3% STS should be kept below 0.5 mL/kg or 20 mL per session.[3] STS can be diluted with normal saline (e.g., 0.5%-1% STS) for injection into cutaneous lesions.

Sclerosing agents may be opacified for fluoroscopic guidance.[13] Detergent sclerosants can be mixed with either oily or water-soluble liquid contrast. Oily contrast medium (Ethiodol or Lipiodol) added in a 1:10 to 3:10 ratio (contrast to sclerosant) results in minimal dilution and, when combined with detergent sclerosant and air mixed through a three-way stopcock, produces relatively stable foam. The injection of opacified sclerosant should be observed by fluoroscopic subtraction (road map); injection must be stopped if extravasation or arterial penetration is seen. Once the sclerosant reaches a small outflow vein, injection should be stopped for a few minutes to allow occlusion of the outflow. Additional opacified sclerosant is injected until the lesion is completely filled as shown by fluoroscopy. With non-opacified sclerosant, roadmap imaging shows washout of previously injected contrast or negative opacification (see Fig. 44-1, *F*). Control of minor documented venous drainage to minimize egress of sclerosant can be accomplished in the head and neck by manual compression, and in the limbs by manual compression or tourniquets. A sterile automated orthopedic tourniquet inflated to a pressure less than mean arterial pressure can be used in the limbs. In lesions with significant venous drainage (confluent VMs), permanent outflow occlusion—accomplished by placing coils or tissue adhesive at sites of communication between the malformation and adjacent conducting veins—is useful in retaining the sclerosant in the VM and minimizing the risk for pulmonary embolism or cardiovascular reaction to the sclerosant (see Fig. e44-2). When sclerosing VMs of the extremities, a peripheral intravenous line should be placed in the affected limb to document venous patency before and after treatment and to infuse heparinized saline during sclerotherapy.

Sclerotherapy for superficial vascular malformations is performed with unopacified (sometimes diluted) sclerosant, with observation of skin color rather than the fluoroscopic image. The injection must be terminated when ischemic changes such as pallor or duskiness become evident. Applying cold sterile saline onto the surface of the skin to induce local vasoconstriction seems to minimize damage.

A double-needle technique in which a venous channel is cannulated with two needles, one for injection and one to release blood and excess sclerosant, has been proposed for added safety (see Fig. 44-3).[17,18]

Adjunctive Techniques
Use of Platinum/Fiber Coils
In the presence of rapid venous drainage or massive venous spaces, direct injection of sclerosant into the VM is both ineffective and risky. In this type of lesion, placement of coils into the malformation or at the junction of the malformation and the draining veins before injection of sclerosant creates a permanent sclerosis and minimizes the risk for pulmonary thromboembolism.[19,20] Microcoils can be placed into the venous pouch directly through the access needle, with or without control by a balloon occlusion catheter introduced via the femoral or internal jugular veins, or a tourniquet. Sclerosant can be injected around the coils. In extensive malformations of the conducting veins, such as the marginal varices in patients with Klippel-Trénaunay syndrome CLVM, a catheter or microcatheter can be placed percutaneously into the vein and advanced to the confluence between the anomalous and deep veins or perforators. After occluding the anastomoses with coils, the sclerosant can be injected along the length of the anomalous vein as the catheter is withdrawn.

Use of Acrylic Polymer
Acrylic polymers such as *N*-butyl-2-cyanoacrylate (NBCA) are not ideal sclerosing agents for VMs. In addition to their high cost, they are absorbed slowly, and a firm painful mass is left in the soft tissues for many months. They are useful when rapid occlusion and minimal swelling are desired, such as for outflow occlusion in conjunction with injection of sclerosant or for hemostasis before resection (see Fig. e44-2). NBCA opacified with oily contrast medium in a ratio of 1:4 to 1:6 appears to be effective in controlling bleeding and improving localization of VMs during resection. Risks include unintended occlusion of major veins and pulmonary embolization. Intraoperative injection of tissue adhesive (NBCA) immediately before surgical excision of VMs of the orbit has been reported.[21] In general, orbital VMs should not be treated by sclerotherapy because of the potential for development of orbital compartment syndrome and subsequent loss of vision.[22] An exception to this rule is use of bleomycin, which causes minimal swelling.[23]

Intralesional Laser Photocoagulation
Diode or Nd:YAG bare laser fibers can be used through catheters or large cannulas to ablate the endothelium of VMs. This procedure is especially useful for treating the long anomalous channels in patients with CLVMs, but it can also be applied to common VMs (see Fig. e44-2).[24] It appears to be most effective when combined with injection of sclerosant. Compared with sclerotherapy alone, endovenous laser therapy (EVLT)/sclerotherapy results in less postprocedural swelling and faster recovery.

Bleomycin
Bleomycin (1 unit/mL, maximum 15 units per procedure) is a useful sclerosant in selected lesions. It results in progressive fibrosis of the VM, without acute thrombosis and with minimal swelling, making it the best agent for VMs in the orbit or airway. As a sole sclerosant, it should be reinjected every 3 weeks for optimal results.[25] Bleomycin can also be used with a small amount of ethanol or foam after outflow occlusion (see Fig. 44-1).[23,26-28] This technique causes lesional thrombosis, so procedures are staged 6 to 8 weeks apart. Side effects of bleomycin include alopecia, pigmentation, nausea, hair loss, pulmonary fibrosis, acute pulmonary reaction (acute respiratory distress syndrome [ARDS]), and anaphylaxis.[29]

Lymphatic Malformations

Sclerosants used for LMs include ethanol, doxycycline, bleomycin, Ethibloc, and OK-432.[30-33] The latter two agents are not approved for use in the United States. OK-432, a solution of killed group A streptococci in a suspension containing penicillin, is undergoing clinical evaluation in a multicenter head and neck trial under the supervision of the University of Iowa.[34] It has been used extensively in Japan, Canada, and Europe. OK-432 causes an inflammation, probably due to an immune response to the agent, and subsequent shrinkage of the cysts (see Fig. 44-4).

Bleomycin is effective in treating LMs, although because of potential systemic toxicity, it is best to reserve its use for LMs that have failed other sclerosants or for microcystic LMs in the orbit or airway. Ethanol can be used for localized macrocystic LMs, but has the highest risk of nerve injury and skin necrosis. Doxycycline is effective in extensive LMs, because large volumes given at one session are well tolerated (see Fig. e44-3).[32,33] It is generally administered as a solution of 10 mg/mL in volumes up to 100 mL. The injection is extremely painful during and for 2 hours after injection. Reconstitution of the drug with a mixture of water and contrast medium results in radiopacity. STS is used for sclerosing microcysts and cutaneous vesicles. Acetic acid has also been reported to be an effective sclerosant for LMs but is not widely used.[35]

Individual macrocysts are cannulated with a needle under sonographic guidance, and fluid is aspirated as completely as possible.[32,33,36] Alternatively, pigtail catheters can be placed and used to inject and drain the cysts sequentially over a period of several days. The cysts can be opacified with a small amount of contrast medium, which is then aspirated, or needle position can be confirmed by ultrasonography alone. Injection of sclerosant can be monitored with ultrasonography or fluoroscopic guidance. For superficial lesions consisting of smaller cysts, sonographic guidance is more practical and effective. The needle, connected to a syringe of sclerosant, is positioned in a cyst or space, sclerosant is injected, and the needle is moved to another cyst and the process repeated. If additional treatment is necessary, injection is usually repeated every 6 weeks. A multiagent technique has also been described in which a pigtail catheter is placed, and a cyst is injected first with STS, then with ethanol.[31] Although effective in sclerosing individual cysts, this technique requires pigtail catheter drainage for several days.

CONTROVERSIES

For a full discussion of this topic, please visit www.expertconsult.com.

OUTCOMES

Objective analysis of the results of sclerotherapy is difficult because "cure" is rarely achieved. Most reviews used patient questionnaires to determine the outcome of treatment. Patient satisfaction with ethanol or STS is high, with more than 75% of patients with facial lesions reporting good or excellent results.[44-46] As expected, patients with diffuse VMs have less improvement than those with focal lesions.[47]

Although patients with facial VMs often seek treatment because of disfigurement, VMs of the limbs are usually treated to alleviate pain. Most published series report successful outcomes of sclerotherapy in terms of pain relief.

The complete discussion of sclerotherapy outcomes can be found at www.expertconsult.com.

COMPLICATIONS

Complications developed in 12% of the procedures and in 28% of patients undergoing a series of sclerotherapy sessions with ethanol (some patients have complications from more than one procedure).[49] Peripheral nerve deficits occur in 1% of procedures and 10% of patients after sclerotherapy with ethanol.[44,49] Most neuropathies recover, but permanent injury to the peroneal and laryngeal nerves has been reported. Neuropathy appears to be less common with microfoam techniques, but delayed loss of nerve function can be seen with excessive swelling, especially in the forearm, calf, and foot, and with extravasation. Skin blistering is common after sclerotherapy, especially if the vascular malformation is superficial, and generally heals uneventfully with appropriate supportive care. When ethanol is used, skin necrosis and scarring develop in about 10% to 15% of patients, usually at the site of cutaneous involvement of the malformation. Marked swelling can result in airway obstruction, feeding difficulty, neuropraxia, and neuropathy but is often followed by a good therapeutic response.[50]

Compartment syndrome must be dealt with early to avoid permanent neurologic and tissue injury. Patients who are at risk should have frequent checks of capillary refill, sensation, and movement of the treated limb for 12 to 24 hours after the procedure. Although some tingling or partial loss of feeling is frequently seen after sclerotherapy in the distal ends of limbs, patients with progression of sensory symptoms should go to the operating room for measurement of compartment pressure and fasciotomy if necessary.

Pulmonary embolization is a recognized complication of sclerotherapy and can manifest in several ways. Embolization of microthrombi or large clots can occur after release of tourniquets, with movement of the patient on awakening from anesthesia, or later, after the patient has been discharged home.[51,52] Pulmonary edema can develop after sclerotherapy for extensive VMs with ethanol (see Fig. e44-3). Reintubation and admission to the intensive care unit may be required, but the edema generally resolves after a few hours.

Acute cardiovascular collapse has been described in patients undergoing ethanol ablation procedures. Collapse is preceded by elevated pulmonary artery pressure. It is postulated that ethanol—or some combination of ethanol and other products of sclerotherapy—causes pulmonary vasoconstriction and acute right heart failure with electromechanical dissociation. The complication usually occurs after more than 0.5 mL/kg has been injected. If the patient is hemodynamically stable, pulmonary hypertension can be treated by infusion of vasodilators into the pulmonary artery; otherwise, routine resuscitation measures are necessary.

Children undergoing ethanol sclerotherapy occasionally demonstrate acute desaturation and bradycardia that is generally reversible with administration of 100% oxygen and interruption of ethanol administration.[13] These events are rarely if ever seen with detergent sclerosants.[53] Complications of LM sclerotherapy occur infrequently. Neuropathy is uncommon with doxycycline or foam sclerosants. Airway compression caused by swelling has been observed with OK-432, and thoracic compartment syndrome occurred with doxycycline in patients with circumferential chest wall LMs.

POSTPROCEDURAL AND FOLLOW-UP CARE

Antibiotic ointment and a loose sterile dressing are applied to needle puncture sites after sclerotherapy, and the treated areas are elevated. Swelling is generally maximal 24 hours after the procedure, so patients at risk for airway obstruction or compartment syndrome are observed in the hospital overnight. Patients with VMs involving the airway or neck are kept intubated with the head elevated until swelling has resolved. With bleomycin as the sclerosant, extubation is often feasible at the end of the procedure. Administration of systemic corticosteroids (dexamethasone, 0.1 mg/kg every 8 hours), elevation, and application of ice packs help minimize swelling. Patients should receive generous amounts of intravenous fluid (generally twice the maintenance amount) during and after VM sclerotherapy, and urine output should be carefully monitored. Hemoglobinuria secondary to hemolysis is an expected effect of sclerosant injection. Gross hemoglobinuria is managed by hydration and alkalization of urine (5% dextrose in water mixed with 75 mEq of sodium bicarbonate per liter and administered at twice the maintenance rate). Hemoglobinuria can be monitored visually and usually clears within 6 hours.

Ketorolac and morphine sulfate are appropriate analgesics; during hospitalization, patient-controlled analgesia is generally used to manage pain. Patients receiving doxycycline for LM sclerotherapy require narcotic analgesia for approximately 2 hours after the procedure. After discharge, VM patients receive a tapering dose of corticosteroids for 1 week, as well as analgesics. LM patients do not require steroids. If there are extensive vesicles, oral antibiotics may be given for 1 week to minimize the risk of infection. If skin injury occurs, patients are reevaluated frequently for evidence of infection. Otherwise, clinical assessment is carried out 2 months after the procedure.

KEY POINTS

- Low-flow vascular malformations amenable to endovascular treatment include venous malformations (VMs), lymphatic malformations (LMs), and combined malformations such as capillary-lymphatic-venous malformation (CLVM) or Klippel-Trénaunay syndrome.
- Useful treatment techniques include sclerotherapy, venous embolization (for outflow occlusion), and endovenous laser ablation.
- Preprocedural imaging and postprocedural care are important components of treatment.

▶ **SUGGESTED READINGS**

Burrows PE, Mason KP. Percutaneous treatment of low-flow vascular malformations. J Vasc Interv Radiol 2004;15:431–4.

Lee BB, Bergan J, Gloviczki P, et al. Diagnosis and treatment of venous malformations. Consensus document of the International Union of Phlebology (IUP)-2009. Int Angiol 2009;28(6):434–51.

Legiehn GM, Heran MK. A step-by-step practical approach to imaging diagnosis and interventional radiologic therapy in vascular malformations. Semin Intervent Radiol 2010;27(2):209–31.

Perkins JA, Manning SC, Tempero RM, et al. Lymphatic malformations: review of current treatment. Otolaryngol Head Neck Surg 2010; 142(6):795–803, 803 e1.

The complete reference list is available online at www.expertconsult.com

CHAPTER 45
Management of High-Flow Vascular Anomalies
James E. Jackson and Alex M. Barnacle

INTRODUCTION

Vascular anomalies are often poorly managed for a number of reasons: they are uncommon (other than the true infantile hemangioma), their mode of presentation is extremely variable, their classification has been very confusing and is still poorly understood by the majority of doctors, and their treatment is challenging. The interested interventional radiologist is in an ideal position to play a major, if not the lead, role in patient management. So many aspects of assessment and treatment require radiologic input, and it is essential that this involvement starts at the time of referral and the patient's first visit to the outpatient clinic. It is not good practice for a radiologist to accept a referral for endovascular treatment of a vascular malformation without first assessing the patient.[1]

For a clinician familiar with these anomalies, the diagnosis is almost always straightforward. A thorough patient history and physical examination usually make it clear which patients require, and are likely to benefit, from treatment. Patients and referrers are invariably keen for definitive intervention to cure what are often highly disfiguring or lifestyle-limiting conditions, but most vascular malformations cannot be cured, and the aim of any intervention is usually long-term symptom control. The radiologist's role is as much that of gatekeeper as interventionalist, stressing the current limitations of medical science, advising against heroic and often fruitless major intervention, and helping patients come to terms with their condition. A holistic approach is key, and the care of a patient with a vascular anomaly is ideally undertaken by a multidisciplinary team.

CLASSIFICATION

In 1982, Mulliken and Glowacki proposed what was at that time a very new way of classifying vascular anomalies.[2] Their system has been modified very little since then, with only minor changes made by the International Society for the Study of Vascular Anomalies (ISSVA) when it was established in 1992. This is now the most widely recognized system in use, encouraging management based on underlying histology and natural history of the lesion subtypes. The dichotomous Mulliken and Glowacki classification separates vascular tumors from vascular malformations. The *vascular tumor* arm includes the common infantile hemangiomas as well as rarer congenital hemangiomas and other vascular tumors, many of which are high flow. The *vascular malformation* arm comprises low-flow venous and lymphatic malformations and high-flow arteriovenous malformations (AVMs).

Vascular Tumors

The majority of vascular tumors are infantile hemangiomas, which occur in up to 12% of Caucasian infants by the age of 1 year. Congenital hemangiomas share some of the characteristics of the common infantile lesions but have very different natural histories. Other tumors in this arm of the classification system are rare but are more likely to involve interventional radiology. These include tufted angiomas and kaposiform hemangioendotheliomas.

Infantile Hemangioma

Infantile hemangiomas are by far the most common lesions in this subgroup. They are not present at birth, appearing at around 2 to 4 months of age. Typically they demonstrate a highly active period of growth and proliferation and then slowly involute, disappearing during school age. It is this natural history that clearly separates them from vascular malformations that, in contrast, are present at birth and grow commensurately with the child. Infantile hemangiomas are usually superficial lesions with a characteristic bright red color and are easily diagnosed clinically, rarely troubling the radiologist. Occasionally, deeper lesions occur that do not exhibit skin staining. Such rapidly growing masses generate consternation and urgent referral. The diagnosis is simple because the imaging features are usually characteristic. Ultrasound demonstrates a well-defined echogenic lesion that is highly vascular with large central feeding arteries and draining veins (Fig. 45-1). The highly arterialized nature of the lesion simply reflects its extremely active proliferation. Occasionally, biopsy may be required to allay concerns. Infantile hemangiomas express glucose transporter-1 (GLUT-1), a simple diagnostic marker. Core needle biopsy, when necessary to exclude more serious pathology, is usually straightforward under ultrasound guidance because lesions are typically superficial. A 16G coaxial technique is advocated in view of the highly vascular nature of these lesions, allowing a single pass through the tumor capsule and plugging of the biopsy track with Gelfoam (Pfizer, New York, N.Y.) pellets; complications in the authors' experience are rare.

Perhaps surprisingly, most of these highly vascular tumors do not cause vascular steal or cardiac compromise and can be managed conservatively. Intervention is indicated when lesions cause significant mass effect or disfigurement. Subglottic lesions and those that obstruct the visual axis are of particular concern. Pharmacologic management is now the mainstay of treatment in this group, with β-blockers the preferred first-line therapy.[3] Novel therapies such as the use of rapamycin to suppress stem cell

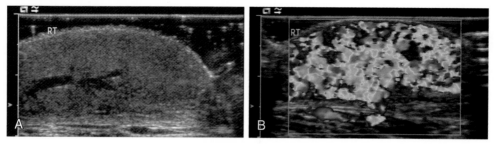

FIGURE 45-1. Ultrasound images of infantile hemangioma. **A,** Well-defined soft-tissue mass with prominent central vessels. **B,** Hypervascularity on color Doppler imaging.

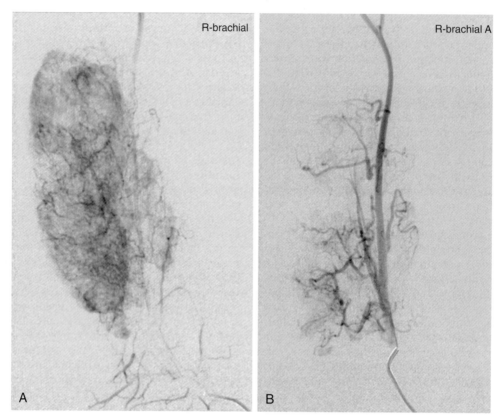

FIGURE 45-2. Angiogram of infantile hemangioma of upper limb in an 8-month-old child who presented with ulceration and recurrent bleeding requiring repeated transfusion. **A,** Preembolization angiogram of right brachial artery shows extensive neovascularity throughout lesion. **B,** Angiography after particle embolization demonstrates significant reduction in arterial supply to lesion.

proliferation are also evolving.[4] Occasionally, high-output cardiac failure occurs in children with very large infantile hemangiomas, particularly those involving the liver, and this requires urgent intervention. Particle embolization of the capillary bed is a simple and effective approach, aiming to reduce the vascularity of the lesion and stabilize the child's cardiovascular status until the natural history of the lesion causes involution (Fig. 45-2). Surgical ligation or coil embolization of the main feeding artery usually fails, the highly angiogenic tumor simply recruiting other arterial feeders. Particle embolization may also be indicated to reduce tissue bulk in rare instances where large lesions cause platelet sequestration and clotting factor consumption, although there is currently no published evidence for this.

Congenital Hemangioma

This hemangioma subgroup merits brief mention because of significant differences in natural history and prognosis when compared with infantile hemangiomas, which influence management decisions. Congenital hemangiomas are fully formed at birth, and this feature alone distinguishes them from the infantile group. They are similar in appearance but have subtle differences in color and contour compared to the classic infantile lesions. Imaging features are not strikingly different from those of infantile hemangiomas, although the lesions are often more heterogeneous, and calcification can be seen.

Congenital hemangiomas form two distinct clinical subgroups defined by their natural history. Some involute very rapidly in the first few months of life and are termed *rapidly involuting congenital hemangioma* (RICH), and others never involute (*noninvoluting congenital hemangioma*, NICH). Both types are histologically and immunophenotypically distinct from infantile hemangiomas.[5] Neither expresses GLUT-1. Biopsy of such lesions is sometimes helpful to allow clinicians to predict outcome. Urgent embolization of very large congenital hemangiomas is often requested but should be avoided if possible, because a proportion of these lesions will involute quickly without intervention.

Other Vascular Tumors

Infantile and congenital hemangiomas make up the vast majority of lesions in the vascular tumor arm of the Mulliken and Glowacki classification of vascular anomalies, but it is important to recognize other much less common lesions. These include the tufted angioma (TA), kaposiform hemangioendothelioma (KHE), hemangiopericytoma, and pyogenic granuloma. Recognition of TAs and KHEs in particular is important for two reasons: they often have a more unusual aggressive appearance despite their benign histology (Fig. 45-3), precipitating direct referral to oncologists, and they are sometimes associated with the Kasabach-Merritt phenomenon (KMP).[6] Both are GLUT-1 negative on biopsy and have characteristic histology, so biopsy is often useful. *Kasabach-Merritt phenomenon* describes a pattern of variable but often severe coagulopathy and thrombocytopenia; it is seen in association with a variety of soft-tissue lesions, but most commonly KHE. Children with vascular tumors who exhibit KMP show a variable response to therapy, and mortality rates are high. Evolving pharmacologic approaches to other vascular tumors may have a role to play in the management of these lesions. Embolization remains an alternative approach in an attempt to reduce tissue bulk and downregulate the drivers for KMP, but evidence is lacking.

Liver Vascular Tumors in Childhood

Vascular tumors of the liver deserve special mention because of the large volume of inaccurate and misleading literature in publication and confusion over their management. Lesions in the adult liver, spleen, and bone that have traditionally been described as hemangiomas almost certainly represent small venous malformations and are entities entirely distinct from true liver hemangiomas of infancy.

Both infantile and congenital hemangiomas occur in the liver in a proportion of children. The infantile lesions are almost always multifocal or diffuse and associated with multiple cutaneous hemangiomas, whereas the congenital lesions are typically solitary. Ultrasound confirms their high-flow nature and can demonstrate shunting at an intralesional level; this simply reflects disorganized neovascularity within these rapidly proliferating lesions (Fig. 45-4). It is important that these are *not* labeled as AVMs because this inevitably leads to high levels of clinical anxiety and the potential for unnecessary intervention. Infantile hemangiomas of the liver have the same natural history as the more common skin lesions, showing slow involution over time. Hepatic congenital hemangiomas are more commonly the RICH subtypes rather than NICH, and involute spontaneously and quickly. As elsewhere, biopsy is diagnostic

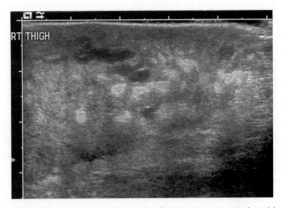

FIGURE 45-3. Ultrasound image of tufted angioma in a 2-day-old child. Internal architecture of lesion is far more heterogeneous than is seen in infantile hemangiomas.

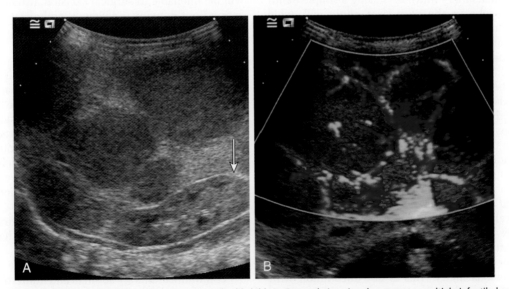

FIGURE 45-4. Ultrasound images of right lobe of liver in a 4-month-old child. **A,** Grayscale imaging demonstrates multiple infantile hemangiomas within liver (arrow indicates right kidney). **B,** Color Doppler confirms extensive irregular neovascularity.

and should guide management. Additionally, serum α-fetoprotein (AFP) should be measured to exclude hepatoblastoma. Because serum AFP concentrations vary widely between individuals in the neonatal period and can be elevated in children with liver hemangiomas, serial measurements are recommended to ensure levels fall rapidly in the first few weeks after birth.

Extensive liver hemangiomas can cause dramatic hepatic enlargement in the neonate, leading to respiratory and cardiac compromise. Thrombocytopenia and coagulopathy can also be seen. In such instances, medical management is often successful.[7] In refractory or fulminant cases, embolization may buy the child some time by reducing lesion size and the volume of blood flow through it. A combination of coil and particle embolization is usually successful. Left axillary arterial access is often a useful approach in the neonate,[8] and carbon dioxide angiography minimizes the volume of fluid and iodinated contrast media required in these hemodynamically unstable children.

Vascular Malformations

Low-flow malformations are discussed in detail in Chapter 44. This chapter will focus on high-flow (arteriovenous) malformations. All malformations are considered to be present at birth, although they may not become apparent until childhood or even adult life. An increase in size during childhood and especially around puberty is common, and many individuals present at this time because of the increasing prominence of the malformation, which may be associated with new or worsening symptoms including pain, ulceration, and hemorrhage. Progression of high-flow malformations may also occur in response to pregnancy or trauma, which may be accidental or iatrogenic—for example, proximal surgical ligation or embolization of feeding arteries and subtotal resection.

On clinical examination, a pulsatile soft-tissue swelling is usually evident, with prominence of draining superficial veins. The high-flow nature of a malformation is often clear on simple palpation, but a deeper-seated lesion may be less obviously pulsatile. In such cases, detection of an arteriovenous signal ("machinery murmur") using a simple handheld Doppler probe in the outpatient clinic will avoid misdiagnosing a high-flow lesion as one that is low-flow; this is clearly an important distinction to make because subsequent imaging and treatment of these two entities is different. The differential diagnosis of a vascular soft-tissue tumor should be considered, although a history of a longstanding preexisting swelling or the clinical finding of an associated overlying cutaneous stain will help make the diagnosis. Biopsy will be necessary in some individuals if doubt exists as to its true nature. Note should be made of any complications of the malformation, such as thinning of the overlying skin, frank ulceration, infection, and bleeding.

An *acquired posttraumatic arteriovenous fistula* may have an identical appearance on clinical examination to that of a high-flow AVM. The diagnosis is usually obvious because of a history of antecedent trauma, but some patients will not volunteer this information and indeed may have forgotten a previous injury. This is not uncommon with scalp lesions where a relatively minor injury, which may or may not have been associated with a cutaneous laceration, can rarely present many years later with a pulsatile soft-tissue swelling due to an enlarging arteriovenous communication. The demonstration of a single fistulous communication at subsequent angiography will sometimes be the first indication of this diagnosis, which is an important one to make because a cure is likely if treated appropriately.

Imaging

Other than Doppler ultrasound—which, as mentioned earlier, may be very helpful during initial clinical assessment of a vascular malformation—other cross-sectional imaging of high-flow malformations, although often performed, is rarely essential. The reason is that the decision regarding whether a high-flow malformation requires treatment is based upon clinical findings and symptoms. Many patients require no more than reassurance about the diagnosis and a frank discussion about its nature and natural history. If treatment is felt to be necessary, magnetic resonance imaging (MRI) is the noninvasive modality of first choice to demonstrate the extent of the AVM. Magnetic resonance angiography (MRA) may be helpful to document its angiographic anatomy, but this is often better visualized by catheter angiography. Bone involvement is best demonstrated on computed tomography (CT). Contrast-enhanced CT is rarely helpful and should not be performed unless there is a contraindication to MRI. Even then it is unlikely to give any more information than catheter angiography, which will be necessary if the decision has been made that treatment is required.

Management

Not all AVMs require treatment. Those that are quiescent, are not associated with significant symptoms, and cause little in the way of cosmetic deformity are often best left alone. Individuals who do not require treatment should be informed that they should request reassessment if the malformation becomes more troublesome.

Patients with high-flow malformations requiring therapy should proceed to angiography, and in many instances this will be combined with embolization. Some of these lesions will be amenable to surgical excision, usually after embolization,[9] but in many individuals, embolization will provide the best form of treatment.

Embolization

The most important aspect of embolization of a high-flow malformation is an understanding of the anatomy of vascular communications within it because these have a bearing both upon the method of vascular occlusion and on the final result. Houdart et al.[10] classified intracranial AVMs into three main types based upon the anatomy of the arteriovenous communications (Fig. 45-5), which they termed:

- Type I: Arteriovenous. These AVMs have a first identifiable venous component that is supplied by three or fewer arterial pedicles.
- Type II: Arteriolovenous. Here the first identifiable venous component is supplied by more than three (often very many) arterial pedicles.
- Type III: Arteriolovenulous. Here the arteriovenous communications are so small and numerous they cannot be separately identified, and the first obviously venous component is often at some distance from them.

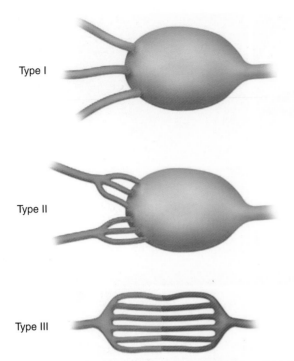

Type I

Type II

Type III

FIGURE 45-5. Diagrammatic representation of classification of high-flow arteriovenous malformations based upon angiographic anatomy of their arteriovenous communications.

These anatomic variations can coexist within the same malformation. In particular, AVMs with a dominant type III anatomy may also contain type II communications.

The general principle of embolization is that occlusion is performed at the site of the abnormal arteriovenous shunts and *not* in the vessel proximal to this point.[11-13] Embolization of arterial feeding vessels, which was performed for many years with metallic coils or particulate matter, is akin to proximal surgical ligation and must be avoided. It has little effect upon symptoms in most individuals, renders subsequent treatment more difficult because the arterial inflow vessels have been occluded, and may indeed paradoxically increase the size and activity of the AVM. If, however, embolization is directed at the AV communications themselves, from the arterial side, by a direct percutaneous puncture or via a retrograde venous approach,[11] and these are totally obliterated—often with a liquid embolic agent such as sodium tetradecyl sulfate (STS) or absolute alcohol—long-term improvement in symptoms can be achieved. Type I and type II lesions are particularly suited to this form of treatment.

A rare example of a type I lesion consisting of a single arteriovenous communication is sometimes described as *truncal AVM*. These have an identical appearance to posttraumatic arteriovenous fistulas and are most commonly found, in the authors' experience, in the kidneys. Such lesions are often very large, with extremely rapid flow into aneurysmal venous sacs; embolization is usually easier from the arterial side. This is the one type of high-flow malformation in which embolization of the arterial side of the malformation can be considered. Balloon occlusion techniques are often helpful to slow flow, and coils or plugs may be placed in the artery (rather than the vein), but it is important to achieve as distal an occlusion as possible to reduce

any risk of continued perfusion of the fistulous communication via collaterals (Fig. 45-6).

Much of the literature on embolization of high-flow vascular malformations discusses the importance of occluding the "nidus," but this term is unhelpful and should, in the current authors' opinion, be avoided. It was originally coined because the tortuous blood vessels seen on angiography when a high-flow vascular malformation is studied can be likened to a nest. Although the term *nidus* was originally used when describing intracranial lesions, it has now been adopted by interventional radiologists treating peripheral AVMs. This "nest" actually consists primarily of feeding arteries, the occlusion of which should be avoided; it has become clear that the best results are achieved when embolization is directed at the first identifiable venous component.

For this reason, the current authors feel that the confusing term *nidus* should no longer be used. High-flow vascular malformations should be thought of as *venous sumps*. In other words, it is the low-pressure first venous component at the site of abnormal arteriovenous communication that drives the AVM. If this is left untouched and only the feeding vessels are occluded, the low-pressure "sump" continues to draw in blood from adjacent collaterals. If the venous component is occluded from the start, however, the low-pressure "drive" disappears, and arteriovenous shunting is obliterated. This can often be performed with no arterial embolization at all, such that follow-up arteriograms appear normal.

No two AVMs are alike, but the general principle of the technique of embolization of a lesion with a type I (arteriovenous) or type II (arteriolovenous) anatomy is as follows (Figs. 45-7 and 45-8):

1. Diagnostic angiography is performed to document the anatomy of the malformation and determine the site of the *first venous component* (see Fig. 45-7, *A* and Fig. 45-8, *A* and *B*).
2. The first venous component is accessed by direct puncture (see Fig. 45-8, *C*) or a retrograde venous approach (see Fig. 45-7, *B*) and less commonly via a major arterial pedicle (Fig. 45-9), although this approach is often necessary when treating intracranial lesions (for obvious reasons).
3. Venous outflow from this first venous component is controlled such that there is contrast medium stasis within it. This may be straightforward when there is a single outflow vein that can be temporarily occluded with an occlusion balloon (see Fig. 45-7, *B*), or with a tourniquet if the AVM involves a limb. It can be considerably more difficult if there are multiple outflow veins, particularly if one or more of these are not easily accessible.
4. Once contrast medium stasis has been achieved in the first venous component, angiography is performed to document the volume of contrast medium required to fill it without retrograde filling of arterial feeding vessels.
5. The venous sac can then be filled with the same quantity of STS or absolute alcohol. The sclerosant is left in situ for a few minutes and then aspirated, if possible, before venous outflow occlusion is released and angiography is performed to check on the progress of embolization (see Fig. 45-8, *D*).

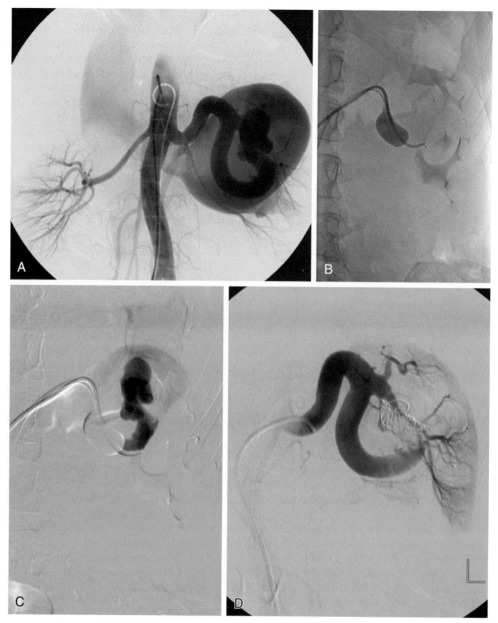

FIGURE 45-6. Massive arteriovenous malformation (AVM) of left kidney with type I arteriovenous angiographic anatomy. **A,** Abdominal aortogram demonstrates rapid flow through AVM into an aneurysmal venous sac and thence the inferior vena cava. **B-C,** Occlusion balloon catheter has been inflated within major feeding pedicle to reduce flow during subsequent embolization, which was performed with combination of coils and glue introduced via separate catheter placed alongside occlusion balloon catheter. **D,** Postembolization selective left renal arteriogram demonstrates obliteration of arteriovenous shunting and preservation of normal renal artery branches.

6. Steps 4 and 5 may have to be repeated. It is essential that step 4 always precedes further introduction of sclerosant into the venous sac because flow dynamics can change subtly during embolization such that retrograde arterial filling might occur with a smaller amount of contrast medium than it initially took to fill the venous sac.

One of the major difficulties faced when attempting this form of embolization is preventing migration of the embolic agent into outflow veins, and subsequently the pulmonary arteries. In the limbs, this may be achieved with a tourniquet inflated to above arterial pressure to provide both arterial inflow and outflow occlusion during embolization. In other territories, such as the pelvis or head and neck,

occlusion balloons and a more frequent use of "glue" is often required.

Onyx (ev3/Covidien, Plymouth, Minn.), a nonadhesive liquid embolic agent composed of ethylene vinyl alcohol, is a helpful agent when the venous component of the AVM can only be satisfactorily catheterized via an arterial pedicle, but this is an unusual situation in a peripheral (as opposed to an intracranial) AVM. If this is the case, it is important to use this agent to occlude the first venous component rather than the feeding arteries (see Fig. 45-9).

AVMs with a largely intraosseous component are especially well suited to treatment by this method of embolization because they usually have a type II (arteriolovenous) anatomy. These are usually best approached by direct

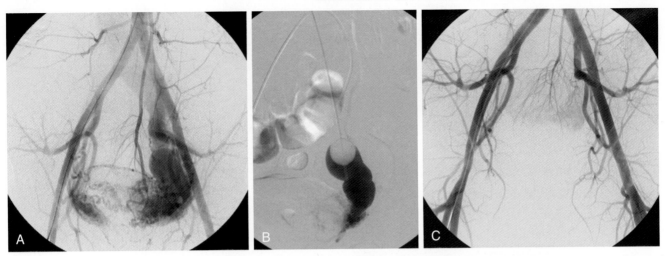

FIGURE 45-7. Large left and smaller right pelvic arteriovenous malformations (AVMs) with type II arteriolovenous angiographic anatomy. **A,** Abdominal aortogram demonstrates anatomy of AVMs, both of which have numerous supplying vessels communicating with a central venous sac. **B,** Dilated first venous component of left pelvic AVM has been catheterized retrogradely from a right internal jugular venous approach, and its outflow has been temporarily occluded with occlusion balloon catheter. Angiogram performed via balloon catheter lumen demonstrates contrast medium stasis within venous sac, without retrograde arterial filling. Embolization was performed with sodium tetradecyl sulfate (see text for technique). Same technique was used to treat right-sided pelvic AVM at a separate procedure. **C,** Follow-up study performed 6 months after final embolization demonstrates obliteration of arteriovenous shunting on both sides, with preservation of normal arterial pelvic branches.

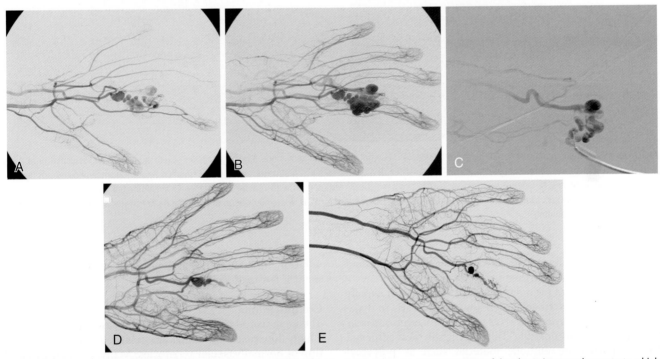

FIGURE 45-8. Left index finger arteriovenous malformation (AVM) with type II arteriolovenous anatomy. **A-B,** Left hand arteriograms demonstrate a high-flow AVM involving left index finger, consisting of a tortuous dilated first venous component supplied by several branches arising from both digital arteries. **C,** First venous component has been punctured percutaneously. Outflow from this venous component was controlled with tourniquet inflated around forearm during embolization with sodium tetradecyl sulfate. **D,** Postembolization arteriogram demonstrates obliteration of arteriovenous shunting. **E,** Follow-up arteriogram performed 6 months after embolization demonstrates some residual digital artery aneurysmal change but no arteriovenous shunting.

transosseous puncture of the dilated venous component of the malformation (Fig. 45-10).

Embolization and Surgery

If surgery is to be performed, the aim should be to totally excise the AVM.[9] Preoperative embolization may be very helpful, but it is very important to understand that this is performed to make surgery easier by reducing the vascularity of the AVM, rather than to reduce the extent of resection. Tissue expansion and muscular flap transfer techniques may be necessary when a large cutaneous defect is likely to result from excision. The full range of surgical techniques

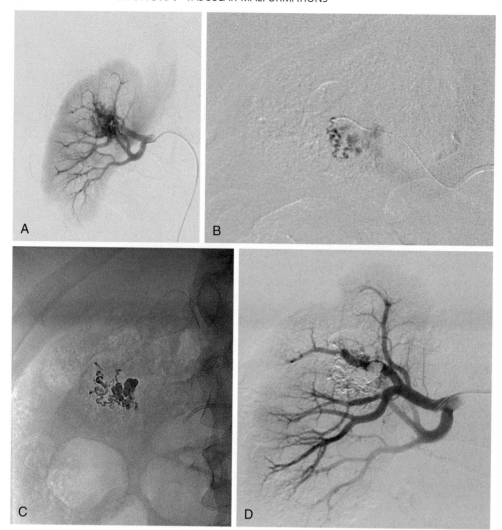

FIGURE 45-9. Right renal arteriovenous malformation (AVM) with type II arteriolovenous anatomy causing severe hematuria. **A,** Selective right renal arteriogram demonstrates complex high-flow AVM. This consisted of a dilated tortuous first venous component supplied by several small pedicles arising from intrarenal artery branches. **B,** One of venous pedicles has been selectively catheterized with coaxial 3F catheter. **C,** Unsubtracted image after embolization demonstrates a cast of Onyx used to fill much of first identifiable venous component. **D,** Postembolization arteriogram demonstrates almost complete obliteration of arteriovenous shunting.

that may be used lies outside the scope of this chapter and will not be discussed further.

The technique of preoperative embolization will usually differ from that described earlier. The aim is clearly to make the malformation avascular so as to give the surgeon as near a bloodless a field as possible. This is generally best achieved with a particulate embolic material such as polyvinyl alcohol, and such embolization is often straightforward, particularly since many AVMs requiring surgery will have a type III (arteriolovenulous) angiographic anatomy. A particle size should be chosen that will allow deep penetration into the malformation without passing through the arteriovenous communications. If some larger communications are present, these may require embolization with other agents (e.g., glue) introduced via a coaxial arterial catheter or a direct puncture route. Coil occlusion alone of feeding arteries is useless because the malformation will remain very vascular via collaterals. Indeed, it is important not to embolize feeding vessels with coils or plugs, even when distal embolization has been performed with particles. This

will only hamper future angiographic assessment or treatment if the malformation recurs.

Complications

The most feared complication of endovascular treatment of a high-flow vascular malformation is inadvertent embolization of normal vascular territories. Many if not all vascular malformations are incurable, and although good long-term results can be obtained, particularly in those with a favorable angiographic anatomy as detailed earlier, it is important to remember that few are life threatening. If, for example, a hand with an AVM is intermittently uncomfortable but otherwise functions normally, it is imperative that it not be converted to one with serious loss of function due to a complication of embolization. To avoid non–target vessel occlusion, it is important to adhere to the general principles of any embolization procedure:

1. Have a thorough understanding of normal anatomy and the potential collateral pathways that occur in different vascular territories.

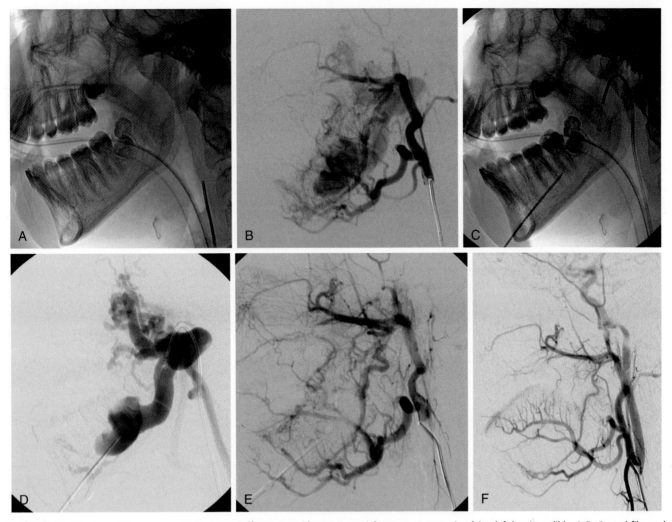

FIGURE 45-10. Large intraosseous arteriovenous malformation with type II arteriolovenous anatomy involving left hemimandible. **A-B,** Control film and subtracted image from selective left external carotid arteriography demonstrates rapid arteriovenous shunting into dilated first venous component in body of left hemimandible. **C-D,** First venous component has been punctured percutaneously through the bone, and angiography has been performed to document venous anatomy. Embolization was performed with glue. **E,** Postembolization arteriogram documents obliteration of arteriovenous shunting. **F,** Follow-up arteriogram at 6 months confirms excellent angiographic result.

2. Perform frequent angiographic runs during the embolization to monitor progress.
3. Be aware of the rapid changes that can occur in flow during embolization.
4. Mix nonopaque embolic agents with contrast medium before their injection.
5. Always inject embolic agents under continuous fluoroscopic guidance.
6. Be aware of your own limitations, and do not proceed if there is any doubt in your mind as to the distribution of any injected embolic material.
7. Avoid doing "that little bit more" to turn a good angiographic result into an excellent one. At the stage when there is a noticeable reduction in arteriovenous shunting, the risk of nontarget embolization increases. It is often best to stop the procedure at this point and arrange a follow-up procedure after 1 to 3 months to assess what further needs to be done. If embolization has been aimed at the first venous component as described earlier, the follow-up study will often show a considerable angiographic improvement, and in some cases further embolization will not be necessary.

These principles should make it clear that embolization of a high-flow AVM is not a procedure that should be undertaken by anyone inexperienced in general embolization techniques. There is a very strong argument that all AVMs should be treated in specialist centers.

CONCLUSIONS

High-flow vascular malformations are very difficult to manage. The best results are undoubtedly achieved in specialist centers that are able to provide multidisciplinary input. When treatment is necessary, long-term symptomatic improvement is achieved in the majority of individuals, and there is no doubt that the radiologic and clinical obliteration of more high-flow malformations has come with a better understanding of their radiologic anatomy and the use of agents directed at the arteriovenous shunts themselves, rather than at the proximal feeding vessels.

KEY POINTS

- It is essential to understand and use Mulliken's classification that divides vascular anomalies into two groups: *vascular tumors*, the most common of which is the infantile hemangioma, and *vascular malformations*.

- Most hemangiomas do not require treatment.

- Not all high-flow vascular malformations require treatment.

- High-flow arteriovenous malformations (AVMs) are divided into three main types based upon their angiographic anatomy.

- Avoid the term *nidus* when describing a high-flow AVM; think of these lesions as *venous sumps*.

- When treating high-flow AVMs by embolization, the best results are obtained when occlusion is aimed at the first venous component immediately beyond the site of arteriovenous communication.

▶ **SUGGESTED READINGS**

Jackson JE, Mansfield AO, Allison DJ. Treatment of high-flow vascular malformations by venous embolization aided by flow occlusion techniques. Cardiovasc Intervent Radiol 1996;19:323–8.

Mulliken JB, Glowacki J. Hemangiomas and vascular malformations in infants and children: a classification based on endothelial characteristics. Plast Reconstr Surg 1982;69:412–22.

Sung KC, Young SD, Dong IK, et al. Peripheral arteriovenous malformations with a dominant outflow vein: results of ethanol embolization. Korean J Radiol 2008;9(3):258–67.

The complete reference list is available online at www.expertconsult.com

CHAPTER 46

Abdominal Aorta and the Inferior Vena Cava

Amber Jones and Monica Smith Pearl

Arterial supply to the abdominal viscera provided by the abdominal aorta and venous return of blood to the right atrium from all structures below the diaphragm via the inferior vena cava (IVC) are the subjects of this chapter. Classic as well as variant anatomy and relevant clinical scenarios are presented because a number of pathologic processes involve these vessels. The abdominal aorta, including its branches, is discussed from the level of the diaphragm to its termination into the common iliac arteries. The IVC, along with its tributaries, is discussed from its origin at the confluence of the common iliac veins to its termination in the right atrium.

ABDOMINAL AORTA

The major blood supply to the abdominal viscera is derived from the aorta, which is constant in location and presence despite extensive variability in the anatomy of its branch vessels. The abdominal aorta begins as a midline structure at the level of the diaphragmatic crura, anterior to the lower border of the 12th thoracic vertebra, and has an average diameter of 1.5 to 2 cm. As it descends through the abdomen, it tapers slightly, with an average diameter of 1.5 cm below the renal arteries. Clinically, the abdominal aorta is often divided into suprarenal and infrarenal arterial segments. The rationale for this division is the higher incidence of atherosclerotic and aneurysmal disease in the infrarenal abdominal aorta and the increased complexity of interventions involving the suprarenal portion. It terminates in a bifurcation into two common iliac arteries at the lower region of the fourth lumbar vertebra, just slightly to the left of midline. On the anterior abdominal wall, this bifurcation may be visualized as a point approximately 2.5 cm below the umbilicus or at the level of a line drawn between the highest points of the iliac crests.

Imaging of the abdominal aorta may be accomplished by ultrasound (US), computed tomography (CT), and magnetic resonance imaging (MRI). Ultrasound is widely available, portable, and lacks ionizing radiation, but it is heavily operator dependent and thus its reproducibility is variable.[1] Other challenges arise when there is excess bowel gas and obesity. Multidetector CT is a noninvasive imaging technique that allows for rapid image acquisition and high spatial resolution, including nearly isotropic submillimeter resolution in the X, Y, and Z planes.[2] Other advantages of multidetector CT include widespread availability, detailed evaluation of the aortic wall and lining mural thrombus, detection of unsuspected extraluminal abnormalities, and multiplanar postprocessing for interventional planning.[2] MRI is another noninvasive imaging modality that has the potential to illustrate the arterial anatomy of the abdominal aorta and its branches. Time-of-flight (TOF) and phase-contrast (PC) magnetic resonance angiography (MRA) are two well-known techniques that rely on flowing blood to image the arterial system. These techniques, however, are prone to artifacts related to disruptions or variations in blood flow, as seen with pulsatile and turbulent flow.[3] Gadolinium (Gd)-enhanced three-dimensional (3D) MRA, introduced in the early 1990s, relies on the T1 shortening effects of circulating Gd-chelate contrast media instead of on flowing blood. The technique is quick, easy to perform, and provides high-resolution 3D images with minimal artifacts related to spin saturation, slow flow, or turbulent flow associated with TOF.[3]

As the aorta descends through the abdominal cavity, it gives off anterior, lateral, and posterior branches. Anterior branches include the celiac trunk, superior mesenteric artery, and inferior mesenteric artery, which supply the gastrointestinal viscera, as well as the phrenic and gonadal arteries (Fig. 46-1).

The bilateral *inferior phrenic arteries* may arise together as a trunk or as independent vessels just above or at the origin of the celiac trunk. They pass upward from the abdominal aorta to the diaphragm and give off multiple branches to the adrenal glands. The inferior phrenic artery also supplies the Glisson capsule of the liver through anastomoses at the bare area of the liver within the triangular ligaments.

The *celiac trunk* is the first wide anterior branch of the abdominal aorta; it arises just below the diaphragmatic hiatus and anterior to the superior part of the first lumbar vertebra. It supplies the foregut, which includes the abdominal esophagus, stomach, duodenum superior to its major papilla, liver, pancreas, and gallbladder. Blood supply to the spleen also develops in relation to that of the foregut region (Fig. 46-2). (See Chapter 52 for further discussion of the celiac trunk and its branches.)

The *common hepatic artery*, a medium-sized branch of the celiac trunk, is directed forward and to the right and divides into its two terminal branches, the hepatic artery proper and the gastroduodenal artery. The *hepatic artery proper*, named from the origin at the gastroduodenal artery to its bifurcation into right and left hepatic branches, ascends toward the liver in the free edge of the lesser omentum. It runs to the left of the bile duct and anterior to the portal vein to the porta hepatis, where it divides into the right and left hepatic arteries. As the right hepatic artery approaches the liver, it gives off the *cystic artery*, which passes downward and forward along the neck of the gallbladder. Alternatively, the cystic artery may arise from

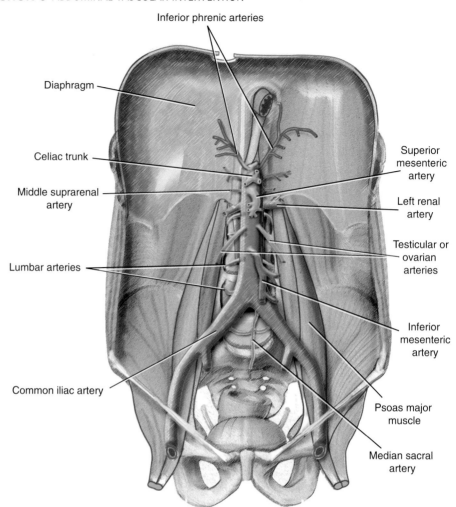

FIGURE 46-1. Abdominal aorta. *(Redrawn from Drake RL, Vogl W, Mitchell AWM. Gray's anatomy for students. Philadelphia: Elsevier/ Churchill Livingstone; 2005.)*

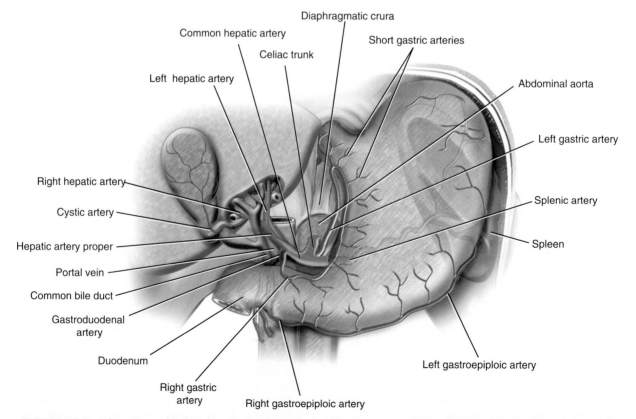

FIGURE 46-2. Celiac artery and its branches. Liver has been raised and lesser omentum and anterior layer of greater omentum removed.

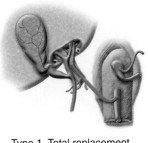

Type 1. Total replacement of CHA

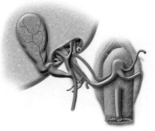

Type 2. Early bifurcation of CHA

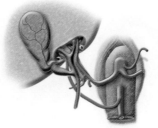

Type 3. Replaced right HA

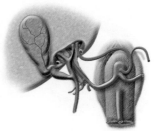

Type 4. Replaced left HA

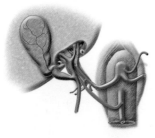

Type 5. Accessory right HA from the superior mesenteric artery

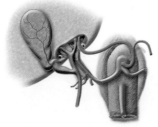

Type 6. Accessory left HA from left gastric artery

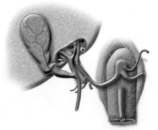

Type 7. Accessory left HA from right HA

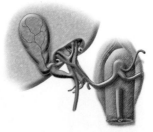

Type 8. Right HA passes anteriorly to the common bile duct

FIGURE 46-3. Hepatic artery variations: types 1 through 8. Most frequent variation is replacement of hepatic artery. Variations occur in about 40% of the population. *CHA,* Common hepatic artery; *HA,* hepatic artery. *(Redrawn from Uflacker R. Atlas of vascular anatomy: an angiographic approach. Baltimore: Lippincott Williams & Wilkins; 1997.)*

the common hepatic, left hepatic, or even the superior mesenteric artery. Additionally, there may be more than one cystic artery. The *right gastric artery* arises from any site along the hepatic artery, before or after the gastroduodenal artery. It descends to the pyloric end of the stomach, passes to the left along its lesser curvature, and anastomoses with the left gastric artery.

In the event of occlusion of the proper hepatic artery, collateral blood supply is provided by small unnamed collateral arteries in the porta hepatis and by reversal of flow in the right gastric artery. If the occlusion involves a proximal hepatic artery branch, intrahepatic collaterals provide additional blood flow, an important consideration during embolization of intrahepatic bleeding.

In general, 45% of patients have some variation in their hepatic arterial supply. Variations may involve a replaced artery that substitutes for the absent normal vessel, or an accessory artery that appears in addition to the one normally present.

Eight different types of variations have been described, the most common being replacement of either the right hepatic artery from the superior mesenteric artery (type 3) or the left hepatic artery from the left gastric artery (type 4). Other replaced variants include the common hepatic artery from the superior mesenteric artery (type 1). Accessory variants include an accessory right hepatic artery from the superior mesenteric artery (type 5) and an accessory left hepatic artery from either the left gastric artery (type 6) or the right hepatic artery (type 7). A type 2 variant involves early bifurcation of a short common hepatic artery or separate origins of the right and left hepatic arteries from the celiac trunk, with the gastroduodenal artery arising from

the right hepatic artery. Additionally, variant anatomy may involve the pathway of the artery, with a type 8 variant involving the right hepatic artery passing anterior to the common hepatic duct instead of posteriorly. These variants can occur in isolation or together (Fig. 46-3).

The *gastroduodenal artery* is a short but large branch of the common hepatic artery that descends near the pylorus between the superior part of the duodenum and the pancreatic neck. (See Chapter 52 for further discussion of the gastroduodenal artery.)

The *superior pancreaticoduodenal artery* divides into anterior and posterior branches as it descends between the duodenum and pancreatic head, and supplies these structures. (See Chapter 52 for further discussion of the superior pancreaticoduodenal artery.) The pancreaticoduodenal arteries enlarge and provide important collateral pathways between the celiac trunk and superior mesenteric artery in the case of stenosis or occlusion of either aortic branch.

Classic celiac trunk anatomy is present in up to only 70% of individuals; a wide range of variants may exist. Awareness of these variations is essential for visceral vascular imaging. Couinaud described eight different types of variations of the celiac trunk (Fig. 46-4). Type 1 involves a classic configuration of the celiac trunk, with all three branches arising as a trunk from the abdominal aorta. The variation exists in the possible subtypes: a hepatosplenic trunk, with the left gastric artery arising from the trunk; a hepatogastrosplenic trunk, with the three arteries arising simultaneously in a trifurcation; or a gastrosplenic trunk in which the splenic artery is dominant and the hepatic artery arises from the splenic artery. Another variant described involves a common trunk for two arteries, the hepatic and splenic

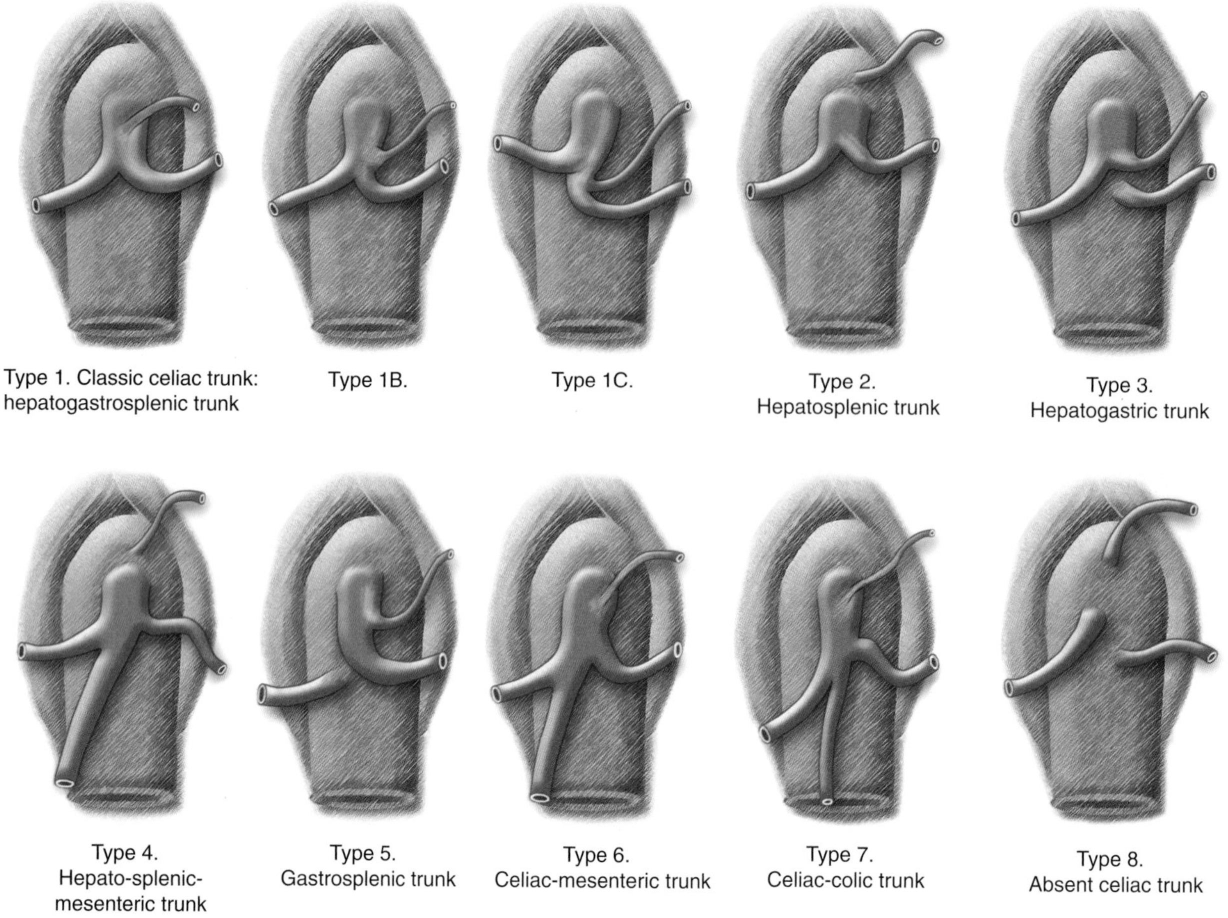

FIGURE 46-4. Schematic drawing showing variations in configuration of celiac trunk. *(Redrawn from Uflacker R. Atlas of vascular anatomy: an angiographic approach. Baltimore: Lippincott Williams & Wilkins; 1997.)*

arteries for type 2 and the hepatic and left gastric arteries for type 3, whereas the third artery, the left gastric artery in type 2 and the splenic artery in type 3, arises directly from the aorta. Alternatively, the splenic artery in type 3 may arise from the superior mesenteric artery. Similar to a type 2 variant is type 4, in which the left gastric artery arises directly from the aorta; however, the common trunk comprises the hepatic, splenic, and superior mesenteric arteries. The most complex configuration is type 5, in which the left gastric and splenic arteries form a common trunk, and the common hepatic artery, when present, may arise from the aorta or superior mesenteric artery. When the hepatic artery does not exist, it is replaced by the right, left, or both hepatic arteries at the same time. Types 6 and 7 involve additional arteries arising from the celiac trunk, including the superior mesenteric artery in type 6 and the left colic or middle colic arteries in type 7. Additionally, the three main arteries may arise directly from the aorta as in type 8.

The *superior mesenteric artery* is the anterior branch of the abdominal aorta supplying the midgut, which includes the entire small bowel from the duodenum inferior to its major duodenal papilla, the cecum, the appendix, the ascending colon, and the right two thirds of the transverse colon. (See Chapter 52 for further discussion of the superior mesenteric artery and its branches, including the inferior

pancreaticoduodenal artery, jejunal and ileal arteries, and middle colic, right colic, and ileocolic arteries.)

The *inferior mesenteric artery* supplies the hindgut, which includes the left third of the transverse colon, the descending colon, the sigmoid colon, the rectum, and the upper part of the anal canal. It is the smallest of the three anterior branches of the abdominal aorta and arises anterior to the body of the third lumbar vertebra a few centimeters above the aortic bifurcation into the common iliac arteries. (See Chapter 52 for further discussion of the inferior mesenteric artery and its branches, including the left colic artery, sigmoid arteries, and superior hemorrhoidal [rectal] artery.)

The *left colic artery*, the first branch of the inferior mesenteric artery, ascends retroperitoneally and divides into ascending and descending branches. The ascending branch supplies the distal part of the transverse colon and proximal descending colon, and anastomoses with the left branch of the middle colic artery at the splenic flexure. The descending branch passes inferiorly to supply the distal descending colon, and anastomoses with the highest sigmoid artery. From the anastomoses between these arteries originates the marginal artery of Drummond, a lateral arcade in the mesentery of the left colon. Anastomosis of the marginal artery with the ascending branch of the left colic artery and distal left branch of the middle colic artery is frequently made through an additional more medial arcade, the arc of Riolan. These arcades provide an important collateral blood supply because the watershed area between the superior and inferior mesenteric arteries at the splenic flexure is extremely vulnerable to ischemia.

The *testicular* and *ovarian arteries* are paired visceral branches of the abdominal aorta that arise anterolaterally below the origin of the renal arteries. They pass inferolaterally, with similar paths in the abdomen but divergent ones in the pelvis. They descend into the pelvis along the anterior surface of the psoas muscles, anterior to the IVC, adjacent to the gonadal veins and ureters, and anterior to the iliac vessels. In the pelvis, the *testicular arteries* take a lateral course and enter the spermatic cord to continue into the scrotum, where they become tortuous and divide into several branches to provide the sole blood supply to the testes. The testicular artery also contributes one or two small branches to the ureter and cremaster muscle. The origin and course of the first part of the *ovarian arteries* are the same as those of the testicular arteries, but they take a more medial path in the pelvis. The ovarian artery travels through the suspensory ligament of the ovary (infundibulopelvic ligament) and provides branches to the ovary and fallopian tubes and small branches to the ureter. The artery then continues medially to the uterus and through the broad ligament, where it anastomoses with the terminal parts of the uterine artery. The ovarian arteries enlarge significantly during pregnancy to augment uterine blood supply. The most common variation in origin of the gonadal artery is from the renal artery, followed less often by the adrenal, lumbar, or even the iliac artery.

Lateral aortic branches include the middle adrenal (suprarenal) and renal arteries. The *middle adrenal arteries* are small and arise just above the renal arteries, one on either side of the aorta, opposite the superior mesenteric artery. They pass laterally and slightly upward over the crura of the diaphragm, where they anastomose with adrenal branches of the inferior phrenic and renal arteries and contribute to the vascular supply of the adrenal gland. As it travels to supply the right adrenal gland, the right middle adrenal artery passes posterior to the IVC. The origins of the middle adrenal arteries may be replaced by the celiac artery or superior mesenteric artery in 2% to 5% of patients.

The *renal arteries*, usually 4 to 6 cm in length and 5 to 6 mm in diameter, arise from the aorta just inferior to the origin of the superior mesenteric artery between the first and second lumbar vertebrae. The renal artery passes laterally and, after giving off the inferior adrenal artery, bifurcates into anterior and posterior branches that supply the renal parenchyma. The anterior division supplies the upper and lower poles and the anterior aspect of the midportion of the kidney. The posterior division primarily supplies the posterior renal parenchyma, with supplemental supply to the upper and lower poles. The divisional arteries then divide into apical, upper, middle, lower, and posterior segmental arteries that give rise to interlobar arteries. At the corticomedullary junction, the interlobar arteries divide into the arcuate arteries. The terminal branches of the renal artery are the interlobular arteries, which ultimately supply the glomeruli. The right renal artery, whose orifice is located on the anterolateral wall of the aorta, is longer than the left

and passes posterior to the IVC, right renal vein, head of the pancreas, and descending part of the duodenum. The left is somewhat higher than the right, originates in a more lateral location, and courses through the retroperitoneum posterior to the left renal vein, body of the pancreas, and splenic vein.

Variations in number, location, and branching patterns of the renal arteries affect more than 30% of people. Accessory renal arteries are commonly present and more prevalent than any other accessory arteries of similar size in other organs. They may originate from the abdominal aorta above or below the primary renal artery or from the iliac (usually common) artery, enter the hilum with the primary artery, or pierce the kidney at some other level. Renal artery origins arising above the origin of the superior mesenteric artery are extremely rare. Congenital renal anomalies are often associated with aberrant locations of renal artery origins and supernumerary vessels. A horseshoe kidney, for example, has a 100% incidence of multiple renal arteries.

The renal arteries are end arteries and have poorly developed collateral pathways, unlike the colonic and hepatic vasculature. In the presence of slowly progressive proximal renal artery stenosis, renal capsular, ureteral, adrenal, and other retroperitoneal arteries may enlarge sufficiently to provide enough collateral blood supply to preserve renal viability, although normal function may not be maintained. In contrast, acute proximal occlusion of a previously normal renal artery results in significant ischemia secondary to inadequate preexisting collateral supply.

The posterior branches include the paired lumbar arteries and the median sacral artery. The *lumbar arteries* are usually four in number, although a smaller fifth pair may arise from the median sacral artery. They run laterally and posteriorly over the lumbar vertebral bodies and pass posterior to the sympathetic trunks and between the transverse processes of adjacent lumbar vertebrae to reach the abdominal wall. From this point onward, they demonstrate a branching pattern similar to a posterior intercostal artery, including segmental branches that supply the spinal cord. A small percentage of patients will have a lower anterior spinal artery, or artery of Adamkiewicz, arising from an L1 or L2 lumbar artery, which becomes clinically important when considering lumbar artery embolization. The lumbar arteries anastomose with one another, as well as with the lower posterior intercostal, subcostal, iliolumbar, deep circumflex iliac, and inferior epigastric arteries. These anastomoses may form the basis of collateral supply to the lower extremities in the event of distal aortic occlusive disease.

The *median sacral artery* is small and arises from the posterior wall of the abdominal aorta, just proximal to its bifurcation. Alternatively, it may arise as a common trunk with the lumbar arteries or occasionally from the common iliac artery. It descends in the midline, anterior to the fourth and fifth lumbar vertebrae, and continues over the anterior surface of the sacrum and coccyx. There are anastomoses with the rectum, lumbar branches of the iliolumbar artery, and the lateral sacral arteries. It may be distinguished angiographically from the superior hemorrhoidal branch of the inferior mesenteric artery by its posterior location and lack of a terminal bifurcation.

The abdominal aorta bifurcates on the left side of the fourth lumbar vertebral body into the two *common iliac arteries* that supply the pelvis and lower extremities. Each is approximately 5 cm in length and 8 to 10 mm in diameter and passes inferiorly and laterally to divide into two terminal branches, the external iliac and internal iliac (hypogastric) arteries. In addition to the terminal branches, the common iliac arteries give branches to the surrounding tissues, peritoneum, psoas muscle, ureter, and nerves. The common iliac artery may be a potential source of an accessory lower pole renal artery, median sacral artery, or iliolumbar artery.

A clinically important pathologic process involving the abdominal aorta is *aneurysm* formation, or fusiform or saccular enlargement 1.5 times greater in diameter than a normal aorta. Generally defined as greater than 3 cm in diameter, the cause of an abdominal aortic aneurysm is multifactorial; however, atherosclerotic changes and intimal calcification are prominent features. Without surgical or endovascular intervention, the aneurysm continues to grow, thereby increasing the risk for rupture, which is considered negligible below a diameter of 5 cm.

INFERIOR VENA CAVA

The IVC and its tributaries are frequent sites of vascular pathology. Caval morphology reflects intravascular volume status and intraabdominal pressure, and caval involvement may be the first manifestation of diseases involving the organs drained by its tributaries. Imaging by US, CT, and MRI plays an important role in diagnosis and management of the diverse conditions affecting the IVC.[4] US, including color Doppler flow imaging, is a useful modality for initial evaluation and helps differentiate artifactual filling defects from true intraluminal thrombus. US, however, is operator dependent, and visualization of the IVC may be impaired by bowel gas or obesity. CT and MRI are essential for staging and treatment planning. The IVC is typically evaluated in the portal venous phase (60-70 seconds after injection of 100-150 mL of nonionic contrast material at a rate of 3-5 mL/s). During this phase, there is denser contrast material in the renal and suprarenal IVC than in the infrarenal portion owing to venous return from the kidneys. Dynamic multiphasic imaging is performed only if indicated (e.g., in renal cell carcinoma). MRI is the most reliable technique for depicting the presence and extent of tumor thrombus, although routine use of this modality is limited by availability and cost considerations. The most robust MRI sequences for imaging the IVC are breath-hold T1-weighted MRI performed after intravenous administration of contrast material and balanced steady-state free precession.[4]

The IVC, a single right-sided structure in 97% of individuals, returns blood from all structures below the diaphragm to the right atrium of the heart. It is formed by the confluence of the two common iliac veins at the level of the fifth lumbar vertebra just to the right of midline. It has an oval shape in cross-section, but given its elastic structure, it is easily deformed by adjacent abdominal or retroperitoneal masses and dilates or collapses in response to changes in intravascular volume and intraabdominal pressure. The IVC, whose infrarenal portion has an average diameter of approximately 23 mm, ascends anterior to the vertebral column through the posterior abdominal region on the right side of the abdominal aorta. Having reached the liver, the retrohepatic IVC resides in a groove on the posterior

surface in the bare area of the liver and continues in a superior direction; it leaves the abdomen by piercing the diaphragm's central tendon at the level of the eighth thoracic vertebra (Fig. 46-5). During its course superiorly, the anterior surface of the IVC is crossed by the right external iliac artery, right gonadal artery, duodenum, pancreatic head, bile duct, portal vein, and liver, which overlaps and occasionally completely surrounds it. The supradiaphragmatic portion of the IVC, only approximately 2.5 cm in length, pierces the fibrous pericardium and passes behind the serous pericardium to open into the inferoposterior part of the right atrium. In front of its atrial orifice is a semilunar valve, termed the *eustachian valve* or *valve of the inferior vena cava*, that is rudimentary in adults. However, it plays an important role during development by directing incoming oxygenated blood through the foramen ovale into the left atrium.

Tributaries to the IVC include the common iliac veins, lumbar veins, right testicular or ovarian vein, renal veins, right adrenal vein, hepatic veins, and inferior phrenic veins. Veins draining the abdominal part of the gastrointestinal tract, spleen, pancreas, and gallbladder constitute the portal venous system and are not tributaries of the IVC.

The external and internal iliac veins join to form the common iliac veins anterior to the sacroiliac articulation. The common iliac veins pass obliquely upward toward the right, unite at an acute angle, and form the IVC at the level of the fifth lumbar vertebra. The right and left common iliac veins differ slightly in their ascent. The right common iliac vein, shorter than the left, has a nearly vertical direction and ascends posterior and then lateral to the right common iliac artery. The left common iliac vein, more oblique in its course, begins medial to its corresponding artery and also becomes posterior to the right common iliac artery more superiorly. Each common iliac vein receives iliolumbar and sometimes lateral sacral veins, whereas the left common iliac vein receives, in addition, the middle sacral vein.

Four to five pairs of lumbar veins drain the lumbar muscles and skin from the abdominal wall, as well as the vertebral venous plexuses. The left lumbar veins are longer than the right and pass posterior to the aorta. These veins may empty into the posterolateral aspect of the IVC at the levels of the first through fourth lumbar vertebral bodies. However, not all lumbar veins drain directly into the IVC. The first and second lumbar veins may empty into ascending lumbar veins, and the fifth lumbar vein generally drains into the iliolumbar vein, a tributary of the common iliac vein (Fig. 46-6).

The ascending lumbar veins are paired longitudinal structures that connect the common iliac, iliolumbar, and lumbar veins. They ascend parallel to the IVC, posterior to the psoas major muscles and anterior to the vertebral transverse processes. Superiorly they join the subcostal veins and turn medially to form the azygos vein on the right and the hemiazygos vein on the left. The ascending lumbar veins become important collateral channels between the lower and upper parts of the body in the event of IVC stenosis or occlusion.

The gonadal veins ascend from the pelvis anterior to the psoas major muscle and accompany the gonadal arteries and ureters. The testicular veins originate from the posterior aspect of the testis and unite to form the pampiniform plexus. They follow the spermatic cord, pass through the

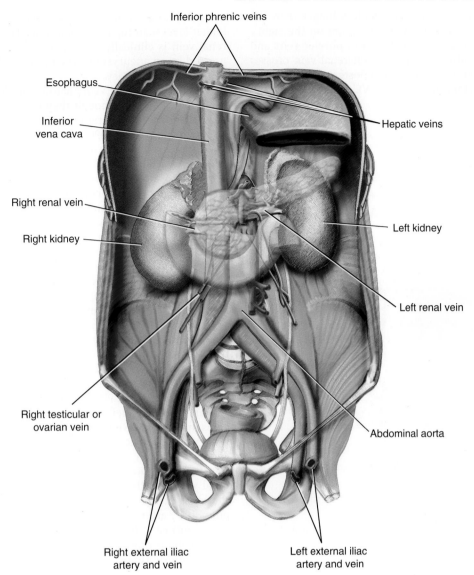

FIGURE 46-5. Inferior vena cava. *(Redrawn from Drake RL, Vogl W, Mitchell AWM. Gray's anatomy for students. Philadelphia: Elsevier/Churchill Livingstone; 2005.)*

inguinal ring, and ascend retroperitoneally to form two or more veins on both sides of the testicular artery. These veins unite to form a single vein, which on the right drains into the IVC at an acute angle just below the right renal vein. On the left side, the testicular vein empties into the left renal vein at a right angle just before the renal vein crosses the aorta. Similarly, two ovarian veins on each side originate from a venous plexus in the broad ligament of the uterus and follow the path of the ovarian artery; they terminate in the same manner as the testicular veins in males.

Variant anatomy includes drainage of the right gonadal vein directly into the right renal vein rather than the IVC, which occurs in less than 10% of individuals. Another more infrequent drainage pattern entails the left gonadal vein emptying directly into the IVC.

Important clinical scenarios involving the gonadal veins are related to their valves and extensive collateral network. The testicular and ovarian veins have several valves, dysfunction or incompetence of which may cause testicular varicoceles or pelvic varices, respectively. Varicoceles are

common and occur in 5% to 17% of males, 10 times more often on the left than on the right. They may be bilateral in less than 10% and are isolated to the right in only 1% to 2%. Varicoceles are associated with pain, infertility, and testicular hypoplasia. Additionally, incompetent ovarian valves may be present in 40% on the left and 35% on the right and result in unimpeded reflux of blood into the pelvis and subsequent distention and engorgement of the ovarian veins. No effective medical treatment exists for either scenario, and management options involve surgical ligation of the gonadal veins or embolization. Multiple small anastomoses between the gonadal veins and other retroperitoneal veins exist along the entire length of the vessels. This must be considered when performing interventions on the gonadal veins, such as embolization for varicoceles because missed collaterals could lead to recurrence.

Multiple renal veins contribute to formation of the left and right renal veins, both of which are anterior to the renal arteries and drain into the IVC (Fig. 46-7). The orifice of a normal left renal vein is anterior, whereas that of the right is posterior. The left renal vein, which is longer than the right and averages 7 cm in length (vs. 3 cm on the right), receives the left gonadal vein, left inferior phrenic vein, and generally the left adrenal vein. The left renal vein crosses the midline anterior to the aorta and posterior to the superior mesenteric artery. It joins the IVC at the level of the second lumbar vertebral body, opposite and at a slightly higher level than the right renal vein. The course of the left renal vein is clinically important because it may be compressed by an aneurysm involving either the aorta or superior mesenteric artery.

Variations in renal vein anatomy are less common than arterial variations, although they may be present in up to 40% of individuals. Persistence of any component of the circumaortic venous plexus formed by the fetal subcardinal and supracardinal veins may result in an anomaly. The most common variant is multiple right renal veins (28%), followed by a circumaortic left renal vein, which has both preaortic and retroaortic components. The retroaortic component may enter the IVC near the level of the normal preaortic vein or as low as the confluence of the left and right iliac veins. More rarely, in 3% of individuals a single left retroaortic renal vein passes posterior to the aorta to reach the IVC.

Clinically relevant scenarios involving the renal veins are related to collateral circulation and tumor invasion. Renal veins commonly anastomose with other retroperitoneal veins such as the lumbar, azygos, and gonadal veins. These connections may become prominent in patients with portal hypertension and enable drainage from the splenic and short gastric veins into the left renal vein. These anastomoses are also important in obstruction; an obstructed right renal vein is drained via lumbar veins and the azygos vein, and an obstructed left renal vein is drained by the lumbar veins, hemiazygos vein, and left gonadal vein. Additionally, renal vein obstruction may be secondary to neoplastic venous extension, which is rare except for renal cell carcinomas. In addition, tumor extension may spread along the renal vein into the IVC and, in rare cases, may grow into the right atrium across the tricuspid valve and into the pulmonary artery.

In contrast to the multiple arteries supplying the adrenal gland, venous drainage is accomplished by a single vein on each side. Multiple adrenal veins may occur, but they are

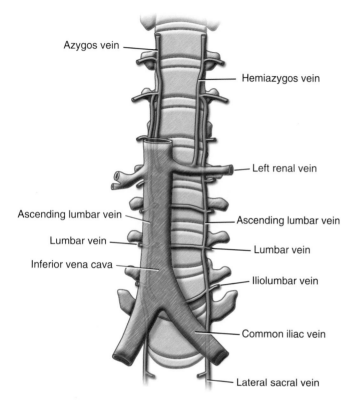

FIGURE 46-6. Lumbar veins. *(Redrawn from Drake RL, Vogl W, Mitchell AWM. Gray's anatomy for students. Philadelphia: Elsevier/Churchill Livingstone; 2005.)*

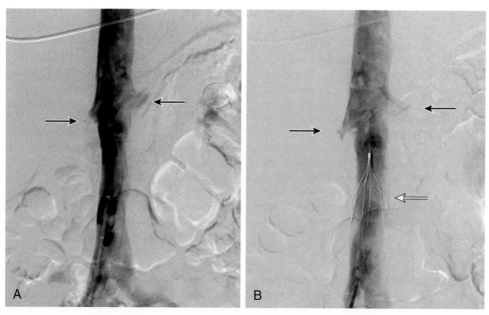

FIGURE 46-7. **A-B,** Conventional venograms of inferior vena cava (IVC). Note location of renal arteries *(black arrows)*, important landmarks for placement of IVC filter *(white arrow)* in **B.**

the exception. The right adrenal vein is short and almost immediately empties into the posterolateral wall of the IVC about 2 to 4 cm above the right renal vein, usually at the level of the 12th rib. The left adrenal vein, after forming a common trunk with the left inferior phrenic vein, passes inferiorly to enter the superior aspect of the left renal vein 3 to 5 cm from the IVC. Both adrenal veins communicate with renal capsular and retroperitoneal veins, which become alternative drainage patterns in the case of adrenal vein obstruction. Variant anatomy of the adrenal veins involves a small accessory hepatic vein draining into the right adrenal vein, or vice versa, and the left adrenal vein draining directly into the IVC.

The inferior phrenic veins follow the course of the inferior phrenic arteries. The right terminates in the IVC above or together with the right hepatic vein, whereas the left, which is often represented by two branches, has one branch ending in the left renal or adrenal vein and the other passing in front of the esophageal hiatus in the diaphragm and draining into the IVC.

The terminal branches of the portal vein and hepatic artery join to perfuse the hepatic sinusoids, which drain into the centrilobular hepatic veins. These veins combine and form the sublobular veins, whose union in the liver parenchyma forms the hepatic veins. The hepatic veins are arranged into upper and lower groups. The *upper group* refers to the right, middle, and left hepatic veins, which exit the posterosuperior surface of the liver and join the hepatic segment of the IVC just before it penetrates the diaphragm approximately 2 cm below the right atrium. The orientation

of the upper group hepatic veins is anterior for the left hepatic vein, anterolateral for the middle hepatic vein, and lateral or posterolateral for the right hepatic vein. In 65% to 85% of individuals, the middle and left hepatic veins form a common trunk before draining into the IVC. The veins of the lower group vary in number, are of small size, and originate from the right and caudate lobes. Inferior right hepatic veins, large-caliber veins from the inferior aspect of the right lobe, may be present in up to 15% of individuals and are usually solitary, but they may be duplicated.

The developmental phase of the IVC is complex and involves paired and segmented structures whose abnormal persistence or regression leads to anomalies of the IVC. The posterior cardinal, supracardinal, and subcardinal veins are three pairs of fetal veins that form the IVC (Fig. 46-8). The *posterior cardinal veins*, which normally involute completely, may give rise to an anomalous retrocaval right ureter if the right posterior cardinal vein persists. The *supracardinal veins* are important in development of the infrarenal IVC and azygos veins. Aberrations in regression of the supracardinal veins give rise to duplication of the infrarenal IVC as a result of persistence of the left supracardinal vein, or a left-sided IVC as a result of regression of the right supracardinal vein. In either case of variant infrarenal IVC anatomy, unless an associated anomaly of the subcardinal veins is present, there is generally a normal suprarenal IVC. In the case of caval duplication, each iliac vein is usually isolated and drains into the ipsilateral IVC. The left side of a duplicated IVC drains into the left renal vein; it crosses the aorta in the expected location to join the

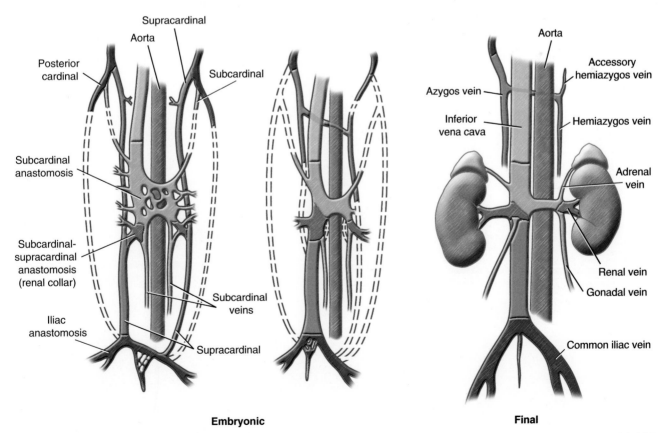

Embryonic

Final

FIGURE 46-8. Development and normal anatomy of inferior vena cava. (*Redrawn from Kadir S. Atlas of normal and variant angiographic anatomy. Philadelphia: Saunders; 1991.*)

right IVC and form a normal single suprarenal IVC. When there is only a single left-sided IVC, both iliac veins drain into the left-sided IVC, which usually crosses the aorta at the level of the left renal vein to form a normally located right-sided suprarenal IVC. The *subcardinal veins* form the intrahepatic IVC and contribute to the renal veins and suprarenal IVC. Regression of the right subcardinal vein results in absence of the intrahepatic segment of the IVC and consequent azygos or hemiazygos continuation of the IVC.

Clinically relevant scenarios involving the IVC are related to thrombosis or occlusion and the extensive collateral network present in such cases. Collateral drainage of the IVC varies with the level of occlusion and involves a superficial or deep venous network. The superficial system includes the epigastric, circumflex iliac, lateral thoracic, thoracoepigastric, internal thoracic, posterior intercostal, external pudendal, and lumbovertebral anastomotic veins. The deep system includes the azygos, hemiazygos, and lumbar veins. The vertebral venous plexus, including the Batson venous plexus, is also included in the collateral venous circuit. Venous drainage of the lower extremities in the case of infrarenal caval obstruction may be accomplished by the ascending lumbar, paraspinal, gonadal, inferior epigastric, and abdominal wall veins. Obstructed or retrograde flow in the internal iliac veins leads to drainage via the gonadal and ureteric veins, as well as the inferior mesenteric vein, through anastomoses with the hemorrhoidal veins. If the occlusion is in the segment between the renal and hepatic veins, drainage may occur through the azygos and hemiazygos veins, as well as through the collateral routes described for infrarenal obstruction.

Obstruction at the level of the suprahepatic IVC results in collateral flow through all of the routes described, except for the inferior mesenteric vein.

KEY POINTS

- Knowledge of variations in classic anatomy involving branches of the abdominal aorta is fundamental for visceral vascular imaging and intervention.
- Extensive anastomoses occur between branches of the abdominal aorta supplying the abdominal viscera and provide collateral blood supply in the event of occlusion or stenosis.
- The inferior vena cava and its tributaries are frequent sites of vascular pathology, and caval involvement may be the first manifestation of diseases involving the organs drained by its tributaries.

▶ **SUGGESTED READINGS**

Drake RL, Vogl W, Mitchell AWM. Gray's anatomy for students. Philadelphia: Elsevier/Churchill Livingstone; 2005. p. 219–362.

Kaufman JA, Lee MJ, editors. Vascular & interventional radiology: the requisites. St Louis: CV Mosby; 2004. p. 246–376.

Uflacker R, editor. With contributions by Feldman CJ. Atlas of vascular anatomy: an angiographic approach. Baltimore: Williams & Wilkins; 1997. p. 405–604, 635–729.

The complete reference list is available online at www.expertconsult.com

CHAPTER 47

Aortic Endografting

Joo-Young Chun, Matthew M. Thompson, and Robert A. Morgan

CLINICAL RELEVANCE

Abdominal aortic aneurysms (AAAs) occur in around 5% to 10% of the male population older than 65 years, and the incidence increases with advancing age. Aortic aneurysms are a significant cause of death in elderly patients. Although the risk of rupture is very low for aneurysms less than 5 cm in diameter, the risk increases substantially with aneurysms larger than 6 cm in diameter and is around 50% per year for aneurysms larger than 8 cm. Mortality rates for traditional open repair of AAAs vary widely, depending on the center. In the United Kingdom, the crude surgical mortality between 2001 and 2005 for elective aneurysm repair was 7.8%. Complication rates of open surgery rise substantially with increasing age and comorbidity.

Endovascular aneurysm repair (EVAR) was initially introduced with the aim of achieving lower mortality and morbidity rates in elderly and unfit patients deemed to be at greater risk for complications from conventional surgery. Since its introduction by Parodi almost 2 decades ago, EVAR has become widely used worldwide and is now the main method used to treat many patients with AAAs, not only the elderly and unfit.[1]

INDICATIONS

Indications for treatment of abdominal aortic aneurysms are:

• *Aneurysm diameter.* Treatment of AAAs is based on the aneurysm reaching a size threshold above which leaving it untreated is more hazardous than treatment. The treatment threshold is based on the perceived annual rupture rate of aneurysms of different diameters. Although rupture rates of small aneurysms are very low, the rate increases to 10% per year once aneurysms reach 6 cm in diameter. The U.K. Small Aneurysm Trial (SAT) and the U.S. Aneurysm Detection and Management (ADAM) study were conducted to discern optimal management of AAAs between 4.0 and 5.5 cm. Both studies concluded that surgery should be performed at a threshold diameter of 5.5 cm, and that surgery for smaller aneurysms provided no survival advantage. It remains controversial whether the 5.5-cm threshold should apply to women, and many interventionalists treat AAAs in women when they reach 5 cm, even less in some centers.[2-4]

• *Symptomatic aneurysms.* Painful or tender AAAs should be treated.

• *Rapidly growing aneurysms.* A diameter increase of 5 mm or greater in 6 months is recognized as an indication for intervention.

Anatomic Inclusion Criteria for Endovascular Aneurysm Repair

Inclusion criteria for EVAR are based mainly on the anatomic features of the aortic neck and iliac arteries because it is imperative that a good seal is achieved at the three attachment points (i.e., the neck and iliac arteries) and that the devices can be passed up the iliac arteries to the aorta.

Neck Inclusion Criteria
Neck Diameter
In general, the maximum aortic neck diameter for conventional EVAR is 33 mm.

Neck Length
The standard required length of aortic neck required for EVAR is 15 mm from the lowest renal artery to the start of the aneurysm. Many operators accept necks shorter than 15 mm for EVAR, but the potential for a proximal leak increases with decreasing neck length. The success of EVAR in shorter necks depends on several factors, such as neck angulation, suprarenal versus infrarenal fixation, and the presence of hooks or barbs on the devices.

Neck Angulation
Increasing angulation reduces the success of fixation and attainment of an adequate seal. The accepted threshold of angulation is 60 degrees. Adequate seal and fixation in angulated necks are also dependent on neck length: the longer the neck, the better the chance of a good seal despite neck angulation. Moreover, EVAR is often successful in necks angulated by more than 60 degrees if neck length is longer than 15 mm.

Neck Conicity
Aortic necks that increase in diameter inferiorly (conical necks) decrease the potential for adequate fixation and seal after EVAR. There is little agreement on the degree of conicity that should be accepted, although in practice this also depends on neck length.

Mural Thrombus and Calcification
In general, increasing amounts of mural thrombus or calcification increases the potential for a proximal leak. Circumferential thrombus or calcification is regarded by many as a contraindication to EVAR for this reason.

Iliac Artery Inclusion Criteria
Diameter and Length
Similar to the neck, the maximum iliac diameter that can act as a distal landing zone for EVAR depends on the maximum device diameter. In practice, this is currently

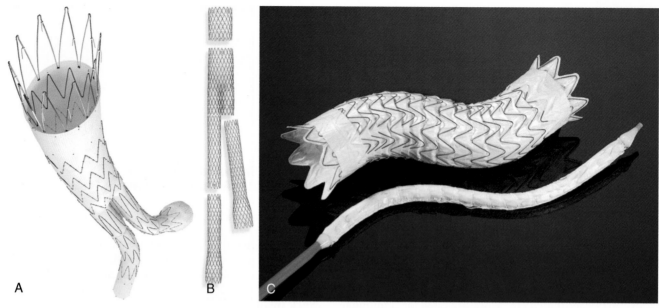

FIGURE 47-1. A, Bifurcated Zenith endograft. **B,** Bifurcated AneuRx endograft. **C,** Excluder endograft constrained in its delivery sheath. (**A** courtesy Cook Inc., **B** courtesy Medtronic Inc., **C** courtesy Gore Medical Inc.)

25 mm (Endurant device maximum limb diameter = 28 mm [Medtronic Inc., Santa Rosa, Calif.]). The iliac arteries must also be of adequate caliber to accept passage of the endo-graft. Device companies are constantly trying to reduce the caliber of their device delivery systems. Currently, 6 to 7 mm is accepted as the minimum iliac artery diameter for passage of most endograft delivery catheters. Finally, the common iliac arteries must be long enough to provide an adequate landing zone to provide a good seal (at least 3 cm long).

Tortuosity and Calcification
It may not be possible to pass the delivery catheter up exces-sively tortuous iliac arteries. However, many noncalcified tortuous iliac arteries can be straightened out by very stiff guidewires, but this is seldom possible if the iliac arteries are heavily calcified.

CONTRAINDICATIONS

There are few absolute contraindications to EVAR; most contraindications are relative:
  • Adverse proximal neck morphology
  • Adverse iliac artery morphology
  • Allergy to radiographic contrast medium, which can be circumvented by the use of alternative contrast agents such as carbon dioxide

EQUIPMENT

Endografts

Currently available devices are constantly undergoing mod-ifications, and new iterations are released on a regular basis. Moreover, new endograft designs are developed by manu-facturers all the time, with the result that the range of endo-grafts changes on an almost annual basis. Most companies manufacture bifurcated and aortouniiliac devices.

The most commonly used devices at this time are the Zenith endograft (Cook Medical, Bloomington, Ind.) (Fig. 47-1, *A*), Endurant endograft (Medtronic), AneuRx Endo-graft (Medtronic) (Fig. 47-1, *B*), Excluder endograft (W.L. Gore & Associates, Flagstaff, Ariz.) (Fig. 47-1, *C*). Other devices include the Aorfix endograft (Lombard Medical, Didcot, UK), Endologix Powerlink endograft (Edwards Life Sciences, Irvine, Calif.), and Anaconda endograft (Terumo Medical Corp., Somerset, N.J.).

Equipment Required for Implantation

The following items are routinely used for implantation of these devices:
  • Single-piece arterial puncture needles
  • Vascular sheaths—6F to 18F, depending on the endo-graft selected
  • Guidewires—standard, hydrophilic, and ultrastiff guide-wires in 180 cm and 260 cm lengths
  • Catheters—aortic flush and selective catheters
  • Balloons—large-caliber balloon catheters to dilate or mold the devices to the aortic neck or iliac arteries (e.g., Coda balloon [Cook Medical])

TECHNIQUE

Anatomy and Approach

Imaging
All patients require comprehensive imaging of the aorta and iliac arteries to assess their suitability for EVAR. The main-stay of imaging is computed tomography (CT), which pro-vides optimal information on the lumen and wall of the aortoiliac segment. Magnetic resonance imaging (MRI) is used preferentially by some centers and is useful in patients who are allergic to iodinated contrast material. Images should be assessed in the axial plane and also via multiplanar reconstruction using maximum intensity projection images.[5]

Device Selection

In most institutions, selection of a particular device is often decided by the personal preference of the operator. The majority of endografts are suitable for most anatomic variations in aneurysm morphology. In general, when selecting a particular device, the endograft should be oversized by 10% to 20% with respect to the diameter of the native vessel from outer wall to outer wall.

If possible, bifurcated endografts should be used, but some patients are unsuitable for bifurcated devices and should be treated with aortouniiliac (AUI) devices. The main indications for the use of AUI devices are:

1. Presence of severely diseased or occluded iliac arteries on one side, with a relatively normal contralateral iliac artery
2. Narrow distal aorta between the aneurysm and the aortic bifurcation in which space is insufficient to accept two limbs of the device

Technical Aspects

Procedure for Device Insertion (Bifurcated Devices)
(Fig. 47-2)

- The procedure may be performed in the angiography suite or operating room. The most important aspect is the quality of the imaging equipment, which outweighs potential benefits in terms of sterility provided by operating rooms.
- The best results of EVAR are achieved by using a team approach consisting of interventional radiologists and vascular surgeons. Each team member contributes different complementary skills to the procedure, enabling even the most difficult problems to be overcome.
- Most procedures are performed under general anesthesia, although regional and local anesthesia are options.
- Access to the arterial system is usually achieved by bilateral femoral arteriotomies. However, percutaneous closure devices are now available for closure of large-caliber access site punctures, and many interventionalists now use these in preference to conventional femoral arteriotomies in suitable patients.
- In most cases, the main body is inserted via the right femoral artery, and the contralateral limb is passed up the left femoral artery. Operators may decide to pass the main body up the left side if the right side is severely diseased and unsuitable for passage of the large-caliber main body delivery system.
- The left femoral artery is punctured, and a 6F sheath is inserted. Via this access, a standard aortic flush catheter is advanced into the abdominal aorta and placed with the catheter tip at the level of L1.
- The right femoral artery is catheterized, and a selective catheter (e.g., Cobra) and a standard guidewire are advanced into the upper thoracic aorta. The standard guidewire is exchanged for an exchange-length very stiff guidewire (e.g., Lunderquist [Cook Medical]), and the catheter is removed.
- The main body is advanced over the Lunderquist guidewire to the level of L1 (to the approximate level of the renal arteries). A flush aortogram is performed with a small amount of contrast medium (e.g., 7-10 mL injected at 10 mL/s). The aim of aortography is to locate the origins of the renal arteries. The CT scan should be scrutinized to assess whether any angulation of the intensifier is required (in either the oblique or craniocaudal projection) to profile the origins of the renal arteries. In general, adequate opacification of the aorta and renal arteries can be achieved with these small amounts of contrast medium. Many patients have impaired renal function, so efforts should be made to limit the amount of contrast medium. Carbon dioxide is a very effective contrast medium for aortography and can be used in lieu of iodinated contrast for all or many parts of the procedure.
- The top of the main body is deployed so that the graft material is positioned immediately below the renal arteries. After deployment of the main body, repeat aortography may be performed to confirm the correct location of the endograft and continued patency of the renal arteries.
- The next step is catheterization of the contralateral limb. The pigtail catheter (which is outside the graft) is withdrawn over a guidewire into the lower aorta and exchanged for an angled-tip catheter such as a Cobra, Vanshee (Cook Medical), or Berenstein (Cordis Corp., Warren, N.J.) catheter. With the aid of an angled-tip hydrophilic guidewire and/or oblique angulation of the image intensifier, the operator cannulates the opening in the main body for the contralateral limb. This step may be straightforward or extremely difficult. Factors that cause difficulty in cannulation include a large aneurysm with little mural thrombus, tortuous iliac arteries, and angulation of the aneurysm in the anteroposterior plane.
- In some cases, retrograde cannulation of the contralateral limb opening may not be possible. The contralateral limb opening can be cannulated antegradely by snaring a wire passed through the opening from the ipsilateral side.
- The contralateral limb is inserted so that the top of the limb overlaps the markers in the contralateral limb opening on the main body. The aim is to deploy the limb so that it lands just proximal to the common iliac bifurcation. If the graft is a type that has limb sections bilaterally (e.g., Zenith), the ipsilateral limb is inserted after the contralateral limb. Limb extensions may be placed if there is a large distance between the lower end of a limb and the common iliac bifurcation.
- If patients have aneurysmal common iliac arteries that cannot provide a sealing zone for the endograft limbs, it is necessary to extend the limbs into the external iliac arteries. Embolization of the internal iliac artery (IIA) is required before this maneuver to prevent retrograde leaks up the IIA after the procedure. Alternatively, branched iliac endografts are now available and may be used in preference to IIA embolization.
- All attachment sites and connections are dilated with large-caliber compliant balloons.
- Finally, completion angiography is performed to assess patency of the endograft, iliac arteries, and renal arteries and absence of a leak into the aneurysm sac.
- It is important to perform completion angiography with all stiff guidewires removed because kinks or stenoses of the limbs may be concealed if the limbs are straightened out by the presence of stiff guidewires. The usual technique is to place a flush catheter up one iliac limb of the device, and leave a catheter or balloon up the other limb so that access to the endograft is maintained from each

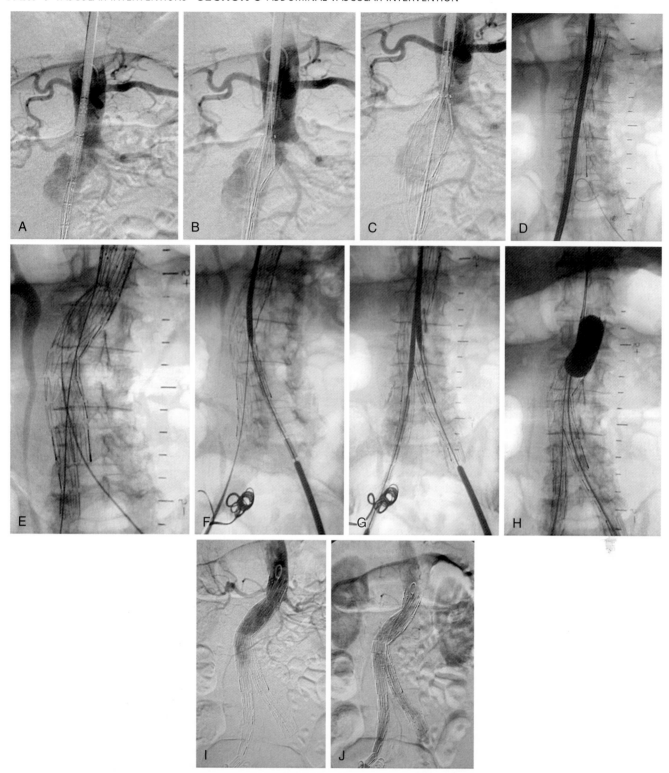

FIGURE 47-2. Insertion of a Zenith bifurcated endograft. **A,** Delivery catheter is advanced to level of renal arteries. **B-E,** Angiography is performed to define renal arteries, and main body of endograft is deployed. **F-H,** After deployment of main body, contralateral limb is cannulated, followed by insertion of limbs of endografts into both iliac arteries. **I-J,** Completion angiography confirms a patent endograft, patent renal arteries, and no visible endoleak.

side of the groin to manage any problems revealed by angiography.
• If type 1 or type 3 endoleaks are visible on completion angiography, they should be treated immediately (see later discussion).

• If completion angiography suggests a kink in one of the endograft limbs as it passes around a curve in the iliac artery, or angulation of the tip of the limb with respect to its attachment to the native iliac artery, the kink or the angulated end of the graft should be supported

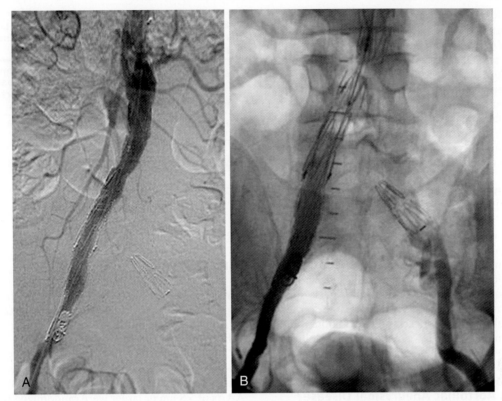

FIGURE 47-3. Aortouniiliac graft has been placed in right common iliac artery, and occluder has been placed in left common iliac artery.

by the insertion of a suitable uncovered self-expanding stent.

Insertion of Aortouniiliac Devices (Fig. 47-3)
- Most but not all AUI devices are two-piece devices with an upper body and a lower limb that are designed to be placed just above the ipsilateral common iliac bifurcation. An occluder or vascular plug is placed in the contralateral common iliac artery to prevent an endoleak from occurring as a result of retrograde flow up the common iliac artery.
- The first part of the procedure is exactly the same as for bifurcated devices until the proximal component of the device has been deployed.
- The distal component is inserted and deployed. The site of the ipsilateral common iliac artery bifurcation is defined by angiography via the pigtail catheter that is left in situ after deployment of the proximal endograft.
- The pigtail catheter is withdrawn over a guidewire, and a Lunderquist guidewire is passed up the contralateral femoral access so that the tip is placed in the aneurysm sac. The sheath containing the occluder is advanced up the contralateral iliac artery, and the occluder is extruded so that it is deployed in the proximal common iliac artery.

CONTROVERSIES

In an evolving treatment such as EVAR, controversies are inevitable. Major controversies include the following.

Who Should Be Treated by Endovascular Repair?

This question remains unanswered despite the increasing amount of data available. The pragmatic view is that EVAR offers lower early and midterm aneurysm-related mortality in the majority of patients compared to open surgery, although the benefit of EVAR over open surgery in young patients, elderly patients, and patients with severe cardiorespiratory comorbidity is not supported at this time by level 1 data.

Should Patients with Aneurysms Smaller Than 5.5 cm Be Treated?

Although the standard threshold for intervention in AAAs is 5.5 cm, some clinicians think that patients with smaller aneurysms should also be treated. Smaller aneurysms with longer necks and less aortic and iliac angulation tend to be morphologically favorable for EVAR. There is some evidence that EVAR for smaller aneurysms is less problematic and associated with improved early outcomes when compared with EVAR for larger aneurysms, thus supporting early reintervention in patients with smaller AAAs.

Two prospective randomized trials for the evaluation of EVAR for small AAAs have recently reported their findings. The PIVOTAL trial (Positive Impact of Endovascular Options for Treating Aneurysms Early) is a U.S. multicenter trial in which 728 patients with 4.0- to 5.4-cm AAAs were assigned to either ultrasound (US) surveillance or early EVAR with the AneuRx endograft.[6] Of the 366 patients assigned to surveillance, 112 patients underwent aneurysm repair during follow-up. The majority of these were due to increase in aneurysm size and aneurysm-related symptoms. After a mean follow-up of 20 months, the overall mortality and aneurysm-related mortality were similar in the two groups. The authors concluded that both rigorous surveillance and early EVAR were safe approaches in the management of small aneurysms.

The CAESAR trial (Comparison of Surveillance versus Aortic Endografting for Small Aneurysm Repair) trial compared early EVAR of small aneurysms with the Zenith endograft with surveillance in 360 patients.[7] At the end of 54 months follow-up, all-cause mortality and aneurysm-related mortality and major adverse events did not differ between the two groups. However, the authors noted that one sixth of small aneurysms under surveillance may lose feasibility for EVAR during this period owing to changes in aneurysm morphology, mainly related to unfavorable proximal aortic neck anatomy.

Should the Anatomic Inclusion Criteria Be Widened?

There is limited evidence that the standard anatomic inclusion criteria regarding neck length (15 mm or greater), neck diameter (33 mm or under), neck angulation (<60 degrees), and minimal neck thrombus might be too rigid, with successful EVAR being possible in patients with neck dimensions outside these parameters. Further data are required before anecdotal reports of successful conventional EVAR in more challenging anatomy can be translated into an alteration of the accepted anatomic inclusion criteria.

Is Internal Iliac Artery Embolization Safe in Patients with Aortoiliac Aneurysmal Disease?

There is continuing debate regarding the safety of IIA embolization if patients have aneurysmal common iliac arteries, because of concerns of pelvic ischemia, especially after bilateral embolization. Branched iliac endografts are relatively novel iliac extension limbs with a side branch for implantation into the IIA. They have the advantage of preserving flow into the IIA but the drawback of adding substantial cost and complexity to the overall procedure. Deployment of iliac branched devices (IBDs) is technically challenging and is reflected by prolonged operating times of up to 390 minutes and relatively low technical success rates.[8] Their patency rates are currently under evaluation, and only short and midterm patency rates are available at present. Of these, a recent systematic analysis reported a 12% occlusion rate, and a further study reported an intraoperative branch occlusion rate of 25%.[9] In addition, there is a significant cost implication when using these devices, because they remain expensive.

We have recently reviewed our data on unilateral and bilateral IIA embolization prior to EVAR. In a series of 88 patients, 65 underwent unilateral and 23 underwent bilateral IIA embolization. The procedure was technically successful in 96%, and there were no cases of severe pelvic ischemic symptoms such as buttock necrosis, colonic ischemia, or paraplegia (unpublished data). Therefore, IIA embolization may be a low-morbidity procedure after all, with the implication that the use of branched grafts may be unnecessary.

OUTCOMES AND COMPLICATIONS

Since the introduction of EVAR, a large body of literature has accumulated worldwide.[10-29] A number of randomized controlled trials (RCTs) comparing EVAR and open repair

TABLE 47-1. Thirty-Day Outcomes of Three Large Randomized Controlled Trials Comparing Endovascular Repair with Open Repair

Study	Number	Endovascular Repair Mortality (%)	Open Repair Mortality (%)	P Value
EVAR-1[30]	1082	1.7	4.7	0.009
DREAM[19]	345	1.2	4.6	0.1
OVER[33]	881	0.5	3	0.004

have been published, including the EVAR-1,[18,30,31] DREAM,[19,32] and OVER[33] trials.

Early Outcomes

Early results of these trials were consistent in demonstrating a significantly lower 30-day mortality following EVAR than open surgery. These outcomes are outlined in Table 47-1.

The EVAR-1 trial was a U.K.-based study that compared the mortality, durability, and cost-effectiveness of EVAR with open surgical repair. A total of 1082 patients with AAAs of 5.5 cm or larger were randomized to endovascular or open repair. The 30-day mortality for the EVAR group was 1.7%, versus 4.7% in the group undergoing open repair ($P = 0.009$). At follow-up 4 years after randomization, this advantage for EVAR was maintained with respect to aneurysm-related deaths (4% in the EVAR group vs. 7% in the open surgery group), but the all-cause mortality was similar in both groups—around 28%. In addition, postoperative complications and reinterventions were more frequent in the endovascular than the open repair group—41% of EVAR patients versus 9% of open repair patients ($P <0.0001$), and 20% of EVAR patients versus 6% of open repair patients ($P <0.0001$), respectively. There was no significant difference in quality of life between the two groups. The cost analysis of both treatment arms revealed higher costs for the EVAR group (£13,257 vs. £9946 for the open repair group).

In the DREAM trial (Dutch Randomized Endovascular Aneurysm Management Trial), 351 patients with AAAs 5 cm or greater were randomized to either endovascular or open repair. Similar to the EVAR-1 trial, the 30-day mortality after EVAR was lower by a factor of 3 than after open repair (1.2% for EVAR vs. 4.6% for open repair), although this difference did not reach statistical significance ($P = 0.1$).[19] Two years after randomization, the early advantage seen after EVAR was lost. At 2 years, the cumulative survival of both groups was equivalent at around 90%. However, also similar to EVAR-1, the incidence of aneurysm-related deaths was lower at 2 years in the EVAR group (2.1% vs. 5.7%; $P = 0.05$). The intervention and complication rates were also higher after EVAR than in the open surgery group. In the first 9 months after aneurysm repair, reintervention rates for EVAR were about three times the rate for surgery. After 9 months, the reintervention rates were roughly similar in the two arms of the trial. Complications occurred in 19.4% of patients in the EVAR group versus 16.9% in the open surgery group, and reinterventions were performed in

14% of EVAR patients versus 5% of those undergoing open repair ($P = 0.03$).

Therefore, both trials reported a threefold reduction in 30-day mortality for EVAR as compared with open repair, which was maintained in terms of aneurysm-related mortality at follow-up. Unfortunately, there was no survival advantage for EVAR in terms of all-cause mortality in either trial at follow-up.

In addition to the RCT data, several prospective registries have contributed a large amount of data that have greatly improved our understanding of the outcomes of EVAR. The EUROSTAR (European Collaborators on Stent-Graft Techniques for Abdominal Aortic Aneurysm Repair) registry is the largest of its kind. It was established in 1996, not long after arrival of the first commercial devices, and contains data on 8345 patients from 177 vascular centers across Europe. The early data involving the first generation devices with their design flaws were removed from the database in 2003, so current data only reflect the endografts in use at present. EUROSTAR analyses have reported a 30-day mortality rate of 2.4% for all patients.[11] Nonfatal systemic complications (mainly pulmonary and renal) occurred in 11% of patients. The rate of conversion from endovascular to open repair was negligible at 0.9%. Early device-related complications such as graft thrombosis and graft migration occurred in 2.6%, and access site complications developed in 6% of procedures. Deterioration in renal function as a result of endograft coverage of the renal artery, thrombotic renal artery occlusion, or distal embolization of the renal artery branches occurred in about 2% of cases.[11]

Late Outcomes

Long-term results of up to 10 years follow-up after EVAR and open repair were published by the EVAR-1 trial collaborators in 2010.[31] This paper confirmed earlier reports that although the EVAR group showed an early benefit with respect to aneurysm-related mortality, the benefit was lost by the end of the study ($P = 0.73$). By the end of follow-up, there was no significant difference between endovascular and open repair with respect to all-cause mortality ($P = 0.72$). In addition, the trial also reported increased rates of graft-related complications in the EVAR group ($P <0.001$), resulting in a higher rate of reinterventions ($P <0.001$) following EVAR. This reflects the increased overall costs in the EVAR group, which has been found to be £3019 more expensive than open repair at 8 years of follow-up.

The DREAM trial has also recently reported long-term follow-up data.[32] Six years after randomization, there was no significant difference in the rate of overall survival between EVAR and open repair ($P = 0.97$). In addition, EVAR was associated with a significantly greater rate of reintervention than open repair ($P = 0.03$). The majority of reinterventions occurred more than 4 years after EVAR and were performed for endograft migration, limb thrombosis, and endoleak (types 1 and 2).

The OVER (Open Versus Endovascular Repair) trial reported midterm outcomes at 2 years that showed the early postoperative benefit of EVAR was not sustained beyond 2 years. All-cause mortality was 7% in the EVAR group and 9.8% in the open repair group ($P = 0.13$), whereas aneurysm-related mortality was 1.4 versus 3%, respectively

TABLE 47-2. Mid- to Long-Term Outcomes of Randomized Controlled Trials Comparing Endovascular Repair to Open Repair

Study	Follow-Up (Years)	Endovascular Repair	Open Repair	P Value
OVER[33]	2	All-cause mortality		
		7	9.8	0.13
		Aneurysm-related mortality		
		1.4	3	0.1
EVAR-1[18]	4	All-cause mortality		
		26	29	0.46
		Aneurysm-related mortality		
		4	7	0.04
		Postoperative complications		
		41	9	0.0001
EVAR-1[31]	10	Total survival		
		54	54	0.72
		Aneurysm-related survival		
		93	93	0.73
		Survival without complications		
		48	85	0.001
		Survival without reintervention		
		72	90	0.001
DREAM[32]	6	Total survival		
		68.9	69.9	0.97
		Survival without reintervention		
		70.4	81.9	0.03

($P = 0.1$).[33] Results of the three RCTs are summarized in Table 47-2.

The EUROSTAR registry collaborators have recently presented 8-year follow-up data.[34] Mortality at the end of follow-up was 9.5%. Major adverse events were reported in 11.1% of patients, and aneurysm rupture was reported in 0.5%. Device migration was seen in 1.8% and reinterventions were required in 19.2%.

Despite repair of the AAA, late rupture of aneurysms still leads to death in a small proportion of patients. However, it is generally difficult to separate death secondary to late rupture from death secondary to other causes in this group of patients with a high degree of cardiorespiratory and renal comorbidity. The best data regarding late mortality are provided by the EUROSTAR registry. A subanalysis evaluated the effect of aneurysm size on delayed outcomes and divided patients into groups with small aneurysms (4-5.4 cm), medium aneurysms (5.5-6.4 cm), and large aneurysms (6.5 cm or larger). Rates of freedom from aneurysm-related death at 4 years were 97%, 95%, and 88% for the small, medium, and large groups, respectively. Cumulative freedom from rupture rates at 4 years were 98.3%, 98.3%, and 90.5%, respectively.[35] Therefore, these results indicate a correlation between the largest aneurysms and late mortality, similar to the correlation between increasing aneurysm size and death before treatment. In a systematic review, the National Institute of Clinical Excellence found an overall mortality rate of 3% for aneurysm-related deaths, whereas the pooled all-cause mortality in patients after EVAR was 15.1% from a follow-up of 7 to 48 months.[36]

The EUROSTAR registry has also provided invaluable information on the mid- to long-term outcomes of the endografts themselves. Multivariate analysis of the data has shown that only type 3 endoleaks and endograft migration are clinically important factors in the cause of late aneurysm rupture. Type 3 leaks and migration are associated with 6- and 7.5-fold increases in the risk for late rupture. The absence of a type 1 endoleak as a risk factor for late rupture may be due to the fact that migration inevitably leads to a type 1 leak immediately before rupture occurs. The significance of migration for late rupture is the impetus for the necessity to perform plain radiographs of the endografts at annual intervals so that migration can be diagnosed early before it leads to rupture. Migration is related to infrarenal fixation and deployment of endografts in short or angulated necks (or both).

Limb occlusion secondary to kinking of the endograft limb, angulation of the limb as it joins the native iliac artery, or the presence of neointimal hyperplasia occurs in 2% to 4% of patients on an annual basis. Threatened limb occlusion can be diagnosed by duplex US evaluation of the limb and iliac artery. Many clinicians perform duplex US evaluation as part of their routine follow-up protocol for this reason. Increased velocity measurements suggesting a significant lesion are an indication for early admission for angiography, with a view to insertion of supporting uncovered stents across the lesion.

Overview of Evidence

The major RCTs reported a significant reduction in 30-day mortality for EVAR as compared with open repair, which was maintained in terms of aneurysm-related mortality at early follow-up, but there was no survival advantage for EVAR in terms of all-cause mortality. Long-term follow-up data show that the early benefit with respect to aneurysm-related mortality is lost. This fact, together with the increased complication and reintervention rates and higher cost of EVAR, prompted critics of EVAR to conclude that it offers no real advantage over open repair in medically fit patients with AAAs.

However, the reduction in aneurysm-related mortality after EVAR is a real benefit, and most patients given the choice between surgery and EVAR would probably opt for EVAR on the basis of the reduced mortality alone. The EVAR-1 and DREAM trials had methodological flaws. One of the main limitations was that a mature procedure (i.e., open surgery perfected over a period of at least 60 years) was being compared with a new, still evolving technique performed by operators with limited experience and using a variety of devices that were still undergoing modification. Therefore, the EVAR results were a summation of the experience of several old and new designs of endografts. There have since been significant developments in commercially available endovascular devices, and several older-generation endografts that were included in the early trial and registry data are now obsolete. Currently available endografts now incorporate suprarenal barb fixation, precision deployment mechanisms, low-profile delivery systems that can be placed percutaneously, and flexible but robust construction for durability.

Another flaw relates to the interpretation of complications and reintervention. In general, complications in the EVAR group are vascular specific and are easier to identify and record. On the other hand, open repair complications such as abdominal hernia and adhesional bowel obstruction are less vascular specific and more likely to result in readmission under another surgical specialty, resulting in underreporting. Furthermore, the practice of reintervention for type 2 endoleaks has changed substantially since the trials began, with most patients who have type 2 leaks now being managed conservatively unless there is evidence of aneurysmal sac enlargement. In view of this, it is arguable whether type 2 leaks should be regarded as a complication unless they are associated with enlarging sac size. In EVAR-1, type 2 leaks contributed to 79 (42%) of the 186 complications, and they almost doubled the overall complication rate of 41%. Similarly, 17 patients who underwent reintervention for type 2 leaks in the EVAR-1 trial may not have undergone reintervention at the current time. Therefore, the reintervention and complication rates of the EVAR group would have been substantially reduced if the significance of type 2 leaks reflected current practice.

The final limitation relates to calculation of the cost of EVAR, which included three CT scans in the first postoperative year, followed by annual surveillance CTs. However, current practice in many units now recommends primary imaging follow-up by duplex US, which reduces exposure to ionizing radiation and reduces overall costs. Surveillance imaging is discussed in more detail later under "Postprocedural and Follow-Up Care."

Endovascular Repair in Unfit Patients

The EVAR-2 trial randomized patients with AAAs of 5.5 cm or larger who were unfit for open repair to EVAR plus best medical therapy or to best medical therapy alone; 338 patients were randomized to either EVAR (n = 166) or conservative (n = 172) management. The 30-day mortality for patients in the EVAR group was 9%. Overall mortality at 4 years was 64%. There was no significant difference in all-cause mortality between the two groups, nor was there a difference in aneurysm-related mortality between the two groups. However, there are several contentious issues concerning interpretation of the data. As a result, many interventionalists now consider the EVAR-2 trial data to be flawed and poorly applicable to current practice. At this time, there are no new conclusive data to guide us on the role of EVAR in patients who are unfit for surgery. Nevertheless, it is true to say that most interventionalists treat patients on an individual basis, and many patients unfit for open repair undergo EVAR worldwide, despite the results of the EVAR-2 trial.

Endoleaks and Management

Endoleaks are defined as leakage of blood into the aneurysmal sac outside the endograft but not leakage outside the vascular compartment. Endoleaks are classified into five types:

- Type 1—attachment site endoleaks that occur at the neck or in the iliac arteries
- Type 2—retrograde leaks into the sac from collateral pathways, such as the inferior mesenteric artery or lumbar arteries
- Type 3—leaks that occur at connections or through tears in the graft fabric

• Type 4—graft porosity

• Type 5—increasing sac size without a definable leak

There is evidence from the EUROSTAR and RETA registries that type 1 and type 3 leaks are independent risk factors for postprocedural aneurysm rupture and late aneurysm-related death, but there is no evidence that type 2 leaks are similarly problematic. The incidence of type 1, 2, and 3 leaks on completion angiography is 4%, 10%, and 2%, respectively.

Any type 1 or type 3 leak present on the completion angiogram should be treated immediately. If type 1 and 3 endoleaks are discovered on follow-up imaging, patients should be admitted for reintervention as soon as possible.[11,13,36-39]

Proximal type 1 endoleaks are due to leakage of blood between the wall of the neck and the outside of the graft. This is generally due to either inadequate coverage of the neck by the device, with persistent room between the upper end of the graft material and the renal arteries, or a suboptimal seal due to a short neck, neck angulation, neck thrombus, or calcification. Inadequate coverage of the neck should be treated by insertion of a cuff to extend the proximal graft coverage to the renal arteries. All manufacturers provide cuffs in a range of sizes to accompany their main body devices. It is sensible to either hold a stock of aortic cuffs for use when required, or to routinely order a cuff for every EVAR procedure.

If graft coverage of the neck is adequate and the endoleak is thought to be due to a poor seal, repeat balloon dilation of the neck should be performed. A persistent proximal type 1 endoleak should be treated by insertion of a giant Palmaz stent inside the endograft in the neck of the aneurysm. If a proximal leak persists despite these measures, interventions such as banding of the neck or embolization of the endoleak with coils or liquid embolic agents may be successful.

Endoleaks at distal attachment sites are also due to inadequate coverage or a poor seal. Similar to aortic cuffs, it is sensible to either stock a range of limb extensions or routinely order suitable iliac extensions for each case. Coverage of the endograft should extend to the common iliac bifurcation, and if this is not the case, limb extensions should be inserted to achieve this goal. Extension of graft coverage with repeat balloon dilation of the limb is successful in treating most distal type 1 leaks. If a distal type 1 endoleak persists despite these measures, it is usually because the common iliac artery is too wide to enable a good seal for the endograft limb. In this situation, the only recourse is to extend the graft coverage to the external iliac artery. Embolization of the ipsilateral IIA is usually performed to prevent a type 2 endoleak caused by retrograde flow from this vessel, although there is no clear evidence that this latter maneuver is necessary.

Type 3 connection endoleaks usually respond to repeat balloon dilation. If they persist despite repeat dilation, an additional endograft should be placed across the connection, although in practice this is seldom necessary. Type 3 endoleaks secondary to tears in the graft fabric are, in general, challenging to diagnose and require treatment by additional endografts.

If a type 2 leak is present, no immediate intervention is necessary. More than 50% of type 2 endoleaks resolve spontaneously over a period of 3 years. Patients should be evaluated routinely, and intervention undertaken only if there is evidence of an increase in size of the aneurysm sac. Treatment of type 2 endoleaks involves embolization of the feeding vessels, either by a transarterial or direct sac puncture route.[40-42]

Endoleaks and their management are discussed more fully in Chapter 50.

POSTPROCEDURAL AND FOLLOW-UP CARE

Most patients are discharged from the hospital a few days after the procedure. During the early days of the technique, most patients would spend a day or so in the intensive care unit, but with increasing experience, it became clear that this was unnecessary unless patients had severe comorbidity. At present, postprocedural care for the majority of patients involves early ambulation and discharge 3 to 7 days after EVAR.

All patients require imaging after EVAR to monitor the integrity of the endograft, patency of the iliac arteries, absence of any endoleaks, and shrinkage or otherwise of the aneurysm sac. The standard imaging protocol after EVAR has involved regular contrast-enhanced CT scans. A typical program includes a CT scan either before discharge or at 6 weeks, and further CT scans at 6 and 12 months and annually thereafter. However, CT follow-up is expensive for hospitals and involves a high cumulative radiation dose for patients. As a result, in recent years many hospitals have moved to a follow-up protocol of US at a similar time interval to the CT protocol described, and annual plain abdominal radiography.[43-46]

> ### KEY POINTS

- The risk of rupture of aortic aneurysms is very low for aneurysms less than 5 cm and increases to around 50% for aneurysms larger than 8 cm.

- Indications for intervention are aneurysm size exceeding 5.5 cm according to body habitus, aneurysm size increasing by 5 mm or more, and a tender aneurysm.

- Standard anatomic inclusion criteria for infrarenal endovascular repair are a neck length of 15 mm or longer, neck diameter of 33 mm or less, neck angulation of 60 degrees or less, minimal neck thrombus, iliac arteries larger than 7 mm, and lack of excessive iliac artery tortuosity and heavy calcification.

- Type 1 or type 3 endoleaks visualized on completion angiography should be treated immediately.

- Type 3 endoleaks and migration are the most important factors in late endograft failure.

- Patients should be monitored indefinitely with a standard imaging and clinical protocol, which may involve computed tomography or ultrasound and plain abdominal radiography.

▶ **SUGGESTED READINGS**

Beebe HG, Kritpracha B. Imaging of abdominal aortic aneurysm: current status. Ann Vasc Surg 2003;17:111–8.

Brewster DC, Cronenwett JL, Hallett JW, et al. Guidelines for the treatment of abdominal aortic aneurysms. J Vasc Surg 2003;37:1106–17.

Drurry D. A systematic review of the recent evidence for the safety and efficacy of elective endovascular repair in the management of infrarenal aortic aneurysms. National Institute for Clinical Excellence. E-publication.

Fowkes F, Greenhalgh RM, Mannick JA, editors. The cause and management of aneurysms. London: WB Saunders; 1990. p. 19–28.

Hellinger JC. Endovascular repair of thoracic and abdominal aortic aneurysms: pre- and postprocedural imaging. Tech Vasc Interv Radiol 2005;8:2–15.

Katzen BT, MacLean AA. Complications of endovascular repair of abdominal aortic aneurysms: a review. Cardiovasc Intervent Radiol 2006;29: 935–46.

Rose J. Stent grafts for unruptured abdominal aortic aneurysms: current status. Cardiovasc Intervent Radiol 2006;29:332–43.

White GH, Yu W, May J, et al. Endoleak as a complication of endoluminal grafting of abdominal aortic aneurysms: classification, incidence. diagnosis and management. J Endovasc Surg 1997;4:152–68.

The complete reference list is available online at www.expertconsult.com.

CHAPTER 48
Fenestrated Stent-Grafting of Juxtarenal Aortic Aneurysms
Mohamad Hamady

INTRODUCTION

Continuous developments in endovascular treatment of abdominal and thoracic aortic aneurysm, together with growing experience and encouraging results, have paved the way for emergence of a new generation of stent-grafts that allow extension of the proximal landing zone and preservation of renal and visceral arteries.

Since the first report of fenestrated endovascular repair of aortic aneurysms (FEVAR) by Park et al. in 1996,[1] several large published series and multicenter studies have demonstrated high technical success and promising short- and midterm results. But FEVAR also represents unique challenges to the endovascular interventionalist. These include appropriate patient selection, accurate endograft planning, and demanding technical skills.

INDICATIONS AND ANATOMIC SUITABILITY

Clinical indications for FEVAR include aneurysm diameter of 5.5 cm or more, rapidly enlarging aneurysm at a rate of 5 mm over 6 months or 1 cm over 1 year, aneurysm neck 15 mm or less, and patients deemed unfit for open surgery. High-risk patients for major vascular surgery include patients with significant pulmonary disease, poor renal function, severe coronary or heart valve disease, and hostile abdomen.[2]

Ideal anatomy for FEVAR includes aortic diameter of 20 to 32 mm at the level of the renal arteries, neck angulation of less than 45 degrees, iliac artery diameter of 7 mm or more, and iliac angulation of 85 degrees or less. The renal arteries should be 4 mm or larger to avoid stent thrombosis. Renal artery or superior mesenteric artery (SMA) ostial stenosis should be handled with great care and is considered an adverse anatomic feature.

CONTRAINDICATIONS

There is no absolute contraindication, but the presence of an adverse anatomic feature could make the procedure difficult and increase procedural comorbidity. If there are three or more adverse anatomic features, the procedure could be extremely difficult or impossible.[3] Symptomatic or ruptured aneurysm is not suitable for this technology because stent-graft manufacture can take at least 6 weeks. Recent development of off-the-shelf devices may enable their use for symptomatic aneurysms, but it is hard to envisage that ruptured aneurysm would be suitable.[4]

DEVICES

The first commercially available fenestrated stent-graft is the Cook device. It is a composite system that consists of a proximal custom-made component, a bifurcated component, and two iliac limbs. The system is based on the original Zenith platform (Cook Medical, Bloomington, Ind.), which is made of woven polyester fabric sutured to stainless-steel Gianturco stents.

The proximal component contains two or three fenestrations and a scallop (Fig. 48-1). Rarely, there are four fenestrations. There are two types of fenestrations, small and large. The small fenestration is 6 mm in width and 6 or 8 mm in height. It is reinforced with a nitinol ring and should be 15 mm or more from the proximal edge of the fabric. The large fenestration is 8 to 12 mm in diameter and should be 10 mm or more from the edge of the graft. The scallop is 6 to 12 mm in depth and 10 mm wide. It is also reinforced with a nitinol ring and has gold radiopaque markers. The bare spring (which contains fixation barbs) is located within the top cap. This, together with one or two posterior diameter reducing ties, assists device orientation until final deployment.

The small fenestrations and scallop have no struts across them. The small fenestrations are intended to be stented. This stenting serves two goals: migration resistance and sealing. The large fenestration can have struts crossing the fenestration.

The proximal fenestrated component has some important radiopaque markers: an anterior check mark, three anterior vertical markers, and three posterior horizontal markers.

Bare metallic stents or covered stents may be used to bridge the gap between the fenestrations and target branch vessels. The choice of side branch stent depends on the distance of the side vessel from the aneurysm and the presence of mural thrombus. Uncovered balloon-expandable stents may be preferred over covered stents if the distance from the renal artery or the SMA to the aneurysm is 5 mm or more and/or if the mural thrombus is not severe enough to cause poor opposition of the stent to the side wall. The nitinol ring and overdilation of the stent after deployment of the side branch stent using an oversized balloon help seal the renal or SMA stent against the graft wall and resist future migration. However, many operators prefer to use covered stents in all cases.

New Devices

At least two new devices have been introduced recently to overcome certain limitations and shortfalls of the existing commercially available Cook device. Although these devices are awaiting full evaluation through multicenter studies and/or randomized trials, they clearly provide the endovascular community with a wider range of options and take endovascular treatment of challenging aneurysms a step further.

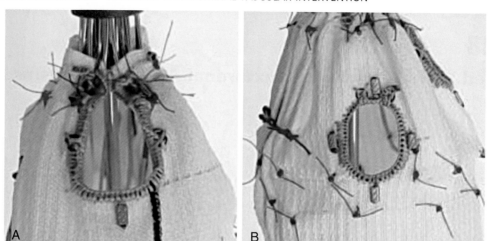

FIGURE 48-1. A, Semioval scallop with reinforced nitinol ring and three gold markers. **B,** Circular small fenestration with reinforced nitinol ring and four gold markers.

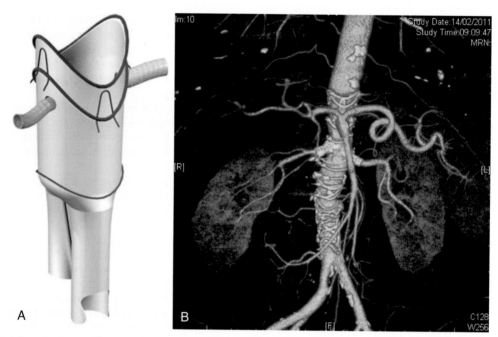

FIGURE 48-2. A, Schematic picture of fenestrated Anaconda device showing fenestrations, hooks, and valley of proximal stent. **B,** Three-dimensional (3D) volume-rendered image following implantation of Anaconda device.

Custom-Made Fenestrated Anaconda Device (Vascutek, Terumo, Japan)

This fenestrated device was developed on the background of the original Anaconda device.[5,6] Its proximal end is positioned suprarenally, and this part of the device provides the seal and fixation by means of hooks and rings. The anterior valley is oriented to cradle the SMA and/or celiac trunk. The fenestrations are made in the unsupported part of the fabric, which gives more flexibility to orient the fenestration according to the circumferential orientation of the renal or SMA vessels. The typical device encompasses two renal fenestrations supported by nitinol rings and marked by four radiopaque markers (Fig. 48-2). However, an SMA fenestration can be added to increase the coverage length in shorter

landing zones. Our initial experience with this device shows that potential advantages include the ability to (1) accommodate more difficult anatomy and angulation and (2) partially reposition the top device after cannulating one vessel so that the device can be reoriented, and the next fenestration faces the second vessel. The device also gives the operator the option of cannulating the fenestration antegradely prior to full device deployment, since there is no closed top cap. However, the delivery system profile is still relatively large, similar to the Cook fenestrated stent.

Ventana Fenestrated System (Endologix, Irvine, Calif.)

The Ventana endograft is based on the conventional Endologix aortic endograft, which is based on a different concept of fixation and seal. Use of the aortic bifurcation as a point of anatomic fixation for the bifurcation of the graft, and the separate seal achieved through placement of a proximal extension that overlaps with the bifurcation graft, allows two separate benefits. The first benefit is fixation, based upon the aortic bifurcation rather than the proximal diseased aorta. This morphology also maintains the aortic bifurcation should interventions across the bifurcation for occlusive disease be required in the future. The second advantage is resistance to migration of the proximal segment because there is no "baffle" for the aortic flow to push against.

Based upon these concepts, the Ventana fenestrated device uses a proximal fenestrated extension that seals with a bifurcation graft seated at the aortic bifurcation. The initial design of the device was produced with the aim of allowing placement in various individuals without the need for specific individual graft creation or off-the-shelf devices. All fenestrations and the scallop are marked with radiopaque markers to allow for ease of visualization, and the stent-graft can be rotated and oriented appropriately in vivo using a highly torquable low-friction delivery system. The delivery system includes prepositioned sheaths through the fenestrations that allow cannulation of the renal branches with catheters prior to graft deployment. After positioning catheters and wires in the renal arteries, the prepositioned sheaths can be advanced into the renal arteries and the graft positioned with the scallop at the level of the SMA. Deployment of the main body is followed by placement of the covered renal stents to complete the procedure.

PROCEDURE PLANNING

Planning is one of the most important prerequisites for successful FEVAR. A thorough understanding of the axial anatomy, stent-graft features, and practical knowledge about the behavior of the graft inside the patient are needed.

Full computed tomographic angiography (CTA) of the aorta should be acquired with 1- to 2-mm slice thickness, using a modern 16 or more multidetector CT scanner. The images are reconstructed using a variety of commercially available three-dimensional (3D) software packages. The center-of-flow line is used to straighten the aorta and correct for angulations.

The following is a guide for planning for the Cook device, although the process is not grossly different for other fenestrated devices.

Several important anatomic measurements are required to decide on the positions of the fenestrations for the visceral arteries. These measurements are (1) the lower border of the celiac trunk, (2) the distance from the celiac trunk to the middle of the SMA ostium, (3) the distance from the lower border of the celiac trunk to the middle of the ostium of the right renal artery, and (4) the distance from the lower border of the celiac trunk to the middle of the ostium of the left renal artery (Fig. 48-3). The internal vessel diameter is measured at the level of each fenestration. The circumferential orientation of the side vessels is determined according to the clock position, allowing for corrected angulation. The clock position of each fenestration is preferred to be 15 minutes anterior to the measured one to compensate for the effect of posterior reducing ties (Fig. 48-4). The diameter of the proximal landing zone is measured from outer to outer wall and is oversized by 15%. The bifurcated device is then planned in a similar manner to the standard Cook intrarenal device, keeping in mind that there must be at least two overlapping stents with the fenestrated device.

TECHNIQUE OF STENT INSERTION

An interventional suite with angiographic facilities to produce high-quality images is important for successful FEVAR. The procedure is usually performed under general anesthesia, although local or spinal analgesia can be used. Following bilateral groin cutdown (or use of large-vessel percutaneous closure devices), access with wire and sheath is gained into each common femoral artery. The ipsilateral side is chosen according to the size of the external iliac artery (>7.5 mm) and the straighter path to the aorta. The contralateral side is accessed with a large sheath, usually 20F. The author uses a Gore DrySeal Sheath (W.L. Gore & Associates, Flagstaff, Ariz.). This sheath has an occlusion balloon that prevents excessive blood loss during the

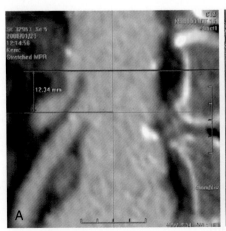 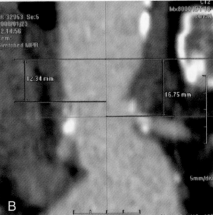 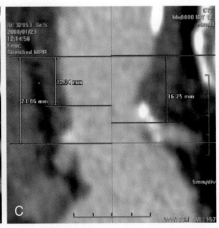

Lower Celiac Axis – Mid SMA	Lower Celiac Axis – Mid Lt. renal A	Lower Celiac Axis – Mid Rt. renal A
12mm	17mm	22mm

FIGURE 48-3. A-C, Measurements that define horizontal position of fenestrations and scallop.

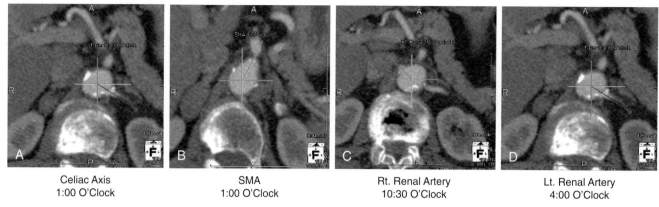

| Celiac Axis | SMA | Rt. Renal Artery | Lt. Renal Artery |
| 1:00 O'Clock | 1:00 O'Clock | 10:30 O'Clock | 4:00 O'Clock |

FIGURE 48-4. A-D, Clock orientation of fenestrations and scallop.

procedure. Once the sheath is positioned in the lower abdominal aorta, two more wires are introduced through the sheath. One of these is used to take a straight flush catheter for diagnostic images in the first instance. The main device with fenestrations should be oriented outside the patient, using the radiopaque markers, then introduced under fluoroscopy into the intended position at the level of the renal arteries. The images obtained at this stage should be acquired in the neutral anteroposterior position to avoid confusion. Following partial deployment of the device, minor adjustment is feasible at this stage, since the device is not completely free because it is still attached to the top cap.

One of the contralateral wires is used to advance a catheter with a curved tip, usually a Cobra catheter, into the lumen of the stent-graft. The Cobra catheter, with the help of a hydrophilic wire, is manipulated to cannulate one of the fenestrations. At this stage, the x-ray tube can be rotated to a plane where all four markers of the fenestration are aligned. The hydrophilic wire and catheter are introduced into the renal artery. The position of the catheter in the target vessel is confirmed by injection of contrast medium. A stiff wire such as a 0.035-inch Jindo wire (Cordis Corp., Hialeah, Fla.) or Rosen (Cook Medical) is parked in a stable position inside the renal artery, taking care not to advance the wire too far to avoid branch rupture or pseudoaneurysm formation. The catheter is exchanged for a suitable size sheath, usually 7F. Advancing the sheath through the fenestration into the target vessel can be facilitated by using 4 mm short balloon (2-4 cm). Similar steps are then repeated to cannulate the opposite renal fenestration. We usually position renal stents inside the sheath before deploying the stent-graft.

Balloon-expandable rather than self-expanding stents are routinely used. Balloon-expandable stents ensure high radial force as well as accurate deployment (Fig. 48-5). Following full aortic endograft deployment by removing the trigger wires and releasing the top cap, the cap is withdrawn carefully into the ipsilateral iliac artery, taking care not to disturb the intrarenal sheaths. The renal stents are deployed at this stage, with a 3- to 4-mm protrusion into the aortic lumen. Subsequently, an oversized balloon is inflated in the ostium of the fenestration to flare the stent, a step important to secure adequate seal and graft wall opposition.

After all fenestrations have been stented, the bifurcated component can be introduced and is deployed in the usual manner as for standard EVAR, followed by deployment of two iliac limbs. There must be overlap of at least two stents, preferably three, between the proximal fenestrated component and the bifurcated device. Balloon molding is performed at all junctions below the level of the fenestrations.

FEVAR represents a particular challenge to the endovascular interventionalist. This procedure is much more complicated than simple EVAR or thoracic EVAR (TEVAR). Hence, there is a need for a harmonic team trained with not only endovascular and open surgical skills, but also in the radiologic interpretation of images.

COMPLICATIONS AND OUTCOMES

The evidence for safety and efficacy of FEVAR continues to evolve. Since the first case published by Park et al.[1] in 1996, several prospective and retrospective studies have been published reporting single and multicenter experience. However, no randomized controlled trial or registry data are available to date, despite existence of this technology for almost 2 decades.

Mortality

Most published series have reported low morality post FEVAR. In a series of 54 patients who underwent the procedure, 30-day mortality was 3.7%.[7] In another series of 45 patients, early mortality was 2.2%.[8] Verhoeven et al. reported mortality as low as 1% in a large single-center series of 100 patients.[9] In the United States multicenter prospective trial of 30 patients published in 2009, there was no aneurysm-related mortality.[10] The retrospective analysis report of the French multicenter experience reported 2.5% early mortality.[11] Those results are favorable compared with those from nonfenestrated EVAR trials and registries.

Similar to 30-day mortality rates, long-term results following FEVAR show low death rates. The reported cumulative survival rates at 24 months range between 79% and 86%.[11,12] These results compare favorably with survival following open repair of juxtarenal aneurysms.[13,14]

Renal Impairment

Transient renal failure, defined as an increase in serum creatinine over 2 mg/dL or by more than 30% compared

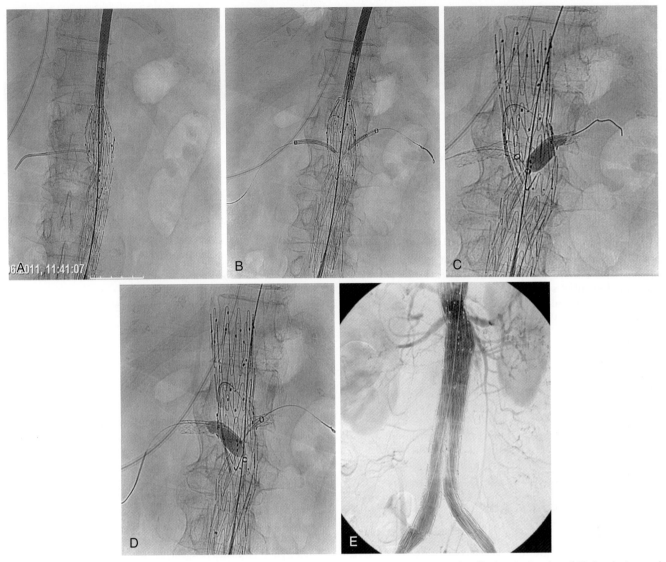

FIGURE 48-5. Steps in cannulating and stenting fenestrations. **A,** Bilateral renal artery cannulation with stiff wires. **B,** Insertion of 6F sheaths into each renal artery. **C-D,** Stent deployment in renal artery, and balloon remodeling with large-size balloon to obtain flared ostium. **E,** Check angiogram to document patency of side vessel and exclude endoleak.

with baseline measurements, is reported to be more common in open repair than FEVAR. In a systematic review of eight studies of FEVAR constituting 368 patients, and 12 studies including 1164 patients who underwent open repair, renal failure was estimated to be 14.9%, (confidence interval [CI] 11.5-18.7) versus 20% (CI 17.9-22.5), respectively.[15] However, there was no significant difference in the incidence of permanent dialysis dependence between the two groups of patients. In the French multicenter experience of 134 patients who underwent FEVAR, there was worsening renal function in 11%, with only 1% of patients needing permanent dialysis.[11] It is likely the deterioration in renal function in those cases was due to cholesterol embolization and contrast nephrotoxicity rather than renal artery occlusion.

Primary Endoleak

Type I and III endoleaks represent a failure to exclude the aneurysm from the systemic circulation and place the sac

at increased risk of expansion and possible rupture. On the other hand, type II endoleaks are considered benign and are treated expectantly. The reported endoleaks in published FEVAR cohort studies is quite low. This is perhaps a reflection of careful selection of patients with appropriate anatomy for this technology.

The type I endoleak rate is estimated to be between 0% and 7%.[16,17] In the French experience, there was an 6% incidence of type I and III endoleaks, the majority of them treated successfully by an endovascular approach.[11] In the multicenter trial in United States, there were no type I or III endoleaks. The reported 20% type II endoleak rate in this latter study showed no apparent effect on aneurysm sac growth.[10]

Target Vessel Patency

All published series of FEVAR have reported high patency rates of stented renal arteries, SMAs, and in some cases celiac trunks, which reflect high technical success rates and device integrity. Primary patency rates range from 91% to 100%.[8,16-22] Reported midterm patency rates are slightly reduced (90%-97%). The pooled estimate of target vessel perfusion was 96.6% (CI 95.4-97.8) during the procedure, and 92% (CI 90.3-94.8) at 1-year follow-up.[15] These results compare favorably with open surgical repair of juxtarenal aneurysms, which was reported to be 85%.[23]

Secondary Reintervention

Reintervention is usually required for endoleak treatment, maintaining vessel patency, rescuing access vessel problems, and laparotomy for mesenteric ischemia. In a systematic review of 368 FEVARs there was a 15% reintervention rate (CI 11.5-18.7). The majority of the reported reinterventions were secondary to endoleaks.[15] In the French multicenter study, there were 10% reinterventions, with endoleak and target vessel problems being the most common indications.[11] Verhoeven et al. reported 11 reinterventions in their large single-center series.[9] These figures are significantly higher than the pooled estimate of reintervention in open repair (relative risk [RR] 0.87; CI 0.83-0.91; $P = 0.0001$).

Sac Growth

Sac shrinkage is a clear sign of successful exclusion of the aneurysm from the systemic circulation. Haulon et al. reported sac size reduction by more than 5 mm in 33% and 73% of patients at 6 months and 2 years, respectively.[11] Greenberg et al. observed a reduction of more than 5 mm in sac diameter in 40% of patients at 6 months and in 53% of patients at 24 months, with no growth in any of the 30 cases included in their study.[10]

POSTPROCEDURE CARE AND FOLLOW-UP

Following the procedure, the patient is usually transferred to a high-dependency unit for 1 to 3 days.

CTA is performed at discharge or at 1 month after the procedure, and subsequently at 6 months, 12 months, and yearly intervals thereafter. The CT images should be evaluated not only for endoleaks and sac size but also for the relative position of the stent components to each other to detect early migration. In addition, the side branch stents should be evaluated for stent fracture and side vessel stenosis.

KEY POINTS

- Patients with short aneurysm necks (<15 mm long) can be treated by fenestrated endovascular aneurysm repair (FEVAR).
- Care assessment of computed tomography images using a workstation is essential to plan an appropriate device.
- Most current devices are custom-made and take time to manufacture, although off-the-shelf devices are under evaluation and development.
- FEVAR is much more technically challenging than conventional EVAR and ideally requires collaborating teams of surgeons and interventional radiologists to optimize success.
- Outcomes and complication rates compare well with open surgery.

► **SUGGESTED READINGS**

Avgerinos ED, Dalainas I, Kakisis J, et al. Endograft accommodation on the aortic bifurcation: an overview of anatomical fixation and implications for long-term stent-graft stability. J Endovasc Ther 2011;18:462–70.

Ehsan O, Murray D, Farquharson F, et al. Endovascular repair of complex aortic aneurysms. Ann Vasc Surg 2011;25:716–25.

Knott AW, Kalra M, Duncan AA, et al. Open repair of juxtarenal aortic aneurysms (JAA) remains a safe option in the era of fenestrated endografts. J Vasc Surg 2008;47:695–701.

Nordon IM, Hinchliffe RJ, Holt PJ, et al. Modern treatment of juxtarenal abdominal aortic aneurysms with fenestrated endografting and open repair–a systematic review. Eur J Vasc Endovasc Surg 2009;38:35–41.

Park JH, Chung JW, Choo IW, et al. Fenestrated stent-grafts for preserving visceral arterial branches in the treatment of abdominal aortic aneurysms: preliminary experience. J Vasc Interv Radiol 1996;7(6): 819–23.

Scurr JR, Brennan JA, Gilling-Smith GL, et al. Fenestrated endovascular repair for juxtarenal aortic aneurysm. Br J Surg 2008;95:326–32.

The complete reference list is available online at www.expertconsult.com.

CHAPTER 49
Management of Thoracoabdominal Aneurysms by Branched Endograft Technology

Mark R. Tyrrell, C. Jason Wilkins, and Stéphan Haulon

INTRODUCTION

This chapter is concerned specifically with the management of aortic aneurysms that involve both the thoracic and abdominal segments of the aorta and its associated visceral branches. The aortic arch, aortic dissection, isolated thoracic, infrarenal, juxtarenal and suprarenal aneurysms are dealt with elsewhere in this book. The reader should note that extensive aortic pathologies commonly require solutions incorporating combinations of open surgery and fenestrated and branched endovascular solutions. It should be recognized that the total endovascular repair of thoracoabdominal aortic aneurysms (TAAAs) is currently a technique and technology in evolution. There is little if any level 1 evidence to support the general use of the solutions that we will discuss.

The majority of patients who have infrarenal aortoiliac aneurysms can now be relatively safely treated, but the prognosis for patients who have large (>6 cm diameter) aortic aneurysms that involve the origins of the abdominal visceral vessels remains grave. The untreated natural history is only 17% survival at 5 years,[1] and the annual combined rupture/dissection/mortality rate is 14%.[2]

Although the first successful open repair was reported 56 years ago,[3] the risks of treatment remain considerable. In the pre-endovascular era, Crawford's considerable experience showed that operative mortality risk and the risk of paraplegia relates to aneurysm extent, leading to the Crawford classification.[4] This classification (now slightly modified)[5] still forms the foundation underpinning the technical approach and risk assessment of TAAA repair. Even in the "best risk" subgroup (Crawford type IV TAAA), the physiologic demands of open surgical repair place considerable stresses on patients that are likely to be beyond the reserve of many, and the recovery time is long in survivors. Endovascular infrarenal aortic aneurysm (AAA) repair results in significantly lower 30-day mortality than anatomically equivalent open surgery.[6-8] Similarly, endovascular repair of isolated thoracic aortic aneurysms (TEVAR) is associated with a lower risk of death than its conventional equivalent.[9-11] Since the first generations of devices available for endovascular aneurysm repair (EVAR) were relatively simple tubes or bifurcated grafts, initial attempts to extend the benefits of EVAR to patients with TAAA led to "hybrid" solutions. These involve laparotomy, extra-anatomic bypass to the visceral vessels, and then extended EVAR to exclude the aneurysmal segment while preserving blood flow to the vital organs. Although initial reports were greeted with enthusiasm,[12-14] good results have not been universal,[15,16] and the approach does not exploit all of the potential advantages of a "pure" endovascular approach (e.g., lesser surgical insult, better physiologic control, rapid recovery). This unmet need, together with rapid technologic advances, has encouraged the development of more ambitious endovascular solutions to extend the principles and potential benefits of EVAR to the challenging TAAA patient group.

Total endovascular repair of a true aortic aneurysm using a branched device was first described in 2001.[17]

PHILOSOPHY

The ultimate therapeutic goal in the treatment of TAAA is the same as that in the endovascular treatment of any aortic aneurysm: exclusion of the aneurysm wall from arterial blood pressure, thereby eliminating the risk of aortic rupture and exsanguination, while preserving distal perfusion. In the special case of endovascular management of TAAA, there is the additional requirement to preserve organ blood flow and function. The latter is achieved by the provision of custom-made branches for extension into the visceral vessel ostia—branched endovascular aneurysm repair (BEVAR).

In common with all varieties of EVAR, the technique relies on adequate proximal and distal aortic or iliac sealing zones. In common with most, it requires intravascular assembly of several overlapping parts, each of which must seal with adjacent components. In common with the use of fenestrated devices used to proximalize the proximal aortic sealing zone in juxtarenal AAA (FEVAR), it requires cannulation of target visceral vessels and extension from the main device into each of these using covered bridging stents.

There is, however, an important philosophic and practical difference between FEVAR and BEVAR. In the case of FEVAR, much of the seal is provided by apposition of the main device against the wall of the (relatively normal) visceral-bearing aorta, with secondary sealing between the (balloon-expandable) extension stent and the device (by internal flaring) and between the extension stent and the target vessel. In the case of BEVAR, there is no visceral vessel level apposition between the main device and the (aneurysmal) visceral vessel–bearing aortic wall. In this case, the branches are an integral part of the main device (and their origins are therefore manufactured as hemostatic), with seal being required within the branch and into the target vessel.

In practice, some aneurysm anatomies require combined FEVAR/BEVAR solutions. In the interests of clarity (and in keeping with the chapter title), this chapter will concentrate on "pure" BEVAR solutions, but the principles are extendable to more complex problems.

For more information on this topic, please visit www.expertconsult.com.

SPECIAL CONSIDERATIONS

It should be borne in mind that BEVAR requires considerably more complex device design and planning than conventional EVAR. Deployment is more technically demanding and takes longer to complete (a greater contrast and radiation burden). It also requires different arterial access (particularly subclavian/axillary/brachial) and has more potential for type III endoleak (because of the large number of overlapping components).

It is self-evident that patient, aneurysm anatomy, and surgical team selection are paramount.

Device design requires high-quality, arterial phase contrast-enhanced computed tomography (CE-CT) imaging and access to software capable of three-dimensional (3D) image manipulation. This permits measurement of the true diameters of the aortic and target vessel landing zones and of the relative true longitudinal and rotational distances between target vessels based on calculated center lines. In designing devices, the following minimum sealing zones should be planned: 20 mm graft/artery (aorta, iliac, or visceral vessel), 40 mm (3 stent overlap) between central components, and full branch length between branches and bridging stents.

For more information on this topic, please visit www.expertconsult.com.

Anatomic Considerations

Successful deployment and aneurysm exclusion require adequate proximal and distal aortic and target vessel sealing zones. Each of these has to be of sufficient length and straightness. For durable patency, the target vessels have to be of a minimum diameter (5 mm). Target vessel cannulation may be problematic, but the limitations concerning target vessel origin proximity are less of a problem than with FEVAR. Good torque and manipulation and passage of relatively long covered stents demand techniques (and anatomy) to achieve reasonably straight routes from access vessels to target vessel ostia. Aortic tortuosity at the visceral bearing segment may preclude use of currently available devices.

TECHNIQUE

Anatomic considerations are most easily explained in the context of an understanding of the steps involved in the deployment of a BEVAR device (the use of mixed FEVAR/BEVAR devices requires modifications to the steps delineated below):

1. Before anesthesia, it is important to check the device against the printed plan and description.
2. The chosen access vessels are cannulated by surgical cutdown and percutaneous access as required. In practice, the most common routes are surgical exposure of one femoral artery (the side associated with the larger diameter and least tortuosity), percutaneous puncture of the contralateral femoral artery, and open exposure of the left distal subclavian, axillary, or brachial.
3. Full anticoagulation is established using sodium heparin. This is monitored, corrected, and maintained until arterial closure is complete (target activated clotting time 300 seconds).
4. If necessary, proximal (tube) extension devices are passed via the iliac system and abdominal aorta and are deployed to seal at the planned proximal landing zone.
5. The main body is prepared, oriented correctly (using the various check markers and other radiopaque markers integral to the device) (Fig. 49-1, *A*), and passed to the planned proximal sealing zone (aorta, proximal TEVAR extension device, or previously placed elephant trunk, according to the case), reoriented if necessary, deployed, and released from the delivery system, which is then withdrawn. We have found the use of a centimeter-marked pigtail catheter is useful in positioning the device accurately—the objective being to "land" with the branch ends 15 to 20 mm superior to (or inferior to in the case of upward-pointing branches) the target vessel.
6. Distal aortic extension devices (tube or bifurcated according to the requirements of each case) are then introduced and deployed to provide a distal seal. All sealing zones are molded using a compliant balloon.
7. All large sheaths occupying the iliac system are removed, and the femoral arteriotomy is closed over a small access sheath to reperfuse the pelvis and lower limbs.
8. At this point, the aorta is effectively relined, the proximal and distal aortic landing zones are sealed, the pelvis and legs have normal blood supply, but the aneurysm sac and its visceral branches are still pressurized and perfused via the open device branches.
9. The use of a "through-and-through" wire is an essential adjunct. This can be achieved by cannulation of the endograft via the upper limb access, passage of a fine 300-cm-long wire, and snaring and retrieving it via the femoral access. This allows a degree of tension and aids passage of the long sheath (10F, 80 cm) inserted from the upper limb access vessel, which might otherwise tend to collapse and coil into the aortic arch.

    For more detail on this step, please visit the accompanying website at www.expertconsult.com.
10. Each branch and target vessel is accessed, stented, balloon-molded, and angiographically checked as a complete sequence before the next vessel is attempted (Fig. 49-2). Most branches are designed in a downward-pointing configuration, mandating that most of the visceral vessel manipulations are conducted via upper limb access. A branch is accessed via the upper limb sheath using soft steerable wire/catheter combinations (or a preloaded catheter). Suitable catheters (100 cm long, beacon tip) are advanced over the (260 cm long) wire. The target vessel is accessed via the branch. Once the catheter is in a stable position as far as possible within the target vessel, the soft wire is withdrawn and replaced with a stiffer supportive wire over which the bridging stent will be passed. A covered self-expanding stent of appropriate diameter and sufficient length to bridge from the branch to the target and provide seal

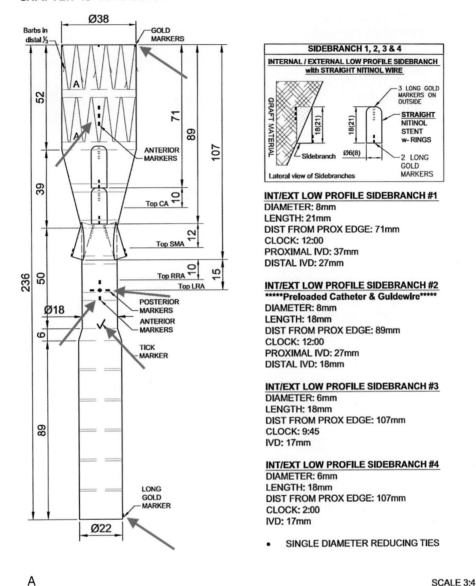

SIDEBRANCH 1, 2, 3 & 4
INTERNAL / EXTERNAL LOW PROFILE SIDEBRANCH
with STRAIGHT NITINOL WIRE

GRAFT MATERIAL

3 LONG GOLD MARKERS ON OUTSIDE
STRAIGHT NITINOL STENT w- RINGS
2 LONG GOLD MARKERS
Sidebranch
Ø6(8)
18(21)
18(21)

Lateral view of Sidebranches

INT/EXT LOW PROFILE SIDEBRANCH #1
DIAMETER: 8mm
LENGTH: 21mm
DIST FROM PROX EDGE: 71mm
CLOCK: 12:00
PROXIMAL IVD: 37mm
DISTAL IVD: 27mm

INT/EXT LOW PROFILE SIDEBRANCH #2
*****Preloaded Catheter & Guidewire*****
DIAMETER: 8mm
LENGTH: 18mm
DIST FROM PROX EDGE: 89mm
CLOCK: 12:00
PROXIMAL IVD: 27mm
DISTAL IVD: 18mm

INT/EXT LOW PROFILE SIDEBRANCH #3
DIAMETER: 6mm
LENGTH: 18mm
DIST FROM PROX EDGE: 107mm
CLOCK: 9:45
IVD: 17mm

INT/EXT LOW PROFILE SIDEBRANCH #4
DIAMETER: 6mm
LENGTH: 18mm
DIST FROM PROX EDGE: 107mm
CLOCK: 2:00
IVD: 17mm

- SINGLE DIAMETER REDUCING TIES

A

SCALE 3:4

FIGURE 49-1. Diagrammatic branched endovascular aneurysm repair (BEVAR) device plans with arrows to show: **A,** Alignment markers.

Continued

at both its ends is positioned, unsheathed, and balloon-molded. The stiff wire is replaced with a soft wire (to unmask any kinking that may exist), and check angiography is conducted via the sheath to establish patency and freedom from endoleak.

11. Once the full sequence has been completed for each target vessel, all catheters, wires, and sheaths are removed and the access vessels closed.

Access Vessels for Main Device Delivery

BEVAR devices are generally larger and less flexible than "simple" EVAR and TEVAR devices. Planning must therefore include consideration of the caliber and tortuosity of the iliac system. We recommend a low threshold for use of iliac conduits. If employed, these require a staged approach to avoid suture line bleeding during the main (anticoagulated) procedure.

Access Vessels for Target Vessel Cannulation and Covered Stent Graft Extension

The principle concern is preservation of adequate wire and catheter torque for manipulation, successful cannulation, support wire exchange, and tracking of covered stents. The greater the distance between the point of manipulation and the target, and the greater the tortuosity (which provides resistance to smooth wire rotation and causes unpredictable catheter torque build up), the greater the degree of difficulty. Using long, trackable coaxial sheaths to provide support, shorten the effective distance and reduce the number of instrument-versus–vessel wall interactions, is an essential adjunct. It does, however, require a reasonably large upper limb access vessel and open access. This generally means proximal access (subclavian/axillary rather than brachial). It also raises the possibility of injury to these relatively fragile vessels. Passage across the left vertebral

DISTAL COMPONENT
(Branched & Fenestrated)

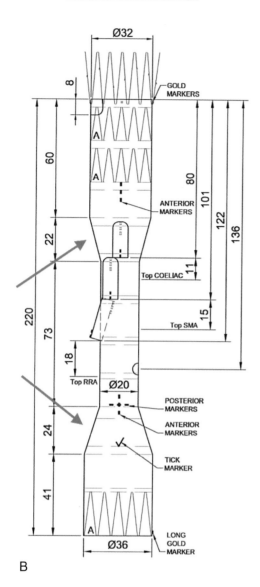

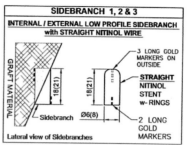

SIDEBRANCH 1, 2 & 3
INTERNAL / EXTERNAL LOW PROFILE SIDEBRANCH
with STRAIGHT NITINOL WIRE

GRAFT MATERIAL
18(21)
18(21)
Sidebranch
Ø6(8)
Lateral view of Sidebranches

- 3 LONG GOLD MARKERS ON OUTSIDE
- **STRAIGHT NITINOL STENT w- RINGS**
- 2 LONG GOLD MARKERS

REINFORCED ACCESS SCALLOP #1
(For Preloaded Catheter & Guidewire)
WIDTH: 10mm
HEIGHT: 8mm
CLOCK: 9:45
IVD: 31mm

INT/EXT LOW PROFILE SIDEBRANCH #1
DIAMETER: 8mm
LENGTH: 18mm
DIST FROM PROX EDGE: 80mm
CLOCK: 12:00
PROXIMAL IVD: 30mm
DISTAL IVD: 20mm

INT/EXT LOW PROFILE SIDEBRANCH #2
DIAMETER: 8mm
LENGTH: 21mm
DIST FROM PROX EDGE: 101mm
CLOCK: 11:00
IVD: 19mm

INT/EXT LOW PROFILE SIDEBRANCH #3
*****Preloaded Catheter & Guidewire*****
DIAMETER: 6mm
LENGTH: 21mm
DIST FROM PROX EDGE: 122mm
CLOCK: 9:45
IVD: 19mm

REINFORCED SMALL FENESTRATION #1
DIAMETER: 6mm
DIST FROM PROX EDGE: 136mm
CLOCK: 3:00
IVD: 19mm

- SINGLE DIAMETER REDUCING TIES

B

SCALE 3:4

FIGURE 49-1, cont'd. B, "Waisted" design to ensure branch opening in relatively narrow aortic lumens. Please visit the website at www.expertconsult.com for additional images.

arterial origin and/or occupation of the subclavian artery incorporates the potential for posterior circulation embolization and stoke.

The tightness of the curve of the arch position of the left subclavian along its greater curvature are responsible for the directness (or otherwise) of the route between the site of the arteriotomy and the descending aorta. Although it is subject to some controversy, this anatomy has been categorized.[20] In short, tightly curved arches with subclavian ostia that arise relatively proximal and inferior to the arch's inner curve (type III) pose the greatest difficulty. The addition of further twists and turns in the descending aorta and the angle between the device main body, side-branch, and target vessel all conspire to amplify the technical challenge. As described earlier, use of through-and-through "body flossing" control to allow

for a degree of tension and shortening of catheters and sheaths that might otherwise tend to collapse and coil is essential.

The addition of preloaded catheters guarantees cannulation of one (or two) side branches and can be a useful step but requires larger-diameter main body delivery devices.

Target Vessel Anatomy

For durable patency, the target vessels should be of a minimum diameter (5 mm). In relatively small vessels, it is important that the "bridge" between the branch and target vessel is composed of a single stent. A system of telescoped short stents risks effective stenosis by occupancy of the available lumen by unnecessary stent and graft material and

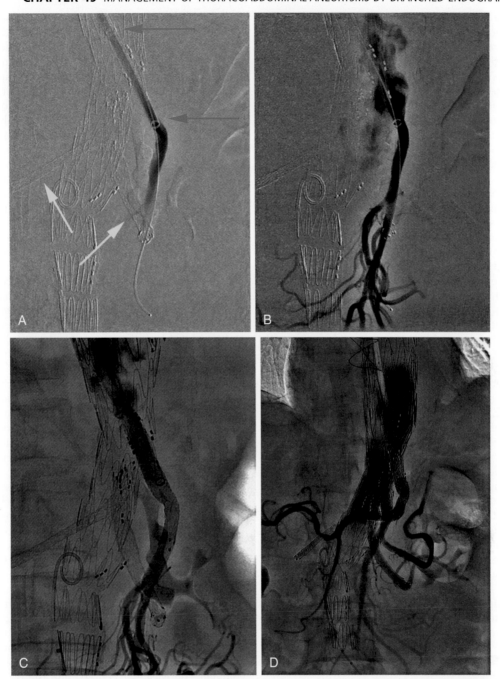

FIGURE 49-2. Each vessel is completed in sequence. **A,** In this series, coaxial sheath system is visible *(red arrows)*, and renal arteries have been stented *(yellow arrows).* **B,** Superior mesenteric artery (SMA) branch is cannulated and a wire passed deep into target vessel. **C,** Self-expanding stent is passed and deployed, stiff wire is removed, and a check angiogram is conducted. Ultimately, all four vessels are completed. **D** shows completion of celiac, SMA, and both renal arteries (contrast has been selectively injected to show gut vessels).

is another potential site for endoleak and disconnection. Depending on aneurysm anatomy, visceral vessels can "point down" or "point up" relative to the aortic wall. Even in the case of upward-pointing (usually renal) vessels, we try to design downward-pointing branches to provide sufficient space for the branches to open. Where opening space is limited, it is possible to design "waisted" branch-bearing segments (see Fig. 49-1, *B*).

For more information on anatomy and stent design, please visit www.expertconsult.com.

Prevention of Paraplegia

Paraplegia is the most feared complication associated with TAAA repair and it occurs with variable incidence irrespective of the method of repair. At tissue level, it is caused by infarction of the spinal cord in the territory of the anterior spinal artery. In many cases, this is likely to be a consequence of hypoperfusion due to an abrupt loss of segmental intercostal/lumbar arterial inflow and poor anterior spinal collateralization. In some, it is likely that there is an embolic mechanism, and its avoidance requires adequate anticoagulation and procedure planning to minimize instrument/device/wire abrasion of the aortic wall.

Addressing the problem of low spinal cord blood flow is more complex and requires attention during both the operative and postoperative phases. In the operative phase, strategies can be directed to reducing neuronal metabolic demand and maintaining effective spinal cord capillary perfusion. The former includes administration of steroids, barbiturates, and other drugs, together with selective, or permissive global hypothermia. Most authors advocate the maintenance of global and local blood flow (and pressure), together with relief of the hydrostatic resistance to effective capillary perfusion—specifically venous and cerebrospinal fluid (CSF) pressures. In addition to careful anesthetic management of blood pressure, operators should plan procedures so as to preserve as much anterior spinal blood flow as possible, and also plan the sequence of the operation to produce brief episodic interruptions to cord flow rather than prolonged ones.

Nevertheless, the incidence of paraplegia is generally comparable with open surgery[17-19,21-28]—this despite the likely loss of a larger number of intercostal vessels with BEVAR (required to achieve adequate aortic sealing zones).

Nonetheless, we would emphasize the importance of preserving intercostal, lumbar, subclavian (vertebral), and internal iliac vessels (collateral anterior spinal artery flow) in planning BEVAR cases. Where necessary, the staged ancillary use of extra-anatomic debranching procedures (e.g., carotid-subclavian bypass to preserve vertebral and supreme intercostal flow) or use of branched iliac devices[29] should be considered.

In the postoperative phase, continued maintenance of high-normal blood pressure and flow, together with close monitoring, is the minimum. Ischemia-reperfusion injury has the potential to cause delayed paraplegia via the mechanism of edema within the fixed constraints of the spinal canal, which raises resistance to effective perfusion. In some cases, the institution/reinstitution of CSF drainage (together with elevation of the systemic perfusion pressure) can reverse the symptoms.

For an expanded discussion of paraplegia prevention following TAAA repair, please see www.expertconsult.com.

OUTCOMES

There are no randomized controlled trial data to compare open and endovascular TAAA repair. All that exists to date are single-center reports detailing outcomes of total endovascular treatments in "pioneer" vascular units. These include centers where the approach has been dominantly FEVAR,[19] those where it has been dominantly BEVAR,[18] and some where a mixture of solutions have been reported.[28] This brings a potential point for confusion: although both technologies are applicable to TAAA (depending on aneurysm anatomy), it is important to distinguish between patients treated for pararenal aneurysms and those treated for true TAAAs. Each aneurysm category likely brings its own preponderance of comorbidities and tolerance to surgery. Large series describing outcomes after open surgical treatment of TAAA indicate a correlation between aneurysm anatomy (and surgical remedy) and the probability of death and major complications (most notably

paraplegia).[4,5] At this early stage, it is important that endovascular reports are similarly categorized and that outcomes are not viewed as being specifically dependent on the use of FEVAR, TEVAR, or a combined approach (pending reported evidence to the contrary). Within these limitations, the technical completion rate is high, and published 30-day mortality rates range from 5.5% to 9.1% in larger series (those describing >20 patients), with rates of 0% to 25% in smaller series. The (temporary and permanent) paraplegia rates vary between 2.7% and 16.7%.[17-19,21-28]

In most series, the number of patients reported are simply too small to allow for meaningful subanalysis according to the modified Crawford classification.[5] The size of the Cleveland Clinic experience remains unique.[31] It confirms that the relationship between aneurysm extent (and previous aneurysm surgery) and mortality holds true for endovascular repair, as it does for conventional surgery. The common observation that the patients treated so far are deemed unfit for the equivalent open operation is likely to have veracity, and it is probably the case that endovascular repair of TAAA does represent a less severe challenge than open surgery, which should translate to a lower 30-day mortality risk (and/or an option to treat patients who would not otherwise be considered). It is intuitively true that fitness for open TAAA repair is a very "high bar," and it does not follow that these are patients are unfit per se, or that they have life-shortening diagnoses. The situation is not analogous to that of infrarenal AAA repair, where the EVAR-2 trial suggested that patients unfit for that operation would gain no survival benefit from intervention by EVAR.[32] However, there is no method for measuring the average impact of any particular type of operation; neither is there a reliable way of measuring tolerance to surgical load for any individual patient or patient group. Finally, current follow-up data are short. There is no good information regarding the impact of BEVAR on long-term survival, late morbidity (particularly that related to long-term target vessel patency), reintervention rate, aneurysm dilatation, or delayed rupture.

At the time of this writing, it is only safe to view the available reports as confirmation of the (short-term) feasibility of total endovascular repair of TAAA and conclude that early results are no worse than those commonly reported with open surgery. The last conclusion comes with the caveat that these reports reflect the experience of pioneer endovascular centers, and the data include a significant learning curve (the former may skew outcomes positively, and the latter negatively).

The "bespoke" nature of the current BEVAR devices brings three inherent problems: manufacturing delay, lack of availability of devices for emergency use, and expense. The first two problems may be remediable by generic designs (which have been proposed for both BEVAR[33] and FEVAR[34] designs). Until "off-the-shelf" designs are available, mortality should be reported both in terms of operations attempted and "intention to treat." Where a device is not available with sufficient exigency, the hybrid option[12-14] may be a useful alternative.

CONCLUSIONS

The management of aneurysms affecting the thoracic and visceral-bearing segment of the abdominal aorta remains a major clinical challenge. Advances in imaging and material science have made total endovascular solutions a practical option in these cases. Although it seems probable this option can be achieved with a lower risk of 30-day mortality than that associated with equivalent open surgery (and also that less physiologically fit patients can be considered for treatment), spinal cord injury rates continue to be a source for concern. This chapter has been written specifically to emphasize and outline use of branched endovascular devices, but we strongly advocate using a mixture of approaches (BEVAR, FEVAR, hybrid, and open surgery), depending on patient fitness, aortic pathology, and urgency.

KEY POINTS

- Experience with use of branched devices for endovascular aneurysm repair is limited worldwide, but use of this technology is increasing.

- Patients with thoracoabdominal aortic aneurysm (TAAA) who are unsuitable for open surgical repair may well be suitable for branched endovascular aneurysm repair (BEVAR).

- A combination of BEVAR and fenestrated endovascular repair (FEVAR) provide a useful solution for many patients.

- Paraplegia and mortality rates are not insignificant but are comparable to surgery.

▶ **SUGGESTED READINGS**

Elefteriades JA. Natural history of thoracic aortic aneurysms: indications for surgery, and surgical versus nonsurgical risks. Ann Thorac Surg 2002;74:S1877–80.

Gawenda M, Aleksic M, Heckenkamp J, et al. Hybrid-procedures for the treatment of thoracoabdominal aortic aneurysms and dissections. Eur J Vasc Endovasc Surg 2007;33 (1):71–7.

Greenberg RK, Lu Q, Roselli EE, et al. Contemporary analysis of descending thoracic and thoracoabdominal aneurysm repair: a comparison of endovascular and open techniques. Circulation 2008;118:808–17.

Resch T, Greenberg RK, Lyden S, et al. Combined staged procedures for the treatment of thoracoabdominal aneurysms. J Endovasc Ther 2006;13:481–9.

Roselli EE, Greenberg RK, Pfaff K, et al. Endovascular treatment of thoracoabdominal aortic aneurysms. J Thorac Cardiovasc Surg 2007; 133:1474–82.

The complete reference list is available online at www.expertconsult.com.

CHAPTER 50

Endoleaks: Classification, Diagnosis, and Treatment

Klaus A. Hausegger

CLINICAL RELEVANCE

Endovascular aneurysm repair (EVAR) of infrarenal abdominal aortic aneurysms (AAA) has become a widespread procedure of late. Two recently published prospective trials have shown that EVAR of AAAs produces clinical results similar to those of open surgery after observation periods of 6 and 10 years, respectively, with EVAR having an advantage in postoperative mortality and morbidity.[1,2] However, despite similar results regarding rupture and survival rates, these treatment concepts have fundamental differences. In traditional open surgical repair, the aneurysm is excluded from the arterial circulation under direct visualization. A surgical graft is sewn in with a tight suture at the proximal and distal ends of the aneurysm. Arterial side branches originating from the aneurysmal sac, such as the inferior mesenteric artery (IMA), lumbar arteries, and accessory renal arteries, are either surgically ligated or reanastomosed to the surgical graft if necessary. In any case, tight sutures and hemostasis must be achieved primarily.

Unlike open repair, perigraft blood flow outside the endoprosthesis but inside the aneurysm sac may occur after EVAR. This phenomenon has been coined *endoleak* (EL) by White et al.[3] In this chapter, the different types of ELs are described and the most rational imaging strategies for the diagnosis of ELs are discussed. The clinical significance and possible treatment options are also covered here.

DEFINITION

The term *endoleak* was introduced by White et al. in 1997 and is well accepted in the current literature.[3] In earlier publications, terms such as *perigraft flow*, *perigraft leak*, or *leakage* were used to describe the same findings.

According to White's definition,[3] endoleak is a condition associated with endoluminal vascular grafts, defined by the persistence of blood flow outside the lumen of the endoluminal graft but within an aneurysm sac or adjacent vascular segments being treated by the graft. Endoleak is due to incomplete sealing or exclusion of the aneurysm sac or vessel segment, as evidenced by imaging studies (e.g., contrast-enhanced computed tomography [CT] scanning, ultrasonography [US], angiography).

CLASSIFICATION OF ENDOLEAKS

White et al. also proposed the first systematic classification of ELs.[3,4] This original classification was modified in a consensus conference of vascular surgeons and interventional radiologists, and the widely accepted classification was established.[5,6]

Primary ELs can be distinguished from secondary ELs according to the timing of development:

- *Primary ELs* occur during the first 30 days after EVAR. These ELs usually develop immediately after EVAR, and the aneurysm was never actually completely excluded from the arterial circulation.
- *Secondary ELs* occur later. Typically, the aneurysm has been excluded from the arterial circulation primarily. However, during follow-up, an EL not seen before is diagnosed. This type of EL is often caused by stent-graft distortion or migration.

Another classification of EL is based on their source and differentiates five types (Table 50-1):

- *Type I ELs:* In this type of EL, inflow occurs from the attachment sites of the endograft, so these ELs are also called *attachment site endoleaks*. If the leak occurs at the proximal attachment site, it is called a *type IA EL* (Fig. 50-1). If the leak is around the distal attachment site, it is a *type IB leak*. If aortouniiliac stent-grafts have been inserted and an EL occurs at the iliac occluder, it is a *type IC EL*.
- *Type II ELs:* These ELs are also called *reperfusion leaks*. The aneurysm sac is partially perfused via arterial side branches originating from the aortic lumen. These side branches can be the IMA, lumbar arteries, or in rare cases, accessory renal arteries (Fig. 50-2). Direct arterial inflow into the sac occurs via this side branch perfusion despite tight sealing at the proximal and distal attachment sites. Typically, an inflow and outflow situation is present in type II ELs. Type II ELs can be further divided into simple single-vessel inflow and single-vessel outflow leaks (*type IIA*) and complex inflow and outflow vessel leaks, typically via multiple lumbar arteries (*type IIB*).
- *Type III ELs:* Type III ELs are caused by graft failure. Typically these types of ELs occur during long-term follow-up and are due to some type of fatigue of the fabric material or fracture of the stent component, or both. The stent-graft is under constant mechanical microstress caused by the steady impact of arterial pulsation. Over time, stent wires may break, and holes can develop in the fabric material. Stent-graft distortion may also lead to a type III EL. Eventually, remodeling of the aneurysm may occur and lead to increased bending of the graft. Again, this can be a reason for wire fracture and perforation of the fabric material. With early modular stent-graft designs, junctional separations were observed and resulted in type III ELs (Figs. 50-3 and 50-4). In these stent-graft designs, the overlapping zones at the junctions were too short. This problem has been addressed in newer stent-graft designs simply by extending the junctional overlapping zones. Type III ELs can also be subcategorized. A *type IIIA EL* is present if the EL is caused by a midgraft hole. A *type IIIB EL* is a junctional leak, and a *type IIIC EL* is caused by any other type of graft failure. Generally speaking, with

TABLE 50-1. Classification of Endoleaks

Type I		Attachment site leak
	A	Proximal
	B	Distal
	C	Iliac plug in aortouniiliac stent-grafts
Type II	A	Reperfusion leak
		Simple single inflow/outflow
	B	Leak
		Complex side branch perfusion
	Hyperdynamic on US	Quick wash-in
	Hypodynamic on US	Slow wash-in
Type III		Device-related leak
	A	Midgraft hole
	B	Junctional separation
	C	Any other leak caused by device failure
Type IV		Porosity leak
Type V		Endotension
	A	Sac enlargement without demonstration of EL with any imaging modality
	B	Sac enlargement, currently no EL discernible, but type I or II EL in previous examinations
	C	Type I or III EL proven at surgery, not shown during follow-up imaging
	D	Type II EL proven at surgery, not shown during follow-up imaging

EL, Endoleak; *US,* ultrasound.
(Modified from Veith FJ, Baum RA, Ohki T, et al. Nature and significance of endoleaks and endotension: summary of opinions expressed at an international conference. J Vasc Surg 2002;35:1029–35; Baum RA, Stavropoulos SW, Fairman RM, et al. Endoleaks after endovascular repair of abdominal aortic aneurysms. J Vasc Interv Radiol 2003;14:1111–7; and Parent FN, Meier GH, Godziachvili V, et al. The incidence and natural history of type I and II endoleak: a 5-year follow-up assessment with color duplex ultrasound scan. J Vasc Surg 2002;35:474–81.)

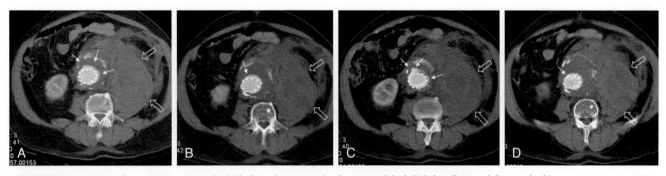

FIGURE 50-1. A-D, Axial computed tomography (CT) slices show a proximal type I endoleak (EL) *(small arrows)* that resulted in aneurysm rupture. Retroperitoneal hematoma can be seen clearly *(open arrows).*

newer stent-graft designs, the incidence of type III ELs has decreased. However, long-term follow-up beyond a period of 10 years is needed to demonstrate whether modern stent-graft designs are durable enough.

- *Type IV ELs:* These types of ELs are caused by graft porosity. The phenomenon of *angiographic blush* can be observed during the immediate postimplantation angiogram. Stent-graft designs differ in graft material composition, and immediately after implantation, some graft materials are temporarily slightly permeable. The degree of graft permeability is influenced by the degree of anticoagulation. This porosity is self-limiting and resolves within hours after EVAR. In most currently available stent-graft designs, graft material porosity has been reduced to a minimum, so type IV ELs are rarely a problem and have no real clinical relevance. The only important issue is that it can sometimes be difficult to differentiate a type IV arterial blush on the postimplantation angiogram from other clinically relevant forms of ELs. Some authors do not even consider a type IV EL to be a true EL.

- *Type V ELs:* Type V ELs are summarized under the term *endotension.* These types of ELs were not described in White's original 1997 classification but were added by the same authors 2 years later.[7] A type V EL, or endotension, is present if the diameter of the aneurysmal sac increases during follow-up without a discernible EL. A subcategorization differentiates type VA, VB, VC, and VD ELs.[6] *Type VA EL* is the actual endotension. Neither dual-phase contrast-enhanced CT nor any other imaging modality is capable of detecting an EL, and no EL has been shown in previous control studies, but the diameter of the sac increases. *Type VB EL* is present if the diameter of the sac increases and no EL is shown at a given follow-up CT, but a type I or II EL was shown on previous studies. Therefore, an EL might be still present but is not apparent on the given CT scan owing to flow dynamics. *Type VC and VD ELs* are surgically proven type I and III or type II ELs that have not been shown on CT or other imaging modalities.

Type I and III ELs are also called *device-related ELs* because a persistent channel of blood flow into the sac is

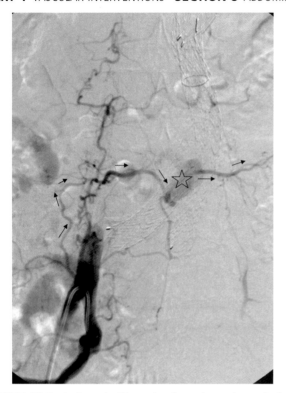

FIGURE 50-2. Angiography 18 months after endovascular repair shows a typical type II endoleak (EL) being fed by right iliolumbar artery. This artery communicates with right lumbar artery at the L5 level. Lumbar artery is perfused in a retrograde fashion *(arrows)*. In contrast, left lumbar artery showed antegrade flow *(arrows)*. An inflow/outflow situation thus occurs, the typical feature of a type II EL. EL itself is marked with a star.

present as a consequence of insufficient sealing of the graft at the proximal or distal attachment site, or at the junction zone of modular stent-grafts.

SIGNIFICANCE AND INCIDENCE OF ENDOLEAKS

Development of an EL is the most common undesired event during or after EVAR. The reason a primary type I EL develops is improper patient selection in most cases. It has been shown that a short aneurysmal neck, severe angulation and calcification, and extensive thrombus lining of the neck are risk factors for a type I EL.[8,9] If patients with these conditions are not considered for EVAR, primary type I ELs are rare events. Type III ELs are related to graft failure and are not under direct influence of the operator. These types of ELs were frequent with first- and second-generation stent-grafts.[10] The incidence decreased significantly with third-generation devices. Type II ELs are not typical complications because their development can hardly be influenced by the operation; they are inherent phenomena of EVAR.[3] Type IV ELs are not true ELs because they represent an angiographic feature without any clinical consequence.[3] Type V ELs seem to be related to type II ELs and can just barely be called complications.

In an analysis of 6787 patients from the registry database of the European Collaborating Groups on Stent-Graft Techniques for Abdominal Aortic Aneurysm Repair (EUROSTAR), the annual incidence of device-related ELs (i.e., type

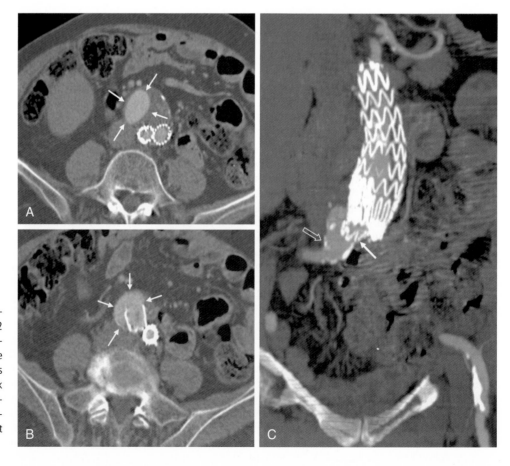

FIGURE 50-3. A-C, Computed tomographic angiography (CTA) follow-up 12 months after endovascular repair. Slippage of the right iliac limb out of the short right common iliac artery (CIA) has resulted in a distal type III endoleak *(white arrows)*. Multiplanar reconstruction **(C)** nicely shows relationship of dislocated iliac limb *(solid arrow)* to parent vessel *(open arrow)*.

DIAGNOSIS OF ENDOLEAKS

Because of their clinical relevance, most authors assume that diagnosis of ELs is important. Adequate follow-up care of patients after EVAR can be provided only if the responsible physician knows whether the patient has an EL and, if such is the case, which type of EL it is. Sufficient information about the morphologic evolution of the aneurysmal sac is vital, whether it be maximum sac diameter or, even better, sac volume.

Imaging modalities used for patient follow-up after EVAR and for diagnosis of ELs are CT, US, magnetic resonance imaging (MRI), intraarterial digital subtraction angiography (DSA), and plain abdominal radiology. As an alternative method of monitoring patients after EVAR, intraluminal sac pressure monitoring has been proposed. Each imaging modality is discussed separately in the following sections.

Diagnosis of Endoleaks with Computed Tomography

In many institutions, CT is still the most commonly used diagnostic imaging modality for post-EVAR patient follow-up. Typically, multiphase examinations are performed with multislice CT scanners, including an unenhanced, arterial, and delayed-phase scan.[17-19] Unenhanced images may be helpful in differentiating small perigraft leaks from areas of calcified thrombus or metallic structures of the stent-graft.[18] Typically the arterial-phase acquisition clearly shows perigraft flow if present. However, Rozenblit et al. showed that a delayed CT acquisition in addition to the arterial-phase scan can help detect additional ELs (Fig. 50-5). These authors also showed that the number of indeterminate findings can be reduced when an additional delayed-phase CT is acquired,[19] so a triphasic CT acquisition protocol, including a delayed-phase scan acquired 50 seconds after injection of contrast material, has now been adopted in many institutions.[20]

The diagnostic CT criterion for an EL is a contrast-enhancing area outside the stent-graft lumen but inside the aneurysmal sac. For correct classification of an EL, the location of the contrast-enhancing area, its relationship to the proximal and distal sealing zones, and the presence of possibly perfused side branches have to be evaluated. Additional desirable information includes stent-graft integrity, deformity, and migration.

In the case of a type I EL, direct communication of the parent vessel with the sac lumen may be depicted. Sometimes this communication can be displayed best in a multiformatted reconstruction (see Fig. 50-1).

The diagnostic clue to a type II EL is seeing contrast-enhancing side branches with direct communication to the area of contrast enhancement in the sac (Fig. 50-6).

In type III ELs, the EL is usually in direct communication with the stent-graft, and direct communication between the lumen of the stent-graft and sac can often be seen. Disintegration of the stent-graft and metallic strut fractures are strong indicators of a type III EL. Although the metallic skeleton of the stent-graft is typically evaluated by plain abdominal films, the same information can be provided by modern multislice CT scanners.[21]

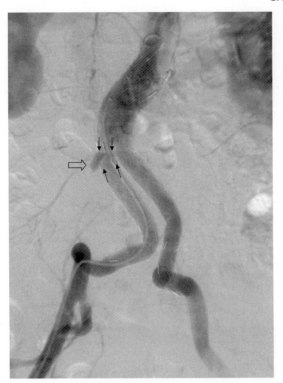

FIGURE 50-4. Angiographic follow-up 18 months after endovascular repair with a first-generation stent-graft. Right iliac limb has separated from stent-graft body *(arrows)*. A type III endoleak (EL) is the consequence *(open arrow)*.

I and III ELs) was 6% and that of type II ELs was 5%.[11] In this analysis, the authors showed a clear difference in performance of different stent-graft designs with regard to EL occurrence. Device-related ELs occur less frequently with second- and third-generation stent-grafts because they provide a better proximal and distal seal and better modular stability.

There is clear evidence that ELs directly influence the clinical outcome of EVAR.[12] It has been shown that type I and III ELs are significant risk factors for rupture after EVAR.[13] The incidence of these types of ELs varies between 0% and 10%[13] and strongly depends on patient selection.

The situation is less clear for type II ELs. Gelfand et al. summarized the results of 10 EVAR trials involving a total of 2617 patients.[14] The incidence of type II ELs was 6% to 17% at 30 days, 4.5% to 8% at 6 months, and 1% to 5% at 1 year. A EUROSTAR database analysis of 3595 patients showed significantly higher rates of secondary interventions in patients with type II ELs than in patients without ELs. However, conversion to open repair or post-EVAR rupture was not significantly associated with type II ELs.[15] In contrast, rupture of aneurysms with a type II EL has been described, although this occurs rarely.

The frequency of type V ELs is less well defined. Mennander et al. reported an incidence of 3.1% in a series of 160 patients; aneurysm rupture occurred in 3 of the 5 patients with endotension they followed. However, no significant intraperitoneal or retroperitoneal bleeding was observed.[16]

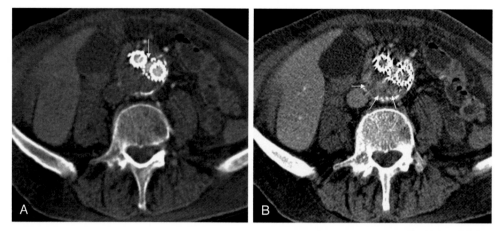

FIGURE 50-5. Computed tomographic angiography (CTA) follow-up 6 months after endovascular repair. This example shows potential benefit of a multiphase CT protocol. **A,** In the early arterial phase, no endoleak (EL) is shown. Contrast-enhancing structure medial to left limb *(arrow)* is inside stent-graft lumen. **B,** In the delayed phase, diffuse contrast enhancement outside stent-graft in dorsal part of aneurysmal sac can be seen, clearly indicative of EL *(arrows).* Because there was no increase in aneurysm size, these findings had no clinical consequence.

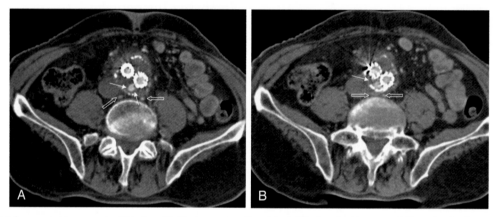

FIGURE 50-6. Axial computed tomography (CT) slices **(A, B)** show a type II endoleak (EL) *(small white arrows).* Note that lumbar arteries of segment L5 are well perfused and therefore permit an inflow/outflow situation *(open arrows).* However, CT is unable to show the direction of flow.

Type IV ELs do not play a clinically significant role, as already mentioned.

Type V ELs, by definition, are characterized by increasing diameter of the sac without a detectable EL.

Although CT has been advocated as the gold standard for EL detection,[19,22] it has several drawbacks. One is that a considerable amount of potentially nephrotoxic contrast medium is required. Depending on the multislice CT scan protocol, 80 to 120 mL of contrast medium per examination is used. Over a 5-year period, Azizzadeh et al.[23] found impaired renal function in 83% of their 398 patients who underwent EVAR. Impaired renal function was defined according to the American Kidney Foundation as a glomerular filtration rate (GFR) of less than 90 mL/h as calculated with the Cockcroft equation. Interestingly, only 16.1% of patients had an abnormal serum creatinine level in this study. The authors found that patients with a preoperative GFR of less than 45 mL/h had significantly worse 48-month survival rates than patients with higher preoperative GFR values, although perioperative mortality was comparable. Based on these observations, it can be stated that repeated application of contrast material may have an adverse influence on the clinical course of at least some patients.

Therefore, the authors conclude that periprocedural renal protection and the use of alternative contrast agents during follow-up might be beneficial in selected patients.

The second drawback of multislice CT is radiation exposure. Although several technical features are implemented in modern CT scanners to reduce radiation exposure, multislice CT remains a radiologic examination responsible for more than two thirds of the total patient radiation dose associated with medical imaging.[24] It is easy to understand that lifelong surveillance with at least annual CTs will lead to non-negligible radiation exposure. Based on an equation published by the International Commission for Radiation Protection, the lifetime risk for induction of cancer is 280 per million patients after a *single* abdominal CT scan.[22] Assuming an observation period of 10 years with 12 CTs, this would roughly mean a risk of inducing cancer in about 1 patient in 300. In this very simplistic calculation, the radiation risk associated with single examinations is merely added; multiplication of risk as a result of accumulation of radiation damage has not been taken into consideration.

Similarly, White and Macdonald estimate a total effective radiation exposure of 145 to 205 mSv for 70-year-old

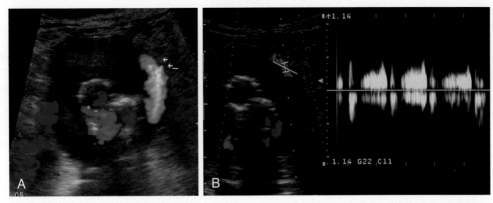

FIGURE 50-7. A, Color-coded ultrasound. Transverse image shows a large communicating type II endoleak (EL) *(arrows)* perfused via fourth lumbar arteries and inferior mesenteric artery. **B,** Spectral Doppler ultrasound shows pulsatile flow in EL. *(Courtesy J. Martin, S. Wallace, and R. McWilliams from the Liverpool Royal Hospital.)*

patients, including planning CT, EVAR, and surveillance CT at 1, 3, 6, and 12 months and yearly thereafter. In their calculation, this leads to a lifetime cancer risk of 0.42%, or 1 in 240. These numbers become more worrisome with decreasing patient age. For a 50-year-old patient, the cancer risk would be 0.73%, or 1 in 140.[25] However, a mitigating factor is that we are dealing with an elderly patient population usually well above the age of 65, and it has been well documented that radiation risk is significantly lower in the elderly.

Nevertheless, contrast medium load and radiation exposure are important concerns when serial CTs are performed for long-term follow-up of patients after EVAR. For this reason, two studies evaluated whether the commonly used multiphase CT protocol can be reduced by eliminating the early arterial phase,[26] or the unenhanced or delayed phase, or both.[27] The authors of the first study concluded that the arterial phase may not be necessary for routine EL detection, whereas the authors of the latter study found that the combination of unenhanced and arterial-phase CT affords the highest positive predictive value for detection of ELs after 1 month, and that the delayed phase does not significantly increase the sensitivity for detection of ELs, although ELs not seen on early-phase CT may be seen on delayed-phase CT.[26,27] In another study, Bley et al. showed that serial volumetric analysis of nonenhanced CT may serve as an adequate screening test to identify ELs that cause a volumetric increase of more than 2%.[28] Recently, dual-energy CT has been evaluated for EL detection after EVAR.[29] With dual-energy CT, only one single delayed scan is acquired with a dual-source CT scanner. From this dataset, a virtual nonenhanced scan is calculated. Compared with a triphasic CT protocol, there was no significant difference in the numbers of ELs detected, but the radiation dose was up to 61% less.

The third drawback of CT is that it cannot display flow dynamics. In some cases, correct EL classification depends on evaluating the direction of perigraft flow and the direction of flow in aneurysmal side branches. This problem is discussed in the sections describing the value of DSA and US in patient follow-up after EVAR.

The ideal CT protocol has not yet been defined. Although it is of utmost importance to apply the CT protocol with the best tradeoff between radiation and contrast medium exposure and diagnostic yield, proper timing and selection of the imaging modality used during follow-up have the largest influence.

Diagnosis of Endoleaks with Ultrasonography

US is being used more frequently as an alternative to multiphase CT in patient follow-up after EVAR. It is less expensive, and no radiation or nephrotoxic contrast material is required (Fig. 50-7).[30,31] The reliability of US in detecting ELs has been evaluated in numerous studies. In an early study, Sato et al. reported a 74% specificity and 97% sensitivity of color-coded US (ccUS) for detection of ELs.[30] Better results were reported by Zannetti et al., who found an encouragingly high 91.7% sensitivity and 98.4% specificity of ccUS for EL detection, with CT serving as the standard of reference.[31] In contrast, Raman et al. found only 42.9% sensitivity of ccUS in detecting ELs. Its specificity was 96%, and the positive predictive value was 53.9%, with only modest correlation of the results of ccUS and CT. Based on their experience with 281 patients, the authors concluded that ccUS cannot effectively replace CT after EVAR.[32]

In more recent studies, contrast-enhanced US (CEUS) has been compared with CT. Encouraging results have been reported by Giannoni et al.[33] and Napoli et al.[34] In both studies, CEUS showed ELs not detected by other imaging modalities. One potential advantage of US over other imaging modalities is its ability to characterize blood flow dynamics. For instance, a persistent EL is typically associated with an inflow and outflow situation. In contrast to CT, these flow phenomena can be evaluated with US. In a small but interesting series of 18 patients, Bargellini et al.[35] used CEUS to analyze the hemodynamic flow pattern of type II ELs and found a correlation of type II EL flow dynamics and AAA size. Type II ELs with wash-in and wash-out times less than 100 and 520 seconds, respectively, were called *hyperdynamic ELs*, in contrast to *hypodynamic ELs*, which had longer wash-in and wash-out times.[35] The authors showed that a volume increase of 1 mL per month or greater might be associated with hypodynamic type II ELs. They hypothesized that insufficient outflow from the sac in a hypodynamic EL could lead to pressurization of the aneurysm and possible enlargement. On the other hand, in hyperdynamic type II ELs, a widely patent inflow and outflow tract might allow free flow through the aneurysm without significant effects on pressure. In a more recent study, Beeman et al. also tried to determine Doppler sonographic flow parameters, which may be associated with the persistence of type II ELs and an increase in AAA sac diameter. In contrast to the Bargellini study, they found no correlation between the intrasac flow velocity and increased AA size after EVAR. However, the presence of multiple type II ELs and a bidirectional intrasac flow were identified as possible predictors of an increase in sac diameter.[36] In another study, Parent et al. showed that a to-and-fro flow pattern in a type II EL is more often associated with spontaneous sealing of the EL than is the case with a monophasic or biphasic flow pattern.[37]

Despite these interesting observations, the roles of ccUS and CEUS are still under evaluation. In a systematic review performed by Ashoke et al. and based on eight published and two unpublished studies, the sensitivity and specificity of US were 69% and 91%, respectively. The authors concluded that US does not have sufficient diagnostic accuracy for detection of all ELs in routine clinical practice.[38] However, this conclusion was only partially confirmed by Mirza et al.,[39] who performed a more recent and more extensive systematic review. Twenty-one studies comparing ccUS with CT and seven studies comparing CEUS with CT were included. Similar to Ashoke's analysis, sensitivity for ccUS (77%) was rather low, but specificity was 94%. However, CEUS had a sensitivity and specificity of 98% and 88%, respectively.[39]

Another important parameter during patient follow-up after EVAR is sac diameter. US was thought to be less reliable than CT for sac measurement, but several recent studies have shown them to be equally reliable.[40]

The fact that CEUS may detect ELs not shown by computed tomographic angiography (CTA) explains why CTA can no longer be considered the standard of reference.[31,34,41] Most endoleaks are shown by both imaging modalities, but some are only seen on CTA and some only by CEUS.

In general, ccUS and especially CEUS are valid methods for patient follow-up after EVAR, and in many centers, US has replaced CTA as the standard method.

Diagnosis of Endoleaks with Magnetic Resonance Imaging

Because lifelong surveillance is necessary after EVAR, a noninvasive imaging tool that does not expose the patient to radiation and nephrotoxic contrast media is desirable. MRI seems to fulfill these demands, and its potential use for post-EVAR patient follow-up has been evaluated in several studies.

It is well known that metallic implants cause artifacts in MRI images, and the metallic skeleton and metallic markers of stent-grafts may certainly do so.[42] Two types of artifacts can be observed. The ferromagnetic components of the stent-graft cause *susceptibility artifacts*. The higher the content of ferromagnetic material, the stronger the artifact. In some stent-grafts, such as the Zenith endoprosthesis (Cook Medical, Bloomington, Ind.) and the Lifepath stent-graft (Edwards Lifesciences, Irvine, Calif.), this type of artifact makes evaluation of the abdomen impossible. Other types of endoprostheses with a skeleton made of nonferromagnetic material (e.g., nitinol) cause only minimal susceptibility artifacts that do not compromise the examination's diagnostic value.

The other type of artifact is caused by radiofrequency shielding as a result of the cage-like structure of the metal component.[43] This *radiofrequency shielding effect* is strongly influenced by the geometric orientation of the stent and conductance of the metal. The shielding effect can lead to a reduction in luminal signal to various degrees.[44]

Several types of stent-grafts have been tested for their MRI compatibility. Generally speaking, it has been shown that stent-grafts with nitinol components cause minor artifacts, whereas stent-grafts with steel or Elgiloy components cause severe artifacts that make diagnosis impossible.

Safety aspects must be considered as well. Two potential safety hazards exist. One is the risk of dislodgement by the strong magnetic field, and the other is heating. van der Laan et al. tested seven different stent-graft designs in an in vitro experiment. They found no attractive or torque force in stent-grafts with a nitinol skeleton, but some force when the Zenith and Lifepath devices were tested. The skeleton of both devices has stronger ferromagnetic properties. However, the authors assume that the MRI safety of these two devices is not very relevant for follow-up because their extensive image artifacts render MRI-based follow-up of these devices senseless.[46]

Heating effects can be caused by the process of resistive dissipation of energy from eddy currents, by currents from conducting loops, and by resonating radiofrequency waves.[44] However, to the best of our knowledge, no adverse effects from any commercially available stent-graft design have been reported in the current literature with the use of a 1.5-T MRI scanner.

Several studies have proved that MRI can be a valuable option for surveillance of nitinol-supported stent-grafts.[45] Although clinical experience with MRI surveillance is still limited, it has been shown that discrete ELs can be shown more clearly with contrast-enhanced MRI than with CT, because MRI is much more sensitive than CT to contrast medium–induced signal changes (Fig. 50-8). In a small series, van der Laan et al. found that dynamic contrast-enhanced MRI is capable of detecting more ELs than multiphasic CT and allows more precise EL classification.[46] These findings have been confirmed by Wieners et al.,[47] who found that diagnostic accuracy was superior to CTA in 66% of their patients. With time-resolved magnetic resonance angiography (MRA), flow direction can be determined.[48] As is the case with US or intraarterial angiography, different types of ELs can be discriminated by demonstration of the flow pattern in a given EL. This specific type of analysis is not possible with CT. Nevertheless, in most institutions MRA is not used as a routine examination for patient follow-up after EVAR. It may, however, be helpful in more difficult cases.

Diagnosis of Endoleaks with Plain Abdominal Films

Endoleaks cannot be detected directly with plain abdominal films. However, change in the integrity of the stent-graft or stent-graft migration (or both) is an indicator of a possible EL. Typically, plain abdominal films are acquired at each control CT examination. Plain radiography can show stent-graft migration, kinking, or other deformities; limb dislocation; strut fractures; separation of stent-graft components; and progressive dilation of components of the graft[49] (Fig. 50-9). However, with 16- and 64-row (and upwards) CT

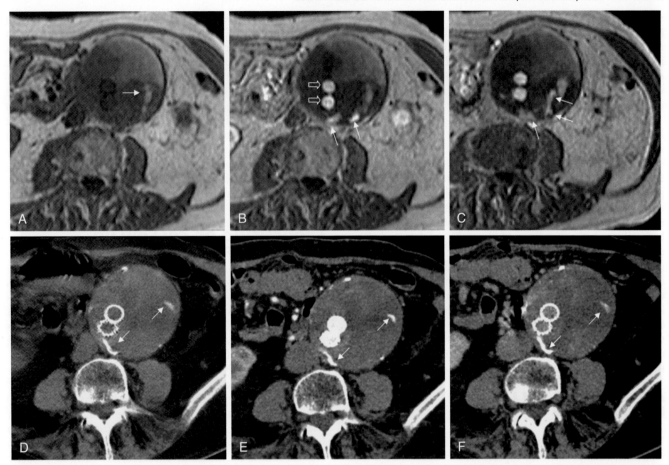

FIGURE 50-8. A-C, Dynamic contrast-enhanced magnetic resonance imaging (MRI) 12 months after endovascular repair with a Gore endoprosthesis. Example nicely shows possible advantages of MRI in detection of endoleaks (ELs). In nonenhanced phase, a faint hyperintense area can be seen in left lateral part of aneurysm *(arrow)* that may be caused by fresh thrombus. In arterial phase, both iliac limbs show intense enhancement with contrast material and are well perfused *(open arrows)*, but there is obvious contrast enhancement in aneurysmal sac *(white arrows)*. In delayed phase, EL is even more obvious *(arrows)*. **D-F,** Multiphase computed tomographic angiography (CTA) in same patient on same day. Aneurysmal sac is filled with inhomogeneous thrombotic material; some flakes of calcium can also been seen *(arrows)*. However, in no phase of examination can EL detected on MRI be seen.

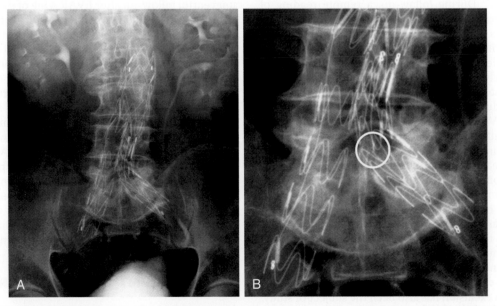

FIGURE 50-9. Plain abdominal film 24 months after endovascular repair with a Talent stent-graft system. Because of obvious kink in left iliac limb, longitudinal connect bar is broken *(inside white ring)*. This had no clinical consequences.

scanners, isovolumetric data acquisition in all three directions has become possible. With these types of CT scanners, the metallic component of the stent-graft is displayed in great detail, so if CTA is performed with a high-resolution multislice CT system, strut fractures and other postinterventional complications can be detected, and plain abdominal films may not be necessary.[21]

Diagnosis of Endoleaks with Intraarterial Angiography

Intraarterial arteriography is not a routine procedure in patient follow-up after EVAR. Nevertheless, some authors consider angiography the standard of reference for EL diagnosis.[6] With arteriography, every single attachment site can be evaluated specifically, and if an EL is detected, flow dynamics can be seen, facilitating proper EL classification (see Fig. 50-2). It is well known that an EL detected by CT in the vicinity of the lumbar arteries can be a type II EL if flow in the lumbar artery is retrograde, or a type I EL if flow is antegrade. However, CT cannot provide this information. Only intraarterial angiography, US, or eventually, dynamic time-resolved MRI may show flow direction.[6] Therefore, in unclear situations, intraarterial angiography is the examination of choice for the further evaluation of ELs.

ALTERNATIVE FOLLOW-UP POSSIBILITIES

The basic principle of EVAR is depressurization of the aneurysm sac, thus preventing rupture. It has been shown that ELs may be associated with increased intrasac pressure. An alternative method to monitor patients after EVAR could be assessment of intrasac pressure. However, until recently, measurement of sac pressure required an invasive procedure, either placement of a catheter into the sac during the insertion procedure or direct puncture of the sac during follow-up. With new technical developments, a miniaturized pressure sensor has become available that can be placed inside the aneurysm sac during the stent-graft insertion procedure.[50] During follow-up, a remote reading of intrasac pressure can be performed via an antenna placed on the patient's abdomen. This device has been tested in animal experiments, and the first human experience is already available. It has been shown that shrinkage of the aneurysm clearly correlates with low intrasac pressure.

In a recent study, 55 patients were monitored with pressure sensors during stent-graft insertion and up to 12 months after EVAR. When the aneurysm was excluded successfully, a significant intraoperative pressure decrease was observed. During follow-up, increased intrasac pressure necessitated treatment of 4 of 14 patients with type II ELs. The authors concluded that noninvasive pressure sensors may provide important information during the insertion procedure and may be of value during follow-up to detect clinically relevant ELs.[51] However, at present the pressure distribution in the aneurysmal sac is not known, and the reliability of the sensor device must be proved in more experimental and clinical studies.

Whether D-dimer assay can be an indicator of incomplete aneurysm exclusion has also been the subject of study. D-dimer is a cross-linked fibrin degradation product released into the bloodstream in the event of an ongoing fibrinolytic process, which is typically activated after a recent thrombotic event. After complete exclusion of an aneurysm, a stable clot is formed in the sac that essentially undergoes organization. However, if blood flow in the sac persists, a steady state of thrombus formation and compensatory fibrinolysis may occur and result in a possible increase in D-dimer. This hypothesis has been evaluated in a multicenter study that included 74 patients after EVAR. It was shown that patients with type I ELs and those with unchanged or increasing sac diameter had significantly higher D-dimer serum levels than patients with decreasing sac diameters.[52] These observations are interesting, but the clinical value of the D-dimer level in patient follow-up after EVAR is unclear.

SEQUENCING OF FOLLOW-UP AFTER EVAR

Until recently, a typical follow-up protocol after EVAR was a CT scan at 1, 3, 6, and 12 months and annually thereafter.[1,2] With increasing experience, however, the requirement for such a rigid follow-up regimen has been questioned. As mentioned earlier, the value of US has been proven, and the potential risks of frequent CTA have been addressed.

In a meta-analysis and systematic review of 32 manuscripts that included 17,987 EVAR cases, Nordon et al.[53] found that 90% of patients received no benefit from surveillance imaging. On the other hand, Jones et al.[54] showed that patients with incomplete follow-up after EVAR have a higher fatal complication rate than patients who undergo regular follow-up imaging. Therefore, as early as possible after the primary intervention, it is important to identify any patients with a high risk of complicated follow-up that may necessitate a secondary intervention or even lead to late rupture; such patients should undergo a strict follow-up regimen. On the other hand, patients with a low risk of aneurysm-related morbidity and mortality after EVAR may be allocated to a less rigid follow-up regimen. This would lead to a risk-adjusted follow-up protocol.[55]

Several factors have been identified as predictors of uneventful follow-up after EVAR. One of these is significant shrinkage of the aneurysmal sac. Houbballah et al.[56] showed that significant sac shrinkage after 12 months is associated with low aneurysm-related mortality and morbidity and good long-term outcome. It has also been shown that a normal 1-month CTA showing no EL is associated with lower aneurysm-related morbidity and mortality compared with patients with an EL; no benefit accrued from a 6-month CTA if the 1-month CTA was normal.[55] Similar results were reported from the U.S. Powerlink system (Endologix, Irvine, Calif) trial. A total of 1591 post-EVAR CTAs performed in 345 patients were analyzed. The negative predictive value of the post-EVAR CTA for a secondary intervention was 96.4%, and if US was included, the value could be increased to 97.6%.[57] These data obviously show that the initial post-EVAR CT is an important parameter for risk stratification. A reasonable risk-adjusted follow-up regimen is shown in Figure 50-10.

MANAGEMENT OF ENDOLEAKS

The indication for treatment of ELs is based on two variables. First, the type of EL must be defined. Type I and III

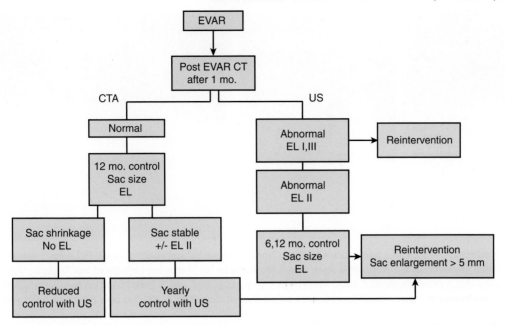

FIGURE 50-10. Flow chart schematic proposing a risk-adjusted follow-up protocol for endovascular aneurysm repair *(EVAR)* using either computed tomographic angiography (CTA) or ultrasound *(US)*. *EL,* Endoleak. *(Modified from Sternbergh WC 3rd, Greenberg RK, Chuter TA, et al. Redefining postoperative surveillance after endovascular aneurysm repair: recommendations based on 5-year follow-up in the US Zenith multicenter trial. J Vasc Surg 2008;48:278–84.)*

TABLE 50-2. Influence of Type of Endoleak and Sac Behavior on Indication for Treatment

Endoleak	Type I	Type II	Type III	Type IV	Type V
Diameter decreasing	++	−	++	−	−
Diameter stable	++	−	++	−	na
Diameter increasing	++	+	++	−	+

++, Treatment highly recommended; −, conservative management recommended; *na,* in type V ELs, the sac increases in size by definition.

ELs are so-called high-pressure ELs and require treatment whenever possible.[58] In contrast, most type II ELs are benign, and treatment becomes necessary only when sac diameter increases.[59]

The second variable is the status of the sac. It has been shown that sac shrinkage is associated with a good long-term outcome.[56] Patients with a stable sac diameter who do not have a high pressure EL (i.e., type I or III EL) are observed regardless of whether there is a type II EL present. An enlarging sac is an indication for treatment. Table 50-2 shows how the combination of these two variables influences the indication for treatment of ELs.

Treatment of Type I Endoleaks

A type I EL is a proximal attachment site leak. As previously mentioned, this is a high-pressure EL and therefore warrants treatment whenever possible. Type I ELs may be caused by stent-graft migration or dilation of the neck,[60] and sometimes by both factors occurring simultaneously. In cases of migration, the proximal leak may be sealed by insertion of an extension cuff.[61] However, because most aneurysms associated with migration have short necks, it may be challenging to place the extension cuff high enough

to seal the leak and also maintain patency of the renal arteries.

If neck dilation is the main reason for the EL, sealing may be achieved by reinforcement of the proximal section of the stent-graft with a large Palmaz stent.[62] Fenestrated and branched stent-grafts may offer an attractive future alternative in instances where the neck is too short or dilated, or in cases of significant mismatch between the diameter of the stent-graft and the aortic neck.

Some authors also report successful embolization of type I ELs with liquid embolization material like Onyx (ev3/Covidien, Plymouth, Minn.).[63] Although initial technical success has been observed in several cases, it must be taken into consideration that the neck is not reinforced, and migration is not prevented.

If endoluminal procedures are unsuccessful, late surgical conversion must be considered. In fact, type I ELs are the most common causes of late surgical conversion after EVAR.[64]

Type IB ELs are usually treated easily by stent-graft extension. If progressive dilation of the distal landing zone makes it impossible to achieve a tight seal in the common iliac artery, it may be necessary to extend the stent-graft into the external iliac artery, which usually has a smaller diameter. If this is the case, to avoid a type II EL due to

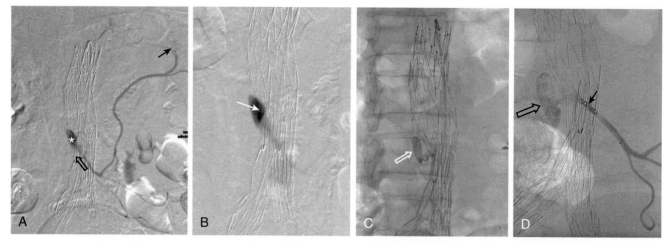

FIGURE 50-11. Transarterial treatment of a type II endoleak (EL). **A,** Typical angiographic appearance of type II EL *(asterisk)* mainly fed by arc of Riolan and retrogradely perfused inferior mesenteric artery (IMA) *(open arrow)*. Microcatheter has already been introduced into Riolan arc *(arrow)*. **B,** Tip of micro-catheter already in center of EL *(arrow)*. Embolization should ideally begin from this position. **C and D,** Embolization has been performed with bucrylate, which was injected into sac, obliterating EL *(open arrows)*. Thereafter, coil embolization of main trunk of IMA has been performed *(solid arrow)*. Flow in EL was abolished.

retrograde flow, the internal iliac artery should be occluded near its origin before insertion of the stent-graft extension.

Treatment of Type II Endoleaks

In most institutions, type II endoleaks are treated if the maximum sac diameter increases by 5 mm or more within a 6-month observation period. Patients with a persistent type II EL but a stable sac diameter may be treated conservatively.

The etiopathologic principle of type II ELs is based on an inflow/outflow dynamic in the sac despite an adequately inserted stent-graft. Arteries contributing to reperfusion of the sac are the IMA, lumbar arteries, and rarely accessory renal arteries. For effective treatment, this inflow/outflow action must be interrupted. Ideally the EL should be embolized in its center, like the nidus of an arteriovenous malformation. This can be accomplished by three methods: a transarterial arterial approach, percutaneous sac puncture, and transcaval sac puncture.

Transarterial Arterial Approach
Many type II ELs are fed by a retrogradely perfused IMA. In most cases, it is relatively straightforward to navigate a microcatheter via the arc of Riolan into the stump of the IMA and directly into the sac. Embolization should be performed directly in the sac at the center of the EL to occlude all in- and outflow vessels (Fig. 50-11). If only the inflow via the IMA is occluded, perfusion of the EL may be maintained by recruitment of other side branches, much like a partially embolized arteriovenous malformation. Embolization can be performed with coils and/or liquid embolic agents like thrombin, bucrylate, or Onyx.

Transarterial embolization can also be performed via the iliolumbar branches of the hypogastric arteries, since these arteries can serve as collaterals to lumbar arteries. However, it is often impossible to reach the lumbar arteries, owing to the tortuous course of the iliolumbar arteries. Again, the

goal must be to reach the sac and not just embolize the side branch.

Percutaneous Sac Puncture
An alternative approach to the EL is direct sac puncture. Percutaneous puncture of the sac can be done via a translumbar or transabdominal approach, depending on the patient's physiognomy and the shape and size of the aneurysm. With the transabdominal approach, puncture can be performed under US guidance, which this author prefers where possible (Fig. 50-12). The translumbar approach might be safer if bleeding complications from the sac are considered. However, no comparative studies have yet been performed measuring the differences in outcome between the two approaches. If the sac is punctured, embolization is performed with coils, thrombin, and/or liquid embolization material.

Transcaval Sac Puncture
A third possibility to approach the sac is via the inferior vena cava. For the transcaval approach, a transjugular intrahepatic portosystemic shunt (TIPS) puncture set is inserted via the common femoral vein into the inferior vena cava, from where the sac is punctured. Embolization is performed as described earlier. This technique has been described by Mansueto et al. in 12 patients, with a success rate of 92%.[65]

In an early study, Baum et al. compared the results of translumbar and transarterial IMA embolization of type II ELs in 33 patients. Translumbar embolization was much more successful, with only 1 technical failure in 13 procedures, whereas transarterial embolization failed in 16 out of 20 patients.[66] However, with a modified technique of transarterial embolization, better results can be achieved. Stravropoulos et al. did not embolize just one feeding artery, but tried to enter the sac with a microcatheter and perform an intrasac embolization, as is done with a translumbar approach. With this technique, the authors achieved results similar to the translumbar technique. The technical success

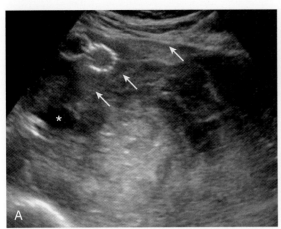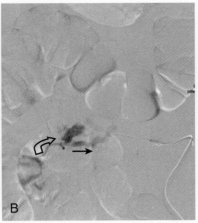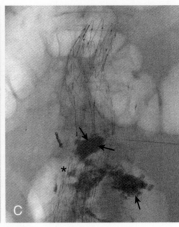

FIGURE 50-12. Treatment of a type II endoleak (EL) by direct sac puncture. **A,** Transabdominal puncture of a type II EL under sonographic guidance. Needle can be seen clearly under US *(arrows).* Tip of needle was guided into center of area of maximum perfusion *(asterisk).* **B,** Direct contrast injection nicely displays EL. Inflow *(open arrow)* and outflow *(solid arrow)* vessels can be clearly seen. **C,** Bucrylate was injected directly into EL via transabdominal approach. Distribution of glue nicely reflects angioanatomic outline of EL *(arrows).* Unfortunately, only a minimal amount of glue reached right lumbar artery *(asterisk).*

rate was 78% in 23 patients treated with a transarterial approach, compared to 72% in 62 patients after translumbar embolization.[67] Sarac et al. reported their experience with 140 embolization procedures in 95 patients with type II ELs and increasing sac size. They used both the transarterial and translumbar techniques, depending on the patient's vascular anatomy. Various combinations of coils, coils and glue, or glue alone were used. They found no long-term difference (after 5 years) in terms of access route or embolized vessel. The only significant factor in the univariable analysis was embolization with coils only. Patients treated in this way were more likely to undergo a second embolization.[68]

There are no clear guidelines for choosing a specific technique. It seems reasonable to take an individualized approach depending on the unique angioanatomic situation. If it seems easy to reach the endoleak via a transarterial approach, whether it is the IMA or one of the iliolumbar arteries, this access should be preferred. However, if the feeding arteries are very small and tortuous, which may be especially true for the iliolumbar vessels, a direct approach to the endoleak should be taken.[68]

Complications of both techniques involve nontarget embolization, which may lead to ischemia of the colon[68] or even skin necrosis.[69] In our experience, we observed one patient who developed ipsilateral sciatic nerve symptoms after embolization via the iliolumbar artery. For translumbar embolization, retroperitoneal hematoma has been reported as a complication.[68]

Treatment of Type III Endoleaks

Type III ELs are high-pressure ELs and require treatment when diagnosed. With third-generation stent-graft designs, this type of EL is infrequent.[62] Typically, stent-graft separation is the cause, although rarely a graft tear can be the reason for the leak. Most type III ELs are treated by insertion of another stent-graft that lines the area of separation or graft tear (Fig. 50-13). In rare circumstances, severe stent-graft distortion may necessitate explantation of the device.

Treatment of Type V Endoleaks

Type V ELs are an exclusion diagnosis. The sac size increases without a discernable EL. Since by definition, no specific leak can be detected, treatment is always nonfocused and has no guarantee of success. Treatment options include stent-graft relining with a coaxial system, most often with a monoiliac device. We treated one patient with repeated sac puncture and evacuation of serous fluid in order to decompress the abdomen. However, this was a purely symptomatic treatment, and the patient was ultimately converted to open surgery.[70]

As for all types of problematic ELs, especially for type V ELs, a surgical solution should always be considered.

SUMMARY

Although stent-graft designs have been improved over the last few years, postinterventional surveillance is still essential for patients after EVAR. The surveillance method varies from center to center and is influenced by local factors (Table 50-3), but in most centers contrast-enhanced CT and US are the imaging methods of choice for follow-up. In recent years, there was a clear shift from CTA to US for routine follow-up, but a gold standard for EL detection has not been clearly defined. Currently, MRI does not play an important role in this field, although this may change in future.

At our institution, we perform the first follow-up CT scan 1 month after stent-graft insertion if the primary procedure was uneventful and no type I EL was seen on a high-quality final completion angiogram during the implantation procedure. In the case of a type I EL that is not fixed during the initial procedure, we perform an early control CT scan while the patient is still in the hospital. Depending on the patient's general condition and the results of the early CT scan, definitive treatment of the EL is performed.

If the 1-month CTA is normal and does not show an EL, the next CTA is performed 12 months after stent-graft

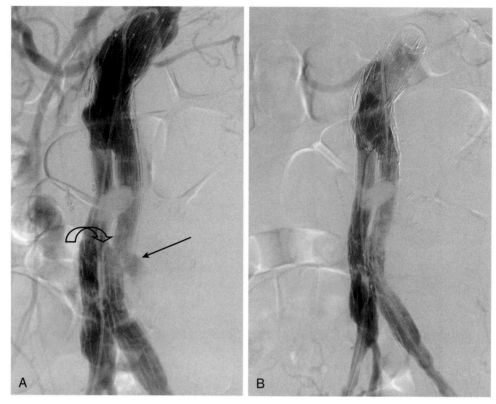

FIGURE 50-13. A, Double type III endoleak (EL) in a patient with detachment of both iliac limbs from main body of prosthesis *(arrows)*. EL on right side is hard to see *(solid arrow)*. **B,** Treatment was relatively easy, with coaxial insertion of two stent-grafts in each limb.

TABLE 50-3. Summary of Diagnostic Value of Currently Applied Imaging Modalities in Follow-Up After Endovascular Repair

Imaging Modality	Advantage	Disadvantage	Current Status
Multiphasic contrast-enhanced CT	Easy to perform Every type of stent-graft can be evaluated	Iodinated CM needed Radiation Uncertain classification of ELs	Standard of reference Routine FU examination in most centers Examination at 3, 6, and 12 months and yearly thereafter
MRI	No iodinated CM needed No radiation Excellent contrast resolution Flow patterns in EL may be shown	Suitable only for certain stent-graft designs Contraindicated in patients with a pacemaker Metal skeleton cannot be evaluated	Good alternative to CT if stent-grafts are MRI compatible
Ultrasound	No radiation No contraindications Shows flow phenomena	Strong operator dependency Metal skeleton cannot be evaluated	Valuable method in experienced hands CM may improve diagnostic value
Plain films	Good overview of metallic parts Migration and distortion well shown	No visualization of the sac EL not shown directly	Part of routine FU in many departments, performed in addition to other examinations
Intraarterial angiography	Specific examination of every attachment and connection site possible Flow dynamics can be shown	Invasive procedure Iodinated CM needed	Not a routine procedure Usually performed if noninvasive imaging modalities provide no clear information
Alternative methods	Completely noninvasive (sac pressure sensor)	Unclear value	Not widely available

CM, contrast material; *CT,* computed tomography; *EL,* endoleak; *FU,* follow-up; *MRI,* magnetic resonance imaging.

insertion. If that examination is also normal, we rely on CEUS during further follow-up in yearly intervals.

If the 1-month CT shows an EL which can be clearly defined as a type II EL, a 12-month CTA is performed, and the future follow-up strategy is dependent on the evolution of the sac diameter. With increasing diameter, we intervene when the sac diameter has increased by at least 5 mm. With a constant sac diameter, we also follow our patients with yearly CEUS examinations.

For CTA we still rely on three-phase contrast-enhanced CT. However, in patients with renal insufficiency, we prefer to insert MRI-compatible stent-grafts and perform MRI studies during follow-up, in addition to plain abdominal films. In rare cases in which neither multiphasic CT nor CEUS is conclusive, we perform intraarterial arteriography.

KEY POINTS

- *Endoleaks* (ELs), defined as the phenomenon of perigraft flow, remain a specific problem after endovascular repair of aortic aneurysms.

- Because the development of ELs, especially type I and III ELs, is associated with a higher frequency of adverse events in long-term follow-up, strict surveillance of all patients after endovascular repair is mandatory.

- The most commonly used imaging modality for follow-up is multiphasic computed tomography (CT). However, CT carries the risk of contrast medium–induced nephropathy, as well as the risks associated with exposure to radiation.

- Doppler ultrasound with or without contrast enhancement has proved to be a valuable tool in follow-up.

- A risk-adjusted follow-up regimen that helps optimize the timing and number of follow-up examinations should be applied.

- Future trends include the use of intrasac pressure sensors, which may allow monitoring of patients after endovascular repair and thus reduce the number of follow-up CT or magnetic resonance imaging (MRI) examinations.

- Type I and III ELs are high-pressure ELs and should be treated whenever possible.

- Type II ELs are often benign and are managed conservatively when the sac size is stable.

- Persistent type II ELs should be treated when the sac diameter increases by 5 mm or more.

► SUGGESTED READINGS

De Bruin JL, Baas AF, Buth J, et al; for the DREAM Study Group. Long-term outcome of open or endovascular repair of abdominal aortic aneurysm. N Engl J Med 2010;362:1881–9.

Mirza T, Karthikesalingam A, Jackson D, et al. Duplex ultrasound and contrast-enhanced ultrasound versus computed tomography for the detection of endoleak after EVAR: systematic review and bivariate meta-analysis. Eur J Vasc Endovasc Surg 2010;39:418–28.

Naughton PA, Garcia-Toca M, Rodriguez HE, et al. Endovascular treatment of type 1 and 3 endoleaks. Cardiovasc Intervent Radiol 2011;34:751–7.

Stavropoulos SW, Park J, Fairman R, et al. Type 2 endoleak embolization comparison: translumbar versus modified transarterial embolization. J Vasc Interv Radiol 2009;20:1299–302.

Sternbergh WC 3rd, Greenberg RK, Chuter TA, et al. Redefining postoperative surveillance after endovascular aneurysm repair: recommendations based on 5-year follow-up in the US Zenith multicenter trial. J Vasc Surg 2008;48:278–84.

The United Kingdom EVAR Trial Investigators. Endovascular versus open repair of abdominal aortic aneurysm. N Engl J Med 2010;362:1863–71.

The complete reference list is available online at www.expertconsult.com.

CHAPTER 51

Endovascular Treatment of Dissection of the Aorta and Its Branches

Matthew D. Forrester and Michael D. Dake

INTRODUCTION

Management of aortic dissection is complex and directed by multiple patient and disease-specific factors requiring a complication-specific approach. Appropriate aortic imaging is paramount for both diagnosis and treatment planning. Initial blood pressure, heart rate control, and monitoring in the intensive care unit setting are critical. Descending aortic dissections (Stanford type B, DeBakey III) complicated by rupture, rapid false lumen expansion, tissue malperfusion, or intractable pain or uncontrollable hypertension are likely to require acute intervention. Conversely, uncomplicated type B dissections are typically treated medically. With the advent and evolution of endovascular techniques, less invasive treatment options are becoming available to the clinician more often. Ultimately, treatment of aortic dissection will likely employ multiple techniques and patient- and disease-specific approaches.

INDICATIONS FOR INTERVENTION

Appropriate treatment for an aortic dissection is determined by a combination of location and extent of the dissection, time from onset of symptoms, comorbid risk factors, and dissection-related conditions such as visceral malperfusion or impending rupture. Although most patients present with acute dissection, up to a third present with symptoms of more than 2 weeks' duration.[1] This distinction between acute and chronic dissection is of therapeutic significance because patients with acute aortic dissections are at highest risk for life-threatening complications. In the current era, treatment options can be divided into three main categories: medical management, surgical intervention, and endovascular intervention. Recommendations for the management of thoracic aortic dissection have been made by the 2010 American College of Cardiology Foundation/American Heart Association (ACCF/AHA) task force for the diagnosis and management of patients with thoracic aortic disease.[2]

Ascending aortic dissections (Stanford type A, DeBakey I, II) account for about 60% of all dissections[3] and are at high risk of acute complications including cardiac tamponade (5%), myocardial ischemia (7%-19%), acute aortic regurgitation (45%), heart failure (5%), stroke (8%), and ultimately death.[4] The mortality rate for acute type A dissections without intervention is estimated at 1% per hour after patients arrive in the hospital, with mortality rates of 38%, 50%, 70%, and 90% at 24 hours, 48 hours, 1 week, and 2 weeks, respectively.[5,6] In general, type A dissections require emergent surgical repair. Presently, there are no U.S. Food and Drug Administration (FDA)-approved endovascular devices for the ascending aorta.[2]

There remains some controversy over the treatment strategy of type B aortic dissections. In 1965, DeBakey et al.

published a large series of 179 aortic dissection patients treated surgically, with an operative mortality of 21% and a 5-year mortality of 50%.[7] In comparison to large series of patients with aortic dissections who had undergone nonoperative treatment, DeBakey et al. concluded that all patients with aortic dissections should undergo surgical intervention.[7,8] Later, Wheat et al.[9] advocated a selective approach based on the observation that surgical intervention carried a 25% early mortality, whereas patients treated pharmacologically had a 16% early mortality.[10] It was not until 1970 when Daily et al.[11] at Stanford introduced the Stanford dissection classification that the importance of distinguishing ascending and descending aortic dissections became apparent. It was widely held that type B dissections ought to be treated medically unless life-threatening complications were present. Though operative mortality for type B dissections significantly improved over time (57%-13% in the Stanford series),[10] several risk factors including visceral ischemia, aortic rupture, and older age portended dramatically increased risk with surgical repair.[8,12] In the current era of endovascular stent-grafts, it seems intuitive that less invasive techniques for stabilizing complicated acute type B dissections, which carry a high risk of mortality with and without surgical intervention, could provide an opportunity to improve outcomes in this very ill patient population.

Although 20% to 50% of uncomplicated type B aortic dissections demonstrate eventual aneurysmal dilatation within 3 to 5 years of diagnosis,[13,14] there is a small risk of rupture in the acute setting, with a 30-day mortality of about 10% in contemporary studies. Most authors advocate medical treatment with blood pressure control and close follow-up with interval imaging.[15] Many of these patients will ultimately require intervention beyond the acute setting, so some authors have suggested that asymptomatic descending aortic dissections be treated with stent-grafts to prevent late complications.[16] However, long-term data comparing medical treatment and stent-grafts in uncomplicated acute type B dissections are insufficient at present to define the appropriate treatment strategy. The INSTEAD trial (Investigation of Stent-Grafts in Aortic Dissection) attempted to answer a similar debate in subacute and chronic type B dissections (within 2-52 weeks of onset) by randomizing patients to either medical therapy or stent-graft placement.[17] The trial found no difference in all-cause and aorta-related mortality at 1-year follow-up, but 91% of those in the stent-graft group demonstrated evidence of aortic remodeling, compared to only 19% of those in the medical group.[17] Even though the INSTEAD trial did not include acute aortic dissections (<2 weeks from onset), the trial did reveal a potential for stent-grafts to promote aortic remodeling and potentially prevent late aneurysmal degeneration. However, it is important to note that based on this trial, it appears that stent-graft treatment of patients with subacute or chronic aortic dissection offers no benefit in terms of reducing the risk of aortic rupture or enhancing life expectancy. Longer follow-up is necessary to understand the true benefit or lack thereof for stent-grafts in asymptomatic type B dissections.

In contradistinction, complicated type B aortic dissections, defined by the presence of visceral or peripheral malperfusion, rupture, rapid false lumen expansion, persistent pain, or uncontrollable hypertension, often require intervention. Despite significant improvement in operative mortality for acute type B dissections, operative mortality in the presence of visceral ischemia and rupture remains as high as 70% to 80%.[8,18] Addition of endovascular interventions has provided an opportunity for a less invasive, more expeditious procedure to stabilize the dissection, prevent rupture, and restore true lumen perfusion.

Endovascular treatment options include aortic stent-graft placement, dissection flap fenestration, and branch vessel stenting.[19] Each technique aims to achieve one or both of the two major goals in treating acute aortic dissection: prevent aortic rupture and restore end-organ perfusion. Current indications for intervention encompass the life-threatening complications of acute aortic dissection,

hence the term "complicated." As mentioned previously, *complicated dissections* are defined by visceral or limb malperfusion, aortic rupture or impending rupture (e.g., rapid false lumen expansion), or evidence of an unstable dissection plane (e.g., persistent pain, uncontrollable hypertension).

In type A dissection, aortic branch vessel obstruction is usually corrected concomitantly with surgical management and repair of the ascending aorta.[20] In type B dissection, branch vessel malperfusion is an indication for intervention. Recently, stent-graft placement over the primary entry tear has been increasingly performed as an alternative to open surgical distal fenestration of the intimal flap, percutaneous radiologic balloon fenestration of the aortic septum, operative replacement of the diseased aorta, or bypass graft reperfusion of ischemic vessels.[21]

The concept of endovascular stent-graft repair is predicated on successful device placement over the primary entry tear to obliterate blood flow into the aortic false lumen (Fig. 51-1). The intent is to mimic the effect of operative repair by isolating the false lumen from the circulation and redirecting all blood flow into the true lumen.

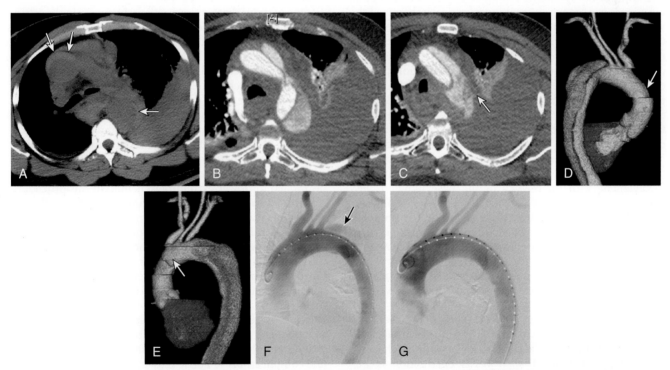

FIGURE 51-1. A 69-year-old man with complicated acute type B aortic dissection managed by thoracic endograft placement. **A,** Axial computed tomography (CT) image at level of carina, without contrast enhancement. Circular rims of high-attenuation tissue density surround both ascending and proximal descending thoracic aorta *(arrows)*, strongly suggesting acute aortic intramural hematoma (IMH). **B,** Patient presented with chest pain and systolic blood pressure over 200 mmHg. After intravenous (IV) contrast is administered, repeat CT imaging shows aortic dissection within aortic arch. **C,** CT image at a level slightly higher in arch demonstrates a large fluid density surrounding the arch and a small wisp of contrast *(arrow)* beyond the expected confines of the aorta—findings diagnostic for aortic rupture. **D,** Three-dimensional (3D) surface-rendered CT image of posterior aspect of thoracic aorta demonstrates descending aorta dissection and a small amount of hematoma surrounding ascending aorta *(arrow)*, without obvious abnormality affecting posterior arch. **E,** Similarly rendered 3D view of anterior side of aortic arch shows obvious involvement of arch, with dissection extending along its anterior surface *(arrow)*. **F,** Left anterior oblique projection of a thoracic aortogram shows location of primary entry tear just distal to left subclavian artery, with opacification of a limited extent of false lumen *(arrow)*. Together the imaging allows a diagnosis of a type IIIa aortic dissection with retrograde proximal extension from a primary entry tear just distal to left subclavian artery origin. False lumen is patent to a limited extent in the arch, but not in ascending aorta, where there is only evidence of IMH. **G,** Aortogram after deployment of endovascular stent-graft across primary entry tear, extending from left subclavian artery origin to mid-segment of descending aorta. After thoracic endovascular aneurysm repair (TEVAR), there is no longer filling of false lumen. Patient was discharged home on third day after procedure.

As demonstrated in experimental models of dissection, coverage of the primary entry tear is the optimal method of relieving true lumen collapse, restoring perfusion to branch arteries off the true lumen, and promoting thrombosis of the aortic false lumen.[22] Interestingly, dissections with a completely thrombosed aortic false lumen are associated with a favorable prognosis.[23-25] In contrast, false lumen patency contributes to progressive aortic dilation and is a predictor of late mortality.[26]

In the typical case of type B dissection, progressive thrombosis of the aortic false lumen after stent-graft placement proceeds distally, irrespective of the location of the primary intimal disruption.[27] The tempo of false lumen thrombosis is variable among individuals and influenced by several factors, such as the size of the false lumen and amount of residual false lumen flow via uncovered additional tears in the septum below the distal margin of the device. Over time, the false lumen progressively remodels and shrinks.[28] Although published results of stent-graft management of patients with acute type B dissection are encouraging, it is important to be aware that the literature for aortic dissection often mixes outcomes from a wide variety of clinical contexts in terms of age of dissection, extent of disease, and presence of complications.

Malperfusion syndrome is defined by obstruction of one or more aortic branches, resulting in critical ischemia of the vascular territory supplied by the obstructed branches.[19] Obstruction may result from either a "static" or "dynamic" obstruction. A *static obstruction* occurs when the dissection directly enters a branch vessel. As the dissection process extends into a branch, it may terminate with false lumen reentry, with a tear in the flap at the distal extent of the false channel, or it may terminate without a reentry tear in the false lumen. The former scenario with branch vessel reentry of the false lumen is more common and results in double-barrel or dual-channel flow to the vascular bed supplied by the involved branch. The other form of static branch vessel involvement with no reentry of the false lumen is less common and is typically associated with tissue malperfusion. Without a reentry tear, there is no flow via the blind sac of the false lumen, which progressively enlarges to its distal extent and may critically obstruct or markedly narrow the true lumen. Thus, the vascular territory supplied by the affected branch is frequently ischemic, and tissue necrosis may occur without expeditious intervention with reperfusion.

Alternatively, *dynamic obstruction* occurs when the aortic true lumen is collapsed and flow to its branches is compromised by the dissection flap and usually much larger false lumen. Dynamic branch vessel obstruction is frequently associated with a large proximal primary entry tear and a relatively circumferential intimal dissection. The extent of true lumen obliteration is commonly greatest at the levels of the distal descending and proximal abdominal segments. A slitlike aortic true lumen below the diaphragm often courses anteriorly to give origin to the celiac trunk and superior mesenteric arteries. In these cases, the true lumen may be barely perceptible as a wafer-thin crescent, with the dissection septum prolapsed over the origins of true lumen branches like a curtain. The severity of dynamic obstruction may be variable owing to constant motion of the dissection flap, particularly in the acute phase, and to hemodynamic changes in blood pressure and heart rate.[22,29]

In an individual patient, both static and dynamic mechanisms of branch vessel involvement with or without resultant ischemia may coexist. Branch vessel malperfusion occurs in 30% to 50% of all aortic dissections[20,30] and yields an almost threefold increase in the risk of in-hospital mortality with acute type B dissection.[31] Given the markedly high operative mortality rate with malperfusion, endovascular options are attractive. Malperfusion syndrome can be treated by thoracic aortic stent-grafting and coverage of the primary intimal tear, distal aortic intimal flap fenestration, branch-vessel stenting, or a combination of all three.

Surgical intervention for rupture or impending rupture in type B dissections also carries an extremely high operative mortality.[18] Acutely, coverage of the intimal tear with an appropriately sized stent-graft may effectively exclude a rupture or stabilize the dissection while improving true lumen flow. Moreover, exclusion of the primary intimal tear and precluding false lumen patency may reduce some of the late sequelae of type B dissections (aneurysmal dilation, rupture, and mortality) by promoting false lumen thrombosis.[28,32,33] The feasibility of successful stent-grafting depends on appropriate selection of patients with suitable aortic anatomy, which ideally includes a sufficient proximal landing zone (usually 15-20 mm) in a relatively disease-free segment of nondissected aorta.

One of the earliest endovascular treatments in the setting of acute type B dissection was performed in 1935 by Gurin, who fenestrated an intimal flap distally to treat lower extremity ischemia.[34] This strategy treats a nonreentry aortic false lumen and dynamic obstruction of the aortic true lumen by decreasing resistance to false lumen outflow rather than treating the proximal tear.[35] Percutaneous balloon fenestration can be used to mitigate the effects of dynamic aortic true lumen obstruction by creating an artificial tear in the dissection septum that enhances communication of flow between true and false lumens.

Similar to Gurin's original attempt, flap fenestration can be applied for lower extremity ischemia. In this procedure, the intimal flap is punctured and transgressed, usually with a needle/sheath combination using fluoroscopic and/or intravascular ultrasound imaging guidance.[35] In most cases, to facilitate easy targeting, the puncture is performed from the smaller aortic true lumen to the larger false lumen. Once the flap is successfully penetrated, a guidewire and balloon catheter are then advanced to a position that bridges the septum. Commonly, a series of successively larger balloons up to 25 or 30 mm in diameter are inflated to create an adequate fenestration. Limitations include continued false lumen flow, which may expose patients to increased late complications of aortic dissection,[23] particularly aneurysm formation. However, fenestration may provide a treatment option in patients with malperfusion who are poor surgical candidates or who have unsuitable anatomy for stent-grafting.

Finally, uncovered stent placement either within the aorta or (more typically) within compromised aortic branch vessels may further improve flow to an ischemic region. Indications for an uncovered stent include inadequate relief of static obstruction of a branch vessel after open aortic surgery, stent-grafting, or septal fenestration.[28,35-37] Uncovered stent placement may also be used alone or as an adjunct to percutaneous balloon fenestration of the dissection septum to increase aortic true lumen diameter.

In a published report, Dake et al. detailed outcomes in patients with acute complicated type B aortic dissection.[28] Eleven presented with symptomatic branch vessel obstruction involving 38 abdominal arterial beds. Of these compromised vessels, 22 were obstructed exclusively by a dynamic process associated with aortic true lumen obliteration, 15 by both dynamic and static mechanisms of branch involvement, and 1 by static obstruction alone. After endograft placement over the primary entry tear, all 22 of the branch vessels obstructed exclusively by a dynamic process and 6 of the 15 arteries with a combination of dynamic and static branch involvement were immediately reperfused. Adjunctive endovascular procedures were used to relieve persistent ischemia in the other obstructed cases.

Dissection variants like intramural hematoma (IMH) and penetrating atherosclerotic ulcer (PAU) add additional complexity to treatment and indications for intervention for acute aortic disease. Some 16% to 36% of IMHs progress to classic aortic dissection.[38] Moreover, because a significant percentage of patients with IMH and no apparent intimal tear on noninvasive imaging actually have a visible tear at the time of operation or autopsy, it is difficult to clearly distinguish IMH and aortic dissection. There is a general consensus that IMH be treated similarly to classic aortic dissection in the corresponding aortic segment.[2,38] PAUs, which are often associated with IMH[39] and pseudoaneurysm, may be amenable to surgical or endovascular intervention, but affected patients are often very ill and have significant atherosclerotic disease throughout the vascular tree that may lead to difficulty with endovascular access and stent-graft deployment.[38]

It is important to note that acute aortic dissection in patients with Marfan syndrome or other connective tissue disorders should be treated uniquely. Although initial management of the acute dissection follows the same overall principles, there is a general consensus that stent-grafts and other endovascular interventions be used with extreme caution if at all.[2,40,41] Not only are these patients often young and the long-term durability of stent-grafts not yet known, there is also significant concern regarding the continuous radial forces on a diseased aortic wall induced by stent-grafts. Further, stent-grafts may promote aortic dissection in some genetic aortopathies. Thus, endovascular intervention in patients with connective tissue disorders is not recommended unless there is a clear indication for intervention and the patient presents with prohibitive operative risk factors.[38]

CONCLUSIONS

Catheter aortography was once considered the gold standard for diagnosis of aortic dissection, now computed tomography (CT) scanning has clearly become the preferred imaging modality for both diagnosis and treatment planning because it is highly sensitive and specific. Many invasive and noninvasive imaging modalities may be useful, however.

Management of aortic dissection is complex and directed by multiple patient and disease-specific factors. Initial blood pressure and heart rate control and monitoring in the intensive care unit setting are critical. Ascending aortic dissections (Stanford type A, DeBakey I and II) generally require emergent surgical intervention, whereas descending aortic dissections (Stanford B, DeBakey III) present a more difficult challenge in terms of management decision making. Type B dissections complicated by rupture, rapid false lumen expansion, tissue malperfusion, or intractable pain or uncontrollable hypertension are likely to require acute intervention. Conversely, uncomplicated type B dissections are typically treated medically. With the advent and evolution of endovascular techniques, less invasive treatment options are becoming available to the clinician, but a clear consensus regarding open surgical repair versus stent-graft and other adjunctive interventions remains elusive. Further clinical investigation is clearly needed and is ongoing. Ultimately, treatment of aortic dissection will likely employ multiple techniques and more patient- and disease-specific approaches.

KEY POINTS

- Aortic dissection is the most calamitous disorder affecting the aorta and is twice as common as aortic rupture.
- Treatment strategies for aortic dissection have been subject to remarkable technologic innovation since 1992.
- Recent investigations have explored endoluminal stent-graft placement as an alternative to surgical repair.
- The ideal prosthesis for treatment of aortic dissection is not yet available—it is unreasonable to expect that one device will be able to address all manifestations of this disease.

▶ SUGGESTED READINGS

Ahmad F, Cheshire N, Hamady M. Acute aortic syndrome: pathology and therapeutic strategies. Postgrad Med J 2006;82:305–12.

Chavan A, Lotz J, Oelert F, et al. Endoluminal treatment of aortic dissection. Eur Radiol 2003;13:2521–34.

Iyer VS, Mackenzie KS, Tse LW, et al. Early outcomes after elective and emergent endovascular repair of the thoracic aorta. J Vasc Surg 2006;43:677–83.

Leurs LJ, Bell R, Degrieck Y, et al. Endovascular treatment of thoracic aortic diseases: combined experience from the EUROSTAR and United Kingdom Thoracic Endograft registries. J Vasc Surg 2004;40:670–9.

Szeto WY, Gleason TG. Operative management of ascending aortic dissections. Semin Thorac Cardiovasc Surg 2005;17:247–55.

Westaby S, Bertoni GB. Fifty years of thoracic aortic surgery: lessons learned and future directions. Ann Thorac Surg 2007;83:S832–4.

The complete reference list is available online at www.expertconsult.com.

CHAPTER 52

Alimentary Tract Vasculature

Nadia J. Khati, Morvarid Alaghmand, Michael J. Manzano, and Anthony C. Venbrux

CLINICAL RELEVANCE

An understanding of the vascular anatomy of the alimentary tract allows a wide range of therapeutic options for patients who traditionally were treated by open surgery. In addition to the use of catheter-directed embolotherapy and pharmacologic vasoconstriction for gastrointestinal (GI) hemorrhage, a knowledge of variant anatomy may prevent complications such as nontarget organ embolization. For example, recognition of variant anatomy during hepatic artery chemoembolization for liver tumors may prevent inadvertent delivery of toxic chemotherapeutic drugs to the upper GI tract (e.g., inadvertent reflux of chemotherapeutic agents into the gastroduodenal artery, with possible resultant duodenal mucosal injury and ulceration).

The venous anatomy in the alimentary tract is also important. The transjugular intrahepatic portosystemic shunt (TIPS) procedure functionally creates a portosystemic shunt that reduces the high pressure in patients with advanced portal hypertension. Such elevated pressure may cause life-threatening esophageal variceal hemorrhage. TIPS, though not perfect, can be lifesaving.

Delayed strictures of the biliary system may occur if the hepatic artery is injured (e.g., clipped) during cholecystectomy in a patient with advanced liver disease. Such ischemic strictures result from inadequate blood flow to the bile ducts, the latter receiving blood supply from the hepatic artery.

Thus, an understanding of alimentary tract vasculature is essential while performing image-guided interventions.

VASCULAR IMAGING OF THE ALIMENTARY TRACT

Evaluation of the gastrointestinal tract vasculature can be performed with different imaging modalities including multidetector-row computed tomography (MDCT), magnetic resonance angiography (MRA), conventional angiography and ultrasound.

The most common indications for imaging of the gastrointestinal (GI) tract vasculature include acute and chronic mesenteric ischemia, median arcuate ligament syndrome, aneurysms and dissections as well as evaluation of the portal venous system either in the assessment of portal hypertension or following a transjugular intrahepatic portosystemic shunt (TIPS) procedure.

Ultrasound

The use of abdominal ultrasound in the evaluation of the gastrointestinal (GI) tract vasculature is limited to visualization of the larger vessels such as the major branches of the aorta (celiac trunk, superior mesenteric artery) and the portal venous system. The many branches of the small

bowel mesentery and inferior mesenteric artery are usually not visualized due to their small. Other limitations of US include patient body habitus, sonographer's degree of experience and overlying bowel gas. The 2 most common clinical situations where US is helpful in making a diagnosis is in the evaluation of chronic mesenteric ischemia due to median arcuate ligament syndrome and when evaluating the portal venous system. Using color and Doppler sonography, both entities can easily be diagnosed by measuring velocities across vessels, direction of flow and patency of vessels.

CT Angiography and MR Angiography

CT angiography (CTA) and MR angiography (MRA) are the 2 most commonly used non-invasive imaging modalities for the diagnosis of mesenteric ischemia in the acute setting. Both exams involve the administration of iodinated contrast for CT and gadolinium for MRI and can only be performed in patients with normal renal function. With the advent of volumetric acquisition of images and three-dimensional (3D) reconstruction algorithms both the mesenteric arterial and venous system can be adequately visualized, especially when using dual-phase imaging (arterial and venous phases). Both CTA and MRA are highly accurate in the diagnosis of acute mesenteric artery thrombosis, mesenteric and portal venous thrombosis by demonstrating either a filling defect within the occluded vessels or an abrupt cut-off of the affected vessels. In addition, these modalities may show secondary signs of ischemia such as bowel wall thickening and mesenteric edema or hemorrhage. In patients with renal impairment, non-contrast enhanced MR angiography using balanced steady-state free precession (SSFP) can be used as an alternative to image the aorta and its branches. Some advantages of using CTA over MRA include greater availability in most institutions, faster acquisition time, and improved spatial resolution allowing better visualization of smaller peripheral vessels of the mesenteric circulation. Furthermore, CTA can evaluate the presence of atherosclerotic disease by visualizing calcified plaque, which is very difficult to perceive on MRA.

Catheter Angiography

Catheter angiography is still considered by many radiologists as the gold standard for imaging the aorta and the mesenteric arteries and veins even though it remains an invasive test, involves the use of ionizing radiation and the administration of iodinated contrast material. It remains the study of choice when non-occlusive mesenteric ischemia is suspected. In patients with renal impairment, carbon dioxide (CO_2) can be safely substituted for iodinated material as the contrast medium. One of the biggest advantages of using conventional angiography over other

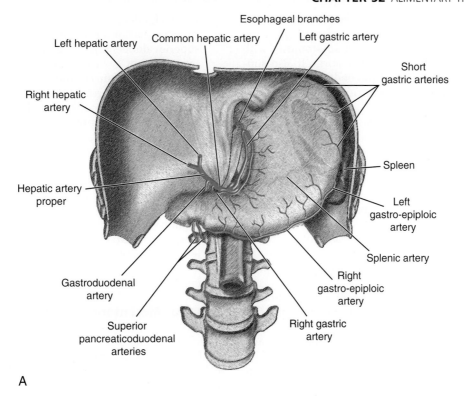

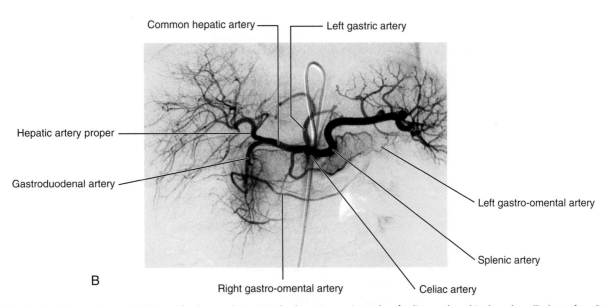

FIGURE 52-1. Celiac trunk. **A,** Distribution of celiac trunk. **B,** Digital subtraction angiography of celiac trunk and its branches. *(Redrawn from Drake RL, Vogl W, Mitchell AWM. Gray's anatomy for students. Philadelphia: Elsevier/Churchill Livingstone; 2005.)*

imaging modalities is that it can serve as a diagnostic and therapeutic tool when necessary. Vasodilators or thrombolytics can be administered at the time of the examination in addition to visualizing possible collateral circulations.

ARTERIAL SUPPLY

Three major arteries that supply the alimentary tract are the celiac axis, superior mesenteric artery (SMA), and inferior mesenteric artery (IMA).

Celiac Trunk

The celiac axis arises from the ventral surface of the aorta at the level of the T12-L1 disc space. It immediately divides into three branches—the left gastric artery, splenic artery, and common hepatic artery—and supplies the liver, spleen, stomach, and pancreas (Fig. 52-1). Both the splenic and left gastric artery can arise directly from the aorta as separate branches, but in over 95% of patients, the common hepatic artery arises from the celiac trunk.

The left gastric artery is the smallest branch of the celiac axis. It supplies the gastroesophageal junction (abdominal part of the esophagus) and anastomoses with esophageal branches from the thoracic aorta. It also supplies the fundus and a portion of the body of the stomach and anastomoses with the right gastric artery, a branch of the hepatic artery.

The splenic artery is the largest branch of the celiac trunk. It has a tortuous course to the left along the superior border of the pancreas and has three branches:

- Pancreatic branches. As the hepatic artery passes along, it gives off small branches to supply the neck, body, and tail of the pancreas.
- Short gastric arteries, which supply blood to the fundus of the stomach
- Left gastroepiploic artery (terminal branch of the splenic artery), which runs along the greater curvature of the stomach and anastomoses with the right gastroepiploic artery

The common hepatic artery is a medium-sized branch of the celiac trunk and runs to the right. It divides into two major branches:

- The hepatic proper, which ascends toward the liver and is located on the left side of the bile duct and anterior to the portal vein. It gives off two branches: the right and left hepatic arteries.

- Gastroduodenal artery, which descends posterior to the superior part of the duodenum. At the lower part of the superior duodenum, the gastroduodenal artery divides into the right gastroepiploic (which supplies both surfaces of the stomach and the greater curvature) and the superior pancreaticoduodenal arteries. The second branch divides into anterior and posterior branches and supplies the head of the pancreas and the duodenum. Other branches of the common hepatic artery include the supraduodenal and right gastric arteries.

Anastomoses in the stomach include:

- Left gastric, right gastric, and short gastric arteries from the spleen. This anastomosis makes an arcade along the lesser curvature of the stomach.
- Right gastroepiploic artery (terminal branch of the gastroduodenal artery), which forms anastomoses with the left gastroepiploic artery (terminal branch of the splenic artery). These vessels form an arcade along the greater curvature of the stomach.

Superior Mesenteric Artery

The SMA is one of the major blood supplies to the lower GI tract (Figs. 52-2 and 52-3). It is located inferior to the celiac axis (usually within 2 cm and at the level of L1). Anatomically, the SMA is crossed anteriorly by the splenic vein

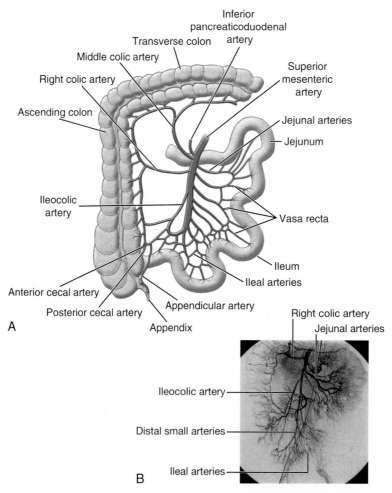

FIGURE 52-2. Superior mesenteric artery (SMA). **A,** Distribution of SMA. **B,** Digital subtraction angiography of SMA and its branches. *(Redrawn from Drake RL, Vogl W, Mitchell AWM. Gray's anatomy for students. Philadelphia: Elsevier/Churchill Livingstone; 2005.)*

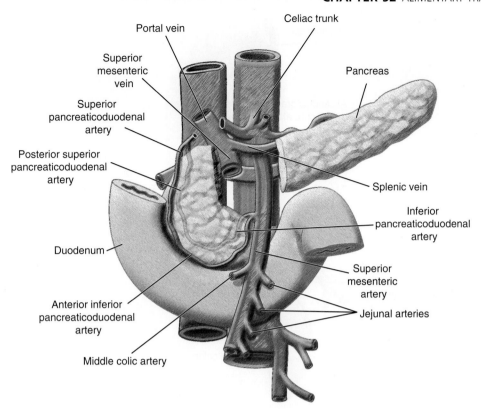

FIGURE 52-3. Initial branching and relationships of superior mesenteric artery. *(Redrawn from Drake RL, Vogl W, Mitchell AWM. Gray's anatomy for students. Philadelphia: Elsevier/Churchill Livingstone; 2005.)*

and the neck of the pancreas, and as it descends, it passes anterior to the left renal vein, the uncinate process of the pancreas, and the inferior part of the duodenum. The SMA supplies the duodenum, pancreas, entire small bowel, appendix, ascending colon, and approximately two thirds to three fourths of the transverse colon. Its branches are the:

- Inferior pancreaticoduodenal artery, the first branch of the SMA. It divides into anterior and posterior branches and, as mentioned earlier, forms an anastomosis with the superior pancreaticoduodenal artery. This arcade supplies the head and uncinate process of the pancreas and the duodenum.
- Jejunal arteries, which arise from the left side of the SMA and supply the jejunum
- Ileal arteries, located on the left side of the SMA. These arteries supply most of the ileum.
- Ileocolic arteries, which arise from the right side and supply the terminal ileum, cecum, and lower ascending colon. The superior branch anastomoses with the right colic artery, and the inferior branch continues toward the ileocolic junction and divides into colic, cecal, appendicular, and ileal branches.
- Right colic artery, which arises from the right side of the SMA and supplies the ascending colon. It divides into ascending and descending branches that anastomose with the middle colic artery.
- Middle colic artery, which arises from the right side of the SMA and divides into right and left branches. The right branch forms an anastomosis with the right colic artery, and the left branch forms an anastomosis with the left colic artery, a branch of the IMA.

Inferior Mesenteric Artery

The IMA is another major blood supply to the lower GI tract (Fig. 52-4). It is located at the level of L2-L4 (most often at the L3-L4 disc space level, 2-3 cm above the aortic bifurcation). The IMA supplies the distal transverse colon, descending colon, sigmoid colon, and rectum. The following are branches of the IMA:

- Left colic artery, with ascending and descending branches. The ascending branch supplies the upper part of the descending colon and the distal part of the transverse colon. The descending branch supplies the lower part of the descending colon and anastomoses with the first sigmoid artery. The left colic artery is absent in approximately 12% of patients.
- Sigmoid arteries, which descend in the sigmoid mesocolon and supply the lowest part of the descending colon and the sigmoid colon. These branches anastomose superiorly with the left colic and inferiorly with the superior rectal artery.
- Superior rectal artery, the terminal branch of the IMA. At the S3 level, this vessel divides into two terminal branches on either side of the rectum and finally anastomoses with the middle and inferior rectal arteries (from the internal pudendal and internal iliac arteries).

Important collateral blood supply of the lower alimentary tract consists of the:

- Marginal artery of Drummond, which anastomoses with the SMA and IMA. It runs along the mesenteric border of the colon and supplies the vasa recta.

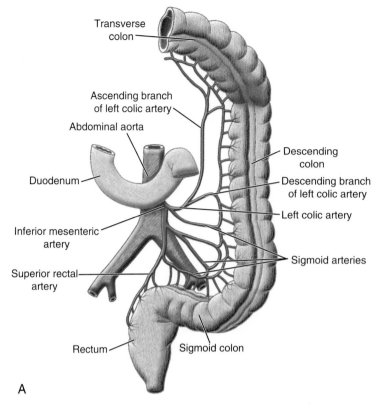

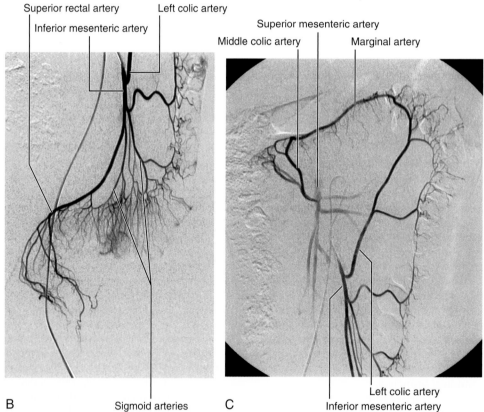

FIGURE 52-4. Inferior mesenteric artery (IMA). **A,** Distribution of IMA. **B,** Digital subtraction angiography of IMA and its branches. *(Redrawn from Drake RL, Vogl W, Mitchell AWM. Gray's anatomy for students. Philadelphia: Elsevier/Churchill Livingstone; 2005.)*

- Arc of Riolan, an intraarterial bridge between the left colic and middle colic arteries
- Superior hemorrhoidal branches, which arteries form anastomoses with the IMA and internal iliac arteries

VENOUS SYSTEM

Venous drainage of the spleen, pancreas, gallbladder, and abdominal part of the GI tract (except the inferior portion of the rectum) is through the portal system. After blood passes through the hepatic sinusoids, it returns to the inferior vena cava through the hepatic veins.

Portal Vein

The portal vein is formed by the confluence of the splenic vein and superior mesenteric vein (SMV) and originates behind the neck of the pancreas at the level of L2. The inferior mesenteric vein, left gastric vein, right gastric vein, and superior pancreaticoduodenal veins are tributaries that empty into the portal vein.

Splenic Vein

The splenic vein originates from vessels in the hilum of the spleen. It courses along with the splenic artery and tail of the pancreas. This vessel drains blood from the short gastric, left gastroepiploic, pancreatic, and usually the inferior mesenteric veins.

Superior Mesenteric Vein

The SMV originates in the right iliac fossa and receives venous blood from the terminal ileum, cecum, and appendix. The SMV ascends on the right side of the SMA, anterior to the right ureter, inferior vena cava, horizontal part of the duodenum, and uncinate process of the pancreas and corresponds to the SMA and its branches. The small intestine, cecum, ascending colon, and transverse colon drain into the SMV. Tributaries are the jejunal, ileal, ileocolic, right colic, middle colic, right gastroepiploic, and inferior pancreaticoduodenal veins.

Inferior Mesenteric Vein

The inferior mesenteric vein originates as superior rectal veins. As the inferior mesenteric vein exits the pelvis and while ascending, it receives blood from sigmoid veins and the left colic vein. Usually this vessel joins the splenic vein posterior to the body of the pancreas. Occasionally it enters at the union of the splenic vein and the SMV. The splenic flexure, descending colon, sigmoid colon, and rectum are drained by the inferior mesenteric vein.

LIVER VASCULATURE

Blood vessels conveying blood to the liver are the hepatic artery (≈30% of the blood circulation) and the portal vein (≈70%) (Fig. 52-5).

Arterial Supply

After the common hepatic artery gives off the gastroduodenal artery, its name changes to the *proper hepatic artery*, and it ascends to the liver porta. It has three branches: the right, middle, and left hepatic arteries.

The hepatic arterial anatomy has many variations. Only in 55% of cases are all branches from the common hepatic artery present. Common variations include:
- Accessory or replaced left hepatic artery arising from the left gastric artery (25%)
- Accessory or replaced right hepatic artery arising from the SMA (17%-22%)
- Entire common hepatic artery replaced by the SMA

Other, less common variations include:
- Right hepatic artery arising from the SMA or left hepatic artery arising from the left gastric artery
- Common hepatic artery arising from the SMA or from the left gastric artery or aorta

Portal Venous System

As mentioned, the portal vein is formed by the confluence of the splenic and superior mesenteric veins. The inferior mesenteric, left gastric, right gastric, and superior pancreaticoduodenal veins are tributaries that empty into the portal vein (Figs. 52-6 and 52-7). The main portal vein has two left and right tributaries that each have their own divisions in the liver. These divisions supply all segmental and subsegmental parts of the liver. The portal venous system has tributaries that make important anastomoses with systemic veins (Figs. 52-8 and 52-9):
- Anastomoses of the left gastric vein (portal vein tributary) and azygous venous system (superior vena cava tributary) (i.e., a cause of esophageal varices)
- Anastomoses of small veins around the ligamentum teres that communicate with the portal system and superficial abdominal veins. These veins drain into either the inferior vena cava or the superior vena cava (i.e., result in caput medusa).
- Anastomoses of the superior rectal tributaries of the inferior mesenteric vein with the middle and inferior rectal branches of the internal iliac veins or inferior vena cava (i.e., a cause of hemorrhoids).
- Anastomoses of the left and right colic veins with tributaries of the renal and lumbar veins of the inferior vena cava.

Venous Blood Supply of the Liver

There are three major hepatic veins: left hepatic, middle hepatic, and right hepatic. These veins drain different segments of the liver.

BILIARY SYSTEM VASCULATURE

Arterial Supply

There is great variation in the arterial supply of the biliary system. In the most common pattern, the common hepatic duct receives blood from the right hepatic artery. Blood to the gallbladder and cystic duct is supplied by the cystic

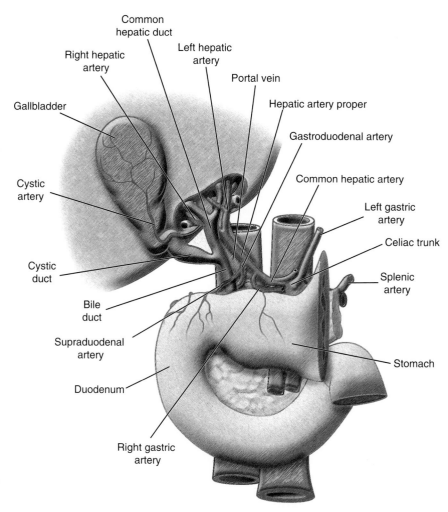

FIGURE 52-5. Distribution of common hepatic artery. *(Redrawn from Drake RL, Vogl W, Mitchell AWM. Gray's anatomy for students. Philadelphia: Elsevier/Churchill Livingstone; 2005.)*

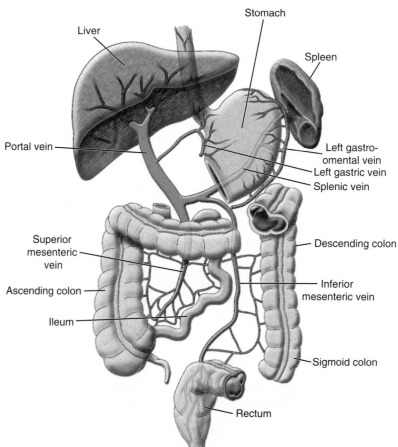

FIGURE 52-6. Venous drainage of abdominal portion of gastrointestinal tract. *(Redrawn from Drake RL, Vogl W, Mitchell AWM. Gray's anatomy for students. Philadelphia: Elsevier/Churchill Livingstone; 2005.)*

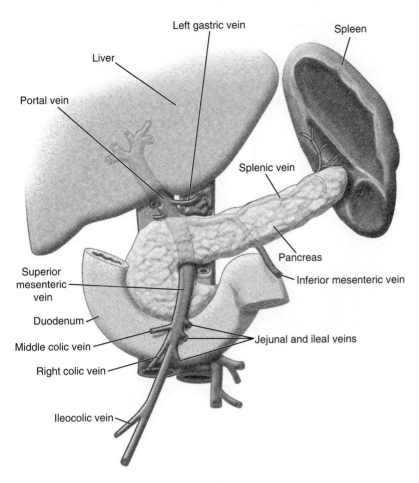

Left gastric vein

Spleen

Liver

Portal vein

Splenic vein

Pancreas

Inferior mesenteric vein

Superior mesenteric vein

Duodenum

Middle colic vein

Jejunal and ileal veins

Right colic vein

Ileocolic vein

FIGURE 52-7. Portal vein. *(Redrawn from Drake RL, Vogl W, Mitchell AWM. Gray's anatomy for students. Philadelphia: Elsevier/Churchill Livingstone; 2005.)*

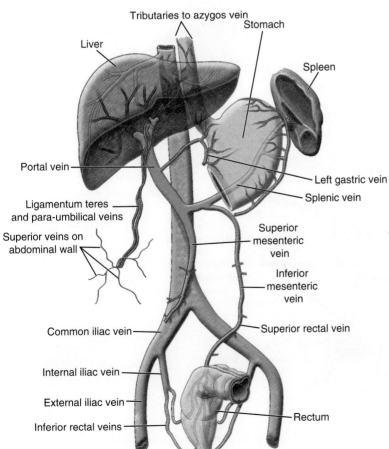

Tributaries to azygos vein

Stomach

Liver

Spleen

Portal vein

Left gastric vein

Splenic vein

Ligamentum teres and para-umbilical veins

Superior mesenteric vein

Superior veins on abdominal wall

Inferior mesenteric vein

Common iliac vein

Superior rectal vein

Internal iliac vein

External iliac vein

Rectum

Inferior rectal veins

FIGURE 52-8. Portosystemic anastomoses. *(Redrawn from Drake RL, Vogl W, Mitchell AWM. Gray's anatomy for students. Philadelphia: Elsevier/Churchill Livingstone; 2005.)*

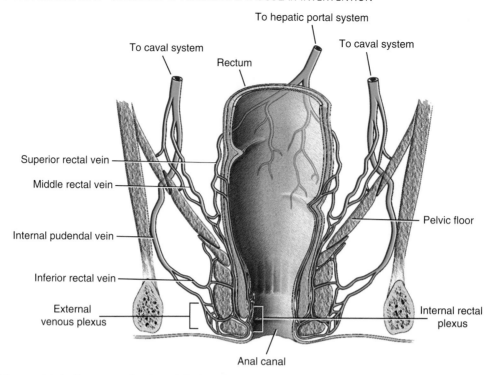

FIGURE 52-9. Veins associated with rectum and anal canal. *(Redrawn from Drake RL, Vogl W, Mitchell AWM. Gray's anatomy for students. Philadelphia: Elsevier/ Churchill Livingstone; 2005.)*

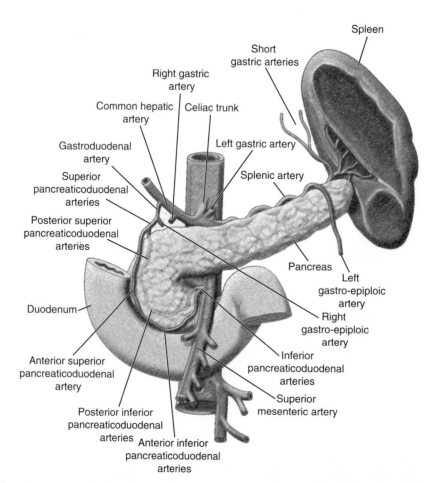

FIGURE 52-10. Arterial supply to pancreas. *(Redrawn from Drake RL, Vogl W, Mitchell AWM. Gray's anatomy for students. Philadelphia: Elsevier/Churchill Livingstone; 2005.)*

artery, a branch of the right hepatic artery. The common bile duct in its upper portions receives branches from the right hepatic, proper hepatic, or gastroduodenal arteries. The lower part of this duct receives blood from the postero-superior pancreaticoduodenal artery.

Venous Supply

Venous blood from the gallbladder enters either directly into the liver or through a cystic vein that joins the portal vein. Venous blood from the common bile duct drains into the beginning of the portal vein.

SPLEEN VASCULATURE

Arterial Supply

The splenic artery, as mentioned previously, is a branch of the celiac artery and supplies blood to the spleen through several branches. This artery passes posterior to the pancreas and is located anterior and superior to the splenic vein.

Venous System

The splenic vein accompanies the splenic artery and then empties into the main portal vein.

PANCREAS VASCULATURE

Arterial Supply

The head of the pancreas is supplied by the pancreaticoduodenal artery (the upper part by the superior pancreaticoduodenal artery and the lower part by the inferior pancreaticoduodenal artery). Anterior and posterior divisions of the superior and inferior pancreaticoduodenal arteries form an arcade in the pancreas. Blood supply to the neck, body, and tail of the pancreas is provided by the great pancreatic, dorsal, and caudal pancreatic branches (from the splenic artery) (Fig. 52-10).

The remainder of the blood supply is derived from the transverse pancreatic artery via the pancreaticoduodenal artery. Some of the small branches to the tail are provided by the left gastroepiploic artery.

Venous Supply

Pancreatic veins drain blood from the body and tail of the pancreas into the splenic vein. In addition, splenic, portal, and superior mesenteric veins drain the rest of the pancreas.

KEY POINTS

- The upper and lower gastrointestinal (GI) tracts are supplied by three major visceral vessels that arise from the abdominal aorta.
- Because of its rich collateral blood supply, embolotherapy in the upper GI tract is generally well tolerated.
- The lower GI tract (SMA and IMA) generally requires (1) superselective catheterization for embolization (use of microcatheters with limited embolization) or (2) therapy with pharmacologic vasoconstrictors (e.g., vasopressin). The latter is accomplished by placing the catheter tip in the main trunk of the artery (i.e., no requirement to be superselective with the catheter).
- The biliary ducts derive their blood supply from the hepatic artery.

▶ **SUGGESTED READINGS**

Drake RL, Vogl W, Mitchell AWM. Gray's anatomy for students. Philadelphia: Elsevier/Churchill Livingstone; 2005.

Horton KM, Fishman EK. CT Angiography of the Mesenteric Circulation. Radiol Clin N Am 2010;331–45.

Kaufman JA, Lee MJ. Visceral arteries. In: Kaufman JA, Lee MJ, editors. Vascular and interventional radiology. Philadelphia: Mosby; 2003.

Khoshini R, Garrett B, Sial S, et al. The Role of Radiologic Studies in the Diagnosis of Mesenteric Ischemia. MedGenMed 2004;6(1):23.

Klar E, Rahmanian PB, Bücker A, et al. Acute Mesenteric Ischemia: A Vascular Emergency. Dtsch Arztebl Int 2012;109(14):249–56.

Ozel A, Toksoy G, Ozdogan O, et al. Ultrasonographic diagnosis of median arcuate ligament syndrome: A report of two cases. Medical Ultrasonography 2012;14(2):154–7.

Shih MCP, Hagspiel KD. CTA and MRA in Mesenteric Ischemia: Part 1, Role in Diagnosis and Differential Diagnosis. AJR 2007;188:452–61.

CHAPTER 53

Management of Upper Gastrointestinal Hemorrhage

Simon J. McPherson and Rafiuddin Patel

Upper gastrointestinal (UGI) hemorrhage is defined as bleeding into the gut proximal to the ligament of Treitz, and its causes fall into three major groups: (1) UGI hemorrhage due to direct bleeding into the gut, which is usually due to primary gut pathology, (2) transpapillary hemorrhage (comprising hemobilia and transpancreatic duct hemorrhage), and (3) variceal hemorrhage (Table 53-1). Management of variceal hemorrhage secondary to portal hypertension is considered separately in Section 14, Intervention in Portal Hypertension.

Spontaneous acute UGI bleeding is common, with an incidence of approximately 100 per 100,000 adults per year and a mortality of 5% to 14% in the United Kingdom and North America.[1,2] Both incidence and mortality increase with age. In the United States, patients with a bleeding peptic ulcer had an average hospital cost of $5000 in 1996.[3] The incidence of UGI bleeding is six times that for hemorrhage distal to the ligament of Treitz.[4] Presentation may be acute with hematemesis and/or melena, or chronic with iron-deficiency anemia.

DIAGNOSIS

In the absence of hematemesis, the source of GI bleeding is uncertain, and determining its precise location from the clinical presentation can be misleading. Approximately 45% of patients presenting to the emergency department with GI bleeding and no hematemesis have a UGI source.[5] Melena is four times more likely to come from UGI bleeding than any other cause, but bleeding from the small bowel or right side of the colon commonly presents with melena. *Hematochezia* is passage of fresh or altered blood per rectum and is frequently due to colonic or rectal bleeding, but profuse UGI bleeding is the cause of severe hematochezia in 15% of patients.[6] These possible sites of bleeding must be differentiated to allow effective intervention.

Endoscopy is the investigation of first choice and allows for rapid identification and treatment of GI bleeding. In a significant minority of patients, endoscopy is negative (normal), fails to achieve a full assessment of the UGI tract, or the presence of copious blood obscures the precise site of hemorrhage. These patients require additional techniques to identify the bleeding source. Newer optical imaging techniques such as wireless capsule endoscopy and push enteroscopy have been developed. However, they are labor intensive, time consuming, and are not widely available. Prolonged imaging time and the patient preparation required for capsule endoscopy precludes its use in the acute setting.

Imaging and radiologic interventions have become pivotal in the evaluation and treatment of GI blood loss when endoscopy is inconclusive or fails to control bleeding. Radionuclide imaging is highly sensitive in detecting active GI bleeding, with threshold sensitivity for sulfur colloid scintigraphy of 0.1 mL/min and for red blood cell scintigraphy of 0.2 to 0.4 mL/min.[7] Prolonged imaging times can also be advantageous in detecting intermittent or obscure GI bleeding. However, imprecise anatomic location of the bleeding point, the requirement to return for sequential imaging over many hours, and its limited availability and applicability in the acute setting largely restricts radionuclide imaging to the investigation of obscure chronic blood loss.

Diagnostic catheter angiography is a sensitive modality for detecting active bleeding, with a reported threshold sensitivity of 0.5 mL/min in animal models, and this may be five to nine times more sensitive with digital subtraction.[8,9] Catheter angiography can accurately localize the site of bleeding and allows definitive therapeutic intervention. However, it is invasive and carries associated risks of vascular access and catheter manipulation. Catheter angiography is also of limited sensitivity and specificity when bleeding is not active. It is usually reserved for definitive treatment of active bleeding resistant to endoscopic treatment or following noninvasive imaging identification of the point or likely cause of active bleeding.

In recent years, computed tomography (CT) has undergone major technologic advances. Development of multidetector computed tomographic angiography (MD-CTA) has provided accurate, sensitive, and rapid diagnosis of hemorrhage in a wide spectrum of clinical scenarios. High speed and narrow collimation allow coverage of large volumes that include the entire abdomen and pelvis in a single breath hold, producing images with reduced respiratory and motion artifact that can be accurately timed to acquire sequentially during arterial and portal venous phases.[10] A recent in vitro study found the threshold for detecting bleeding with MD-CTA to be 0.35 mL/min.[11] A recent meta-analysis of the use of CT in diagnosing acute GI bleeding confirmed the accuracy of MD-CTA, with a pooled sensitivity of 82% to 94% and a specificity of 74% to 92%.[12] The sensitivity of MD-CTA has been shown to be higher in patients with active hemorrhage (91%) than in those with obscure GI bleeding (50%-81%).[13,14] The drawbacks of MD-CTA are the associated radiation exposure and iodinated contrast requirements, particularly if repeat scans are required for intermittent bleeding. Preexisting high-attenuation material within the bowel lumen may also limit the diagnostic value of the study.

MD-CTA is rapidly and widely available and easy to perform. Even when active bleeding is not seen, it may demonstrate the bleeding site owing to high-attenuation thrombus, pseudoaneurysm formation, possible arterioenteric fistulas, or vessel irregularity. MD-CTA also aids in the planning of transarterial embolization, reducing subsequent angiographic radiation dose, contrast volume, and procedure time. Additional advantages of MD-CTA include depiction of extravascular and extraluminal pathology. MD-CTA is now established as the imaging investigation of choice in cases of suspected GI bleeding with negative or failed endoscopy (Figs. 53-1 and 53-2).

MANAGEMENT

Interventional radiologic treatment and conventional surgery are usually reserved for those patients who have

failed endoscopic management. Embolotherapy for UGI hemorrhage was first introduced by Rosch et al. in 1972.[23] Since its initial role in the management of poor surgical candidates, transcatheter embolization has expanded to become the preferred treatment when endoscopic intervention fails.[24-27] Surgery is now generally reserved for patients who have failed endoscopic and radiologic treatments.

For more information on morbidity and mortality in patients from both treatment groups, including an extensive table of outcomes, please visit the accompanying website at www.expertconsult.com.

INDICATIONS

UGI hemorrhage is usually intermittent. Even patients with acute massive GI bleeding may have episodes of temporary hemostasis. If this coincides with acquisition of the CT or angiographic runs, the examination may be negative.[36] Identifying the site of bleeding most commonly requires the patient to be actively bleeding. A useful indicator of active bleeding is the degree of hemodynamic compromise (systolic blood pressure < 100 mmHg and heart rate > 100 beats/min or clinical shock).[27] Patients who have been aggressively resuscitated may not show hemodynamic changes, and the rate of fluid resuscitation required to maintain a stable pulse and blood pressure (the "metastable" patient) should also influence the decision to perform angiography. In general, the more hemodynamically unstable a patient is, the greater the chance of identifying the source of hemorrhage. For this reason, angiography, which is both diagnostic and therapeutic, is best performed in endoscopy-refractory acute UGI hemorrhage while the

TABLE 53-1. Common Causes of Nonvariceal Upper Gastrointestinal Hemorrhage

Direct Hemorrhage
Peptic ulceration (gastric and duodenal)
Mallory-Weiss tear
Gastritis/esophagitis
Angiodysplasia
Dieulafoy lesion
Post-anastomotic (marginal) ulcer
Arterioenteric fistula (aneurysms and pseudoaneurysms)
Tumors (particularly large primary leiomyosarcomas and pancreatic neuroendocrine tumors)
Duodenal diverticular disease

Transpapillary Hemorrhage
Endoscopic sphincterotomy
Hemobilia (trauma, hepatic abscesses, hepatic surgery, liver biopsy, biliary drainage procedures, tumors)
Transpancreatic duct (postpancreatitic pseudoaneurysms, tumors)

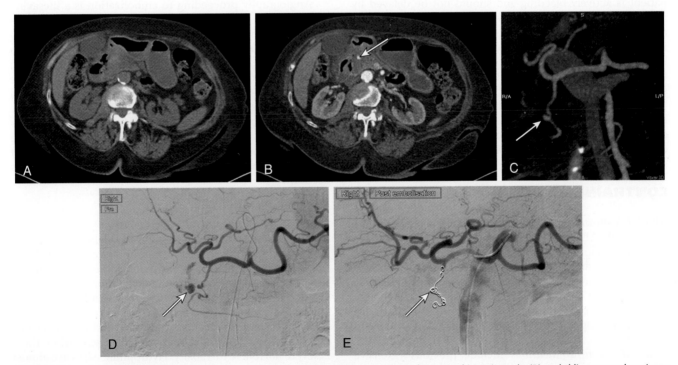

FIGURE 53-1. Axial unenhanced **(A)**, arterial-phase contrast-enhanced multidetector computed tomographic angiography **(B)**, and oblique coronal maximum intensity projection **(C)** demonstrate active bleeding from gastroduodenal artery *(arrows)* in a patient who presented with melena. Upper gastrointestinal endoscopy was incomplete owing to a duodenal stricture. Corresponding catheter angiogram **(D)** and successful coil embolization *(arrow)* distal and then proximal to site of hemorrhage **(E)**.

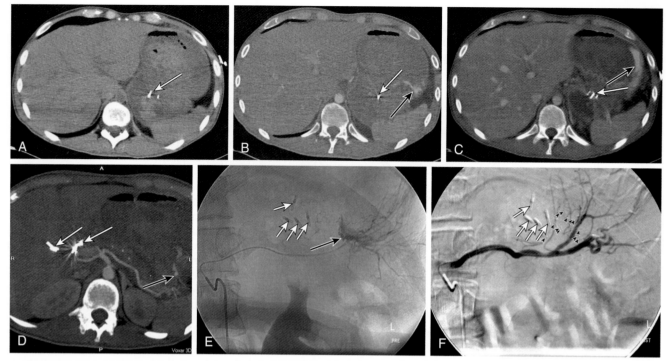

FIGURE 53-2. Patient with a history of chronic pancreatitis and recurrent hematemesis due to peptic ulcer disease previously treated by endoscopy. On this admission, upper gastrointestinal endoscopy could not identify bleeding site, owing to extensive hematoma within stomach. Axial unenhanced **(A)**, arterial phase **(B)**, and delayed portal venous phase **(C)** images confirmed active bleeding into stomach *(black arrows)*. Endoscopic clips relate to previous episodes of hematemesis *(white arrows)*. Axial thick-section maximum intensity projection **(D)** demonstrates bleeding is from the short gastric arteries via the splenic artery *(black arrow)*. Previous gastroduodenal artery embolization coils are also demonstrated *(white arrows)*. Subsequent catheter angiography correlation **(E)** and successful glue embolization **(F)**. Active bleeding *(black arrow)* and glue cast is outlined *(arrowheads)*. Previous endoscopy clips are also marked *(white arrows)*.

patient is actively bleeding and should not be delayed by resuscitation maneuvers, which can be continued in the angiography department. The endoscopist can assist the interventionist by placing multiple endoscopic clips at the site of endoscopically uncontrollable hemorrhage to facilitate embolization, even if the patient has temporarily stopped bleeding at the time of angiography.[37]

Recurrent UGI bleeding with no cause seen at repeated endoscopy or on MD-CTA (arterial and delayed phase) is a difficult clinical problem. In such patients, a transpapillary cause or reflux from brisk lower GI bleeding should be suspected.

CONTRAINDICATIONS

Absolute contraindications to embolization are rare, if they exist at all. Alternative contrast agents (carbon dioxide [CO_2] and gadolinium) can be used in patients with severe reactions to iodinated contrast media (ICM). Severe bleeding diatheses are usually correctable over time, and access sheaths can be left in situ until this is achieved. Although successful vessel occlusion with embolization is more difficult in the coagulopathic patient, it is usually preferable to open surgery.

Relative contraindications include previous extensive UGI surgery or radiotherapy in which embolization is associated with an increased risk of gastric or duodenal infarction. Patients with severe visceral artery atherosclerosis also warrant increased caution.

Angiography proceeding to embolization is a lifesaving procedure. It is rarely indicated in low-volume non–life-threatening acute hemorrhage. Traditionally, intermittent low-volume bleeding has been investigated with scintigraphy. MD-CTA is increasingly being used to guide the further investigation and management of these patients. MD-CTA is also useful in patients who have had a large UGI hemorrhage but show no clinical or endoscopic evidence of active bleeding, where low-volume active contrast extravasation may be demonstrated (Fig. 53-3), the underlying cause, or other CT features suggestive of active bleeding (as previously discussed in the diagnosis section).

EQUIPMENT

A wide variety of catheter shapes are available for catheterizing the celiac axis or superior mesenteric artery (SMA). Cobra, sidewinder, and visceral hook catheters are among the most popular. As with all embolizations, the catheter should have no side holes. There is a tradeoff between tip control (torquability) and trackability. The 4F systems generally have better trackability than their 5F equivalents. Larger catheter systems are occasionally useful when there is severe aortoiliac tortuosity. Hydrophilic wires are almost essential, and hydrophilic catheters are often useful. When arteries smaller than the gastroduodenal artery (GDA) require catheterization, microcatheter systems are usually required.

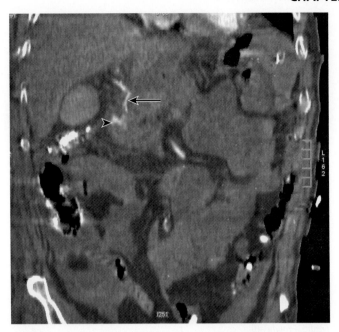

FIGURE 53-3. Oblique coronal reformatted arterial-phase, multislice computed tomography image showing active gastroduodenal *(arrowhead)* bleeding in a hemodynamically stable patient. Gastroduodenal artery is marked *(arrow)*.

The choice of embolic agent depends on a combination of the abnormality being treated, vascular anatomy, achievable catheter position, and operator preference. The most common embolic agents are metallic coils (both standard 0.035-inch and platinum microcoils must be available) and polyvinyl alcohol (PVA) particles (300- to 500-μm particles are probably the most commonly used). Temporary occlusion can be achieved with gelatin sponge (Gelfoam or Spongstan) cut into pledgets of 1 to 2 mm to form a slurry or injected as separate "torpedoes" (Fig. 53-4). The powder form should not be used because the much smaller particles occlude at or close to the capillary level, making tissue necrosis highly likely.

Cyanoacrylate ("glue") is a useful liquid embolic agent in situations where the active bleeding point in the vessel cannot be traversed with a catheter to prevent back bleeding from collateral sources, and a stable catheter position without compromise of nontarget vessels is achieved. Cyanoacrylate causes permanent embolization with almost instant polymerization when placed in contact with blood and does not rely on the coagulation process, so it is also advantageous in severely coagulopathic patients. However, cyanoacrylate should be used with caution and only by the adequately trained/experienced; uncontrolled delivery resulting in nontarget embolization may have catastrophic consequences. Additional risks include gluing a

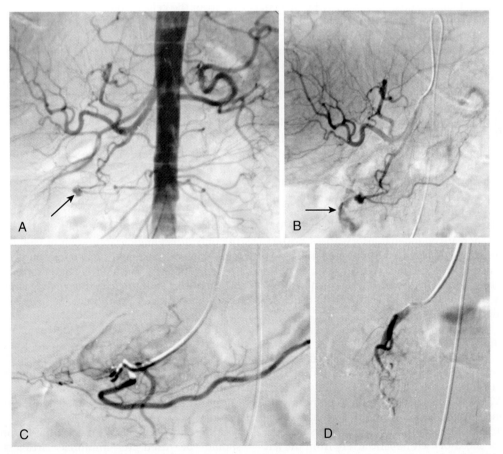

FIGURE 53-4. Gelfoam embolization of gastroduodenal artery (GDA) hemorrhage, via a 5F catheter. This procedure was performed before availability of microcatheters. **A,** Aortic flush run showing pseudoaneurysm *(arrow)*. **B,** Active extravasation *(arrow)* on a selective GDA injection. **C,** Catheter could not be advanced beyond the bleeding point. **D,** Completion angiogram post Gelfoam embolization with technical and clinical success.

microcatheter in a vessel. Detachable-tip microcatheters are a way of circumventing this potential complication.

TECHNIQUE

Anatomy and Approaches

Awareness of the normal arterial anatomy and possible anatomic variations is essential.

Normal Anatomy

The celiac axis and SMA arise from the anterior abdominal wall at T12 and L1-2, respectively. The first branch of the celiac axis is the left gastric artery. It divides after 1 to 2 cm into the splenic and common hepatic arteries. The dorsal pancreatic artery or inferior phrenic artery sometimes arise from the trunk. The common hepatic artery becomes the proper hepatic artery after the origin of the GDA. The characteristic cystic artery is a branch of the right hepatic artery. The right gastric artery, which supplies the pylorus and lesser curve of the stomach, arises from the common, proper, or left hepatic artery but is often difficult to identify on angiography. The left gastric artery runs cranially, supplying the distal esophagus and fundus of the stomach. It communicates with the right gastric artery, the branches of the gastroepiploic arteries, the short gastric branches of the splenic artery, and often the inferior phrenic artery.

The splenic artery runs along the superior surface of the pancreas. This accounts for it being the most common site of pancreatitic pseudoaneurysms. It supplies the spleen, stomach, and pancreas. It provides the dorsal pancreatic artery, pancreatica magna, and short gastric arteries. Its terminal branches are the splenic hilar superior and inferior divisions, with the left gastroepiploic artery arising from the latter and supplying the greater curve of the stomach.

The first branch of the GDA is the *posterior superior* pancreaticoduodenal artery, which supplies the duodenum to the right and the pancreas to the left. The terminal divisions of the GDA are the *anterior superior* pancreaticoduodenal and the right gastroepiploic arteries. The latter anastomoses with the left gastroepiploic artery, which is a branch of the splenic artery. The *superior* pancreaticoduodenal arteries form a rich arterial network in the pancreatic head and neck, with numerous anastomoses with the *inferior* pancreaticoduodenal branch of the SMA (Fig. 53-5).

The *inferior* pancreaticoduodenal artery arises posteriorly from the proximal SMA or the first jejunal arteries. Catheters that face to the rear in the SMA (e.g., a cobra) permit easier catheterization of the inferior pancreaticoduodenal artery than forward-facing catheters in the SMA (e.g., a sidewinder).

Variant Anatomy

In a dissected cadaver study, the classically described branching pattern of the celiac artery, SMA, and inferior mesenteric artery were present in only 22%, 24%, and 16%, respectively.[38] Variant anatomy is therefore common, and the interventionist should be familiar with common variations and alert to their presence. Common variants include:
- A replaced or accessory left hepatic artery from the left gastric artery
- A replaced proper, replaced right, or accessory right hepatic artery from the SMA

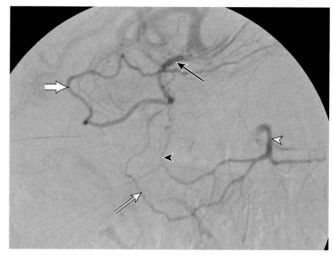

FIGURE 53-5. Pancreaticoduodenal arcade. Note gastroduodenal artery *(black arrow)*, posterosuperior pancreaticoduodenal artery *(black arrowhead)*, right gastroepiploic *(white block arrow)*, anterior superior pancreaticoduodenal artery *(white arrow)*, and inferior pancreaticoduodenal artery *(white arrowhead)*.

- The left gastric, hepatic, or splenic arteries (or all three) arising independently from the aorta
- A common celiac-mesenteric trunk
- The dorsal pancreatic or inferior phrenic arteries arising from the celiac trunk
- The GDA arising from the right or left hepatic artery
- The arc of Buehler, which is a persistent embryonic connection between the celiac trunk and proximal SMA

The extensive UGI vascular supply makes embolization in this territory very safe, but there is a tradeoff. It also makes hemostasis more difficult to achieve. Bleeding points must be occluded distally ("closing the back door") as well as proximally (see Fig. 53-1). As the dominant feeder to a bleeding point is occluded, alternative collateral pathways to that bleeding point will often quickly become apparent.

Technical Aspects

Extravasation of contrast medium into the bowel lumen is the only *direct* angiographic sign of UGI bleeding. *Indirect* signs include false and (less commonly) true aneurysms, vessel irregularity (Fig. 53-6), vessel cutoff and arteriovenous/arterioportal shunting, neovascularity, and increased vascularity from dilated arterioles (as seen in angiodysplasia). It is important to image into the venous phase. Caution should be exercised when vessel truncation or possible small pseudoaneurysms are seen in patients who have undergone previous UGI surgery (Fig. 53-7).

Arterial access is via the common femoral artery in the vast majority, but occasionally brachial or radial approaches are required for sharply angulated, stenosed, or tortuous vessels.

Antiperistaltic agents (hyoscine butylbromide/glucagon) should be used to minimize artifacts from bowel movement.

Multiple mask images should be obtained in uncooperative patients or those unable to breath hold. If possible,

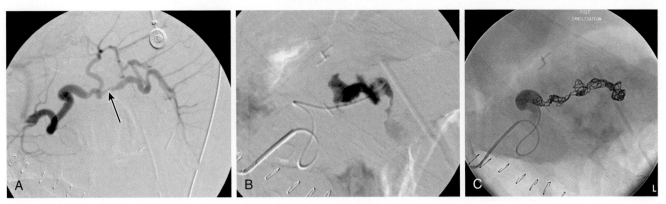

FIGURE 53-6. Vessel irregularity is an indirect indicator of source of upper gastrointestinal hemorrhage. **A,** Irregularity of mid-splenic artery *(arrow)*. **B,** Microcatheter injection at site of irregularity demonstrates active bleeding. **C,** Post coil embolization of distal splenic artery, with cessation of hemorrhage. No evidence of splenic infarction on ultrasound follow-up.

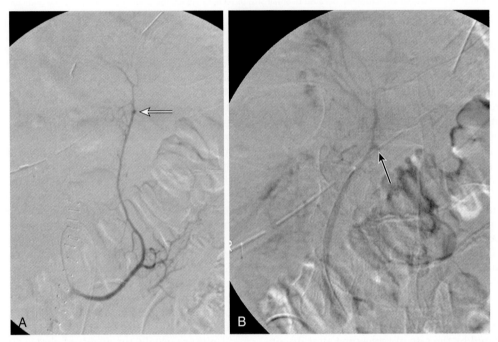

FIGURE 53-7. Hematemesis 1 week post gastroesophagectomy. **A,** Possible pseudoaneurysm *(arrow)* close to the pull-through anastomosis but superselective microcatheter injection with catheter tip at level of "abnormality" showed no active bleeding. **B,** Venous-phase image demonstrates an identical venous abnormality *(arrow)*. Appearances are due to ligated vessels. Hemorrhage was subsequently shown to be from a jejunal diverticulum that was successfully embolized.

these should be obtained during shallow respiration to maximize the chance of a suitable mask.

Patients who are too uncooperative, often because they are also hemodynamically unstable, will require *anesthetic support.*

Local *vasodilators,* such as tolazoline or glyceryl trinitrate, are useful if the hemodynamic state allows their use. Vasospasm is a common cause of intermittent bleeding. Vasodilators can also reverse catheter-induced spasm, which may impair angiographic demonstration of the bleeding point (or its underlying cause) or prevent catheter access to an active bleeding site.

Superselective angiograms of small vascular territories are often necessary to demonstrate active bleeding. These usually require use of microcatheters. Pump injections of

undiluted ICM can be performed through most microcatheters at flow rates of 3 mL/s and a pressure limit of 700 psi, which is considerably faster than achievable by hand injection and increases the diagnostic yield.

An isoosmolar nonionic ICM such as iodixanol (Visipaque) should be considered. Patients will often already have a degree of prerenal failure from intravascular volume depletion. This will be compounded by the high volumes of ICM often required. Iodixanol has been shown to be less nephrotoxic than nonisoosmolar agents, but its benefit has not been specifically demonstrated in this clinical context.[39]

CO_2 angiography is a useful adjunct if available. Simple noncommercial delivery systems are safe and easy to use, but dedicated angiographic inversion opacification software is required, along with faster acquisition frame rates

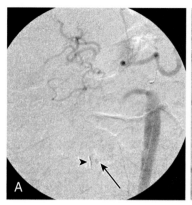 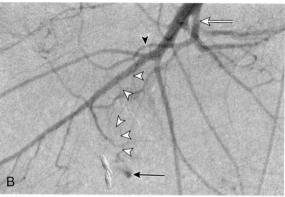 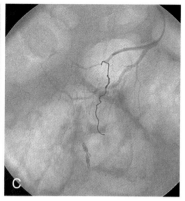

FIGURE 53-8. Recurrent upper gastrointestinal bleeding with multiple duodenal ulcers previously controlled endoscopically. Endoscopy was nondiagnostic. **A,** Carbon dioxide aortic injection shows a small "bubble" *(arrow)* at site of previously clipped D3 ulcer *(arrowhead).* Superior pancreaticoduodenal arcade could not be catheterized via celiac axis. **B,** Superselective microcatheterization of posterior pancreaticoduodenal artery (PPDA) *(black arrowhead)* via superior mesenteric artery and inferior pancreaticoduodenal artery *(white arrow)* confirms active bleeding *(black arrow)* from a duodenal branch *(white arrowheads)* of the PPDA. **C,** Appearance post microcoil embolization. Because of small size of feeding vessel, the 2-mm coils are oversized and straightened.

of 3 to 6 frames per second.[40] It will often demonstrate the site of bleeding with flush or selective runs, unlike ICM, which more commonly requires superselective catheter positions to demonstrate active bleeding. This increases the speed of the procedure, which is an obvious advantage in the hemodynamically unstable patient. CO_2 has a very low viscosity, expanding at the site of hemorrhage to fill the luminal space and producing a prominent "bubble."[41] It also acts as a vasodilator, which is an advantage in a patient with intermittent hemorrhage. Back et al. reported on 27 patients with suspected GI bleeding, and hemorrhage was detected in 44% of patients with CO_2, versus 14% with ICM.[42] The absence of any nephrotoxic effect is of further benefit. Disadvantages of CO_2 include the failure to precisely define the feeding vessel owing to bolus fragmentation, additional procedural complexity, and intolerance in some patients (Fig. 53-8).

Vasopressin infusion was introduced in the 1970s and remained popular through the 1980s, although it was more widely adopted in the United States than in Europe. Enthusiasm was tempered by the rate of rebleeding after discontinuation of the infusion, cardiovascular complications (e.g., myocardial ischemia, dysrhythmias, visceral infarction, puncture site occlusions), and the difficulty in maintaining a selective catheter position. The superiority of embolization over vasopressin infusion was established when Gomes et al. reported in 1986 that the probability of success in major GI hemorrhage was 52% for vasopressin infusion versus 88% for embolization.[43]

Similarly, *autologous blood clot*, which was also popular in the 1970s and 1980s, is now rarely used.

Embolization Technique

During the embolization, catheters are flushed with non-heparinized saline. "Check" arteriograms are obtained frequently. A stable catheter position must be confirmed before embolization by test passage of the coil-pushing wire or test injection for particulate agents.

Although microcoils are more easily delivered by the injection technique, this is not usually applicable in small or end arteries.

Nonradiopaque particulate embolic material (e.g., gelatin sponge and PVA particles) must be mixed with 50% ICM and injected under continuous high-quality fluoroscopy on a small field size to minimize reflux of the embolic agent into nontarget vessels.

In the hemodynamically unstable patient, volume depletion results in reduced vessel size. Coil embolization in this setting can result in undersized coils, with recanalization once the intravascular volume is restored. A degree of coil oversizing is recommended in this setting. The temptation to pack the sac of a pseudoaneurysm with coils must be avoided because this is usually ineffective, with recurrence almost inevitable.

Occasionally, intentional arterial dissection with a guidewire may be employed, but permanence of the created occlusion is difficult to determine because severe guidewire-induced spasm will have an identical appearance.

In *gastric and duodenal hemorrhage*, the rich supply from the pancreaticoduodenal arcade makes embolization safe but sometimes challenging.

Coils are usually the agents of choice. They can be combined with particulate agents or glue to achieve thrombosis, particularly in the setting of coagulopathy (Fig. 53-9). Particulate agents or glue may be used as sole agents when hemorrhage is from small vessels that cannot be selectively catheterized or when the distal vessels are too small or tortuous to be catheterized (see Fig. 53-4).

Diffuse hemorrhagic gastritis or duodenitis is more difficult to manage endovascularly than a single large eroded artery from a peptic ulcer. The latter can be isolated from the circulation with coils distally and proximally (Fig. 53-10). Diffuse bleeding requires sufficient reduction in perfusion pressure in all the vessels contributing to the bleeding to allow thrombosis to occur without causing necrosis. Gelfoam slurry or larger PVA particles are the usual agents of choice in this scenario.

All potential feeding arteries to the site of hemorrhage must be imaged. Recurrent bleeding may occur, even despite effective initial embolization; thorough exclusion of further feeding vessels, owing to rapid collateral development, is vital. In the pancreaticoduodenal arcade, this usually requires postembolization "check" angiograms from

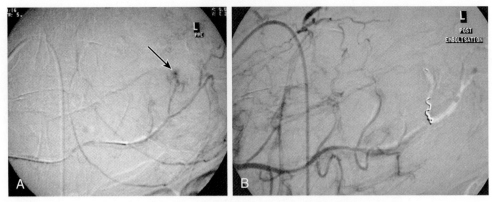

FIGURE 53-9. Gastric ulcer hemorrhage with coagulopathy and multiorgan failure. **A,** Bleeding gastric ulcer *(arrow)* supplied by right gastroepiploic artery. No contribution from left gastric artery was seen on selective catheterization. **B,** Hemostasis required Gelfoam particles in addition to coils in the feeding vessel.

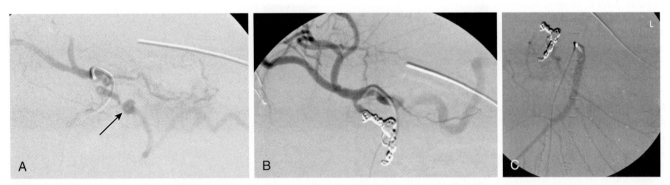

FIGURE 53-10. A 65-year-old woman presented with failure to control upper gastrointestinal hemorrhage at laparotomy. Twenty units of packed red blood cells were transfused. **A,** Mid-gastroduodenal artery pseudoaneurysm *(arrow).* **B,** Hepatic artery injection after embolization via a 4F Cobra catheter. **C,** Superior mesenteric artery injection demonstrates no retrograde collateral reconstitution of pseudoaneurysm.

both the celiac axis and SMA sides (Fig. 53-11; also see Fig. 53-10).

When the region of bleeding is known from endoscopy, but there is no angiographic abnormality, particulate material can be used to reduce the perfusion pressure. In the duodenum, this often requires protection of the normal circulation by placement of coils in the proximal right gastroepiploic artery and the pancreaticoduodenal arteries (to protect the SMA) before injection of particles into the GDA.

Gastric bleeding requires catheterization of the left gastric artery. A sidewinder catheter advanced into the splenic (or sometimes the hepatic) artery and then gradually withdrawn until it engages in the left gastric artery origin is one of the more reliable techniques for achieving this.

In *hemobilia,* embolization is the primary treatment modality when conservative management fails or is inappropriate.[44] It is superior to surgery. The abnormality, whether due to trauma, iatrogenic injury, or tumor, is usually intrahepatic. Surgical treatment is to ligate the extrahepatic vessels, but this carries a risk of failure. If proximal vessel ligation induces a sufficient reduction in perfusion pressure, thrombosis may occur, but in many patients bleeding will continue owing to recruitment of distal intrahepatic collateral vessels. The bleeding vessel must be embolized both distal and proximal to the bleeding point

to prevent this. This additional capability to block distally is the reason why embolization is superior to surgery. Coils are most commonly used, but if the vessel distal to the bleeding point cannot even be catheterized with a microcatheter, it should be blocked distally with glue or particulate agents such as 300- to 500-μm PVA (Fig. 53-12).

Postpancreatitic true aneurysms, pseudoaneurysms, or pseudocyst hemorrhages warrant separate consideration. Approximately 10% of patients with acute pancreatitis develop such complications, and it is reported that mortality exceeds 90% with conservative management.[45,46] Rupture and decompression of the pseudoaneurysm or pseudocyst into the stomach or duodenum results in UGI hemorrhage. A less common scenario is rupture into the pancreatic duct with transpapillary bleeding (hemosuccus pancreaticus) (Fig. 53-13).

The most commonly involved vessel is the splenic artery, but any upper abdominal vessel may be involved. The phlegmonous pancreas makes open surgical exposure of the relevant feeding vessels or the alternative extirpation of diseased pancreatic tissue very difficult. This is reflected in mortality rates of up to 56%.[47,48] Radiologic treatment is the treatment of choice for these patients. A classification of aneurysms and pseudoaneurysms associated with pancreatitis has been proposed.[49] This suggests that true aneurysms from a named major artery are best treated by proximal and distal embolization or stent-graft placement

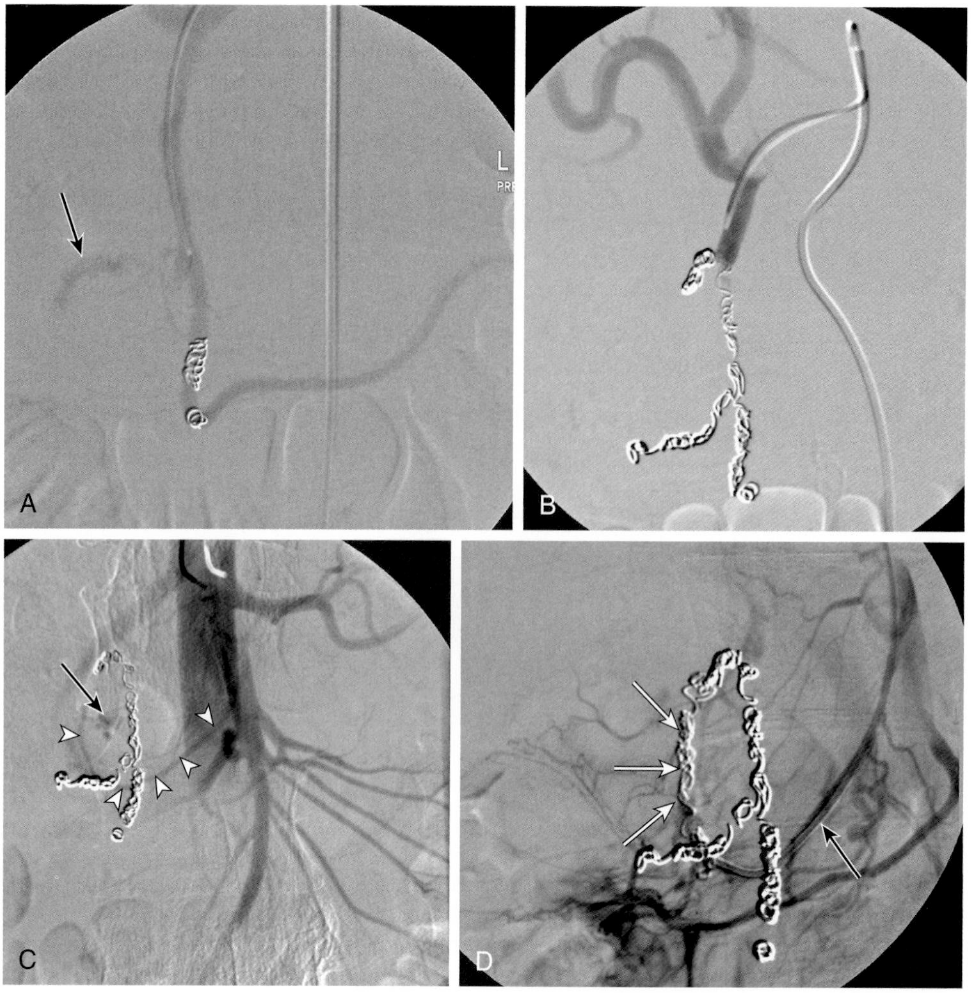

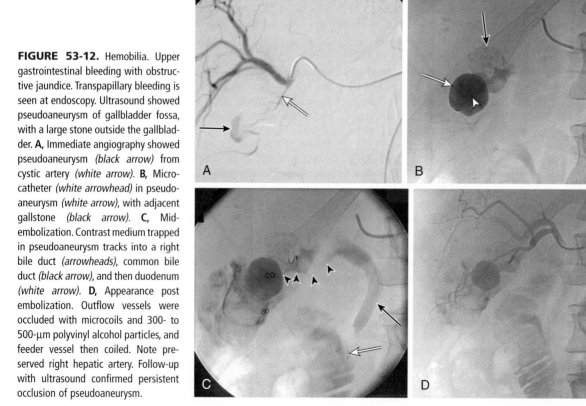

FIGURE 53-11. Bleeding duodenal ulcer with failed endoscopic treatment. **A,** Active bleeding from gastroduodenal artery (GDA) *(arrow)* territory, with initial distal coils. **B,** Patient became hemodynamically stable post coil embolization of the GDA and its proximal branches. Inferior pancreaticoduodenal artery (IPDA) was not examined; 2 days later, hematemesis recurred. **C,** Arteriography shows active bleeding *(black arrow)* via the IPDA *(white arrowheads)*. **D,** Permanent hemostasis achieved after coil occlusion of bleeding site *(white arrows)* via the IPDA *(black arrow)*.

FIGURE 53-12. Hemobilia. Upper gastrointestinal bleeding with obstructive jaundice. Transpapillary bleeding is seen at endoscopy. Ultrasound showed pseudoaneurysm of gallbladder fossa, with a large stone outside the gallbladder. **A,** Immediate angiography showed pseudoaneurysm *(black arrow)* from cystic artery *(white arrow)*. **B,** Microcatheter *(white arrowhead)* in pseudoaneurysm *(white arrow)*, with adjacent gallstone *(black arrow)*. **C,** Midembolization. Contrast medium trapped in pseudoaneurysm tracks into a right bile duct *(arrowheads)*, common bile duct *(black arrow)*, and then duodenum *(white arrow)*. **D,** Appearance post embolization. Outflow vessels were occluded with microcoils and 300- to 500-μm polyvinyl alcohol particles, and feeder vessel then coiled. Note preserved right hepatic artery. Follow-up with ultrasound confirmed persistent occlusion of pseudoaneurysm.

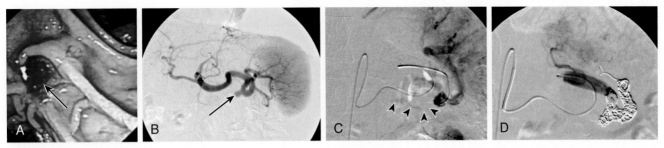

FIGURE 53-13. **A,** Transpapillary bleeding at endoscopy showing a clot at the ampulla *(arrow)*. **B,** Saccular aneurysm *(arrow)* of distal splenic artery. Embolization at this level carries increased risk of splenic infarction due to occlusion of collateral supply from collateral pathway via the short gastric arteries. **C,** Contrast injection into pseudoaneurysm confirms it to be the source of hemorrhage, with opacification of pancreatic duct *(arrowheads)*. **D,** Coil embolization of distal splenic artery. Minor infarction of upper and lower pole of spleen that required no intervention.

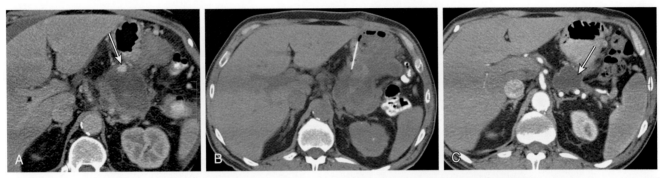

FIGURE 53-14. A 55-year-old man presented with acute-on-chronic alcoholic pancreatitis and hematemesis. **A,** Arterial-phase computed tomography (CT) scan showed a small pseudoaneurysm *(arrow)* apposed to posterior wall of stomach. No abnormality was evident on superselective arteriography. Pseudoaneurysm was designated as "low flow." **B,** CT-guided transgastric placement of a 22-gauge Chiba needle into pseudoaneurysm, with injection of 1000 IU of thrombin, resulted in thrombosis of pseudoaneurysm. **C,** Arterial-phase CT scan 6 months later. Pseudoaneurysm remains occluded, with a small, well-defined residual pancreatic pseudocyst *(arrow)*.

if anatomically appropriate. "High-flow" pseudoaneurysms, which fill early on angiography and arise from a named artery, are best treated by proximal and distal coiling. "Low-flow" pseudoaneurysms identified on contrast-enhanced CT, but that only fill in the late venous phase of angiography or are not seen at all, are best treated by percutaneous thrombin injection under CT or ultrasound guidance (Fig. 53-14). Patients with active pancreatitis treated in this way require close CT follow-up, and repeated treatments are often necessary but ultimately successful.

Pancreaticoduodenal arcade true aneurysms may also occur, owing to increased flow to supply an occluded celiac axis due to trauma, median arcuate ligament compression, or atherosclerosis (Sutton-Kadir syndrome).[50] Embolization is usually via the inferior pancreaticoduodenal artery when there is active bleeding, but there is a risk of celiac territory necrosis if insufficient additional collateral vessels are present. Alternative strategies in patients who are not actively bleeding include celiac artery stenting when appropriate, followed by coil embolization of the inferior pancreaticoduodenal artery or, if the aneurysm is saccular, packing of the aneurysm alone with detachable neuroradiologic coils or the slowly polymerizing liquid embolic agent ethylene-vinyl alcohol (Onyx [ev3/Covidien, Plymouth, Minn.]) (Fig. 53-15).[50]

Cooperation between the endoscopist, interventional radiologist, and surgeon is essential. It relies on good communication and a thorough knowledge of the therapeutic options. For example, when endoscopy successfully identifies the cause of UGI bleeding but is unable to treat it, the endoscopist can place a series of metal clips as a target, which allows embolization even in the absence of an angiographic abnormality.[37] A single clip is unreliable because it might detach in the interval between endoscopy and angiography. Therefore, several clips are preferable.

Similarly, "blind" embolization of the appropriate territory is an option when there is no angiographic abnormality, if the endoscopist has accurately identified the site of bleeding.[27]

In a small number of patients, angiography will demonstrate the cause of bleeding, but embolization will be impossible or inappropriate. Subsequent surgery can be assisted, particularly in patients who have had previous UGI resective surgery, by placing a single coil at the site of hemorrhage as a target (which can be identified by intraoperative fluoroscopy) or by leaving a microcatheter in situ for injection of methylene blue dye or saline (which causes blanching of the segment of bowel) at operation.

CONTROVERSIES

The preference to perform angiography while the patient is actively bleeding is not uniformly accepted. Some authors still advocate that the patient should be hemodynamically stable at the time of angiography.[26]

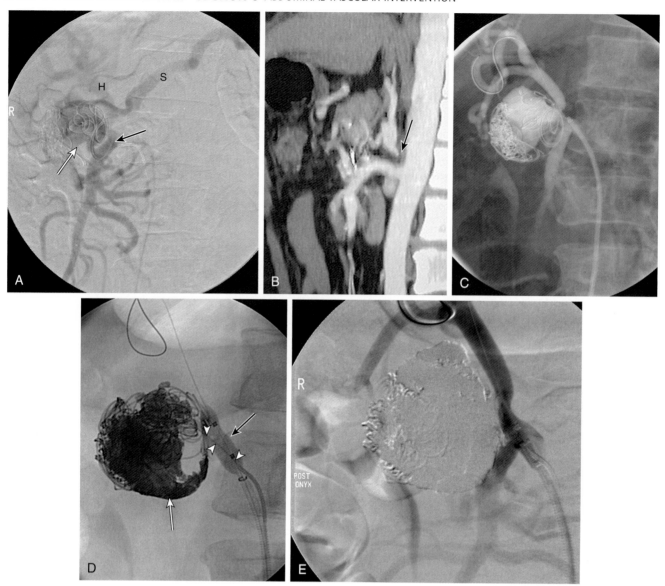

FIGURE 53-15. A 40-year-old man presented with a history of two previous major motor vehicle accidents and a 10-year history of a high-flow pancreaticoduodenal arcade aneurysm (PDAA) with recent expansion. There had been two previous unsuccessful attempts at coil embolization. **A,** Superior mesenteric artery (SMA) injection *(black arrow)* shows 4-cm PDAA *(white arrow)* with retrograde hepatic *(H)* and splenic *(S)* supply. **B,** Sagittal CT reformatted image shows the presumed posttraumatic celiac origin occlusion *(arrow)*. **C,** Preembolization angiogram. **D,** Embolization using ethylene-vinyl alcohol (Onyx) *(white arrow)* via a microcatheter *(arrowheads)* and a protection balloon *(black arrow)* across the wide neck. **E,** Complete occlusion of aneurysm, with preservation of SMA and pancreaticoduodenal arcade.

MD-CTA, with its high-contrast sensitivity, has a critical role to play in the diagnosis of UGI bleeding,[10,51] but its role is not emphasized or clearly delineated in recently published guidelines.[52,53] Current practice in our institution is for patients with an active bleeding point not controlled at the time of endoscopy to undergo emergency catheter angiography and embolization. Patients suspected of bleeding actively with no endoscopic visualization of a bleeding point or following recent endoscopic treatment (deemed a failure to respond to endoscopic treatment) undergo triple-phase (unenhanced, arterial, and delayed-phase) contrast-enhanced MD-CTA with no bowel contrast media and proceed to angiography only if active bleeding or a potential source is identified (see Fig. 53-3).

OUTCOMES

For a full discussion of the clinical success rates in UGI bleeding following embolization, please visit the website at www.expertconsult.com.

COMPLICATIONS

The general complications of angiography apply and include access site hematoma, femoral artery pseudoaneurysms, arterial dissection and perforation, and ICM allergic reactions and nephrotoxicity. These complications are more frequent in patients undergoing UGI embolization because

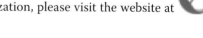

they are commonly volume depleted, coagulopathic, and poorly cooperative.

Specific postembolization complications include gastric or duodenal critical ischemia, resulting in strictures, ulceration, and necrosis, but these fortunately are rare. They are predisposed to by damage to potential collateral vessels from previous upper abdominal surgery or radiotherapy and by severe atherosclerosis.

Infarction of the spleen is usually caused by a distal splenic artery embolization resulting in inadequate collateral supply. When embolization at this site is unavoidable, splenic infarction remains unpredictable. Even if this does occur, it is easier to deal surgically with the sequelae of splenic infarction than active UGI bleeding from the splenic artery. Hepatic infarction after hepatic artery embolization almost invariably occurs in patients with portal vein occlusion. Extreme caution should be exercised in performing embolization in such patients. Patients with hepatic transplants are unusually dependent on their hepatic arterial supply for liver viability, and similar caution should apply to these patients.

POSTPROCEDURAL AND FOLLOW-UP CARE

Active follow-up is integral to the success of embolization for UGI hemorrhage. It should include daily rounds for all postinterventional patients who remain hospitalized. This allows early detection and treatment of recurrent bleeding and complications. Ideally, follow-up should continue for at least 30 days after the procedure. A prospective record of procedures should be kept and audited against reference standards of care, such as those in Table 53-2. Postembolization ischemic strictures only warrant treatment if they are symptomatic. On this basis, routine imaging to detect postembolization UGI tract stenoses is not indicated.

KEY POINTS

- The safety and efficacy of embolization in life-threatening upper gastrointestinal (UGI) hemorrhage is well established.
- Embolization has largely replaced surgery in endoscopy-refractory gastroduodenal bleeding.
- It is the treatment of choice in transpapillary bleeding and the vascular complications of pancreatitis.
- Diagnostic success is dependent on the best achievable image quality and a thorough knowledge of normal and variant anatomy.
- Multidetector computed tomographic angiography (MD-CTA) is a reliable and accurate imaging technique to identify bleeding and plan transcatheter UGI therapy in patients who are clinically suspected of bleeding, but endoscopy is negative or incomplete.
- Timing is critical. Most UGI hemorrhage is intermittent.
- Therapeutic success depends on diagnostic success, underlying pathology, and meticulous embolization technique.

TABLE 53-2. Success Rates for Transcatheter Embolization in Upper Gastrointestinal Bleeding

Site	Reported Rates (%)	Threshold (%)*
UGI bleeding (overall)	62-100	75
Focal gastroesophageal (gastric ulcer, Mallory-Weiss tear)	71-100	90
Hemorrhagic gastritis	25-78	70
Duodenal ulcer (benign)	72-100	—
Technical success[†]	—	90
Clinical success[‡]	—	60

*Thresholds are the minimum acceptable success rates for clinical audit/quality improvement programs.
[†]Technical success equates to immediate angiographic success.
[‡]Clinical success extends to 30-day follow-up.
UGI, Upper gastrointestinal.
Adapted from Drooz AT, Lewis CA, Allen TE et al., for the Society of Interventional Radiologists Standards of Practice Committee. Quality improvement guidelines for percutaneous transcatheter embolization. J Vasc Interv Radiol 1997;8:889–95.

▶ SUGGESTED READINGS

Frisoli JK, Sze DY, Kee S. Transcatheter embolization for the treatment of upper gastrointestinal bleeding. Tech Vasc Interv Radiol 2005;7: 136–42.

Geffroy Y, Rodallec MH, Boulay-Coletta I, et al. Multidetector CT angiography in acute gastrointestinal bleeding: why, when, and how. Radiographics 2011;31:E35–E46.

Green MHA, Duell RM, Johnson CD, et al. Haemobilia. Br J Surg 2001; 88:773–86.

Hastings GS. Angiographic localization and transcatheter treatment of gastrointestinal bleeding. Radiographics 2000;20:1160–8.

Jackson JE, Stabile B. Visceral embolization. In Dyet JF, Ettles DF, Nicholson AA, Wilson SE, editors. Textbook of endovascular procedures. Philadelphia: Churchill Livingstone; 2000. p. 328–40.

Ledermann HP, Schoch E, Jost R, et al. Superselective coil embolization in acute gastrointestinal hemorrhage: personal experience in 10 patients and review of the literature. J Vasc Interv Radiol 1998;9:753–60.

Mirsadraee S, Tirukonda P, Nicholson A, et al. Embolization for non-variceal upper gastrointestinal tract haemorrhage: a systematic review. Clin Radiol 2011;66:500–9.

The complete reference list is available online at www.expertconsult.com.

CHAPTER 54

Management of Lower Gastrointestinal Bleeding

Michael D. Darcy

CLINICAL RELEVANCE

Lower gastrointestinal bleeding (LGIB) is much less common than upper gastrointestinal (GI) tract bleeding; the incidence of LGIB is only around 20.4 cases per 100,000 adults per year. However, it is associated with a 10% mortality rate,[1] and though less common than upper GI bleeding, it more often demands the specialized skills of the interventional radiologist. These cases are not as easily managed by endoscopic techniques, and many gastroenterologists will not attempt endoscopy while the patient is actively bleeding, owing to the difficulty in clearing blood and achieving visualization. Interventional techniques afford the opportunity to localize hemorrhage more precisely and stop bleeding less invasively than surgery.

INDICATIONS

LGIB is frequently self-limiting, so the first task is to determine whether the patient is bleeding actively enough to make it likely an arteriogram will be positive. Actual output of blood is not always the best criterion. The patient can be grossly bleeding but not have hematochezia because of the large holding capacity of the colon. Alternatively, bloody output from the rectum can continue long after bleeding has stopped as old blood is expelled. Feingold et al.[2] found that using pulse and blood pressure assessment alone was very predictive of a positive tagged red blood cell (TRBC) scan. In this study, 62% of unstable patients (defined as a heart rate >100 or systolic blood pressure <100 mmHg) had a positive TRBC, but only 21% of hemodynamically stable patients had positive scans. Similarly, an analysis of 88 patients showed three clinical factors that correlated with positive angiography.[3] Angiograms were significantly more positive when (1) blood pressure was less than 90 mmHg (87% positive vs. 12% positive when blood pressure was higher), (2) transfusion requirements were 5 or more units of blood (84% vs. 15% for fewer transfused units), and (3) hemoglobin dropped more than 5 g/dL from prior readings (85% vs. 26% for lesser hemoglobin drops).

On the other hand, angiography should not be delayed until the patient is severely hypotensive. By the time a patient goes into shock, close to 40% of blood volume has been lost.[4] The threshold for deciding to do angiography should also be modified by the patient's cardiovascular and resuscitation history. An elderly patient with moderate cardiovascular disease may need a higher perfusion pressure to avoid end-organ ischemia and thus may poorly tolerate even mild hypotension. End-organ ischemia can also be exacerbated by the decreased oxygen-carrying capacity of blood hemodiluted by resuscitation fluids.

When patients are massively bleeding and hypotensive, the decision to proceed directly to angiography is fairly clear. When uncertain whether there is active bleeding, a TRBC scan may be worthwhile, since it is 5 to 10 times more sensitive than angiography at detecting bleeding. A review of over 600 TRBC scans showed that only 45% were positive.[5] However, if a TRBC is negative, its higher sensitivity to bleeding provides evidence that an arteriogram will be very unlikely to demonstrate bleeding. Thus a negative scan is useful in determining the advisability of an arteriogram. Although sensitive to the presence of bleeding, TRBC scans are not as effective at localizing the bleeding site. Zuckerman et al.[6] noted that TRBCs were falsely negative or provided incorrect localization in 3% to 59% of cases.

In recent years, computed tomographic angiography (CTA) has been proposed as a minimally invasive way to document and localize active bleeding, with several advantages over TRBC scans. Experimental work in a swine model has shown that CT can detect bleeding at a rate as low as 0.3 mL/min.[7] Early studies[8-11] demonstrated the ability of CTA to document active extravasation and localize LGIB. Subsequently, CTA was shown to have 79% to 91% sensitivity, 85% to 99% specificity, and 91% to 98% accuracy for detection of GI bleeding.[12-14] CTA trumps TRBC scans in that CTA can define the bleeding pathology in 52% to 75% of cases.[10,15] This allows formulation of a therapeutic plan better tailored to the patient's pathology (see Fig. e54-1). Another advantage of CTA is its ability to depict arterial anatomy (Fig. 54-1). This should facilitate subsequent arterial catheterization as well as increase the ability to localize the bleeding site. In fact, the exquisite depiction of arterial anatomy allowed one sigmoid diverticular bleed to be embolized empirically, which previously would never have been considered in the LGI tract.[16] Practical advantages of CTA over TRBC scans are that they tend to be more readily available and more rapidly performed.

Although generally reserved for acute active bleeding, angiography can occasionally be useful in patients with chronic low-grade bleeding in whom multiple endoscopies and other tests have failed to yield the diagnosis. Rollins et al.[17] reported that in patients with chronic LGIB, angiography revealed either structural lesions that could account for the bleeding or actual extravasation in 44% of their patients.

CONTRAINDICATIONS

Many of the contraindications to elective angiography become relative contraindications when weighed against the need to manage life-threatening bleeding.

Frank discussion about these risks and possible benefits should occur during the informed consent process. History of a life-threatening contrast allergy is a fairly firm contraindication to immediate angiography. Time can be taken to

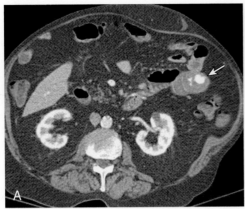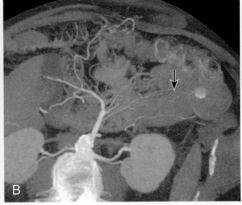

FIGURE 54-1. A, Computed tomography shows extravasation of contrast *(arrow)* into small bowel. **B,** Computed tomographic angiogram done at same time shows proximal jejunal branches *(arrow)* supplying the bleed. Atherosclerotic plaque is shown near superior mesenteric artery (SMA) origin, suggesting caution during attempts to catheterize SMA.

pretreat with steroids if bleeding is not massive, but the magnitude of the reaction must be weighed against the risk of exsanguination in each individual case. Similarly, the risk of renal failure in patients with preexisting renal insufficiency must be balanced against the need for possible life-saving embolization. Vigorous intravenous hydration can be started to reduce the risk of contrast nephropathy, but the patient's cardiopulmonary status must be monitored to avoid fluid overload and pulmonary edema.

Coagulopathy is a relative contraindication because it increases the risk of access site bleeding. Even with severe coagulopathy, angiography can still be done with a plan to leave a sheath in the arterial access site until the coagulopathy has been corrected. The sheath can also be used to continuously monitor arterial pressure in the postprocedure period. Alternatively, closure devices can be used to manage the arteriotomy. Another reason coagulopathy is a relative contraindication is that it significantly lowers the efficacy of embolization.[18] This is because emboli usually reduce blood flow, but complete cessation of flow requires formation of some thrombus around the emboli.

EQUIPMENT

Equipment commonly used in LGIB procedures is listed in Table 54-1. An in-depth discussion of this topic can be found at www.expertconsult.com.

ANATOMY AND APPROACH

A full discussion of LGI tract anatomy and best surgical approaches can be found at www.expertconsult.com.

TECHNICAL ASPECTS

Generally, arteriography for LGIB should start with selective catheterizations (see Table 54-1). Aortography is usually not necessary.

Without a lateral aortogram, it is usually not possible to ascertain the orientation of the vessel origins prior to engaging them with a catheter, so often physicians will start with their favorite catheter and then switch to another shaped

TABLE 54-1. Common Equipment

Equipment	Options/Examples	Manufacturer
6F sheath	Multiple versions	Multiple options
5F catheter for SMA	SOS Omni	AngioDynamics Queensbury, N.Y.
	Cobra	Multiple options
	Lev 1	Cook Medical Inc. Bloomington, Ind.
5F catheter for IMA	RIM	Cook Medical Inc. Bloomington, Ind.
	Rarely, SOS or Cobra	See above
3F microcatheter	Progreat	Terumo Medical Inc. Somerset, N.J.
	Mass Transit	Cordis Corp. Miami, Fla.
Wire for microcatheter	Glidewire GT	Terumo Medical Inc. Somerset, N.J.
	Transcend	Boston Scientific Miami, Fla.
Embolic agents	Microcoils	Multiple options
	0.025 in Glidewire to push microcoils	Boston Scientific Natick, Mass.
	PVA (>300 micron)	Multiple options

IMA, Inferior mesenteric artery; *PVA,* polyvinyl alcohol; *SMA,* superior mesenteric artery.

catheter if the first selection fails to adequately engage the target artery. The selective catheter should be advanced far enough into the vessel to prevent recoil out into the aorta, but it should not be advanced so far as to be injecting beyond proximal side branches.

If hemorrhage is identified, repeat arteriograms in different obliquities may be needed to define which specific branch the hemorrhage is arising from. If bleeding is not identified, provocative angiography can be done, which involves infusing a vasodilator or thrombolytic drug into the artery suspected to be the source of bleeding (Fig. 54-2). The goal is to stimulate bleeding to allow visualization of the extravasation on repeat digital subtraction angiography (discussed further in Controversies section).

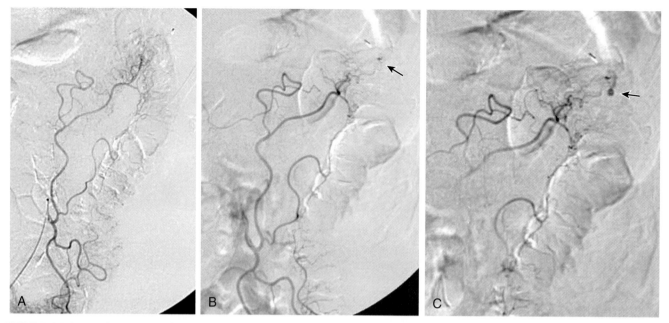

FIGURE 54-2. A, Inferior mesenteric artery (IMA) arteriogram of patient who had a positive tagged red blood cell scan in splenic flexure region. No abnormality was seen on this arteriogram. **B,** Because patient had numerous studies to locate bleeding source, provocative angiography was performed. Repeat arteriogram after infusion of tissue plasminogen activator (tPA) into IMA reveals a point of extravasation *(arrow).* **C,** Magnified later phase more clearly shows extravasation *(arrow).* Defining source of bleeding allowed placement of a microcoil and effective hemostasis.

Once the bleeding vessel has been localized, the 5F angiographic catheter is left in the main vessel ostium, and a 3F microcatheter is advanced coaxially through the 5F catheter. The microcatheter is necessary because of the small size (especially if the patient is vasoconstricted) and tortuosity of the mesenteric branches. Roadmapping can be useful to guide passage of the microcatheter but may be of limited value if there is excessive respiratory motion. Occasional contrast injections through the microcatheter are usually needed to insure that the correct branch is being entered. The microcatheter should be advanced as close to the point of extravasation as possible, even out into the vasa recta in the bowel wall. Once the microcatheter has been advanced to the desired site, embolization can be performed.

An expanded discussion of the technical aspects involved in arteriography can be found at www.expertconsult.com.

CONTROVERSIES

There are several controversies in the interventional management of LGIB. One is the role of provocative angiography. Although first introduced in 1988,[27] this procedure has not been widely used because questions exist regarding its utility and safety. The yield of stimulating bleeding has ranged from 29% up to 89%.[28-31] This wide range of results is most likely due to wide variation in the protocols used. In addition to extravasation, provocative angiography has occasionally demonstrated angiodysplasias or hypervascular tumors not evident on the original nonprovocative arteriograms. The goal is to identify the source of bleeding to allow definitive therapy. Kim et al. noted definitive treatment was made possible by provocative angiography in 31% of those who underwent the procedure.[30] However, most series report no hemorrhagic complications resulting from

the thrombolytic infusions,[29-31] so even the relatively modest yield is probably warranted, given that this technique is usually applied to patients who have undergone multiple other procedures that have failed to find the source of bleeding.

In the early 1990s, one of the main areas of contention was whether to embolize or infuse pitressin. As the safety of modern embolization techniques was established, this controversy faded.[32] Immediate control of bleeding, the fact that maintaining a catheter for 12 to 24 hours is not necessary, and the lack of systemic effects all favor use of embolization. However, even though it is becoming a more common first-line therapy, there is still uncertainty whether there are specific lesions or anatomic regions that should be treated by methods other than embolization. This will be discussed more fully in the Outcomes section.

Which embolic agent is best is another controversy; in most series, a mixture of approaches is used. Microcoils are the most common embolic agent, but PVA or gelfoam (either as sole embolic agent or to augment coils) are often used in some studies. NBCA has been used in a few small series, with good results[33,34]; 100% technical success was achieved, with rebleeding rates of 14% to 15% and no ischemic complications. However, late intestinal stricture has been reported as a complication.[35] The main potential benefit of NBCA is that it is more mechanically occlusive and does not rely on formation of thrombus on the embolic nidus, so it should work better in coagulopathic patients. Glue must be used with caution. A study done in a swine model nicely demonstrated that ischemic changes were minimal if three or fewer colonic vasa recta were embolized, but full-thickness circumferential ischemic changes were seen in the animals when five or more vasa recta were embolized with glue.[36] To date, there has been no randomized trial comparing these various embolic agents.

Another point of debate is at what level to embolize—at the marginal artery or beyond. In a letter,[37] Nicholson and Ettles compared two studies[38,39] in which emboli were deposited at different levels. Initial control of bleeding was controlled in 71% to 86% of patients in both studies, but long-term clinical success varied. With emboli deposited at or proximal to the marginal artery, 52% of the patients developed recurrent bleeding.[39] When emboli were deposited beyond the marginal artery, the rate of recurrent hemorrhage was 0%.[38] However, Bandi et al. reported moderate recurrent hemorrhage despite vasa recta–level embolization.[22] Aside from efficacy, safety is also is also a concern, since there are cases where it is not technically possible to embolize distal to the marginal artery (see Fig. e54-5). Funaki[40] described cases where long segments of the marginal artery were embolized without ischemia, but this is not commonly accepted therapy. Thus the optimal level of embolization has not clearly been defined, and larger clinical trials are needed to clarify this point.

OUTCOMES

Outcomes should be evaluated for both technical success (successful occlusion of the desired vessel) and clinical success (termination of bleeding). Results from modern series are shown in Table 54-2. For LGIB, the range of technical success for embolization is 73% to 100%, with an average of 93%.[18,22,38,39,41-61] Vessel spasm and tortuosity are the most common causes of technical failure. Despite improvement in catheters and wires, technical success figures have not changed much over the past 30 years. However, this simply reflects the changing goals of embolization. Previously, flow-directed emboli were injected from a selective position in a major visceral branch. Modern microcatheters, on the other hand, are advanced into the marginal artery or beyond into the vasa recta before embolizing. Thus in more modern series, the definition of technical success is simply more stringent and difficult to achieve.

Clinical success (termination of bleeding) is more difficult to achieve than technical success because bleeding may continue even after successful occlusion of the target artery. A diffuse blood supply to the bleeding lesion (as with tumors or inflammatory conditions), having significant collateral flow around the target artery, and coagulopathy (with continued flow through the target artery) can all cause continued bleeding after embolization. Clinical success therefore occurs at a slightly lower rate (60%-100%, average 81%) than technical success (see Table 54-2).

Just looking at initial clinical success may overestimate the benefit of embolization, since bleeding will recur in 0% to 52% of patients. This wide variance is likely due to different follow-up periods, with rebleeding rates being

TABLE 54-2. Outcomes of Embolization for Lower Gastrointestinal Bleeding

Author	Year	No. of Patients	Site	Technical Success (%)	Initial Clinical Success (%)	Major Ischemic Complications (%)
Guy[50]	1992	9	Mixed	100	100	0
Gordon[49]	1997	17	Mixed	82	77	6
Peck[39]	1998	21	Mixed	81	71	0
Ledermann[61]	1998	7	Mixed	86	86	0
Nicholson[38]	1998	14	Colon	100	86	0
Bulakbasi[18]	1999	10	Mixed	90	60	0
Evangelista[46]	2000	17	Mixed	88	76	0
Luchtefeld[41]	2000	17	Mixed	82	82	6
Bandi[22]	2001	48	Mixed	73	69	0
Funaki[47]	2001	27	Colon	93	96	4
Kuo[53]	2003	22	Mixed	100	86	0
Khanna[51]	2005	12	Mixed	92	75	0
Neuman[57]	2005	23	Mixed	100	78	4
d'Othee[45]	2006	19	Mixed	89	68	11
Sheth[58]	2006	63	Mixed	97	83	0
Lipof[55]	2008	75	Mixed	97	84	7
Kickuth[52]	2008	20	Mixed	100	90	5
Tan[60]	2008	32	Mixed	97	63	3
Kwak[54]	2009	17	SB	100	88	0
Maleux[56]	2009	39	Mixed	100	85	10
Gillespie[48]	2010	37	Mixed	100	95	5
Tan[59]	2010	23	Colon	100	78	0
AVERAGES				93	81	3

underestimated in studies with shorter follow-up. Delayed recurrent bleeding has been reported to occur at the original site of embolization as long as 4 years later.[56] However, recurrent bleeding has been documented to arise from a site different from the originally treated lesion in as many as 50% to 66% of cases.[18,46] This should not cause one to discount the potential long-term benefit of LGIB embolization. A recent study found that embolization could be the definitive therapy in over 50% of colonic diverticular bleeds.[59]

Subgroup analysis of outcomes has not been extensively investigated; instead, most studies lump together different pathologic lesions. Also, small-bowel and colonic sources are usually included together in series despite their significantly different anatomy. The jejunum and rectum have much greater potential for collateral flow, so theoretically embolization should be less effective in these regions. Peck et al.[39] suggested that these regional anatomic differences do alter efficacy, although there were few patients in each group. Subsequently, Tan et al. showed that embolization was far more effective in the colon, with only a 15% rebleeding rate compared to a 60% rate of rebleeding after embolization of small-bowel hemorrhage.[60] No large series have studied specific pathologic lesions. Some case reports have focused on angiodysplasias,[62,63] and whereas some report clinical success, others suggest that angiodysplasias are prone to rebleeding after embolization.[22,39] A meta-analysis of 25 studies revealed that the rate of recurrent bleeding was only 15% for diverticular bleeding, but was 45% for angiodysplasias and other lesions.[51] More work is needed in analyzing outcomes for specific lesions.

COMPLICATIONS

Patients undergoing LGI embolization may sustain the typical complications associated with angiography, including puncture site hematomas, arterial occlusion, contrast reactions, and contrast-induced renal failure.

Since embolization for LGIB requires superselective catheterization, complications of spasm or dissection can occur in the target vessel. If this occurs in a proximal branch, it may lead to bowel ischemia in that distribution. If it occurs very peripherally, the only result may be that it prevents completion of embolization. On the other hand, spasm or dissection may decrease blood flow to the site of bleeding enough to arrest hemorrhage. In fact, vigorous manipulation of the guidewire to purposely induce spasm has been described as a way to stop LGIB.[64]

Bowel ischemia is the most concerning complication of LGI embolization, but this is also the area where the greatest progress has been made. Early series of LGI embolization using larger catheters and emboli reported infarction rates of 10% to 33%.[19-21,65,66] With newer microcatheters and microembolic agents, the rate of major ischemic complications (defined as complications requiring therapy) is approximately 3% (range 0%-11%).[18,22,38,39,41-61] The overall ischemic complication rate in some modern series[18,38,39,41,46,49,50] ranges from 5% to 70% (average 21%); however, one must realize that the vast majority of these complications are not clinically significant. Included are self-limited abdominal pain not requiring treatment and minor asymptomatic patches of ischemic mucosa discovered only on endoscopy done for other indications. These minor "ischemic complications" rarely require any therapy.

One concern is that minor ischemic changes could cause delayed stricture formation. Bandi et al.[22] reported on 48 patients with follow-up out to 10 years. No clinically significant complications were seen. Postprocedure endoscopy or surgical pathology was available in 25 of their patients; 6 had minor signs of ischemia identified at endoscopy, but none of these patients were symptomatic. In another study,[67] Horiguchi et al. described one patient (out of 14 embolization patients) who developed some circular muscular fibrosis identified on histologic exam. However, this patient also had an extensive embolization procedure with embolization of the proximal SMA arcade using numerous gelfoam pledgets, which is essentially the older embolization technique used 20 to 30 years ago. More recently, Neuman et al.[57] reported 2 of 23 (8.7%) LGI embolization patients requiring dilation or surgical correction of postischemic strictures. Although longer follow-up is warranted, it appears that with modern superselective techniques, most significant ischemic complications can be safely avoided.

Please visit www.expertconsult.com for an expanded discussion of possible complications.

POSTPROCEDURE AND FOLLOW-UP CARE

Whether or not to leave the arterial sheath in place is the first clinical decision that must be made. Leaving it in place is useful if the patient has a coagulopathy or if intraarterial monitoring is desired. If there is significant concern that early rebleeding may occur, leaving the sheath in place can also allow rapid repeat angiography.

Intravenous fluid and blood product administration should continue, with quantities determined by careful monitoring of postprocedure pulse, blood pressure, and hematocrit. The rectal output should be monitored, along with vital signs and complete blood cell counts to look for evidence of ongoing bleeding.

With each vital sign check, the abdomen should also be evaluated for tenderness, rigidity, rebound, or other signs of bowel ischemia. Supplemental oxygen is critical. Loss of red blood cells and hemodilution by intravenous fluids all contribute to reduced oxygen-carrying capacity. Administering oxygen via nasal prongs or mask will help compensate for this. Once the bleeding has stopped and the patient is stabilized, plans should be made for definitive therapy. If the etiology of the bleeding was not clear at angiography, colonoscopy should be done to define the pathology. It can also be useful to survey for postembolization ischemic changes.

SUMMARY

Angiography is an important tool for diagnosis and localization of LGIB. Advances in catheters and embolization materials have made the risk of significant ischemic complications so low that embolization should be considered a reasonable first-line therapy for LGIB.

▸ SUGGESTED READINGS

Darcy M. Treatment of lower gastrointestinal bleeding: vasopressin infusion versus embolization. J Vasc Interv Radiol 2003;14(5):535–43.

Kuo WT. Transcatheter treatment for lower gastrointestinal hemorrhage. Tech Vasc Interv Radiol 2004;7(3):143–50

Wu LM, Xu JR, Yin Y, Qu XH. Usefulness of CT angiography in diagnosing acute gastrointestinal bleeding: a meta-analysis. World J Gastroenterol 2010;16(31):3957–63. Epub 2010/08/17.

The complete reference list is available online at www.expertconsult.com.

CHAPTER 55

Acute Mesenteric Ischemia

Louis Boyer, Agaicha Alfidja, Lucie Cassagnes, Anne Ravel, and Pascal Chabrot

Acute mesenteric ischemia (AMI) is a life-threatening vascular emergency that requires early diagnosis and intervention to adequately restore mesenteric blood flow and prevent fatal bowel necrosis. Causes include arterial embolus, which occurs most frequently (40%-50%),[1] arterial thrombosis (20%-30%), venous obstruction (5%-18%),[2-4] and nonobstructive causes (20%-30%).[4] Clinical signs vary considerably and are nonspecific. Regardless of the cause, patients present with severe abdominal pain that is initially out of proportion to any physical findings.[5] Risk factors and clinical course differ according to underlying physiopathology.

Arterial embolism occurs in patients with cardiac conditions that predispose to emboli (thrombi, tachyarrhythmia), but can also complicate aortic catheterization procedures. Onset of symptoms is rapid, with intense and unrelenting abdominal pain that is disproportionate to physical examination findings. Associated symptoms include nausea and diarrhea, with bloody stools in some cases. Symptoms related to emboli in other locations are not uncommon. Patients who develop acute abdominal pain after arterial interventions in which catheters traverse the visceral aorta or who have arrhythmias (e.g., atrial fibrillation) or recent myocardial infarction should be suspected of having AMI.[5]

Arterial thrombosis occurs in patients at risk for atherosclerosis. Thrombosis can also complicate aortic aneurysm or dissection. In most cases, symptom onset is insidious, sometimes preceded by symptoms of chronic mesenteric ischemia (e.g., intermittent postprandial abdominal pain, food avoidance, weight loss). Patients often have evidence of atherosclerotic occlusive disease elsewhere, such as coronary or peripheral artery disease. The frequency with which chronic intestinal ischemia progresses to AMI, presumably by acute-on-chronic thrombosis, is unknown.[5]

AMI as a complication of aortic dissection is discussed elsewhere in this book.

Mesenteric venous thrombosis often affects much younger patients, many of whom have a history of one or more risk factors for hypercoagulability. Symptoms may present later than acute arterial thrombosis, sometimes after as long as 30 days, and are frequently less dramatic.

Nonocclusive mesenteric ischemia generally occurs in older individuals with severe clinical conditions and splanchnic vasoconstriction; these patients are sometimes unable to express abdominal pain. In the intensive care unit setting, acute respiratory distress syndrome or severe hypotension from cardiogenic or septic shock may precede nonocclusive mesenteric ischemia. Here, AMI is the result of severe and prolonged intestinal arterial vasospasm. Symptoms typically develop over several days, and patients may have experienced malaise and vague abdominal discomfort. The diagnosis is more often made when infarction occurs: patients develop increased pain associated with vomiting and may become hypotensive and tachycardic, with loose bloody stools. In this setting, the diagnosis of nonocclusive mesenteric ischemia is highly probable, especially if patency of the superior mesenteric vein (SMV) has been demonstrated.[6]

Nonocclusive mesenteric ischemia should be suspected in patients receiving vasoconstrictive substances and medications (e.g., cocaine, ergot, vasopressin, norepinephrine) who develop abdominal pain.[5] It should also be suspected in patients who develop abdominal pain after coarctation repair or surgical revascularization for intestinal ischemia due to arterial obstruction.[5]

AMI is an uncommon cause of acute abdominal pain (<1% among abdominal emergencies, according to Bergan et al.).[7] The diagnosis should be considered in patients with the following risk factors: age older than 60 years, previous history of vascular disease or valvular heart disease, cardiac arrhythmia, emboli, hypotension, recent heart failure, or hypercoagulability. Laboratory evaluation most frequently shows leukocytosis and lactic acidosis, and the amylase value is elevated in approximately 50% of patients; approximately 25% of patients have occult blood in the stool.

Although challenging, the diagnosis of AMI must be rapidly confirmed by a sensitive and specific imaging technique. Abdominal radiographs often show nonspecific dilated bowel loops. In contrast to chronic intestinal ischemia, duplex ultrasonography of the abdomen is not an appropriate tool for suspected AMI.[5]

Computed tomographic angiography (CTA) is the current best imaging tool for diagnosing AMI. Taourel et al.[8] found that when dynamic contrast-enhanced CT was used in cases of suspected AMI, presence of at least one sign (arterial or venous thrombosis, intramural gas, portal venous gas, focal lack of bowel wall enhancement, liver or splenic infarcts) resulted in diagnostic sensitivity of 64%, specificity of 92%, and accuracy of 75%. CTA is highly sensitive for the diagnosis of SMV thrombosis, with 100% sensitivity versus 70% for angiography and Doppler ultrasonography[3] (Fig. 55-1).

Conventional angiography is accurate for the diagnosis and characterization of AMI, but has been superseded in most institutions by CTA. However, if endovascular revascularization seems possible, angiography must be performed without delay.

Ideally, treatment must be undertaken early at the reversible ischemic stage, before bowel infarction (the common endpoint of all etiologic processes), which is characterized by onset of signs of peritoneal irritation.

INDICATIONS

Although surgical treatment is still in many cases considered the standard of care even in the absence of peritoneal signs,[9,10] mortality rates remain as high as 50%.[11] Therefore, transarterial techniques are a valuable alternative to

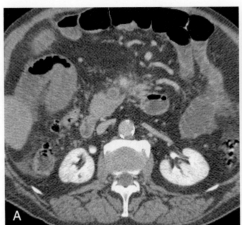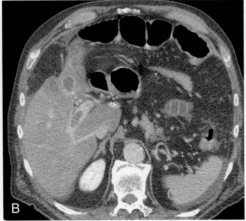

FIGURE 55-1. A-B, Computed tomographic angiography showing acute thrombosis of superior mesenteric and portal veins in a patient with worsening abdominal pain, treated by intensive intravenous heparin therapy because of a contraindication to thrombolysis.

surgical treatment in selected cases. It is during the early stages of AMI that medical and endovascular techniques can be most effective.[12] Patients so treated may still require surgery. If symptoms do not regress or bowel infarction occurs, surgical exploration can be undertaken by laparotomy or laparoscopy. A multidisciplinary approach is mandatory, with collaboration among gastroenterologists, anesthetists, surgeons, and radiologists.

Nonocclusive Mesenteric Ischemia

Arteriography is indicated in patients suspected of having nonocclusive mesenteric ischemia whose condition does not improve rapidly with treatment of their underlying disease.[5] Angiography can demonstrate the characteristic mesenteric arterial vasospasm and allow direct intraarterial instillation of a vasodilator. Treatment of the underlying shock is the most important initial step. Transcatheter administration of a vasodilator into the area of vasospasm is indicated in patients who do not respond to systemic supportive treatments and also patients with intestinal ischemia due to cocaine or ergot poisoning. Abdominal symptoms that persist after relief of intestinal vasospasm are an indication for laparotomy and resection of necrotic intestine.

Arterial Thromboembolism

Standard treatment for patients with acute obstructive mesenteric embolus or thrombosis is a laparotomy with embolectomy or revascularization and, if indicated, resection of infarcted bowel.

Vasodilators are considered a valuable supportive treatment option. They have been used preoperatively and postoperatively to reduce associated vasospasm in cases with complete occlusion.[6,13]

When thrombolytics are rapidly administered within a few hours after symptom onset before bowel infarction occurs, they may limit or even reverse bowel ischemia. Their use has been advocated to treat distal emboli, reserving proximal lesions for surgical treatment.[14] However, good results have also been obtained with thrombolysis of proximal emboli.[15] Angioplasty can still be performed on

any underlying stenoses should arterial recanalization be insufficient.[16]

Percutaneous transluminal angioplasty (PTA) and/or stenting, a commonly employed treatment for chronic mesenteric ischemia, remains a valuable option in the acute setting. Successful use of PTA and/or stenting has been reported in patients without bowel infarction, as well as in patients with signs of peritoneal irritation.[16-18]

Despite limited data, percutaneous treatment (lytic therapy, PTA, and/or stenting) of acute arterial obstruction is a reasonable option given the high mortality associated with open surgery.[5]

Venous Thrombosis

The mainstay of therapy for patients with mesenteric venous thrombosis is anticoagulation with surgical resection of affected bowel.[1,19] Thrombolytic therapy is reserved for mildly symptomatic thromboses diagnosed early, in the absence of contraindications to thrombolysis. In situ thrombolysis associated with PTA or mechanical methods to clear the obstruction have also been reported.[19,20]

CONTRAINDICATIONS

- Contraindications related to angiography include those related to iodine contrast injection, such as allergy and renal or cardiac failure.
- In the presence of infarcted bowel or markedly elevated lactic acid levels, the decision to perform percutaneous treatment versus surgery should be questioned.[5] For some authors, whenever bowel infarction is suspected with peritoneal signs, surgery is mandatory.
- Other contraindications to percutaneous treatment include uncontrollable bleeding disorders and septic shock.
- Precipitation has been reported when papaverine is mixed with heparin, lactated Ringer's solution, thrombolytic agents, or ioxaglate contrast.[21] Papaverine is also contraindicated in patients with complete ventricular block.
- Standard contraindications to thrombolysis.

EQUIPMENT

Developments in catheter and guidewire technology, as well as in other angiographic equipment (flat panels, rotational angiography, road mapping), fibrinolytic medications, and contrast media, allow interventional radiologists to treat acute intestinal ischemia safely and effectively by selective and superselective catheterization.

TECHNIQUE

Anatomy and Approaches

AMI is usually due to pathology in the superior mesenteric artery (SMA) or SMV territory. Obstruction of the inferior mesenteric vessels often causes less severe symptoms because of better collateral circulation. Among all visceral arteries, the SMA is the most susceptible to emboli (90%) because of its acute angle of origin with respect to the aorta and high blood flow. In 50% of cases,[22] emboli lodge 6 to 8 cm beyond the SMA origin at a relative narrowing near the origin of the middle colic artery; in 18% at the origin of the SMA; in 25% at the origin of the right colic artery and the ileocolic-appendicular artery. The inferior mesenteric artery (IMA) is seldom the landing site of an embolus because of its smaller lumen.

After improvement of the cardiovascular status by intravenous fluid resuscitation, pain control, and administration of broad-spectrum antibiotics, anteroposterior and lateral aortography with a 4F pigtail catheter is performed. The origins of the celiac trunk, SMA, and IMA are assessed on lateral aortograms. Collateral vessels and possible associated aortic or other visceral arterial pathologic processes are best analyzed on anteroposterior angiograms. The SMV is best seen on late acquisition images.

Because of the caudal orientation of the SMA, a brachial access can be useful, with a long introducer sheath to cannulate the SMA. If a femoral access is used, stiff guidewires are required to provide support to aid passage of catheters into the SMA. Shepherd's hook–type catheters allow selective catheterization of the SMA via the femoral approach. When using brachial or axillary access, a multipurpose or Cobra catheter are valuable tools.

An embolus usually appears as a sharp, round filling defect and abrupt cutoff of flow near the origin of the middle colic artery, with frequently associated severe vasospasm and other systemic arterial emboli.[23] Thrombosis appears as a more tapered occlusion near the origin of the SMA and is often associated with diffuse atheroma and a partially developed collateral circulation. Typical findings of mesenteric venous thrombosis include visible thrombus in the SMV, reflux of contrast into the aorta, a prolonged arterial phase with accumulation of contrast agent, thickened bowel walls, extravasation of contrast agent into the bowel lumen, and a filling defect in the portal vein or a complete lack of a venous phase. Nonocclusive mesenteric ischemia is characterized by slow flow and narrowing of the origins of multiple SMA branches, alternating dilation and narrowing of the intestinal branches (i.e., "string of sausages" sign), spasm of the mesenteric arcades, and impaired filling of the intramural vessels. SMV patency must be proved to confirm this diagnosis.

Technical Aspects

Various percutaneous techniques can be carried out immediately after diagnostic angiography.

Angiographically Infused Vasodilator Medications

Papaverine is dissolved in normal saline to a concentration of 1 mg/mL, although a higher concentration can be used. Usually a bolus of 60 mg of papaverine is administered selectively into the SMA through the angiographic catheter (downstream from an accessory or replaced right hepatic artery if it exists) immediately after diagnostic angiography. Bolus injection is followed by an infusion at 30 to 60 mg/hr; the dose is adjusted for clinical response for at least 24 hours. Papaverine infusion can be continued for up to 12 to 24 hours after surgery. In most cases, the papaverine infusion is maintained for 24 hours. The catheter is then flushed with normal saline for 30 minutes, and angiography is repeated. If vasospasm persists, the cycle should be repeated every 24 hours for a maximum of 5 days.[24]

Recently, other vasodilators have been used in the treatment of nonocclusive mesenteric ischemia. Ernst et al.[25] reported use of a bolus administration of 20 g of alprostadil into the SMA, followed by intraarterial perfusion of 60 µg/day for 3 days in four patients. Huwer et al.[26] treated 23 patients with intraarterial bolus injection and subsequent intraarterial infusion of tolazoline combined with heparin sodium.

Angiographically Infused Thrombolytic Agents

Various intraarterial thrombolytic agents have been used through an angiographic catheter. The first case was described by Jamieson et al.[27] in 1979, using streptokinase and heparin. Reports of successful use of several different thrombolytic agents, using a variety of methods of administration, have been published: streptokinase,[28] urokinase,[29] recombinant tissue plasminogen activator (rtPA),[15] and combinations of thrombolytic agents such as streptokinase and rtPA.[30] We prefer to use rtPA, with an initial 20-mg bolus by transcatheter administration directly into the embolus/thrombus, followed by a more distal bolus of 20 mg if partial lysis is obtained (Fig. 55-2). Heparin is administered concomitantly using a 4000-unit intraarterial bolus, followed by continuous intravenous infusion. If symptoms do not improve within 4 hours or if peritonitis develops, surgery must be performed. When using rtPA, thrombolytic activity is negligible after 4 hours. Roberts[31] advocates rapid delivery, such as the pulse spray method at a high dose during a short infusion time, using a short-acting thrombolytic agent.

Angioplasty

There have been several case reports of angioplasty for the treatment of AMI.[17] Recanalization of an occluded segment may be obtained with an angled 0.035-inch, 260-cm-long hydrophilic (Terumo Medical Corp., Somerset, N.J.) guidewire after a femoral approach. Angiography is performed through a 5F Simmons or Michaelson catheter tip, and then catheter exchange with a balloon catheter allows dilation and stenting (Figs. 55-3 and 55-4). Without predilation, a low-profile self-expandable stent is preferable to a balloon-expandable stent.[17] Completion aortography can then be obtained with an aortic flush catheter. Heparin therapy is

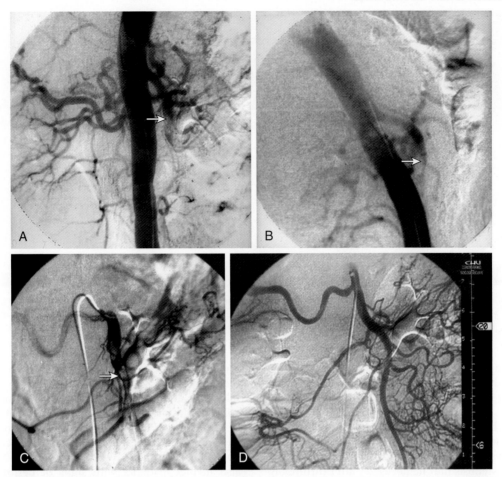

FIGURE 55-2. A 66-year-old man treated with Coumadin for atrial fibrillation was admitted after acute abdominal pain and lower gastrointestinal hemorrhage. There was no sign of peritoneal irritation and no contraindication to thrombolysis. Oblique aortography (**A**), lateral aortography (**B**), and selective mesenteric arteriography (**C**) show a round filling defect 3 cm distal to superior mesenteric artery (SMA) origin, occluding SMA *(arrows)*. Intraarterial thrombolysis with recombinant tissue plasminogen activator (rtPA) was performed (to a dose of 30 mg rtPA). At day 2, abdominal pain had disappeared, and selective SMA angiography (**D**) showed complete recanalization of all SMA branches.

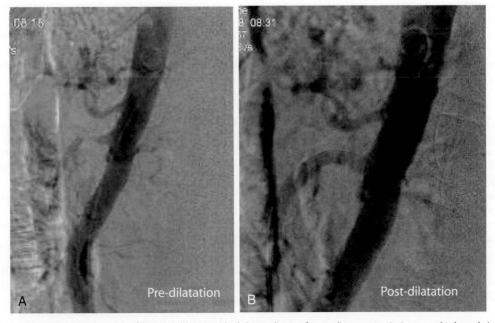

FIGURE 55-3. Pre- and postdilatation imaging of 73-year-old man with abdominal pain after cardiac surgery. **A,** Aortography, lateral view, showing superior mesenteric artery obstruction. **B,** Satisfactory patency after balloon angioplasty and stenting.

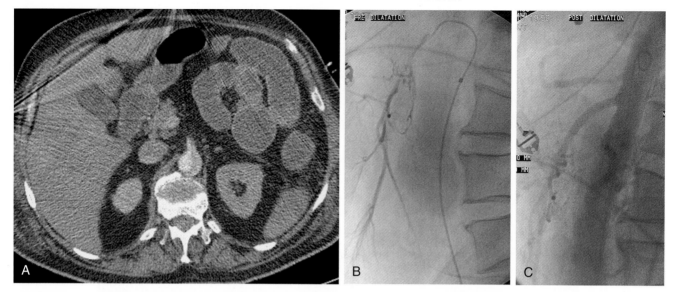

FIGURE 55-4. **A,** Computed tomographic angiography of superior mesenteric artery (SMA), showing clinically symptomatic obstruction by a static extension of aortic dissection in a 79-year-old man. **B,** Aortography, lateral view, showing selective SMA injection, confirming severe obstruction. **C,** Control aortography after balloon angioplasty, showing satisfactory patency of SMA; during follow-up, there was rapid relief of abdominal pain.

administered during the procedure, followed by low-molecular-weight heparin for 2 days and oral antiplatelet therapy with acetylsalicylic acid and ticlopidine.

Combined Techniques for Arterial Recanalization

Intraarterial mechanical fragmentation combined with local thrombolysis has been described. Angioplasty to treat any underlying stenosis may be necessary after thrombolysis of an occluded artery. Wakabayashi et al.[32] reported two successful subsequent PTA procedures 30 minutes after lytic therapy with urokinase. The balloon was inflated at a low pressure for a short period (30 seconds) to reduce adverse effects. Simonetti et al.[33] reported treating seven patients with occlusive AMI by PTA and/or thrombolysis.

Venous Recanalization

Cases of successful treatment with intravascular thrombolytic agents have been reported by Rivitz et al.[34] (transjugular urokinase infusion). Using a percutaneous transhepatic approach, Yankes et al.[20] described successful recanalization of the SMV using a urokinase infusion and an occlusion balloon. Rosen and Sheiman[35] described successful treatment of a patient with SMV and portal vein thrombosis using an AngioJet catheter and infusion of tPA into the SMA. Goldberg and Kim[19] reported recanalization of SMV thrombosis via a transhepatic approach using a combination of AngioJet (Possis Medical, Minneapolis, Minn.) and Amplatz (Cook Medical, Bloomington, Ind.) thrombectomy devices, balloon angioplasty, and pulse spray rtPA fibrinolysis. More recently, Takahashi et al.[36] reported percutaneous transhepatic mechanical thrombectomy with transcatheter urokinase. Crouch[37] used intraarterial mesenteric infusion of urokinase to treat venous mesenteric thrombosis.

CONTROVERSIES

Angiography remains the gold-standard diagnostic technique, but CT is very useful for the diagnosis of AMI,

especially for SMV thrombosis. Because interventional radiology may have a significant role in the management of selected patients with a poor surgical prognosis, we believe angiography should be performed in all patients suspected of having AMI. Early angiography confirms the diagnosis and helps to plan treatment if the nonsurgical endovascular option is still possible. Whenever possible, this strategy can also include patients with signs of peritoneal irritation. Indeed, there is often a tendency to take patients with peritonitis straight to the operating room, without performing angiography. However, if angiography is rapidly available, it can help identify those patients who may require embolectomy or vascular reconstruction, but it also allows transcatheter treatment of vasospasm in the perioperative period.

Indications for percutaneous treatment and choice of specific technique remain controversial. Concerning the use of thrombolytics, there is no consensus concerning the choice of optimal agent, dose and method of delivery, length of treatment, or the role of adjunctive anticoagulation. In patients with signs of peritoneal irritation, percutaneous treatment versus surgery is very controversial.

OUTCOMES

To our knowledge, there are no controlled trial data regarding the optimal method to diagnose or treat AMI.

Although the efficacy of intraarterial papaverine has not been proven by randomized controlled studies, decreased mortality rates (46%) have been reported when using papaverine versus traditional management (70%-80%) (Table 55-1).[38]

Initial clinical success was obtained and mesenteric ischemia resolved in all four patients who were treated with aprostadil[25]: one patient recovered completely; three patients recovered from mesenteric ischemia but died subsequently due to complications of their primary diseases. When using tolazoline,[26] the overall mortality rate was 30% (7 of 23 patients).

TABLE 55-1. Outcomes

Technique	Patients	Outcome	References
Intraarterial papaverine	35 patients	Mortality rates 46% vs. 70%-80% by traditional management	Boley et al.[38]
Intraarterial thrombolytics	8 patients	Resolution of abdominal pain in 70% of patients within 1 hour	Simo et al.[39]
Angioplasty and/or thrombolysis	4 patients 8 patients	Satisfactory clinical outcome in 80% Favorable clinical outcome in 5 patients (62.5%) without surgery	Simonetti et al.[33] Gagnière et al.[42]
Thrombolysis of SMV obstruction	11 patients	Favorable outcome in 10 patients (90.9%)	Kim et al.[44]

SMV, Superior mesenteric vein.

To the best of our knowledge, no study has ever compared different thrombolytic agents. Intraarterial infusion is better than intravenous administration (fewer complications, higher drug concentration in contact with thrombus, and angiographic monitoring of clot lysis). The largest series of intraarterial mesenteric thrombolysis using urokinase was reported by Simo et al.[39] in 10 patients. In 90% of patients, intraarterial thrombolysis was angiographically successful, and resolution of abdominal pain occurred in 70% of patients within an hour. This latter sign is believed to be the most significant factor in predicting success of fibrinolysis. Results of thrombolysis are better with SMA emboli than with thrombosis.[15] Clinical success was observed in 5 of 8 patients with AMI after thrombolysis.[40] At follow-up of 2 to 7 years, 4 patients were still alive, with another embolic episode in a lower limb in 1 patient. One patient died of an unrelated cause without recurrence of emboli. Most cases involving successful use of thrombolytic agents have been in hemodynamically stable patients without signs of bowel infarction.[33] In comparison, Bingol et al.[41] performed surgical embolectomy in 24 patients with acute SMA embolism (within 6 hours after onset of symptoms in 15 patients, 6 to 12 hours in 9 patients, and over 12 hours in 3 patients). After selective low-dose administration of rtPA, segmental intestinal resection was necessary in 4 patients, and extended resection was required in 5 patients who consequently died. Favorable results were observed in the remaining 19 patients.

Simonetti et al.[33] successfully treated 5 of 7 patients with occlusive AMI by PTA and/or thrombolysis. Remission of clinical signs was observed in 4 patients (80%). More recently, Gagnière and al. successfully treated 8 patients with acute thrombotic mesenteric ischemia, with a good clinical outcome in 5 patients who did not require additional surgery.[42]

Treatment by anticoagulation has been shown to be effective, although the rate of recanalization is not as high as with intraarterial thrombolysis.[43] In a review of 11 patients treated with percutaneous thrombectomy/thrombolysis for SMV thrombosis in the absence of peritoneal signs, Kim et al.[44] reported successful recanalization in 10 patients, with no recurrence of thrombosis within 42 months' follow-up.

COMPLICATIONS

Overall mortality of AMI remains high even after surgery (60%-80%).[2] The chief complication of intraarterial papaverine is hypotension, which can occur if the infusion

catheter slips into the aorta. It can be detected with close monitoring of vital signs and confirmed by angiography. When using tolazoline,[26] the overall mortality rate was 30% (7 of 23 patients).

Complications of percutaneous thrombolysis include bleeding at the puncture site, distal embolization, allergic reactions with streptokinase (sometimes with urokinase), post-revascularization syndrome, and catheter thrombosis, especially with urokinase, which can be prevented by adjunctive heparinization.

The leading complication of PTA is risk of embolization. It is considered less important when the occlusion is short.[42] Embolization is strongly suggested angiographically if there is a delay in forward flow of contrast medium despite a good technical result in recanalizing an obstruction. Subsequent thrombolysis is believed to be effective in those cases.[32]

Complications of venous recanalization include bleeding and refractory thrombosis.[44]

POSTPROCEDURAL AND FOLLOW-UP CARE

Postprocedural management includes clinical monitoring of abdominal pain, monitoring of vital functions, and laboratory assessment of serum electrolytes and anticoagulation. Parenteral nutrition can be started early, with monitoring of liver function. When bowel resection is performed, inpatient recovery can be prolonged, and patients may experience "short bowel syndrome." In this situation, patients may require dietary modification, such as small, frequent meals. When a proximal obstruction has been treated, we perform CTA 1 month after the procedure, even if the patient's clinical status is satisfactory. When a stent has been implanted, a further follow-up CTA is performed 6 months later to detect any early restenosis.

KEY POINTS

- Acute mesenteric ischemia is a life-threatening emergency requiring early treatment before bowel infarction.
- Computed tomographic angiography is very useful for diagnosis and has a key role in the diagnosis of superior mesenteric vein thrombosis and prognosis.
- Early angiography remains the gold standard for diagnosis.
- Local intraarterial thrombolysis should be performed for acute mesenteric obstruction.

► **SUGGESTED READINGS**

Hirsch AT, Haskal ZJ, Hertzer NR, et al. ACC/AHA 2005 guidelines for the management of patients with peripheral arterial disease (lower extremity, renal, mesenteric, and abdominal aortic): executive summary: a collaborative report from the American Association for Vascular Surgery/Society for Vascular Surgery, Society for Cardiovascular Angiography and Interventions, Society for Vascular Medicine and Biology, Society of Interventional Radiology, and the ACC/AHA Task Force on Practice Guidelines (Writing Committee to Develop Guidelines for the Management of Patients With Peripheral Arterial Disease) endorsed by the American Association of Cardiovascular and Pulmonary Rehabilitation; National Heart, Lung, and Blood Institute; Society for Vascular Nursing; TransAtlantic Inter-Society Consensus; and Vascular Disease Foundation. J Am Coll Cardiol 2006;47:1239–312.

Kozuch PL, Brandt LJ. Review article: diagnosis and management of mesenteric ischaemia with an emphasis on pharmacotherapy. Aliment Pharmacol Ther 2005;21:201–15.

Lock G. Acute intestinal ischaemia. Best Pract Res Clin Gastroenterol 2001;15:83–98.

Oldenburg WA, Lau LL, Rodenberg TJ, et al. Acute mesenteric ischemia: a clinical review. Arch Intern Med 2004;164:1054–62.

Roberts A. Thrombolysis: clinical applications. In: Baum S, Pencost MJ, editors. Abrams' angiography interventional radiology, 2nd ed. Philadelphia: Lippincott Williams & Wilkins; 2006. p. 233–56.

Sreenarasimhaiah J. Diagnosis and management of intestinal ischaemic disorders. BMJ 2003;326:1372–6.

The complete reference list is available online at www.expertconsult.com.

CHAPTER 56

Chronic Mesenteric Ischemia

Ulku C. Turba, H. Omur Sildiroglu, and Alan H. Matsumoto

Although chronic mesenteric ischemia (CMI) is a relatively uncommon entity owing to the robust mesenteric arterial collateral circulation, detection of intestinal angina and CMI is of critical importance. If the diagnosis is overlooked or missed, acute mesenteric ischemia can result. Once acute mesenteric ischemia develops, patient mortality rates become very high. In addition, an accurate diagnosis and pretreatment noninvasive evaluation will facilitate treatment planning and affect optimal clinical outcomes (Fig. 56-1).

INDICATIONS

The natural history of mesenteric arterial disease is not well defined. In the only study published to date, a retrospective analysis revealed that 23% of asymptomatic patients who were noted to have disease of all three mesenteric arteries at the time of aortography (performed for other reasons) developed symptoms of, or sequelae related to, mesenteric ischemia during a 7-year period of follow-up.[1] Therefore, given the paucity of data about the natural history of mesenteric arterial occlusive disease, the most common indication for treatment of stenoses or occlusions of the mesenteric arteries is the presence of ischemic symptoms. Based on the surgical literature, during aortic reconstruction for aneurysmal or occlusive disease, mesenteric arterial reconstruction should be routine even in asymptomatic patients because these patients have a worse postoperative course if their mesenteric vascular disease is not corrected at the time of their aortic surgery.[1,2] The topic of aggressive treatment in asymptomatic patients with mesenteric arterial occlusive disease when there is no need for aortic reconstruction is where the controversy begins. We believe that even in asymptomatic patients, the presence of significant three-vessel mesenteric arterial occlusive disease warrants strong consideration for revascularization, especially if endovascular therapy is feasible. An isolated asymptomatic mesenteric arterial stenosis should be managed on a case-by-case basis because many of these patients may never become symptomatic, especially those with an isolated stenosis of the celiac or inferior mesenteric arteries.

CONTRAINDICATIONS

Symptomatic median arcuate ligament (MAL) compression of the celiac artery is best treated by surgical release of the ligament; use of a stent is this situation is not advised. Balloon-expandable stents placed in an artery compressed by the MAL may be crushed and/or fractured by extrinsic compression of the stent by the ligament. Self-expanding stents do not have enough hoop strength to resist external compression and are likely to fracture over time. More importantly, symptoms related to the MAL are most likely neurogenic, owing to compression of the celiac ganglion. Therefore, placement of a stent in the celiac artery may actually exacerbate the symptoms.

Patients who have severe atheromatous disease of the aorta and are at risk for cholesterol embolization during an endovascular procedure should be considered for an extra-anatomic surgical bypass procedure.

EQUIPMENT

- 50 to 100 mL of iodine-based contrast. Alternatively, CO_2 may be used judiciously in patients at risk for contrast-induced nephropathy.
- A multi-sidehole catheter for aortography and selective catheters (RC 1, Simmons 1, Rosch Inferior Mesenteric [RIM], or SOS Omni 2 [AngioDynamics, Glen Falls, N.Y.]), depending on the anatomy, are used for selective catheterization of the mesenteric arteries.
- A guiding sheath or guiding catheter of proper size and shape will facilitate delivery of a balloon catheter and/or stent (Fig. 56-2, A, B, and D) and allow for contrast injections to assess results of the intervention. In mesenteric arteries that have an acute caudal orientation off the aorta, an 8F tip-deflecting catheter (Morph catheter [Biocardia Inc., Mountain View, Calif.]) has been employed to aid the intervention for a femoral access.
- Pressure transducers for translesion pressure gradient measurements, as needed, to determine the hemodynamic significance of questionable stenoses will be useful.
- A variety of 0.035-inch, 0.018-inch, or 0.014-inch guidewires and compatible balloon and stent platforms are recommended.
- Heparin, nitroglycerin, conscious sedation medications, oral antiplatelet agents, prophylactic antibiotics prior to stent placement, and possibly a closure device for the arteriotomy are often used or administered before, during, or after completion of the endovascular procedure.
- High-resolution angiography equipment that allows for multiplanar imaging, an experienced interventionalist, a nurse dedicated to patient monitoring during the procedure, and a well-trained technologist are also essential for procedural success.

TECHNIQUE

Anatomy and Approaches

Once the clinical indication is established, treatment planning becomes crucial. Computed tomographic angiography (CTA) and magnetic resonance angiography (MRA) are excellent roadmaps for treatment planning (Fig. 56-3, A). With the availability of preshaped guide sheaths and guiding catheters (see Fig. 56-2), most patients can be treated from

387

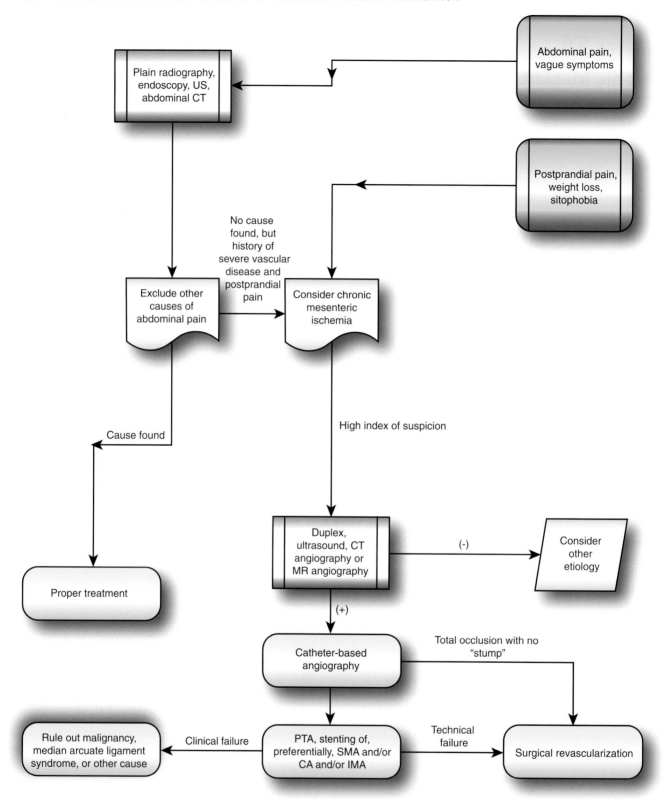

FIGURE 56-1. A diagnostic and treatment algorithm for chronic mesenteric ischemia. *CA,* Celiac artery; *CT,* computed tomography; *IMA,* inferior mesenteric artery; *MR,* magnetic resonance; *PTA,* percutaneous transluminal angioplasty; *SMA,* superior mesenteric artery; *US,* ultrasound.

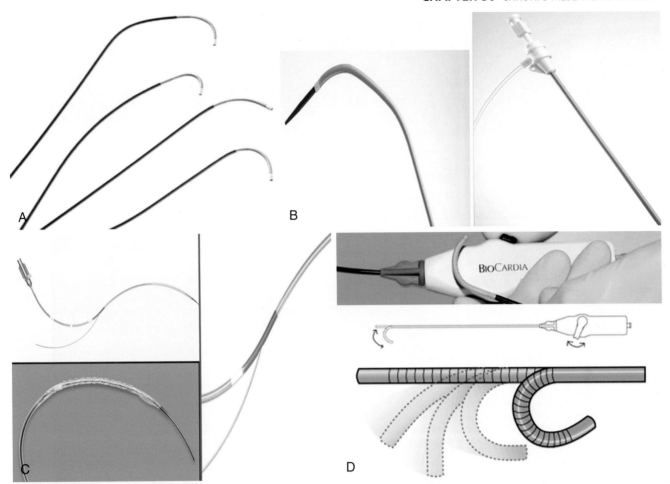

FIGURE 56-2. **A,** A variety of styles and sizes of preshaped guide sheaths are commercially available. These preshaped, reinforced sheaths facilitate delivery of 0.035-inch or smaller balloon catheter and stent systems while allowing for the performance of angiograms via their side ports. **B,** A variety of styles and sizes of preshaped guide catheters are commercially available. These preshaped, reinforced catheters are very torquable and facilitate delivery of 0.014- to 0.018-inch balloon catheter and stent systems, while allowing for the performance of angiograms via their side ports or check flow valves. **C,** A premounted 0.018-inch rapid exchange (monorail) balloon system can be used with a nonexchange-length guidewire. These low-profile balloon and stent systems allow for better trackability and traversal of tight lesions. **D,** An 8F reinforced deflecting catheter (Morph catheter [Biocardia, Mountain View, Calif.]) can be manually controlled to a variety of curves while providing a "backbone" through which to advance the balloon and stent system when the angle of vessel from the aorta is challenging. This guiding catheter may reduce the need for using a brachial artery approach for mesenteric artery stent procedures. (**A** *courtesy Cook Medical, Bloomington, Ind.;* **B** *and* **C** *courtesy Cordis Endovascular, Warren, N.J.;* **D** *courtesy Biocardia, Mountain View, Calif.*)

a femoral artery approach. In the presence of an infrarenal aortic occlusion, an approach from an upper extremity may be necessary, and the profile of the system used should be minimized. There is one observational study that suggests that an upper extremity versus a femoral approach to mesenteric artery stenting may be associated with better outcomes.[8] However, these findings have not been corroborated by other investigators.

Lateral aortography should be performed to confirm the findings of the pretreatment noninvasive imaging studies and further delineate the lesion(s). Occasionally, the celiac artery originates from the aorta in a slightly left anterior projection (i.e., in a 1 o'clock location), necessitating a slight oblique projection. The inferior mesenteric artery (IMA) usually originates off the aorta in a left anterior oblique orientation (i.e., in a 2 o'clock location), requiring a 60-degree right anterior oblique projection to best profile its origin. Previous CTA and/or MRA images should be reviewed to determine the best "working projection" for

each mesenteric artery before endovascular treatment, thereby minimizing procedure time, radiation to the patient, and contrast volume used.

Technical Aspects

The technique of mesenteric artery angioplasty and stenting for chronic intestinal ischemia is similar to that for renal artery angioplasty and stenting. Operators performing these procedures should be experienced in endovascular techniques in order to minimize the risk for a complication that leads to the development of acute mesenteric ischemia.

A reverse-curve catheter such as an SOS Omni 2, RC 1, or Simmons 1 catheter is typically used to catheterize the celiac artery or superior mesenteric artery (SMA) from the femoral artery approach, and a selective angiogram is obtained to better define the arterial anatomy and ensure an intraluminal location prior to proceeding to an

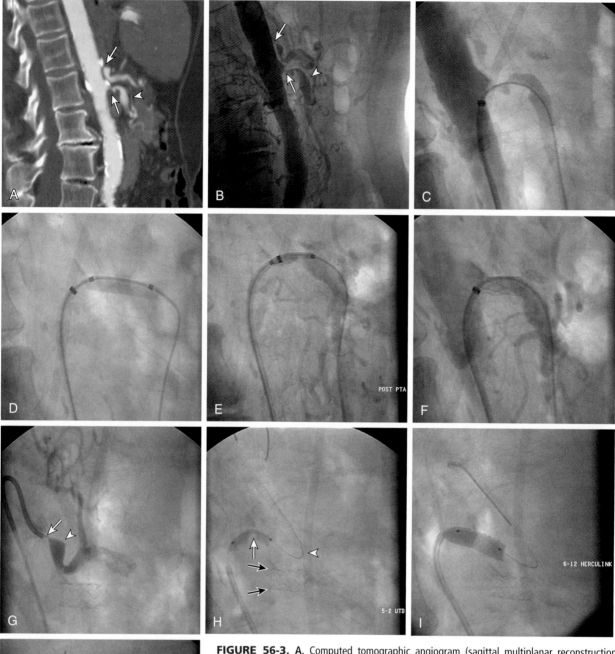

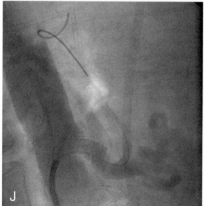

FIGURE 56-3. A, Computed tomographic angiogram (sagittal multiplanar reconstruction) demonstrates severe celiac artery and superior mesenteric artery (SMA) stenoses *(arrows)*, with poststenotic dilation of SMA *(arrowhead)*. **B,** Lateral aortogram demonstrates severe celiac artery and SMA stenoses *(arrows)*, with poststenotic dilation of SMA *(arrowhead)*. **C,** Guiding catheter is positioned at SMA orifice, and a 0.035-inch guidewire is positioned across lesion. **D,** Percutaneous transluminal angioplasty (PTA) of SMA was performed using a 5 × 20 mm balloon. **E,** Postangioplasty angiogram during stent positioning reveals suboptimal PTA result. **F,** After deployment of a 5 × 15 mm Genesis balloon-expandable stent (Cordis Corp., Hialeah, Fla.) a widely patent SMA is noted. **G,** Selective angiogram of celiac artery demonstrates severe stenosis *(arrow)* and poststenotic dilation of vessel *(arrowhead)*. (Note extrinsic luminal effect of median arcuate ligament [MAL] distal to poststenotic dilation.) **H,** Balloon angioplasty of celiac artery with a 5 × 20 mm balloon shows "waist" on balloon *(white arrow)* due to severe stenosis. The 0.014-inch guidewire remains in celiac artery *(white arrowhead)*. SMA stent is also demonstrated *(black arrows)*. **I,** A 6 × 12 mm Herculink balloon-expandable stent (Guidant Corp., Indianapolis, Ind.) was deployed in celiac artery after suboptimal PTA result. **J,** After stent deployment, celiac artery is now widely patent. (Note that stent has been placed proximal to extrinsic effect of MAL on celiac artery.)

intervention. For catheterization of the IMA, a RIM or SOS 2 catheter is preferred. An appropriately shaped guiding sheath or catheter is then advanced over the guidewire to the level of the origin of the mesenteric artery. The angioplasty and stenting procedure can then be performed in a similar fashion to a renal revascularization procedure, using 0.035-inch, 0.018-inch, or 0.014-inch guidewire platforms. Because of the resistant nature of many ostial mesenteric arterial stenoses, balloon-expandable stents are preferred. For truncal lesions, either balloon-expandable or self-expandable stents are used, depending on the length and configuration of the lesion (Fig. 56-4; also see Fig. 56-3). Covered stents (iCast [Atrium Medical, Hudson, N.H.]) may be used in a selected subgroup of CMI patients where aortic/ostial soft plaque might be at risk for causing cholesterol emboli, or in small mesenteric arteries at risk for developing in-stent restenosis. However, these theoretical advantages of using covered stents have not been established with data from well-designed clinical trials. We do use covered stents in the subgroup of CMI patients who present with restenosis in an existing mesenteric artery stent or in mesenteric arteries less than 6 mm in diameter, owing to high rates of in-stent restenosis in arteries less than 6 mm in diameter. Devices compatible with 0.014-inch guidewires are typically more flexible, easier to deliver, and track better in acutely oriented arteries compared with 0.035-inch platform devices. However, 0.014-inch balloons tend to be more compliant and tend to "dog bone" within a resistant lesion, and 0.014-inch stents do not have as much hoop strength and are less visible than 0.035-inch stents. Therefore, 0.014-inch balloon and stent systems are less likely to provide optimum luminal diameters in very resistant ostial mesenteric artery lesions.

In cases in which advancement of the balloon and stent across the lesion into the parent SMA, IMA, or celiac artery is not possible owing to tortuous iliac arteries, acute angulation of the artery from the aorta, and the presence of a tight stenosis or chronic total occlusion, use of a deflectable braided 8F guide catheter (Morph catheter) may be helpful. Its shape can be manually changed to optimize the catheter angle and provide stability within the aorta to allow for advancement of the balloon and stent across the lesion (see Fig. 56-2, D).

Translesion pressure gradients may be obtained if there is any question about the hemodynamic significance of a stenosis or the results of the angioplasty/stenting procedure. Pressures should be obtained simultaneously from the aorta and beyond the lesion of concern. In general, a peak-to-peak systolic pressure gradient above 20 mmHg and/or a 10% gradient of the mean arterial pressures are considered significant. A systolic pressure gradient less than 10 mmHg is considered insignificant. Systolic pressure gradients between 10 and 20 mmHg are managed on a case-by-case basis. There are no outcomes data upon which these measurements and parameters are based; cited gradients are derived from experience with renal artery stenting.

Whenever possible, multiple vessels are treated in one setting. In the presence of an occlusion *and* a stenosis, we usually treat the stenosis initially and then treat the occlusion if the patient is tolerating the procedure. The other option is to have the patient return for treatment of the occlusion if the symptoms do not resolve after treating the stenotic vessel. In almost all atherosclerotic lesions, stents are used either primarily or after predilation with an undersized balloon. Provisional stenting can be performed after percutaneous transluminal angioplasty (PTA) due to the lesion recoiling, a flow-limiting dissection, and/or a suboptimal result.

An empirical intravenous bolus of 3000 to 5000 units of heparin is administered prior to the intervention, or heparin is given to keep the activated clotting time (ACT) above 220 seconds (typically 70 units/kg body weight). Intraarterial nitroglycerin is given in 100 to 200 μg aliquots to reduce or minimize vasospasm. Whenever possible, patients are started on aspirin and clopidogrel the day before the procedure. If withheld for a medical reason, the patient may be given aspirin (325 mg) and clopidogrel (300 mg) orally in the recovery/holding area immediately before the procedure. The patient is maintained on 81 to 325 mg of aspirin for life and also treated with 75 mg of clopidogrel for at least 30 days.

CONTROVERSIES

Extensive collateral networks between the mesenteric arterial beds make the incidence of symptomatic CMI relatively uncommon. Given the poorly defined natural history of occlusive mesenteric arterial disease and the increasing number of asymptomatic patients with mesenteric arterial stenoses detected on CTA and MRA obtained for other reasons, the discussion around mesenteric revascularization in asymptomatic patients remains controversial.[1-3] Having said that, there is a consensus among vascular specialists that mesenteric revascularization should be performed on patients with asymptomatic mesenteric arterial disease who will be undergoing reconstruction of their abdominal aorta, especially if the IMA is likely to be sacrificed. However, whether revascularization of a critical stenosis of the SMA should be performed in an asymptomatic patient who is otherwise having no vascular issues remains controversial, with no proven benefit or clinical outcomes studies.

Although some authors suggest that surgery for the treatment of patients with CMI is a better option than endovascular therapy, the risk of significant postoperative morbidity and mortality favors an endovascular approach as the first treatment option.[4] Primary assisted clinical success rates with endovascular therapy approach 90% at 5 years, with 5-year survival rates of 76%.[5,6] In addition, failure of angioplasty and stenting does not eliminate surgery as a therapeutic option. For some patients, initial treatment with stenting may provide a good bridge therapy so that open surgery can be performed at a later date when nutritional status is better and other surgical risk factors are minimized.[7] In most institutions, endovascular therapy is now considered the primary choice for stenotic lesions of the mesenteric arteries when the risk of cholesterol embolization is not too great. Whether all atherosclerotic lesions should be treated with stenting, versus angioplasty alone, is not well defined owing to limitations in the literature. In our initial experience with 33 patients in which 12 patients received stents and 21 patients underwent PTA alone,[5] there was a trend toward better outcomes with stenting, although the difference was not statistically significant ($P = 0.073$). In our current experience (166 patients as of 2011), PTA seems to have better primary patency rates than

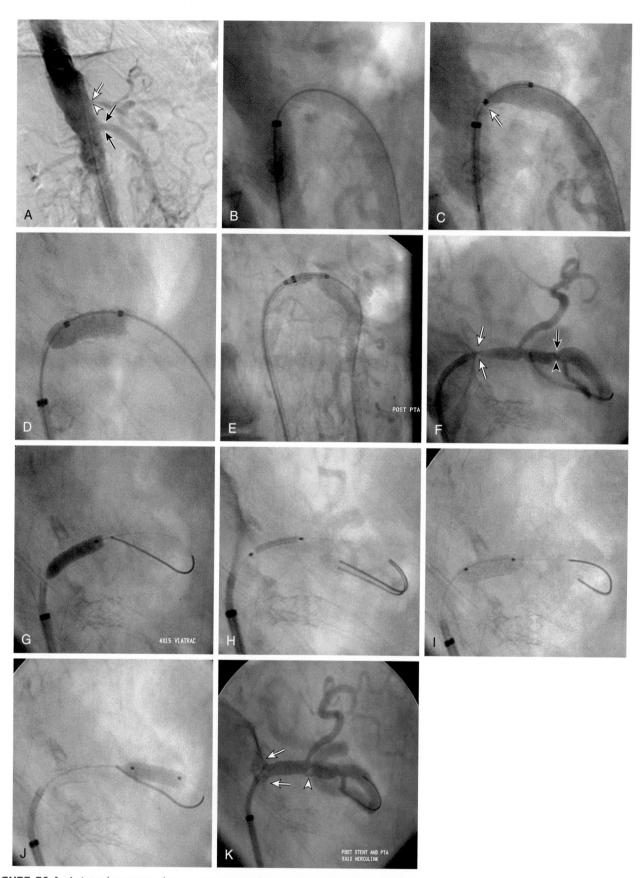

FIGURE 56-4. A, Lateral aortogram demonstrates severe celiac artery stenosis *(white arrows)* and moderate superior mesenteric artery (SMA) stenosis *(black arrows).* **B,** SMA lesion was crossed with 0.035-inch guidewire. Pressure measurements showed a 30 mmHg systolic gradient between aorta and SMA. **C,** Decision was made to primarily stent the lesion with a 7 × 15 mm balloon-expandable stent. Positioning of stent across ostium of artery is seen *(arrow).* **D,** Deployment of stent shows full expansion of balloon. **E,** SMA stent is in good position, and SMA is widely patent. **F,** Severe proximal celiac artery stenosis *(white arrows)* is seen, with tandem stenoses noted more distally *(black arrows).* **G,** Percutaneous balloon angioplasty of celiac artery origin stenosis was performed using a 0.014-inch platform, with a suboptimal result. **H,** A 5 × 12 mm Herculink stent was positioned at origin of celiac artery. **I,** Balloon-expandable stent was successfully deployed. **J,** Angioplasty using a 6 × 15 mm balloon was performed on the more distal stenoses. **K,** After percutaneous transluminal angioplasty (PTA) and stent deployment, angiogram depicts anterior wall of aorta *(arrows)* and proper stent location across ostium. Additionally, a nonocclusive dissection of celiac artery more distally at one of the sites of PTA is seen *(arrowhead).*

TABLE 56-1. Chronic Mesenteric Ischemia: Comparison of Endovascular Study Results

Study (1996-2012)	No. Patients (No. Vessels)*	Technical Success (%)	Early Symptom Relief (%)	Long-Term Symptom Relief (%)	Mean Follow-Up (Months)
Allen et al.[13]	19 (24)	95	79	79	39
Maspes et al.[14]	23 (41)	90	77	75	27
Sheeran et al.[15]	12 (13)	92	92	75	16
Kasirajan et al.[4]	28 (32)	100	N/A	66	36
Matsumoto et al.[5]	33 (47)	88	88	84	38
AbuRahma et al.[16]	22 (24)	96	95	61	26
Razavi et al.[17]	70 (N/A)	97	98.5	90	36
Landis et al.[6]	29 (63)	97	90	79	28
Lim et al.[18]	5 (9)	100	80	40	52
Silva et al.[10]	59 (79)	96	88	83	38
Schaefer et al.[19]	19 (23)	96	95	54	17
Piffaretti et al.[20]	9 (10)	100	89	78	31
Lee et al.[21]	31 (41)	98	70	56	6
Sarac et al.[8]	65 (87)	N/A	85	75	31
Peck et al.[22]	49 (66)	88	90	61	37
Malgor et al.[23]	101 (125)	98	98	91	41
Aksu et al.[24]	15 (18)	100	87	71	16
Fioole et al.[25]	51 (60)	93	78	67	25
Turba et al.[42]	166 (221)	94	88	71	34

*Publications less than 9 vessels treated were excluded.

stenting in the treatment of the SMA ($P = 0.014$) but no significant difference in the IMA or celiac artery. Therefore, there may be some basis for using provisional stenting after suboptimal PTA. For stenotic lesions, Landis et al.[6] found higher restenosis rates after PTA than after stenting, but this group also demonstrated good results with *either* PTA or stenting for total occlusions, despite the belief of most interventionalists that stents are associated with better outcomes in total occlusions. Sarac et al.[8] also found no difference in outcomes and recurrence rates in patients with CMI due to occluded versus stenotic mesenteric arteries. Lastly, patients have experienced good clinical outcomes after treatment of an isolated IMA or celiac artery stenosis in the presence of an SMA occlusion.[5,9] Therefore, in patients with CMI, treatment of the SMA is not crucial to relieve symptoms of mesenteric ischemia. Most recently, Silva et al.[10] published a series of 61 stent revascularization procedures, with results that suggest a benefit to primary stent placement. However, there is no prospective randomized study that compares the use of stents to PTA alone in patients with CMI. Because of individual patient differences in disease severity and distribution, the type of endovascular treatment should be determined on a case-by-case basis.

Similar to renovascular lesions, the exact role of translesion pressure measurements has not been defined. In addition, the role of antiplatelet agents after an endovascular intervention has not been clearly delineated in this patient population. Although there is no consensus, after the angioplasty/stenting procedure, indefinite therapy with aspirin and a minimal duration of 30 days of clopidogrel therapy have been recommended.[3-5]

OUTCOMES

Published results for patients with CMI treated with angioplasty with or without stent placement are difficult to compare, owing to the continued evolution of devices and techniques and variability in the patient populations studied. Since the initial reports of successful PTA of the SMA in 1980 by Uflacker et al.[11] and Furrer et al.,[12] dramatic improvement in symptoms after balloon angioplasty has been consistently reported (Table 56-1). When compared with surgery, 30-day mortality rates are lower after angioplasty/stenting, in large part because of postoperative cardiopulmonary and renovascular complications seen with open surgical repair. Endovascular approaches do not expose patients to the risks inherent in general anesthesia because endovascular procedures are usually performed with conscious sedation alone. Compared to open surgery, postprocedural hospitalization after endovascular treatment is much shorter, and patients are more likely to be discharged home rather than to an intermediate care facility.

Technical success rates after endovascular revascularization for treatment of CMI range from 88% to 100%, with an average of about 95%. Higher success rates are seen in more recently published series, likely owing to improved devices and better technique. Immediate clinical benefit ranges from 70% to 98%, with most series reporting a long-term

TABLE 56-2. Chronic Mesenteric Ischemia: Comparison of Endovascular Treatment to Open Surgery Results

Study (1995-2011)	No. Patients ET/OS (No. Vessels ET/OS)	Technical Success ET/OS (%)	Early Symptom Relief ET/OS (%)	Long-Term Symptom Relief ET/OS (%)	Mean Follow-Up ET/OS (Months)
Rose et al.[27]	8/9 (9/16)	30/100	75/100	67/100	9/34
Kasirajan et al.[4]	28/85 (32/130)	100/100	N/A / N/A	66/87	60/24
Brown et al.[7]	14/33 (18/33)	N/A /93	N/A / N/A	N/A / N/A	13/34
Sivamurthy et al.[28]	19/41 (21/46)	95/100	33/71	22/59	19/25
Biebl et al.[29]	23/26 (47/30)	N/A / N/A	79/100	75/89	10/25
Atkins et al.[30]	31/49 (42/88)	97/100	87/90	74/91	15/42
Zerbib et al.[31]	14/15 (14/19)	93/100	N/A / N/A	71/93	15/21
Davies et al.[32]	15/17 (18/26)	93/100	86/100	73/100	34/34
Oderich et al.[33]	83/146 (105/265)	95/100	93/95	69/94	30/36
Rawat et al.[34]	36/40 (45/75)	N/A / N/A	83/90	70/82	22/41

ET, Endovascular treatment; *N/A,* not available; *OS,* open surgery.

clinical benefit in 40% to 91% of patients with a mean follow-up period of 16 to 52 months (see Table 56-1).[4-6,8,10,13-25]

Restenosis rates after PTA and/or stenting appear to be higher than with renal artery angioplasty and stenting (15%-60% at 1-5 years). The primary patency rate has been reported to be between 60% and 85% at 1 year, with primary assisted patency rates approaching 90% to 100%. In our experience with 166 patients, we have been using both 0.014-inch and 0.035-inch platforms since 2005. A retrospective analysis of these two subgroups of patients treated with stents for CMI at our institution revealed no difference in primary patency rates when comparing the two platforms.

Open surgery has been the classic treatment for CMI. However, more recently, Schermerhorn et al.[26] demonstrated that as of 2002, endovascular therapy was being used more often than open surgery to treat patients with CMI. A compilation of single-institution comparisons of surgical mesenteric revascularization to endovascular therapy is shown in Table 56-2.[4,7,27-34] Most investigators agree that patient selection bias is a significant limitation in trying to make a direct comparison of the demographics, risk factors, and outcomes in the surgical versus endovascular treatment subgroups. In the past, patients referred for endovascular therapy were not good surgical candidates, so endovascular therapy might have been their only option. Patients are now referred for endovascular procedures as first-line treatment because it is less invasive and associated with less morbidity than open surgery. Moreover, patients may still be able to undergo surgical revascularization if endovascular therapy fails. In the follow-up of patients who have undergone endovascular intervention, if there is an in-stent restenosis or recurrence after PTA alone, a repeat endovascular intervention can be safely performed, with good clinical benefit in almost all patients. Interventions in the celiac artery appear to be associated with more symptomatic recurrences, possibly owing to the presence of a component of MAL compression.

In our experience with 166 patients, PTA has had better primary patency rates than stents in the SMA, although we did not find significant differences in the celiac artery or IMA. In the medical literature, there is no consensus on this issue because of the limited number of patients reported in each series (see Tables 56-1 and 56-2). Unfortunately, there are no data from randomized controlled trials comparing patency rates after mesenteric revascularization with PTA versus stenting versus open surgery. In addition, many studies provide follow-up based on clinical symptoms. Because continued relief of pain may not necessarily be synonymous with widely patent mesenteric vessels, actual arterial patency rates are difficult to assess in most studies.

COMPLICATIONS

The frequency of adverse events is similar to other endovascular procedures, ranging from 0% to 16% in larger series, and is most often related to access site complications.[5,17,19] Newer low-profile stent platforms and the use of arterial closure devices will likely further reduce this complication rate. In our experience, we have seen a decline in access-related complications during the past 5 years.

In addition to general complications associated with catheter-based angiography (e.g., puncture site hematomas, contrast-induced nephropathy), PTA-induced flow-limiting dissections have been reported. However, the routine use of stents will likely minimize the occurrence of this complication.[13,35] Two cases of post–PTA-induced acute mesenteric ischemia have been reported.[6,13] However, the occurrence of this complication seems less common with endovascular therapy than with open surgery.

In some cases of very severe and long-standing CMI, revascularization may be associated with reperfusion injury to the bowel, manifested by abdominal pain, mucosal edema, and ascites. There is no consensus about the treatment of reperfusion injury. However, in a rat model, SMA occlusions were surgically created for 1 hour, followed by reperfusion for 4 hours. Prophylactic use of nitroglycerin delivered within the lumen of the small bowel was associated with a decrease in intestinal injury. Oxygen free radicals and hydroxyl radicals are possible byproducts of reperfusion injury. Therefore, allopurinol, a xanthine oxidase inhibitor and thus an indirect inhibitor of oxygen free radical production, may in theory be useful for preventing reperfusion injury and is currently under investigation.[36] Whether agents such as sodium bicarbonate or

N-acetylcysteine provide a clinical benefit by reducing oxidative reactions is also not known.

Because postprocedural renal failure is associated with poor outcomes after mesenteric revascularization,[19,37] efforts to minimize contrast-induced nephropathy should be employed. Pretreatment evaluation with MRA (in patients with an estimated glomerular filtration rate [eGFR] >30 mL/min), use of alternative contrast agents during the procedure (i.e., CO_2), preprocedural hydration, and pretreatment with sodium bicarbonate may help minimize the occurrence of postprocedural renal failure.[38]

POSTPROCEDURAL AND FOLLOW-UP CARE

Patients with technically successful revascularization procedures should be kept either nil by mouth or on clear liquids for the first 12 hours or so. Diet can usually be advanced as tolerated the morning after the procedure. Patients can generally leave the hospital 1 to 3 days after the procedure, depending on the complexity of their presentation and clinical situation. We commence patients on therapy with aspirin and clopidogrel the day before the procedure. On occasion, 300 mg of clopidogrel and 325 mg of aspirin are given to the patient on the morning of the procedure. Hydration with intravenous normal saline is initiated as soon as possible (preferably 12 hours before the procedure, but at minimum of 1 hour before the procedure). In patients at risk for contrast-induced nephropathy, initiation of a sodium bicarbonate infusion may be beneficial.[38]

The medical regimen in these patients, including risk factor modification, administration of lipid-lowering agents, and aggressive blood pressure and glucose control, should be optimized. The patient remains on aspirin, 81 to 325 mg/day for life (as tolerated), and a minimum of 75 mg/day of clopidogrel for 30 days. If the patient has advanced cardiovascular disease, the clopidogrel regimen may be extended based on cardiovascular risk factors. Careful symptomatic and noninvasive imaging follow-up for signs of recurrent disease is mandatory. Once recurrent symptoms develop or significant recurrent stenosis (i.e., > 70% diameter narrowing) is documented, the patient should undergo repeat intervention.

KEY POINTS

- Postprandial abdominal pain, weight loss, and anorexia are the classic clinical symptoms of chronic mesenteric ischemia (CMI). Patients may also present with diarrhea, gastroduodenitis unresponsive to pharmacotherapy, gastroparesis with vomiting, and/or postprandial heaviness. There are reports documenting the reversible nature of the gastrointestinal symptoms after successful revascularization.[3,39,40] The goal is to make the diagnosis of CMI before the symptoms become too debilitating and before progression to acute mesenteric ischemia occurs.

- The diagnosis of CMI is primarily based on a careful medical history and exclusion of other causes of the symptoms. Primary and secondary malignancies, median arcuate ligament compression syndrome, gastric and duodenal ulcers, chronic pancreatitis, and aneurysmal disease are several entities that can mimic the clinical presentation of CMI. At least 50% of patients have risk factors associated with, and/or symptoms of, atherosclerotic cardiovascular disease. Atherosclerotic disease is the primary etiology for occlusive mesenteric arterial disease, but chronic mesenteric ischemia may be caused by nonatheromatous lesions such as Takayasu arteritis, fibromuscular dysplasia, aortic dissections, and radiation-induced arteritis.

- There are numerous anatomic variants and collateral pathways in the mesenteric vascular bed, and these variations play a significant role in determining which patients develop ischemic symptoms.[41] Although symptoms of chronic mesenteric ischemia generally occur when at least two of the three main mesenteric vessels are narrowed or occluded, there are exceptions to this rule. Because of the variability in vascular anatomy and collaterals, disease of all three vessels may or may not cause symptoms, or sometimes single-vessel involvement may lead to symptoms.

- Although catheter-based angiography is the gold standard for evaluating the mesenteric vascular system, with the availability of multidetector computed tomography (CT) scanners and dedicated cardiovascular magnetic resonance (MR) systems, catheter-based angiography is primarily reserved for the setting of endovascular treatment or in cases of equivocal noninvasive studies. In general, when there is a high index of clinical suspicion, we proceed with a noninvasive vascular imaging study (see Fig. 56-1).

- The accuracy of computed tomographic angiography (CTA) in evaluating chronic mesenteric ischemia approaches 95% to 100%.[36,41] However, extensive calcification may limit CTA's diagnostic value. Contrast-enhanced magnetic resonance angiography (MRA) is another excellent diagnostic modality for screening for chronic mesenteric ischemia.

- Duplex ultrasonography is often used for screening for proximal mesenteric arterial stenosis or occlusion. For the superior mesenteric artery (SMA), a peak systolic velocity greater than 275 cm/s and an end-diastolic velocity greater than 45 cm/s is highly specific for a significant stenosis.[3]

► SUGGESTED READINGS

Behar JV, Matsumoto AH, Angle JF, et al. Endovascular interventions for chronic mesenteric ischemia. In: Matsumura JS, Pearce WH, Yao JST, editors. Trends in vascular surgery. Los Angeles: Precept Press; 2002. p. 237–47.

Cognet F, Ben Salem D, Dranssart M, et al. Chronic mesenteric ischemia: imaging and percutaneous treatment. Radiographics 2002:22: 863–79.

Leung DA, Matsumoto AH, Hagspiel KD, et al. Endovascular interventions for acute and chronic mesenteric ischemia. In: Baum S, Pentecost MJ, editors. Abrams' angiography: interventional radiology, 2nd ed. Philadelphia: Lippincott Williams & Wilkins; 2005. p. 398–414.

Matsumoto AH, Angle JF, Spinosa DJ, et al. Percutaneous transluminal angioplasty and stenting in the treatment of chronic mesenteric ischemia: results and long-term follow-up. J Am Coll Surg 2002;194 (1 Suppl):S22–S31.

Razavi M, Chung HH. Endovascular management of chronic mesenteric ischemia. Tech Vasc Interv Radiol 2004;7:155–9.

Uflacker R. Atlas of Vascular Anatomy: An angiographic approach, 2nd ed. Philadelphia: Lippincott Williams & Wilkins; 2006. p. 405–605.

The complete reference list is available online at www.expertconsult.com.

CHAPTER 57

Renal Vasculature

Nadia J. Khati, Morvarid Alaghmand, Ali Noor, Aaron Reposar, Rishabh Chaudhari, Ramy Khalil, and Anthony C. Venbrux

INTRODUCTION

Understanding the vascular anatomy of the kidneys, ureters, adrenals, and bladder is essential for image-guided therapy. For example, a patient with a traumatic fistula between the renal artery and vein may benefit from transcatheter embolotherapy. Such a procedure would spare the renal parenchyma and avoid emergent surgery.

Understanding the arterial blood supply to the ureters is important. In the clinical setting of reimplantation of the ureters into a neobladder, delayed distal ureteral strictures may develop secondary to ischemia. Such problematic lesions are due to disruption of the blood supply.

It is also important to have knowledge of the venous anatomy of the kidneys and adrenals. Sampling of renin levels from the renal veins may help determine a cause of hypertension (i.e., renovascular). Similarly, sampling from the adrenal veins may localize an aldosterone-producing tumor.

RENAL VASCULAR ANATOMY

Arterial Supply

The renal artery originates from the aorta at the area between L1 and L2, just inferior to the origin of the superior mesenteric artery (SMA). These arteries are typically posterior to the renal veins and anterior to the renal pelvis. The left renal artery arises at a higher level than the right renal artery and follows an upward course, but the right one is longer and passes posterior to the vena cava, with a downward course to the right kidney (Fig. 57-1).

As each renal artery approaches the hilum, it divides into anterior and posterior segmental arteries (Fig. 57-2). The posterior branch, which arises first, supplies a large portion of the posterior part of the kidney. Next, the four anterior divisions at the renal hilum arise as apical, upper, middle, and lower anterior segmental arteries. The apical and lower anterior divisions supply the anterior and posterior surfaces of the upper and lower renal poles. The upper and middle divisions supply the remaining parts of the anterior surface. The other divisions after the segmental arteries are the lobar, interlobar, arcuate, intralobular, and glomerular arteries. The renal artery gives off small branches to the renal capsule and adrenal gland (inferior adrenal artery).

Accessory renal arteries, which are the most common variant, can originate from the lateral aspect of the abdominal aorta, iliac, or renal artery (or rarely from the lower thoracic aorta or lumbar or mesenteric artery). They usually enter above or below the hilum. Perihilar arteries are other variations.

Of all documented renal vascular variants, accessory renal arteries are the most common and most clinically important. They are seen in up to one third of patients. Multiple accessory renal arteries are unilateral in 30% of patients and bilateral in approximately 10% of patients. Accessory arteries typically originate from the aorta or iliac arteries between the levels of T11 and L4 or rarely from the lower thoracic aorta, lumbar, or mesenteric arteries or a more proximal portion of the abdominal aorta above the origin of the SMA. Most accessory arteries flow into the renal hilum to perfuse both the upper and lower poles and are typically equal in size to a single renal artery. Less frequently, smaller accessory vessels are found to course directly into the renal parenchyma from the renal cortex and are thereby classified as polar arteries.

Perihilar arterial branching—branching of main renal arteries into branches at a point more proximal than the renal hilum—is also a common variant and especially important to note in preoperative mapping of renal transplant donors. In general, kidneys do not have efficient collateral circulation.

Venous System

As mentioned earlier, the renal veins are anterior to the renal arteries (see Fig. 57-1). The left renal vein is longer and crosses the midline anterior to the abdominal aorta and posterior to the SMA. This vein receives the left testicular or ovarian vein from below, the left suprarenal vein from above, and the lumbar vein before joining to the inferior vena cava (IVC; Fig. 57-3).

Ureteric Vasculature

As the ureters pass toward the bladder, they receive branches from adjacent vessels (Fig. 57-4). The renal arteries supply the upper end of the ureters, abdominal aorta, and testicular or ovarian arteries. The common iliac arteries supply the middle part, and the rest are supplied by branches from internal iliac arteries. There is anastomosis between these branches.

Bladder Vasculature

The superior and inferior vesical arteries, which arise from the anterior trunk of the internal iliac artery and small branches from the obturator and inferior gluteal and uterine and vaginal arteries, all supply the bladder (Fig. 57-5).

ADRENAL SUPRARENAL VASCULATURE

Arterial Supply

There are three primary sources for adrenal gland arterial supply (Fig. 57-6):

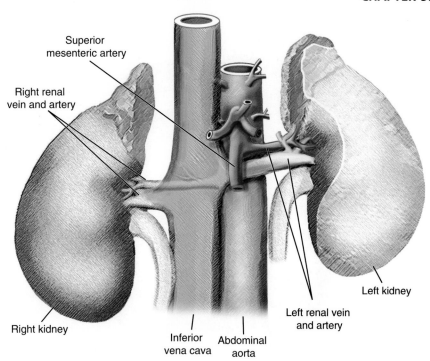

FIGURE 57-1. Renal vasculature. *(Redrawn from Drake RL, Vogl W, Mitchell AWM, editors. Gray's anatomy for students. Philadelphia: Churchill Livingstone; 2005.)*

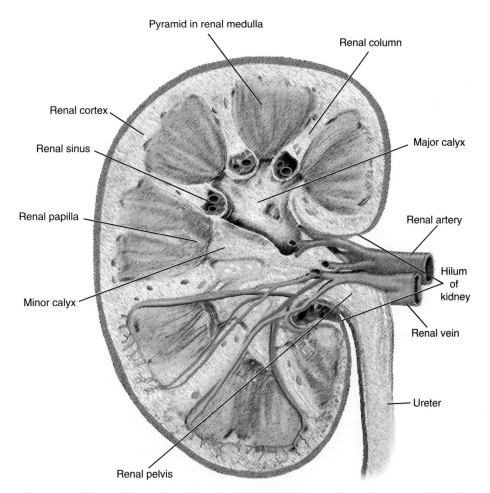

FIGURE 57-2. Internal structure of kidney. *(Redrawn from Drake RL, Vogl W, Mitchell AWM, editors. Gray's anatomy for students. Philadelphia: Churchill Livingstone; 2005.)*

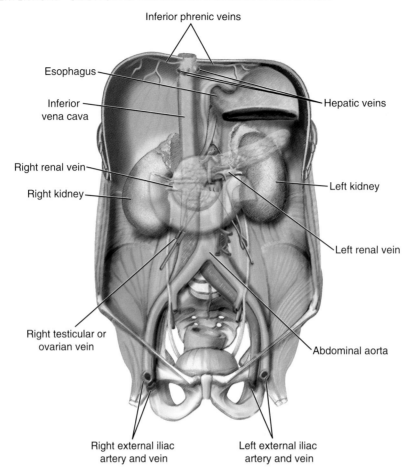

FIGURE 57-3. Inferior vena cava. *(Redrawn from Drake RL, Vogl W, Mitchell AWM, editors. Gray's anatomy for students. Philadelphia: Churchill Livingstone; 2005.)*

1. Superior adrenal arteries, which arise from the inferior phrenic artery (from aorta, celiac, renal, or left gastric artery)
2. Middle adrenal artery, which arises directly from the aorta or less commonly from the celiac artery or SMA
3. Inferior adrenal artery, which arises from the renal arteries

Venous Supply

Adrenal venous drainage consists of a single vein. The right adrenal vein enters the IVC, and the left adrenal vein enters the left renal vein.

VASCULAR IMAGING OF KIDNEYS AND ADRENAL GLANDS

Assessment of the renal vasculature can be performed using varying imaging modalities including ultrasound (US), conventional angiography (Figs. 57-7 and 57-8), computed tomography (CT), magnetic resonance imaging (MRI), and nuclear medicine (Table 57-1).

The most common indications for imaging the renal vessels include evaluation of renal artery stenosis or occlusion, aneurysms and dissections, arteriovenous fistulae, and renal vein thrombosis. Preoperative imaging of the kidneys and their vasculature may also be indicated for potential renal donors and for surgical planning of renal tumors. Lastly, follow-up and evaluation of renal vascular stents is a common indication for diagnostic imaging.

Ultrasound

Color Doppler sonography is an easily performed examination, can be done portably, and is relatively inexpensive and widely available. It is a noninvasive test and can be done on patients with renal failure and patients who have a history of allergies to iodinated contrast. It also has the advantage of not using ionizing radiation. However, its limitations include non-visualization of main renal arteries, which can occur in approximately 42% of patients, and the inability to document the presence of accessory renal vessels. These limitations can be due to the patient's body habitus, overlying bowel gas obscuring the renal vasculature, or the sonographer's lack of experience. The main indication for using US is evaluation of renovascular hypertension, by measuring peak systolic velocities through the main renal arteries and obtaining renal/aortic velocity ratios. Visualizing the stenotic segment itself can be challenging. This can be overcome by documenting a dampened tardus-parvus waveform found downstream from the stenosis. Duplex Doppler sonography can also evaluate the renal vein, looking for intraluminal thrombus or extrinsic compression.

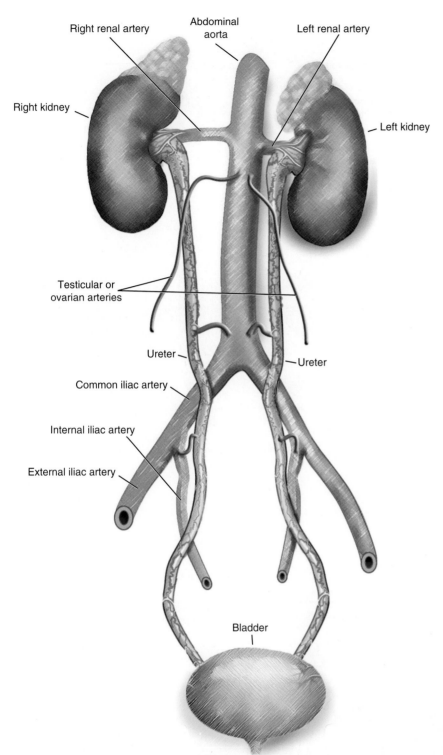

Right renal artery

Abdominal aorta

Left renal artery

Right kidney

Left kidney

Testicular or ovarian arteries

Ureter

Ureter

Common iliac artery

Internal iliac artery

External iliac artery

Bladder

FIGURE 57-4. Ureters. *(Redrawn from Drake RL, Vogl W, Mitchell AWM, editors. Gray's anatomy for students. Philadelphia: Churchill Livingstone; 2005.)*

Computed Tomographic Angiography and Magnetic Resonance Angiography

When US is unavailable or its results are equivocal, computed tomographic angiography (CTA) or magnetic resonance angiography (MRA) can be performed. Both exams are noninvasive but involve administration of iodinated contrast for CTA and gadolinium for MRA (Figs. 57-9 and 57-10). Thus they can only be performed in patients with normal renal function. With the advent of volumetric

acquisition of images and three-dimensional (3D) reconstruction algorithms, the normal and variant renal vascular anatomy of native and transplanted kidneys can be accurately displayed. In patients with renal impairment, noncontrast-enhanced MRA using balanced steady-state free precession (SSFP) can be used as an alternative to image the renal vessels (Fig. 57-11). Compared to conventional MRA with gadolinium, unenhanced MRA provides excellent anatomic images. In addition, the sensitivity and specificity for detecting clinically relevant renal artery

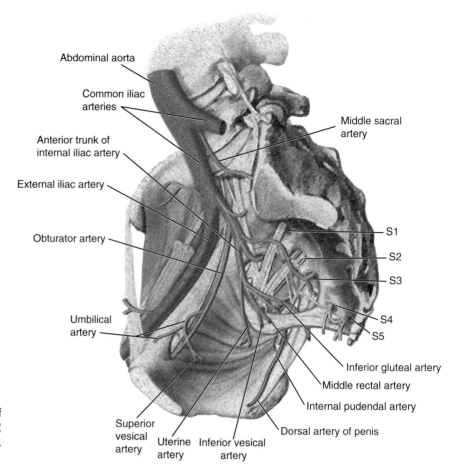

FIGURE 57-5. Branches of anterior trunk of internal iliac artery. *(Redrawn from Drake RL, Vogl W, Mitchell AWM, editors. Gray's anatomy for students. Philadelphia: Churchill Livingstone; 2005.)*

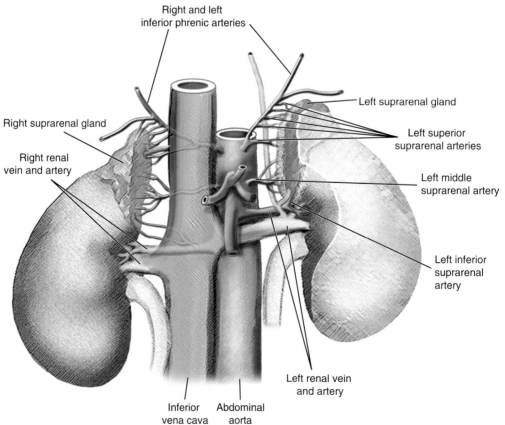

FIGURE 57-6. Arterial supply to suprarenal glands. *(Redrawn from Drake RL, Vogl W, Mitchell AWM, editors. Gray's anatomy for students. Philadelphia: Churchill Livingstone; 2005.)*

TABLE 57-1. Comparison of Imaging Modalities for Renal Vascular Anatomy

Modality	Advantages	Disadvantages
US	Readily available Inexpensive No contrast No ionizing radiation	Operator dependent Bowel gas (20% nondiagnostic), obesity Lower sensitivity than MRA and CTA
MRA	Accurate No ionizing radiation	Expensive Limited availability Risk of nephrogenic systemic fibrosis with gadolinium contrast Contraindicated in patients with pacemakers and implants Tends to overestimate high-grade renal artery stenoses
CTA	Readily available Moderate cost High sensitivity	Iodinated contrast material required Contraindicated in renal insufficiency Ionizing radiation

CTA, Computed tomographic angiography; *MRA,* magnetic resonance angiography; *US,* ultrasound.

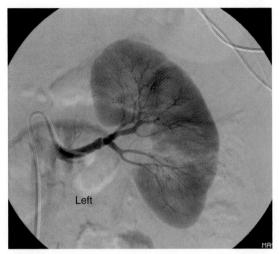

FIGURE 57-7. Anteroposterior digital subtraction selective left renal arteriogram in patient who sustained blunt trauma to left kidney during a motorcycle accident. Note irregularity of distal main left renal artery, with irregularity and a small intimal flap.

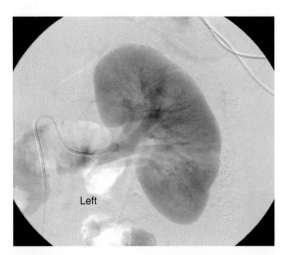

FIGURE 57-8. Anteroposterior digital subtraction image during venous phases of a selective left renal arteriogram (same patient as Fig. 57-7). Note renal vein emptying into inferior vena cava.

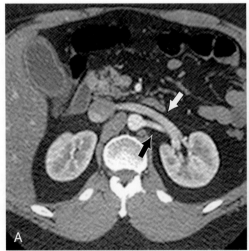
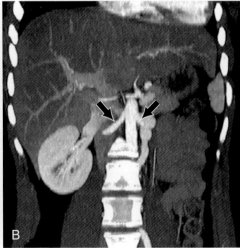

FIGURE 57-9. Axial **(A)** and coronal **(B)** contrast-enhanced computed tomographic angiograms at level of renal vessels. Renal arteries *(black arrows)* and left renal vein *(white arrow)* are shown.

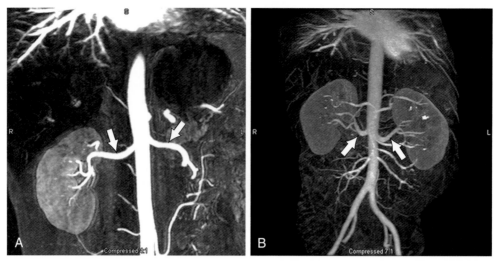

FIGURE 57-10. Reconstructed coronal magnetic resonance angiograms of abdominal aorta and renal arteries *(arrows)*. Kidneys are also nicely depicted.

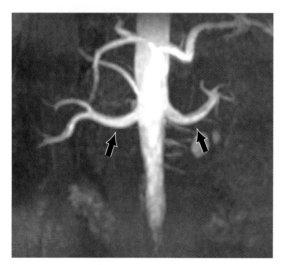

FIGURE 57-11. Coronal magnetic resonance angiogram without gadolinium, showing normal renal arteries *(arrows)*.

stenosis are similar to contrast-enhanced MRAs. Both CTA and MRA provide excellent evaluation of the renal arteries and veins as well as the renal parenchyma.

Nuclear Medicine Imaging

Nuclear medicine renography using an angiotensin-converting enzyme (ACE) is limited to the diagnosis of renal artery stenosis. This test is noninvasive, safe, and can be performed on patients with abnormal renal function. It does not, however, depict the normal renal vascular anatomy and is not a very dependable test in cases of bilateral renal artery stenosis.

Catheter Angiography

Many radiologists still consider catheter angiography the gold standard for imaging the renal vessels, even though it remains an invasive test and involves using ionizing radiation and administering iodinated contrast material. In patients with renal impairment, carbon dioxide (CO_2) can be safely substituted for iodinated material as the contrast medium to visualize the renal vessels. CO_2 usually identifies main renal artery lesions well, but when used as a substitute for iodinated contrast, CO_2 has inferior visibility of anatomic detail in the peripheral renal artery branches.

One of the biggest advantages of using conventional angiography when evaluating renal vascular disease is that it allows diagnosis and potential treatment when necessary. For example, balloon angioplasty or stenting can be performed in cases of renal artery stenosis or dissection, and embolization of renal artery aneurysms or renal artery transection due to trauma can be done. The renal venous system can also be imaged to detect renal vein thrombosis or perform renal venous sampling to evaluate renovascular hypertension.

Adrenal Vein Sampling

Imaging of adrenal gland vasculature is nowadays limited to venous sampling. This test is performed in patients with primary hyperaldosteronism and is used to differentiate bilateral hyperplasia from aldosterone-secreting adrenal adenomas. Distinguishing between these two entities is important because adrenal adenomas are treated surgically, whereas patients with hyperplasia are managed medically. Adrenal vein sampling is an invasive test, involves using iodinated contrast material, and can be a challenging procedure even in experienced hands. Finding the right adrenal vein for sampling can be difficult because of its small size and its orientation draining along the midposterior wall of the IVC. The left adrenal vein is usually easier to find because it drains into the left renal vein. Despite all these hurdles, this procedure is reported to be technically successful in 97% of cases when performed by skilled interventional radiologists.

▶ SUGGESTED READINGS

Daunt N. Adrenal vein sampling: how to make it quick, easy, and successful. Radiographics 2005;25:S143–S158.

Drake RL, Vogl W, Mitchell AWM, editors. Gray's Anatomy for Students. Philadelphia: Elsevier Churchill Livingstone; 2005.

Hazirolan T, Oz M, Turkbey B, et al. CT angiography of the renal arteries and veins: normal anatomy and variants. Diagn Interv Radiol 2011;17:67–73.

Kahn SL, Angle JF. Adrenal vein sampling. Tech Vasc Interv Radiol 2010;13(2):110–25.

Kaufman JA, Lee MJ, editors. Vascular and interventional radiology: the requisites. St. Louis: Mosby; 2004.

Khoo MM, Deeab D, Gedroyc WM, et al. Renal artery stenosis: comparative assessment by unenhanced renal artery MRA versus contrast-enhanced MRA. Eur Radiol 2011;21(7):1470–6.

Spinosa DJ, Matsumoto AH, Angle JF, et al. Safety of CO2- and gadodiamide-enhanced angiography for the evaluation and percutaneous treatment of renal artery stenosis in patients with chronic renal insufficiency. AJR Am J Roentgenol 2001;176:1305–11.

Sutter R, Nanz D, Lutz A, et al. Assessment of aortoiliac and renal arteries: MR angiography with parallel acquisition versus conventional MR angiography and digital subtraction angiography. Radiology 2007;245:276–84.

Thurston W, Wilson SR. The urinary tract. In: Rumack CM, Wilson SR, Charboneau JW, editors. Diagnostic ultrasound. 3rd ed. Elsevier: Philadelphia; 2004.

Urban BA, Rather LE, Fishman EK. Three-dimensional volume-rendered CT angiography of renal arteries and veins: normal anatomy, variants and clinical applications. Radiographics 2001;21:373–86.

CHAPTER 58

Renovascular Interventions

John H. Rundback and Joshua L. Weintraub

EPIDEMIOLOGY

Renal artery stenosis (RAS) is a well-characterized condition caused by narrowing of one or both renal arteries due to atherosclerosis, fibromuscular dysplasia, or arteritis. Atherosclerotic disease is the predominant cause of RAS, and it is likely worldwide prevalence will continue to grow as average life expectancy rises.[1] RAS is both a sequela of generalized atherosclerosis and a marker for subsequent atherosclerotic clinical events.[2,3] Although some degree of RAS is extremely prevalent in elderly patients, patients with peripheral or coronary artery disease,[4,5] or in autopsy samples,[6] the clinical presentation is variable and often unpredictable. As a result, there is currently tremendous debate regarding the role of imaging and intervention in patients with RAS.

The intrinsic physiologic alterations occurring in experimental RAS were first described by Harry Goldblatt in 1934.[7,8] Over the past decade, there has been an increasing appreciation that the pathophysiology of RAS may involve activation of a much more complex neurohumoral response than originally described.[8-10] RAS may be a silent "asymptomatic" finding or be associated with several related and overlapping clinical syndromes including renovascular hypertension (RVH), impaired renal function (also called *ischemic nephropathy*), and cardiac decompensation.[11] Investigation is ongoing, but as yet, no reliable biomarkers for RVH have been identified. Measurements of elevated serum brain natriuretic peptide (BNP > 80 pg/mL) have been reported as predictive of a blood pressure response to revascularization,[12] although this has not been consistently reproduced in clinical studies.[13,14]

RVH is the most common correctable form of hypertension and is estimated to occur in 12% to 25% of the hypertensive population.[3] Clinical clues suggestive of RAS are used to define individuals warranting more detailed evaluation with noninvasive imaging or arteriography: onset of hypertension prior to age 30 (suggestive of renal artery fibromuscular dysplasia) or over age 50; accelerated, malignant, or multidrug resistant hypertension; and hypertension associated with recurrent episodes of heart failure (Table 58-1). Asymmetric renal atrophy may also be noted. Clinical prediction rules have been applied to identify a cohort of patients with approximately 30% likelihood of RAS, using an algorithmic evaluation of clinical variables that include smoking history, gender, age, presence of dyslipidemia, body mass index, serum creatinine (SCr), presence of an abdominal bruit, and existence of known atherosclerosis in other vascular beds.[15] There is a linear correlation between severity of coronary artery disease (CAD) found during coronary angiography and the presence of RAS, as well as overall mortality risk.[16] In patients undergoing cardiac catheterization, factors associated with concurrent RAS include peripheral arterial disease, a widened pulse pressure, dyslipidemia, older age, renal insufficiency, and more severe CAD.[17] In particular, the presence of right CAD may be a marker for RAS.[18]

RAS is also a well-known cause of ischemic nephropathy and has been cited as a putative cause of declining renal function in 25% to 58% of patients.[19] Although difficult to determine with certainty, ischemic nephropathy may also be a relatively common and treatable cause of end-stage renal disease. Earlier studies in which patients initiating renal replacement therapy were audited for renovascular disease found RAS in 27% to 45%.[20-22] Characteristics suggestive of underlying RAS in this population include angiotensin inhibitor–induced renal failure, unexplained rapid declines in renal function, and an absence of proteinuria.[23]

Finally, RAS is a known cause of recurrent heart failure[24-26] and may also contribute to poorly controlled angina in patients with nonreconstructable CAD.[27] Magnetic resonance angiography has shown significant unilateral or bilateral RAS in nearly half of all patients presenting with flash pulmonary edema.[28] In these individuals, the presence of predominantly diastolic dysfunction and elevated serum endothelin levels may be suggestive.[29,30]

CLINICAL INDICATIONS

Indications for imaging and intervention for RAS have been reported in a consensus document published by the Society of Interventional Radiology[31] and the American College of Cardiology.[32] The document also offers guidelines for appropriate use of screening renal angiography at the time of coronary angiography[33] for patients in whom clinically important RAS is suspected. Incidental nonselective or selective renal angiography without a clinical indicator is not recommended.

In general, three criteria should be fulfilled to support an indication for renal revascularization: a suitable clinical scenario, anatomic stenosis of at least 50% with measurement of a trans-stenotic pressure gradient of 20 mmHg in uncertain cases, and safe and reasonable anatomic conditions for access and therapy. Proper patient selection has been shown to optimize outcomes[34]; conversely, nonrigorous adherence to the treatment of patients with appropriate indicators has been a principal source of criticism for both cohort and randomized trials failing to show benefit from renal intervention.[35,36] In particular, lack of adherence to trans-stenotic pressure measurements as a determinant for intervention in hypertensive patients is a major failing in many reported studies. In this regard, it is important to realize that the visual estimate as well as quantitative angiography of stenosis is often unreliable for evaluating the hemodynamic relevance of a lesion. While other methods have been proposed for assessing lesion severity, trans-stenotic gradients have been repeatedly validated as the simplest and most reliable technique. In a recent study comparing hyperemic

404

TABLE 58-1. Indications for Renal Angiography

History
Onset of hypertension at <30 or >55 years of age
Malignant, accelerated, drug-resistant hypertension
Smoking
Systemic atherosclerosis
No family history of hypertension
ACEI- or ARB-induced renal failure
Unexplained or rapidly progressive renal failure
Recurrent flash pulmonary edema or heart failure
Physical Examination
Epigastric bruit
Retinopathy
Asymmetric renal atrophy
Laboratory
Hypokalemia
Mild or absent proteinuria
Elevated plasma renin activity

ACEI, Angiotensin-converting enzyme inhibitor; *ARB*, angiotensin receptor blocker.

systolic gradient (HSG), fractional flow reserve (FFR), quantitative angiography, and intravascular ultrasound, HSG had the best receiver operating characteristic curve for predicting blood pressure response to renal artery stenting.[37] Although it is impossible in any individual to know the exact magnitude of a pressure difference across a renal artery lesion that is hemodynamically relevant and has clinical effect, a resting or hyperemic (after intrarenal vasodilator administration) trans-stenotic gradient of at least 20 mmHg has been validated in experimental and clinical trials to be associated with a greater likelihood of improved clinical outcomes.[38-40]

TECHNICAL DETAILS

The techniques of renal artery stenting have evolved over the past decade. Modern methods incorporate specially shaped guides and sheaths that better align with the renal ostium, lower-profile wires for lesion traversal, pressure-sensing wires for measuring trans-stenotic gradients, and dedicated stents.[41] Renal artery stents are balloon expandable and embedded into their delivery balloons, facilitating a low profile, and have structural variation producing proximal reinforcement to better efface resistant aorto-ostial lesions. Both over-the-wire and monorail stent delivery systems are available.[42] Drug-eluting stents show trends toward reduced restenosis but have not been widely accepted for routine use,[43] although they have demonstrated clinical value for small and branch RAS.[44]

Careful preintervention planning is necessary to assure the highest possible technical success. The best route for crossing the lesion should be carefully assessed, and flush aortography is recommended to assess the severity of aortic atherosclerosis as a determinant of both the safety of intervention (due to cholesterol or plaque embolization) and selection of technique and guiding catheters optimized to the renal artery anatomy. Arteries with a sharp caudal angulation from the aorta may be approached from an upper extremity access.[45,46] For mild or equivocal lesions, trans-lesional pressure measurements should be performed to confirm the hemodynamic significance prior to intervention.

Pharmacologic adjuncts are important for preventing procedure-related complications. Patients should be adequately hydrated. Oral or intravenous *N*-acetylcysteine or parenteral bicarbonate saline infusions may be of value for preventing contrast-induced nephropathy in patients with renal insufficiency.[47] In these patients, carbon dioxide (CO_2) angiography can also be used to augment or replace conventional contrast arteriography to decrease iodinated contrast exposture.[48] Antiplatelet therapy, generally with clopidogrel loading, is initiated prior to the procedure. Heparin sulfate or bivalirudin should be administered to provide full anticoagulation prior to crossing the RAS, as well as periodically during prolonged catheter and device manipulation; if available, measuring activated clotting time is useful to ensure adequate levels of anticoagulation. Intraarterial nitroglycerin, verapamil, dopamine, or papaverine can be administered into the renal artery both for measurements of the hyperemic systolic gradient and to limit wire- and catheter-induced vasospasm. Verapamil (1-2.5 mg) should be used with caution in patients with first-degree heart block.

There are several basic steps for aorto-ostial renal artery stenting. Once a stenosis is identified by aortography, the lesion is carefully and atraumatically crossed using a floppy-tipped 0.014- to 0.035-inch guidewire and an appropriately shaped angled-tip catheter. The goal is to have the guiding sheath or catheter aligned with the aortic ostium to prevent inadvertent scraping and dislodgment of cholesterol plaque from the aortic wall. In patients with markedly atherosclerotic or ecstatic aortas, a "no touch" technique may be used, utilizing a second stiffer wire to stabilize the guide away from the aortic wall while the working wire is passed across the RAS.[49] Depending upon the balloon or stent system used, predilation or placement of a second "buddy" wire may be needed to allow the stent to pass across the stenosis. The shortest possible stent that will cover the target lesion plus 1 to 2 mm on each side and with a diameter equal to the normal width of the target renal artery is positioned across the stenosis and is slowly inflated, with care taken to avoid balloon sliding that may risk dissection.

It is essential that the renal artery is imaged in the proper oblique projection so that the lesion is exactly in profile, especially if the lesion is ostial. The goal is to place the stent so that it covers the lesion and extends 1 to 2 mm past it on both sides. For ostial lesions, the proximal end should extend 1 to 2 mm into the aorta to ensure that it covers the ostium adequately. After deflation, the balloon is removed while maintaining guidewire position across the treated site. Completion angiography is performed via the guiding catheter or sheath. If there is a satisfactory angiographic appearance and no residual transstenotic gradient, the guidewire is carefully removed (Fig. 58-1).

COMPLICATIONS

A total complication rate as high as 35% has been reported for renal interventions, although most events are minor.[50] Serious complications usually occur in less than 5%,[31] although major adverse events can occur in 8% to 13% of patients with advanced azotemia or severe aortic disease.[51] The most common complications are puncture site related (1%-2% transfusion risk) and worsening renal insufficiency.

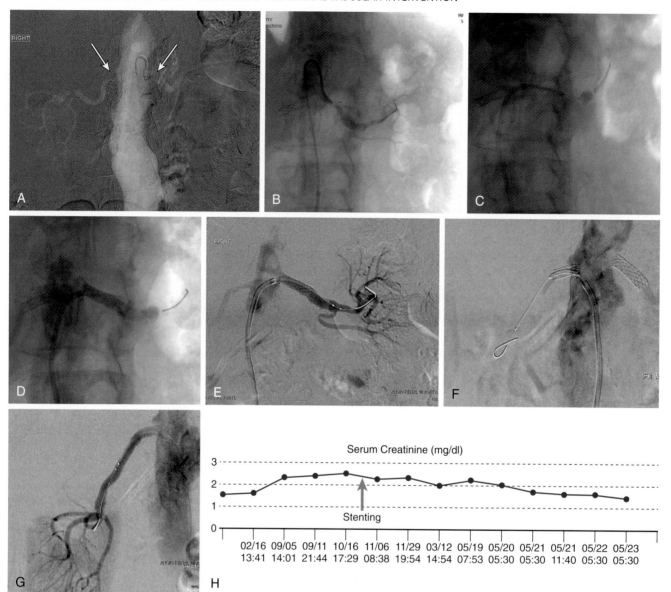

FIGURE 58-1. A, Carbon dioxide (CO_2) renal arteriography in patient with renal insufficiency and prior right renal artery stenting demonstrates severe bilateral ostial stenosis *(arrows).* **B,** Selective left renal arteriography confirms severe ostial stenosis. Balloon occlusion distal embolic protection (DEP) device (Guardwire [Medtronic, Santa Rosa, Calif.]) has been advanced across lesion. **C,** Stent positioning is performed after inflation of DEP balloon and during control angiography performed through aortic guide sheath. **D,** Contrast injection immediately after stent deployment shows adequate ostial positioning and successful occlusion of intrarenal flow by DEP device. An aspiration catheter (Export [Medtronic]) is then used to suction embolic debris that may have accumulated proximal to DEP balloon. **E,** Completion angiography on left shows resolution of stenosis and preserved intrarenal flow. An in-stent right RAS is noted that was subsequently confirmed to be hemodynamically significant. **F,** Stent-in-stent revascularization of right renal artery is performed with distal balloon occlusion. **G,** Completion digital subtraction angiography on right also shows resolution of ostial stenosis after repeat stenting. **H,** Plotted curve of serum creatinine prior to and following procedure shows worsening renal function before intervention but continued gradual improvement in the 6 months following treatment.

This latter event occurs in approximately 5% with normal renal function, and up to 25% of patients with extant renal insufficiency. Progressive renal insufficiency may be due to progression of intrinsic renal pathology, contrast-induced nephropathy, or embolization. Development of overt renal infarction is rare, occurring in approximately 1% of patients. Guidewire perforations are almost always self-sealing, and peripheral perforations that do not stop bleeding can be treated by subsegmental transcather occlusion using coils or gelfoam. Renal artery rupture after balloon inflation or stenting occurs in less than 1% of cases and can potentially cause renal loss or death. Prompt recognition and reinflation of a percutaneous transluminal angioplasty balloon or an occlusion balloon across the site of rupture is critical until definitive therapy is undertaken. The availability of stent grafts allows most cases to be salvaged by endovascular therapy.

DISTAL EMBOLIC PROTECTION

There is uncertainty as to the value of routinely using distal embolic protection (DEP) devices during renal artery stenting. Embolization of both atherosclerotic debris and cholesterol crystals has been identified during all stages of renal artery interventions using both ex vivo modeling and intraprocedural duplex sonography.[52,53] In one report, microembolic Doppler signals were seen in all cases of renal artery intervention and were especially prominent when stenting was performed compared with percutaneous transluminal renal angioplasty (PTRA) alone; the most striking embolization occurred with poststent dilation and flaring.[53] Clinical series have described captured debris in 100% of procedures when using occlusion balloon protection systems (Guardwire [Medtronic, Santa Rosa, Calif.]) and 80% with filter-type DEPs,[54] with 99% stabilization or improvement in renal function observed out to 2 years after stenting with the use of DEP. However, other reports have been less favorable, and there are considerable limitations to the regular use of DEPs.

Since no DEP has been specifically designed for use in the renal arteries, the available configuration of the devices and the need for a relatively long "landing zone" for filters precludes their use in many cases. In addition, protection devices tend to have a larger crossing profile that may not easily traverse highly stenotic lesions, and they further tend to be relatively bulky and rigid, with a perceived risk of associated renal artery spasm or dissection. New devices with unique designs allowing shorter overall filter lengths and improved embolic capture have been described but are not routinely used or yet indicated for use in renal intervention.[55]

For more information on these future directions, please visit the accompanying website at www.expertconsult.com.

REPORTED OUTCOMES AND PREDICTORS

Hypertension

Overall, 12% of the U.S. population has treatment-resistant hypertension,[62] and it is estimated that up to one quarter of these have RAS. Overall, blood pressure response after renal artery stenting (RAST) is seen in approximately two thirds of patients.[63] Meta-analysis of earlier cohort series,[64] as well as the five completed industry premarket approval RAST trials, have shown both early and sustained blood pressure benefit (Table 58-2).[65-69] In a recent Swedish study of 234 patients undergoing RAST, both systolic and diastolic blood pressure (SBP/DBP) were improved on follow-up out to 4 years.[70] Characteristics of patients experiencing hypertension benefit include higher baseline stenosis and trans-stenotic gradient,[39] more elevated initial SBP and DBP, preserved parenchyma, and a shorter duration of hypertension.[71,72] Better long-term blood pressure response has been described in men and patients with a glomerular filtration rate (GFR) above 40 mL/min.[73] A contemporary evaluation of 149 patients followed over a course of 9 years found drug-resistant hypertension (patients receiving $\geq$ 4 antihypertensive medications), use of clonidine, DBP greater than 90 mmHg, and larger renal volume to be the best determinants of favorable blood pressure after treatment.[74] However, randomized trials have not consistently demonstrated better blood pressure outcomes in patients treated by RAST compared with medical therapy alone.[75-77] In light of this controversy, one strategy that has been proposed is to reserve intervention for patients with RAS and evidence of accelerated or malignant hypertension or end-organ injury including heart failure, stroke, or declining renal function.[78]

Renal Failure (Ischemic Nephropathy)

Renal insufficiency may be seen with global or unilateral RAS, and progression to dialysis is not uncommon.[79] Once on dialysis, patients with RAS have a worse prognosis than other dialysis groups.[80] Functional response to stenting has a linear correlation with the baseline SCr,[81] and the absolute level of renal function remains a strong predictor of mid- to long-term survival despite revascularization.[82,83] Overall, stabilization or improvement of renal function is reported

TABLE 58-2. Primary Outcomes from Prospective Clinical Trials of Renal Artery Stenting

Trial	Year	Patients/Lesions	Follow-Up	Baseline (Mean Values)			Follow-Up (Mean Values)			Restenosis
				SBP*	DBP*	SCr (GFR)	SBP*	DBP*	SCr (GFR)	
Premarket Approval Studies										
RENAISSANCE[66]	2008	100/117	3 yr	157	75	1.39 (51.49)	139[†]	71[†]	1.40 (53.68)	21.3%
ASPIRE-2[67]	2005	208/244	2 yr	168	82	1.36	149[†]	77[†]	1.46	16.8%[‡]
SOAR[68]	2010	188/188	11 mo	160	77	1.15	135[†§]	74[§]	1.29[§]	12.6%[‡]
REFORM[69]	NP	100/115	2 yr	150	74	1.3	136[†]	73	N/A	8.1%[‡]
HERCULES[70]	NP	202/241	9 mo	162	78	1.2 (58)	145[†]	75[†]	N/A (57)	10.5%[‡]
Randomized Controlled Trial										
ASTRAL (med)	2009	403	34 mo	152	76	2.02	140	71	2.02	N/A
ASTRAL (stent)		403		149	76	2.02	140	73	2.26	

*Blood pressures represent mean values recorded as mmHg.
[†]Statistically significant ($P \leq 0.05$).
[‡]Nine-month angiographic assessment.
[§]Three-year follow-up (available on 36% of study cohort).
ASTRAL, Angioplasty and Stenting for Renal Artery Lesions trial; *DBP,* diastolic blood pressure; *GFR,* glomerular filtration rate measured in mL/min/1.73 m²; *(med),* medical therapy alone; *N/A,* not available; *NP,* not yet published; *SBP,* systolic blood pressure; *SCr,* serum creatinine measured in mg/dL.

in approximately 75% of patients, with a better functional response noted following global revascularization (treatment of bilateral RAS or RAS in a solitary functional kidney) in some but not all series.[83-86] Renal intervention has been repeatedly demonstrated to slow the rate of renal decline in patients with RAS,[87,88] but it is not clear whether improving renal function after revascularization is associated with decreased overall mortality, although this has been noted in limited series.[89,90] The presence of metabolic syndrome is associated with higher restenosis rates and reduced preserved clinical benefit in the long term.[91] The best results are seen in patients with rapidly declining function[92,93] (see Fig. 58-1). In this patient group, renal intervention may further improve renal function beyond the gains seen by discontinuing renin-angiotensin system blockade alone.[94] In contrast, the presence of proteinuria portends a worse functional response to intervention,[95] most likely reflecting the development of tubulointerstitial fibrosis and glomerular injury that has been pathologically demonstrated with long-standing RAS.[96] In addition, the benefits of intervention must be weighed against the risk of acute functional injury in up to 20% of patients following RAST, with associated worse outcomes and a potential earlier need for hemodialysis.[97,98]

The ASTRAL trial (Angioplasty and Stenting for Renal Artery Lesions) randomized 806 patients with RAS to medical therapy or RAST,[99] with a primary endpoint of inverse SCr over 5 years of follow-up. There was a trend towards less functional decline in patients who were stented, although this did not reach statistical difference ($P = 0.06$) and was not noted within the first 2 years of enrollment. In addition, there was no difference in overall mortality or a composite endpoint of renal-related events, even in a subgroup of patients with stenosis greater than 70% and global ischemia.

Notwithstanding, the ASTRAL trial has been broadly criticized[100,101] for an unusual design in which only patients with uncertainty regarding clinical benefit from revascularization were enrolled. In the busiest participating centers, only 25% of patients with a hemodynamically significant RAS were included in the trial. Because of this schema, the results cannot be generalized to all patients with RAS. Further compromising interpretation of ASTRAL data is that only three quarters of the stent-randomized patients actually received the prescribed treatment, potentially mitigating any observed benefit from stent therapy. In a separate report from an ASTRAL site describing outcomes in 127 patients with RAS who were treated outside of the study, 62% demonstrated slowing of renal decline after RAST and were deemed "responders."[102] Responders were less likely to require renal replacement therapy than nonresponders (6% vs. 29%), or had renal replacement therapy later (median 3.6 vs. 0.7 years); mortality was similar in both groups.

Renal Salvage

An interesting extension of renal revascularization is for patients with pending or recently initiated hemodialysis. Although the functional response to RAST inversely correlates with GFR prior to intervention across the broad range of mild to moderate azotemia,[103] there is recent evidence suggesting a paradoxical benefit in patients with predialysis levels of renal dysfunction.[104,105] In a prospectively collected dataset of 908 patients from Germany and the United Kingdom treated by RAST, individuals with stage 3 chronic kidney disease (CKD) and stage 4/5 CKD had odds ratios for at least a 20% postprocedural improvement in GFR of 2.69 and 6.72, respectively, both of which were highly statistically significant. A similar effect was not seen in patients with milder stages of CKD.[104] In the 251 patient Italian ODORI registry, in which changes in mean estimated GFR following intervention were stratified according to baseline values, the most dramatic results were seen in patients with an initial GFR between 15 and 20 mL/min/1.73 m^2. In this group, there was almost a 13 mL/min/1.73 m^2 increase in GFR at 1-year follow-up.[105] The concept of renal revascularization to remove patients from hemodialysis has not been well studied but is conceptually possible.[106-108] In an earlier surgical series,[106] 16 of 20 patients with dialysis-dependent ischemic nephropathy were able to discontinue dialysis, with global revascularization and prehemodialysis estimated GFR progression predictive of outcomes. Complete removal of patients from renal replacement therapy following RAST has also been reported.[108] A recent series by Thatipelli et al.[108] described removal of hemodialysis in 8 of 16 patients with both chronic and acute renal failure as the cause for renal replacement therapy; in this study, renal size and absence of proteinuria were found to be associated with dialysis cessation.[110]

Notably, renal recovery and salvage is observed with equal likelihood following unilateral or bilateral intervention in patients with advanced CKD,[109] most likely as a result of the RAS being nephroprotective in patients with long-standing disease, unilateral RAS, and contralateral advanced nephrosclerosis.[107,110]

Heart Failure and Cardiovascular Risk

There is a direct association between RAS and cardiovascular events, with RAS as an independent predictor of events.[111] More than 40% of patients with heart failure (HF) have underlying RAS, and these patients are characterized by higher diuretic and lower angiotensin-converting enzyme use, more frequent and prolonged admissions for HF, and higher mortality.[112] Although left ventricular hypertrophy in patients with RAS improves after RAST,[113,114] left ventricular function prior to intervention is predictive of late mortality.[115] Percutaneous transluminal renal stenting (PTRS) in patients with congestive HF results in reduced HF severity, fewer hospitalizations, and substantial increases in the time between HF admissions.[116] In this population of patients, both short- and long-term benefits have been repeatedly demonstrated following RAST.[117]

RAS is an independent predictor of major cardiac events and stroke. Investigators have demonstrated a graded relationship between RAS severity and the observed risk of cardiovascular mortality.[16] Additional observational studies have found co-linearity between renal ischemia and cardiovascular events.[118] There is not only an observed reduced 4-year survival in patients with CAD and RAS compared with CAD alone,[16] but RAS may be a stronger predictor of cardiovascular mortality than severity of hypertension.[118,119] Although renal revascularization improves left ventricular performance,[113] there is conflicting evidence that there is an associated reduction in cardiovascular events and improved

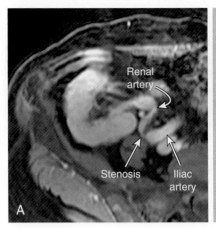 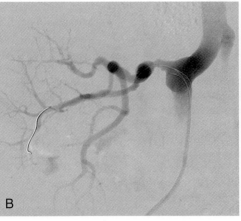 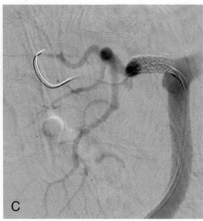

FIGURE 58-2. A, Contrast-enhanced liver acquisition with volume acceleration magnetic resonance angiography (LAVA MRA) sequence in transplant patient with worsening renal function shows anastomotic stenosis *(arrow)*. **B,** Corresponding catheter arteriogram from ipsilateral femoral approach confirms severe stenosis at end-to-side anastomosis of graft renal artery to donor external iliac artery. **C,** After stenting, stenosis resolved and patient's renal function improved.

survival. Early surgical series by Hunt and colleagues,[120] as well as observational angioplasty and stent data,[89,90] noted reduced cardiovascular mortality after renal revascularization. However, two other reports failed to demonstrate diminished cardiac events following percutaneous renal intervention.[121,122] The Cardiovascular Outcomes in Renal Artery Lesions (CORAL) trial, currently near completion, will provide much needed level 1 evidence regarding this effect.[123]

TRANSPLANT RENAL ARTERY STENOSIS

Renal artery stenosis is the most common vascular complication of a renal transplant, generally occurring within the first year after surgery,[124] and may present as renal dysfunction, peripheral edema, and new-onset or uncontrolled hypertension. Confirmation of the diagnosis is usually made by duplex sonography with color-flow Doppler. Different duplex velocity parameters exist for the diagnosis of transplant RAS (TRAS), depending on the type of arterial anastomosis.[125] There is a belief that TRAS may in many cases represent a form of vascular rejection,[126] but mechanical factors, such as arterial kinking and clamp injury,[124] and metabolic conditions[127] may also be responsible. There is a threefold risk of TRAS in kidneys with an end-to-end anastomosis (to the hypogastric artery) when compared to grafts having an end-to-side anastomosis to the recipient external iliac artery.[124] Most mechanical stenoses are anastomotic, whereby stenoses due to presumed acute rejection may be noted within the main donor renal artery. In addition, occlusive disease of the donor iliac artery due to atherosclerosis or arterial trauma may be encountered.

Angiography remains the gold standard for definitive determination of TRAS and allows simultaneous therapy with PTRA or PTRS as first-line therapy in most cases. Technical challenges are similar to native RAS treatment, although a prior knowledge of the site of anastomosis is critical for determining the optimal access site for initial arterial puncture. For transplants with end-to-end anastomoses, a contralateral femoral approach is recommended

to allow easy entry into the donor hypogastric artery; in contrast, an ipsilateral femoral approach is preferred for end-to-side anastomoses. Upper extremity access is rarely needed but can on occasion offer an advantage for crossing a severely kinked or ecstatic stenosis. Angioplasty alone may be used for segmental or mid-arterial stenosis. For anastomotic lesions or lesions with recoil after PTRA, stenting is preferred[128-130] (Fig. 58-2). Drug-eluting stents have been described for treatment of smaller-caliber TRAS.[131] Complication rates vary widely from 0% to 25%, with few serious difficulties in most series, and the most common adverse event being progressive loss of renal graft function due to contrast nephropathy or progressive acute or chronic rejection.[132] Technical success in larger series is in the 88% to 100% range, with most series reporting the higher rates.[132]

Reported outcomes for hypertension control, reduction in antihypertensive medications, renal function, and graft preservation following renal angioplasty or stenting are varied,[133] with most current studies describing a predominantly beneficial effect for all parameters.[128-130,133-136] However, two randomized trials failed to show improvements in either blood pressure or SCr out to 3 years,[137,138] possibly related to the inclusion of patients with severe renal dysfunction. This latter factor has been shown to be a predictor of poor results, with patients in the lowest tertile of renal function less likely to preserve their grafts than patients with lesser degrees of renal decline.[139] In a review of PTRS results encompassing 351 total patients from 14 series over the last decade, overall clinical benefit occurred in a median of 79% of patients (interquartile range 76%-86%).[132] In general, categorical outcomes for renal function and blood pressure benefit have not been described, although Peregrin et al. noted better blood pressure control in 65% of patients, with renal function improvements in 45% and stabilization in 21%; complete resolution of hypertension did not occur.[133] Following PTRS, graft preservation has been reported in 91% and 86% of patients at 1 and 5 years, respectively.[134] Restenosis can be as high as 28% following PTRA alone[132] but appears to occur in approximately 5% of patients after either primary or secondary stenting.[128,133]

CONCLUSIONS

Stenosis of native and transplant renal arteries is a well-recognized cause of hypertension and renal failure, with associated risks of cardiovascular events and renal replacement therapy. There is firm and evolving evidence that atherosclerotic RAS is independently associated with worse survival, but the value of percutaneous intervention in mitigating this risk is not established; ongoing studies will address the issue. However, in light of highly disparate results from published trials, and despite apparent flaws in the experimental design of recently failed randomized controlled trials, the role of RAST remains to be fully elucidated. Clearly, some patients will benefit and others will be harmed by this or any intervention. Studies aimed at determining the best utilization of PTRS and identifying markers for optimal patient selection are needed.

KEY POINTS

• Careful patient selection is critical to assuring optimal results from renal artery stenting; outcomes are best in patients with shorter duration and higher degrees of systolic hypertension, rapidly declining renal function, and recurring heart failure.

• There is emerging evidence that patients with advanced chronic kidney disease (GFR < 30 mL/min/1.73 m^2) have the potential to delay or avoid hemodialysis after renal artery stenting, and that the use of distal embolic protection devices as well as glycoprotein 2B3A inhibitors may contribute to preserved renal function.

• Careful technique and revascularization based on a measurement of a hyperemic or resting trans-stenotic gradient of greater than 20 mmHg using pressure wires are important for achieving satisfactory results.

• Transplant renal artery stenosis may be immunologically mediated. Most series report hypertension and renal function benefit in the majority of patients, and graft salvage in up to 85% of patients 5 years after treatment.

► SUGGESTED READINGS

Colyer WR, Eltahawy E, Cooper CJ. Renal artery stenosis: optimizing diagnosis and treatment. Prog Cardiovasc Dis 2011;54(1):29–35.

Holden A. Is there an indication for embolic protection in renal artery intervention? Tech Vasc Interv Radiol 2011;14(2):95–100.

Lao D, Parasher PS, Cho KC, Yeghiazarians Y. Atherosclerotic renal artery stenosis–diagnosis and treatment. Mayo Clin Proc 2011;86(7):649–57.

Ritchie J, Chrysochou C, Kalra PA. Contemporary management of atherosclerotic renovascular disease: before and after ASTRAL. Nephrology (Carlton) 2011;16(5):457–67.

Seddon M, Saw J. Atherosclerotic renal artery stenosis: review of pathophysiology, clinical trial evidence, and management strategies. Can J Cardiol 2011;27(4):468–80.

The complete reference list is available online at www.expertconsult.com.

CHAPTER **59**

Acute Renal Ischemia
Andrew Hugh Holden

Acute renal ischemia is defined as diminished renal excretory function as a result of acutely impaired renal perfusion.[1] The common etiologies causing acute renal ischemia are listed in Table 59-1. Patients present with acute renal insufficiency if they suffer acute bilateral renal hypoperfusion or acute hypoperfusion to a solitary functional kidney. Acute renal artery occlusion may also present with acute loin pain and hematuria, particularly if due to traumatic or embolic etiologies. The degree of renal parenchymal ischemia is influenced by the severity and chronicity of renal artery occlusion. These parameters may also influence management decisions. For example, patients with a background history of atherosclerotic renal artery stenoses and well-formed collaterals may benefit from recanalization of a chronic complete renal artery occlusion. Patients with acute renal artery occlusion without collateral formation are less likely to benefit from delayed revascularization. Endovascular revascularization techniques are not commonly used for most causes of acute renal ischemia but may provide major benefits for the patient in certain specific situations.

INDICATIONS

The indications for endovascular intervention in the setting of acute renal ischemia are listed in Table 59-1 and will be described separately.

Renal Artery Trauma

Renal artery trauma is a rare complication of blunt abdominal trauma (0.08% of blunt trauma hospital admissions), but is increasingly recognized with routine use of computed tomography (CT) in the trauma setting.[2] It is frequently associated with other injuries.[3] The most common arterial injury is traumatic dissection, which is often associated with partial or complete arterial occlusion. Complete arterial avulsion is less common. Hemodynamically stable patients with unilateral renal artery trauma may be managed conservatively, with a 6% risk of development of renovascular hypertension.[2] Surgical repair of main renal artery injuries should only be undertaken if there is bilateral injury or a solitary kidney[4] and should be performed urgently to preserve renal function. Open surgical revascularization techniques include thrombectomy, direct arterial repair, and bypass grafting using synthetic or vein grafts. The results of surgical revascularization have been poor, with preservation of renal function achieved in only a minority of patients.[5] Endovascular techniques, including thrombolysis[6,7] and stenting,[7,8,9] have been described but have been used sparingly. The proposed indications include patients with unilateral renal artery trauma or in whom open surgical repair is contraindicated. Frequently these patients are undergoing catheter-directed intervention to

manage traumatic injuries elsewhere.[10] The most common reported technique is stenting of an occluded or dissected (but patent) renal artery, either with a bare metallic or covered stent. In the setting of a totally occluded renal artery, it is unclear whether there is complete avulsion or traumatic dissection with intact arterial wall layers. In the event of free arterial bleeding after stenting, the interventionalist should be prepared to embolize the artery.[10]

Renal Artery Thromboembolism

Renal arterial thromboembolism is uncommon, with most emboli of left atrial origin in patients with atrial fibrillation.[11] Patients usually present with colicky loin pain.[11] Revascularization should occur urgently because acute complete renal ischemia can produce irreversible kidney damage in 60 to 90 minutes. However, treatment may be worthwhile after 90 minutes because embolic occlusion may be incomplete in some cases.[11] Endovascular techniques have only been described in sporadic case reports[12] and have included aspiration thrombectomy and thrombolysis.

Acute Ischemia in Renal Artery Atherosclerosis

The causes of acute renal ischemia in a setting of renal artery atherosclerosis are listed in Table 59-2. Hemodynamically significant renal artery stenoses frequently progress, with risk factors for progression including severe stenoses, high systolic blood pressure, and diabetes mellitus.[13,14] Progression to occlusion is associated with loss of renal mass and decreased renal function.[15] Rapid progression of an atherosclerotic stenosis usually occurs secondary to plaque dissection, resulting in a critical stenosis or total occlusion. In this situation, renal artery revascularization is indicated, particularly if the relevant renal artery supplies a solitary functional kidney (Fig. 59-1). It is useful to have any recent imaging available that demonstrates a patent renal artery and reasonable renal size.[16]

A more common cause of acute renal ischemia in patients with atherosclerotic renal artery stenosis is the institution of an angiotensin-converting enzyme inhibitor (ACEI) or angiotensin receptor blocker (ARB). It is normal for patients to experience a minor rise in serum creatinine (<20% above baseline) once an ACEI/ARB is introduced. However, patients with significant underlying renal hypoperfusion may suffer a more severe acute decline in renal function.[17] These patients are ideal candidates for revascularization (Fig. 59-2).[18]

Aortic Dissection with Renal Hypoperfusion

Early experience of endografting for acute type B aortic dissection has proved promising for reducing false lumen

411

TABLE 59-1. Etiology of Acute Renal Ischemia

- Trauma with renal artery dissection/avulsion
- Renal artery thromboembolism
- Acute ischemia in renal artery atherosclerosis
- Aortic dissection with renal hypoperfusion
- Renal artery occlusion after endovascular intervention

TABLE 59-2. Etiology of Acute Renal Ischemia in Renal Artery Atherosclerosis

- Acute occlusion of a renal artery stenosis in a solitary functional kidney
- Unilateral acute arterial occlusion in a patient with bilateral renal artery stenosis
- Plaque ulceration/dissection causing an acute critical renal artery stenosis
- Patients with critical renal artery stenosis begun on angiotensin-converting enzyme inhibitor therapy

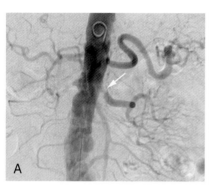 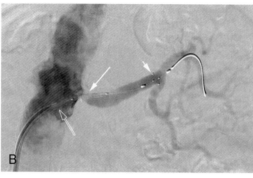 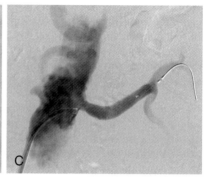

FIGURE 59-1. Acute ischemia in renal artery atherosclerosis. This 68-year-old man with known long-standing right renal artery occlusion presented with acute renal failure due to rapid progression of a left renal artery atherosclerotic lesion, presumably from plaque ulceration. **A,** Abdominal aortography confirms a right renal occlusion and a high-grade left renal artery stenosis *(arrow).* **B,** Primary stenting of left renal artery stenosis. Note balloon-expandable stent *(long arrow)* with guide catheter for angiographic control *(open arrow).* Embolic filter *(short arrow)* is positioned in distal main renal artery. **C,** Appearance after stent deployment.

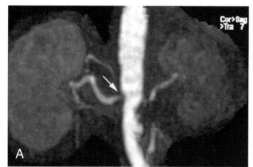 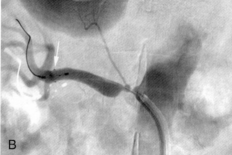 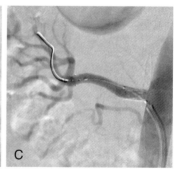

FIGURE 59-2. Acute renal ischemia in a patient recently commenced on an angiotensin-converting enzyme inhibitor (ACEI). **A,** Contrast-enhanced magnetic resonance angiography shows critical ostial stenosis of right main renal artery *(arrow).* Note atrophic left kidney. **B,** Right renal angiography via a guide catheter. Note distal embolic filter *(arrow).* **C,** Angiography after stenting. ACEI was restarted in this patient, without a decline in renal function.

perfusion and pressurization, particularly in the thoracic aorta.[19] The primary treatment goal of endoluminal repair is to exclude the primary inflow intimal tear. Type B aortic dissection frequently involves the renal arteries, but significant acute renal ischemia is less common. This may be due to dynamic obstruction due to compression of the aortic true lumen (Fig. 59-3) or static renal artery obstruction where the dissection extends into the renal arteries themselves. These patients present with ongoing hypertension and acute renal impairment. Renal ischemia usually responds to endograft closure of the proximal main entry tear, although other procedures such as renal artery stenting may also be required to restore renal perfusion.

Renal Artery Occlusion After Endovascular Intervention

Stenting of atherosclerotic stenoses of the renal artery ostium is associated with improved procedural success, patency, and reduced restenosis rates[20,21] when compared with angioplasty alone. For this reason, primary stenting of ostial atherosclerotic renal artery stenosis is considered the treatment of choice, with angioplasty reserved for non-ostial atherosclerotic stenoses and stenotic disease due to other pathologies such as fibromuscular dysplasia.[22] If angioplasty is performed, complications such as arterial dissection or elastic recoil with residual stenosis are

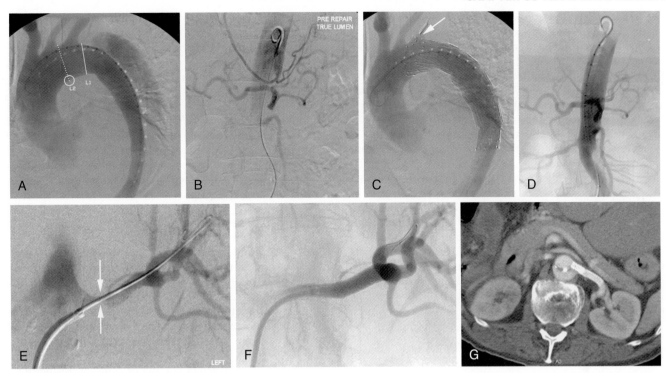

FIGURE 59-3. Stanford type B acute aortic dissection with acute renal ischemia. **A,** Arch aortogram demonstrates a type B dissection arising distal to left subclavian artery. **B,** Abdominal aortogram with catheter in true lumen. Note that visceral arteries are poorly perfused, and there is no renal artery perfusion. **C,** Stent-graft repair of inflow fenestration, with exclusion of false lumen in thoracic aorta. Left subclavian artery ostium has been covered (arrow). **D,** Abdominal aortogram after thoracic aortic repair. Note improved visceral artery perfusion. Right kidney is now perfused. **E,** A guidewire is manipulated from aortic true lumen into left renal artery. Note that proximal left renal artery is compressed by false lumen (arrows). **F,** A combination of covered and uncovered stents is used to recanalize left renal artery. **G,** Computed tomography after left renal artery revascularization.

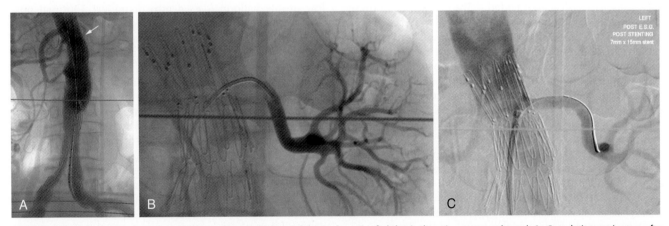

FIGURE 59-4. Inadvertent coverage of left renal artery during endoluminal repair of abdominal aortic aneurysm (arrow). **A,** Completion angiogram after endoluminal aneurysm repair. Note that ostium of left renal artery has been covered (arrow). **B,** A catheter is manipulated above graft material into left renal artery. **C,** After stenting of left main renal artery, perfusion to left kidney has been reestablished.

important indications for secondary stenting.[23] Complications after renal artery stenting may also result in acute renal ischemia. These include arterial rupture, stent fracture,[24] dislocation of mural thrombus,[25] and incomplete stent deployment with residual stenosis and thrombosis.[26] All of these conditions require secondary intervention.

A rare complication of endovascular abdominal aortic aneurysm repair is proximal malposition of the endograft, resulting in inadvertent coverage of the main renal artery ostium and acute renal ischemia. This can often be managed by endovascular techniques (Fig. 59-4).[27]

CONTRAINDICATIONS

The major contraindication to attempted revascularization in the acute renal ischemia setting is when significant irreversible ischemic parenchymal damage has already occurred. In this situation, the patient is unlikely to benefit in terms of renal preservation or blood pressure control.

This may be difficult to assess noninvasively. Renal size is frequently used as a predictor, with a renal length above 9 cm considered worth attempting revascularization in the open surgical literature.[28] Given the reduced morbidity associated with endovascular techniques, it is reasonable to reduce the size threshold to 7 to 8 cm. It is important to review serum creatinine levels because a recent decline in renal function is an excellent predictor of improved outcome with revascularization.[29,30] In semi-elective and elective situations, Doppler ultrasound, CT, or magnetic resonance imaging (MRI) assessment of intrarenal perfusion may be useful to identify patients whose renal function may potentially improve after revascularization.[16] In the acute causes of complete arterial occlusion (e.g., traumatic renal injury, thromboembolism), patients are unlikely to benefit from revascularization occurring more than 24 hours after the occlusion. Traumatic occlusion involving bilateral renal arteries or an artery to a single functional kidney is best managed surgically.

EQUIPMENT

Appropriately shaped guide catheters or guide sheaths (e.g., renal double curve, multipurpose) are recommended. These provide stability at the renal artery ostium for intervention and also facilitate selective contrast injections during the intervention for optimum placement of angioplasty balloons and stents. In most renal artery interventions, the use of low-profile angioplasty balloons and high radial force balloon-expandable stents delivered on 0.014- or 0.018-inch guidewires is recommended.[31] The low profile of these systems improves technical success, and the rapid exchange monorail systems decrease procedure time. There is some evidence that embolic protection devices improve outcome in chronic atherosclerotic renal artery stenosis,[32,33] but there is no reported experience with these devices in acute renal ischemia. In the situation of inadvertent coverage of renal artery ostia during endovascular aneurysm repair, more robust 0.035-inch guidewire–compatible angioplasty balloons and stents are recommended.

Optimal periprocedural care is important during renal artery revascularization procedures. Adequate pre- and postintervention intravenous hydration are essential.[34] There are conflicting reports regarding the nephroprotective value of N-acetylcysteine.[35,36] Intraarterial gadolinium chelates appear to be less nephrotoxic[37] in the doses used[38] than iodinated contrast agents, but the lower radiopacity[37] of gadolinium means that this is of limited value in the setting of acute renal artery revascularization. Carbon dioxide can also be used,[39] but the careful use of iodinated contrast medium is recommended for most interventions.

TECHNIQUE

Anatomy and Approaches

Noninvasive imaging of renal artery anatomy with contrast-enhanced magnetic resonance or computed tomographic angiography (MRA/CTA) is recommended before any endovascular renal artery procedure if possible. This enables selection of the optimal approach and equipment such as selective catheters, guide catheter, or guide sheath. An ipsilateral femoral approach allows best access in most cases because the secondary curve of the guide catheter can stabilize against the contralateral wall of the abdominal aorta. Most renal arteries arise with either a perpendicular or slightly downsloping orientation to the long axis of the aorta. Renal double curve or multipurpose shapes are well equipped to deal with this orientation. Occasionally a renal artery with a very steep inferior orientation will require a downward-seeking catheter such as a Simmons shape or even a brachial artery approach.

Technical Aspects

Flush abdominal aortography using a small volume of contrast agent is initially recommended to assist in accurate localization of the renal artery ostium relative to bony landmarks.

An appropriately shaped guide catheter is then positioned at the relevant renal artery ostium, and intraarterial heparin and glyceryl trinitrate are administered via this catheter.

In cases of renal artery trauma or acute occlusion of an atherosclerotic stenosis, a 0.014- or 0.018-inch guidewire is manipulated through the lesion, with the tip of the guidewire placed in a lobar or segmental branch. Care should be taken to keep the guidewire from advancing into a more peripheral location and causing renal artery perforation.

In most cases, a low-profile, rapid-exchange, balloon-expandable stent can be delivered over this guidewire. Occasionally, preliminary angioplasty is required with a low-profile balloon (e.g., 4-mm diameter). Optimal positioning of the stent to treat the renal artery lesion can be achieved by using anteroposterior and oblique projections, with contrast agent injected via the guide catheter. The stent can then be deployed.

In the renal artery trauma setting with partial or complete renal artery thrombosis, catheter-directed thrombolysis can be performed.[6,7] If traumatic arterial dissection is demonstrated, this may be treated by primary stenting,[7-9] possibly with the use of a covered stent. In the trauma setting, the patient should be closely monitored during thrombolysis or after stenting to avoid decompensation due to retroperitoneal bleeding from an injured renal artery. Renal artery embolization may be required.

In the setting of acute renal artery embolism, catheter-directed thrombolysis has been performed.[11] Transcatheter aspiration thrombectomy has also been described.[11] This is a more appealing technique for emboli of left atrial origin because these emboli are frequently incompletely lysed with thrombolytic therapy.

In patients with acute deterioration in renal function due to ulceration of atherosclerotic plaque, an embolic protection device should be considered because of the embolic potential of the lesion. Patients who experience an acute deterioration in renal function after commencing therapy with an ACEI or ARB may also benefit from embolic protection (see Fig. 59-2). A distal filter or occlusion balloon may be used. A "primary passage" technique is usually possible via the guide catheter, but a low-profile "buddy wire" is occasionally required.

In the type B aortic dissection complicated by acute renal ischemia, the first recommended endovascular approach is reperfusion of the abdominal aortic true lumen by stent-grafting the inflow intimal tear in the thoracic aorta (see Fig. 59-4). This will often dramatically improve renal perfusion. On occasion, there is persistent renal ischemia. This may be due to extrinsic compression of the renal artery by the aortic false lumen or extension of the dissection flap into the renal artery. Revascularization can be achieved by reconnecting the aortic true lumen to the renal true lumen with stents. Covered stents may be required to exclude the aortic false lumen component. An alternative approach to stent-graft repair of type B dissection is to improve true luminal perfusion (and branches perfused by the true lumen) using intraarterial fenestration techniques.

Careful completion angiography after renal artery angioplasty is important to identify suboptimal results including significant residual stenosis or postangioplasty arterial dissection. Rapid frame rate angiography and measurement of translesional arterial pressure gradients (using a 4F catheter or a pressure wire) are important techniques to detect these complications. Secondary stenting can usually adequate treat postangioplasty residual stenosis and dissection.[40]

Complications after renal artery stenting include arterial rupture, stent fracture, dislocation of mural thrombus,[41] and incomplete stent deployment with residual stenosis and thrombosis. Arterial rupture and stent fracture may be managed with covered stenting,[42] but incomplete stent deployment with renal artery occlusion usually requires surgical bypass. Dislocated mural thrombus has been treated with aspiration thrombectomy and thrombolysis.[41]

The first maneuver with a malpositioned endograft partially or completely covering a main renal artery ostium is to attempt to pull the proximal attachment site of the graft below the renal artery ostia. This can be achieved using a number of techniques, including a balloon inflated into the body of the graft or pulling a guidewire that has been passed across the graft bifurcation and snared via the contralateral groin. If the renal artery ostium has been incompletely covered, the kidney can usually be revascularized by manipulation of a guidewire into the renal artery and primary stenting the renal artery ostium open, which displaces the graft material below the renal artery ostium (see Fig. 59-3).

CONTROVERSIES

Endovascular techniques are not well established for most causes of acute renal ischemia and are therefore controversial. Open surgery remains the standard of care in the settings of renal artery trauma and thromboembolism. Endoluminal repair for all forms of type B aortic dissection has not been validated, although early evidence suggests that this technique has therapeutic benefit in complicated aortic dissection. The selected use of renal embolic protection devices appears beneficial, but experience is limited to single-center reports.

OUTCOMES

The results of endovascular revascularization in long-standing atherosclerotic renal artery stenosis have been mixed. Meta-analyses of available randomized controlled trial data (see Suggested Readings) have failed to show benefit of renal artery angioplasty in improving or preserving renal function. However, the subgroups of patients with a recent decline in renal function or a deterioration after commencing therapy with an ACEI/ARB form a better prognostic group. Endovascular recanalization of occluded renal arteries secondary to atherosclerotic stenoses has been described in case reports,[43] including the use of embolic protection.[44] In such cases, collateral circulation is crucial to preserve renal parenchyma despite inflow occlusion. In one study of 21 attempted recanalizations, 13 were successful,[45] although two arteries reoccluded in the first 6 months. All 11 patients with patent arteries showed a significant improvement in renal function, and hemodialysis was discontinued in 3 patients. One predictive factor of success was a delay between occlusion and revascularization of less than 90 days. This improvement in renal function has not been confirmed by others.[46]

The data on endovascular treatment in trauma and thromboembolism are limited, but preliminary results appear promising. Similarly, there are little published data on the efficacy of techniques for renal artery revascularization in type B aortic dissection, although early results are promising. Most complications encountered after endovascular intervention can be successfully managed with further endovascular techniques.

COMPLICATIONS

Complications encountered during renal artery revascularization include postangioplasty dissection, arterial rupture, residual stenosis, and distal atheroembolization. Access artery complications include hematoma, false aneurysm, and arteriovenous fistula.

POSTPROCEDURAL AND FOLLOW-UP CARE

Early postprocedural aftercare after renal artery intervention should include ongoing intravenous hydration, preferably for 12 to 24 hours. Long-term antiplatelet therapy is advised, but anticoagulation in patients successfully revascularized is not normally necessary. Renal artery patency after endovascular intervention is usually monitored by Doppler ultrasonography, with a baseline study usually performed approximately 1 month after intervention.

KEY POINTS

- Endovascular techniques in the setting of acute renal ischemia are uncommon.
- Endovascular revascularization may provide major benefits in selected cases.
- Acute renal ischemia in the setting of atherosclerosis is usually on the basis of plaque ulceration or patients treated with an angiotensin-converting enzyme inhibitor or angiotensin receptor blocker (ACEI/ARB). These patients may benefit from revascularization.
- Acute renal ischemia as a complication of endovascular intervention can usually be managed with further endovascular techniques.

▸ SUGGESTED READINGS

The ASTRAL Investigators. Revascularization versus medical therapy for renal artery stenosis. N Engl J Med 2009;361:1953–62.

Cwikiel W, Midia M, Williams D. Non-traumatic vascular emergencies: imaging and intervention in acute arterial conditions. Eur Radiol 2002;12:2619–26.

Davies MG, Saad WE, Peden EK, et al. Implications of acute functional injury following percutaneous renal artery intervention. Ann Vasc Surg 2008;22(6):783–9.

Leertouwer TC, Gussenhoven EJ, Bosch JL, et al. Stent placement for renal artery stenosis: where do we stand? A meta-analysis. Radiology 2000;216:78–85.

Nordmann AJ, Woo K, Parkes R, Logan AG. Balloon angioplasty or medical therapy for hypertensive patients with atherosclerotic renal artery stenosis? A meta-analysis of randomised controlled trials. Am J Med 2003;114:44–50.

The complete reference list is available online at www.expertconsult.com.

CHAPTER 60

Renal Artery Embolization

Dierk Vorwerk

CLINICAL RELEVANCE

Embolotherapy of the renal arteries was introduced into the portfolio of the interventional radiologist many years ago. It was most popular around 25 years ago when preoperative embolization of kidneys containing a renal cell carcinoma (hypernephroma) was widely used as a routine procedure in the belief that preoperative embolization might avoid tumor seeding during surgery. Since no oncological benefit has since been proven by this strategy, and blood loss is no longer a major problem in renal surgery, preoperative embolization is now limited to a few uncommon circumstances. Nevertheless, many different techniques were developed, resulting in the current array of indications for renal embolotherapy.

INDICATIONS

Tumor Embolization

Total renal embolization is indicated for inoperable hypernephromas in patients with persistent hematuria or severe paraneoplastic symptoms such as hypercalcemia (Stauffer syndrome). In these patients, complete embolization of the tumor-bearing kidney is indicated if a functioning contralateral kidney is still present. Some groups prefer tumor embolization even without symptoms to reduce tumor bulk in combination with immunostimulating therapies. In total embolization not followed by nephrectomy, embolization should be performed by particles of small diameters or bucrylate–ethiodized oil mixed in a ratio of 1:3 to 1:5 to allow deep deposition into the tumor tissue.

Preoperative embolization is still indicated in a small subset of tumors, especially those that have developed extensive venous involvement. Preoperative embolization may be indicated as a safety procedure in patients who refuse blood transfusions, such as Jehovah's witnesses. In preoperative embolization, the technique is modified because only occlusion of the main renal artery is necessary. This can be achieved by coils, Amplatzer plugs, or bucrylate–ethiodized oil mixed in a ratio of 1:1 to 1:3 to achieve rapid occlusion of the main renal artery.

Partial tumor ablation by embolization (Fig. 60-1) is preferred in patients who have a tumor in a single functioning kidney. Partial embolization has also been used as a preparation for thermal ablation of a circumscribed peripheral malignant tumor to reduce the risk of postprocedural bleeding after radiofrequency ablation or to enhance its efficacy.[1]

There is more published experience of renal artery embolization for ruptured or bleeding benign renal tumors such as angiomas and particularly angiomyolipomas.[2] The latter have a tendency to grow during pregnancy, and prophylactic embolization may be performed in women who wish to become pregnant to prevent major bleeding during pregnancy. In benign lesions, a partial embolization is preferable whenever possible.

As an alternative to partial embolization, advanced surgical techniques such as partial nephrectomy—either open or laparoscopic—and radiofrequency ablation have been described.

Defunctionalization

Total renal embolization, including bilateral embolization in some cases, may be indicated in patients with massive protein loss in nephrotic syndrome or other complications of end-stage renal failure such as intractable hypertension. Other indications for total renal embolization are failing kidney transplants, as an alternative to surgical removal in cases of graft intolerance syndrome, and persistent urinary leaks in failing kidneys.[3]

Very rarely, partial defunctionalization has been described in cases with segmental arterial stenosis and hypertension where the responsible segmental artery was embolized.[4] Alternatively, these patients may undergo intrarenal percutaneous transluminal angioplasty (PTA) using small balloons.

Bleeding Control

Blunt or direct trauma may cause renal bleeding due to renal laceration or renal artery rupture. Trauma may also cause renal artery pseudoaneurysms, arteriovenous (AV) fistulas combined with hematuria, direct hemorrhage into the pelvicalyceal system, or development of perirenal hematomas.

Unfortunately, the main causes of traumatic renal hemorrhage are iatrogenic in origin and represent the majority of cases of traumatic renal hemorrhage in Europe. They include renal biopsies in native and transplant organs, percutaneous techniques such as percutaneous nephrostomy (Fig. 60-2), nephrolithectomy, and percutaneous transluminal renal angioplasty (PTRA), where direct arterial perforation by the guidewire tip has been described.[5] Also, indirect methods such as shockwave lithotripsy can lead to renal trauma requiring embolotherapy.

Although iatrogenic hemorrhage is relatively common, few cases require treatment (0.3%-1% of percutaneous renal interventions[6] and 0.5% of percutaneous biopsies[7]). Moreover, although hemorrhage that requires treatment is unusual, temporary and self-limiting bleeding or AV fistulas occur in up to one third of percutaneous renal procedures.[7] Since the introduction of partial nephrectomy techniques, bleeding after partial surgery has become a significant cause of iatrogenic hemorrhage. Approximately 2% of patients

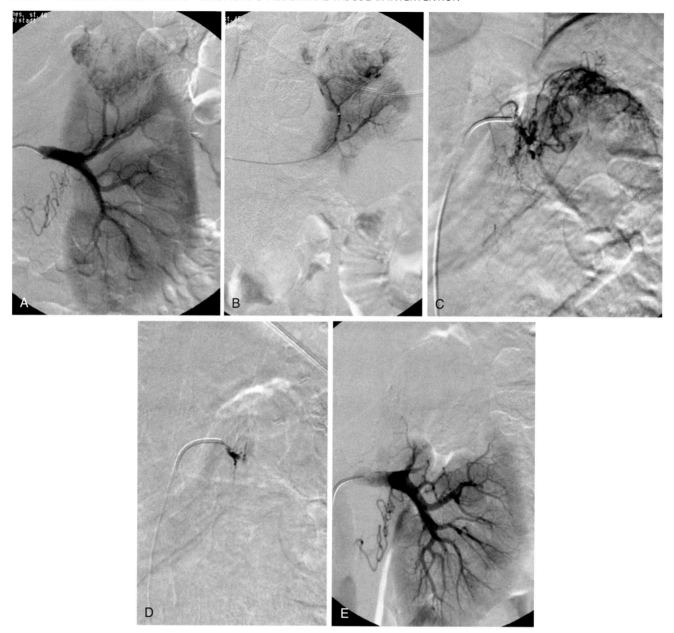

FIGURE 60-1. Selective tumor embolization in patient with single kidney. **A,** Angiography shows pathologic arteries at upper pole, indicating a hypernephroma. **B,** Superselective angiography of tumor-feeding branch before particle embolization. **C,** Selective angiography of suprarenal artery shows additional tumor vascularization. **D,** After particle embolization, this branch is completely excluded. **E,** After embolization, upper pole is devascularized, but lower pole parenchyma is preserved.

who undergo partial nephrectomy develop postsurgical bleeding, and most of them require percutaneous embolization.[8]

Direct stab wounds, bullet wounds, and motor vehicle accidents are other traumatic causes of renal injury. Embolotherapy is the treatment of choice in patients who are (1) not controlled by conservative management and (2) do not have complete central laceration of the renal arteries, which requires surgery.

Rarely, benign tumors such as angiodysplasias, angiomas, or angiomyolipoma (Fig. 60-3) may cause spontaneous—sometimes substantial—bleeding (Wunderlich syndrome)[9] and may undergo embolization. In a few cases, they may also develop hypertension.

Renal Artery Aneurysms

As a special problem, true and false aneurysms of the mainstem renal artery[10] may occur that may be prone to rupture or serve as an embolic source for renal infarction. There is a general consensus that a diameter of 20 mm is a threshold for treatment; smaller aneurysms may undergo treatment if severe hypertension is present and difficult to treat. Central renal artery aneurysms require treatment by coil placement or, if possible, exclusion by the use of stent grafts. Peripheral (pseudo)aneurysms may be due to trauma or systemic diseases such as polyarteritis nodosa. Peripheral aneurysms are best treated by exclusion, coil placement, or medical adhesive (cyanoacrylate, "glue") deposition. The most

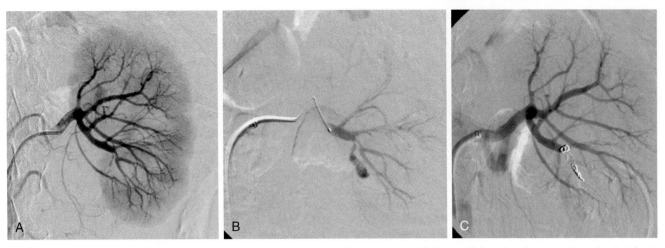

FIGURE 60-2. Traumatic bleeding after nephrostomy. **A,** Left renal angiogram shows narrowing of a lower pole branch and some extravasation. **B,** Selective angiography clearly demonstrates extravasation. **C,** After coil embolization combined with glue, sealing of bleeding site has been achieved.

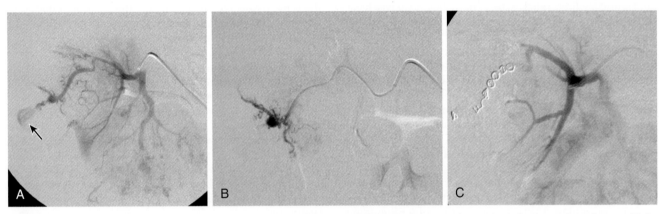

FIGURE 60-3. Acute bleeding from a tumor (angiomyolipoma). **A,** Right renal angiography shows irregular arteries, indicating angiomyolipoma with free bleeding at upper lateral portion *(arrow).* **B,** Bleeding branch is selectively catheterized by a microcatheter. **C,** After placing several coils, branch is interrupted and bleeding stopped.

difficult location for treatment of renal artery aneurysms is at the site of a renal artery bifurcation (or trifurcation), because exclusion of the aneurysm may require occlusion of one or more segmental arteries. A combination of bare metallic stents with coils, glue, Onyx (ethylene vinyl alcoholic copolymer [ev3/Covidien, Plymouth, Minn.]), or flow-diverting stents may be an option in these challenging locations.[10-14]

CONTRAINDICATIONS

There are few absolute contraindications to total or selective renal artery embolization. Embolization should be avoided in the presence of acute infection to avoid superimposed infection of the devascularized territories.

Relative contraindications are impaired global renal function, allergic reactions to contrast media, acute hyperthyroidism, planned radioiodine therapy, and single kidneys. In the latter, embolization may be performed if no other nephron-sparing surgical alternative exists.

EQUIPMENT

A modern angiographic unit (preferably with the possibility of pulsed fluoroscopy) and experience with coaxial catheters, microcatheters, and a variety of different embolization agents (e.g., glue, particles, coils) are required.

TECHNIQUE

Anatomy and Approaches

Depending on the underlying disease, a complete or partial embolization is performed. Classical indications for complete renal embolization are embolotherapy before tumor nephrectomy, total renal ablation in tumors where there is a contraindication to surgery, or defunctionalization for benign causes either in native kidneys or transplants.

Partial embolization is performed to preserve renal function when it is possible to treat a localized lesion, and can be used in traumatic or iatrogenic lesions as well as in single kidneys with renal artery tumors. Whereas in total renal artery embolization, complete destruction of functioning renal tissue is the aim of treatment, when partial renal embolization is performed, the aim is to minimize loss of normal renal parenchyma.

Technical Aspects

Many materials have utility for renal arterial embolization. For total renal embolization, absolute ethanol is a common embolic agent used. Other liquid embolics such as glue (bucrylate [Histoacryl; Braun, Melsungen, Germany]) may be used after mixing with ethiodized oil (Ethiodol, Lipiodol [Guerbet USA, Bloomington, Ind.]). Total embolization with embolic microspheres (e.g., polyvinyl alcohol [PVA] particles), using a small particle size between 20 and 500 µm, has also been described.

In partial embolization, the choice of embolic agent depends on the purpose of treatment. In selective tumor embolization, the tumor bed is preferentially embolized using small particles after superselective catheterization of the tumor-feeding renal artery branches. Alternatively, embolization with glue mixed with ethiodized oil may be performed. If the main feeding branch can be identified, it can be additionally occluded by coil placement or a bucrylate–ethiodized oil mixture. If the patient is being treated for a vascular complication such as AV fistula, pseudoaneurysm, or blunt traumatic hemorrhage, a very localized embolization is desired, either by coil embolization or local application of glue (bucrylate–ethiodized oil).

Technique of Renal Artery Embolization

To increase safety and avoid complications, a coaxial technique is generally required for renal artery embolization. This may be achieved with a combination of a 6F guiding catheter in a suitable configuration (e.g., renal double curve or multipurpose configuration) in combination with a smaller coaxial inner catheter (e.g., 4F selective 0.035- or 0.038-inch catheter). This relatively inexpensive combination allows the application of macrocoils, particles, and glue and is suitable for embolization of larger parts of the kidney, including total renal embolization.

For embolization of smaller target arteries, the coaxial approach may be modified by using smaller catheter combinations. For example, a 4F guiding catheter (0.035- or 0.038-inch) may be used in combination with a coaxial microcatheter that is advanced as close as possible to the point of embolization. This latter combination enables embolization with microcoils (0.014- to 0.18-inch diameter), glue, and particles, whereas the size of particles that are deliverable depends on the inner diameter of the microcatheter used and also the outer shape of the individual particle. This more advanced approach is preferred in challenging situations.

Total Renal Embolization

Total renal embolization may be performed using absolute ethanol 95%. Ethanol embolization may be performed by either of two techniques. The single-dose technique requires temporary blockade of the main renal artery by an occlusion balloon. Then 10 to 15 mL of ethanol is injected into the renal artery beyond the occluding balloon. After 10

minutes, contrast medium is injected carefully to assess for the presence of distal renal arterial thrombosis after deflating the occlusion balloon. If complete distal thrombosis has not yet occurred, a repeat injection of ethanol using the same technique may be performed. The other technique does not involve use of an occlusion balloon; smaller volumes of 4 to 10 mL are injected slowly over a few minutes, followed by injection of contrast medium. For both techniques, no more than 20 mL of ethanol on average, or an absolute maximum of 50 mL, should be used; individual dosage is approximately 0.5 mL/kg body weight. The endpoint of both techniques is total cessation of flow in the main and peripheral renal arteries.

If glue is used to perform total renal embolization, it is also desirable to use a balloon occlusion catheter to avoid dislodgement of embolic material into nonrenal arteries. Alternatively, embolization using small particles (20-300 µm) followed by glue injection into the segmental arteries and the main renal artery may be performed.

Use of coils alone or large particles does not usually lead to complete devascularization and defunctionalization of the renal tissue, which is generally the treatment endpoint. Coil embolization alone might be an alternative if preoperative embolization is performed.

Pain Management in Total Renal Embolization
Complete renal embolization is usually followed by development of postembolization syndrome, with abdominal pain, nausea, and fever. Sometimes symptoms can become very profound, and prophylaxis is mandatory. Besides general treatment with intravenous fluids, antipyretics, and antiemetics, pain can be controlled either by an epidural catheter for 24 to 48 hours or by on-demand patient assisted analgesia delivered by an automated pump system. Selective embolization does not usually cause general symptoms.

Selective Renal Embolization
Again, selection of the appropriate embolic agent generally depends on the underlying disease. Standard coils, microcoils, glue, or Onyx may be used for selective renal embolization. Glue (bucrylate–ethiodized oil) is a relatively inexpensive agent and is used for many applications. The speed of precipitation is influenced by the amount of ethiodized oil that is mixed with bucrylate and may vary between 1:1 and 1:5.

There are two application techniques for bucrylate–ethiodized oil. One is the "sandwich" technique, where after having flushed the catheter with 40% glucose solution, a portion of 0.05 to 0.1 mL of bucrylate–ethiodized oil is injected through the catheter, followed by careful flushing with the 40% glucose solution. The other technique is an en bloc technique; the catheter is flushed with 40% glucose, then the bucrylate–ethiodized oil solution is continuously injected through the microcatheter until the desired amount has been delivered. The microcatheter is then quickly withdrawn to avoid its tip being stuck at the delivery site, and it is removed through the guiding catheter. The microcatheter must be discarded because its lumen becomes occluded by glue. The en bloc technique may be used if only a single application is necessary, whereas the sandwich technique is helpful when the catheter has to be used for multiple applications in the same area, or passage of a catheter to the desired location is difficult and cumbersome.

In some cases of renal hemorrhage, the bleeding site is not detectable despite adequate selective angiography. In this situation, the vascular sheath should remain in situ, and repeat angiography should be performed 6 to 12 hours later if the patient continues to show evidence of renal hemorrhage. Alternatively, when there is arterial trauma after insertion of a nephrostomy catheter, the catheter can be withdrawn over a guidewire that remains in the renal collecting system. Then the bleeding source is more likely to be detected because the nephrostomy catheter no longer tamponades the puncture tract.

Renal Artery Aneurysms

In aneurysms of small segmental arteries, coil embolization or glue application is the embolization technique of choice. In aneurysms of the main renal artery, a stent graft, either balloon-expandable or self-expanding (e.g., Graftmaster [Jomed], Fluency [Bard], etc.) is recommended[15] to exclude the aneurysm if this is technically possible. Alternatively, coil embolization, preferably by detachable coils, may be performed after placement of a supporting bare metallic stent across the aneurysm neck.

A relatively new technique is available using flow-dividing stents, which have a knitted body with small interspaces that keep branch arteries open while the flow inside the aneurysm is drastically reduced, resulting in aneurysm thrombosis. Only a few cases have been reported to date.[14]

Arteriovenous Fistulas

AV fistulas may be of cryptogenic origin[16] or more commonly are due to trauma (often iatrogenic) or malignant renal tumors. Long-standing AV fistulas may become very large and then become technically very challenging to treat. Small fistulas may be occluded by coils of suitable size, but larger fistulas generally have high flow and therefore coils may be dislodged into the venous circulation. Under these circumstances, detachable coils are preferable because of the ability to retrieve the coil if it is not possible to achieve a stable coil position within the fistula. Large-diameter fistulas may also be occluded by detachable balloons or Amplatzer plugs. For safety reasons, the venous outflow tract may be blocked during embolization by a balloon-occlusion catheter. However, the interventional radiologist should always be prepared to perform retrieval of any coils or other embolic devices from the pulmonary circulation if distal device migration occurs.

CONTROVERSIES

There are no major controversies regarding the efficacy of selective embolization for traumatic hemorrhage of bleeding from other causes. Total renal embolization usually is a palliative treatment. There has been some debate regarding the usefulness of preoperative total renal artery embolization before total nephrectomy to reduce blood loss. With the evolution of renal surgery, most groups have given up this option as a routine procedure but reserve it for specific circumstances (e.g., if blood transfusion is not possible in the case of Jehovah's witnesses).

OUTCOMES

Total Embolization

Palliative tumor embolization is usually very successful at controlling hemorrhage if an appropriate embolic agent has been used. However, recurrent bleeding due to ongoing tumor growth is possible. Some authors have reported an increased survival time in patients undergoing renal embolization in inoperable tumors,[17] but the data are not consistent[18] or randomized. Preoperative tumor embolization is nowadays restricted to specific cases (see previous section), since there are no proven major benefits.

Defunctionalization is also technically successful in most instances. Peregrin et al. reported success in six of eight patients with intractable hypertension and end-stage renal disease.[19] Golwyn et al.[20] reported 11 patients with uncontrolled hypertension and/or nephrotic syndrome and end-stage renal disease who underwent complete defunctionalization by absolute ethanol. Hypertension was controlled in nine of ten patients, and nephrotic syndrome was controlled in four of four patients.[20] Mitra et al.[21] reported 15 patients with end-stage renal disease and flank pain due to consistent hydronephrosis, of whom 14 were pain free after treatment.

Ubara et al.[22] treated 64 patients with enlarged polycystic kidneys by bilateral renal embolization. In all patients, renal size decreased considerably ($\approx 50\%$) after 1 year, and the nutritional status of their patients improved significantly.

Perez Martinez et al.[23] performed successful defunctionalization of nonfunctioning renal allografts in seven patients, using microparticles of 300 to 500 µm. Delgado et al.[24] performed total graft embolization in 48 patients with graft intolerance syndrome. Treatment was successful in 31 of 48 cases. Eleven out of 48 patients underwent transplantectomy secondary to persistent intolerance or graft infection. They recommended graft embolization as a first-line treatment in cases of graft intolerance syndrome, although 25% will need to undergo secondary transplantectomy.[24] Similar results were achieved by Atar et al.[25] in 25 patients (26 grafts) with graft intolerance; technical and clinical success was achieved in 24 of 26 events, and nephrectomy was performed in one patient.

Partial Renal Embolization

Many series exist on the treatment of iatrogenic and traumatic injuries by embolization. Maleux et al.[26] reported 13 cases with renal injury due to renal biopsies who underwent successful embolization with subsequent control of hemorrhage. Angiographically, seven AV fistulas, six pseudoaneurysms, and two cases of perinephric contrast extravasation were found. However, renal function at least temporarily deteriorated in all patients, with progressive renal function loss in three.

Sam et al. followed 50 patients with iatrogenic injuries and embolization over a period of 12 years.[27] Technical success was achieved in 98%. Clinical success was also 98%, with a primary clinical success rate of 83% within the first 24 hours after treatment. They could not find significant changes in renal function or blood pressure in patients available for follow-up. Perini et al.[28] reported the results of embolization in 21 patients with renal allografts, with technical success in 95%. In our own series with a mixed group of mainly iatrogenic indications, treatment was immediately successful in 21 of 22 cases, and permanent success was achieved in 18 of 21 patients (86%).[29]

In patients with partial nephrectomy, renal artery embolization is safe.[8] Hyams et al. found 20/998 patients with bleeding after partial nephrectomy, 4 of them requiring conservative treatment and 16 undergoing selective embolization, with successful cessation of hemorrhage in all patients.[8] Sofocleous et al.[30] reported 22 patients with bleeding due to trauma by motor vehicle accident (n = 10), auto/pedestrian accident (n = 1), gunshot (n = 4), stab wounds (n = 6), and a fall in 1 patient. Angiographic findings yielded extravasation,[11] arterial rupture,[5] AV fistulas,[3] pseudoaneurysms,[3] or bleeding into the calyceal system.[2] Embolization was successful in all patients, with no major complications.

Chatziioannou et al.[31] analyzed the renal function in six consecutive patients with renal trauma and embolization who presented with elevated creatinine levels and found that the serum creatinine returned to normal levels within 1 week after embolization. Hagiwara et al.[32] analyzed 22 patients who presented with grade 3 renal trauma or higher on computed tomography (CT) imaging and underwent subsequent renal angiography. Only one patient had laceration of the main renal artery and underwent nephrectomy, eight required embolization, and all other patients were treated conservatively. They concluded that in the vast majority of severe renal trauma, nephrectomy is avoidable.

Results of renal embolization for bleeding angiomyolipomas are encouraging. Stoica et al. analyzed 11 patients who underwent emergency embolization for bleeding tumors, with clinical and technical success in all patients.[33]

There are now a few larger series available reporting on clinical outcomes after embolization of renal angiolipomas as a therapeutic approach. Kothary et al.[34] analyzed 19 patients with 30 angiolipomas. Technical success was achieved in all patients. Recurrence occurred in 43% of patients with tuberous sclerosis, but not in patients with sporadic angiolipomas. Recurrence occurred after 79 months on average.

COMPLICATIONS

Selective Embolization

Very rarely, complications may occur in selective embolization and are mainly due to nontarget embolization of the embolization material. There are very few reports on development of severe hypertension after segmental embolization.[35]

Total Embolization

Postembolization syndrome is an almost constant finding after total renal embolization, and prophylactic treatment is a mandatory component of the procedure. However, symptoms may become severe despite appropriate measures. Low-grade fever may last up to 6 weeks after embolization. On CT, gas may be seen within the embolized tissue but is not generally a sign of superinfection.

Other complications include nontarget embolization. In particular, ethanol may cause severe complications due to reflux into the aorta, with necrotic damage of the skin, adrenals, colon, or spinal cord. The safety of ethanol embolization may be improved by the use of occlusion balloons and mixing the ethanol with contrast medium.

The complication rate in 1146 preoperative and palliative renal embolization procedures was 4%, with a mortality of 0.07%.[36] Besides nontarget embolization, transvenous embolization, thromboembolism, acute hypertension, or arterial injuries occurred in this large series.

POSTPROCEDURE AND FOLLOW-UP CARE

As already noted, complete renal embolization is usually followed by development of postembolization syndrome, with abdominal pain, nausea, and fever. Sometimes symptoms can become severe, and prophylaxis is mandatory. Besides general treatment with antipyretics, antiemetics, and intravenous fluid infusion, pain can be controlled either with an epidural catheter over 24 to 48 hours or by a patient-controlled analgesia intravenous automated pump system. Antibiotic therapy is recommended.

Selective embolization usually does not cause general symptoms, and no specific follow-up measures are required. If large segments of renal vascular territory have been embolized, oral antibiotic therapy may be considered.

KEY POINTS

- Selective or complete renal embolization depends on the clinical situation. Nephron-sparing techniques are preferred. Embolization can be helpful in palliative and emergency situations and variant agents are used depending on the individual case.

▸ **SUGGESTED READINGS**

Maleux G, Messiaen T, Stockx L, et al. Transcatheter embolization of biopsy-related vascular injuries in renal allografts. Long-term technical, clinical and biochemical results. Acta Radiol 2003 Jan;44(1):13–7.

Perini S, Gordon RL, LaBerge JM, et al. Transcatheter embolization of biopsy-related vascular injury in the transplant kidney: immediate and long-term outcome. J Vasc Interv Radiol 1998 Nov-Dec;9(6):1011–9.

Sofocleous CT, Hinrichs C, Hubbi B, et al. Angiographic findings and embolotherapy in renal arterial trauma. Cardiovasc Intervent Radiol 2005 Jan-Feb;28(1):39–47.

The complete reference list is available online at www.expertconsult.com

CHAPTER 61
Management of Renal Angiomyolipoma
Ghassan E. El-Haddad and Deepak Sudheendra

CLINICAL RELEVANCE

Angiomyolipoma (AML) is the most common benign mesenchymal neoplasm of the kidney. It is characterized by proliferation of varying amounts of dysmorphic thick-walled blood vessels, smooth muscle, and mature adipose tissue.[1] AMLs account for 0.3% to 3% of renal masses and 1% of surgically resected tumors,[2-5] although these numbers probably underestimate the prevalence of this tumor. Malignant transformation does not occur except in rare cases.[6] Around 50% to 70% of AMLs are sporadic, more commonly unilateral and single, right-sided (two thirds of lesions), and occur almost exclusively in adult females (fourth to sixth decade, with a 4:1 female/male ratio).[7-10] Some 30% to 50% of AMLs are bilateral, multiple, develop early in life (third to fourth decade), have no sex predilection, and are usually associated with tuberous sclerosis complex (TSC).[10,11] TSC (Bourneville disease) is a syndrome with autosomal dominant inheritance and includes variable expressions of mental retardation, seizures, facial angiofibroma, subungual fibroma, retinal hamartomas, renal cysts, and AMLs. Approximately 20% of patients with AMLs have TSC, and up to 80% of patients with TSC have AMLs.[12] In addition, AMLs associated with TSC are far more likely to be larger than the sporadic form, which increases the risk of hemorrhage.[7]

The classic treatment of AMLs that are symptomatic, show progressive growth on follow-up imaging studies, or are larger than 4 cm has been nephron-sparing partial nephrectomy.[13] However, since the first embolization of a bleeding AML with gelfoam in 1977,[14] selective renal artery embolization, which spares normal renal parenchyma, has become increasingly popular and is gradually replacing partial or total nephrectomy.

In adults, a renal mass containing fat is diagnostic of AML,[15] and cross-sectional imaging with computed tomography (CT) or magnetic resonance imaging (MRI) are the best diagnostic imaging modalities to detect subtle fat within a tumor.[16-18] Since approximately 5% of AMLs have no detectable fat on imaging, AMLs without demonstrable fat require tissue diagnosis to exclude renal cell carcinoma.[17] AMLs may occasionally extend into the inferior vena cava, but that does not imply malignant transformation.[19] CT angiography (CTA) may show numerous, often aneurysmal, vessels within and around the tumor. If a solid-appearing lesion is detected in a patient with TSC, fluorodeoxyglucose positron emission tomography (FDG-PET) can be helpful because AMLs are generally not FDG-avid.[20,21] Angiography is generally performed for intervention rather than diagnosis. The angiographic findings of AML are consistent with a highly vascular tumor, sacculated pseudoaneurysms, lack of normal vessel tapering, tortuous vessels, absence of arteriovenous shunting, "sunburst" appearance of capillary nephrogram, and "onion-peel appearance" of peripheral vessels in the venous phase.[22-24]

INDICATIONS

The most serious complication of renal AML is tumor rupture and acute hemorrhage, which can be massive (Wunderlich syndrome) and life threatening.[8,25] Patients with AML and TSC are also at increased risk for tumor invasion of the adjacent normal renal parenchyma, causing chronic kidney disease and even end-stage-renal failure.[26]

Treatment of AML depends on the presence of symptoms, size and number of tumors, and presence or absence of TSC. AMLs smaller than 4 cm in maximum diameter that are discovered incidentally in asymptomatic patients do not require treatment.[8,27] There is controversy as to when to perform follow-up imaging, but this is usually done by annual CT or ultrasound. Symptomatic presentations of AML include abdominal or flank pain, a palpable mass, hematuria, fever, anemia, and hypertension, with the most common symptoms being acute flank pain and hematuria.[28,29] There is a direct correlation between AML size and symptoms. About 80% of AMLs smaller than 4 cm in maximum diameter are usually asymptomatic, whereas nearly 80% of tumors larger than 4 cm cause symptoms.[25] Of the latter, 80% to 90% are symptomatic, and 50% to 60% bleed spontaneously.[8,30]

In addition to size, the likelihood of AML hemorrhage depends on the presence of intratumoral aneurysms larger than 5 mm.[22] The relation between pregnancy and AML rupture is not clearly defined, but a review of the reported cases in the literature suggests that pregnancy could increase the risk of renal AML rupture.[31] AMLs that are larger than 4 cm in asymptomatic patients may be observed using short follow-up intervals. However, in view of the significantly increased risk for a potentially catastrophic hemorrhage, either spontaneously or after minimal trauma, partial nephrectomy or renal arterial embolization is warranted in these patients.[30]

A variety of embolic materials have been used, including particles (<500 μm), but these do not penetrate to the capillary level. Absolute ethanol is advocated by some interventionalists to be the embolic agent of choice for selective embolization of AML because it causes complete occlusion of the peripheral renal arteries. Ethanol is mixed with ethiodized oil (Ethiodol [iodized poppyseed oil]; Savage Laboratories, Melville, N.Y.) to make it radiopaque. It is very important to inject the mixture slowly to prevent reflux and nontarget embolization into the rest of the renal arterial circulation. Selective renal artery embolization can also be performed on AMLs larger than 10 cm, since resection of these tumors would require that a greater percentage of the kidney be removed.[32]

CONTRAINDICATIONS

An absolute contraindication to selective renal artery embolization is ongoing renal sepsis. Nephron-sparing partial nephrectomy rather than selective renal artery embolization should be considered in the case of severe allergy to contrast media, single kidney, or when a skilled interventional radiologist is unavailable.

Relative contraindications include mild to moderate allergy to iodinated contrast material, renal dysfunction, or planned radioiodine therapy.

EQUIPMENT

The following equipment is required to perform transcatheter renal artery embolization:
- Angiographic unit with digital fluoroscopy (preferably pulsed fluoroscopy to reduce radiation dose)
- Contrast material
- 5F Pigtail catheter
- Standard 5F to 6F vascular sheath
- Standard 4F or 5F selective angiographic catheters (Cobra-2, Simmons-1) with 0.035-inch guidewires
- High-flow coaxial microcatheters (0.025- to 0.028-inch lumen) with appropriate microwires
- Embolization agent: ethanol and ethiodized oil, or polyvinyl alcohol particles (<500 μm)
- Polycarbonate syringes and metal three-way stopcocks

TECHNIQUE

Anatomy and Approaches

In about two thirds of individuals, each kidney is supplied by a single artery that originates from the aorta below the superior mesenteric artery at approximately the level of L1-L2 intervertebral disc space. About 25% to 30% of people have variations in the number, location and branching patterns of the renal arteries. The kidneys may directly receive second, third, and even fourth supernumerary arterial branches from the aorta or the iliac arteries. The right renal artery orifice is usually located at the anterolateral aspect of the aorta. The left renal artery orifice is usually located at a more lateral position. Typically the renal artery divides into five branches at the level of the renal pelvis, each supplying a segment of the kidney (apical, anterosuperior, anteroinferior, inferior, and posterior). The segmental arteries are end arteries that give rise to the interlobar arteries. The interlobar arteries divide into the arcuate arteries at the corticomedullary junction. The interlobular arteries are the terminal branches that ultimately supply the glomeruli. A small branch arises from the proximal portion of each renal artery, supplying the adrenal gland and renal capsule.

Technical Aspects

Renal embolization is generally performed under conscious sedation. Antibiotic prophylaxis is recommended within 1 hour from the procedure. An abdominal aortogram is usually performed via a common femoral artery approach to determine the possible presence of accessory renal arteries and the number of vessels feeding the tumor (Fig. 61-1). The proximal renal arteries are best seen using a contrast

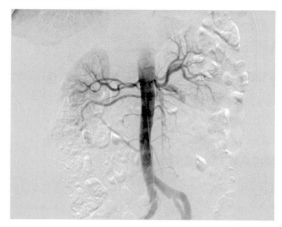

FIGURE 61-1. Flush aortogram demonstrating three accessory right renal arteries.

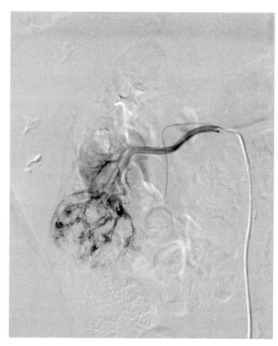

FIGURE 61-2. Selective catheterization of a second accessory renal artery predominantly supplying a highly vascular lower-pole right renal angiomyolipoma with abnormal tortuous vessels and small sacculated pseudoaneurysms.

injection of 15 to 25 mL/s for 2 seconds and rapid filming (3-6 frames/s). Selective arteriogram is then performed to evaluate the arterial branches and renal masses (Figs. 61-2 and 61-3). Many selective catheters can be used for that purpose, but the basic choices are a curved selective catheter such as a 5F Cobra-2 catheter (Cook Medical, Bloomington, Ind. [when renal artery arises at an angle close to 90 degrees]) or a reversed-curve catheter such as a Simmons-1 or SOS Omni catheter (when renal artery arises at an acute angle). A transbrachial or even a transradial approach can also be used if access from the common femoral artery is not possible.[33] Injection rates of 5 to 6 mL/s for 2 to 3 seconds (3-6 frames/s) are generally used for optimal

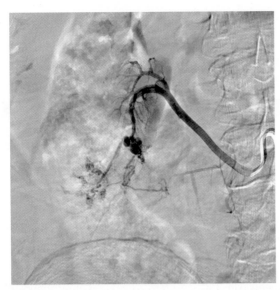

FIGURE 61-3. Selective catheterization of a third accessory right renal artery partially supplying inferior portion of lower-pole hypervascular angiomyolipoma. Upper portion of tumor demonstrates tumor staining from prior embolization.

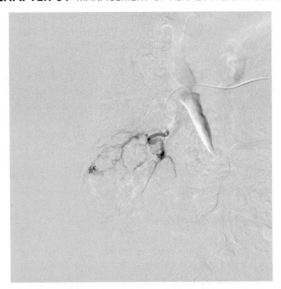

FIGURE 61-4. Superselective catheterization of right renal artery third-order branch supplying lower-pole angiomyolipoma with injection of ethanol/Ethiodol mixture. Tumor staining is seen.

imaging of intrarenal arterial branches. Oblique views are used to best image the renal vasculature (ipsilateral oblique shows the kidney en face).

Once a decision to embolize is made, a high-flow microcatheter (Renegade HI-FLO [Boston Scientific, Natick, Mass.]) is used to select the vessel to be embolized, distal to the branches supplying normal renal parenchyma. For selective renal artery embolization, several embolic agents have been used. For the embolization of AMLs, we prefer a mixture of ethanol and ethiodized oil (Ethiodol [Savage Laboratories]). Ethanol is mixed with ethiodized oil in a 7:3 ratio, using polycarbonate syringes and a three-way metal stopcock. Just enough iodized oil is added to be able to visualize the flow of the embolic fluid and monitor when stasis is achieved to avoid nontarget embolization (Fig. 61-4). The endpoint is occlusion of the arterial branches supplying the tumor and nonopacification of the tumor itself (Fig. 61-5). If there is residual vascularization, additional embolic mixture is delivered until stasis is achieved. All branches supplying the tumor should be embolized. Patients are closely monitored overnight for management of postembolization syndrome. Alternatively, the tumor bed can be embolized with particles (<500 μm) if there is concern for nontarget embolization. However, particles do not penetrate to the capillary level, whereas ethanol causes permanent occlusion at the arteriolar and capillary level, leading to tumor necrosis.[34,35] Coils are not used in the setting of selective arterial embolization because collaterals can form around the occlusion site.

CONTROVERSIES

Small series have reported aneurysmal rupture during embolization of AMLs using an occlusion balloon, attributed to increased intravascular pressure or erosion of the thin aneurysm wall by ethanol.[36,37] It is recommended to use small particles for embolization in cases of intratumoral

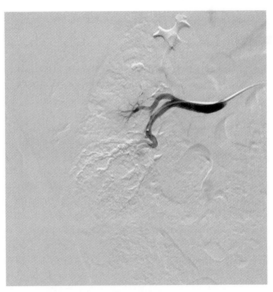

FIGURE 61-5. Postembolization control arteriogram demonstrating occlusion of the arterial branches supplying the tumor, and nonopacification of the tumor itself.

aneurysm, or injecting the ethanol/Ethiodol mixture slowly without an occlusion balloon.[3]

OUTCOMES

Partial Renal Embolization

The few retrospective analyses of small series of patients with AML who have undergone emergency embolization have demonstrated high technical success rates close to 100%.[38] One of the larger series available reporting on long-term results (3 months to 7 years) of preventive embolization for AML also showed complete technical success. The overall recurrence rate of AML was found to be 36.1%

(median time interval from embolization to recurrence was 6 to 7 years) in patients with tuberous sclerosis, but not in patients with sporadic AML.[39] Despite these results, embolotherapy remains the treatment of choice for AML in patients with TSC. Because of the nature of TSC, closer follow-up is recommended to identify patients who require repeat embolization. In a more recent retrospective case series with long-term follow-up of 34 patients, selective arterial embolization with alcohol for AML was found to be a safe and effective method for improving clinical symptoms (85%) and preventing tumor progression (97%).[40]

COMPLICATIONS

Selective Embolization

The complications of selective embolization are very rare. Almost all patients develop a low-grade fever and flank pain, likely related to postembolization syndrome, and are treated conservatively with antipyretics, antiemetics, and analgesics. Severe complications can occur from nontarget embolization of ethanol. Other complications include those encountered in any arterial catheterization (e.g., hematoma, pseudoaneurysm, etc.).

POSTPROCEDURE AND FOLLOW-UP CARE

Hydration, analgesics, antiemetics, and antipyretics are used to control postembolization syndrome, which is much more prevalent in total renal than partial renal embolization. Patients are usually admitted overnight for management of postembolization syndrome and discharged once he/she has resumed adequate oral intake, no longer needs parenteral narcotics for pain control, and has voided. In patients with TSC, a postembolization imaging protocol consists of a baseline contrast-enhanced CT scan at 1 month, 6 months, 1 year, and then annually for life. MRI may be an alternative to CT if there is contrast allergy, renal failure, or to minimize radiation exposure. For patients with sporadic AML, CT images are obtained at 1 month and 12 months; lifelong surveillance is *not* required. Decrease in AML size following embolization is variable. Regardless

of changes in size, any increase in enhancement or vascularity should be considered suspicious and warrants close follow-up or angiography, with possible repeat embolization.[39]

KEY POINTS

- Renal angiomyolipoma (AML) is a benign tumor that may cause pain, hematuria, and more importantly, massive bleeding when larger than 4 cm. It can be sporadic or associated with tuberous sclerosis complex (TSC).

- Selective renal artery embolization is a successful nephron-sparing treatment for large or symptomatic AML.

- Absolute ethanol mixed with ethiodized oil is the preferred embolic agent. Alternatively, particles can be used. Coils should be avoided.

- Long-term surveillance following embolization is needed in patients with TSC, owing to a high rate of recurrence.

▶ **SUGGESTED READINGS**

Chick CM, Tan BS, Cheng C, et al. Long-term follow-up of the treatment of renal angiomyolipomas after selective arterial embolization with alcohol. BJU Int 2010;105(3):390–4.

Han YM, Kim JK, Roh BS, et al. Renal angiomyolipoma: selective arterial embolization–effectiveness and changes in angiomyogenic components in long-term follow-up. Radiology 1997;204(1):65–70.

Kothary N, Soulen MC, Clark TW, et al. Renal angiomyolipoma: long-term results after arterial embolization. J Vasc Interv Radiol 2005;16(1):45–50.

Oesterling JE, Fishman EK, Goldman SM, et al. The management of renal angiomyolipoma. J Urol 1986;135(6):1121–4.

Soulen MC, Faykus MH, Jr, Shlansky-Goldberg RD, et al. Elective embolization for prevention of hemorrhage from renal angiomyolipomas. J Vasc Interv Radiol 1994;5(4):587–91.

Steiner MS, Goldman SM, Fishman EK, et al. The natural history of renal angiomyolipoma. J Urol 1993;150(6):1782–6.

The complete reference list is available online at www.expertconsult.com

CHAPTER 62

Transvenous Renal Biopsy

Anthony F. Watkinson

CLINICAL RELEVANCE

Renal histopathologic examination remains the diagnostic gold standard for most renal parenchymal diseases[1,2] and is therefore essential for clinical management of renal diseases such as proteinuria, hematuria, and renal failure.[3,4] The conventional technique for obtaining renal tissue involves percutaneous puncture of the kidney. This is a safe technique when performed in low-risk patients by experienced operators.[5] The first description of renal tissue sampling by percutaneous needle biopsy was published in 1951.[6] Improved technology and ultrasound guidance have considerably reduced the risk of complications with renal biopsy techniques and improved safety and efficacy.

Nevertheless, significant risk still attends renal biopsy, and serious complications have been reported. Even under ideal circumstances, overt complications occur in up to 3.5% of cases,[7] and the incidence of perirenal hematoma has been reported to be 57% to 85%.[8,9] Percutaneous renal biopsy is therefore considered high risk in patients with abnormal clotting or low platelets. Furthermore, a number of other clinical conditions such as solitary, small, or obstructed kidneys, uncontrolled hypertension, horseshoe kidney, mechanical ventilation, and uncooperative patients present relative contraindications to percutaneous approach. An aging population, diabetes, and more widespread use of anticoagulant and antiplatelet drugs have led to more frequent clinical encounters with high-risk biopsy candidates.

Some novel techniques have been developed in the last decade as alternatives to percutaneous biopsy in patients with contraindications.[10-12] They include performing renal biopsies through an open surgical approach, transvenous approaches using transjugular and transfemoral access, and laparoscopic techniques. Development of a cutting core biopsy needle has made transjugular renal biopsy the most important of these.

Open biopsy has the added risk of general anesthesia and its associated morbidity and mortality. Transjugular biopsy is theoretically safer because the needle is advanced as distally as possible into the medullary interlobar veins; the needle then passes through the vein wall into the surrounding parenchyma, directed away from the larger blood vessels. When bleeding does occur, it will do so back into the venous system, limiting extravascular blood loss.[13] Another theoretical advantage of the transjugular approach is a lower likelihood of capsular perforation with the inside-out approach, in comparison to the 100% capsular perforation rate with percutaneous biopsy. Furthermore, if capsular perforation occurs and there is significant extravasation, elective coil embolization of the biopsy track can be performed during the same procedure.

Transjugular renal biopsy technique was developed as a modification of the classical transjugular liver biopsy[14] and

described in 1990 by Mal et al.[15] Authors first reported using a modified 9F liver core biopsy needle in 50 patients for transjugular renal cortical biopsies,[15] and then in 200 patients with contraindications to percutaneous biopsy.[10] In a recent comparison of 400 transjugular transvenous renal biopsies to an equal number of percutaneous biopsies, similar results were reported for both.[7] This is a significant finding because 75.8% of patients in the transjugular renal group had bleeding disorders.

In clinical practice, the proportion of patients with contraindications to percutaneous biopsy is small (≈7%).[16] In high-risk patients, transjugular renal biopsy provides clinicians with expanding opportunities for obtaining renal histologic samples. Clinical utility of this procedure is also emphasized by the fact that diabetic patients undergoing renal biopsy frequently have nondiabetic renal disease.[17,18] It has been established that transjugular renal biopsies, especially in patients with acute renal failure, affects patient management.[19]

The initially feared potential disadvantage of low diagnostic yield (owing to the need to first traverse the medulla to reach the cortex) was shown to be unfounded in various studies.

INDICATIONS

- Patients with a bleeding diathesis or on oral anticoagulation that cannot be stopped
- Concomitant hemodialysis catheter placement[19]
- Patients with concurrent renal and liver disease who warrant both renal and hepatic biopsies
- Morbidly obese patients
- Patients on mechanical ventilation
- Failed percutaneous renal biopsy

RELATIVE CONTRAINDICATIONS

- Absent right kidney
- Occluded central veins such that venous access from above is not possible

EQUIPMENT

Initial studies used a modified Colapinto aspiration needle for the biopsy. More recently, transjugular 19G Quick-Core side-cut biopsy needle systems (Cook Medical, Bloomington, Ind.) have been popular, with good cortical sampling.[7,20] However, there is a higher incidence of capsular perforation.[20]

The Quick-Core side-cut biopsy needle system consists of a 7F, 50.5-cm transjugular sheath with a 14G inner stiffening cannula; a 5F, 80-cm multipurpose curved catheter; and a 60-cm, 19G biopsy needle with a 2-cm throw length. The biopsy needle has an inner stylet and a 2-cm specimen notch with a beveled end. The biopsy needle is enclosed in a 5F straight angiographic catheter and cut to length to ease advancement through the transjugular sheath. An Arrowflex vascular sheath (Arrow International Inc, Reading, Pa., USA) can be used as an alternative to the Quick-Core transjugular vascular sheath. The stiffness of the Quick-Core system makes a left jugular approach challenging.

The blunt-tipped Quick-Core biopsy needle is a modification of the device that has been shown to not only provide sufficient cortical tissue for histopathologic diagnosis but also possibly reduce capsular penetration and hence significant bleeding in an animal study[21] and a subsequent study of seven patients.[22]

TECHNIQUE

The procedure is usually performed in a supine patient in an angiographic suite with a biplane or single-plane fluoroscopic machine. Prothrombin time (or International Normalized Ratio [INR]), partial thromboplastin time, platelet count, and serum creatinine level are obtained before the procedure. Attempts should be made to correct any coagulopathy (INR > 1.5, platelets < 50,000/μL) before the procedure.

The patient's head is turned away from the side of puncture. The skin is cleaned with an iodine solution or chlorhexidine. The patient is then covered with a surgical drape. Right internal jugular vein access is preferred to the left because the former has a relatively direct continuation into the superior and inferior venae cavae. The right internal jugular vein is punctured after local anesthesia under ultrasound guidance. A 7F to 9F transjugular vascular sheath (or Arrowflex sheath) is inserted. A hydrophilic guidewire (Terumo Medical Corp., Somerset, N.J.) or standard Bentson wire (Cook Medical) is then advanced into the inferior vena cava. The renal vein is then selectively catheterized using a 5F Cobra (Cordis Corp., Hialeah, Fla.) or multipurpose curved catheter introduced through the sheath. The catheter is manipulated into the posterior lower branch of the right renal vein. The hydrophilic wire or Bentson wire is then exchanged for a 145-cm Amplatz Super Stiff Wire (Boston Scientific Corp., Natick, Mass.). Subsequently, the vascular (or Arrowflex) sheath is advanced over a stiff guidewire into the renal vein under fluoroscopic guidance.

Once the sheath is advanced into the renal vein, a transvenous Quick-Core biopsy needle with its protective outer straight catheter sheath is inserted. This catheter should be gently advanced as distally as possible into a peripheral cortical vein of the lower pole of the right kidney. An optimal peripheral position is confirmed by flushing with a small amount of contrast medium through the vascular sheath. The position is judged to be satisfactory when a wedge of cortical parenchyma is enhanced (Fig. 62-1, *A*). In such a position there is little likelihood of damaging a large central vein or artery. Furthermore, more glomeruli are obtained per pass when parenchymal enhancement is obtained.[7]

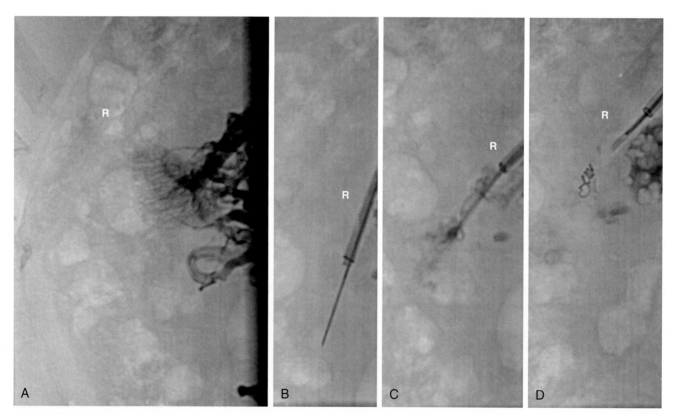

FIGURE 62-1. **A,** Unsubtracted image after introduction of a 7F Arrowflex sheath into right *(R)* renal vein over a stiff guidewire. After removal of guidewire, sheath has been wedged and a venogram performed with gentle injection to outline extent of renal cortex. **B,** Biopsy needle has been fired to take biopsy sample. **C,** Outer 5F covering catheter has been advanced along tract, and needle withdrawn. Gentle contrast infusion demonstrates extravasation and that capsule has been breached. **D,** Coil has been placed along this catheter to seal the tract.

When the straight catheter is withdrawn, it exposes the 19G biopsy needle. Tissue samples can then be taken with the aid of a spring-loaded gun (Fig. 62-1, *B*). Alternatively, the inner stylet with the specimen notch can be advanced first into the renal cortex, and the outer cutting cannula advanced over it. The straight catheter is then advanced back over the needle into the biopsy track. The needle containing the tissue specimen is removed. Contrast is injected through the straight catheter to identify any capsular perforation (Fig. 62-1, *C*).

If capsular perforation is present, the biopsy track can be prophylactically embolized with coils at the discretion of the operator (Fig. 62-1, *D*). Though embolization coils are used in general, some operators prefer gelfoam to plug the tract.[24] Usually only a small volume of contrast is used during the procedure (<30 mL of iodinated contrast [strength 300 mg/mL]), which should reduce the risk of any renal dysfunction. Tissue samples are processed in a standard manner for evaluation by light microscopy, immunofluorescence, and electron microscopy. An average of 4 to 6 passes are made to obtain a sufficient sample for histologic analysis.[16,23]

The right kidney is preferentially biopsied because the right renal vein is shorter and its angle allows for easier access to the kidney. The left renal vein is longer and tends to form a right angle with the inferior vena cava. The left may be biopsied in the case of a single kidney or unfavorable venous anatomy of the right kidney.

The critical step in performing transjugular renal biopsy is positioning the needle in a subcortical location and allowing enough distance from the capsule to avoid capsular penetration.[21]

All biopsy devices are then removed. The catheter, its stiffeners, and sheath are all removed, and hemostasis is obtained with manual compression.

OUTCOMES

Transjugular biopsy provides renal tissue in 92% of patients.[16] Tissue adequacy for histologic examination (i.e., number of glomeruli obtained) is excellent (range 94%-100%).[7,10,24] The average number of glomeruli per sample ranges from 10 to 19, comparable to percutaneous kidney biopsies.[16,23,25] The overall diagnostic success of the procedure ranges from 89% to 97%.[23,25] This is comparable to the yield of percutaneous biopsy, which generally ranges from 95% to 98.8%.[5,7,26] Furthermore, transjugular biopsies yield better samples for immunofluorescence. The amount of tissue retrieved increases with the number of passes up to three to four passes, and decreases thereafter with poorer-quality samples.[13,24]

It is a safe procedure in patients with coagulopathy.[25] The small amount of iodinated contrast (<30 mL) used for the procedure is unlikely to result in contrast-induced nephropathy.[19,27] As opposed to percutaneous biopsy, perforation of the renal capsule and therefore the risk of perirenal hematoma are less likely.

However, transjugular renal biopsy may not be feasible in the following conditions:
- Congenital absence or thrombosis of the right internal jugular vein
- Thrombosis of the inferior vena cava and/or renal vein
- Recurrent course of the renal vein

Transjugular renal biopsy requires relatively high operator skills, technical equipment, and occupation of the radiology fluoroscopy suite. In inexperienced hands, it can be a time-consuming and costly procedure compared to percutaneous biopsy. These limitations mean that percutaneous renal biopsy will not be routinely replaced by transjugular biopsy. However, transjugular biopsy has a vital role in providing tissue samples to clinicians when a percutaneous route is contraindicated.

COMPLICATIONS

The rates of complications with transjugular kidney biopsy are likely to be influenced by patient selection and local policy regarding contraindications to percutaneous biopsy and operator experience. The complication rate of transjugular renal biopsy performed in patients with clotting disorders is comparable to percutaneous biopsy.[27]

Major complications with transjugular renal biopsy, such as bleeding requiring resuscitation or intervention, occur in only 1% to 2% of patients.[7,23] It is important to appreciate that these patients are in general at high risk for bleeding due to their coagulation status. More commonly, patients experience a transient microscopic hematuria.

Major bleeding into either the perirenal space or pelvicalyceal system can occur. Gross hematuria due to puncture of the renal pelvis or calyces is a recognized complication of transjugular kidney biopsy. Puncture of the renal pelvicalyceal system can result in a fistula between a blood vessel and renal calyx. Patients might need resuscitation, blood transfusion, transarterial embolization, or surgery, similar to patients with a major bleed into the perirenal space.

An arteriocalyceal communication may be identified by injection of contrast through the protective catheter immediately following biopsy. Performing peripheral cortical biopsies may avoid this complication.

Capsular perforation occurs in 74% to 90% of cases.[16,24] The overall incidence of perirenal hematoma is less than 30%, compared to 57% to 85% reported for percutaneous approach.[8,9,25]

POSTPROCEDURE AND FOLLOW-UP CARE

The procedure is usually well tolerated, and most patients return to their baseline activity the day following the procedure.[23] In view of evidence in the percutaneous biopsy literature that delayed bleeding after 8 hours may occur in up to 20% of patients,[28] caution is required with regard to the length of postprocedural observation. After the procedure, patients remain on bed rest for 12 hours, and standard hemodynamic monitoring is carried out for 24 hours. Vital signs should be monitored every 15 minutes in the first 6 hours post procedure. Hematocrit is usually assessed within 4 to 6 hours post biopsy. The patient is usually discharged the next day.

CONCLUSIONS

Transjugular renal biopsy is a useful procedure in patients with contraindications to conventional percutaneous renal biopsy. A combination of advanced technology and increased experience with the technique in the past decade has enabled transjugular renal biopsy to become an efficacious, well-tolerated, and relatively safer alternative to percutaneous renal biopsy in certain clinical situations.

Transjugular renal biopsy, at least in current practice settings, is unlikely to become a high-volume procedure, but despite this can be effectively and safely done by interventional radiologists with transjugular liver biopsy experience and equipment.

The role of this procedure is to enable histologic diagnosis in patients with contraindications to percutaneous biopsy. The tissue sample obtained is adequate in over 90% of cases to make a confident diagnosis and influence management[16] by excluding important factors from differential diagnosis, instilling confidence in instituting specific treatments, and providing valuable prognostic information. Transjugular renal biopsy should be reserved for patients in whom the biopsy result could influence the therapeutic strategy, particularly those with rapidly progressive renal disease and contraindications to percutaneous biopsy.

KEY POINTS

- Transjugular renal biopsy provides tissue samples for histology in patients with contraindications to percutaneous renal biopsy.

- It is theoretically a safer procedure because postprocedure hemorrhage remains intravenous, limiting extravascular blood loss.

- The safety and efficacy of transjugular renal biopsy in patients with abnormal clotting is comparable to percutaneous renal biopsy in patients with normal clotting.

- Transjugular renal biopsy in patients with renal dysfunction affects patient management.

▶ SUGGESTED READINGS

Meyrier A. Transjugular renal biopsy: update on hepato-renal needlework. Nephrol Dial Transplant 2005;20:1299–302.

The complete reference list is available online at www.expertconsult.com

CHAPTER 63

Transjugular Liver Biopsy

Sebastian Kos, Deniz Bilecen, Augustinus Ludwig Jacob, and Markus H. Heim

CLINICAL RELEVANCE

Despite tremendous achievements in diagnostic imaging, laboratory studies, and clinical medicine, it is still valuable and often mandatory to acquire liver tissue samples for further histopathologic characterization of infectious, metabolic, and neoplastic diseases and/or their course.

Historically, Paul Ehrlich, a German pioneer of immunology, was the first to perform a percutaneous liver biopsy. In 1883, he determined the hepatic glycogen content in a diabetic patient.[1] In the following years, Lucatello applied the technique on a liver abscess (1895). Schüpfer et al. had already documented its potential in the diagnosis of chronic cirrhotic liver disease in a series of rat experiments and clinical studies. After Menghini propagated the "1-second needle biopsy of the liver" 50 years later, this procedure was broadly implemented in the management of chronic and acute hepatic diseases.[2]

Since the early days when blind biopsies were performed, a tremendous evolution of the biopsy procedure has taken place. Approaches, materials used (true cutting needles, fine-needle aspiration), and guided imaging techniques (e.g., fluoroscopy, sonography, computed tomography) have been improved, applied, and evaluated.

Meanwhile, percutaneous liver biopsy has been well proven to allow fast, safe, and adequate tissue sampling. It therefore has become the gold standard to obtain liver specimens. However, because it by definition penetrates the hepatic capsule, there is a significant risk for intra- and perihepatic hematoma and consequent relevant blood loss. This technique must not be used in patients with a known or suspected bleeding diathesis or those receiving oral anticoagulation. Further factors like an uncooperative patient, severe obesity, or high-volume ascites have been shown to increase the complication rate and may lead to puncture failure.

Therefore, alternative approaches (laparoscopic, transfemoral, transjugular) were established, enabling hepatic tissue sampling after failure of, or in the presence of contraindications for, the biopsy procedure.[3] Given their higher mortality and morbidity, the use of laparoscopic biopsies is reduced to special cases, such as when an abdominal operation under general anesthesia is mandatory otherwise.[3]

As a pioneer, Dotter was the first to biopsy dog livers using a transvenous jugular approach in 1964.[4] Weiner and Hanaffe used the same access to catheterize the hepatic veins in 1967, and in 1970 published their initial experience with transjugular hepatic biopsy in a series of humans.[5,6] By 1973, Rosch had already performed the technique on 44 patients, showing the need for the procedure.[7] Unlike percutaneous access, it approaches the liver through the right jugular vein, through the vena cava, and most often the right hepatic vein. The biopsy is then performed directed away from major vessels into the parenchyma (inside-out). The capsule is not injured, minimizing the risk of intra- or perihepatic hematoma. Blood leakage into the biopsy channel immediately drains into the access vein, thereby avoiding significant extravascular blood loss and hemodynamic alterations.

Today the transjugular liver biopsy is well accepted and broadly established as the first-line backup for the percutaneous approach.[8] In the hands of an experienced interventional radiologist, it is safer than the latter and well tolerated. Since many patients with liver disease consequently suffer from coagulopathy and/or ascites, there is huge potential for the technique.

Optional concomitant measurement of the hepatic venous pressure gradient (HVPG) is calculated as the difference between wedged (WHVP, an estimate of portal venous pressure) and free hepatic venous pressure (FHVP). It was shown that the HVPG provides relevant information to assess the risk of esophageal varix bleeding in patients with known portal hypertension. Furthermore, it may help document the efficacy of drug treatment in those patients by its changes over time.[9] The risk of variceal bleeding is zero with HVPG lower than 12 mmHg, whereas an HVPG of more than 20 mmHg in cirrhotic patients is predictive of early rebleeding and death.[9]

INDICATIONS

General Indications for Liver Biopsy in Diffuse Nonfocal Liver Disease

The following general indications for liver biopsy in diffuse nonfocal liver disease were modified from Bravo et al.[3]:

- Diagnosis, grading (inflammatory activity), and staging (degree of fibrosis/cirrhosis) of noninfectious liver diseases (e.g., nonalcoholic steatohepatitis [NASH], alcoholic liver disease, autoimmune hepatitis)
- Grading and staging of infectious liver diseases (e.g., chronic hepatitis B or C)
- Diagnosis of hemochromatosis, with quantitative analysis of iron levels
- Diagnosis of Wilson disease, with quantitative analysis of copper levels
- Diagnosis of primary biliary cirrhosis and primary sclerosing cholangitis
- Detection of adverse effects occurring under drug treatment (e.g., methotrexate)
- Evaluation of abnormal biochemical tests in combination with negative or inconclusive serologic testing
- Evaluation of liver status after transplantation and of the donor liver before transplantation
- Fever of unknown origin
- Clinical presentation of acute liver failure[10]

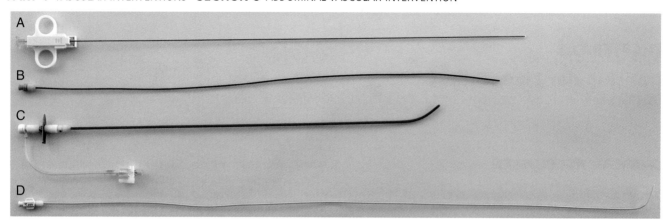

FIGURE 63-1. Key equipment. **A,** Biopsy device. **B,** 5F straight catheter. **C,** 7F catheter with stiffening metal cannula. **D,** 5F multipurpose catheter.

Specific Indications for Transjugular Liver Biopsy

Transjugular liver biopsy is indicated in the following specific circumstances:
- Severe coagulopathy (thrombocytopenia < 70,000; prothrombin time < 60% of normal level)
- Massive ascites
- Massive obesity
- Suspected vascular tumor or peliosis hepatic
- Need for additive vascular procedures like transjugular intrahepatic portosystemic shunting
- Need for additive biopsies (e.g., kidney)
- Need for additive diagnostics (e.g., venography, HVPG)
- Failure of prior percutaneous liver biopsy
- Patients on mechanical ventilation

CONTRAINDICATIONS

Relative Contraindications

Patients with known severe renal impairment, hyperthyroidism, and/or known allergy to iodinated contrast media should not undergo the procedure, owing to the possible adverse effects of the contrast media used.

If necessary in children and pregnant women, the need for the procedure should be discussed interdisciplinarily and with the patient, owing to the use of radiation.

As in any transjugular approach, occlusion, obstruction, and even more rare, congenital absence of the right jugular vein, inferior vena cava, and/or hepatic veins may limit accessibility.

EQUIPMENT

For transjugular liver biopsy, different biopsy needles have been designed. Corr et al. reported a series of 200 cases which were biopsied with a modified Ross needle (Cook Medical, Bloomington, Ind.). This was placed through a 9F curved sheath.[11]

More often encountered are side-cutting needles like the Quick-Core needle (Cook Medical), which is inserted using a 7F curved sheath with a stiffening and guiding metal cannula. The cutting needles available (18 and 20 gauge) provide a semiautomated springfire mechanism to acquire tissue. This, according to our own experience and the literature, is relatively easy to use and has a high diagnostic yield. In 43 patients, Little et al. performed successful biopsy in 98% (42/43 patients)[12]; 118 biopsies were obtained, with an average of 2.8 passes per patient. Mean maximum sample lengths lay between 1.1 and 1.5 cm. Other studies showed successful biopsy rates of 100%, with 100% diagnostic histologic core specimens.[13]

Recently a new aspiration needle device (Hakko Co. Ltd., Nagano, Japan) was evaluated in Niigata, Japan, with promising initial results compared to the Quick-Core needle (less fragmentation, longer specimens, more portal triads, shorter intervention) but is not yet commercially available.[13]

Key equipment (Fig. 63-1) includes:
- 7F catheter with stiffening metal cannula
- 5F straight catheter
- 5F multipurpose catheter
- Hydrophilic guidewire, standard Bentson wire, and an Amplatz super-stiff wire
- Quick-Core biopsy needle (18-20 gauge)

TECHNIQUE

Anatomy and Approaches

Prior to the procedure, written informed consent is obtained. International Normalized Ratio (INR) or prothrombin time, partial thromboplastin time, platelet count, and serum creatinine level as well as clearance are obtained before the procedure. Apparent coagulopathies (INR > 1.5, platelets < 50,000/µL) should be corrected before the procedure. Conscious sedation and antibiotic prophylaxis may be used at the discretion of the operator.

The procedure is then most often performed with the patient in a supine position under fluoroscopy guidance in an angiography suite under cardiac and blood pressure monitoring. In the commonly used approach, the right neck of the patient is exposed and the head turned away from the side of puncture. Iodine solution or chlorhexidine are then used for skin disinfection, and the skin is covered with a sterile drape. Access via the right internal jugular vein is common because this vein, in contrast to the left internal jugular vein, or even more rarely the external jugular veins, offers almost direct continuation into the superior vena cava, right atrium, and inferior vena cava.[14-16] Access

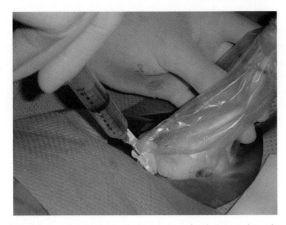

FIGURE 63-2. Ultrasound-guided puncture of right internal jugular vein.

through the femoral vein is rarely used, technically more difficult, and will not be discussed here.

After local anesthesia, the vein is then punctured under ultrasound guidance, following the technique of Seldinger (Fig. 63-2).[17] For better venous filling during puncture of the internal jugular vein, the table is placed in moderate Trendelenburg position. Via a 7F transjugular vascular sheath, a hydrophilic guidewire (e.g., Glidewire [Terumo Medical Corp., Somerset, N.J.]) or a standard Bentson wire (Cook Medical) is then advanced into the inferior vena cava. A 5F multipurpose curved catheter (Cook Medical) is introduced through the sheath and guided into the right hepatic vein.

At this point, measurement of the HVPG may be performed. For this purpose, the catheter is brought into the wedge position. This is ascertained by: (1) the absence of venous reflux, (2) parenchymal filling (Fig. 63-3) after the injection of 2 mL of iodinated contrast media (concentration 300 mg/mL), and (3) a slurping noise occurring due to air suction into the distally sealed/wedged catheter upon removal of the guidewire.

The inserted wire is then exchanged for a 180-cm, 0.035-inch Amplatz Extra Stiff Guidewire (Cook Medical) or, in cases with a more acute angle between the inferior vena cava and liver vein, for a 260-cm Lunderquist guidewire (Cook Medical). Then the 7F catheter with stiffening metal cannula is inserted under fluoroscopic guidance. Through this, a 5F straight catheter is intermittently used to guide the more rigid 7F catheter into the liver vein (Fig. 63-4). The correct position (≈3-4 cm from the inferior vena cava) is documented using a single flush of 5 or 6 mL of iodinated contrast (concentration 300 mg/mL) through the catheter. Because of the favorable orientation of the vessel, mostly the right hepatic lobe is punctured through the right hepatic vein.

With the catheter in place, the transvenous Quick-Core biopsy device is inserted until its tip is flush with the catheter. The tip of the catheter is then turned out of the vein's axis, and the biopsy device is advanced for about 5 mm into the parenchyma. The specimen is acquired using the semi-automated springfire mechanism. Of tremendous importance is a deep puncture site to avoid perforation of the capsule. Up to three samples are obtained and immediately processed for further histologic, cytologic, immunohistochemical, and/or microbiological evaluation as needed.

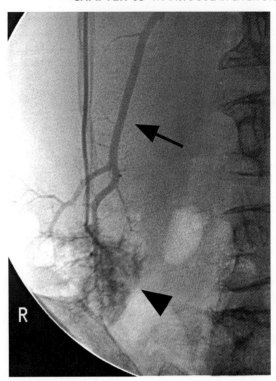

FIGURE 63-3. Fluoroscopic documentation before measuring hepatic venous pressure gradient. Catheter is wedged and 2 mL of contrast media applied. Note resulting parenchymal filling *(arrowhead)* and draining vein *(arrow)*.

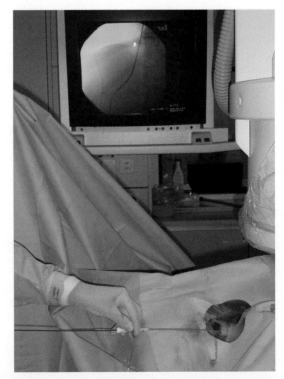

FIGURE 63-4. With 7F catheter and stiffening cannula in right hepatic vein, 5F straight catheter is removed.

The needle containing the tissue specimen is removed. Contrast is injected through the straight catheter to rule out any possible capsular perforation. Catheter, cannula, and sheath are then removed, and local hemostasis is obtained by manual compression.

Technical Aspects

- The right internal jugular vein is by far the most common access vessel. Rarely the left internal jugular vein, external jugular veins, or even femoral veins are used for catheterization.
- For success and especially to avoid potential complications like perforation of the Glisson capsule, careful positioning of the biopsy device in the hepatic vein is mandatory.
- Biopsies are commonly taken out of the right hepatic vein.
- By using limited amounts (<10 mL) of iodinated contrast media (concentration 300 mg/mL), the risk of inducing nephropathy can be minimized.

CONTROVERSIES

Because major bleeding is the most significant and feared complication of percutaneous liver biopsies, so-called plugged biopsy, with immediate embolization of the puncture channel, is performed. Different plugging materials, such as fibrin glue, coils, absorbable gelatin sponge, and Tisseel/Tissucol Fibrin Sealant (Baxter International Inc.; not approved by the U.S. Food and Drug Administration [FDA]), have been used worldwide. In a few studies, plugged biopsy has been shown to be as safe and successful as the transjugular technique.[18] However, stratified prospective comparative studies are lacking. Sawyerr et al. reported a 3.5% (2/56) rate of relevant transfusion-requiring bleeds in the plugged biopsy group, compared to 0% (0/44) in the transjugular access group.[19] Some authors therefore recommend the plugged biopsy only as a backup in cases with impossible or failed transvenous access.[1]

Regarding measurement of HVPG, recent data suggest that comparison of FHVP and WHVP may better reflect prognosis and therapeutic outcome of cirrhosis than the traditional comparison of right atrial pressure with WHVP.[20]

OUTCOMES

- Transjugular liver biopsies successfully obtain liver specimens in 80% to 100% of cases.[13,21,22] Sampled tissue only represents about 1/50,000 of the total liver mass.[3]
- It is mandatory to define standardized criteria, allowing representative tissue sampling. Existing data in the literature offer a broad range of recommendations for optimal tissue sampling. In general, transjugular liver biopsies are diagnostic in 85% to 100% of cases using 18G to 19G needles.[13,21,22] A single study proved that with a single-core and two-core assessment, grading and staging of liver cirrhosis and inflammation was underestimated compared with three-core analysis.[23] Colloredo et al. and Bedossa et al. found liver biopsies of at least 20-mm in size and containing 11 complete portal tracts (CPTs) necessary for evaluation of hepatitis activity.[24,25] However, Cholongitas

et al. were able to gain adequate histologic diagnosis in 89% of cases with smaller specimens (>14 mm) and containing fewer CPTs (>5 CPTs).[26] Regarding optimal specimen size, in a review of 11 series of transjugular liver biopsies, mean core length fell between 10 and 20 mm.[26,27] According to our synthesis of the data, adequate histologic interpretation with reduced sampling errors should be achievable with: (1) 2 to 3 nonfragmented cores, (2) 6 to 11 CPTs, and (3) 15- to 20-mm sample size.

- The duration of transjugular liver biopsies varies between 30 and 60 minutes.[3]
- Using the percutaneous approach, redundant passes with consecutive additional capsular damage are associated with an increased risk of complications.[28] The latter may be reduced by using a coaxial technique. Transjugular liver biopsies with multiple passes, in contrast, can be performed without an increase in complication rate.[29]
- The rate of associated complications is between 1.3% and 20%, with mortality of up to 0.5%.[30,31]

COMPLICATIONS

The mortality rate varies between 0% and (in a few studies) 0.5%.[9,30] The general complication rate varies between 0.1% and 20%.[9,30] Complications most often encountered include neck hematoma, accidental carotid puncture, transient Horner syndrome, and transient dysphonia. Local complications can be minimized with ultrasound guidance.[17] Abdominal pain (13%), transient fever, pneumothorax, and cardiac arrhythmias (10%) may also occur.[3] Rarely, capsular perforation, intraperitoneal hemorrhage, and creation of a fistula between the hepatic vein, hepatic artery, portal vein, or biliary tree are seen.[1,28]

Comparison with the percutaneous approach is difficult because in current practice, patients who undergo transjugular biopsy are often sicker, most often having a relevant coagulopathy.

POSTPROCEDURE AND FOLLOW-UP CARE

Transjugular liver biopsies performed under local anesthesia are well tolerated by the patient. During usual postprocedure care, the patient remains supine for 4 to 6 hours, and vital signs are taken every 30 minutes during this period. If the patient is hemodynamically stable, follow-up creatinine and hemoglobin are obtained the next day before discharge. Results of biopsy specimen analysis (histologic, cytologic, immunohistochemical, and/or microbiological) must be shared with the patient's primary healthcare provider for ongoing follow-up.

KEY POINTS

- Transjugular liver biopsy is a safe and highly effective procedure to obtain diagnostic liver specimens from patients with diffuse liver disease.

- The procedure demands more time and entails greater costs than the gold-standard percutaneous approach. Therefore, in routine practice it functions as a backup procedure for cases in which the percutaneous approach is not feasible or failed.

- Adequate sample size (15-20 mm) and number (2-3 cores) are crucial for successful diagnosis, grading, and staging of the underlying disease.
- The right-sided transjugular approach is superior to access routes via the femoral veins, left internal jugular vein, and external jugular veins.
- Patients undergoing liver biopsies are often suffering from advanced liver disease or malignancy. The overall mortality in one study was 19% within 3 months. This was not influenced by the actual liver biopsy.
- Concomitant measurement of the hepatic venous pressure gradient (HVPG) provides relevant information to assess the risk of esophageal varix bleeding and determine the efficacy of drug treatment in portal hypertension.

▸ **SUGGESTED READINGS**

Bravo AA, Sheth SG, Chopra S. Liver biopsy. N Engl J Med 2001;344: 495–500.

Edmison JM, McCullough AJ. How good is transjugular liver biopsy for the histological evaluation of liver disease? Nat Clin Pract Gastroenterol Hepatol 2007;4:306–7.

McAfee JH, Keeffe EB, Lee RG, Rosch J. Transjugular liver biopsy. Hepatology 1992;15:726–32.

Senzolo M, Burra P, Cholongitas E, et al. The transjugular route: the keyhole to the liver world. Dig Liver Dis 2007;39:105–16.

Sheela H, Seela S, Caldwell C, et al. Liver biopsy: evolving role in the new millennium. J Clin Gastroenterol 2005;39:603–10.

Strassburg CP, Manns MP. Approaches to liver biopsy techniques–revisited. Semin Liver Dis 2006;26:318–27.

The complete reference list is available online at www.expertconsult.com

CHAPTER 64

Chemoembolization for Hepatocellular Carcinoma

Michael C. Soulen

CLINICAL RELEVANCE

Hepatocellular carcinoma (HCC) is a leading cause of morbidity and mortality, ranking fifth for men and eighth for woman as source of primary malignancy.[1,2] The highest incidences of HCC are found in sub-Saharan Africa and Eastern Asia, with age-adjusted incidence rates of 17.43 and 6.77 per 100,000 in men and women of developing countries, compared to 8.71 and 2.86 per 100,000 in men and women of developed regions of the world.[1] However, the incidence of HCC in developed countries, including the United States, has risen significantly in the past 2 decades, in part attributed to the increased prevalence of hepatitis B and C during this same period.[3] Establishing generalizable standards of practice for treatment in HCC is confounded by wide variations in prognostic features present at diagnosis, severity of underlying liver disease, and access to medical services around the world.

Three curative options of resection, liver transplant, and ablation exist as first-line treatment modalities for early HCC, achieving 5-year survival rates of 50% to 70%.[4] Arterial embolization techniques are primary therapy for more advanced stages of HCC in patients who are nonsurgical candidates. At these advanced stages of HCC, chemoembolization has been shown to be an effective palliative therapy that can also improve patient survival.[5,6]

Chemoembolization combines the effects of targeted ischemia with high local chemotherapeutic drug concentration and prolonged drug dwell time in the tumor. Hepatic cancers receive blood primarily from the hepatic artery, in contrast to normal liver, which derives the majority of its blood flow from the portal circulation.[7,8] This is the basis for targeted chemoembolization of tumor cells via the hepatic artery. Lipiodol, a brand of iodized esters of poppyseed oil used as a contrast agent, is selectively retained within tumor cells and serves as the delivery vehicle of the chemotherapy agents. Particle embolization after infusion of the chemotherapy emulsion increases the dwell time of the cytotoxic agents by slowing the rate of their efflux from the hepatic circulation. In addition, ischemia causes cell death directly and potentiates intracellular drug uptake by impeding the function of metabolically active cell membrane pumps that normally function to clear cytotoxic chemicals from the cytosol. Because the liver metabolizes most of the chemotherapeutic agents, systemic toxicity is reduced.

Use of traditional iodized oil–drug emulsions in the United States has been challenged in recent years by severe shortages of the powered forms of the drugs used to make the emulsions. Commercial solutions are not concentrated enough for this purpose. An alternative delivery platform uses polymeric embolic microspheres formulated to be able to adsorb chemotherapeutic drugs from solution, then elute them into the liver following tumor embolization. These new drug-eluting beads have been approved for chemoembolization in Europe and can be loaded off-label in the United States. The safety and efficacy of this delivery platform is still under investigation.

Another alternative to Lipiodol chemoembolization is radioembolization with yttrium-90 microspheres. There are no prospective comparative studies of radioembolization and chemoembolization, but retrospective analyses show similar safety and efficacy profiles.

INDICATIONS

Chemoembolization is the most widely used primary treatment for unresectable HCC, with the best outcomes in patients with reasonably preserved liver function (Child-Pugh class A-B [Table 64-1]), Eastern Cooperative Oncology Group (ECOG) performance status of 0 to 1 (Table 64-2), and without macrovascular invasion or extrahepatic spread.[9,10]

There is an additional neoadjuvant role for chemoembolization as a therapy for those awaiting liver transplantation. Neoadjuvant treatment may decrease the risk of tumor progression outside of criteria that would preclude liver transplantation.[5,11,12]

CONTRAINDICATIONS

The only absolute contraindication to chemoembolization is decompensated baseline liver function. Patients at high risk of acute liver failure include those with greater than 50% replacement of liver by tumor, a lactate dehydrogenase level above 425 IU/L, aspartate aminotransferase (AST) level above 100 IU/L, and total bilirubin level above 2 mg/dL.[13] Relative contraindications include those unlikely to benefit from therapy due to poor prognosis, such as widely metastatic disease, Child-Pugh class C liver disease, or decompensated performance status (ECOG 3-4). Patients at risk for liver failure include those with markedly elevated bilirubin, hepatic encephalopathy, transjugular intrahepatic portosystemic shunt (TIPS), main portal vein occlusion, or hepatofugal portal blood flow.[6] In these settings, segmental or subsegmental chemoembolization may be performed. Chemoembolization in the setting of biliary stenting, sphincterotomy, or bilioenteric anastomosis increases the risk of abscess formation.[14] Portal vein thrombosis can be managed by adjustment of the embolization protocol to limit the degree of embolization and distribution of chemotherapeutic agent[15] or by documenting sufficient hepatic collateral flow is present to compensate for lack of portal flow.[16] Contraindications to the angiographic procedure include anaphylactoid contrast media allergy, renal insufficiency, uncorrectable coagulopathy, and peripheral vascular disease preventing establishment of arterial access. Contraindications to chemotherapy such as

TABLE 64-1. Child-Pugh Classification of Liver Disease

Parameter	Points Assigned		
	1	*2*	*3*
Ascites	Absent	Slight	Moderate
Bilirubin, mg/dL	≤2	2-3	>3
Albumin, g/dL	>3.5	2.8-3.5	<2.8
Prothrombin time:			
Seconds over control	1-3	4-6	>6
INR	<1.8	1.8-2.3	>2.3
Encephalopathy	None	Grade 1-2	Grade 3-4

Total score of < 7 considered grade A (well-compensated disease), total score of 7-9 considered grade B (significant functional compromise), and total score > 9 considered grade C (decompensated liver disease). *INR*, International normalized ratio.

TABLE 64-2. ECOG Performance Status

Grade	Description
0	Fully active, able to carry on all predisease performance without restriction
1	Restricted in physically strenuous activity but ambulatory and able to carry out work of a light or sedentary nature
2	Ambulatory and capable of self-care but unable to carry out any activities; up and about > 50% of waking hours
3	Capable of only limited self-care, confined to bed or chair > 50% of waking hours
4	Completely disabled; cannot carry on any self-care; totally confined to bed or chair
5	Dead

ECOG, Eastern Cooperative Oncology Group.
From Tuite CM, Sun W, and Soulen MC. General assessment of the patient with cancer for the interventional oncologist. J Vasc Interv Radiol 2006;17:753–8.

severe cytopenias, renal insufficiency, and cardiac dysfunction may preclude treatment.[6,17]

EQUIPMENT

- Fluoroscopic unit capable of digital subtraction angiography (DSA) of sufficient quality to carefully evaluate the visceral vasculature, preferably equipped with cone-beam computed tomography (CT) capability
- Visceral catheters/wires:
  - A 4F hydrophilic Cobra catheter and hydrophilic guidewire suffice for about half of procedures.
  - Standard reverse-curve visceral catheters (Simmons, SOS, Rosch)
  - Microcatheters 105 to 130 cm in length with 0.025- to 0.027-inch inner lumen are specifically designed for chemoembolization.
  - 0.014- to 0.018-inch guidewires for use with microcatheters
- Contrast agent and oil suspension: Lipiodol
- Chemotherapy agents (e.g., doxorubicin, epirubicin, cisplatin, mitomycin-C)
- Embolization agents: 100- to 300-μm spherical embolic particles

TABLE 64-3. Sample Admission Orders

ADMIT TO: Interventional Radiology
DIAGNOSIS:
CONDITION:
VITAL SIGNS: Per routine
ACTIVITY: Ad lib
DIET:
FOLEY TO GRAVITY
STRICT I/O
ADMIT LABS: CBC, PT, PTT, PLATELETS, LIVER FUNCTION TESTS, ELECTROLYTES
IV: Start NS @ 200 mL/h
MEDS:
 Benadryl (diphenhydramine) 50 mg IV × 1
 Ancef (cephazolin) 1 gm IV × 1 (if allergy to PCN, use ciprofloxacin 400 mg IV × 1)
 Flagyl (metronidazole) 500 mg IV × 1
 Zofran (ondansetron) 24 mg IV × 1
 Decadron 10 mg IV × 1

TECHNIQUE

Preoperative Evaluation

- Diagnosis by tissue biopsy or markedly elevated serum α-fetoprotein (AFP) associated with a growing mass in a cirrhotic liver with imaging characteristics of HCC (arterial enhancement, venous washout, pseudocapsule)
- Cross-sectional imaging of the liver with dynamic contrast enhancement to define the size and segmental location of tumor(s) within the liver and evaluate the hepatic vasculature and biliary tree
- Exclusion of significant extrahepatic disease with chest, abdomen, and pelvic cross-sectional imaging
- Laboratory studies including complete blood cell count (CBC), international normalized ratio (INR), creatinine, hepatic function, and AFP level
- Clinical assessment for performance status, comorbidities, and informed consent

Preprocedure

In the 12 hours prior to surgery, patients are given nothing by mouth and can be admitted the morning of the procedure. Sample admitting orders can be found in Table 64-3. A Foley catheter may be inserted, and hydration is initiated with normal saline at 200 to 300 mL/h. Prophylactic antibiotics (cephazolin 1 g and metronidazole 500 mg), antiemetics (ondansetron 24 mg), Decadron 10 mg, and diphenhydramine 50 mg are administered intravenously. In the setting of a bilioenteric anastomosis or biliary stent, the patient receives 2 days of oral levofloxacin and metronidazole and a preprocedure bowel prep with oral neomycin-erythromycin.

Procedure

Thorough diagnostic visceral arteriography—including celiac, superior mesenteric, and selective right hepatic, left hepatic, and (if needed) left gastric arteriogram—is performed to define the hepatic vasculature and document portal vein flow to the liver.[18] Visualization of the celiac

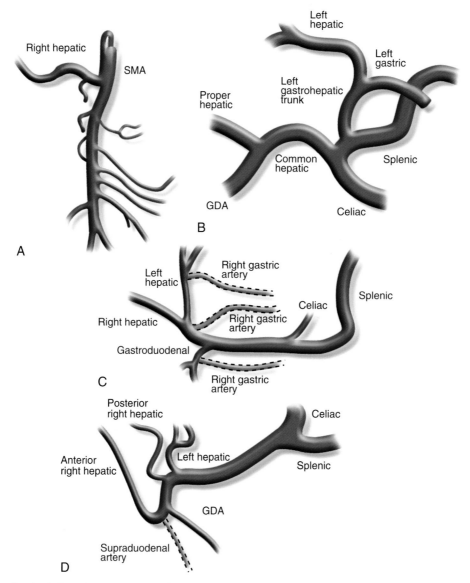

FIGURE 64-1. **A,** Replaced right hepatic artery originating from superior mesenteric artery *(SMA)* axis. **B,** Accessory left hepatic artery originating from left gastric artery. **C,** Right gastric artery origination from variable anatomic locations. **D,** Variable gastroduodenal and supraduodenal artery origination from right hepatic branch. *GDA,* Gastroduodenal artery. *(Redrawn from the Society of Interventional Radiology 2004 Annual Scientific Meeting Workshop Book, p. 402.)*

artery and superior mesenteric artery (SMA) distributions, particularly the right gastric and supraduodenal arteries, is essential to avoid infarction of the stomach or small bowel. Figure 64-1 shows several celiac artery and SMA anatomic variations. Accessory or replaced hepatic arteries are common and must be selectively catheterized beyond any gastric or mesenteric branches in the process of embolization (Fig. 64-2, *A*). The cystic artery often originates off the right hepatic artery (Fig. 64-2, *B*), and chemoembolization proximal to its takeoff may cause a sterile ischemic and/or chemical cholecystitis, which is a risk factor for increased severity and duration of a postembolization syndrome.[19] Hypervascular tumors may lead to reversal of flow in the gastroduodenal artery (GDA), such that SMA injection will fill the hepatic artery via the enlarged GDA, mimicking a replaced right hepatic artery, whereas celiac injection will fail to opacify the GDA because of the flow reversal. It is essential to place the catheter tip past the origin of the GDA

to avoid nontarget embolization of the bowel once the tumor is embolized and direction of flow normalizes. Peripheral hypervascular tumors may parasitize blood supply from extrahepatic collaterals originating from the inferior phrenics, intercostals, lumbars, internal mammaries, mesenteric, epiploic, splenic, pancreatic, and cystic arteries. Prior hepatic embolization predisposes to this. Clues would be failure of the tumor to completely opacify during hepatic angiography, and oily embolization or follow-up cross-sectional imaging showing viable tumor. Chemoembolization can be performed through these collaterals so long as superselective catheterization can be obtained with avoidance of nontarget tissues normally supplied by the vessels. Alternatively, given the high risk of nontarget embolization, bland embolization can be performed.

The next step is superselective catheterization of the hepatic artery supplying the tumor. A 4F hydrophilic Cobra catheter used with a hydrophilic guidewire is successful in

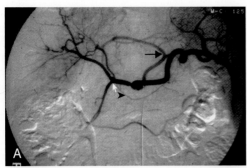
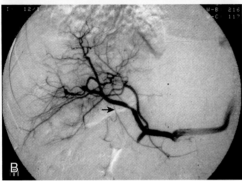

FIGURE 64-2. A, Celiac injection in a patient with metastatic colon cancer illustrates critical anatomic variants and nontarget structures: a large accessory left hepatic arising from left gastric artery *(black arrow)*, trifurcation of common hepatic artery, with no proper hepatic segment *(white arrow)*, and right gastric artery arising from segment IV branch *(black arrowhead)*. **B,** Catheter has been advanced selectively into right hepatic artery for chemoembolization. Selective injection now shows a prominent cystic artery not seen on celiac injection *(black arrow)*. Catheter should be advanced beyond this prior to injecting chemoembolic emulsion.

about half of the cases. The standard 0.035- to 0.038-inch lumen catheter rapidly injects the chemoembolic emulsion and is unlikely to clog with particles. However, its use should be restricted in vessels of less than twice this diameter to avoid partial occlusion of the vessel by the catheter and subsequent pseudostasis. There are microcatheters with slightly larger lumens and shorter overall length designed for hepatic chemoembolization of small vessels and branches that cannot be accessed with standard-sized angiographic catheters.

Repeat arteriography is done once the catheter tip is positioned in the vessel to confirm the anatomy prior to injection of chemoembolic material. Selective injection may reveal anatomy previously not noted, such as cystic, right gastric, or falciform arteries arising from the target hepatic artery, or guidewire-induced spasm in the target artery. For this purpose, high-flow microcatheters can be power injected at 5 mL/s after lowering the pressure threshold on the injector to 800 psi. Cone-beam CT can be a useful adjunctive imaging technique at this stage to better define the perfused territory, identify feeding vessels, and evaluate for both the completeness of coverage of the target tumor volume and the presence of nontarget perfusion.

With the anatomy defined, the next step is injection of the chemotherapy emulsion, followed by injection of embolic particles. Although no chemotherapeutic agent has proven superiority, an example regimen is 100 to 150 mg

cisplatin, 50 mg doxorubicin, and 10 mg mitomycin-C dissolved in 10 mL of radiographic contrast. Typically, 2.5 mL of chemotherapy solution is emulsified with 2.5 mL of oil to create 5-mL aliquots to be injected into the hepatic vessel. This can be done using polycarbonate or glass syringes and a metal stopcock. The exact ratio of chemotherapeutic solution and oil can be adjusted depending upon the size and vascularity of the target tumor(s). For very vascular tumors, a ratio of two parts oil to one part chemo solution maybe appropriate. By breaking up the total dose in to 3 to 4 aliquots of 5 mL each, the oil/chemo ratio can be adjusted so as to deliver the entire dose while achieving the desired level of flow reduction. Intraarterial lidocaine (30 mg boluses up to 200 mg total) is injected before and after each aliquot to alleviate pain and spasm during the embolization. The chemoembolization emulsion is injected until slowing of blood flow is achieved, at which point embolic particles (typically 1-2 mL of 100- to 300-μm spherical embolics) are added to the final 5-mL aliquot. The endpoint is a "tree in winter" appearance, with elimination of the tumor blush but preservation of flow in the lobar and segmental arteries to allow repeat treatment in the future. The catheter itself holds 1 to 1.5 mL of emulsion, so the final flush of the catheter must be taken into account when assessing the desired endpoint to avoid complete stasis.

The technique for chemoembolization with drug-eluting beads is in evolution, but current recommendations include slow infusion (1 mL/min) of a very dilute suspension (20-30 mL), with avoidance of complete stasis. Since the beads are not radiopaque, extra caution must be employed to avoid nontarget embolization.

Postprocedure Care

After the procedure, hydration is continued with normal saline (3 L/24 h), and intravenous antibiotic and antiemetic therapies are continued. Narcotics, chlorpromazine, and acetaminophen are additionally supplied to control pain, nausea, and fever, respectively. If employed, the Foley catheter is removed early the next morning, assuming urine output is adequate. Discharge can occur once the patient has resumed adequate oral intake, parenteral narcotics are no longer required for pain control, and he/she has voided after catheter removal. Some 60% to 90% of patients suffer from a postembolization syndrome of pain, fever, nausea, and vomiting lasting from several hours to a few days.[13] About 50% of patients can be discharged within 1 day, and almost all by 2 days. Oral antibiotics are continued for an additional 5 days (2 weeks for patients with biliary-enteric anastomosis or stent), as are antiemetics and oral narcotics as needed. Laboratory studies are repeated in 3 weeks to assess recovery of liver function, hematologic or renal toxicity, and change in tumor markers when appropriate.

Repeat Embolization

Depending on the location of the tumor and the hepatic arterial anatomy, repeat procedures can occur in other segments or lobes within 3 to 4 weeks in patients with preserved liver function. A patient typically undergoes 2 to 4 chemoembolization procedures to treat the entire tumor burden, after which response is assessed by repeat imaging, clinical assessment, and tumor markers.

COMPLICATIONS

The complication rate of chemoembolization is reported at approximately 4%.[9] Major complications include hepatic insufficiency or infarction, hepatic abscess, biliary necrosis, tumor rupture, surgical cholecystitis, and nontarget embolization. Rarer toxicities include cardiac events, renal insufficiency, and anemia, with incidences of less than 1% each. Thirty-day mortality is approximately 1%.

OUTCOMES

The primary outcome assessed following chemoembolization is patient survival time, but secondary outcomes have been analyzed as measures of success, including objective response (size reduction, fraction of tumor necrosis, Lipiodol retention rate), biological response (decrease in AFP), quality of life, and symptomatic improvement. Case-control retrospective and longitudinal cohort studies have demonstrated the benefit of chemoembolization on patient survival, but there is a paucity of randomized controlled trials (RCTs) to confirm definitive clinical value. Two randomized trials[5,6] found a modest survival benefit with chemoembolization treatment of HCC and a meta-analysis of RCTs from 1978-2002 comparing chemoembolization to conservative treatment[20] concluded there was a significant benefit in 2-year survival with chemoembolization but none with embolization alone. The best survival benefits in chemoembolization are achieved when patients are well selected, as delineated in the indications for treatment given earlier. Three-year survival in these patients may exceed 50%.[4]

CONTROVERSIES

No consensus exists on the most efficacious chemotherapeutic or embolic agents for chemoembolization. Doxorubicin, mitomycin, and cisplatin are the commonly used antitumoral drugs. Centers in the United States most often use cisplatin alone or a mixture of cisplatin, doxorubicin, and mitomycin-C (CAM). The two RCTs that demonstrated increased survival benefit administered doxorubicin in one trial and cisplatinum in the other. However, RCTs directly comparing cytotoxic agents have shown no significant increases in survival relative to each other.[21,22] For the embolization arm of the procedure, no evidence supports the use of one particulate agent or size over another.

Optimal retreatment schedule remains an area of debate. A 2- to 3-week interval between treatment sessions is ideal for prevention of tumor regrowth, but there is risk of ischemia-induced liver failure with such a short treatment interval. The RCTs that demonstrated survival benefit used a mean retreatment schedule of 1 to 4.5 treatments, and current recommendations are for 3 to 4 chemoembolization sessions per year in patients with preserved liver function.[4]

In the controversy of the efficacy of chemoembolization versus embolization alone, the meta-analysis done by Llovet and Bruix[20] showed survival benefit with chemoembolization but not embolization alone. However, studies directly comparing the two treatment modalities have not shown survival advantages in the chemoembolization arm of treatment.[23,24] This suggests the modest survival advantages produced in current studies have to be strengthened with additional RCTs with larger patient populations to achieve the necessary power to establish definitive results and recommendations.

KEY POINTS

- Hepatocellular carcinoma (HCC) is prevalent worldwide, with increasing incidence in developed nations.
- Chemoembolization has a role in the treatment of unresectable HCC as a palliative therapy with potential to increase survival time and as neoadjuvant therapy to prevent tumor progression in patients awaiting liver transplantation.
- Further randomized controlled trials are needed to address the issue of the most advantageous intraarterial therapy and treatment course for advanced HCC.

▶ **SUGGESTED READINGS**

Bruix J, Sherman M. AASLD guideline: management of hepatocellular carcinoma: an update. Hepatology 2011;53:1020–2.

Liu DM, Salem R, Bui JT, et al. Angiographic considerations in patients undergoing liver-directed therapy. J Vasc Interv Radiol 2005;16: 911–35.

Llovet JM, Bruix J. A systematic review of randomized trials for unresectable hepatocellular carcinoma chemoembolization improves survival. Hepatology 2003;37:429–42.

The complete reference list is available online at www.expertconsult.com.

CHAPTER 65

Radioembolization for Hepatocellular Carcinoma

Eleni Liapi and Jean-François H. Geschwind

INTRODUCTION

Conventional external radiotherapy has been limited and unsatisfactory for hepatocellular carcinoma (HCC), primarily because the liver has a low irradiation tolerance.[1] The introduction of three-dimensional conformal radiotherapy (3D-CRT) and other computerized treatment planning techniques have significantly increased the use of radiation therapy in patients with unresectable HCC; however, radiation-induced liver disease (RILD) remains a major complication even when using 3D-CRT.[2,3]

Intraarterial injection of radioembolic microspheres into the tumor vessels has evolved as a promising answer to the challenge of delivering high-dose radiation to liver tumors while limiting dose to the uninvolved liver. By exploiting HCC's preferential blood supply by the hepatic artery, radioembolization combines delivery of internal radiation to the tumor and concomitant microembolization of small intratumoral blood vessels. This chapter is focused on the two most commonly employed radioembolization methods for palliation of unresectable HCC: yttrium-90 (^{90}Y) microsphere embolization and iodine-131 (^{131}I)-Lipiodol embolization.

YTTRIUM-90 (^{90}Y) RADIOACTIVE MICROSPHERES

Clinical Relevance

The treatment of unresectable liver cancer with intraarterial injection of ceramic ^{90}Y microspheres was first introduced in the 1960s.[4,5] Early studies focused mainly on treating colorectal liver metastases, but further experience and encouraging results led to the application of ^{90}Y microsphere embolization in patients with HCC.[6-8] Currently, there are two types of commercially available radioactive microspheres:

- ^{90}Y glass microspheres (TheraSphere [Nordion Inc., Ottawa, Ontario, Canada.])
- ^{90}Y glass resin-based microspheres (SIR-Spheres [Sirtex Medical Inc., Lake Forest, Ill.])

They both contain ^{90}Y as the active particle but differ in the type of carrier. ^{90}Y can be produced by bombardment of stable ^{89}Y with neutrons in a nuclear reactor. This radioactive product is a pure β emitter (937 kiloelectron volts [keV]) that decays to stable ^{90}Zr, with a half-life of 64.2 hours. Emitted electrons have an average tissue penetration of 2.5 mm (effective max. 10 mm). One gigabecquerel (27 millicuries [mCi]) of ^{90}Y per kilogram of tissue provides a dose of 50 Gy.

^{90}Y glass microspheres (TheraSphere) are nonbiodegradable insoluble microspheres that contain ^{90}Y in a glass matrix. ^{90}Y cannot leak out from this glass matrix.

TheraSphere microspheres have a mean diameter of 25 ± 10 μm and 1 mg contains between 22,000 and 73,000 microspheres (Fig. 65-1). TheraSphere is supplied in 0.6 mL of sterile, pyrogen-free water contained in a 1-mL V-bottom vial secured within a clear acrylic vial shield. TheraSphere is available in six dose sizes: 3 GBq (81 mCi), 5 GBq (135 mCi), 7 GBq (189 mCi), 10 GBq (270 mCi), 15 GBq (405 mCi), and 20 GBq (540 mCi). Each dose of ^{90}Y microspheres is supplied with an administration set that facilitates infusion of the microspheres from the dose vial (see later discussion). The intended dose of radiation to the targeted area ranges between 125 and 150 Gy (12,500-15,000 rads). Following intraarterial injection, TheraSphere microspheres embolize at the arteriole level. Histologic studies have shown increased accumulation of ^{90}Y microspheres along the vascular periphery of the hepatic tumor, and up to 50 or 60 times more than in normal liver parenchyma.[9] After lodging in the distal arteriolar circulation, the microspheres emit β radiation that penetrates tissue a maximum effective 10 mm, thereby sparing normal liver parenchyma beyond this limit. Radiation essentially ceases 10 days after embolization, but even before that it poses no threat to others.

Utilization of ^{90}Y glass microspheres for intraarterial treatment of hepatic malignancies was initially approved in Canada in 1991. In 1999, a Humanitarian Device Exemption (HDE) was granted by the U.S. Food and Drug Administration (FDA) for treatment of unresectable HCC with ^{90}Y microspheres, and their clinical use was initiated in the United States; some 800 patients with HCC have been treated since then.

The second type of ^{90}Y microspheres (SIR-Spheres) is biocompatible, non degradable, and resin-based, with a diameter of 29 to 35 μm (Fig. 65-2). SIR-Spheres have an average activity of 40 Bq per sphere and can be suspended in sterile water and contrast media to the desired total activity. Compared with glass microspheres (specific activity of 2467 Bq per glass microsphere), resin microspheres have much lower specific activity per sphere. SIR-Spheres were granted premarket approval by the FDA in 2002 for treating unresectable metastatic liver tumors from primary colorectal cancer, in conjunction with adjuvant floxuridine-based chemotherapy administered via the hepatic artery. Most clinical trials for treatment of unresectable HCC with SIR-Spheres have been conducted in Australia, Hong Kong, and Europe.[10-12] Since the radioactive element is the same as that of glass microspheres, tissue penetration and decay characteristics are identical. Characteristics of the two devices are compared in Table 65-1. The radioactivity of ^{90}Y delivered is dependent on the volume of liver and adjusted for shunting to the gastrointestinal (GI) tract and lungs based on estimates of flow from a technetium-99 (^{99}Tc)-macroaggregated albumin scan.

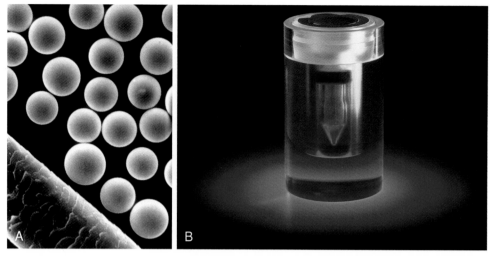

FIGURE 65-1. A, Magnified view (EM picture) of ^{90}Y glass microspheres (TheraSphere) compared to size of a hair. ^{90}Y glass microspheres are non-biodegradable microspheres that contain ^{90}Y in a glass matrix from which the yttrium is unable to leak out. Their mean diameter is 25 ± 5 μm and 1 mg contains between 22,000 and 73,000 microspheres. **B,** The ^{90}Y glass microsphere dose is supplied in 0.6 mL of sterile pyrogen-free water contained in a 1-mL vial with a V-shaped bottom secured within a clear acrylic vial shield. *(Courtesy Nordion Inc., Ottawa, Ontario, Canada.)*

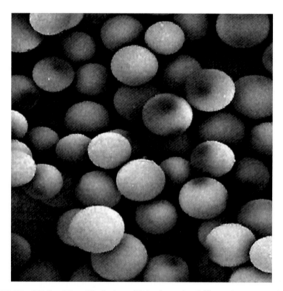

FIGURE 65-2. Magnified view (EM picture) of ^{90}Y resin microspheres (SIR-Spheres). *(Courtesy SIR-Spheres, Sirtex Medical Inc., Lake Forest, Ill.)*

TABLE 65-1. Characteristics of ^{90}Y Microspheres (Glass vs. Resin)

	Glass Microspheres	Resin-Based Microspheres
Mean number of spheres per dose	4×10^6	50×10^6
Specific gravity	3.7 g/cm^{-3}	1.6 g/cm^{-3}
Specific activity	2467 Bq/microsphere	40 Bq/microsphere
FDA approval category	HDE	Premarket approval
Dose variation with tumor volume	No	Yes
Hepatopulmonary shunt upper limit (%)	10	20
Suspension medium	Normal saline	Sterile water

FDA, U.S. Food and Drug Administration; *HDE,* Humanitarian Device Exemption.

PATIENT SELECTION AND PREPARATION

In an institutional setting, a multidisciplinary panel consisting of interventional radiologists, medical and surgical oncologists, radiation oncologists, hepatologists, pathologists, and transplant surgeons may review patients' eligibility for treatment with ^{90}Y microspheres. Pretreatment evaluation always includes a routine clinical history, physical examination, complete blood cell count, blood biochemical analysis (including liver and renal function), and an α-fetoprotein assay. Selection criteria are similar to those for transcatheter arterial chemoembolization (TACE) and are listed in Table 65-2. Functional status is assessed by the Eastern Cooperative Oncology Group (ECOG)

TABLE 65-2. Selection Criteria for Radioembolization

Adequate hematologic profile (granulocyte count ≥ 1.5×10^9/L; platelets ≥ 60×10^9/L)
Adequate renal function (creatinine < 2.0 mg/dL)
Adequate liver function (serum bilirubin < 2.0 mg/dL; aspartate aminotransferase, alanine aminotransferase, and alkaline phosphatase values < 5 times the upper limit of normal)
Bulk disease representing < 70% tumor replacement of liver
Tumor representing < 50% replacement of liver with an albumin level < 3.0 g/dL
Lymph node–limited extrahepatic HCC metastases
Eastern Cooperative Oncology Group score of 0 to 2
Uncompromised pulmonary function
No prior external beam radiation therapy

HCC, Hepatocellular carcinoma.

performance status. Okuda stage and Child-Pugh score should also be obtained before treatment. Pretreatment imaging may include a triple-phase contrast-enhanced spiral computed tomography (CT) scan of the abdomen, chest, and pelvis and/or contrast-enhanced magnetic resonance imaging (MRI) of the abdomen and pelvis to identify extrahepatic disease and calculate tumor and liver volumes. At our institution, the standard imaging workup includes a baseline gadolinium-enhanced MRI scan of the liver and abdomen, with diffusion/perfusion sequences for thoroughly assessing baseline tumor imaging characteristics as well as disease status.

Prophylactic therapy with gastric acid inhibitors on the day of treatment is highly recommended and has resulted in substantial reduction of associated GI symptoms.

Preoperative Planning

Pretreatment Visceral Angiography and ^{99m}Tc-Labeled Macroaggregated Albumin Injection

The purpose of performing baseline celiac and hepatic angiography is to define the vascular anatomy, plan a tailored treatment, and detect possible extrahepatic shunting. Prophylactic coil embolization of the gastroduodenal artery (GDA)—and/or any other collateral vessel or gastric variant (e.g., right gastric artery and its pancreaticoduodenal branches) that may result in microspheres being lodged into the GI area—is of no clinical consequence and highly recommended, since nontargeted delivery of ^{90}Y microspheres to the GI tract can cause substantial morbidity. If the radioactive microspheres are planned to be injected from either the right or left hepatic artery (lobar treatments) and the tip of the catheter is placed far enough from the origin of the GDA, prophylactic GDA occlusion may not be necessary.

Accessory branches that contribute to the tumor vascular bed should also be readily identified because more treatments may be necessary, and the amount of radioactivity to be delivered must be calculated to include the relative contribution of each vessel to the liver volume to be treated. For instance, in the presence of a middle hepatic artery, which usually arises from the right hepatic artery, delivery of ^{90}Y to the segment supplied by the middle hepatic artery may be precluded despite accurate catheter placement, given the flow dynamics. Therefore, three treatments (one each to the right, middle, and left hepatic arteries) may be necessary to cover the entire liver. Another example might include a patient with an accessory right hepatic artery, necessitating a third treatment (left hepatic [segments II-IV], right hepatic [segments V/VIII], and accessory right hepatic [segments VI/VII]).

Direct arteriovenous intratumoral shunting is common in HCC, so ^{90}Y microspheres may shunt to the lungs, resulting in radiation-induced pneumonitis, with significant morbidity and possible mortality when the total lung dose approaches 30 to 50 Gy. Assessment of possible shunting to the lungs is therefore crucial *before* initiating treatment. A metastable technetium-99 (^{99m}Tc) macroaggregated albumin (^{99m}Tc-MAA) scan is performed after injecting ^{99m}Tc-MAA through the relevant hepatic artery (where treatment will be targeted) at the time of the pretreatment angiogram to calculate the percent radiation that might go to the lungs.

The size of these albumin microspheres is 30 to 50 μm, which closely resembles the size of ^{90}Y microspheres, so their injection may be similar to the distribution of ^{90}Y microspheres. If activity is noted in the lungs, a *shunt fraction* is calculated as the ratio of the lung counts to the total counts. ^{99m}Tc-MAA scans cannot effectively demonstrate flow to the GI tract, and this drawback has been attributed to the much lower density of MAA particles ($\approx$1.3 g/cm^{-3}) than glass microspheres (3.7 g/cm^{-3}). Overall, ^{99m}Tc-MAA provides a better simulation for resin-type microspheres (density 1.6 g/cm^{-3}) than the glass type.

Radiation Dosimetry

It bears noting here that patients in whom the hepatopulmonary shunt fraction is greater than 10% of the injected dose with glass microspheres and greater than 20% with resin-based microspheres, or in whom the shunt fraction indicates potential exposure of the lung to an absorbed radiation dose of more than 30 Gy should *not* be considered for treatment with ^{90}Y microspheres (Fig. 65-3).

For the complete discussion of radiation dosimetry and the calculations involved, please visit www.expertconsult.com.

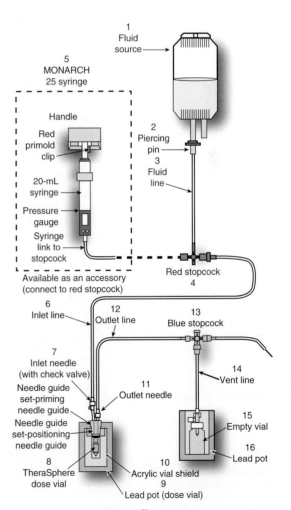

FIGURE 65-3. Diagram showing ^{90}Y glass microspheres administration set. Essential components (listed as numbers) of the ^{90}Y glass microspheres administration system are listed in Table 65-4.

CONTRAINDICATIONS

^{90}Y microsphere embolization is contraindicated in patients who present with:

- Concurrent malignancy
- Vascular abnormalities, bleeding diathesis, or portal vein thrombosis (PVT) (contraindications for catheterization)
- Severe liver dysfunction or pulmonary insufficiency
- History of prior external beam radiation
- Evidence of any uncorrectable flow to the GI tract
- Predicted risk of over 30 Gy (0.61 GBq, 16.5 mCi) from a single treatment or an accumulated dose of 50 Gy to be delivered to the lungs

Pretreatment high-risk factors have recently been identified and include:

- Infiltrative type of tumor
- Bulk disease representing at least 70% tumor replacement of liver
- Tumor representing at least 50% replacement of liver with an albumin level below 3.0 g/dL
- Aspartate aminotransferase (AST) or alanine aminotransferase (ALT) higher than 5 times upper normal limit
- Bilirubin higher than 2 mg/dL

A recent study has shown that ^{90}Y microspheres can be used safely in patients with portal circulation compromised at the level of the first-order portal branches.[13] Prior intraarterial liver-directed treatment or systemic chemotherapy is not considered a contraindication to radioembolization.

EQUIPMENT

The catheterization set used for radioembolization is listed in Table 65-3. The TheraSphere Administration Set consists of a sterile disposable tubing set and one empty sterile vial. The tubing set is made of preassembled sterile components and is for single use only. The preassembled tubing set contains a needle plunger assembly and an integrated 20-mL syringe. The essential components of the ^{90}Y glass microspheres administration system are listed in Table 65-4. The syringe and red stopcock control the flow of the fluid carrier to the dose vial, causing the microspheres to be transported through the outlet line to the catheter. The blue stopcock permits the delivery system to be purged of air and primed with fluid in preparation for the infusion of microspheres. It is crucial to carefully assemble the delivery kit; any error during setup may lead to misadministration. It is also very important to ensure that the connections to the saline bag, syringe, and inlet and outlet lines are tight so the system is sealed and can maintain a constant pressure.

TECHNIQUE

Anatomy and Approach

^{90}Y microspheres can be delivered through the hepatic artery segmentally, subsegmentally, regionally, or to the whole liver, depending on the distribution of HCC, making this approach suitable for focal and diffuse HCC, as well as for patients with prior hepatectomy.

After informed consent is obtained, access is achieved into the right (or left) common femoral artery, and an aortogram and celiac and superior mesenteric arteriograms are performed to delineate the vascular supply to the tumor and select the relevant feeding artery. The superior mesenteric arteriogram is carried well into the venous phase to check for patency of the portal vein. Anatomic variants such as an accessory and/or replaced right or left hepatic artery or a common origin of the left hepatic and left gastric artery are common (up to 20%-30%) and may become complicating factors because they increase the risk of nontarget embolization (Fig. 65-5). If ^{90}Y microsphere treatment cannot be given safely because of left or right gastric or gastroduodenal vascular anatomic relationships, one should consider coil embolizing these vessels and then proceed with ^{90}Y microsphere embolization. After the catheter is accurately positioned within the hepatic artery corresponding to the desired treatment target area, the ^{90}Y

TABLE 65-3. List of Materials Needed for Radioembolization

Item
5F vascular sheath
Bentson wire
5F pigtail catheter
5F Simmons-1 catheter, glide
0.35 Terumo Glidewire
3F microcatheter (i.e., Renegade) if needed
Microcatheter wire (i.e., Transend)
Chemotherapy-resistant three-way stopcocks

TABLE 65-4. ^{90}Y Glass Microsphere Administration Set

Item	Number Corresponding to Fig. 65-3
Fluid source	1
Piercing pin	2
Fluid line	3
Red stopcock	4
MONARCH 25 syringe	5
Inlet line	6
Inlet needle (with check valve)	7
TheraSphere dose vial	8
Lead pot (dose vial)	9
Acrylic vial shield	10
Outlet needle	11
Outlet line	12
Blue stopcock	13
Vent line	14
Empty vial	15
Lead pot	16
Needle guide set-priming needle guide	17
Needle guide set-positioning needle guide	18
Pinch clamp	19

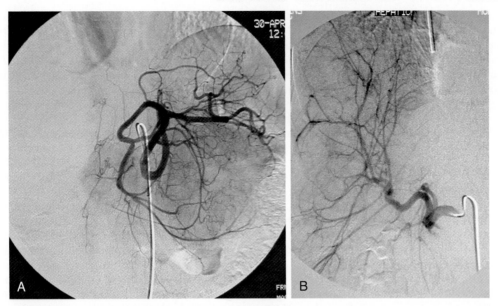

FIGURE 65-5. Digital subtraction angiographic views of celiac axis **(A)** and proper hepatic artery **(B)** during an evaluation angiogram of a radioembolization candidate demonstrate a replaced proper hepatic artery arising separately from the aorta.

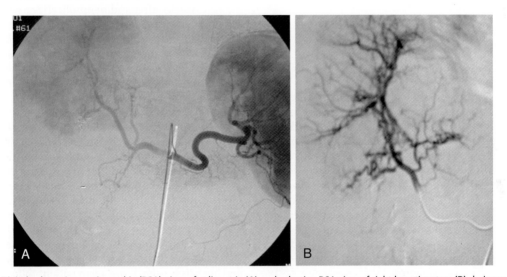

FIGURE 65-6. Digital subtraction angiographic (DSA) view of celiac axis **(A)** and selective DSA view of right hepatic artery **(B)** during a radioembolization procedure in a patient with HCC. After catheter was accurately positioned within right hepatic artery in proximity to tumor, ^{90}Y microspheres were safely administered.

microspheres can be safely administered (Fig. 65-6). Sufficient pressure should be applied to maintain the spheres in suspension, allowing unimpeded passage through the catheter to the intended target. If necessary, a 3F coaxial system (0.0325 inches or larger) may be used, but use of smaller microcatheter systems is not encouraged because there may be too much outflow resistance to injection, preventing adequate flow rates and particle suspension.

Technical Aspects

Important key points for ^{90}Y glass microspheres administration:
- A catheter with an internal diameter of 0.5 mm (0.020 inch) or greater is required to deliver the

radiospheres to the liver. Excessive resistance to flow in the administration system due to a smaller catheter diameter may cause microspheres to be retained in the blue stopcock of the administration set and in the catheter.
- The catheter should not occlude the vessel in which it is placed.
- For 3F catheters, a syringe pressure of 40 to 60 psi should be maintained for the duration of each flush. Flushing should be continued until optimal delivery of the TheraSphere is achieved. A minimum flush of 160 mL is recommended. Using a flow rate of less than 20 mL/min (i.e., appropriate to the flow of the native vessel) may decrease delivery efficiency of the administration system.

- For 5F catheters, initial flushing using two to three flushes (40-60 mL) at a syringe pressure of 15 to 25 psi may be used. This should be followed by additional flushes, maintaining a syringe pressure of 30 to 50 psi. Flushing should be continued until optimal delivery of ^{90}Y glass microspheres is achieved. A minimum flush of 100 mL is recommended.
- Radiation monitoring of the TheraSphere administration set and catheter must be used to verify when optimal delivery has been achieved.

Radiation Issues

Radiation safety is always of utmost importance. Areas of increased vulnerability are the eyes, skin, and hands. Beta radiation from ^{90}Y can typically travel more than a meter in air but is substantially reduced by less than a centimeter of acrylic. Throughout the administration procedure, the ^{90}Y glass microspheres dose vial remains sealed within the clear acrylic vial shield in which it is supplied. Although the dose vial is shielded in acrylic, the outlet line and catheter are not. Typical surface radiation dose rates from the patient are 4 to 12 mrem/h. These dose ranges are well within the accepted radiation levels for outpatient radiation treatments, and no special precaution is necessary for either inpatients or outpatients.

CLINICAL OUTCOMES

Toxicities and Early Mortality

Post-radioembolization syndrome consists of fatigue, nausea, vomiting, anorexia, fever, abdominal discomfort, and cachexia. The most common adverse effects associated with ^{90}Y microsphere treatment are elevation of bilirubin (34.7%), pain (17.4%), ascites (16.5%), hyperglycemia (16.5%), and transient elevations in liver enzyme levels (16.5%) as a result of tumor lysis, with return to baseline within 2 to 3 weeks after treatment. Other adverse effects include hepatic decompensation and edema, decrease in platelet counts, GI symptoms—including gastritis—and occasionally gastric and duodenal ulcerations (3.8%-13%).[14] Most of the more serious side effects occur after whole-liver administration of ^{90}Y microspheres.

Goin et al. have published two initial studies on risk factors associated with toxicity and early mortality after hepatic administration of arterial ^{90}Y for HCC.[15,16] These studies showed toxicity rates in 118 patients with HCC treated with hepatic arterial ^{90}Y between 1986 and 2003. Interestingly, most of these patients had advanced disease and impaired liver function. Twenty-five patients (21%) were reported to have a major complication resulting in death; 12 were judged to be treatment related. Specific treatment-related toxicities included liver toxicity, pneumonitis, and GI bleeding, with a higher incidence and severity than that suggested by other reports. Risk factors associated with 90-day mortality were also reported in these studies. Seven variables were studied: five liver reserve variables (infiltrative tumor, tumor volume > 70% of liver, tumor volume > 50% of liver, albumin level ≤ 3 g/dL, bilirubin level ≥ 2 mg/dL, AST/ALT levels ≥ 5 times the normal upper limit) and two non–liver reserve variables (lung dose > 30 Gy, non-HCC diagnosis). Patients who had at least one adverse variable (27%) were labeled as being at high risk.

Ninety-day mortality rates were 49% and 7% in the high-risk and low-risk groups, respectively ($P < .001$), and median survival times for the high-risk and low-risk groups were 3.6 months and 15.5 months, respectively ($P < .001$). Of the 12 fatal toxicities related to treatment, 11 were in patients in the high-risk group.

A more detailed analysis of liver toxicities that occurred in the patients at low risk showed that 45% of these patients had bilobar disease, 16% had more than 50% of their liver replaced with tumor, 17% had portal vein compromise, 14% had ascites at presentation, 10% had Child-Pugh class B disease, 33% had Okuda stage II disease, and 16% had CLIP scores greater than 2. Almost half of these patients (42%) developed grade 3 or greater liver toxicity, as defined by the Southwest Oncology Group criteria, but the majority of them (78%) were transient. The most frequent toxicities were ascites, increased bilirubin levels, and increased aminotransferase levels. Increased pretreatment bilirubin levels and radiation dose were associated with increased risk of liver toxicity ($P = .001$ and $P = .08$, respectively). In addition, shorter time between treatments in 23 patients who had two or more ^{90}Y courses was associated with an increased risk of liver toxicity ($P = .05$).

Radiation-induced liver disease usually occurs between 4 and 8 weeks after radioembolization, with an incidence ranging between 0% and 4%. Classic and non-classic RILD may be seen after radioembolization. It has been shown that a single liver radiation dose of 150 Gy is associated with an increased risk of liver toxicities. The biochemical toxicity rates after radioembolization have ranged between 15% and 20%.[17]

The incidence of biliary sequelae after radioembolization is reported to be less than 10%. Atassi et al. reported that less than 2% of patients required intervention for biliary toxicities induced by radioembolization.[18] Radiation-induced cholangitis has also been reported.

A long-term complication of radioembolization is liver fibrosis, resulting in contraction of the hepatic parenchyma and portal hypertension.[19] Liver fibrosis with concurrent portal hypertension is more evident radiologically than clinically, since the clinical signs of portal hypertension (e.g., reduced platelet counts [<100,000/dL], variceal bleeding) are rarely seen. Long-term patient follow-up for clinical evidence of portal hypertension is recommended because this is not an acute process. This finding is more commonly seen with bilobar treatment, and its incidence is increased in patients who have chemotherapy-associated steatohepatitis. The presence of preexisting cirrhosis leading to portal hypertension in most HCC patients makes them more susceptible to aggravation of this complication.

Tumor Response to Treatment

Tumor response to treatment and tumor progression can be assessed by applying the World Health Organization (WHO) tumor response criteria,[20] the Response Evaluation Criteria in Solid Tumors (RECIST),[21] the European Association for the Study of the Liver (EASL) criteria,[22] and National Cancer Institute (NCI) amendments that define how to take tumor necrosis into consideration of response.[23]

Radioembolization has been shown to limit HCC progression. This may help as a bridge to transplantation, allowing patients to wait longer for donor organs.[24] In a study by Hilgard et al., the partial response, stable disease, and progressive disease rates for a group of 62 patients with HCC treated with ^{90}Y glass microsphere radioembolization using the conventional RECIST criteria after 3 months was 16%, 74%, and 10%, respectively.[25]

Overall Survival and Time to Progression

Please visit www.expertconsult.com for the full discussion of outcomes.

POSTPROCEDURE AND FOLLOW-UP CARE

Following ^{90}Y microspheres embolization, patients are transferred to the recovery area for 4 to 6 hours of postangiogram observation and then to the floor for overnight admission. Mild pain and minimal nausea may be controlled with medication and should not prevent the patient's discharge. Upon discharge, patients receive a packet of information containing prescheduled follow-up appointments, prescriptions, emergency and scheduling contact numbers, and radiation safety precautions. Prescribed drugs include ciprofloxacin 500 mg twice daily × 7 days; Compazine 5 to 10 mg every 8 hours as needed for nausea and vomiting; oral oxycodone (20-mg tablets), one tablet twice daily for pain; gastric acid inhibitors; and stool softeners. Mild and self-limiting liver enzyme elevation may be noted but usually is of no clinical significance. A physician assistant or research coordinator typically contacts the patients initially by phone 2 weeks after treatment. At approximately 4 to 6 weeks, the patient is asked to obtain a follow-up imaging study as well as laboratory and tumor marker tests (Figs. 65-7 and 65-8). A brief clinical encounter is then scheduled to evaluate tumor response to treatment and assess the patient's liver function and performance status. Tumor response, performance status, and liver function are the main factors dictating whether further treatment is necessary.

RADIOLABELED LIPIODOL

Clinical Relevance

Lipiodol is a mixture of iodized ethyl esters of the fatty acids of poppyseed oil, containing 37% iodine by weight. It is selectively taken up by hepatic tumors when administered via the hepatic artery and retained by HCC patients for many weeks, even up to a year, whereas it is cleared from the normal or cirrhotic liver within 4 weeks. When injected into the hepatic artery, it traverses the peribiliary plexus to the portal veins, resulting presumably in a dual embolization.[33] Early in the course of investigating Lipiodol's unique features, addition of a radionuclide to this substance gave a new dimension to its clinical use. So far, most clinical research has been performed using ^{131}I-labeled Lipiodol, which is commercially available as Lipiocis (CIS Bio International, Gif sur Yvette, France). [131]I is a β-emitting radionuclide with a physical half-life of 8.04 days. This long half-life has limited use of ^{131}I, since patients must be kept in isolation during initial decay of the radionuclide. The maximum and mean β energies are 0.61 MeV and 0.192 MeV, respectively. [131]I emits a principal γ photon of 364 keV

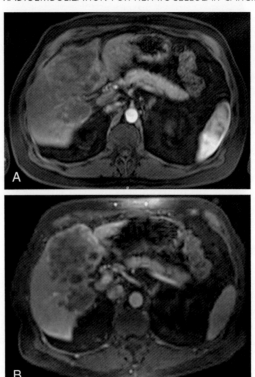

FIGURE 65-7. Magnetic resonance imaging (T1 sequence, arterial phase) before **(A)** and 1 month after **(B)** radioembolization with ^{90}Y glass microspheres in a patient with hepatocellular carcinoma. Note decrease in enhancement of treated lesion following radioembolization, corresponding to favorable response to treatment (50% necrosis without change in size).

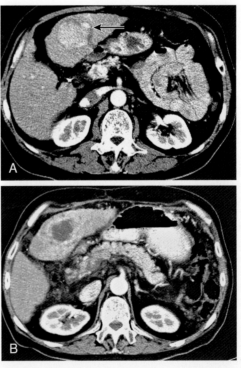

FIGURE 65-8. A, Pretreatment computed tomography (CT) illustrating a 6.8 × 5.8 cm hypervascular lesion *(arrow)*. **B,** CT 3 months post treatment. Lesion exhibits significant necrosis and moderate size decrease. *(From Geschwind JF, Salem R, Carr BL, et al. Yttrium-90 microspheres for the treatment of hepatocellular carcinoma. Gastroenterology 2004;127:S194–S205.)*

(81%). Most (75%-90%) of the administered activity is trapped within the liver 24 hours post administration. It has been reported that after 24 hours, tumor-to-liver uptake ratios range between 2.3 and 12. Tumor and normal liver effective half-lives are 5.5 and 3.5 days, respectively.

Contraindications

Absolute contraindications include pregnancy, breastfeeding, life expectancy less than a month, hepatic encephalopathy, Okuda stage III, and allergy to contrast media. Relative ones are unacceptable medical risk for isolation, uncontrollable coagulopathy, and acute or severe renal failure (creatinine clearance < 30 mL/min).

Equipment

The angiographic set that can be used for injection of ^{131}I-Lipiodol is the same as the one used for radioactive microspheres embolization and is listed in Table 65-2. ^{131}I-Lipiodol is supplied in solution for use at room temperature and may be diluted with 2 to 10 mL unlabeled Lipiodol to increase the total injected volume. A standard activity of 2.22 GBq (60 mCi) ^{131}I-Lipiodol is usually injected slowly via a protected glass or plastic syringe. The activity can be modified according to tumor load or other medical reasons.

Technique

Anatomy and Approach
As in radioembolization with ^{90}Y microspheres, an aortogram and celiac and superior mesenteric arteriograms are initially performed to delineate the vascular supply to the tumor and select the relevant feeding artery. After the catheter is positioned within the hepatic artery corresponding to the desired treatment target area, ^{131}I-Lipiodol can safely be administered. If necessary, a 3F coaxial system (0.0325 inches or larger) may be used.

Technical Aspects
It has been shown that exposure of fingers to radiation is not significantly increased during compression of the puncture site after the procedure. However, if desirable and feasible, a closure device can be used to minimize compression time. The dose to the fingers can be reduced by using a protected syringe with a volume that exceeds the volume of Lipiodol and by holding the syringe at its cold end. The radiologist should stand at the left side of the patient, and compression should be carried out while alternating hands or by a mechanical device if available.

Outcomes

Please visit www.expertconsult.com for the full discussion of outcomes.

Side Effects and Complications

Most reports using ^{131}I-Lipiodol agree on its good tolerance. Early side effects that are observed fairly frequently consist

of moderate and temporary fever (29%), moderate and temporary disturbances of liver function tests (20%), and pain on injection (12.5%). Moderate and reversible leukopenia (7%) and serious diffuse infiltrative pneumopathies (2%) are observed more rarely. These diffuse infiltrative pneumopathies appear about 1 month after the injection and most frequently after the second injection. They are clinically manifested by the appearance of dyspnea, which is sometimes associated with dry cough and bilateral crepitations. The CT scan may show infiltrates that have the appearance of frosted glass, are bilateral, are surrounded by septal thickenings, and may evolve into fibrosis with some honeycomb-like appearance.

Postprocedure and Follow-Up Care

Patients should be admitted to an approved isolation unit with an appropriately shielded room and an in-unit bathroom and must be advised to avoid unnecessary radiation exposure to family members and the public. Pregnancy should be avoided for at least 4 months after treatment. Nursing personnel must be advised on radiation safety. Quantitative whole-body imaging 1 week after treatment is recommended to confirm the distribution of ^{131}I-lipodol. Local and whole-body activity can be expressed as percentage of administered activity and compared with a ^{131}I standard for dosimetry calculations. Based on data from total body scans, the mean decay-corrected percentage of ^{131}I uptake in the total body at 7 days after administration is 72.8%, while uptake in the normal liver, tumor, and lungs is 26.1%, 17.2%, and 11.7%, respectively. After 2 weeks, the total body uptake is 53.1%, and the percentage uptake for normal liver, tumor, and lungs drops to 14.4%, 14.5%, and 7.4%, respectively.

CONCLUSIONS

The efficacy and safety of radioembolization, as with all locoregional and oncology treatments, are dependent on the objectives of treatment, patient selection, the experience of the treating physician, and the periprocedural and continuing clinical care. Current data suggest that radioembolization may show potential clinical benefit in carefully selected patients with unresectable HCC.

KEY POINTS

- Direct intraarterial administration of radioactive embolic material to the feeding vessels of a hepatocellular carcinoma can result in increased effective radioactivity within the tumor without significantly affecting the surrounding liver parenchyma.

- The most commonly used radioembolization materials are ^{90}Y radioactive glass or resin microspheres and ^{131}I-Lipiodol.

▶ **SUGGESTED READINGS**

Geschwind JF, Salem R, Carr BI, et al. Yttrium-90 microspheres for the treatment of hepatocellular carcinoma. Gastroenterology 2004; 127(5 Suppl 1):S194–S205.

Goin JE, Salem R, Carr BI, et al. Treatment of unresectable hepatocellular carcinoma with intrahepatic yttrium 90 microspheres: a risk-stratification analysis. J Vasc Interv Radiol 2005;16(2):195–203.

Goin JE, Salem R, Carr BI, et al. Treatment of unresectable hepatocellular carcinoma with intrahepatic yttrium 90 microspheres: factors associated with liver toxicities. J Vasc Interv Radiol 2005;16(2):205–13.

Lambert B, Van de Wiele C. Treatment of hepatocellular carcinoma by means of radiopharmaceuticals. Eur J Nucl Med Mol Imaging 2005; 32(8):980–9.

Lewandowski RJ, Geschwind JF, Liapi E, Salem R. Transcatheter intraarterial therapies: rationale and overview. Radiology 2011;259(3):641–57.

The complete reference list is available online at www.expertconsult.com.

CHAPTER 66

Embolotherapy for the Management of Liver Malignancies Other Than Hepatocellular Carcinoma

Constantinos T. Sofocleous and Allison S. Aguado

Bland hepatic transcatheter arterial embolization (HAE) and chemoembolization (TACE) are routinely used to treat inoperable hepatocellular carcinoma (HCC)[1,2] and other primary and secondary hepatic malignancies.[2-42] Embolic treatment of hepatic metastases is undertaken when liver disease is dominant, with no or stable extrahepatic disease. The liver is an ideal organ for arterial embolization in managing tumors supplied by the hepatic artery because it affords selective treatment of the tumor and preserves the blood supply to the organ, at least 70% of which originates from the portal system.[1,2] Selective embolization of arterial feeders to the tumor results in ischemia and selective necrosis while sparing the normal liver parenchyma supplied by the portal vein.[1-3] HAE used as sole treatment or combined with chemotherapeutic agents (TACE) is targeted to the hepatic arterial branches feeding the tumor. This is achieved using embolic agents (particles) small enough to reach and occlude the capillaries to the tumor. Addition of chemotherapy to embolization (TACE) was based on the theoretic advantage of delivering concentrated drug to a tumor sensitized by the ischemia caused by embolization. Chemotherapeutic dwell time in the tumor is significantly prolonged, and systemic effects are minimized.[38] To date, no randomized trial has shown any advantage of TACE over HAE,[43] suggesting that the main mechanism of tumor death is the ischemia caused by embolization. Drug-eluting bead (DEB) TACE has been used to treat metastatic colorectal carcinoma, metastatic neuroendocrine tumor, and cholangiocarcinoma. However, there is a lack of standardized comparative data regarding response.[44] A small retrospective single-center series by Ruutiainen et al. concluded that there is a trend (not statistically significant) toward improved survival and tumor and symptom control with TACE when compared to hepatic arterial embolization (HAE).[45] However, the small numbers, the retrospective nature of the study, a significant patient crossover between the groups, and the relatively larger size of the embolic material used for HAE raise important questions regarding the validity of any meaningful interpretation of that study.

Proximal arterial occlusion is not desirable because it will lead to development of intrahepatic collateral vessels that will resupply the tumor.[46] Permanent proximal arterial occlusion (surgical ligation or catheter coil embolization) should never be performed in the management of hepatic tumors because it not only provokes intrahepatic collateral formation but also precludes repeat intervention and embolization (Table 66-1).

INDICATIONS

In general, the selection criteria for patients with HCC apply to patients with other liver malignancies when determining candidates for embolotherapy.[1-3] Patients with unresectable malignant tumors supplied by the hepatic arterial tree will benefit from embolization. The purpose of hepatic embolization is either symptomatic relief or improvement of survival. Indications for HAE include rapid progression of liver disease (in the face of stable or absent extrahepatic disease), symptoms related to tumor bulk, and symptoms related to hormonal excess, especially in the case of neuroendocrine tumors (NETs).[47] In patients with hepatic metastases from colon, breast, and renal cell carcinoma, melanoma, gastrointestinal tumors or sarcomas, or other primaries, embolization is used for control of tumor load involving the liver to improve outcomes. Control of hepatic metastases may allow prolonged survival when compared with patients who do not undergo embolization.[43,46] With the exception of NETs, patients with secondary hepatic disease who have no symptoms related to the hepatic disease but have extrahepatic disease are probably poor candidates for embolization.

CONTRAINDICATIONS

There are a limited number of contraindications to hepatic embolization for treating liver malignancies. Advanced cirrhosis and liver failure are contraindications to embolization in patients with HCC but are relatively rare in patients with other primary or secondary liver malignancies. Extensive and progressive extrahepatic disease is a contraindication to embolization of hepatic malignancies (with the exception of NETs, where embolization is aimed at controlling hormonal symptoms or pain). Involvement of more than 75% of the liver parenchyma by tumor makes a patient vulnerable to embolization and at high risk for development of liver failure. Although this finding is not an absolute contraindication to treatment, caution should be used and embolization should be performed in stages (one sector at a time).[6,16,47]

Though rare, severe atherosclerotic disease precluding safe performance of arteriography and embolization is a contraindication. Renal insufficiency is a contraindication unless the patient is already undergoing hemodialysis and plans have been made for hemodialysis before and after the procedure. Mild renal insufficiency (creatinine > 1.5 mg/dL) can be managed with good hydration and infusion of sodium bicarbonate (3 mL/kg/h of a solution of sodium bicarbonate, 154 mEq/L administered over a 1-hour period before procedure, and 1 mL/kg/h infused for 6 hours after procedure) to prevent deterioration in renal function. We advise the minimum possible use of contrast material in this population; iodixanol (Visipaque 320) is our contrast agent of choice.

Allergy to contrast material is a rare contraindication. Patients can be premedicated with steroids. Additional contraindications to doxorubicin or other chemotherapeutics and thus TACE include hyperbilirubinemia (>3 mg/dL), leukopenia (<3000 cells/mm^3), and coagulopathy (international normalized ratio [INR] > 2). Pregnancy is a contraindication, and females of childbearing age and potential should have a negative serum pregnancy test before undergoing treatment.

EQUIPMENT

To optimally perform embolization, a dedicated angiography suite is required and must have the capability of digital subtraction angiography (DSA) with the application of road mapping techniques. A fully equipped suite will also have available the appropriate angiographic catheters and microcatheters and corresponding guidewires. A 6F sheath is always needed to make the necessary catheter exchanges with the minimal possible trauma to the common femoral artery. The most commonly used catheters for angiography are 4F and 5F selective Cobras, which nowadays are available in hydrophilic form. Frequently, a 3F microcatheter is used coaxially for superselective embolization. An extensive inventory of guidewires and selective catheters should be available (Table 66-2) for cases in which catheterization cannot be achieved with the Cobra catheter and a 0.035-inch Glidewire. Our contrast agents of choice are iohexol 140 and 300.

TECHNIQUE

Anatomy and Approach

It is essential that the operator be very familiar with hepatic arterial anatomy and variations (Fig. 66-1, A-C). Before undertaking any type of hepatic embolization, a triphasic contrast-enhanced computed tomography (CT) examination is essential to demonstrate tumor size, location, and arterial supply. It is common to identify replaced or accessory hepatic arterial branches that feed the target tumor and must therefore be embolized. During arteriography and after imaging the celiac axis with selective injections, one should always image the proximal superior mesenteric artery in search for accessory and replaced hepatic arteries (see Fig. 66-1, B and C). It is important to remember that phrenic branches are frequently tumor feeders, particularly in patients who have undergone multiple previous embolization sessions. Embolized tumors frequently recruit the phrenic arteries as an alternative feeding pathway after embolization of the hepatic branches. Before embolization, it is important to assess portal vein status, which can be accomplished with contrast-enhanced CT before the procedure, and arterial portography during arteriography before embolization. Arterial portography is routinely performed with the angiographic catheter in the splenic or superior mesenteric artery and delayed filming, so that the portal vein is opacified and imaged (Fig. 66-1, D).

Preprocedural Preparation

It is imperative that before any embolization procedure, optimal imaging of the liver be performed to depict the anatomy and characteristics of the tumor to be embolized. In our institution, the preferred imaging study before any embolization procedure is a triphasic CT scan. This allows depiction of the arterial anatomy, including the identification of anatomic variations, which is extremely important before any attempt at embolization. It also demonstrates portal vein status. A good triphasic CT scan will also provide information about the vascularity and distribution of the tumor or tumors to be treated (Fig. 66-2, A and B). Angiography and embolization are performed in standard fashion via the femoral artery, with angiography used to depict the hepatic arterial anatomy and variations, as well as the distribution of vascular masses throughout the liver (Fig. 66-2, C).

Technical Aspects

Celiac axis and hepatic arteriography is always performed before embolization. Selective arteriography is necessary to identify tumors with a poor vascular component and, rarely, even hypervascular tumors that were not visualized on the celiac arteriogram. The catheter is advanced over a guidewire in the vessels expected to be supplying the target tumor, based on prior triple-phase CT information. When treating patients with multifocal bilobar disease (see Fig. 66-2, C), we select the lobe with the most disease for treatment at the first sitting. Initially, we perform arteriography with the catheter positioned selectively in the right or left hepatic artery, followed by embolization (Fig. 66-2, D).

TABLE 66-1. Malignant Liver Tumors Other Than Hepatocellular Carcinoma

Primary	Metastatic
Cholangiocarcinoma	Neuroendocrine tumor
Angiosarcoma	Sarcoma, gastrointestinal stromal tumors
	Melanoma and ocular melanoma
	Colorectal cancer
	Breast cancer
	Renal cell cancer

TABLE 66-2. Technical Aspects: Key Equipment for Hepatic Arteriography and Embolization

Wires	Catheters	Microcatheters	Embolic Agents
0.035 inch:	5F:	0.018-0.025 inch:	Polyvinyl alcohol, 50-300 μm
Benson	C2 Cobra	Tracker	Embospheres, 40-300 μm
Angle Glidewire	Simmons 2	Renegade	Contour SE, 50-300 μm
Shapeable Glidewire	SOS 2	Progreat	BeadBlock, 100-300 μm
	4F Glide		

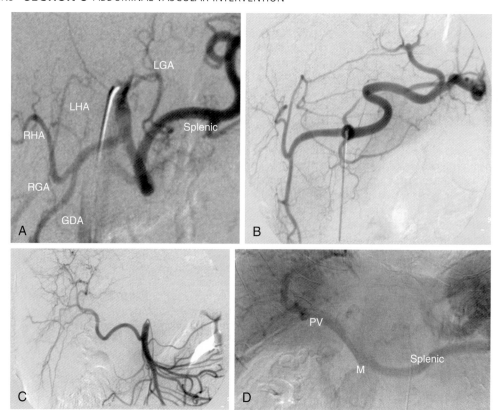

FIGURE 66-1 A, Celiac arteriogram demonstrating normal anatomy. **B,** Celiac arteriogram showing that common hepatic artery divides into left hepatic and gastroduodenal arteries. There is no identification of a right hepatic artery. **C,** Evaluation of proximal superior mesenteric artery in same patient as in **B** demonstrates a replaced right hepatic artery. **D,** Arterial portography. Delayed filming during arteriography (catheter tip in splenic artery) shows portal vein. *GDA,* Gastroduodenal artery; *LGA,* left gastric artery; *LHA,* left hepatic artery; *M,* superior mesenteric vein; *PV,* portal vein *RGA,* right gastric artery; *RHA,* right hepatic artery.

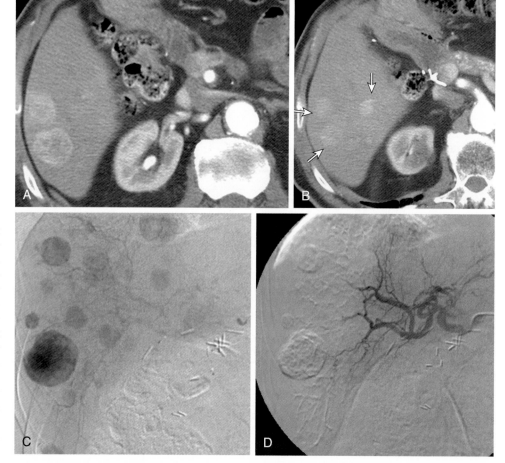

FIGURE 66-2 A-B, Two different arterial-phase computed tomography slices through liver of a patient with known metastatic neuroendocrine tumor show multiple hypervascular masses *(arrows)*. **C,** In same patient, delayed phase of catheter arteriography (catheter tip in common hepatic artery) shows innumerable vascular masses throughout both liver lobes. Right lobe has a larger tumor load. **D,** Postembolization arteriography demonstrates stasis in right hepatic artery and branches, with characteristic "pruned tree" appearance. Left hepatic artery remains patent.

Several embolic agents are used for treatment, and even more regimens for the administration of TACE. In the following section, we describe the technique of bland embolization we routinely use in our institution.

Selection of the embolic agent for treatment is based on the preference of the interventional radiologist. We always start by using the smallest size of the desired particles (see Table 66-2). A vial of the smallest particle is poured into a small glass or stainless steel cup, and the vial is rinsed of residual particles by filling it with contrast material and then pouring the contents into the cup containing the particles. The suspension is made and then drawn into a syringe for administration into the target vessel under continuous fluoroscopic control to confirm antegrade flow toward the tumor until stasis is evident or until 10 mL of the embolic agent has been used. We evaluate flow after the administration of 10 mL of the smallest particles, and if antegrade flow is still evident, we continue embolization with the next smallest particles. Once again, 10 mL of these particles is administered, and if antegrade flow persists, the next size particles are used, again injecting up to 10 mL of the particles, and so on. When stasis (defined as lack of antegrade flow, with evidence of reflux on injection of even small amounts of contrast material) is achieved, we terminate the embolization and perform arteriography to document occlusion of the target vessel and identify any supply to the target tumor from other vessels, which we may then select and embolize. Finally, arteriography will show stasis in the embolized vessel, which will have a "pruned tree" appearance (see Fig. 66-2, *D*), and preservation of antegrade blood flow to nontarget vessels such as the gastroduodenal and, if visualized, the cystic artery (Fig. 66-3).

Though rare in the treatment of secondary hepatic malignancies, pooling of contrast material within the target tumor during embolization may be noted. This is known as an *embolization sink*, and it is accompanied by an endless capacity for contrast material and particles and maintains antegrade flow. In our experience, using small amounts of

50-µm polyvinyl alcohol particles at this point will cause cessation of flow into the sink and stasis. Rarely, accessory vessels of the right or left hepatic artery must be embolized superselectively with a coil before undertaking tumor embolization to avoid embolization of nontarget tissue.

We recommend and try to embolize solitary tumors (Fig. 66-4, *A* and *B*) superselectively with a coaxial technique and 3F microcatheters, again administering up to 10 mL of the smallest particle size available and following the same algorithm as described in the previous paragraph for lobar embolization. We repeat the same procedure until all vessels supplying the tumor are occluded according to our standard protocol, beginning with the smallest particles and continuing until stasis. As with any type of embolization, we perform a final arteriogram when stasis has been achieved in all target branches (Fig. 66-4, *C*). At this point we consider evaluation of vessels that have not been embolized, and if appropriate, we also perform angiography of nonhepatic vessels supplying the tumor (e.g., phrenic or internal mammary arteries). Provided the patient is doing well, excessive contrast agent has not been administered, and embolization of additional vessels is considered safe, embolization continues. When stasis has been achieved in all vessels supplying the target tumor or the hemiliver, embolization is concluded, and when necessary, a future treatment plan for repeat embolization of residual disease is devised.

Tumors Smaller Than 5 cm
Patients with up to three tumors less than 5 cm in size (see Fig. 66-4, *A*) usually undergo ablation after embolization. Radiofrequency ablation (RFA) is performed unless contraindicated due to proximity (<1 cm) to structures that may be in danger from thermal injury. This clinical protocol aims to achieve "double kill" of the tumor. We believe combining the two methods increases the possibility of achieving 100% tumor cell death. The combination of arterial embolization and thermal ablation makes sense in that

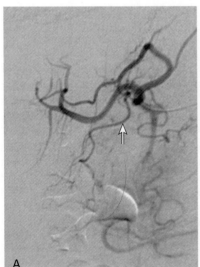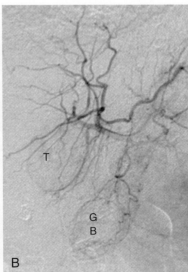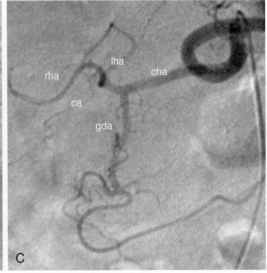

FIGURE 66-3 **A-B,** Arteriography before embolization in a patient with a solitary neuroendocrine metastasis in liver. Study clearly demonstrates cystic artery *(arrow)* originating from right hepatic artery. In **B,** vascular tumor *(T)* and gallbladder *(GB)* are also visualized. **C,** Postembolization of right hepatic artery *(rha)* shows preservation of flow to cystic artery *(ca)*, gastroduodenal arteries *(gda)*, left hepatic arteries *(lha)*, and common hepatic arteries *(cha)*.

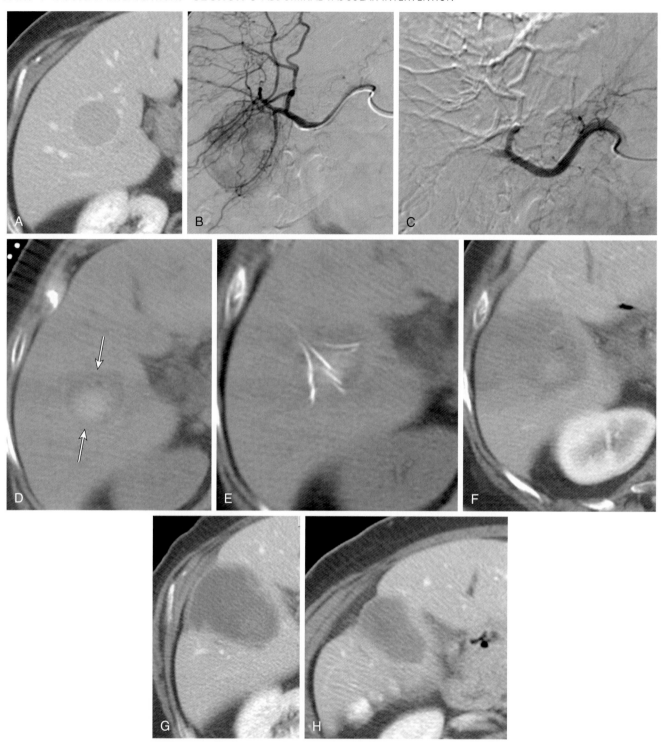

FIGURE 66-4 **A,** Solitary neuroendocrine tumor in a triple-phase computed tomography (CT) examination before embolization and radiofrequency ablation (RFA). **B,** Arteriography before embolization demonstrates solitary vascular mass. **C,** Postembolization arteriogram showing "pruned tree" appearance of right hepatic artery and no further visualization of vascular mass. **D,** Twenty-four hours after embolization, limited CT examination before RFA shows embolized lesion *(arrows)* containing radiopaque contrast material and embolic agent, and thus facilitates placement of RFA probe. **E,** RITA starburst 5-cm probe placed with tines expanded to show coverage of lesion before RFA. **F,** After two overlapping 5-cm RFA sessions, immediate triple-phase CT shows changes consistent with necrosis, with a good margin around lesion. **G,** A 6-week follow-up triple-phase CT scan shows no enhancement around or within lesion, consistent with successful embolization and RFA. **H,** A 3-month follow-up triple-phase CT scan shows no local tumor progression and expected shrinking of necrotic region.

embolization eliminates the arterial blood supply, thereby removing at least the arterial "heat sink" and allowing the maximum effect of RFA. In addition, bland embolization frequently results in dense opacification (Fig. 66-4, *D*) of the treated tumor by the combination of particles mixed with contrast material that remains within the treated tumor, very similar to what is seen after TACE with Lipiodol. This facilitates targeting of the lesion by CT the day after embolization, and coverage of the entire lesion with the appropriate-size RFA probe (Fig. 66-4, *E*), as well as performance of additional overlapping treatment to provide a clear margin of necrosis around the treated lesion (Fig. 66-4, *F-H*).

CONTROVERSIES

The most common controversial issue regarding hepatic embolization of hepatic malignancies is probably the value of addition of chemotherapy to the embolic agent. To date, no prospective randomized trial comparing HAE and TACE for the treatment of hepatic malignancies has been conducted, and therefore there is no definite answer to this question.

In the case of embolotherapy for NET, many authors favor TACE over HAE, in part because of early reports demonstrating greater and more durable regression in a subgroup of patients who underwent systemic chemotherapy after HAE than in those who received HAE alone.[46] To the contrary, however, higher response rates in patients with carcinoid tumor metastatic to the liver were reported after HAE than after TACE.[12] On the other hand, when reviewing the results of islet cell carcinoma as a separate group, it appears that TACE may be more beneficial than HAE, as reported by the same authors.[12] However, as commented in their discussion, these results should be interpreted with caution because this retrospective study resulted in a higher percentage of patients with unresected primary and higher metastatic liver loads in the population who underwent HAE.[12] Another study suggests that morbidity, mortality, symptom improvement, and overall survival are similar in patients with hepatic neuroendocrine metastases managed by TACE or HAE.[48]

It is, of course, extremely difficult to make any objective comparison between the reported results of several series because of the large heterogeneity in study groups, treatment protocols, and methods used to evaluate response rates. No study to date has demonstrated a clinical benefit of adding either chemotherapeutic agents or Lipiodol, and in at least one previous series, severe complications were recorded when chemotherapeutic agents and Lipiodol were added to the embolic agent and used to treat carcinoid tumors.[42]

In the case of colorectal metastases, a randomized study comparing TACE and HAE demonstrated no advantage of one technique over the other.[36]

Randomized controlled trials comparing HAE and TACE are very much needed to provide true scientific evidence of the value of adding chemotherapy to the embolization of hepatic malignancies.

An additional question is which type of particle should be used for HAE and TACE. In our practice, where we perform bland HAE with particles only (see Table 66-2), we always start with the smaller particle and proceed as we have explained in detail in the previous section. We believe that small particles provide terminal vessel blockade and result in profound ischemia and cell death. In view of the lack of evidence that the addition of chemotherapy is associated with any survival benefit and, at least in some series, the finding of increased toxicity and risk with chemotherapy, we currently consider HAE the embolization treatment of choice for all hepatic malignancies.

OUTCOMES

In this section we review the natural history, specific indications, and outcomes of HAE for the treatment of specific metastatic and primary malignancies involving the liver.

Neuroendocrine Hepatic Metastases

Neuroendocrine tumors are frequently found when the disease becomes metastatic.[46,49,50] These tumors have been described by Moertel as "cancers in slow motion"[49] because they are indolent. NETs are the most common secondary hepatic malignancies managed with HAE and TACE.* The metastatic deposits in the liver frequently exceed the primary neoplasm in size, making the liver the organ with the most tumor load. Development of hepatic metastases is accompanied by synthesis and release of hormonal substances in the circulation that lead to a constellation of symptoms (rash, hypertension, diarrhea, and electrolyte disorders) known as the *carcinoid syndrome*. At this stage, the liver becomes the most desirable target for treatment and palliation of the developing symptomatology.† Surgical resection of liver metastases is desirable, but less than 10% of patients are initially seen with resectable tumors.[51-54] Progressive pain and discomfort, as well as dyspnea, develop in the latest stages of the disease because significant hepatomegaly causes compression of the diaphragm. Hepatic embolization is undertaken to reduce the hormone-producing liver tumor and decrease symptomatology and, in particular, pain.[5] Inoperable tumors can be managed by administration of pharmacologic antagonists of tumor metabolites,[46,49-56] HAE, TACE, or a combination of these treatments. The increased availability of somatostatin analogs has allowed relatively good medical treatment of NETs. To maximize the effect of embolization on tumor control and relief of symptomatology, many authors recommended hepatic embolization as early as a metastasis develops and when the symptomatology is the result of hormone production. For solitary or relatively small (<5 cm) and not more than three localized tumors, HAE and TACE can be combined with RFA or other ablation techniques to maximize tumor necrosis and improve local disease control.[30] Embolization can also be applied in advanced disease scenarios and when all other treatments have failed, especially in selected symptomatic cases. In these patients, the psychological effect of the treatment is important.[46]

Rarely, embolization can be used in patients with large hepatic deposits to decrease the tumor load and render a previously inoperable patient a surgical candidate. This is particularly important in cases where large metastatic

---

*References 3, 4, 6, 8-10, 12-14, 16, 18, 19, 21, 22, 24, 28, 30-32, 34, 35, 39, 41, 42.
†References 8, 10, 13, 16, 18, 19, 30, 39, 42.

masses compress vital structures such as large hepatic veins, the inferior vena cava, and the portal vein. With tumor reduction, the effects of compression are decreased, and a previously inoperable or borderline case may become a surgical candidate.[46]

Outcomes are inversely related to the degree of liver replacement by tumor. Overall median survival for patients with carcinoid tumor metastatic to the liver is only 3 years, with greater than 70% mortality within 5 years after diagnosis.[49] The best results are documented in patients with the least tumor load in the liver. A common finding of most series of HAE and TACE for the management of NET is a morphologic response as documented by imaging; however, partial or complete response rates have been reported in the available literature and widely range from 6.7% to 100%.[45] Median survival of 13 to 80 months has been reported for patients with NET after embolization.[‡] If one looks at the results of embolization for carcinoid tumor and islet cell carcinoma separately, it is clear that patients with carcinoid have significantly prolonged survival after embolization.[16,50,52]

The issue of pain relief in patients with NET was addressed directly in a series of HAE procedures, and it was noted that more extensive tumor burden is likely to be present when the primary symptom is pain rather than symptoms of hormonal excess. This was consistent with the findings that symptomatic relief of pain was of shorter duration than control of hormonal symptoms, and that 40% of patients treated for pain alone died within an average follow-up period of 13.7 months, whereas only 6% of patients treated for hormonal symptoms died within an average follow-up period of 24 months.[6] It is possible pain develops in patients farther along in the natural history of the disease, which would explain the poorer results of treatment in this subgroup.

It is common knowledge that patients with more than 75% of the liver replaced by tumor are poor candidates for embolization in general. Poor outcomes and response rates have been documented in this population. In contrast, patients with less than 50% involvement have a trend for longer survival. A large percentage of (and in some series all) patients with greater than 75% involvement died within 30 days to 6 months after HAE or TACE. Some authors recommend a tumor burden greater than 50% and others greater than 75% as an exclusion criterion for embolization. Others, including our institution, undertake embolization of patients with greater than 50% tumor load as a palliative treatment, especially when severe symptomatology impedes quality of life. In these high-risk patients, embolization should be performed in stages, with only a part of the vascular tumor embolized at each session, frequently not more than one sector at a time.[47] Using this approach, one series[6] treated patients with greater than 75% replacement of the liver by tumor. They reported response rates of 43% and 25% and overall survival of 20.1 and 16 months for patients with carcinoid tumor and islet cell carcinoma, respectively. In our experience, patients with metastatic carcinoid had significantly longer hepatic progression-free survival (HPFS) than patients with islet cell tumor (median HPFS: 10 vs. 5.9 months, respectively; $P = 0.003$). Median primary (after single embolization) symptom-free survival was

similar between the groups (5 months for carcinoid vs. 6.5 months for islet cell tumor; $P = 0.41$).

Sarcomas and Gastrointestinal Stromal Tumors

Traditional treatment of nonresectable metastatic sarcoma of the liver is limited to chemotherapy or palliative radiation therapy. Some patients receive only supportive care. The majority of patients with liver-dominant metastases do not have resectable disease, and current treatment options are limited. Systemic chemotherapy has variable response rates and provides marginal improvement in overall survival in comparison to supportive measures. The up-to-date limited experience in the treatment of liver-dominant metastatic disease from visceral sarcoma suggests that the hepatic malignant volume may seriously affect survival. Based on the results of very few series and small numbers of patients with metastatic sarcoma treated by liver resection, a median survival of almost 40 months can be expected in patients who undergo complete resection, versus 8 to 12 months in those who undergo partial resection.[57-59] Unresectable patients have very limited treatment options. A small number of series have used TACE and HAE to treat sarcoma and gastrointestinal stromal tumor (GIST).[57-59] In a previous series of 15 patients with leiomyosarcoma metastatic to the liver,[36] a response rate of 70% was achieved with a mixture of polyvinyl alcohol, cisplatin, and vinblastine administered in two sessions 4 weeks apart. Similar results were demonstrated in a second small series by Rajan et al.[33] This series, which involved 16 patients with liver-dominant metastatic sarcoma, demonstrated a partial response rate of 69%, with a median survival of 20 months from the time of diagnosis and 13 months from the initial TACE procedure.

In a series[25] using bland particle embolization (without addition of any chemotherapeutic agent), we demonstrated a radiographic response rate of 60%, comparable to that reported in the TACE series, and a median survival of 24 months, which compares favorably with the median survival of 8 to 12 months in patients with liver-dominant disease who are unable to undergo complete resection. In the same series from our institution, no survival difference was documented between patients with liver-dominant versus liver-only disease, between patients with synchronous versus metachronous liver disease, or between patients with less than five tumors versus those with multifocal liver metastases. This may suggest that liver failure is fatal in most patients with liver-dominant metastases from sarcoma. A significant survival benefit was documented in patients who had a demonstrable radiographic response (median of 63 vs. 19 months), and therefore we encourage aggressive regional therapy with HAE in patients who show response to initial embolization, whereas in patients demonstrating no radiographic response, other locoregional treatment options, including RFA, microwave ablation, or cryotherapy, should be considered for local control, depending on the extent of disease. In the same small series from our institution, a significant improvement in survival in patients with GIST versus leiomyosarcoma was observed.[25] When analyzing the results of the study, one can observe that patients who survived to 2001 and received the then-available STI571 or imatinib (Gleevec) had longer survival. This was attributed to the ability of embolization to control

‡References 4, 6, 9, 12-14, 16, 18, 19, 21.

the disease until an effective systemic therapy became available. Currently at our institution, embolization is used in patients with GIST that failed or became resistant to Gleevec. Resistance develops at a median of 2 years after initiation of treatment.[25]

In summary, based on the natural history of the disease and the limited results available for HAE and TACE, it is reasonable to consider embolization an effective treatment option because it can improve survival beyond 12 months. Adding chemotherapeutic agents and Lipiodol to the embolic regimen is controversial, since there is no evidence either improves outcomes.

Metastatic Ocular Melanoma

Ocular melanoma develops in 3500 to 4000 individuals annually.[15] Up to 40% of patients will have liver metastases at initial evaluation, and the liver becomes involved in up to 95% of patients in whom metastatic disease develops. The liver is the sole site of metastasis in more than 80% of patients. Many systemic treatments, including immunotherapy, chemotherapy, and even the antiangiogenic agent thalidomide, have been used in patients with metastatic disease.[15] There are extremely few reports of resection of ocular melanoma metastatic to the liver, but relatively good results were achieved in a selected population with a limited number of metastases and probably indolent disease. The same guidelines for eligibility for TACE and HAE apply to this population as for HCC and other secondary hepatic tumors.

Uveal melanoma metastatic to the liver has been treated by TACE to increase accumulation of chemotherapeutic agent in the tumor and prolong the dwell time of the agent; systemic effects are minimal when compared with arterial chemoinfusion and systemic chemotherapy. The largest series reporting on TACE for ocular melanoma metastatic to the liver retrospectively reviewed 201 patients, 44 of whom were treated with TACE plus cisplatin and polyvinyl sponge,[5] and concluded that only TACE combining embolotherapy with cisplatin-based regimens resulted in a meaningful response rate (36% = 16/44).[5] These results were similar to those of a previous study reporting a 46% response rate and median overall survival of 11 months in a group of 30 patients treated by the same regimen.[29] At our institution, we have treated a very small number of patients with ocular melanoma metastatic to the liver by HAE or arterial chemoinfusion.

Metastatic Colon Cancer

Colon cancer is the second leading cause of cancer-related death in the United States, with more than 50,000 deaths and 150,000 new cases reported annually. The most desirable and the only possible cure for hepatic metastases from colon cancer is surgical resection; however, less than 30% of patients have resectable disease at initial evaluation. Systemic chemotherapy remains the standard of care for this population. Recent developments in chemotherapeutic agents have resulted in improved overall median survival to just over 20 months. When progression of hepatic disease is noted during chemotherapy, palliative treatment is desired. A limited number of series have reported on use of TACE and HAE to treat patients with hepatic metastases

from colon cancer that failed systemic chemotherapy. In one series, it was documented that a mean survival of at least 12 months was necessary to justify the cost of TACE in this population.[60] Other trials have documented that survival rates are significantly improved in patients with good performance status, no extrahepatic disease, and solitary lesions.[36,37] Sequential TACE in patients with four or fewer tumors up to 8 cm each was performed to reduce tumor size to 5 cm or less and then treat them with laser-induced thermal ablation; this regimen resulted in a mean survival of more than 26 months, versus 12.8 months for patients treated by TACE only.[61] It is therefore reasonable to consider embolization, especially when combined with ablation, a viable treatment option for managing hepatic-dominant disease that has failed systemic chemotherapy, and stable or no extrahepatic disease.

One study using DEB-TACE reported an overall response rate at 1 month of 80%. Another publication studied response rates at 1 month and reported an overall response rate of 100%, but did not clarify the criteria used.[44] Radioembolization for these typically hypovascular tumors is beyond the scope of this chapter but is covered elsewhere (see Chapters 64 and 65).

Cholangiocarcinoma

The natural history of unresectable cholangiocarcinoma is 5 to 8 months' survival. Resectable disease also has poor outcomes, with at best a 50% survival rate 3 years after surgery. Limited published data on embolization of cholangiocarcinoma are available. One series using TACE documented 23-month median survival in nonresectable patients. It is noteworthy that in this study, 2 of 17 patients had a significant decrease in tumor load in the liver and became resectable after TACE.[7]

Other Malignancies

Embolization has been used to treat liver metastases from breast, renal, thyroid, thymus, ovarian, lung, pancreatic, gastric, and small bowel cancer and tumors from an unknown primary. Even so, no large study has addressed any of these tumors separately to allow any meaningful interpretation and specific conclusions regarding the value of the technique. It is not, however, unreasonable to consider treatment of such metastases with HAE or TACE, based on the available experience and results of treatment of HCC and secondary tumors, as well as the knowledge that liver tumors in general are supplied by the hepatic artery. Selection of candidates for treatment should be based on their performance status and the presence of no or stable extrahepatic disease and solitary lesions. In this last group, the combination of embolization with ablation is beneficial.[30,61]

COMPLICATIONS

Complications after hepatic embolization of non-HCC tumors have been reported in 7% to 17%, with serious complications occurring in approximately 5%.[2-43] Severe complications include liver abscesses requiring drainage or, in nonresolving cases, even resection. Such abscesses have been reported in approximately 2% of cases. The same rate has been observed for liver infarction.[43] Liver abscess formation is usually noted 10 or more days after embolization and manifests as high fever, leukocytosis, and pain. Patients who do not have an intact sphincter of Oddi because of previous bilioenteric anastomosis or sphincterectomy are at higher risk for abscess development. In this population, a biliary-excreted antibiotic such as Zosyn (piperacillin plus tazobactam) rather than the usual cefazolin (Ancef) should be used prophylactically. The most serious complication of embolization is inadvertent occlusion of nontarget vessels (nontarget embolization), which, however, is very rare if a diagnostic arteriogram has been carefully performed and the appropriate technique of embolization has been followed. Even in the most careful hands, occasional nontarget embolization of the cystic artery (which is often not visualized on the arteriogram) may occur and be accompanied by a prolonged postembolization syndrome, but it is extremely rare that cholecystectomy will be required.

In general, it has been noted that patients with extensive hepatic replacement by tumor (>75%) have a tendency toward a less favorable outcome and an increased rate of severe complications, including death due to postembolization liver failure. The 30-day mortality rate is about 1%.[43]

Minor complications reported after embolotherapy for liver tumors include cholecystitis, transient contrast agent–induced transient renal failure, peripheral arterial emboli, postprocedure infections such as pneumonia, and local hematoma at the puncture site requiring no treatment.

Side Effects

Virtually all patients who undergo HAE suffer a degree of postembolization syndrome, consisting of fever, pain, nausea, and vomiting; severity is variable between patients and between different treatments in the same patient. In its mildest form, the syndrome lasts no longer than 48 hours, and patients can even be managed as outpatients with oral medication for pain relief. In more severe forms, patients cannot tolerate oral medication and require intravenous hydration, antiemetics, and pain relief medication. Thus, the degree of postembolization syndrome influences the patient's hospital stay, which can vary from 2 to 10 days.

POSTPROCEDURAL AND FOLLOW-UP CARE

Close monitoring for several hours after the procedure is performed in the recovery room. Bed rest is recommended for 2 to 4 hours to prevent inadvertent bleeding at the puncture site. We recommend 4 hours of bed rest for patients in whom hemostasis was achieved by digital compression, and 2 hours for those who underwent successful deployment of a closure device. Hydration plus pain management, as well as encouragement of early mobilization, is the typical care after any embolization procedure. During recovery, vital signs are stabilized and the level of pain is monitored and controlled with intravenous morphine sulfate. When the patient is ready to be transferred from the recovery room to the regular floor unit, pain is assessed again, and if necessary, patient-controlled analgesia with morphine sulfate is initiated. Intravenous antibiotics (Ancef, 1 g) are administered before the procedure and continued for 24 hours. Temperature is monitored, and if fever (>38.5°C) develops, blood is drawn for culture, and intravenous antibiotic coverage continued as needed. Antipyretics are administered accordingly. Clear liquids are encouraged as soon as possible after the procedure. Nausea and vomiting are controlled with antiemetics, and when oral intake is good, without any need for intravenous medication, patients are discharged from the hospital. For patients who undergo RFA after embolization, the same recovery routine is followed.

A follow-up triple-phase CT examination is performed for 4 to 6 weeks after the procedure to evaluate the radiologic response to treatment and plan additional embolization as needed (see Fig. 66-4, *F-H*). If local or distant intrahepatic tumor progression is noted, repeat embolization is performed. If there is no evidence of tumor progression and the treated tumor appears necrotic, follow-up continues with triple-phase CT every 3 months for the first year and every 6 months afterward. Patients who have bilobar disease and receive unilateral treatment return for embolization of the other lobe within 6 to 8 weeks after the initial treatment. Follow-up continues in the same manner.

KEY POINTS

- Hepatic arterial embolization (HAE) is effective in the treatment of liver malignancies other than hepatocellular carcinoma and should be considered along with other available treatments.

- Hepatic arterial embolization has the best results when combined with ablation in patients with up to three lesions under 5 cm each.

- Indications and outcomes of HAE vary for each type of tumor treated.

► **SUGGESTED READINGS**

Brown KT, Koh BY, Brody LA, et al. Particle embolization of hepatic neuroendocrine metastases for control of pain and hormonal symptoms. J Vasc Interv Radiol 1999;10:397–403.

Carter S, Martin Ii RC. Drug-eluting bead therapy in primary and metastatic disease of the liver. HPB (Oxford) 2009;11(7):541–50.

Dodd GD 3rd, Soulen MC, Kane RA, et al. Minimally invasive treatment of malignant hepatic tumors: at the threshold of a major breakthrough. Radiographics 2000;20:9–27.

Gupta S, Johnson MM, Murthy R, et al. Hepatic arterial embolization and chemoembolization for the treatment of patients with metastatic neuroendocrine tumors: variables affecting response rates and survival. Cancer 2005;104:1590–602.

Madoff DC, Gupta S, Ahrar K, et al. Update on the management of neuroendocrine hepatic metastases. J Vasc Interv Radiol 2006;17:1235–50.

Maluccio MA, Covey AM, Schubert J, et al. Treatment of metastatic sarcoma to the liver with bland embolization. Cancer 2006;107:1617–23.

Pitt SC, Knuth J, Keily JM, et al. Hepatic neuroendocrine metastases: chemo- or bland embolization? J Gastrointest Surg 2008;12(11):1951–60.

Rajan DK, Soulen MC, Clark TW, et al. Sarcomas metastatic to the liver: response and survival after cisplatin, doxorubicin, mitomycin-C, Ethiodol, and polyvinyl alcohol chemoembolization. J Vasc Interv Radiol 2001;12:187–93.

Salman HS, Cynamon J, Jagust M, et al. Randomized phase II trial of embolization therapy versus chemoembolization therapy in previously treated patients with colorectal carcinoma metastatic to the liver. Clin Colorectal Cancer 2002;2:173–9.

Sanz-Altamira PM, Spence LD, Huberman MS, et al. Selective chemoembolization in the management of hepatic metastases in refractory colorectal carcinoma: a phase II trial. Dis Colon Rectum 1997;40: 770–5.

Sullivan KL. Hepatic artery chemoembolization. Semin Oncol 2002;29: 145–51.

The complete reference list is available online at www.expertconsult.com.

CHAPTER **67**

Radioembolization of Liver Metastases

Khairuddin Memon, Robert J. Lewandowski, and Riad Salem

CLINICAL RELEVANCE

Metastatic disease to the liver is the most common form of hepatic malignancy, the colon being the most common primary tumor location.[1] At presentation, most of these oncology patients are not candidates for operative cure, and many have failed systemic chemotherapeutic regimens. The safety and efficacy of radioembolization with yttrium-90 (^{90}Y) in these patients with liver-dominant disease and good performance status have been reported in the literature.[2-7] Radioembolization is performed using percutaneous transarterial techniques in the interventional radiology suite. By definition, *radioembolization* is injection of micron-sized embolic particles loaded with a radioisotope; an interdisciplinary team is crucial to the success of a ^{90}Y radioembolization program. This team should be well represented with members from interventional radiology, medical, radiation and surgical oncology, transplant surgery, nuclear medicine, radiation oncology, hepatology, and radiation safety.

INDICATIONS

^{90}Y can be delivered to the hepatic tumor as either a constituent of a glass microsphere, TheraSphere (Nordion Inc., Ottawa, Ontario, Canada), or as a biocompatible resin-based microsphere, SIR-Spheres (Sirtex Medical Inc., Lake Forest, Ill.).

Please visit www.expertconsult.com for more information on these therapies.

In general, indications for treatment of liver tumors using ^{90}Y include: (1) unresectability, (2) adequate hematologic and hepatic functions, (3) correctable gastrointestinal (GI) flow on technetium-99m–labeled macroaggregated albumin (^{99m}Tc-MAA) scan, (4) cumulative lung dose for all treatments less than 50 Gy, and (5) liver-dominant disease and adequate performance status.

CONTRAINDICATIONS

Appropriate patient selection is critical to avoid morbidity and mortality from radioembolization. Irrespective of liver tumor etiology, evaluating a patient for possible treatment with ^{90}Y should be driven by the patient's Eastern Cooperative Oncology Group (ECOG) performance status (Table 67-1) rather than their clinical stage. From a practical standpoint, patients with ECOG 0, 1, or 2 status (equivalent to Karnofsky score of 60% or higher) should be considered for therapy. For patients who do not fulfill this criterion (ECOG > 2), there is a relative contraindication to radioembolization. Decision to treat these patients should be based on individual patient evaluation and clinical judgment and intent. Besides performance status, prothrombin time (PT), albumin, and total bilirubin should be scrutinized because they have been shown to be the best indicators of overall

liver function.[11] If these values are abnormal, greater care must be taken in treating, given the relative higher risk for radiation-induced liver disease and failure. Once the patient is clinically deemed a candidate for radioembolization, angiography and ^{99m}Tc-MAA infusion are performed. These tests may reveal further contraindications to treatment, which include uncorrectable flow to the GI system and excessive pulmonary shunting.[12]

The lungs can tolerate 30 Gy per treatment session and 50 Gy cumulatively.[13] Therefore, when treatment planning is undertaken and lung shunting is identified, the total cumulative pulmonary dose must be calculated. Patients may be treated if their cumulative pulmonary dose will not exceed 50 Gy cumulatively for all planned infusions of ^{90}Y. However, in patients with compromised pulmonary function, such as chronic obstructive pulmonary disease or previous lung resection, caution must be taken when approaching total cumulative doses. In these instances, the decision to treat must be individualized and based on overall clinical status.

EQUIPMENT

The TheraSphere administration set consists of one inlet set, one outlet set, one empty vial, and two interlocking units consisting of a positioning needle guide and a priming needle guide, all contained behind a Lucite shield. A MONARCH 30-mL syringe (Merit Medical, South Jordan, Utah) is used to infuse saline through the system. The saline solution containing the TheraSphere ^{90}Y microspheres is infused through a catheter placed in the hepatic vasculature. Once the catheter is positioned at the treatment site and the authorized user verifies the integrity of the delivery system, the catheter is connected to the outlet tubing. Delivery of TheraSphere is accomplished by pressurizing the MONARCH syringe.

The SIR-Spheres administration set consists of a Perspex shield, the dose vial, and inlet and outlet tubing with needles. Standard 10- or 20-mL injection syringes preloaded with sterile water are required to infuse the microspheres into the delivery catheter. Pressure gauges are not available when infusing SIR-Spheres.

TECHNIQUE

Anatomy and Approaches

All radioembolization patients initially undergo mesenteric angiography and a ^{99m}Tc-MAA lung shunting scan.[12,14-16] The angiographic evaluation required has been described by Liu et al.[14] An abdominal aortogram facilitates proper visceral catheter selection as well as assesses aortic tortuosity and mural atherosclerotic disease. The superior mesenteric artery is studied to assess any variant vessels to the

TABLE 67-1. Performance Status Criteria

ECOG Scale	Characteristics	Equivalent Karnofsky Score
0	Asymptomatic and fully active	100%
1	Symptomatic, fully ambulatory, restricted in physically strenuous activity	80%-90%
2	Symptomatic, ambulatory, capable of self-care, more than 50% of waking hours are spent out of bed	60%-70%
3	Symptomatic, limited self-care, spends more than 50% of time in bed	40%-50%
4	Completely disabled, no self-care, bedridden	20%-30%

ECOG, Eastern Cooperative Oncology Group.

liver (accessory or replaced right hepatic), as well as for visualization and identification of a patent portal vein. The celiac artery is injected to study the hepatic branch anatomy. Subsequently, selective left hepatic (flow to segments 2, 3, 4A, and 4B), right hepatic (flow to segments 1 [caudate lobe may have other blood supply], 5, 6, 7, and 8), and gastroduodenal (flow to the pancreas, stomach, small bowel, and omentum) arteriograms are performed. To visualize small vessels as well as vessels that may demonstrate reversal of flow (e.g., result of flow shunt, sumping secondary to hypervascular tumor), dedicated microcatheter injection with relatively high rates (2-3 mL/s for 8-12 mL) should be performed.[14] Without adequate contrast bolus, many ancillary vessels (which have profound effect on hemodynamics and directed therapy) may go unnoticed. Although it may be argued that high injection rates may represent supraphysiologic flow dynamics, the potential changes induced as a result of regional therapy with radioembolization (spasm, ischemia, stasis, and vessel injury) may result in altered physiologic states and thus reflux into these vessels.

Aggressive prophylactic embolization of vessels prior to therapy is highly recommended, such that all hepaticoenteric arterial communications are completely eliminated. These vessels include the falciform, accessory or left phrenic, right or accessory gastric arteries (from the left hepatic artery), supraduodenal, retroduodenal, and accessory right hepatic artery feeding segment 6 (from gastroduodenal artery [GDA]). Reflux of microspheres into the GDA or gastric arterial circulation may result in grave clinical consequences that include severe ulceration, GI bleeding, or pancreatitis. Given the serious clinical risks of microsphere reflux into nontarget organs and the lack of clinical consequences of prophylactic embolization of the GDA/right gastric, the latter approach is strongly favored.[7,14,16,17] Figure 67-1 demonstrates the principles of prophylactic embolization before radioembolization.

At the conclusion of the initial angiographic evaluation of a patient for ⁹⁰Y radioembolization, 4 to 5 mCi of ⁹⁹mTc-MAA is injected in the proper hepatic artery, followed by imaging for lung shunt fraction. This step is required, given the arteriovenous connections that exist in liver tumors that shunt blood from the liver to the lungs. This permits calculation of lung dose prior to radioembolization. *Lung shunt*

fraction (LSF) is defined as (total lung counts)/(total lung counts + total liver counts).

Once a patient has been deemed a candidate for ⁹⁰Y radioembolization through rigorous review of their medical history, functional status, pertinent imaging, laboratory values, angiographic imaging with aggressive prophylactic embolization, and lung shunt analysis, they return to the interventional radiology clinic on a separate date to have their therapy. ⁹⁰Y radioembolization is performed on an outpatient basis. The selected catheter is advanced into the treatment vessel of choice as determined by pretreatment angiography and either the TheraSphere or SIR-Spheres administration device is used for microsphere infusion. The dose delivered is calculated according to the following formulas:

TheraSphere[12]:

$$A\,(GBq) = [D\,(Gy) \times M\,(kg)]/50$$

where A is activity delivered to the liver, D is the absorbed delivered dose to the target liver mass, and M is the target liver mass. Liver volume (mL) is estimated with computed tomography (CT) and then converted to mass using a conversion factor of 1.03 kg/mL.

SIR-Spheres[18]:

$$A\,(GBq) = BSA\,(m^2) - 0.2 + (\%\text{ tumor involvement}/100)$$

where *BSA* is body surface area; or by recommended dose according to % tumor burden:

- Greater than 50% tumor burden, 3.0 GBq
- 25% to 50% tumor burden, 2.5 GBq
- Less than 25% tumor burden, 2.0 GBq

Technical Aspects

TheraSphere Infusion Technique

- Infusions should be performed using 3F systems. This includes standard lobar infusions as well as cases with difficult anatomy, small vessels, or subselective catheterizations. In these instances, the required pressures are greater, usually 20 to 40 psi. Although discouraged, the use of 4F or 5F systems should allow for constant low-pressure (10-20 psi) infusion throughout the administration.
- Irrespective of the size of the catheter system, it is necessary to ensure that the rate of infusion mimics the rate of hepatic arterial flow. This rate is assessed by visual inspection of a test dose of contrast infusion prior to TheraSphere administration. In some patients (e.g., elderly with diminished cardiac function, celiac stenoses), slower hepatic arterial flow may be apparent. In such cases, the infusion rate of TheraSphere must mimic this slower flow. Injecting TheraSphere at an infusion rate faster than the vessel will tolerate can result in reflux and administration to nontarget sites.
- Delivery of TheraSphere is dependent upon blood flow through the hepatic vasculature distal to the catheter tip. Therefore, it is necessary to make certain the catheter does not occlude the vessel in which it is placed, since doing so will result in vessel spasm and reflux as the infusion proceeds.

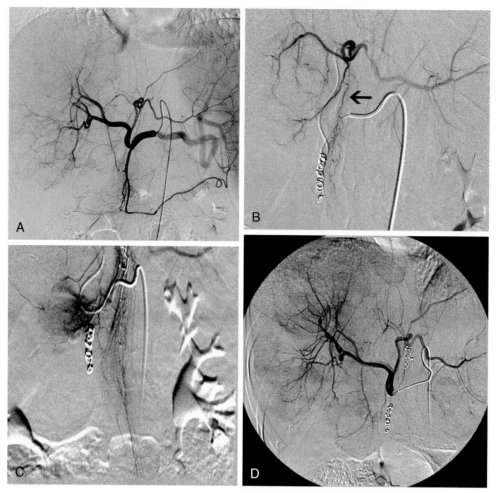

FIGURE 67-1. A, Celiac angiogram demonstrates patent gastroduodenal artery (GDA) and patent right and left hepatic arteries. **B,** In anticipation of radioembolization, GDA has been embolized. Left hepatic angiogram demonstrates a falciform artery *(arrow).* **C,** Delayed injection of left hepatic artery confirms "falciform complex," a tangle of vessels traveling through falciform ligament that has anastomosed with anterior abdominal wall (musculophrenic, superior epigastric arteries). **D,** Completion common hepatic angiogram demonstrates completely embolized GDA and falciform arteries. Patient's anatomy has been prepared for radioembolization.

SIR-Sphere Infusion Technique

- Most SIR-Spheres infusions should be performed through 3F catheter systems. Although smaller catheter systems result in the need to generate higher pressures for microsphere delivery, they create a safety mechanism preventing the forceful and unimpeded advancement of microspheres that might occur with larger 5F catheters.
- There is no pressure gauge on the SIR-Spheres delivery kit, so pressure cannot be monitored.
- Delivery of SIR-Spheres is dependent on blood flow through the hepatic vasculature distal to the catheter tip. Given the embolic load of SIR-Spheres, it is necessary to make certain the catheter does not occlude the vessel in which it is placed in order to prevent reflux. Flushing should be continued until optimal delivery is achieved.
- It is essential that the vascular bed providing blood flow to the liver be altered in a manner comparable to that achieved using surgical techniques when placing surgical pumps. This includes prophylactic embolization of the GDA and right gastric arteries as well as the supraduodenal, falciform, accessory left gastric, and accessory inferior phrenic (extrahepatic). Once this is achieved, given the fact that metastatic cancer is usually multifocal and bilobar, treatment using a lobar approach is favored, thereby minimizing the risk of hepatic decompensation.
- Given the large number of microspheres (40-80 million) and lower activity of SIR-Spheres (50 Bq per microsphere), the delivery of SIR-Spheres is distinctly different than that for TheraSphere. Fluoroscopic guidance is essential during the infusion. The technique of SIR-Spheres infusion involves the alternating infusion of sterile water and contrast, never allowing direct SIR-Spheres contact with contrast. This allows the authorized user to adequately monitor the injection and ensure that vascular saturation has not been reached.
- The infusion is complete if either: (1) the entire intended dose has been infused without reaching stasis, or (2) stasis has been reached and only a portion of the dose has been infused. Given the risk of reflux and nontarget radiation once stasis has been reached, continued infusion of SIR-Spheres is not recommended.

CONTROVERSIES

The role of radioembolization for treatment of liver tumors continues to be defined as patient selection criteria are refined. Although the safety of this therapy is well established, comparisons with other therapies require further inquiry, including chemoembolization, bland embolization, radiofrequency ablation, and cryotherapy. Controlled comparative randomized trials would aid in answering these questions. Furthermore, tumor size, location, and imaging characteristics ideal for radioembolization require further investigation. Finally, patients with portal vein thrombosis represent a population that may significantly benefit from radioembolization.

OUTCOMES

The efficacy and safety of radioembolization with ^{90}Y is well supported in the medical literature with phase 2 and level 1 randomized data.[1,2,18-20] Specifically, TheraSphere and SIR-Spheres have been used in treating patients with HCC and liver-dominant metastatic disease (colon, neuroendocrine, breast, cholangiocarcinoma, and other liver metastases).

Herba and Thirlwell performed a dose escalation study in 37 CRC patients with TheraSphere, starting at 50 Gy and escalating in 25-Gy increments to 150 Gy.[21] There was a positive response observed by CT. Stabilization or decrease in tumor size was observed in 22/30 patients (73%). Because of the small sample size of the study, no statistically significant relationship between dose and clinical or radiologic beneficial effects was observed.

A second dose escalation study was completed in 43 CRC patients with TheraSphere.[22] There were no life-threatening or fatal toxicities. Median survival was 408 days. Two patients had a complete response, 8 had a partial response, and 35 (81%) were at least stable. Higher doses were associated with greater tumor response and increased survival ($P = 0.05$). In addition, tumor hypervascularity ($P = 0.01$), higher baseline performance status ($P = 0.002$), and less liver involvement ($P = 0.004$) were associated with enhanced response or survival. Clinical toxicities included duodenal/gastric ulcers in 6 patients (14%) that resolved with medical management.

In another study of 19 patients with unresectable chemotherapy-refractive hepatic metastatic disease of various origins treated with SIR-Spheres, by positron emission tomography (PET) criteria, 15 (79%) of the patients demonstrated response to therapy at 3 months while 4 (21%) demonstrated no response. The authors again concluded that there is a significant reduction of hepatic metastatic load as evaluated by PET following radioembolization.[6]

Seventy-two patients with unresectable metastatic CRC were treated with TheraSphere using a targeted dose of 120 Gy on a lobar basis. Partial tumor response by World Health Organization (WHO) criteria was 40.3%. Median time to hepatic progression and overall survival from first treatment was 15.4 months and 14.5 months, respectively. ECOG score of 0, tumor replacement 25% or less, absence of extrahepatic disease, response to therapy, and earlier stage at diagnosis of primary were related to improved survival. Treatment-related toxicities included mild fatigue (61), nausea (21%), and abdominal pain (25%). Grade 3 and 4 bilirubin toxicities were observed in 9 of 72 patients (12.6%).[25]

Sato et al. reported on a large cohort of patients (137) with liver metastases treated with TheraSphere. Primary sites included colon (n = 51), breast (n = 21), neuroendocrine (n = 19), pancreas (n = 6), lung (n = 5), cholangiocarcinoma (n = 7), melanoma (n = 5), renal (n = 4), esophageal (n = 3), ovary (n = 2), adenocarcinoma unknown primary (n = 3), and one each from adrenal, angiosarcoma, bladder, cervical, duodenal, gallbladder, gastric, lymphoma, parotid, squamous cell carcinoma, and thyroid. Clinical toxicities included fatigue (56%), abdominal pain (26%), and nausea/vomiting (23%). On imaging follow-up, WHO, Response Evaluation Criteria in Solid Tumors (RECIST), European Association for the Study of the Liver (EASL), and PET responses of 42.8%, 29%, 67%, and 79% were obtained, respectively. Median survival from first treatment for all patients was 300 days. One-year survival was 47.8%, and 2-year survival was 30.9%. The authors concluded that TheraSphere hepatic treatments can be performed safely on an outpatient basis in patients with unresectable liver neoplasia.[26]

A randomized phase 3 clinical trial of 74 patients was conducted to assess whether a single injection of SIR-Spheres in combination with intrahepatic FUDR could increase the tumor response rate, time to disease progression in the liver, and survival compared to FUDR alone.[2] Patients in the trial had a diagnosis of adenocarcinoma of the large bowel, with unresectable metastases limited to the liver and lymph nodes in the porta hepatis. Both treatment arms received 12-day cycles of continuous-infusion FUDR. The SIR-Spheres treatment arm also received a predetermined quantity of ^{90}Y that varied (2 GBq, 2.5 GBq, or 3 GBq) depending on tumor size. ^{90}Y microspheres were administered one time only within 4 weeks of insertion of the hepatic artery access port. Mean SIR-Spheres dose administered was 2.156 ± 0.32 GBq. Six of 34 patients (18%) in the hepatic artery chemotherapy (HAC) arm had at least a partial response, and 16/36 patients (44%) in the HAC + selective internal radiation therapy (SIRT) arm had at least a partial response.

A total of 208 patients who had failed irinotecan and/or oxaliplatin-based chemotherapy were treated with SIR-Spheres on a lobar and whole-liver basis. The most common clinical toxicities were constitutional (fatigue, fever, weight loss), GI (nausea, vomiting, gastric ulcers), and bilirubin elevations, which occurred in 45%, 30%, and 4.5%, respectively; 5% of patients experienced GI ulceration. There were no cases of radiation-induced liver disease. Imaging response was 35%, and PET response was 91%. Survival was 10.5 months and 4.5 months for responders and nonresponders, respectively. The authors concluded that for patients with metastatic CRC, resin microspheres provide acceptable clinical toxicities, significant objective imaging responses, and promising survival rates.[30]

Jakobs et al. reported results on 41 salvage patients with unresectable hepatic colorectal metastases. The mean activity delivered was 1.9 GBq. Some 71% reported mild to moderate postembolization syndrome. There were 2 cases of gastric ulceration and 1 case of cholecystitis. The mean CEA decrease was 32% for the entire cohort of colorectal patients. By RECIST criteria, partial response, stable disease, and progressive disease were observed in 7, 25, and

4 patients, respectively, at a median interval of 2.9 months. Median overall survival was 10.5 months; improved survival was observed for patients with CAE and imaging response (19.1 vs. 5.4 months and 29.3 vs. 4.3 months, respectively, $P = 0.0001$).[31]

In a recent multicenter phase 2 trial, Cosimelli et al. found that radioembolization produced meaningful responses and disease stabilization in patients with advanced unresectable and chemorefractory metastatic CRC. By RECIST criteria, complete response, partial response, stable disease, and progressive disease were noted in 22%, 24%, 44%, and 8% of patients, respectively. Median overall survival was 12.6 months.[32]

In addition to the studies described, various studies have reported combining ^{90}Y microspheres with chemotherapeutic drugs to manage hepatic metastases from CRC. Sharma et al. performed a phase 1 study analyzing the combination of radioembolization with modified FOLFOX4 systemic chemotherapy in patients with unresectable CRC liver metastases in a series of 20 patients, with the primary endpoint of toxicity. Five patients experienced grade 3 abdominal pain (two of whom had microsphere-induced gastric ulcers); grade 3 or 4 neutropenia was recorded in 12 patients; one episode of transient grade 3 hepatotoxicity was noted. Partial responses were demonstrated in 18 patients and stable disease in 2. Median progression-free survival was 9.3 months, and median time to progression in the liver was 12.3 months. They concluded that this chemoradiation regimen merits investigation in a phase 2-3 trial.[33]

In a recent multicenter phase 3 randomized trial comprising 46 patients with unresectable liver-limited metastatic CRC, Hendlisz et al. compared intravenous fluorouracil (FU) alone (arm A) with combined radioembolization and intravenous fluorouracil (arm B). Median overall survival was 7.3 and 10.0 months in arms A and B, respectively ($P = 0.80$). Median time to tumor progression (TTP) was 2.1 and 4.5 months, respectively ($P = 0.03$). Grade 3 or 4 toxicities were recorded in six patients after FU monotherapy and in one patient after radioembolization plus FU treatment ($P = 0.10$). They concluded that combination therapy is well tolerated and significantly improves time to progression compared with fluorouracil alone, and that this procedure is a valid therapeutic option for chemotherapy-refractory liver metastases from CRC. Low accrual and follow-up longer than planned led to early closure of the trial, with 46 patients included in the study rather than the anticipated 58 required to obtain an estimated 90% power.[34]

Bangash et al. investigated ^{90}Y radioembolization in 27 patients with progressive liver metastases from breast cancer on standard polychemotherapy. The response rate was 39.1%; stable and progressive disease was seen in 52.1% and 8.8%, respectively, and response on PET was noted in 63%. Median survival was 6.8 and 2.6 months in patients with ECOG 0 vs. 1, 2, and 3. Grade III bilirubin toxicity affected 11% of patients. The authors concluded that ^{90}Y may be a viable option for treating patients with breast cancer metastases to the liver who have progressed on standard polychemotherapy.[36]

Recently the role of radioembolization for hepatic metastases from uveal melanoma has been investigated. Up to 90% of these patients die with hepatic metastases, and without treatment, survival after development of metastases ranges between 2 and 7 months.[37] Golsalves et al. reported a 32-patient analysis where they investigated the role of radioembolization after failure of chemoembolization and immunoembolization in patients with hepatic metastases from uveal melanoma. The authors reported a median overall and hepatic progression-free survival of 10 and 4.7 months, respectively. Patients with local disease control and baseline tumor burden less than 25% had longer overall and hepatic progression-free survival than those who had progressive disease or tumor burden over 25%. They concluded that radioembolization is a safe and effective salvage therapy .[37]

Yttrium-90 for metastatic neuroendocrine cancer has been investigated. The high embolic load coupled with low specific activity makes this an ideal therapeutic option for this condition.

In a multicenter phase 2 study of 42 patients with hepatic neuroendocrine tumor metastases, Rhee et al. investigated the efficacy and safety of ^{90}Y radioembolization. They observed that 92% and 94% of patients treated with glass and resin microspheres, respectively, showed either partial response or stable disease at 6 months, and median survival was 22 and 28 months, respectively. Complete response was not observed in any patient. Grade 3 toxicities were recorded in 6 patients, which included bilirubin toxicity (n = 1), alanine aminotransferase (ALT) toxicity (n = 1), aspartate aminotransferase (AST) toxicity (n = 1), and alkaline phosphatase (ALP) toxicity (n = 3). They concluded that ^{90}Y is a viable therapy with acceptable toxicity for hepatic metastases of neuroendocrine tumors.[39]

Recently, Benson et al. presented results from a multi-institutional single-arm prospective trial investigating the role of TheraSphere in patients with hepatic metastases from CRC, neuroendocrine (NE) tumors, and non-CRC/non-NE (mixed tumors).[40] Grade 3 toxicities included pain (n = 17, 11.4%), fatigue (n = 4, 2.7%), vomiting (n = 5, 3.4%), ascites (n = 5, 3.4%), lymphopenia (n = 5, 3.4%), alkaline phosphatase toxicity (n = 12, 8.1%), hyperbilirubinemia (n = 6, 4%), hypoalbuminemia (n = 4, 2.7%), and hypokalemia (n = 3, 2%). Two patients (1.3%) had grade 4 hyperbilirubinemia, infection, and thrombocytopenia. Grade 5 toxicities included death in 11 patients (7.4%) and infection, liver dysfunction, and thrombosis/embolism in 1 patient each (0.7%). Partial response, stable disease, and progressive disease were seen in 10.2%, 60%, and 30% patients, respectively. Median hepatic progression-free survival was 89 days in CRC patients, 536 days in NE patients, and 88 days in non-CRC/non-NE patients. Median progression-free survival was 88 days in CRC patients and 85 days in non-CRC/non-NE patients. Median overall survival was 263 days in CRC and 313 days in CRC and non-CRC/non-NE groups. The authors concluded that TheraSphere demonstrated excellent tolerability and safety profile in patients with advanced metastatic liver disease.[40]

Please visit www.expertconsult.com for a review of additional studies on outcomes of these treatments.

COMPLICATIONS

Radioembolization with ^{90}Y has a low toxicity profile. The most common side effect of radioembolization is fatigue, with over 80% of patients experiencing transient fatigue and vague flulike symptoms. This is related to short-lived, low-dose radiation effects on the normal hepatic parenchyma.[1,7,19] There are several other potential complications that may be encountered:

1. Postembolization syndrome: patients (50%) often experience mild abdominal pain following radioembolization, reversible with narcotics.[7,28] This syndrome seen with radioembolization is not as severe as that observed with chemoembolization, and usually is dominated by fatigue and constitutional symptoms.[19,20,28]

2. Radiation gastritis/GI ulcer/pancreatitis: attenuated radiation to adjacent structures is another theoretical concern, such as may be imparted to the right colon or gallbladder following treatment. Treatment to the left lobe of the liver may cause radiation gastritis secondary to its proximity to the stomach. GI ulceration and nontarget administration of microspheres should be minimized using the angiographic techniques previously described.[7,14,16,41] Aggressive prophylactic embolization is recommended to minimize the risk of ulceration or pancreatitis.[10,42]

3. Radiation pneumonitis: proper lung shunting studies and incorporation of this information in dosimetry models should be practiced universally. The risk of radiation pneumonitis is mitigated if cumulative lung dose is limited to 50 Gy.[13]

4. Radiation hepatitis: another possible complication of radioembolization is radiation hepatitis. Classic findings of anicteric ascites, elevated ALP, thrombocytopenia, and veno-occlusive disease may occur following treatment.[43] More recently, investigators studied the tolerance of liver using external beam radiation. Patients with HCC were able to tolerate 39.8 Gy, and patients with liver metastases could tolerate 45.8 Gy without inducing radiation hepatitis.[44] Caution should be exercised in patients undergoing combination radiosensitizing chemotherapy and radioembolization.

5. Lymphopenia is another possible clinical sequela of ^{90}Y infusion. This is not surprising, given the exquisite sensitivity of lymphocytes to radiation. Although this tends to occur more commonly in glass microsphere patients, there have not been reports of opportunistic infection.[19,45]

6. Biliary injury: given the microspheres size of 20 to 60 microns being quite similar to the blood supply to the peribiliary plexus, microspheres may lodge in this plexus and cause microscopic injury.[14] Possibilities include abscess formation, biliary necrosis, bilomas and radiation cholecystitis.[46]

7. Hepatic fibrosis/portal hypertension: injection of ^{90}Y into the hepatic arterial system may cause hepatic fibrosis, resulting in portal hypertension. Investigators have reported this as a possible complication of ^{90}Y therapy.[47] Patients were explored surgically pre- and post-^{90}Y infusion. At repeat laparotomy, increased portal pressures and venous congestion was noted. The author concluded that ^{90}Y therapy might have contributed to this surgical finding.

8. Radiation cholecystitis: radioembolization may cause radiation cholecystitis. Although clinically relevant radiation cholecystitis requiring cholecystectomy is uncommon, imaging findings of gallbladder injury (enhancing wall, mural rent) are quite common.[7,46]

POSTPROCEDURE AND FOLLOW-UP CARE

Radioembolization can be performed on an outpatient basis. Postprocedurally, patients recover in the holding area according to standard postangiography protocol. They are discharged within 6 hours of the procedure (2 hours if an arterial closure device is used). Our protocol recommends routine use of prophylactic antiulcer medications and proton pump inhibitors in all patients at the time of discharge to minimize risks of GI irritation.[41] In some cases, a 5-day steroid dose pack is also given to counteract fatigue.

For the full discussion of clinical follow-up in the early postprocedure weeks, please visit www.expertconsult.com.

Thirty days following the first treatment, assessment of response to the first infusion is undertaken, and the overall clinical status of the patient is evaluated. Liver function tests, complete blood cell count with platelets and tumor markers, and cross-sectional imaging are obtained. In the majority of cases, overall liver function (total bilirubin) in liver metastases patients should be unchanged. Thirty-day imaging follow-up assesses response of the first lobe and establishes the second lobe baseline prior to treatment. Once all lobes have been treated, patients undergo follow-up CT/PET at 90-day intervals.

If patients continue to exhibit chronic abdominal pain, nausea, vomiting, or bleeding following radioembolization, endoscopic evaluation may be indicated to exclude GI ulceration. Despite using the prophylactic drug regimens described, it is possible to develop radiation gastritis and ulceration, both of which may require surgery for definitive treatment. Radiation-induced liver disease is also a possibility, particularly in patients with compromised liver function at initial treatment. Response to steroids in this condition is variable.

KEY POINTS

- Hepatic metastases are common, most typically from colorectal and neuroendocrine primaries.

- Radioembolization for hepatic metastatic disease is safe and effective in appropriately selected patients.

- Developing a radioembolization program requires an interdisciplinary team including medical, surgical, radiation oncology, interventional radiology, nuclear medicine, and radiation safety professionals.

▶ SUGGESTED READINGS

Liu DM, Salem R, Bui JT, et al. Angiographic considerations in patients undergoing liver-directed therapy. J Vasc Interv Radiol 2005;16(7): 911–35.

Salem R, Thurston KG. Radioembolization with ⁹⁰yttrium microspheres: a state-of-the-art brachytherapy treatment for primary and secondary liver malignancies. Part 1: technical and methodologic considerations. J Vasc Interv Radiol 2006;17(8):1251–78.

Salem R, Thurston KG. Radioembolization with ⁹⁰yttrium microspheres: a state-of-the-art brachytherapy treatment for primary and secondary liver malignancies. Part 2: special topics. J Vasc Interv Radiol 2006; 17(9):1425–39.

Salem R, Thurston KG. Radioembolization with ⁹⁰yttrium microspheres—a state-of-the-art brachytherapy treatment for primary and secondary liver malignancies. Part 3: comprehensive literature review and future direction. J Vasc Interv Radiol 2006;17(10):1571–93.

The complete reference list is available online at www.expertconsult.com.

CHAPTER 68

Bland Embolization for Hepatic Malignancies

Karen T. Brown

Although surgery remains the best hope for cure in patients with most primary and metastatic liver cancers, many patients are not candidates for resection at presentation. This may be due to extent or distribution of disease, underlying liver function, or general medical condition of the patient. The basic physiologic principle that makes hepatic intraarterial therapy feasible is the dual blood supply to the liver. The portal vein provides more than 75% of blood flow to the normal hepatic parenchyma and is the primary trophic blood supply. Conversely, studies performed in the early 1950s established that the primary blood supply to liver tumors was from the hepatic artery.[1] Malignant tumors may be targeted by delivering treatment intraarterially, sparing normal hepatic parenchyma and diminishing or eliminating systemic effects of treatment.

In the last 30 years, many papers have been published describing myriad different techniques for performing hepatic embolotherapy. Many of the studies used chemotherapeutic agents and Lipiodol, despite the lack of convincing pharmacokinetic data. Studies clearly demonstrating an increased concentration of the chemotherapeutic agent(s) used for embolization within the embolized tumor(s) were performed with mitomycin C, doxorubicin, and aclarubicin dissolved in hydrocarbon solvents and then in Lipiodol[2] or with a lipophilic agent,[3] methods that are not used clinically. When the chemotherapeutic agent was dissolved in water and then mixed with Lipiodol and administered as an emulsion, the concentration of drug in the tumor was high immediately but low at 6 hours, 1 day, and 7 days.[2] In a study by Raoul and colleagues,[4] doxorubicin was given to patients intraarterially, either alone as an infusion, emulsified with Lipiodol, or with Lipiodol and gelatin sponge. There was no significant difference in total amount of doxorubicin released into circulating blood, but patients in whom gelatin sponge was used had less released within the first hour of treatment. In a prospective randomized clinical study evaluating the effect of Lipiodol added to intraarterial cisplatin and doxorubicin, no difference in response was noted between the groups given only intraarterial chemotherapy and those who received chemotherapy emulsified with Lipiodol.[5] Another study of intraarterial doxorubicin versus doxorubicin with Lipiodol found no difference in the area under the concentration time curve (AUC) or the terminal half-life, and no difference in pharmacokinetic or systemic toxicity in the same dose schedule as in patients who received intravenous doxorubicin.[6] It seems that the pharmacokinetic data supporting the use of intraarterial chemotherapy or chemotherapy plus Lipiodol, at least when given with the hydrophilic chemotherapeutic agents commonly used today and administered as an emulsion, are not robust.

What has been demonstrated in both pharmacokinetic and clinical studies[4,7,8] is the benefit derived from addition of an embolic agent, even Gelfoam, to the transarterial chemoembolization (TACE) cocktail. Some authors even postulate that the primary effect of embolotherapy is derived from the embolic agent and not the chemotherapy or Lipiodol.[8] If indeed the primary effect of TACE results from ischemia-induced cell death, the goal must be to induce terminal vessel blockade, inasmuch as we know that more proximal vessel occlusion within the liver leads to the almost immediate development of flow distal to the occlusion via myriad collateral vessels, as demonstrated by Michels in 1953.[9] Bland embolization with small particles is an effective method of intraarterial treatment of hypervascular primary and metastatic tumors to the liver that can be used instead of TACE, thereby avoiding the added expense and systemic toxicity of chemotherapy.

INDICATIONS

Bland embolization is indicated for treatment of unresectable "hypervascular" hepatic neoplasms and can be used to treat both benign[10] and malignant[11] processes, but malignant lesions are most commonly treated. It is important to define "hypervascular" hepatic tumors. Malignant tumors in the liver derive primary blood supply from the hepatic artery, whereas normal hepatic parenchyma is primarily supplied by the portal vein. The term *hypervascular* does not simply mean the tumor has arterial blood supply, but rather that the tumor is more "arterialized" than normal liver. This encompasses tumors that demonstrate enhancement on the arterial phase of a triple-phase computed tomography (CT) scan even if these same tumors appear to be low density on the equilibrium phase.

The most common indication is for treatment of unresectable primary hepatocellular cancer (HCC), based on anatomic distribution of disease, vascular invasion, underlying hepatic function, or a combination of these factors. The majority of patients with HCC have underlying liver disease with resultant cirrhosis. Patients with normal liver function and, presumably, normal hepatic parenchyma may undergo resection of 75% to 80% of their liver without developing postoperative hepatic failure. Patients with underlying liver disease require a greater volume of liver remnant to maintain hepatic function, so tumors that might be resectable in patients with normal liver parenchyma may not be resectable in the presence of cirrhosis. In addition, patients with Child class C cirrhosis may be more likely to die of their underlying liver disease than of their HCC and are unlikely to tolerate arterial embolization well. For this reason, embolotherapy is indicated in patients with Child A or B cirrhosis.

Patients with hepatic metastatic disease from neuroendocrine tumors, gastrointestinal stromal tumors, other sarcomas, ocular melanoma, and a variety of other "hypervascular" metastases (e.g., from breast or renal cell cancer) may also be candidates for bland embolization, assuming the liver is the only site of disease, or when the procedure is being performed for palliation of symptoms. In the case of typically indolent neuroendocrine tumors metastatic to the liver, the diagnosis may first be established when patients present with symptoms related to hepatic metastases because the primary tumors are often small and whatever vasoactive or hormonal peptides they produce are excreted into the portal vein and then deactivated by the liver. It is only when the hormonally active tumor metastasizes to the liver and hormone is secreted directly into the systemic circulation that symptoms occur. Similarly, nonfunctional neuroendocrine tumors may first be diagnosed when hepatic metastatic disease results in abnormal liver function test results picked up on routine screening or cause "bulk-related" symptomatology. Hypervascular metastases from other primary tumors such as breast, renal cell, or even prostate cancer are not uncommon, and these tumors also respond to bland embolization. Given the pattern of metastatic dissemination of disease with these cancers, isolated hepatic metastases are less common, and liver-directed therapy is less often indicated.

Since the purpose of hepatic embolization is to either treat symptoms or extend survival, patients who are asymptomatic from their secondary hepatic disease and who have disease elsewhere should probably not be considered candidates. Intraarterial therapy based on ischemia induced by terminal vessel blockade should not be expected to be efficacious in patients with hypovascular tumors and has no proven role in the treatment of typical metastatic adenocarcinoma from most gastrointestinal malignancies.

CONTRAINDICATIONS

Although there are no absolute contraindications to hepatic arterial embolization, in general, patients with Child class C cirrhosis should not undergo embolization as a primary method of treatment; their survival is much more likely to be determined by their liver disease, not their tumor. If embolization is warranted, such as to stop bleeding, embolization should be limited in scope. When evaluating a patient for embolization, one should consider the severity of the underlying liver disease as well as the extent of the tumor being treated. Several methods of classification have been developed in an effort to weigh both these factors, the simplest being the Okuda stage. In this scheme, patients are given points for the presence or absence of ascites, serum bilirubin and albumin levels, and tumor extent. In 1999, Llovett et al.[12] proposed the BCLC (Barcelona Clinic Liver Cancer) staging classification as a means of both classifying patients and linking their stage to a specific treatment. Although selective embolization of a solitary well-circumscribed HCC in a patient with Child class B cirrhosis might be well tolerated, embolization of a hemiliver in a Child A patient with multifocal hepatoma involving more than 75% of the liver and with portal vein tumor thrombus may result in hepatic failure and even death.

Patients with HCC and cirrhosis may have thrombocytopenia and coagulation disorders. If the platelet count is less than 50,000/mm³, we give 1 unit of platelets during the procedure. It is less common to have to correct a liver-related coagulopathy because patients with that degree of synthetic liver impairment are typically not candidates for embolization. We do not routinely administer fresh frozen plasma if the International Normalized Ratio (INR) is less than 2.0.

Noncirrhotic patients with metastatic disease from neuroendocrine or other tumors should be embolized with caution if more than 75% of the liver is replaced by tumor; if they are treated, embolization should be staged. Instead of treating a hemiliver, either the anterior _or_ posterior division of the right liver, _or_ the lateral segment of the left liver could be treated initially, and after seeing how this treatment is tolerated by the patient, further embolization could be performed.

If the creatinine level is greater than 1.5 ng/dL, patients receive 3 mL/kg/h of a solution of sodium bicarbonate (154 mEq/L) administered over a 1-hour period before the procedure. They are then maintained on a 1 mL/kg/h infusion for 6 hours after the procedure. The volume of contrast material should be kept to a minimum. Patients with allergies to contrast agents are premedicated with prednisone 13, 8, and 1 hour before the procedure.

EQUIPMENT

Bland hepatic arterial embolization does not require anything not traditionally found in the usual angiography suite. Selective catheters, such as 4F or 5F Cobras and reverse-curve catheters (Simmons or SOS catheters), are used through a vascular sheath placed in the right external iliac artery. Coaxial microcatheters are used when necessary for subselective embolization. Conventional nonionic contrast material is typically used. Since treatment depends on terminal tumor vessel blockade, we use the smallest particles commercially available. Until the late 1990s, 50-µm polyvinyl alcohol (PVA) particles (Cook Medical, Bloomington, Ind.) were the smallest particles available, then Embospheres (BioSphere Medical, Rockland, Mass.), a hydrophilic trisacryl gelatin microsphere, became available in 100- to 300-µm sizes. Despite the larger sphere size, the fact that the microspheres were spherical and hydrophilic meant they did not "clump" like PVA and were capable of penetrating more distally into the terminal vasculature.[13-15] Eventually, 40- to 120-µm Embospheres became available, and we began to use graduated sizes of Embospheres almost exclusively. Use of Embospheres is associated with preservation of arterial patency,[16] an important consideration in patients who are expected to need repeated treatment.

TECHNIQUE

Preprocedure Preparation

Patients should take nothing by mouth after midnight. They are admitted to the hospital the morning of the procedure and have an intravenous line started. Patients with impaired renal function receive sodium bicarbonate (see earlier discussion). Hydration is begun with normal saline in all patients. Those with allergies to contrast receive 50 mg of prednisone orally 1 hour before the procedure (they have already received two other doses of prednisone [see earlier discussion]). All patients are given 4 mg of ondansetron (Zofran) and 1 g of cefazolin (Ancef) intravenously. Patients who do not have an intact sphincter of Oddi receive 2 g of cefotetan (Cefotan) intravenously.

Anatomy and Approach

As part of the preprocedure workup, every patient has a triple-phase CT scan within 1 month of the scheduled embolization. Triple-phase CT is essential for documenting the extent of disease, demonstrating arterial anatomy, evaluating the portal venous system, and looking for nonhepatic blood supply to the tumor. This study serves as the basis for a treatment plan. The extent and distribution of the tumor are laid out (Fig. 68-1, *A*), arterial blood supply to the tumor is evident (Fig. 68-1, *B*), and any contribution from the extrahepatic vasculature, such as the phrenic (Fig. 68-2, *A* and *B*) or internal mammary arteries, should be seen. On the day of the procedure, the plan needs only to be executed.

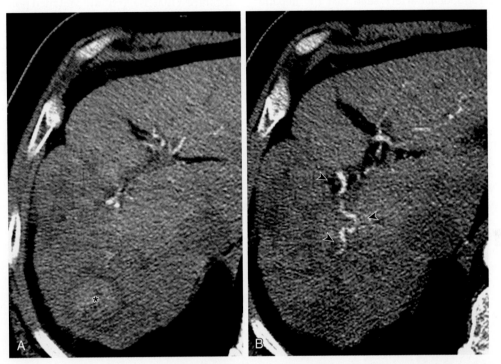

FIGURE 68-1. **A,** Arterial phase of a triple-phase computed tomography (CT) scan demonstrates solitary hypervascular hepatocellular carcinoma (HCC) in segment VI *(asterisk).* **B,** Adjacent image from arterial-phase CT shows primary supply to HCC is a segment VI branch *(arrowheads),* seen coursing toward tumor.

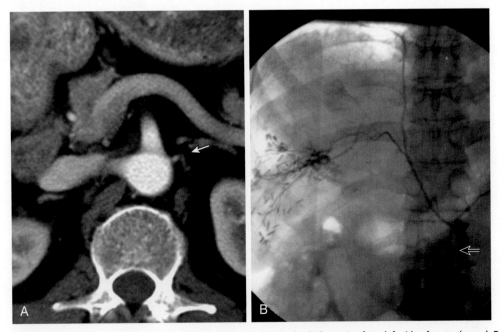

FIGURE 68-2. **A,** Right phrenic artery is shown on triple-phase computed tomography (CT) to arise from left side of aorta *(arrow).* **B,** Arteriogram taken through a Cobra catheter selectively placed in right phrenic artery *(arrow).* Information from arterial-phase CT makes finding and catheterizing the vessel much easier.

Technical Aspects

Celiac and superior mesenteric angiography is performed to document arterial anatomy, demonstrate the hypervascular tumor, and evaluate the direction of blood flow, which cannot be determined by conventional triple-phase CT. Hemodynamically significant stenosis of the celiac or hepatic artery origin results in retrograde blood flow through the gastroduodenal artery such that the hepatic arteries are opacified on the superior mesenteric angiogram (Fig. 68-3, *A-C*). Similarly, significant portal venous hypertension results in hepatofugal flow on the portal venous phase of the angiogram, even though the portal vein may be opacified as well. All this information is integrated into the treatment plan for the patient. Even hypervascular tumors may not be evident on celiac angiography (Fig. 68-4, *A*), so selective arteriography should be undertaken by injecting the vessels known to supply the tumor by previous triple-phase CT (Fig. 68-4, *B*).

If multifocal bilobar disease is present, one side of the liver is selected for treatment at the first sitting, usually the side with the most tumor. The catheter is placed selectively into the right or left hepatic artery, and arteriography is performed. A 2-mL syringe of 40- to 120-μm Embospheres (or the smallest particle of the operator's choice) is poured into a small glass or stainless steel cup, and the syringe is rinsed of residual spheres by filling it with an equal volume of contrast material (≈5 mL) and then pouring the contents into the cup containing the spheres. The target vessel is subsequently embolized with the Embospheres suspended in contrast material until stasis is evident, or until 10 mL of 40- to 120-μm particles have been used. Stasis is defined as lack of antegrade flow, with evidence of reflux on injection of even small amounts of contrast material.

When stasis occurs, the procedure is terminated, and a final arteriogram is performed to document occlusion of the target vessel and preservation of blood flow to nontarget vessels. If antegrade flow persists after 10 mL of the

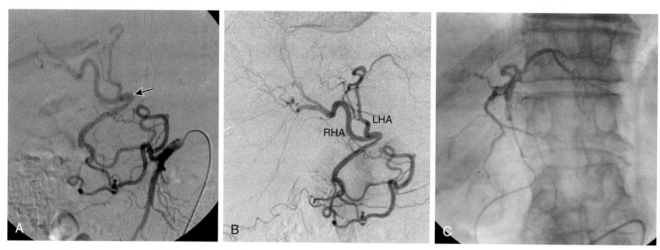

FIGURE 68-3. A, Superior mesenteric arteriogram showing extensive pancreaticoduodenal collaterals reconstituting common hepatic artery *(arrow)* secondary to hepatic arterial occlusion. **B,** Hepatic artery occlusion could not be crossed from the celiac artery, so a 4F Cobra catheter was selectively placed into a collateral vessel. Arteriography demonstrates reconstitution of proper hepatic artery and right *(RHA)* and left *(LHA)* hepatic branches. **C,** Through the Cobra catheter, a coaxial catheter was advanced selectively into left hepatic artery in preparation for embolization.

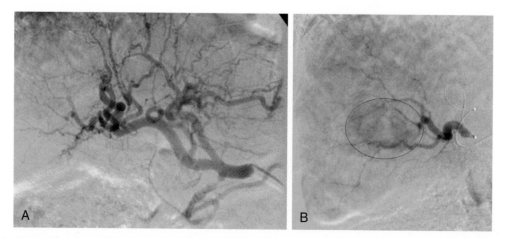

FIGURE 68-4. A, Common hepatic arteriogram in same patient as in Figure 68-1. No definite evidence of tumor neovascularity. **B,** Selective arteriogram of a segment VI branch demonstrates hypervascular tumor *(ellipse)*.

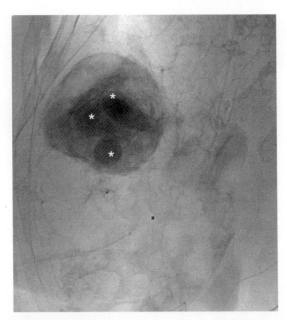

FIGURE 68-5. Example of "embolization sinks," with pooling of contrast material in what appear to be large spaces *(asterisks)* within the tumor after occlusion of the small vasculature.

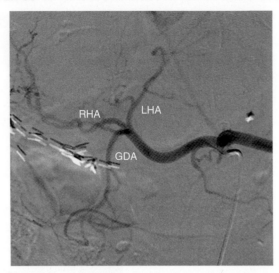

FIGURE 68-6. In this case, common hepatic artery branches into left hepatic artery *(LHA)*, anterior division of right hepatic artery *(RHA)*, posterior division of RHA, and gastroduodenal artery *(GDA)*. One must be very careful in this situation to not reflux embolic material into GDA.

smallest particles have been used, embolization is continued with the next size of particles (100-300 μm in the case of Embospheres). Once again, up to 10 mL of these particles are infused. If antegrade flow persists, the next size particles are used, once again injecting up to 10 mL of these particles, and so on. Occasionally, *embolization sinks* develop (Fig. 68-5), which are areas where contrast material seems to pool after the tumor vasculature has been embolized. These sinks seem to have an endless capacity for contrast agent and particles and thus maintain antegrade flow. When one of these sinks is evident, the operator will often switch to 100-μm PVA particles. It usually takes only a small amount of conventional PVA to arrest flow into the sink, at which point antegrade flow ceases.

Sometimes branches of the left or right hepatic artery are embolized superselectively, either because one is treating a solitary tumor, arterial anomalies (accessory vessels with an aberrant origin) are present, or to avoid nontarget embolization (e.g., when there is a trifurcation of the common hepatic artery into right and left hepatic arteries and the gastroduodenal artery (Fig. 68-6). In these cases, a coaxial catheter is placed selectively into each branch supplying the target territory. After arteriography is performed, embolization is begun with the smallest particles. If stasis does not occur after 10 mL of that size particle are used, the next size particle is injected, and so on, until stasis is evident, at which point the catheter is repositioned in the next branch to be embolized, and once again embolization is begun with the smallest-size particle.

For solitary tumors, an attempt is made to embolize the tumor as selectively as possible. The initial arteriogram is reviewed to determine which vessel or vessels are feeding the tumor. Each vessel is then selected, typically with a coaxial 2F to 3F catheter, and that vessel is embolized with up to 10 mL of the smallest-size particle. If antegrade flow persists after 10 mL of the smallest particle have been used, treatment is continued with the next size particle, and so

on, until stasis occurs and persists. If additional vessels are identified supplying the tumor, these vessels are sequentially catheterized and treated according to our standard protocol, beginning with the smallest particle and continuing until stasis is evident.

When embolization of the target vessel or vessels is complete, a final angiogram is performed to document the result. When appropriate, angiography of nonhepatic vessels potentially supplying the tumor (e.g., phrenic, internal mammary, or intercostal arteries) is performed. If the patient is doing well, use of contrast material has not been excessive, and embolization of additional vessels is thought to be safe, the procedure continues. If the entire tumor has been treated or a hemiliver has been treated, the procedure is terminated, and the treatment plan for the next embolization (should that be necessary) is outlined. An immediate CT scan is then performed. This scan will demonstrate uptake of contrast in the treated tumor with circumferential coverage (Fig. 68-7, *A* and *B*), assuming appropriate vessels have been targeted. Tumor contrast retention seems to correlate with development of tumor necrosis by imaging[17] (Fig. 68-7, *C*).

Solitary Tumors Smaller Than 5 cm

Patients with solitary HCC may be ablated immediately after embolization. Thermal ablation is preferred, barring some contraindication (adjacent bowel or other structure thought to be susceptible to thermal damage). The idea here is to "double-kill" the tumor. In other words, by combining two methods that when used alone may incompletely treat the tumor, we hope to achieve 100% tumor cell death. The combination of arterial embolization and thermal ablation makes sense, since embolization takes away the arterial blood supply. Thermal ablation is then performed on a tumor that has already been deprived of its arterial blood supply, allowing the thermal method to work more effectively by at least removing the arterial "heat sink." After bland embolization, there is typically dense opacification of the treated tumor because the particles mixed with contrast

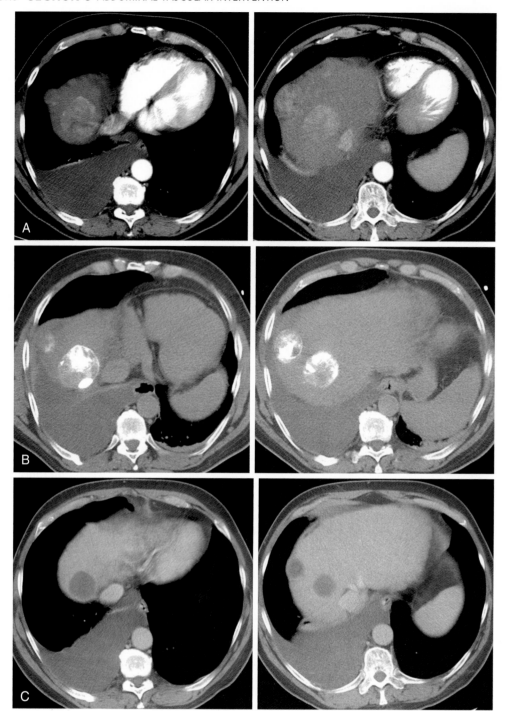

FIGURE 68-7. **A,** Arterial-phase computed tomography (CT) prior to embolization; two enhancing masses are identified in segment VIII. **B,** CT obtained immediately after embolization shows circumferential uptake of contrast by tumors. **C,** Venous-phase CT 3 months after embolization demonstrates imaging findings of tumor necrosis.

agent remain within the treated tumor (Fig. 68-8), analogous to what is seen after TACE with Lipiodol. This allows easy targeting of the lesion by CT. If a portion of the tumor appears incompletely treated by bland embolization, this area is evident on CT (Fig. 68-9) and can be targeted by thermal or chemical methods. Our results using this method to treat tumors smaller than 7 cm are comparable to surgical resection.[18]

Summary of Technical Aspects
• Preprocedure road map from triple-phase CT is very important.
• Anticipate nonhepatic arterial supply and look for it.

• Move up to the next size particle after every 10 mL of one size particle is used in each vessel.
• When an embolization sink is encountered, use 50- or 100-μm PVA particles to arrest antegrade flow.
• Tumor contrast retention on immediate postembolization CT correlates with subsequent imaging findings of tumor necrosis.

CONTROVERSIES

The main controversy with regard to hepatic arterial embolization of primary and secondary hepatic malignancies revolves around the use of chemotherapeutic agents.

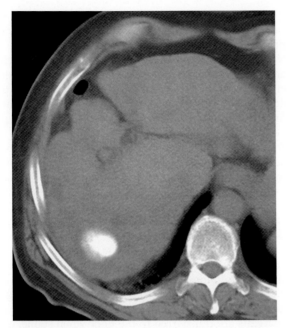

FIGURE 68-8. Computed tomography the day after embolization of tumor demonstrated in Figures 68-1 and 68-4. Before radiofrequency ablation, contrast material and particles retained within tumor are making it very "dense."

Although the concept of delivering high-dose chemotherapy to the tumor or tumors is sound, there is a paucity of evidence-based findings supporting routine use of chemoembolization. Because TACE is more complicated to perform, adds the expense of chemotherapy, has the potential for systemic side effects, and may have a higher incidence of postembolization vessel occlusion, there are barriers to its routine use. If indeed the primary effect of TACE as currently practiced is due to ischemia, particle embolization would make more sense, be less expensive, not have chemotherapy's side effects, and might be more readily practiced in the community setting.

OUTCOMES

In a series of 322 patients undergoing bland embolization for HCC at our institution between 1997 and 2005, with a median follow-up of 20 months, 1-, 2-, and 3-year overall survival rates were 66%, 46%, and 33%, respectively.[11] When patients with extrahepatic disease or portal vein involvement by tumor were excluded (similar to patients reported by Lo[19] and Llovet[20] and their colleagues, two seminal studies), overall 1-, 2-, and 3-year survival rates rose to 84%, 66%, and 51%, and median survival to 40 months. Subgroups of patients being treated for solitary HCC who also underwent thermal ablation the day after embolization had survival results that paralleled those seen after surgical

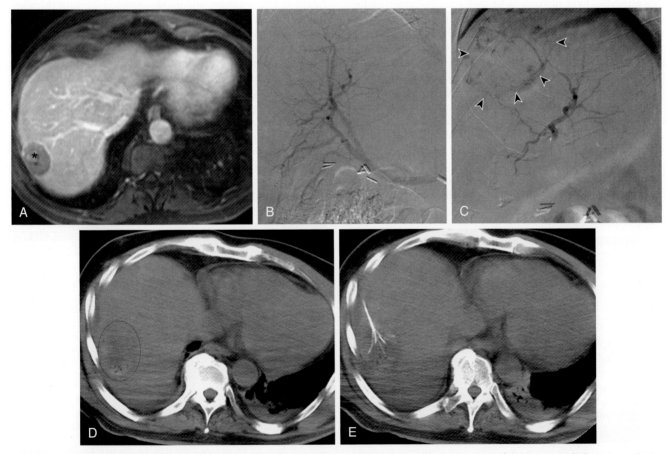

FIGURE 68-9. A, Magnetic resonance imaging of a solitary hepatocellular carcinoma *(asterisk)* in segment VIII of the liver. **B,** Right hepatic arteriogram with no discernible hypervascularity. **C,** Selective injection of a segment VII branch shows hypervascular tumor *(arrowheads)*. **D,** Computed tomography the day after embolization at the time of radiofrequency ablation (RFA), with deposition of contrast material and particles predominantly in posterior aspect of tumor *(ellipse)*. **E,** RFA multitined electrode is targeted to anterior part of tumor, which contains less contrast material and particles.

resection in a case-control study at our institution.[18] We have reported the results of treating patients with metastatic neuroendocrine tumor[21] and metastatic sarcomas[22] that parallel those reported by others using TACE.

COMPLICATIONS

Postembolization syndrome (PES) occurs in approximately 80% of patients and consists of pain, fever, nausea, and vomiting. PES should be considered a side effect and not a complication of embolotherapy. We think of it as a type of tumor lysis syndrome. After abrupt ischemic tumor cell death, the tumor cells lyse and release their intracellular material into the bloodstream. This is analogous to what happens when patients with lymphoma are treated with chemotherapy. Intracellular toxins may cause fever, nausea, and vomiting. PES is treated with analgesics, antipyretics, and antiemetics and typically subsides after 24 to 72 hours. Occasionally, one or more components of PES persist. As long as the symptoms are controlled with oral medications and core temperature is lower than 38.5°C, the patient may be discharged from the hospital.

Liver abscess is a rare complication of hepatic embolization, so the typical postembolization appearance of a low-density lesion with scattered gas bubbles should not be confused with a liver abscess (Fig. 68-10). We avoid scanning patients in the immediate postembolization period to avoid raising the issue of liver abscess. Similar to postoperative patients, liver abscess does not usually occur earlier than 7 to 10 days after embolization. It is seen most commonly in patients who have undergone bilioenteric bypass or who for any reason (e.g., sphincterotomy) do not have an intact sphincter of Oddi.[23] In a review of almost 1000 patients undergoing over 2000 embolization procedures, the risk of liver abscess in patients with a contaminated biliary tree was found to be up to 300 times higher than the baseline risk.[23] Patients with a liver abscess will have an elevated white blood cell count and fever and appear ill. Patients without an intact sphincter of Oddi are treated prophylactically with an antibiotic expected to cover biliary flora (e.g., cefotetan) before embolization, rather than the customary Ancef. Cefotetan is given intravenously for as long as these patients are in the hospital, and they are sent home on 1 week of metronidazole (Flagyl) and ciprofloxacin (Cipro). Despite this, liver abscess may occur.

Nontarget embolization is one of the most dreaded complications of hepatic embolotherapy but occurs infrequently when strict attention is paid to arterial anatomy. The gallbladder is probably the most commonly involved nontarget organ. Inadvertent gallbladder embolization results in prolonged PES with fever, pain, and nausea/vomiting, but rarely requires surgical intervention. In our practice, despite some nasty-looking gallbladders, few patients have required intervention. Rarely a cholecystostomy catheter is placed that can be removed in 2 to 3 weeks.

POSTPROCEDURAL AND FOLLOW-UP CARE

After embolization, patients are observed in the postanesthesia care unit for several hours. Requirement for pain medication is monitored, and patient-controlled analgesia is initiated when warranted. Blood pressure is stabilized, and patients are transferred to the floor when stable. Clear liquids are allowed for the first 24 hours, and the diet is advanced as tolerated. Intravenous antibiotics are administered for 24 hours when the sphincter of Oddi is intact or for the duration of hospital stay when not. Antipyretics are administered as needed; if the temperature exceeds 38.5°C, blood is drawn for culture. Patients are discharged from the hospital when taking adequate nutrition by mouth, when pain is adequately controlled with oral narcotics, and when the temperature is lower than 38.5°C for 24 hours.

Follow-up triple-phase CT is performed 2 to 4 weeks after treatment is complete. In the case of patients requiring more than one embolization for complete treatment, this is 2 to 4 weeks after the final treatment. The follow-up CT scan is reviewed for any evidence of persistent untreated disease. If there is no evidence of enhancement of the treated tumor, these patients are monitored with triple-phase CT every 3 months for the first year and every 6 months thereafter. When there is evidence of untreated disease, recurrent disease, or new disease elsewhere within the liver, the patient is scheduled for retreatment.

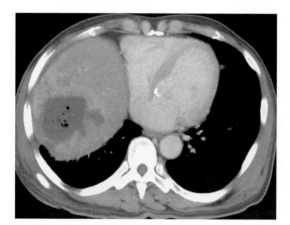

FIGURE 68-10. On contrast-enhanced computed tomography, tumor has low density and scattered "gas bubbles." This appearance is fairly typical after embolization when imaged within first few weeks after treatment and should not be confused with an abscess.

KEY POINTS

- Embolization with particles alone, when performed to effect terminal vessel blockade, is an effective method of treating hypervascular primary and secondary hepatic malignancies.

- No study to date has demonstrated a survival advantage of chemoembolization over particle embolization.

- Embolization with particles alone is easy to perform with items on hand in the interventional radiology suite, is performed selectively or superselectively to treat existing tumor, and has a reproducible endpoint.

- Although postembolization syndrome occurs in the majority of patients treated by particle embolization, it typically resolves within 48 hours, and there are no systemic effects of chemotherapy to contend with.

- Using particles alone for hepatic arterial embolization does not seem to result in as high a rate of permanent occlusion of the native vessels as is seen after chemoembolization.

► **SUGGESTED READINGS**

Brown DB, Geshwind JFH, Soulen MC, et al. Society of Interventional Radiology position statement on chemoembolization of hepatic malignancies. J Vasc Interv Radiol 2006;17:217–23.

Brown KT, Koh BY, Brody LA, et al. Particle embolization of hepatic neuroendocrine metastases for control of pain and hormonal symptoms. J Vasc Interv Radiol 1999;10:397–403.

Brown KT, Nevins AB, Getrajdman GI, et al. Particle embolization of hepatocellular carcinoma. J Vasc Interv Radiol 1998;9:822–8.

Llovet JM, Real MI, Montana X, et al. for the Barcelona Clinic Liver Cancer Group. Arterial embolisation or chemoembolisation versus symptomatic treatment in patients with unresectable hepatocellular carcinoma: a randomized controlled trial. Lancet 2002;359:1734–9.

Lo CM, Ngan H, Tso WK, et al. Randomized controlled trial of transarterial Lipiodol chemoembolization for unresectable hepatocellular carcinoma. Hepatology 2002;35:1164–71.

Madoff DC, Gupta S, Ahrar K, et al. Update on the management of neuroendocrine hepatic metastases. J Vasc Interv Radiol 2006;17:1235–50.

Maluccio M, Covey AM, Ghandi R, et al. Comparison of survival rates after bland embolization and ablation versus surgical resection for treating patients with solitary hepatocellular carcinoma up to 7 cm. J Vasc Interv Radiol 2005;16:955–61.

The complete reference list is available online at www.expertconsult.com.

CHAPTER 69

Portal Vein Embolization

Thierry de Baère and Alain Roche

One of the prerequisites for partial hepatic resection is the presence of enough remaining functional liver parenchyma to avoid life-threatening postoperative liver failure. Therefore, the possibilities of curative resection of liver tumors are strongly dependent on the volume of the future remnant liver (FRL). In clinical practice, these possibilities are frequently limited when an extended hepatectomy is mandatory because the FRL is too small. The more frequent case is need for a right extended hepatectomy with a small left lobe. Major liver surgery is indicated in some patients with impaired liver function, whatever the cause (e.g., cirrhosis, cholestasis, fibrosis, steatosis), and this further limits the possibility of surgery because larger FRL volume is needed. It has long been demonstrated that liver trophicity closely depends on hepatic portal blood flow, and consequently portal branch ligation results in shrinkage of the corresponding lobe and hypertrophy of the contralateral one.[1] In the same manner, liver atrophy occurs after surgical or spontaneous portocaval shunting, hypertrophy of the remnant liver occurs after partial hepatectomy, and the Spiegel lobe hypertrophies in Budd-Chiari disease when the caudate lobe remains the only one to still have hepatopetal portal blood flow.

It was established in the 1970s that portal venous blood flow promoted hepatic cell regeneration, and that blood arising from the duodenopancreatic area had strong hepatotropic properties. Insulin and glucagon were then soon recognized as growth regulatory factors that, when infused concomitantly, synergistically stimulated hepatic regeneration.[2] More recently, hepatocyte growth factor (HGF) could be isolated in different laboratories and described to rise after partial hepatectomy.[3] Multiple other peptides such as transforming growth factor (TGF)-α or serotonin have also been demonstrated to play a role in hepatic regeneration.

The aim of portal vein embolization (PVE) is to selectively induce hypertrophy of the FRL during the preoperative period. This is achieved by embolization of the intrahepatic portal branches of the future resected liver, leading to distribution of the entire portal blood flow containing hepatotropic factors exclusively toward the FRL.

INDICATIONS

Limits for hepatic resections, and consequently indications for PVE, depend on multiple factors, but FRL/total functional liver ratio for a given patient (according to age and liver function) is the main factor that determines possibilities for a safe resection. Depending on the authors, PVE is considered when this ratio is expected to be less than 25% to 40% in patients with normal liver function, and less than 40% to 50% in patients with liver dysfunction.[1-3]

Many studies have demonstrated that computed tomography (CT) estimations of liver volumes were correctly correlated to real volumes, despite partial volume effect, respiratory phase, or interobserver variations. Consequently, liver CT volumetry is a key examination to determine surgical possibilities and need for PVE. Because tumors do not contain functional hepatocytes, tumor volume must be subtracted from that of liver during CT volumetry. In the same manner, when radiofrequency ablation (RFA) is planned simultaneously with the hepatectomy for treating a tumor located in the FRL, one should pay attention to subtracting the volume of the future RFA lesion (tumor volume + safety margin) from the FRL volume. CT volumetry should be performed 1 month after PVE to evaluate hypertrophy of the FRL (Fig. 69-1).

Hepatocellular Carcinoma

PVE was initially proposed for controlling retrograde tumor thrombus invasion in the portal vein in hepatocellular carcinoma (HCC), but today there is little evidence to support this indication. Most HCCs occur in patients with compromised liver, which dramatically increases the risk of severe postoperative complications and limits possibilities for major curative liver resections. Consequently, PVE is actually proposed in selected cases to extend indications for curative surgery and increase its safety. Apart from increasing FRL volume and function, minimizing the sudden increase in portal pressure at resection in these cirrhotic patients may also be an advantage of preoperative PVE.

Liver Metastases

Curative resection of liver metastases is mainly performed in patients presenting with colorectal primary cancer. Liver metastases are found in 40% to 70% of patients with colorectal cancer. In about one third of cases, the liver is shown to be the only site of cancer spread, even at autopsy. There is no spontaneous long-term survival in untreated patients, whose median survival time ranges from 6 to 24 months. At the time of diagnosis, the majority of patients present with unresectable tumors, and resection can be performed in less than 20% of all patients with colorectal liver metastases. The main limitation for resectability is the impossibility to be curative while leaving a sufficient residual amount of functional liver parenchyma. Consequently, preoperative PVE may dramatically improve the possibilities for a curative resection of liver metastases by increasing the volume and function of the FRL.

Other Indications

Portal vein embolization has been reported before resection of hilar cholangiocarcinoma, multiple benign adenomas whose dissemination in the liver parenchyma impeded curative surgery, and of a huge benign adenoma. It has also allowed resection in primary sclerosing cholangitis.

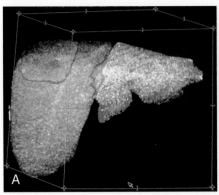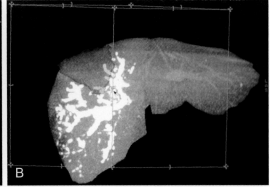

FIGURE 69-1. Three-dimensional computed tomography (CT) volumetry of the liver before **(A)** and 1 month after **(B)** portal vein embolization. Left lobe (future remnant liver [FRL]), highlighted in green, hypertrophied in the month between the two images. Liver to be resected is shown in blue, and tumor is in red. Note glue inside right portal branch seen in **B**.

CONTRAINDICATIONS

PVE is a neoadjuvant preoperative therapy with indications and contraindications closely resembling those for hepatic resection. Usual contraindications or high-risk conditions for performing the percutaneous transhepatic approach (e.g., massive ascites, severe blood coagulation disorders) are contraindications or limits to liver surgery as well. Consequently, in practice, they do not have a real impact on PVE.

A biliary obstruction contraindicates the transhepatic approach through any sector of the liver affected by bile duct dilatation. Nevertheless, because biliary drainage of the FRL is necessary to promote hypertrophy, access through the FRL will be obtained.

EQUIPMENT

Ultrasound guidance is necessary for puncture of a small peripheral portal vein branch. We use a 27-cm 5F needle catheter (Transhepatic chlangiography catheter, DPLTH-5.0-27-ST, Cook Medical, Bloomington, Ind.) or a 20-cm 18-gauge EchoTip needle (Temno chiba needle, CHI1815, Carefusion, McGraw Park, Ill.) for entering the portal vein.

The procedure requires a digital subtraction angiography (DSA) suite with possible angulation of the C-arm that will aid intraportal navigation when venous anatomy is unusual and in atypical PVE before complex resections. In such complex embolization or atypical resection, three-dimensional (3D) reconstruction from cone beam CT acquisition and 3D roadmap renders catheterization easier (Fig. 69-2). On demand catheter tip can be shaped, alternatively Cobra shape can be used when approach is contralateral, or short sidewinder catheter can be used when approach is ipsilateral. Usually, a 0.035-inch hydrophilic guidewire suffices for the entire procedure. Microcatheters are used by some operators for particle embolization through ipsilateral access.

Embolic agents vary from center to center. We use cyanoacrylate (Histoacryl, B. Braun Medical, Bethlehem, Pa.) mixed with Lipiodol Ultra Fluid, 10 mL (Guerbet, Villepinte, France). Others use spherical embolic material ranging from 300 to 500 to 500 to 700 µm.

When cyanoacrylate is used, a 3-way stopcock resistant to Lipiodol is needed, as well as isotonic glucose solution for the sandwich technique. In addition, 1-mL syringes are needed for cyanoacrylate injection, and a 20-mL syringe is needed for flushing.

TECHNIQUE

Anatomy and Approaches

A thorough knowledge of hepatic segmentation and portal venous anatomy is essential before performing PVE. The most frequent variation is slipping from right to left of segment V and VIII branches, separately or together. Therefore, two main variations are frequently encountered: (1) trifurcation of the portal vein into the left branch, segments V + VIII branch and segments VI + VII branch, when the slipping is limited and (2) bifurcation of the portal vein into a right vein limited to segments VI + VII, and left vein also giving rise to segments V + VIII branch, when the slipping is complete (Fig. 69-3). Besides knowledge of the anatomy, a clear knowledge of the plane of the hepatectomy is necessary before starting the procedure because the extent of PVE must mimic the extent of surgery, and because more and more atypical surgery is performed, many different types of PVE are possible[4] (Fig. 69-4).

Technical Aspects

The procedure may be performed under intravenous sedation and analgesia, but most teams prefer general anesthesia, which provides more comfort for the patient and the operator.

Access can be obtained from a contralateral approach (i.e., puncture of the left portal branch and embolization of right portal branches) or an ipsilateral approach (i.e., puncture of the right to embolize right portal branches). The advantage of the contralateral approach is easier catheterization of the right lobe branches, but there is a risk of damage to the FRL. An ipsilateral approach allows for easier catheterization of segment IV branches when needed. The drawbacks of the ipsilateral approach are the difficulty of access to right portal branches in a retrograde fashion and difficulty in obtaining a good final portography, since the catheter has to pass through embolic material to be placed in the portal vein for the final contrast medium injection. Choosing the access also depends on the embolic material

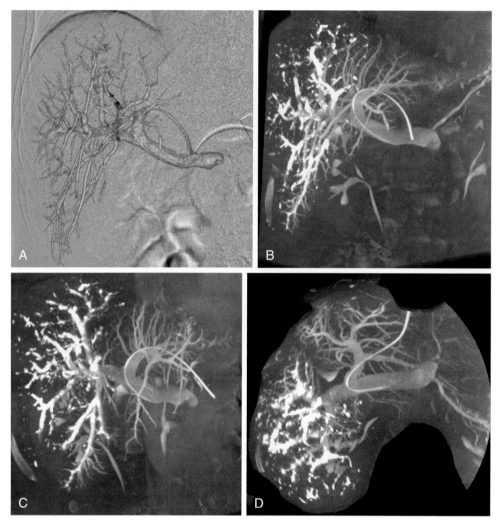

FIGURE 69-2. **A,** Three-dimensional reconstruction of portal tree from cone beam computed tomography acquisition. Multiplanar reconstruction in frontal **(B)**, frontal oblique **(C)**, and axial plane **(D)** obtained after portal vein embolization of right liver, where glue is demonstrated in branches feeding segments V, VI, VII, and VIII. Note segment III contralateral puncture without embolization of segment IV.

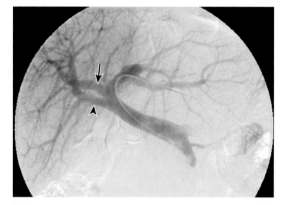

FIGURE 69-3. Digital subtraction angiographic portography obtained after puncture of a segment III portal branch shows an anatomic variation: bifurcation of the portal vein into a right vein limited to segments VI and VII *(arrowhead)*, and left vein giving rise to segment V and VIII branches *(arrow)*.

used. Glue can hardly be manipulated from the ipsilateral side, but large embolic materials like plugs require large-diameter access, which is less risky when obtained on the ipsilateral side. Ultimately, the choice between the ipsilateral and contralateral route should be based on their respective complication rates, which are similar and mainly related to puncture of unexpected structures like biliary branches or hepatic arteries. The largest series of contralateral PVE reviewed 188 cases performed in different centers using contralateral access as well as N-butyl cyanoacrylate as an embolic material.[5] In the literature, the only factor increasing complications is puncture of the right posterior segment versus puncture of the right anterior segment,[6] thus advocating puncture of the anterior segment when compatible with the location of the PVE to be performed.

When the goal of PVE is occlusion of right branches, we preferred access of the portal vein with the contralateral anterior subxiphoid left route, which allows antegrade catheterization of all right branches to be occluded and free-flow embolization, thereby enabling safe maneuvers. The puncture is achieved under ultrasonographic guidance with a 5F needle catheter. When branches for segment IV do not

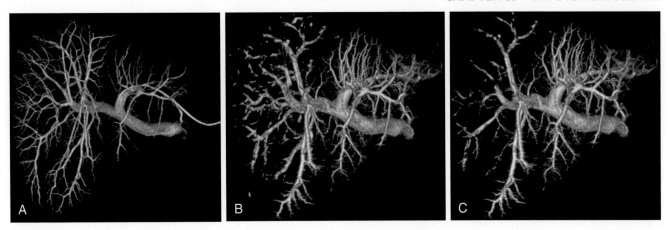

FIGURE 69-4. A, Frontal view of three-dimensional reconstruction of the portal tree from cone beam computed tomography (CT) acquisition before portal vein embolization (PVE) demonstrates portal branch anatomy. **B,** Atypical PVE to right posterior segment (segments VI and VII) has been performed, and right anterior oblique reconstruction obtained from cone beam CT portography shows glue in yellow and patent branches in brown. **C,** Right anterior oblique reconstruction where glue is subtracted shows patent branches to all liver except right posterior segment.

have to be occluded, the entry point in portal veins may be the Rex recess. If segment IV is affected by PVE, entering a peripheral segment III branch is recommended to facilitate catheterization of segment IV branches. Retrograde catheterization of the main portal trunk for performing portography is the first step of the procedure to identify individual intrahepatic branches and anatomic variations. In all patients with a known or suspected compromised liver, the portal pressure must be measured before embolization because it represents a prognostic parameter. Catheterization of every branch to be embolized is then performed with the 5F catheter of the needle catheter device. Depending on individual anatomy, a 1- to 2-cm length and 30- to 90-degree angulated tip is then shaped with steam in order to make further maneuvers easier. Every main trunk to be occluded is selectively catheterized for performing a distal and free-flow embolization.

The degree of selectivity (sectorial, segmental, or subsegmental) before each embolization depends on individual anatomy and local hemodynamics. It is chosen for each vein to ensure a stable selective positioning of the catheter, providing best conditions for free-flow embolization and preventing inadvertent reflux of embolic material. Massive reflux of embolic agent into the FRL would annihilate its hypertrophy or induce almost total portal occlusion and thereby fatal portal hypertension when the rest of the portal vasculature has already been totally embolized. Consequently, right branches originating close to the portal bifurcation should be superselectively catheterized. Caution should also be exercised to avoid reflux into left lobe veins when occluding veins in segment IV. Because of this potential risk, segment IV portal veins should be occluded first for added safety, and a particulate embolic agent must be preferred to cyanoacrylate.

We mostly perform embolization with a mixture of cyanoacrylate and Lipiodol. Safe use of this embolic agent necessitates following a very strict technique but presents multiple advantages. It allows for complete and durable occlusion. Its radiopacity increases safety at the time of embolization. Histoacryl and Lipiodol are mixed in a ratio of 1 part Histoacryl for 1 to 3 parts Lipiodol; the more Lipiodol in the mixture, the longer the polymerization time of

the glue. Consequently, it allows distal embolization in every case because the polymerization time can be adapted to individual and instant hemodynamic variations. Furthermore, the cyanoacrylate induces a very strong inflammatory reaction involving vessels as well as bile ducts, which is thought to increase production of hepatotropic factors. The mixture is pushed with isotonic glucose, following the "sandwich technique," with the volume of every injection of mixture being lower than the catheter content. The total dose of Histoacryl will be 1 to 3 mL administered in 4 to 10 successive injections of mixture. Catheter occlusion with repetitive injections of glue is a risk of this technique. Pushing the 0.035-inch Glidewire through the catheter, still in position, immediately after each injection of glue minimizes this risk. This cleans the inner wall of the catheter from the residual glue/Lipiodol mixture and gently pushes it out in the embolized vein under fluoroscopic control. A control portography is performed at the end of the procedure, and postembolization portal pressure is registered. In our experience, the transhepatic tract does not require embolization.

CONTROVERSIES

Approaches

Before complex hepatectomies, PVE may concern the left and right portal branches. A transhepatic access may then be chosen, giving preference to entering a vein not to be occluded.[4] The transjugular approach has been successfully used when it was impossible to perform the conventional transhepatic technique because of tumor interposition or severely impaired hemostasis.[7] The surgical transileocolic approach requires laparotomy but allows tumor extension staging during the same procedure. Nevertheless, most teams prefer transhepatic approaches.

Distal Embolization or Proximal Ligation?

Distal embolization is achieved with particulate agents, cyanoacrylate, or other liquid agents. Proximal ligation is surgically performed or may be done percutaneously with steel coils or detachable balloons. Considering that the intrahepatic portal vasculature was classically considered as terminal type, interest in performing a distal embolization rather than a proximal surgical ligation has been contested. Nowadays there are strong arguments for preferring a distal occlusion. The efficacy of PVE versus right portal vein ligation before extended right hepatectomy has been demonstrated.[8] Increase in FRL volume was significantly higher with PVE (188 ± 81 mL vs. 123 ± 58 mL; $P = .012$). A strictly proximal occlusion allows distal reentry through the intraparenchymatous vascular shunt opening.[9] After having achieved control with a previous proximal ligation, we also encountered antegrade portoportal collateral circulation bypassing the ligation and supposed it to be from parabiliary veins that were acting as a homolog to the parabiliary arteries, which are well known to play a predominant role in development of intrahepatic arterial collateral circulations.

Choice of Embolic Agent

Many embolic agents have been used and compared, either in animal experiments or in clinical use. In animals, cyanoacrylate seems more efficient than spherical particles,[10] although never compared in human randomized trials. There is no definitive argument in the clinical literature in favor of one specific type of agent, except that it must provide a distal occlusion. Among particulate and liquid agents, the actual tendency is to favor agents inducing complete distal and durable occlusion, as well as a strong inflammatory reaction. Four weeks after embolization, we obtained hypertrophy of 68%, 53%, or 44% when using, respectively, cyanoacrylate, gelatin sponge, or coils.[11]

Absolute ethanol has also been experimentally assessed and clinically used by several teams.[9,12] Fifteen to 65 mL of ethanol had to be injected to induce adequate occlusion, either in the right portal vein or at a segmental or subsegmental level. Technical ease of use and its efficacy in inducing hypertrophy are clear advantages of ethanol. In contrast, the clinical and hepatic biological tolerance of ethanol appeared to be much poorer than that of cyanoacrylate. Consequently, one should be very careful in using this embolic agent, especially in patients with a compromised liver.

When particles are used, embolization with small spherical particles provides improved hypertrophy and resection rates compared with larger nonspherical particles.[13] Coils do not induce distal occlusion and are generally used for proximal occlusion when combined with a distal embolic such as particles or alcohol.[9,13] Plugs should probably be similarly used for proximal occlusion when the distal portal vein is occluded with small-size material or liquid agent.

Combined Transcatheter Arterial Chemoembolization and Portal Vein Embolization

Combining PVE with transcatheter arterial chemoembolization (TACE) has been explored recently in HCC treatment and provides very interesting results. Yamakado et al. demonstrated 57% hypertrophy by combining TACE and PVE, whereas hypertrophy was 36% for PVE alone.[14] Similar benefit has been reported in another publication.[15] Delay between conventional TACE (Lipiodol + drug + Gelfoam)

and PVE was 3 to 6 weeks. This waiting time between TACE and PVE seems reasonable to avoid complications linked with concomitant arterial and portal occlusion. In one comparative study, postoperative mortality was the same in the TACE plus PVE group as in the PVE-alone group. The 4 deaths among the 36 patients occurred in patients (2/18) with hypertrophy of the FRL below 10% after PVE, but there was no death when hypertrophy was above 10%.[15] These data are in accordance with previous reports that demonstrated increased complications in patients who do not demonstrate sufficient hypertrophy.

Does Portal Vein Embolization Accelerate Growth Rate of Liver Metastases?

Our group studied volumetry of the FRL and that of liver metastases located in the FRL in five cases.[16] Volume measurement before PVE and 1 month later showed that increase of the normal liver varied from 59% to 127%, compared with 60% to 970% for the metastases. The ratio between the growth rate of the left lobe and the liver metastases varied from 1.0 to 15.6. However, the spontaneous growth rate of metastases before PVE, which should be subtracted from the total tumor growth to define the exact potential enhancement by PVE, was unknown in this study. Kokudo et al. demonstrated an increase in proliferative activity of intrahepatic colorectal metastases in patients who underwent PVE compared with a control non-PVE group.[17] The Ki-67 labeling index of metastatic lesions was significantly higher in the PVE group. Long-term survival was similar in the two groups, but disease-free survival was significantly poorer in the PVE group. To overcome this potential adverse effect, some have proposed a two-stage hepatectomy, with PVE being performed after a primary resection of metastases that are present in the FRL. RFA of lesions located in the FRL, before or simultaneously with PVE, is also a reported alternative option.[18] To conclude, complementary studies are still needed, but it is logical to consider that PVE accelerates tumor growth in some patients and some tumors. However, clinical experience demonstrates that this rare and probably limited adverse effect remains negligible when compared with the advantages of PVE in widely extending indications for curative surgery.

OUTCOMES

Liver Regeneration After Portal Vein Embolization: Mechanisms and Effects

PVE redistributes the totality of portal blood flow and its hepatotropic contents toward the FRL. Moreover, liver cell lesions in the embolized liver produce regenerating factors.[19] PVE dilates the portal branches in the FRL, exposing liver vasculature to stretch stress, which acts as a trigger for release of interleukin-6 (IL-6) from endothelial cells and contributes to activation of the regenerative cascade in the FRL. Induction of heat-shock protein in the nonembolized lobe is supposed to have similar effects. PVE also acts through two potentially complementary pathways specifically related to embolization: ischemia and inflammation. With most embolic agents, PVE induces a mild ischemia, apoptosis or necrosis of some hepatocytes, and intercellular disjunction. Moreover, injection of embolic material induces a foreign body reaction and a cascade of inflammatory phenomena with production of cytokines and liver growth factors by Kupffer cells and granulocytes. This pathway may be more or less predominant, depending on the intensity of the inflammatory reaction induced by the embolic agent used for PVE. Consequently, embolic agents inducing a strong inflammatory reaction, such as cyanoacrylate[13] or ethanol, should induce more hypertrophy than others.

Functional Increase Parallels Volume Increase

Volume increase of the FRL after PVE was demonstrated by early studies; thereafter, it was shown that volume increase did parallel functional increase. Indeed, PVE produces a significant increase in bile volume and biliary indocyanine green (ICG) concentration in the FRL. Histologic examination of the FRL and assessment of volumetric, cell kinetic, and morphometric parameters attributed to PVE a gain of functional hepatocyte mass and early induction of hepatocyte proliferation after hepatectomy.[20] Levels of erythrocyte polyamine, which is known to be related to liver regeneration, increase in the 7 days after PVE. Hepatic energy charge levels in the FRL remain comparable to those of normal liver; hepatic plasma clearance of sorbitol and antipyrine was stable after PVE, whereas the percentage of FRL to total liver volume increased, thereby demonstrating that the functional reserve of FRL increased. Functional improvement after PVE has also been demonstrated through evaluation of first-pass lidocaine extraction and ^{99m}Tc-galactosyl serum albumin scintigraphy.

Liver Hemodynamic Effects of Portal Vein Embolization

When performed on a normal liver, right PVE induces an immediate mild increase in portal pressure, from 2 to 5 cm of saline.[11] However, some minutes or even seconds after embolization, the portal pressure comes back to its initial value. In patients with abnormal liver parenchyma, portal pressure increase tends to be greater and more durable. Interestingly, in both cases, the portal pressure registered immediately after PVE is similar to levels registered after hepatectomy, and subsequently may be of diagnostic interest in predicting the hemodynamic surgical outcome. The hypertrophy rate has a significant correlation with the absolute value of portal blood flow velocity on day 1 after PVE,[21] and Doppler evaluation of left portal branch velocity in the post-PVE period seems to easily predict the hypertrophy rate of the nonembolized left lobe.[22] Measurement of portal pressure is not routinely performed in patients with normal liver, but in cirrhotic patients, measuring the portal pressure and central venous pressure is useful to determine whether the patient has a portosystemic gradient above 12 mmHg, in which case he/she is at major risk of complications occurring during surgery.

Induced Hypertrophy

We reported on 108 PVE procedures, 43 before right hepatectomy, 58 before right extended hepatectomy, and 7 before more complex hepatectomy, with a mean increase of 70% in FRL volume and an increase in FRL/total liver volume by 12.4%, with an overall value of 32% at 4 weeks after PVE.[2] Major series reported increases in volume of 30% to 42% and FRL/total liver ratio increases from 19% to 36% to 31% to 59%. Disparities may be explained by different delays before surgery (2-4 weeks), use of diverse embolic agents, and different proportions of patients with compromised liver in the respective studies, knowing that hypertrophy is diminished in patients with cirrhotic livers.[23-26] Almost all patients with normal liver experience hypertrophy after PVE, whereas only 86% of patients with chronic liver disease develop hypertrophy, and patients who did not demonstrate hypertrophy had a poor surgical outcome.[25] Induced hypertrophy is linked to FRL volume, with higher hypertrophy in a small initial FRL,[26,27] thus indicating PVE even when the FRL has a very small volume. Indeed, we were able to provide enough hypertrophy to convert patients to surgery with an FRL as low as 6.9%.[27] In addition, pre-PVE chemotherapy regimens can affect the degree of hypertrophy—namely, a platin-based regimen that induces portal sinusoid dilation, also known as *blue liver*, can lower or slow down hypertrophy of the FRL.[28] Targeted therapies that aim at inhibition of vascular endothelial growth factor (VEGF) or VEGF receptor can also affect the degree of hypertrophy, as demonstrated by Abdalla et al.[29] when more than 6 courses of bevacizumab have been delivered. In clinical practice, it is wise to observe a 4- to 6-week "chemo-holiday" before PVE and decrease the number of preoperative courses as much as possible. Delivery of chemotherapy during the waiting period after PVE remains very controversial.

Delay to Surgery

Delay between PVE and surgery should be as short as possible to preclude any tumor growth. In our experience, all patients reached the critical FRL/total functional liver volume ratio of 25% after 4 to 5 weeks. Consequently, like several other teams, we consider a 4- to 5-week delay before surgery to be a good compromise between hepatic hypertrophy and tumor dissemination. Other teams consider the hypertrophy gain negligible after 2 to 3 weeks and prefer to perform resection earlier. Effect of PVE before large resections was evaluated through retrospective[29-31] or prospective[25] comparisons with non-PVE series. In all retrospective studies, the FRLs were significantly smaller at presentation in the PVE group, and thanks to PVE were similar at surgery.

Follow-Up After Surgery

Risk of Liver Failure After Surgery

Postoperative liver failure appears to be more severe in patients with high portal pressure and low hypertrophy of the FRL (<20%).[25,26] It was also found that portal pressure and serum level of hyaluronate measured before and after PVE were the most useful parameters in predicting outcome after hepatectomy.[32] The cutoff points of significance for serum hyaluronate were 130 ng/mL and 160 ng/mL before and after PVE, respectively. Cutoff for portal pressures was 16 cm and 25 cm of saline, measured before and immediately after PVE, respectively. Consequently, high initial portal pressure and important elevation after PVE both

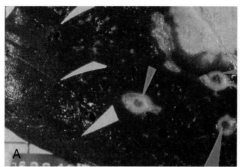 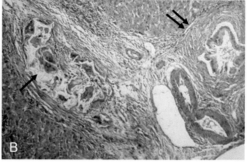

FIGURE 69-5. Effects of cyanoacrylate embolization. A, Macroscopic view after liver resection shows strong inflammatory reaction involving portal spaces in embolized area *(blue arrowheads),* compared to normal unembolized territory *(yellow arrowheads).* **B,** Histologic view (saffron stain) of embolized liver shows cyanoacrylate in portal vein *(arrow)* and intense peribiliary duct sclerosis *(double arrow),* with biliary epithelium remaining normal.

indicate limited resection, and an initially elevated pressure should be considered a poor indication for PVE. Preoperative ^{99m}Tc-galactosyl serum albumin has been reported to be a useful tool for predicting residual liver function before hepatectomy.[33]

Long-Term Results and Survival

Abdalla et al. reported equivalent median survival durations with or without PVE before extended hepatectomy (or ≤ 5 segments resected) at 40 and 52 months, espectively.[29] We have reported 5-year survival and 5-year disease-free survival of 34% and 24%, respectively, in 60 patients who underwent PVE for liver metastases, which was comparable with the survival rates obtained after resection without PVE.[34] Long-term results from the literature in specific groups of patients presenting with liver metastases from colorectal tumors[34,35] demonstrate the same survival in patients operated with and without PVE, with 40% 5-year overall survival in the PVE group and 38% in the non-PVE group in our institution,[34] and 37.3% and 38.1% for Azoulay et al.[36] In hepatocellular carcinoma, 5-year survival is not significantly different with and without PVE for Azoulay et al., with 44% in the PVE group and 53% in the non-PVE group.[37] The same was reported by Wakabayashi et al., with 39.9% and 44.1%.[32] These impressive results were obtained even though it is likely that patients in the PVE groups had more extensive disease. Oussoultzoglou et al. reported equivalent 5-year survival for PVE (44%) and non-PVE (35%) patients, but surprisingly, the intrahepatic recurrence rate was 26% in the PVE group, while it was significantly higher in the non-PVE group (76%).[38] This low recurrence rate could provide an increase in safety margins for the surgeon at the time of surgery, knowing that sufficient liver reserve was present and there was less chance of tumor seeding through the portal vein.

POSTPROCEDURAL AND FOLLOW-UP CARE

Clinical tolerance is generally excellent, with only mild abdominal pain or discomfort and slight fever, which disappears in less than 3 days. During the post-PVE period, the prothrombin time remains above 70% of the baseline value. Serum aspartate transaminase and alanine transaminase values slightly increase and may reach a maximum value of three times the normal value on the first day after PVE, except when using ethanol, which induces a greater cytolysis. Alterations in the total bilirubin level are insignificant. Normally, the total duration of hospitalization for the procedure does not exceed 3 days.

At histopathologic study in patients embolized with Histoacryl, portal vein walls are damaged, with their lumens filled with embolic material and macrophage cells, and periportal inflammatory reaction and fibrosis are constantly associated. A massive peribiliary fibrosis, as encountered in sclerosing cholangitis, is also observed in most cases treated with cyanoacrylate[11] (Fig. 69-5). Specimens contain very rare and small foci of necrotic tissue, except in ethanol embolization, where these foci are more evident.

COMPLICATIONS

The overall complication rate reported in a large multicenter study was 28%,[5] 14% of which entailed incidental imaging findings of small cyanoacrylate fragments in the FRL not precluding hypertrophy and surgery. The remaining 14% included one complete portal vein thrombosis, two major migrations of embolic material in the FRL that required angioplasty, one hemoperitoneum, one hemobilia, and six cases of transitory hepatic insufficiency. It is noteworthy that five of the six cases of transitory hepatic insufficiency occurred in 30 cirrhotic livers, while only one transitory hepatic insufficiency occured in 157 noncirrhotic livers. In the literature from experienced teams, the major complication rate rarely exceeds 1.5%, without any reported mortality. Except for inadvertent embolization, most complications will occur in the punctured lobe, which is an argument in favor of an ipsilateral approach. However, complication rates reported for ipsilateral and contralateral approaches are the same. In the literature, the only factor increasing complications is puncture of the right posterior segment versus puncture of the right anterior segment,[39] thus advocating puncture of the anterior segment when compatible with the location of the PVE to be performed. In patients who underwent a duodenopancreatectomy and who present with a chronically infected biliary tree, the PVE can be done without risk of hepatic abscess, contrary to that which occurs after intraarterial chemoembolization or after RFA.

KEY POINTS

- Indications for portal vein embolization (PVE) are based on the ratio of the volume of: (future remnant liver – planned ablation or resection in the future remnant liver [FRL])/(total liver volume – tumor volume).

- When complementary radiofrequency ablation (RFA) of a lesion located in the FRL is foreseen during surgery, do not forget to subtract the supposed volume of the future necrotic RFA lesion when calculating FRL volume.

- When liver function is compromised, ratios below 40% to 50% are an indication for PVE.

- In nonaltered liver, ratios below 25% to 40% are an indication for PVE; 40% corresponds to patients who received chemotherapy, namely with oxaliplatin.

- Access the portal system in a peripheral branch.

- When segment intravenous (IV) embolization is required (before right hepatectomy extended to segment IV), access to the portal system through a segment III vein, upstream to the Rex recess, or contralateral to the FRL will allow easy catheterization of segment IV pedicles.

- Distal embolization is required. Our preference is Histoacryl glue mixed with Lipiodol, but small-sized spherical embolic material can be used.

- PVE is not indicated in patients with portal hypertension greater than 20 cm of saline.

- Long-term survival of patients who can undergo resection after PVE is comparable to survival of those who do not need PVE before surgery.

▶ SUGGESTED READINGS

Abdalla EK, Hicks ME, Vauthey JN. Portal vein embolization: rationale, technique and future prospects. Br J Surg 2001;88:165–75.

de Baere T, Denys A, Madoff DC. Preoperative portal vein embolization: indications and technical considerations. Tech Vasc Interv Radiol 2007;10:67–78.

Denys A, Bize P, Demartines N, et al. Quality improvement for portal vein embolization. Cardiovasc Intervent Radiol 2010;33(3):452–6.

Madoff DC, Abdalla EK, Vauthey JN. Portal vein embolization in preparation for major hepatic resection: evolution of a new standard of care. J Vasc Interv Radiol 2005;16:779–90.

The complete reference list is available online at www.expertconsult.com.

CHAPTER 70

Vascular Intervention in the Liver Transplant Patient

Julien Auriol, Philippe Otal, Marie Agnès Marachet, Thomas Lemettre, Bogdan Vierasu, Francis Joffre, and Hervé Rousseau

Since the first clinical attempt by Thomas E. Starzl in 1963, liver transplantation is now accepted as the gold standard treatment of advanced chronic liver disease, irreversible hepatocellular failure, and a selected group of patients with hepatocellular carcinoma.

There were 74,497 liver transplants performed in the United States from 1988 to 2005 according to the Organ Procurement and Transplantation Network (OPTN). Actual 1-, 3-, and 5-year survival rates based on OPTN data as of February 17, 2006, are 85%, 78%, and 72%, respectively (Liver Kaplan-Meier Patient Survival Rates for Transplants Performed: 1995-2002). Long-term survival rate (10 years) is 57% in a 2000 publication of over 4000 transplantations.

The improving survival rates during the past 10 years are based on progress in surgical techniques, improvement in immunosuppression, and early diagnosis and treatment of complications.

TECHNICAL FEATURES

Orthotopic liver transplantation (OLT) consists of removing the damaged liver and replacing it with a graft in the recipient's native bed.[1] *Heterotopic liver transplantation* is when the graft is placed in an extrahepatic site, usually at the root of the mesentery, but is no longer used, owing to poor outcomes. *Auxiliary liver transplantation* is placement of the donor liver in the presence of the native liver. Such transplants may be either orthotopic (after removal of part of the native liver and placement of a portion of the donor liver) or heterotopic.

Segmental liver transplantation uses a portion of the donor liver. These segmental grafts can be cadaveric or living donor. In the case of cadaveric segments, the graft can be a *split liver graft*, in which the cadaveric whole liver is reduced into two smaller grafts, each retaining its own venous drainage, portal venous inflow, hepatic artery inflow, and biliary drainage. Living donor segmental liver transplantation is similar to split livers in technical issues and complications. The conventional hepatectomy for OLT requires subdiaphragmatic clamping of the inferior vena cava (IVC) and resection of the retrohepatic IVC along with the recipient liver. This clamping of the IVC decreases venous return to the heart and often results in hemodynamic instability, metabolic alterations, and low renal blood flow. To limit hemodynamic consequences, a venovenous bypass was developed to allow diversion of blood from the recipient IVC and portal vein directly to the patient's superior vena cava during the anhepatic phase. Restoration of venous continuity during implantation is achieved by an upper subdiaphragmatic and a lower end-to-end donor-to-recipient IVC anastomosis.

Since 1989, another technique known as the *piggyback technique* is more and more used. The major hepatic veins of the recipient are clamped and interconnected, forming a cuff that can then be anastomosed to the suprahepatic vena cava of the donor liver in an end-to-end or end-to-side fashion (Fig. 70-1). This technique preserves the recipient retrohepatic vena cava and avoids vena caval clamping, preserving venous return during the operation and avoiding venovenous bypass.

Perhaps the most significant potential disadvantage of the piggyback technique is the increased risk of hepatic venous outflow obstruction, a technical complication that leads to stenosis of the recipient suprahepatic IVC/recipient hepatic vein anastomosis and/or suprahepatic thrombosis. The donor-to-recipient portal vein anastomosis is performed in an end-to-end fashion.

Arterial anastomosis between the donor and recipient arteries is usually end to end. The site usually varies depending on the arterial anatomy of donor and recipient and on the surgeon's preference. One must recognize that patients with anomalous hepatic arterial anatomy may not have a large enough common hepatic artery to use as inflow. Patients with celiac axis stenosis may also have inadequate inflow. The median arcuate ligament syndrome has been described as affecting arterial inflow in liver transplantation. In these circumstances, use of a donor iliac arterial conduit from the infrarenal (or occasionally supraceliac) aorta to the allograft may be necessary. However, artificial conduits should be avoided, owing to the risk of thrombosis and infection. Biliary connections involve either a primary duct-to-duct technique (choledochocholedochostomy, the most common used) or require a choledochojejunostomy (to a Roux-en-Y defunctionalized intestinal loop). Duct-to-duct anastomosis is usually done over a T-tube. Advantages of leaving a T-tube are (1) observation of bile production and its quality as a sign of hepatic allograft function and (2) easy cholangiographic access to the biliary system in cases of abnormalities in liver function tests. The disadvantage of the T-tube is the risk of bile leak after removal of the tube, requiring emergency endoscopic retrograde cholangiopancreatography and decompression of the duct. Other types of biliary reconstructions, including choledochoduodenostomy and cholecystoduodenostomy, have been used through the years. Biliary complications of liver transplants are discussed more fully in Chapter 139.

ARTERIAL COMPLICATIONS

Hepatic artery complications after liver transplantation are uncommon but represent an important cause of morbidity, mortality, and retransplantation. In native liver, the biliary

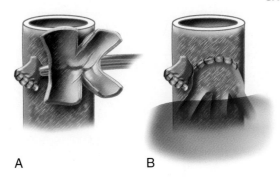

FIGURE 70-1. A-B, Schematic drawing of "piggyback" hepatic vein reconstruction. A common cuff from confluence of left and middle hepatic veins of recipient is created and anastomosed to donor suprahepatic inferior vena cava.

tree is protected from ischemia by a rich arterial network coming from choledochal branches originating from the posterior pancreaticoduodenal arcade but also from the capsular branches. The liver graft parenchyma receives oxygen both from the portal vein and hepatic artery, but the biliary tree is fed only by the hepatic artery. Thus, arterial stenosis or occlusion may induce severe biliary complications, such as biliary necrosis, biliary leak, or liver abscesses.

In children, hepatic artery complications are more frequent but have fewer consequences. In pediatric recipients, revascularization of the transplant through the adhesions to the diaphragm and other adjacent organs may protect the graft from ischemic complications.

There are four types of arterial complications: hepatic artery stenosis, hepatic artery thrombosis, hepatic artery pseudoaneurysm, and splenohepatic arterial steal syndrome.

Hepatic Artery Stenosis

Hepatic artery stenosis occurs in 5% to 13% of transplants (one third in the first month), with a mean delay between diagnosis and transplantation of 100 to 126 days. The mechanisms and predisposing factors for this complication are failure of the surgical technique related to a small (children) or diseased artery, excessive vessel length with kinking and angulations, retransplantation, anatomic variation of the hepatic artery, and arterial reconstructions.[2-4]

Excluding conduits, the majority of hepatic artery stenoses are anastomotic (46%-75%), with distal stenoses representing 40% to 46%. In 3% to 8% of cases, stenoses are proximal to the anastomosis in the recipient artery. Multiple stenoses are found in 5% to 25%, and in the majority of cases (77%) anastomotic stenosis coexists with distal stenosis.[2-5]

Clinical presentation is variable and goes from asymptomatic with minimal increase in liver function test results (20% of cases) to acute liver failure or biliary complications. Laboratory findings are nonspecific and insidious.[2] Doppler ultrasonography can allow early diagnosis. Values considered indicative of hepatic artery stenosis are a resistive index less than 0.5 and a systolic ascending time greater than 100 ms, or both. The right and left hepatic arteries must be evaluated to detect distal stenosis.

Indications
A protocol for management of hepatic artery stenosis has been proposed by Saad et al.,[5] who recommend a combination of surgery and percutaneous transluminal angioplasty (PTA). Hepatic artery PTA is reserved for solitary focal stenosis and nonsurgical candidates with other types of lesions (tandem lesions, arterial kinking). Repetitive endoluminal therapy is also required for post-PTA restenosis. Surgical revision is proposed for technical failure of PTA and hepatic artery thrombosis.

Contraindications
Hepatic artery stenosis with associated kinks (tandem lesions) can be considered a relative contraindication and should be managed surgically.

Equipment
- Basic angiography set
- Long 5F introducer sheath
- Hydrophilic 5F cobra (or Simmons) catheter
- Hydrophilic 0.035-inch guidewire
- 0.014- or 0.018-inch guidewire
- Balloon size range: 4 to 6 mm
- Stent size range: 4 to 6 mm

Technique
Angiography is performed with standard catheter technique, mostly from a transfemoral approach, with 5F catheter (Simmons or cobra). A long sheath up to the origin of the feeding vessel may be useful. The size of the balloon ranges from 4 to 6 mm and can be chosen according to the automatic measurement, using the sheath as a reference. Heparin is administered after crossing the lesion with a 0.014- to 0.018-inch guidewire. Some authors advocate primary stenting to reduce the risk of acute thrombosis or dissection.[3] Recent technical improvements make the procedure safer, such as monorail material or use of coronary stents (Fig. 70-2).

Controversies
Traditionally, the treatment of symptomatic hepatic artery stenosis was surgical and included revascularization and even retransplantation. In the past 20 years, numerous authors have described endoluminal treatment.[2,3] Nevertheless, treatment of hepatic artery stenosis is debated because large numbers of patients are asymptomatic. In fact, if not treated, hepatic artery stenosis doubled the rate of biliary complications, thus reducing graft life expectancy. Furthermore, there is a progression from stenosis to thrombosis: the hepatic artery thrombosis rate for untreated significant hepatic artery stenosis is 65% at 6 months,[5] and hepatic artery thrombosis is associated with higher morbidity and mortality than hepatic artery stenosis. Patency of the hepatic artery is crucial because vascularization of the biliary tree of the transplanted liver relies only on it, as opposed to the native liver in which a rich network of collateral arteries may compensate for hepatic artery occlusion. Improvements in symptoms and results of liver function tests have been demonstrated after treatment of the stenosis.[2-4,6-9] Graft survival and complication rates in those patients treated by radiologic or surgical interventions matched those with normal arterial inflow.[2] As mentioned earlier, kinking of the hepatic artery contraindicates hepatic artery PTA.

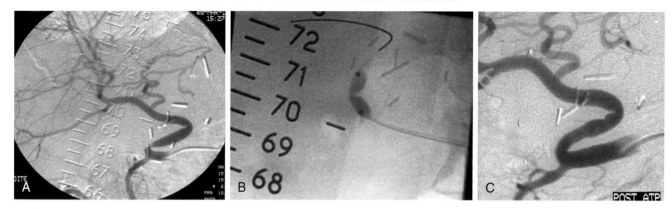

FIGURE 70-2. Percutaneous transluminal angioplasty of anastomotic hepatic artery stenosis. **A,** Selective hepatic artery angiogram confirms Doppler diagnosis of stenosis at origin of donor artery. **B,** Balloon catheter is advanced over 0.018-inch guidewire and inflated. **C,** Angiogram after procedure depicts satisfactory result. No stent was deployed, and hepatic artery is patent at 3-year follow-up.

Outcomes

Hepatic artery angioplasty has a technical success rate up to 81%.[4,5] Causes of failure are hepatic artery tortuosity and inability to cross the lesion.

Restenosis rates after hepatic artery PTA and stent placement are the same (≈30%), but restenosis of stents usually occurs later than restenoses in patients treated with balloon dilatation alone. Primary restenosis occurred at a mean interval of 2.7 months from initial PTA and 5.3 months after stent placement.[5] All the data about follow-up patency rates are based on Doppler ultrasonography, which is not the gold-standard test for evaluation of hepatic artery stenosis.

Complications

The rate of immediate complications (rupture and dissection) ranges between 7% and 9.5%.[4,5] Hepatic artery thrombosis rates at 30 days and 1 year are 5% and 19%, respectively.[5] Postprocedural anticoagulation and antiplatelet therapy may be beneficial in reducing this rate, but further investigations are required.[5]

Postprocedural and Follow-up Care

A monthly Doppler sonogram is recommended in the immediate 6 months after angioplasty.

Hepatic Artery Thrombosis

Hepatic artery thrombosis is a rare but serious complication after liver transplantation, requiring retransplantation in almost 50% of patients.[10] It occurs in 2.5% to 6.8% after OLT,[10-12] and this incidence increases 5.8-fold when the donor hepatic artery was reconstructed with an interposition graft to the supraceliac aorta.[10] Risk is increased in children (11%-26%) but is claimed to have less consequence, mainly if it occurs late after transplantation.[13-17] Celiac trunk compression by the median arcuate ligament and hepatic artery stenosis are also described as predisposing factors for hepatic artery thrombosis. Hepatic artery thrombosis is classified as early or late by its occurrence within or beyond 30 days after OLT. Early hepatic artery thrombosis represents 33% to 46%[10,11] of patients and may have a mortality rate as high as 55%, whereas it decreases to 15% if thrombosis occurs after this period.[11] Clinical presentation of hepatic artery thrombosis ranges from an increase in serum transaminase levels with or without cholestasis to liver abscess and biliary complications, including cholangitis and bile duct stenosis or necrosis; liver dysfunction and hepatic failure may also be seen. Impairment of graft function is observed in patients with early hepatic artery thrombosis, whereas biliary tract destruction is seen more often in patients with late hepatic artery thrombosis. Biliary ischemia may have very discrete presentation limited to anastomotic stenosis or leak. In rare cases, hepatic artery thrombosis can be clinically asymptomatic.

The key diagnostic technique is Doppler ultrasonography (potentially supplemented by microbubble contrast medium) and in many centers is confirmed with contrast-enhanced computed tomography (CT).

Indications

Emergency revascularization is of paramount importance to prevent the consequences of ischemia, in particular biliary ischemia. Retransplantation was initially considered the treatment of choice, but postoperative survival rates were poor. More recently, endovascular treatment of hepatic artery thrombosis has emerged as an alternative procedure in the early phase after transplantation. Rapid intervention limits the consequences of ischemia and is more likely to be effective because the clot is fresh.

Contraindications

There are no contraindications except those related to all angiographic procedures (i.e., severe abnormal clotting, severe iodine allergy, renal failure).

Equipment

- Basic angiography set
- Long 5F introducer sheath
- Hydrophilic 5F cobra (or Simmons) catheter
- Hydrophilic 0.035-inch guidewire
- 0.014- or 0.018-inch guidewire
- Urokinase or recombinant tissue plasminogen activator
- ± Balloon and stent (size range: 4-6 mm) in case of underlying abnormality

Technique

After selective angiography and confirmation of the diagnosis, the catheter is advanced inside the thrombus if possible. The dose and timing of thrombolysis vary. For example,

Zhou et al.[12] recommend administering a 100,000- to 250,000-IU (international units) bolus of urokinase during the first 15 minutes, followed by a second perfusion (250,000-750,000 IU) given over the next 30 minutes in case of an unsatisfactory result, and then a continuous perfusion of urokinase (50,000-100,000 IU/h) is given for 12 to 24 hours. During perfusion, an arteriogram is repeated to monitor the outcome and interrupt treatment as soon as the clot is dissolved and the peripheral branches of the hepatic artery are perfused. If an underlying hepatic artery stenosis is revealed after reperfusion, a PTA with or without stent placement helps prevent rapid recurrence of thrombosis. Some authors also recommend leaving the catheter in place for 2 to 3 days to reintroduce thrombolysis in case of thrombus recurrence. Antibiotic therapy is usually prescribed, aiming at reducing the risk of liver abscess.

Outcomes
In the largest published series,[12] successful revascularization was obtained in all eight cases. Two patients died of unrelated reasons, and the six others remained in good health during the follow-up period.

Complications
No severe complications are reported. In particular, no anastomotic or intraabdominal bleeding were noted despite the short delay from surgery.

Hepatic Artery Pseudoaneurysm

Pseudoaneurysm is a rare occurrence after liver transplantation. Most pseudoaneurysms occur within the first month after surgery, and the presenting signs include hemobilia, unexplained fever or graft dysfunction, and hepatic artery occlusion. Intrahepatic aneurysms are often related to percutaneous intervention (biopsy, biliary procedures). Extrahepatic aneurysms are commonly mycotic, are secondary to fungal septicemia, and often arise at the anastomosis. These are associated with high mortality if not treated.[18]

Indications
All hepatic artery pseudoaneurysms should be treated, even mycotic ones. The risk of rupture outweighs the potential risk of infection of embolic agents or stent.

Technique
Hepatic artery pseudoaneurysm can be managed successfully by transcatheter or percutaneous embolization with the use of embolic agents such as coils, detachable balloons, thrombin, and Gelfoam.

Transcatheter management uses microcoils to pack the aneurysm and maintain downstream hepatic arterial perfusion.

Direct percutaneous puncture of the aneurysm under image guidance (ultrasonography preferably) with delivery of coils and/or thrombin (thrombin can be used as an adjunct to coil embolization) is an alternative strategy but should be reserved for those cases in which a conventional approach is not technically possible.[19] In that situation, inflation of a balloon in the hepatic artery at the level of the aneurysm neck during occluding material injection helps reduce the risk of distal intrahepatic embolization.

Treatment by placement of an expanded polytetrafluoroethylene (ePTFE)-covered coronary stent graft has been described with success.

Equipment
For endovascular approach:
- Basic angiography set
- Long 5F introducer sheath
- Hydrophilic 5F cobra (or Simmons) catheter
- Hydrophilic 0.035-inch guidewire
- A coaxial microcatheter
- Microcoils
- ePTFE-covered coronary stent graft

For percutaneous approach (using ultrasound and fluoroscopic guidance):
- Ultrasound system
- 18-gauge needle if coils are used
- 22-gauge needle if thrombin is used
- ± Balloon (size range: 2-6 mm) in case of combined endovascular and percutaneous approach

Complications
There is a risk of distal intrahepatic embolization by coil migration and occlusion of the hepatic artery branch that supplies the pseudoaneurysm. The potential risk of hepatic infarction is very low in patients with a patent portal vein, as opposed to stenosis secondary to ischemia of the ductal wall, which is supplied exclusively by the hepatic artery.

Migration of coils into the biliary tract is also a rare but described complication and can cause cholangitis and pancreatitis.

Controversies
The treatment of hepatic artery pseudoaneurysms with coil embolization of the hepatic artery proximal and distal to the pseudoaneurysm should be avoided in patients who have undergone hepatic transplantation. Lack of collateral vessels makes the transplanted liver more prone than the native one to develop bile duct stenosis of ischemic origin.

Splenohepatic Arterial Steal Syndrome

Splenohepatic arterial steal syndrome is a rare arterial complication after liver transplantation and is characterized by decreased arterial perfusion of the hepatic graft due to diverted blood flow in a large splenic or gastroduodenal artery; this leads to ischemic damage of the graft. Its role in liver ischemia is still debated.

The treatment is complex, with a high rate of complications after splenic or gastroduodenal artery ligation or coil embolization requiring retransplantation in 18% of cases.[20,21]

PORTAL COMPLICATIONS

The portal complication rate is very low. The incidence of portal vein thrombosis is less than 2%,[22] and the portal vein stenosis rate has been reported at 7% in adults.[23] In pediatric recipients with reduced-size liver transplant, the rate of delayed portal venous stenosis or occlusion is reported to be as high as 19%.[24] The risk is increased by a preexisting portal vein thrombosis or hypoplasia, large portocaval collateral vessel, anastomotic stenosis by surgical technique failure, procoagulant disorder, and use of an interposition graft (e.g., reduced-size liver transplant, transplant using segments II and III from a living-relative donor).

If adequate collateral vessels develop, portal stenosis or thrombosis may be asymptomatic, and graft function is usually unaffected. However, in most cases hepatic dysfunction or symptoms of portal hypertension such as variceal bleeding, ascites, or splenomegaly lead to the diagnosis. Diagnosis is confirmed by Doppler ultrasonography. Portal vein stenosis criteria are a portal vein corrected velocity greater than 1 m/s or threefold of the velocity upstream in the portal vein, and/or the appearance of collateral vascularization.[25] In children, a portal vein 2.5 mm or less in diameter is also a criterion used to identify portal vein stenosis.[26]

Portal Vein Stenosis

Indications
The main indication for treatment of portal vein stenosis is the presence of portal hypertension symptoms (i.e., variceal bleeding, ascites, splenomegaly).

Contraindications
There are no specific contraindications. Abnormal clotting (INR > 1.5) or platelet count less than 50,000/mm^3 should be corrected before the procedure.

Ascites at the puncture site is a relative contraindication and should be drained first to reduce the risk of postprocedural bleeding.

Equipment
• Ultrasound system
• 6F or 7F sheath
• Hydrophilic 0.035-inch guidewire
• Pigtail catheter
• Multipurpose catheter
• Balloon (size: 8-14 mm)
• Self-expanding stent

Technique
Percutaneous venoplasty has been established in many teams as the treatment of choice for portal vein stenosis. This procedure is usually performed under general or local anesthesia, with a transhepatic approach. The transplanted liver is punctured under ultrasound and then fluoroscopic guidance, and the needle is targeted to the right portal branch for a full-sized liver or to the left portal branch for a reduced liver. Portal venograms with portal venous pressure measurements are performed. After administering a bolus of heparin directly into the portal vein, the stenotic segment is dilated, pressure gradient is measured, and portal venography is performed (Fig. 70-3). Metallic stent placement is reserved for elastic stenosis recoil, in cases with a persistent gradient of 5 mmHg or greater, or recurrent lesions.

To limit postprocedural bleeding risk through the portal puncture tract, some authors recommend embolization with Gelfoam.

Use of a transjugular intrahepatic portocaval shunt–type approach has also been reported by some to avoid this type of complication, particularly in a patient with a coagulopathy or ascites. Another option is to embolize competitive native shunts with coils to avoid recurrent thrombosis.[27-30]

Outcomes
Percutaneous venoplasty is effective and has long-term success in 76% of patients.[23,26] Long-term results seem to be improved with stents, with a 3-year patency rate of 100% reported,[26] but no controlled study is available.

Complications
No case of anastomosis rupture has been reported, even when venoplasty was performed in the early postoperative period.

Portal Vein Thrombosis

Cases of portal vein thrombosis have also been treated with good success by a combination of chemical thrombolysis, stent placement, and mechanical fragmentation.[24,31] A transhepatic or transjugular approach can be used, and thrombolysis can be safely performed even in the perioperative setting. Using local intraclot infusions, thrombolytic doses can be kept relatively low, limiting the risk of bleeding complications.

CAVAL COMPLICATIONS

Orthotopic liver transplantation preserving the retrohepatic IVC, the so-called piggyback technique, is the most commonly used because it avoids caval cross-clamping during the anhepatic phase of surgery and has a low rate of complications. Thanks to development of this technique, the rate of caval complications is low (<1%).[32] A higher incidence is reported in living-relative and other partial liver reconstruction (up to 3.9%).[33]

Stenosis

A stenosis may develop at the suprahepatic or infrahepatic anastomoses in the standard orthotopic technique or involve the hepatic vein orifices or cavocaval anastomosis in the piggyback technique.

In the early postoperative period, these complications are thought to be secondary to technical factors such as a tight suture line, donor/recipient size discrepancy, kinking of a redundant hepatic vein, or caval compression from a large graft. Torsion of the IVC has also been reported. Chronic obstructions are thought to be caused by fibrosis around the anastomotic site, intimal hyperplasia, or compression from a hypertrophic graft.

Clinical presentation depends on stenosis location. A Budd-Chiari–like syndrome with ascites, portal hypertension, and graft failure is present in the case of suprahepatic stenosis because of hepatic venous outflow obstruction. In this case, biopsy demonstrates marked centrilobular congestion. Peripheral edema and renal dysfunction may occur if there is a significant transanastomotic infrahepatic caval gradient, but infrahepatic stenosis usually causes fewer clinically significant symptoms or objective findings.

Diagnosis is usually obtained by Doppler ultrasonography and CT:
• In suprahepatic obstruction, hepatic vein stenosis is suspected when Doppler ultrasonography shows monophasic hepatic venous waveform or slowed hepatic venous velocity with decreased portal vein velocities. Thrombosis of the hepatic vein can also be found.

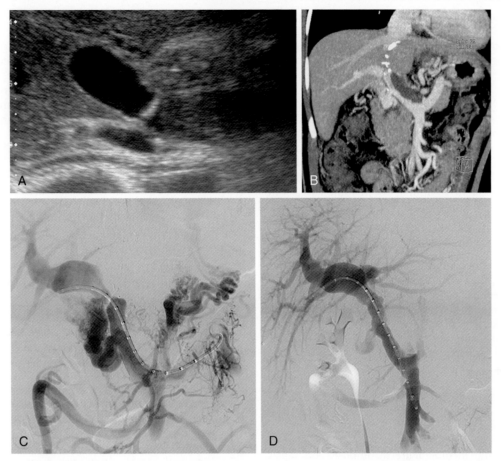

FIGURE 70-3. Percutaneous transluminal angioplasty of anastomotic stenosis of portal vein, revealed by bleeding of an esophageal varix 9 months after orthotopic liver transplantation. **A,** Doppler ultrasonography shows tight stenosis of anastomosis and cruoric material in receiver portal vein. **B,** Computed tomographic coronal multiplanar reformatted image of portal system confirms ultrasound information. **C,** Transhepatic portography depicts preocclusive anastomosis and importance of collateral pathway, in particular in left gastric vein territory. Transstenotic pressure gradient was measured at 19 mmHg. **D,** Angiogram after procedure confirms complete restoration of portal venous flow and normalization of flow direction in collateral pathway. At 1-year Doppler follow-up, stenosis did not recur.

Enhanced CT can show narrowing of the hepatic venous anastomosis or lack of opacification of the hepatic vein, with ill-defined low-attenuating areas in the transplanted liver similar to those commonly depicted in Budd-Chiari syndrome.
• In cavocaval stenosis, Doppler ultrasonography shows the direct sign of increased velocities at the caval anastomosis.

In both cases, venography with pressure measurements remains the gold standard for diagnosing caval abnormalities.

Indications
Nowadays, endovascular repair has widespread acceptance because surgical repair is very complex. Symptomatic stenosis—caval or hepatic—might be treated percutaneously. When asymptomatic hepatic vein stenosis is depicted by follow-up Doppler ultrasonography, percutaneous angioplasty should be considered to prevent occlusion.

Equipment
• Basic angiography set
• Hydrophilic 0.035-inch guidewire
• Pigtail catheter

For a hepatic vein stenosis:
• Hydrophilic 5F cobra (or Simmons) catheter
• Balloon (size: 6-10 mm)
• Self-expanding stent (size: 6-10 mm)
For a cavocaval stenosis:
• Self-expanding stent, 15 to 30 mm in diameter, with adapted introducer sheath

Technique
The procedure is performed using local anesthesia. A femoral approach is usually preferred for side-to-side caval anastomosis; for end-to-side or cavoatrial anastomosis, a jugular approach seems to be more convenient. After catheterization, pressure gradient measurements are performed to estimate the hemodynamic consequences of the stenosis. When hepatic venous outflow obstruction is present, stents are almost systematically used because the fibrotic tissues often immediately recoil after angioplasty. Balloon-expandable stents are usually preferred because their placement is precise and they may be redilated in case of a residual significant pressure gradient.

For significant cavocaval anastomosis stenosis, IVC compression, or torsion, stent placement is required. The stents used must have a large diameter to avoid migration. Creation of a "pull-through" wire system via combined transjugular and transfemoral access has also been reported to facilitate precise and safe placement of a venous stent.

Controversies

There is no consensus regarding the degree of hepatic vein pressure gradient that is hemodynamically significant. Nevertheless, symptoms usually develop when the pressure gradient exceeds 5 to 6 mmHg. For cavocaval stenosis, any gradient over 10 mmHg is usually considered abnormal,[8] but gradients less than 10 mmHg are in some cases sufficient to induce symptoms.

Complications

The most common complication of caval angioplasty is stent migration; they tend to become lodged in the right atrium, right ventricle, or pulmonary arterial bed. To prevent migration, the stent diameter has to exceed the unobstructed diameter of the target vessels.[33] Wittich et al.[34] reported an anchoring method with use of a T-fastener commonly used for performing percutaneous gastrostomy. In this instance, a transhepatic approach combined with ultrasonography and fluoroscopic guidance allows safe percutaneous insertion of the T-fastener into the intracaval stent. Its suture line is secured in the subcutaneous tissue of the anterior abdominal wall.

Other complications related to venous stent placement are uncommon but include acute thrombosis and sepsis. There has been no documented report in the literature of disruption of caval anastomosis after percutaneous intervention, even in the early postoperative period.[33]

BILIARY COMPLICATIONS

Bile duct complications are an important cause of postsurgical morbidity and graft survival. They occur in as many as 25% of recipients after cadaveric OLT[35,36] and in 34% of recipients after living left lobe transplantation, owing to the small size of the segmental duct anastomosed with the intestinal loop.[37] This subject is discussed in Chapter 139.

KEY POINTS

- Hepatic artery percutaneous transluminal angioplasty (PTA) is reserved for solitary focal stenosis and nonsurgical candidates.
- Endovascular treatment of hepatic artery thrombosis has emerged as an alternative procedure, even in the early phase after transplantation.
- Percutaneous PTA is effective in treating portal vein stenosis but has to be reserved for patients with symptoms of portal hypertension.
- Endovascular treatment of hepatic venous outflow obstruction relies almost systematically on stents because the fibrotic tissues often immediately recoil after angioplasty.

► **SUGGESTED READINGS**

Denys A, Chevallier P, Doenz F, et al. Interventional radiology in the management of complications after liver transplantation. Eur Radiol 2004; 14:431–9.

Karani JB, Yu DF, Kane PA. Interventional radiology in liver transplantation. Cardiovasc Intervent Radiol 2005;28:271–83.

The complete reference list is available online at www.expertconsult.com.

CHAPTER 71

Management of Trauma to the Liver and Spleen

Robert F. Dondelinger

Clinical examination is unreliable in both establishing the diagnosis of hepatic or splenic contusion and evaluating its severity. In the most severe injuries, during the initial phase of *compensated hemorrhagic shock*, clinical signs are subtle until 40% of the blood volume is lost. The ensuing bradycardia can be puzzling in that it may be observed as a result of vagal stimulation. Because of their rich vascularization, both the liver and spleen can bleed profusely and be responsible for rapidly progressive hypotension or shock. If blood volume is not corrected quickly, *uncompensated hemorrhagic shock* occurs, followed by metabolic acidosis, myocardial depression, diffuse intravascular coagulation, and death. Polytransfusion and hypothermia further contribute to the metabolic acidosis and wash-out coagulopathy that can jeopardize the result of arterial embolization.

In patients with less severe hepatic or splenic injury, abdominal pain, either diffuse or localized to the right or left upper quadrant, is the most frequent complaint. Localized abdominal symptoms are found in 27% and nonspecific abdominal symptoms in 41%. Pain in the right shoulder (Kehr sign) or its equivalent on the left side is indicative of phrenic, hepatic, or biliary injury on the right and splenic injury on the left and is specific if no trauma to the shoulder has occurred. The presence of three or more lower rib fractures increases the relative risk for hepatic or splenic injury significantly and is an indicator for thorough imaging. Respiratory difficulty caused by limited diaphragmatic excursion due to pain or phrenic irritation is a symptom suggestive of underlying liver or spleen injury. Occasionally, hemothorax is a sign of splenic rupture because a lacerated spleen is likely to herniate through a phrenic tear and bleed into the thorax. It should be stressed that clinical symptoms can be absent in up to 19% of patients with documented liver injury and in 35% with splenic contusion. Elevation of serum transaminase levels in excess of 130 IU/L is an indication of liver injury, even in the absence of clinical complaints. Posttraumatic hemobilia and bilhemia are of particular interest for the management of patients with liver injury.

Hemobilia is a sign of intrahepatic hemobiliary fistula and is estimated to develop in 2.5% of patients with hepatic injuries. Posttraumatic hemobilia is generally caused by an intrahepatic vascular lesion, such as a pseudoaneurysm or arteriovenous fistula (AVF) that has eroded a bile duct wall. Therefore, hemobilia often coexists with biloma or a bile fistula. In some patients, persistent discrete extrahepatic hemorrhage is responsible for development of hemorrhagic ascites some time after the trauma. Persistent mixing of bile with blood from a liver contusion prevents healing and explains recurrences of hemobilia. Significant bile duct obstruction due to clot and causing jaundice can occur but is a rare event. Bleeding is quite variable: profuse, causing shock and requiring urgent treatment, or moderate or occult. With persistence of the lesion, which often goes

unrecognized, hemobilia has a tendency to recur, sometimes for decades. The mean reported interval between injury and hemobilia is about 1 month, but a considerable time interval may separate the injury from onset of symptoms. The classic clinical triad consists of gastrointestinal hemorrhage, obstructive jaundice, and biliary colic. The triad is incomplete in about 60% to 70% of cases.

The diagnosis of hemobilia is indirectly established by endoscopy. Endoscopic retrograde cholangiopancreatography (ERCP) confirms bleeding from the papilla in only a minority of cases, but it shows intraluminal choledochal defects corresponding to clots, also occasionally seen in the pancreatic ducts, and provides evidence of proximal biliary obstruction (Fig. 71-1). ERCP does not show the intrahepatic bleeding site or the nature of the vascular lesion responsible for the hemobilia. Overall, ERCP is diagnostic of hemobilia in about a third of cases and can rule out a gastroduodenal bleeding source. Bile duct dilation often remains moderate because the clots are not totally obstructive. Endoscopic ultrasound (US) may be more contributory than ERCP by more precisely showing mobile hyperechoic material without acoustic shadows in the gallbladder and common bile duct, indicative of an endoluminal clot. Sphincterotomy with choledochal flushing removes clot from the bile ducts and exposes fragmented clot to the fibrinolytic activity of bile, thereby accelerating regression of the bile duct obstruction. Most often, the intrinsic fibrinolytic properties of bile cause clots to dissolve spontaneously. US, computed tomography (CT), and magnetic resonance imaging (MRI) can also suggest the diagnosis of hemobilia by showing echoic material in the bile ducts or hyperdense material and extra- and intrahepatic bile duct dilation and sometimes the intrahepatic vascular lesion. Blood pool scintigraphy may show accumulation at the site of an intrahepatic vascular lesion, but arteriography is definitive for both diagnosis and treatment. It locates the bleeding source in more than 90% of cases by demonstrating either an underlying vascular lesion—a pseudoaneurysm or an arterioportal fistula—or, in a minority of cases, extravasation of contrast material into the bile ducts. Spontaneous definite resolution of hemobilia without any type of intervention occurs in only a minority of patients.

Bilhemia results from a posttraumatic communication established between a bile radicle and an intrahepatic vein and is a rare event after blunt hepatobiliary injury, with only a limited cohort of patients being reported. Because of low pressure in the hepatic venous system, bile drains into the vascular system. Jaundice caused by bilhemia cannot always be distinguished from that caused by hemobilia. It may well happen that a patient has a massive increase in direct bilirubin early after trauma, as well as later in the course of follow-up for hemobilia, thus indicating that bilhemia and hemobilia may occur in the same patient. In contrast to hemobilia, in bilhemia ERCP is able to show passage of bile

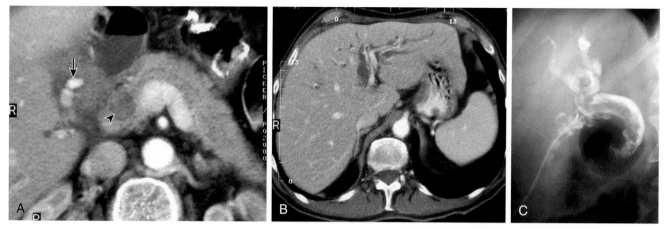

FIGURE 71-1. This patient exhibited upper gastrointestinal hemorrhage (hemobilia) after cholecystectomy. Computed tomography showed **(A)** a pseudoaneurysm located in the gallbladder fossa *(arrow)*, a dilated choledochus filled with hyperdense material *(arrowhead)*, and **(B)** dilation of intrahepatic bile ducts, predominantly in left lobe. **C,** Opacification through a surgical biliary drain showed massive intraluminal defects within dilated intrahepatic and extrahepatic bile ducts, corresponding to duct obstruction with blood clots. The postoperative pseudoaneurysm was treated by selective arterial embolization.

in hepatic veins, and hepatic arteriography is usually nondiagnostic.

Surgical treatment has shown that simple débridement and tamponade of the biliovenous fistula is therapeutic, and hepatic resection can be avoided. Bilhemia can be treated nonsurgically by selective endoscopic intrabiliary balloon placement to tamponade the leak within the liver for several days, or by sphincterotomy and bile duct stenting for decompression. If biliary obstruction is present and responsible for elevated pressure in the bile ducts, balloon dilation or stenting of a stricture should be performed.

INDICATIONS

Indications for hemostatic arterial embolization of hepatic or splenic posttraumatic injuries are not based on scientific evidence but rather on pragmatic grounds according to local logistics. Isolated hepatic and splenic injuries are most often considered in adults and in children.

In a hemodynamically stable or rapidly stabilized patient after resuscitation, the observation on CT of dense extravasation of contrast material or a localized blush of contrast material within the liver or spleen parenchyma or diffusing through the capsule and diluting in the hemoperitoneum in the subphrenic, perihepatic, or perisplenic space is an unequivocal sign of ongoing bleeding or free intraperitoneal hemorrhage (Figs. 71-2 to 71-6). Inside the liver or spleen parenchyma, contrast material may line the capsule or layer in a hematoma. Extravasated contrast material shows characteristic attenuation values of 80 to 130 Hounsfield units (HU) and might be surrounded by hematoma with lower density. The density of extravasated contrast material is similar to that measured in large opacified vessels. Clotted blood, in the absence of extravasation, has density values around 60 HU, and unclotted free intraperitoneal blood, not mixed with contrast material, has values of 35 to 45 HU (Fig. 71-7). Extravasation of contrast material usually appears rapidly at the arterial phase of opacification. Massive and rapid accumulation of contrast material in the perihepatic or perisplenic spaces without continuity from an intravisceral contusion indicates rupture

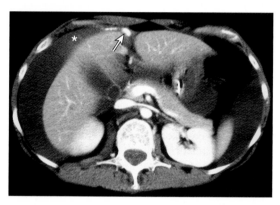

FIGURE 71-2. Contrast-enhanced computed tomography shows no intrahepatic parenchymal injury. On arterial-phase scan, extravasation of contrast medium is seen originating from ligamentum teres *(arrow)* and progressively seeping into anterior perihepatic peritoneal space *(asterisk)*. Massive supramesocolic hemoperitoneum is distending abdominal cavity.

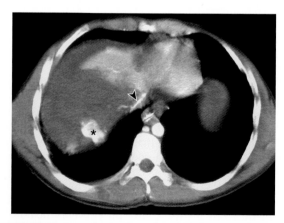

FIGURE 71-3. On contrast-enhanced computed tomography, extensive contusion and laceration of right lobe of liver are seen, along with massive extravasation of contrast material *(asterisk)*. Inferior vena cava is flattened and shows irregular margins *(arrowhead)*. At laparotomy, laceration of retrohepatic caval wall was confirmed.

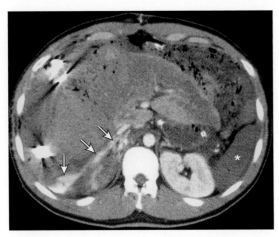

FIGURE 71-4. Contrast-enhanced computed tomography scan obtained after emergency laparotomy for massive hepatic posttraumatic laceration. Note faint enhancement of liver parenchyma, absence of splenic enhancement *(asterisk)* caused by severe vasoconstriction, and massive extravasation of contrast material *(arrows)* originating from bare area of liver around the inferior vena cava. Liver is compressed by operative perihepatic packing. Multiple air bubbles are seen within packing material and within liver parenchyma at laceration site.

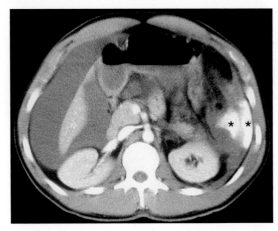

FIGURE 71-6. Computed tomography scan obtained after admission of 37-year-old man following car accident. Contrast material *(asterisks)* that extravasated as a result of splenic rupture has accumulated in left paracolic gutter. Also note massive perihepatic hemoperitoneum and blood in left anterior and posterior pararenal space.

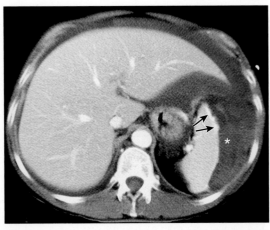

FIGURE 71-5. This 42-year-old woman was admitted after a traffic accident. Flattening of spleen by a subcapsular hematoma *(asterisk)* was noted. Subcapsular deposit of contrast medium *(arrows)* is in contact with splenic tissue. Note absence of intrasplenic contusion and massive perisplenic hemoperitoneum.

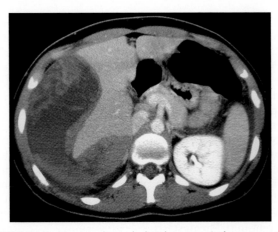

FIGURE 71-7. Massive subcapsular liver hematoma is shown on contrast-enhanced scan, with a scalloped border of underlying parenchyma. Mixed densities correspond to fresh clots and fluid content within hematoma.

of a hilar vessel. Rarely, extravasation appears only on delayed scans.

Indications for hepatic or splenic arteriography and embolization can be extended to patients with evidence of continuous hemorrhage who remain borderline after resuscitation. Today, because of rapid scanning by multidetector CT, all trauma patients suspected of sustaining abdominal injury undergo CT examination at admission. Such management requires optimal organization and skills in the radiology department. Patients with early ongoing bleeding after primary surgical hemostasis and those who are referred after crash laparotomy should also undergo arteriography without delay, being transferred immediately from the operating room to the angiography suite. Patients who

rebleed after initially successful embolization should be treated again angiographically. After the initial posttraumatic phase, cross-sectional imaging is also able to demonstrate mature nonacutely bleeding vascular lesions such as pseudoaneurysms or AVFs in the liver or spleen. Because of their relatively high risk of delayed bleeding, these vascular injuries are likewise treated by selective embolization during a scheduled procedure.

CONTRAINDICATIONS

A contraindication to hemostatic arterial embolization of the liver or spleen is a hemodynamically unstable patient who requires urgent regular or damage-control laparotomy.

There might be several pitfalls in recognizing extravasation of contrast material on CT. In the case of severe hypovolemic shock, the arteries contract as a result of the output of vasoconstrictive agents. Severe arterial vasoconstriction is called *hypoperfusion complex* on CT images and may

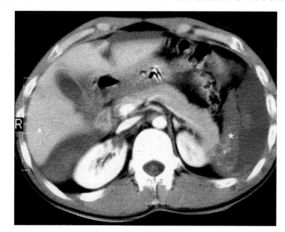

FIGURE 71-8. This 32-year-old man was admitted after blunt abdominal injury involving deceleration force. On contrast-enhanced computed tomography, spleen *(asterisk)* is not enhanced because of arterial vasoconstriction and is displaced medially by massive perisplenic hemoperitoneum. Bleeding originated from a mesenteric laceration.

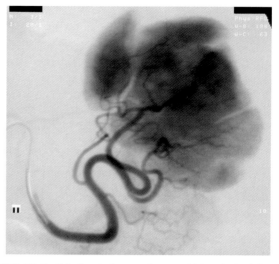

FIGURE 71-9. Splenic arteriogram shows multiple splenic clefts or fissures at splenic convexity that are separating territories with different arterial supply. These fissures may simulate a posttraumatic splenic fracture on cross-section imaging.

simulate disruption of the splenic artery by decreased enhancement or complete absence of splenic enhancement (Fig. 71-8; also see Fig. 71-4). This syndrome occurs in 0.01% to 2% of cases of major abdominal trauma in children with hypovolemic shock and may lead to unnecessary laparotomy. The CT appearance is particularly puzzling when no splenic enhancement at all is seen, but other solid organs are normally enhanced. The liver with its dual vascular supply is not usually affected, but the pancreas can be affected as an isolated organ in the same way as the spleen. When vasoconstriction resolves, progressive splenic enlargement may be seen on repeat CT examination. A sudden increase in intrasplenic blood inflow in an injured vessel may be responsible for early rebleeding despite apparent initial hemostasis.

Theoretic causes of erroneous interpretation of hepatic or splenic injury on angiography include a false-positive diagnosis suggested by a splenic fissure; a nonopacified splenic polar artery; early venous return in the spleen caused by massive injection of contrast medium; superimposition of the gastric fundus, pancreatic tail, accessory spleen, or left adrenal; and preexisting hepatic or splenic infarct (Fig. 71-9). Because of the large projection area of the liver, false-positive results on arteriography are rare. False-negative diagnoses are due mainly to minimal parenchymal injury. False-negative findings of persistent hemorrhage are estimated to occur in 1% to 2% of patients. A multicenter survey found that arteriography is used today as a diagnostic modality in only 2% of patients being treated by observation.

EQUIPMENT

Standard angiographic equipment is required, and a combined CT and angiographic unit allows rapid diagnosis and treatment of polytrauma patients. For catheterization of the hepatic or splenic artery, preshaped Sidewinder or Cobra angiographic catheters are used. Gelfoam pledgets or coils are routinely used as hemostatic embolization agents. Microcoils can be delivered selectively to the

bleeding site through coaxial microcatheters (Microferret, Radifocus).

TECHNIQUE

Anatomy and Approach

Hepatic arterial anatomy and variants must be kept in mind to obtain a complete arteriographic workup. As a reminder, the right hepatic artery, right lateral hepatic artery, or celiac artery may originate from the superior mesenteric artery, and the left hepatic artery or branches of the left lateral sector may originate from the left gastric artery. Vascular anatomy and variants of the liver should be known to correctly diagnose any parenchymal filling defect due to a nonopacified aberrant hepatic artery. The origin of the cystic artery should be recognized because inadvertent embolization should be avoided. Rarely, bleeding from the cystic artery requires hemostatic embolization.

The spleen is usually vascularized through a single splenic artery that branches at the hilum. A polar artery, most often directed to the upper pole, may originate from the main artery proximal to the hilar branches. An accessory spleen has its own independent small artery originating from the main splenic artery at the hilum. Occasionally the hepatic and splenic arteries may have a separate ostium originating from the abdominal aorta.

Angiographic access is gained by either a femoral or left axillary approach.

Technical Aspects

Arteriographic Findings

Arteriography was used to evaluate hepatic or splenic injury in the past, but rapidly became obsolete with the advent of US and CT. For many years, arteriography was a reliable method for diagnosing subcapsular hematoma, large parenchymal contusion, posttraumatic vascular lesions, and extravasation of contrast medium. Typical arteriographic

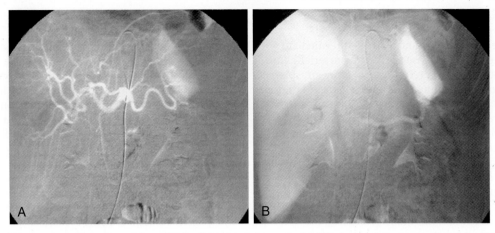

FIGURE 71-10. Celiac arteriography performed immediately after computed tomography (CT) shows splenic compression and medial displacement by a hematoma but fails to demonstrate extravasation of contrast medium into the spleen, obvious on CT.

findings of hepatic or splenic injury include a parenchymal defect at the site of vascular interruption or contusion, a parenchymal blush of contrast medium, an arterioportal fistula, early venous return or displacement of intraparenchymal arteries, enlargement of the spleen, detachment of the liver or spleen from its contact with the diaphragm or the lateral abdominal wall, and spastic arterial contraction. In the liver, an avascular zone with marked displacement of vessels and dense parenchymal staining caused by compression usually corresponds to hematoma or biloma. Definitive angiographic signs are extravasation of contrast material or demonstration of a vascular injury (pseudoaneurysm or AVF) without extravasation of contrast material (Figs. 71-10 to 71-12).

Hepatic or splenic vein injury is demonstrated by angiography only in exceptional circumstances. Delayed arteriography obtained in the first days after liver injury has shown arterial hypervascularization and disruption of portal flow in the contused areas. Posttraumatic arterioportal flow may also be seen in the absence of a gross posttraumatic arterioportal fistula. These phenomena are transient and not related to the severity of the injury.

Embolization Technique
Hepatic or splenic arteriography is usually performed with preshaped 5F Sidewinder-type catheters for demonstration of the site of contrast material extravasation or a vascular lesion already seen on CT. Hemostatic embolization is generally performed with coaxial 2F to 3F microcatheters and Gelfoam pledgets, particles, or microcoils as embolization agents, either alone or in combination. When using coils, each coil should be tightly packed individually, without residual coil elongation in the bleeding artery, and all coils should be tightly packed together (without interstices) to avoid late recanalization and coil migration. When treating arterial pseudoaneurysms, coils should *not* be placed inside the aneurysmal sac because late rupture has been described in extraparenchymal arterial segments. The so-called sandwich technique, consisting of coil placement proximal and distal to the aneurysmal sac, should be used. Complete and persistent vaso-occlusion of the parent vessel proximal and distal to the pseudoaneurysm so revascularization by backflow cannot occur should be documented angiographically before catheter withdrawal.

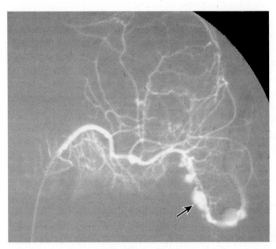

FIGURE 71-11. This 30-year-old man was admitted after abdominal contusion. Splenic arteriography shows extravasation of contrast material *(arrow)* at lower pole of spleen and poor recognition of normal intrasplenic vasculature as a result of severe vasoconstriction.

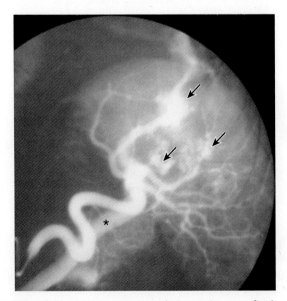

FIGURE 71-12. Posttraumatic intrasplenic arteriovenous fistula with early venous return *(asterisk)* and several pseudoaneurysmal lesions *(arrows)*. Treatment consisted of selective arterial embolization.

CONTROVERSIES

Surgeons are relatively reluctant to treat intermediate- or high-grade splenic injury conservatively by arterial hemostatic embolization. They prefer splenectomy or spleen-preserving surgical techniques because, in their opinion, conservative treatment is costly and there is still a risk of secondary splenic rupture. Surgeons also argue that CT is unable to provide direct information about intrasplenic vascular injuries, and that the risk for secondary bleeding by progressive hematoma development cannot be reliably identified. There is no classification system that shows in the individual patient whether a splenic injury has to be monitored with imaging techniques, whether embolization of a segmental artery or the main branch of the splenic artery is indicated, or whether surgery is the safest form of therapy.

Surgeons are more inclined to adopt conservative treatment of blunt hepatic injuries, provided intensive monitoring, including cross-section imaging, is applied. They consider that selective arterial embolization carries a definite risk of liver and gallbladder necrosis and septic complications. In the most complex situations, initial or delayed liver resection can be accomplished with low mortality and liver-related morbidity.[1] At the present time, it is not yet clear what role can be assigned to embolization techniques in the conservative treatment of liver trauma.

Most surgeons would advocate angiographic visualization of the hepatic arteries in patients who do not undergo emergency laparotomy and who have higher-grade hepatic injuries on CT in Moore's classification.

OUTCOMES

Posttraumatic Hemostasis of the Liver and Spleen on an Emergency Basis

Surgical management of liver injuries is more complex than that for splenic trauma. Hepatic artery embolization was shown to be a valuable adjunct in managing severe hepatic hemorrhage, although scientifically based results are lacking. Embolization on an emergency basis and as a primary hemostatic treatment, including management of

hemoperitoneum, was reported in small series of patients. Other reports have illustrated the value of arterial embolization for ongoing or recurrent hemorrhage despite initial laparotomy and reintervention.[2-4] In one study, arterial embolization was shown to be 100% effective in treating extravasation of contrast medium in the liver after blunt hepatic injury in a cohort of hemodynamically stabilized patients with 52% grade 3 and 4 injuries.[5] In another study, 16 of 30 markedly unstable patients with blunt liver injury underwent arterial hemostatic embolization. The patients were stabilized after embolization, and no major complication was observed.[6] In yet another study of 24 patients with posttraumatic vascular lesions, transcatheter occlusion was successful in 88%.[7] Patients with grade 4 and 5 hepatic injury who remained hemodynamically stable only with continued resuscitation could undergo hepatic arteriography and embolization to bridge the therapeutic option of nonoperative intervention and surgery. Treatment was effective in 10 of 11 patients[8] (Fig. 71-13, A-C).

The role of arterial embolization in splenic injury is much debated, and it was reported to be successful, without any need for subsequent splenic surgery, in 87% to 95% of cases.[9] In one study, an intrasplenic blush of contrast material was seen on CT in 8% of patients and confirmed to be a pseudoaneurysm on arteriography; 20 of 26 patients successfully underwent embolization, and 6 underwent splenectomy for technical failure of embolization.[10] Patients with coagulation abnormalities (e.g., disseminated intravascular coagulation) can still be treated selectively with arterial embolization, but arteriography must document complete and permanent vascular occlusion at completion of the procedure (Fig. 71-14, A-C). Overall, liver-related mortality, treatment failure, and complications seem to remain constant despite an increase in nonoperative management. High-grade liver injuries have greatly benefited from arterial hemostatic embolization.[11]

Posttraumatic Vascular Lesions in the Spleen

In practice, it is much more common to treat an intrasplenic posttraumatic vascular injury with some delay than acute splenic bleeding with documented extravasation of contrast material at admission. A pseudoaneurysm, AVF, or

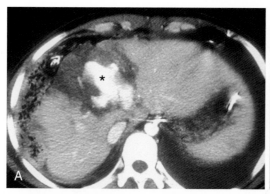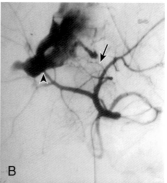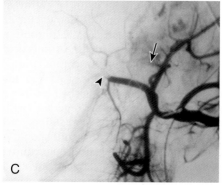

FIGURE 71-13. This patient underwent crash laparotomy at another hospital, where he was admitted after a car accident. **A,** Computed tomography obtained after transfer shows perihepatic packing and massive extravasation of contrast medium *(asterisk)* within the zone of extensive hepatic contusion. **B,** Immediate hepatic arteriography confirmed massive extravasation originating from right *(arrowhead)* and left *(arrow)* intrahepatic arterial branches. **C,** Embolization was achieved by selective occlusion of left hepatic arterial branches *(arrow)* and more proximal embolization of the right hepatic artery *(arrowhead)* with Gelfoam pledgets. Patient survived and required additional embolization 24 hours later for contrast material oozing from arterial branches in left lobe.

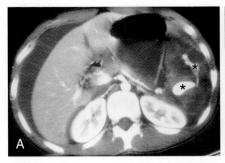 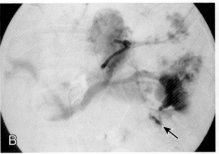 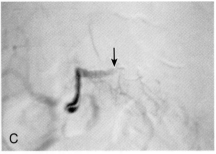

FIGURE 71-14. This patient was admitted in shock after blunt abdominal trauma. **A,** Computed tomography (CT) at admission showed a shattered spleen with multiple sites of extravasation of contrast material *(asterisks)*, intrasplenic and perisplenic hematoma, and perihepatic hemoperitoneum. **B,** Without patient transfer, splenic arteriography was performed in an integrated CT angiography unit. Parenchymal phase showed a fragmented spleen and extravasation of contrast material at lower pole of spleen *(arrow)*. **C,** Embolization of splenic artery with large Gelfoam fragments was accomplished at the level of hilar bifurcation *(arrow)* for immediate and definitive hemostasis.

a combination of both may develop after organ-preserving management of posttraumatic splenic injury. Their real frequency, which is unknown, may increase with general acceptance of conservative nonoperative management in which higher grades of splenic injury are included. In the past, persistent intrasplenic pseudoaneurysm only rarely evolved to clinical significance, with occasional rupture requiring emergency laparotomy. Intense imaging with CT, echocardiography, Doppler ultrasound, or MRI at admission and during follow-up will give a more precise indication of the real frequency of splenic vascular lesions, but at present the literature is limited, and only a few reports on imaging have been published. The fate of these lesions is still unknown, and it is unclear whether they might really lead to delayed rupture of the spleen in all cases. Delayed pseudoaneurysm rupture is hypothesized to occur in 3% to 46% of patients, depending on size, location, maturity of the capsule, and hemodynamic parameters. Posttraumatic pseudoaneurysms and AVFs can also regress spontaneously and thrombose after several weeks or months, similar to posttraumatic intrarenal lesions. The frequency of spontaneous thrombosis is also unknown.

Systematic CT examination with optimal bolus injection technique detects more of these lesions and allows preventive arterial embolization before hemorrhagic complications arise. It is of major importance to recognize that almost 75% of false aneurysms of the spleen are detected only on follow-up CT examinations and not at admission. Persistent AVFs probably have a lower risk of late bleeding than pseudoaneurysms do, but they may occasionally lead to high-flow portal hypertension or acute myocardial ischemia. In practice, catheter arterial occlusion should be performed when the vascular lesion is persistent, increases in size, or is symptomatic. Selective arterial embolization of an intrasplenic pseudoaneurysm or AVF has only occasionally been reported.[10,12] The presence of a splenic pseudoaneurysm during follow-up should be considered a predictor of failed nonoperative management until more precise figures on their evolution are available.

Posttraumatic Vascular Lesions in the Liver

Pseudoaneurysm

Posttraumatic hepatic pseudoaneurysm occasionally occurs in adults and children. Its frequency is estimated to be 2%

to 3%, and it predominates in patients with grade 4 injury. A pseudoaneurysm forms at the site of arterial injury and results from a self-limited blood cavity that is surrounded by liver parenchyma, contained by a pseudo-wall, and still connected to a ruptured vessel. Pseudoaneurysms may arise from a lobar or segmental intrahepatic artery or from an extrahepatic artery. They predominate in the right lobe. Persistent bilomas or bile fistulas are probably responsible for some of these pseudoaneurysms because of the erosive potential of bile on the vascular wall.[13] Posttraumatic stenosis of the bile ducts may also be associated with pseudoaneurysm, thus emphasizing the correlation between biliary and arterial injury in liver trauma. Color-flow Doppler imaging, CT, and MRI should be able to reveal all significant pseudoaneurysms unless they are of small size with a diameter less than 1 cm. Noninvasive imaging is indicated first when unexplained sepsis or gastrointestinal hemorrhage occurs in the posttraumatic phase.

Similar to the spleen, the fate of these posttraumatic hepatic pseudoaneurysms is not well known. Some, the smaller ones, may thrombose spontaneously; others may remain patent, persist, or enlarge rapidly. Enlargement up to 9 cm in diameter in 10 years has occasionally been reported. Pseudoaneurysms may become complicated when they rupture into the biliary system and are responsible for hemobilia. They may also be due to recurrent septic complications or rupture secondarily inside the liver parenchyma, erode into a vein, or perforate through the liver capsule into the upper gastrointestinal tract.

Currently accepted treatment of hepatic pseudoaneurysm is selective angiographic coil embolization, including extraparenchymal pseudoaneurysms located on the proper hepatic artery.[7,14] Placement of coils in the parent artery at the site of the pseudoaneurysm or use of the sandwich embolization technique is standard practice. Pseudoaneurysms located in the periphery of the liver parenchyma and difficult to reach because of the small size of arteries, spasm, thrombosis, or previous embolization or ligation can be treated by intrasaccular embolization through direct percutaneous transhepatic needle placement in the aneurysmal sac under cross-sectional imaging guidance. Embolization techniques are 90% effective in occluding pseudoaneurysms or AVFs in elective interventions.[6,15] Recurrence of a vascular lesion after correct vaso-occlusion is rare.

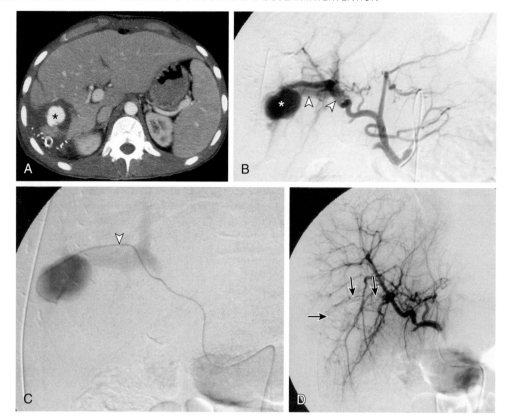

FIGURE 71-15. This patient, admitted after a traffic accident, underwent immediate surgery for repair of a liver laceration. Peripheral sutures and a surgical drain were placed. Continuous oozing of blood through surgical drain was observed after surgery. **A,** Computed tomography showed a 2-cm-diameter pseudoaneurysm *(asterisk)* within area of contusion in right lobe of liver. **B,** Hepatic arteriography confirms a pseudoaneurysm *(asterisk)* and arterioportal fistula. Note opacified right hepatic portal vein *(arrowheads)*. **C,** Selective catheterization of feeding artery of pseudoaneurysm with a microcatheter *(arrowhead)*. **D,** Embolization was achieved by placement of microcoils within the feeding artery *(arrows)*. Postembolization hepatic arteriography shows minimal intrahepatic vascular amputation.

Arterioportal and Arteriovenous Fistula

Arterioportal fistulas or AVFs result from arterial rupture into an adjacent portal or hepatic vein. This type of post-traumatic vascular injury is said to occur after 5% to 20% of percutaneous transhepatic procedures. In fact, after blunt hepatic injury, AVF is seen with a frequency equal to that of pseudoaneurysm during conservative management (Fig. 71-15, *A-D*). Arterioportal, arteriovenous (hepatic vein), or complex arterioportovenous fistulas or portovenous communications can be seen. Small and peripherally located arterioportal fistulas and those with low-flow or purely venous shunts can close spontaneously because of the low-pressure system, whereas fistulas with a high pressure gradient involving a segmental or lobar artery usually grow and enlarge to a certain point. Some may remain quiescent for long periods, up to many years. AVFs also usually show a pseudoaneurysm component, or they may coexist together with a separate pseudoaneurysm.

Intrahepatic or extrahepatic rupture of an arterioportal fistula or AVF can occur. Rupture into the bile ducts with hemobilia is the most classic complication. Large AVFs can result in overload of the right heart, and a large hepatic arterioportal fistula can lead to dynamic portal hypertension with gastroesophageal varices, variceal bleeding ascites, or mesenteric ischemia, which in turn produce symptoms, sometimes many years after the trauma. Hepatic infarct or abscess, as may be seen with diffuse arteriohepatic vein shunting in hepatic vascular malformations, is uncommon after trauma.

COMPLICATIONS

Delayed Hemorrhage in the Spleen

Before the era of CT examination of trauma patients, rebleeding or delayed rupture of the spleen was highly overestimated and limited the acceptance of conservative therapy. Today, a 1% incidence of rebleeding necessitating reoperation is anticipated after operative repair or partial splenectomy. When nonoperative management is applied, delayed bleeding within the first week is reported in up to 6% of cases. Delayed splenic rupture does not necessarily occur only with major trauma treated conservatively without surgery. Minor injury, particularly subcapsular, probably more than central splenic hematoma is prone to delayed rupture. Delayed or so-called secondary splenic rupture is a potential cause of mortality after blunt abdominal trauma and prompted systematic splenectomy in the past. Extended splenic lacerations were found at surgery in 5% to 15% of patients with delayed bleeding versus 1% of those with acute rupture. In the early literature, 15% to 30% of splenic injuries were reported to be secondary ruptures, but the literature after the use of cross-sectional imaging in trauma patients reported a drop in secondary splenic rupture to 1%. In the past, scintigraphy and arteriography had shown that so-called delayed splenic rupture was merely a missed diagnosis in most patients.

Delayed bleeding from a ruptured spleen occurs within a week in half the patients; in 75%, the "latent period" described by Baudet was less than 2 weeks. The presence of subcapsular hematoma is not an accurate predictor of secondary rupture per se, but rather an increase in volume of a splenic hematoma. True secondary splenic rupture with an initially intact capsule is a rare posttraumatic occurrence, with secondary bleeding from a preexisting capsular tear being a more frequent event. The spleen may rebleed when massively revascularized after an initial period of arterial vasoconstriction, as a result of hemostatic clot lysis by endogenous fibrinolysis, or after decompression of a subcapsular hematoma by catheter drainage or in situ injection of thrombolytic drugs into a hematoma. Rupture may also be due to infectious perisplenitis. Delayed splenic rupture has a worse prognosis than an immediately recognized injury and carries a higher mortality rate than repair of a primary splenic rupture. Delayed rupture is treated more often by splenectomy than primary rupture with similar severity is. Surgeons remain reluctant to perform angiographic embolization as a hemostatic alternative to splenectomy for delayed bleeding or rebleeding.

Delayed Hemorrhage in the Liver

In the liver, ongoing internal hemorrhage or oozing of blood through a surgical drain may be seen after an initial laparotomy in a small number of cases. These patients either undergo another operation or are investigated with arteriography, and subsequent embolization is performed. Patients who underwent a crash laparotomy and are transferred to a referral center should systematically undergo angiography before reoperation if their hemodynamic status is favorable. Delayed hemorrhage in patients treated conservatively can occur within days or a week but is seldom reported. The literature suggests that nonsurgical expectant or angiographic management of delayed hemorrhage in the liver is safe in these patients and more readily accepted by surgeons than such management for the spleen. However, in patients with the most severe grades of liver injury, postoperative lethal complications are caused by delayed hemorrhage in 50%. Expanding hematomas should be managed without delay, either surgically or, in selected cases, by arterial embolization.

Hepatic Necrosis

Severe and extensive hepatic necrosis has been recognized in the recent past as a major and frequent complication following arterial hemostatic embolization in high-grade liver injury.[16-18] It can occur after a burst or crush injury with arterial occlusion or after combined arterial and portal occlusion. In one report, major hepatic necrosis occurred in 41% of severe liver injuries treated with arterial hemostatic embolization.[16] Thrombosis of an intrahepatic portal branch is not sufficient to induce necrosis. CT shows a nonenhanced lobe or a well-demarcated segmental hypodense area without enhancement. Later, gas bubbles or intravascular branching gas patterns develop within the infarcted parenchyma (Fig. 71-16). Arterial hemostatic

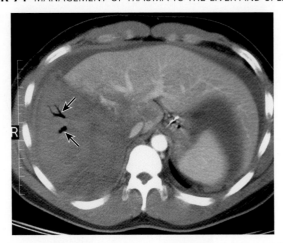

FIGURE 71-16. Large hemorrhagic contusion with mixed densities is seen in right lobe of liver. Liver capsule is interrupted. Gas has accumulated in peripheral portal vein branches *(arrows)* in area of contusion. Massive hemoperitoneum is present.

embolization can further contribute to parenchymal necrosis. When unrecognized, abscess formation, sepsis, and multiorgan failure are dreadful complications of hepatic tissue necrosis. The radiologist should be aware of complete nonenhancement of a liver lobe in the posttraumatic period; in such cases, liver resection is indicated in selected patients to prevent escalation of complications (Fig. 71-17). Postembolization morbidity is greatly related to liver and gallbladder necrosis.[18]

Hepatic Abscess

Posttraumatic liver abscess is twice as common as persistent biloma and three times more common than chronic hematoma. Abscesses may develop several months or 1 or 2 years after trauma. Secondary pyogenic abscess may form on the background of an ischemic contusion and lead to parenchymal necrosis, particularly after conservative treatment without débridement. A persistent biloma, hematoma, or mixed fluid collection may become infected at any time. In patients treated by systematic laparotomy for blunt liver injury, particularly after major trauma, a 7% abscess rate is found. In patients treated conservatively, the risk for the development of liver abscess should not be underestimated; an incidence of 1.4% is still reported.[19] Massive nonselective arterial embolization has to be avoided in trauma patients to minimize necrosis and superinfection of hepatic tissue. Posttraumatic liver abscesses can usually be treated by image-guided percutaneous aspiration or drainage techniques, but they have a higher failure rate than abscesses that develop in normal liver parenchyma because bile fistulas and vascular lesions can coexist.

Splenic Pseudocyst and Abscess

An intrasplenic or subcapsular hematoma that is undrained may resolve incompletely and evolve into a chronic blood collection, also called a *chronic pseudocyst* (Fig. 71-18). Posttraumatic splenic pseudocysts are observed frequently in some reports after nonoperative treatment and are almost absent in others, depending on the intensity of

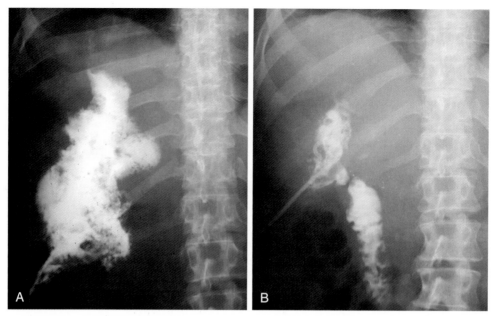

FIGURE 71-17. A, Opacification of a posttraumatic necrotic cavity in the liver with contrast material through a drainage catheter showed no biliary or extrahepatic fistula. **B,** After 3 weeks of external catheter drainage, opacification through catheter showed an extrahepatic fistula between necrotic cavity and duodenum, which subsequently closed after prolonged drainage.

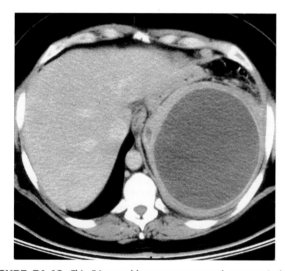

FIGURE 71-18. This 54-year-old man was managed conservatively for splenic contusion. Computed tomography scan obtained during follow-up showed a large fluid collection that was limited by a thick wall and had almost completely replaced normal splenic tissue. Old blood was aspirated from this chronic posttraumatic hematoma.

imaging during follow-up. Large subcapsular splenic hematomas are prone to developing such persistent fluid collections, which contain brownish old blood. Isolated case reports advocate open or celioscopic decapsulation as treatment. At surgery, a chronic hematoma may have an invasive, apparently neoplastic character. Pathologic examination shows a well-encapsulated mass with a thick fibrous wall around the organized hematoma within or around the spleen, without epithelial cell lining. Pathology suggests that delayed rupture from an organized chronic hematoma is not more frequent than rupture of a pseudocyst of pancreatic origin, although it may occur several years after injury. In some patients it may not be possible to differentiate between a hemorrhagic pancreatic pseudocyst and a chronic hematoma. Chronic splenic hematomas may enlarge because of an osmotic pressure gradient more than 1 month after injury and become symptomatic; they are known as *chronic expanding hematomas*. Usual surgical treatment is conservative and consists of pseudocystectomy, which preserves the cyst wall and spleen. Conservative laparoscopic treatment of posttraumatic splenic cysts is advised in selected patients. Splenectomy is the treatment of choice for cysts of unknown cause or uncertain diagnosis. Surgery can be replaced by percutaneous aspiration or short-term catheter drainage under US or CT guidance.[20] A chronic persistent intrasplenic hematoma may occasionally exhibit a calcified wall, which is indicative of its nature.

When conservative management of chronic hematoma or pseudocyst is adopted, imaging should demonstrate regression and persistent healing after percutaneous aspiration or short-term catheter drainage. Chronic splenic hematic cysts are at risk for superinfection and abscess formation when they do not regress spontaneously or are left untreated. Posttraumatic splenic abscess, which classically develops after spleen-preserving treatment, can be drained with a percutaneously placed catheter. Prognosis for unilocular splenic abscesses is generally better than for multiloculated collections.

Biloma

Biloma or bile fistula may develop after any type of hepatic intervention or expectant nonsurgical treatment. After surgery, the rate of prolonged bile leak is 3%. After conservative treatment with restrictive patient inclusion, biloma develops in 11.5% of patients, and a free peritoneal bile leak

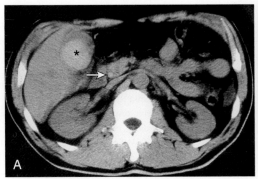
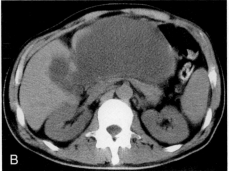

FIGURE 71-19. This 41-year-old man was admitted after blunt trauma from a car accident. **A,** Non–contrast-enhanced computed tomography (CT) at admission showed a high-density fresh clot in gallbladder lumen *(asterisk)* and intrapancreatic choledochus *(arrow)*. An area of moderate liver contusion was seen in segment IV (not shown). Conservative treatment was applied. **B,** During the following days, patient became febrile and complained of upper abdominal discomfort. CT performed 6 days after percutaneous aspiration showed a large fluid collection extending from gallbladder fossa to left subhepatic space.

in 8%.[21] Biliary cysts may develop secondary to hepatic infarction, arterial trauma, or arterial hemostatic embolization. Usually they resolve after repeated percutaneous aspiration or short-term catheter drainage (Fig. 71-19).

Posthepatectomy Biliary Stricture

A biliary stricture may occur in the intrahepatic or extrahepatic biliary tract several months or more than 1 year after hepatectomy for traumatic rupture, without evidence of bile duct injury at the time of trauma. Proposed mechanisms include anatomic distortion of the bile duct wall secondary to hepatic resection and subsequent regeneration, followed by inflammation and fibrosis. Repeated percutaneous transhepatic balloon dilation or metal stent placement for this type of benign bile duct stricture proved successful in only 50% of patients.[22]

Other

Hepatic US examination may be abnormal in 22% of cases in the posttraumatic phase, with capsular retraction, calcifications, or segmental bile duct obstruction being observed. These findings may persist for many months. Cholelithiasis may develop in the long term after hemobilia in children and adults. Coagulopathy may be seen in 5% of cases. Ectopic nodules of hepatic tissue not connected to the liver may grow independently, as in "splenosis" after blunt liver trauma.

POSTPROCEDURAL AND FOLLOW-UP CARE

Follow-up imaging studies are necessary after hemostatic arterial embolization in the liver and spleen. Patients who underwent hemostatic arterial embolization in the liver at admission should undergo repeat CT imaging within a minimum of 3 weeks because pseudoaneurysm and recurrent bleeding due to delayed rupture may develop in a small percentage of cases, despite arterial embolization. Generally, US and CT allow adequate follow-up of liver injury. On US, hyperechoic hemorrhage changes to hypoechoic and then to a normal hepatic echo pattern within several weeks because of resorption of blood and edema and granulation tissue formation. Central hematomas show a similar pattern of regression. On CT, hematomas change to a hypodense area with progressive enlargement at the phase of liquefaction, followed by slow regression in diameter. Patients with central or subcapsular hematoma should be monitored for at least 1 month, and those who receive anticoagulants should be observed particularly closely. Hepatic contusion regresses faster than hematomas (≈2 weeks) and may result in localized capsular retraction and scar calcification or a decrease in the volume of a sector or lobe secondary to vascular compromise. Patients with grade 4 or 5 injury usually need closer clinical follow-up and more imaging than those with lower grades because complications requiring treatment are more frequent. CT evidence of healing may take 1 to 6 months. Complete healing of the most severe liver injuries on CT may require 12 to 15 months, even in children.

In the spleen, serial CT examinations have shown that perisplenic fluid resolves completely in 1 to 4 weeks, and intrasplenic hematoma takes several months. Complete return to normal appearance of the spleen may require up to 4 months for low-grade injury and 1 year for multifocal and extended contusion. Patients who undergo conservative nonoperative treatment of splenic injury should be observed closely for 1 month with subsequent CT examinations. Intrasplenic pseudoaneurysm or AVFs might have been overlooked during arteriography at admission or may develop later. The fate of these lesions is still unknown, and it is unclear whether they might really favor delayed rupture of the spleen in all cases. Delayed rupture of pseudoaneurysm is hypothesized to occur in 3% to 46% of patients. Posttraumatic pseudoaneurysms and AVFs can also regress spontaneously and thrombose after several weeks or months, similar to posttraumatic intrarenal or intrahepatic vascular lesions. The rate of spontaneous thrombosis is also unknown. Probably, regular CT examinations with optimal bolus injection technique would detect more of these lesions and allow preventive arterial embolization before hemorrhagic complications arise. It is of major importance to note that almost 75% of false aneurysms of the spleen are detected only on follow-up CT examinations.

KEY POINTS

- Conservative treatment of blunt liver or spleen injury should be based on complete computed tomography (CT) examination of the abdomen, pelvis, and thorax to detect associated injuries that need repair. Expectant nonoperative treatment of liver or spleen injury should not be based exclusively on CT features or CT grading of liver or spleen contusion.

- Extravasation of contrast material or an intrahepatic or intrasplenic high-density blush on CT suggests persistent hemorrhage, and in most cases requires hemostatic intervention with either arteriography and selective embolization or surgery.

- Hemostatic arterial embolization should be performed in hemodynamically stable patients in whom CT has shown extravasation of contrast material or an intrahepatic or intrasplenic vascular lesion. In addition, marginally stable patients with ongoing arterial bleeding can be treated in centers where radiologists are part of the trauma team and specialized in hemostatic embolization in acute trauma victims.

- Tissue necrosis is a major complication following arterial embolization in high-grade hepatic and splenic injuries.

- Conservative management of splenic injury, including low grades, carries a risk of delayed bleeding and thus necessitates close observation and repeated imaging.

► **SUGGESTED READINGS**

Emery KH. Splenic emergencies. Radiol Clin North Am 1997;35:831–43.

Kluger Y, Paul DB, Raves JJ, et al. Delayed rupture of the spleen, myths, facts, and their importance—case reports and a literature review. J Trauma 1994;36:568–1.

Mirvis SE, Shanmuganathan K. Abdominal computed tomography in blunt trauma. Semin Radiol 1992;27:150–83.

Rees CR. Blunt splenic trauma and the angiographer: will we go back to the future? Radiology 1991;181:12–4.

Sclafani SJ, Shaftan GW, Scalea TM, et al. Nonoperative salvage of computed tomography-diagnosed splenic injuries: utilization of angiography for triage and embolization for hemostasis. J Trauma 1995;39:818–25.

The complete reference list is available online at www.expertconsult.com.

CHAPTER 72
Splenic Embolization in Nontraumatized Patients
Robert F. Dondelinger

INDICATIONS

Arterial embolization of the spleen may have two different objectives: interruption of arterial flow to the splenic artery or one of its branches, or ablation of splenic tissue by infarction. Depending on the aim of the procedure, splenic embolization may be considered an alternative to either splenectomy or ligation of the splenic artery. A typical indication for interruption of flow in the splenic artery or one of its branches is posttraumatic hemorrhage.

Splenic artery embolization has also been advocated to treat bleeding due to ruptured gastroesophageal varices, but portal hypertension has not been proven to be significantly influenced in all cases by arterial splenic embolization when portal pressure was recorded.

Catheter-mediated infarction of splenic tissue may be advocated as an alternative to splenectomy in various pathologic conditions. The volume of the spleen may be subnormal, but in the vast majority of cases, splenomegaly is obvious. Because intrasplenic arterial vascularization is represented by terminal vessels, efficient infarction of splenic tissue is regularly achieved after embolization of the intrasplenic branches.

Hypersplenism due to portal hypertension is certainly the primary indication for embolization of arterial splenic tissue.[1,2] Causes of hypersplenism vary. Most patients have alcoholic or postnecrotic liver cirrhosis, with a platelet count of less than $60,000/mm^3$ and at least one major episode of bleeding from ruptured gastroesophageal varices. Embolization of the spleen has the advantage of retaining the organ in place, and a distal splenorenal shunt is still possible after correction of the anemia and thrombocytopenia.

Children with gastroesophageal bleeding as a sign of hypersplenism secondary to Gaucher disease, atresia of the intrahepatic bile ducts, or portal vein thrombosis have also been treated by splenic embolization.

Splenic embolization is also indicated in patients being maintained on hemodialysis who have pancytopenia and splenomegaly, and in renal transplant patients in whom intolerance to immunosuppressive medications after renal transplantation had to be corrected.[3]

Thalassemia is also responsible for progressive hypersplenism, which requires an increase in the number of blood transfusions.[4,5] Partial splenic embolization is a valid alternative to splenectomy in this group of patients, in whom the risk for infections and lethal complications is particularly high after splenectomy.

Idiopathic thrombocytopenic purpura may also be corrected by splenic embolization.[6,7] The procedure is well tolerated in these patients because the spleen is of normal volume or only moderately enlarged. The physiopathologic mechanism of correction of thrombocytopenia has not been completely elucidated. Infarction of splenic tissue probably decreases sequestration of platelets in the spleen and reduces intrasplenic production of autoantibodies directed against platelets.

Splenic embolization has been used in a variety of other pathologic conditions, such as splenic lymphoma, chronic lymphatic leukemia, myeloid leukemia, myelofibrosis, hairy cell leukemia, polycythemia vera, hereditary spherocytosis, autoimmune hemolytic anemia, idiopathic hypersplenism, and Felty syndrome, as well as in patients with hypersplenism and cytopenia induced by anticancer chemotherapy.[8-11]

Preoperative partial splenic embolization has also been advocated before laparoscopic splenectomy,[12,13] in a tumorous spleen when correction of hypersplenism and reduction of tumor mass are expected, and in patients with hypersplenism, those at high operative risk, and those who refuse blood transfusion (Jehovah's Witnesses).[14]

CONTRAINDICATIONS

There are no absolute contraindications to embolization of the spleen. When massive splenomegaly is present, as occurs in malignant hemopathy, it is advisable to perform two or three sequential embolization procedures to improve tolerance and minimize the risk for complications secondary to infarction of a large volume of tissue.

EQUIPMENT

Arterial splenic embolization requires only standard angiographic equipment. For catheterization of the splenic artery, Sidewinder type I or II catheters are best suited. Stiff and soft hydrophilic guidewires are used routinely. Coaxial microcatheters, such as the Microferret or Radifocus, are useful for distal delivery of the embolization agent to the splenic artery at the splenic hilum. As embolization material, pledgets of gelatin sponge (Gelfoam) are most commonly used.

TECHNIQUE

Anatomy and Approach

For anatomy of the celiac trunk and splenic vessels, refer to Chapter 52.

Splenic embolization is performed after selective catheterization of the splenic artery via a femoral or (more rarely) axillary or brachial approach.

Technical Aspects

Antibiotic Prophylaxis

To avoid septic complications after splenic embolization, the patient undergoes antiseptic preparation before the procedure. A bath of povidone-iodine is given the day before embolization and the puncture site is prepared. Systemic antibiotics are administered starting on the day of embolization according to different protocols, which should be adapted to local preference:

• Intramuscular injections of 1,000,000 units of penicillin G with 3 mg/kg of gentamicin for 5 days after embolization
• A dosage of 0.5 g of cephalothin administered as four injections per day for 15 days after embolization
• Tobramycin (1 mg/kg) and oxacillin (1 g) intravenously 30 minutes before the procedure
• In children, gentamicin (10 mg/kg/day) and cefoxitin sodium (100 mg/kg/day) intravenously for 5 days or longer
• A 14-valent pneumococcal polysaccharide vaccine administered a few days before embolization

Catheterization Technique

In the vast majority of cases, standard preshaped 5F Cobra or Sidewinder catheters allow optimal catheterization of the splenic artery, with the tip of the catheter being advanced a sufficient distance from the ostium into the splenic artery. It is recommended that the splenic artery be catheterized as distally as possible to reduce any possible reflux of embolic material into the gastric and pancreatic arteries originating from the splenic artery, into other branches of the celiac artery, or into the abdominal aorta. A coaxial technique may be used in a tortuous splenic artery to optimize distal catheterization, but antegrade flow should be maintained in the splenic artery during embolization to prevent reflux of embolization agents. The risk of inadvertent embolization of caudal pancreatic arteries by migrant embolic material is not clinically significant when large particles are used as the embolization material. A branch of the splenic artery that usually originates proximal to the hilar branches and is directed to the upper pole of the spleen may be overlooked by catheterization that is too distal.

Embolization Technique and Material

Gelatin pledgets ($1 \times 1 \times 5$ mm) prepared by the operator during the procedure are the most commonly used material for splenic embolization. Use of Gelfoam powder may be associated with potential complications, such as pancreatitis and necrosis of the gastric wall secondary to thrombosis of many small terminal arteries. Particles of different size are injected, smaller particles first to block the most distal intrasplenic arteries, and large particles at the end to block the arteries at the splenic hilum. Formation of a plug of gelatin particles early in the procedure has to be avoided because it may preclude further correct embolization of the distal branches. Between 20 and 40 gelatin pledgets are necessary, depending on the volume of the spleen. Gelfoam pledgets are soaked in an antibiotic solution before injection.

The use of large steel coils lodged in the splenic artery does not induce infarction of splenic tissue. Coils are a safe embolization material, but the best long-term positive results are obtained when the coils are lodged in branches at the splenic hilum.

The extent of infarction has to be assessed during the procedure. When a significant reduction in flow of contrast medium is observed in the splenic artery, embolization is stopped. At that moment, the extent of infarction generally corresponds to 70% to 80% of the splenic volume (Fig. 72-1). Angiography can be performed during the procedure to assess the progression and extent of embolization. Angiographic catheter exchange is avoided during the procedure to prevent septic complications.

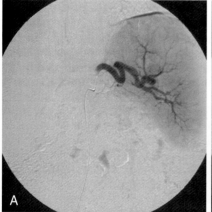 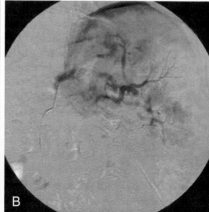 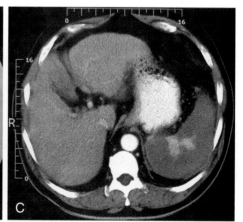

FIGURE 72-1. This 61-year-old male Jehovah's Witness awaiting liver transplantation for hepatitis C virus–related end-stage cirrhosis refused blood transfusion. Platelet count was low (22,000/mL^3) secondary to portal hypertension and subsequent hypersplenism. **A,** Selective pre-embolization splenic arteriography shows moderately enlarged spleen. **B,** Selective splenic arteriography performed after embolization with Gelfoam pledgets shows a heterogeneous spleen with stasis of contrast material in intrasplenic arterial branches and disruption of peripheral splenic parenchyma. Extent of infarction is estimated at 80%. **C,** Platelet count increased to 400,000/mL^3 4 days after splenic embolization. Contrast-enhanced computed tomography shows extended infarction of spleen and small persistent areas of viable tissue close to splenic hilum.

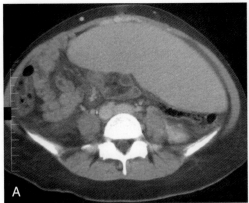
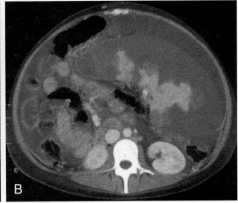

FIGURE 72-2. This 51-year-old woman awaiting liver transplantation for end-stage liver cirrhosis secondary to autoimmune liver disease had hypersplenism and a low platelet count (16,000/mL^3). **A,** Pre-embolization contrast-enhanced computed tomography (CT) shows large homogeneous splenomegaly. **B,** CT performed after extended splenic embolization shows massive tissue infarction and residual viable splenic tissue at hilum. Note peritoneal effusion as a complication of splenic embolization.

CONTROVERSIES

Controversies may be linked to the rationale for indications, choice of embolization material, extent of embolization, and alternative medical therapy.

Many other substances have been described as alternatives to Gelfoam: autologous clot, polyvinyl alcohol, silicone microspheres, isobutyl-2-cyanoacrylate, and ethanol. However, these materials do not offer significant advantages over the ease of use of Gelfoam.

Embolization of a large spleen may be associated with significant complications when extensive infarction is produced. Celioscopic splenectomy after rapid arterial embolization is an alternative with little hemorrhagic risk in such a case.

No evidence-based published results have demonstrated how much splenic tissue must be infarcted to achieve correction of hypersplenism. Experience suggests that embolization of 70% to 80% of splenic tissue yields more consistent improvement than infarction of 30% to 50%.

In patients with idiopathic thrombocytopenic purpura, high-dose steroids may correct the thrombocytopenia and render partial splenic embolization unnecessary.

Finally, estimation of the extent of infarction in the spleen is approximate during the angiographic procedure itself and can be assessed precisely only during follow-up with cross-section imaging (Fig. 72-2).

OUTCOMES

It is difficult to assess the clinical benefit gained from arterial embolization of the spleen; the number of clinical trials is limited, and most studies are based on a small number of patients. Individual reports and small series of patients treated by embolization of the splenic artery for traumatic bleeding or aneurysm are available in the literature and are discussed in Chapter 71.

Experimental studies in animals have shown that injection of gelatin particles into the splenic arteries induces persistent obliteration of the vessels 8 weeks after embolization.[15] At the early phase, 24 hours, and 2 weeks after embolization, irregular zones of hemorrhagic infarction coexist with areas of normal splenic tissue. At the late phase, fibrosis replaces the areas of intrasplenic infarction. Leukocyte values were increased in all animals 24 hours after embolization, and the hematocrit decreased by 20% during the first week after embolization. Experimental data in animals with a normal spleen show no influence on the lifespan of erythrocytes and no significant increase in circulating thrombocytes.

Among the clinical studies reported, only a few contain a significant number of cases. Generally, partial embolization of the spleen varying from 30% to 80% is performed. Most of the patients reported earlier in the literature were treated for hypersplenism. Platelet count increases rapidly after splenic embolization in humans, and a temporary hyperthrombocytosis is often observed. A normal platelet count can be observed 1 to 2 years after the procedure. The frequency of bleeding episodes from gastroesophageal varices was shown to be reduced in adults and in children to 0.4 per year after splenic embolization.[16,17] An increase in platelets was achieved in 96% of patients, even when coils were used.[18] Spigos et al.[19] reported on the effect of splenic embolization in 13 patients, 7 of them receiving immunosuppressive therapy; a significant increase in white cell and platelet counts was noted 2 weeks after embolization. Similar results were observed by Gerlock et al.[3] in a study consisting of six patients undergoing hemodialysis and one transplant patient. These early results have been confirmed by later experience. Pringle et al.[5] reported on six patients with thalassemia and hypersplenism who were treated by splenic embolization. All patients showed correction of hypersplenism, reduction of the need for blood transfusions, and an obvious positive effect on growth in children who underwent the procedure. In eight patients treated for idiopathic thrombocytopenic purpura, long-term normalization of the platelet count was observed in six in our early experience and was confirmed in larger patient series.[20,21] In the other reported cases where embolization was performed for idiopathic thrombocytopenic purpura or another surgical intervention, normalization of platelet count was achieved.

A small number of splenic embolization procedures have been performed in patients with splenomegaly secondary to a malignant hemopathy. In this group, splenectomy may be indicated in the late phase of the disease. Most patients at initial evaluation have a considerably enlarged spleen that is causing abdominal compression and organ displacement, signs of hypersplenism, and inadequate response to chemotherapy. Debulking is probably the most beneficial effect gained from splenectomy or embolization. The hematologic response to surgery or embolization is unpredictable, and life expectancy remains unchanged. We have treated patients with chronic lymphatic leukemia, myeloid splenomegaly, leukemic lymphosarcoma, hairy cell leukemia, and polycythemia vera, as well as one patient with autoimmune hemolytic anemia in whom an accessory spleen was left after splenectomy and was embolized. Positive effects have been noted to some degree in all patients with hypersplenism or with a need for blood transfusions, except for the patient who had an accessory spleen embolized.[21] The reduction in splenic volume is, however, less in tumorous spleens after arterial embolization than in congestive or normal spleens. Regeneration of splenic tissue from the hilum to the periphery occurs in almost all cases when viable splenic tissue is left in place.

COMPLICATIONS

Surgical splenectomy is not free of untoward side effects; it is associated with a number of complications and a mortality rate varying according to the underlying disease. Splenectomy performed for treatment of spherocytosis carries a morbidity rate of 3.52% and a mortality rate from sepsis of 2.23%, versus rates of 24.8% and 11%, respectively, when splenectomy is performed for cure of thalassemia. This risk of dying of fulminant sepsis after splenectomy increases 200 to 800 times when splenectomy is performed in a patient with hemopathy.[18,22] Splenorrhaphy, partial splenectomy, and peritoneal implantation of fragments of splenic tissue after splenectomy significantly lower the risk of infectious postoperative complications. Splenectomized patients are at risk for overwhelming septicemia, bacterial meningitis, and pneumonia. In half the cases, *Streptococcus pneumoniae* is identified as the responsible microbe; in 30% of cases, *Haemophilus influenzae* or *Neisseria meningitidis* is present. In the majority of cases, fatal septicemia occurs during the 2 years after the spleen has been removed.

Arterial splenic embolization may also be associated with serious complications, similar to those after surgery.[23] Furthermore, the occurrence of a splenic abscess can be explained by the persistence of infarcted and necrotized splenic tissue, arrest of opsonizing function of the spleen after circulation in the spleen has stopped, and backflow of digestive bacteria through the splenic vein into the spleen. Total embolization of the spleen induces a non-negligible postembolization mortality rate, whereas partial splenic embolization carries a mortality rate of about 9% in published reports containing a limited number of patients.[16] Partial splenic embolization leaves functional splenic tissue in situ, which protects the patient from infection, but the minimal volume of splenic tissue necessary to maintain opsonic and immunologic function of the spleen has not been determined. Experience is certainly an important factor in reducing complications, as shown by the low or absent mortality reported in studies containing a significant number of patients.[3,17-19,22-24]

Among other major postembolization complications, rupture of the spleen, necrosis of the gastric wall, renal insufficiency, acute pancreatitis, pneumonia, and thrombosis of the splenic vein have been described. Minor complications are represented by abdominal pain in the left upper quadrant, slight fever, nausea and vomiting, paralytic ileus, pleural and peritoneal effusions, and plate-like atelectasis in the left lower lobe. Children may have an elevated temperature after splenic embolization for a longer time than adults. Strict aseptic angiographic technique, preventive systemic antibiotics, and partial or repetitive splenic embolization, which has replaced total infarction of the spleen, have significantly diminished local complications after splenic embolization. In a group of renal transplant patients, who are at particular risk for complications, Spigos observed one splenic abscess after partial embolization in 76 cases.[25] Among 18 cirrhotic patients with portal hypertension studied by Owman et al.,[24] 2 suffered a splenic abscess after subtotal embolization of the spleen, 1 patient died, and 4 had thrombosis of the splenic vein. In the six immunosuppressed patients who underwent embolization by Gerlock et al.,[3] no abscesses developed.

POSTPROCEDURAL AND FOLLOW-UP CARE

Pain Control

Clinical tolerance of splenic embolization depends on the volume of the spleen, extent of embolization, embolization material used, and the underlying disease. Intraarterial 2-chloroprocaine hydrochloride has been used during the procedure to control abdominal pain. Postembolization abdominal pain is usually well controlled by medication. Continuous epidural analgesia has been used after embolization, but it may complicate an otherwise easy procedure. A short hospital stay ranging from 4 to 6 days is necessary for patients who undergo embolization of a hematologic disorder when the spleen is not or only moderately enlarged. In contrast, patients with an enlarged spleen or a complex underlying disease may need a longer hospitalization.

Assessment of the Extent of Embolization

After completion of the procedure, the local effect of arterial embolization on the spleen may be assessed by nuclear medicine studies, ultrasound, computed tomography (CT), or magnetic resonance imaging (MRI). Technetium-99 (^{99m}Tc) sulfur colloid scans and ultrasound are limited in their ability to precisely demonstrate the extent of embolization. CT and MRI allow precise assessment of the volume of infarcted zones in the spleen and reflect the transformation of infarcted tissue to fibrosis by increases in density values on subsequent CT examinations or corresponding MR signals (see Fig. 72-2). Both imaging modalities show zones of liquefaction in the early phase after embolization and detect early complications such as bleeding, intrasplenic or perisplenic abscess, and perisplenic effusions, as well as late complications such as thrombosis of the splenic vein and intrasplenic growth of the remaining splenic tissue. MRI is particularly able to differentiate embolized areas in the spleen from persistently vascularized tissue and demonstrates transformation of infarcted zones to fibrous tissue.

KEY POINTS

- Partial splenic arterial embolization, in which a portion of the splenic parenchyma is left viable, preserves the immunologic function of the spleen.

- Partial embolization of 50% to 70% of splenic tissue produces effects similar to those of total splenic tissue infarction in correction of hematologic disorders and hypersplenism, but it is associated with a lower rate of complications.

- The risk for complications after splenic embolization should be prevented by prophylactic antibiotic therapy and strict aseptic angiographic technique.

► **SUGGESTED READINGS**

Jonasson O, Spigos DG, Mozes MF. Partial splenic embolization: experience in 136 patients. World J Surg 1985;9:461–7.

Kimura F, Itoh H, Ambiru S, et al. Long-term results of initial and repeated partial splenic embolization for the treatment of chronic idiopathic thrombocytopenic purpura. AJR Am J Roentgenol 2002;179:1323–6.

Madoff DC, Denys A, Wallace MJ, et al. Splenic arterial interventions: anatomy, indications, technical considerations, and potential complications. Radiographics 2005;25:S191–S211.

Mozes MF, Spigos DG, Pollak R, et al. Partial splenic embolization, an alternative to splenectomy: results of a prospective, randomized study. Surgery 1984;96:694–702.

Nio M, Hayashi Y, Sano N, et al. Long-term efficacy of partial splenic embolization in children. J Pediatr Surg 2003;38:1760–2.

Papidimitriou J, Tritakis C, Karatzas G, Papaionnou A. Treatment of hypersplenism by embolus placement in the splenic artery. Lancet 1976;2:1268.

The complete reference list is available online at www.expertconsult.com.

CHAPTER 73

Management of Visceral Aneurysms

James E. Jackson

False aneurysms (pseudoaneurysms) of the visceral arteries represent an area of contained hemorrhage and are relatively uncommon but at high risk of rupture, with subsequent acute gastrointestinal or retroperitoneal hemorrhage. They always require treatment regardless of their size. Many are related to acute or chronic pancreatitis but may also occur after surgery or without an obvious cause. There should be a high index of suspicion for the presence of a pseudoaneurysm in a patient with a history of pancreatitis in whom upper gastrointestinal bleeding subsequently develops, although other causes (e.g., segmental portal venous hypertension secondary to splenic venous occlusion or unrelated peptic ulceration) are still more likely. However, if the episodes of hemorrhage in such patients are related to severe epigastric pain radiating to the back, a pseudoaneurysm communicating with the pancreatic duct and causing *hemosuccus pancreaticus* is likely.[1]

True aneurysms of the visceral arteries are rare. The splenic artery is the vessel most commonly involved, and the majority of aneurysms are an incidental finding on cross-sectional imaging. Their risk of rupture is not clear, but if less than 2 cm in diameter, they are unlikely to cause problems, except perhaps during pregnancy. A combination of atheromatous disease and aneurysm formation may be seen in association with enlargement of the pancreaticoduodenal arcade vessels as a result of either atheromatous stenosis of the celiac axis or, more commonly, compression of the celiac axis origin by the median arcuate ligament of the hemidiaphragm. These aneurysms may rarely rupture into the retroperitoneum.

INDICATIONS

All visceral artery pseudoaneurysms require treatment, and the vast majority can be managed successfully by embolization, which should be the procedure of first choice.[2-4] Surgery should be reserved for patients in whom complex anatomy precludes an endovascular approach.

Indications for treatment of true visceral artery aneurysms are less clear-cut because prospective data on the risk of rupture are lacking. The splenic artery is the vessel most frequently involved, and aneurysms, when present, are commonly related to branch origins. Those less than 2 cm in size can probably be ignored. The American College of Cardiology and American Heart Association guidelines for management of patients with peripheral arterial disease[5] conclude that:

1. "Open repair or catheter-based intervention is indicated for visceral aneurysms measuring 2.0 cm in diameter or larger in women of childbearing age who are not pregnant and in patients of either gender undergoing liver transplantation."

2. "Open repair or catheter-based intervention is probably indicated for visceral aneurysms measuring 2.0 cm in diameter or larger in women beyond childbearing age and in men."

Although few would disagree with the first of these guidelines, the wording of the second is less helpful. There are undoubtedly patients in whom an asymptomatic visceral artery aneurysm measuring up to 2.5 cm in size is found on imaging performed for other reasons and can be managed conservatively. Indeed, some authors suggest that 2.5 cm rather than 2 cm should be the size above which therapy is required.[6] There is no doubt, however, that symptomatic aneurysms or those that show a gradual increase in size on follow-up will require treatment. An additional indication for treatment of renal artery aneurysms is renovascular hypertension.

The decision whether to proceed with open surgical or endovascular repair of a true visceral artery aneurysm depends on a number of factors, including the size and site of the aneurysmal disease. In the context of acute rupture, the patient may stabilize after the initial hemorrhage because of tamponade of the ruptured aneurysm by surrounding hematoma, especially when the hemorrhage occurs into the retroperitoneum, and such individuals may be treated by embolization. Patients who are hemodynamically compromised are more likely to need to proceed straight to open surgery.

CONTRAINDICATIONS

The only absolute contraindications to an endovascular approach are those that apply to any angiographic technique—namely, a bleeding diathesis that cannot be corrected and a history of life-threatening anaphylaxis to iodinated contrast medium.

TECHNIQUE

Anatomy and Approach

Thorough knowledge of conventional and variant visceral arterial anatomy is essential, as is recognition of the many collateral pathways that can develop via normal anastomoses in response to visceral artery occlusive or stenotic disease.[7] This rich collateral supply to most of the abdominal viscera means that embolization of major visceral vessels can often be performed without causing organ infarction. Lack of appreciation of the extent of this collateral network can, however, result in failure of endovascular therapy. For example, a pseudoaneurysm involving a right hepatic artery branch should be definitively treated by placing embolization coils on either side of the arterial defect to exclude it

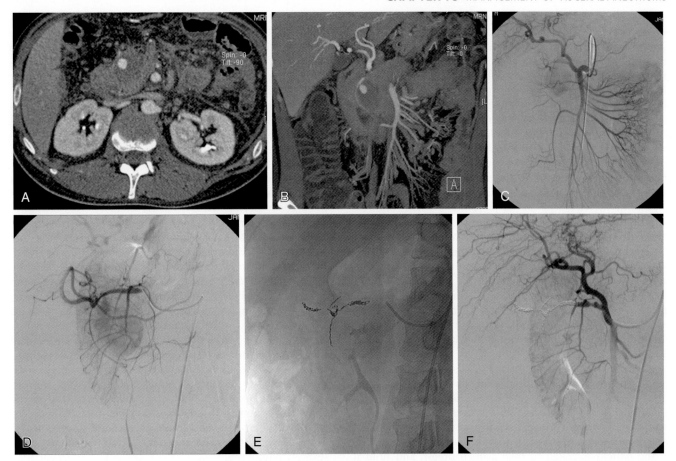

FIGURE 73-1. Gastroduodenal artery (GDA) pseudoaneurysm in chronic pancreatitis. **A,** Axial computed tomography (CT) demonstrates GDA pseudoaneurysm consisting of a small patent lumen surrounded by a large amount of thrombus. **B,** Coronal reconstruction CT showing same GDA pseudoaneurysm. Other images (not shown) demonstrated variant visceral artery anatomy, with the GDA arising from a replaced common hepatic artery arising from superior mesenteric artery. **C,** Selective superior mesenteric arteriogram demonstrates anatomy and also shows pseudoaneurysm. Note that patent lumen of pseudoaneurysm is considerably larger than on CT scan performed 24 hours previously, demonstrating the rapid changes that can occur. **D,** Selective GDA angiogram demonstrates a jet of contrast medium filling aneurysmal sac immediately proximal to trifurcation into right gastroepiploic, anterior superior pancreaticoduodenal, and supraduodenal arteries. **E,** Control film after embolization with platinum microcoils. Note that coils have been placed in each of the three vessels beyond pseudoaneurysm neck, as well as proximal to it within distal GDA to ensure its exclusion from circulation. **F,** Selective common hepatic arteriogram after embolization confirms exclusion of pseudoaneurysm and shows preservation of supply to duodenum.

completely from the circulation. An angiographer who fails to recognize that intrahepatic arterial branches will receive a collateral supply from several possible sources (e.g., other hepatic, internal mammary, and inferior phrenic arteries) *immediately* after proximal hepatic artery occlusion is more likely to perform an inadequate embolization by placing coils only proximal to the pseudoaneurysm neck.

Multislice computed tomography (CT) performed during the arterial phase of contrast medium enhancement will usually provide exquisite images, in a variety of planes, of both true and false aneurysms, which can be of great help in documenting the anatomy and planning endovascular therapy (Fig. 73-1). Most visceral arterial aneurysmal disease that requires therapy will be approached via a common femoral artery puncture. Occasionally an axillary or brachial artery approach will provide a more favorable route, such as when the aneurysmal disease involves a superior mesenteric artery that has a very acute origin from the aorta, or when there is marked compression of the origin of the celiac axis by the median arcuate ligament of the hemidiaphragm.

Technical Aspects

Visceral Angiography

It is essential that high-quality diagnostic angiographic images be obtained to document completely the anatomy of the diseased segment of the vessel so that treatment is successful. Considerable experience is necessary to routinely acquire high-quality diagnostic images of the visceral arteries. Unfortunately, it is increasingly difficult to obtain sufficient experience, because the indications for visceral angiography have decreased substantially over the last decade as alternative noninvasive imaging studies and ready access to endoscopy have become available. It is not the purpose of this chapter to discuss the technique of diagnostic visceral angiography, but it is such an important part of the procedure that some of the most useful technical points will be mentioned briefly. Interested readers are referred to other texts for a more detailed description.[8]

One of the major problems with digital subtraction angiography, currently the method of image acquisition used almost exclusively for visceral angiography, is that of movement artifact; this is the most common cause of serious image degradation during abdominal imaging. There are two sources of movement during visceral angiography. The first, bowel peristalsis, can easily be abolished in the majority of patients by the administration of smooth muscle relaxants, but a common mistake, and one that is often the cause of poor-quality images, is to rely on a single dose of drug. For example, many radiologists will give 20 mg of hyoscine butylbromide (Buscopan) intravenously at the beginning of the procedure and rely on this dose to provide bowel paralysis for much of the study; this will very rarely suffice. A starting dose of 40 mg is recommended and should be increased by 20-mg increments when required. It is common to administer 100 mg during an arteriogram taking between 45 and 60 minutes to complete. Complete bowel paralysis may occasionally not be produced by hyoscine butylbromide alone, and the addition of glucagon in 1-mg aliquots may be necessary.

The second type of movement, which may be much more difficult to deal with, is that of respiration. Several techniques may be used to obtain diagnostic images. Very few individuals are able to hold their breath without *any* abdominal movement for more than about 15 seconds, and most will manage less than 10. This means that severe image degradation commonly occurs during the late arterial/early venous phase, which is often the most important part of the angiogram for determining the site of pathology in patients being investigated for gastrointestinal bleeding. Movement is likely to be even more pronounced if the patient is asked to take a deep breath and hold it during image acquisition. It is better to ask the patient to stop "at a comfortable position" in the middle of respiration and try to stop breathing at the same position for each run. A substantial improvement in abdominal stillness can also be achieved by simply pinching the nose (with a nose clip) during breath-holding. It is always worthwhile to practice these techniques with the patient before obtaining images.

In many individuals, considerable movement persists on early images, despite use of the aforementioned techniques, and it is rare, even with the fittest of patients (indeed, it is usually the younger, fitter patients who experience the most difficulty keeping still during breath-holding), to find an individual who is able to hold the abdomen completely still to allow good-quality venous images. The technique that is useful in practically all patients is that of acquisition of images during normal respiration. More than 90% of visceral arteriograms performed at this author's institution include at least one run (and sometimes all) acquired during normal breathing. This underused technique often produces the best diagnostic images. It relies on regular breathing and the acquisition of several images before the injection of contrast medium, each of which may then be used as a mask for the subsequent angiographic images. When performed in this manner, a different mask will usually be available for each stage of the respiratory cycle, and perfectly subtracted images will be obtained throughout the run in the arterial, capillary, and venous phases. The best results are obtained if images are acquired at one frame per second, and two (and sometimes more) full respiratory cycles are imaged before contrast medium is injected.

Embolization

Although the endovascular techniques used to treat false and true visceral artery aneurysms are often similar, each will be discussed separately because there are some important differences.

False Aneurysms (Pseudoaneurysms)

The success of treatment depends on complete, persistent thrombosis of the pseudoaneurysm sac. There are several possible methods by which this may be achieved, each of which will be discussed.

EMBOLIZATION OF THE DISEASED VESSEL ON EITHER SIDE OF THE ARTERIAL DEFECT This technique, which is most easily performed by placing metallic coils on either side of the arterial defect (Figs. 73-2 to 73-4; also see Fig. 73-1), is one that has been used more than any other and, when performed correctly, will be curative with little risk of recurrence. The catheter chosen to obtain a sufficiently distal position to allow embolization will obviously depend on the anatomy (and personal preference of the angiographer), but in many situations a coaxial catheter will be necessary.

It is essential that *complete* occlusion of the vessel beyond the pseudoaneurysm be achieved before proximal embolization is performed so that the possibility of recanalization via collaterals is prevented. Clearly, if bleeding were to recur via this route because of inadequate distal embolization, the chance of successfully reembolizing the pseudoaneurysm will have been markedly reduced because access to the vessel beyond the arterial defect is likely to have been severely hampered.

PACKING THE PSEUDOANEURYSM SAC WITH COILS The pseudoaneurysm sac lacks a wall and is contained only by surrounding hematoma. Filling this sac with embolic material, especially metallic coils, should therefore be avoided because it will usually cause expansion of the sac and may cause its rupture. This method of embolization should certainly never be performed as a sole method of inducing pseudoaneurysm thrombosis. Although it may initially produce a satisfactory angiographic result, with sac thrombosis and preserved patency of the parent vessel, subsequent lysis of the surrounding hematoma will almost invariably cause the "coil ball" to fall away from the arterial defect, and the pseudoaneurysm will then recanalize and be at the same risk of hemorrhage as it was before attempted treatment.[9]

PLACEMENT OF A COVERED STENT ACROSS THE PSEUDOANEURYSM NECK Placement of a covered stent ("endograft") across the neck of a pseudoaneurysm involving a large-caliber vessel such as the splenic, hepatic, or superior mesenteric artery[10,11] is, at first sight, an attractive option because it will completely exclude the aneurysm while maintaining patency of the parent vessel. It is rarely used for the treatment of visceral artery pseudoaneurysms, however, for the following reasons:

1. Insertion of a covered stent usually requires use of a guiding sheath, and it may not be possible to introduce the sheath into a suitable position because of unfavorable anatomy of the visceral artery origin or arterial tortuosity or both. This is especially true of the splenic artery.
2. Manipulation of the large catheters and sheaths used for insertion of covered stents in a diseased vessel

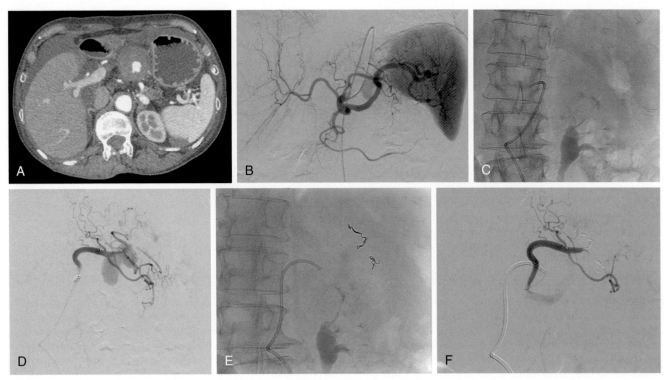

FIGURE 73-2. Pseudoaneurysm of left gastric artery after an episode of acute pancreatitis. **A,** Axial computed tomography demonstrates a large upper abdominal pseudoaneurysm closely applied to lesser curvature of stomach. **B,** Celiac axis angiogram shows a large pseudoaneurysm cavity superimposed between splenic and left gastric arteries. Control film **(C)** and selective left gastric arteriogram **(D)** show coaxial catheter and a large pseudoaneurysm arising from left gastric artery immediately beyond a bifurcation. **E,** Control film after embolization demonstrates platinum microcoils across pseudoaneurysm neck and within inferior gastric branch vessel, which arises immediately proximal to arterial defect. **F,** Selective left gastric artery angiogram after embolization, confirming complete exclusion of pseudoaneurysm from circulation.

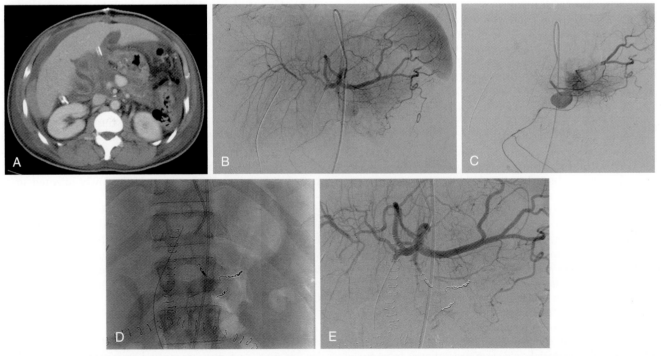

FIGURE 73-3. Transverse pancreatic artery pseudoaneurysm causing massive hemorrhage 1 week after Whipple operation. **A,** Axial computed tomography demonstrates contrast medium filling aneurysmal cavity in retroperitoneum immediately anterior to superior mesenteric artery. Free fluid of varying attenuation is present within abdomen, consistent with recent hemorrhage. **B,** Celiac axis angiogram demonstrates faint filling of pseudoaneurysm cavity lying beneath transverse pancreatic artery. Note that right hepatic artery is occluded as a result of recent surgery, with its more distal branches reconstituted via collaterals. **C,** Selective dorsal pancreatic arteriogram demonstrates a large pseudoaneurysm arising from a transverse pancreatic artery immediately proximal to a posterior omental branch. **D,** Control film after embolization shows platinum microcoils within transverse pancreatic and omental branches beyond pseudoaneurysm, as well as within parent vessel proximal to arterial defect. **E,** Celiac axis angiogram after embolization confirms complete exclusion of pseudoaneurysm from circulation.

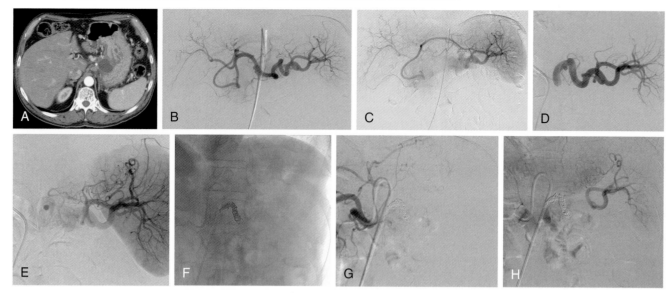

FIGURE 73-4. Splenic artery pseudoaneurysm in a patient with chronic pancreatitis causing episodes of life-threatening gastric hemorrhage. **A,** Axial computed tomography through upper part of abdomen demonstrates a pseudocyst intimately related to lesser curvature of stomach; no pseudoaneurysm could be identified on this study. **B,** Early arterial-phase image from a celiac axis angiogram shows no abnormality. **C,** Later arterial-phase image from a celiac axis angiogram demonstrates small rounded cavity filled with contrast material, consistent with pseudoaneurysm. **D,** Oblique selective splenic arteriogram shows pseudoaneurysm arising from main trunk of midsplenic artery. **E,** Later image shows persistent opacification of aneurysmal sac. **F,** Control film after embolization shows platinum microcoils packed within main splenic artery across pseudoaneurysm neck. **G,** Postembolization celiac axis angiogram confirms splenic artery occlusion. **H,** Later-phase image from same arteriogram shows reconstitution of distal splenic artery branches, which occurred predominantly via gastric artery collaterals.

close to a pseudoaneurysm poses a greater risk of periprocedural rupture than do the smaller catheters generally used for embolization.

3. Although the neck of the pseudoaneurysm may appear small, it should be remembered that the disease process causing the vessel defect (e.g., pancreatitis) is likely to be involving a greater length of arterial wall than is apparent angiographically. In such situations, placement of a balloon-expandable covered stent may be associated with a high risk of arterial rupture.

4. If the neck of the pseudoaneurysm involves a vessel bifurcation, a covered stent may not cover the arterial defect completely and can present a subsequent risk of continued sac perfusion secondary to retrograde filling of the branch not stented.

5. Covered stents may occlude normal branch vessels arising close to the pseudoaneurysm neck, but this is often not a contraindication to their use in visceral vessels because there is usually an excellent collateral supply from adjacent arteries.

COMBINATION OF AN UNCOVERED STENT AND EMBOLIZATION An alternative therapeutic option that may be useful in certain circumstances where anatomy precludes use of the methods just discussed is the combination of an uncovered ("bare-mesh") stent placed across the arterial defect and packing the pseudoaneurysm sac with coils (or other embolic material) via a microcatheter introduced through the stent mesh (or placed within the sac before deployment of the stent). This technique may be helpful when preservation of the visceral arterial lumen is essential and a covered stent cannot be used for one reason or another. The problems associated with sac packing and the risk of subsequent clot lysis and pseudoaneurysm

recanalization, mentioned earlier, should be borne in mind if this method of treatment is used, and for these reasons it is less likely to be successful than use of a covered stent.

PERCUTANEOUS THROMBIN INJECTION Thrombin injection has become the accepted method for treating postcatheterization femoral artery pseudoaneurysms,[12-14] and this has resulted in its use to manage pseudoaneurysms at other sites. Its description for the treatment of visceral artery pseudoaneurysms is limited to only a few case reports. The technique involves introducing a fine-bore needle (usually 22 gauge) into the patent lumen of the pseudoaneurysm under CT, ultrasound, or fluoroscopic guidance (or any combination of these modalities). Once a suitable needle position has been confirmed, thrombin (at a concentration between 500 and 1000 units/mL) is slowly injected until sac thrombosis is achieved, in exactly the same way as performed when treating pseudoaneurysms involving the femoral artery. Only small volumes of the thrombin solution should be injected (thrombosis will often be achieved with < 1 mL) to reduce the risk of spillage of this agent into the parent vessel, with the possible complication of end-organ thrombotic infarction (see later discussion under Controversies).

True Aneurysms

As mentioned earlier, true aneurysms of the visceral arteries are rare, and those requiring treatment are much less common than visceral artery pseudoaneurysms.

SPLENIC ARTERY ANEURYSMS These are the most common visceral artery aneurysms and are often located near the splenic hilum and involve vessel bifurcations.[15] The methods of embolization discussed earlier for pseudoaneurysms are the same:

1. Exclusion of the aneurysm from the circulation requires embolization of both branch vessels beyond the sac and then occlusion of the parent vessel. Because of the usual proximity of these aneurysms to the splenic hilum, some end-organ infarction is almost inevitable when this technique is used, but the amount of splenic substance that will be lost depends on the anatomy.
2. Filling the sac with coils or other embolic agents is much less likely to cause expansion or rupture of the aneurysm because, unlike pseudoaneurysms, the sac has a containing wall. It is difficult in many cases, however, to achieve complete aneurysm thrombosis because turbulent flow at the diseased vessel bifurcation is likely to maintain sac patency. Liquid polymers injected into the aneurysm during protection of the main vessel lumen and distal branches by a balloon inflated across its neck may provide a more successful, permanent method of treatment in certain situations (see Renal Artery Aneurysms, next).

For these reasons, surgery may be preferred in some individuals for distal splenic artery aneurysms that fulfill the criteria for treatment.[16]

RENAL ARTERY ANEURYSMS Like splenic artery aneurysms, those involving the renal artery often involve bifurcations. Embolization on either side of the aneurysm neck is rarely an option because it will cause a varying degree of renal parenchymal infarction. In patients in whom treatment is required, surgery is often preferred.[6,17] There have been a number of case reports, however, of successful treatment by embolization, which is usually performed by packing the aneurysm sac with coils or other embolic material.[18-20] There is often a problem in achieving complete sac thrombosis with coils, for the same reasons discussed earlier when treating true aneurysms of the distal splenic artery, but some success has been achieved with liquid polymers injected into the aneurysmal cavity during temporary inflation of a balloon across its neck to avoid migration of the embolic material into the distal renal vessels.[21,22] A similar technique involving balloon protection may be used when packing with coils.[23]

OTHER VISCERAL VESSELS True aneurysms involving other visceral vessels are exceptionally uncommon, but when they do occur, treatment can often be performed with endovascular techniques. The method of treatment, whether it be by parent vessel occlusion, use of a covered stent, or packing the sac with or without a covering bare stent, will depend on the anatomy of each individual aneurysm.

CONTROVERSIES

Although some authors are enthusiastic about the use of thrombin to treat visceral artery pseudoaneurysms, there are several important points to consider before recommending this technique as a first-line procedure:
1. Complete exclusion of the pseudoaneurysm from the circulation by distal and proximal vessel occlusion with coils has a proven track record and, if performed correctly, will result in complete sac thrombosis and prevention of hemorrhage in all cases.
2. The reason why thrombin injection works so well for postcatheterization femoral artery pseudoaneurysms is that there is generally a small vascular injury to an

otherwise normal and straight vessel. Arterial injury in a visceral artery pseudoaneurysm secondary to pancreatitis, for example, may be much larger. This not only increases the likelihood of sac reperfusion but also enhances the risk for spillage of thrombin into the parent vessel and end-organ infarction. End-organ damage is probably more likely to occur when the pseudoaneurysm arises from a small vessel because a lesser amount of spilled thrombin would be required to produce normal vessel thrombosis (see Figs. 73-1, D and 73-3, C). The tortuosity of visceral vessels—in particular, the splenic artery—also increases the risk of sac reperfusion secondary to turbulent flow across the pseudoaneurysm neck.
3. If sac recanalization were to occur, the patient would be at the same risk for hemorrhage (which may be life threatening) as before attempted treatment.
4. Because sac recanalization can occur after thrombin injection, regular inpatient follow-up in the days following this form of therapy is essential to confirm that sac thrombosis is maintained. The length of time follow-up should continue and the frequency at which it should occur vary between individuals but will obviously have implications on both inpatient stay and cost of investigations.

For these reasons, thrombin injection for visceral artery pseudoaneurysms should be reserved for unusual cases in which definitive treatment by embolization is not possible, such as unfavorable anatomy precluding complete exclusion of the pseudoaneurysm or the necessity for maintenance of patency of the injured vessel.

COMPLICATIONS

Complications after embolization of visceral artery aneurysmal disease are infrequent.

Partial or Complete Splenic Infarction

Infarction becomes increasingly more likely the closer the pathology to the splenic hilum (Fig. 73-5). Complete occlusion of the proximal splenic artery rarely results in infarction because of the presence of an excellent collateral supply via vessels such as the left gastric, right gastroepiploic, and dorsal pancreatic arteries. Embolization of a splenic branch close to the splenic hilum, however, is likely to result in a segmental splenic infarct. Complete infarction of the spleen may necessitate surgical splenectomy.

Pancreatitis

Pancreatitis is uncommon but may result from occlusion of short pancreatic artery branches during splenic artery embolization.

Hepatic Ischemia/Infarction

Complete occlusion of the common or proper hepatic artery is likely to cause some derangement in liver function test results for a few days, but is very unlikely to result in permanent liver damage unless the portal venous supply is also compromised, as it may occasionally be in severe liver trauma.

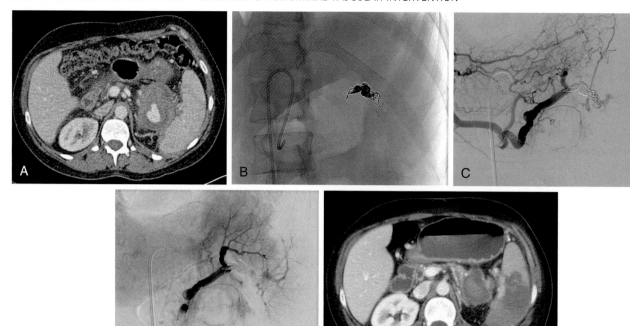

FIGURE 73-5. Splenic artery pseudoaneurysm close to splenic hilum in a patient with acute pancreatitis; embolization was complicated by partial splenic infarction. **A,** Axial computed tomography (CT) demonstrates large pseudoaneurysm close to splenic hilum. **B,** Control film after embolization shows metallic coils packed within distal splenic artery. **C,** Celiac axis angiogram after embolization demonstrates occlusion of splenic artery and early reconstitution of splenic artery branches beyond embolization coils by multiple collaterals arising from left gastric artery. **D,** Later image from same angiogram demonstrates better filling of distal splenic artery branches. **E,** Axial CT performed several days after embolization demonstrates partial splenic infarction despite good collateral supply to spleen seen on postembolization angiogram. High-density thrombus is present in embolized pseudoaneurysm.

Stomach, Duodenal, or Small Intestinal Infarction

Because of the rich collateral supply to the bowel, such infarction is extremely unusual but is more likely to occur in patients after previous surgery or embolization, or in those with severe visceral artery atheromatous disease.

Contrast Medium–Related Complications

As with any procedure that involves the use of iodinated contrast medium, there is a risk of renal impairment, which is obviously greater in individuals who are unwell, dehydrated, or septic.

POSTPROCEDURAL AND FOLLOW-UP CARE

Follow-up after the procedure depends on the method of endovascular treatment and the underlying pathology. Visceral artery pseudoaneurysms that have been treated by coil embolization on either side of the arterial defect and in which sac exclusion was documented at the time of angiography do not generally require routine imaging follow-up. It is common, however, for some form of cross-sectional imaging to be performed because of the underlying disease process (e.g., pancreatitis) and for confirmation of pseudoaneurysm thrombosis. As discussed earlier, however, early and repeated follow-up imaging of pseudoaneurysms treated by percutaneous thrombin injection will be

necessary until the chance of recanalization is thought to be very small.

True aneurysms that have been treated by embolization are more likely to require longer-term imaging follow-up, but again, this will depend on the endovascular technique that was used. In patients in whom the sac was packed with coils to preserve patency of the parent vessel, regular cross-sectional imaging, usually with ultrasound or CT, will normally be required to confirm that the size of the aneurysm remains stable. Patients with true aneurysms that have completely thrombosed, with a decrease in sac size, can be safely discharged from further follow-up.

KEY POINTS

- Visceral artery pseudoaneurysms are at high risk of rupture and always require treatment regardless of size.

- True visceral artery aneurysms are rare, and the majority are incidental findings on cross-sectional imaging and do not require treatment.

- True aneurysms measuring 2.0 cm in diameter or larger in women of childbearing age who are not pregnant and in patients of either gender undergoing liver transplantation require treatment.

- Embolization is the procedure of first choice for the treatment of visceral artery pseudoaneurysms, and the majority will be successfully managed in this manner.

► **SUGGESTED READINGS**

Mendelson RM, Anderson J, Marshall M, Ramsay D. Vascular complications of pancreatitis. Aust N Z J Surg 2005;75:1073–9.

Pilleul F, Beuf O. Diagnosis of splanchnic artery aneurysms and pseudoaneurysms, with special reference to contrast enhanced 3D magnetic resonance angiography: a review. Acta Radiol 2004;45: 702–8.

The complete reference list is available online at www.expertconsult.com.

CHAPTER 74

Intraarterial Ports for Chemotherapy

Thierry de Baère, Ernst-Peter Strecker, and Irene Boos

Radiologically guided implantation of port catheter systems (also known as *portacaths*) has become an accepted method for long-term venous access, with procedure success being as good as or better than ports implanted by open surgery. Because of improved materials, equipment, and technical skills, catheter placement is more accurate when performed by interventional radiologists under fluoroscopy combined with angiography than in the surgical suite, and detecting anatomic variants in vascular anatomy can be considered better under fluoroscopy and angiography.

Also, intraarterial infusion therapy can be performed easily and safely using a port catheter system. Ports with long-term indwelling catheters have a low rate of thrombotic and infectious complications and offer more comfort for the patient, good cosmetic results, and lower costs when compared with repeated arterial catheterization. Port catheter systems have proven to be safe and efficient for local chemotherapy arterial access, with the main applications described here for liver tumors and intrapelvic gynecologic cancer.

Regional Chemotherapy for Liver Tumors

Thierry de Baère

INDICATIONS

Because intraarterial hepatic chemotherapy (IAHC) is a local treatment, it is used in cases of liver metastases without or with very limited extrahepatic disease. It is often used as a rescue after failure of intravenous (IV) therapies for metastases, and provides a high response rate even using drugs that were or became inefficient with IV administration. Because it is highly efficient, IAHC might also be used as inductive therapy in chemo-naive patients with nearly resectable liver metastases. In such settings, the goal is to obtain the highest tumor response possible as early as possible in the disease to downstage a nonsurgical candidate to a surgical candidate. Indeed, it has been demonstrated that the increase in response rate of colorectal liver metastases (CRLM) to treatment is linearly correlated with an increase in resection rate, and consequently with an increased chance of cure.[1]

For primary tumors, particularly hepatocellular carcinoma (HCC), IAHC is less used owing to the high efficacy of transarterial chemoembolization (TACE). Consequently, this chapter will deal only with colorectal cancer liver metastases.

CONTRAINDICATIONS

Obviously, the hepatic artery must be patent to allow for IAHC, so occlusion or severe stenosis of this artery are contraindications. In the same manner, retrograde flow due to severe stenosis of the celiac trunk does not allow for the standard technique of port catheter placement. The artery chosen for access (femoral or axillary) must be patent and free of any stenosis or severe atherosclerotic disease to avoid thrombosis after insertion of the indwelling catheter. Because material will be implanted, the patient must not have local or generalized sepsis before catheter placement, or complications of sepsis may occur. Patency of the portal system is not mandatory, but one should be aware that if the indwelling catheter induces hepatic artery thrombosis, there is a risk of hepatic necrosis. In the era of targeted therapy, particularly extensive use of bevacizumab in colorectal cancer, one must know that this drug might affect bleeding and scarring processes. A time window without bevacizumab is thus recommended to allow for IAHC port catheter placement. We usually do not deliver bevacizumab within 15 days after port implantation.

EQUIPMENT

Standard Implantation

- 5F catheter and guidewire for visceral angiography
- *To avoid blood leak after indwelling catheter insertion, introducer sheath must not be used.*
- Microcatheter (2.4F) plus 0.016-inch guidewire
- Microcoils (0.018 inch; 2/5 mm to 4/8 mm in diameter)
- Exchange stiff 0.018-inch guidewire (Muso [Terumo Medical Corp., Somerset, N.J.] or V18 [Boston Scientific, Natick, Mass.])
- Indwelling catheter tapered from 5F to 2.7F, with a side hole (ST-305C, [B. Braun Medical, Center Valley, Pa.]). The kit has a subcutaneous port.

TECHNIQUE

Until recently, the unique route of catheter insertion was by laparotomy with retrograde cannulation of the gastroduodenal artery (GDA). The most often described access route for percutaneous technique is the axillary or femoral artery, with a port positioned on the chest wall or lower abdominal wall.[2-4] We prefer the femoral route for implantation because this access is always necessary for flow remodeling, which is always needed as a first step before indwelling catheter insertion. Flow remodeling is needed to infuse chemotherapy in the complete liver, and only in the liver, through a single artery. *Single artery* means that replaced hepatic arteries, if present, must be occluded proximally with stainless steel coils to maintain a patent single artery for indwelling catheter insertion (Fig. 74-1, *A-C*). In the case of replaced hepatic arteries, the hepatic artery that will be kept patent and selected for indwelling catheter insertion will be the one that bears the GDA or the largest one (Fig. 74-1, *D* and *E*). Infusion of drug *only in the liver* means that every single artery arising from the hepatic

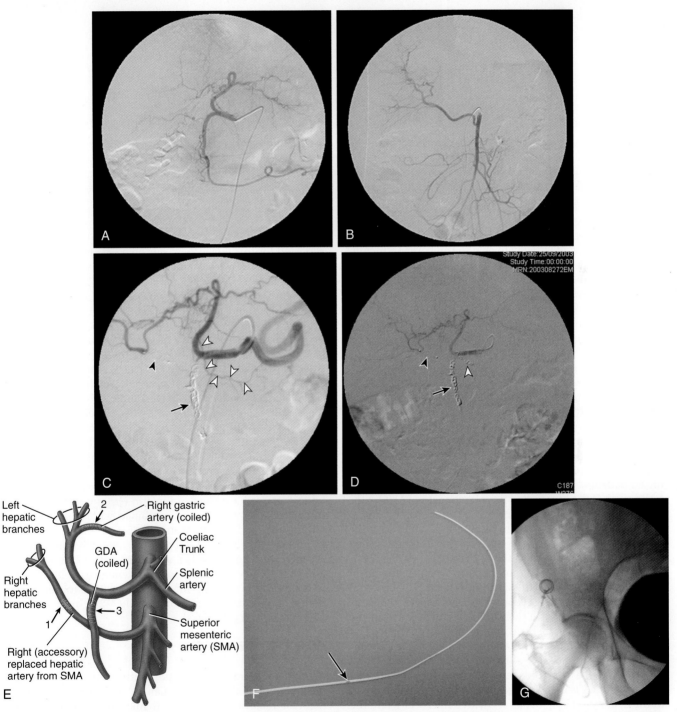

FIGURE 74-1. **A,** Angiogram obtained in main hepatic artery shows vascularization of left lobe of liver. **B,** Angiogram in superior mesenteric artery (SMA) shows a replaced right hepatic artery from SMA feeding right lobe of liver. **C,** Angiogram obtained after occlusion of replaced right hepatic artery *(black arrowhead)* shows vascularization of complete liver through main hepatic artery. The gastroduodenal artery (GDA) has been occluded with coils *(black arrow),* but right gastric artery (RGA) is still patent *(white arrowheads).* **D,** Final angiogram obtained through side hole of implanted catheter shows replaced right hepatic artery *(black arrowhead)* and GDA *(black arrow),* which are occluded. Coils can be seen in RGA *(white arrowhead).* **E,** Schematic drawing of **D** shows coils in replaced right hepatic artery *(arrow 1),* in RGA *(arrow 2),* and in GDA *(arrow 3).* Chemotherapeutic drug is flowing through side hole of catheter in hepatic artery. **F,** Catheter side hole *(black arrow)* is seen 20 cm from distal tip. Catheter will be shortened before insertion to have side hole 7 cm from tip. **G,** Plain film of port inserted inside anterior iliac crest.

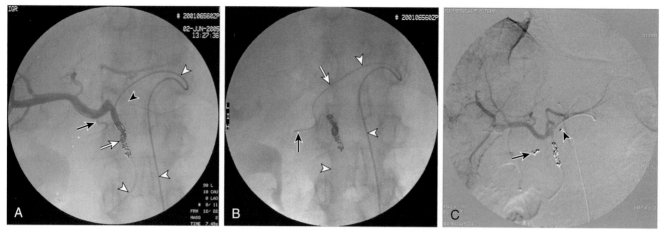

FIGURE 74-2. **A,** Angiogram obtained through side hole of catheter *(white arrowheads)* implanted in gastroduodenal artery, which has been coiled *(white arrow)*, shows patent right gastric *(black arrowhead)* and supraduodenal *(black arrow)* arteries. **B,** Microcatheter tip *(black arrow)* is in supraduodenal artery and has been introduced through side hole *(white arrow)* of implanted catheter *(white arrowheads)*, which is barely seen. **C,** Final angiogram obtained through side hole of implanted catheter shows opacification of liver arteries and coils in supraduodenal *(arrow)* and right gastric *(arrowhead)* arteries.

artery downstream of the infusion hole in the catheter must be occluded to avoid infusion to neighboring organs, including the stomach, duodenum or pancreas. In clinical practice, the GDA and right gastric artery (RGA) are the arteries that nearly always require an endovascular occlusion because it is rarely possible to place the perfusion hole of the catheter downstream of them (see Fig 74-1, *D*). The absence of reported toxic effects on the gallbladder make it unnecessary to systematically occlude its feeding vessels, but a very large cystic artery should probably be occluded. Indeed, even though cholecystectomy has been described as a necessary step in preventing cholecystitis secondary to drug diffusion to the gallbladder through the cystic artery at the time of surgical catheter placement, it is worth emphasizing that *no* cholecystitis has been reported in four series that studied over 250 patients with percutaneously implanted port catheters, including only 11 cholecystectomized patients.[2,4-6]

Because of the high risk of tip migration, the IAHC catheter must not be placed floating in the hepatic artery lumen. The indwelling catheter has to be inserted deeply into the GDA to provide stability of tip location. This indwelling catheter has a side hole that allows drug delivery (Fig. 74-1, *F*); it is placed in the common hepatic artery upstream of the arising of the GDA.[6] The side hole is located 20 cm from the tip when the catheter is provided, and usually the catheter is shortened to have the side hole 7 to 8 cm from the tip as a compromise between pushability over the wire at time of insertion and stability after placement of the indwelling catheter. In practice, after the initial angiogram and occlusion of the replaced hepatic artery (if present) and RGA, the GDA is catheterized as distally as possible down to the distal right epiploic artery with a microcatheter. The microcatheter is fed with a 0.018-inch stiff exchange wire that will be used to insert the indwelling catheter. To increase pushability of the indwelling catheter over the 0.018-inch exchange wire, the microcatheter can be placed inside the indwelling catheter over the wire. The GDA will then be occluded around the indwelling catheter, using the side hole of the indwelling catheter to insert a microcatheter that will allow occlusion of the GDA with 0.018-inch

coils. Although the use of cyanoacrylate glue has been reported for this purpose, in our own experience, we never use glue because we have found coils much safer than liquid embolic in the GDA. The goal of coil/glue occlusion of the proximal GDA is to provide both fixation of the catheter and occlusion of the GDA (see Fig. 74-1, *D* and *E*).

When the GDA cannot be catheterized, does not exist, or has been ligated, the tip of the indwelling catheter can be placed in a peripheral branch of the hepatic artery, and the side hole is left in the hepatic artery. After angiographic control of the correct location of the catheter, providing complete and unique liver perfusion (Fig. 74-2), the catheter is tunnelized and linked to a port placed either on the chest wall or the pelvic wall, according to access route. Catheter maintenance means flushing with heparin solution (5000 units/10 mL) after completion of chemotherapy until the next course.

In our experience treating liver metastases from colorectal cancer, we have used oxaliplatin (100 mg/m^2) delivered intraarterially over 2 hours combined with IV folinic acid (40 mg/m^2) and a 5-fluorouracil (5-FU) bolus at day 1, extended with 5-FU (1200 mg/m^2) over 48 hours. More recently we reported IAHC with oxaliplatin (100 mg/m^2 in 2 hours) plus IV 5-FU–leucovorin (leucovorin, 400 mg/m^2 in 2 hours; FU, 400 mg/m^2 bolus then 2400 mg/m^2 in 46 hours), and cetuximab (400 mg/m^2 then 250 mg/m^2/wk, or 500 mg/m^2 every 2 weeks).

CONTROVERSIES

Using the femoral artery for port catheter insertion is technically more challenging but can be achieved nowadays in the vast majority of patients thanks to improvements in catheter and materials designs. Femoral access will most often be needed for endovascular flow remodeling, even if the indwelling catheter is inserted through the axillary route. Since the first report of percutaneous port implantation for IAHC by Arai et al.[7] in 1982, the axillary route has been much more used than the femoral route. It is preferred because it allows easier insertion of the catheter into the hepatic artery, which usually has a descending orientation in the initial part of the celiac trunk. One thus avoids the sharp angulation encountered when using femoral access. The main disadvantage of the axillary route is a higher rate of overall and severe complications, including up to 3% of aneurysms requiring arterial stents for treatment. It may also induce axillary artery thrombosis[4] and a 0.5% to 1% rate of stroke.[2,3,8] Aneurysms are caused by the difficulty of accessing and manually compressing the axillary artery. This leads some teams to access the axillary artery by surgical exposure and cutdown of a small branch, such as the thoracoacromial artery.[3] Strokes occur when the body of the catheter lies in front of the origin of the left vertebral artery. For some authors, the retrieval or exchange of such catheters is risky enough to make them recommend that such a maneuver be performed through a femoral access if possible.[3]

OUTCOMES

The technical success rate of catheter insertions is very high in our experience and close to 100% in most series, including the largest recently reported one.[3,9] Even if it is more time consuming, the catheter-blocking technique must be preferred to free-floating catheters; the risk of tip dislodgement is reported to be over 20% with a free-floating catheter in the hepatic artery.[10] The largest series of percutaneous catheter implantations reported patency rates of 91%, 81%, and 58%, respectively, at 6 months, 1 year, and 2 years, allowing 3 to 102 courses of chemotherapy (mean = 35).[3]

A study comparing percutaneously and surgically placed port catheters reported the same rate of complications, with significantly shorter hospital stay and lower analgesic requirements for the percutaneous group (1.8 ± 0.7 days and 2 ± 0.9 doses) versus the surgical group (8.2 ± 22 days and 9.7 ± 3.2 doses).[5] We recently compared percutaneous and surgical insertion of port catheters for IAHC and demonstrated that the success rates of implantation were 97% (65/67) for percutaneous placement and 98% (58/59) for surgical implantation.[6] Among 107 patients, primary functionality was not different for percutaneous placement (n = 4.80 courses) versus surgical implantation (n = 4.82 courses), but functionality after revision was significantly higher for percutaneous versus surgical placement (9.18 vs. 5.95 courses, $P = 0.004$). This increased secondary functionality is due to easier revision of percutaneously placed ports versus surgical ones. The rates of discontinuation of IAHC linked to complications of the port catheters were 21% for percutaneous and 34% for surgical implantation.[6] Overall, the rate of reintervention to maintain patency of the port catheter system varies from 20% to 30% according to reports. The reinterventions are most often due to gastric pain and the need for embolization of a previously nonoccluded RGA or occlusion of a collateral vessel to an occluded right gastric. The main complication of IAHC through percutaneous implanted ports is gastric ulceration occurring in patients in whom the RGA could not be occluded.

We reported that intraarterial oxaliplatin and systemic 5-FU resulted in an objective response rate of 64% in colorectal cancer metastases that developed in chemonaive patients, and 45% in patients resistant to IV oxaliplatin or irinotecan.[11,12] The dramatic incidence and amplitude of response after intraarterial oxaliplatin led us to operate on 20% of initially unresectable patients by combining radiofrequency ablation and hepatectomy.[12] Nevertheless, IAHC greatly affects liver function, reflected by impaired indocyanine green clearance, with rates up to 60% at 15 minutes. Interrupting IAHC allows a progressive normalization of this clearance within 2 to 4 months. Additionally, the macroscopic and microscopic aspects of the liver parenchyma are greatly modified, with infraclinical sclerosing cholangitis, central vein fibrosis, and moderate hepatocellular necrosis or cholestasis in the centrolobular area.[13]

More recent IAHC regimens have combined IV chemotherapy and even targeted therapies to provide very impressive results. Recently, 49 patients with unresectable CRLM (53% previously treated with chemotherapy) received IAH floxuridine and dexamethasone plus systemic chemotherapy with oxaliplatin and irinotecan.[14] In this study, more than five CRLMs were present in 73% of patients; 98% had bilobar disease, and 86% had six or more segments involved. Of the 49 patients, 92% had complete (8%) or partial (84%) response, and 47% (23/49) were able to undergo resection in a group of patients with extensive disease. For chemotherapy-naive and previously treated patients, the median survival from the start of IAH therapy was 50.8 and 35 months, respectively. In our center, we treated 36 patients with extensive nonresectable CRLM (≥4 LM in 86%; bilobar LM in 91%) using IAHC with oxaliplatin (100 mg/m² in 2 hours) plus IV 5-FU–leucovorin (leucovorin, 400 mg/m² in 2 hours; FU, 400 mg/m² bolus then 2400 mg/m² in 46 hours), and cetuximab (400 mg/m² then 250 mg/m²/wk, or 500 mg/m² every 2 weeks) as first-line treatment.[15] Overall response rate was 90% (95% confidence interval [CI], 70-99), disease control rate was 100% (95% CI, 84-100), and 48% of patients were downstaged enough to undergo R0 resection and/or radiofrequency ablation. After a median follow-up of 11 months, median progression-free survival (PFS) was 20 months (median overall survival [OS] not reached; 12- and 18-month OS, 100%).

COMPLICATIONS

Catheter tip dislodgement is reported in more than 20% of catheters that have been left free-floating in the hepatic artery,[10] and such technique must be avoided. Thrombosis of the hepatic artery is rare and seems to be related to the size of the indwelling catheter (e.g., when catheters > 5F are placed in the hepatic artery). Some authors have reported that free-floating catheters are more prone to induce thrombosis due to the moving tip, which can damage the arterial wall.

The most frequent and severe complications of IAHC are related to extrahepatic perfusion of the anticancer drug, including gastric ulceration occurring in patients in whom the RGA could not be occluded. Indeed, a rate of 36% of acute gastric mucosal lesions has been reported in patients undergoing IAHC without embolization of the RGA, but this rate decreased to 3% in patients with an embolized right gastric artery.[16] We have had the same experience without and with RGA embolization—30% and 5% ($P = 0.019$) rates of ulceration, respectively. It is worth noting that success rates with RGA embolization significantly improved from 17% among the first 23 patients to 66% (n = 16) among the last 24 ($P = 0.0006$) because of the learning curve of the interventional radiologist.[9] When comparing surgical placement and percutaneous implantation for gastroduodenal misperfusion, Aldrighetti et al. reported 7.1% in the percutaneous group and 17.8% in the surgical group,[5] while we reported the reverse, with 35% in the percutaneous group and 9% in the surgical group.

POSTPROCEDURE FOLLOW-UP

Postprocedure follow-up includes clinical examination of the lower limb when femoral access has been used. Femoral thrombosis is rare but must be detected early. Some authors systematically used aspirin or clopidogrel in patients with implanted arterial ports. Hemorrhage at the puncture site is also rare so long as the diagnostic catheter used for placement is the same size as the implanted catheter, and no sheath has been used during the procedure. The port and the catheter itself are flushed with heparin after placement and every chemotherapy perfusion in order to avoid thrombosis of the system. Catheter patency is checked with digital subtraction angiography (DSA) imaging before chemotherapy perfusion. During this pre-chemotherapy testing, DSA is used to verify that the catheter is *only* perfusing the liver and no extrahepatic structures such as the stomach, pancreas, or duodenum. If an extrahepatic branch is found, it must be embolized through a contralateral femoral access.

CLINICAL RELEVANCE

Nonresectable hepatic metastases and primary liver cancers can be cured in only a few patients. Some 60% of colorectal cancer patients will present with liver metastases, and only 20% of them will undergo a surgical resection, which is the only curative treatment available. Median survival of patients with CRLM is 10 to 14 months when treated with 5-FU and leucovorin[16] and up to 16.2 and 14.8 months, respectively, when adding oxaliplatin or irinotecan,[17] and even a slight improvement when combined with epidermal growth factor receptor (EGFR) and vascular endothelial growth factor (VEGF) inhibitors.

Regional chemotherapeutic techniques have the primary advantage of increasing drug concentrations in tumor deposits. Most of them display a steep dose/response curve, resulting in a significant increase in response rates. If the classical results of intraarterial liver chemotherapy are rather disappointing, recent chemotherapeutic regimens allow hope that a new era is beginning for this regional approach.

The rationale for IAHC is that the liver has a dual blood supply. Liver metastases are perfused almost exclusively by the hepatic artery, whereas the normal liver derives most of its blood supply from the portal vein and little from the hepatic artery. Furthermore, in 30% of patients, the liver is the only site of metastatic disease. Some drugs undergo hepatic extraction, resulting in high local concentrations with minimal systemic toxicity. This is especially true for fluoropyrimidines and floxuridine (FUDR). FUDR has been extensively used intraarterially because it is extracted by the liver at more than 95% during the first pass. The estimated increase in liver exposure by IAHC for cisplatin is four to sevenfold compared to IV perfusion. IAHC could also allow delivery of a larger dose of drugs. This is particularly interesting for drugs with a steep dose/response curve. Finally, IAHC could decrease the toxicity of drugs by means of a high total body clearance and good liver extraction, resulting in a better efficacy/toxicity ratio.

KEY POINTS

- Intraarterial hepatic chemotherapy (IAHC) through a percutaneous implanted port is highly feasible.
- Accessory hepatic arteries (if present) must be occluded.
- Extrahepatic branches arising from the hepatic artery must be occluded.
- Response rate of intraarterial oxaliplatin is around 40% in patients not responding to intravenous oxaliplatin and around 90% in chemo-naive patients.

Locoregional Chemotherapy for Gynecologic Pelvic Cancer

Ernst-Peter Strecker and Irene Boos

Transcatheter arterial chemotherapy is not a standard treatment, but one of the treatment options for gynecologic cancer (e.g., uterine, cervical, or endometrial carcinoma). With local intraarterial chemotherapy (IAC), a high drug concentration can be achieved in the region infused and in the tumor tissue,[18,19] and thus total drug dosage and the possible incidence of systemic toxic effects or other side effects can be reduced. New concepts combine IAC chemotherapy with intravenous (IV) chemotherapy[20] because locally advanced carcinoma, suitable for IAC, is a potentially systemic disease.

Intraarterial regional chemotherapy is not a new method, but it has never gained widespread use. Because results from clinical comparative studies are lacking, this kind of therapy is not being recognized for inclusion in current therapy guidelines, even though surprisingly good results can be observed in some cases. Given the good results obtained in other anatomic regions (e.g., locally advanced breast cancer),[21] IAC in general should be reevaluated.[22]

INDICATIONS

Port implantation for IAC is useful as a means for repeated intraarterial access, which is necessary when several cycles of chemotherapy are planned and/or one chemotherapy cycle lasts for several days. Thus, complex procedures with repeated arterial puncture and repeated selective catheter placements can be avoided, as well as long-term indwelling external catheters. Clinical indications for IAC follow those for IV chemotherapy.

Chemotherapy in general is efficacious in squamous cell carcinoma and in adenocarcinoma of the uterine cervix,[23] but a curative effect is proven only for combined radiochemotherapy, which simultaneously combines intracavitary and percutaneous radiotherapy with cisplatin as a radiosensitizer. As a primary therapy, radiochemotherapy has a better outcome than radiotherapy alone, and the long-term outcome in patients with stage IB or II cervical carcinoma is comparable to that of primary surgery, but with different types of side effects.

Because postsurgical adjuvant radiotherapy alone is not efficacious in terms of local recurrence and intrapelvic or extrapelvic progression in all patients, combined radio-chemotherapy is recommended when there is no contraindication for cisplatin, especially in patients with special risk factors such as involvement of lymphovascular tissue, lymphangiosis, large tumor, parametrial invasion, or remaining tumor tissue after surgical resection. Disease-free survival time can be improved significantly by adjuvant radiochemotherapy when compared with radiotherapy alone.

Chemotherapy is efficacious as neoadjuvant therapy for locally advanced cervical cancer that is considered inoperable, including stage IIB bulky cervical carcinoma and stage III-IV malignancies, and as a presurgical or pre-radiotherapeutic procedure applied for downstaging. However, the results of clinical studies are contradictory in terms of survival time and risk of local recurrence.[24]

Chemotherapy is indicated as a palliative procedure in advanced, metastatic, or recurrent cervical carcinoma that is considered inoperable and in which radiation therapy is not possible or expected to show poor results, as well as in patients with distant metastases. However, efficacy of chemotherapy is reduced in previously radiated tissue.

For endometrial cancer, chemotherapy plays a less important role because surgical tumor resection and radiation therapy are the more efficacious options. The effects of adjuvant systemic chemotherapy are not promising in general and do not justify an indication. At the present time, an eventual exception is discussed for cases of serosal papillary adenocarcinoma, which has a poor prognosis even in low-stage disease. However, this indication has not been proven so far, and at present remains a point of discussion while results of further clinical studies are evaluated. Recent studies suggest, however, that adjuvant chemotherapy may be superior to percutaneous abdominal radiotherapy in patients with successfully resected stage III or IV endometrial carcinoma, including those with high-risk features.

Chemotherapy eventually combined with radiotherapy may be indicated when local tumor recurrence or metastases cannot be treated surgically or with radiotherapy and the patient is clinically ill.

Chemotherapy also is an option for patients who suffer from tumor progression under systemic endocrine therapy, with the latter being the favored systemic treatment for palliation of recurrent, metastatic, or high-risk endometrial carcinoma.[25]

CONTRAINDICATIONS

Apart from the contraindications for chemotherapy in general, contraindications for IAC are:
- Patient has signs of local or systemic infection or coagulopathic disease.
- Access vessel or target vessel is not suitable for catheterization (e.g., high-grade stenosis or occlusion of common femoral artery or iliac arteries or aorta, which, however, is rare in this group of patients).
- Patient is in a condition not suited for antiplatelet or antithrombotic medication, which is necessary to prevent catheter or arterial thrombosis.
- Patient has a known intolerance to individual components of the port catheter system, such as titanium, silicone, or another material.

EQUIPMENT

Optimal conditions for performing this procedure are present in the angiographic suite, which is equipped with laminar air flow. When there is no possibility of air filtration, the air conditioning system should be turned off during the intervention. As for any minor surgical intervention, sterile material is required, and the intervention has to be performed under aseptic conditions. For implantation of materials into the patient's body, the requirements for aseptic conditions and sterility are much stronger than for simple angiography.

Specific materials needed include:
- Seldinger needle
- Guidewire, 0.035-inch or other size according to the inner lumen of the indwelling catheter
- Permanently indwelling catheter to be combined with subcutaneous port chamber. Useful catheter characteristics include radiopacity, good visibility under fluoroscopy, pliability, nonthrombogenic properties, and being made of a material that is compliant with the eventually aggressive drugs to be infused. We use a low-profile titanium port system (T-Port Low Profile, PFM, Germany) that comprises a port chamber, a 4.8F catheter, and a noncoring puncture needle.
- Contrast medium: standardized iodine contrast as used for angiographic procedures
- Inflatable tourniquets to be applied to the lower limbs during drug infusion, including pressure-measuring device
- Perfusor system

TECHNIQUE

Anatomy and Approaches

The patient is prepared as for conventional angiography or angiographic intervention.

Arterial Access
Commonly, a femoral arterial access is used to access the arteries feeding the gynecologic pelvic cancer. With the use of local anesthesia and via a unilateral percutaneous approach in the groin, the femoral artery is punctured using the Seldinger method. The indwelling catheter is then introduced immediately over a guidewire and advanced into the abdominal aorta. An arterial introducer sheath should *not* be used because it creates a larger arterial puncture hole that increases the risk of bleeding into the subcutaneous pocket. Orienting aortoiliac angiography of the pelvic arteries is then performed using the digital subtraction technique.

Technical Aspects

Target Vessels
To combine repeated bilateral infusion with a permanently indwelling port catheter system, bilateral ports would be necessary. To avoid bilateral ports, in our experience the infusion catheter is inserted unilaterally and then placed up into the distal abdominal aorta, thus providing the option of bilateral intraarterial infusion. With this catheter position, the primary pelvic tumor site is treated, including local

lymph node metastases within the pelvis and near the aorta. Selective catheterization of the internal iliac arteries does not appear to be advantageous. The catheter tip should be placed in the lower half of that part of the aorta extending between the renal artery ostium and aortic bifurcation. The catheter tip should not be placed in the close vicinity of a single lumbar artery or the inferior mesenteric artery to avoid toxic effects to spinal nerves or bowel. The catheter should not be placed in a straight fashion through the patient's vasculature (to avoid catheter dislodgement due to body movements) but also not too curved (to prevent catheter dislocation). Last, the catheter tip should be placed in such a manner that the chemotherapeutic agent will be distributed equally to both iliac arteries. This is confirmed by digital subtraction angiography with slow low-pressure contrast medium injection (4 mL contrast media injected within 1 second), mimicking the route the chemotherapeutic agent will take when it is administered.

Port Catheter System

After removal of the guidewire, the catheter is shortened at its outward end and connected to the port, and a subcutaneous tunnel is created, localized laterally and distally to the puncture site. Some ports require creation of only minimal subcutaneous space (e.g., with a large dilator) rather than a surgical procedure to form a large subcutaneous pocket. The patency of port and catheter are reconfirmed with contrast medium and fluoroscopy, and the port system is flushed with heparinized saline (give about 1000 units from a mixture of approximately 5000 units in 10 mL normal saline). We restrict overall use of heparin because it increases the risk of subcutaneous bleeding at the port implantation site, which would interfere with early use of the device for chemotherapy. The port is then introduced into the subcutaneous tunnel using a needle holder designated for this purpose, and the skin wound is closed thoroughly and securely by sutures. For suturing we prefer a vertical mattress stitch for secure closure of both deep and superficial skin layers. Finally a dressing is applied. Usually, compression of the arterial puncture site is not necessary because there is no bleeding. The patient is told to rest in bed for 24 hours and avoid extensive movement of the groin area during this period.

Drug Infusion

Chemotherapy is begun the day after port implantation. After local skin disinfection, the port membrane is punctured under sterile conditions with a noncoring needle. Before use of the port catheter system for drug infusion, the location of the catheter tip, patency of the system, and absence of leaks have to be checked under fluoroscopy with a small amount of contrast medium. Tourniquets are applied at both thighs and inflated to above suprasystolic blood pressure to redistribute the blood flow to the pelvic organs. The chemotherapeutic agent is administered via a perfusor system. Because infusion time may last some 6 to 7 minutes, intolerable leg pain is treated with IV administration of an analgesic agent. After termination of the infusion, we wait 1 minute before we remove the tourniquets. Within this period, owing to normal body circulation, the small pelvic organs will be supplied repeatedly with blood and chemotherapeutic agent, whereas the lower limbs are spared.

After use, the system has to be flushed with a saline-heparin mixture to remove any possible remnants of the chemotherapeutic agent and prevent occlusion or thrombosis. Flushing is also recommended during withdrawal of the needle to avoid reflux of blood or remaining drug into the catheter or port chamber, or even into the subcutaneous tissue, all of which would induce catheter damage or thrombosis, or even tissue necrosis. If more than one drug is to be administered, flushing is recommended between individual drug infusions to prevent drug interactions. To avoid damaging seals, we use a 10-mL syringe and manual injection to keep pressures below 10 atm; intrasystem pressures exceeding 15 atm can produce leaks that make further use of the system impossible because extravasation of the chemotherapeutic agent may result.

Repeated infusion is performed several times in 3- or 4-week intervals, depending on the patient's condition and the chemotherapeutic regimen. Before, during, and after infusion of chemotherapy, IV saline is infused to maintain urinary output. The chemotherapeutic regimen also includes agents for prevention of chemotherapy-related side effects.

Removal of Port System

Usually the port catheter system can be explanted easily if it is no longer needed or in case of irreversible dysfunction, inflammation, or infection of the surrounding tissue. Under local anesthesia, a small incision is made distal to the palpable puncture window, the port chamber is grasped with a forceps or a needle holder designated for this purpose, and under rotating movements, the port and catheter are eventually retrieved as a whole after local mobilization of the port chamber within the subcutaneous tissue. Bleeding from the access artery site is stopped by manual compression, the skin is sutured, and a dressing is applied.

CONTROVERSIES

Intraarterial versus Intravenous Chemotherapy

With intraarterial application of the chemotherapeutic agent, local concentration at the target site is significantly increased as compared with IV infusion. Intraarterial infusion takes advantage of the first-pass effect: cisplatin especially binds to tumor tissue at the earliest time after arterial infusion, owing to its high affinity to tissue proteins. Thus, a high local drug concentration can be achieved, and systemic toxic side effects can be significantly reduced.[26] This effect is to be postulated for other chemotherapeutic agents as well. Clinical superiority of regional IAC over systemic therapy was proven in patients with other types of malignancy such as pancreatic cancer[27]; thus this effect can also be postulated for uterine, cervical, and endometrial cancer.

Regional Drug Infusion versus Selective Infusion

Bilateral internal iliac infusion eventually combined with balloon occlusion has been suggested to improve local drug efficacy,[28] as well as selective infusion into the uterine artery. The latter may be technically difficult and time consuming, and it requires alteration of intrapelvic blood flow.[29] The

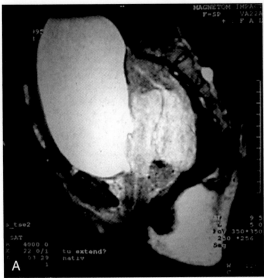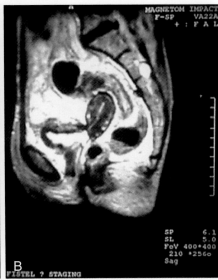

FIGURE 74-3. A, Magnetic resonance image of a 44-year-old patient with inoperable squamous cell carcinoma of uterine cervix, FIGO (International Federation of Gynecology and Obstetrics) stage IV. Status before neoadjuvant locoregional intraarterial chemotherapy via distal aorta and both iliac arteries for downstaging. **B,** Status after four cycles of intraarterial chemotherapy indicates successful downstaging. Patient now is suited for surgical resection.

infusion catheter is nearly as large as the vessel diameter, and the risk of arterial spasm, thrombosis, and arteritis is high in such small arteries. To avoid complications such as sciatic nerve palsy, coil embolization of the superior gluteal artery has to be performed.[30] There is a considerable risk that the chemotherapy drug will enter the inferior gluteal artery and induce gluteal skin necrosis.

However, both techniques are not suited in combination with a permanently indwelling port system because there is only one possible arterial target site per port system. Thus, bilateral infusion would require bilateral ports.

Selective catheterization techniques are complex but are not necessary when applying the more simple regional infusion technique described earlier, comprising less selective catheter placement in the aorta and bilateral tourniquets at both thighs.

Another advantage of regional IAC is that it reaches the primary tumor and the sites of intrapelvic extension and intrapelvic and pelvic lymph nodes. The inguinal lymph nodes especially would not be reached with more selective catheter placement. Moreover, this technique is easy to perform and less time consuming, without the need of additional interventional procedures, such as arterial occlusion by embolization.

In our experience, selective or superselective infusion is performed only rarely in cases revealing strongly unilateral tumors, such as clinically significant recurrent inoperable vulvovaginal cancer requiring palliation. In such cases, the infusion catheter may be placed superselectively in the tumor feeding the artery.

OUTCOMES

For intraarterial application in particular, neoadjuvant IAC for downstaging of pelvic gynecologic malignancy proved to be successful in up to 95% of patients with advanced cancer[31,32] and is effective in reducing tumor volume, increasing the clinical and pathologic complete response rate, and improving operability[31,33,34]; a survival benefit is suggested[35,36] (Figs. 74-3 and 74-4).

Some of our patients with locally advanced cancer presented with hydronephrosis due to tumor encasement of the ureters. In some patients, this clinical condition was reversed with reduction of intrapelvic tumor mass, which could be achieved by regional IAC.

Adjuvant chemotherapy has not thus far improved survival time in general but is a valuable adjunct when used as part of combined radiochemotherapy and for palliation when there is no other treatment option.

For intraarterial application in particular, there are no randomized studies in patients with pelvic gynecologic malignancy in whom IAC resulted in a survival benefit as compared with systemic IV chemotherapy. However, intraarterial application at least offers the option of reducing systemic toxic side effects and may play an important role in terms of quality of life in patients in whom an individual treatment regimen is mandatory.

COMPLICATIONS

Our technical success is nearly 100%. Intervention-related local complications at the femoral access site, such as subcutaneous hematoma, occur rarely. Femoral artery thrombosis or thromboembolization to runoff arteries has never been observed in our patients, who usually are in good vascular health.

Most of the complications with port catheter systems arise from a malfunctioning device and are due to catheter-related problems and infection, with an incidence of up to 0.1 event per 100 catheter-days.

Dislodgement of the catheter and catheter kinking can usually be avoided with proper implantation technique.

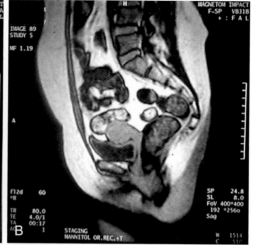

FIGURE 74-4. A, Magnetic resonance image of 42-year-old patient with advanced adenocarcinoma of uterine cervix shows inoperable cervical carcinoma, with tumor invading parametrial region, vaginal wall, and bladder. Status before neoadjuvant locoregional intraarterial chemotherapy via distal aorta and both iliac arteries for downstaging. **B,** Appearance at 5-month follow-up. Status after 5 cycles of intraarterial chemotherapy reveals successful downstaging. This enabled surgery to be performed. Resected organs no longer showed evidence of metastatic disease or regional extension of primary neoplasm. *(From Strecker EP, Heber R, Boos I, et al. Preliminary experience with locoregional intraarterial chemotherapy of uterine cervical or endometrial cancer using the Peripheral Implantable Port System [PIPS™]: a feasibility study. Cardiovasc Intervent Radiol 2003;26:118–22.)*

Catheter occlusion due to remnants of antiblastic substance or thrombosis can be treated by flushing the system, the latter combined with instillation of thrombolytic active substances. For removal of thrombus from the catheter lumen, a small amount of recombinant tissue plasminogen activator is instilled via a syringe and is moved back and forth until the catheter has reopened.

Dislocation, migration, or rotation of the port chamber within the subcutaneous tissue usually also induces kinking or dislocation of the catheter and is more likely to occur in obese patients. This situation eventually requires fixation of the chamber to the surrounding tissue by surgical sutures.

Leakage at the connection site between catheter and port chamber, or leakage of the self-sealing puncture membrane, occurs rarely but can usually be avoided with proper implantation and puncture technique and with proper handling during flushing and infusion, avoiding too-high pressures within the system.

In our experience, the incidence of thrombotic or infectious complications was 0.06 per 100 catheter-days and 0.03 per 100 catheter-days, respectively.[37]

The interventional radiologist should also be aware of complications due to the chemotherapeutic agent infused:

- General complications due to antiblastic drugs include myelosuppression leading to leukocytopenia or thrombocytopenia.
- Local complications due to chemotherapeutic drugs include local neurotoxicity and occlusion of the target vessel.
- Toxic damage to the target vessel may result. Aortitis due to chemical vasculitis of the vasa vasorum has been described in one case[38] and was due to slight displacement of the tip of a permanently indwelling catheter; this can be prevented by monitoring the catheter location before each infusion.

POSTPROCEDURAL AND FOLLOW-UP CARE

- Administer a broad-spectrum antibiotic for prophylaxis against infectious complications.
- Give aspirin, 100 mg, for 4 weeks to prevent thrombotic complications.
- Check skin wound at the port implantation site in the groin for infection.
- At long-term follow-up, check the skin at the port implantation site in the groin for infection, inflammation, thinning and atrophy, or necrosis.
- Flush port catheter system after any use.
- Perform IV hydration with infusion of saline after chemotherapy to maintain urinary output.

KEY POINTS

- Locoregional intraarterial chemotherapy should be performed as an interdisciplinary treatment regimen that includes oncologists, gynecologists, pathologists, interventional radiologists, and radiotherapists.

- Patients undergoing chemotherapy are prone to infection. Take care! Modern antibiosis is not suited to substitute for aseptic conditions during the intervention.

- To avoid complications with the port catheter system, verify correct catheter placement and proper function of the system before closing the skin after port implantation and before each use of the system for infusion of antiblastic drugs. Flush the system before use, after use, during withdrawal of the puncture needle, and in between drugs when more than one drug is to be infused. *Do not* use the port catheter system for blood withdrawal.

▶ SUGGESTED READINGS

Elias D, de Baère T, Sideris L, Ducreux M. Regional chemotherapeutic techniques for liver tumors: current knowledge and future directions. Surg Clin North Am 2004;84:607–25.

Fiorentini G, Poddie DB, Cantore M, et al. Locoregional therapy for liver metastases from colorectal cancer: the possibilities of intraarterial chemotherapy, and new hepatic-directed modalities. Hepatogastroenterology 2001;48:305–12.

Power DG, Healey-Bird BR, Kemeny NE. Regional chemotherapy for liver-limited metastatic colorectal cancer. Clin Colorectal Cancer 2008;7: 247–59.

Strecker EP, Boos I. Improved vessel access widens therapy options. Diagn Imaging Eur 1999;15(6):25–31.

The complete reference list is available online at www.expertconsult.com.

CHAPTER 75

Vascular Anatomy of the Pelvis

Elizabeth A. Ignacio, Naomi N. Silva, Nadia J. Khati, Andres Krauthamer, Venkatesh Krishnasamy, Emily J. Timmreck, Emily M. Tanksi, and Jordan Ruby

The rich vascular supply of the pelvis not only supports the structures contained within it, including the bladder, rectum, and reproductive organs, but also extends to the lower extremities. For a complete understanding of vascular anatomy as it pertains into the endovascular procedures of interventional radiology, it is useful to discuss the vascular structures in sections, from the bifurcation of the aorta and the inferior vena cava to the level of the common femoral arteries and veins. We will also review the anatomy of the iliac vessels, including their branches, common variants, and various collateral pathways (Fig. 75-1).

ARTERIES

Abdominal Aorta

The abdominal aorta terminates at the bifurcation into a right and left common iliac artery. This bifurcation is usually at the lower border of the L4 vertebral body (Fig. 75-2). On physical examination, this site corresponds to a point approximately 2.5 cm below the umbilicus, or at the level of a line drawn between the highest points of the iliac crests. Although the false pelvis (greater pelvis) has its superior border at the S1 level (first sacral vertebral body), it is important to consider the aortic bifurcation in any arterial evaluation of the pelvis (Fig. 75-3).

Aortoiliac Bifurcation

As mentioned, the aorta bifurcates into a right and left common iliac artery. These two arteries pass anterior and slightly to the left of the L5 vertebra and superior sacrum before branching into the right and left external iliac and internal iliac (hypogastric) arteries (Figs. 75-4 and 75-5; also see Fig. 75-3). The external/internal iliac bifurcation occurs above the pelvic inlet of the true pelvis (lesser pelvis).

An important pathologic process that can occur at the aortic bifurcation is an associated common iliac vein compression disorder called *May-Thurner syndrome* or *iliac compression syndrome* (Fig. 75-6). In brief, this syndrome involves compression of the right common iliac artery on the left common iliac vein against the spine and pelvic brim. This compression may clinically manifest as left lower extremity edema, pain, and/or iliofemoral deep vein thrombosis.

External Iliac Artery

The external iliac arteries (right and left) course inferiorly and laterally but remain above the pelvic inlet. The inguinal ligament, found between the two points of the anterior-superior iliac spine (Fig. 75-7) and the pubic tubercle, marks the anatomic boundary of the trunk and lower limb. At this level there are two terminal branches of the external iliac arteries: the inferior epigastric artery and the deep circumflex artery (see Fig. 75-7). These branches provide arterial supply to the inferior abdominal wall. Beyond this point, the external iliac arteries become the common femoral arteries (Fig. 75-8).

Internal Iliac Artery

The internal iliac artery and its branches constitutes the major arterial supply to the pelvic viscera, the wall, and the perineum, including the erectile tissues of the clitoris and penis as well as nerves extending into the gluteal region of the lower limb (Figs. 75-9 to 75-11). The main trunk of the internal iliac artery runs anteromedial to the sacroiliac joint before it divides into the anterior and posterior trunks just above the greater sciatic foramen (Fig 75-12; also see Fig. 75-9).

Anterior Division

The anterior trunk of the internal iliac artery usually has six major branches, three parietal and three visceral. At this level the branching pattern is subject to many anatomic variations. By the most common order of their origin, these include the umbilical artery, obturator artery (see Fig. 75-10), inferior vesical artery, middle rectal artery (see Fig. 75-10), internal pudendal artery, and inferior gluteal artery (Figs. 75-13 and 75-14). These arterial branches supply the pelvic viscera, perineum, gluteal region, adductor region of the thigh, and in the fetus, the placenta. The uterine artery (see Fig. 75-10) also generally arises from the anterior division of the internal iliac artery, but several variations in its origin have been described in the literature.

The first branch of the anterior trunk, the umbilical artery (Fig. 75-15), leaves the true pelvis and ascends to the umbilicus. In utero, this artery is large and carries blood from the fetus back to the placenta. Eventually this terminal branch involutes after birth, and its fibrous remnant is the medial umbilical ligament. Unlike the umbilical artery, the

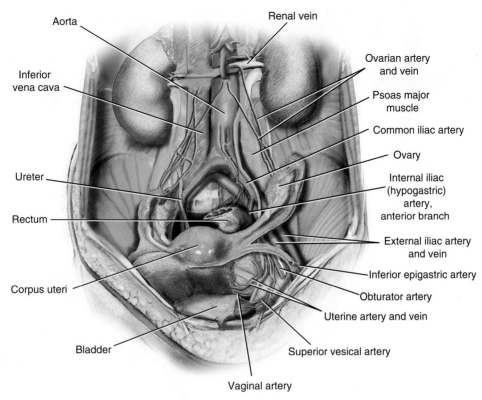

FIGURE 75-1. Blood supply of the pelvis. *(From Townsend CM, Beauchamp RW, Evers BM, Mattox KL. Sabiston textbook of surgery. 17th ed. Philadelphia: Saunders; 2004. p. 2238.)*

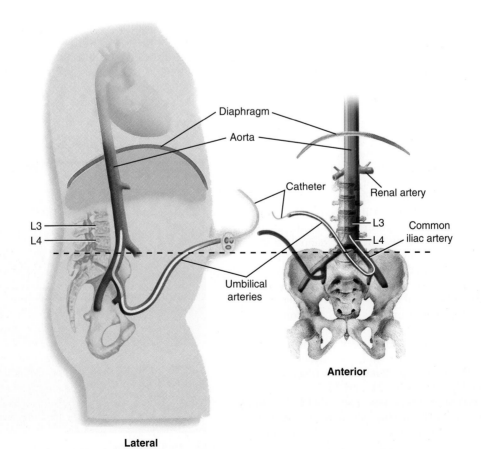

FIGURE 75-2. Lateral and anterior location of abdominal aortic bifurcation with reference to L3 and visualization of umbilical arteries and common iliac arteries. *(From Roberts J, Hedges J. Clinical procedures in emergency medicine. 4th ed. Philadelphia: Saunders; 2004. p. 379.)*

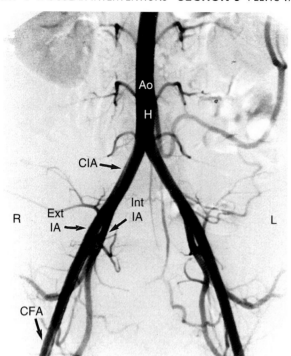

FIGURE 75-3. Digital subtraction angiogram in anteroposterior projection shows distal abdominal aorta *(Ao)* with small lumbar branches, common iliac artery *(CIA)*, internal and external iliac arteries *(Ext IA, Int IA)*, and common femoral artery *(CFA)*. *(From Mettler F, Guiberteau M. Essentials of radiology. 2nd ed. Philadelphia: Saunders; 2005. p. 379.)*

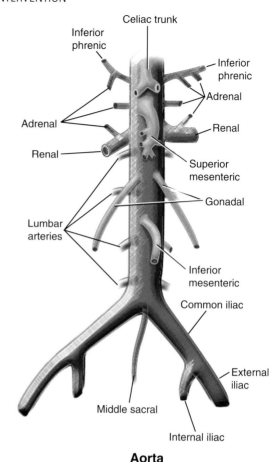

Aorta

FIGURE 75-4. Abdominal aorta with major branches, bifurcation into common iliac arteries, and their split into external and internal iliac arteries. Middle sacral artery is included. *(From Wein AJ, Kavoussi LR, Novick AC, et al., editors. Campbell's urology. 9th ed. Philadelphia: Saunders; 2007. p. 6.)*

more proximal branch, the superior vesical artery, persists and courses inferiorly and medially to bring blood to the distal segment of the ureter and the superior aspect of the bladder (see Fig. 75-15). In addition, it can provide arterial supply to the ductus deferens in men.

The obturator artery (see Figs. 75-1, 75-10, 75-13, and 75-14) is usually the second branch of the anterior trunk. It extends along the pelvic side wall and exits the true pelvis anteriorly through the obturator canal. It is the main arterial supply for the adductor muscles of the thigh.

In men, the inferior vesical artery (Fig. 75-16) is the third branch off the anterior trunk. From its anterior course it supplies the bladder, distal part of the ureter, seminal vesicle, and prostate. In women, the equivalent is the vaginal artery (see Fig. 75-15), which supplies arterial blood flow to the vagina and rectum as well as the bladder.

The fourth branch from the anterior trunk of the internal iliac artery is the middle rectal artery (Fig. 75-17; also see Figs. 75-10 and 75-13). A network of arterial anastomoses join this artery medially to supply the rectum, with contributions from both the superior rectal artery, a branch of the inferior mesenteric artery above, and the inferior rectal artery, a branch of the internal pudendal artery (Figs. 75-18 and 75-19; also see Figs. 75-13, 75-21, and 75-27).

The internal pudendal artery (see Figs. 75-13, 75-18, 75-19, 75-21, and 75-27) exits inferiorly from the true pelvis through the greater sciatic foramen inferior to the piriformis muscle. The artery travels lateral to the ischial spine and then through the lesser sciatic foramen. There, the artery enters the perineum and brings arterial flow to the erectile

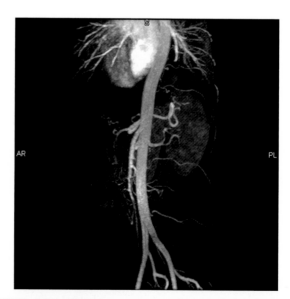

FIGURE 75-5. Magnetic resonance angiogram of abdominal aorta, oblique view. Aorta bifurcates into common iliac arteries. These two arteries pass anterior to L5 vertebral body and superior sacrum.

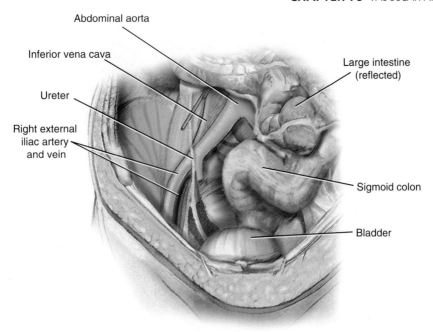

FIGURE 75-6. Anatomic visualization of abdominal aorta lying over inferior vena cava. *(From Townsend CM, Beauchamp RW, Evers BM, Mattox KL. Sabiston textbook of surgery. 17th ed. Philadelphia: Saunders; 2004. p. 2043.)*

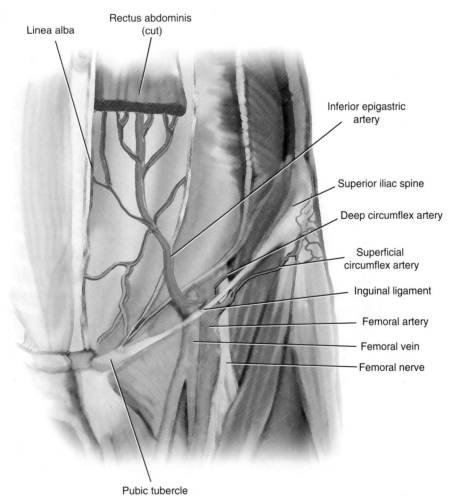

FIGURE 75-7. Visualization of inferior epigastric artery, deep circumflex artery, femoral artery, and superior iliac spine. *(From Townsend CM, Beauchamp RW, Evers BM, Mattox KL. Sabiston textbook of surgery. 17th ed. Philadelphia: Saunders; 2004. p. 1176.)*

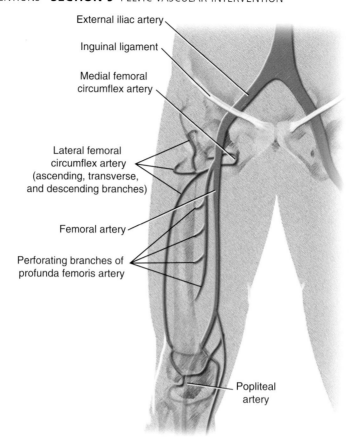

FIGURE 75-8. Visualization of external iliac artery becoming common femoral artery. *(From Marx J. Rosen's emergency medicine: concepts and clinical practice. 6th ed. St Louis: Mosby; 2006. p. 540.)*

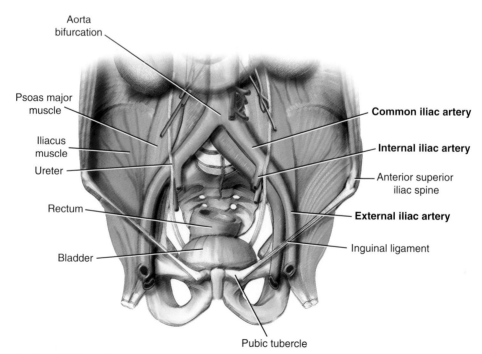

FIGURE 75-9. Anterior view of abdominal aorta splitting into common iliac arteries, and common iliac arteries splitting into internal and external iliac arteries. *(From Gabbe SG, Niebyl JR, Simpson JL. Obstetrics—normal and problem pregnancies. 4th ed. Edinburgh: Churchill Livingstone; 2002. p. 1372.)*

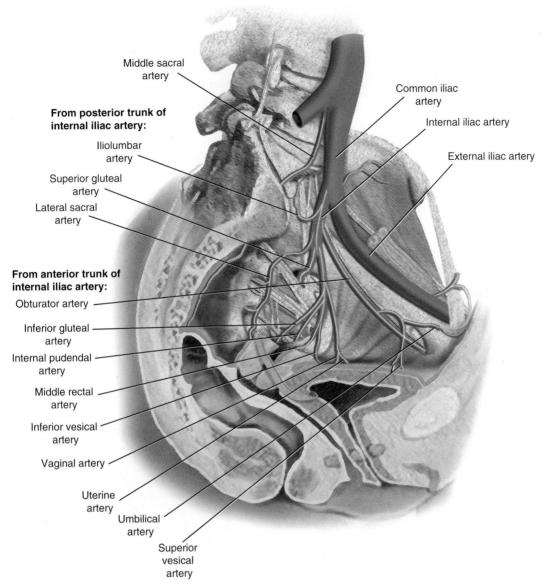

Middle sacral
artery

Common iliac
artery

Internal iliac artery

External iliac artery

**From posterior trunk of
internal iliac artery:**

Iliolumbar
artery

Superior gluteal
artery

Lateral sacral
artery

**From anterior trunk of
internal iliac artery:**

Obturator artery

Inferior gluteal
artery

Internal pudendal
artery

Middle rectal
artery

Inferior vesical
artery

Vaginal artery

Uterine
artery

Umbilical
artery

Superior
vesical
artery

FIGURE 75-10. Lateral view of common iliac artery splitting into external and internal iliac arteries and major vessels of anterior and posterior trunk of internal iliac artery. *(From Gabbe SG, Niebyl JR, Simpson JL. Obstetrics—normal and problem pregnancies. 4th ed. Edinburgh: Churchill Livingstone; 2002. p. 1373.)*

tissues of the penis and clitoris (see Figs. 75-18 and 75-19).

The terminal branch of the anterior trunk is the inferior gluteal artery (see Figs. 75-13 and 75-14). This artery courses medially between the anterior rami of S1 and S2 (or S2 and S3) and exits the true pelvis through the greater sciatic foramen inferior to the piriformis muscle. The inferior gluteal artery not only provides arterial blood to the gluteal region but also contributes to the arterial supply of the hip joint via arterial anastomoses.

Of clinical significance, the inferior gluteal artery (see Figs. 75-13 and 75-14) is the vestige of the embryonic sciatic artery. Early in utero, the sciatic artery is the primary axial artery of the lower extremity. This artery normally regresses to form the proximal inferior gluteal artery after development of the femoral artery system (see Figs. 75-7 and 75-8) from the external iliac artery. If that system fails to develop

or develops only partially, the sciatic artery persists as the dominant arterial supply to the lower extremity. A persistent sciatic artery, a rare anomaly, may be subject to aneurysm formation and produce pain and a pulsatile gluteal mass.

The uterine artery (Figs. 75-20 to 75-22; also see Fig. 75-15) frequently originates from the medial aspect of the anterior branch of the internal iliac artery. The artery takes a medial and anterior path in the base of the broad ligament of the cervix. Beyond this transverse segment, it ascends along the lateral aspect of the uterus and can anastomose with the ovarian artery (see Figs. 75-1, 75-20, and 75-22). The uterine artery is the main arterial blood supply to the uterus and also provides flow to the ovary and vagina via anastomoses (see Fig. 75-22). Some investigators have noted an origin of the uterine artery directly off the internal iliac artery. Other variations encountered include (1) the

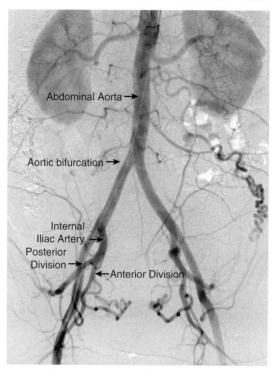

FIGURE 75-11. Aortogram. Internal iliac arteries provide major arterial supply to pelvic walls and viscera.

uterine and internal pudendal arteries sharing a common trunk (see Figs. 75-13, 75-18, 75-19, 75-21, and 75-27), (2) the uterine and vaginal arteries sharing a common trunk (see Figs. 75-10, 75-15, 75-20, and 75-21), and (3) the uterine and vesical arteries sharing a common trunk.

Posterior Division

There are three branches of the posterior trunk of the internal iliac artery: the iliolumbar artery, the lateral sacral artery (see Fig. 75-10), and the superior gluteal artery (see Fig. 75-10). These arteries contribute blood supply to the lower posterior abdominal wall, posterior pelvic wall, and gluteal region.

The iliolumbar artery (see Fig. 75-10) is the first branch of the posterior trunk; it follows a superior and posterior course and divides into a lumbar branch and an iliac branch. The lumbar branch provides arterial blood flow to the posterior abdominal wall, psoas muscle, and lumbar paraspinal muscles. The iliac branch travels along the side wall of the false pelvis into the iliac fossa and provides blood supply to the associated muscle and bone.

Typically, two lateral sacral arteries (see Figs. 75-10 and 75-14) arise from the posterior division. These arteries run medially and inferiorly and branch into the anterior sacral foramina to sustain the surrounding musculoskeletal structures and sacral canal.

Text continued on p. 538

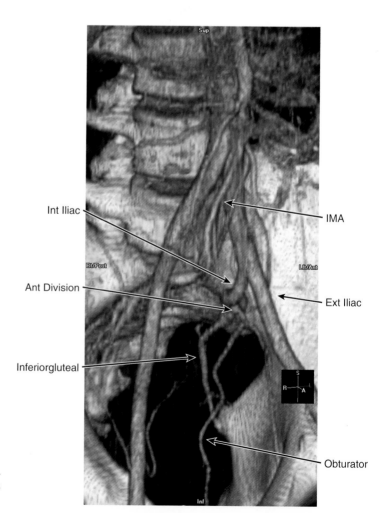

FIGURE 75-12. Three-dimensional rendering of aortic bifurcation. Internal iliac artery runs anterior to sacroiliac joint and then divides into anterior and posterior branches.

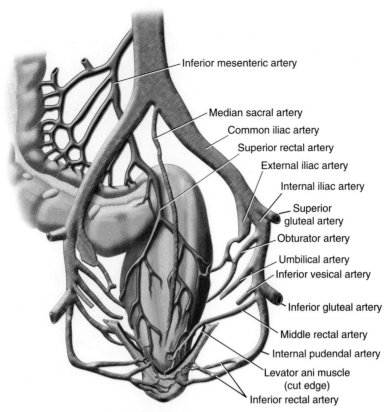

FIGURE 75-13. Anterior view of obturator artery, middle rectal artery, internal pudendal artery, inferior gluteal artery, and median sacral artery. *(From Townsend CM, Beauchamp RW, Evers BM, Mattox KL. Sabiston textbook of surgery. 17th ed. Philadelphia: Saunders; 2004. p. 1407.)*

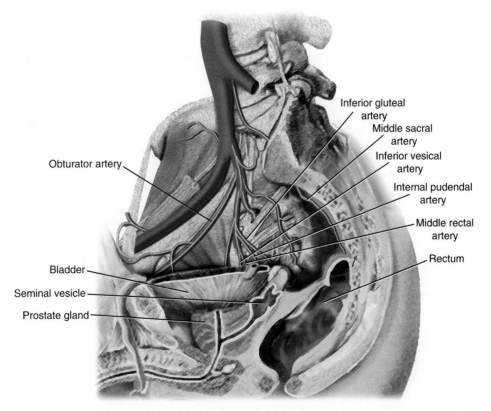

FIGURE 75-14. Lateral view of obturator artery, inferior vesical artery, middle rectal artery, internal pudendal artery, inferior gluteal artery, and middle sacral artery. *(From Wein AJ, Kavoussi LR, Novick AC, et al., editors. Campbell's urology. 9th ed. Philadelphia: Saunders; 2007. p. 49.)*

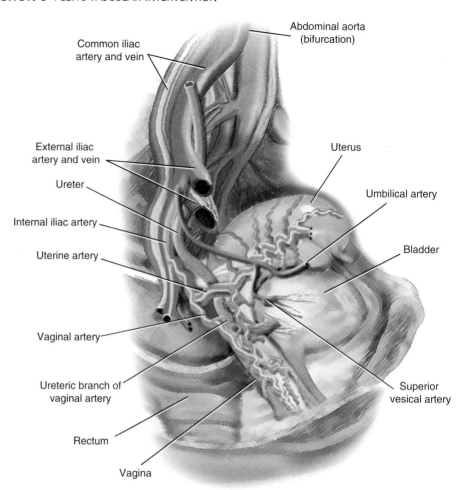

FIGURE 75-15. Lateral view of umbilical artery, uterine artery, superior vesical artery, ureter, and bladder. *(From Stenchever MA, Droegmueller W, Herbst A, Mishell D. Comprehensive gynecology. 4th ed. St Louis: Mosby; 2001. p. 63.)*

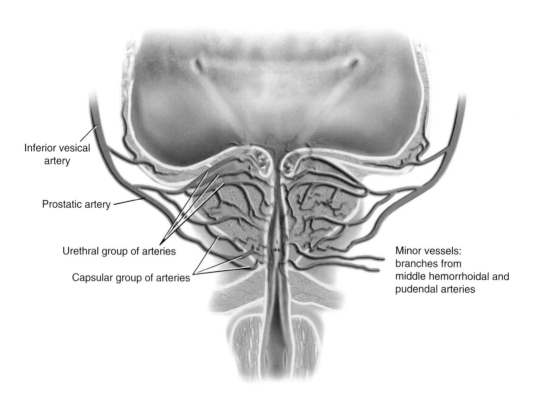

FIGURE 75-16. Visualization of inferior vesical artery, prostatic artery, and prostate. *(From Wein AJ, Kavoussi LR, Novick AC, et al., editors. Campbell's urology. 9th ed. Philadelphia: Saunders; 2007. p. 65.)*

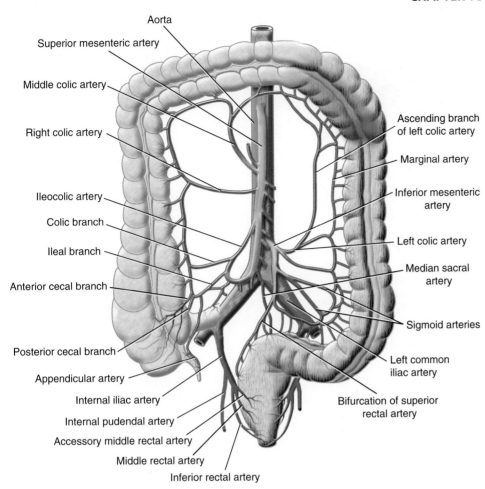

Aorta

Superior mesenteric artery

Middle colic artery

Right colic artery

Ileocolic artery

Colic branch

Ileal branch

Anterior cecal branch

Posterior cecal branch

Appendicular artery

Internal iliac artery

Internal pudendal artery

Accessory middle rectal artery

Middle rectal artery

Inferior rectal artery

Ascending branch
of left colic artery

Marginal artery

Inferior mesenteric
artery

Left colic artery

Median sacral
artery

Sigmoid arteries

Left common
iliac artery

Bifurcation of superior
rectal artery

FIGURE 75-17. Complete view of lower gastrointestinal arterial supply. In particular, middle rectal artery, superior rectal artery, inferior mesenteric artery, internal pudendal artery, and median sacral artery are seen. *(From Townsend CM, Beauchamp RW, Evers BM, Mattox KL. Sabiston textbook of surgery. 17th ed. Philadelphia: Saunders; 2004. p. 2290.)*

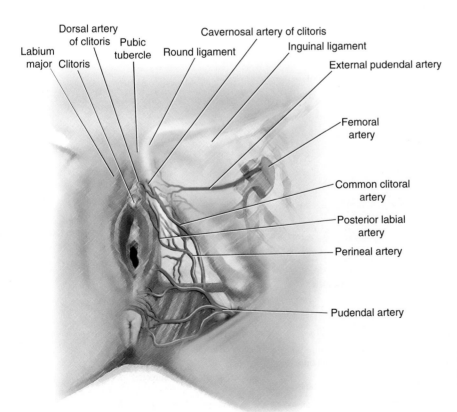

Dorsal artery
of clitoris Pubic
tubercle

Labium
major Clitoris

Cavernosal artery of clitoris

Round ligament

Inguinal ligament

External pudendal artery

Femoral
artery

Common clitoral
artery

Posterior labial
artery

Perineal artery

Pudendal artery

FIGURE 75-18. Sacral view of female pelvis showing internal pudendal artery and its clitoral branch. *(From Wein AJ, Kavoussi LR, Novick AC, et al., editors. Campbell's urology. 9th ed. Philadelphia: Saunders; 2007. p. 78.)*

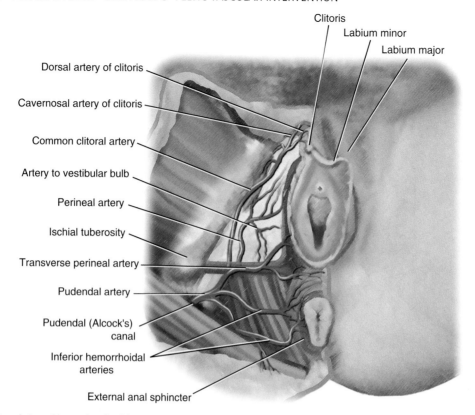

FIGURE 75-19. Sacral view of internal pudendal artery exiting pudendal canal and branching to supply perineum of external female genitalia and internal anal sphincter. *(From Noble J. Textbook of primary care medicine. 3rd ed. St Louis: Mosby; 2001. p. 1444.)*

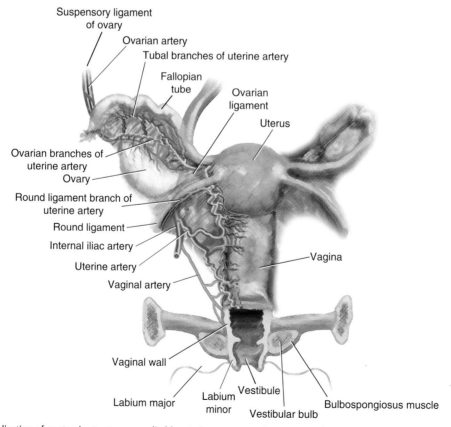

FIGURE 75-20. Visualization of anatomic structures supplied by uterine artery, ovarian artery, and vaginal artery. *(From Noble J. Textbook of primary care medicine. 3rd ed. St Louis: Mosby; 2001. p. 1448.)*

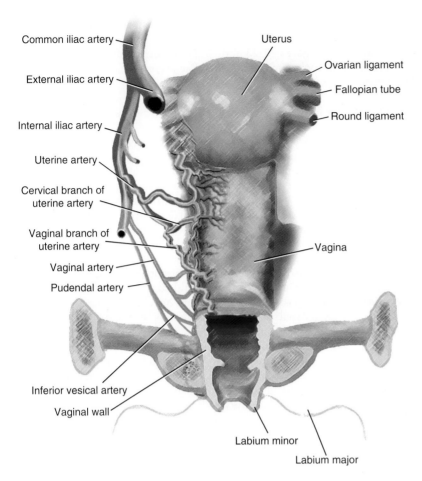

Common iliac artery

External iliac artery

Internal iliac artery

Uterine artery

Cervical branch of uterine artery

Vaginal branch of uterine artery

Vaginal artery

Pudendal artery

Inferior vesical artery

Vaginal wall

Uterus

Ovarian ligament

Fallopian tube

Round ligament

Vagina

Labium minor

Labium major

FIGURE 75-21. Visualization of female organs being supplied by uterine artery, vaginal artery, and internal pudendal artery. *(From Gabbe SG, Niebyl JR, Simpson JL. Obstetrics—normal and problem pregnancies. 4th ed. Edinburgh: Churchill Livingstone; 2002. p. 1374.)*

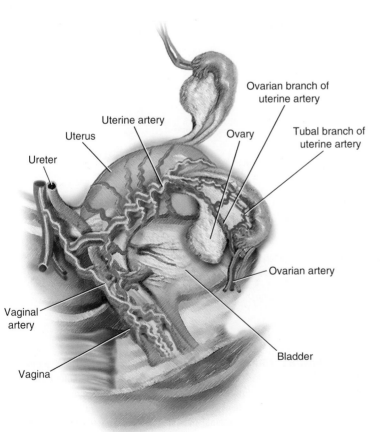

Uterine artery

Uterus

Ureter

Ovarian branch of uterine artery

Ovary

Tubal branch of uterine artery

Ovarian artery

Bladder

Vaginal artery

Vagina

FIGURE 75-22. Visualization of ovarian artery and its anastomosis with uterine artery and its branches. *(From Gabbe SG, Niebyl JR, Simpson JL. Obstetrics—normal and problem pregnancies. 4th ed. Edinburgh: Churchill Livingstone; 2002. p. 1373.)*

The terminal branch of the posterior trunk is the superior gluteal artery (see Figs. 75-10 and 75-13). The artery dives deep and anterior to the S1 ramus and exits the true pelvis via the greater sciatic notch above the piriformis muscle. Providing supply to the gluteal region of the lower extremity, this artery also supplies branches to the pelvic wall.

In the discussion of pelvic vascular anatomy, it is important to include the ovarian artery (see Figs. 75-1, 75-20, and 75-22) and the median sacral artery (see Figs. 75-4, 75-13, 75-14, and 75-17)—vessels of abdominal origin that also supply the pelvis. The ovarian artery arises from the abdominal aorta and then descends to the pelvic inlet, where it courses through the infundibulopelvic ligament to the ovary proper. The ovarian artery is a primary source of blood flow for both the ovary and uterus via arterial anastomoses.

The median sacral artery (see Figs. 75-4, 75-13, 75-14, and 75-17) originates just above the aortic bifurcation and then descends along the anterior sacrum and coccyx to provide the terminal pair of lumbar arteries. This artery anastomoses with the iliolumbar and lateral sacral arteries (see Fig. 75-10) to support the posterior structures of the pelvis.

Figures 75-23 and 75-24 are angiographic images of the branches of the internal iliac artery.

VEINS

The two common iliac veins come together at the L5 vertebral level to form the inferior vena cava just right of midline. In general, all named pelvic veins follow the course of their arterial counterparts, and the common iliac veins to the inferior vena cava bifurcation are no exception. They are found to the right of the aortic bifurcation and the corresponding iliac arteries. These iliac veins represent the primary venous drainage of the true pelvis (Fig. 75-25; also see Fig. 75-1).

An extensive venous network of interconnected plexuses is associated with the visceral structures contained within the pelvis (Fig. 75-26). More specifically, the rectum and anal canal involve three venous systems, delineation of which has important clinical significance. The rectum and anal canal drain via the superior rectal veins, tributaries of the inferior mesenteric veins, and into the hepatic portal venous system (see Fig. 75-26). The same territory is also served via venous drainage from the middle and inferior rectal veins into the caval system. With portal hypertension and resulting reversal of portal venous flow, the pelvic plexus is an important portocaval shunt.

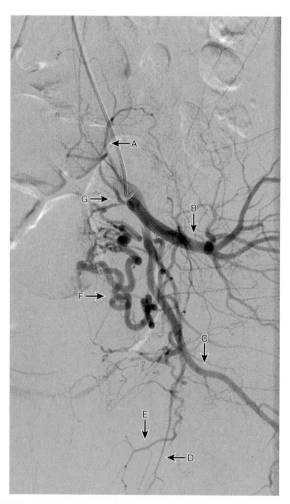

FIGURE 75-23. Selective left internal iliac artery digital subtraction angiographic injection using 5F Roberts uterine artery catheter (RUC [Cook Medical, Bloomington, Ind.) in patient with uterine fibroids. *A,* Iliolumbar artery; *B,* superior gluteal artery; *C,* inferior gluteal artery; *D,* obturator artery; *E,* internal pudendal artery; *F,* enlarged uterine artery; *G,* lateral sacral artery.

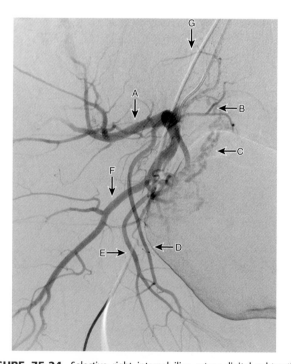

FIGURE 75-24. Selective right internal iliac artery digital subtraction angiographic injection using 5F Roberts uterine artery catheter (RUC [Cook Medical, Bloomington, Ind.) in patient with uterine fibroids. *A,* Superior gluteal artery; *B,* lateral sacral artery; *C,* enlarged broad ligament artery; *D,* obturator artery; *E,* internal pudendal artery; *F,* inferior gluteal artery; *G,* iliolumbar artery.

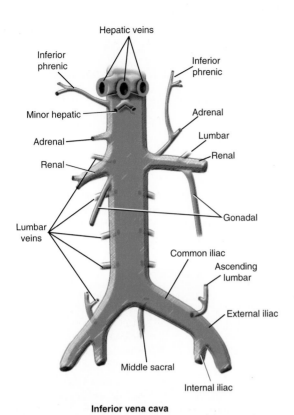

FIGURE 75-25. Inferior vena cava, its split into common iliac veins, and their split into internal and external iliac veins. *(From Wein AJ, Kavoussi LR, Novick AC, et al., editors. Campbell's urology. 9th ed. Philadelphia: Saunders; 2007. p. 6.)*

The rectal venous plexus around the anal canal has two parts. The internal rectal plexus is located between the internal anal sphincter and the epithelial lining and drains via the superior rectal vein. Internal hemorrhoids (Figs. 75-27 and 75-28) result from enlargement of these plexus branches. Internal hemorrhoids are covered with colonic mucosa and are located above the pectinate line. The external rectal plexus is subcutaneous and involves the external anal sphincter. External hemorrhoids (see Figs. 75-27 and 75-28) result from enlargement of these vessels.

Of notable exception to the rule, the single deep dorsal vein (Fig. 75-29) that drains the erectile tissues of the penis and clitoris does not follow the course of the internal pudendal artery (see Figs. 75-13, 75-18, 75-19, 75-21, and 75-29) into the true pelvis. Rather, this vein passes through a gap between the arcuate ligament and the anterior margin of the perineal membrane. In men, this vein drains to the prostatic venous plexus; in women, it drains to the vesical venous plexus.

The median sacral vein (see Fig. 75-26) and the ovarian vein (see Fig. 75-1) are mentioned here to complete the discussion of venous drainage in the pelvis, although their courses parallel the associated arteries and drain through the inferior aspect of the abdomen. The median sacral veins converge into a singular vein that empties into the left common iliac vein (see Fig. 75-26) or the inferior vena cava junction. The ovarian veins follow their arterial complements and empty into the abdomen at the renal vein on the left and the inferior vena cava on the right.

The ovarian and internal iliac veins may give rise to painful varices in women, and the spermatic vein is

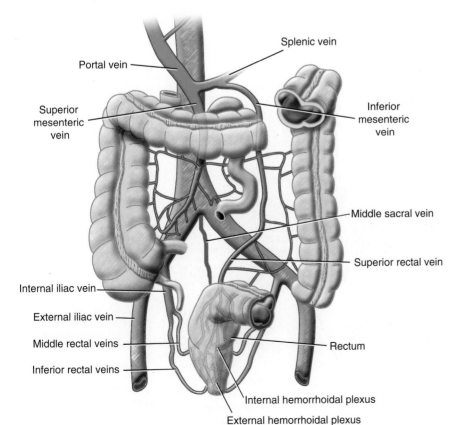

FIGURE 75-26. Extensive venous network of pelvis, including superior rectal vein, inferior mesenteric vein, portal vein, middle rectal vein, and inferior rectal vein. *(From Townsend CM, Beauchamp RW, Evers BM, Mattox KL. Sabiston textbook of surgery. 17th ed. Philadelphia: Saunders; 2004. p. 1411.)*

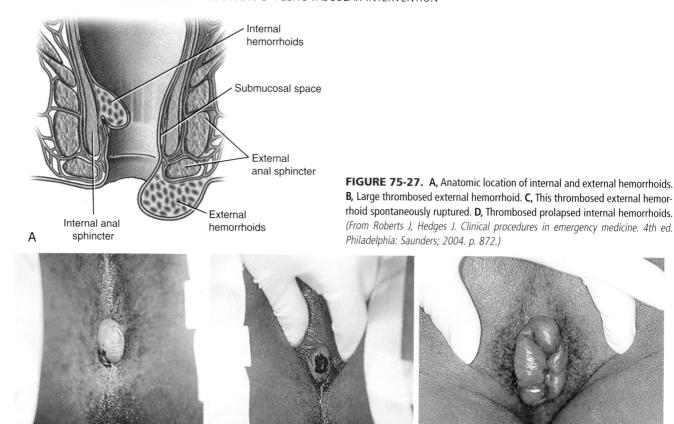

FIGURE 75-27. A, Anatomic location of internal and external hemorrhoids. **B,** Large thrombosed external hemorrhoid. **C,** This thrombosed external hemorrhoid spontaneously ruptured. **D,** Thrombosed prolapsed internal hemorrhoids. *(From Roberts J, Hedges J. Clinical procedures in emergency medicine. 4th ed. Philadelphia: Saunders; 2004. p. 872.)*

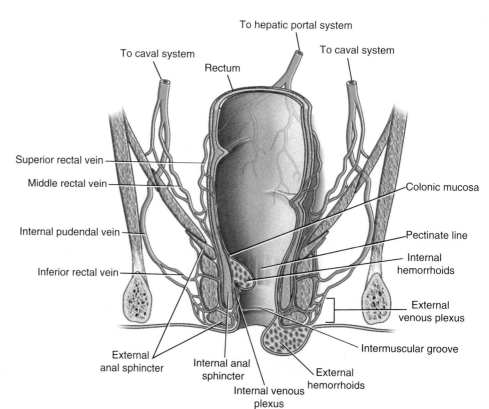

FIGURE 75-28. Comparison of anatomic locations of internal versus external hemorrhoids. *(From Ferri F. Ferri's clinical advisor: instant diagnosis and treatment. 8th ed. St Louis: Mosby; 2006. p. 369.)*

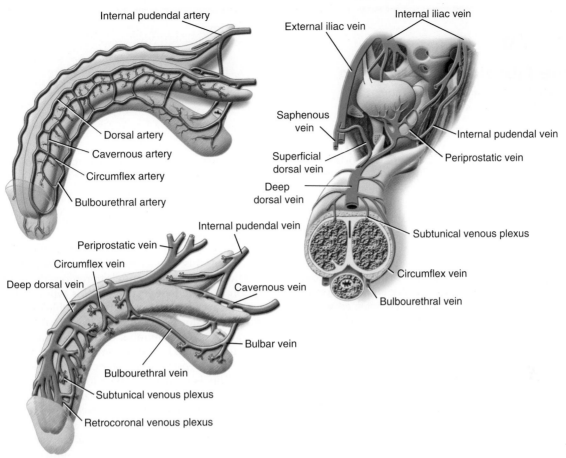

FIGURE 75-29. Comparison between location of internal pudendal artery and deep dorsal vein on penis. *(From Wein AJ, Kavoussi LR, Novick AC, et al., editors. Campbell's urology. 9th ed. Philadelphia: Saunders; 2007. p. 1593.)*

associated with varicoceles in men (see Chapters 79 and 80 in this book).

KEY POINTS

- The two major branches of the common iliac arteries are the internal (hypogastric) and external iliac arteries.
- The anterior division of the internal iliac artery has six branches: the umbilical artery, obturator artery, inferior vesical artery, middle rectal artery, internal pudendal artery, and inferior gluteal artery.
- The uterine artery generally arises from the anterior division of the internal iliac artery, but several variations in its origin have been described.
- The posterior division of the internal iliac artery has three branches: the iliolumbar artery, lateral sacral artery, and superior gluteal artery.

► **SUGGESTED READINGS**

Ferri F. Ferri's clinical advisor: instant diagnosis and treatment. 8th ed. St Louis: Mosby; 2006.

Gabbe SG, Niebyl JR, Simpson JL. Obstetrics—normal and problem pregnancy. 4th ed. Edinburgh: Churchill Livingstone; 2002.

Marx J. Rosen's emergency medicine: concepts and clinical practice. 6th ed. St Louis: Mosby; 2006.

Mettler F, Guiberteau M. Essentials of radiology. 2nd ed. Philadelphia: Saunders; 2005.

Noble J. Textbook of primary care medicine. 3rd ed. St Louis: Mosby; 2001.

Roberts J, Hedges J. Clinical procedures in emergency medicine. 4th ed. Philadelphia: Saunders; 2004.

Stenchever MA, Droegmueller W, Herbst A, Mishell D. Comprehensive gynecology. 4th ed. St Louis: Mosby; 2001.

Townsend CM, Beauchamp RD, Evers BM, Mattox KL. Sabiston textbook of surgery. 17th ed. Philadelphia: Saunders; 2004.

Wein AJ, Kavoussi LR, Novick AC, et al., editors. Campbell's urology. 9th ed. Philadelphia: Saunders; 2007.

CHAPTER 76

Uterine Fibroid Embolization

James B. Spies and Ferenc Czeyda-Pommersheim

Uterine fibroid embolization (UFE) was first reported in the United States in 1997 as a minimally invasive alternative to hysterectomy and myomectomy for treatment of fibroids.[1] Since that time, its effectiveness has been confirmed by other investigators, including in two major randomized comparative trials,[2,3] and it has rapidly been incorporated into practice. In 2008, the American College of Obstetricians and Gynecologists, based on good and consistent scientific evidence (level A), concluded that "based on long- and short-term outcomes, uterine artery embolization is a safe and effective option for appropriately selected women who wish to retain their uteri."[4] With this acknowledgment, uterine artery embolization is now widely accepted as an alternative to hysterectomy.

INDICATIONS

Despite the very high incidence of uterine fibroids, many patients are asymptomatic. The most common symptom associated with uterine fibroids is heavy menstrual bleeding. Other symptoms include dysmenorrhea, pelvic pain and pressure, urinary frequency, and hydronephrosis. Fibroids have also been implicated in reduced fertility, infertility, and complicated pregnancies.

Most patients with symptomatic fibroids are candidates for UFE, and it is indicated for those who wish to avoid major surgery or definite loss of reproductive capacity. Although there are no well-established guidelines for UFE patient selection, in general, the size and extent of fibroids determine a patient's suitability for embolization.

Fibroid location is also a consideration in patient selection, since there is some evidence that location may impact outcome[5] (Fig. e76-1). Submucosal fibroids shrink more rapidly than intramural fibroids, and intramural fibroids shrink more rapidly than those on the serosa. There are some fibroid locations that are likely less favorable, and these are discussed further under Contraindications.

CONTRAINDICATIONS

UFE is contraindicated in patients who are pregnant or if uterine, cervical, or endometrial malignancy is suspected. Thus, patients with fibroids and imaging findings suggestive of malignant degeneration or patients with indeterminate adnexal masses merit further evaluation prior to proceeding with embolization.

Postmenopausal bleeding is rarely due to fibroids and always warrants endometrial biopsy to rule out malignancy. Similarly, we believe patients with marked irregularity of menstrual bleeding, which we define as vaginal bleeding more frequent than every 21 days or lasting longer than 10 days, should be considered for endometrial biopsy. Although continuous or frequent bleeding may occur with

intracavitary or partially intracavitary fibroids, this type of bleeding pattern may also be caused by endometrial hyperplasia, polyps, endometrial malignancy, or other nonfibroid causes.

There are some specific subtypes of fibroids that may be best managed with surgery. Intracavitary fibroids, particularly when less than 3 cm, may be resectable using hysteroscopic methods. If a gynecologist skilled in hysteroscopic resection is unavailable or fails to remove the fibroid, embolization is certainly effective for this type of fibroid. Large serosal fibroids are often easily resectable by myomectomy, and the decision whether embolization or surgery is preferred depends on a number of factors. In most cases where the patient would like to become pregnant and when there has not been a previous myomectomy, surgery may be preferred. This is particularly true for very large fibroids that are mostly outside the uterine wall. The extreme example of a large narrow-based, completely pedunculated serosal fibroid is usually best treated surgically. This type of fibroid is likely to have relatively less shrinkage than other fibroids and is prone to adhesion formation. Similarly, for a woman with a massive uterus (>24 weeks size), the degree of shrinkage in the uterus may not be sufficient to provide long-term patient satisfaction, and these patients may have a better long-term outcome with surgery.[6] Finally, there are some specific fibroid locations, notably broad ligament fibroids and cervical fibroids that anecdotally do not respond to UFE or respond poorly. These fibroids can be a therapeutic conundrum, since they are not easily treated surgically if the uterus is to be spared.

EQUIPMENT

One of the advantages of uterine embolization for interventional radiologists is that the procedure requires no equipment that is not usually on the shelves of any well-stocked interventional suite.

The first requirement is for an angiographic unit with a digital roadmapping or similar digital guidance system, essential if this procedure is going to be performed in a safe manner with a minimal fluoroscopic dose. Pulsed fluoroscopy is also very important to reduce patient radiation dose, and the pulse rate should be no higher than 15 pulses per second to minimize radiation exposure.

Standard 4F or 5F selective angiographic catheters are typically used for entry into the hypogastric arteries. Large-bore (0.025- to 0.028-inch lumen) microcatheters with appropriate microwires are required in patients with small or very tortuous uterine arteries, and many operators use them in all cases.

Embolic material is the central requirement of the procedure. Although Gelfoam pledgets or slurry have been used in rare cases, there is relatively little study of the effectiveness of the material outside Japan. The vast majority of fibroid embolizations in Western countries have been performed using particulate or spherical embolic materials.[7] These are discussed later in the section on technical controversies.

TECHNIQUE

Anatomy and Approach

The internal iliac artery provides the majority of the blood supply to the pelvis and inner thigh. The internal iliac artery bifurcates to an anterior and posterior division in 57% to 77% of the general population.[8,9] Uterine fibroid tumors derive their main peripheral blood supply almost exclusively from the uterine artery.[10] The uterine artery is the first or second branch of the anterior division of the internal iliac artery in 51% of the general population. The contralateral anterior oblique view is best used to image this variant. The uterine artery arises from a trifurcation of the internal iliac in approximately 40%, which is best imaged by the ipsilateral anterior oblique projection. In approximately 1% of the population, the uterine artery is absent; in these cases, it is often replaced by the ipsilateral ovarian artery.[10]

Technical Aspects

Once femoral access is obtained, a catheter is advanced over the aortic bifurcation to the opposite hypogastric artery. Most practitioners use a single catheter to treat both uterine arteries (first one side, then the other). The first vessel usually catheterized is the one opposite the puncture site. A Waltman loop is often used to enter the ipsilateral uterine artery,[11] although there are interventionalists who use a Rosch inferior mesenteric (RIM) catheter for both sides, with the catheter pulled back from the left to the right to "hang" the catheter in the origin of the ipsilateral hypogastric artery, using it as a conduit to advance a microcatheter and wire into the right uterine artery. Another approach is use of the Roberts catheter (Cook Medical, Bloomington Ind.), which has a larger preformed loop similar to a Waltman loop.

An alternative is to use a two-catheter approach, one from each common femoral artery. This has the advantage of allowing simultaneous embolization, reducing the fluoroscopy and procedure time substantially.[12] It has the disadvantage of a second femoral puncture.

Regardless of whether single or double puncture is used, once a catheter is in the hypogastric artery, a roadmap image is obtained to demonstrate the origin of the uterine artery so that it can easily be entered with the catheter or microcatheter. Once an adequate view of the origin has been obtained, an angiographic wire (or microwire) can be advanced into the uterine artery and a catheter advanced over it. A 4F or 5F catheter may be used, but if it causes spasm, a microcatheter should be used coaxially, and the outer catheter retracted into the hypogastric artery. If the vessel is not excessively tortuous, the catheter is advanced to the major medial turn of the vessel and placed in the proximal portion of the transverse segment of the uterine artery, preferably beyond the origins of any visible side branches. If the vessel is tortuous, the catheter may be

advanced until it is just proximal to the first severely angulated segment to avoid spasm. Embolization should not proceed unless the catheter is well seated in the uterine artery because misembolization to other branches may occur, with potentially disastrous results. Prior to embolization, angiographic imaging is used to confirm catheter position and demonstrate the fibroid blood supply (Fig. e76-2, A). As mentioned, there are several choices for embolic material, and these are discussed in greater detail under Controversies.

Historically, the endpoint of embolization was complete occlusion of the uterine artery with coil or gelatin sponge plug adjuncts, but this has changed to subtotal occlusion in recent years. There are two endpoints of embolization in current use. The first is embolization until there is stasis or near stasis in the uterine artery, corresponding with complete occlusion of all its major branches. This endpoint is best achieved with polyvinyl alcohol (PVA) particles and other spherical embolics, with the exception of trisacryl gelatin microspheres (TAGM). For TAGM, less complete occlusion of the uterine arteries is effective and preferred, with the embolic injected slowly until the forward flow slows to sluggishness within the uterine artery. This corresponds to an angiographic image in which the fibroid feeding branches are distally occluded, but the uterine arteries and the proximal portions of its branches are patent, sometimes called the "pruned tree" appearance[13] (Fig. e76-2, B). Regardless of the embolic material used, it is important to wait a few minutes after the apparent conclusion to be sure there is no early recanalization, which may allow for reperfusion of the fibroids.

CONTROVERSIES

The primary current controversy in UFE is the choice of embolic material. The efficacy of traditional PVA particles (Contour [Boston Scientific, Natick Mass.], Ivalon [Cook Medical], other manufacturers) has been well established in numerous clinical trials, both the early large case series[14-17] and subsequent randomized trials.[2,3] Similarly there are now considerable data to document the effectiveness of TAGM (Biosphere Medical, Rockland Mass.).[18,19] A randomized comparative study compared TAGM to PVA particles and demonstrated comparable rates of symptom improvement and fibroid infarction.[20]

Despite an early presumption that the choice of embolic material was unlikely to impact outcome, this has not proven to be the case. In a randomized comparison of spherical PVA (sPVA, Contour SE, Boston Scientific, Watick, Mass.) and TAGM, there was a markedly poorer rate of fibroid infarction with the spherical PVA.[13] These outcomes have subsequently been confirmed in two randomized comparisons of sPVA particles to other embolics, noting both poorer infarction rates[21] and poorer long-term clinical outcomes.[22] These findings taken together confirm a poorer outcome with spherical PVA and suggest they should not be used as an embolic for this procedure.

At this time, there are no published data from randomized trials assessing two newer embolics, PVA hydrogel (BeadBlock Microspheres [Terumo Medical Corp., Somerset, N.J.]) or Polyzene F–coated hydrogel (Embozene Microspheres, CeloNova BioSciences, San Antonio, Tex.) microspheres for UFE, although at least one nonrandomized comparative study raises similar questions of effectiveness of PVA hydrogel particles.[23]

OUTCOMES

UFE is most commonly performed to control symptoms such as menorrhagia, dysmenorrhea, and urinary and pelvic pain and pressure, and one measure of success is the degree of improvement it can offer for these symptoms. Over the past decade, many series have been published, but among the largest was the FIBROID Registry sponsored by the Society of Interventional Radiology (SIR) Foundation to evaluate UFE in a broad range of settings; 72 practices enrolled patients in the Registry, including all U.S. geographic regions, as well as international sites.[24]

Thirty-day follow-up was completed in 2729 patients,[7] and short-term outcomes focused on adverse events. These are presented in the section on Complications. At 1 year after treatment,[25] 87% had a significant improvement in symptom scores, with fewer than 6% having had no symptomatic improvement; 82% in this group reported they were satisfied with the procedure at 12 months. Similar outcomes were found 2 and 3 years after treatment,[26] with the mean scores in the range of normal at both 24 and 36 months post procedure. By 3 years after treatment, 9.8% of patients had undergone hysterectomy, 2.9% had had a myomectomy, and 1.8% repeat embolization. Over 85% of patients still in follow-up 3 years after treatment remained satisfied with the outcome.

Randomized Trials

There have been a number of randomized trials, but the two most important in terms of the comparative symptom and quality-of-life outcomes are the EMMY Trial and the REST Trial, both published in recent years.

The EMMY Trial was a multicenter trial performed in the Netherlands, comparing embolization to hysterectomy.[27] At 2 years after treatment, there were similar levels of symptom control, health-related quality of life, and patient satisfaction with outcome, although 24% of UFE patients had either failure of symptom control or recurrent symptoms leading to hysterectomy. By 5 years after treatment, most patients had continued symptom control, although an additional 4% of uterine artery embolization patients, or 28% of patients in total, had undergone hysterectomy after treatment.[28]

Similar results were found in the REST Trial, a multicenter trial from the United Kingdom, with results first published in 2007.[2] The study compared patients randomly assigned to either UFE or surgery, with the choice of surgery (either hysterectomy or myomectomy) the choice of the surgeon or patient. The primary outcome was health-related quality of life, and the outcomes were very similar between surgery and embolization. There was a greater likelihood of reintervention with uterine embolization, with 20% of patients undergoing reintervention after UFE by the median initial follow-up interval of 32 months. By 5 years after treatment, symptoms, quality of life, and satisfaction were very high in both groups, although reintervention was higher with UFE (32%) than with surgery (4%). There were no differences in complications between the two groups.[29]

Fertility and Pregnancy After Uterine Fibroid Embolization

One important question for patients considering UFE is whether it will have an impact on fertility and pregnancy outcomes. Recent studies have shed some light on both issues.

The only randomized trial to compare the reproductive outcomes of myomectomy and UFE was completed in Prague. The investigators randomized 121 patients to either UFE or myomectomy and reported the reproductive short-term outcomes of symptoms and ovarian function[30] and the early reproductive outcomes 2 years after treatment.[31] In the latter report, there were clear advantages for myomectomy in terms of reproductive outcomes. UFE patients were less likely to become pregnant (relative risk [RR] .45), less likely to deliver a full-term pregnancy (RR .64), and more likely to miscarry (RR 2.79). Yet despite the advantages of myomectomy, patients who had UFE still had a 50% chance of getting pregnant within 2 years.

One additional question regarding reproductive outcomes is the frequency of complications related to pregnancy and delivery. Homer and Saridogan have published a systematic review of pregnancy risks after UFE.[32] The authors gathered all the published outcomes of pregnancies after UFE and compared them to controls derived from several published studies. The review showed that UFE patients did not have increased odds of preterm delivery, malpresentation, or intrauterine growth retardation. They were at greater risk of miscarriage (odds ratio [OR] 2.8), cesarean section (OR 2.1), and postpartum hemorrhage (OR 6.4).

Despite the limitations of these studies, they provide the best evidence we have to guide our counseling of patients. Based on the studies reviewed, we favor myomectomy for patients who are interested in pregnancy (particularly within 2 years), who have fibroids that can be safely removed, and who have not had a prior myomectomy. For those with extensive disease, prior surgery, or no clear plans for pregnancy, UFE may be an option, although each patient's circumstances should be considered individually. Without a large comparative study assessing pregnancy outcomes, more specific recommendations cannot be made. For women considering pregnancy, it is important to have a discussion of the knowns and unknowns regarding reproductive outcomes after both myomectomy and UFE.

COMPLICATIONS

Complications after UFE are uncommon, and serious complications are rare. In the FIBROID Registry, there was a major adverse event rate of 0.66% in the hospital, and 4.8% within 30 days of the procedure. A *major adverse event* is defined as one in which the initial hospitalization is prolonged beyond 48 hours, or there is a need for an emergency room visit or readmission to the hospital or reintervention (surgical or interventional). In the Registry, only 1.1% of patients required surgical intervention within 30 days of the procedure.

An earlier study of 400 consecutive patients found an overall morbidity rate of 5%, with a major adverse event rate of 1.25%.[33] Among these patients, there was only one hysterectomy required for a complication, and there were no permanent injuries or deaths. In the randomized comparative trials, there were no overall differences in major complications.[2,34] These findings were confirmed in a recent comparative study of hysterectomy, myomectomy, and UFE that showed no difference in adverse events (minor or major) among the three treatments.[35]

If one excludes pain requiring additional management, the most common serious complication occurring after uterine embolization is fibroid passage, which is often associated with pain, bleeding, or infection. It only occurs in fibroids that are intracavitary, partially intracavitary, or have an interface with the endometrial cavity. On occasion, a fistulous tract may form from the myometrium to the endometrial cavity and cause chronic vaginal discharge as the treated fibroid slowly is expelled.[36] Fibroid passage usually occurs within the first 3 to 6 months after embolization, although it has been reported up to 3 years after the procedure.[37] The manifestations of fibroid passage are varied; for some patients it is minor, causing only cramping, while for others it can lead to major bleeding or infection. Careful follow-up is required and the patient should be instructed about the potential symptoms associated with fibroid passage. If symptoms suggestive of passage occur, the patient requires evaluation, both with pelvic examination and magnetic resonance imaging (Fig. e76-3). Management may include nonsteroidal antiinflammatory drugs (NSAIDs), oral narcotics, oral or intravenous (IV) antibiotics, and potentially hospitalization and dilatation and curettage or extraction.

Severe infections can occur in the short term after uterine embolization, and these early infections may not be associated with fibroid passage. They appear to represent a variant of pyometrium and may rapidly progress to sepsis. There have been two deaths due to early sepsis reported.[38,39]

Puncture site injuries may occur, with either arterial or nerve injuries, but are quite rare. Perhaps owing to this population's age range, most of these patients have normal vessels. In the Registry, vessel injuries occurred in 0.1% of cases.[7]

Venous thromboembolic events (VTE) after UFE have been estimated to occur in 0.25% of patients.[40] There are several factors that may predispose to VTE in the patient population undergoing UFE, including obesity and oral contraceptive use. The embolization procedure itself has also been shown to induce a temporary hypercoagulable state.[41] Each patient should be considered at risk for VTE and should be considered for prophylactic measures. In our practice, we use sequential compression devices on the legs and, for high-risk patients, use prophylactic low-molecular-weight heparin.

One of the early observations about UFE was that a small proportion of women transitioned into menopause after the procedure, leading to questions about whether uterine embolization has a negative impact on ovarian reserve. This issue was addressed in the EMMY Trial, where ovarian reserve was assessed for both patients treated with hysterectomy with ovarian preservation and UFE.[42] Both procedures were associated with a modest reduction in ovarian reserve on average. One important caveat in this study is that the women treated had a median age in the mid-40s; it is not clear that ovarian reserve is affected to the same extent or at all in women younger than 40, who are more likely to attempt pregnancy.

The risk of ovarian failure after UFE is age related, with highest rates occurring in patients older than 45.[15] The FIBROID Registry investigators reported on the frequency of amenorrhea after UFE. Of the 1701 UFE patients who completed 12 months of follow-up, 125 (7.3%) had amenorrhea; 2% of these patients were 35 to 39 years old, 12% were 40 to 44, 42% were 45 to 50, and 43% were older than 50.[25] These findings may be explained by nontarget embolization, since there is evidence that in some patients, embolic material may pass to the ovarian arteries via tubal branches.[43] This nontarget embolization may be more likely to affect patients with diminished ovarian reserve (older patients).

PERIPROCEDURE AND FOLLOW-UP CARE

For any therapy to be successful, there has to be a care plan that provides for (1) management of symptoms routinely encountered during recovery and (2) monitoring for potential complications that might occur. UFE results in ischemic infarction of fibroids and may also cause transient myometrial ischemia, both of which may result in short-term pelvic pain and nausea. However, with an appropriate care management plan, recovery after this procedure is well tolerated.[44] In a study of 100 patients treated and evaluated prospectively, the mean in-hospital peak visual analog scale (VAS) score on an appropriate regimen was 3.03, and the mean maximum outpatient score during the first week was 4.89 (scale 0 = no pain, to 10 = worst imaginable pain). Only 11 patients had pain scores greater than 7 at any time after the procedure in the hospital, and only 19 had such pain in the first week after treatment. Of those patients who were employed, 93.8% missed fewer than 10 days of work, and 62.3% of patients reported returning to complete normal activity within 14 days after the procedure.

The procedure is usually performed with the patient under conscious sedation with midazolam (Versed [Baxter, Glendale, Calif.]) and fentanyl (Sublimaze [Baxter]). In most practices, patients are admitted for an overnight stay, although some practitioners are performing the procedure as a "same-day" procedure.[45]

Pain typically will start at the conclusion of the procedure or shortly thereafter. While hospitalized, patients are usually are given narcotics administered via an IV patient-controlled analgesia (PCA) pump, with morphine sulfate, fentanyl, or hydromorphone the typical medications used. Patients often will need supplemental doses of the PCA narcotics ("clinician boluses") in the first few hours after the procedure. The operating physician or another qualified practitioner should be available to evaluate patients in pain and provide the medication needed during the early post-procedure period. In addition to PCA, patients also receive ketorolac (Toradol [Roche, Nutley, N.J.]) 30 mg IV every 6 hours.

For nausea, IV antiemetic agents are given as needed, and in some practices are given prophylactically. Some physicians use ondansetron (Zofran [GlaxoSmithKline, Research Triangle Park, N.C.]) 4 to 8 mg IV given as needed every 6 hours. Others use metoclopramide (Reglan [Robins, West Eatontown, N.J.]) 5 to 10 mg IV every 4 to 6 hours, or promethazine (Phenergan [Elkins-Sinn, Cherry Hill, N.J.]) 12.5 to 25 mg orally every 4 to 6 hours.

On the morning of discharge, usually the day after the procedure, the PCA and other IV medications are discontinued, and an oral regimen is instituted. Patients are discharged with prescriptions for NSAIDs, oral narcotics, and an antiemetic.

Beyond just medications, each patient should be given detailed written discharge instructions. They are instructed to call the interventional radiologist on call for persistent or severe pain, high fever, or any other symptoms of concern. Many practices follow up with patients by telephone the day after discharge and again within the first 2 weeks by phone or with an office visit to ensure uneventful recovery. Most practices also obtain follow-up imaging and an office evaluation of the patient at 3 to 6 months after the procedure to assess outcome.

KEY POINTS

- Based on level 1 data, uterine fibroid embolization (UFE) is now established as an effective therapy for uterine fibroids, with the large majority of patients experiencing symptom relief.
- UFE is safe, with a major complication rate of less than 3%.
- Most patients with symptomatic fibroids are candidates for UFE.
- Based on limited comparative studies, women seeking to become pregnant who have not have had prior fibroid intervention may on average have better reproductive outcomes after myomectomy. Nonetheless, women may become pregnant after embolization, and the decision about whether embolization or myomectomy is a better choice must be made after consideration of an individual patient's circumstances.

► **SUGGESTED READINGS**

Goodwin S, Spies JB. Uterine fibroid embolization. N Engl J Med 2009; 361:690–7.

Mara M, Maskova J, Fucikova Z, et al. Midterm clinical and first reproductive results of a randomized controlled trial comparing uterine fibroid embolization and myomectomy. Cardiovasc Intervent Radiol 2008; 31(1):73–85.

Moss J, Cooper KG, Khaund A, et al. Randomised comparison of uterine artery embolisation (UAE) with surgery treatment in patients with symptomatic uterine fibroids (REST trial): 5 year results. BJOG 2011;118(8):936–44.

Spies JB, Pelage JP, editors: Uterine artery embolization. Philadelphia: Lippincott Williams & Wilkins; 2005.

van der Kooij S, Hehenkamp WJ, Volkers NA, et al. Uterine artery embolization vs. hysterectomy in the treatment of symptomatic uterine fibroids: 5-year outcome from the randomized EMMY trial. Am J Obstet Gynecol 2010;203:e1–e13.

Worthington-Kirsch R, Spies J, Myers E, et al. The Fibroid Registry for Outcomes Data (FIBROID) for uterine artery embolization: short term outcomes. Obstet Gynecol 2005;106:52–9.

The complete reference list is available online at www.expertconsult.com.

CHAPTER 77

Peripartum Hemorrhage

Elizabeth A. Ignacio and Kiang Hiong Tay

INTRODUCTION

Peripartum hemorrhage (PPH) is reported as the most common maternal morbidity in developed countries and a major cause of death worldwide. Globally, postpartum hemorrhage may account for 25% of delivery-associated deaths.[1] The incidence may be up to 20% of pregnancies beyond 18 weeks' gestation. In the United States, PPH may occur in 1% to 5% of deliveries.[2]

Figures vary widely depending on the precise definition of PPH. Generally *postpartum hemorrhage* is defined as a blood loss of 500 mL during a vaginal delivery or more than 1000 mL blood loss with a cesarean delivery. Clinicians may add the specification of a 10% drop in hemoglobin, although the laboratory findings may lag significantly behind the patient's true blood loss status. Over 99% of PPH will occur within 24 hours of delivery.

The use of embolization to control pelvic hemorrhage was first described in 1972.[3] As a treatment for pelvic fractures, the technique was successful and later applied to the treatment of PPH as described by Brown et al. in 1979.[4] With several refinements over the years, this procedure has emerged as a safe and highly effective option for treating PPH.

PATHOPHYSIOLOGY

The etiologies for PPH can be summarized in the 4Ts mnemonic: tone, trauma, tissue, and thrombin (Table 77-1).

Uterine atony is the most common cause of PPH, accounting for 70% to 80% of cases.[5] This occurs when there is decreased contraction of the myometrium. The postgravid uterus is floppy or flaccid and unable to provide adequate compression for hemostasis. Risk factors for atony include multiple gestation, fetal macrosomia, and prolonged labor.

Possibly related to uterine atony, uterine inversion is a rare condition that can cause PPH. The incidence is around 0.05%. The myometrium of the inverted uterus is unable to contract and retract, resulting in severe blood loss. The mechanism for development of uterine inversion is unclear but may be related to combined factors of uterine atony, fundal placenta, increased fundal pressure, and undue cord traction.

Birth trauma leading to lacerations and hematomas may be the cause of significant PPH, with an incidence of about 20% in these patients.[5] Injuries to the vagina, cervix, and uterus leads to hemorrhage, given the highly increased vascularity that has developed during pregnancy. Risk factors that increase the trauma of delivery include fetal macrosomia, any instrumentation (e.g., forceps, vacuum), vaginal birth after cesarean section, or episiotomy.[2]

A small subset of patients with birth trauma may sustain substantial injury to the uterus classified as uterine rupture.

The incidence is 0.6% in patients who undergo vaginal birth after cesarean section.[6] The risk for uterine rupture increases with classical cesarean incisions, short interval between pregnancy, and a history of multiple cesarean deliveries, especially in women with no previous vaginal delivery. The use of pharmaceutical induction and/or augmentation of labor can increase the rate of uterine rupture as well.

On average the placental delivery occurs within 10 minutes following the fetus. The diagnosis of *retained placenta* is defined as the absence of placental expulsion by 30 minutes. In about 10% of patients with PPH, retained placental tissue is the primary etiology.[5] The operator may attempt several manipulations to retrieve the retained tissue and/or treat the ensuing blood loss. However, in a fraction of these patients, the tissue plane between the uterine wall and the placenta cannot be identified or separated, and the diagnosis of abnormal placentation or invasive placenta should be considered. Risk factors for retained placenta include any events that may have damaged the endometrial lining before becoming pregnant, multilobed placenta, prior uterine surgery, or cesarean section delivery.

The presence of invasive placenta can be life threatening. In the United States, the overall incidence is 1 in 533 deliveries, a rate that appears to be increasing and likely secondary to the increased rate of cesarean section.[7] There are three different types of invasive placenta with reference to the depth of invasion: (1) *placenta accreta*, which adheres to the myometrium, (2) *placenta increta*, which invades the myometrium, and (3) *placenta percreta*, which penetrates the myometrium to or through the serosa.

Coagulation disorders may result in PPH and may be the causal etiology in 1% of patients.[5] Preexisting disease may be discovered prior to delivery and allow for preparation and appropriate prophylaxis. Examples include idiopathic thrombocytopenic purpura (ITP), thrombotic thrombocytopenic purpura (TTP), factor X deficiency, familial hypofibrinogenemia, and von Willebrand disease. Disseminated intravascular coagulation (DIC) can occur in the setting of sepsis, placental abruption, and amniotic fluid embolism.

IMAGING

The diagnosis of PPH is a clinical one defined by the amount of blood loss and the hemodynamic status of the patient. No preprocedure imaging is required to make the diagnosis.

For patients with suspected PPH, ultrasound may show hematoma, retained placental fragments, or possibly abnormal placental invasion. Color flow Doppler images are especially helpful to identify the vascularity of any products of conception and demonstrate the abnormal lacunae of an invasive placenta (Fig. 77-1).

TABLE 77-1. Peripartum Hemorrhage Etiologies

The Four Ts

Tone:
  Uterine Atony
  Uterine Inversion
Trauma:
  Laceration of uterus, cervix, or vagina
Tissue:
  Retained placenta
  Abnormal or Invasive placentation
Thrombin:
  Disseminated intravascular coagulation (DIC)
  Platelet dysfunction
  Coagulopathy

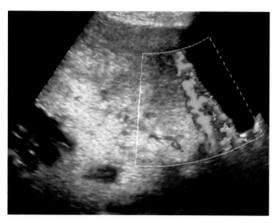

FIGURE 77-1. Pelvic ultrasound with color flow Doppler showing invasive placentation. Note presence of placental vascularity in myometrium abutting and possibly penetrating serosal surface into bladder.

Computed tomography (CT) scan with intravenous contrast findings are nonspecific. Magnetic resonance imaging (MRI) is usually not possible in the acutely hemorrhaging patient.

INDICATIONS

When hemorrhage persists despite resuscitative efforts, vasopressors, and/or surgical intervention, pelvic arterial embolization is indicated. (See Additional or Adjunctive Therapy.) The decision to proceed with endovascular therapy is usually multidisciplinary, with input from the obstetric surgeon and the interventional radiologist as well as the intensivist and anesthesiologist.

CONTRAINDICATIONS

Few absolute contraindications to endovascular therapy exist in the face of persistent life-threatening PPH. If a patient has a history of severe anaphylaxis to iodinated contrast, endovascular therapy may not be possible unless alternative contrast media are used (e.g., carbon dioxide, gadolinium). However, if the contrast allergy is relatively mild, pretreatment with diphenhydramine and steroids may be sufficient to avoid a reaction from contrast exposure.

Preexisting renal insufficiency is a relative contraindication to embolization therapy. Because the patient may be in

extremis, the risk for renal failure must be weighed against the morbidity and mortality of continued PPH.

The desire to maintain fertility may be a relative contraindication to pelvic arterial embolization. The pelvis has a rich and varied arterial supply, optimal for collateral arterial supply and support of the uterus following embolization.[8] However, the risk for temporary or even permanent menopause post embolization exists, given the common occurrence of anastomoses between the ovarian and uterine arteries.[9] Additionally, there may be increased risk for subsequent pregnancy complications such as spontaneous abortion, preterm delivery, and abnormal placentation after uterine artery embolization.[9,10] Although future fertility is an important consideration for all patients who undergo pelvic embolization, in the face of ongoing hemorrhage, this may not be the clinical priority.

METHODS AND MATERIALS

Pelvic Arterial Embolization

Embolic Agents

Several embolic agents are available. Most operators will choose absorbable gelatin sponge or Gelfoam (Pharmacia & Upjohn/Pfizer, New York, N.Y.). A gelatin slurry may be mixed relatively quickly with small cut cubes of gelatin sponge and dilute contrast homogenized through a three-way stopcock. Gelatin sponge particles of varying sizes are usually the materials of choice because they are safe, inexpensive, and easy to use. In addition, they have the potential for recanalization. Some operators will choose microcoils for embolization in PPH, particularly if there is a pseudoaneurysm present, if hemorrhage is refractory to gelatin sponge embolization and/or definitive devascularization is necessary. Caution should be taken in the use of coils because their presence proximally in an artery may preclude reentry should new hemorrhage recur.

Particle embolics such as polyvinyl alcohol (PVA), Embosphere (BioSphere Medical, South Jordan, Utah), and Embozene microspheres (CeloNova BioSciences, Peachtree City, Ga.) are another choice in the treatment of PPH. The gelatin microspheres are U.S. Food and Drug Administration (FDA) approved and used frequently for uterine artery embolization; microspheres are considered permanent embolic agents. Particles are more costly than gelatin sponges, and there is some controversy over the increased likelihood for ischemia or necrosis.[11]

N-butyl cyanoacrylate (NBCA) glue has also been described as an effective embolic for pelvic hemorrhage.[12] The delivery of glue is more technically challenging, but it is a viable option if the use of other embolic materials is unsuccessful.

Catheters and Microcatheters

Most interventional radiologists will use a 4F or 5F vascular sheath for access. A nonselective flush catheter may be used initially (e.g., pigtail catheter). Many selective catheters are available, and the choice is operator dependent. Examples of commonly used selective catheters include a Cobra-shaped catheter, a nontapered angled catheter, and the Roberts uterine curve catheter (RUC [Cook Medical, Bloomington, Ind.]). A microcatheter may be used when necessary; it should have a sufficient inner diameter to

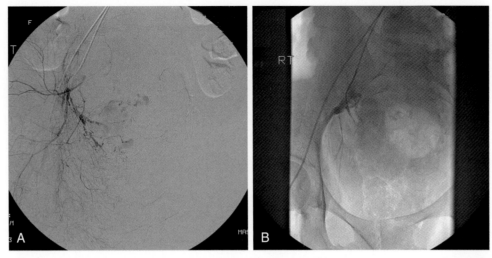

FIGURE 77-2. This patient had peripartum hemorrhage that presented with massive vaginal hemorrhage. **A,** Several sites of active hemorrhage were seen on selective uterine arteriogram. Despite selective placement of catheter tip, there was contrast reflux to anterior pelvic arteries and visualization of severe vasoconstriction. **B,** Adequate hemostasis was achieved with gentle gelfoam embolization. Contralateral side was also embolized (not shown).

accommodate the embolic agent of choice. Examples include the 2.4F to 3F Renegade HI-FLO Microcatheter (Boston Scientific, Natick, Mass.), with a 0.027-inch inner diameter, and the 2.4F to 2.8F Progreat microcatheter (Terumo Medical, Somerset, N.J.), with a 0.027 diameter.

Preoperative Intraarterial Balloon Placement

Occlusion Balloon Catheter
A standard occlusion balloon catheter may be used. This is preferred over an angioplasty balloon catheter because the balloon is soft, compliant, and less likely to damage the artery if it is left inflated for a period of time. An example is the 5F Boston Scientific Occlusion Balloon Catheter, which can be inflated up to a diameter of 8.5 mm.

ARTERIOGRAM AND EMBOLIZATION

Technique

Access is obtained into the common femoral artery, and a 4F or 5F vascular sheath is placed under local anesthesia. One may map out the arterial anatomy of the pelvis using a flush catheter in the distal aorta and a nonselective arteriogram. In the interest of saving time, many operators do not routinely obtain this nonselective contrast injection. However, it can be helpful to initially survey all pelvic arteries for any active hemorrhage, especially in patients who may have already undergone surgical arterial ligation.

In the clinical setting of PPH, the most likely source of hemorrhage is the uterine artery.[13] A selective catheter is used to access each uterine artery for arteriogram. Depending on the temporal occurrence of the PPH, the postgravid uterus may show extensive uteroplacental neovascularization. Bleeding may be intermittent, so empirical embolization therapy may be delivered even in the absence of active extravasation. The catheter should be advanced over a wire into the transverse or horizontal segment. Care should be taken to avoid any cervicovaginal branches, since such nontarget embolization can result in labial necrosis. The uterine

artery is embolized with the embolic agent of choice. For most operators, the desired endpoint for embolization may be complete stasis with a standing column of contrast in the artery over a 3 to 5 count of arterial beats, versus "pruning" of the vascular bed, but there are no randomized data to prove which course is superior (Figs. 77-2 and 77-3).

A follow-up nonselective pelvic arteriogram is important to evaluate for any new sites of active hemorrhage or collateral arterial supply to the uterus that may lead to recurrent hemorrhage. Successful arterial embolization for PPH requires occlusion of bilateral uterine arteries because cross-filling can result in recurrent hemorrhage. Collateral arterial supply that may lead to persistent hemorrhage may often be found from other branches of the internal iliac artery (e.g., internal pudendal, obturator, vesical arteries, etc.), uterine-ovarian arterial anastomoses, and the external pudendal artery.

Clinical Pitfalls and Pearls

Usually, gelatin sponges are easily accessible, safe, and effective embolic agents for PPH, but large amounts of absorbable gelatin sponges may still not be effective if there are markedly dilated vessels and high-pressure perfusion blood flow caused by extensive uteroplacental neovascularization (e.g., in severely invasive placentation). Changing hemodynamics and withdrawal of vasopressors may also lead to rebleeding following gelatin sponge embolization.

Vasoconstriction and vasospasm are often encountered during the procedure, especially in young or hemodynamically unstable patients. Advancing a selective catheter into the uterine artery may prove challenging if not impossible. Care should be taken to avoid forcing the catheter too far; dissection and arterial rupture may occur. If the catheter cannot safely be seated in the uterine arteries, nonselective embolization of the internal iliac arteries bilaterally may be necessary. At this site, gelatin sponges are the preferred embolic agent.

If tamponade devices such as packing or an occlusion balloon in the cervix or vagina have to be removed, these

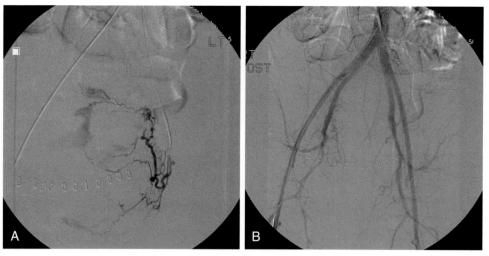

FIGURE 77-3. Peripartum hemorrhage in a patient with sickle cell anemia who underwent cesarean section. Uterine compression sutures had been placed for severe atony, but patient continued to hemorrhage. **A,** Arteriogram showed several sites of active contrast extravasation on selective uterine arteriogram. **B,** Patient had selective bilateral uterine artery embolization with Embosphere microspheres (500-700 μm and 700-900 μm). Follow-up arteriogram showed adequate hemostasis.

maneuvers should be performed while the patient is still in the interventional radiology suite, with arterial access maintained at the groin. Should rebleeding then occur, additional endovascular therapy may more easily be achieved.

PREOPERATIVE INTRAARTERIAL BALLOON PLACEMENT

Technique

If a diagnosis of invasive placentation is known prior to delivery, perioperative planning for endovascular therapy is possible. Prophylactic preoperative placement of internal iliac artery balloon catheters prior to surgery (e.g. cesarean section and/or hysterectomy) has been described and may be a useful adjunct for these high-risk patients.[14,15,16]

The procedure can be done in the standard interventional radiology suite with low-dose fluoroscopic capability and partial shielding to limit the radiation exposure of the patient and fetus.

Access is obtained into each common femoral artery, and a 4F or 5F vascular sheath is placed under local anesthesia. One may map out the internal iliac arterial anatomy and obtain measurements using a flush catheter in the distal aorta and a nonselective arteriogram. A selective catheter such as a Cobra-shaped catheter may be used to advance access into the contralateral internal iliac artery. A 0.035-inch wire of choice is advanced. A standard occlusion balloon catheter may be advanced over the wire into the proximal portion of the internal iliac artery, just beyond the bifurcation. The procedure is repeated for both internal iliac arteries. One should measure, test, and record the occlusion balloon volume on each side for the reinflation that will occur immediately post delivery.

The catheter and sheath on each side is then secured at the groin, and the patient may be transferred to the obstetrical operating room (Fig. 77-4). Once the baby is delivered, the balloons may be inflated immediately. Operators should

track the time duration for balloon inflation and be mindful of the risk for pelvic end-organ ischemia. Occlusion balloons may be deflated after delivery of the placenta, once the obstetrical surgeon has definitively achieved hemostasis. The interventional radiologist can remove balloon catheters and vascular sheaths at the end of the surgery, provided the patient's coagulation status is adequate.

ADDITIONAL OR ADJUVANT THERAPIES

In the multidisciplinary care of PPH patients, it is helpful for the interventional radiologist to be aware of adjuvant therapies and specific tools used by other specialties (Table 77-2).

A detailed discussion of these methods and materials can be found at www.expertconsult.com.

OUTCOMES OF ENDOVASCULAR THERAPIES

The clinical outcomes for perioperative arterial interventions prior to, during, and after delivery—specifically in patients with known abnormal placentation—including different protocols of arterial embolization and/or balloon occlusion have been described with good results.[14,20,21] However, these studies lack standardization in patient selection to allow for direct comparison or do not have numbers large enough for analysis of variables that may impact clinical success or failure. Kirby et al. assessed previously published series with 10 or more patients from 1992 to 2009 and found initial success rates as low as 58% and final success rates ranging from approximately 70% to 100%.[11] In a retrospective analysis of 43 patients, this group reported a technical success rate of 100% for arterial embolization in PPH. The primary clinical success rate was 79% (33 of 42 patients).[11] Five patients required a second embolization procedure, and there was cessation of hemorrhage in four of these patients, with the resulting final clinical success 88%.

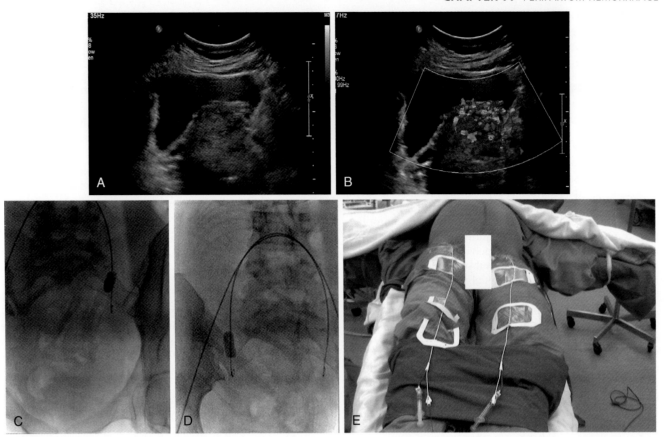

FIGURE 77-4. Intraarterial balloon placement in patient with placenta percreta. Ultrasound **(A-B)** showed placental invasion through uterine myometrium into bladder wall. Patient underwent preoperative placement of bilateral internal iliac artery balloon catheters **(C-E)**. Note faintly visible fetal long bones on fluoroscopic images.

TABLE 77-2. Peripartum Hemorrhage Adjuvant Therapies

Uterotonics
Compression sutures
Tamponade balloon
Hematologic therapy:
    Infusion of recombinant activated factor VII (rFVIIa)
    Intraoperative blood salvage, autotransfusion

In another recent study including 76 patients, Ganguli et al. also reported a technical success rate of 100%.[22] The clinical success rate was 95% overall. Results were stratified with respect to primary PPH (hemorrhage within the first 24 hours of delivery) and secondary PPH (hemorrhage occurring more than 24 hours after delivery), and each group had clinical success rates of 98% and 88%, respectively.[22] Management of PPH in the particular clinical setting of abnormal placentation continues to evolve.

Sivan et al. reviewed outcomes for 30 patients with presumed placenta accreta who underwent prophylactic pelvic artery catheterization of the internal iliac arteries.[21] Accreta was confirmed in 25 cases (83.3%). Twenty-three of the patients (76.6%) had embolization and 2 (8%) had hysterectomy. The authors reported a decreased median estimated blood loss and no major catheterization-related complications in patients with placenta accreta.[21] Additionally, three women had subsequent pregnancies as well as

uncomplicated cesarean section delivery. The authors postulated that in these high-risk patients, this endovascular protocol may prevent hysterectomy and preserve fertility.

In a study by Tan et al., 11 patients with placenta accreta or its variants underwent perioperative internal iliac balloon occlusion for cesarean delivery. They reported 39.4% less intraoperative blood loss ($P = 0.042$) and 52.1% less mean blood volume transfused ($P = 0.005$) in patients with known placenta accreta or variants.[14]

In separate reports, Timmermans et al. and Alkazaleh et al. described "conservative" management of patients with abnormal or invasive placentation (e.g., cesarean section in which the placenta remained) and then postoperative arterial embolization to promote involution and shedding of the placenta.[23,24] In the Timmermans review, there were 12 patients in whom the diagnosis of invasive placenta was made antepartum, and the placenta was left completely in situ. Endovascular therapy failed in 3 of the 12 patients (25%); conversely, embolization treatment was successful in 75%.

However, Bodner et al. reported on 28 patients with placenta accreta/percreta, 6 of whom underwent balloon occlusion, cesarean section, transcatheter embolization, and cesarean hysterectomy.[25] They could find no significant difference in intraoperative blood loss. Similarly, a retrospective case-control comparison by Shrivastava et al.[16] also reported that prophylactic intravascular balloon catheters did not benefit patients with placenta accreta undergoing cesarean hysterectomy in terms of overall blood loss, operative time, or hospital days.

COMPLICATIONS

Overall complication rates for PPH embolization have been reported as 6% to 7%.[13,26] Identifying the precise causality of complications in these patients may be quite complex, since problems may be compounded by the hemorrhage itself and the associated medical and surgical therapies.

Minor postprocedure complications related to groin access can occur. Postembolic syndrome (PES) may be the most common minor complication. The major complication of end-organ ischemia is quite rare, given the robust arterial environment of the pelvis. Conflicting reports debate the use of PVA and the subsequent development of ischemic complications. Kirby et al. advise that nonabsorbable particles should be avoided.[11]

Temporary or permanent menopause may occur after arterial embolization, but the exact incidence in patients with PPH and embolization treatment is unknown. Patients should be counseled that despite the high rate of technical and clinical success, retention of fertility is not guaranteed, and urgent or emergent hysterectomy may still be required if persistent hemorrhage occurs, particularly in patients with invasive placentation.

KEY POINTS

- Patients with peripartum hemorrhage (PPH) may be triaged to embolization treatment when other medical or surgical therapies fail.
- Embolization is straightforward, with a high rate of clinical success and low complication rate.
- Arterial embolization may be coordinated with other obstetrical manipulations and surgeries to decrease the morbidity and mortality of PPH patients.
- The perioperative use of endovascular techniques in patients with abnormal placentation is still controversial.

► **SUGGESTED READINGS**

Brown BJ, Heaston DK, Poulson AM, et al. Uncontrollable post-partum bleeding: a new approach to hemostasis through angiographic arterial embolisation. Obstet Gynecol 1979;54:361–5.

Kirby JM, Kachura JR, Rajan DK, et al. Arterial embolization for primary postpartum hemorrhage. J Vasc Interv Radiol 2009;20(8):1036–45.

Schuurmans N, MacKinnon C, Lane C, Etches D. SOGC Clinical Practice Guidelines: Prevention and management of postpartum haemorrhage. J Obstet Gynaecol Can 2000;88:1–11. Accessed at www.sogc.org/guidelines/public/88E-CPG-April2000.pdf

The complete reference list is available online at www.expertconsult.com.

CHAPTER **78**

Management of Pelvic Hemorrhage in Trauma

Patrick C. Malloy

In most major trauma centers, angiography and transcatheter embolization have become the standard of care for managing pelvic hemorrhage, either as primary treatment or an as adjunct to open surgery and orthopedic stabilization techniques. Dynamic contrast-enhanced multidetector computed tomography (CT) imaging can rapidly detect the site of hemorrhage, whereas modern endovascular techniques can often allow embolization by selective catheterization in a timely fashion. A wide array of embolic agents are available, from traditional Gelfoam administration for proximal nonselective embolization to microcoils and fibered detachable coils for selective or superselective deployment. Optimal patient outcome requires a team effort so other concomitant serious injuries can be actively treated during the endovascular procedure. This effort often involves active participation from trauma surgery, intensive care medicine, subspecialty-trained radiology technologists, critical care and trauma nursing, perfusion therapy, and respiratory therapy. Current-day angiographic suites are equipped for monitoring and managing an actively bleeding patient. Optimal treatment frequently requires the interventionalist to identify the site of active bleeding, but the clinical team must ensure there will be no lapse in ongoing therapy during the embolization procedure. With this team-based approach, patients are often able to safely undergo endovascular therapy for pelvic hemorrhage and avoid open surgery, the results of which can be compromised by difficult operative exposure, complex vascular anatomy, and active hemorrhage at the time of the procedure, resulting in excessive operative mortality.

INDICATIONS

Angiography and possibly endovascular intervention are indicated in the setting of known or suspected pelvic hemorrhage due to blunt or penetrating pelvic trauma.[1-4] Preprocedural dynamic contrast-enhanced CT, with acquisitions in both the arterial and venous phases, is extremely useful in selecting patients and planning the procedure. CT findings of vascular injury in the setting of pelvic trauma may range from normal or nearly normal to signs of previous or active bleeding, such as intraperitoneal and retroperitoneal blood, vascular pseudoaneurysms, and frank extravasation. In addition, the soft tissue and skeletal injuries accurately depicted on CT frequently provide a clue to the site of the injured vessel. CT is accurate in demonstrating intraabdominal solid organ visceral trauma that may require open exploration before angiography. Despite the accuracy of CT, however, it is useful to remember that these images represent merely a snapshot in time in the evolution of injury in a trauma patient. Angiography may therefore be indicated because of the mechanism of injury or clinical deterioration in a previously stable patient in whom CT did not demonstrate active hemorrhage. Vascular injury in

patients undergoing angiography in the setting of pelvic trauma may include the gamut of small- to medium-vein and small arteriole and capillary transection or injury, often not seen on angiography, to medium- to large-artery pseudoaneurysms, stretch injuries, dissections, and vascular truncations. These larger arterial injuries may produce a complicated clinical course that is often characterized by alternating periods of relative stability and rapid destabilization. These patients may require emergency angiography and intervention without repeat CT imaging.

To summarize, indications for angiography and embolization in the setting of pelvic trauma include[5]:

1. Major pelvic fracture with signs of bleeding, and ongoing transfusion requirements in patients in whom nonpelvic sources of bleeding have been excluded.
2. Major pelvic fracture, with or without other associated injury, in patients in whom pelvic bleeding cannot be controlled at surgery.
3. Pelvic trauma with evidence of active extravasation of contrast material on CT.
4. Pelvic trauma with hemodynamic instability in patients in whom other nonpelvic sources of bleeding are excluded, even without evidence of active extravasation on CT.

CONTRAINDICATIONS

Contraindications to angiography and endovascular intervention may include acutely unstable patients with multisystem trauma. Such patients may have multiple sites of potential hemorrhage, including the pelvic vessels and solid organs such as the spleen, liver, and kidney. These unstable patients may have such overwhelming acute blood loss that they may best benefit from acute operative exploration or "damage-control surgery," followed by angiography and endovascular intervention. Adjunctive pelvic packing, as part of a damage-control protocol, may be effective in achieving rapid hemostasis in hemodynamically unstable patients with pelvic ring injuries and may either preclude the need for embolization or play a complementary role with subsequent endovascular treatment.[6,7] In addition, in patients with acute intraperitoneal hemorrhage, the peritoneal cavity may be rapidly distended with blood and result in an abdominal compartment syndrome that may severely inhibit blood return via the inferior vena cava and perfusion to visceral organs, and restrict ventilation secondary to diaphragmatic elevation and the resultant reduction in tidal volume and high airway pressure. These patients may require open exploration and intraperitoneal clot extraction for stabilization before the endovascular procedure.

Patients with altered vascular anatomy due to previous vascular surgery (e.g., aortobifemoral bypass, interventions such as endovascular repair for abdominal aortic aneurysm) may represent a relative contraindication because of severely altered anatomy. In general, however, these patients typically may present challenges with respect to vascular access and selective catheterization, but endovascular therapy is not precluded because of the frequent preservation of pelvic vessels.

In the setting of trauma and acute blood loss, patients can suffer loss of coagulation proteins, platelet deficits, and other associated factors such as hypothermia that can lead to rapid development of an acquired coagulopathy. Even though the degree of coagulopathy can be severe, it remains more of a management challenge than a contraindication. Access site complications can be minimized by using closure devices when appropriate, or by leaving a vascular sheath in place until the coagulopathy can at least be partially corrected.

Some patients may have a relative contraindication to the use of iodinated contrast material, either because of a previous history of a severe contrast agent reaction or because of marginal renal function, particularly in the setting of long-standing insulin-requiring diabetes mellitus. In clinical practice in the acute setting, it is rare that we have sufficient history to document a previous life-threatening reaction to iodinated contrast material. Use of iodixanol (Visipaque), an iodinated monomeric isoosmolar contrast agent, may minimize the potential for reaction to contrast media and for contrast medium–induced nephropathy.[8]

In the setting of femoral neck fracture, embolization of the ipsilateral superior gluteal artery or the ipsilateral posterior division of the internal iliac artery may be associated with delayed bone healing after orthopedic interventions on the femur or with avascular necrosis.[9] In these situations, however, it is unclear whether there is a clinical difference between permanent coil occlusion or Gelfoam embolization of posterior division vessels.

EQUIPMENT

Fixed equipment for diagnosis and intervention in patients with pelvic hemorrhage includes an angiographic system, typically equipped with a large–field of view flat-panel detector or image intensifier capable of high–frame rate 1024×1024 digital subtraction angiography and high-quality magnification fluoroscopy. These systems are discussed in more detail in previous chapters. Newer systems equipped with flat-panel detectors are capable of rotational acquisitions that produce CT-like cross-sectional data. In the setting of pelvic hemorrhage, this capability may be useful in confirming treatment of a site of hemorrhage seen on preprocedural CT. Refinement of the use of these flat-panel CT acquisitions will require further clinical study. In addition, the system should be equipped with barrier radiation protection devices for both the patient and operator, and dose-saving technology such as last image hold, variable frame rate, and variable-dose fluoroscopy.

Typical catheters used for pelvic angiography and interventions include 4F and 5F pigtails, reverse-curve Simmons 1 and SOS catheters, and angled catheters such as the Cobra C2, Berenstein, and vertebral curve catheters. Most diagnostic angiography will be done via pigtails or 0.035/0.038-inch (inner diameter) catheters because of the need for injections at relatively high flow rates. Coaxial microcatheters are often used for selective and superselective applications. We prefer 0.018- to 0.021-inch (inner diameter) microcatheters because of the ability to deploy embolization microcoils, the newer detachable coils, and Gelfoam slurry or small pledgets if needed. Larger-lumen, 0.027-inch (inner diameter) microcatheters offer the advantage of higher contrast material flow rates but may be suboptimal for microcoil deployment because of their larger lumen, which at times does not adequately constrain the coil and results in difficulties in deployment.

Embolization procedures generally involve the use of coils or Gelfoam for vascular occlusion. Spherical embolic material is available in a wide range of sizes and may occasionally be used (discussed later). Embolization coils may include 0.035-inch-diameter stainless steel or fibered platinum coils or 0.018-inch-diameter fibered platinum or fibered detachable coils. When a discrete area of extravasation or pseudoaneurysm is identified and the patient's clinical condition permits, selective coil embolization is preferable to regional particulate embolization. Gelfoam pledgets or slurry may be used as an adjunct to selective distal coil embolization or may be used as primary treatment to achieve rapid vascular occlusion in the setting of severe hemodynamic instability.

As mentioned previously, nonionic contrast material is used exclusively for both diagnosis and intervention in pelvic hemorrhage. In the acute posttraumatic setting, iodixanol, a monomeric isoosmolar agent, is used because of a slightly lower incidence of contrast medium–induced nephropathy. In a stable, non–volume-depleted adult, dimeric nonionic agents such as iohexol may be used. In patients with marginal renal function, iodixanol is our iodinated contrast agent of choice. Carbon dioxide may be substituted in these settings to reduce the total load of iodinated contrast material, but it is usually limited to large-vessel injections and proximal internal iliac arteries. (Note: In trauma patients, CO_2 should only be used below the level of the diaphragm because of the potential risk of stroke.) We prefer the use of iodinated contrast agents for selective and superselective pelvic angiography to confirm the site of vessel injury and guide the deposition of embolic material.

TECHNIQUE

Anatomy and Approach

Vascular access sites for pelvic angiography and intervention follow the guidelines for diagnostic angiography of the abdominal aorta, as outlined in previous chapters, with the inclusion of some special considerations. Arterial access is typically gained in the right or left common femoral artery. Selection of the right or left side may be dictated by (1) findings on preprocedural cross-sectional imaging, (2) in conjunction with operator experience and preference, or (3) in the possible presence of concomitant injuries, stabilization devices, or previously placed vascular catheters. Despite the fact that a patient with acute pelvic hemorrhage has often sustained recent pelvic trauma and may have a concomitant femoral/acetabular fracture, groin hematoma, or unstable pelvis requiring placement of a binder or external fixation device, access can most often be effectively gained in the common femoral artery without complication. Axillary or brachial access is rarely necessary. Some interventionalists find it technically easier to catheterize the internal iliac artery and its branches from a contralateral femoral approach. Because of the frequent presence of cross-pelvic collaterals, selective bilateral internal iliac angiography is most often necessary for a complete study in the setting of blunt trauma. In the majority of cases, however, the study can be performed from a single common femoral entry access.

Technical Aspects

Initial angiographic evaluation of the pelvis in the setting of trauma is optimally performed with a flush catheter placed in the midportion of the infrarenal abdominal aorta. The importance of the flush run is to visualize the entire pelvic arterial vasculature, including the median sacral, iliolumbar, inferior epigastric, and deep circumflex iliac vessels, which would not be visualized on selective internal iliac angiography. In addition, internal iliac branch vessels will be visualized before catheter and guidewire manipulations, which might otherwise lead to temporary spasm. Selective arteriography of the internal iliac arteries follows the flush examination, the initial side being dictated by the most significant pathology shown on CT or flush angiography. Further subselective catheterization is dictated by abnormalities seen on the initial angiograms or on preprocedural CT. Superselective catheterization of anterior or posterior division branch vessels often requires the use of a microcatheter to avoid spasm or restriction of flow. Use of 4F catheters with a 0.038-inch lumen may allow superselective catheterization and treatment of internal iliac branch vessels while retaining the option of coaxial microcatheter placement if needed. At least two views separated by 45 to 60 degrees should be obtained on each side. The ipsilateral anterior oblique view visualizes the proximal to mid–superior gluteal artery as it exits the pelvis via the sciatic notch, a frequent site of injury in "open-book" fractures of the pelvis. The contralateral anterior oblique view separates the anteroposterior ramifications of the branches of the anterior division.

Coil embolization is most frequently accomplished by placing the catheter tip just proximal to the area of injury and occluding the upstream vessel. In many cases it is impractical to negotiate a catheter distal to the site of injury and coil back across the injured vessel. In the case of dissection or transection of a larger vessel, as may be seen in the superior gluteal artery at the sciatic notch, coils are placed in the proximal portion of the vessel and then deployed back to just beyond the origin of the vessel. Coil pushers are preferable to injecting coils. Figures 78-1 through 78-6 demonstrate the findings from a patient after a severe pelvic crush injury. Despite preexistent vascular disease, the vessels are significantly narrowed because of shock and ongoing blood loss. Active extravasation is easily seen from the mid- to distal portion of a branch of the left anterior internal iliac artery, which is selectively catheterized and embolized.

Gelfoam may be used as a primary embolic agent or as an adjunct to coil embolization. Both Gelfoam slurry (a gelatinous suspension of small pledgets) and discrete larger pledgets are used. Gelfoam powder should be avoided

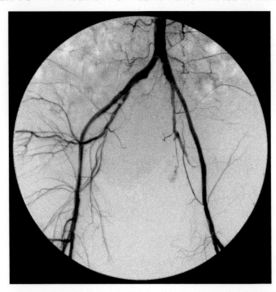

FIGURE 78-1. Rollover crush pelvic injury. A flush pelvic arteriogram demonstrates active extravasation from left anterior division.

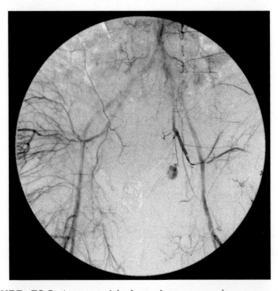

FIGURE 78-2. Later arterial phase shows a pseudoaneurysm. Note marked pelvic vasoconstriction secondary to hypotension.

because of its tendency for embolization of far distal vascular beds, which may lead to ischemic complications. Gelfoam embolization can be a rapid, highly effective means of attaining hemodynamic control in an acutely bleeding patient and may be the preferred agent in an unstable patient in whom subselective catheterization of the bleeding vessel appears to be a technically demanding and time-consuming task. Gelfoam slurry, mixed with full- to half-strength contrast material to allow visualization during deployment, may be introduced through both 4F/5F catheters and microcatheters. Larger Gelfoam pledgets may be deployed through catheters with a 0.038-inch lumen and are particularly effective for rapid occlusion of a large vessel such as the anterior or posterior division vessels or the main internal iliac artery.

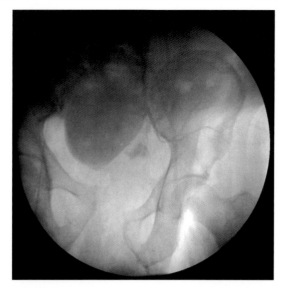

FIGURE 78-3. Unsubtracted view shows "open-book" pelvic fracture.

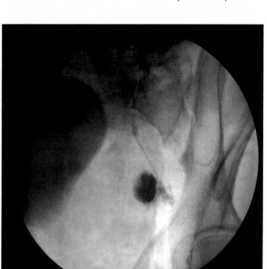

FIGURE 78-4. Superselective catheterization with a microcatheter.

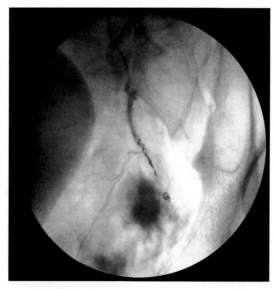

FIGURE 78-5. Result after selective embolization.

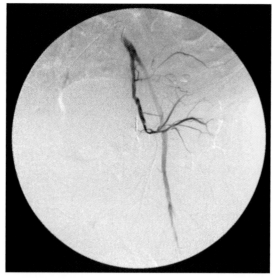

FIGURE 78-6. Result after nonselective embolization.

CONTROVERSIES AND SPECIAL CONSIDERATIONS

Nonselective embolization of the internal iliac artery in the absence of active extravasation is controversial despite localizing CT findings suggesting previous pelvic bleeding. There have been reports of fatal gluteal necrosis[10] and avascular necrosis of the femoral head[9] after internal iliac artery embolization. Particulate embolization of the posterior division of the internal iliac artery in the absence of documented vascular injury on angiography should therefore be avoided or approached with extreme caution.

Pediatric and pregnant patients require special consideration. Although pelvic fractures are uncommon in children, several associated factors in the setting of trauma have been found to be associated with pelvic fractures. In a study of all blunt trauma patients at the Johns Hopkins Children's Center from 1990 to 2005, in the setting of blunt trauma, four factors were associated with a higher incidence of pelvic fractures: being Caucasian, age between 5 and 14 years, being struck as a pedestrian, or a motor vehicle crash occupant. These data may aid in selecting patients for more advanced imaging and possible intervention.[11] Use of newer 3F or 2F catheters enables safe, effective vascular access for intervention when surgery is contraindicated or impractical.[12]

Pelvic and acetabular fractures during pregnancy are associated with high maternal (9%) and fetal (35%) mortality rate. Pedestrian/automobile trauma is associated with a higher maternal mortality rate, and automobile collisions are associated with a higher fetal mortality, compared to falls or other trauma. Although injury severity correlates with both maternal and fetal outcomes, mortality has not been found to correlate with trimester of pregnancy, fracture classification (simple vs. complex), or fracture type (acetabular vs. pelvic).[13] Angiography and embolization is technically feasible in the pregnant patient regardless of fetal age, and often superselective techniques can be employed to avoid occlusion of the uterine vessels. The primary goal is to quickly stop the bleeding, however, and larger-vessel damage control–type embolization may be necessary as a lifesaving measure for either the mother or fetus in the unstable patient.

OUTCOMES

Continued refinement of modern guidelines for care has resulted in significantly better outcomes for patients with pelvic hemorrhage after trauma than those of historical controls (before the advent of embolization and use of CT for diagnosis and triage). Today's paradigm involves open exploration, orthopedic stabilization, and angiography with embolization. Before the use of angiography in pelvic trauma, Hawkins et al. published a series of 192 patients over a 3-year period from 1966 to 1969; 35 underwent open laparotomy for hemorrhage, and 7 (20%) died as a result of massive hemorrhage and unsustainable transfusion requirements.[14] In 1979, Matalon et al. reported a series of 28 patients who underwent angiography after pelvic trauma; 20 showed active extravasation, and 18 underwent successful embolization. Of the 18, all demonstrated angiographic control, and 17 demonstrated clinical control, which led the authors to conclude that angiography with embolization facilitates the management of patients with pelvic trauma.[1] Panetta et al. reported a series of 31 patients with extensive pelvic fractures and large retroperitoneal hematomas who underwent embolization. Successful embolization was achieved in 27 patients (87.1%), leading the authors to conclude that embolization was the "procedure of choice" for treating significant pelvic hemorrhage.[3] Agolini et al. reviewed the experience at a level I trauma center over a 5-year period in which 806 patients were evaluated for pelvic fractures; 35 required pelvic angiography for suspected hemorrhage, 15 of whom required embolization. Treatment of all 15 was successful, and no deaths from continued hemorrhage occurred in the embolization group.[4] Velmahos et al. reported a series of 100 consecutive patients over a 2-year period who underwent angiography for major pelvic fractures (n = 65) or visceral trauma (n = 35). Fifty-seven of these patients were treated by embolization for active extravasation, and 23 underwent embolization for indirect signs of vascular injury. Embolization was found to be effective in 95%. Four patients had recurrent bleeding, three of whom were treated by repeat embolization. In this series, embolization in the setting of acute blunt pelvic injury was found to be highly effective in the permanent control of acute pelvic hemorrhage.[15] Embolization has been demonstrated to be equally as effective for penetrating pelvic trauma.[16]

CT has played a major role in shaping the care of patients with pelvic trauma. Advancements in CT, with the capability of rapid-bolus arterial imaging techniques, have resulted in accurate diagnosis and localization of active pelvic hemorrhage. Shanmuganathan et al. reported a series of 26 patients in whom CT was able to accurately distinguish active hemorrhage from blood clot and demonstrate the anatomic location and cause of the bleeding.[17] Stephen et al. subsequently reported a series of 111 patients who underwent CT after pelvic trauma, 11 of whom required angiography for signs of clinical deterioration. In these patients, the positive predictive value of extravasation seen on CT was 80%, and the predictive value of a negative test was 98%.[18] Rapid advances in CT technology have solidified the central role of multislice CT in evaluating patients after pelvic trauma. CT has replaced angiography in the diagnostic evaluation of pelvic trauma. In patients stable enough to undergo CT, this modality serves to appropriately triage patients between conservative therapy, orthopedic stabilization and angiography, and open surgery.

Overall patient outcomes have been positively influenced by the emergence of transcatheter embolization as part of the standard of care in current management of pelvic hemorrhage associated with trauma. This clinical paradigm still requires difficult decision making, which can be a challenge for even the most skilled clinician. Newer techniques and products for embolization may improve the procedure, but the historical literature has documented pelvic embolization in the setting of pelvic trauma to be safe and highly effective from its inception. Overall mortality in the setting of pelvic trauma, however, is significantly influenced by associated injuries.[19] In a study of 16,630 blunt trauma registry patients, 1545 (9.3%) had a pelvic fracture, and 16.5% of these patients had associated abdominal injuries. Those with severe pelvic fractures and an Abbreviated Injury Scale (AIS) of 4 or above had a 30.7% incidence of associated intraabdominal injuries, most commonly involving the bladder, urethra, and liver. Although only 0.8% of these patients died as a result of the pelvic fracture, the overall mortality of the pelvic fracture group was 13.5%.[20] Other studies have similarly documented the frequent association of chest and head trauma with severe pelvic fractures, and these associated injuries often had the greatest impact on the eventual outcome of the patient.[21,22]

COMPLICATIONS

There have been few reported complications with pelvic embolization for traumatic hemorrhage. A case of bladder necrosis secondary to pelvic embolization in the trauma setting was reported.[23] Takahira et al. reported gluteal muscle necrosis in 5 of 151 patients after embolization for pelvic trauma.[10] A case of avascular necrosis of the femoral head was reported in a 41-year-old woman after embolization for pelvic trauma.[9] A small series reported three patients who experienced lower extremity paresis after pelvic embolization for pelvic tumor.[24] Bilateral internal iliac embolization has been found in one study to have no impact on male sexual function. Sexual dysfunction, in this series, was found to be due to the effects of the pelvic fracture alone.[25] In comparison, bladder, gluteal, rectal, scrotal, and perineal necrosis has been reported in surgical series of internal iliac artery ligation for pelvic hemorrhage and in oncologic series.[26,27]

POSTPROCEDURAL AND FOLLOW-UP CARE

Embolization patients should follow standard guidelines for access-site monitoring after arterial interventions, as outlined in earlier chapters. Although it is tempting to allow vascular sheaths to remain in place for arterial pressure monitoring and management of the presumed coagulopathy associated with rapid volume resuscitation, it is often wise to remove these devices as soon as possible to avoid complications of distal embolization and access-site complications. A variety of vascular closure devices are now available that may be appropriately used in this clinical scenario.

In a successful embolization patient after pelvic trauma, hemodynamic parameters should stabilize rapidly. Transfusion requirements should decrease shortly after the procedure, although fluid shifts and equilibration from rapid volume resuscitation may prompt further transfusion, despite the absence of sustained active extravasation. Continued close hemodynamic monitoring is warranted after embolization. If a patient destabilizes after successful pelvic embolization, repeat abdominal and pelvic CT should be performed to identify the site of bleeding, which may be recurrent in the pelvis or at a previously unrecognized site of vascular trauma.

► **SUGGESTED READINGS**

Lang EK. Transcatheter embolization of pelvic vessels for control of intractable hemorrhage. Radiology 1981;140:331–9.

Savage C, Cohen AM, Moore FA. Invited commentary. Radiographics 2004;24:1605–6.

Tomacruz RS, Briston RE, Montz FT. Management of pelvic hemorrhage. Surg Clin North Am 2001;81:925–48.

Yoon W, Kim JK, Jeong YY, et al. Pelvic arterial hemorrhage in patients with pelvic fractures: detection with contrast-enhanced CT. Radiographics 2004;24:1591–605.

The complete reference list is available online at www.expertconsult.com.

KEY POINTS

- Pelvic angiography plus embolization is part of the standard of care for patients with traumatic pelvic hemorrhage.

- Contrast medium–enhanced multidetector computed tomography imaging is effective in detecting and localizing active pelvic hemorrhage.

- Pelvic embolization has a high rate of both technical and clinical success in treating active pelvic hemorrhage.

- Pelvic embolization has few relative contraindications and a low complication rate.

CHAPTER 79

Management of Male Varicocele

Bryan Grieme, Andrew Akman, Ali Albayati, Emily J. Timmreck, Emily M. Tanski, and Anthony C. Venbrux

INTRODUCTION

Although relatively uncommon, male varicocele often affects otherwise healthy men with symptoms such as pain and infertility. The concept of treating a male varicocele was first developed by Dr. Paré in the 16th century, primarily to treat symptoms such as pain and swelling. The British surgeon Dr. Barfield first proposed a link between male infertility and varicoceles in the 19th century. In recent years, research has suggested a strong association with men who have symptomatic varicoceles and infertility. Today, interventional radiology offers a minimally invasive catheter-directed approach to embolize varicoceles. This chapter will review the diagnosis, etiology, treatment indications, and techniques of managing the male varicocele.

INCIDENCE

Varicocele is most commonly diagnosed in the adult male population at a rate between 15% and 17%. The incidence occurs in less than 1% in boys younger than age 10 and then plateaus at 15% in late adolescence. Approximately 90% of varicoceles occur on the left side. The remaining 10% occur bilaterally. Gat et al. found an unusually high incidence of bilateral varicocele (80.7%; 210 of 255) in infertile men with varicocele, but only 21 of 210 (10%) right-sided varicoceles were palpable.[1] The incidence of unilateral right-sided varicocele is 0.4%.[2] The finding of an isolated right-sided varicocele warrants further evaluation. It can be associated with situs inversus, as well as with retroperitoneal and abdominal tumors such as lymphoma and metastases.[3,4]

DIAGNOSIS

Varicocele diagnosis is primarily made by clinical presentation and physical exam. The simple grading system of Dubin and Amelar[5] is most commonly used: grade 0, not palpable; grade 1, palpable only with the patient standing and performing a Valsalva maneuver; grade 2, palpable without a Valsalva maneuver; and grade 3, visible.

High-resolution real-time ultrasound and color-flow Doppler ultrasound may be used to either confirm the diagnosis or detect subclinical (nonpalpable) varicoceles. The significance of subclinical varicocele with regard to infertility is currently controversial.[6-9] Doppler ultrasound may further distinguish between types of varicoceles and their blood flow characteristics.[10] Because only palpable varicoceles have been documented to be associated with infertility, the *Report on Varicocele and Infertility* (published jointly by the Male Infertility Best Practice Committee of the American Urological Association and the Practice Committee of the American Society for Reproductive Medicine, September 2004) recommends that routine evaluation of infertile men with varicoceles include a medical and reproductive history, physical examination, and a minimum of two semen analyses, but imaging studies are only indicated if the physical exam is inconclusive.[11]

Spermatic venography is another imaging technique. It is generally reserved for venous mapping in preparation for transcatheter embolotherapy or surgical ligation[12] (Fig. 79-1).

Varicocele is seen in about 40% of men seeking evaluation for infertility. There is some controversy regarding the causal relationship of varicocele and infertility (e.g., 85% of men with varicoceles are fertile, and reports of improvement in pregnancy rate are inconsistent[2,13-17]). Significant evidence in the literature supports the hypothesis that varicoceles have a negative effect on the testis and fertility and that varicocele repair can reverse or prevent these effects.[1,18-24]

In a prospective trial, Laven et al. randomized 67 young adults with varicoceles to treatment (percutaneous embolotherapy) and nontreatment groups; 21 healthy male volunteers without varicoceles served as controls. One year after treatment, left testis volumes were measured and found to be comparable to those of the control group and significantly different (larger) ($P < .001$) from the untreated group. Semen quality (sperm concentration) increased significantly ($P < .01$) in the treated group and was unchanged in the untreated and control groups.[25]

INDICATIONS

The three primary indications for treatment of a varicocele are (1) subfertility or infertility in adult men, (2) varicocele and testicular atrophy in adolescent or pediatric-aged patients, and (3) pain. Recurrence of varicocele after surgical ligation is also an indication. The most common indication for treatment of a varicocele in an adult male is infertility/subfertility. Criteria for treatment in this group should include: (1) abnormal semen parameters, (2) absence of any other identifiable or correctable causes of male infertility, and (3) a female partner with normal fertility or treated infertility. Adult men with a palpable varicocele and abnormal semen analysis but who are not currently attempting to conceive should also be offered varicocele repair. Adolescents and young men with a varicocele but a normal-sized ipsilateral testicle or normal semen analysis, or both, should be offered annual follow-up monitoring.[11]

CONTRAINDICATIONS

Surgical ligation rather than percutaneous embolotherapy should be chosen in patients with a history of severe allergy to contrast media or when a skilled interventional radiologist is unavailable.

559

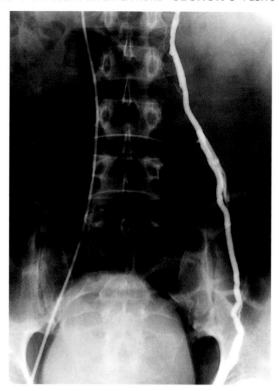

FIGURE 79-1. Left gonadal venography. *(From Kim SH. Uroradiology. In: Eisenberg RL, editor. Radiology: an illustrated history. Philadelphia: Mosby-Year Book; 1995.)*

EQUIPMENT

The following equipment is required to perform transcatheter embolization:
- High-resolution digital fluoroscopy
- Standard catheters and guidewires
- Ultrasound for vascular access
- Contrast material
- 7F or 8F vascular sheaths
- Hockey stick–shaped catheters
- Guide catheters with Simmons- and Hopkins-type (i.e., modified Cobra) curves
- Microcatheters and guidewires
- A selection of standard and hydrophilic wires, such as Bentson, Rosen, Terumo, Roadrunner
- Embolization coils and, when appropriate, microcoils
- Appropriate procedural and postprocedural staffing

TECHNIQUE

Anatomy and Approach

Venous blood drains from each testicle into multiple venous sinuses called the *pampiniform plexus* or the *spermatic venous plexus*. This plexus coalesces at approximately the level of the femoral head to form the internal spermatic vein (ISV), the primary draining vein. Classically, the left ISV drains into the left renal vein, and the right ISV into the inferior vena cava (IVC) anterolaterally, just caudal to the right renal vein. This classic anatomic pattern is seen on the right in 78% of patients and on the left in 79%.

Variations from the classic pattern seen on the right are termination of the ISV in the renal vein in 8% and multiple veins terminating in the IVC and the renal vein in 16%. On the left, multiple veins terminating in the renal vein are seen in 20%. Rarely, one of multiple branches may terminate in the infrarenal IVC.[26]

Three other veins arise from within the pampiniform plexus: the external pudendal, vasal, and cremasteric veins. The external pudendal vein forms at the level of the superior pubic ramus and drains into the great saphenous vein. The vasal or ductus deferens vein forms just above the testicle, joins the inferior or superior vesicle vein, and ultimately drains into the internal iliac vein. The cremasteric (external spermatic) vein forms at the level of the superior pubic ramus and drains via the inferior epigastric vein into the external iliac vein. Based on the results of an intraoperative surgical venography study performed by Wishahi,[27] venous drainage of the testes is mainly via the ISV, followed by the external pudendal, vasal, and cremasteric veins in decreasing order of significance.

The number of valves in spermatic veins is reported to vary between zero and three. The relationship of valves to the formation of a varicocele is uncertain. Absence of valves has been demonstrated in autopsy series in men without varicoceles. Furthermore, the cause-and-effect relationship is uncertain in that venous dilation may cause valves to become incompetent.

In addition to drainage to the systemic circulation through the external pudendal, vasal, and cremasteric veins, additional collateral communication between testicular venous drainage and the systemic circulation exists in a significant number of men. These collaterals communicate with the retroperitoneal, peritoneal, ureteral, and adrenal veins and with the portal circulation through the splenic, superior mesenteric, and sigmoid colonic veins. Wishahi,[27] using gradual pressure venography (simulating physiologic conditions), demonstrated no cross-communication between the left and right internal spermatic venous plexuses in the scrotum or pelvis, but did show cross-communication between the ISVs at the L3 level and the medial spermatic vein divisions in 55%. Such communications can create aberrantly fed varicoceles and contribute to recurrence or lower the technical success rate (or both). Wishahi also contends that the lack of intrascrotal or pelvic cross-communication supports the theory that elevated scrotal temperature rather than retrograde flow of renal or adrenal metabolites is the more likely cause of the bilateral effect of varicocele on testicular dysfunction.[27]

The primary etiologic factor for development of a varicocele appears to be a right-angle entry of the left spermatic vein into the high-pressure system of the left renal vein. This creates a hydrostatic column of pressure against which the pampiniform plexus must function to allow testicular venous outflow in the upright position.[28] Compression of the left renal vein between the aorta and superior mesenteric artery (nutcracker syndrome) has been described as a cause of left-sided varicocele.[29] The presence of left renal vein entrapment was found by Pallwein et al. to be associated with a significantly higher recurrence rate after surgical repair. In their study, 16 of 84 patients (19%) with left-sided varicocele had left renal vein entrapment. Within 19 months (standard deviation, 11.7 months), 27 patients (32.1%) demonstrated recurrence of varicocele. All 16 patients with left renal vein entrapment experienced recurrence.[30]

Technical Aspects

Patients undergoing transcatheter embolotherapy are generally treated on an outpatient basis with intravenous conscious sedation. In patients without a history of heart disease, atropine may be administered to reduce the incidence of vagal reactions. Gonadal and buttock shielding is provided, and fluoroscopy is limited to minimize the gonadal radiation dose. A femoral vein or jugular venous[31] approach may be used. With the femoral approach, the right common femoral vein is accessed, followed by placement of a 7F or 8F vascular sheath. An internal spermatic venogram is then performed. If using the femoral approach, a 7F or 8F Hopkins curved catheter (modified Cobra catheter) is used to selectively catheterize the left renal vein and then the orifice of the left ISV. For right-sided varicoceles treated from a femoral approach, a nontapered 7F Simmons-1 guide catheter is used to select the origin of the right ISV, which is usually located on the right anterolateral surface of the vena cava just below the right renal vein. Infrequently, the origin of this vessel is found along the inferior surface of the right renal vein. With the ISV orifice engaged, approximately 10 to 20 mL of contrast material is injected while the patient performs a Valsalva maneuver. One or two radiographs are taken, the images spanning from the level of the orifice of the ISV to the pubic symphysis. Careful collimation, limiting the number of images, and appropriate gonadal and buttock shielding are imperative to minimize the testicular radiation dose. If the ISV is identified and found to be incompetent, transcatheter embolotherapy may proceed.

A variety of agents have been used to occlude the ISV. Mechanical agents include embolization coils (Nester Coils [Cook Medical, Bloomington, Ind.], Interlock coils [Boston Scientific, Cork, Ireland]), Penumbra PC 400 detachable coils (Penumbra Inc., Alameda, Calif.), microcoils, tissue adhesives, compressed Ivalon plugs (Ivalon Inc., San Diego, Calif.), and woven nitinol wire plugs (Amplatzer Vascular Plug [Saint Jude Medical, St. Paul, Minn.]). Other occlusive agents have been used. Sclerosing agents include 3% sodium tetradecyl sulfate (Sotradecol), sodium morrhuate (55 mg/mL; no longer available in the United States), hypertonic glucose (70%-80%), absolute ethanol, hot contrast material, and others.

A recent development for occlusion of the spermatic vein is a self-expanding nitinol occlusion device covered with polytetrafluoroethylene (PTFE) (ArtVentive Endoluminal Occlusion System [ArtVentive Medical Group Inc., Carlsbad, Calif.]). This device is not yet commercially available in the United States but has undergone initial human clinical trials elsewhere with favorable initial clinical results.

When using coils, a 5F nontapered straight end-hole catheter is advanced coaxially through the guide catheter to the distal ISV just above the pubic symphysis. Embolization then proceeds from this level to the ISV origin. The embolic end point is complete occlusion of the ISV and collaterals. If the collateral veins are large, selective catheterization plus embolization is recommended. After left ISV embolization, selective catheterization of the right should be attempted.

If venous incompetence is present, embolization should be performed even in the absence of a clinically apparent varicocele on this side. For right ISV embolization from the femoral approach, a microcatheter may be necessary and is coaxially directed through a Simmons-1 diagnostic catheter.

Microcoils may then be deployed in the same manner as on the left. When using the right internal jugular approach, a gently curved or hockey stick–shaped catheter such as a JB1 or H1H (Benston-Hanafee-Wilson 1 [Terumo Interventional Systems, Somerset, N.J.]), may be used to select the right or left spermatic vein. A microcatheter is not usually required when using the angled diagnostic catheter.

Embolization with a sclerosing agent may be performed with the use of an occlusion balloon catheter positioned in the ISV above the superior pubic ramus. With the balloon inflated caudally, a test injection of contrast material at the cranial end of the ISV is performed to determine the appropriate volume of sclerosing agent needed to fill the vein. An alternative to using an occlusion balloon is to occlude the distal aspect (caudal aspect) of the spermatic vein with a "nest" of coils before injection of the sclerosing agent. To further reduce the risk of reflux of sclerosant into the scrotum, manual compression of the inguinal canal with a leaded glove during injection and for approximately 10 minutes after injection of the sclerosing agent is recommended. Reflux of sclerosing agent into the scrotum may be associated with pampiniform plexus phlebitis and should be scrupulously avoided. Occasionally, collaterals may make embolization challenging (Fig. 79-2).

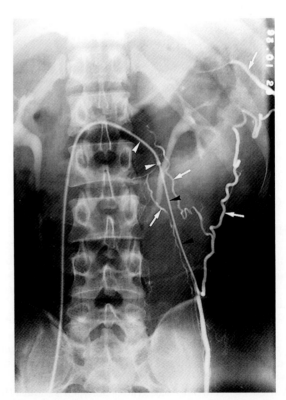

FIGURE 79-2. Left varicocele in 27-year-old man. Note collaterals *(white arrows)*, which may contribute to embolotherapy treatment failures or recurrence. *(From Kim SH. Uroradiology. In: Eisenberg RL, editor. Radiology: an illustrated history. Philadelphia: Mosby-Year Book; 1995.)*

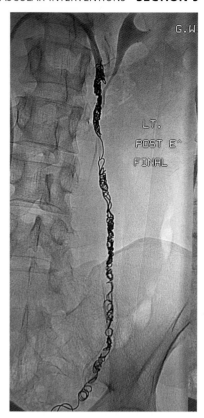

FIGURE 79-3. Digital subtraction completion venogram documenting coil occlusion of left spermatic (gonadal) vein.

OUTCOMES

Technical success rates range between 90% and 97%.[5,14,32] Improvement in semen parameters (sperm count and sperm motility) ranges from 27% to 78% after embolotherapy, and 24% to 84% after surgical corrections.[33,34] In a study of 86 men with varicocele, Steckel et al. found that in men with large varicoceles (grade 3), baseline semen parameters were significantly worse than in those with smaller varicoceles, but showed much greater improvement after varicocelectomy.[35] Improvement in sperm count and motility takes approximately 3 months.[27] Success rates when performing surgical varicocele repair for pain range from 48% to 86% (Fig. 79-3).[36]

COMPLICATIONS

Complications related to percutaneous varicocele embolization are uncommon, occurring in less than 5% of cases, and include nausea, groin hematoma, reaction to contrast material, and femoral vein thrombosis (occurring at the same rate as with any percutaneous femoral vein procedure, i.e., < 1%). As mentioned earlier, significant thrombosis of the pampiniform plexus can occur when sclerosing agents are used; reported incidence is between 1% and 4% and may be associated with significant pain, swelling, or both.

Varicocele recurrence rates range between 4% and 11%.[37] Recurrence rates are generally considered lower in patient cohorts treated by embolotherapy than in patients treated by surgery. Recurrence is usually related to dilation of collaterals not seen at the time of the procedure. Recurrence after surgical ligation is most easily treated with transcatheter techniques, whereas recurrence after embolotherapy is more difficult to treat. Halden and White[38] were able to successfully treat 96% of varicoceles recurring after surgical ligation but only 61% recurring after embolotherapy.

Transcatheter embolotherapy is generally performed in healthy young men with normal life expectancy. Therefore, minimizing the radiation dose is critical. Chalmers et al. calculated the lifetime fatal cancer risk to be about 0.1% in a retrospective series. In a small prospective series, the same investigators showed they could, with meticulous attention to technique, achieve a sevenfold reduction in median radiation dose.[39]

POSTPROCEDURAL AND FOLLOW-UP CARE

After embolization, the sheath and catheter or catheters are removed, and hemostasis is achieved by manual compression. Patients are typically observed for 4 to 6 hours before discharge, with intravenous fluids continued until the patient can tolerate oral fluids. Rest is encouraged for the remainder of the day, with resumption of normal activities the next day. Postprocedural symptoms may include nausea, testicular or back pain (or both), and low-grade fever. Pain is generally treated with nonsteroidal antiinflammatory drugs. Heavy lifting and sports may be resumed in 2 to 3 weeks.

KEY POINTS
• Varicocele is an abnormal dilation of the scrotal pampiniform plexus. It is the most common abnormality found in men evaluated for infertility.
• Treatment options include surgical repair (inguinal, subinguinal, and retroperitoneal approaches) or percutaneous transcatheter embolotherapy.

► **SUGGESTED READINGS**

Benoff S, Gilbert BR. Varicocele and male infertility: part I. Preface. Hum Reprod Update 2001;7:47–54.

Diamond DA. Adolescent varicocele: emerging understanding. BJU Int 2003;92(Suppl 1):48–51.

Evers JLH, Collins JA. Assessment of efficacy of varicocele repair for male subfertility: a systematic review. Lancet 2003;361:1849–52.

Jarow JP. Effects of varicocele on male infertility. Hum Reprod Update 2001;7:59–64.

Kass EJ. Adolescent varicocele. Pediatr Clin North Am 2001;48:1559–69.

Redmon JB, Carey P, Pryor JL. Varicocele—the most common cause of male factor infertility? Hum Reprod Update 2002;8:53–8.

Silber SJ. The varicocele dilemma. Hum Reprod Update 2001;7:70–7.

The complete reference list is available online at www.expertconsult.com.

CHAPTER 80

Management of Female Venous Congestion Syndrome

Darren D. Kies, Judy M. Lee, Anthony C. Venbrux, and Hyun S. Kim

CLINICAL RELEVANCE

Chronic pelvic pain, characterized by non-cyclic pelvic pain for longer than 6 months, is a common medical problem among women.[1] The condition is potentially debilitating, and it afflicts millions of women worldwide. It has been reported that up to 39.1% of women have suffered chronic pelvic pain at some period in their lives.[2]

Pelvic congestion with pelvic varices has been the focus of clinical and research interests for many years since its first description by Richet in 1857[3] and its first association with chronic pelvic pain by Taylor in 1949.[4] Physical symptoms of pelvic congestion causing chronic pelvic pain have been well documented,[5] but with no clear consensus in diagnosis and treatment.

Common therapies for pelvic congestion include medroxyprogesterone acetate (Provera [Pfizer Inc., New York, N.Y.])[6] and goserelin (Zoladex [AstraZeneca Pharmaceuticals, Wilmington, Del.])[7] to suppress ovarian function, and hysterectomy with or without bilateral salpingo-oophorectomy (TAH/BSO).[8] Despite its curative intent, hysterectomy studies reported residual pain in 33% of patients and a 20% recurrence rate.[8,9] To improve clinical efficacy and reduce peri- and postoperative morbidity, percutaneous pelvic vein embolization treatment has been introduced.

INDICATIONS

Venogram and embolization are indicated for patients who are suffering from chronic pelvic pain, and pelvic congestion is suspected to be the cause of the pain. Symptoms and signs of pelvic congestion have been well documented,[5,10] but because several symptoms can overlap with those of other conditions, the diagnosis can be overlooked. The diagnosis of pelvic varices can be challenging even with advanced imaging studies such as ultrasound (US), computed tomography (CT) (Fig. 80-1, A), or magnetic resonance imaging (MRI) (Fig. 80-1, B). Even with direct visualization with laparoscopic evaluation, the diagnosis can be missed in up to 80% of patients[10] (Fig. 80-1, C).

Thus, thorough clinical evaluation is imperative. Affected patients are typically in their late 20s or early 30s. Pelvic congestion with varicosities in the infundibulopelvic and broad ligaments draining via ovarian and internal iliac vein tributaries can cause dull, aching, unilateral pain in the pelvis. The pain can be worsened by walking and postural changes. It can be cyclic with dysfunctional bleeding and dysmenorrhea, or accompanied by dyspareunia or postcoital ache that may last for hours or days[5,11] (Table 80-1).

CONTRAINDICATIONS

Frequently, pelvic embolization is performed in patients who have exhausted many surgical procedures, and there are few contraindications. Patients who have active pelvic inflammatory disease or any other significant infections should be treated for such prior to embolization. Patients with prior allergic reactions to iodinated contrast should be premedicated prior to embolization. Finally, venogram and embolization cannot be performed in patients without safe venous access.

EQUIPMENT

The procedure is performed in an angiography suite under high-quality fluoroscopic guidance. Sterile environment is a requirement. A fluoroscopic table with tilt function may be helpful, but a technique described in the following section can be used instead, and successful embolization with excellent outcome can be expected without the tilt table. Iodinated contrast (Omnipaque 350 [Nycomed, Princeton, N.J.]) is used for optimal visualization.

TECHNIQUE

Anatomic Aspects

Venous drainage from the pelvis is via common iliac, external iliac, and internal iliac veins and ovarian veins. The ovarian veins originate in the pelvis and course cephalad to empty into the left renal vein from the left ovarian vein and the inferior vena cava just inferior to the right renal vein from the right ovarian vein. Multiple trunks and communication to the inferior mesenteric vein can be seen, particularly on the left. There could be communications existing between right and left ovarian veins, ovarian veins to iliac veins, and left pelvic veins to right pelvic veins. Such communications may serve as a cause for potential recurrences after resection and a basis for transcatheter treatments of varices and incompetent ovarian veins.

Diagnostic criteria for pelvic varices on venogram include 5 mm or greater diameter of the ovarian vein, uterine vein, and utero-ovarian arcade; free reflux in the ovarian vein, with incompetence of the valve; filling of contrast material across midline; vulvar or thigh varices; and stagnant clearance of contrast material from the pelvic veins.[10,12,13]

Technical Aspects

For optimal visualization of ovarian vein incompetency and pelvic varices, a direct venogram of the renal veins,

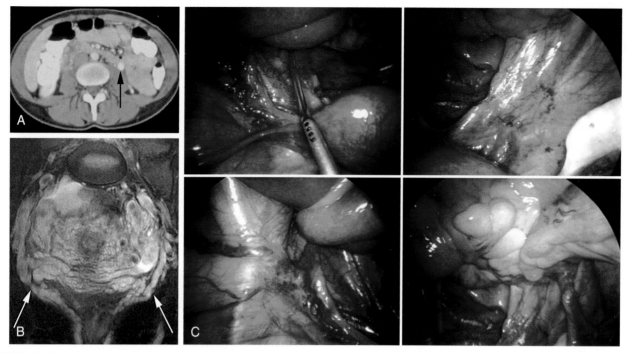

FIGURE 80-1. **A,** Postcontrast axial computed tomography image shows dilated incompetent left ovarian vein *(arrow).* **B,** Coronal T2-weighted magnetic resonance image shows significant pelvic varices *(arrows)* around uterus. **C,** Images from direct laparoscopic examination show pelvic varices around uterus.

TABLE 80-1. Signs and Symptoms of Chronic Pelvic Pain Suggestive of Pelvic Congestion

Symptoms

Dull, aching pelvic pain, worse with standing, activity, or Valsalva maneuver
Pain in right or left lower quadrant, dyspareunia
Postcoital ache
Secondary dysmenorrhea
Dysfunctional uterine bleeding
Urinary frequency/urgency with negative cystoscopy and urine culture
Gastrointestinal symptoms without a cause or irritable bowel syndrome
Low back pain
Migraine headache
Family history of varicosities

Signs from Physical Examination

Ovarian point tenderness on abdominal examination
Cervical motion tenderness
Adnexal tenderness

Diagnostic Studies

Polycystic ovaries on US
Varices may be visualized on laparoscopic study; US, CT, and MRI helpful but not a necessity.

CT, Computed tomography; *MRI,* magnetic resonance imaging; *US,* ultrasound.
From Beard RW, Reginald PW, Wadsworth J. Clinical features of women with chronic lower abdominal pain and pelvic congestion. Br J Obstet Gynaecol 1988;95:153–61.

preferably selective ovarian venograms, should be performed. After informed consent, the patient is prepared and draped for a sterile procedure. Moderate conscious sedation is employed and intravenous (IV) antibiotic with gram-positive coverage is administered. Similar to diagnostic venography and embolotherapy procedures for male varicocele,[14] diagnostic venography is performed via a transfemoral or transjugular approach. We prefer the transfemoral approach. The common femoral vein is accessed using the Seldinger technique and an 18- or 21-gauge single-wall needle. A 7F vascular sheath (Cordis Corp., Miami Lakes, Fla.) is placed in the right femoral vein, and a 7F Hopkins-customized guiding catheter (Cordis Corp.) is advanced into the left renal vein, pointing to the origin of the left ovarian vein. A left renal venogram is performed through the guiding catheter (Fig. 80-2, *A*). The left ovarian vein is selected with a 4F or 5F Glide Bentson-Hanafee-Wilson JB-1 or hockey stick–shaped catheter (Terumo Medical, Somerset, N.J.) over a 0.035-inch-diameter Glidewire (Terumo Medical), and a proximal left ovarian venogram is performed by hand-injection using iodinated contrast (Fig. 80-2, *B*). Performance of the Valsalva maneuver in an attempt to increase intraabdominal pressure and accentuate the pelvic varices may be useful. In our experience, variable duplex waveforms of the pelvic veins are seen with the Valsalva maneuver in patients with pelvic congestion syndrome (PCS).[13] We perform venography and embolization with the patient supine for the needs of conscious sedation.

After confirming incompetence of the valves in the left ovarian vein, the hydrophilic-coated catheter is further advanced to the distal ovarian vein over the Glidewire. Once the catheter is advanced to the pelvic level, a distal ovarian venogram is performed (Fig. 80-2, *C* and *D*). Hand-injection of the contrast to assess the volume of blood in the cross-pelvic varices is performed. Subsequently, embolotherapy of the deep pelvic varicosity is performed with a slurry of sodium morrhuate (5% [American Regent Laboratories, Shirley, N.Y.]) and Gelfoam (Pharmacia & Upjohn, Kalamazoo, Mich.) that was prepared on the tabletop before

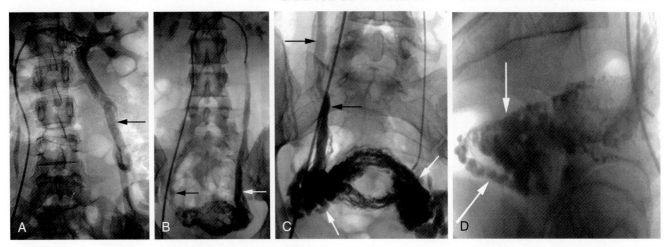

FIGURE 80-2. A, Direct venogram with injection from left ovarian vein origin shows significantly dilated tortuous left ovarian vein *(arrow)*. Note absence of competent valve. **B,** Direct venogram of left ovarian vein shows dilated incompetent left ovarian vein *(white arrow)*, with filling of pelvic varices and cross-filling of right pelvis draining via right internal iliac vein *(black arrow)*. Direct venograms of left ovarian vein on frontal **(C)** and lateral **(D)** views show significantly dilated pelvic varices *(white arrows)* draining via right ovarian vein *(black arrows)*.

embolotherapy. This sclerosant solution causes denaturation of proteins at the cell surfaces, causing thrombosis of pelvic varices at the tributaries. Subsequently, the entire course of the left ovarian vein is embolized with 0.035-inch-diameter stainless steel or platinum coils (Cook Medical, Bloomington, Ind.).

Subsequently, the origin of the right ovarian vein is selected with the same guiding catheter heat-shaped into a Simmons 2 contour, and a proximal right ovarian venogram is performed. Then, the distal portion of the right ovarian vein is selected with a 4F or a 5F Glide JB1 or hockey stick–shaped catheter coaxially through the Simmons 2–shaped guiding catheter over a 0.035-inch-diameter Glidewire. Contrast material is injected by hand into the cross-pelvic varices to estimate the volume of contrast material that can be injected until reflux into the contralateral internal iliac vein or ovarian vein occurs. The same amount of the sodium morrhuate/Gelfoam slurry is injected slowly into the pelvic varices. Five minutes are allowed for protein denaturation and thrombosis to take effect. Subsequently, the entire length of the right ovarian vein is embolized with 0.035-inch-diameter stainless steel or platinum coils.

We perform embolotherapy of pelvic varices from the internal iliac vein approach to reduce the risk of recurrence of the varices, given the free communication between the ovarian varices and internal iliac vein tributaries visualized during the ovarian venogram (Fig. 80-3, *A*). During the second treatment, a 7F vascular sheath is placed in the right femoral or right jugular vein and a 7F Berman wedge catheter (Arrow International, Reading, Pa.) is used to select the left internal iliac vein. Once the balloon on the catheter is inflated, a balloon-occluded left internal iliac venogram is performed by hand-injection of contrast. If further study is necessary, the catheter is advanced into tributaries off the internal iliac vein, and a subselective balloon-occluded venogram is performed, searching for residual pelvic varices in the pelvic, vulvar, or thigh regions. If varices are diagnosed, the volume in the cross-pelvic varices is assessed with hand contrast injection, estimating the contrast volume until it refluxes into the contralateral internal iliac vein. The same amount of the sodium morrhuate/Gelfoam slurry

combination is injected slowly into the pelvic varices while the balloon is inflated to occlude the main internal iliac vein. The balloon is inflated for approximately 5 minutes during the embolization to prevent reflux of embolic material into the common iliac vein or inferior vena cava. Subsequently, a Waltman loop is created with a 7F Berman wedge catheter, and the right internal iliac vein is selected for balloon-occluded venogram (Fig. 80-3, *B*). The same treatment technique is used for treatment of the right pelvic varices (Fig. 80-4).

EQUIPMENT

- Imaging:
  - C-arm image intensifier (high-quality angiographic suite)
- Medications and contrast:
  - Lidocaine 1%
  - Midazolam, fentanyl
  - Iodinated contrast
- Access:
  - 18G single-wall percutaneous needle and 0.035-inch-diameter wire <u>or</u>
  - 21G micropuncture needle and 0.018-inch-diameter wire
- Catheters and wires:
  - 7F Hopkins-customized guiding catheter (Cordis Corp.)
  - 4F or 5F Glide Bentson-Hanafee-Wilson JB-1 or hockey stick–shaped catheter (Terumo Medical)
  - 7F Berman wedge catheter (Arrow International)
  - 0.035-inch-diameter glide wire (Terumo Medical)
- Embolization materials
  - Sodium morrhuate (5% [American Regent Laboratories]) and Gelfoam (Pharmacia & Upjohn)
  - 0.035-inch-diameter stainless steel or platinum coils (Cook Medical)

CONTROVERSIES

Ovarian varices may be present in asymptomatic patients, particularly in parous patients.[15] Direct venogram alone is

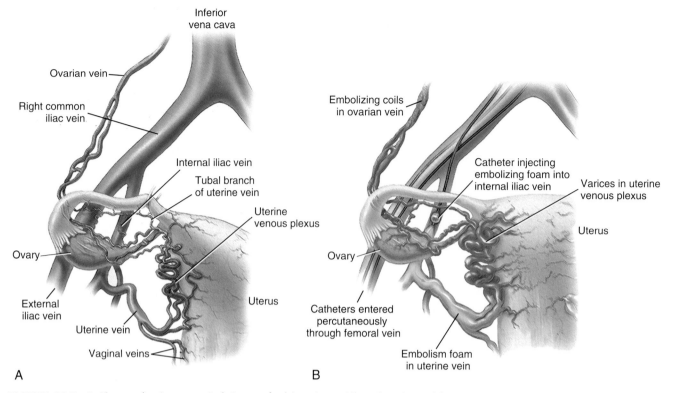

FIGURE 80-3. A, Diagram showing anatomic drainages of pelvic varices to bilateral ovarian and iliac veins. **B,** Diagram showing embolization of right ovarian vein with coils and right internal iliac vein varices with sclerosant and Gelfoam combinations.

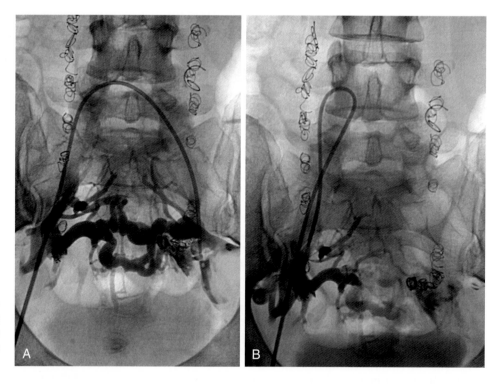

FIGURE 80-4. Balloon-occluded venograms of left (**A**) and right (**B**) internal iliac veins show residual pelvic varices after bilateral ovarian vein embolization with coils.

unable to differentiate patients with chronic pelvic pain due to pelvic varices from patients with chronic pelvic pain not due to PCS, with incidental pelvic varices. Thus, thorough clinical evaluation prior to embolization is imperative.

Though we believe the technique just presented is safe, efficient, and durable, there is no consensus regarding optimal technique. Review of the literature demonstrates variable use of different embolic agents, including coils, sodium morrhuate/Gelfoam slurry, sodium tetradecyl sulfate, and *N*-butyl cyanoacrylate (Table 80-2). There is also variability among interventionalists with regard to the necessity of bilateral ovarian vein embolization and routine

TABLE 80-2. Literature Review

Study	No.	Embolization	Material	Mean Follow-up (mo)	Clinical Outcome
Edwards et al., 1993[20]	1	Bilateral ovarian	Coils	6	Significant relief in 100%
Sichlau et al., 1994[21]	3	Bilateral ovarian	Coils	1 at 14 months, 2 long term	Significant relief in 100%
Tarazov et al., 1997[22]	6	4 left ovarian, 1 bilateral ovarian	Coils	12-48	Significant relief in 66.6%, partial relief in 33.3%
Capasso et al., 1997[23]	19	13 unilateral ovarian, 6 bilateral ovarian	Coils	15.4	Significant relief in 57.9%, partial relief in 15.8%, no relief in 26.3%
Cordts et al., 1998[24]	9	4 left ovarian, 4 bilateral ovarian, 1 obturator	Coils	13.4	Significant relief in 66.7%, partial relief in 22.2%, no relief in 11.1%
Maleux et al., 2000[25]	41	32 unilateral ovarian, 9 bilateral ovarian	Glue	19.9	Significant relief in 58.5%, partial relief in 9.7%, no relief in 31.8%
Venbrux et al., 2002[19]	56	56 bilateral ovarian, 43 bilateral internal iliac	Sclerosant (SM/GF slurry) and coils	22.1	Significant/partial relief in 96%, no relief in 4%
Pieri et al., 2003[26]	33	1 right ovarian, 11 left ovarian, 21 bilateral ovarian	Sclerosant (3% STS)	6 and 12	Significant relief in 100%
Bachar et al., 2003[27]	6	3 left ovarian, 3 bilateral ovarian	Coils	7.3	Significant relief in 50%, partial relief in 33.3%, no relief in 17.7%
Kim et al., 2006[16]	127	106 bilateral ovarian, 20 unilateral ovarian, 108 internal iliac	Sclerosant (SM/GF slurry) and coils	45	Significant relief in 85%, no relief in 12%, 3% worsened
Kwon et al., 2007[17]	67	64 left ovarian, 1 right ovarian, 2 bilateral ovarian	Coils	44.8	Significant relief in 82%, no relief in 15%, 3% worsened
Gandini et al., 2008[28]	38	Bilateral ovarian	Sclerosant (3% STS)	12	Significant relief in 100%

embolization of the internal iliac veins. Further randomized studies are needed to determine optimal technique to maximize treatment efficacy.

OUTCOMES

Percutaneous embolotherapy has revolutionized PCS treatment, and although there are no large-scale prospective randomized control trials comparing embolotherapy with traditional medical and/or surgical therapies, it has become the treatment of choice owing to its low morbidity, effectiveness, and durability. A review of the literature regarding percutaneous embolotherapy for the treatment of PCS is summarized in Table 80-2. Numerous small studies have consistently reported clinical success rates between 50% and 100%. In the largest cohort of patients to date, Kim et al. demonstrated that 83% of patients experienced statistically significant improvement in pain symptoms at a mean long-term follow-up of 45 months.[16] A subset of patients that had previously undergone hysterectomy also demonstrated significant improvement in pain symptoms (Fig. 80-5). Kwon et al. demonstrated similar results in a series of 67 patients, but coils were used as the exclusive embolic agent, embolization was largely unilateral (96% left ovarian), and the internal iliac vessels were not treated.[17]

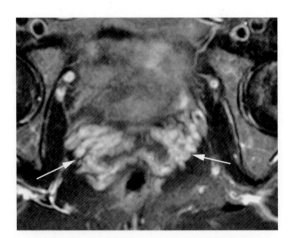

FIGURE 80-5. Axial T2-weighted magnetic resonance image of pelvis in patient with prior hysterectomy shows dilated pelvic varices (arrows).

COMPLICATIONS

Direct pelvic venogram and embolization is generally a low-risk procedure. Minor complications may include hematoma formation in the access site, pain, and nausea and vomiting associated with medications during the procedure. Allergic reactions to iodinated contrast should also be taken into consideration, and constant monitoring during and after the procedure is imperative. Major complications may include pulmonary embolism (PE), deep venous thrombosis (DVT), or embolic material embolization to the lung, all of which were not reported to be significant. Long-term study showed no symptomatic PE, DVT, or symptomatic distal embolization of embolic materials.[18] A recurrence rate of 5% among those who improved after embolization was reported in a long-term study.[18] No significant changes in female hormonal levels or menstrual cycles were noted.[18,19] Successful pregnancies and deliveries have been reported,[18] but further study is indicated to fully evaluate for any possible impact on fertility.

POSTPROCEDURE AND FOLLOW-UP CARE

After the procedure, patients are admitted for overnight observation and pain control; a mild to moderate degree of pain is expected after embolization. Although patients can be discharged on the same day with oral medications, patients often receive IV patient-controlled analgesia (PCA) with morphine (1 mg demand) or fentanyl (20 µg demand), necessitating admission to the hospital. The IV PCA is ready for patient use immediately upon completion of the procedure. All patients also receive 30 mg of IV ketorolac every 6 hours during the first 24-hour period. For patients receiving inadequate pain relief with IV PCA, an additional IV dose of the respective regimen of opioid is given every 15 minutes until the pain is improved. After embolization treatments, patients are followed at 3 months, 6 months, 1 year, and then yearly.

▶ **SUGGESTED READINGS**

Beard RW, Highman JH, Pearce S, Reginald PW. Diagnosis of pelvic varicosities in women with chronic pelvic pain. Lancet 1984;2(8409):946–9.

Beard RW, Reginald PW, Wadsworth J. Clinical features of women with chronic lower abdominal pain and pelvic congestion. Br J Obstet Gynaecol 1988;95(2):153–61.

Hobbs JT. The pelvic congestion syndrome. Br J Hosp Med 1990;43(3):200–6.

Kim HS, Malhotra AD, Rowe PC, et al. Embolotherapy for pelvic congestion syndrome: Long-term results. J Vasc Interv Radiol 2006;17:289–97.

Robinson JC. Chronic pelvic pain. Curr Opin Obstet Gynecol 1993;5:740–3.

Venbrux AC, Chang AH, Kim HS, et al. Pelvic congestion syndrome (pelvic venous incompetence): Impact of ovarian and internal iliac vein embolotherapy on menstrual cycle and chronic pelvic pain. J Vasc Interv Radiol 2002;13:171–8.

The complete reference list is available online at www.expertconsult.com.

CHAPTER 81
Treatment of High-Flow Priapism and Erectile Dysfunction

Tiago Bilhim, João M. Pisco, Max Kupershmidt, and Kenneth R. Thomson

Superselective embolization of terminal branches of the male internal pudendal artery is a highly successful procedure in the treatment of high-flow arterial priapism. Vascular imaging and treatment in patients with erectile dysfunction (ED) using cavernosography and internal pudendal artery angiography and angioplasty remains a controversial topic.

PRIAPISM

Priapism is a pathologically persisting erection of the penis not associated with sexual stimulation. It is a result of imbalance of arterial inflow and venous outflow involving the corpora cavernosa. The incidence in the general population is low, between 0.5 and 2.9 per 100,000 person-years, and is higher in patients with sickle cell anemia and in men using intracorporal injections.[1,2]

There are two types—low-flow/ischemic and high-flow/arterial—and these are grouped based on the pathophysiology, with implications for subsequent treatment options and outcomes.

Low-Flow/Ischemic/Veno-occlusive Priapism

Incidence
• This is the most common type.

Etiology
• Any prothrombotic state
• Intracavernous vasodilator injections for treatment of ED
• Postembolization or surgery for venous leak
• Neurogenic
• Drugs
• Idiopathic

Pathophysiology
Low-flow priapism is caused by decreased outflow of blood due to venous thrombosis; thus there results a compartment syndrome–like pathophysiology, with the risk of gangrene.

Clinical Presentation
Acute onset of severe pain, rigidity, and other compartment syndrome clinical findings are noted. Venous blood is evident on aspiration of the corpora cavernosa. Doppler studies show no or low velocities in cavernosal arteries.

Management
Priapism is a medical emergency, and if not treated within 24 hours, leads to irreversible ischemia and tissue necrosis. This type of priapism is usually treated by a consultant urologist.

First-line treatment is aspiration that confirms the diagnosis and at the same time decompresses. This is followed by irrigation with a sympathomimetic pharmaceutical agent and, if necessary, a surgical shunt. The management is slightly different but follows the same principles for the sickle cell anemia variant of veno-occlusive priapism.[3,4]

High-Flow/Nonischemic/Arterial Priapism

Incidence
• Less common than the low-flow type; in adults, 80% to 90% have a single fistula causing the priapism, but in children, 50% have multiple fistulas.[3-5]

Etiology
• Mostly traumatic
• Typically a straddle injury to the perineum
• Sometimes results from complications of low-flow priapism
• Can be idiopathic without a recognizable event

Pathophysiology
There is unregulated blood flow in an arteriolacunar (not arteriovenous) fistula between one of the terminal branches of the internal pudendal artery (most commonly the cavernosal artery) and lacunar spaces of the corpora cavernosa. The bulbar and dorsal penile arteries are less frequently involved. Venous outflow is not restricted, because there is no compression of subtunical veins, normally produced by neural stimulation; hence, there is a constant state of inflow/outflow without pooling of blood. Shearing forces on the endothelium cause release of increased levels of nitric oxide and activation of the cyclic guanosine monophosphate pathway, resulting in relaxation of smooth muscle.[6-8]

Clinical Presentation
Unlike the low-flow/occlusive type, there is no ischemia or pain, and hence it is not an emergency. The onset is usually delayed after injury, but typically it is clinically evident within 72 hours.[9] Aspiration of the cavernosa reveals arterial blood. Doppler studies show normal or high velocities in cavernosal arteries. The actual site of the arteriolacunar fistula can usually be accurately determined.[3,4]

Management
American Urological Association (AUA) guidelines[4] suggest initial conservative management, with 62% of cases resolving spontaneously. However, we believe early interventional radiology management with embolization of the fistula provides a better outcome for high-flow fistulas.

ERECTILE DYSFUNCTION

Erectile dysfunction is defined as inability to reach or maintain erection sufficient for satisfactory sexual performance.[10] ED is commonly associated with diabetes mellitus (threefold increased risk of ED), hypertension, vascular disease, dyslipidemia, hypogonadism, and depression.

Incidence

- ED affects up to one third of men throughout their lives and over 150 million men worldwide.
- Prevalence increases with age: 12% are younger than 59 years, 22% are 60 to 69, and 30% are older than 69.[11]

Etiology

- ED may result from organic causes, psychological causes, or a combination of both.
- Possible organic causes: vascular, neurogenic, hormonal, anatomic, drug-induced.[12]

Pathophysiology

A normal sexual erectile response results from the production of nitric oxide from endothelial cells after parasympathetic stimuli. Nitric oxide causes smooth muscle relaxation, which leads to arterial influx of blood into the corpus cavernosum, followed by compression of venous return, producing an erection. This neurovascular function must be integrated with sexual perception and desire.[12] Other smooth muscle relaxants (e.g., prostaglandin E_1 analogs and α-adrenergic antagonists) can cause sufficient cavernosal relaxation to result in erection. Many of the drugs that have been developed to treat ED act at this level.[13]

Vascular causes of ED may be arterial and/or venous, and these are the ones amenable to endovascular treatment. Generalized penile arterial insufficiency may result from stenotic arterial lesions of the internal pudendal arteries or from microangiopathy of the arteries of the corpora cavernosa. Failure of the veins to close completely during an erection (veno-occlusive dysfunction) may occur in men with large venous channels that drain the corpora cavernosa, and may be studied by cavernosography.[13] Evidence is accumulating in favor of ED as a vascular disorder in the majority of patients.[14]

Clinical Presentation

Up to 70% of men with ED remain undiagnosed and untreated.[15] ED has an effect equal to or greater than the effects of family history of myocardial infarction, cigarette smoking, or measures of hyperlipidemia on subsequent cardiovascular events.[16] All patients with ED should be considered for screening for undetected cardiovascular disease.

Management

The AUA recommends that the initial evaluation of ED include a complete medical, sexual, and psychosocial history.[17] History and physical examination are sufficient to make an accurate diagnosis of ED in most cases.[12] The five-item version of the International Index of Erectile Function Questionnaire (IIEF-5) is a validated survey instrument that can be used to assess the severity of ED symptoms.[18]

Vascular Studies in the Patient with Erectile Dysfunction

Although erectile function can improve after vascular reconstructive surgery or endovascular angioplasty of the internal pudendal/penile arteries,[20-23] there is still very little evidence to recommend vascular imaging studies and therapies for ED in the general population. More rigorous trials are needed to prove short- and long-term effectiveness.[19]

Duplex sonography with pulsed Doppler analysis (with and without dynamic erection studies with vasoactive substances) and nocturnal penile tumescence (NPT) are usually performed as first-line studies. Evaluation of these vasculogenic factors ultimately depends on cavernosography and internal pudendal angiography.[24]

RELEVANT ANATOMY

For a brief discussion of the arterial and venous anatomy relevant to these procedures, visit www.expertconsult.com.

TREATMENT OF HIGH-FLOW/ NONISCHEMIC/ARTERIAL PRIAPISM

Contraindications

There are no specific contraindications to treatment.

Equipment

- Standard angiographic access with 5F access sheath
- Pigtail and Cobra-2 5F catheters (for internal iliac catheterization) or the Roberts uterine artery catheter (RUC [Cook Medical, Bloomington, Ind.])
- Terumo angled Glidewire, 0.035-inch (Terumo Medical Corp., Somerset, N.J.)
- Terumo Progreat microcatheter, 2.7F (Terumo)
- Nitroglycerin injection (10 µg/mL)
- Nonionic contrast medium (iodine, 300 mg/mL)
- Gelfoam sheet (hand-cut pledgets from sheet) or 2- to 3-mm-diameter microcoils

Technical Aspects

The fistula is usually unilateral, and unilateral embolization is performed to avoid the risk of cavernosal gangrene and ED. Preferably the side of the fistula is identified with duplex ultrasonography[3] or computed tomography (CT)[28] before the procedure. If not possible, a pelvic aortogram with a pigtail catheter usually is sufficient to show the side of bleeding (Fig. 81-1).

Both the external and internal pudendal arteries should be catheterized and angiography performed (Fig. 81-2). With the use of microcatheters, deep catheterization of the internal iliac artery is not required. Better angiography will be obtained with use of a vasodilator, such as 10-µg aliquots of nitroglycerin injected intraarterially.

Embolization should be performed in a highly selective position in the minor arterial branches as close to the site of bleeding as possible; this can prevent ischemic

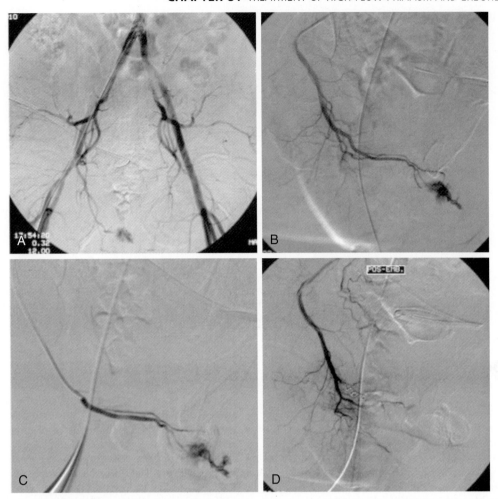

FIGURE 81-1. A, Pigtail pelvic arteriogram showing a right-sided large arteriolacunar fistula. **B,** Selective digital subtraction angiography (DSA) (6 mL; 3 mL/seg) of right internal pudendal artery with steep oblique view (35° RAO; −10° caudal-cranial angulation), better depicting fistula. **C,** DSA after selective catheterization. **D,** Control angiogram after embolization with 2- and 3-mm microcoils.

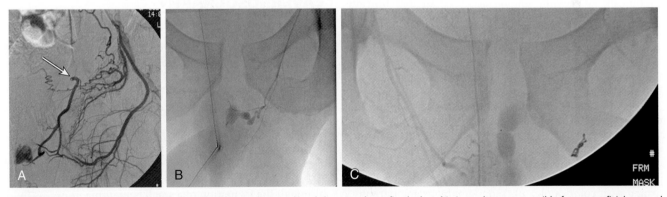

FIGURE 81-2. A, Internal pudendal artery has been catheterized, and there is a large fistula, but this is much more accessible from superficial external pudendal artery *(arrow)* in this steep oblique view. **B,** Superficial external pudendal arising from external iliac artery has been catheterized, providing easy access to fistula. **C,** Fistula has been occluded with a small pledget of Gelfoam. Further injection through internal pudendal artery shows no filling of fistula. Patient's sexual function returned to normal within 30 days.

complications and preserve blood supply to the corpora cavernosa, with preservation of erectile function. The most accepted embolic agents are microcoils or Gelfoam. Gelfoam (Baxter Healthcare Corp., Hayward, Calif.) is used in very small pledgets inserted through the microcatheter. Angiography should be performed after each pledget is inserted to ensure that the emboli are in the correct place.

In a large fistula, 2- to 3-mm-diameter microcoils may be used instead of or in addition to Gelfoam, but they may be palpable afterward (Fig. 81-3).

Bilateral embolization is rarely required even when bilateral fistulas are present (treat the larger one)[7,29,30] and is typically used only in cases where unilateral embolization has not worked.

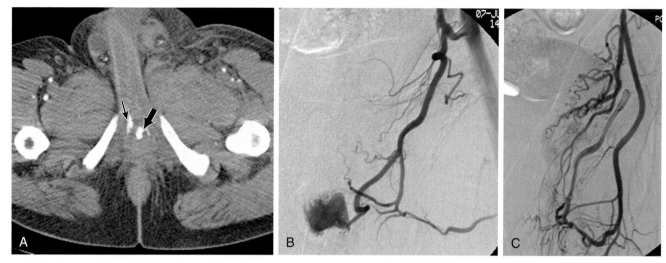

FIGURE 81-3. **A,** Status post trauma, with cavernosal extravasation shown on computed tomography *(thick arrow)*; normal blush within corpus spongiosum *(thin arrow).* **B,** Pudendal arteriogram shows fistula site. Note that in this view, pudendal artery crosses obturator foramen, a useful indicator for catheterizing correct artery. No vasodilators were used. **C,** Artery just proximal to site of fistula has been occluded by coils (this was an acute trauma case). Note contrast medium in corpora cavernosa. Angiogram of right pudendal artery shows no further filling.

Timing of Procedure

Although more than two thirds of the cases of arterial priapism may eventually resolve spontaneously without treatment, the patient's life may be adversely affected by the condition. Prolonged priapism has also been shown to result in permanent changes in the lacunae and endothelium, with a worsening prognosis for erectile recovery.[5,31,32] Hence, we believe embolization should be performed sooner rather than later, preferably within weeks of diagnosis.

Outcomes

Technically successful embolization is angiographically apparent during the procedure, with 74% to 90% resolution of high-flow priapism and 3% to 9% of subsequent ED.[4,5,35] After one side is embolized, a fistula on the other side may become apparent even if one was not seen initially, because the pressure gradient across the capillary bed between the two sides changes.[33]

Priapism resolves with detumescence of the corpora cavernosa at some time within 24 hours of the procedure, most within 4 to 6 hours. Recurrence of priapism usually occurs within the first 24 hours.[6]

Failure of resolution after 24 hours should raise the suspicion of failure of the embolization, which may be confirmed with color duplex ultrasonography or angiography.

Complications

Complications common to any angiogram may occur. Spasm of the pudendal arteries is common unless antispasmodic drugs are used.

The most important complication is nontarget embolization. One trap for the unwary is the normal capillary blush seen within the spongiosa (see Fig. 81-3). This may appear localized and suggest a bleeding point, but this does not persist into the venous phase of an angiogram.[17] Impotence or at least some ED may occur if a penile artery is occluded.

Postprocedural and Follow-Up Care

Recanalization of fistulas occurs in 10% to 30%[5,34] and is successfully treated with repeated embolization. It is more common when nonpermanent embolization agents such as Gelfoam are used. The use of coils rather than Gelfoam results in longer recovery times of erectile function.[19] Recovery of erectile function occurs on average between a few weeks and 3 months.[35]

Case reports of bilateral embolization indicate preserved erectile function after bilateral embolization.[7]

CAVERNOSOMETRY AND CAVERNOSOGRAPHY

Many patients with organic ED do not have abnormalities of the penile arterial system and may have abnormalities of the venous system in erection, which can be studied with cavernosography.

For a full discussion of the equipment and technical aspects of this procedure, please visit www.expertconsult.com.

Complications

There are few complications from cavernosography, although the formation of a small hematoma or excess fluid administration may occur. Priapism and thrombosis of the corpora cavernosa have been reported but are very rare. No special postprocedural care is necessary.

Outcomes

Cavernosography with cavernosometry can demonstrate venous leakage, which is of prime importance, since surgical techniques and eventually sclerotherapy or administration of vasoactive drugs seem very effective in restoring erectile function.[36] The main drawback is an unknown positive predictive value and the possibility of frequent false-positive results.[37]

INTERNAL PUDENDAL ANGIOGRAPHY AND ANGIOPLASTY IN ERECTILE DYSFUNCTION

Angiography or computed tomographic angiography (CTA) studies[38] may be performed in patients with suspected vascular ED after an abnormal Doppler study or DICC. The main goal is to assess the anatomy, patency, and distribution of arterial lesions in patients who are candidates for penile revascularization (Fig. 81-4). Surgical reconstruction may be performed, with few studies showing good results from internal pudendal artery angioplasty.[20-23]

Contraindications

• If psychogenic, neurogenic, and hormonal factors of ED have not been eliminated

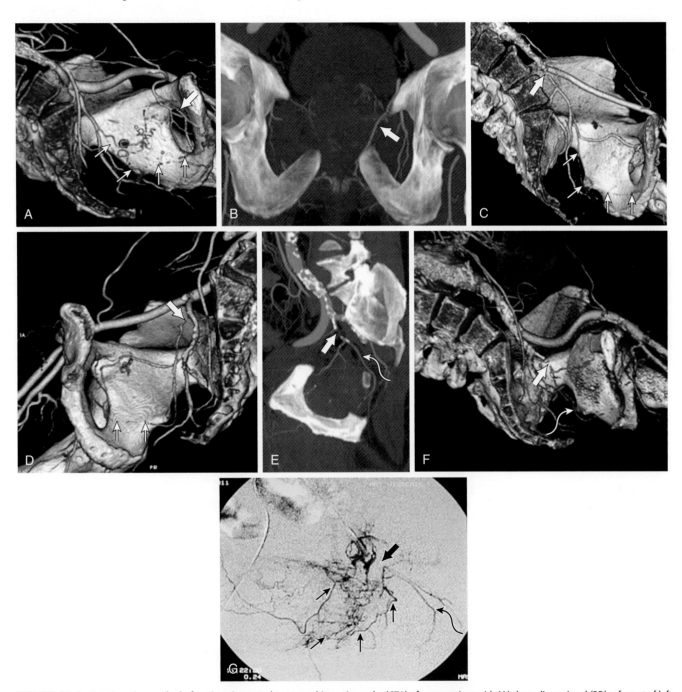

FIGURE 81-4. Arteriogenic erectile dysfunction. Computed tomographic angiography (CTA) of same patient with **(A)** three-dimensional (3D) reformat of left pelvic side and **(B)** coronal maximum intensity projection (MIP) reformat. Long occlusion of internal pudendal artery *(arrows)*, with collateral blood flow to penis through obturator branches *(thick arrows)*. **C,** CTA 3D reformat of left pelvic side, showing focal occlusion of origin of internal iliac artery *(thick arrow)* and multiple stenoses of internal pudendal artery *(arrows)*. **D,** CTA 3D reformat of right pelvic side, showing subocclusive stenosis of origin of internal pudendal artery *(thick arrow)* and distal occlusion of internal pudendal artery *(arrows)*. Occlusion of left proximal anterior division in another patient *(thick arrow)*. **E,** CTA with sagittal MIP reformat. **F,** 3D reformat. **G,** After selective catheterization. Note repermeabilization of internal pudendal artery distal to occlusion *(curved arrow)* via vesical and prostatic collaterals *(arrows)*. *(E and G, from Bilhim T, Pisco J, Rio Tinto H, et al. Unilateral versus bilateral prostatic arterial embolization for lower urinary tract symptoms in patients with prostate enlargement. Cardiovasc Intervent Radiol 2012;Dec 12. [Epub ahead of print]. Used with permission.)*

• Absence of previous duplex sonography and nocturnal penile tumescence (relative contraindications)

Equipment

• Standard angiographic access with 5F access sheath; long hydrophilic sheaths, 6F
• Cobra-2 5F catheters (for internal iliac catheterization) or the Roberts uterine artery catheter (RUC [Cook Medical]).
• Terumo angled Glidewire, 0.035-inch (Terumo)
• Torquable 0.018-inch guidewires
• Intracorporal papaverine (30-60 mg); nitroglycerin injection (50-200 µg)
• Nonionic contrast medium (iodine, 300 mg/mL)
• Angioplasty balloons (2-5 mm in diameter)

Technical Aspects

Venous outflow should be minimized and arterial inflow maximized with injection of intracorporal papaverine (30-60 mg) to induce an erection before angiography. During the filming sequence, intraarterial nitroglycerin (50-200 µg) mixed with 30 mg of papaverine may be used. Selective anterior division internal iliac angiography, with an injection of 6 mL at 3 mL/min, with ipsilateral oblique projections (35°) and caudal-cranial angulation (−10°) is performed. This enables visualization of the internal pudendal artery and identification of accessory pudendal arteries (seen in up to 7% of patients).

For stenoses of the common iliac arteries, standard transluminal angioplasty techniques are used. Torquable 0.018-inch guidewires may be helpful, and 3- to 5-mm balloons may be used for proximal lesions and 2- to 3-mm balloons for distal lesions. Heparin, 5000 to 10,000 units, are administered intravenously as the guidewire traverses the stenosis.

Outcomes

Lesions may be found in the iliac or internal pudendal arteries in 31% to 44% of patients, and at the base of the penis in 29% to 58% of patients. In younger patients, disease is concentrated in the cavernosal arteries (62% of patients). Asymmetry of disease is common. Clearly, selection of patients will determine the angiographic results.[24] There are very limited studies proving the efficacy of angioplasty in the treatment of ED, with clinical success ranging from 12.5% to 100%. Improper patient evaluation, with only routine peripheral arteriography without cavernosography, so that small penile artery disease and/or venogenic ED has not been excluded, might well explain many of the failures.[24]

Complications

Complications common to angioplasty and endovascular procedures affect this procedure.

Postprocedural and Follow-Up Care

Antiplatelet agents (aspirin [100 mg/day] and clopidogrel [75 mg/day]) should be given pre- and postdilation for 2 days prior to the procedure. Double platelet inhibition is recommended for 3 months thereafter, and aspirin may be maintained lifelong. Lifestyle modification and pharmacotherapy for comorbid cardiovascular diseases should be addressed.

Patients should be evaluated previously, and response to treatment measured with the use of the IIEF-5, a simple and validated questionnaire that quantifies erectile function. Cavernosometry and cavernosography, if not performed previously, should be considered afterwards, especially in those patients where erectile function does not improve after angioplasty. Patients with proven distal arterial disease not amenable to endovascular treatment may be offered surgical repair.

KEY POINTS

• There are two types of priapism: low flow and high flow.
• Only the high-flow type is suitable for embolization therapy.
• An unregulated arteriolacunar fistula is the cause of high-flow priapism.
• Superselective embolization with Gelfoam or microcoils is effective.
• Organic vascular erectile dysfunction (ED) is becoming more frequently recognized.
• Venogenic ED may be diagnosed by cavernosography and treated surgically.
• Arteriogenic ED may be diagnosed by selective pelvic arteriography and treated by angioplasty or surgery.

► **SUGGESTED READINGS**

Bookstein JJ. Penile angiography: the last angiographic frontier. AJR Am J Roentgenol 1988;150:47–54.

Sadeghi-Nejad H, Seftel AD. The etiology, diagnosis, and treatment of priapism: review of the American Foundation for Urologic Disease Consensus Panel Report. Curr Urol Rep 2002;3:492–8.

Savoca G, Pietropaolo F, Scieri F, et al. Sexual function after highly selective embolization of cavernous artery in patients with high-flow priapism: long-term follow-up. J Urol 2004;172:644–7.

The complete reference list is available online at www.expertconsult.com.

CHAPTER 82

Vascular Anatomy of the Thorax, Including the Heart

Kean H. Soon, Robert C. Heng, Kevin W. Bell, Yean L. Lim, and Antony S. Walton

SYSTEMIC ARTERIES

The *thoracic aorta* is conventionally described as consisting of three segments: the *ascending aorta*, *aortic arch*, and *descending aorta*. Conceptually, they may be regarded as the segmental supply to the heart; the head, neck, and upper limbs; and the thorax, respectively.

Ascending Aorta and Its Branches

The ascending aorta arises from the aortic orifice, which in life is closed by the aortic valve. Just above its origin, it is in the midline of the chest, almost central within the heart, with the right atrium to its right, the right ventricular outflow tract anteriorly, the left part of the coronary groove and the transverse sinus on its left, and the left atrium posteriorly. It passes superiorly and to the left, with a gentle anterior convexity, and ends at the level of the second costal cartilage (manubriosternal junction) by becoming the aortic arch. The pulmonary trunk lies on its left throughout its course. The proximal 15 to 20 mm of the ascending aorta has a characteristic bulbous appearance at catheter angiography because of the three sinuses of Valsalva. At two of these sinuses, the ascending aorta gives rise to its only branches, the coronary arteries.

Radiologic Observations
Although the ascending aorta is classically described as being 2.5 cm in diameter and 5 cm in length, these dimensions are highly variable in practice when measured on axial computed tomography (CT) images (Fig. 82-1). Aortic diameter can exceed 30 mm at its origin in young patients with no clinical history or features of any cardiac disease. This is undoubtedly partly due to the oblique angle of measurement and pulsation artifact, but it may partly reflect the difference between an elastic living vessel filled with blood at high pressure and a rigid, empty cadaveric specimen. Dilation and elongation also occur with age and disease.

Coronary Arteries
The heart receives blood supply from two major epicardial arteries, the left and right coronary arteries (LCA, RCA). These two coronary arteries originate from the aortic sinuses (coronary sinuses of Valsalva). There are normally three aortic sinuses: right anterior, left posterior, and right posterior. These sinuses are bordered by three leaflets of the aortic valve that form an inverted "Mercedes sign" on cross-sectional view of the aortic root (Fig. 82-2, *A*). The LCA originates from the left posterior aortic sinus, whereas the RCA originates from the right anterior aortic sinus

(Fig. 82-2, *B*). The right posterior sinus is normally free of coronary arteries. Volume-rendered three-dimensional (3D) images of CT coronary angiography are used in this section to illustrate the courses of the coronary arteries.

The LCA courses lateral to the aorta and posterolateral to the pulmonary artery for a variable length (a few millimeters to 2 cm). It then bifurcates into two main branches, the left anterior descending (LAD) and the left circumflex (LCx) arteries. The segment of the LCA proximal to its bifurcation is commonly known as the *left main coronary artery* (LMCA). Occasionally the LCx has a separate origin from the LAD. In this situation, the LMCA is nonexistent.

Clinical Importance
The LMCA supplies approximately 75% of the left ventricle. Severe disease (≥70%) in the LMCA puts the patient at high risk of cardiac death. The finding of severe LMCA disease should call for immediate attention from the treating cardiologist. Severe LMCA disease is normally treated by coronary artery bypass graft (CABG) surgery. Percutaneous coronary intervention (PCI) of LMCA disease is normally reserved for those who are considered inoperable, high-risk patients, or those with protected left main disease (i.e., a patent bypass graft to the LAD or LCx). With the increasing use of drug-eluting stents in PCI, more LMCA disease is now being treated with PCI, particularly ostial or mid-LMCA disease. Distal LMCA disease that involves both the origins of the LAD and LCx is usually considered less favorable for PCI. So far, 10-year data for PCI to treat unprotected LMCA disease (i.e., the LAD or LCx is not grafted) show no significant difference in mortality rate or composite endpoint of death, myocardial infarction, or stroke between PCI and CABG. Nonetheless, PCI of the LMCA is associated with an increased risk of target-vessel revascularization despite the use of drug-eluting stents.[1]

Of the two main branches of the LCA, the LAD is usually the larger and more important one; it supplies the anteroseptum, anterior, anterolateral, and anteroapical walls of the left ventricle. The LAD runs along the interventricular groove on the anterior surface of the heart toward the apex of the heart (Fig. 82-3, *A*). It gives off medial branches known as *septal branches*, and lateral branches known as *diagonal branches*. Septal branches come off the LAD almost perpendicularly and supply the anterior two thirds of the muscular interventricular septum. The first septal branch is usually the largest, and it supplies the atrioventricular (AV [His]) bundle and proximal bundle branches.

In the setting of acute anterior myocardial infarction, occlusion of the proximal LAD may be complicated by bundle branch block and hemiblock, pump failure, and

575

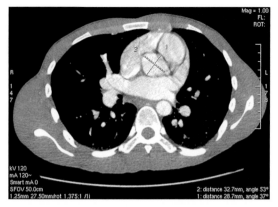

FIGURE 82-1. Contrast-enhanced axial computed tomography image of chest of young man, just above aortic valves. Ascending aorta is central in the heart, slightly to left of midline in this case. It is oval in shape, with a long-axis diameter of 33 mm. Ostium of left coronary artery is just visible at one end of caliper 2. Patient had no history or clinical features of cardiac disease.

ventricular tachycardia or fibrillation. The finding of severe disease in the LAD should attract prompt attention from the treating cardiologist. In patients with symptomatic hypertrophic obstructive cardiomyopathy (HOCM), transcoronary ablation of septal hypertrophy (TASH) with infusion of ethanol into septal branch(es) can be performed to reduce the septum nonsurgically.[2]

Lateral to the LAD, the first or second diagonal branches are sometimes of significant size and supply the high anterolateral wall of the left ventricle. Beyond the diagonal branches, the LAD reaches the apex of the heart. Sometimes the LAD wraps around the apex and continues its course along the interventricular groove onto the diaphragmatic surface of the heart for a variable length.

The LCx is usually the smaller branch of the LCA, supplying the lateral and posterior wall of the left ventricle. The LCx comes off the LMCA stem posterolaterally and runs beneath the left auricle. It runs along the left AV groove toward the posterior surface of the heart (Fig 82-3, *B*). The

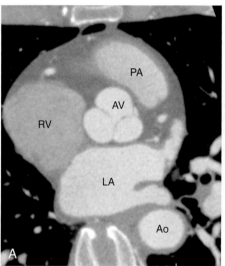

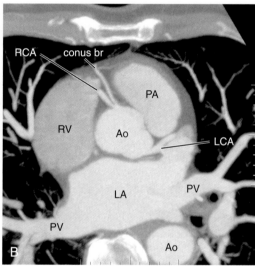

FIGURE 82-2. A, Axial image of a gated computed tomography (CT) scan of heart, showing three aortic sinuses (sinuses of Valsalva). **B,** Thick slab of maximal intensity projection CT coronary angiography showing origins of right coronary artery *(RCA)* and left coronary artery *(LCA)*. Conus branch of RCA shares same origin of its parental artery RCA. *Ao,* Aorta; *AV,* aortic valve; *LA,* left atrium; *PA,* pulmonary artery; *PV,* pulmonary vein; *RV,* right ventricle.

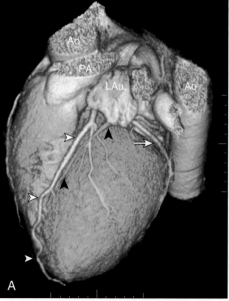

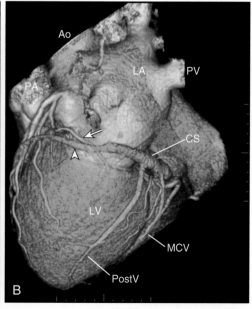

FIGURE 82-3. A, Three-dimensional (3D) volume-rendered computed tomography (CT) coronary angiography image showing branches of left coronary artery, left anterior descending artery *(three vertical arrowheads on left)*, and left circumflex artery *(arrow)*. **B,** 3D volume-rendered CT coronary angiography image showing course of left circumflex artery *(arrow)* and great cardiac vein *(right arrowhead)*, which continues on as coronary sinus *(CS)*. CS receives tributaries from posterior vein *(PostV)* of left ventricle and middle cardiac vein *(MCV)*. *Ao,* Aorta; *LA,* left atrium; *LAu,* left auricle; *PA,* pulmonary artery; *PV,* pulmonary vein.

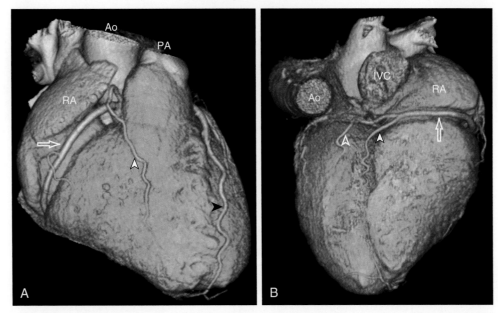

FIGURE 82-4. **A,** Three-dimensional (3D) volume-rendered image showing right coronary artery *(open arrow)* and its conus branch *(middle arrowhead)* and a small marginal branch. Right black arrowhead points to left anterior descending artery. **B,** 3D volume-rendered image showing posterior aspect of heart and course of right coronary artery (RCA) *(open arrow)* and its terminal branches, posterior descending artery *(arrowhead)*, and posterolateral branch of RCA *(open arrowhead)*. *Ao,* Aorta; *IVC,* inferior vena cava; *PA,* pulmonary artery; *RA,* right atrium.

main branches of the LCx are the obtuse marginal arteries that come off tangentially to the LCx and run along the lateral aspect of the left ventricle. Beyond the edge of the left ventricle, sometimes there are more branches coming off the LCx, supplying the posterolateral aspect of the left ventricle; these are the posterolateral branches of the LCx.

Occasionally there is a branch coming off the LMCA between the LAD and the LCx that is known as the *ramus intermediate artery*. The ramus intermediate artery can be of considerable size, supplying the anterolateral aspect of the left ventricle. Thus, it functionally replaces the first diagonal branch of the LAD or first obtuse marginal branch of LCx.

The RCA comes off the right anterior sinus of Valsalva and runs downwards in the right AV groove posterolaterally to the pulmonary artery and beneath the right atrial auricle (Fig. 82-4, *A*). The RCA gives off branches to supply the right atrium, right ventricle, posteroseptum, and to a variable degree the inferior and posterior aspects of the left ventricle. The earliest atrial branch of the RCA is normally the sinoatrial (SA) nodal artery. The SA nodal artery comes off the RCA underneath the right auricle and runs posteriorly toward the left of the superior vena caval ostium to supply the SA node. There is considerable variation in the distribution of the SA nodal artery. In about 59% of hearts, the SA nodal artery comes from the RCA. However, in about 38% of hearts, the SA nodal artery is a continuation of a large left atrial branch of the LCx. In the remaining 3%, the SA node receives dual blood supply.[3]

An early branch of the RCA that courses anteriorly and around the right ventricular infundibulum is the conus branch of the RCA. It may anastomose with an analogous branch from the LAD. In about 20% of hearts, the conus branch originates separately from the right anterior sinus of Valsalva instead of its parent artery, the RCA (see Fig. 82-2, *A*).[4] As the RCA runs along the right AV groove

toward the inferior border of the right ventricle, there is a branch coming off the RCA obliquely to supply the anterior surface of the right ventricle, known as the *marginal branch* of the RCA. Beyond the bifurcation of this marginal branch, the RCA wraps around the edge of the right ventricle and runs along the posterior AV groove to reach the crux of the heart, where the AV groove meets with the posterior interventricular groove. At the crux, the RCA gives off a branch superiorly into the interatrial septum to supply the AV node in 90% of cases. Inferior to the crux along the posterior interventricular groove, the RCA gives off a branch known as the *posterior descending artery* (PDA) in about 85% of patients (Fig. 82-4, *B*). The PDA supplies the posteroseptum and inferior wall of the right and left ventricles. A dominant RCA by definition supplies the PDA and continues beyond the crux along the left posterior AV groove to terminate into one or several posterolateral branches. In 10% of patients, the PDA is a continuation of the left coronary system (predominantly the LCx, i.e., the left dominant coronary system). In about 5% to 10% of hearts, the RCA and LCx share the same blood supply to the diaphragmatic surface of the heart (i.e., a co-dominant coronary system).[5]

In the right dominant system, occlusion of the proximal RCA in acute inferior myocardial infarction may lead to right heart failure, hypotension, and AV nodal block (second- or third- degree AV block).

Coronary Artery Nomenclature

The definition of coronary segments is important, especially in reporting the results of CT coronary angiography. Sometimes it can be difficult to define a particular segment of the coronary artery tree or the branches of the main coronary segments. Specifying the exact location of the disease and the segment involved as precisely as possible is important in communicating with the treating physicians, especially in coronary arteries with multiple lesions. Several

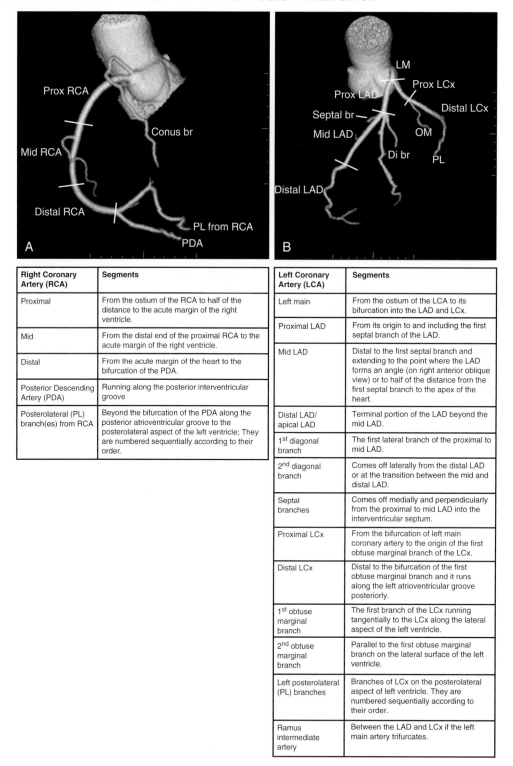

Right Coronary Artery (RCA)	Segments
Proximal	From the ostium of the RCA to half of the distance to the acute margin of the right ventricle.
Mid	From the distal end of the proximal RCA to the acute margin of the right ventricle.
Distal	From the acute margin of the heart to the bifurcation of the PDA.
Posterior Descending Artery (PDA)	Running along the posterior interventricular groove
Posterolateral (PL) branch(es) from RCA	Beyond the bifurcation of the PDA along the posterior atrioventricular groove to the posterolateral aspect of the left ventricle; They are numbered sequentially according to their order.

Left Coronary Artery (LCA)	Segments
Left main	From the ostium of the LCA to its bifurcation into the LAD and LCx.
Proximal LAD	From its origin to and including the first septal branch of the LAD.
Mid LAD	Distal to the first septal branch and extending to the point where the LAD forms an angle (on right anterior oblique view) or to half of the distance from the first septal branch to the apex of the heart.
Distal LAD/ apical LAD	Terminal portion of the LAD beyond the mid LAD.
1st diagonal branch	The first lateral branch of the proximal to mid LAD.
2nd diagonal branch	Comes off laterally from the distal LAD or at the transition between the mid and distal LAD.
Septal branches	Comes off medially and perpendicularly from the proximal to mid LAD into the interventricular septum.
Proximal LCx	From the bifurcation of left main coronary artery to the origin of the first obtuse marginal branch of the LCx.
Distal LCx	Distal to the bifurcation of the first obtuse marginal branch and it runs along the left atrioventricular groove posteriorly.
1st obtuse marginal branch	The first branch of the LCx running tangentially to the LCx along the lateral aspect of the left ventricle.
2nd obtuse marginal branch	Parallel to the first obtuse marginal branch on the lateral surface of the left ventricle.
Left posterolateral (PL) branches	Branches of LCx on the posterolateral aspect of left ventricle. They are numbered sequentially according to their order.
Ramus intermediate artery	Between the LAD and LCx if the left main artery trifurcates.

FIGURE 82-5. A, Three-dimensional (3D) volume-rendered coronary tree of right coronary artery *(RCA)*, showing segments of RCA and its branches. **B,** 3D volume-rendered coronary tree of left anterior descending *(LAD)* artery. *br,* Branch; *Di br,* diagonal branch; *LCx,* left circumflex artery; *LM,* left main; *OM,* obtuse marginal; *PDA,* posterior descending artery; *PL,* posterolateral; *Prox,* proximal.

classifications are used to define coronary segments, such as the 26-segment Coronary Artery Surgery Study (CASS) system and 15-segment American Heart Association (AHA) system.[6,7] Figures 82-5, *A* and *B* illustrate the nomenclature of coronary arteries based on a modified 16-segment AHA classification.[8]

Anomalous Coronary Arteries

Coronary arteries with aberrant origins are known as *anomalous coronary arteries* (ACA). The frequency of ACA varies from 0.3% to 5.6% depending on the definition of ACA in each individual study.[9] Studies with more stringent criteria only accept coronary arteries as anomalies if they

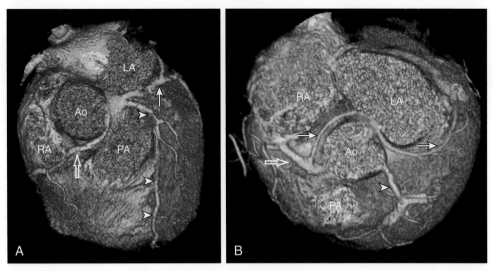

FIGURE 82-6. A, Superior view of three-dimensional (3D) volume-rendered image showing an anomalous right coronary artery (RCA) *(open arrow)* with an interarterial course between aorta *(Ao)* and pulmonary artery *(PA)*. Left anterior descending (LAD) *(arrowheads)* and left circumflex (LCx) arteries *(solid arrow)* have separate origins at left coronary sinus. **B,** Superior view of 3D volume-rendered image showing an anomalous LCx *(solid arrows)* with a benign course. Anomalous LCx originates from RCA *(open arrow)* and courses posterior to aorta before resuming its normal path down in left atrioventricular groove. Arrowhead points to LAD. *Ao,* Aorta; *LA,* left atrium; *PA,* pulmonary artery; *RA,* right atrium.

originate from the opposite coronary sinuses of Valsalva. The less stringent studies may include coronary arteries with ectopic origins at their respective coronary sinuses. The most frequent forms of ACAs in descending order are an RCA originating from either the right or left sinus of Valsalva (Fig. 82-6, *A*), an LCx arising from the right coronary sinus or RCA (Fig. 82-6, *B*), and an LCA arising from the right sinus of Valsalva.[9]

CLINICAL SIGNIFICANCE OF ANOMALOUS CORONARY ARTERIES The clinical outcome of ACAs is not always benign. Just like any coronary artery, ACAs may undergo atherosclerosis and become the culprit artery for ischemic heart disease.[10] Failure to adequately identify and assess ACAs may lead to misdiagnosis and failure to appropriately treat the culprit artery.

More significantly, ACAs are associated with sudden death. It has been reported that 12% to 31% of all cases of sudden death in young athletes/military recruits in the North American population may be associated with ACAs.[9,11-14] Most sudden deaths associated with ACA occur during or after physical exercise. Although the exact mechanism of cardiac ischemia in such cases is unclear, it has been postulated that interarterial ACAs with a proximal course between the aorta and pulmonary arterial trunk (so-called malignant coronary anomaly) may be compressed during or after physical exercise (see Fig. 82-6, *A*). ACAs with an interarterial course can be corrected by surgical reimplantation of coronary arteries to their respective coronary sinuses of Valsalva.[15] Therefore, early detection of malignant ACA may lead to prevention of sudden death in adolescents or young athletes with this condition.

Cardiac Veins

The cardiac veins, in general, follow the distribution of the coronary artery system, running parallel and superficial to the coronary arteries and their branches. The great cardiac vein runs parallel but in opposite direction to the LAD in the anterior interventricular groove (see Fig. 82-3, *A*). The great cardiac vein continues its course in the left anterior AV groove along with the LCx artery (see Fig. 82-3, *A*). Throughout it course, the great cardiac vein receives its tributaries from the left ventricle and atrium. In the left posterior AV groove, the great cardiac vein becomes a larger venous structure known as the *coronary sinus* (see Fig. 82-3, *B*). The coronary sinus is about 3 to 5 mm in diameter and 2 to 5 cm in length and receives blood from most cardiac veins before it empties into the right atrium. One of its major tributaries is the middle cardiac vein, which runs superiorly in the posterior interventricular groove along the PDA (see Fig. 82-3, *B*). It empties into the coronary sinus at the crux of the heart. The lateral, posterolateral, and posterior cardiac veins of the left ventricle receive blood from their respective aspects of the left ventricle before emptying into the coronary sinus along the left AV groove. There are multiple anterior cardiac veins that receive blood from the right ventricle and drain into the small cardiac vein. The small cardiac vein runs along the right AV groove downward toward the crux, where it subsequently empties into the coronary sinus. Some of anterior cardiac veins drain directly into the right atrium.

Identification of the coronary sinus and its tributaries are important in the electrophysiologic study of the cardiac conduction system. The coronary sinus is a frequent site for placing a pacing catheter or electrode in an electrophysiologic study. In patients with heart failure and dyssynchrony between the right and left ventricles, cardiac resynchronization therapy (CRT) with biventricular pacing can help resynchronize the right and left ventricles and hence improve cardiac output, heart failure symptoms, and survival.[16,17] Biventricular pacing involves placement of a pacing electrode into one of the anterolateral tributaries of the great cardiac vein or posterior vein of the left ventricle via the coronary sinus.

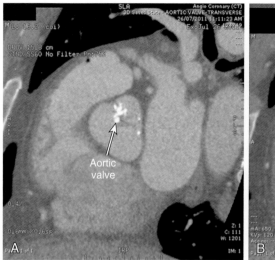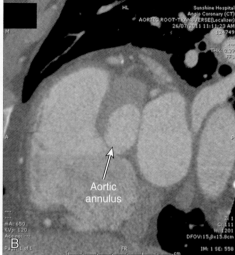

FIGURE 82-7. A, Transverse view of aortic valve. **B,** Transverse view of aortic annulus reveals its oval shape.

Transcutaneous Aortic Valve Implantation (TAVI)

Aortic valve replacement has hitherto been performed via open heart surgery. Rapid advances in catheter-based treatment for valvular heart disease makes the less invasive catheter-based transcutaneous aortic valve implantation (TAVI) a reality. Currently there are two widely used TAVI systems, a balloon-expandable Edwards SAPIEN valve (Edwards Lifesciences, Irvine, Calif.) and a self-expandable CoreValve system (Medtronics Inc., Minneapolis, Minn.) (Fig. e82-1).[18,19] Both systems are bioprosthetic valves mounted on a catheter-based delivery system.

Still in its early stages of clinical use, TAVI is currently indicated only for those patients with aortic stenosis with high surgical risks, such as age older than 80 years, or for younger patients (>65 years) with severe comorbidities such as severe respiratory disease, liver cirrhosis, or previous cardiac surgery. The large multicenter Placement of Aortic Transcatheter Valves (PARTNER-A) Trial, comparing TAVI using the Edwards SAPIEN valve to surgical valve replacement, showed very promising results, with a non-inferiority of TAVI in comparison with surgery in terms of its procedural success and mortality rates.[20] In 30 days, TAVI had a lower mortality rate (3.4% vs. 6.5%), and at 1 year, TAVI's mortality rate was as good as the surgical mortality rate (24.2% vs. 26.8%, respectively). TAVI has the advantages of shorter hospital stay and shorter recovery time. Nonetheless, TAVI was associated with a higher stroke rate (5.5% vs. 2.4% at 30 days and 8.3% vs. 4.3% at 1 year). In the PARTNER-B trial, where TAVI was compared to best medical therapy for severe aortic stenosis in patients unfit for surgical aortic valve replacement, TAVI was associated with a 45% relative risk reduction in all-cause mortality rate at 1 year (30.7% vs. 50.7%).[21] In view of PARTNER-A and PARTNER B's encouraging results, it is expected that TAVI's indications would be extended to include younger, lower-surgical-risk patients or patients not suitable for surgery across all age groups.

Accurate sizing of the aortic annulus and careful selection of patients are crucial to the success of TAVI. Various imaging modalities are currently in use to evaluate a

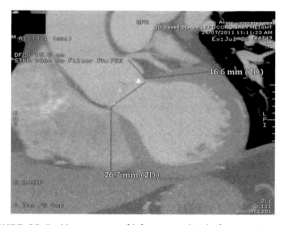

FIGURE 82-8. Measurement of left coronary height from aortic annulus.

patient's aortic valve, aortic root, and suitability for TAVI. An echocardiogram is necessary to diagnose and determine the severity of aortic stenosis, aortic valve two-dimensional (2D) morphology (with or without concurrent aortic valve incompetence), degree of calcification, and aortic annular and sinotubular diameters. Similarly, fluoroscopic measurements of aortic annular diameter, aortic sinus diameter, diameter of sinotubular junction, height of the coronary ostium from the aortic annulus, and diameter of the ascending aorta are important measurements to obtain prior to acceptance of TAVI candidates.

Because the aortic annulus is often oval in shape rather than round, as we commonly thought, a proper assessment of the aortic annulus may require a multi-imaging modality approach. Hence, 2D echocardiography (transthoracic and transesophageal) and fluoroscopy may be limited in showing the oval nature of the aortic annulus. Further assessment with CT may help visualize the annular shape and measure the size of the aortic annulus to reduce any chance for error or inter-reader variability (Figs. 82-7 and 82-8).[22] Common planes used to assess the aortic root are coronal (Fig. 82-9, *A*), saggital (Fig. 82-9, *B*), and transverse planes of the aortic valve and aortic root (see Fig. 82-7). At present, a small

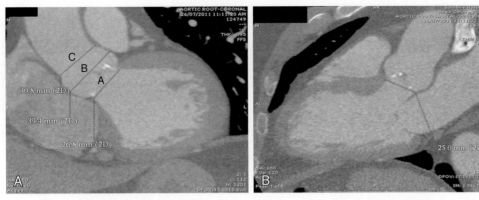

FIGURE 82-9. A, Aortic root measurements in coronal view, which is similar to left anterior oblique view on fluoroscopic working view. Letters *A, B, C* correspond to aortic annular diameter, aortic sinus diameter, and sinotubular diameter, respectively. **B,** Aortic annular diameter in saggital view (corresponding to three-chamber view of echocardiography).

aortic annulus (diameter < 18 mm for Edwards SAPIEN valve; < 20 mm for CoreValve) or a large aortic annulus (diameter > 25 mm for Edwards SAPIEN valve; > 27 mm for CoreValve), a dilated ascending aorta with a sinotubular diameter larger than 43 mm, or a low left coronary origin from the aortic annulus (height < 14 mm) (see Fig. 82-8), may exclude patients from TAVI. These guidelines may change when larger-sized valves become available. The value of aortic annular planimetry on CT is still being investigated.

A CT aortogram is also useful to evaluate the status of the aorta, femoral-iliac, and subclavian arteries to determine whether the peripheral arteries can accommodate the catheter of the TAVI delivery system (i.e., access vessel has to be > 6 mm). If peripheral access via the femoral or subclavian artery is unsuitable owing to small size, tortuosity, or extensive atherosclerosis with concentric calcification, an apical approach through a small thoracotomy is possible with the Edwards SAPIEN valve system.[23]

In a suitable patient, access is obtained via the femoral artery or subclavian artery with an 18G sheath (size of delivery system is expected to decrease with advances in catheter technology). The stenotic aortic valve is first crossed and predilated with a balloon saddled between the aortic valve leaflets. The heart is often paced at 160 to 180 bpm to stop the balloon from being pushed out of its position. Once the stenotic valve is properly dilated, a prosthetic valve is positioned carefully to the ideal location and deployed under the guidance of a fluoroscopic aortogram. After deployment, a fluoroscopic aortogram is obtained to recheck the position of the prosthetic valve and assess for any aortic incompetence. If the valve is deployed too high, there is increased risk of aortic injury, device migration, paravalvular leak, and coronary occlusion. If the valve is deployed too low, there is increased risk of mitral valve dysfunction, heart block, and paravalvular leak.[22]

Aortic Arch and Its Branches

The aortic arch is the part of the aorta that lies in the superior mediastinum. Both its origin and termination are at the *sternal plane*, which is classically defined as the horizontal plane that passes from the manubriosternal junction to the T4/T5 intervertebral disc. It lies just above the level of the pulmonary trunk. At its origin, the arch is in the midline of the chest, with the thymic bed anteriorly, the superior vena cava to its right, a thin rim of fat and small lymph nodes to its left, and the trachea posteriorly. It arches superiorly over the *right* pulmonary artery, the aortopulmonary window, and the *left* main bronchus, in that order, toward the left side of the vertebral body of T4 in a direction that roughly parallels the proximal left pulmonary artery. About two thirds of the way along its course, just beyond the origin of the left subclavian artery, are three important but radiologically occult relationships: the left vagus nerve, which crosses its left side; the recurrent laryngeal branch of the left vagus nerve, which hooks under it and then passes up along its right side; and the ligamentum arteriosum, which joins the undersurface of the arch to the superior surface of the left pulmonary artery. At its highest, a normal arch reaches midway up the manubrium, or about one vertebral body level above its origin. The arch typically ends left anterior to the body of T4.

Radiologic Observations

The diameter of the arch progressively decreases as it gives off its three major branches such that, barring significant aneurysmal dilation, its termination is some 25% to 30% narrower than its origin. The position of its termination is also highly variable and ranges from directly anterior to left posterior to the vertebral body. The latter position is more commonly seen in elderly patients, probably because of elongation of the vessel, which "pushes" the descending aorta posteriorly and leftward (Fig. 82-10). The horizontal level of the sternal plane and the height to which the arch rises are also highly variable and dependent on body habitus (Figs. 82-11 and 82-12).

The curvature of the aortic arch and the angle of origin of its branches vary with age. In young patients, the origins of all three arch branches tend to be at almost the same horizontal level at the apex of the arch. In advanced age, the aorta is elongated with a more acute curvature, which has two effects on the arch: (1) it "pushes" the origins of the arch branches anteriorly, away from the vertebral column, and (2) it raises a "new" and higher arch apex caudal (posterior) to the arch branches, which places their origins on a slope. Together, these effects increase the acuity of the

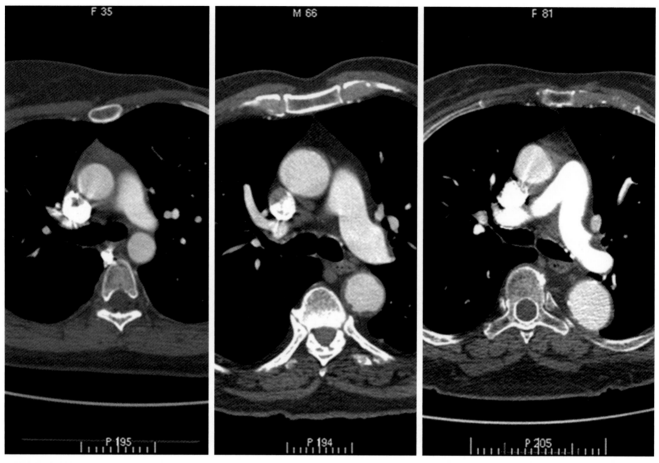

FIGURE 82-10. Contrast-enhanced axial computed tomography images of chest of a young woman *(left)*, an older man *(middle)*, and an elderly woman *(right)* at level of carina. Note differences in position of descending aorta relative to vertebral body, and diameter of ascending aorta relative to descending aorta (which is aneurysmal in elderly patient on right).

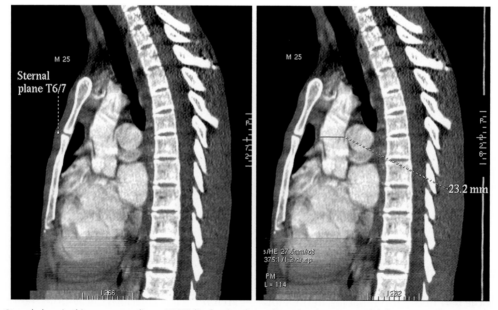

FIGURE 82-11. Sternal plane in this young man lies at T6/T7 disc level and cuts through pulmonary trunk bifurcation rather than aortopulmonary window (note his unusually tall vertebral bodies). Arch apex rises almost to top of manubrium (see also Fig. 82-12). "Jagged" appearance of ascending aorta is a pulsation artifact.

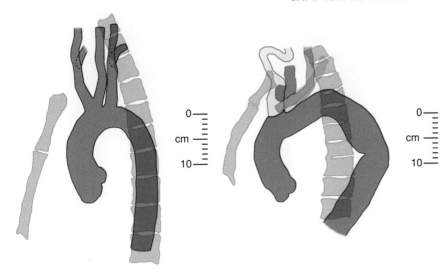

FIGURE 82-12. Left anterior oblique "catheter angiogram" arch views reconstructed from computed tomography scans. Left image is drawn from young man in Figure 82-10, and right image from an 81-year-old woman. Note common origin of brachiocephalic trunk and left common carotid artery in both patients, unusually low origin of right common carotid artery in elderly woman, different relative positions of branch origins to sternal plane and arch apex, and striking difference between the two patients in vessel tortuosity and arch curvature, length, and height.

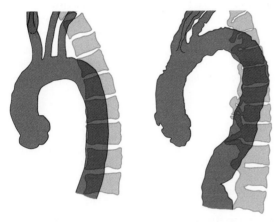

FIGURE 82-13. Left anterior oblique "catheter angiogram" arch views reconstructed from computed tomography scans. In left image from a 35-year-old woman, arch branches arise at same axial (horizontal) level, perpendicular to apex of arch. In right image from a 78-year-old man, aorta is elongated, with a "new" and higher apex caudal to arch branches such that their origins are on a slope. This elongation also "pushes" origins of great vessels anteriorly (compare their distances from vertebral column with those in younger patient). Because their destinations at thoracic inlet remain fixed, these changes result in arteries being "bent backward" on the arch.

Brachiocephalic Trunk (Innominate Artery)

This branch is the first and largest branch of the aortic arch, with a typical diameter of 13 to 15 mm and a length of 5 to 6 cm. At its origin it is in the midline of the chest, directly anterior to the trachea, with the superior vena cava to its right and the origin of the left common carotid artery to its left. The left brachiocephalic vein crosses it anteriorly. It courses superiorly, curves gently toward the right, and terminates by branching into the right subclavian and right common carotid arteries, just deep to the right sternoclavicular joint.

Left Common Carotid Artery

The left common carotid is the second and longest branch of the aortic arch; it ascends from the apex of the arch to the left carotid bifurcation in the neck, which typically occurs between the third and fourth midcervical vertebral bodies. The left brachiocephalic vein crosses it anteriorly as it passes to the left anterolateral aspect of the trachea. It lies immediately anteromedial to the left subclavian artery throughout its course in the chest, a distance of about 6 to 7 cm. Its usual diameter of about 10 mm is significantly less than the diameter of the brachiocephalic trunk.

Left Subclavian Artery

The last and most posterior of the large branches of the thoracic aorta takes origin from the apex of the arch, left lateral to the trachea. It passes superior and slightly lateral to the thoracic inlet and gives off the left vertebral artery as it enters the neck. It abuts the left mediastinal pleura laterally throughout its course and thus forms the left superior mediastinal border on chest radiographs. Its diameter is typically slightly larger than that of the left common carotid artery at about 12 mm.

Variations in Aortic Arch Branching Pattern

The "conventional" branching pattern of the aortic arch just described is seen in about two thirds of the population. Many variations occur, both individually and in combination. The single most prevalent variant is a common origin for the brachiocephalic trunk and left common carotid artery, said to be present in about 25% of the population

angles of origin of the arch branches and cause them to be "bent backward" on the arch (Fig. 82-13; also see Figs. 82-12 and 82-14 for more illustrations of the same phenomenon). Thus, although selective cannulation of the arch branches in young patients is readily achieved with a catheter that has a tip angled at 45 degrees, such as a Hinck catheter, an S-tipped catheter (i.e., reverse curve catheter) such as a Simmons is often required in elderly patients.

The aortic arch gives rise to the three great vessels of the head, neck, and upper limbs: the brachiocephalic (innominate) trunk, the left common carotid artery, and left subclavian artery. None has a sizable or named intrathoracic branch in the "normal" anatomic configuration. It therefore follows that their diameters remain essentially constant throughout their course.

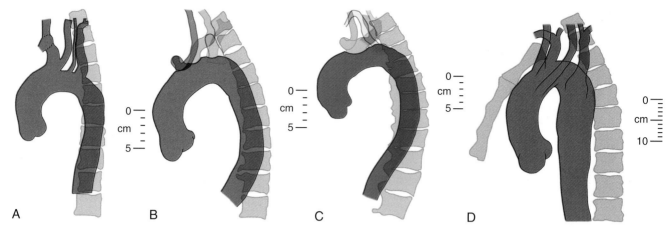

FIGURE 82-14. A, Left anterior oblique "catheter angiogram" arch view reconstructed from computed tomography (CT) scan. This 23-year-old man has a common origin of brachiocephalic trunk and left common carotid artery, as well as a direct arch origin for left vertebral artery. Note similar level of origin for all three arch branches at apex. **B,** Left anterior oblique "catheter angiogram" arch view reconstructed from CT scan. This 68-year-old man has direct arch origins for both right and left common carotid and subclavian arteries. Right subclavian artery arises as fourth branch just distal to left subclavian artery and passes behind esophagus. Note infundibular origin of retroesophageal right subclavian artery, almost 20 mm in diameter, which is commonly seen with this configuration. **C,** Left anterior oblique "catheter angiogram" arch view reconstructed from CT scan. In this 84-year-old woman, a common origin gives rise to right and left common carotid and left subclavian arteries. Right subclavian artery arises distal to this trunk and is retroesophageal—again note its infundibular origin, measuring about 15 mm in diameter in this case. **D,** Left anterior oblique "catheter angiogram" arch view reconstructed from CT scan. In this unusual configuration in a 49-year-old man, there is a right-sided aortic arch with levocardia and a retroesophageal left subclavian artery. Isolated left common carotid artery is the first and lowest branch and arises from left wall of aorta, rather than its convexity, 3 cm below manubriosternal junction. Right common carotid and subclavian arteries arise next and mirror their "standard" left counterparts. Retroesophageal left subclavian artery arises from a dome-shaped aneurysmal infundibulum 5 cm in diameter. (Distances and dimensions were measured from source CT images.)

(see Fig. 82-12). Other common patterns are (1) a direct arch origin for the left vertebral artery, usually just proximal to the left subclavian, (2) a common origin for all three great vessels, and (3) a direct arch origin for the right subclavian artery as a fourth vessel distal to the left subclavian (a "retroesophageal right subclavian artery" or "replaced right subclavian artery"). Figure 82-14 illustrates the appearance of several variants produced from oblique sagittal reconstructions of thin-section contrast-enhanced CT scans that the authors have personally documented in clinical practice.

Descending Aorta and Its Branches

The last and longest segment of the thoracic aorta begins at the T4/T5 intervertebral disc level as a continuation of the aortic arch. At its origin it is anterolateral or directly lateral to the vertebral column. It runs inferiorly and medially toward the aortic hiatus of the diaphragmatic crura and ends by entering the abdomen through the hiatus in the midline, immediately anterior to the spine and usually at the T12/L1 disc level. Its normal diameter ranges from about 20 to 30 mm, slightly larger at its origin than at its termination. Its length varies greatly with body height and age and may range from under 20 to more than 40 cm. It has four major longitudinal relationships throughout its course: the esophagus on its right anterior aspect, the azygos vein on its right or right posterior aspect, the hemiazygos vein on its left posterior aspect, and the thoracic duct posteriorly between the azygos and hemiazygos veins.

There are no large branches in the descending aorta. Instead, there are numerous small branches that can be divided into two groups: somatic branches, which supply the chest wall, diaphragm, spine, and mediastinal "packing tissues"; and visceral branches, which supply the airways, lungs, esophagus, and pericardium.

Key Somatic Branches of the Descending Aorta
Intercostal Arteries
The intercostal arteries are arranged in two groups, anterior and posterior. The anterior intercostal arteries are branches of the internal thoracic (upper six spaces) and musculophrenic (seventh to ninth spaces) arteries. The lowest two spaces do not receive an anterior supply. The posterior intercostal arteries are branches of the superior intercostal artery (upper two spaces) and the descending aorta (lower nine spaces). They supply the chest wall, parietal pleura, and, through their dorsal branches, the skin and muscles of the back and the spine and its contents.

Spinal Arteries
A spinal artery arises from the dorsal branch of each posterior intercostal artery. It takes a recurrent course through the adjacent neural exit foramen into the spinal canal. It supplies the bones, meninges, nerves, and cord. Most spinal arteries are tiny and form a rather tenuous anastomotic network with their contralateral, cranial, and caudal counterparts. Some, however, are large enough to join one of the three major longitudinal spinal arteries directly. These are termed the *segmental medullary feeders*, the largest of which is the arteria radicularis magna, or great anterior segmental medullary artery (of Adamkiewicz). Though classically described as a branch of the left 10th posterior intercostal artery, it may arise on either side anywhere from the T8 to the L2 level.

RADIOLOGIC OBSERVATIONS The advantage of localizing the artery of Adamkiewicz before thoracoabdominal aortic surgery is self-evident. When shown at catheter angiography, it joins the anterior spinal artery at a characteristic hairpin turn. Noninvasive demonstration of this tiny vessel (0.5 mm) remains challenging, although angiographic techniques with magnetic resonance imaging (MRI) and multidetector-row CT have recently been shown to be effective.[24,25] It is also occasionally visible on routine multidetector CT scans (Fig. 82-15).

Esophageal Arteries

Esophageal branches from the descending aorta and the bronchial arteries supply the middle third of the esophagus. The upper third of the organ is supplied by the inferior thyroid artery, and the lower third by the left gastric and phrenic arteries.

Key Visceral Branches of the Descending Aorta
Bronchial Arteries

These small arteries are highly variable in number, size, origin, and course. They arise from the aorta just below the arch, roughly at the level of the carina, and there are usually two on the left and one on the right. On each side, they supply the adjacent lymph nodes before entering the pulmonary hilum. They supply the bronchial tree and visceral pleura and give branches to the pericardium and esophagus. Bronchial arteries are normally occult to catheter aortography but are often partly visible on CT imaging (Fig. 82-16).

SYSTEMIC VEINS

Venous drainage of the thorax may be broadly divided into four groups: (1) visceral return from abdominal viscera through the inferior vena cava, (2) somatic return from the abdomen through both the inferior vena cava and the azygos system, (3) somatic and visceral return from the chest, mostly through the azygos system but also through the brachiocephalic veins via the internal thoracic and first posterior intercostal veins, and (4) venous return from the head, neck, and upper limbs through the brachiocephalic veins. Only the inferior vena cava enters the heart directly; the azygos and brachiocephalic systems drain into the superior vena cava.

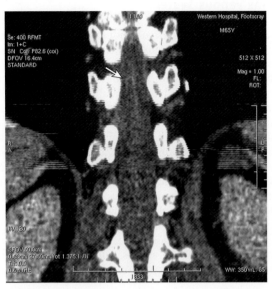

FIGURE 82-15. Coronal reconstruction of routine contrast-enhanced chest computed tomography scan shows tiny vessel with characteristic hairpin turn in right side of lower thoracic spinal canal, consistent with artery of Adamkiewicz *(white arrow)*. It could not be traced contiguously into an exit foramen in this case, but apex of hairpin turn is at level of T10 exit foramen; artery is thus likely to be from right 11th posterior intercostal artery.

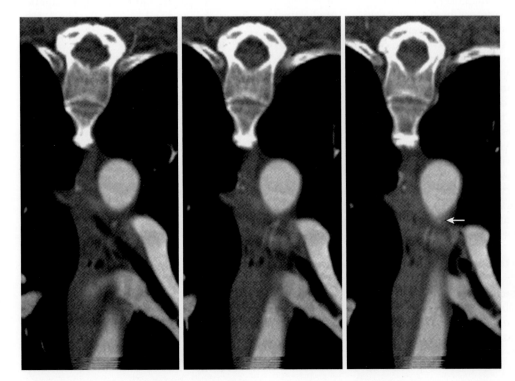

FIGURE 82-16. Three contiguous images from coronal reconstruction of contrast-enhanced chest computed tomography scan (left image, anterior; right image, posterior). Arrow on most posterior image shows origin of superior left bronchial artery. It gives off a large branch to esophagus and then turns to enter left pulmonary hilum inferior to left main bronchus.

Inferior Vena Cava

The thoracic segment of the inferior vena cava enters the posteroinferior aspect of the right atrium almost immediately after it passes through the diaphragm and is thus a very short vessel (15 to 20 mm). It has no tributaries. Unlike the infrahepatic segment, it is held rigidly open by the liver parenchyma and the fibrous skeleton of the right atrium and is oval in shape with a diameter of about 30 to 40 mm.

Azygos Venous System

The azygos system has three major components: the azygos vein proper, the hemiazygos vein, and the accessory hemiazygos vein. The azygos and hemiazygos veins arise respectively from the right and left sides of the retroperitoneal compartment of the abdomen, usually from a confluence of the ascending lumbar and subcostal veins. They enter the chest either by accompanying the aorta and thoracic duct through the aortic hiatus or through separate perforations in the diaphragmatic crura. They ascend more or less vertically in the posterior mediastinum. The azygos ends by arching forward over the right main bronchus to enter the superior vena cava. The azygos arch valve may sometimes be demonstrable on contrast-enhanced CT imaging.[26] The hemiazygos ends at about T8 by joining the azygos vein. The accessory hemiazygos vein is the left-sided equivalent of the upper half of the azygos vein; it ends inferiorly by joining either the hemiazygos or the azygos vein.

Somatic Venous Drainage of the Chest

Chest drainage is asymmetric and highly variable. The first, or supreme, posterior intercostal vein on each side drains into the brachiocephalic or vertebral vein. The superior intercostal vein on each side drains the second and third intercostal spaces; on the right, it joins the azygos vein, and on the left, it usually enters the brachiocephalic vein but often communicates with the accessory hemiazygos vein. The lowest eight right posterior intercostal veins drain directly into the azygos. The accessory hemiazygos and hemiazygos respectively receive the upper and lower four of the remaining eight left posterior intercostal veins.

The posterior intercostal veins drain most of the chest wall. They also receive the thoracic intervertebral veins that accompany the spinal nerves as they exit the neural foramina, thereby draining the valveless and richly anastomosing internal and external vertebral venous plexuses. The much smaller and often paired anterior intercostal veins drain into their respective internal thoracic vein, which accompanies the internal thoracic artery and ends by joining the brachiocephalic vein. In its course it lies 10 to 20 mm from the lateral margin of the sternum. Two internal thoracic veins may accompany each artery.

Visceral Venous Return of the Chest

Venous drainage of the thoracic esophagus is through numerous small unnamed tributaries. From the upper third, these tributaries drain into the brachiocephalic veins; from the middle third into the azygos system; and from the lower third into the left gastric vein. The latter establish a portosystemic anastomosis that, in portal hypertension, results in variceal dilation of the distal esophageal veins, which are commonly seen on CT imaging in patients with advanced cirrhosis.

Venous drainage from the lungs and airways is accomplished by two groups of veins. The superficial system is a confluence of vessels at the pulmonary hilum that drain the larger airways and nearby visceral pleura. They form the bronchial veins, usually two on each side, which drain into the azygos system but also communicate with the pulmonary veins. The deep system drains the lung parenchyma and most of the visceral pleura and forms the pulmonary veins. There is thus an admixture of systemic and pulmonary venous return into the left atrium.

Brachiocephalic Veins

The brachiocephalic vein on each side is formed by the confluence of the internal jugular and subclavian veins, which generally occurs deep to the medial end of the clavicle, lateral to the common carotid artery. The right brachiocephalic vein is usually no more than 3 cm in length and passes straight down in the upper right superior mediastinum. The left brachiocephalic vein takes an oblique course through the anterior mediastinum; it crosses the left common carotid artery and brachiocephalic trunk and joins its right counterpart to form the superior vena cava. It is typically 6 to 7 cm in length.

Superior Vena Cava

The superior vena cava is normally between 6 and 8 cm in length and about 30 to 35 mm in diameter. It is formed from the confluence of the right and left brachiocephalic veins, roughly a third to halfway down the manubrium. About 15 to 20 mm below its origin, it is joined by its major tributary, the azygos vein, which arches forward from its right prevertebral position. It ends by entering the superior aspect of the right atrium. It forms the radiologic right superior mediastinal border.

PULMONARY VESSELS

Pulmonary Trunk and Arteries

The pulmonary trunk arises from the right ventricular outflow tract above the pulmonary valve at a slightly higher level than the aortic origin. It arches posteriorly on the left of the ascending aorta and bifurcates in the concavity of the aortic arch, anterior to the left main bronchus, into the right and left pulmonary arteries. At its bifurcation, the diameter of the trunk is similar to that of the adjacent ascending aorta. The right pulmonary artery lies anterior to the bronchus intermedius. It gives off its upper lobe branch as it passes under the azygos arch before entering the right pulmonary hilum. The left pulmonary artery arches over the left main bronchus and gives off its upper lobe branch as it enters the left pulmonary hilum behind the lobar bronchi.

Pulmonary Veins

The pulmonary veins are formed from the capillary network of the lungs and return oxygenated blood to the systemic circulation. However, they also communicate with and drain the bronchial veins. There are usually two pulmonary veins from each lung, one draining the upper lobe and one draining the lower lobe. They are the most anterior vessels at the pulmonary hila; the right pulmonary veins lie immediately anterior to the pulmonary artery, whereas the left pulmonary veins lie immediately anterior to the main bronchus. They generally enter the left atrium through separate orifices.

LYMPHATIC DRAINAGE

As occurs elsewhere in the body, lymphatic drainage of the thorax follows the vascular supply and can therefore be broadly divided into somatic and visceral components, although there is significant cross-drainage and communication between the two.

Somatic lymphatic drainage of the chest wall is into chains of nodes that lie adjacent to the azygos and hemiazygos veins posteriorly (posterior mediastinal nodes) and the internal thoracic vessels anteriorly (parasternal nodes). These nodes drain into the right lymphatic duct or the thoracic duct.

Visceral lymphatic drainage is mainly into nodes around the trachea, pulmonary hila, and the aortic arch, particularly the tracheobronchial nodes. These nodes drain into the right and left bronchomediastinal trunks, which communicate freely with the posterior mediastinal channels. They usually join their respective brachiocephalic veins directly, but may also end in the right lymphatic duct or thoracic duct.

The thoracic duct enters the chest through the aortic hiatus immediately anterior to the vertebral column. As it passes superiorly, it drains the posterior mediastinal nodes and communicates freely with the bronchomediastinal trunks. It exits the thoracic inlet on the left of the esophagus and ends in either the left subclavian, jugular, or brachiocephalic veins as one or multiple channels.

The right lymphatic duct drains the right posterior chest wall and usually ends in the confluence of the right jugular and subclavian veins. It is short and highly variable in size, course, and position.

KEY POINTS

- The left main coronary artery supplies approximately 75% of the left ventricle, and thus severe disease of this vessel puts the patient at high risk for cardiac death.
- Anomalous coronary arteries are associated with sudden death.
- The largest spinal artery, the arteria radicularis magna, or great anterior segmental medullary artery (of Adamkiewicz), may arise on either the right or left side anywhere from the T8 to L2 levels.
- In advanced age, the aorta is enlarged and has a more acute curvature. These effects increase the acuity of the angles of origin of the arch branches. This poses technical challenges during selective catheterization of the vessels.
- As it courses superiorly in the chest, the thoracic duct of the lymphatic system drains the posterior mediastinal nodes and communicates freely with the bronchomediastinal trunks. It exits the thoracic inlet on the left side of the esophagus and ends in either the left subclavian, jugular, or brachiocephalic veins as one or multiple channels.

▶ **SUGGESTED READINGS**

Bergman RA (curator). Anatomy Atlases: A Digital Library of Anatomy Information. Available at http://www.anatomyatlases.org/.
McMinn RMH, editor. Last's anatomy: Regional and applied. 8th ed. Edinburgh: Churchill Livingstone, 1990.
Netter FH. Atlas of human anatomy. 3rd ed. Teterboro, NJ: Icon Learning Systems, 2003.
Standring S, editor. Gray's anatomy: The anatomical basis of clinical practice. 39th ed. London: Elsevier/Churchill Livingstone, 2005.

The complete reference list is available online at www.expertconsult.com.

CHAPTER 83

Thoracic Aortic Stent-Grafting and Management of Traumatic Thoracic Aortic Lesions

Nina M. Bowens, Edward Y. Woo, Mark A. Farber, and Ronald M. Fairman

Treatment of descending aortic aneurysms has been the most common application for thoracic endovascular aortic repair (TEVAR) (Fig. 83-1). However, thoracic stent-grafts are preferentially used for repair of traumatic injuries to the aorta, acute type B dissections complicated by malperfusion, rupture, and failure of medical therapy, and virtually all thoracic aortic pathology when anatomically feasible. This is not surprising given that open surgery mandates a thoracotomy, single-lung ventilation, aortic cross-clamping, typically partial cardiopulmonary bypass, and for very proximal thoracic aortic lesions, circulatory arrest (Fig. 83-2). In the United States, three commercially available devices, including the Gore (Flagstaff, Ariz.) TAG and more recently the conformable TAG (CTAG), the Cook Medical (Bloomington, Ind.) TX2, and the Medtronic (Minneapolis, Minn.) Talent and Valiant, have U.S. Food and Drug Administration (FDA) approval and labeling for treatment of thoracic aortic aneurysms (TAAs). The pivotal trials evaluating these devices clearly demonstrated improved 1-year outcomes compared to open surgery (Table 83-1), and the 5-year TEVAR data are now available and continue to indicate freedom from aneurysm-related mortality.[1-8]

There has been widespread acceptance and utilization of endovascular therapy whereby it has become the preferred approach for thoracic aortic transections and complicated type B dissections at most centers of excellence. Furthermore, it is remarkable that even in the absence of FDA approval, physicians have recognized the broader applications of an endovascular approach and embraced off-label use of TEVAR to treat various thoracic aortic pathologies.[9-22]

INDICATIONS

Thoracic aortic stent-grafting evolved from abdominal aortic stent-grafting. Initial reports of TEVAR involved using "homemade devices" or abdominal components in an off-label manner. Dedicated thoracic components have been commercially available in the United States since 2005, and device iteration continues to progress beyond the first generation.[23-25] The historical indication for operative intervention has been an aneurysm size of 6.5 cm, based on studies demonstrating significantly increased rupture rates.[9] However, with the widespread availability of thoracic endografts, this rigorous anatomic selection criteria may be evolving in real-world practice to earlier intervention for smaller aneurysms. Fusiform and saccular aneurysms have been the most commonly treated pathology, but worldwide, thoracic stent-grafts have been increasingly used for aortic dissection (acute and chronic), penetrating ulcers, aortic (airway and gastrointestinal) fistulas, aortic rupture, and blunt traumatic injury, which has recently received FDA approval in the United States.[19-26]

Management of traumatic injury to the thoracic aorta or great vessels is often complex. Arterial injury is confined to the thoracic aorta in 81% of cases, affects the aortic branch vessels alone in 16%, and involves both the thoracic aorta and great vessels in 3%.[27,28] Penetrating injuries involving these structures frequently results in rapid exsanguination and death. Common causes of penetrating thoracic trauma include stab wounds and medium-velocity bullet wounds. The anatomic location and extent of intrathoracic vascular injury secondary to penetrating trauma is difficult to anticipate, owing to variant depth and trajectory of the penetrating object. Blunt thoracic trauma, although less common, may result in injury to the ascending aorta, aortic arch, descending thoracic aorta, or great vessels.

Establishing the diagnosis of injury to the thoracic aorta or great vessels usually begins with considering the mechanism of injury. Frequently, especially in the setting of blunt trauma, multisystemic injury and depressed levels of consciousness limit acquisition of historical data. In these circumstances, algorithmic protocols such as the Advanced Trauma Life Support (ATLS) guidelines allow coordinated assessment, diagnostic evaluation, and resuscitation. As in the elective setting, computed tomographic angiography (CTA) has become the diagnostic study of choice, given its widespread availability and rapid image acquisition time (Fig. 83-3).[29,30]

CONTRAINDICATIONS

An absolute contraindication to thoracic stent-grafting is anatomic ineligibility. Absence of proximal or distal landing zones prevents treatment with a standard thoracic stent-graft. Successful exclusion of the pathology depends on achieving a satisfactory proximal and distal seal. Current commercially available thoracic stent-graft devices have a maximal postdeployment diameter of 46 mm, thereby prohibiting successful achievement of seal zones in vessels with diameters greater than 42 mm. At the other end of the spectrum, the smallest current-generation thoracic devices have a postdeployment diameter of 21 mm, prohibiting successful seal zone achievement in vessels with diameters less than 16 mm. More complex endovascular options, including branched grafts and hybrid reconstructions with aortic debranching, can be performed in anatomically complex cases, but these options will not be discussed in this chapter; such procedures play a limited role in emergency management of thoracic catastrophes.

Relative contraindications to endovascular repair of the thoracic aorta also exist. Long-term durability of TEVAR has not yet been established, so its applicability in the young patient remains controversial. Historically, open repair was used for unstable patients who were unable to undergo preoperative imaging. However, the Vascular Group at

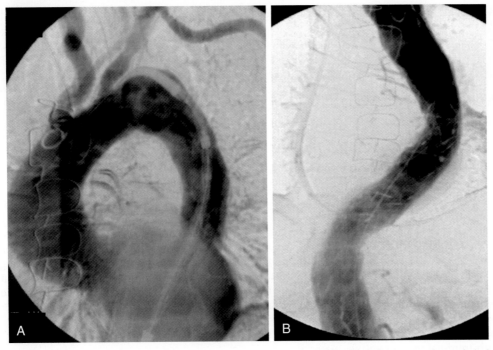

FIGURE 83-1. A, Large aneurysm of mid-descending thoracic aorta. **B,** Successfully excluded aneurysm after graft deployment.

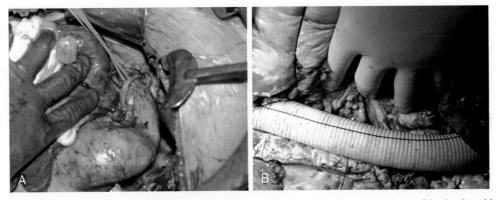

FIGURE 83-2. A, Open thoracotomy demonstrating thoracic aortic aneurysm (TAA), uninflated lung, vagus nerve *(blue loop)*, and left subclavian artery *(blue loop)*. **B,** Dacron interposition graft in place of TAA.

TABLE 83-1. Summary Data of Pivotal Trials

Trial	Authors	Subjects	MAE (30-day)	TDM	ARM	ACM	SAT	Endoleak
VALOR Talent	Fairman et al.[1]; unpublished data	195 endovascular, 189 retrospective open surgical cases	41% (vs. 84.4%, *P* < .001)	2% (vs. 8%, *P* < .01)	1 yr: 3.1% 5 yr: 3.9%	1 yr: 16.1% (vs. 20.6%, *P* = ns) 5 yr: 41.5%	1 yr: 91.5% 5 yr: 91.4%	1 yr: 12.2%
Gore TAG	Bavaria et al.[42] Makaroun et al.[8]	140 endovascular (+51 following graft revision), 94 open controls	28% (vs. 70%, *P* < .001)	2.1% (vs. 11.7%, *P* < .001)	5 yr: 2.8%	5 yr: 32% (vs. 33%, *P* = .433)	5 yr: 81% (initial TAG) 2 yr: 87.1% (revised)	5 yr: 10.6%
Zenith TX2	Matsumura et al.[4]	160 endovascular, 70 open controls	41.9% (vs. 68.6%, *P* < .01)	1.9% (vs. 5.7%, *P* < .01)	1 yr: 5.8%	1 yr: 8.4% (vs. 14.5%)	1 yr: 92.9%	1 yr: 3.9%

ACM, All-cause mortality; *ARM,* aneurysm-related mortality; *MAE,* major adverse events; *SAT,* successful aneurysm treatment; *TDM,* 30-day mortality.

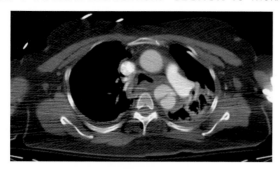

FIGURE 83-3. Computed tomographic angiogram demonstrating findings consistent with aortic transection.

Albany established the safety of stent-grafting in traumatic rupture of the thoracic aorta, and practice guidelines developed by the Society for Vascular Surgery continue to support the use of TEVAR for traumatic thoracic aortic injury.[31,32] The concern of contrast-induced nephropathy in patients with concomitant thoracic aortic pathology and renal insufficiency can be successfully circumvented by using intravascular ultrasound (IVUS), allowing TEVAR to be performed with minimal use of contrast material.

PREOPERATIVE EVALUATION

Preoperative imaging is critical for successful endovascular repair of the thoracic aorta. Cross-sectional imaging, preferably CTA with thin slices focused on the aorta, is required. Three-dimensional reconstructions, such as the MMS (Medical Metrix Solutions Inc., West Lebanon, N.H.) or TeraRecon system (DuPont, Wilmington, Del.), are then important for determining accurate centerline measurements. Contrast-enhanced angiograms are rarely indicated before the procedure.

For many years, arch aortography with visualization of the great vessels has been the gold standard for diagnosing arterial injuries of the thoracic aorta and great vessels. Liberal application of multidetector CTA in the setting of thoracic trauma has increased the ability to rapidly diagnose injuries of the thoracic aorta and great vessels and provided adequate information on which to base therapeutic treatment algorithms. Although somewhat controversial, CTA in many circumstances obviates the mandatory requirement for diagnostic arteriography, even in the setting of traumatic injury. Many physicians now opt for selective utilization of traditional arteriography, reserving this option for indeterminate findings on CTA, or more commonly using arteriography as an adjunct to percutaneous therapeutic intervention.

Successful exclusion of an arterial defect—whether aneurysm, dissection, or injury—with a stent-graft fundamentally relies on achieving a seal between the device and the vessel wall both proximal and distal to the site of pathology. Achieving a satisfactory seal in these locations depends on several factors. Of critical importance is correct device sizing. An undersized device results in inadequate apposition between the stent-graft and vessel wall, resulting in incomplete exclusion. Slight oversizing ($\approx$10%) allows circumferential transmission of postdeployment radial forces from the device to the aortic wall, thereby facilitating device/vessel apposition and seal zone achievement.

Unfortunately, zealous oversizing may result in crimping of graft material, predisposing to type I endoleak. Exaggerated oversizing may precipitate potentially life-threatening intimal dissection or arterial injury induced by the stent-graft itself.

Achieving a proximal seal is frequently more challenging than obtaining a distal seal. This is due to several factors, including angulation of the distal aortic arch and proximity of the great vessels. In most patients, the likelihood of achieving satisfactory proximal and distal seal zones can be determined by carefully evaluating preprocedural CT images, correlating this information with intraprocedural angiographic data, and having a low threshold for performing partial (or complete) over-stenting of the left subclavian artery. Coverage of the left subclavian artery remains a controversial subject because the literature is devoid of randomized prospective data. Most would support coverage of the left subclavian in the emergency setting, with selective revascularization based on vertebral anatomy following TEVAR. However, guidelines in the elective setting remain in evolution.[32,33]

ANATOMY AND APPROACH

Preprocedural abdominal and pelvic CTA (performed simultaneously with chest CTA) allows accurate evaluation of the anatomic features of the abdominal aorta and iliac arteries. Primary considerations include identifying stenotic or occlusive lesions and determining the degree of arterial tortuosity. The minimal iliac arterial diameter required to allow retrograde passage of the device varies with the size and type of stent-graft selected. Current commercially available devices make use of large-caliber introducer sheaths (20F to 24F) that generally require an iliac arterial diameter of at least 7 to 8 mm. Further consideration is also given to the patient's surgical history and physical examination findings in an effort to avoid unnecessary dissection through scar tissue from prior surgical procedures. This information is then used to formulate an appropriate target strategy for surgical access.

EQUIPMENT

The process of optimal device selection can be complicated. In addition to the basic considerations of device diameter and length, the importance of device conformability, trackability, deployment accuracy, availability, and operator familiarity should not be underestimated.

The Gore TAG was the first FDA-approved device for the treatment of thoracic aneurysms. Design revisions in 2004 (spine removal) simplified its use and significantly decreased late graft-related complications. Five-year results comparing endovascular treatment using the Gore TAG with open surgical repair demonstrated significantly reduced mortality and major adverse events (MAEs) in patents undergoing TEVAR.[8] Medtronic completed its pivotal VALOR trial of the Talent thoracic stent-graft, demonstrating TEVAR superiority to open surgical repair.[1] Trials evaluating the Valiant, which involves modifications and enhancements to the Talent graft, similarly published favorable early and midterm results for stent use in a wide variety of thoracic aortic pathologies.[2,3] The FDA approved the Medtronic Valiant device in 2011. The Cook Medical

TABLE 83-2. Thoracic Endovascular Graft Device Iterations

Device		Original	Current	Next Generation
Gore TAG (W.L. Gore Flagstaff, Ariz.)	FDA approval	2005	2009	2011 Conformable TAG (CTAG)
	Features	• Flexible PTFE • Nitinol exoskeleton	• Strong, low-porosity PTFE • No longitudinal spine	• No barbs or springs • Increased flexibility • Compression resistant • Enables device oversizing
Talent (Medtronic Vascular, Minneapolis, Minn.)	FDA approval	2008	2011	2011 Valiant
	Features	• Polyester • Nitinol wire frame • Modular design	• No connecting bar • 8-peak radial proximal fixation	• No connecting bar • 8-peak radial proximal fixation
Zenith TX2 (Cook Medical, Bloomington, Ind.)	FDA approval	2008	2009 TX2 Pro-Form	Pending TX2 Low Profile
	Features	• Dacron • One- or two-piece modular system • Self-expanding stainless steel Z-stents • Distal and proximal barbs	• Improved proximal graft control	• Decreased-caliber delivery system

FDA, U.S. Food and Drug Administration; *PTFE*, polytetrafluoroethylene.

Zenith TX2 trial also succeeded in demonstrating non-inferiority of TEVAR over open surgical repair.[4,5] Moreover, it is important to recognize that following initial FDA approval, these devices undergo further iteration over time as industry responds to physician feedback (Table 83-2).

Common aspects among these devices that separate them from abdominal grafts include a long shaft to deliver the endograft to the proximal thoracic aorta from the groin, larger diameters and lengths to accommodate the thoracic aorta, and a tubular nonbifurcated design. Increased flexibility and conformability to account for the often tortuous thoracic aorta, as well as the aortic arch, is likewise important.

The various grafts have design features that make them unique. Each has a different release mechanism during endograft deployment. The Valiant (Medtronic) offers a proximal self-expanding polished nitinol wire frame for fixation and is available in larger diameters that allow treatment of aortas up to 42 mm. This graft has been modified to include the addition of an eight-peak spring (compared to a five-peak spring in the Talent system) to allow for improved proximal fixation and elimination of the connecting bar for increased flexibility. The proximal bare spring remains constrained following deployment of the stent-graft and is released subsequently. The Zenith (Cook) device uses a completely covered proximal stent and an uncovered stent distally, with barbs both proximally and distally for improved fixation; in the regular graft sizes, it also has a tapered graft. This graft may be used as a one- or two-component system. Two-year data examining use of the TX2 Zenith graft suggest that the two-component system is employed in more complex patients and thus associated with increased perioperative morbidity.[5] The recently improved conformable TAG (Gore CTAG) device incorporates a short uncovered stent proximally for better wall apposition and an unflared straight distal configuration. The enhanced device has improved compression resistance and is manufactured in smaller diameters and tapered designs. In addition, a novel trilobed balloon to allow continuous aortic flow during balloon inflation is also available as an accessory. Moreover, the choice of endograft should

TABLE 83-3. Suggested Equipment for Endovascular Management of Traumatic Thoracic Aortic Injuries

- 0.035-inch Bentson guidewire (150 cm)
- 0.035-inch Newton-J guidewire (150 cm)
- 0.035-inch Amplatz Super Stiff guidewire (260 cm)
- 0.035-inch Meier guidewire (300 cm)
- 0.035-inch LES-3 Lunderquist guidewire (260 cm)
- 0.018-inch Mandril guidewire
- 18-gauge, 7-cm access needle
- 21-gauge, 7-cm access needle
- 5F micropuncture set
- 5F, 10-cm vascular sheath
- 8F, 20-cm vascular sheath
- 20F, 22F, and 24F vascular sheaths
- Vascular instrument tray
- C-arm fluoroscopy unit, or fluoroscopically equipped procedure room
- Range of aortic stent-grafts (22-46 mm diameter, 10-15 cm length)
- Aortic molding balloon
- 10-mm Dacron conduit

certainly be tailored to individual patient specifications such as aneurysm anatomy and access availability.

Despite the tubular design, thoracic endografting can often be more challenging than abdominal endografting, so it is critical to have the necessary equipment, facilities, and personnel during procedures. Standard wires and catheters are necessary for obtaining access. Stiff wires, such as the Lunderquist (Cook), are important for device tracking. The devices of all manufacturers can be quite stiff and difficult to track through a tortuous aorta or around the aortic arch. All wires must be at least 260 cm for access from the groin. Marker pigtail catheters can be helpful for intraprocedural length measurements. Balloons used for graft effacement are generally device specific. At times, a noncompliant aortic balloon may be necessary (Table 83-3).

Ideally, these procedures should be performed in an endosuite within a fully functional operating room. Certainly, a mobile system can suffice, but the resolution with a fixed platform is superior. Operating room capabilities are important because most of these procedures require at least one femoral exposure, and retroperitoneal access to the iliac artery is often needed.[7,34] Notably, gender analysis of the Talent system revealed that iliac conduits are required significantly more often in women than men.[35] In addition to vascular access concerns, emergency situations requiring an open operative procedure can arise, necessitating operating room capabilities.

Assembly of an appropriate operative team is paramount for successful aortic repair and patient outcomes. Technicians familiar with the devices, equipment, and procedural steps are helpful, and anesthetic support is critical. Patients often need invasive monitoring for strict hemodynamic control, especially when working around the arch. Moreover, spinal drains may be necessary to decrease intraspinal pressure and help prevent paraplegia. Neurologic support is also indicated and may be in the form of monitoring motor or somatosensory evoked potentials. Studies have clearly shown that monitoring of such potentials can help manage the incidence of paraplegia, at least during open repair.[36-39]

TECHNIQUE

Thoracic stent-grafting usually requires access for delivery of the device, as well as intraprocedural angiography. Current thoracic stent-graft devices are usually introduced in a retrograde fashion from a femoral approach through the iliofemoral system into the abdominal aorta, before being advanced to the thoracic aorta.

To facilitate endoluminal repair of the thoracic aorta, the patient is positioned in a supine fashion on a fluoroscopy-compatible table, with the right upper extremity tucked parallel to the right flank, and the left upper extremity extended on an arm board. This enables access of a C-arm fluoroscopy unit from the patient's right side, allows percutaneous access to the left brachial artery (if required), and provides adequate operator access to the bilateral femoral regions. The left upper arm is selectively prepped and draped in circumstances where it is suspected that retrograde brachial artery access will be required. Access through the arm is helpful because the catheter will mark the location of the subclavian artery at all times. In addition, with aortic dissection it can be very helpful in obtaining access to the true lumen (see Chapter 51).

An oblique skin incision approximately 5 cm in length is created over the midportion of the primary common femoral artery. The subcutaneous tissues and fascial layers are then divided using electrocautery to the level of the femoral sheath. The femoral sheath is opened, and the common femoral artery is encircled with vessel loops. An 18-gauge needle is then used to access the anterior aspect of the common femoral artery. A Bentson guidewire is advanced through the needle and then through the iliac arterial system under fluoroscopic visualization. The needle is then exchanged for a short 7F vascular sheath.

Retrograde percutaneous access of the contralateral common femoral artery is performed at this time, with or without the assistance of ultrasound guidance. A 10-cm, 5F sheath is then positioned within the contralateral common femoral artery. In selected patients, percutaneous insertion of the device through the primary common femoral artery can also be accomplished with minimal complications.[32]

A significant number of adjunctive procedures, specifically access conduits, were performed when abdominal endografting was started.[34] This has decreased significantly with the advent of smaller devices and sheaths. Nevertheless, thoracic devices are still quite large, usually in the range of 22F to 25F to accommodate the thoracic aorta. In the setting of severe aortoiliac occlusive disease or small-caliber iliac arteries, retrograde arterial passage of stent-graft devices from the femoral region may not be technically feasible. The points of limitation are usually the common femoral artery and the origin of the external iliac artery. Unilateral iliac occlusive disease can be circumvented by selecting the nondiseased contralateral iliofemoral system as the site of arterial access. Although a nondiseased artery will generally stretch somewhat, any plaque/calcification will limit stretching and lead to potential injury. Device-specific guidelines should be followed in terms of required access diameter.

Techniques to circumvent access limitations include common iliac artery conduits or direct common iliac artery puncture. Direct aortic puncture is rarely needed and is not discussed in this chapter. In circumstances of bilateral external iliac artery stenosis (<7 mm) or occlusion, a suprainguinal extraperitoneal dissection may be used to expose the common iliac artery.

Exposure of the iliac artery is generally quite straightforward and adds only several minutes to the procedure. A curvilinear incision is made along the flank. The muscles are divided, and the peritoneal contents are swept cephalad and medially to gain access to the retroperitoneum. Care must be taken to avoid injuring the ureter. Control of the common, internal, and external iliac arteries is achieved. Direct punctures can be closed primarily with a purse-string suture or patch. Conduits are generally used when significant disease of the common iliac artery prevents direct puncture. A 10-mm graft is then sewn into the artery, which is ligated at the end of the procedure if there is no iliac injury requiring bypass. Regardless of whether a conduit is used, tunneling to the ipsilateral groin may allow easier passage of the devices, especially in larger patients, in whom the common iliac artery can be quite deep.

In cases where the size is close, it is recommended that one electively proceed with common iliac artery exposure to prevent arterial injury. The most common injury usually involves an avulsion or tear of the external iliac artery and common femoral artery on sheath removal and less often on sheath entry (Fig. 83-4). In such circumstances, wire access should be maintained, and a large aortic balloon should be inflated for proximal control. Expeditious arterial

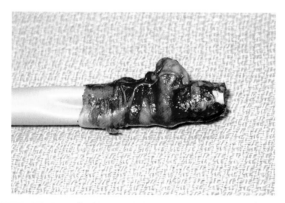

FIGURE 83-4. Avulsed external iliac artery on an endograft delivery sheath after sheath withdrawal.

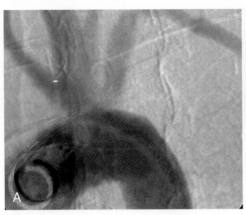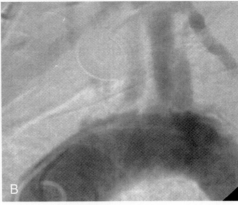

FIGURE 83-5. A, Arch vessels seen as a conglomerate mass because of inadequate rotational obliquity of image intensifier. **B,** Well-splayed arch with increased obliquity.

exposure and repair should then proceed, which most commonly entails a bypass from the common iliac artery to the common femoral artery. Significant blood loss and hypotension can occur during this time, and in such cases, rapid intervention by the surgeon, interventionalist, and anesthesiologist is critical. In addition to systemic complications such as myocardial infarction, renal ischemia, and others, a major concern during this period is spinal cord injury, which often occurs in the setting of retroperitoneal hemorrhage and associated hypotension.

In the setting of traumatic injury of the thoracic aorta, concomitant pelvic injury with associated disruption of the iliohypogastric vessels is generally considered a contraindication to iliofemoral access on the side of injury, mandating an individualized approach to aortic access in these patients. In many circumstances, the decision regarding in which groin to perform primary surgical cutdown is inconsequential; however, careful consideration of the previous factors is mandatory.

After establishing bilateral femoral access, an individualized decision regarding the risks and benefits of systemic anticoagulation has to be considered. If no contraindication to anticoagulation exists, the patient is systemically heparinized. The bilateral guidewires are then advanced to the level of the ascending aortic arch under fluoroscopic guidance, with the assistance of a 100-cm, 5F Kumpe catheter. A 100-cm, 5F pigtail marker catheter is advanced over the percutaneous guidewire and positioned within the ascending aortic arch, proximal to the site of injury. Guiding the wires through a tortuous aorta can at times be difficult. Furthermore, with large aneurysms the wire can sometimes get convoluted in the sac, and care must be taken to not create a dissection or rupture the aneurysm. Ultimately, a stiff wire, such as a Lunderquist (Cook), is advanced through the Kumpe catheter in the primary access site and positioned within the ascending aortic arch. It is best to retroflex the soft tip of the wire off the aortic valve to ensure that damage to the coronary ostia or heart does not occur.

Once appropriate access is achieved, the device is introduced into the thoracic aorta where it will be deployed. It is critical to bring the device to its appropriate position before obtaining a road map image because the aortic architecture will change as a result of the stiffness of the device. The table is then rotated right side down, and the fluoroscopy C-arm is rotated laterally, thereby achieving a left

anterior oblique projection of the aortic arch. All angiograms should be performed with significant obliquity (full lateral for viewing the visceral vessels) to correctly splay the thoracic aorta, especially the arch (Fig. 83-5).

The subsequent procedure varies according to the type of thoracic stent-graft used. Some devices (e.g., Gore TAG) have a large-caliber access sheath (20F-24F) that is advanced over the primary guidewire through the iliofemoral system into the abdominal aorta. The device is subsequently advanced through the sheath into the thoracic aorta. Other devices, such as the Medtronic Talent device, are preloaded within a sheath that is advanced as a single unit through the iliofemoral system into the aorta. Deployment of the endograft should proceed as per the manufacturer's instructions for use. Postdeployment ballooning depends on the device. Notably, ballooning should be avoided when TEVAR is used for the treatment of aortic dissection (see Chapter 51). If ballooning is performed, careful hemodynamic control is important because aortic pulse pressure can shift the graft.

The number of modular pieces necessary is dependent on aortic anatomy and the choice of graft. An overlap of at least 5 cm is usually desirable to prevent a junctional endoleak. Careful preoperative planning is critical when the aorta tapers proximally to distally. In such circumstances, the graft has to be built up distally to proximally so the larger component intussuscepts into the smaller component. The Zenith (Cook) does offer a tapered endograft that can somewhat accommodate for this.

IVUS is useful in minimizing contrast material load by reducing the number of runs. Aortic anatomy and the exact location of branch vessels can be determined, and measurements of diameter can be confirmed if preoperative measurements are unclear. In aortic dissections, IVUS is most useful in differentiating the true lumen from the false lumen (see Chapter 51) and can ensure that all wires and catheters are in the lumen of choice.

Completion digital subtraction aortography is routinely performed after deployment of the thoracic device. This study serves to confirm luminal patency of the stent-graft, the absence of device kinking, and evaluates for the presence of endoleak. Complete discussion of the management of endoleaks is beyond the scope of this chapter, but often intervention with balloon molding of the device or deployment of additional device components is required to achieve satisfactory exclusion in the setting of traumatic injuries.

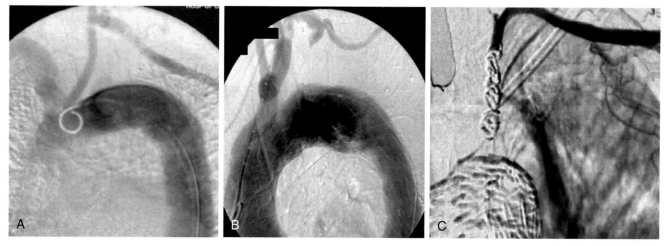

FIGURE 83-6. A, Transposition of left subclavian artery to left common carotid artery. **B,** Left common carotid artery–to–left subclavian artery bypass with proximal ligation of subclavian artery. **C,** Left common carotid artery–to–left subclavian artery bypass with coil embolization of proximal subclavian artery.

When performing TEVAR, it is often necessary to extend the graft into the distal arch. Although discussion of hybrid arch procedures and full arch devascularization is beyond the scope of this chapter, techniques for coverage and revascularization of the left subclavian artery are important to know because this is not uncommon. In patients with proximal aneurysm extension or a severely angulated arch, the device may have to be extended to the origin of the left common carotid or innominate artery (bovine arch). Although acute arm ischemia rarely occurs with left subclavian artery coverage, ischemic events of the posterior circulation and spinal cord ischemia can result. Cases of chronic arm claudication have been reported.[33,40]

Revascularization of the left subclavian artery is usually performed via left subclavian–to–left common carotid artery transposition or bypass between these vessels in elective cases prior to repair of the thoracic aorta (Fig. 83-6). Preoperative duplex ultrasound of the carotid arteries is necessary to rule out any concomitant flow-limiting common or internal carotid artery disease. Interruption of retrograde flow via the proximal left subclavian artery is important to prevent a type II endoleak. In cases of transposition, this is performed by closing the stump of the proximal vessel. If a bypass is performed, ligation of the proximal subclavian artery or coil embolization of the proximal vessel can be performed.[33,41]

As stated previously, acute arm ischemia does not usually occur after coverage of the subclavian artery, so the decision to revascularize the artery is based on the risk of cerebral and spinal ischemia. Preoperative imaging of the vertebral arteries and basilar artery is helpful to determine the need for revascularization. In patients with a dominant left vertebral artery, right vertebral artery lesion, absent right vertebral artery, or incomplete collateral pathways via the basilar artery, revascularization is indicated. Some patients will have previously undergone left internal mammary artery bypass to the left anterior descending coronary artery, and in this setting coverage of the left subclavian artery would be contraindicated. In addition, when coverage of the entire thoracic aorta is planned, revascularization should be performed to minimize spinal cord ischemia. Nevertheless, under emergency circumstances such as rupture, dissection, or traumatic injury, coverage of the left subclavian artery may be necessary, and time may not permit revascularization. This is usually well tolerated by the patient.

POSTPROCEDURAL AND FOLLOW-UP CARE

Postprocedural management after stent-graft repair of the thoracic aorta is significantly influenced by the extent and nature of the repair, and by the associated injuries when dealing with trauma. Patients with aortic transection secondary to blunt trauma often have multisystemic injuries that require coordinated surgical prioritization and intervention as indicated. Management of non–life-threatening injuries is usually temporarily deferred. Following thoracic aneurysm repair, the patient is transferred to an intensive care unit for monitoring, stabilization, and resuscitation.

Interval surveillance is required for patients who have undergone stent-graft repair. At our institution, repeat CTA of the chest is obtained during hospitalization following stabilization and/or recovery from other injuries in the setting of traumatic aortic repairs. For all patients treated with TEVAR, follow-up CT angiograms and multiplanar chest radiographs are obtained at 1, 6, and 12 months after the procedure, with yearly studies thereafter. Follow-up radiologic evaluation enables identification of endoleak, assesses stent-graft position and integrity, and allows timely reintervention if required.

PIVOTAL TRIALS

The Gore TAG was the initial endoprosthetic device to receive FDA approval. Trials have consistently demonstrated improved outcomes when compared to open repair. The pivotal trial identified a total of 234 patients, of which 140 were treated with TEVAR and 94 by standard open repair. Early data demonstrated 30-day operative mortality of 2.1% versus 11.7% ($P = .004$) in the TEVAR and surgical groups, respectively. Spinal cord ischemia in the endograft group was 2.9% versus 13.8% ($P = .003$) in the control population. Patients undergoing TEVAR experienced reduced rates of respiratory failure and renal failure but higher rates of peripheral vascular complications.[42]

Midterm data with mean 2-year follow-up demonstrated comparable survival in the endograft and surgical groups. Incidence of endoleak was demonstrated at 11% and 9% for 30-day and 2-year follow-up, respectively. The majority of endoleaks were documented as type I. With regard to TEVAR efficacy, approximately 90% of aneurysms decreased in size or remained stable at 2-year follow-up, with no cases of aneurysm rupture. Stent fractures were identified in 14% of patients having undergone TEVAR, prompting device revision in 2001 with removal of the longitudinal spine and conversion to the graft's current iteration, including a stronger polytetrafluoroethylene (PTFE) material with decreased porosity, introduced in 2004.

Five-year results of TEVAR using the Gore TAG device, including the additional 51 patients enrolled using the new device iteration, continued to demonstrate superiority in aneurysm-related mortality and MAEs when compared with open repair.[26] Data successfully addressed concerns regarding morbidity from reintervention and graft failure. MAEs were considered to include events that resulted in prolonged treatment, hospitalization, major disability, or death. At 5 years, aneurysm-related mortality was significantly reduced in patients treated with the TAG device compared to patients treated with open surgical repair (2.8% vs. 11.7%, P = .008). All-cause mortality between the two groups at 5 years was similar, although high: 32% in the TAG group and 33% in the open surgical repair group. MAEs were more prevalent in the open surgical repair group, occurring predominantly in the immediate postoperative period (28% vs. 70%) and persisting through 5-year follow-up (57.9% vs. 77%). The majority of MAEs occurring in TEVAR patients consisted of peripheral vascular complications, compared to respiratory, renal, wound, and neurologic complications in the open surgical repair group.[42]

At 5 years, endovascular repair with the TAG outperformed open surgical repair. Endoleaks were identified in 10.6% of patients and were predominantly type I, occurring at sites of attachment. However, the rate of aneurysm-related intervention remained low at 3.6% in the TAG group and 2.1% for the open surgical group. Distinct from the shorter-term follow-up, at 5 years, 19% of patients treated with TAG had 5 mm or more of sac enlargement, of which only a minor percentage (9.1%-12.5%) could be attributed to endoleak. Analysis of the confirmatory arm using the revised TAG with low-porosity fabric demonstrated no sac enlargement at 1 year, while 2.9% experienced enlargement at 2 years. However, neither of these figures was significant when compared to patients repaired with the original TAG device iteration. There was only one event of stent migration in the TAG group, no aneurysm rupture, and no graft collapse.[8] Although the FDA recently approved the CTAG device for aneurysmal disease and isolated thoracic aortic lesions, detailed data from these trials have not been released.

The Pivotal VALOR I trial investigating the Medtronic Vascular Talent thoracic stent-graft system was initiated shortly after the TAG and similarly demonstrated favorable results and efficacy for endoprosthetic treatment of TAAs. This trial lacked a concurrent open surgical arm and instead used retrospective open surgical data. The trial enrolled 195 patients and identified 189 retrospective open surgical controls. The Talent device consisted of a polyester fabric with self-expanding nitinol frame using a modular design. Early data demonstrated a significant decrease in 30-day

mortality in the VALOR group compared to controls (2% vs. 8%, P < .01). At 1 year, all-cause mortality was similar and non-significant, but aneurysm-related mortality was significantly lower in the VALOR group than the surgery group (3.1% vs. 11.6%, P < .002). At 1 year, MAEs occurred in 41% of VALOR patients and 84.4% of open surgical controls. Again, vascular complications accounted for the majority of MAEs in the group treated with endovascular repair. At 30 days, 25.9% percent of patients were found to have an endoleak, the majority of which were type II. At 1 year, endoleaks were identified in 12.2% and evenly distributed between type I and type II. Four events of stent-graft migration were identified, with only one requiring intervention during the 1-year follow-up. Aneurysm diameter was stable or decreased in 91.4% of VALOR patients, and endoleak accounted for more than half of patients who experienced aneurysm expansion.[1]

The 5-year data for the VALOR I trial are currently emerging and remain favorable. Similar to the Gore TAG trial, all-cause mortality over the 5-year period was high (43.9%), with the majority of deaths due to cardiovascular, pulmonary, and cancer-related causes. Freedom from aneurysm-related death remained high at both 1 year (96.9%) and 5 years (96.1%), with the majority of deaths attributable to aneurysms occurring during the first year (86%). There were four aneurysm ruptures, and four patients converted to open repair during the 5-year follow-up. Both type I and type II endoleak occurred in the VALOR group but remained less than 10%. At 5 years, aneurysm size was stable or reduced in 90.8% of patients with stent-graft. The majority of secondary interventions were performed during the first year after graft placement and performed to treat endoleak. There was no graft collapse or loss of patency, and less than 2% of patients experienced graft migration. In summary, the 5-year results using the Talent thoracic stent-graft have demonstrated sustained protection from aneurysm-related mortality, aneurysm rupture, and conversion. Device integrity was maintained over the 5 years, and most secondary interventions were performed to treat endoleak; half of these interventions occurred during years 1 to 5 (submitted data).

Preliminary data are emerging from the VALOR II trial, which is an extension of the VALOR I trial using the modified Talent graft, the Valiant. For improved flexibility, the Valiant lacks a longitudinal connecting bar and contains an 8-peak proximal spring configuration for improved distribution of radial force; it is also available in longer lengths. The multiinstitutional study investigated TAA of degenerative etiology in 160 patients. It is notable that the VALOR II trial contained a sicker population with more comorbid illness than the VALOR I. At 30-days, all-cause mortality and aneurysm-related mortality were 3.1%, while 38.1% experienced one or more MAEs. There were no aneurysm ruptures or conversions to surgery. Aneurysms were successfully treated in 97.4% of patients. At 1-year, endoleak was identified in 13% of patients, with secondary procedures required for 3.0% of type I and 1.0% of type III endoleaks. At 1 year, the Valiant system of the VALOR II trial proved noninferior when compared to the Talent device used in the VALOR I trial, with an odds ratio of 0.70 (unpublished data).

The pivotal Zenith TX2 trial evaluated endoprosthetic treatment of TAAs, in addition to large ulcers; 1-year data successfully demonstrated noninferiority.[4] The device has undergone several iterations and consists of polyester sewn to self-expanding Cook Z-stents containing fixation barbs at the distal and proximal ends of the device. The study consisted of 160 patients in the endovascular arm and 51 retrospective open controls. Among the TX2 patients, 40.5% received a two-piece graft, and 38% received a one-piece. All-cause mortality at 30 days and 1 year in the TX2 groups compared to open controls was determined noninferior (98.1% vs. 94.3% and 91.6% vs. 85.5%, respectively). Freedom from aneurysm-related mortality was 94.2% in the TX2 group, compared to 88.2% in the open surgical controls. MAEs were significantly lower in patients treated with TEVAR: 9.4% versus 33% in surgical controls. The rate of endoleak at 30 days and 1 year were 13% and 3.9%, respectively. Secondary interventions were similar in both groups, with the majority occurring in the initial 30 days and due to type I endoleak. Stent migration was identified in 2.8% of patients. There were no identified cases of stent fracture, barb separation, component separation, or device collapse.

TEVAR has been increasingly adopted for off-label indications. A multicenter trial of the Gore TAG device to treat complicated type B dissection, traumatic aortic tear, and ruptured degenerative aneurysms demonstrated significant advantages over open repair. Endograft deployment was successful in all 59 patients enrolled, and data were compared against 800 literature-matched open controls. Both mortality and paraplegia were reduced in patients treated with the TAG, compared to literature-based controls. MAEs occurred in 81% of patients. Endoleak was identified in 29% of patients who underwent TEVAR, the majority classified as type I.[43]

Comparative meta-analysis evaluating effectiveness of TEVAR in the setting of thoracic aortic transection demonstrated decreased mortality in patients treated with endovascular repair compared to open repair (9% vs. 19%). MAEs including spinal cord ischemia and renal failure were significantly reduced in patients treated endovascularly. However, the rate of procedural failure was increased in the endovascular group, but consisted predominantly of endoleak.[43]

Based on this systematic review and meta-analysis of 7768 patients from 138 studies, the Society for Vascular Surgery has successfully formulated guidelines for the use of endovascular repair in the setting of traumatic aortic injury. While acknowledging the overall poor quality and nonuniformity of the data, several recommendations were made and include: (1) repair of thoracic injury urgently or immediately following correction of concomitant serious nonaortic injuries, (2) repair of intramural and ruptured aortic hematomas, (3) considering TEVAR for all age groups unless anatomic constraints prevent endovascular repair, (4) selective revascularization based on vertebral anatomy, (5) systemic heparinization based on individual patient risk factors, (6) placement of spinal drainage only in the setting of spinal cord ischemia, (7) use of general anesthesia, and (8) open femoral exposure for endovascular access. An overall consensus addressing the issue of optimal device selection or sizing strategies was not reached. However, the Society did advise against excessive endograft oversizing to prevent device failure, including endoleak, device infolding, collapse, or occlusion. Opinions were varied with regard to optimal long-term postoperative follow-up and ranged from recommendations similar to those for elective TEVAR

to every 2 to 5 years in the absence of abnormalities in the initial 3 years.[32]

Several next-generation devices have emerged and are presently undergoing trials, with data awaiting publication. The Medtronic Valiant endograft system is still undergoing follow-up beyond 1 year in the VALOR II trial. Similarly, clinical trials are being conducted on the latest Gore device, the CTAG, with purported increased arch conformability and greater amenity to graft oversizing. Additionally, Cook has developed the Pro-Form system to address issues of arch conformability. The TX2 LP (low-profile) system has been designed to reduce the diameter of the delivery system to accommodate a larger range of access vessel calibers. Continued advancement in graft technology should lead to even greater improvement in outcomes, graft durability, reduced reintervention rates, and broader applications of TEVAR.

CONTROVERSIES

Because randomized controlled trials are lacking, several questions remain regarding the ideal application of TEVAR. Currently there are no universally accepted guidelines defining which patients are ideal candidates for endoluminal repair.[12] Use of TEVAR should be based on an operative risk that is comparable or at least lower than that for open repair or medical management. Factors including patient age, life expectancy, comorbidities, aortic anatomy, and operator experience must be carefully considered prior to intervention. Moreover, the all-cause mortality demonstrated in the pivotal trials is sobering and indicates the serious comorbidities from which this population suffers.

Existing data demonstrate decreased morbidity and mortality for TEVAR compared to conventional open repair, but the longer-term applicability of stent-grafting must be considered. This is an especially valid concern in the trauma patient, who is often young, as well as for patients with a significant life expectancy. Over time, the potential for late complications unique to endovascular repair (e.g., endoleak, graft migration, stent fracture) may result in significant morbidity and overall expense secondary to the need for frequent follow-up and reintervention.[12,44] Notably, most stent-grafts are evaluated for product durability of 10 years, and data on graft efficacy beyond this point are currently unavailable.

Compared with older patients, young patients typically have fewer comorbidities and higher physiologic reserve and are therefore more likely to tolerate an open thoracic surgical procedure. In addition, there are several anatomic features that increase the technical difficulty of TEVAR in younger patients, including the narrow aortic luminal caliber and a more acute angle between the distal aortic arch and descending aorta. These factors may predispose to proximal endoleak, partial luminal obstruction, device kinking, and device collapse (compression).[45-47] Proponents of traditional open surgical intervention contend that these factors, in combination with known long-term outcomes, favor continued application of the open surgical technique. Moreover, independently considering age, patients older than 75 stand to realize the most benefit following TEVAR as compared to open repair.[12]

Much of the data for application of TEVAR remain undefined, but there are a handful of applications where decision between open repair and TEVAR is clear. Given the highly invasive nature of open repair, including thoracotomy with single-lung ventilation, patients with severe pulmonary disease are likely to incur significantly less morbidity with endovascular repair. On the other hand, open repair is recommended for patients with connective tissue disorders including Ehlers-Danlos and Marfan syndromes and polycystic kidney disease, given the young age at presentation and the significant risk of aortic dissection upon device deployment.[12]

The preponderance of evidence suggests that TEVAR is a viable option for treating a wide variety of aortic pathologies. Treatment of degenerative aneurysms remains the only on-label indication for the application of endovascular stent-grafting. However current practice patterns suggest that off-label use, including repair of aortic dissection, traumatic aortic transection, and other aortic pathologies, may approach as high as 50%.[6,17] Safe and effective use of TEVAR requires thorough consideration of individual patient factors and the relative risk/benefit ratio compared to other viable treatment modalities such as medical management or open surgery. Based on such considerations, TEVAR may avail itself as the preferred option for treatment of certain pathologies of the thoracic aorta more than others.

OUTCOMES

Results of thoracic stent-grafting thus far have been excellent; procedure-specific morbidity and mortality are low, midterm results have been promising, and favorable long-term results are starting to emerge.[7,14,17,48-54] By avoiding a large incision, single-lung ventilation, partial bypass, and significant blood loss, morbidity is reduced. Paraplegia, one of the more dreaded complications, seems to be reduced with stent-grafting as well.[36,52,55,56]

Analysis of both on- and off-label applications of TEVAR demonstrate increased mortality for variables including urgent/emergent operations, type A dissection, type C aortic coverage, hybrid arch repair, aortic transection, perioperative spinal cord ischemia, and chronic renal failure.[17,57] However, current data confirm that endovascular repair of traumatic injuries and other catastrophes of the thoracic aorta can be performed emergently, with high rates of primary technical success and low rates of procedure-related morbidity and mortality, and may be favored over open repair.[1-5,7,16]

Complications associated with stent-graft repair of the thoracic aorta include endoleak, renal failure, stroke, device migration, paraplegia, infection, and death. However, early and midterm results indicate that combined morbidity and mortality for TEVAR is significantly lower than that associated with open surgical repair.[8,43,56-60]

The low rate of paraplegia after stent-graft intervention compares favorably to open surgical techniques. Despite recent improvements, reported rates of paraplegia after open repair of thoracic aortic transaction vary from 3% to 33%.[55] The incidence of paraplegia after stent-graft repair of thoracic aortic dissection and thoracic aneurysm ranges from 0% to 7%, but no reported cases of paraplegia have been documented after stent-graft deployment for aortic transection.[14] This is likely related to the focal nature of the pathologic process with transection injuries, thereby allowing successful exclusion of the injury with devices of relatively small length.

In addition to decreased procedure-related mortality, the majority of studies demonstrate a reduction in MAEs in patients undergoing TEVAR when compared with open repair. Morbidity and mortality are most influenced by the urgency of the case, patient age, comorbidities, and operator experience.[17,43,60] Patients undergoing TEVAR were less likely to have bleeding, renal, pulmonary, neurologic, or wound complications.[4,8,43,59,60] Vascular complications were more common in the TEVAR group, which is likely secondary to the various methods of vascular access and complications unique to endovascular repair. It is noteworthy that MAEs related to underlying comorbidities that did occur in the TEVAR population tended toward later time points when compared to open surgical controls.[8] This highlights the overall sick population undergoing thoracic aortic repair, as well as the significant physiologic stress of open surgical repair. Despite good results, there has been no difference in overall survival between endovascular and open repair, thus reflecting the serious comorbidities of the population for which surgery is indicated. Nevertheless, TEVAR offers a favorable risk-to-benefit profile when compared to open surgery.

SUMMARY

Thoracic stent-grafting has evolved significantly over the last several years. TEVAR offers minimally invasive treatment of various aortic pathologies. Traditional treatment options entailed the potential for significant morbidity, which is reduced with endografting. Although initial clinical trials were instituted for the treatment of descending thoracic aneurysmal disease, these devices are now being applied to a broad range of pathologies, including aortic dissection and rupture, traumatic transection, and arch aneurysms. With the continued evolution of these devices, their applicability will only increase.

KEY POINTS

- Preoperative imaging (multidetector computed tomographic angiography [CTA] plus three-dimensional modeling) is critical, but preoperative angiography is not usually required.
- Successful performance of TEVAR requires a highly skilled multidisciplinary team.
- Although aneurysms have been the most treated lesion, thoracic stent-grafts have also been used for aortic dissection, penetrating ulcers, traumatic transections, aortic fistulas, and aortic rupture.
- Even in circumstances where operative therapy may be tolerated, thoracic stent-grafting is quickly becoming the treatment of choice.
- Intravascular ultrasound is useful in minimizing contrast material load.
- Thoracic stent-grafts may reduce the incidence of paraplegia when compared with open surgery, but the risk of paraplegia remains.
- Successful performance of stent-graft repair relies on accurate delineation of the location of injury or aortic pathology, characterization of vascular anatomy, and appropriate sizing of the device.

▸ **SUGGESTED READINGS**

Desai ND, Pochettino A, Szeto WY, et al. Thoracic endovascular aortic repair: evolution of therapy, patterns of use, and results in 10-year experience. J Thorac Cardiovasc Surg 2011;142:587–94.

Fairman RM, Criado F, Farber M, et al. Pivotal results of the Medtronic Vascular Talent thoracic stent graft system: the VALOR trial. J Vasc Surg 2008;48:546–54.

Lee WA, Matsumura JS, Mitchell RS, et al. Endovascular repair of traumatic thoracic aortic injury: clinical practice guidelines of the Society for Vascular Surgery. J Vasc Surg 2011;53:187–92.

Melissano G, Kahlberg A, Bertoglio, L, Chiesa R. Endovascular exclusion of thoracic aortic aneurysms with the with the 1- and 2- component

Zenith TX2 TAA endovascular grafts: analysis of 2-year data from the TX2 pivotal trial. J Endovasc Ther 2011;18(3):338–49.

Svensson LG, Kouchoukos NT, Miller, CD, et al. Expert consensus document of the treatment of descending thoracic aortic disease using endovascular stent-grafts. Ann Thorac Surg 2008;85:S1–S41.

Torsello GB, Torsello GF, Osada N, et al. Midterm results from the TRA-VIATA registry: treatment of thoracic aortic disease with the Valiant stent graft. J Endovasc Ther 2010;17(2):137–50.

The complete reference list is available online at www.expertconsult.com.

CHAPTER 84
Bronchial Artery Embolization
Zubin D. Irani and Frederick S. Keller

Hemoptysis has many causes (Table 84-1). Worldwide, disease states causing chronic lung inflammation arising from tuberculosis are the most common cause of hemoptysis. In the developed world, cystic fibrosis is the corresponding common culprit, leading to bronchiectasis requiring bronchial artery embolization. Regardless of the pathologic process, disease chronicity leads to hypertrophy in the respiratory mucosa of the bronchial circulation in response to occlusion of the pulmonary arterioles from hypoxia secondary to underlying pulmonary disease. These hypertrophied vessels are under systemic pressures, and rupture of these vessels leads to bleeding that "floods" the air spaces. It is the hypertrophy of these vessels that allows them to be amenable to transcatheter embolotherapy, resulting in a clinical benefit.

Obtaining and reviewing the history, physical examination, and tests, especially prior imaging studies, may help provide useful information before the procedure (Table 84-2). Try to ascertain the etiology and side of bleeding to help focus attention during the case to that side. Patients may describe a gurgling sensation on the side of the bleeding. If the pathologic process is limited to one side, imaging will show this and allow for targeted angiograms of that area. Contrast-enhanced chest computed tomography (CT) can offer a diagnosis in which chest radiography and bronchoscopy may be nondiagnostic.[1,2] CT can help localize the site of bleeding in over half of cases of hemoptysis[3] while also revealing hypertrophic vessels in the mediastinum along with their site of origin—key information to help with catheterization. CT can also suggest the presence of nonbronchial systemic arteries supplying the lung via thickened pleura,[4] and this can help reduce instances of incomplete embolizations. When imaging is not helpful, bronchoscopy performed early in the course of the presentation can help localize the site of bleeding and/or pathologic process.

Table 84-3 lists some measures to consider in massive hemoptysis. A neurologic examination of the lower extremities is a must before any angiogram and/or embolization to help monitor for spinal cord complications. This should be repeated after the procedure to look for any changes and may also have to be repeated during the case if there is any concern for spinal cord compromise. If there is a history of recent Swan-Ganz catheter use, a pulmonary artery pseudoaneurysm should be considered and, if possible, computed tomographic angiography (CTA) of the lungs performed. In such a case, one can proceed straight to pulmonary angiography. A pulmonary arteriovenous malformation may also present as hemoptysis and can be seen on chest CT. Again, starting with a pulmonary angiogram is appropriate.

INDICATIONS

The typical indication is massive hemoptysis, defined as 300 mL or more of expectorated blood within a 24-hour period.[5-7] Hemoptysis reduces the available surface area for gas exchange. Depending on the severity of the underlying pathologic process, the available lung surface area will vary between patients, and some may experience respiratory distress with a volume of hemoptysis of less than 300 mL. Thus, a functional assessment is also useful in patient selection. Lesser amounts of bleeding (Table 84-4), especially if recurrent and debilitating, may also qualify patients to be candidates for this procedure. Patients with cystic fibrosis typically fall into this latter group, and the availability of lung transplantation has lowered the threshold to use bronchial artery embolization as a palliative measure to build a bridge to lung transplantation.

CONTRAINDICATIONS

Bronchial artery embolization is not indicated in the uncommon case in which hemoptysis arises from a nonbronchial source (systemic collateral artery or pulmonary artery). If there is concern that nontarget embolization may occur, especially to the spinal cord, leading to permanent neurologic deficit, embolization should be deferred.

EQUIPMENT

Table 84-5 lists recommended equipment for bronchial artery embolization. Adequate imaging equipment is a prerequisite. The initial catheter is one that allows for injection of an adequate volume of contrast agent. We prefer a 6F pigtail catheter positioned in the distal aortic arch to obtain a descending thoracic aortogram. The subsequent selection of guidewire and catheter equipment depends on the anatomy. In general, we prefer "pull down"–shaped catheters because they offer a secure and stable selection method of the desired vessel. Microcatheters used in a coaxial fashion through the previously positioned catheter allow for superselective catheter positioning within the vessel of interest to avoid nontarget embolization. The chosen embolic agent (our preference: 350- to 500-μm particles) can then be delivered via the catheter. Coils should be avoided because they preclude access into the same vessel at a later date when repeat embolization may be necessary. Liquid agents penetrate into the capillary level within the mucosa, creating necrosis. Furthermore, they may pass through any shunts and return to the heart for systemic distribution. Nonionic contrast agents should be used to

TABLE 84-1. Causes of Hemoptysis

Chronic inflammations
Infections
Tuberculosis
Fungal infections (e.g., aspergillosis)
Abscess
Pneumonia
Inflammatory states
Sarcoidosis
Wegener granulomatosis
Cystic fibrosis
Bronchiectasis (any cause)
Pulmonary artery causes
Pulmonary artery stenosis/occlusions: congenital or acquired
Pulmonary arteriovenous malformation
Pulmonary artery pseudoaneurysm (traumatic, e.g., Swan-Ganz catheter)
Neoplasms

NOTE: Make sure expectorated blood is not arising from gastrointestinal tract or oropharyngeal source.

TABLE 84-2. Preprocedural Issues to Address in Workup

• Etiology of hemoptysis: imaging will be useful; if known history of Swan-Ganz catheter use, consider pulmonary artery source, obtain pulmonary CT angiogram if possible, and proceed to pulmonary angiogram first.
• Side of bleeding: imaging may show unilateral lung disease; review results of bronchoscopy if done.
• Correct any coagulopathy.
• Any previous bronchial artery embolization? Consider searches for variant anatomy and nonbronchial vessels and obtaining a pulmonary angiogram.

TABLE 84-3. Therapy for Massive Hemoptysis

• Selectively intubate nonbleeding lung to protect it from filling up with blood.
• Place patient with bleeding side dependent.
• Perform bronchoscopy with view to intrabronchial balloon tamponade.
• Obtain bronchial angiogram once patient's condition has stabilized.

TABLE 84-4. Indications for Bronchial Artery Embolization

Massive hemoptysis	300 mL or more in 24 hours
Moderate hemoptysis	Three or more episodes of 100 mL or more within 1 week
Mild hemoptysis	Chronic or slowly increasing episodes

TABLE 84-5. Equipment for Bronchial Artery Embolization

Catheters

"Pull down" (reverse) shapes (Mikaelson, shepherd's hook, Simmons 1)
Forward-looking shapes (Cobra, Rosch celiac, Headhunter 1)

Microcatheters

Nonionic contrast

Embolic agents

Particles (polyvinyl alcohol, 300-500 μm)
Coils (for emergent proximal embolization)
Gelfoam (temporary agent; deliver as a slurry)
Avoid liquid agents, glue.

TABLE 84-6. Systemic (Nonpulmonary) Arteries in Hemoptysis

Bronchial arteries (course along bronchi, enter lung via hilum)
Conventional origins: T5-T6 level, lateral/anterolateral off descending aorta
Cauldwell patterns:
  40%—2 left, 1 right as intercostal bronchial trunk
  21%—1 left, 1 right as intercostal bronchial trunk
  20%—2 left, 2 right (one as intercostal bronchial trunk)
  10%—1 left, 2 right (one as intercostal bronchial trunk)
  Common bronchial trunk (unknown incidence)
  Intercostal bronchial trunk often arises posterolaterally.
Variant origins:
  Aortic arch
  Internal mammary artery
  Thyrocervical trunk
  Subclavian artery and branches (internal mammary artery, thyrocervical trunk, costocervical trunk)
  Brachiocephalic artery
  Abdominal aorta
  Inferior phrenic artery
Nonbronchial systemic vessels (course does not parallel bronchi; enter lung by penetrating pleura and thus are associated with pleural thickening)
  Intercostals
  Subclavian artery branches (e.g., internal mammary artery)
  Axillary artery branches
  Inferior phrenic artery

From Cauldwell EW, Siekert RG, Liniger RE, et al. The bronchial arteries: an anatomic study of 105 human cadavers. Surg Gynecol Obstet 1948;86:395–412 (now J Am Coll Surg).

minimize any chances of transverse myelitis occurring from injections of contrast media.

TECHNIQUE

Anatomy and Approach

By definition, bronchial arteries course along the central airways, entering the lungs via the hilum. Their origins can

be diverse (Table 84-6). Conventional origin is from the anterolateral aspect of the descending thoracic aorta at the T5 and T6 levels. Thus, the tracheobronchial air column is a useful fluoroscopic guide; the left mainstem bronchus level is a good starting position to begin probing with the catheter tip directed laterally or anterolaterally in search of the bronchial arteries. The left and right bronchial arteries can have separate or common origins (Fig. 84-1). Variant anatomy/origins (Fig. 84-2) have been described (see Table 84-6). Systemic collateral vessels have a course that does not follow the central airways. Compared with bronchial arteries, such nonbronchial arteries directly penetrate the pleura to supply the lung and can be recruited from various systemic arteries (Fig. 84-3). A search for these vessels is crucial in cases of "failed" bronchial artery embolization. The anterior spinal artery can derive supply from

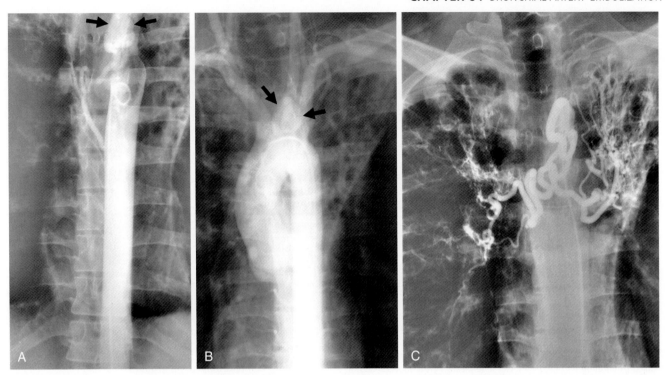

FIGURE 84-1. Value of thoracic aortogram. **A,** Thoracic aortogram showing vascular structure outlined by arrows. **B,** Catheter advanced into aortic arch to get better view of this structure. Arch injection confirms this vessel to be located between origins of great vessels *(arrows)*. **C,** Catheterization of this vessel shows it to be a common bronchial trunk having a variant origin from top surface of aortic arch. Note bronchial arteries coursing along airways and supplying hypervascular lung tissue in both upper lungs.

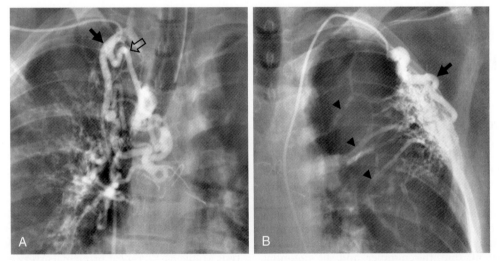

FIGURE 84-2. Systemic arterial supply causing hemoptysis. **A,** Variant bronchial artery *(open arrow)* origin from right internal mammary artery *(black arrow)*. Note axillary approach used for catheterization. Bronchial artery is tortuous. with central course along airways. **B,** Nonbronchial systemic supply from thoracodorsal artery *(black arrow)*. Note groin approach used for catheterization. There is extensive penetration into lung via pleura, with marked shunting into pulmonary circulation *(arrowheads)*.

the bronchial vessels. To prevent embolic agents from going to the spinal artery, a meticulous search should be made in all cases for the medullary spinal artery, which has a characteristic hairpin loop and supplies a vertical midline vessel (anterior spinal artery) and, when present, typically arises from the right intercostal bronchial trunk.

In general, a femoral approach is employed. In cases of tortuous iliac vessels, a sheath can be placed into the aorta to negate the effect of the curves on catheter manipulations. Axillary or high brachial approach may be used to help catheterization of the vessels arising from the subclavian or its branches, such as the internal mammary.

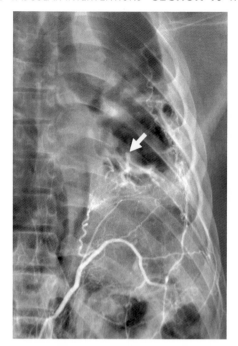

FIGURE 84-3. Nonbronchial systemic supply. Left phrenic injection shows marked penetration into lung via lower lobe pleura. Arrow shows filling of pulmonary artery branch, indicating shunting.

TABLE 84-8. Reasons for Failed Bronchial Artery Embolization/Recurrent Hemoptysis

Incomplete embolization
Recanalization of embolized vessel
Revascularization by collateral vessels
Recruitment of nonbronchial systemic arterial supply
Progression of lung disease
Incomplete treatment of underlying disease

TABLE 84-9. Complications of Bronchial Artery Embolization

Embolization related (i.e., nontarget embolization)
Chest pains (nontarget embolization to intercostals, typically transient)
Dysphagia (nontarget embolization to esophageal branches, transient)
Lower extremity neurologic deficit (nontarget embolization to anterior spinal artery)
Aortic necrosis
Bronchial necrosis
Bronchoesophageal fistula
Pulmonary infarction
General angiography related
Access site complications (e.g., groin hematoma)
Vessel injury; dissections from guidewire, catheter manipulations
Contrast related (e.g., reactions, nephropathy)

TABLE 84-7. Angiographic Findings in Hemoptysis

Neovascularity
Hypervascularity
Hypertrophic and tortuous bronchial arteries
Shunting from bronchial to pulmonary systems
Bronchial artery pseudoaneurysms
Extravasation (rare)

Technical Aspects

Several findings (Table 84-7) may be present on the bronchial angiogram in massive hemoptysis. Extravasation is rarely seen (Fig. 84-4), and embolization is carried out even in its absence.

A thoracic aortogram is performed first. The value of a preliminary descending thoracic aortogram is that not only will the abnormal bronchial arteries be visualized in the majority of patients but the number and all potential sites of bronchial artery origins also will be revealed (see Fig. 84-1). This road map then guides selective catheterization. The tip of a 5F or 6F catheter of choice is used to engage the vessel origin. A microcatheter introduced coaxially allows for a stable and safe catheter position well beyond any possible spinal cord branches, because the microcatheter can usually be navigated well beyond the vessel origin. Bronchial angiography is performed with hand injections of contrast medium before, during, and after embolization. It is scrutinized for the findings seen in massive hemoptysis, along with the presence of any spinal cord branches. The anterior spinal artery is a vertical midline structure, whereas the contributing anterior medullary artery has a characteristic hairpin loop before joining it. After successful embolization, the final angiogram should show stasis of flow.

In the absence of bronchial artery supply, other potential sources of systemic supply (see Table 84-6) should be studied. Finally, if these are unrevealing, one should study the pulmonary arteries as a source for the hemoptysis (Figs. 84-5 and 84-6).

OUTCOMES

Acutely, there is good control of hemoptysis, with nonrecurrence rates of 73% to 98% up to 1 month after the procedure.[8,9] These rates have improved in recent years because of improvement in microcatheter technology, allowing superselective embolization. Long-term recurrence rates of 10% to 52% have been reported with up to a 46-month follow-up.[5,10] In such cases of recurrent hemoptysis (Table 84-8), repeat bronchial artery embolization can be done.

Bronchial artery embolization is not definitive treatment for the underlying lung disease but rather offers symptomatic control, after which the patient can be offered further medical and/or surgical treatment. Reasons for recurrent hemoptysis are listed in Table 84-8. Certain causes show higher recurrence rates and include chronic tuberculosis, aspergilloma, cystic fibrosis, and neoplasms.

COMPLICATIONS

The complications of bronchial artery embolization are listed in Table 84-9. Chest pain and dysphagia[11,12] both tend

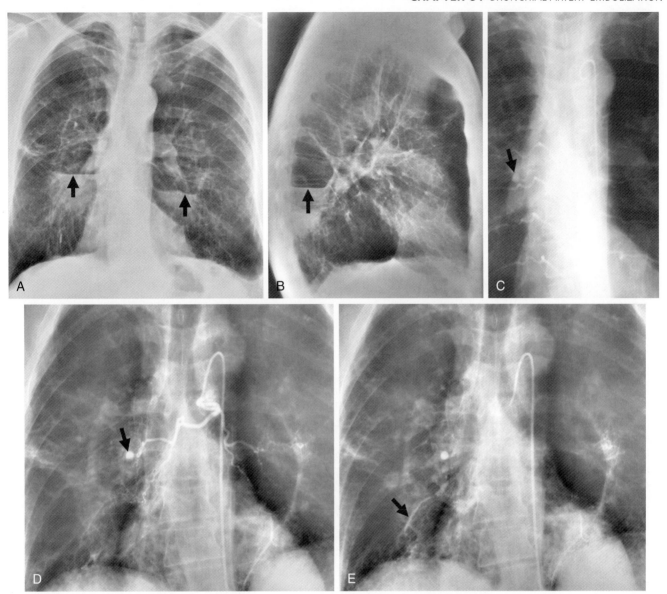

FIGURE 84-4. Patient with massive hemoptysis. **A,** Posteroanterior radiograph showing large cavities with air/fluid (blood) levels *(arrows)*. **B,** Chest radiograph showing large cavities with air/fluid (blood) levels *(arrow)*. **C,** Late-phase thoracic aortogram showing contrast medium pooling in a pseudoaneurysm *(arrow)*. **D,** Early phase of common bronchial trunk injection shows pseudoaneurysm *(arrow)*. Note bronchial arteries coursing along airways. **E,** Late phase of same injection shows contrast extravasation into lower lobe airway *(arrow)*.

to be transient and are related to nontarget embolization of the chest wall (intercostals) and esophageal branches, respectively. Subintimal dissection of the aorta and bronchial vessels is of no clinical significance and is related to guidewire and/or catheter manipulation.

Spinal cord ischemia is a disastrous complication, arising either from the contrast agent causing transverse myelitis, which these days with newer contrast agents is rare, and/or nontarget embolization of the anterior medullary artery. Great caution must be exercised when this artery is present, and positioning the catheter well beyond (distal to) the origin of this vessel is critical to minimize the chances of this complication.

POSTPROCEDURAL AND FOLLOW-UP CARE

Immediate postprocedural care is as for any patient who has had an angiogram, including checking the access site for bleeding. Relating to the embolization itself, a neurologic examination should be performed to look for any deficits in the extremities, which may be a sign of nontarget embolization to the spinal artery. Clinical follow-up is needed to ensure cessation of hemoptysis, and patients should be informed that a repeat procedure may be needed as further collateral vessels get recruited, especially in nonmalignant diseases such as cystic fibrosis. The underlying

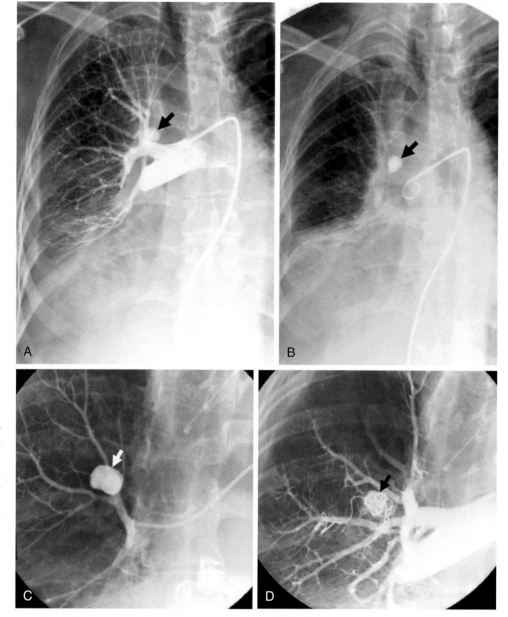

FIGURE 84-5. Pulmonary artery pseudoaneurysm coiling. Patient with Swan-Ganz catheter–induced pulmonary artery pseudoaneurysm causing massive hemoptysis. Early **(A)** and late **(B)** phase of right pulmonary angiogram, with arrow showing pseudoaneurysm. **C,** Selective upper lobe branch angiogram shows pseudoaneurysm *(arrow).* **D,** Arrow shows coils filling up pseudoaneurysm and no filling of the pseudoaneurysm. Patient did well, with no further episodes of hemoptysis.

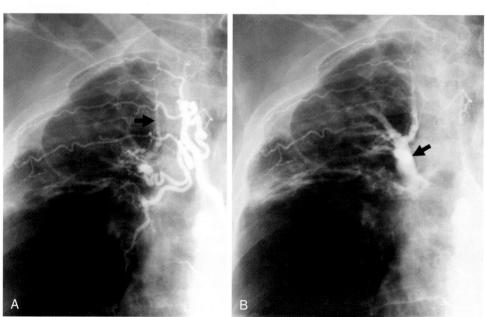

FIGURE 84-6. Bronchial artery–to–pulmonary circulation shunting. Early **(A)** and late **(B)** phase from injection of right intercostal bronchial trunk. Arrow in both phases shows progressive filling of right upper lobe pulmonary vein, indicating shunting.

cause should also be addressed, if possible, by more definitive means.

► **SUGGESTED READINGS**

Fernando HC, Stein M, Benfield JR, et al. Role of bronchial artery embolization in the management of hemoptysis. Arch Surg 1998;133: 862–6.

Jean-Baptiste E. Clinical assessment and management of massive hemoptysis. Crit Care Med 2000;28:1642–7.

Najarian KE, Morris CS. Arterial embolization in the chest. J Thorac Imaging 1998;13:93–104.

The complete reference list is available online at www.expertconsult.com.

KEY POINTS

- Hemoptysis, which is the typical presenting problem leading to bronchial artery embolization, has many causes.

- With hemoptysis, asphyxiation more than exsanguination causes death as blood fills the air spaces in the lung and "drowns" the patient.

- Typically, the bronchial and/or recruited systemic collateral (nonbronchial) circulation is responsible for the hemoptysis; less commonly, the pulmonary artery is the culprit vessel.

- Embolization of these vessels is an efficacious palliative treatment option acutely in such patients, who typically are poor surgical candidates at the time.

- Particles are the embolic agent of choice rather than liquid agents or coils.

- An uncommon yet dreaded complication is spinal cord injury resulting in a permanent neurologic deficit.

CHAPTER 85

Pulmonary Arteriovenous Malformations: Diagnosis and Management

Jeffrey S. Pollak, Katharine Henderson, and Robert I. White, Jr.

Pulmonary arteriovenous malformations (PAVMs) are an important cause of stroke and transient ischemic attack (TIA), as well as brain abscess and other systemic infections due to loss of pulmonary capillary circulation filtering capacity.[1] They may also spontaneously rupture and can be a cause of serious if not lethal hemoptysis and hemothorax, particularly in women during the third trimester of pregnancy and in children and adults with large PAVMs.[2,3]

Patients with large or multiple PAVMs often present with significant hypoxemia resulting in dyspnea and fatigue. A particularly difficult group to treat is a small set of patients with diffuse pulmonary malformations, a category less well recognized.[4,5]

Hereditary hemorrhagic telangiectasia (HHT), the underlying genetic disorder in most patients with PAVM, is common among rare diseases (200 per million people), and of these patients, approximately a third will have PAVM. Worldwide centers now exist for management of PAVM and the other organ manifestations of HHT (www.hht.org).

Screening of affected families for PAVM is most easily done by contrast echocardiography. If positive, noncontrast thin-section computed tomography (CT) of the chest is done to size the PAVM (Fig. 85-1).[6,7]

INDICATIONS

Screening for PAVM should be done periodically in affected children by pulse oximetry and, after age 12, by contrast echocardiography.[3] Large PAVMs in children younger than 12 years of age should be treated because of the risk of pulmonary hemorrhage.[3] In adolescents and adults, all PAVMs with arteries 3 mm or greater in diameter should be treated.[8,9] Recently we developed an algorithm for screening and management of children under 12. Based on our experience at the Yale HHT Center, neither embolic stroke due to paradoxical embolus nor brain abscess have occurred in the children we have examined who had standing oxygen saturation greater than 97%. In a recent study,[10] we found exercise stress testing to be a highly reproducible test in children and adults with PAVM. Although not yet accepted by others, it is our hope that the use of exercise stress testing in patients with HHT will replace the perceived need for early contrast echocardiography and excessive use of CT.[10] This is important because early treatment of small PAVMs in children leads to collateral reperfusion, irrespective of the device used to close the PAVM. Collateral reperfusion requires additional treatment and radiation exposure at a vulnerable age.[10]

CONTRAINDICATIONS

Although there are no absolute contraindications for embolotherapy of PAVM, there are some aspects of the closure

technique that require special attention. First, in patients with secondary or primary pulmonary hypertension, care should be taken so that PAVM closure does not raise pulmonary artery pressures to a level that poses a risk of right-sided heart failure. Measurement of pulmonary artery pressures is essential before occluding PAVMs. Patients with symptomatic liver malformations will have moderate elevations in pulmonary artery pressure (40-60/20-30 mmHg). Also, there is an association between HHT and primary pulmonary hypertension.[11]

Second, in patients with high-flow arteries less than 2.5 cm in length, closure of the sac connecting the artery to the vein should be considered, and special techniques are required.[12] Sac closure with oversized or detachable coils is expensive and time consuming, and at our institution was necessary only 6 times in more than 1000 consecutive patients. Recently, with the introduction and short-term experience with the detachable HydroCoil system (Terumo Medical Corp., Somerset, N.J.) and the Amplatzer II Vascular Plug (St. Jude Medical, St. Paul, Minn.), we believe sac closure will be needed much less often.

Third, in patients with contrast allergy, special attention should be given to the type of contrast material used and the type of allergy. In most instances, an alternative contrast material is selected, and premedication and monitoring or general anesthesia with an anesthesiologist in attendance will allow the procedure to be performed rather than surgical resection.

EQUIPMENT

Our standard techniques have been outlined in recent articles.[9,13] We feel that pushable coils suffice for treating most PAVMs, although detachable coils like the AZUR HydroCoil (Terumo), which is fully retractable before final deployment, as well as the Amplatzer plug, will have a role in managing some PAVMs (Fig. 85-2). Interventional radiologists treating PAVMs should have familiarity with both of these techniques and the standard techniques described.[14,15]

Standard equipment used for 90% of PAVMs includes:
- A 7F sheath placed in either femoral vein and connected to heparinized saline after careful exclusion of all air bubbles
- A 5F pigtail catheter for diagnostic pulmonary angiography
- A 7/5F coaxial LuMax (Cook Medical, Bloomington, Ind.) guide catheter is exchanged for the pigtail, using a reinforced exchange wire. The 100-cm, 5F angled end-hole catheter that comes with the set is used for most occlusions. The 80-cm, 7F guide catheter is placed just proximal to the 5F catheter and provides stability

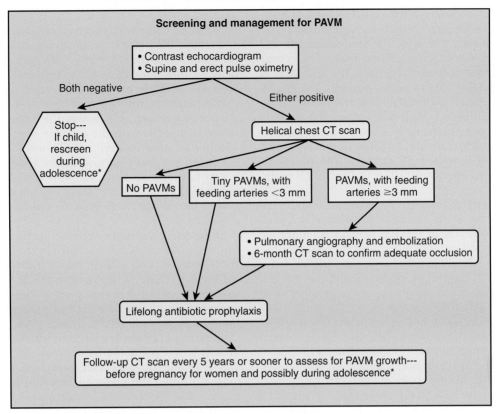

FIGURE 85-1. Current Yale Hereditary Hemorrhagic Telangiectasia (HHT) Center algorithm for diagnosis, treatment, and follow-up of a patient with pulmonary arteriovenous malformation. *(Courtesy Yale HHT Center.)*

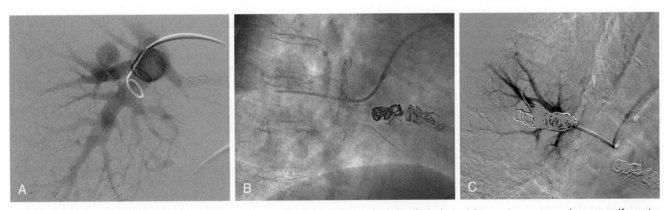

FIGURE 85-2. Use of AZUR HydroCoil in a 61-year-old woman. Five years earlier, we had identified a large right superior segment pulmonary malformation. Because we could not secure a satisfactory position with the guide catheter, we elected to not treat this pulmonary arteriovenous malformation (PAVM) at that time. In 2011, greater familiarity with the AZUR detachable HydroCoil enabled us to occlude PAVM. **A,** Lateral view of right pulmonary angiogram that demonstrates a short high-flow PAVM of superior segment and coils in a right middle lobe PAVM that had been occluded 5 years earlier. **B,** A 5F catheter is seen in a peripheral branch beyond origin of PAVM. We achieved this position in 2006, but exaggerated heart motion prevented safe anchoring of platinum coils, and short uneven caliber of superior segment prevented use of scaffold technique. **C,** In 2011, with availability of a detachable and fully retractable 0.035-inch AZUR HydroCoil, we anchored the first 12-mm HydroCoil and occluded PAVM with seven additional HydroCoils varying from 10 to 6 mm in diameter.

for deployment of tightly packed coils either by the "anchor" or "scaffold" technique (see Anatomy and Approaches).
- The same coaxial catheter approaches apply when using a detachable coil; Amplatzer II plugs up to 12 mm can be placed through the guiding catheter.

Specialized Equipment for Other Anatomy and Physiology

A variety of other 5F catheters can be placed coaxially through the 7F guide catheter. End-hole 100-cm soft hydrophilic catheters (Glidecath [Terumo]) may be useful for occluding small PAVMs where soft catheters are less traumatic than standard 5F ones. Lingula and right middle lobe access can be achieved with a 5F, 100-cm Judkins left (JL) coronary catheter (Cordis Corp., Miami Lakes, Fla.). Once the right middle lobe or lingula is entered, the 7F LuMax is advanced over the JL 3.5 into a secure position. The PAVM is then closed, either with 0.018-inch microcoils (e.g., MicroNester or Tornado coils [Cook]) through a triaxial-placed microcatheter, particularly if the feeding artery is small, or the JL 3.5 coronary catheter is removed and exchanged for the standard 5F catheter. The occlusion would then be completed with 0.035- or 0.038-inch pushable fibered coils.

For patients with pulmonary hypertension (>1/2 systemic pressure), an occlusion balloon catheter is useful for temporary occlusion of the PAVM while monitoring pressures with a small catheter introduced from the contralateral femoral vein for 30 minutes. In our experience, temporary occlusion of the PAVM for 30 minutes has not led to significant elevations in pulmonary artery pressure, and we then proceed with the occlusion.

Double-lumen occlusion balloon catheters (Boston Scientific, Natick, Mass.) are sometimes used for occluding high-flow large-lumen PAVMs (>10 mm diameter). This is particularly true if there is not a good "anchor" vessel present. Oversized MReye coils (Cook) can be placed through the occlusion balloon catheter to form a "scaffold" proximal to the sac. Once several high-radial-force coils are placed, the occlusion balloon is removed, and we complete cross-sectional occlusion of the PAVM by "nesting" soft platinum coils within the scaffold, using the standard 7/5F LuMax system.

For patients with short high-flow arteries (i.e., < 2.5 cm long), embolization is performed through the occlusion balloon catheter (Boston Scientific) with a double-marker Renegade 0.021-inch microcatheter (Boston Scientific) and deployment-suitable pushable, and perhaps detachable, 0.018-inch coils. The resultant coil mass should be at least twice the diameter of the draining pulmonary veins and should fill the aneurysmal sac. Once the sac is filled with oversized microcoils, the occlusion balloon catheter is withdrawn and the occlusion completed with the 7/5F LuMax system and standard 0.035- or 0.038-inch fibered coils.[12]

TECHNIQUE

Anatomy and Approaches

Most PAVMs consist of a variable-length single segmental artery, but 10% are complex, with more than one segmental artery connecting the aneurysmal sac to the draining veins.[9,16,17]

Despite the magnificent images provided by high-resolution multidetector CT scanners, as well as similar images from magnetic resonance angiography (MRA), we still depend on multiprojection diagnostic pulmonary angiography before embolotherapy. It is particularly important to be confident of the morphology of the artery as it enters the sac. The goal of therapy is to occlude the feeding artery as close to the sac as possible, thereby limiting reperfusion from adjacent branches in the lungs of children[3] and

limiting reperfusion from the bronchial circulation, which is known to occur with proximal occlusions.[18,19]

Perhaps the most important aspect of imaging occurs just before deployment of coils. We perform a small series of hand injections of contrast material into the feeding artery in multiple projections, settling on the projection that provides us with the best view of the morphology of the feeding artery as it enters the aneurysmal sac. This image is preserved on the monitor next to our real-time monitor to guide us during deployment of coils. In many instances, the artery narrows before entering the sac. This is very favorable anatomy, and pushable fibered coils 2 mm larger than the diameter of the artery are simply placed and nested into a tight coil mass to produce cross-sectional occlusion.

If the artery widens before entering the sac, a small adjacent artery that would be occluded by the coil mass is selectively entered, and a long Nester coil or stainless steel MReye coil (Cook) is deployed so that at least 2 cm of the first coil is anchored in this "anchor" branch. By using the anchor approach, we have not had a paradoxical embolization of a pushable fibered coil since 1994.[9,17]

Because of self-limited pleurisy, which occurs in approximately 15% of patients after occlusion of single or multiple PAVM in one lung, we tend to perform occlusion of one lung at a time. We prefer to have the patient return for treatment of the other side within 6 weeks. This also allows us to detect recanalization on the earlier occluded side. This is easier on the patient as well as the interventional radiologist.

Figures 85-3 and 85-4 show various views of the anchor and scaffold techniques.

Technical Aspects

Morphology of the artery as it enters the sac is a critical determinant of occlusion method (to anchor or not to anchor).

Patients with a single PAVM receive heparin (50 units/kg) during the occlusion. If the procedure is for multiple PAVMs, patients are fully heparinized (100 units/kg).

All guidewires should be withdrawn under water to void a vacuum effect. Inadvertent air in the catheter can result in angina as a result of air paradoxically embolizing and entering the coronary circulation as the next coil or guidewire is introduced.

The *anchor technique* describer earlier provides a safe method for deploying pushable fibered coils. If there is no suitable anchor vessel adjacent to the sac, and one is uncomfortable with the control of pushable oversized coils placed coaxially, the first coil can be a detachable coil followed by packing pushable coils to create cross-sectional occlusion.

Use of a 7F guide catheter proximal in the feeding artery allows control of the inner 5F catheter so that pushable fibered coils can be packed into a dense "nest," thus achieving cross-sectional occlusion.

For high-flow arteries 10 mm in diameter or larger, the *scaffold technique*, consisting of building an endoskeleton close to the sac with oversized stainless steel or MReye coils is used. Cross-sectional occlusion is achieved by finishing the occlusion with Nester coils. We also use Amplatzer II plugs for larger feeding arteries (Fig. 85-5).

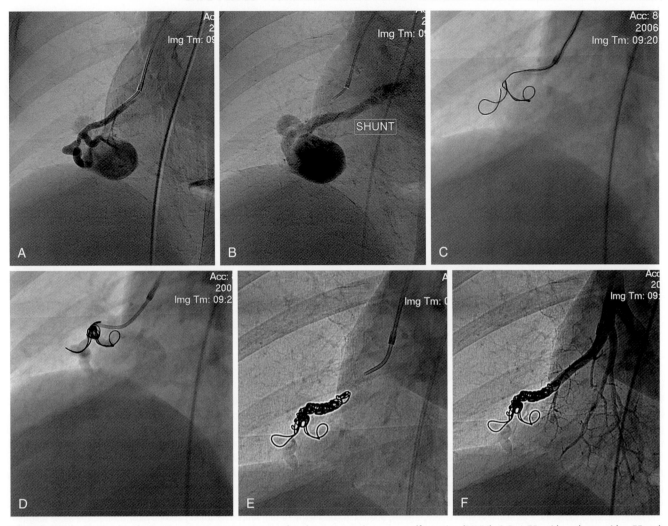

FIGURE 85-3. "Anchor" technique in asymptomatic patient with pulmonary arteriovenous malformation (PAVM). **A-B,** A 7F guide catheter with a 5F end-hole catheter has been advanced into segmental artery to PAVM. Shallow left anterior oblique view best demonstrates entry of artery into aneurysmal sac. Because artery bifurcates immediately before entering sac, one branch is selected to anchor the first 2 cm of a 14-cm, 6-mm-diameter fibered coil; rest of coil is deposited in the other branch and proximal artery **(C-D)**. Key to control of fibered coil placement is having a guide catheter held steady in feeding artery, which allows precise deployment of coils through the 5F end-hole catheter. **E-F,** Final placement of two additional 6-mm coils is demonstrated; they are tightly packed (nested). This prevents recanalization and again is facilitated by having a guide catheter proximal in the feeding segmental artery.

Because occlusion of PAVM is usually elective and there are a great number of anatomic variants, complete diagnostic angiography is required, as well as considering referring a patient with difficult anatomy to an experienced center.

CONTROVERSIES

Although there is no worldwide consensus yet about which PAVMs should be occluded or exactly how to occlude them, consensus in North America and Europe is beginning to be achieved. For example, there is one report of a stroke event via a paradoxical embolus through a 2.8-mm-diameter artery,[20] but for the most part in Great Britain, Canada, Denmark, Netherlands, and France, as well as in North America, the 3-mm-diameter artery appears to be the "threshold size" that warrants occlusion.[21-28]

With regard to occlusion devices, results equal to those obtained with pushable fibered coils had been achieved with detachable silicone balloons (Boston Scientific), but since they were discontinued in 2002, we are occluding most PAVMs with standard pushable fibered coils, facilitated by use of a coaxial guide catheter system.[9,29]

Some authors have favored routinely occluding the aneurysmal sac with detachable coils.[30,31] We have rarely needed detachable coils for occluding PAVMs, and their expense is a downside. In addition, occluding the sac of a PAVM removes our primary anatomic outcome of the procedure (i.e., thrombosis and disappearance of the sac).[32]

In 2006, the nitinol plug developed by Amplatz and associates was reported for occluding the feeding artery to the PAVM.[9,33,34] Over the last 6 years, a number of reports of success using the Amplatzer I plug with coils or the Amplatzer II plug alone have been reported.[14,15] We believe that to adequately treat patients with PAVMs, the interventionalist must be familiar with a variety of approaches, and ideally patients should be referred to experienced centers with a commitment to management and follow-up of patients with HHT/PAVM.[35]

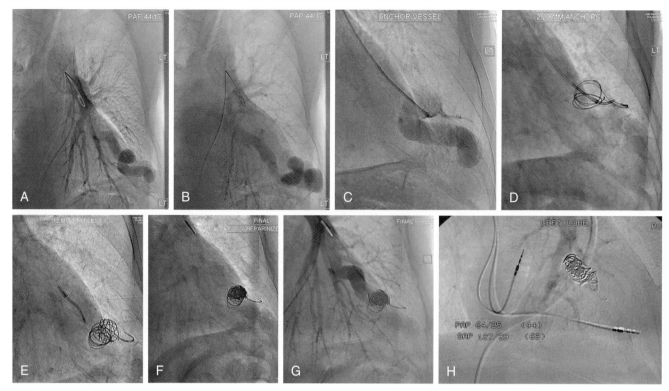

FIGURE 85-4. "Scaffold" and "anchor" techniques for large pulmonary arteriovenous malformation (PAVM) in 78-year-old woman with significant liver AVM as well as mild pulmonary artery hypertension (44/17 mmHg), and 6-year follow-up. **A-B,** Arterial and venous phase of a selective left pulmonary angiogram demonstrate a large PAVM with aneurysmal sac and no immediate evidence of a good anchor artery next to sac. **C,** A good anchor artery is demonstrated by a selective hand injection through guide catheter. It was decided to use anchor technique with oversized 20-mm stainless steel coils to form a scaffold. Main artery to PAVM measured 17 mm in diameter. **D,** Two 20-mm-diameter high-radial-force stainless steel coils have been sequentially anchored and allowed to reform in feeding artery. **E,** Additional 12- and 15-mm-diameter coils have been placed in scaffold. **F,** Final cross-sectional occlusion has been obtained by packing long fibered platinum coils within scaffold. **G,** Final selective angiogram demonstrates cross-sectional occlusion. **H,** Six-year follow-up angiogram (2008) demonstrated that left lung AVM remains occluded. We now use MReye coils to form a scaffold; they are compatible with magnetic resonance imaging and have the same radial force as stainless steel coils. Currently, one could consider a 20-mm Amplatzer II Plug and possibly achieve the same long-term result.

OUTCOMES

Outcomes from multiple single-center series have been reported, and recently we reported our prospective outcomes of 155 patients observed closely for a mean of 6.5 years.[9] All series have demonstrated reduction in shunt measured by radionuclides or 100% oxygen studies. We have maintained and demonstrated that anatomic as well as physiologic outcomes are necessary. In our series, similar to the Dutch series,[8] there were a few recurrences due to reperfusion of incompletely occluded arteries or accessory arteries. Reperfusion can also occur through collateral perfusion from adjacent normal arteries, particularly in children and adolescents, as well as hypertrophy of bronchial arteries, the latter more common in the small subset of patients with diffuse PAVMs.[4,34,35] All recurrences can be relatively easily reoccluded at the 1-year follow-up visit.

Most importantly in the Dutch and our series, enlargement of unoccluded PAVM was demonstrated by thin-section noncontrast CT assessment at 1 year and every 5 years. When PAVMs were multiple or if there was any doubt about reperfusion, often an outpatient pulmonary angiogram was performed and, at the same time, reocclusion of any reperfused PAVM.

Since a small risk of infection remains from unoccluded small or tiny PAVMs, prophylactic antibiotics continue to be recommended prior to procedures that may cause a bacteremia, such as dental work. Stroke or TIA events were reduced and often found to be due to other causes than paradoxical embolus through a PAVM (e.g., atrial fibrillation or other cardiac events).[9] Similar results were obtained by Mager et al. from the HHT center in The Netherlands.[8]

COMPLICATIONS

Those complications occurring during the procedure are due in most part to inadvertent air traversing the PAVM during flushing or passing wires, coils, or other devices. In addition, bland thrombus occurring on catheters can pass through a PAVM and cause serious downstream events. Angina and/or a TIA are now rare events, occurring in no more than 1% of patients treated by experienced teams. In most instances they can be prevented by withdrawing all wires under water and by heparinization during the procedure.

The most feared complication is paradoxical embolization of a device, and these occurrences have been well

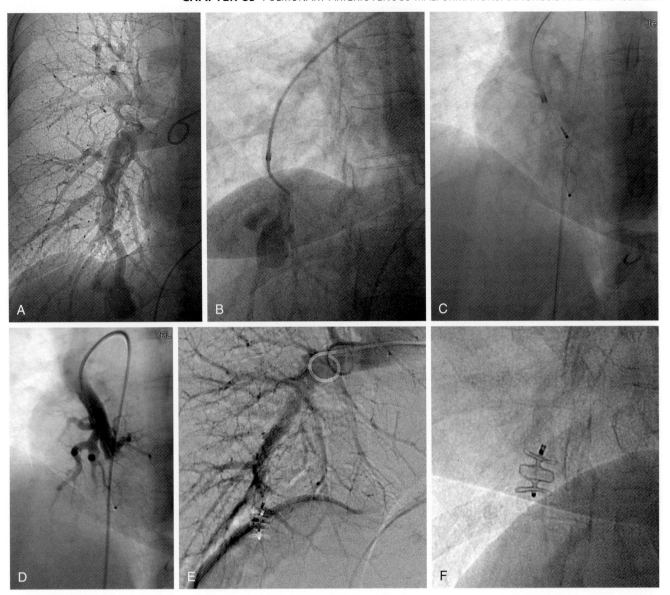

FIGURE 85-5. Amplatzer II Vascular Plug in medium-sized pulmonary arteriovenous malformation (PAVM) without good anchor vessel in 57-year-old with long-standing history of dyspnea and fatigue. **A,** Right lower lobe PAVM is identified. **B,** We did not identify a suitable anchor artery, and a 10-mm Amplatzer II device was temporarily placed (**C**). **C-D,** Amplatzer plug in place before detachment; control angiogram demonstrates excellent occlusion. **E-F,** Four months later, patient returned for treatment of other PAVMs. Magnification view shows Amplatzer occluder in excellent position and confirms PAVM occlusion.

described.[17,36] Now that we have adopted the anchor technique, we have not encountered any paradoxical embolization of a device. Groups treating PAVM should be familiar with "snare devices" for retrieval of misplaced coils.

Although not strictly considered a complication, self-limited pleurisy occurs in 10% to 20% of patients, usually beginning 48 to 96 hours after the procedure. It is thought that this occurs by thrombosis of the aneurysmal sac when adjacent to visceral pleura. Irritation of the visceral pleura is associated with pain. This is typically self-limited and can be treated with ibuprofen for 2 to 3 days. Patients should be warned about this and encouraged to follow up with the treatment center.

In a very small percentage of patients, there may be late pleurisy occurring 2 to 4 months after a successful procedure, which we attribute to delayed thrombosis of the sac. This may be associated with high fever, and in addition to ibuprofen we often give a short course of oral antibiotics.

POSTPROCEDURAL AND FOLLOW-UP CARE

Most patients are seen in our interventional clinic the day before the procedure, and we obtain a history and perform a thorough physical examination. Embolotherapy is performed as a same-day procedure, with discharge 4 to 5 hours after it is finished. All patients call our office or are contacted for 2 days after the procedure to check their progress.

Most important is the follow-up noncontrast CT of the chest 6 months to 1 year after treatment. If the patient cannot return for an outpatient visit at this time, the chest CT is sent for review; after reviewing the CT, we dictate a letter to the referring doctor outlining our findings and follow-up recommendations. In patients with multiple PAVMs in both lungs, it is our impression that follow-up pulmonary angiography at 1 year is more helpful in excluding recurrences than non–contrast enhanced CT.

It is recommended that all patients be seen every 5 years after their occlusion for follow-up clinical evaluation for growth of unoccluded PAVMs and for other organ manifestations of HHT.

- Permanent ablation of PAVMs is possible, with a high success and low complication rate in experienced HHT centers with an interventional radiologist performing these embolizations once or twice per week.
- Most patients with HHT and PAVM have small PAVMs remaining after closure of large ones, and follow-up is important to detect recurrences and monitor growth of small PAVMs to the size when treatment is needed.

KEY POINTS

- Pulmonary arteriovenous malformation (PAVM) is a marker for a relatively common genetic disorder, hereditary hemorrhagic telangiectasia (HHT).
- Treatment of PAVM is performed by embolotherapy techniques using guiding catheters and pushable fibered coils, and in some instances with detachable coils, fully retrievable before final deployment, and Amplatzer II plugs.

► SUGGESTED READINGS

Gossage J, Kanj G. State of the art: pulmonary arteriovenous malformations. Am J Respir Crit Care Med 1988;158:643–77.

Guttmacher AE, Marchuk DA, White RI Jr. Hereditary hemorrhagic telangiectasia. N Engl J Med 1995;333:918–24.

Shovlin CL, Guttmacher AE, Buscarini E, et al. Diagnostic criteria for hereditary hemorrhagic telangiectasia. Am J Med Genet 2000;91: 66–7.

The complete reference list is available online at www.expertconsult.com.

CHAPTER 86

Percutaneous Interventions for Acute Pulmonary Embolism

William T. Kuo

Venous thromboembolism (VTE) is a global health problem that encompasses acute deep venous thrombosis (DVT) and acute pulmonary embolism (PE). Although the true incidence of PE is unknown, it is recognized as a significant cause of morbidity and mortality in hospitalized patients.[1] In the United States alone, it is estimated there are between 500,000 and 600,000 cases per year,[2] and approximately 300,000 people die every year from acute PE.[3] Indeed, acute PE is believed to be the third most common cause of death among hospitalized patients.[4]

Common risk factors for acute PE are related to underlying genetic conditions (e.g., factor V Leiden mutation, prothrombin 20210A mutation, and multiple other thrombophilias), acquired conditions (e.g., cancer, immobilization, trauma, surgery, prior DVT), and acquired hypercoagulable states (e.g., oral contraceptive use, nephrotic syndrome, antiphospholipid syndrome, disseminated intravascular coagulation, hyperestrogenic states, obesity).

There are three basic categories of acute PE: (1) *simple PE* with no associated heart strain and no hypotension, (2) *submassive PE* with associated right heart strain, (3) *massive PE* with associated right heart strain and hemodynamic shock. Patients with simple acute PE require treatment with therapeutic anticoagulation alone. Patients with submassive PE may require treatment escalation beyond anticoagulation; and patients with massive PE certainly require treatment escalation beyond anticoagulation alone.[5] The immediate mortality rate related to simple PE is less than 8% when the condition is recognized and treated with anticoagulation.[1,6,7] However, patients with submassive PE have a higher cumulative mortality rate, reaching approximately 20% over a 90-day period.[8] Patients with massive PE have the highest mortality rate, which can exceed 58%, including a high risk of sudden death.[9]

The pathophysiology of PE consists of direct physical obstruction of the pulmonary arteries, hypoxemic vasoconstriction, and release of potent pulmonary arterial vasoconstrictors that further increase pulmonary vascular resistance and right ventricular (RV) afterload. Acute RV pressure overload may result in RV hypokinesis and dilation, tricuspid regurgitation, and ultimately RV failure. RV pressure overload may also result in increased wall stress and ischemia by increasing myocardial oxygen demand while simultaneously limiting its supply. Ultimately, cardiac failure due to acute PE results from a combination of the increased wall stress and cardiac ischemia that compromise RV function and impair left ventricular (LV) output, resulting in life-threatening hemodynamic shock.[9] Depending on underlying cardiopulmonary reserve, patients with acute massive PE may deteriorate over the course of several hours to days and develop systemic arterial hypotension, cardiogenic shock, and cardiac arrest. Owing to the risk of sudden death, these critically ill patients with massive PE should be quickly identified as candidates for rapid endovascular treatment as a lifesaving procedure.[5]

INDICATIONS

Because of the high mortality associated with acute massive PE, successful management requires prompt risk stratification and decisive early intervention (Table 86-1). Confirmation of hemodynamic shock attributed to central obstructing embolus should be present to justify treatment escalation beyond anticoagulation. The American College of Chest Physicians has recommended that percutaneous catheter-directed therapy (CDT) be considered in acute massive PE patients who are unable to receive systemic thrombolytic therapy because of bleeding risk.[10] In addition, global meta-analytic data has demonstrated that percutaneous CDT can be considered as a first-line treatment option in lieu of intravenous (IV) tissue plasminogen activator (tPA) for patients with massive PE.[11]

Pulmonary angiography was once considered the gold standard for diagnosing PE, but it has largely been replaced by the wide availability of cross-sectional imaging. Historically, many types of imaging studies have been used in diagnosing acute pulmonary embolism, including ventilation/perfusion (V/Q) scanning, magnetic resonance angiography (MRA), and computed tomographic angiography (CTA). CTA is the preferred modality and has proven to be advantageous thanks to its wide availability, superior speed, characterization of nonvascular structures, and detection of venous thrombosis. CTA has the greatest sensitivity and specificity for detecting emboli in the main, lobar, or segmental pulmonary arteries. Systematic reviews and randomized trials suggest that outpatients with suspected pulmonary embolism and negative CTA studies have excellent outcomes without therapy.[12]

If a patient has either acute or chronic renal insufficiency and contrast administration is undesirable, echocardiography may be used to evaluate for right heart dysfunction as an indication for underlying acute PE. The echocardiogram can be performed at bedside, and the study may reveal findings that strongly support hemodynamically significant pulmonary embolism,[13] offering the potential to guide treatment escalation to thrombolytic and/or endovascular therapy. Large emboli moving from the heart to the lungs are occasionally confirmed with this technique. In addition, intravascular ultrasonography has also been used at the bedside to visualize central pulmonary emboli.[14]

Although the diagnosis of submassive PE follows a similar workup to evaluating massive PE, these patients do not present with systemic arterial hypotension, and particular attention must be paid to detecting the presence of right heart strain, which clinches the diagnosis of submassive PE. Identifying right heart strain allows risk stratification for

TABLE 86-1. Risk Stratification and Indications for Aggressive Intervention to Treat Massive Pulmonary Embolism

At least one of the following criteria must be present:
1. Arterial hypotension (<90 mmHg systolic or drop of > 40 mmHg)
2. Cardiogenic shock with peripheral hypoperfusion and hypoxia
3. Circulatory collapse with need for cardiopulmonary resuscitation

From Uflacker R. Interventional therapy for pulmonary embolism. J Vasc Interv Radiol 2001;12:147–64.

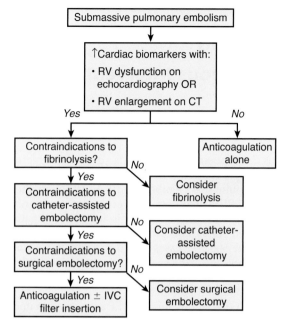

FIGURE 86-1. Algorithm for management of submassive pulmonary embolism patients. According to the algorithm, catheter-directed therapy should be considered in particular when there are contraindications to systemic thrombolysis. *CT,* Computed tomography; *IVC,* inferior vena cava; *RV,* right ventricle. *(From Piazza G, Goldhaber SZ. Management of submassive pulmonary embolism. Circulation 2010;122:1124–9.)*

possible treatment escalation beyond anticoagulation in normotensive PE patients.[5] Echocardiography is the best imaging study to detect RV dysfunction in the setting of acute PE. Characteristic echocardiographic findings in patients with submassive PE include RV hypokinesis and dilatation, interventricular septal flattening and paradoxical motion toward the LV, abnormal transmitral Doppler flow profile, tricuspid regurgitation, pulmonary hypertension as identified by a peak tricuspid regurgitant jet velocity over 2.6 m/s, and loss of inspiratory collapse of the inferior vena cava (IVC).[15] An RV-to-LV end-diastolic diameter ratio of 0.9 or greater, assessed in the left parasternal long-axis or subcostal view, is an independent predictor of hospital mortality.[16] Detection of RV enlargement by chest CTA is especially convenient for diagnosis of submassive PE, because it uses data acquired during the initial diagnostic scan. Submassive PE can be diagnosed when RV enlargement on chest CT, defined by an RV-to-LV diameter ratio greater than 0.9, is observed[17]; RV enlargement on chest CTA also predicts increased 30-day mortality in patients with acute PE.[17,18] Even if shock and death do not ensue, survivors of acute submassive PE remain at risk for developing chronic PE and thromboembolic pulmonary hypertension.[19]

Additionally, monitoring cardiac troponin T (cTnT) identifies the high-risk group of normotensive patients with submassive PE.[20] A persistent increased cTnT level (>0.01 ng/mL) in PE patients with right heart strain predicts a significant risk of a complicated clinical course and fatal outcome, and these patients therefore require more aggressive treatment.[20] Identifying submassive PE for treatment escalation is important because these normotensive PE patients demonstrate increased short-term mortality and high risk of adverse outcomes when the degree of heart strain results in elevations in levels of cardiac troponins and brain-type natriuretic peptide.[21,22] The optimal protocol for treatment of acute submassive PE is still in evolution, but a proposed algorithm for managing submassive PE has been published[23] describing treatment escalation beyond anticoagulation (Fig. 86-1).

Based on the history, angiographic findings, and outcomes of patients undergoing CDT for acute PE, three groups of patients have been identified[24]:

• Type I patients with fresh clots that have recently embolized should respond well to mechanical thrombectomy with increased peripheral flow and oxygenation. In general, 2 to 3 weeks is the upper age limit of thrombus when considering the option of CDT.

• Type II patients with older and more organized clots respond less effectively to mechanical thrombectomy

alone. Although more chronic clots are likely to remain, there is a chance for pulmonary flow improvement if pharmacologic thrombolysis of overlying acute thrombus can be achieved.

• Type III patients with organized chronic PE do not respond well to the effects of CDT.

CONTRAINDICATIONS

Because of the risk of major hemorrhage, aggressive anticoagulation, systemic thrombolysis, and local catheter-directed thrombolysis may be contraindicated in patients with recent major general or intracranial surgery. In such cases, mechanical methods of percutaneous catheter-directed thrombectomy, fragmentation, and/or aspiration should be considered without pharmacologic agents. Since pulmonary hypertension is a relative contraindication to pulmonary angiography, the degree of pulmonary hypertension and underlying cardiopulmonary reserve are important considerations prior to performing pulmonary angiography. These factors must be used to determine a safe rate and volume of contrast injection into the pulmonary circulation. For instance, when systolic pulmonary artery pressure (PAP) exceeds 55 mmHg, or right ventricular end diastolic pressure (RVEDP) is greater than 20 mmHg, the mortality associated with pulmonary angiography using large-volume power injection has been reported to be as high as 3%.[2,3] Therefore, such patients with massive PE should only receive a limited rate of power injection, controlled by hand. In the submassive PE patient, a selective contrast injection into the main left or right PA should not exceed a 20-mL volume at a rate of 10 mL/s. Lower injection parameters by hand may be considered depending on

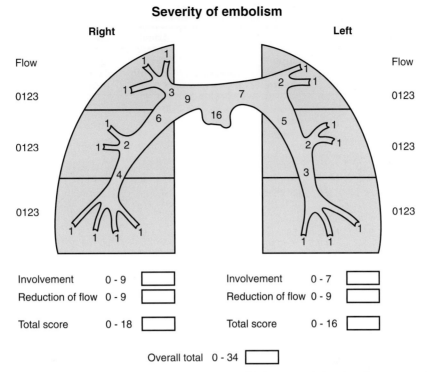

FIGURE 86-2. Schematic of pulmonary arterial segments used to grade severity of pulmonary embolism based on angiographic findings before and after treatment with thrombolytic and/or catheter-directed therapy. Segmental clot involvement and reduction of flow are scored separately. *(From Miller GAH, Sutton GC, Kerr IH, et al. Comparison of streptokinase and heparin in treatment of isolated acute massive pulmonary embolism. BMJ 1971;2:681–4.)*

degree of heart failure, as determined by the operator's judgment, to achieve adequate vessel opacification without endangering the patient. Pulmonary angiography can be used to calculate the degree of pulmonary obstruction before and after treatment, using the calculated Miller Index (Fig. 86-2). Finally, in PE patients with contraindications to anticoagulation and/or thrombolytic agents, placement of an IVC filter should be considered for prophylaxis of recurrent PE.

EQUIPMENT

Modern CDT for massive PE has been defined according to the following criteria: use of low-profile catheters and devices (≤10F), catheter-directed mechanical fragmentation and/or aspiration of emboli, and intraclot thrombolytic injection if a local drug is infused.[11] Therefore, a variety of devices can be successfully used to treat PE, so long as they meet criteria for modern CDT (Table 86-2).

Depending on anticipated bleeding risk, CDT may be performed with either no or low-dose local tPA injection. The initial goal of all these techniques is rapid debulking of central thrombus to relieve life-threatening heart strain, immediately improve pulmonary perfusion, and improve oxygenation (Fig. 86-3).[5]

In contrast to CDT for massive PE, which requires mechanical methods, the protocol for submassive PE consists of gentle image-guided infusion catheter placement and overnight pharmacologic thrombolysis without aggressive mechanical intervention. This treatment may be offered to patients who present primarily with submassive PE (Fig. 86-4), or as adjunctive treatment in patients with prior

massive PE who have been "downstaged" via central clot debulking to submassive PE. For at least one of the access sites, it is preferable that the sheath be sized at least 2F larger than the infusion catheter to allow subsequent central pulmonary artery (PA) pressure measurements through the sheath. An 8F to 10F vascular sheath (e.g., Flexor sheath [Cook Medical, Bloomington, Ind.]) is recommended, and the sheath should be long enough to reach from the access point to the main pulmonary trunk. If a second sheath is placed for dual catheter infusions, the operator can decide on the specific diameter and length, based on vessel tortuosity, sufficient to provide stability for the second infusion catheter.

TECHNIQUE

Anatomy and Approaches

Solid catheter-based skills along with knowledge of the cardiopulmonary anatomy are important for safe intravascular placement and manipulation of catheters and thrombectomy devices. Catheterization of the PA can be performed using a variety of methods, depending on the operator's preference and experience. An example via the transfemoral approach is using a 5F or 6F pigtail catheter in conjunction with a hydrophilic Glidewire (Terumo Medical Corp., Somerset, N.J.) and torque control device. An example via the right transjugular approach is using a C2 catheter (Cook Medical) in conjunction with a Glidewire and torque control device. Regardless of technique used, the electrocardiogram should be continuously monitored by trained nursing staff. Catheterization should be meticulously performed to

TABLE 86-2. Catheter-Directed Therapy for Massive Pulmonary Embolism in 594 Patients

Author, Year (Reference)	Country	Patients, n	Sex- n	Age: Mean, Range	Technique- n	Local Intraclot Lytic During CDT-n	Local Intraclot Lytic, Extended Infusion-n	Minor Cxs	Major Cxs	Clinical Success (%)
Prospective Studies										
Schmitz-Rode et al. 1998[48]	Germany	10	M-6, F-4	54 (36-70)	PF-10	8	1	0	0	8/10 (80)
Schmitz-Rode et al. 2000[49]	Germany	20	M-10, F-10	59 (48-60)	PF-20	0	0	1	0	16/20 (80)
Muller-Hulsbeck et al. 2001[50]	Germany	9	M-4, F-5	55 (27-85)	ATD-9	0	5	0	0	9/9 (100)
Prokubovsky et al. 2003[51]	Russia	20	na	51 (32-75)	PF-20	0	16	0	0	14/20 (70)
Tajima et al. 2004[52]	Japan	25	M-8, F-17	61 (35-77)	PF & AT-25	25	21	0	0	25/25 (100)
Barbosa et al. 2008[53]	Brazil	10	M-7, F-3	57 (39-75)	PF-10, (ATD-na)	0	0	0	0	9/10 (90)
Retrospective Studies										
Brady et al. 1991[54]	England	3	M-0, F-3	36 (18-71)	PF-1, MC-2	2	2	0	0	3/3 (100)
Rafique et al. 1992[55]	South Africa	5	M-1, F-4	35 (21-47)	MC-5	5	5	1	0	5/5 (100)
Uflacker et al. 1996[24]	U.S.A.	5	M-4, F-1	45 (25-64)	ATD-5	1	1	0	1	3/5 (60)
Fava et al. 1997[32]	Chile	16	M-8, F-8	49 (20-68)	PF-16, (BA-na)	16	16	3	0	14/16 (88)
Stock et al. 1997[56]	Switzerland	5	M-3, F-2	50 (21-80)	PF & BA-5	5	5	0	2	5/5 (100)
Basche et al. 1997[57]	Germany	15	na	na (21-73)	PF & BA-2, BA-13	na	na	0	0	12/15 (80)
Hiramatsu et al. 1999[58]	Japan	8	M-4, F-4	58 (42-87)	AT & WD-8	0	8	0	0	7/8 (88)
Wong et al. 1999[59]	England	4	M-2, F-2	33 (18-46)	PF-1,PF & G-1, G-2	0	4	0	1	3/4 (75)
Murphy et al. 1999[60]	Ireland	4	M-2, F-2	60 (46-66)	MC & WD-4	4	4	0	0	4/4 (100)
Voigtlander 1999[61]	Germany	5	M-4, F-1	57 (25-72)	RT-5	0	0	4	0	3/5 (60)
Fava et al. 2000[62]	Chile	11	M-3, F-8	61 (37-79)	Hy-11	0	4	0	0	10/11 (91)
Egge et al. 2002[63]	Norway	3	M-2, F-1	49 (40-54)	PF-3	3	3	0	0	3/3 (100)
De Gregorio et al. 2002[33]	Spain	59	M-25, F-34	56 (22-85)	PF-52, PF & BA-4, PF & DB -3	59	57	8	0	56/59 (95)
Zeni et al. 2003[36]	U.S.A.	16	M-9, F-8	52 (30-86)	RT-16	0	10	2	1	14/16 (88)

TABLE 86-2. Catheter-Directed Therapy for Massive Pulmonary Embolism in 594 Patients—cont'd

Author, Year (Reference)	Country	Patients, n	Sex-n	Age: Mean, Range	Technique-n	Local Intraclot Lytic During CDT-n	Local Intraclot Lytic, Extended Infusion-n	Minor Cxs	Major Cxs	Clinical Success (%)
Reekers et al. 2003[64]	Netherlands	7	M-2, F-6	46 (28-76)	Hy-6, Oa-1	7	0	0	0	6/7 (86)
Tajima et al. 2004[65]	Japan	15	M-4, F-11	60 (27-79)	AT-15	9	0	0	0	15/15 (100)
Fava et al. 2005[66]	Chile	7	M-3, F-4	56 (30-79)	Hy-4, Oa-3	3	3	1	1	6/7/ (86)
Siablis et al. 2005[37]	Greece	6	M-4, F-2	59 (42-76)	RT-6	4	0	2	0	5/6 (83)
Yoshida et al. 2006[67]	Japan	8	M-4, F-4	61 (47-75)	PF & AT-8	na	na	0	1	7/8 (88)
Li J-J et al. 2006[68]	China	15	M-11, F-4	56 (19-73)	PF & ATD-13, PF & Hy-1, PF & Oa-1	6	0	0	0	15/15 (100)
Pieri and Agresti. 2007[69]	Italy	164	na	68 (35-78)	PF-164	164	164	0	0	138/164 (84)
Chauhan et al. 2007[70]	U.S.A.	6	M-2 F-4	64 (49-78)	RT-6	2	0	5	2	4/6 (67)
Krajina 2007[71]	Czech Rep	5	M-1, F-4	67 (52-80)	PF-3, PF & AT-2	3	0	0	0	2/5 (40)
Yang 2007[72]	China	19	M-13, F-6	62 (22-87)	PF-10, PF & AT-5, PF+SR-4	19	na	0	0	18/19 (95)
Margheri 2008[73]	Italy	20	M-12, F-8	66 (32-85)	RT-20	na	0	8	8	17/20 (85)
Vecchio et al 2008[38]	Italy	13	na	68 (54-80)	RT-13	na	0	6	8	8/13 (62)
Chen et al 2008[74]	China	26	M-15, F-11	53 (36-71)	ATD-17, SR-9	21	0	1	0	26/26 (100)
Eid-Lidt et al. 2008[35]	Mexico	18	M-6, F-12	51 (47-55)	PF-5, PF & SR-13	2	0	0	0	16/18 (90)
Kuo et al. 2008[31]	U.S.A.	12	M-7, F-5	56 (21-80)	PF & AT-6, PF & AT & BA-2, RT & AT-2, AT & IC-2	8	na	1	0	10/12 (83)
TOTAL = 35		594		53 (18-87)		356/535 67%	329/552 60%	(7.9%)* [5.0-11.3%]	(2.4%)* [1.9-4.3%]	(86.5%)* [82.2-90.2%]

*Pooled estimates from random effects model.
[%], 95% confidence intervals; AT, aspiration thrombectomy; ATD, Amplatz thrombectomy device (Microvena, White Bear Lake, Minn.); B, Dormia basket (Cook Europe, Bjaeverskov, Denmark); BA, balloon fragmentation; Cxs, complications; G, Gensini (Cordis Corp., Miami, Fla.); Hy, Hydrolyzer (Cordis Corp., Miami, Fla.); IC, infusion catheter; MC, multipurpose catheter; na, data not available; Oa, Oasis (Boston Scientific, Galway, Ireland); PF, pigtail fragmentation; RT, rheolytic AngioJet thrombectomy (Possis Medical, Minneapolis, Minn.); SR, Straub Rotarex (Straub Medical, Wangs, Switzerland); WD, wire disruption.
From Kuo WT, Gould MK, Louie JD, et al. Catheter-directed therapy for the treatment of massive pulmonary embolism: Systematic review and meta-analysis of modern techniques. J Vasc Interv Radiol 2009;20:1431–40.

minimize wire contact with cardiac structures to reduce the risk of ventricular tachycardia and vascular perforation while passing through the right heart and into the pulmonary trunk. Once the pulmonary outflow has been selected, depending on operator preference, the hydrophilic wire can be exchanged for a non-hydrophilic wire such as a 0.035-inch Rosen wire (Boston Scientific, Natick, Mass.) to provide stability for subsequent vascular sheath placement. Selective catheterization of the main right and left PAs is routinely performed, but selective and subselective

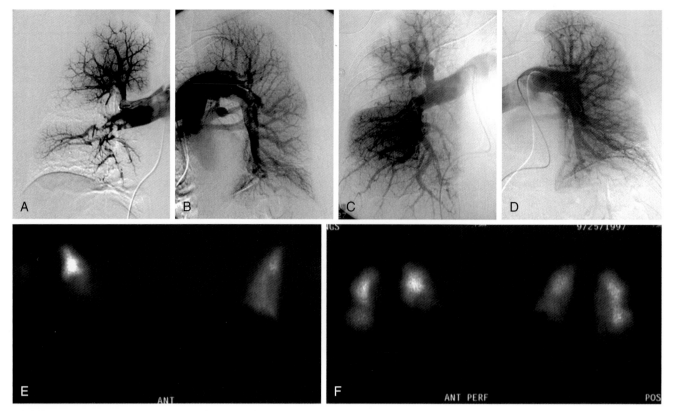

FIGURE 86-3. This patient with massive pulmonary embolism presented with syncope. **A,** Right pulmonary angiogram showed a large central embolism, with thrombus occluding most of the artery and sparing just a portion of the right upper lobe. **B,** Left pulmonary angiogram showed a large filling defect in main left pulmonary artery (PA). Catheter-directed therapy was initiated first to debulk central emboli. An infusion catheter was then wedged into main thrombus in the right PA, and urokinase was started at 100,000 IU/h for 36 hours, with alternating catheterization of the left PA for 12 hours. **C-D,** Posttreatment angiography showed significant improvement of bilateral pulmonary circulation. Patient experienced dramatic clinical improvement along with reduction of PA pressures. **E-F,** Pre- and post-treatment lung perfusion scans showed marked improvement in right lung perfusion, with some improvement in left lower lobe.

catheterization of pulmonary segments is often necessary for further treatment.

The femoral approach is preferred in most patients who are candidates for catheter-directed pulmonary thrombolysis or thrombectomy, but the right internal jugular approach is also feasible and may be preferred in the presence of IVC or iliofemoral thrombus. Most thrombectomy devices are easily passed from the right internal jugular vein into the right ventricle and PA.

Anticoagulation
Initial IV administration of heparin is the therapy of choice to treat all forms of acute pulmonary thromboembolism. Heparin binds to and accelerates the activity of antithrombin III, prevents additional thrombus formation, and permits endogenous fibrinolytic mechanisms to thrombolyse the clot that has already formed. During CDT for massive PE, full heparin anticoagulation may be continued during the clot debulking procedure. However, once the massive PE has been converted to submassive PE and overnight catheter-directed thrombolytic infusion is initiated, full heparin anticoagulation should be discontinued to minimize the risk of bleeding complications. During concomitant low-dose tPA infusion, a subtherapeutic heparin dose is desirable (partial thromboplastin time [PTT] < 60 seconds) to minimize risk of peri-sheath clot formation. To achieve this, the heparin infusion rate is typically between

300 and 500 units/h through a peripheral IV site. Once the patient has completed a course of catheter-directed thrombolytic therapy, full therapeutic anticoagulation can be resumed with full-dose IV heparin or low-molecular-weight heparin (LMWH). Full heparin anticoagulation should be maintained for 7 to 10 days as a bridge to subsequent oral anticoagulation.

Systemic Thrombolysis
Current approved medical therapy for acute massive PE consists of systemic thrombolysis with 100 mg of alteplase (Activase [Genentech, South San Francisco, Calif.]) infused IV over 2 hours,[3] and the most widely accepted indication for thrombolytic therapy in these patients is cardiogenic shock from acute PE. However, contraindications prevent many patients from receiving systemic thrombolysis. Even when patients with acute PE are prescreened for absolute contraindications, the rate of major hemorrhage from systemic thrombolytic administration is still about 20%, including a 3% to 5% risk of hemorrhagic stroke.[8,25] Furthermore, there may be insufficient time in the acute setting to infuse a full dose of IV thrombolytic.

In some instances, in appropriate candidates, it may be desirable to initiate IV tPA while simultaneously activating the interventional team to perform CDT. For example, in selected patients who are in extremis from PE and deemed candidates for any thrombolytic treatment, some clinicians

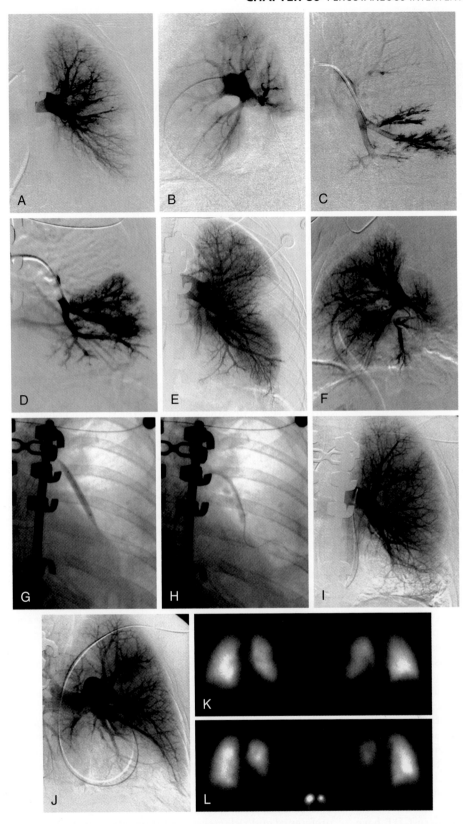

FIGURE 86-4. This 45-year-old woman with lymphoma presented with chest pain and dyspnea but remained hemodynamically stable; the diagnosis was acute submassive pulmonary embolism. **A,** Left pulmonary angiography showed occlusion of the posterior basal segment of the left lower lung. **B,** Lateral view of arteriogram showed occlusion of the posterior basal segment. Note patency of superior, anteromedial, and lateral basal segments, with a wedge of the posterior basal segment missing. **C,** An infusion catheter was carefully advanced into the posterior basal segment artery, and contrast medium injection showed extensive thrombosis. A catheter was wedged, and urokinase infusion was started. **D,** Follow-up angiography 12 hours into treatment showed restored patency of peripheral branches of the posterior basal segment, with persistent proximal occlusion of the posterior basal segment artery. **E-F,** Anterior and lateral views of a 24-hour follow-up angiogram showed persistent proximal occlusion and increased volume of a pleural effusion, with further collapse of the superior segment and left upper lung. **G-H,** Balloon angioplasty and occlusion balloon thrombectomy was performed in the persistently occluded segment of the posterior basal segment resulting in recanalization. **I-J,** Follow-up left pulmonary angiogram 1 month after treatment showed a patent posterior basal segment. **K,** Pretreatment lung perfusion scan showed reduced perfusion of the left lower lobe. **L,** Posttreatment scan showed persistent reduced perfusion of the left lung base due to an underlying pleural effusion.

may wish to initiate urgent "medical" treatment in the form of IV thrombolytic as a bridge to escalation "surgical" treatment with CDT. When used in this fashion, IV tPA could also be less risky. For instance, the amount of IV thrombolytic could be reduced by at least 50% (from the standard 100 mg tPA dose infused over 2 hours) if catheter intervention is initiated promptly, allowing discontinuation of IV tPA within 30 to 60 minutes.[26]

Catheter-Directed Thrombolysis
Under the definition of modern CDT,[11] two basic protocols of catheter-directed thrombolysis have emerged for

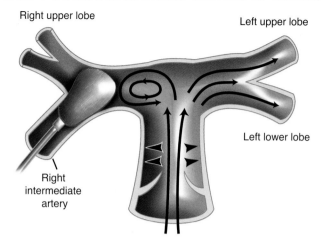

FIGURE 86-5. Schematic drawing of a pulmonary arterial flow model showing vortex formation immediately proximal to the level of obstruction. Note prominent vortex near the occlusion causing most circulating fluid to flow toward the nonoccluded left pulmonary artery. There is minimal fluid contact with the occluding embolus (the balloon). *(From Schmitz-Rode T, Kilbinger M, Günther RW. Simulated flow pattern in massive pulmonary embolism: Significance for selective intrapulmonary thrombolysis. Cardiovasc Intervent Radiol 1998;21:199–204.)*

treatment of massive and submassive PE, respectively. For massive PE, a catheter-directed bolus of thrombolytic drug is used in conjunction with mechanical clot fragmentation and/or aspiration to achieve central clot debulking. Depending on anticipated bleeding risk, CDT may be performed with either no or low-dose local tPA injection. The goal of these techniques is rapid central clot removal to relieve life-threatening heart strain and immediately improve pulmonary perfusion. Catheter intervention is important not only for creating an immediate flow channel through the obstruction, but also for exposing a greater surface area of thrombus to the effects of locally infused thrombolytic drug. If thrombolysis is performed without intraclot drug injection, and if the thrombolytic is instead infused proximal to the target embolus (as performed in older studies), there is little added benefit compared to systemic IV infusion.[27] Schmitz-Rode et al. demonstrated with in vitro and in vivo flow studies[28] that an obstructing embolus causes proximal vortex formation that prevents a drug infused upstream from making rapid contact with the downstream embolus, and the eddy currents instead cause washout of thrombolytic into the unobstructed pulmonary arteries (Fig. 86-5). These flow studies emphasize the importance of direct intrathrombus injection as an adjunct to embolus fragmentation to achieve rapid and effective catheter-directed thrombolysis.[28]

Several devices meeting criteria for modern CDT have been used effectively, but the most common technique is rotating pigtail fragmentation, which has been used either alone or in combination with other methods in 70% of patients worldwide receiving CDT.[11] Although pigtail clot fragmentation appears to effectively debulk proximal emboli, in some instances it has resulted in distal embolization with PAP elevation, requiring adjunctive aspiration

thrombectomy to complete treatment.[29] Aspiration can be performed with virtually any end-hole catheter, such as an 8F JR4 catheter (Cook Medical). Additional clot fragmentation may also be achieved with insertion and inflation of an angioplasty balloon sized below the target arterial diameter (Fig. 86-6). Thus it is important to have adjunctive methods available to use in conjunction with pigtail rotation. The main advantage of the rotating pigtail is its wide availability and low cost relative to the mechanically-driven thrombectomy devices.

For treatment of submassive PE, or once massive PE has been downstaged to submassive PE, further mechanical debulking is usually unnecessary, and the protocol consists of careful image-guided infusion catheter placement into thrombosed segments for overnight pharmacologic thrombolysis.[5] Once the infusion catheters have been properly positioned and connected to IV pumps, catheter-directed thrombolysis should be initiated using alteplase at a rate of 0.5 mg/h through the drug lumen of each catheter if bilateral catheters are used. If only one catheter has been placed for unilateral treatment, the rate may be increased to 1 mg/h through the single infusion catheter. The recommended total tPA infusion rate should be 1 mg/h. To achieve the infusion dose, the reconstituted drug can be diluted in normal saline solution to yield a concentration of 0.1 mg tPA/mL of solution, and the pump can be set accordingly to deliver the prescribed dose. An alternative to catheter-directed tPA is urokinase infusion. The regimen consists of a bolus infusion of 200,000 to 500,000 IU followed by an infusion of 100,000 IU/h of urokinase for 12 to 36 hours.[30] Fibrinogen levels can be monitored, particularly in those patients at greater risk of bleeding or if the infusion will be continued beyond 24 hours. When fibrinogen levels drop below 150 to 200 mg/dL, the infusion should be reduced, discontinued, or alternatively continued with transfusions of fresh frozen plasma if further thrombolysis is desired.[5]

Catheter-Directed Embolectomy, Fragmentation, and Thrombolysis

Contrary to invasive open surgical thrombectomy, which has been associated with high perioperative morbidity and mortality, percutaneous CDT represents a safe, less invasive option for treating patients with acute massive PE.[11] As mentioned, the rationale for using percutaneous devices in the pulmonary circulation is rapid central clot debulking to relieve life-threatening heart strain and immediately improve pulmonary perfusion, which can be immediately verified by follow-up angiography and hemodynamic assessments. Percutaneous embolectomy, clot fragmentation, and mechanical thrombolysis also serve to expose a greater surface area of thrombus to the effects of locally infused thrombolytic drug. However, depending on anticipated bleeding risk, CDT may be performed with either no or low-dose local tPA injection, depending on operator preference and risk assessment. Regardless of the decision to use thrombolytic drug, CDT can be used effectively when full-dose thrombolytic therapy is contraindicated or fails to resolve hemodynamic shock.[3,5,11]

An ideal percutaneous thrombectomy device for treating PE should have these characteristics:

- Low profile (≤10F) and long enough to reach the PA from a peripheral venous access site

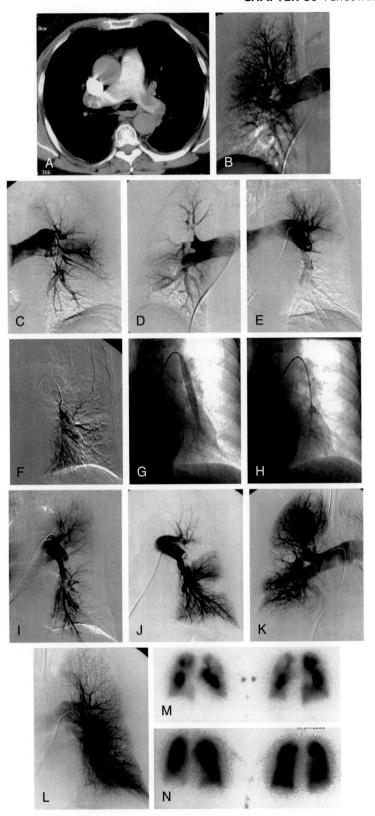

FIGURE 86-6. This 78-year-old woman with chronic obstructive pulmonary disease and history of myocardial infarction 1 month earlier presented to the emergency department with symptoms of deep vein thrombosis, chest pain, shortness of breath, and congestive heart failure. Chest computed tomographic angiography (CTA) was positive for acute pulmonary embolism. Ventilation/perfusion scan showed massive perfusion defects. Patient was transferred to our hospital, and a pulmonary arteriogram was requested for possible catheter-directed treatment. **A,** Chest CT scan showed large filling defects in both main pulmonary arteries. After hemodynamic stabilization, a pulmonary arteriogram was performed. **B,** Right pulmonary angiogram showed severe obstruction at the bifurcation of the right main pulmonary artery (PA). There was reduced perfusion of the right upper lobe and marked hypoperfusion of the right lower lobe. **C,** Left pulmonary angiogram showed a large embolism involving the left lower lobe with marked reduction in peripheral perfusion. Pulmonary artery pressure (PAP) was 39 mmHg. **D,** Follow-up right pulmonary angiogram after 15 hours of catheter-directed thrombolytic infusion showed marked improvement of the obstruction, with some residual clots involving the right upper and middle lobes. There was interval improvement in right lower lobe perfusion. **E,** Follow-up left pulmonary angiogram showed progressive occlusion of the left lower lobe likely from distal migration of a proximal thrombus. PAP was 46 mmHg. **F,** Selective catheterization of the left lower lobe branch through the clot was performed and showed total occlusion of the lower lobe artery. **G,** A 10-mm balloon catheter was advanced into the lower lobe branches over a wire and used to fragment clot. **H,** An occlusion balloon was trawled back several times to further fragment the clots. **I,** An angiogram after mechanical balloon thrombectomy showed improved lower lobe segment patency. A catheter was placed within the partially occluded artery, and thrombolytic infusion was continued. **J,** Follow-up left pulmonary angiogram after 15 hours of local thrombolytic infusion showed significant improvement in left lung perfusion. **K,** Final right pulmonary angiogram showed significant improvement in right pulmonary perfusion. **L,** Final left pulmonary angiogram showed near complete patency of the left PA and peripheral branches. Mean PAP after treatment was 33 mmHg. The patient improved clinically, was weaned off the ventilator, and successfully extubated. **M,** Pretreatment perfusion scan showed multiple wedge-shaped areas of segmental hypoperfusion. **N,** Perfusion scan 3 days after catheter-directed thrombolytic therapy showed remarkable improvement in bilateral pulmonary perfusion. After discharge from the intensive care unit, the only complication was acute renal failure that eventually resolved after 5 days, with return of creatinine to normal levels. The patient was discharged home within 1 week after receiving catheter-directed therapy.

- Adequate flexibility for facile insertion and navigation in the pulmonary circulation
- Capable of achieving embolectomy, clot fragmentation, and/or mechanical thrombolysis in a large vessel
- Allows concomitant intraclot thrombolytic drug injection if desired
- Safe in the central circulation, with low risk of vascular perforation, no widespread distal embolization, and no hemolytic side effects

Since no current device possesses all these characteristics, a combination of devices and methods can be used to achieve effective CDT.

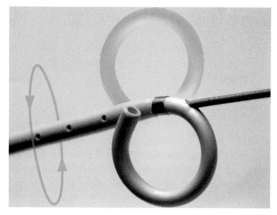

FIGURE 86-7. Photo diagram of the rotating pigtail method most commonly used to treat acute massive pulmonary embolism. *(From Schmitz-Rode T, Janssens U, Duda SH, et al. Massive pulmonary embolism: Percutaneous emergency treatment by pigtail rotation catheter. J Am Coll Cardiol 2000;36:375–80.)*

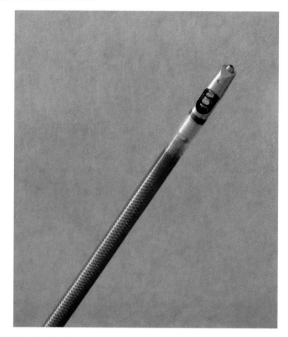

FIGURE 86-8. Close-up photo of the Aspirex device tip. *(Courtesy Straub Medical AG, Wangs, Switzerland.)*

Percutaneous Devices and Methods

Rotating Pigtail Clot Fragmentation

The most common technique currently used is rotating pigtail fragmentation (Fig. 86-7), which has been used either alone or in combination with other methods in 70% of patients worldwide receiving CDT.[11] Although a robust pigtail has been manufactured in Europe specifically for treating PE (Cook Europe, Bjaeverskov, Denmark), virtually any type of pigtail catheter can be used. The pigtail catheter and its distal side holes can also be used to inject local thrombolytic drug directly into the thrombus. Although pigtail clot fragmentation appears to effectively debulk central emboli, in some instances it has resulted in distal embolization with PAP elevation, requiring adjunctive aspiration thrombectomy to complete treatment.[29]

Balloon Angioplasty for Clot Fragmentation

Additional clot fragmentation may also be achieved with insertion and inflation of an angioplasty balloon sized below the target arterial diameter. Specifically, mechanical clot fragmentation has been described using angioplasty balloons between 6 and 16 mm in diameter. When used in conjunction with local pharmacologic thrombolysis for massive PE, these methods have been very successful, with an 87.5% recovery rate, as measured by PAPs, blood O_2 values, and clinical outcomes.[32,33]

Simple Aspiration Thrombectomy

Aspiration can be performed with virtually any end-hole catheter, such as an 8F JR4 catheter (Cook Medical) or 10F Pronto catheter (Vascular Solutions, Minneapolis, Minn.). This method works best on central occlusive thrombus and should be used in conjunction with the methods already mentioned.

Electronic Aspiration Thrombectomy

The Aspirex (Straub Medical, Wangs, Switzerland), has shown promising results for acute PE thrombectomy.[34,35] This device works on the principle of a rotating Archimedes screw that resides within a low-profile catheter lumen (Fig. 86-8). The metallic spiral is connected to an electric motor drive and control unit. Electronic activation of the spiral coil produces aspiration from the open catheter tip, transporting material down the catheter shaft and into a collecting system.

High-Rpm Mechanical Thrombectomy

The Helix Clot Buster (ev3/Covidien, Plymouth, Minn.), formerly known as the *Amplatz thrombectomy device* (ATD), has been used to treat acute PE. The device is a 75- or 120-cm-long, 7F reinforced polyurethane catheter with a distal metal tip containing an impeller connected to a drive shaft. The catheter is connected to an air source turbine that generates up to 140,000 rpm at pressures between 30 and 35 psi during operation. Although little data are available on the new version of this device for treatment of PE, data from off-label use of the older 8F version have been published, with use in conjunction with a 10F guide catheter.[24] The possibility of hemolytic complications exists, but so far the degree has not been shown to be clinically significant.[24] Despite promising results, production of the Helix device is currently on hold by the manufacturer, with possible plans for a product re-release.

Rheolytic Thrombectomy

The mechanism of rheolytic thrombectomy is a high-pressure saline jet in conjunction with aspiration. This creates a Venturi effect that causes fragmentation and aspiration of the clot. The AngioJet (Possis Medical, Minneapolis, Minn.) is a double-lumen system with diameters ranging from 4F to 6F. Although results were promising in early small series of patients with massive PE,[36-38] recent meta-analytic data revealed higher procedure-related complications associated with AngioJet rheolytic thrombectomy (ART), including bradyarrhythmia, heart block, hemoglobinuria, renal insufficiency, major hemoptysis, and procedure-related death. Several deaths related to the AngioJet have been recorded in the U.S. Food and Drug Administration's (FDA's) MAUDE (Manufacturer and User

Facility Device Experience) database.[39] As a result, the FDA has issued a black-box warning on the device label.[40] For all these reasons, the AngioJet device should probably be avoided as the initial mechanical option in CDT protocols for acute massive PE.[26,41]

Pulmonary Artery Stent Placement

Case reports have described the use of metallic stents in critically ill patients with persistent central obstruction from presumed chronic emboli resistant to catheter-directed thrombolysis. The stents have been placed alongside organized PA emboli in which the patients presented with cor pulmonale, profound arterial hypoxemia, and hypotension that did not respond to other therapies.[42,43] The paucity of evidence should make use of stents only considered when there is life-threatening PE refractory to CDT (described earlier).

Ultrasound-Assisted Catheter-Directed Thrombolysis

The EKOS infusion catheter (EKOS Corp., Bothell, Wash.) uses microsonic energy designed to help loosen and separate fibrin to enhance clot permeability while increasing availability of more plasminogen activation receptor sites for tPA. The microsonic energy is also intended to drive the thrombolytic agent deep into the blood clot to accelerate thrombolysis.[44] If successful, it has the potential to shorten the duration of infusion and lower the total dose of thrombolytic drug in submassive PE patients.[44]

CONTROVERSIES

In 1988, Verstraete et al. published a study[27] comparing the recanalization effects of intrapulmonary versus IV infusion of rtPA and showed that transcatheter intrapulmonary delivery did not offer a significant benefit over the IV route. The major flaw in the study was that intrapulmonary drug delivery was performed proximal to the target clot, without intraclot thrombolytic injection and without mechanical intervention. As noted earlier, subsequent in vitro and in vivo flow studies[28] confirmed that an obstructing embolus causes proximal vortex formation that prevents a drug infused upstream (even via catheter) from making rapid contact with the downstream embolus, and the eddy currents instead cause washout of thrombolytic into the unobstructed pulmonary arteries (see Fig. 86-5). This emphasizes the importance of *direct* intrathrombus injection as an adjunct to embolus fragmentation to achieve rapid and effective catheter-directed thrombolysis.[28]

Despite the complications associated with AngioJet rheolytic thrombectomy and the FDA black box warning, some interventionalists continue to use this device to treat acute PE.[26] A meta-analysis of data on CDT[11] revealed that the highest complication rates occurred in patients treated with ART, including a 40% rate of minor complications and 28% rate of major complications that included procedure-related death.[11] Cumulative data indicate that most modern CDT (89%) has been performed worldwide with a high degree of safety and efficacy *without* using ART.

OUTCOMES

In a systematic review and meta-analysis of 594 patients with acute massive PE treated with modern CDT, clinical success was achieved in 86.5% (Fig. 86-9), where success was defined as stabilization of hemodynamics, resolution of hypoxia, and survival to hospital discharge.[11] In the same study, 96% of patients received CDT as the first adjunct to heparin, with no prior systemic tPA infusion, and 33% of cases were initiated with mechanical treatment alone without local thrombolytic infusion.[11] The data were derived across 18 countries from 35 studies—six prospective, 29 retrospective—and pooled results were similar in prospective versus retrospective studies, with no statistically significant difference. The pooled frequency of success was higher in studies in which at least 80% of participants received local thrombolytic therapy during the procedure (91.2% vs. 82.8%). The pooled frequency of success was also higher in studies in which at least 80% of participants received extended local thrombolytic therapy for treatment of residual submassive PE (89.2% vs. 84.2%).[11]

Modern CDT continues to be used worldwide. In 2011, another large-scale study of 111 PE patients confirmed that modern catheter-directed thrombolysis with mechanical fragmentation achieves rapid normalization of the pulmonary pressure and is a safe and effective method for treating acute massive PE.[30] Patients in extremis from massive PE require emergent treatment escalation beyond anticoagulation, and if IV tPA is contraindicated or there is insufficient time for full-dose tPA, CDT may be the only viable treatment option. Indeed, at experienced centers, the use of modern CDT has proven to be a lifesaving treatment in patients dying from acute massive PE.[11,30]

Submassive Pulmonary Embolism

There is growing evidence that aggressive treatment of submassive PE is beneficial. The Management Strategies and Prognosis of Pulmonary Embolism Trial-3 (MAPPET-3) randomized 256 patients with submassive PE to receive 100 mg of IV tPA over a 2-hour period, followed by unfractionated heparin infusion, versus placebo plus heparin anticoagulation.[45] Compared with heparin anticoagulation alone, thrombolysis resulted in a significant reduction in the primary study endpoint of in-hospital death or clinical deterioration that required escalation of therapy (defined as catecholamine infusion, rescue thrombolysis, mechanical ventilation, cardiopulmonary resuscitation, or emergency surgical embolectomy).[45] The difference was largely attributable to a higher frequency of open-label thrombolysis (breaking randomized trial protocol to offer medically necessary thrombolysis) due to clinical deterioration as determined by the treating clinician.[45]

In a prospective study of 200 patients with submassive PE,[19] echocardiography was performed at the time of diagnosis and after 6 months to determine the frequency of pulmonary hypertension between two groups—one group treated with heparin and another group treated with IV tPA and heparin. The median decrease in PA systolic pressure was only 2 mmHg in patients treated with heparin alone, compared with 22 mmHg in those treated with tPA plus heparin.[19] At 6 months, the PA systolic pressure increased in 27% of patients who had received heparin alone, and nearly half of those patients were moderately symptomatic.[19] These data suggest that thrombolytic therapy may reduce the likelihood of developing chronic thromboembolic pulmonary hypertension.[19]

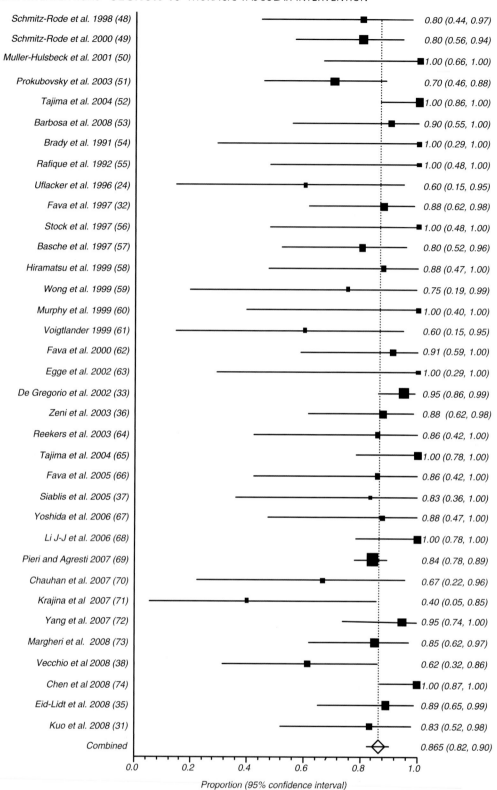

FIGURE 86-9. Forest plot shows clinical success rates from CDT and confidence intervals (CIs) from reported studies encompassing 594 patients with acute massive pulmonary embolism. Percentage clinical success is denoted along x-axis. Extended lines represent 95% CIs. Squares are proportional to study weight. Width of diamond corresponds to 95% CI for pooled clinical success rate of 86.5%. *(From Kuo WT, Gould MK, Louie JD, et al. Catheter-directed therapy for the treatment of massive pulmonary embolism: Systematic review and meta-analysis of modern techniques. J Vasc Interv Radiol 2009;20:1431–40.)*

However, for patients who are not good candidates for systemic tPA, the next logical step to consider is catheter-directed intervention. That is why the incorporation of a CDT protocol with targeted drug delivery and a lower overall thrombolytic dose could further improve outcomes while reducing hemorrhagic risk in the submassive PE group.[5] Indeed, when low-dose (≤30 mg) local tPA was administered to acute massive PE patients—a group at higher risk for bleeding than submassive PE patients[12]—there were no major hemorrhagic complications.[10,11] Furthermore, when patients with massive PE are downstaged to submassive PE via initial catheter-directed treatment of central clot, the overall clinical success was higher when these patients also received extended local thrombolytic therapy.[11] Such results strongly suggest that use of endovascular treatment in the form of local thrombolytic infusion appears to be a promising option for reducing both acute and chronic complications from PE, while avoiding the bleeding risks associated with full-dose systemic thrombolysis.

COMPLICATIONS

From the global meta-analysis on CDT,[11] the pooled risk of major complications was only 2.4%. Among 594 patients, major procedural complications occurred in 25 patients, including 11 groin hematomas (requiring transfusion), five noncerebral hemorrhages (sites unspecified, requiring transfusion), two cases of massive hemoptysis requiring transfusion, one renal failure requiring hemodialysis, one cardiac tamponade treated with surgical repair, one death from bradyarrhythmia and apnea, one death from widespread distal embolization, one death associated with cerebrovascular hemorrhage, and two procedure-related deaths (mechanism unspecified). The highest complication rates occurred in the 68 patients who underwent CDT with the rheolytic AngioJet device, including 27 minor complications (40%) and 19 major complications (28%).[11] The complications of bradyarrhythmia, heart block, hemoglobinuria, temporary renal insufficiency, one minor hemoptysis, one major hemoptysis, five major hemorrhages, and five procedure-related deaths were all associated with the AngioJet device. Interestingly, 76% of the recorded major complications (19/25) in the study were directly attributed to ART, despite the fact that it was used in only a small percentage (11%) of the 594 patients evaluated.[11] Conversely, the data indicated that most modern CDT (89%) was performed worldwide with a high degree of safety and efficacy without using ART.

Overall, compared to the high rate of major hemorrhagic complications from systemic tPA of 20%,[8,25] the rate of major complications from modern CDT has proven to be only 2.4%.[11] Since most of these complications were attributed to ART, elimination of AngioJet from the CDT protocol could further improve the overall safety of modern CDT.

POSTPROCEDURAL ANTICOAGULATION AND FOLLOW-UP CARE

Therapeutic anticoagulation is the primary medical treatment for all patients diagnosed with acute VTE, and it should be prescribed for at least 3 to 6 months or indefinitely, depending on careful assessment of several factors.[10]

If VTE is associated with a major irreversible risk factor such as cancer, these patients have at least a 15% risk of recurrence during the first year after stopping anticoagulation.[46] Consequently, patients with active cancer and a first episode of VTE usually receive treatment indefinitely.[10] Conversely, if VTE is provoked by a major reversible risk factor such as recent surgery, the risk of recurrence is about 3% in the first year if anticoagulation is discontinued after 3 months.[46] Between these two extremes are patients who have suffered acute VTE associated with a minor reversible risk factor (e.g., estrogen therapy or soft-tissue leg injury) and those who have had an unprovoked or idiopathic VTE.[47] For patients with a minor reversible risk factor, the risk of recurrence is about 5% in the first year after stopping anticoagulant therapy.[47] This is considered low enough to justify stopping anticoagulant therapy at the end of 3 months.[10] However, an unprovoked proximal DVT or PE has a higher risk of recurrence (about 10% in the first year after stopping therapy).[46] Continuing anticoagulant therapy beyond 3 months confers a greater than 90% risk reduction for preventing recurrence among these patients; however, if anticoagulants are subsequently stopped after 6 or 12 months of treatment, the risk of recurrence appears to be the same as if anticoagulants had been stopped after 3 months.[10] This high risk of recurrence is indirect evidence that patients with a first unprovoked proximal DVT or acute PE should receive anticoagulant therapy indefinitely. However, after all the major risks and benefits of long-term anticoagulation therapy have been explained, patient preference should also influence the decision.[46] Because of all these complexities, consultation with a hematologist or physician experienced in treating VTE is essential in determining the optimal anticoagulation regimen.

If there are contraindications to immediate anticoagulation for acute VTE, IVC filtration may be indicated. For those patients who have suffered near death from massive PE, IVC filter placement should be considered in addition to anticoagulation. For those diagnosed with submassive PE, it is unclear whether additional filter placement is necessary in addition to anticoagulation. If caval filtration is desired, a retrievable filter is often preferable, since it has the option to be removed. When lifelong filtration is not intended, such patients should be followed closely and scheduled for timely filter removal (e.g., once they are stabilized on therapeutic anticoagulation). Once filtration is no longer indicated, successful IVC filter removal can spare patients the potential risks associated with long-term filter implantation.

KEY POINTS

- Rapid risk stratification by identifying acute massive and acute submassive pulmonary embolism (PE) patients is essential in determining appropriate treatment escalation beyond anticoagulation.

- For patients with less severe or submassive PE (defined by right heart strain), endovascular treatment in the form of local thrombolytic infusion appears to be a promising option for reducing both acute and chronic complications from PE while avoiding the bleeding risks associated with full-dose systemic thrombolysis.

- For patients in extremis from massive PE (defined by hemodynamic shock), emergent treatment escalation is necessary in the form of catheter-directed therapy (CDT) for rapid debulking of central obstructive emboli, especially if systemic tissue plasminogen activator (tPA) is contraindicated.

- CDT may be the only viable option for rapid restoration of pulmonary arterial flow if intravenous systemic tPA is contraindicated or has already failed to resolve hemodynamic shock.

- Rheolytic thrombectomy with the AngioJet device has been associated with a high rate of major complications, including procedure-related death, so to improve the overall safety of modern CDT, it should probably be avoided in future protocols.

- The major complication rate from CDT is only 2.4%, versus the 20% rate of major hemorrhage associated with systemic tPA infusion.

- At experienced centers, the use of modern CDT has proven to be a lifesaving treatment for acute massive PE, with an overall clinical success rate of 86.5%.

- Following intervention, therapeutic anticoagulation should be continued as the ongoing medical treatment, and duration of therapy must depend on careful assessment of several risk factors.

► **SUGGESTED READINGS**

Konstantinides S, Geibel A, Heusel G, et al. Heparin plus alteplase compared with heparin alone in patients with submassive pulmonary embolism. N Engl J Med 2002;347:1143–50.

Kuo WT, Gould MK, Louie JD, et al. Catheter-directed therapy for the treatment of massive pulmonary embolism: systematic review and meta-analysis of modern techniques. J Vasc Interv Radiol 2009;20: 1431–40.

Kuo WT. Endovascular therapy for acute pulmonary embolism. J Vasc Interv Radiol 2012;23:167–79.

Piazza G, Goldhaber SZ. Management of submassive pulmonary embolism. Circulation 2010;122:1124–9.

The complete reference list is available online at www.expertconsult.com.

CHAPTER 87

Craniocervical Vascular Anatomy

Diego San Millán Ruiz, Bradley P. Barnett, and Philippe Gailloud

CRANIOCERVICAL ARTERIES

Cerebral blood flow is provided by the paired internal carotid arteries (ICAs) and vertebral arteries (VAs). The intradural branches of the ICA supply the anterior cerebral circulation (i.e., cerebral hemispheres, including basal ganglia) and the orbit; these branches include the ophthalmic artery (OA), posterior communicating artery (PComA), anterior choroidal artery (AChoA), and anterior and middle cerebral arteries (ACA, MCA). The vertebrobasilar system, formed by fusion of the VAs into the basilar artery (BA), supplies the posterior cerebral circulation, including the brainstem, cerebellum, and posterior aspect of the cerebral hemispheres via the posterior cerebral arteries (PCAs). Connections between the anterior and posterior circulations occur through the circle of Willis (CW) and its branches or through occasionally persistent embryologic carotid-vertebral and carotid-basilar connections (i.e., persistent trigeminal, hypoglossal, and proatlantal arteries). Cortical (or leptomeningeal) anastomoses also exist over the surface of the cerebral convexity and connect the ACA, MCA, and PCA. These anastomoses may provide important collateral pathways in patients with steno-occlusive disorders such as atheromatous disease or moyamoya syndrome. Finally, so-called watershed areas exist between the terminal vascular territories of the principal cerebral arteries. Watershed areas represent zones at risk for ischemic injury in patients with hemodynamically significant stenosis of the ICA, low cardiac output, or severe prolonged hypotension.

The anatomy of the intracranial arterial system is discussed in detail in the following sections, which have been organized into the anterior and posterior circulations, the CW, and major branches of the anterior and posterior circulations (Table 87-1).

Anterior Circulation

Common Carotid Artery

The left and right common carotid arteries (CCAs) have a different origin pattern. The right CCA generally arises from the brachiocephalic trunk (also known as the *innominate artery*). When the brachiocephalic trunk is absent—for instance, in the presence of an aberrant right subclavian artery (SubcA), or arteria lusoria—the right CCA comes directly from the aortic arch. Rarely, the right and left CCAs originate from a common trunk called a *bicarotid trunk*, a pattern usually observed in association with an aberrant right SubcA. The left CCA generally originates directly

from the aortic arch, in between the brachiocephalic trunk and left SubcA. The left CCA is therefore usually longer than the right. A common origin for the left CCA and the brachiocephalic trunk is observed in approximately 13% of cases.[1] This variation is commonly referred to as a "bovine arch," a misnomer because the typical bovine arch consists of a single aortic trunk that provides all the supraaortic branches.[2] In about 9% of cases, the left CCA arises from the brachiocephalic trunk itself.[1] Rarely, the left CCA may share a common origin with the left SubcA and form a left brachiocephalic artery.[3]

Although the CCA does not normally have branches, variations may include variant origins of the superior thyroid, ascending pharyngeal, and vertebral arteries (Fig. 87-1). In rare instances, bronchial arteries can arise from the proximal portion of the CCA.[4]

Carotid Bifurcation

The carotid bifurcation is most commonly located at the level of the superior border of the thyroid cartilage between the C3 and C5 vertebral levels, but extreme positions ranging from C1 to T4 may be encountered. Intrathoracic bifurcations are rare but represent a potential pitfall during angiography, when the ICA or external carotid artery (ECA) may be unintentionally catheterized because of their low origin. Intrathoracic carotid bifurcations may be more frequent in patients with Klippel-Feil anomaly.[5] Both carotid bifurcations are generally found at the same level (28%) or within one vertebral level (65%).[6]

Immediately distal to the bifurcation, the ICA is lateral and posterior to the ECA. The ICA then bends medially to reach the outer opening of the carotid canal at the skull base, whereas the ECA ascends laterally toward the parotid gland, where it divides into its terminal branches. The ICA may infrequently arise medial (4%) or posteromedial (8%) to the ECA.[7] The carotid bulb is a normal widening of the carotid bifurcation that extends from the distal CCA to the proximal ICA. It may also involve the proximal ECA.

External Carotid Artery

The ECA divides into numerous branches along its course between the carotid bifurcation and its termination in the maxillary and superficial temporal arteries in the parotid gland region. The classic ECA description includes eight main branches (described later) that supply the superior aspect of the thyroid gland, the viscerocranium (soft and bony structures of the face), the scalp, and a large part of the neurocranium (skull and meninges) (Fig. 87-2). Because of the existence of an extensive collateral network, selective

TABLE 87-1. Abbreviations

Acronym	Expanded
ACA	Anterior cerebral artery
AChoA	Anterior choroidal artery
AComA	Anterior communicating artery
AG	Arachnoid granulation
AICA	Anterior inferior cerebellar artery
BA	Basilar artery
BVR	Basal vein of Rosenthal
CCA	Common carotid artery
CS	Cavernous sinus
CW	Circle of Willis
ECA	External carotid artery
ICA	Internal carotid artery
ICV	Internal cerebral vein
IJV	Internal jugular vein
IVVP	Internal vertebral venous plexus
MCA	Middle cerebral artery
OA	Ophthalmic artery
PCA	Posterior cerebral artery
PComA	Posterior communicating artery
PICA	Posterior inferior cerebellar artery
PTA	Persistent trigeminal artery
SubcA	Subclavian artery
SCA	Superior cerebellar artery
SMCV	Superficial middle cerebral vein
SSS	Superior sagittal sinus
VA	Vertebral artery
VAVP	Vertebral artery venous plexus
VG	Vein of Galen
WS	Vertebral venous system

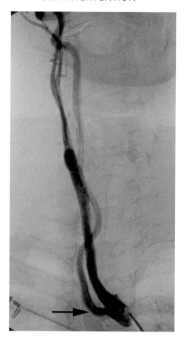

FIGURE 87-1. Digital subtraction angiogram, right innominate injection, anteroposterior view showing a right vertebral artery (VA) *(arrow)* originating from right common carotid artery (CCA). This variant is generally associated with an aberrant right subclavian artery (arteria lusoria). Proximal origin of VA makes it easy to overlook during selective angiography of CCA. *(©2012, Philippe Gailloud, MD.)*

embolization with occlusion of branches of the ECA or the ECA itself is generally well tolerated. Connections between the ECA and ICA or VA are often referred to as "dangerous anastomoses." These anastomoses may play an important role as sources of collateral supply in patients with steno-occlusive disorders, but they also represent important pitfalls during embolization procedures within the ECA territory. These dangerous collateral pathways include (1) anastomoses between external carotid branches (mainly from the facial, maxillary, and superficial temporal arteries) and branches of the distal ICA, including the OA, inferior-lateral trunk, and meningohypophyseal trunk, and (2) anastomoses between external carotid branches (mainly the occipital artery) and muscular branches of the VA. The eight branches of the ECA are as follows:

1. The superior thyroid artery principally supplies the superior pole of the ipsilateral thyroid lobe. The superior and inferior thyroid arteries are connected through a bilateral anastomotic network that can play an important role in collateral cerebral supply.[8] The superior thyroid artery also vascularizes the larynx (superior and inferior laryngeal arteries), as well as the infrahyoid and sternocleidomastoid muscles.

2. The lingual artery arises between the superior thyroid and facial arteries, although in about 20% of cases it forms a common trunk with the facial artery (linguofacial trunk). The lingual artery gives off branches for the hyoid bone, the muscles forming the floor of the mouth, the sublingual gland (sublingual branch), and the muscles of the tongue (deep lingual artery).

3. The facial artery courses over the body of the mandible toward the angle of the mouth and then ascends toward the medial epicanthus (angular artery), where it anastomoses with branches of the OA. The facial artery has numerous branches including the ascending palatine artery (for the tonsils, soft palate, and oropharynx), artery of the submandibular gland, submental artery, inferior and superior labial arteries (for the lips), lateral nasal branch, and angular artery (for the eyelids). Through its connection with the OA, the facial artery may provide collateral flow to the ICA in cases of severe stenosis or occlusion of the ICA. This pathway can be demonstrated by sonography or angiography as reversal of flow within the OA.

4. The ascending pharyngeal artery supplies the pharynx, palate, and tympanic cavity (inferior tympanic artery). Its terminal branches are meningeal arteries for the posterior fossa (clivus and posterior surface of petrous bone) that enter the cranium through the foramen lacerum, foramen jugulare, or hypoglossal canal. These branches may also participate in collateral supply of the distal ICA.

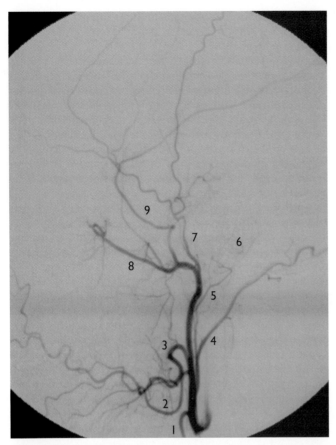

FIGURE 87-2. Digital subtraction angiogram, selective external carotid artery (ECA) injection, lateral view. Main branches of ECA are *(1)* superior thyroid artery, *(2)* lingual artery, *(3)* facial artery, *(4)* occipital artery, *(5)* ascending pharyngeal artery, and *(6)* posterior auricular artery. ECA terminates in *(7)* superficial temporal artery and *(8)* maxillary artery, which provides *(9)* middle meningeal artery. *(©2012, Philippe Gailloud, MD.)*

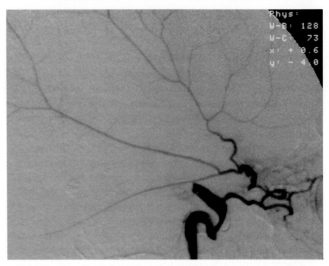

FIGURE 87-3. Digital subtraction angiogram, internal carotid artery (ICA) injection, lateral view showing occlusion of ICA distal to origin of ophthalmic artery (OA). Middle meningeal artery originates from OA via its lacrimal branch. *(©2012, Philippe Gailloud, MD.)*

5. The posterior auricular artery ascends posteriorly between the auricular cartilage and the mastoid process. It may arise as a common trunk with the occipital artery. It gives rise to several muscular branches for surrounding muscles (digastric, stylohyoid, and sternocleidomastoid muscles), the parotid gland, and the auricle. It also provides a small stylomastoid branch that enters through the stylomastoid foramen into the facial canal and ends in the tympanic cavity.

6. The occipital artery courses over the mastoid process toward the suboccipital region and divides into terminal branches at the level of the external occipital protuberance. It provides a sternocleidomastoid branch, an auricular artery (with a meningeal branch entering the cranium through the mastoid foramen), and a descending branch to the suboccipital region. The latter branch is connected to the vertebral and deep cervical arteries and constitutes the suboccipital carrefour or "knot of Bosniak," an important source of collateral supply in cases of steno-occlusive disease involving the VA or ICA.[9] At the same time, this anastomotic network represents a significant pitfall during embolization procedures involving the occipital artery (dangerous anastomosis), and one has to be particularly vigilant for transient opacification (sometimes visible on one frame only) of a portion of the VA during selective occipital angiography. The terminal branches of the occipital artery supply the scalp of the occipital region.

7. The maxillary artery originates behind the neck of the mandible and courses through the pterygomaxillary fissure into the pterygopalatine fossa. The maxillary artery has numerous branches:
   • The deep auricular artery, which often arises with the anterior tympanic artery, courses through the parotid gland and pierces the cartilaginous or bony wall of the external acoustic meatus. It supplies the outer surface of the tympanic membrane and the temporomandibular joint.
   • The anterior tympanic artery enters the tympanic cavity through the petrotympanic fissure and supplies the tympanic membrane.
   • The middle meningeal artery is the largest branch of the maxillary artery. It takes a short vertical extracranial course before it enters the middle cranial fossa through the foramen spinosum. It then takes a characteristic horizontal course anteriorly and laterally toward the pterion. A posterior branch arises in the middle cranial fossa and courses along the inner surface of the temporal and parietal bones. An anterior branch reaches the pterion, where it divides into lateral and medial branches. The lateral branch courses along the inner surface of the frontal bone toward the vertex. The medial branch courses under the lesser sphenoid wing and anastomoses with a recurrent branch of the lacrimal artery (branch of the OA), usually through the meningolacrimal foramen. In some cases, a branch of the middle meningeal artery or the entire artery may arise from the OA (Fig. 87-3). Conversely, the OA may originate partially or completely from the middle meningeal artery and enter the orbit through the superior orbital fissure (see later discussion). The clinical importance of the latter variant lies in the potential risk for blindness during endovascular procedures within the ECA territory.

- The accessory meningeal artery may arise from the middle meningeal artery or from the maxillary artery directly. Despite its name, its main supply is to the pterygoid and tensor veli palatini muscles, with a meningeal contribution representing only about 10% of its territory.[10] The meningeal branch, which is inconstant, enters the middle cranial fossa through the foramen ovale and supplies the dura adjacent to the sella turcica and trigeminal ganglion.
- The inferior alveolar artery enters the mandibular foramen and courses with the inferior alveolar nerve through the mandibular canal. One of its terminal branches, the mental branch, crosses the mental canal and anastomoses with the submental and inferior labial arteries (branches of the facial artery).
- The anterior and posterior deep temporal arteries, the pterygoid branches, and the masseteric and buccal arteries supply the muscles of mastication and the buccinator muscle.
- The posterior superior alveolar artery originates (like all the following branches) from the pterygopalatine segment of the maxillary artery, either directly or from a common trunk with the infraorbital artery. It supplies the mucosa of the maxillary sinus and the teeth.
- The infraorbital artery enters the orbit through the inferior orbital fissure, runs forward along the roof of the maxillary sinus within the infraorbital canal (along with the infraorbital nerve), and exits the skull through the infraorbital foramen. It supplies the mucosa of the maxillary sinus, the cheek, lower eyelid, upper lip, lacrimal sac, upper incisors and canine teeth, and the side of the nose. It anastomoses with the facial artery and posterior superior alveolar artery.
- The descending palatine artery courses down the pterygopalatine canal and gives off a large anterior branch, the greater palatine artery, that crosses the greater palatine foramen, runs forward along the alveolar border of the hard palate, crosses through the incisive canal, and then anastomoses with the sphenopalatine artery, thus supplying the mucosa of the palate, the palatine glands, and the gums. Lesser palatine branches from the descending palatine artery descend into the lesser palatine canals and supply the soft palate and palatine tonsils.
- The sphenopalatine artery supplies the nasal mucosa after passing through the sphenopalatine foramen. The sphenopalatine artery is the targeted vessel in superselective embolization for epistaxis.[11] In patients with inflammation of the nasal cavity (e.g., those with a common cold), a prominent mucosal blush with early venous drainage toward the superior ophthalmic vein and cavernous sinus may be observed and represents a diagnostic pitfall.
- The artery of the pterygoid canal, or the vidian artery, extends backward along the pterygoid canal with the vidian nerve into the cartilage of the foramen lacerum. It supplies the upper part of the pharynx and auditory tube and the tympanic cavity through a small tympanic branch.
- The pharyngeal artery leaves the pterygopalatine fossa through the pharyngeal canal and supplies the upper part of the nasopharynx and auditory tube.

- The artery of the foramen rotundum anastomoses with branches of the inferior lateral trunk through the foramen rotundum.
8. The superficial temporal artery arises within the parotid gland, crosses the zygomatic process, where its pulsations may be felt anterior to the auricle, and then divides into terminal anterior (frontal) and posterior (parietal) branches supplying the muscles, integument, and pericranium of these regions. The transverse artery of the face arises from the superficial temporal artery in the parotid gland and crosses forward between the zygomatic arch and parotid duct to the soft tissues of the cheek.

Internal Carotid Artery

The ICA arises from the carotid bifurcation, most frequently around the C3-C5 vertebral level. The ICA is divided into cervical, petrous, cavernous, and supraclinoid (or cisternal) segments. The course of its proximal cervical segment is closely related to that of the internal jugular vein (IJV) and vagus nerve; it follows a more or less straight trajectory from its origin to the outer opening of the carotid canal. The sharp transition between the mobile distal portion of the cervical ICA and its fixed petrous segment at the skull base represents a zone at risk for traumatic injuries such as arterial dissection[12] (Fig. 87-4). Marked but

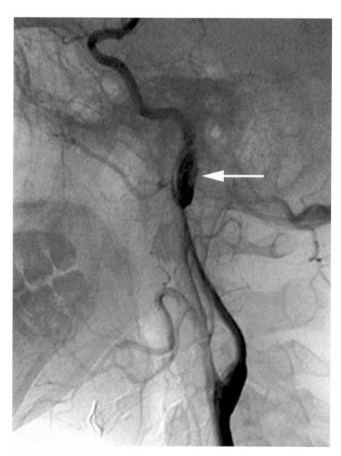

FIGURE 87-4. Digital subtraction angiogram, common carotid artery injection, unsubtracted lateral view showing arterial dissection with pseudoaneurysm formation at junction between mobile cervical and fixed petrous segments of internal carotid artery *(arrow)*. *(©2012, Philippe Gailloud, MD.)*

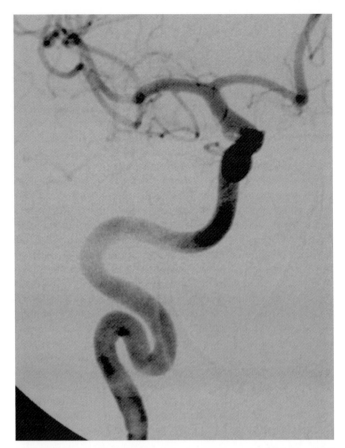

FIGURE 87-5. Digital subtraction angiogram, internal carotid artery (ICA) injection, oblique view showing smooth congenital sinuosity of ICA. (©2012, *Philippe Gailloud, MD.*)

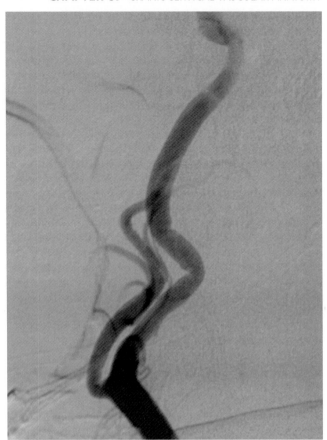

FIGURE 87-6. Digital subtraction angiogram, common carotid artery injection, lateral view showing an acquired dolichoectatic internal carotid artery with a "lead-pipe" appearance and kinking. (©2012, *Philippe Gailloud, MD.*)

smooth sinuosity of the cervical ICA, which may even lead to a 180-degree turn, can be seen in individuals of any age, including young children, and constitutes an anatomic variant. This variant, classically termed *coiling*, more frequently involves the distal portion of the cervical ICA[13] (Fig. 87-5). Coiling does not generally produce significant lumen narrowing but seems to represent a risk factor for arterial dissection.[14] In contrast, the irregular tortuosity that predominates in the proximal portion of the cervical ICA develops with advancing age (generally after 50 years), arteriosclerosis, and high blood pressure. It is often termed *kinking*, especially when associated with arterial hypertension, in which case it acquires a classic "lead-pipe" appearance (Fig. 87-6). The cervical portion of the ICA does not normally give off angiographically detectable branches. Its average caliber is about 6 mm, and in the absence of unusual secondary branches, it remains constant throughout its course.[15] Unusual branches of the cervical ICA include the ascending pharyngeal artery (8%) and less frequently the occipital artery (<0.1%). The so-called aberrant course of the ICA in which it crosses the middle ear cavity is in fact a collateral pathway established between the ICA and ECA branches in the case of cervical ICA agenesis.[16] The branches involved are the inferior tympanic branch of the ascending pharyngeal artery and the caroticotympanic branch of the ICA. An aberrant ICA is a potential hazard during middle ear surgery. Constitutional ICA hypoplasia or agenesis may

be differentiated from acquired lesions (e.g., atheromatous occlusion, dissection, and even congenital thrombosis) by looking at the caliber of the carotid canal on a CT scan. An absent or narrowed carotid canal suggests the constitutional nature of the ICA agenesis or hypoplasia. Acquired or congenital absence of an ICA is associated with a higher incidence of cerebral aneurysms, probably because of increased collateral flow through vessels such as the anterior communicating artery (AComA).[17]

Intracranial Segments of Internal Carotid Artery

The petrous segment of the ICA begins as the vessel enters the carotid canal. The petrous segment is divided into a 1-cm-long vertical portion followed by a horizontal portion that passes forward and medially, crosses over the foramen lacerum, and continues as the cavernous segment beyond the petrous apex. Normal branches of the petrous segment of the ICA include small periosteal rami, the caroticotympanic artery, and the vidian artery. The caroticotympanic artery arises from the lateral aspect of the vertical portion and anastomoses within the tympanic cavity with the anterior tympanic branch of the maxillary artery and the stylomastoid artery. The vidian artery (artery of the pterygoid canal) originates from the anterior aspect of the horizontal portion and courses through the pterygoid canal into the pterygopalatine fossa, where it anastomoses with the maxillary artery. The vidian artery can derive its main supply from either the maxillary artery or ICA.

The cavernous segment of the ICA extends from the petrous apex to the anterior clinoid process, where the ICA crosses the dura mater and forms the roof of the cavernous sinus (dural ring). The cavernous segment of the ICA is intracranial but extradural, located within the laterosellar compartment, and surrounded by the cavernous venous plexus, which continues posteriorly as the carotid artery venous plexus (venous plexus of Rektorzik). The sixth cranial nerve (abducens nerve) abuts the lateral aspect of the cavernous ICA. The cavernous segment corresponds to the proximal portion of the carotid siphon (segments C5-C3).

The cavernous segment provides numerous branches usually described as "trunks," although they often arise separate from the ICA. The meningohypophyseal trunk originates from the superior and posterior aspect of the ICA at the junction between the C5 and C4 cavernous segments (ascending and horizontal segments) (Fig. 87-7). Its branches include (1) the inferior hypophyseal artery, which is responsible for the angiographic blush of the posterior lobe (neurohypophysis) (Fig. 87-8); (2) the medial clival artery, also known as the *dorsal meningeal branch of the ICA*, which anastomoses with clival branches of the ascending pharyngeal artery; (3) the marginal tentorial artery (called the *artery of Bernasconi and Cassinari* when it

vascularizes a tentorial meningioma), which courses along the free margin of the tentorium cerebelli; and (4) the basal tentorial artery, which runs laterally along the petrous edge.

The inferolateral trunk (or inferior cavernous artery of Parkinson) comes off the lateral and inferior aspect of the ICA (see Fig. 87-8). Its branches include (1) the artery of the foramen rotundum (anastomosis with the anterior deep temporal artery), (2) the artery of the foramen ovale (anastomosis with the accessory middle meningeal artery), (3) the artery of the foramen lacerum (anastomosis with the carotid branch of the ascending pharyngeal artery), (4) the lateral clival artery, and (5) anastomotic branches to the OA (deep recurrent OA) and middle meningeal artery.

The inferior capsular and anterior capsular arteries of McConnell arise from the C5 and C4 segments of the cavernous ICA, respectively.[18] The capsular arteries do not contribute significantly to vascularization of the gland itself but send branches to the floor of the sella turcica. They are not usually angiographically detectable.

The supraclinoid or cisternal portion of the ICA (C2 and C1 segments) courses cranially until it bifurcates into the ACA and MCA within the carotid cistern. Immediately after crossing the dural ring, the ICA provides several superior hypophyseal arteries that vascularize the posterior end of the optic nerves, optic chiasm, pituitary stalk, and anterior lobe of the hypophysis.[18] Three important arteries branch off the supraclinoid ICA: the OA, the PComA, and

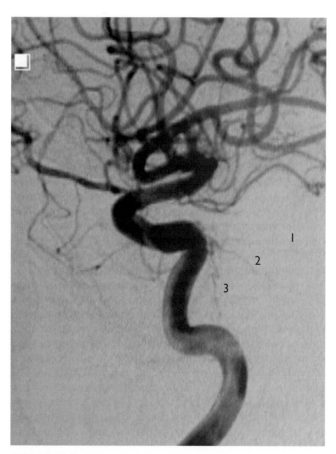

FIGURE 87-7. Digital subtraction angiogram, internal carotid artery injection, lateral view. Main branches of meningohypophyseal trunk are *(1)* marginal tentorial artery, *(2)* basal tentorial artery, and *(3)* dorsal clival artery. (©2012, Philippe Gailloud, MD.)

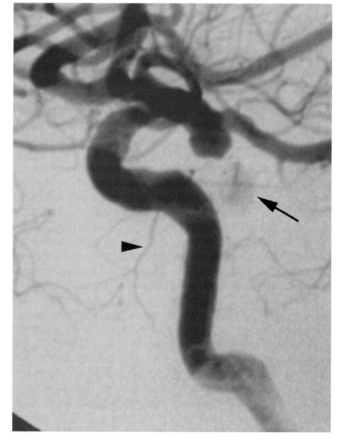

FIGURE 87-8. Digital subtraction angiogram, internal carotid artery injection, lateral view. Arrow points at blush of posterior hypophysis. Inferolateral trunk shows typical "inverse Y" appearance *(arrowhead)*. (©2012, Philippe Gailloud, MD.)

the AChoA. The posterior communicating artery (PComA) is discussed in the CW section.

The OA is divided into intracranial, intracanalicular (within the optic canal), and intraorbital segments. Its origin is located on the intradural portion of the ICA in 89% of cases, but it may also be extradural on the cavernous portion or within the dural wall of the cavernous sinus itself.[13] The OA presents numerous anastomoses with branches of the facial, maxillary, and superficial temporal arteries. A particularly interesting connection is established between the recurrent meningeal branch of the lacrimal artery and the orbital branch of the middle meningeal artery. This anastomosis corresponds to a remnant of the primitive orbital artery and allows an explanation for two clinically significant anatomic OA variants: the OA providing the middle meningeal artery and a complete or partial middle meningeal origin of the OA (Fig. 87-9). Exceptional variants of the OA include origin from the ACA (persistent ventral OA)[19,20] and from the BA.[21] The OA has numerous branches, as summarized in Table 87-2.

The AChoA is a small (0.5-1.5 mm) but functionally important artery that originates from the posterior surface of the ICA in the vast majority of cases, 2 to 4 mm distal to the origin of the PComA (Fig. 87-10). The AChoA usually arises as a single trunk but may be duplicated or triplicated. It courses through the carotid, crural, and ambient cisterns (cisternal segment), enters the choroidal fissure, and terminates within the choroidal plexus of the temporal horn (plexal segment), which it supplies in conjunction with the posterior lateral choroidal artery. There is a reciprocal relationship between the territories vascularized by the AChoA, PComA, PCA, and MCA. The AChoA supplies the uncus, anterior hippocampal and dentate gyri, posterior medial amygdala, and tail of the caudate nucleus through its uncal

TABLE 87-2. Branches of Ophthalmic Artery

Group	Branches
Ocular	Central retinal artery Ciliary arteries Collateral branches for optic nerve (cranial nerve II)
Orbital	Lacrimal artery Muscular arteries Arteries for periosteum and areolar tissue
Extraorbital	Posterior/anterior ethmoidal arteries Supraorbital/supratrochlear arteries Medial palpebral, dorsal nasal arteries

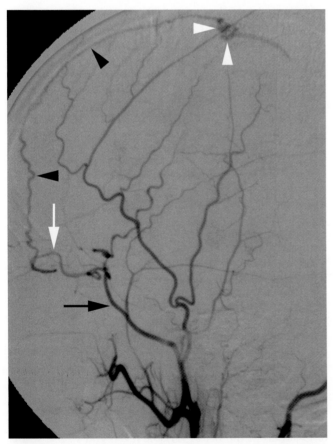

FIGURE 87-9. Digital subtraction angiogram, external carotid artery injection, lateral view. Middle meningeal artery *(black arrow)* provides ophthalmic artery (OA) *(white arrow)* through its orbital branch. A dural arteriovenous fistula of superior sagittal sinus *(white arrowheads)* is fed by anterior meningeal artery *(black arrowheads)*, a branch of OA. If this anatomic configuration is not recognized, embolization may result in major ocular complications. *(©2012, Philippe Gailloud, MD.)*

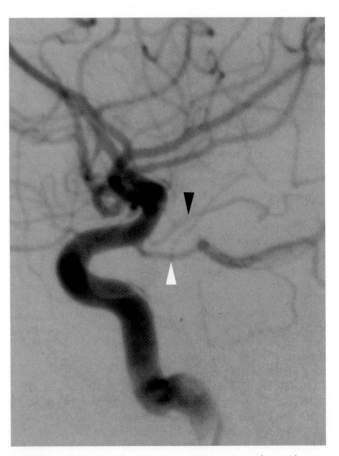

FIGURE 87-10. Digital subtraction angiogram, internal carotid artery injection, lateral view showing origin of posterior communicating artery *(white arrowhead)* and anterior choroidal artery *(black arrowhead)*. *(©2012, Philippe Gailloud, MD.)*

branch. Branches from the cisternal segment of the AChoA supply the inferior aspect of the optic chiasm and posterior two thirds of the optic tract, part of the globus pallidus, the cerebral peduncles, genu of the internal capsule, substantia nigra, red nucleus, and the ventral anterior and ventral lateral thalamus. The plexal segment supplies the choroid plexus of the temporal horn, part of the lateral geniculate body, the posterior limb and retrolenticular portion of the internal capsule, and the optic radiations.

Vertebrobasilar System

The VA generally originates from the posterior superior aspect of the first segment of the SubcA as the first branch of the SubcA. The VAs are frequently asymmetric, the left VA being dominant in 60% of cases and the right one in 20%. Possible variations in the origin of the VA include direct origin from the aortic arch (most frequently on the left side), from a common trunk with other subclavian branches (e.g., thyrocervical trunk), or from the CCA. The latter case occurs most frequently on the right and is usually associated with an ipsilateral aberrant SubcA (arteria lusoria). Dual origin of the VA can occur, generally from the SubcA and aortic arch on the left side or from the SubcA and innominate artery on the right side (Fig. 87-11). These dual origins may mimic VA dissection.[22]

The VA is divided into four segments (V1-V4). The V1 segment extends from the VA origin to the orifice of the transverse foramen of the sixth cervical vertebra. The V2 segment courses cranially through the transverse foramina (in effect, a connective and osseous canal) until it reaches the transverse foramen of the axis (C2). The VA then continues as the V3 segment until it crosses the dura mater in the atlanto-occipital space immediately below the foramen magnum. The V4 segment starts at the point of dural passage (which can usually be identified angiographically as a small reduction in VA caliber), courses through the foramen magnum, and joins the contralateral VA over the anterior aspect of the medulla oblongata to form the BA. The V4 segment is therefore strictly intradural. The V3-V4 junction (dural perforation) and the proximal V4 segment (along the edge of the foramen magnum) represent zones at risk for traumatic injury such as dissection. The V4 segments often have different diameters, thereby resulting in asymmetric contribution to BA flow. The VA sometimes fails to join the contralateral VA and terminates as a posterior inferior cerebellar artery (PICA).

Branches of the VA include (1) muscular branches (see Alternative Collateral Circulation); (2) anterior and posterior meningeal branches; (3) anterior and posterior radiculomeningeal arteries, including a prominent anterior spinal contributor at the midcervical level, usually around C4-C5 (artery of the cervical enlargement); (4) an anterior spinal root, which arises from the V4 segment and fuses with the contralateral root to form the cranial end of the anterior spinal axis; (5) nonfused posterior lateral spinal arteries (from the V4 segment or PICA); and (6) the PICA. Through its vermian and hemispheric branches, the PICA supplies the medulla, inferior portion of the fourth ventricle, tonsils, inferior vermis, and inferior aspect of the ipsilateral cerebellar hemisphere.

The BA results from fusion of the two VAs at the level of the pontomedullary sulcus (Fig. 87-12). It courses

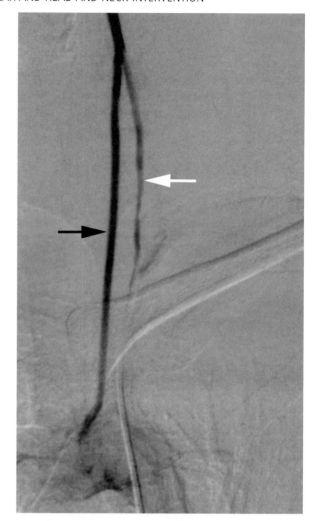

FIGURE 87-11. Digital subtraction angiogram, left vertebral artery (VA) injection, anteroposterior view. Selective injection of left VA *(white arrow)* shows a slightly irregular artery that connects with a second VA root *(black arrow)* to form definitive VA. Second root, which arises directly from aortic arch, is opacified retrogradely. *(©2012, Philippe Gailloud, MD.)*

cranially along a median shallow groove on the anterior surface of the pons within the prepontine cistern, and ends within the interpeduncular cistern above the oculomotor nerves (cranial nerve III) as it bifurcates into paired superior cerebellar or posterior cerebral arteries (or both). Incomplete fusion of the left and right VAs may result in fenestration or duplication of the BA. Fenestrations behave like an arterial bifurcation and are associated with BA aneurysms. With age, marked size asymmetry of the VA, and atheromatous disease, the BA becomes more tortuous and may adopt a pronounced S-shaped course.

Angiographically visible branches of the BA include (1) the anterior inferior cerebellar artery (AICA), which can originate from the BA at variable levels and whose size is inversely proportional to the size of the PICA; (2) the superior cerebellar artery (SCA), which arises from the BA a few millimeters proximal to the origin of the PCA (but can also branch off the PCA itself) and supplies portions of the midbrain, superior aspect of the cerebellar hemisphere, and vermis; and (3) the internal auditory artery, which is usually a branch of the AICA but can also originate directly from

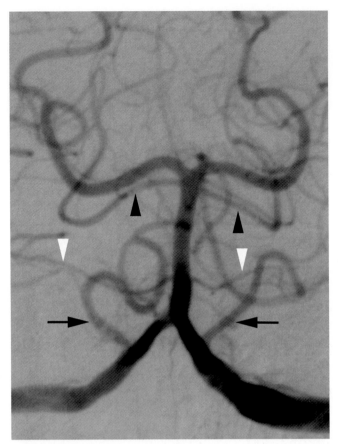

FIGURE 87-12. Digital subtraction angiogram, left vertebral artery (VA) injection, anteroposterior view. Basilar artery is formed by junction of the two VAs. It ends in proximal portion of both proximal cerebral arteries (PCAs) (P1 segment). Posterior inferior cerebellar artery *(black arrows)*, anterior inferior cerebellar artery *(white arrowheads)*, and superior cerebellar artery (SCA) *(black arrowheads)* are documented. Note duplication of left SCA, which in fact corresponds to separate origins of its vermian and hemispheric branches. *(©2012, Philippe Gailloud, MD.)*

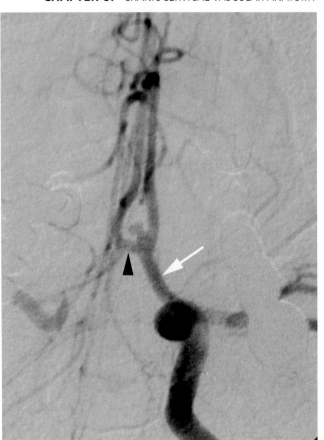

FIGURE 87-13. Digital subtraction angiogram, left internal carotid artery injection, submentovertical view. Left A1 segment *(arrow)* is dominant, with a relatively large anterior communicating artery (AComA) *(arrowhead)*. Small saccular aneurysm is seen at left A1-A2-AComA junction. *(©2012, Philippe Gailloud, MD.)*

the BA. Basilar perforating arteries may sometimes be seen during angiography. Short and long basilar perforating arteries are divided into caudal, middle, and rostral groups. Contrary to a commonly held view, anastomoses among these perforating arteries exist in up to 66.6% of individuals.[23] In rare cases the BA may provide a middle meningeal branch or even the OA.[21] Persistent embryonic connections between the vertebrobasilar circulation and the ICA or ECA are discussed later (see Alternative Collateral Circulation).

Circle of Willis

The CW is an anastomotic network that interconnects the left and right anterior carotid axes to the vertebrobasilar circulation. The CW is located within the subarachnoid cisterns at the base of the brain. The "ideal" CW consists of a complete anastomotic ring with a well-developed AComA, symmetric and well-developed PComAs, the terminal segments of both ICAs, and the proximal segments of both the ACA and PCA (A1 and P1 segments).

The CW represents the most important anastomotic system of the brain circulation, and its efficacy depends on its "completeness" (i.e., essentially the degree of development of the AComA and PComA). The CW plays a determinant role in providing collateral supply to the brain. Anatomic variations of the CW, such as aplasia, hypoplasia, or duplication of its constituents, may therefore have an impact on the potential for collateral flow in pathologic conditions. For instance, a small (<1 mm) or absent PComA has been demonstrated to be a risk factor for ipsilateral ischemic cerebral infarction in patients with ICA occlusion.[24] The angiographic anatomy of the ICA, ACA, and PCA is discussed elsewhere; this section concentrates on the AComA, PComA, and perforators of the CW.

Anterior Communicating Artery

The AComA is 1 to 2 mm long and connects the two ACAs. Frequent variations of the AComA include absence, hypoplasia, duplication, or triplication (embryonic disposition). The presence of a wide AComA is generally associated with marked proximal asymmetry of the ACA (A1 segments) and represents a risk factor for development of berry aneurysms at the junction between the AComA and the A1 and A2 segments (classically labeled *AComA aneurysms*) (Fig. 87-13). In some rare instances, the AComA may be replaced by a broad "en passant" attachment of the two ACAs. The AComA provides perforating arteries (see later discussion).

Posterior Communicating Artery

The PComA arises from the posterior aspect of the supra-clinoid portion of the ICA, proximal to the origin of the AChoA. The PComA connects the anterior and posterior circulation. It can in fact be understood as the most cranial of the carotid-basilar anastomoses.[25] When the proximal PCA (P1 segment) is hypoplastic or absent, the PComA serves as the only or dominant source of blood supply to the PCA territory. This variant, encountered in about 10% of cases unilaterally and 7% bilaterally, is often wrongly termed a "fetal" PCA. This term should be reserved for the situation in which the AChoA, which vascularizes the PCA territory at the fetal stage, keeps that role in the adult con-figuration.[17] The PComA often shows ampullar dilation at its origin from the ICA, which is referred to as an *infun-dibulum*. This must be distinguished from distal ICA sac-cular aneurysms typically located at or near the PComA origin (PComA aneurysms). Distinguishing features include a size of 3 mm or less and a smooth ampullar shape cen-tered by the PComA itself.

Branches of Circle of Willis

Two types of branches arise from the CW: (1) arteries aimed at structures adjacent to the CW (e.g., pituitary stalk; optic nerves, chiasm, and tracts; and some cranial nerves [e.g., oculomotor nerve]) and (2) perforating arteries sup-plying the basal ganglia, thalamus, and cerebral peduncles. These small arteries are terminal branches that may be affected by degenerative changes such as arteriosclerosis/arteriolosclerosis. Perforators of the CW are divided into medial, lateral, and posterior groups. The medial group arises from the posterior superior aspect of the A1 segment and from the PComA. The A1 segment gives off a smaller inferior group that supplies the superior aspect of the optic nerve and chiasm, as well as a superior group of medial striate arteries that penetrate the anterior perforated sub-stance. The recurrent artery of Heubner is one of the larger medial striate arteries; it arises from the A1 segment close to the PComA. The recurrent artery of Heubner can some-times remain a large branch participating in vascularization of cortical tissue within the territory of the MCA. The medial striate arteries supply the anterior hypothalamus, septum pellucidum, medial portion of the anterior commis-sure, pillars of the fornix, and anterior inferior part of the striatum. The artery of Heubner also supplies part of the head of the caudate nucleus, the putamen, the anterior segment of the internal capsule, and inconstantly, the orbital aspect of the frontal lobe. Except for the recurrent artery of Heubner, the medial group of perforators is usually too small to be clearly visualized during digital subtraction angiography (DSA). When visible, these branches are best seen in the anteroposterior projection.

Several small arteries may arise from the PComA, includ-ing branches that supply the infundibulum, optic chiasm, and the preoptic area of the hypothalamus.

Although they are not direct branches of the CW, the perforators arising from the M1 segment of the MCA may be included in this section by analogy with the territory they supply. The M1 segment provides 2 to 15 lateral striate arteries that arise from its inferior medial aspect as a single trunk (40%) or two large proximal trunks (30%) or directly from the M1 segment as individual small arteries (30%). The

lateral striate arteries have a free cisternal course during which they frequently divide into smaller branches before entering the lateral portion of the anterior perforated sub-stance. On a lateral projection, the lateral striate arteries are seen to fan out over the internal capsule. These branches supply the substantia innominata, the lateral portion of the anterior commissure, most of the putamen and lateral segment of the globus pallidus, the superior half of the internal capsule and adjacent corona radiata, and the head of the caudate nucleus. The areas of supply of the medial and lateral striate artery and the AChoA abut each other and are reciprocal in size.

The posterior perforators arise from the PComA and the P1 segment of the PCA. The PComA gives off small thalamic perforators (the anterior thalamo-perforating arteries) that supply the posterior chiasm, optic tract, and posterior hypothalamus, as well as part of the cerebral peduncles, caudate nucleus, oculomotor nerve, and ante-rior and ventroanterior nuclei of the thalamus.

The posterior thalamo-perforating arteries usually arise from the central portion of the P1 segment, either as sepa-rate branches or from a common stem, even when the P1 segment is hypoplastic. The posterior thalamo-perforating arteries enter the posterior perforated substance and supply parts of the thalamus, the posterior limb of the internal capsule, the hypothalamus and subthalamus, the substantia nigra, the red nucleus, and portions of the deep rostral mesencephalon.

Alternative Collateral Circulation

Extensive anastomotic connections exist between the ECA, ICA, and VA. These connections ("dangerous anastomo-ses") have significant implications with regard to thera-peutic embolization involving ECA branches or during angioplasty and stenting procedures performed with distal ICA balloon protection techniques. Some of these collateral pathways become prominent under pathologic conditions, whereas others are visible as normal anatomic variants. The anastomotic pathways linking (1) the ICA and vertebrobasi-lar system, (2) the ECA and ICA, and (3) the ECA/SubcA and VA are considered in the following paragraphs.

Anastomoses between the ICA and vertebrobasilar system represent patent remnants of presegmental dorsal arteries (persistent carotid-basilar and carotid-vertebral anastomoses) that fail to regress as the PComA develops. They include the persistent trigeminal artery (PTA) (Fig. 87-14) and the persistent hypoglossal artery. The existence of a persistent otic artery remains debated. The PTA is the most frequently encountered (0.1%).[27] It connects the prox-imal cavernous ICA with the BA or the cerebellar arteries (in which case it is called a *PTA variant* [PTAV]). A persis-tent proatlantal artery (of Padget) may also be observed connecting the cervical segment of the ICA to the V4 segment of the VA through the foramen magnum. A so-called type II proatlantal artery linking the ECA to the VA is often described; this variant in our opinion is a classic suboccipital collateral pathway (node of Bosniak [see later discussion]) rather than a persistent primitive vessel.

Anastomoses connecting the ECA to the ICA have a significant role in the case of ICA flow impairment (e.g., patients with carotid bifurcation disease). Potential

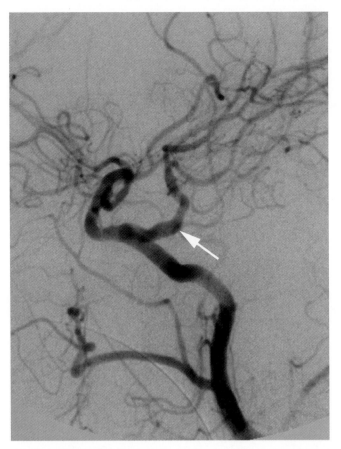

FIGURE 87-14. Digital subtraction angiogram, common carotid artery injection, lateral view. Prominent branch *(arrow)* from cavernous segment of internal carotid artery feeds upper half of basilar artery. This branch corresponds to a persistent embryonic vessel, a persistent trigeminal artery. *(©2012, Philippe Gailloud, MD.)*

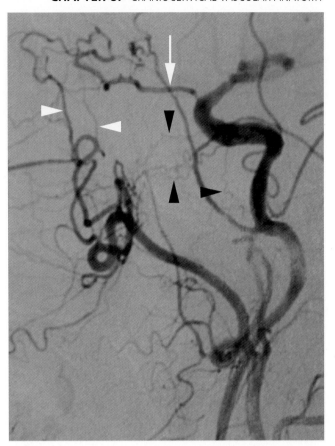

FIGURE 87-15. Digital subtraction angiogram, common carotid artery injection, lateral view. There is severe stenosis of internal carotid artery (ICA) origin at carotid bifurcation. As a consequence, collateral pathways between external carotid artery and distal ICA have become prominent, including connections to ophthalmic artery *(arrow)* through ethmoidal arteries *(white arrowheads)* and to cavernous ICA via arteries of inferolateral trunk *(black arrowheads)*. *(©2012, Philippe Gailloud, MD.)*

collateral routes to the distal ICA include numerous cavernous branches such as the arteries of the foramen rotundum or foramen ovale (connections with the maxillary artery) (Fig. 87-15). Other potential collateral pathways involve the caroticotympanic and petrous arteries (see earlier section Intracranial Segments of Internal Carotid Artery).

The OA is a classic, almost constant source of collateral supply for the distal ICA by way of direct or indirect connections with the facial artery and the maxillary artery (ethmoidal branches) (see Fig. 87-15). When this collateral pathway is in use, flow within the OA is reversed, a finding that can also be documented by sonography. Again, abnormal origin of part or all of the OA from the middle meningeal artery represents an increased risk for complications during procedures within the ECA territory (see Intracranial Segments of Internal Carotid Artery and Fig. 87-9). Visualization of a choroidal blush during preprocedural assessment of the ECA territory is a crucial finding in this regard.

A rich network of collateral channels exists between the VA, the ECA, and several subclavian branches and form the so-called node of Bosniak in the suboccipital region (Fig. 87-16). These anastomoses principally involve muscular branches of the cervical VA, the occipital artery, and branches of the deep cervical and ascending cervical arteries.

Cerebral Arteries

Anterior Cerebral Artery

The ACA is divided by its connection with the AComA into a proximal portion (or precommunicating ACA, A1 segment) and a distal portion (or postcommunicating ACA, A2 to A5 segments). The A1 segment is subject to frequent variation and may be absent, hypoplastic, short, fenestrated, or multiple. Hypoplasia of an A1 segment is a hemodynamic risk factor for the development of AComA aneurysms. Branches from the A1 segment were discussed in the section on CW perforators.

The A2 segments are most commonly symmetric and follow an ascending course in front of the lamina terminalis toward the interhemispheric fissure. The ACA then curves backward around the genu of the corpus callosum (A3 segment) and continues dorsally within the pericallosal cistern (A4 and A5 segments). Along its course, the ACA gives off branches to the medial frontal, parietal, and occipital lobes and to the corpus callosum itself. In about 2% of cases, the A2 segment may be unpaired, with a single median trunk continuing beyond the AComA. An ACA with unpaired A2 segments is often called an *azygos ACA*, although this term should in our opinion be reserved for

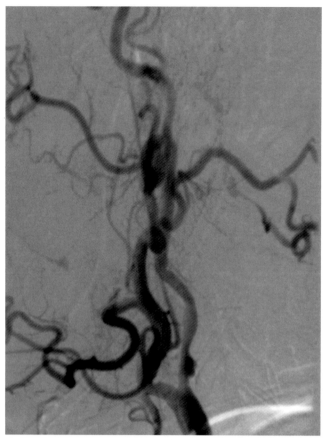

FIGURE 87-16. Digital subtraction angiogram, right common carotid artery injection, lateral view. In this patient with an occluded right vertebral artery (VA), collateral flow to distal right VA was established through muscular branches of occipital artery (knot of Bosniak). (©2012, Philippe Gailloud, MD.)

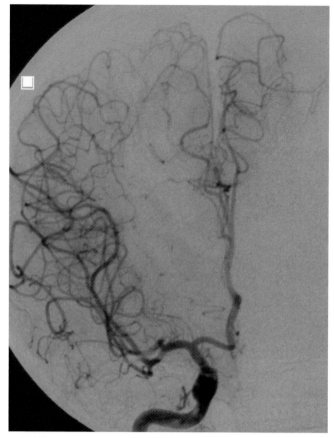

FIGURE 87-17. Digital subtraction angiogram, right internal carotid artery injection, anteroposterior view. A prominent A2 segment provides both pericallosal arteries (bihemispheric anterior cerebral artery), whereas a smaller left A2 segment (not seen) opacifies both callosomarginal arteries. (©2012, Philippe Gailloud, MD.)

the true single ACA seen in children with holoprosencephaly.[26] A pseudo-azygos ACA can also be seen in cases where a prominent A2 segment provides bilateral branches (bihemispheric ACA) (Fig. 87-17). Conversely, an additional branch may originate from the AComA and parallel the A2 segments. It is referred to as the *third A2 segment* or *median ACA* and was encountered in about 9% of cases by Yasargil.[28] The main branches of the ACA are summarized in Table 87-3.

Middle Cerebral Artery

The MCA arises as the largest branch from the ICA bifurcation, and its origin is related to the anterior perforated substance posteriorly, the olfactory stria anteriorly, the optic chiasm medially, and the medial end of the lateral (sylvian) fissure laterally. The proximal portion of the MCA (M1) extends into the lateral fissure and bifurcates into superior and inferior trunks (M2) at the limen insulae. Rarely, an accessory MCA arises either from the portion of the ICA between the AChoA and the ICA termination or directly from the PComA or ACA. The first type probably represents a separate origin of the superior and inferior divisions (Fig. 87-18), whereas the latter represents a prominent recurrent artery of Heubner[27] (Fig. 87-19). A fenestrated M1 segment is found in about 0.5% of patients.

TABLE 87-3. Branches of A2 Segment of Anterior Cerebral Artery

Branches	Distribution
Orbital artery (frontobasilar)	Origin: infracallosal segment or common trunk with frontopolar artery Course: forward on inferior surface of frontal lobe adjacent to anterior cranial fossa; supplies gyrus rectus, medial part of orbital gyri, and olfactory bulb and tract
Frontopolar artery	Origin: infracallosal segment or common trunk with frontopolar artery or with callosomarginal artery Course: anterior in medial surface of cerebral hemisphere; supplies anterior portion of medial and lateral surfaces of superior frontal gyrus
Callosomarginal artery	Origin: either a distinct artery or arising as branches from pericallosal artery Course: when well formed, it lies in sulcus above cingulate gyrus and is parallel to pericallosal artery. It gives ascending branches (anterior, middle, and posterior internal frontal arteries) and the paracentral artery, which may all originate directly from pericallosal artery

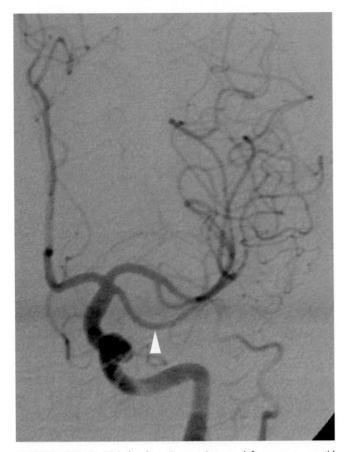

FIGURE 87-18. Digital subtraction angiogram, left common carotid artery injection, anteroposterior view showing an accessory left middle cerebral artery (MCA) *(arrowhead)*. This variant represents separate origins of inferior and superior divisions of MCA. *(©2012, Philippe Gailloud, MD.)*

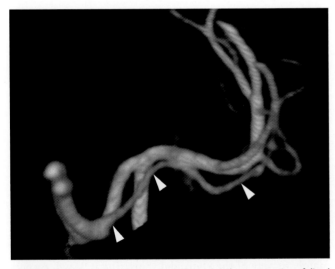

FIGURE 87-19. CT angiogram, three-dimensional reconstruction of distal left internal carotid artery showing accessory middle cerebral artery *(arrowheads)* arising from A1-A2 junction of left anterior cerebral artery. This variant represents a prominent artery of Heubner. *(©2012, Philippe Gailloud, MD.)*

Branches of the M1 segment may be divided into superior lateral and anterior medial groups.

The superior lateral group most frequently gives off a temporopolar artery and an anterior temporal artery and, in some cases, an uncal artery. Variations include the presence of a common temporal trunk providing the temporopolar and anterior temporal branches, which may be mistaken for the MCA bifurcation (false early bifurcation). The inferior medial group of branches from the M1 segment includes the lenticulostriate arteries discussed earlier (see Branches of Circle of Willis).

Impression of a pseudotrifurcation or even a quadrifurcation of the M1 segment may occur if the superior or inferior M2 trunks (or both) divide very proximally. The major trunks diverge at the M1 bifurcation but converge further along the lateral fissure, where they give off their cortical branches. The arterial branches of the superior and inferior trunks supply the regions of the inferior frontal cortex, the frontal opercular cortex, the parietal and central sulcus territories, the middle and posterior temporal cortex, the temporal occipital regions, and the angular and posterior parietal regions.

Posterior Cerebral Artery

The PCA arises as paired terminal branches of the BA as it bifurcates within the interpeduncular fossa (see Fig. 87-12). Variants of PCA origin were discussed earlier (see Posterior Communicating Artery). The proximal segment of the PCA (P1) extends from the BA bifurcation to its junction with the PComA at the anterior margin of the cerebral peduncle. The P1 segment and its branches (thalamo-perforating arteries) were discussed in previous sections (see Posterior Communicating Artery; Branches of Circle of Willis). The PCA is further divided into a P2 segment (ambient, post-communicating, or perimesencephalic) and a P3 segment (quadrigeminal).

The P2 segment courses around the cerebral peduncles within the ambient cistern and extends from the junction with the PComA to the origin of the inferior temporal arteries. The P3 segment courses around the mesencephalic tectum into the quadrigeminal cistern and extends from the origin of the inferior temporal arteries to the P3 terminal division into the parieto-occipital and calcarine arteries. The main branches of the P2 and P3 segments are summarized in Table 87-4. The terminal cortical branches supply the occipital poles, the medial and inferior portions of the occipital lobes, and the inferior portions of the temporal lobes.

CRANIOCERVICAL VEINS

The cerebral veins may be classified into superficial and deep venous systems. The superficial venous system comprises veins that drain the cortex and superficial white matter (1 cm of subcortical white matter). These vessels collect into the superficial pial cortical veins, subarachnoid or bridging veins, and finally the dural venous sinuses. The deep venous system is mainly involved in draining the deep white matter and the diencephalic structures through the tributaries of the internal cerebral vein (ICV) and the basal vein of Rosenthal (BVR), which are the major tributaries of the vein of Galen (VG). The parenchymal veins draining the deep white matter of the brain are called *medullary veins*;

TABLE 87-4. Branches of Posterior Cerebral Artery

Segment	Branches *(Supply)*
P1	Thalamo-perforating arteries *(anterior and part of posterior thalamus, posterior limb of internal capsule, hypothalamus and subthalamus, substantia nigra, red nucleus, portions of deep rostral mesencephalon)* Quadrigeminal artery *(cerebral peduncle, geniculate bodies, tegmentum)*
P2	Peduncular perforating arteries *(corticospinal and corticobulbar tracts, substantia nigra, red nucleus, tegmentum)* Medial posterior choroidal artery *(peduncle, tegmentum, geniculate bodies and colliculi, choroid plexus and roof of third ventricle, pineal gland, pulvinar, habenula, dorsal-medial thalamus)* Lateral posterior choroidal artery *(choroid plexus of lateral ventricle, glomus of choroid plexus, pulvinar, posterior commissure, body of fornix, dorsal-medial thalamus)* Thalamogeniculate perforators *(thalamus, geniculate body)* Inferior temporal arteries *(inferior-medial portions of temporal lobe)*
P3	Parieto-occipital artery Calcarine artery

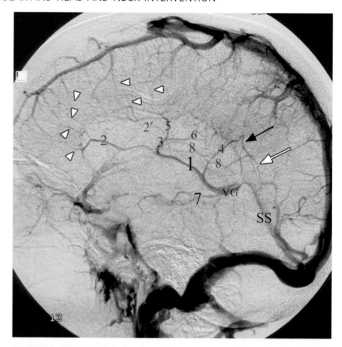

FIGURE 87-20. Digital subtraction angiogram, internal carotid artery injection, venous phase, lateral view. Anterior septal vein *(2)*, thalamostriate vein *(3)*, and superior choroidal vein *(8)* join at level of foramen of Monro ("venous angle") to form *(1)* internal cerebral vein (ICV). Thalamostriate vein is formed by *(5)* anterior caudate vein and *(6)* posterior terminal vein. A more posteriorly located septal vein *(2')* joins ICV behind venous angle. Note how this septal vein and thalamostriate vein cross each other, a useful angiographic sign to distinguish between two structures that course in different planes. Medial atrial vein *(4)* joins terminal portion of ICV and receives a vein from medial wall of atrium *(black arrow)* and a vein from roof of occipital horn *(white arrow)*. *SS*, Sagittal sinus; *VG*, vein of Galen. *(©2012, Philippe Gailloud, MD.)*

they converge into the subependymal veins located in the superior lateral aspect of the lateral ventricles.[29]

The bulk of encephalic venous drainage reaches the transverse and sigmoid sinuses, the largest dural venous sinuses of the posterior cranial fossa. From there, venous outflow into the neck will occur either through the IJV or through the vertebral venous system (VVS), depending on the position of the body.[30,31] In the supine position, the IJVs represent the main encephalic venous outflow pathway. Conversely, in the upright position, the IJVs appear collapsed, and drainage is preferentially redirected into the VVS.

Because of its high spatial and temporal resolution, DSA remains the most powerful imaging technique for appreciating the morphology of the intracranial vasculature and its circulation. Emerging technologies in multirow detector high-resolution computed tomography (CT) or the development of new sequences in magnetic resonance imaging (MRI), such as time-resolved three-dimensional imaging, are promising but do not yet offer the same spatial and temporal resolution as DSA and must not replace catheter angiography when seeking a precise morphologic and hemodynamic appreciation of intracranial vascular lesions.

Cerebral Veins

Deep Venous System

The major collecting veins of the deep venous system are the ICVs, BVR, VG, and straight sinus. Both the ICA and BA supply structures drained by the deep venous system. Structures drained by the deep venous system include the deep white matter of the cerebral hemispheres, diencephalon, corpus callosum, ependyma and choroid plexuses of the lateral and third ventricles, cortex of the internal and inferior aspect of the occipital lobes, mesiotemporal lobe,

tectum of the mesencephalon, pineal gland, and superior vermis and cerebellum. The subependymal veins are mainly involved in draining the medullary veins of the deep white matter. Thrombosis of the deep cerebral venous system may have catastrophic consequences if left untreated because of the lack of efficient collateral pathways.

Internal Cerebral Veins

The paired ICVs arise in the region of the foramen of Monro of the lateral ventricles from convergence of the anterior septal, superior choroidal, and thalamostriate veins (Fig. 87-20). From this point, which is named the "venous point," they course posteriorly within the roof of the third ventricle, cross over the pineal body, and open into the VG under the splenium of the corpus callosum. The ICVs have little capacity for collateralization, because their major outflow is the VG, although connections with the BVR may exist, mainly by way of the choroidal veins. The ICV will receive several lateral and medial subependymal tributaries along its course toward the VG, including the anterior and posterior septal veins, thalamostriate vein, direct lateral vein (inconstant), and medial atrial veins (see Fig. 87-20).

Basal Veins of Rosenthal

The BVR are also paired and display great variability, in keeping with the secondary longitudinal anastomosis of its

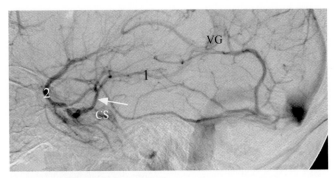

FIGURE 87-21. Digital subtraction angiogram, right internal carotid artery injection, venous phase, lateral and anteroposterior projections. A basal vein of Rosenthal *(1)*, complete type, drains anteriorly into superficial middle cerebral vein (SMCV) *(2)* by way of an uncal vein *(arrow)* and posteriorly into vein of Galen *(VG)*. Uncal vein often joins SMCV, but it may be seen to drain directly into cavernous sinus *(CS)* or into a laterocavernous sinus. *(©2012, Philippe Gailloud, MD.)*

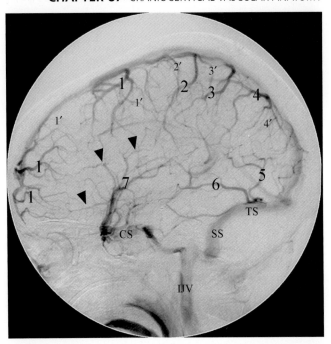

FIGURE 87-22. Digital subtraction angiogram, internal carotid artery injection, venous phase, lateral view showing superficial cerebral veins. *1 and 1'*, lateral and medial ascending cortical veins; *2 and 2'*, lateral and medial perirolandic veins; *3 and 3'*, lateral and medial parietal veins; *4*, a common trunk draining lateral veins from parietal and occipital lobes; *5*, a descending lateral occipital vein and a lateral temporal vein converge into a lateral tentorial sinus on their way to transverse sinus *(TS)*; *7*, a superficial middle cerebral vein (SMCV) that drains into cavernous sinus *(CS)*. Descending frontal cortical veins *(arrowheads)* converge in SMCV. Note absence of connections between perirolandic and lateral temporal veins with SMCV. *IJV,* Internal jugular vein; *SS,* sigmoid sinus. *(©2012, Philippe Gailloud, MD.)*

primitive constituents.[32] When the three segments (anterior or striate segment, middle or peduncular segment, and posterior or mesencephalic segment) that form the adult BVR are connected, the BVR is said to be of the "complete type" (Fig. 87-21). The BVR is formed under the anterior perforated substance, mainly from union of the deep middle cerebral vein (draining the insular veins) and the inferior striate veins (exiting the brain through the anterior perforated substance). The BVR then courses posteriorly around the cerebral peduncles in the crural and ambient cisterns and finally runs backward, upward, and medially through the quadrigeminal cistern into the VG. The deep middle cerebral vein drains several insular veins that occupy the different sulci of the insula.[33]

Unlike the ICV, the BVR offers collaterals with other supratentorial and infratentorial veins: (1) anteriorly, the first segment may connect with the cavernous sinus, the superficial middle cerebral vein, or any of its drainage pathways in the middle cranial fossa by way of an uncal vein; (2) with each other through the peduncular veins when these veins interconnect in the depth of the interpeduncular fossa; (3) infratentorially with the anterior and lateral pontomesencephalic veins by way of the peduncular vein; (4) infratentorially with the superior petrosal vein through the lateral mesencephalic vein; and (5) with the straight sinus or transverse sinus by way of an inconstant dural venous sinus coursing along the tentorium cerebelli.

Superficial Venous System

The superficial venous system comprises the cortical veins that drain the surface of the cerebrum. The pial cortical veins receive veins from the cortex and the underlying subcortical or superficial white matter and then follow a subarachnoid course toward the dural venous sinuses. A typical pattern of cortical veins is difficult to establish because of their highly variable disposition and connections. Cortical veins are named after the lobe they drain and may be further subdivided according to whether they drain the lateral surface (veins of the cerebral convexity), medial surface (interhemispheric veins), or basal surface (inferior veins in relation to the anterior and middle cranial fossae and the tentorium cerebelli) (Fig. 87-22). Most cerebral cortical

veins join the superior sagittal sinus (SSS), although the transverse sinus will receive tributaries from the temporal (lateral and basal surfaces), parietal (lateral surface), and occipital lobes (basal and lateral surfaces).

The brain surrounding the lateral or sylvian fissure is drained superficially by one or several fairly constant superficial middle cerebral veins (SMCVs) that usually drain into a dural venous sinus in the middle cranial fossa.[34]

The SMCV courses anteriorly over the surface of the lateral fissure, crosses over the pole of the temporal lobe, and joins a dural sinus of the middle cranial fossa under the lesser sphenoid wing. The most frequent termination of the SMCV is into a paracavernous sinus (Fig. 87-23), followed by a laterocavernous sinus and finally, following the "textbook" description, into the cavernous sinus.[35,36] Contrary to widespread opinion, the SMCV does not connect with the sphenoparietal sinus of Breschet under the lesser sphenoid wing. The sphenoparietal sinus of Breschet, more correctly referred to as the *venous sinus of the lesser sphenoid wing*, drains only the meningeal and diploic veins.[37]

Connections of functional importance between the veins of the lateral convexity of the cerebrum may exist and usually involve the SMCV on the surface of the transverse fissure (Fig. 87-24). A connection between the SMCV and the SSS by way of a perirolandic vein is commonly referred to as the *great* or *superior anastomotic vein of Trolard*, although Trolard's original description included the

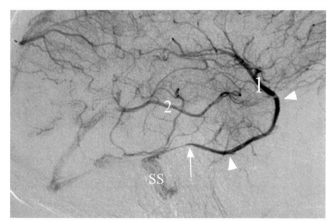

FIGURE 87-23. Digital subtraction angiogram, lateral view showing a paracavernous sinus. Superficial middle cerebral vein *(1)* joins paracavernous sinus *(arrowheads)* under lesser sphenoid wing and then courses over floor of middle cranial fossa before draining into transverse sigmoid sinus *(SS)* junction by way of a superior petrosal sinus *(arrow)*. *2,* Basal vein of Rosenthal. *(©2012, Philippe Gailloud, MD.)*

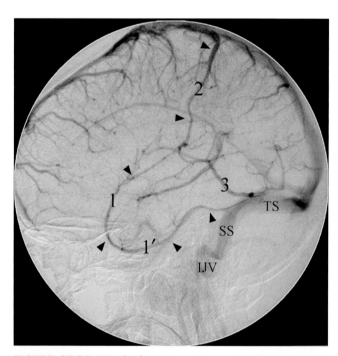

FIGURE 87-24. Digital subtraction angiogram, internal carotid artery injection, lateral view showing cortical anastomoses between *(1)* superficial middle cerebral vein, *(2)* perirolandic vein (great anastomotic vein of Trolard), and *(3)* prominent lateral temporal vein (lesser anastomotic vein of Labbé). *IJV,* Internal jugular vein; *SS,* sigmoid sinus; *TS,* transverse sinus. *(©2012, Philippe Gailloud, MD.)*

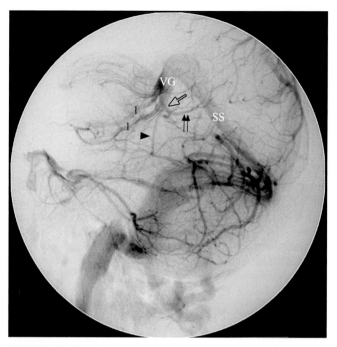

FIGURE 87-25. Digital subtraction angiogram, vertebral artery injection, venous phase, lateral view showing separate drainage into vein of Galen *(VG)* of superior vermian vein *(open arrow)* and a precentral vein *(black arrowhead)*. Internal occipital vein or calcarine vein *(double black arrows)* drains into posterior portion of one of basal veins of Rosenthal *(1)*. *SS,* Straight sinus. *(©2012, Philippe Gailloud, MD.)*

Veins of Posterior Fossa

The veins of the posterior cranial fossa may be subdivided into three groups based on their drainage pattern[39]:

1. A superior or galenic group (Fig. 87-25) consisting of the precentral and superior vermian vein.
2. An anterior or petrosal group (Fig. 87-26) of veins that drain into the superior petrosal vein and superior petrosal sinus. The radiologically demonstrable tributaries of the superior petrosal vein include the (1) lateral pontomesencephalic veins, (2) lateral mesencephalic encephalic vein, (3) transverse pontine veins, (4) vein of the great horizontal fissure of the cerebellum, and (5) vein of the lateral recess of the fourth ventricle, which may be used as an angiographic landmark.
3. A posterior or tentorial draining group includes the inferior vermian veins (generally emptying into the inferior surface of the straight sinus or torcular Herophili) and the inferior hemispheric cerebellar veins (generally emptying into the transverse sinus by way of a medial tentorial sinus [see Fig. 87-26]).

The longitudinal veins of the anterior surface of the brainstem are of clinical importance. These veins are found at every level of the brainstem, may connect cranially with the BVR (by way of the lateral mesencephalic vein and the anterior and lateral pontomesencephalic veins), and may form a continuous network all the way down to the conus medullaris. An intracranial arteriovenous fistula with perimedullary venous drainage and congestion may, through this venous network, be manifested as a venous hypertensive myelopathy (Foix-Alajouanine syndrome).[40]

perirolandic vein and the SMCV and its variable drainage pathways in the middle cranial fossa.[38] The posterior segment of the SMCV may also drain into the transverse sinus by way of a lateral temporal vein, which is then referred to as the *lesser* or *inferior anastomotic vein of Labbé.*

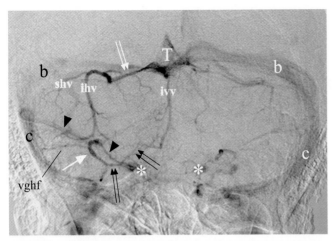

FIGURE 87-26. Digital subtraction angiogram, vertebral artery injection, venous phase, Towne projection. Superior petrosal vein *(white arrow)* drains into superior petrosal sinus *(black arrowheads)*, which in this case connects both medially with cavernous sinus *(asterisks)* and laterally with distal transverse sinus *(b)*. Superior petrosal vein receives vein of lateral recess of fourth ventricle *(black double arrow)* and vein of great horizontal fissure of cerebellum *(vghf)*. Inferior vermian vein *(iw)* drains into torcular Herophili *(T)*. An inferior hemispheric vein *(ihv)* runs upward over posterolateral margin of cerebellum, where it is joined by a superior hemispheric vein *(shv)*. A medial tentorial sinus *(double white arrow)* is seen to collect these veins and drains into torcular Herophili. (©2012, Philippe Gailloud, MD.)

Dural Venous Sinuses

Dural venous sinuses are contained within the layers of dura mater. They receive all the venous blood from the brain and a large part of the blood drained from the neurocranium. There are no dural venous sinuses in the anterior cranial fossa, which is not normally involved in encephalic drainage. The walls of the dural venous sinuses are formed by a single layer of endothelium surrounded by fibrous layers of dura mater.

Cavernous Sinus and Its Venous Connections

The laterosellar compartment is an intracranial extradural space bounded laterally by a wall composed of two dural layers and medially by the body of the sphenoid bone and the meningeal coverings of the pituitary gland. Anteriorly, the laterosellar compartment opens into the orbit through the superior and inferior orbital fissures, whereas posteriorly it is continuous with the clival extradural space.[41] The laterosellar compartment contains the intracranial and extradural portion of the ICA, which is surrounded by a venous plexus commonly referred to as the cavernous sinus (CS) (Fig. 87-27). The CS is primarily involved in draining the orbit through the superior orbital vein, which joins the anterior and superior aspect of the CS. Its major outflow pathways are the emissary veins of the middle cranial fossa into the pterygoid plexus, the carotid artery venous plexus (of Rektorzik), the inferior petrosal sinus, and inconstantly, the superior petrosal sinus. The CS may be connected to the SMCV or the anterior portion of the BVR (or both), in which case it participates in cerebral venous drainage. A connection between the CS and the middle cerebral veins occurs late in development if at all and results in the various possible drainage pathways of the middle cerebral veins in

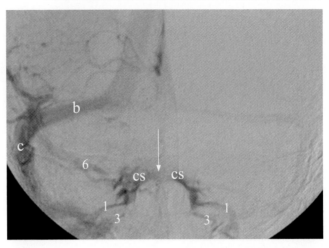

FIGURE 87-27. Digital subtraction angiogram, internal carotid artery injection, venous phase, anteroposterior view showing cavernous sinus *(CS)*. Its main affluent in this case is superficial middle cerebral vein *(6)*. Inferior petrosal sinus *(3)* is a constant outflow of CS and connects with internal jugular vein extracranially at a variable distance from jugular foramen, *(b)* transverse sinus, and *(c)* sigmoid sinus. Arrow points at coronary sinus through which left CS is opacified. An emissary vein of foramen ovale is visible bilaterally *(1)*. (©2012, Philippe Gailloud, MD.)

the middle cranial fossa discussed previously. Other affluences of the CS include the dural sinus of the lesser sphenoid wing, frequently referred to as the *sphenoparietal sinus of Breschet*. Finally, on both sides the CS is interconnected by way of the coronary sinus. Except for the carotid artery venous plexus, all the affluences and effluences of the CS are readily demonstrated by DSA and computed tomographic angiography (CTA).

Superior Sagittal Sinus

The SSS begins at a variable distance from the foramen caecum (of the anterior cranial fossa) and courses along the fixed margin of the falx cerebri in the midline. The SSS is classically described as joining the torcular Herophili, although it most frequently drains preferentially into the right transverse sinus, thus explaining the larger size of the right transverse sinus. The SSS drains cortical veins from the medial and lateral surfaces of the cerebrum and the meningeal and diploic veins.

The SSS may be duplicated, typically in its distal third, or its lumen may be divided by a septum. Hypoplasia of the proximal third of the SSS (Fig. 87-28) is frequently encountered and must not be mistaken for thrombosis. Distinction between hypoplasia of the proximal SSS and thrombosis relies on identifying a pair of large frontal cortical veins that course parallel to the midline on each side and join the SSS close to the coronal suture.

Inferior Sagittal Sinus

The inferior sagittal sinus usually begins in the anterior third of the falx cerebri and courses posteriorly along its free margin. Tributaries are usually anterior pericallosal veins that may delineate the genu of the corpus callosum, small interhemispheric frontal and cingulate tributaries, and anterior callosal veins.[42] The inferior sagittal sinus is hypoplastic in 10% of cases.

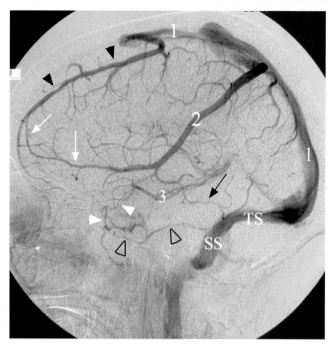

FIGURE 87-28. Digital subtraction angiogram, internal carotid artery injection, lateral view. Anterior portion of superior sagittal sinus (SSS *[1]*) is hypoplastic, and its absence is compensated by a prominent frontal vein coursing parallel to midline on its way to SSS. This vein is characteristically very prominent and present bilaterally in cases of anterior SSS hypoplasia. Its presence is a useful sign for distinguishing hypoplasia from dura sinus thrombosis. This case also shows an interesting alternative drainage pathway in the absence of a superficial middle cerebral vein (SMCV). Large perirolandic vein *(2)* drains normal territory of SMCV. It connects anteriorly with a large frontal vein and inferiorly with a small inferior anastomotic vein of Labbé *(black arrow)*. An uncal vein *(white arrowheads)* drains into a latero-cavernous sinus *(open arrowheads)*, which courses along floor of middle cranial fossa and into transverse sinus *(TS)*. *SS,* Sigmoid sinus. *(©2012, Philippe Gailloud, MD.)*

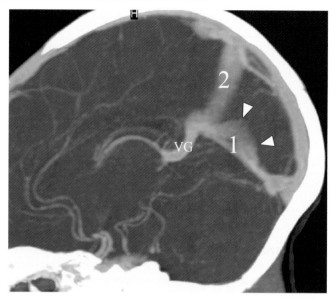

FIGURE 87-29. CT angiogram, sagittal reconstruction showing straight sinus *(1)* in an infant. A prominent falcine sinus *(2)* connects proximal portion of straight sinus to superior sagittal sinus. Note venous lacuna capping straight sinus *(arrowheads)*. *VG,* Vein of Galen. *(©2012, Philippe Gailloud, MD.)*

Straight Sinus

The straight sinus is classically formed by union of the VG and the inferior sagittal sinus on the tentorial incisura behind the splenium of the corpus callosum, and it courses along the tentorium cerebelli. It drains into the torcular Herophili or more frequently directly into one of the transverse sinuses with a left-sided predominance.[38,43] Distal tributaries of the straight sinus include the inferior vermian and occasionally veins from the internal occipital surface. On rare occasion the straight sinus may be absent, in which case it is most often replaced by an intradural channel coursing within the falx cerebri and connecting the VG with the posterior third of the SSS, called a *falcine sinus*. A normal straight sinus and a falcine sinus may coexist (Fig. 87-29).

Transverse and Sigmoid Sinuses and Torcular Herophili

The bulk of cerebral drainage reaches the transverse and sigmoid sinuses by way of the SSS, straight sinus, and superior petrosal sinus. In a little more than half the cases there is a dominance of the right side over the left, in keeping with preferential drainage of the SSS to the right and the straight sinus to the left. The most frequently encountered

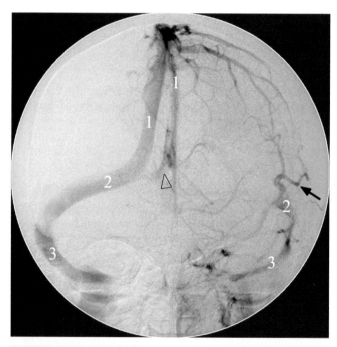

FIGURE 87-30. Digital subtraction angiogram, left internal carotid artery injection, venous phase, anteroposterior projection showing severely hypoplastic proximal left transverse sinus. Both superior sagittal sinus *(1)* and straight sinus *(arrowhead)* drain into right transverse sinus. Left transverse sinus begins at point where it receives a lateral temporal vein *(arrow)*. *2,* Transverse sinus; *3,* sigmoid sinus. *(©2012, Philippe Gailloud, MD.)*

segmental variation is isolated hypoplasia of the proximal portion of the transverse sinus (Fig. 87-30), which may be completely atretic. In such cases, the diameter of the middle portion of the transverse sinus generally becomes increased on receiving the lateral temporal vein and other supratentorial and infratentorial tributaries, with the contralateral transverse sinus draining both the SSS and the straight sinus. This anatomic disposition may represent a pitfall and must be distinguished from thrombosis of the transverse sinus. Hypoplasia of the sigmoid sinus in the presence of a normal transverse sinus is rare, and it is generally coupled with compensatory rerouting of venous blood into a prominent mastoid emissary or posterior condylar emissary vein.[43] Alternatively, an occipital sinus may convey venous blood from the torcular Herophili to the bulb of the IJV in association with either normal, hypoplastic, or absent transverse and sigmoid sinuses.[44]

Vertebral Venous System, Emissary Veins, and Veins of Craniocervical Junction

Blood drained through the transverse and sigmoid sinuses will flow into the IJV in the supine position and into the VVS in the upright position. The VVS is composed of the external and internal vertebral venous plexuses, which have a craniocaudal course and run parallel to each other and the IJV[45] (Fig. 87-31). The external vertebral venous plexus consists of (1) the vertebral artery venous plexus (VAVP), which starts at the cervical level of C1 and engulfs the portion of the VA that runs inside the transverse foramina; caudally, the VAVP exits the C7 transverse canal and usually joins the brachiocephalic veins; and (2) the deep cervical vein, which starts in the suboccipital region and drains either into the VAVP distally or into the brachiocephalic veins. The internal vertebral venous plexus (IVVP) occupies the epidural space at every spinal level and is formed by anterior (more conspicuous) and posterior (less conspicuous) epidural components. The VAVP and IVVP are anastomosed by way of intervertebral veins that follow the emerging spinal roots out of the spinal canal and through the vertebral body and posterior spinal veins.

Venous outflow from the posterior cranial fossa into the VVS occurs through the anterior, lateral, and posterior condylar veins and the mastoid emissary vein.[46,47] The posterior condylar vein typically arises from the distal portion of the sigmoid sinus or from the junction of the sigmoid sinus and jugular bulb, courses through the posterior condylar canal, and drains into the VAVP. The anterior condylar vein, or vein of the hypoglossal canal, is usually plexiform and surrounds the hypoglossal nerve. It connects with the anterior IVVP intracranially and with the anterior condylar confluent extracranially. The anterior condylar confluent is located extracranially in front of the aperture of the hypoglossal canal[38,47] and, through its connections with the anterior condylar vein, inferior petrosal sinus, lateral condylar vein, and IJV, plays an important role as a venous crossroad. The mastoid emissary vein connects the vertical portion of the sigmoid sinus with the retroauricular, suboccipital, or deep cervical veins. The lateral condylar vein usually arises from a small vein that connects the anterior condylar confluent and the IJV.[47] It opens into the VAVP and is therefore not an emissary vein because it is purely extracranial. An occipital emissary vein, though rare, is often mentioned in the literature and connects the torcular Herophili with a suboccipital vein. These veins may be very prominent, especially if they represent the major venous outflow pathway for the posterior cranial fossa, as may be observed in cases of

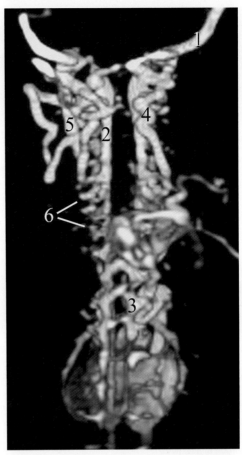

FIGURE 87-31. Magnetic resonance venogram, maximum intensity projection reconstruction of cervical and thoracic venous system in a 2-year-old girl with bilateral internal jugular vein thrombosis leading to prominent venous return through vertebral venous system. Anterior internal vertebral venous plexus (IVVP *[2]*) connects vertebral artery venous plexus (VAVP *[5]*) (incompletely demonstrated in this case) by way of intervertebral veins *(6)* at every level. Posterior IVVP *(3)* is particularly conspicuous at thoracic level. Deep cervical vein (4) joins VAVP. *1*, Sigmoid sinus. *(©2012, Philippe Gailloud, MD.)*

thrombosis or severe hypoplasia of a portion or the entire sigmoid sinus or the IJV. Because of postural variations in encephalic venous drainage, DSA may fail to demonstrate all or any connections between the dural venous sinuses of the posterior cranial fossa and the VVS in the supine position, where the IJV pathway is favored.

Other emissary veins are regularly mentioned in the literature. For instance, the emissary vein of the foramen caecum of the anterior cranial fossa, which connects the veins of the nasal mucosa with the SSS, is classically described in the anatomic and radiologic literature, although it has not to this day been demonstrated radiologically, and its existence in adults is questioned. Recently, however, a vein analogous to the emissary vein of the foramen caecum but coursing through the cribriform plate has been demonstrated on angiography.[48] Finally, the double and symmetric parietal emissary veins (of Santorini) provide a connection between the SSS and the veins of the scalp.[32] Although they are of little functional significance in normal conditions, if present, they may provide an important collateral pathway in cases of distal occlusion of the SSS.

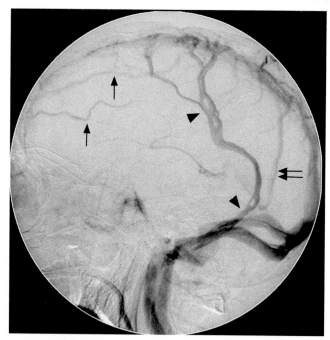

FIGURE 87-32. Digital subtraction angiogram, internal carotid artery injection, late venous phase showing a prominent posterior parietotemporal diploic vein *(arrowheads)* connecting superior sagittal sinus (SSS) with sigmoid sinus. A contralateral posterior parietotemporal diploic vein *(double arrows)* drains into transverse sinus. Note how these vessels cross over sutures as they go from one bone to another. Frontal diploic veins *(arrows)* are also recognized by their tortuous and irregular caliber and drain to anterior portion of SSS. *(©2012, Philippe Gailloud, MD.)*

Veins of the Neurocranium

Veins that drain the neurocranium include the diploic and meningeal veins (Fig. 87-32). The diploic veins run in the diploë of all the bones forming the calvaria and become increasingly prominent with age. The course of the diploic veins is variable and highly asymmetric, but a frontal, one or several parietal, and posterior temporal diploic veins are often demonstrated angiographically. The diploic veins are proximally connected to the dural venous sinuses, mostly the SSS, and may act as important collateral pathways in the case of dural sinus occlusion or other vascular conditions leading to venous hypertension. On DSA, the diploic veins have typical irregular contours and a tortuous course and fill late in the venous phase of a CCA injection, thus allowing easy distinction from cortical or meningeal veins.

Meningeal veins are embedded in the dura mater and should be considered dural venous sinuses.[32,38] The most prominent meningeal veins are the middle meningeal veins, whose sphenoidal portion along the floor of the middle cranial fossa is often demonstrated on DSA. The middle meningeal veins connect caudally with the pterygoid plexus through the veins of the foramen ovale and cranially with the SSS by way of their parietal portion.

Pitfalls

Arachnoid or pacchionian granulations are a frequent source of erroneous diagnosis of thrombosis. Pacchionian

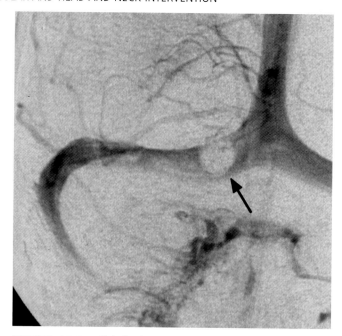

FIGURE 87-33. Digital subtraction angiogram, internal carotid artery injection, venous phase showing prominent arachnoid granulation in proximal third of right transverse sinus *(arrow).* *(©2012, Philippe Gailloud, MD.)*

granulations are invaginations of the subarachnoid space into a dural venous sinus, typically at the point where a cortical vein crosses the dura mater of a dural venous sinus.[48,49] Arachnoid granulations are frequently located in the transverse sinuses in particular, although they may be found in other locations such as the SSS and the straight sinus, around the torcular Herophili, or in the CS.[50] Radiologically, arachnoid granulations appear as a well-circumscribed filling defect on all imaging techniques delineating vessel anatomy (Fig. 87-33). Unenhanced CT may demonstrate a liquid density of the filling defect observed on enhanced scans. T2-weighted images may show high intensity within the arachnoid granulation on MRI, which corresponds to invaginated cerebrospinal fluid. Unequivocal radiologic diagnosis of an arachnoid granulation relies on identification of a vein entering and crossing the filling defect within the dural venous sinus.

Hypoplasia of a dural venous sinus is frequently encountered, especially with the SSS and transverse sinuses, and may also be mistaken for thrombosis, as mentioned earlier.

Hypoplasia of a sigmoid sinus in the presence of a normal transverse sinus must be distinguished from a steno-occlusive process. In cases of severe sigmoid hypoplasia, the pars vascularis of the jugular foramen will also be hypoplastic, and the jugular foramen will be composed of only a pars nervosa. High-resolution CT is the best imaging modality for demonstrating the emissary foramina of the base of the skull. When the sigmoid ends in a pouch, a large mastoid emissary vein may be the major outflow pathway for the ipsilateral transverse sinus. Alternatively, the superior petrosal or petrosquamosal sinus may provide outflow for the transverse sinus in cases of atresia of the entire sigmoid sinus[43] and be very prominent.

The inferior petrosal sinus usually drains into the IJV around the jugular foramen and offers a connection to the anterior condylar confluent. Occasionally the termination of the inferior petrosal sinus in the IJV may be found up to 4 cm below the jugular foramen.[51] This anatomic variation has to be known by neuroradiologists attempting to navigate into the inferior petrosal sinus through the IJV and must be sought if catheterization of the inferior petrosal sinus around the jugular foramen is impossible.

KEY POINTS

- The cerebral circulation is provided by four main arterial axes: the carotid and vertebral arteries. The circle of Willis, located at the base of the brain, interconnects these vessels and can act as a source of collateral supply.

- The circle of Willis is a site of frequent variations. Some of these variants may predispose to the formation of aneurysms (e.g., a hypoplastic A1 segment with a prominent anterior communicating artery). Others, such as the absence of a posterior communicating artery, may be associated with a higher risk of ischemic stroke.

- The main cerebral branches—the anterior, middle, and posterior cerebral arteries—are also linked at the pial level, but the capacity of these pial anastomoses to provide collateral supply declines with age.

- Multiple small anastomoses link the external carotid, internal carotid, and vertebral arteries. These connections, which are not always angiographically visible, can act as collateral pathways in steno-occlusive disorders but also represent a significant pitfall during therapeutic embolization. The operator should keep in mind that these "dangerous anastomoses" might become conspicuous or reverse flow direction during the progress of an embolization.

- The cerebral venous system is divided into superficial and deep components. Variants of the cerebral draining system, such as proximal hypoplasia of the transverse or superior sagittal sinuses, must be differentiated from pathologic conditions, in particular sinus thrombosis.

► SUGGESTED READINGS

Yasargil MG. Microneurosurgery, vol. 1. New York: Thieme Stratton; 1984.

The complete reference list is available online at www.expertconsult.com.

CHAPTER 88

Arterial Anatomy of the Spine and Spinal Cord

Philippe Gailloud

INTRODUCTION

Spinal digital subtraction angiography (SpDSA) is the gold standard imaging modality for evaluating vascular anomalies of the spine and spinal cord. Endovascular treatment of spinal vascular lesions was pioneered in the late 1960s[1-3] shortly after the introduction of selective spinal angiography itself.[4] Performing diagnostic and therapeutic SpDSA requires a solid understanding of the relevant vascular anatomy. This chapter offers an introduction to the arterial anatomy of the spine and spinal cord and discusses the basic principles of SpDSA.

DEVELOPMENTAL ANATOMY

Each primitive dorsal aorta provides three groups of branches aligned in ventral, lateral, and dorsal rows. The dorsal rami start emerging early at the 6-somite stage, shortly after the still-unfused aortas have branched off the first ventral (or vitelline) arteries and slightly before the appearance of the first lateral branches.[5] The dorsal branches stem from the primitive aortas in between somites, adopting an intersegmental rather than segmental distribution. These intersegmental arteries (ISAs) initially consist of capillary loops established between a dorsal aorta and the ipsilateral posterior cardinal vein. Later, the arterial and venous sides of the loops develop into the ISAs per se and their corresponding veins (Fig. 88-1, A-B).[5] Rami sprouting from the arterial limb of the loops connect to similar vessels coming from contiguous ISAs to form longitudinal capillary plexi along the ventrolateral surface of the neural tube (Fig. 88-1, C). These plexi soon extend dorsally to cover the lateral surfaces of the neural tube as well.[5] Transverse channels developing within this network form the primitive anterior and posterior radicular arteries, which are the first and, at this time, only branches of the ISAs. Capillaries extending further medially from each ventrolateral plexus establish a second set of longitudinal chains along the lateral edges of the floor plate of the neural tube. These chains correspond to the primitive anterior spinal arteries (ASAs), which will later coalesce more or less completely into a single ventromedian channel, the basilar artery cranially and the ASA caudally. In view of this developmental history, the dorsal branches and their capillary plexi for the spinal cord represent the fundamental anatomy of the ISA. At the adult stage, they correspond to the ISA stem and the spinal component of the dorsospinal artery (DA). Later-appearing branches include a dorsal branch (dorsal component of the DA) and a lateral branch (intercostal or lumbar arteries of the adult nomenclature) (see Fig. 88-1, C). The final configuration of the ISA depends upon the branching pattern of these secondary arteries; in particular, a DA exists only when the origin of the lateral branch is proximal to the takeoff of the spinal branch (Fig. 88-2).

An understanding of the ISA based on its developmental anatomy is applicable at any vertebral level. Figures 88-3 and 88-4 show the typical configuration of thoracic and lumbar ISAs. Caudally, the median sacral artery (MSA) is the true continuation of the abdominal aorta beyond the takeoff of the common iliac arteries, derived themselves from the umbilical arteries[6,7] (Fig. 88-5). The MSA remains temporarily connected with the capillary network supplying the hindgut and with the primary metanephric plexus.[8,9] Through these connections, the MSA occasionally provides branches normally arising from the abdominal aorta,[8] such as a renal artery (Fig. 88-6, A) or a superior rectal artery (Fig. 88-6, B). At the cervical level, longitudinal anastomoses linking the first six ISAs form the vertebral arteries (VA)[10] (Fig. 88-7). According to Bracard, the VA is better described as a hemodynamic solution than a true artery.[11] The distal V3 and V4 segments of the VA are formed by the enlarged spinal branch accompanying the first cervical nerve,[12,13] a persistent segment of the proatlantal artery.[14] The original intersegmental configuration, fairly apparent in children, accounts for the typical sources of collateral supply observed at the adult stage (Fig. 88-8).

Arteries of the Vertebral Body

The vertebral body is vascularized by anterolateral and posteromedian osseous branches (Fig. 88-9). The anterolateral arteries originate from the stem of the ISA; they are divided into ascending, descending, and recurrent branches. Because of the leftward position of the aorta, they are more numerous on the right side than on the left.[15] Ascending and descending branches connect with corresponding vessels from adjacent levels; these anastomoses often act as collateral supply pathways. They also participate in several anatomic variations described later in this chapter. After a short ascending course, the recurrent branch curves medially with a typical 90-degree angle to establish an anastomosis with the contralateral recurrent artery[15] (Fig. 88-10).

The spinal branch of the ISA usually divides into a radicular artery, coursing medially along the corresponding nerve root, and a retrocorporeal artery that provides the posteromedian osseous branches. Over the posterior aspect of the vertebral body, the retrocorporeal artery participates in the formation of a rich anastomotic network by joining analogous branches from adjacent levels. The retrocorporeal artery is frequently targeted during preoperative spinal embolization, so the presence of dangerous anastomoses within this network has to be kept in mind (Fig. 88-11). The cluster of posteromedian osseous branches is often associated with a prominent blush that can mimic a vascular

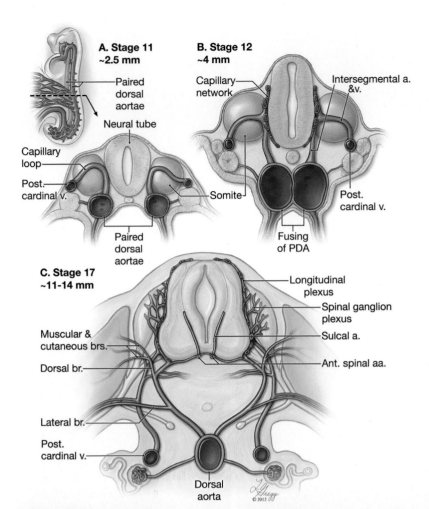

A. Stage 11
~2.5 mm

Paired
dorsal
aortae

Neural tube

Capillary
loop

Post.
cardinal v.

Somite

Paired
dorsal
aortae

B. Stage 12
~4 mm

Capillary
network

Intersegmental a.
&v.

Post.
cardinal v.

Fusing
of PDA

C. Stage 17
~11-14 mm

Longitudinal
plexus

Spinal ganglion
plexus

Muscular &
cutaneous brs.

Sulcal a.

Dorsal br.

Ant. spinal aa.

Lateral br.

Post.
cardinal v.

Dorsal
aorta

FIGURE 88-1. Intersegmental artery (ISA) development in human embryo (adapted from Evans[5]). Upper left inset identifies reconstruction levels. Simple capillary loop is present in 2.5-mm embryo (*A. Stage 11*). A capillary network then appears along anterior and lateral aspects of neural tube (*B. Stage 12*). Midline fusion of primitive aortae has started. In 11/14-mm embryo (*C. Stage 17*), a ventral radicular branch has developed and forms anastomotic chain along anterior aspect of neural tube, with vessels coming from adjacent levels. First sulcal arteries are identified. Secondary dorsal and lateral branches that will develop into spinal and intercostal/lumbar arteries of adult ISA are now visible. (©2012, Lydia Gregg, CMI.)

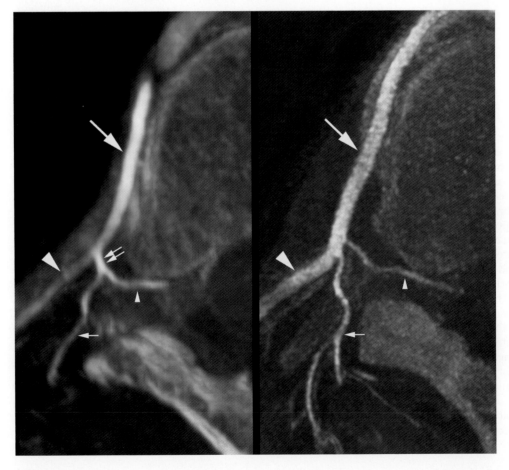

FIGURE 88-2. Branching pattern of intersegmental arteries (ISAs) shown by flat-panel catheter angiotomography (FPCA). Left side shows classic branching pattern, including aortic stem (*arrow*), lateral (or intercostal) branch (*arrowhead*), and dorsospinal artery (DA) (*double arrow*), with its spinal (*small arrowhead*) and dorsal (*small arrow*) components. On right, spinal and dorsal branches originate separately from intersegmental stem; there is therefore no DA. Fundamental constituents of ISA are aortic stem and its spinal branch. Lateral and dorsal musculocutaneous branches develop later. (©2012, Philippe Gailloud, MD.)

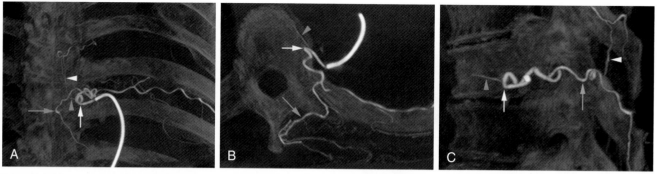

FIGURE 88-3. Flat-panel catheter angiotomography (FPCA) of left T6 showing thoracic internal segmental artery (ISA) anatomy. Typical anatomy of left thoracic ISA in coronal **(A)**, sagittal **(B)**, and axial **(C)** planes. Two-dimensional nature of angiography results in superposition of many branches that can at times be difficult to distinguish (e.g., prominent dorsal muscular branch *(white arrowhead)* may adopt course reminiscent of spinal contributor). Because of leftward position of thoracic aorta, ISAs are longer on right side than on left, in particular at upper thoracic levels, where left ISAs adopt an initial recurrent course before curving sharply backward to pass behind mediastinal attachment of endothoracic fascia *(white arrow)*. Recurrent osseous branch is stretched over lateral aspect of vertebral body *(gray arrowhead)*. Gray arrow points at dorsal branch of ISA (or dorsal component of dorsospinal artery) as it divides into its terminal musculocutaneous branches. *(©2012, Philippe Gailloud, MD.)*

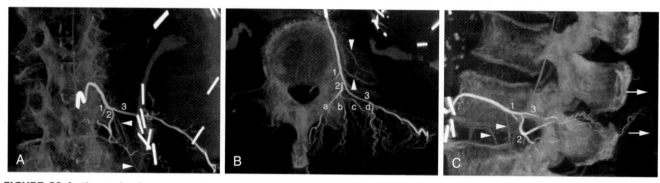

FIGURE 88-4. Flat-panel catheter angiotomography (FPCA) of left L3 showing lumbar internal segmental artery (ISA) anatomy. Typical anatomy of left lumbar ISA in coronal **(A)**, axial **(B)**, and sagittal **(C)** planes. White arrowheads point at two prominent branches for psoas muscle (note muscular blush in **B**). White arrows in **C** indicate terminal subcutaneous arterial network. Note that spinal branch *(1)*, which provides the artery of Adamkiewicz, arises from ISA trunk proximal to its bifurcation into dorsal *(2)* and lateral *(3)* branches. Medial *(a)*, intermediate *(b)*, and lateral *(c)* muscular branches of dorsal component of the ISA are shown in **B**, as well as a posterior perforating artery *(d)* of lateral branch, which participates in vascularization of paravertebral musculature. *(©2012, Philippe Gailloud, MD.)*

anomaly (Fig. 88-12). Similarly, an enhancing Schmorl's node can simulate a more aggressive pathology such as a metastasis (Fig. 88-13). The three branches of the ISA passing through the neural foramen are also known as the *anterior, intermediate,* and *posterior spinal canal arteries.*[15] The anterior and intermediate branches are the retrocorporeal and radicular arteries, the posterior one is the prelaminar artery.[16] These branches can have a common origin (i.e., the spinal branch in its complete form[16]) or originate separately (Fig. 88-14). The left and right prelaminar arteries establish an anastomotic network along the anterior aspect of the posterior vertebral arch that is often difficult to differentiate from the retrocorporeal network on angiographic projections. A modification of the retrocorporeal anatomy is seen at the level of the odontoid process, which is principally vascularized by two branches of the VA, the anterior and posterior ascending arteries[17,18] (see Fig. 88-7). The posterior ascending artery is a cranial extension of the C2 retrocorporeal artery that courses upward within the anterior epidural space. It assumes a typical ogival shape around the odontoid process as it connects with the contralateral

posterior ascending artery to form the apical arcade[17,20] (see Fig. 88-29, *B*). The odontoid process receives additional supply from the ascending pharyngeal artery, notably a branch joining the apical arcade via the hypoglossal canal.[19]

A selective ISA angiogram usually results in visualization of a hemivertebral blush. The extent and conspicuity of that blush varies among individuals. Anastomoses linking osseous branches from adjacent/opposite ISAs explain the common visualization of partial or even complete hemivertebral blushes in adjoining vertebrae, or of a bilateral blush at the studied level. In children, the vertebral blush appearance depends upon the maturation of the growth plate and the progressive dominance of the anterolateral group of osseous branches over the posterior median one (Fig. 88-15) (Gailloud, unpublished data). The evolution of the blush also reflects the transition of the vertebral vascularization from the rich arterial network seen in children to the end-artery configuration of adults, a switch completed at about age 15.[20] The conspicuity of the hemivertebral blush decreases with age as bone marrow is progressively replaced with fat.

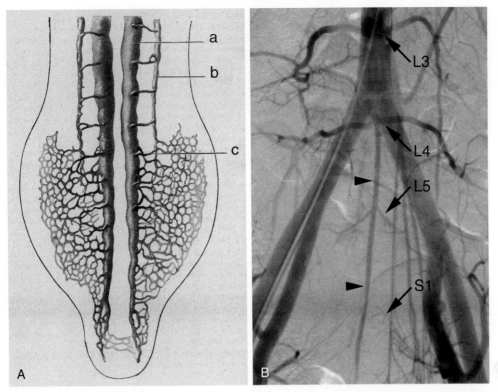

FIGURE 88-5. Anatomy of internal segmental artery (ISA) at sacral level. **A** shows posterior view of capillary network associated with early leg buds of a chick (network originates from lateral aortic branches rather than dorsal ones).[7,67] The portion of dorsal aortas distal to origin of iliac arteries will fuse into a single midline vessel, the median sacral artery (MSA). For convenience, original legends have been replaced with single letters: *a,* right dorsal aorta; *b,* right posterior cardinal vein; *c,* 27th dorsal intersegmental vessel. In **B**, posteroanterior projection of a pelvic angiogram illustrates adult equivalent of structures shown in **A**. Note that MSA *(arrowheads)* exhibits intersegmental pattern typical of primitive dorsal aortas, providing L4 ISAs completely, L5 ISAs partially, and connecting laterally with superior lateral sacral artery at S1. (**A** *from Evans HM. The development of the vascular system. In: Keibel F, Mall FP, editors. Manual of human embryology. Vol 2. Philadelphia and London: J.B. Lippincott; 1912. p. 570–708;* **B** *©2012, Philippe Gailloud, MD.)*

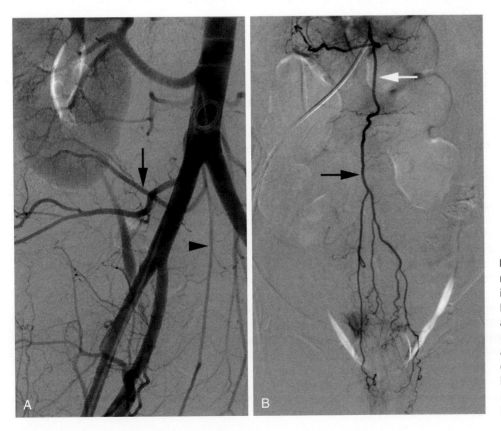

FIGURE 88-6. Anomalous branches of median sacral artery (MSA). **A** shows an inferior polar artery *(arrow)* coming from MSA *(arrowhead)*. In **B**, superior rectal artery *(black arrow)* originates from MSA *(white arrow)*. Although rare, these variants must be kept in mind when seeking elusive sources of hemorrhage from kidney or bowel. (**A** *courtesy Dr. Ali Sultan, University of Miami, Coral Gables, Florida;* **B** *©2012, Philippe Gailloud, MD.)*

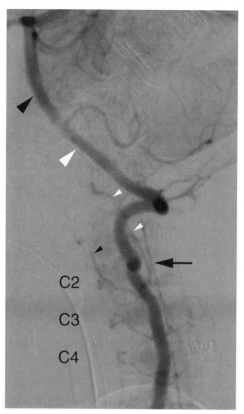

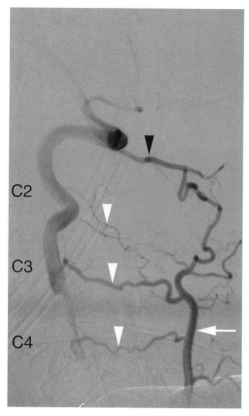

FIGURE 88-7. Anatomy of internal segmental artery (ISA) at cervical level. In this vertebral artery (VA) injection, intersegmental anatomy remains apparent at *C2, C3,* and *C4* (ISA 1-3). VA is made of a chain of longitudinal anastomoses, connecting caudally with subclavian artery and cranially with proatlantal artery. Residual portions of proatlantal artery constitute, among other things, V3 and V4 segments of VA. V4 segment corresponds to ascending ramus of anterior radicular branch of C1 *(large white arrowhead)*. Basilar artery *(large black arrowhead)* is the fusion of primitive anterior spinal axes at brainstem level. Arrow points at anterior spinal artery (ASA), connected cranially to descending ramus of anterior radicular branch of C1 (V4 segment at adult stage). Note anterior *(small black arrowhead)* and posterior *(small white arrowheads)* ascending arteries, two branches of VA derived from first ISA that supply odontoid process. *(©2012, Philippe Gailloud, MD.)*

FIGURE 88-8. Vertebral collateral supply via primitive internal segmental arteries (ISAs). Original intersegmental pattern is not always apparent at adult stage, but inconspicuous primitive vessels remain patent and can play important roles later in life. In this patient with proximal left vertebral artery (VA) occlusion, collateral supply is provided by left deep cervical artery *(white arrow)* via dorsal branches of proatlantal artery *(black arrowhead)* and first three ISAs *(white arrowheads)*. *(©2012, Philippe Gailloud, MD.)*

anatomic variations and represent potential dangerous anastomoses during endovascular procedures.

Intersegmental Artery Trunks

ISA trunks can be ipsilateral (i.e., involving arteries from two or more consecutive vertebral levels) or bilateral (i.e., providing the left and right ISAs for a single level). Bilateral trunks are most common in the lower lumbar region but exceptional in the mid- and upper thoracic regions (except in the Japanese population, according to Adachi[21]) (Fig. 88-17). A bilateral trunk is often falsely suggested by the origin of L4 or L5 ISAs from the MSA (see Fig. 88-5, *B*); a bilateral trunk must show a common stem arising from the MSA itself (Fig. 88-18).

Ipsilateral trunks can be seen at any vertebral level. They are common in the upper thoracic region. Caudally, they are generally seen at L3, L4, or L5; they can involve several consecutive levels, with a complex interplay of spinal and muscular branches. The most extreme form of trunk reported so far consists of a single ascending midline vessel providing bilateral ISAs from T12 to T3.[22] Ipsilateral trunks are divided into complete and incomplete types. To be complete, an ipsilateral trunk must have a full set of branches for each vertebral level it supplies. These include (1) an

Muscular and Cutaneous Branches

The stem of lumbar ISAs gives several superficial and deep branches to the psoas muscle (see Fig. 88-4, *B*).[15] The paraspinal musculature is principally vascularized by the dorsal component of the DA via its medial, intermediate, and lateral muscular branches. Posterior perforators of the lateral branch of the ISA also contribute, either directly or by anastomosing with the lateral muscular branch of the DA (see Fig. 88-4, *B*). Despite extensive interconnections, the muscular branches continue to exhibit a segmental pattern at the adult stage. The terminal skin arteries, on the other hand, have less predictable territories owing to cutaneous shifting and vascular redistribution.[5] Anastomoses between the osseous, muscular, and cutaneous branches of adjacent or opposite ISAs offer a wide range of potential collateral pathways. Figure 88-16 illustrates some typical connections, in particular the anterior and posterior laterovertebral anastomoses, which are commonly involved in

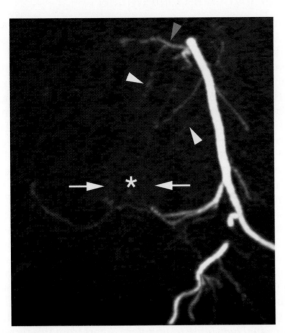

FIGURE 88-9. Arteries of vertebral body. Subtracted axial reconstruction of three-dimensional digital subtraction angiography (3D-DSA) acquisition of left L3 documents two main groups of branches vascularizing vertebral body: anterolateral *(white arrowheads)* and posteromedian *(white arrows)* osseous arteries. Posteromedian arteries are branches of retrocorporeal artery that penetrate posterior wall of vertebral body through basivertebral foramen *(asterisk)*. Gray arrowhead points at recurrent osseous branch, splayed over anterior wall of vertebra. *(©2012, Philippe Gailloud, MD.)*

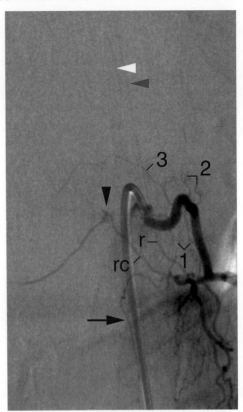

FIGURE 88-10. Angiographic appearance of osseous arteries. Posteroanterior projection of a left T9 angiogram shows inferior *(1)*, superior *(2)*, and recurrent *(3)* osseous branches of internal segmental artery (ISA), as well as retrocorporeal artery *(rc)* and its tufts of posteromedian branches entering basivertebral foramen *(black arrowhead)*. Black arrow points at a paramedian dorsal musculocutaneous branch; letter *r* refers to radicular artery of T9, which provides both anterior *(white arrowhead)* and posterior *(gray arrowhead)* spinal contributors. *(©2012, Philippe Gailloud, MD.)*

anterior component (or stem) providing the anterolateral osseous branches, (2) a lateral component (i.e., the lumbar, subcostal, or intercostal artery), (3) a dorsal component supplying the paraspinal musculature, and (4) a spinal component branching off the radicular artery (Fig. 88-19). The dorsal and spinal components, when sharing a common origin, form a DA.

In the classic form of incomplete unilateral trunk, a DA missing at one of the levels supplied by the trunk arises separately from the aorta. This configuration, reported by Chiras and Merland in 1979,[23] is known as an *isolated DA* or direct emergence of the DA from the aorta[23-26] (Fig. 88-20). Isolated DAs frequently contribute to the vascularization of the spinal cord.[24,26] A subtler variant in which only the ISA stem and its spinal branch originate separately from the aorta can be observed[27] (Fig. 88-21). The incomplete nature of this trunk is more difficult to identify because the presence of a dorsal branch falsely suggests a complete configuration. Absence of vertebral blush at one of the levels supplied by the trunk is an important clue, but one must remember that a blush is not always observed, in particular in older patients. Identifying the spinal component of the ISA or one of its branches, a radicular or a retrocorporeal artery in particular, remains the most reliable angiographic criterion to distinguish between complete and incomplete unilateral trunks.

Longitudinal Arterial Chains of the Spinal Cord

Each primitive ISA sends capillary twigs toward the neural tube. Capillaries from contiguous ISAs connect to form a dense plexus over the surface of the developing cord. The blood supply of the adult spinal cord depends on several primary and secondary longitudinal anastomotic chains derived from this primitive capillary plexus (Fig. 88-22, *A*). Two principal longitudinal chains develop on each side, an anterolateral one first and a posterolateral one slightly later. The posterolateral chains remain separate and turn into the left and right posterior spinal arteries (PSAs). The anterolateral chains become interconnected by an anteromedian anastomotic network from which will emerge a single longitudinal vessel, the ASA. As noted by Evans in 1908, "one of the most beautiful and evident instances of the conversion of a capillary mesh into an arterial channel is afforded in the history of the anterior spinal artery"[9] (Fig. 88-23). A single ASA is present in the human embryo as early as the second month of gestation (15-22 mm, Carnegie stages 18-21).[28,29] It may form by selection of a preferential path within the primitive network,[9,30] by fusion of the two primitive anterolateral chains,[28] or by a combination of these mechanisms. Either process can result in tortuosity, fenestration, or duplication; a long duplication of the ASA is frequently observed at the cervical level but rarely extends below C6[31] (Fig. 88-24). The persistence of plexiform segments, while rare along the ASA, is part of the normal

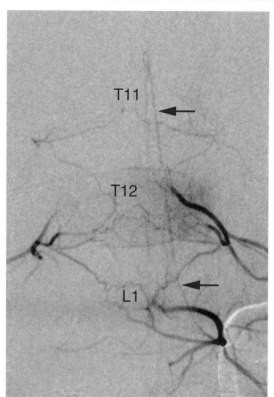

FIGURE 88-11. Retrocorporeal network in a 3-year-old boy. Left T12 injection shows diamond-shaped retrocorporeal network over three levels *(T11, T12, L1)*. A prominent posterior spinal contributor originating from left L1 *(arrows)* is opacified through the network. Visibility of retrocorporeal network decreases with age, so dangerous connections must always be looked for during spinal embolization. *(©2012, Philippe Gailloud, MD.)*

anatomy of the PSAs (named *posterior plexiform channels*[32] by Gillilan). The posterolateral chains remain unfused, vary markedly in diameter, alternate between single-vessel and plexus configuration, and keep multiple small transverse connections (Fig. 88-25). The cervical and thoracolumbar portions of the ASA are not discontinuous, as occasionally reported, but form an unbroken axis extending from its cervicomedullary origin down to the conus medullaris, beyond which it continues as the artery of the filum terminale (Fig. 88-26). It remains true, however, that the caliber of certain ASA segments decreases with age, in particular in the mid-thoracic region, where short interruptions may be noted.[33] Near its caudal end, the ASA branches off two rami that curve sharply backward to reach the dorsal aspect of the conus and continue cranialward as the PSAs[12] (Fig. 88-27). The functional significance of this anastomosis, named *arcade cruciale* by Charpy,[34] was emphasized by Bolton, who noted that blood flow was craniocaudal in the distal ASA and caudocranial in the lumbosacral segments of the PSAs.[35] Lazorthes emphasized the constancy of this anastomosis, for which he proposed the now accepted term of *terminal loop (anse terminale)*.[36] Apart from this terminal loop, there are few large anastomoses between the anterior and posterior longitudinal chains, even in the fetus[37]; an example is seen in Figure 88-25.

The ASA and paired PSAs remain interconnected at the adult stage through a vascular mesh that covers the surface of the spinal cord, the pial or coronary plexus (or vasocorona[38]), within which several secondary longitudinal channels can be identified (see Fig. 88-22, *A*). Corbin listed three secondary chains on each side of the spinal cord.[39] Two of them, the anterolateral and posterolateral chains of Kadyi, are discontinuous channels respectively coursing along the

FIGURE 88-12. Prominent cluster of posteromedian osseous branches. In early arterial phase *(left)*, retrocorporeal artery *(arrowhead)* and its associated cluster of posteromedian osseous branches *(arrow)* are easily identified. Later in arterial phase *(right)*, median capillary blush falsely appears to be connected with anterior spinal artery, and retrocorporeal artery is no longer visible. Location of blush, which projects over basivertebral foramen, provides a useful clue regarding its nature. *(©2012, Philippe Gailloud, MD.)*

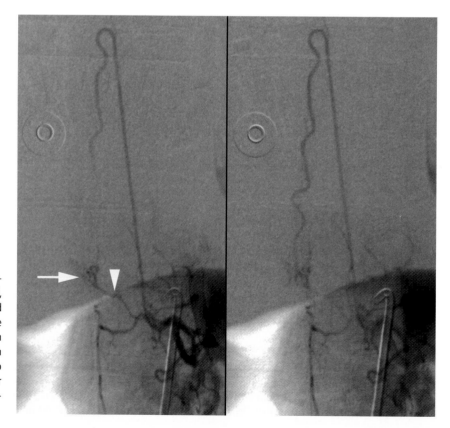

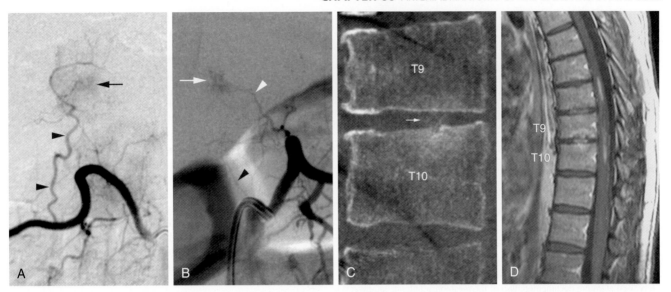

FIGURE 88-13. Abnormal vertebral blushes. **A,** Right L1 angiogram in patient with renal cell carcinoma. Paravertebral longitudinal anastomosis *(arrowheads)* opacifies metastatic lesion in lower aspect of T12 *(arrow)*. **B,** Similar image obtained during left T10 injection in patient with spinal cord hemorrhage. Here, abnormal blush *(arrow)* is opacified by superior osseous branch from internal segmental artery stem *(white arrowhead)* and corresponds to a Schmorl's node. **C,** Left T10 flat-panel catheter angiotomography confirms location of blush within T9-T10 intervertebral space *(small arrow)*, correlating with a Schmorl's node, documented by magnetic resonance imaging **(D)**. Blush can be distinguished from normal cluster of posteromedian osseous branches by its location (away from basivertebral foramen) and by its feeding artery, distinct from retrocorporeal artery. *(©2012, Philippe Gailloud, MD.)*

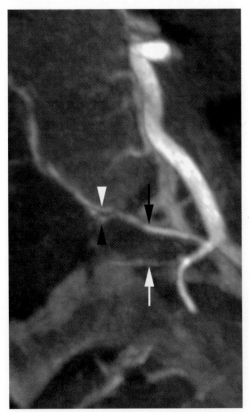

FIGURE 88-14. Spinal canal arteries, including prelaminar artery. Common configuration of the three spinal canal arteries is shown in this axial reconstruction of a selective thoracic flat-panel catheter angiotomogram. Black arrow points at an anterior trunk (spinal branch of internal segmental artery [ISA]) dividing into retrocorporeal artery (or anterior spinal canal branch) *(white arrowhead)* and radicular artery (or intermediate spinal canal branch), which gives a prominent anterior spinal artery contributor *(black arrowhead)*. White arrow identifies prelaminar artery, or posterior spinal canal branch, arising separately from dorsal branch of ISA. *(©2012, Philippe Gailloud, MD.)*

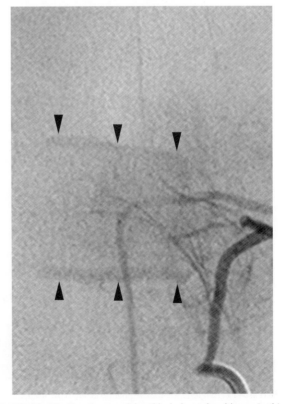

FIGURE 88-15. Prominent endplate blush *(arrowheads)* seen in this left T6 angiogram in an 8-year-old boy is typical for children and should not be interpreted as an abnormal finding. *(©2012, Philippe Gailloud, MD.)*

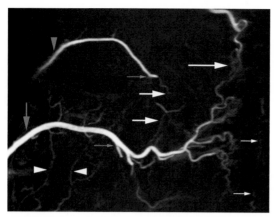

FIGURE 88-16. Principal paravertebral arterial anastomotic pathways. Sagittal reconstruction of three-dimensional digital subtraction angiography (3D-DSA) of left L1 *(gray arrow)* illustrates several paravertebral anastomotic pathways. Ascending and descending osseous branches of internal segmental artery (ISA) stem are documented; two of them establish anterior laterovertebral anastomoses with ascending branches of L2 *(white arrowheads)*. Stem of T12 *(gray arrowhead)* is opacified via posterior laterovertebral anastomosis *(short white arrows)*. Dorsal muscular arteries of L1 form retrovertebral anastomotic network with corresponding branches from T11 *(long white arrow)*. Small gray arrows designate radicular arteries of T12 and L1; small white arrow points at cutaneous network of L1. *(©2012, Philippe Gailloud, MD.)*

dorsal aspect of the ventral nerve roots and the ventral aspect of the dorsal nerve roots. The third one, the lateral (or interradicular) chain, is the most constant of the secondary longitudinal chains.[39] Parke et al. have simplified the nomenclature of these chains by applying the criteria of anatomic constancy and functional significance; their terminology is adopted here[40] (see Fig. 88-22). Although present in the lumbosacral region of fetuses,[41] the posterolateral chain is only seen with constancy in the adult at the cervical level; it was therefore named the *lateral cervical spinal artery* (LCSA) by Parke et al.[40] (see Fig. 88-22, *B*). The LCSA, already described by Kadyi,[12] is equivalent to the lateral spinal artery of the upper cervical spinal cord reported by Lasjaunias.[42] The LCSA is sometimes considered a variation of the course of the PSA above C4, passing in front rather than behind the posterior spinal nerve roots, but the two vessels can be documented simultaneously.[12,43] The division of the descending ramus of the PSA, originating from the distal VA into two branches, one in front and one behind the posterior rootlets, was known to classical anatomists.[44] The PSA and LCSA seem to provide alternate vascular solutions within the arterial network supplying the posterior and lateral surfaces of the upper cervical cord, with reciprocal functional importance, as suggested by Kadyi's original illustration (Fig. 88-28). The prominence of the LCSA in the upper cervical region above the level of the

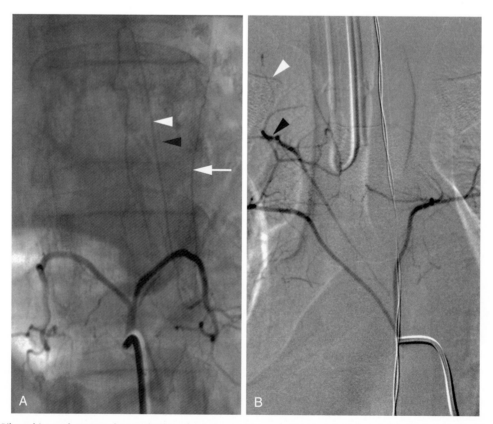

FIGURE 88-17. Bilateral internal segmental artery (ISA) trunks. **A** documents a common trunk for left and right L1. Left L1 provides prominent anterior *(white arrowhead)* and posterior *(black arrowhead)* spinal contributors, as well as adrenal branch *(white arrow)*. In **B**, a common trunk for left and right T4 is shown. In this 12-year-old girl, common trunks for T6 and T7 were observed as well. Note collateral opacification of right T3 *(black arrowhead)* and T2 *(white arrowhead)*. *(©2012, Philippe Gailloud, MD.)*

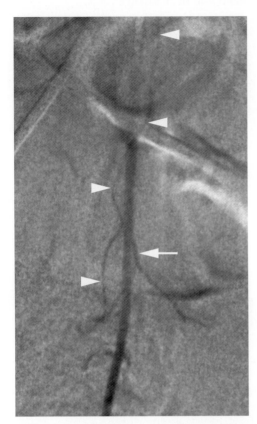

FIGURE 88-18. Bilateral S1 trunk from the median sacral artery (MSA). The trunk includes a short common stem *(arrow)*, separate from the MSA itself, which divides into left and right S1 branches. Note a prominent ASA contributor from right S1 *(arrowheads)*. Compare with Figure 88-5, *B,* in which normal L4 and L5 internal segmental arteries (ISAs) arise separately from the MSA. *(©2012, Philippe Gailloud, MD.)*

brachial plexus, where the amount of white matter is the largest, appears consistent with a metabolic adaptation (Fig. 88-29, *A*). The LCSA, implicated in the formation of several vertebrobasilar variations,[42] can be difficult to distinguish angiographically from the posterior ascending artery of the odontoid process (Fig. 88-29, *B*).

The anterolateral chain of Kadyi, now named the *lumbosacral anterolateral spinal artery* (LALSA), courses behind the line of emergence of the anterior lumbosacral nerve roots[40] (see Fig. 88-22, *D*). The LALSA is made of anastomotic connections linking small lateral branches coming from the ASA itself or, more often, from the proximal portion of the sulcal arteries.[40] Besides vascularizing the underlying white matter, the LALSA supplies the proximal portion of the anterior nerve roots of the cauda equina ("true radicular arteries").[40] For Parke's group, the distance separating the ASA from the anterior nerve roots explains the presence of this secondary anterolateral chain. Finally, the lateral spinal arteries (LSA) are two constant chains extending over the entire length of the spinal cord, alternatively in front or behind the line of attachment of the dentate ligament or on either side simultaneously[40] (see Fig. 88-22, *C-D*). The LSA, equivalent to the *chaînes latérales* (lateral chains) mentioned by Corbin,[39] supply the underlying lateral funiculus.[40]

Radicular Arteries

The primary longitudinal chains initially receive contributions from each ISA; the blood supply of the embryonic spinal cord is therefore ubiquitous. Later, the vascularization depends on a reduced number of radicular arteries (8 anterior and 16 posterior radicular branches on average,

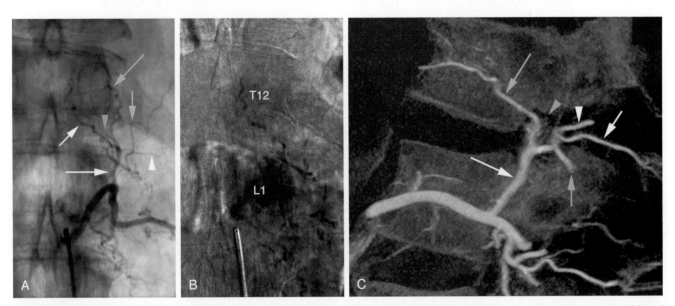

FIGURE 88-19. Complete ipsilateral trunk for L1 and T12. **A** shows left L1 injection, with concomitant opacification of various structures at T12: (1) branch running anteriorly along lateral aspect of T12 vertebral body *(long gray arrow)*, corresponding to left T12 stem; (2) left T12 dorsal branch with its musculocutaneous arteries *(short white arrow)*; (3) left T12 spinal branch *(gray arrowhead)*; and (4), small lateral branch (i.e., left subcostal artery) *(white arrowhead)*. These branches form a complete left T12 internal segmental artery (ISA), opacified via robust posterior laterovertebral anastomosis *(long white arrow)* that continues as inferior phrenic artery *(short gray arrow)*. **B,** Capillary phase of injection, with parameters set to emphasize complete hemivertebral blushes at L1 and T12. **C,** Sagittal flat-panel catheter angiotomography reconstruction confirms presence of complete T12 ISA, with its four components: stem *(long gray arrow)*, spinal branch *(gray arrowhead)*, dorsal branch *(short white arrow)*, and lateral branch *(white arrowhead)*, opacified by posterior laterovertebral anastomosis *(long white arrow)*. *(©2012, Philippe Gailloud, MD.)*

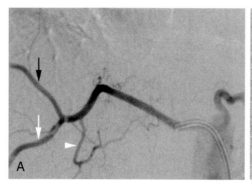
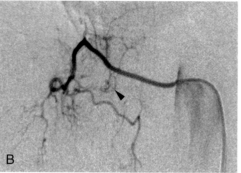

FIGURE 88-20. Incomplete ipsilateral trunk with isolated dorsospinal artery (DA) at right T10. **A** documents ipsilateral trunk for right T11 and T10, which includes lateral branches for both T10 and T11 *(white and black arrows)*, but a DA at T11 only *(white arrowhead)*. This incomplete trunk warrants search for an isolated DA at T10, shown in **B**, with its dorsal and spinal components, including medial, intermediate, and lateral muscular branches, as well as a visible retrocorporeal artery *(black arrowhead)*. *(©2012, Philippe Gailloud, MD.)*

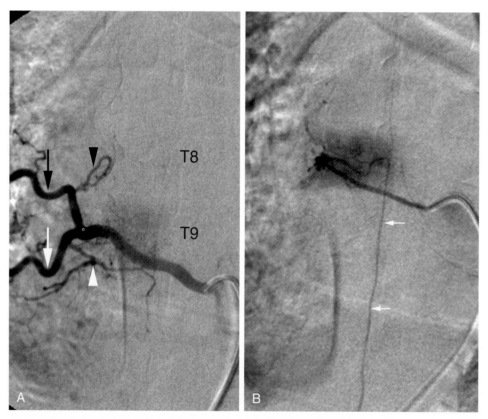

FIGURE 88-21. Incomplete ipsilateral trunk with isolated spinal artery at right T8. **A** shows ipsilateral trunk for right T9 and T8, which includes lateral branches for both T9 and T8 *(white and black arrows)* and a dorsospinal artery at T9 *(white arrowhead)* but only a dorsal branch at T8 *(black arrowhead)*. Although this variant simulates a complete ipsilateral trunk, absence of a hemivertebral blush at T8 while one is clearly seen at T9 strongly suggests an incomplete type. **B,** Injection of diminutive right T8 internal segmental artery (ISA) that only consists of stem with spinal branch, the latter providing artery of Adamkiewicz *(small arrows)*. This configuration represents ISA in its simplest form, equivalent to embryonic ISA (see Fig. 88-1, *C*). *(©2012, Philippe Gailloud, MD.)*

according to Kadyi[12]), a process resulting in large part from a vascular adaptation to the metabolic demand of the gray masses forming the cervical and lumbosacral enlargements.[45] The adult configuration of the longitudinal chains and their radicular contributors reflects a combination of this adaptive mechanism, with the apparent ascent of the conus medullaris within the spinal canal resulting from the differential growth of the spinal cord and vertebral column and from regression of the coccygeal segment of the cord[46] (Fig. 88-30).

The marked predominance of the arteries of the cervical and lumbosacral enlargements at the adult stage has been emphasized.[12,45,47-50] However, it must be remembered that any ISA can participate in the spinal cord supply under

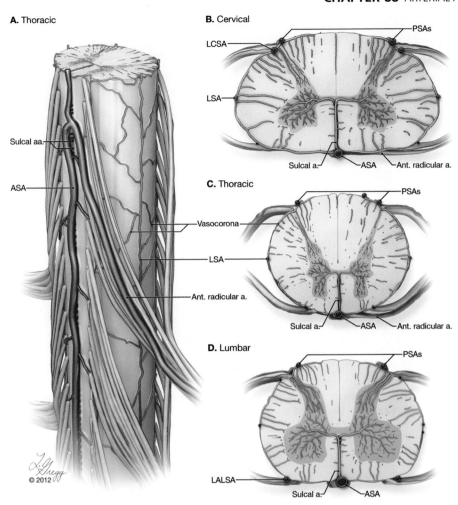

FIGURE 88-22. *Left,* Primary and secondary longitudinal chains and their "meshlike" interconnections. *Right,* Chains are illustrated at cervical *(B),* thoracic *(C),* and lumbar levels *(D).* Lateral spinal artery *(LSA)* is small but can be seen throughout cord. Lateral cervical spinal artery *(LCSA)* and lumbosacral anterolateral spinal artery *(LALSA)* are prominent at cervical and lumbar levels, respectively. *ASA,* Anterior spinal artery; *PSAs,* posterior spinal arteries. *(©2012, Lydia Gregg, CMI.)*

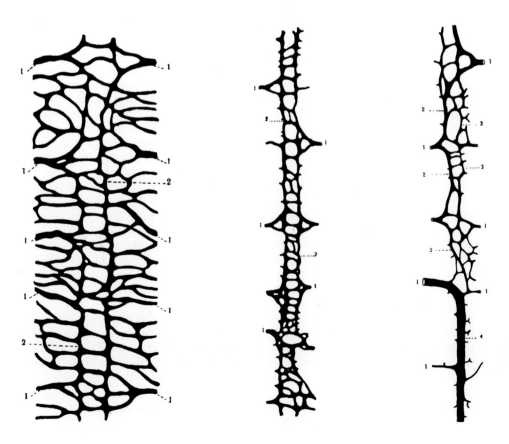

FIGURE 88-23. Development of anterior spinal artery (ASA) in the ox. *Left (9.5-mm embryo),* Two primitive anterolateral chains *(2)* linked by numerous transverse anastomoses and supplied by numerous anterior radicular rami *(1). Center,* Consolidation of rami into anterior radicular arteries (12.5-mm embryo). *Right (20.5-mm embryo),* ASA has reached its adult configuration caudally *(4)* but network is still apparent cranially, where early differentiation of ASA *(2)* and ongoing involution of a segment of primitive anterolateral chain *(3)* can be observed. *(From Sterzi G. Die blutgefässe des rückenmarks. Untersuchungen über ihre vergleichende anatomie und entwickelungsgeschichte. Anat Hefte 1904;24:1–364.)*

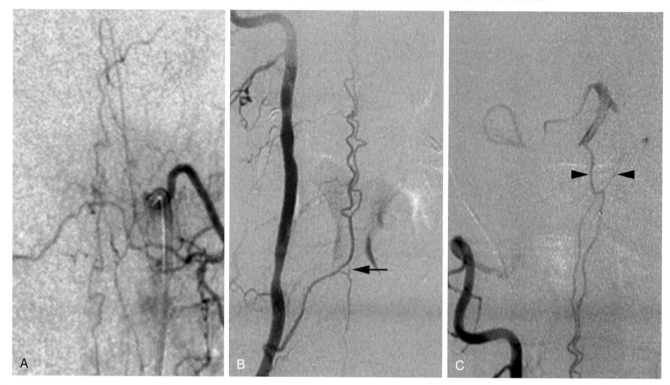

FIGURE 88-24. Tortuosity, fenestration, duplication of anterior spinal artery (ASA). **A,** Normal but tortuous segment of ASA. Cervical **(B)** and cranial **(C)** projections of right vertebral artery (VA) injection in patient with critical V4-segment stenosis. ASA, which here serves as collateral pathway for basilar artery, is duplicated from C5 up to connection with its vertebral roots *(arrowheads in C)*. Note small fenestration at point of bifurcation of artery of cervical enlargement *(arrow in B)*. *(©2012, Philippe Gailloud, MD.)*

normal or pathologic conditions[51] (Fig. 88-31). The principal ASA contributor was named *arteria spinalis magna* by Adamkiewicz,[47] *arteria radicularis magna* by Kadyi,[12] and *artery of the lumbosacral enlargement* by Tanon.[45] This vessel, commonly referred to as the *artery of Adamkiewicz*, is typically found between T8 and L1, with a left-sided prevalence.[49,50] In a recent evaluation of 302 consecutive spinal angiograms, 294 arteries of Adamkiewicz were identified between T6 and L4; 169 (53.0%) were located between T9 and L1 on the left side, and 53 (16.7%) on the right.[52]

The artery of the cervical enlargement usually originates from one of the VAs or costocervical trunks. The distal V3 and V4 segments of the VA correspond to the radicular artery of C1.[12,34,53] As any radicular artery, it divides into anterior and posterior radicular branches, each giving ascending and descending rami. Anteriorly, the left and right ascending rami form the basilar artery, while the descending rami constitute the cranialmost segment of the ASA.[34] As Charpy suggested, the basilar artery can be seen as the intracranial continuation of the ASA.[34] The vertebral roots of the ASA vary in size and origin. One may be absent, one or both can arise from a transverse anastomosis linking the V4 segments, or a single trunk may originate from the angle of junction of the VAs; occasionally, two roots come from the same V4 segment, with or without an additional root from the contralateral VA.[54] The descending rami of the posterior radicular arteries of C1 constitute the vertebral origins of the PSAs, while the ascending rami supply the dorsal aspect of the medulla and establish small connections between the PSAs and the posterior inferior cerebellar arteries (PICA).[43] When this

latter anastomosis prevails, the PSA appears to originate from the PICA.[43] Stopford found this PICA origin to be dominant[54]; for other authors, the PSA most often comes from the VA itself, usually proximally to its passage through the dura.[37,43]

A smaller spinal contributor, illustrated by von Haller in 1754,[55] is almost constantly found at the upper thoracic level, most commonly at or around T5 on the left side. This radicular branch is of particular concern during embolization of upper intercostal or intercostobronchial arteries (Fig. 88-32). Again, it is crucial to remember that contributors to the anterior and posterior spinal chains may exist at any vertebral level, including the small intersegmental branches stemming from the MSA (see Fig. 88-18). The left-sided prevalence of thoracic and lumbar spinal contributors, the artery of Adamkiewicz in particular, appears to be related to geometric factors (selection of the shortest path). Hassler found radicular arteries to be "more common on the left side, especially at the levels at which the aorta was situated distinctly to the left of the midline."[56] On the other hand, no correlation was found between ISA diameters and the likelihood to provide a significant spinal contributor.[57]

Anterior and posterior spinal contributors are usually easily distinguished (Fig. 88-33). Yet spinal cord edema, external compression, or vertebral rotation may at times render the distinction difficult or impossible in the antero-posterior angiographic projection. The term *artery of Lazorthes* is used for a radicular artery that provides significant contributors to both the anterior and posterior spinal chains[36] (see Fig. 88-10).

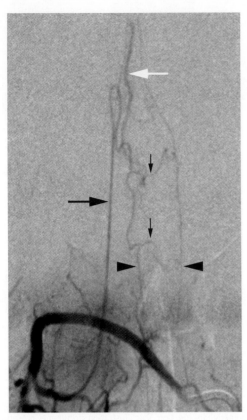

FIGURE 88-25. Posterior spinal network. Posterior spinal arteries (PSAs) are more irregular than anterior spinal arteries (ASAs). Combination of pronounced tortuosity, caliber changes, and transverse interconnections results in network-like morphology. Right L1 angiogram shows prominent posterior contributor *(black arrow)* that opacifies both PSAs *(arrowheads)* through multiple transverse anastomoses *(small arrows)*. Note visualization of short segment of ASA *(white arrow)* through small PSA-to-ASA anastomosis. *(©2012, Philippe Gailloud, MD.)*

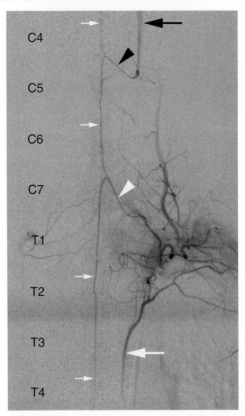

FIGURE 88-26. Artery of cervical enlargement and continuity of anterior spinal axis. Selective injection of left supreme intercostal artery *(left T1)* originating from subclavian artery. Anterior spinal artery (ASA) *(small arrows)* receives two prominent contributions, one from supreme intercostal artery at C7/T1 *(white arrowhead)*, second from left vertebral artery (VA) at C4/C5 *(black arrowhead)*. VA is faintly opacified retrogradely *(black arrow)*. This illustrates two possible origins of artery of cervical enlargement, as well as continuity of ASA across cervicothoracic region. Note also retrograde opacification of left T2 *(white arrow)* through small collaterals. *(©2012, Philippe Gailloud, MD.)*

INTRINSIC ARTERIAL VASCULARIZATION

Adamkiewicz divided the intrinsic arterial vascularization of the cord into centrifugal (or central) and centripetal (or peripheral) systems.[38] The central system depends upon the sulcal arteries stemming from the ASA. The peripheral system is supplied by the PSAs, the secondary longitudinal chains (LCSA, LSA, LALSA), and the network linking these chains, the pial arterial plexus or vasocorona.[38] The territories of the central and peripheral systems overlap to create a narrow intermediate zone of joint supply.[58] Although the two systems are connected through the intramedullary capillary network, the penetrating arteries are considered from a functional standpoint as end arteries.[33] The ability of the pial network to function as a source of collateral supply is limited.[33]

The sulcal arteries stem from the dorsal aspect of the ASA and course within the anteromedian fissure, in the depth of which they divide into the sulcocommissural arteries.[38] The distribution of the sulcal arteries has classically been considered strictly unilateral, aiming alternatively to the left or right side of the cord.[12,59] Although this fact generally remains valid, short common trunks branching

off paired bilateral sulcocommissural branches are not infrequent.[56] The prevalent location of these trunks, which divide in the sagittal plane, remains controversial (lumbosacral for Hassler,[56] cervical and thoracic for Zhang et al.[60]); sulcal trunks providing several ipsilateral branches are less frequent.[60] The sulcal arteries have thus been organized into three types: type 1, undivided unilateral supply; type 2, branched bilateral supply; and type 3, branched unilateral supply.[60] Unsurprisingly, sulcal arteries originating from a duplicated segment of the ASA supply only the corresponding side of the spinal cord.[58] The complex anatomy of the intrinsic vascularization, the unpredictability of the spinal cord collateral supply, and the variety of potential injury sites along the spinal arterial tree from the aorta to the sulcal arteries account for the proteiform nature of medullary ischemic disease. Thus, a focal injury to an artery of Lazorthes can lead to a clinical picture of cord transection in an elderly patient, while the same lesion in a child may remain asymptomatic. The density of sulcal arteries per unit of length is higher in the lumbosacral cord than in the cervical or thoracic cord.[28,48,56,60] Hassler counted 3 to 8 sulcal arteries per centimeter in the cervical cord, 2 to 6 in the

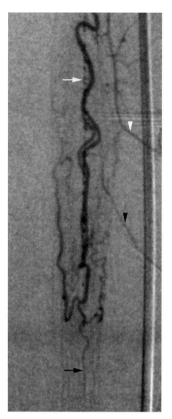

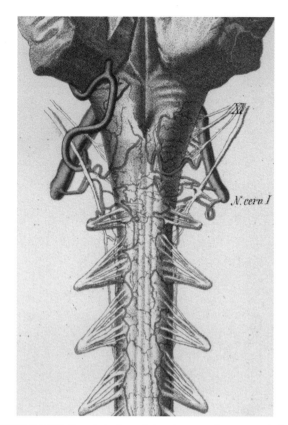

FIGURE 88-27. Terminal loop and artery of filum terminale. Termination of anterior spinal artery (ASA) and its connection with both posterior spinal arteries (PSAs) (i.e., terminal loop) is well seen in this angiogram. Note continuation of ASA as artery of filum terminale *(small black arrow)*, paralleled by multiple small arterial branches accompanying nerve of cauda equina. Prominence of sulcal arteries *(small white arrow)*, imaged here along their anteroposterior axis and therefore projecting along midline as small dots, is unusual; these branches are typically not seen in a normal spinal angiogram.[49] Small anterior *(black arrowhead)* and posterior *(white arrowhead)* contributors are opacified retrogradely. *(©2012, Philippe Gailloud, MD.)*

FIGURE 88-28. Vascularization of dorsal aspect of upper cervical cord and cervicomedullary junction. This illustration documents presence of longitudinal spinal chains in front (lateral cervical spinal artery) as well as behind (posterior spinal artery) dorsal nerve roots of C1, C2, and C3. Both trunks show caliber variations and multiple anastomotic connections; their respective sizes seem inversely proportional. *(Modified from Kadyi H. Über die Blutgefässe des Menschlichen Rückenmarkes. Lemberg, Poland: Gubryonowisz & Schmidt; 1889.)*

FIGURE 88-29. Longitudinal spinal axes at cervical level. **A,** Anteroposterior projection of left vertebral artery angiogram shows well-developed lateral cervical spinal artery *(short black arrows)* extending from V4 segment down to C6. Anterior spinal artery *(short white arrows)* and left posterior spinal artery *(white arrowheads)* are clearly opacified below C4 but only faintly apparent above. Long black arrow points at posterior-inferior cerebellar artery of low origin (variant of lateral spinal system[42]), and black arrowhead shows apical arcade. **B,** Lateral view depicts anterior *(long white arrow)* and posterior *(short white arrow)* ascending arteries of axis, as well as apical arcade *(black arrowhead)*. *(©2012, Philippe Gailloud, MD.)*

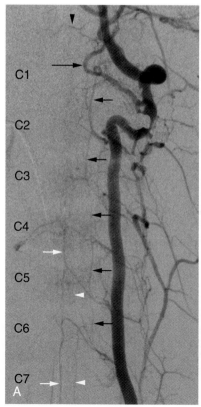

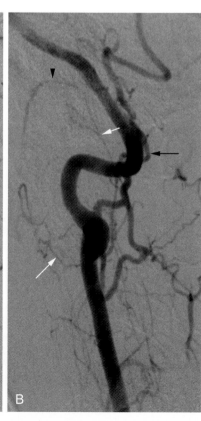

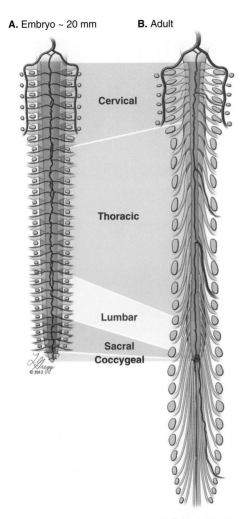

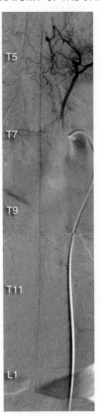

FIGURE 88-31. T5 origin of artery of Adamkiewicz. Early (top half) and late (bottom half) arterial phases of this left T5 injection have been combined to show the only anterior spinal contributor in this 54-year-old patient, with opacification of anterior spinal artery between T4 and L1. *(©2012, Philippe Gailloud, MD.)*

FIGURE 88-30. Functional adaptation and adult morphology of spinal cord supply. Initially, spinal cord fills entire length of spinal canal *(A. Embryo).* As embryo grows, spinal cord elongates proportionally less than spine; conus medullaris ends at about L1/L2 in full-term neonate, and T12/L1 at adult stage[68] *(B. Adult).* This apparent spinal cord shortening is responsible for development of cauda equina and increasingly sharper caudocranial course of radicular arteries, which parallel nerve roots from cervical to lumbosacral regions. Spinal cord segments also grow at different rates. More pronounced stretching of thoracic cord influences distribution and morphology of sulcal arteries, and ultimately sensitivity of this segment to ischemic injuries. *(©2012, Lydia Gregg, CMI.)*

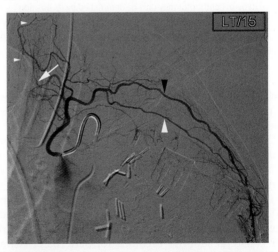

FIGURE 88-32. Upper thoracic spinal contributor. Left T3 injection in patient with hemoptysis after left upper lobectomy shows distal contrast extravasation from both T3 posterior intercostal artery *(black arrowhead)* and its supracostal branch for fourth rib *(white arrowhead).* Most critical finding of this angiogram is detection of anterior spinal contributor *(white arrow)* supplying anterior spinal artery *(small white arrowheads).* Great care must be taken in identifying such branches during endovascular procedures in upper thoracic region. It should also be remembered that flow pattern alterations resulting from ongoing embolization can render dangerous branches more conspicuous, or even reveal dangerous collateral pathways initially not detectable.[69] Iterative control injections through guiding catheter help reduce risk of untoward passage of embolization material into undetected spinal contributors. *(©2012, Philippe Gailloud, MD; and courtesy Kelvin Hong, MD, Interventional Radiology Center, Johns Hopkins Hospital, Baltimore, Maryland.)*

thoracic cord, 5 to 12 in the lumbar cord, and 5 to 11 in the upper sacral cord.[56] These variations are consistent with the fact that although the number of sulcal arteries remains fixed in each cord segment, the thoracic segment—and to a lesser extent the cervical one—are subjected to a more pronounced elongation that results in increased spacing between their perforating branches.[36] For the same reason, cervical and thoracic sulcal branches tend to have an oblique course rather than the transverse disposition seen in the lumbar and sacral regions.[56,60,61] The distance separating significant radicular contributors is also greater at the thoracic level.[61] Hassler noted that thoracic sulcal arteries have a smaller diameter, but their ascending and descending terminal rami cover longer longitudinal distances within the anteromedian fissure (more noticeably in taller subjects). These features offer an anatomic substrate to the increased

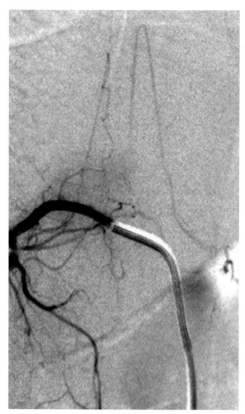

FIGURE 88-33. Angiogram showing direct opacification of a right posterior contributor and simultaneous visualization of a contralateral anterior contributor. Note tighter curve, more tortuous course, and paramedian position of posterior contributor, and more opened curve, smoother course, and median position of anterior one. These features are not always as pronounced; type of contributor may only be determined by its position in regard to midline (see Fig. 88-10). If only one contributor is present, x-ray tube angulation becomes critical; any obliquity in projection may prevent definite identification. (©2012, Philippe Gailloud, MD.)

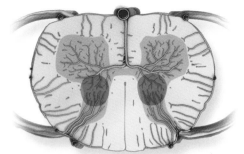

A. Watershed stroke

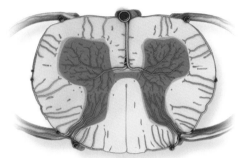

B. Gray matter stroke

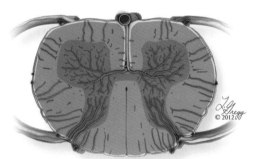

C. Whole cord stroke

sensitivity of the thoracic spinal cord to ischemia, despite the near-constant presence of an ASA contributor in the upper thoracic region.[56,59,61]

Zhang et al. found that branches of the sulcocommissural arteries rarely extend beyond the gray matter, in particular at the lumbosacral level.[60] This characteristic, combined with the selective sensitivity of the spinal gray matter to ischemia, lack of functionally significant intramedullary anastomoses between the superficial and deep systems, and limited ability of the pial arterial network to offer collateral supply,[33] accounts for patterns of ischemic injury limited to the gray matter (Fig. 88-34).

Anatomic Intersegmental Stenoses

Proximal ISA stenoses produced by a specific anatomic configuration are seen in the upper lumbar and left upper thoracic regions. At the lumbar level, compression results from passage of the ISA through the tendinous portion of the diaphragmatic crus.[62] The most commonly involved branches are L1 and L2 on the right and L1 on the left; less often, T12 or L3. Spinal cord ischemia may occur when the compressed vessel provides a spinal artery contributor (Fig. 88-35).[63]

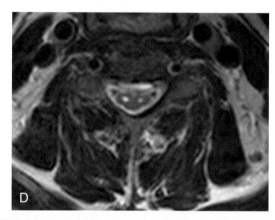

FIGURE 88-34. Variability of spinal cord ischemic injuries. Combination of multiple potential injury sites with ill-predictable collateral supply accounts for variability of spinal ischemic injuries, including limited "watershed-like" infarcts likely involving base of posterior column (**A**), whole gray matter infarcts (**B**), or whole-cord "transection-like" lesions (**C**). **D**, Magnetic resonance imaging manifestation of selective ischemic injury to spinal cord (axial T2-weighted image), with typical "snake-eyes" appearance.[70] (**A-C** ©2012, Lydia Gregg, CMI; **D** (©2012, Philippe Gailloud, MD.)

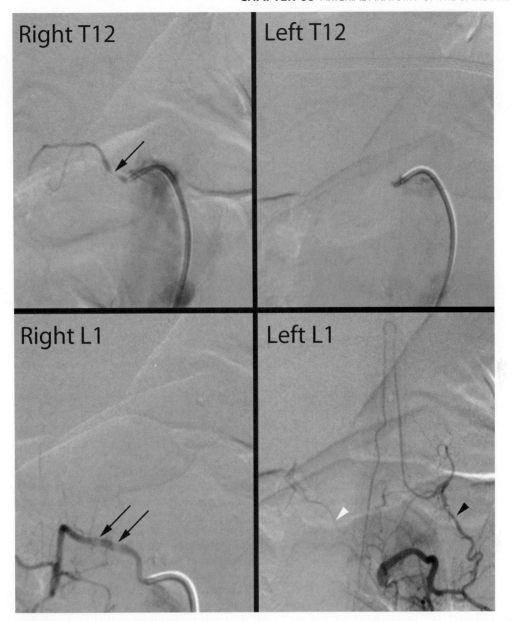

FIGURE 88-35. Lumbar internal segmental artery (ISA) compression by crus of diaphragm. Note typical appearance of compression by diaphragmatic crus at right T12 and L1 *(arrows)*. Left T12, which was originally providing artery of lumbosacral enlargement (artery of Lazorthes), is occluded. Spinal cord supply has been taken over by left L1 via a prominent laterovertebral anastomosis *(black arrowhead)*. Left L1 also provides collateral supply to left T12 via retrocorporeal anastomotic network *(white arrowhead)*. *(©2012, Philippe Gailloud, MD.)*

The second type of "anatomic stenosis" involves the left upper thoracic ISAs, most commonly between T3 and T6, with a frequency of about 25%.[64] In this case, the narrowing appears to derive from the combination of the recurrent proximal course of the upper left thoracic ISAs, related to the leftward position of the aorta at that level, with the fixed passage of the ISAs behind the reinforced medial edge of the endothoracic fascia (Fig. 88-36).[64] In its most pronounced form, the kinked segment can be severely narrowed or occluded. Medullary ischemia may occur when the involved ISA contributes significantly to the cord supply. In that regard, the near-constant presence of an ASA contributor in the upper thoracic region may play a role in the apparent sensitivity of the thoracic cord to ischemia.

SPINAL ANGIOGRAPHY

SpDSA is the gold-standard imaging technique for evaluating spinal vascular disorders. Its safety and accuracy have been enhanced by improved equipment (softer diagnostic catheters, safer contrast agents, better angiography suites) and introduction of new angiography techniques such as flat-panel catheter angiotomography (FPCA) (see Fig. 88-4, for example).[65] In spite of the negative reputation it inherited from its early days, SpDSA is safe when performed by adequately trained angiographers and does not expose patients to large doses of radiation or contrast agent. It is routinely performed under conscious sedation, with the exception of children and patients unable to

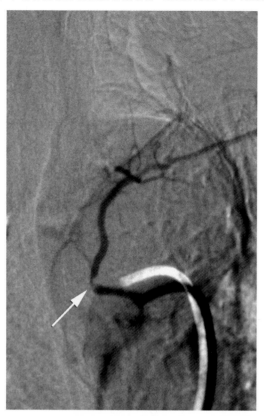

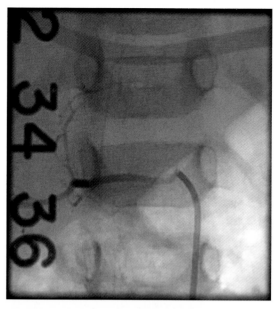

FIGURE 88-37. Use of a ruler, tight collimation, and dose reduction. Unsubtracted image of a right L1 angiogram in a child documents use of ruler to identify investigated vertebral level and tight positioning of collimators. Image was obtained with a dose per frame of 1.82 µGy (standard dose 3.6 µGy). A posterior spinal contributor is seen. (©2012, Philippe Gailloud, MD.)

FIGURE 88-36. Upper left thoracic internal segmental artery (ISA) kink. Left T4 angiogram shows typical appearance of upper thoracic kink, with moderate stenosis *(white arrow)*. Kink occurs as artery turns around medial edge of endothoracic fascia, which is fixed to lateral aspect of vertebral column. Recurrent course of ISAs and their sharp bends are accentuated by lateral deviation of upper thoracic aorta. (©2012, Philippe Gailloud, MD.)

cooperate or lie flat. SpDSA carries extremely low risk of complications.[52]

Basic Spinal Digital Subtraction Angiography Principles

The first part of the procedure consists in carefully labeling the vertebral levels using a radiopaque ruler (Fig. 88-37). The value corresponding to each vertebra is reported on a dedicated sheet on which progression of the study will be documented. This routine prevents losing track of the levels investigated during the procedure, which is time consuming, increases fluoroscopy time, and carries the risk of overlooking or mislabeling an ISA. To reduce radiation exposure to patients and operators, a high angiography table position, short patient-detector distance, and tight collimation are used, while fast frame rates are avoided. High magnification factors and oblique views are associated with increased radiation doses. We routinely perform SpDSA with fluoroscopy rates of 2 or 3 pulse/s. Runs are acquired with a variable frame rate technique (2 f/s for 4 seconds, followed by 1 f/s). The dose per frame is adapted to patients' morphologic characteristics. We are routinely using low-dose protocols, most commonly

a dose of 2.4 µGy/f (1.82 µGy/f for pediatric patients) and only occasionally the standard dose of 3.6 µGy/f (see Fig. 88-37). The choice of catheters depends in part, as for any angiographic procedure, on operators' experience and preferences. A Cobra 2 shape is used for most selective ISA catheterization, supplemented at times by a Simmons-1 or Mickelson. For therapeutic procedures, the shape of the guide is chosen on a case-by-case basis to match the morphology of the targeted ISA. For example, MPA catheters may be useful for right thoracic arteries, whereas Simmons or Mickelson catheters work well for lumbar ISAs with a sharp caudal course. Contrast is injected by hand using a 20-mL syringe. Patients receive a bolus dose of heparin after arterial access is obtained, usually 3000 units (or 50 units/kg in children). Complete spinal angiography includes a pelvic flush angiogram supplemented by selective injections of the internal iliac arteries; an aortic arch injection (anteroposterior projection) is performed at times (although infrequently in our current practice). Thoracic or lumbar aortograms, of very limited value, are not routinely performed. Selective injections of the subclavian arteries and their branches (VAs, costocervical, and thyrocervical trunks) are obtained as well. Although these vessels are usually investigated last, it may be advantageous to start with them and include carotid angiograms when one suspects a posterior fossa or skull-base vascular anomaly (e.g., in the presence of cervical myelopathy). The following principles simplify performing SpDSA:

- Selective injections of ISAs can provoke discomfort and sometimes a painful burning sensation (particularly in smaller ISAs). Adding heparinized saline to the contrast agent (5 mL of saline for 15 mL of contrast) helps prevent discomfort.

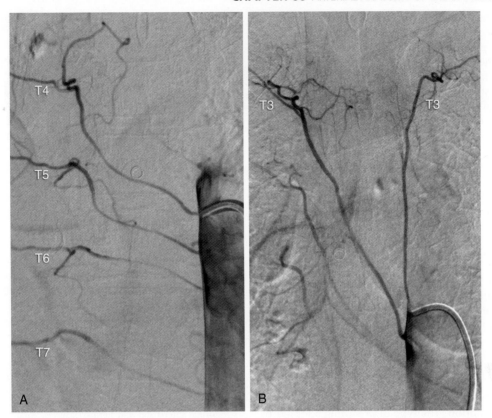

FIGURE 88-38. Distribution of intersegmental ostia. **A,** Internal segmental arteries (ISAs) are aligned craniocaudally, but with irregular interostial distances. T4 injection documents origin of three other intercostal arteries by reflux, showing their uneven distribution. **B,** Likewise, origins for left and right ISAs of a given level are often asymmetric. *(©2012, Philippe Gailloud, MD.)*

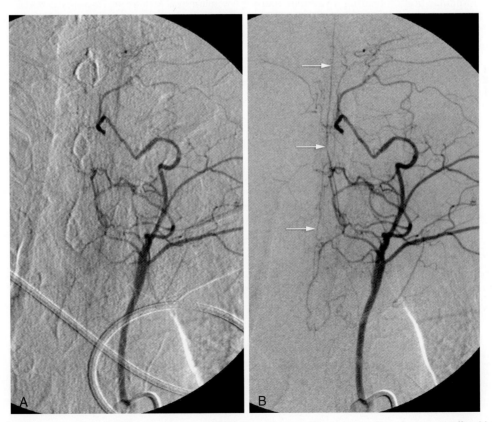

FIGURE 88-39. Mask selection and pixel shifting. Angiogram of left T2-T3 trunk exemplifies image quality enhancement offered by modern electronic image correction. **A,** Image quality suffers from significant motion artifact. **B,** After remasking and pixel shifting, a previously undetected spinal contributor is documented *(arrows)*. *(©2012, Philippe Gailloud, MD.)*

- Patients being studied under general anesthesia must be paralyzed so ventilation can be briefly interrupted during each selective ISA injection.
- Adopt a catheterization routine that keeps studies systematic and fast. We generally study one side at a time, proceeding in a craniocaudal direction by moving from one ISA ostium to the next. This approach is consistent with the anatomy of the ISAs, which are distributed along a longitudinal axis but with varying interostial distances and left-to-right asymmetry (Fig. 88-38).
- Avoid (as much as possible) seeking vessels' ostia by puffing contrast agent, a practice that significantly increases the load of contrast material. Instead, a little experience will help in recognizing that a vessel is selectively engaged by visualizing a slight deflection of the catheter tip. Similarly, once an ISA is selected, resist the urge to check the catheter tip position by injecting contrast. The catheter may temporarily impair flow within small ISAs, resulting in contrast stagnation. If flow is compromised, gently pull the catheter back during the angiographic run to adequately study the selected ISA.

Technical Pitfalls

SpDSA is sensitive to patient-related artifacts such as respiratory or bowel motion. The type of breathing adopted by the patient during the angiographic run, for example Valsalva versus simple breath hold, can result in significant hemodynamic alterations. A small spinal contributor coming from the radicular branch feeding a vascular malformation may be apparent or not, depending on the breathing mode.[66] Bowel-motion artifacts can be decreased by administration of an antiperistaltic agent (e.g., 1 mg glucagon). Motion artifacts can to some extent be reduced with electronic correction methods such as mask selection and pixel shifting. The importance of these methods cannot be emphasized enough, in particular when planning an endovascular procedure (Fig. 88-39).

<hr>

KEY POINTS

- The arterial vascularization of the spine and spinal cord shows an intersegmental pattern inherited from the fetal architecture.
- The presence of a few dominant radicular arteries at the adult stage (in particular, the artery of Adamkiewicz) results from a vascular adaptation to the metabolic need of the gray matter masses forming the cervical and lumbar enlargements of the spinal cord.
- Any intersegmental artery can contribute to spinal cord vascularization or feed a vascular malformation. To be complete, a spinal angiogram must therefore address the whole series of intersegmental branches, including the pelvic and cervical arteries.
- Contributors to the anterior and posterior spinal arteries often originate from branches such as the thyrocervical or intercostobronchial trunks. To avoid spinal cord injuries, extreme care must be taken when evaluating such branches for transarterial embolization procedures.

<hr>

▶ **SUGGESTED READINGS**

Chen J, Gailloud P. Safety of spinal angiography: complication rate analysis in 302 diagnostic angiograms. Neurology 2011;77:1235–40.

Chiras J, Morvan G, Merland JJ. The angiographic appearances of the normal intercostal and lumbar arteries. Analysis and the anatomic correlation of the lateral branches. [Article in English, French] J Neuroradiol 1979;6:169–96.

Herren RY, Alexander L. Sulcal and intrinsic blood vessels of the human spinal cord. Arch Neurol Psychiatry 1939;41:678–87.

Parke WW, Settles HE, Bunger PC, et al. Lumbosacral anterolateral spinal arteries and brief review of "accessory" longitudinal arteries of the spinal cord. Clin Anat 1999;12:171–8.

Zhang Z-A, Nonaka H, Hatori T. The microvasculature of the spinal cord in the human adult. Neuropathology 1997;17:132–42.

The complete reference list is available online at www.expertconsult.com.

CHAPTER 89
Use of Skull Views in Visualization of Cerebral Vascular Anatomy

M. Reza Taheri, Wendy A. Cohen, Basavaraj V. Ghodke, Danial K. Hallam, and Kathleen R. Fink

Selective catheter-guided digital subtraction angiography (DSA) remains a critical step in the characterization and treatment of intracranial aneurysms, vascular malformations, vasospasm, vascular injury, vasculitis, and arterial/venous occlusive disease. It also provides clear visualization of the vascular supply of intracranial masses. DSA offers unique information about vascular pathology, including high spatial resolution, selective vascular characterization, and the ability to evaluate hemodynamics. Neurologic complications of angiography are rare but are more likely to occur in patients of advanced age and with prolonged procedure time.[1] An understanding of the technical components of the procedure, along with a knowledge of basic vascular anatomy and relevant bony landmarks improve visualization of certain pathologies and decrease potential complications.

There are no absolute contraindications for this procedure,[2] but relative contraindications include coagulopathy, renal insufficiency, history of significant allergic reaction to iodinated contrast, severe hypertension, hypotension, and congestive heart failure. For these reasons, laboratory workup may include measurements of coagulation parameters, creatinine, hemoglobin, platelet count, and electrolytes. Risks inherent in this procedure include a roughly 1% chance of neurologic complications such as stroke,[1] bleeding at the puncture site, vascular injury, potential allergic reaction to the iodinated contrast medium, and the risk associated with radiation exposure. The emphasis on these factors can be modulated based on the cross-sectional imaging appearance of the vasculature, as available.

The arterial puncture site (not the skin puncture site) must be below the inguinal ligament.[3] Once the catheter is introduced into the femoral artery, it is advanced to the descending thoracic aorta and double flushed. The arch is subsequently crossed and (depending on the specific pathology, vascular anatomy, and atherosclerotic burden) the common, external carotid, internal carotid, and vertebral arteries are selectively catheterized. Prior to injection, it is essential to position the patient and the image intensifier in such a way that the region or pathology of interest is ideally highlighted. Positioning is typically based on bony landmarks.

For a full range of angiographic skull views, please visit www.expertconsult.com. These user-friendly presentations illustrate specific vascular anatomies and relevant bony landmarks used to highlight certain regions. Common angiographic views of the intracranial vessels are described, along with descriptions and examples of normal and pathologic processes.

The complete reference list is available online at www.expertconsult.com.

CHAPTER 90

Cerebral Functional Anatomy and Rapid Neurologic Examination

Batya R. Radzik and Rafael H. Llinas

The role of interventional neuroradiology has expanded in the past decades as the safety of cerebral angiogram has improved. Not only is the use of diagnostic angiography increasing, the role of intervention in neurologic injury has increased dramatically as well. Angiography is not solely a means of diagnosis; an increasing number of interventions are now being used to treat injuries such as acute stroke, intracranial stenosis, cerebral aneurysms, and cerebral vasospasm through a variety of modalities including intraarterial medications, stents, and embolizations. Even though the safety of cerebral angiography and neurointerventional procedures has improved, the most common neurologic complication remains stroke. This chapter is designed to serve as a primer in clinical neurologic examination.

The literature reports various rates of complications from 0% to 28%[1]; however, the technology for cerebral angiography has gone through extensive improvement over the course of this time. Dion et al. found that in patients undergoing cerebral angiography for any cause, within the first 24 hours there was a 1.3% neurologic complication rate.[2] In the ischemic stroke/transient ischemic attack population there was a 4% neurologic complication rate, with 1% of those deficits being permanent.[1] Additionally, 23% of patients undergoing cerebral angiography were found to have silent infarctions on diffusion weighted imaging.[3] This is important when considering the overall disease burden a patient will accumulate.

The expanding role of the neurointerventionalist in the realm of diagnosis and treatment of patients with acute neurologic diseases requires that he or she the ability to perform a rapid and comprehensive neurologic assessment. All interventional radiologists are proficient at examination of the cerebrovascular system and any abnormalities therein. However, many are not versed in the most basic of neurologic exams to evaluate for complications arising from these procedures. Early detection of strokes can lead to rapid intervention and possible reversal of symptoms. The purpose of this chapter is twofold: to introduce a rapid neurologic examination that can be done by the interventionalist during and after the procedure to detect strokes, and to assist him or her in learning how to proceed in the event that a cerebrovascular event is suggested.

REVIEW OF CEREBRAL CIRCULATION

Knowledge of cerebral circulation at a physical and functional anatomic level is essential to the practitioner, whether performing a two- or four-vessel cerebral angiogram. It is critical to understand the flow of blood upstream from the location of injury. Knowledge of the functions of each of the cerebral hemispheres is essential in understanding the presenting symptoms and localizing the sites of any neurologic damage. Here we discuss the neurovascular anatomy and

functional neuroanatomy to make the reasons behind the focused neurologic examination more clear.

Neurovascular Anatomy

The anterior circulation is derived from the internal carotid arteries. The primary branches are the anterior cerebral artery (ACA) and the middle cerebral artery (MCA). The ACA supplies most of the anterior medial surface of the brain's cortex. The MCA divides into three major branches. The superior division supplies the frontal lobe cortex above the sylvian fissure and the perirolandic cortex. The MCA inferior division supplies the temporal and parietal lobe cortex behind the sylvian fissure. The MCA territory supplies most of the cortex on the dorsolateral convexity of the brain (Fig. 90-1).

The posterior circulation is derived from the vertebral arteries, which merge into the basilar artery and then form the posterior cerebral arteries (PCAs). The vertebral arteries are divided into four segments, of which the fourth segment is completely intracranial. The two vertebral arteries merge into the basilar artery at the pontomedullary junction. The basilar artery travels up to the pontomesencephalic junction, where it splits to form the PCAs. The basilar artery feeds the pons and midbrain through small perforator arteries. The PCA feeds the medial occipital cortex and medial temporal lobe. The vertebral arteries feed the cerebellum, specifically the posterior inferior cerebellar arteries (PICAs), and the basilar artery gives rise to the anterior inferior cerebellar arteries (AICAs) and the superior cerebellar arteries (SCAs) (Fig. 90-2).

Functional Anatomy

The cerebral hemispheres are each divided into four lobes. The frontal, parietal, temporal, and occipital lobes are each responsible for distinct functions. The frontal lobe directs eye movements, motor speech, and orientation. The parietal lobe controls speech and sensation. The temporal lobe is responsible for speech, and the occipital lobe is the primary visual center (Fig. 90-3).

The ACA supplies blood to the anterior frontal lobes and the superior parietal lobes. The superior MCA supplies the lateral portion of the frontal lobe. The inferior division supplies the lateral temporal lobe and a section of the parietal lobe. The PCA feeds the inferior and medial temporal lobe as well as the occipital lobe. The left and right sides of the brain are each responsible for different functions.

Left Middle Cerebral Artery Strokes

Given the different roles of the right and left MCA territories, we will be discussing right and left MCA stroke syndromes separately. It is useful to bear in mind that all the discussion regarding aphasias in left MCA strokes are

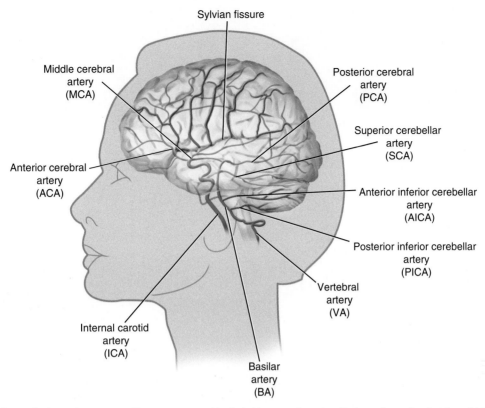

FIGURE 90-1. Cerebral vascular anatomy. Shown are areas of brain fed by named arteries. *(Redrawn from a handout from Bristol-Myers Squibb.)*

applicable in right-handed people; left-handed people may have their language centers in right MCA territory. Additionally, right MCA territory strokes may be much less apparent on a basic neurologic exam if there is no accompanying weakness because they tend to present as "neglects." The MCA divides into the superior, inferior, and deep territory branches.

Left MCA strokes that affect the superior division cause right-sided face and arm weakness and an expressive or nonfluent aphasia; occasionally the inability to move both eyes toward the weak side is also present. In right-handed people, Broca aphasia presents as an inability to speak or express language well, but with understanding intact. This is also true of written speech. A severe dysarthria and aphasia can be differentiated by the aphasic patient's inability to write. A person with severe dysarthria secondary to facial weakness will be able to read and write normally.

Left MCA inferior division strokes cause fluent aphasia, sensory loss on the same side, and a right visual field defect. In right-handed people, the fluent aphasic or receptive aphasic will speak fluent gibberish, making little sense. The basic lesion is one of comprehension. They are unable to "receive" information through speech. Therefore, if asked to perform a command or follow an instruction, they will be unable to understand. Such patients cannot be asked for consent for procedures. Never ask the patient to imitate when trying to determine a patient's ability to comprehend spoken language; this does not test language function. The visual problems will manifest as an inability to see objects on one side or another. It is important to remember that patients will often not realize they are unable to see or

attend to one side. A visual field cut is usually found on examination and not found as a result of a patient complaint.

Strokes affecting the deep territory cause a motor weakness (hemiparesis) involving the face, arm, and leg all on the same side. In the event the proximal left MCA is occluded, a patient will develop a stroke involving all three branches. This syndrome will combine all the symptoms with a right hemiplegia, hemianesthesia, homonymous hemianopia, and global aphasia (receptive and expressive) with a left gaze preference (Table 90-1).

Right Middle Cerebral Artery Strokes

Strokes of the right MCA superior division cause a left face and arm weakness and a left hemineglect. Neglects are a complex topic beyond the scope of this text. Patients with neglects ignore one half of the universe; they will not see you if you stand on the left (most commonly), and they may not respond if you speak to them from the left. They may eat only the right half of their food and may vehemently deny their own deficit. Right frontal stroke will also have forced gaze deviation away from the side of weakness, just like left MCA frontal strokes.

The right MCA inferior division causes a profound left hemineglect. Although frontal neglects can be subtle, right inferior division temporal parietal strokes result in profound neglects. There will be visual field loss and sensory loss (somatosensory deficits) owing to parietal and occipital lobe damage. The right MCA deep territory causes a pure left motor hemiparesis. A stroke of the right MCA stem combines all elements of any of the branch occlusions. Patients will have a left weakness (hemiplegia), sensory loss

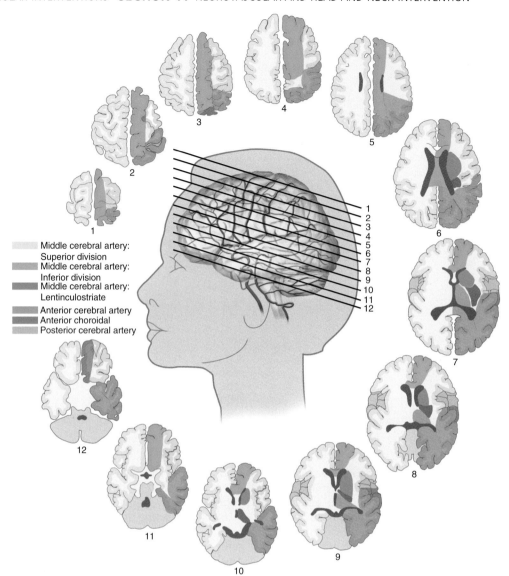

FIGURE 90-2. Vascular anatomy related to areas of brain. Occlusion of named arteries will present as complete or incomplete strokes in these vascular distributions. *(From Baird AE. Anterior circulation stroke. E-medicine. Available at* **http://www.emedicine.com/neuro/topic16.htm**. *Accessed 10-25-06.)*

(hemianesthesia), visual field loss (homonymous hemianopia), hemineglect, and a right gaze preference.

Anterior Cerebral Artery Strokes

Strokes of the ACA primarily affect the legs. A left ACA stroke will cause right leg and some arm weakness and sensory loss, but the leg is much more affected than the arm. It may also cause a grasp reflex, behavioral abnormalities, and transcortical aphasia. This form of aphasia is tricky, but it basically looks like an expressive or Broca aphasia, except the patient may be able to repeat normally. Right ACA strokes cause the same symptoms as left ACA strokes to the left side. The only difference is that instead of developing an aphasia, the patient tends to develop a left hemineglect.

Posterior Cerebral Artery Strokes

PCA strokes will primarily cause a visual field loss or homonymous hemianopia to the opposite side. This large

occipital or PCA stroke causes people to be "blind" on one side of the visual field. This is the most common symptom of a large occipital lesion or PCA stroke. Rarely, larger PCA strokes on the left side can cause an aphasia, right hemiparesis, and hemisensory loss. Larger right-sided strokes will cause a left hemiparesis and hemisensory loss. A PCA stem stroke will cause a hemiparesis, ocular motility disorder, and disturbances in consciousness, memory, and language. Bilateral strokes or lesions of the occipital lobe will lead to the patient appearing blind. Interestingly, such patients may not realize they are blind, and this is a fascinating syndrome referred to as *cortical blindness*. Patients with visual field loss may complain of hallucinations in the abnormal field. The complaint of visual hallucinations, especially only on one side after a procedure, should be followed by a basic assessment of visual field function. These lesions are extremely easy to miss if not tested for because patients often will not notice the visual field loss.

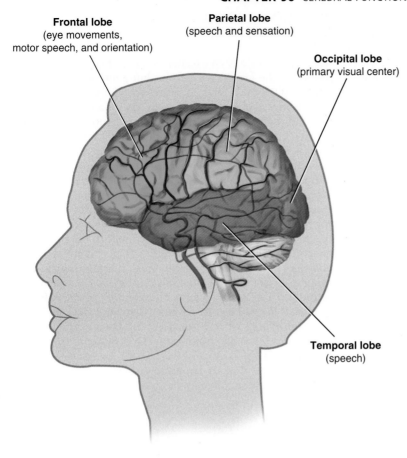

Frontal lobe
(eye movements,
motor speech, and orientation)

Parietal lobe
(speech and sensation)

Occipital lobe
(primary visual center)

Temporal lobe
(speech)

FIGURE 90-3. Frontal lobe *(green)*: eye movements, speech/motor, orientation, neglect. Temporal lobe *(purple)*: speech. Parietal lobe *(blue)*: speech, sensation, neglects. Occipital lobe *(red)*: vision. *(Redrawn from a handout from Bristol-Myers Squibb.)*

TABLE 90-1. Artery, Cerebral Localization, and Physical Examination Correlations

Artery	Lobe	Sign
Right ACA	Frontal, parietal	Left leg weakness
Right MCA: superior division	Frontal, parietal	Left arm/face weakness, hemineglect
Right MCA: inferior division	Temporal, parietal	Profound hemineglect, right gaze preference
Right PCA	Temporal, occipital	Left homonymous hemianopia
Left ACA	Frontal, parietal	Right leg weakness
Left MCA: superior division	Frontal, parietal	Right face/arm weakness, nonfluent aphasia
Left MCA: inferior division	Temporal, parietal	Fluent aphasia, right visual field cut
Left PCA	Temporal, occipital	Right homonymous hemianopia

ACA, Anterior cerebral artery; *MCA,* middle cerebral artery; *PCA,* posterior cerebral artery.
From Blumenfeld H. Neuroanatomy through clinical cases. Sunderland, Massachusetts: Sinauer Associates; 2002.

Basilar Artery Strokes

Ischemia of the basilar artery causes a number of symptoms ranging from changes in the motor system, to visual changes, to coma. Recall that the basilar artery is the only normally unpaired cerebral artery. Thus, occlusion or stroke involving the basilar artery can produce bilateral strokes. The basilar artery is formed by the vertebral arteries and gives off the PCAs. It directly or indirectly feeds the entire brainstem. The basic concept is that the brainstem is the origin of most of the cranial nerves, and thus basilar artery lesions will present with multiple cranial nerve problems unilaterally or bilaterally. Additionally, the midbrain and thalamus are the seats to arousal; therefore, bilateral damage to these structures due to complete basilar artery occlusions can result in coma. Almost all cases of occlusion of the basilar artery have a motor component that is either fixed or transient and can occur on either side of the body. In more severe occlusions, patients may develop decerebrate posturing. Locked-in syndrome is an uncommon presentation that primarily occurs with profound ischemia to the pons bilaterally.

Visual findings can be as simple as nystagmus. The type of nystagmus depends on the location of the lesion. Other findings such as ocular bobbing, skew deviations, intranuclear ophthalmoplegia, one-and-a-half syndrome, ptosis, and pupillary changes have all been described. A variety of sensory changes can occur. Most importantly, the basilar artery system should be considered in patients with acute issues with arousal, double vision, problems swallowing, or eye function and movement changes, especially if the patient has undergone angiographic evaluation or treatment of the vertebral or basilar arteries (see Table 90-1).

RAPID NEUROLOGIC ASSESSMENT

The most expeditious neurologic examination is the Cincinnati Stroke Scale,[4] which was designed to allow first responders to diagnose a stroke so they might appropriately triage patients. This exam is most commonly used in the field by emergency medical technicians and paramedics, as well as by triage nurses in the emergency department. This scale is a derivative of the much more detailed and cumbersome National Institutes of Health Stroke Scale (NIHSS). The NIHSS is designed to assist neurologists in localizing stroke and determining its severity and appropriateness for intervention; as such, it is beyond the scope of this chapter. The Cincinnati Stroke Scale is a rapid exam with three simple elements that allow for a diagnosis of a new stroke. It is performed in three steps:

1. Ask the patient to repeat a sentence, such as "The sky is blue in_____" (add city of choice).
2. Ask the patient to show his or her teeth or smile broadly.
3. Have the patient hold up both arms in front and wait for 10 seconds.

Abnormal patient responses include inability to repeat the sentence exactly, or with slurred speech; asymmetry in part of the face when the patient smiles; or falling or drifting of one arm after 10 seconds. When all three elements of the scale are abnormal in a patient, there is an 88% specificity and 100% sensitivity for a new stroke. Furthermore, results were shown to be highly reproducible between physicians and prehospital providers (Table 90-2).[5]

THE 60-SECOND NEUROLOGIC EXAMINATION

This stroke scale is an excellent tool for first responders to assess for the presence of stroke, but a physician should be able to perform a more comprehensive exam to assist in diagnosing strokes and localizing the anatomy. However, the full neurologic examination is complex and often unwieldy to perform. We have designed a 60-second neurologic examination that will assist the neurointerventionalist in determining whether a stroke has occurred and, almost as importantly, where the stroke has occurred so rapid intervention may be undertaken (Table 90-3). This examination is appropriate before and after procedures and for basic evaluation of fluctuating and neurologically unstable patients. This will allow the examiner to obtain a basic assessment of neurologic function that encompasses the anterior and posterior circulation in approximately 1 minute. It will give information on the arterial circulation of the brain as well as assist in localization of the deficit.

1. **Ask the patient to repeat a sentence such as "It's a sunny day in Baltimore."** It has been estimated that about 25% of stroke patients develop a significant aphasia.[6] It is imperative that an assessment of language be first. If language is abnormal, the rest of the examination may be difficult. In a right-handed

TABLE 90-2. Cincinnati Prehospital Stroke Scale

1. Have the patient show his/her teeth or smile.
2. Have the patient close his/her eyes and hold both arms out, palms either up or down.
3. Have the patient say "The sky is blue in Cincinnati."

Patients with one of these findings: 72% probability of an acute stroke if symptoms are new
Patients with all three findings: 85% probability of an acute stroke if symptoms are new

TABLE 90-3. Six-Point Neurologic Screen: What Lobes Each Test Evaluates and Major Artery Serving That Lobe

Check box for whether test is normal or abnormal before and after operation. Abnormal tests should include which side is abnormal.

Test	Lobe Evaluated	Feeding Artery	Before Surgery Normal	Before Surgery Abnormal	After Surgery Normal	After Surgery Abnormal
Repeat sentence	L Frontal lobe L Temporal lobe L Parietal lobe	Left MCA				
Follow with eyes	R/L Frontal lobe Brainstem	Right/left anterior MCA Basilar artery				
Show teeth	R/L Frontal lobe Brainstem	Right/left MCA Basilar artery				
Touch 4 Fs	R/L Parietal lobe	Right/left MCA	R L	R L	R L	R L
Lift arms/legs	R/L Parietal lobe Thalamus	Right/left MCA Right/left PCA	R L	R L	R L	R L
Finger wiggle	R/L Occipital lobe R/L Parietal lobe R/L Temporal lobe	Right/left PCA Right/left MCA				

4 Fs, Face, forearm, femur, foot; *L,* left; *R,* right.

person, this will test the frontal, temporal, and parietal speech centers on the left. The superior temporal lobe and the inferior parietal lobe form the language cortex. This assists in language recognition and interpretation. Broca's area is found primarily in the left frontal cortex. Occasionally in left-handed people, it is on the right. It will also help the examiner pick up dysarthria, which primarily localizes to the posterior circulation and brainstem. The arteries that supply these regions are both the inferior and superior divisions of the MCA.

2. *Follow my fingers with your eyes.* The first step is having the patient follow the examiner's finger across the vertical plane from left to right and then return. It is important to keep the finger at least 12 to 18 inches away from the patient's face. This tests the function of the frontal eye fields. Inability to move the eyes in one direction typically is the result of damage to the frontal lobe subserved by the ACA or the superior division of the MCA. If one eye moves well but the other eye does not, that is suggestive of a brainstem process referable to the posterior circulation. Jerking eye movements can be normal after anesthesia, but coarse shaking of the eyes can suggest a brainstem or cerebellar problem. Dysconjugate gaze with eye movement when one eye follows poorly suggests brainstem injury if it is new. Patients with a "lazy eye" will have abnormalities on this test, but this is why we examine patients before and after a procedure and document the findings.

3. *Ask the patient to smile or show the teeth.* Note a loss of symmetry. A subtle finding may include a flattened nasolabial fold. A facial droop or weakness typically can occur with strokes that affect the motor system in the frontal lobe or subcortical white matter, as well as the brainstem. It is important to have a baseline sense of what the face looks like. If after a procedure in a patient with new neurologic issues is the first time this is tested, it can be unclear whether there is a baseline asymmetry or deficit.

4. *Touch the patient on the right and left sides of the face, arm, and leg.* The examiner should touch right and left independently to include the four Fs: face, forearm, femur, and foot. Each side should be tested separately, and the patient should be asked if both sides feel the same. Then the examiner should touch both sides of the forearms simultaneously and ask which side was touched. The parietal lobe mediates sensation on the contralateral side. There will be sensory loss with parietal lobe as well as thalamic stroke. Touching the two sides simultaneously tests for neglect and is referred to as *double simultaneous stimulation.* In neglects, the patient will feel the touch on each side, but when both sides are touched at the same time, it will be felt only on the normal side, a classic finding of a parietal lobe lesion.

5. *Have the patient lift both arms in the air and hold them 10 seconds, and then individually lift each leg off the bed for 5 seconds.* Have the patient lift both arms simultaneously and watch for one arm drifting down toward the bed. Each leg should be tested separately. Remember that the leg where the arterial puncture was performed will be tender, and care should be taken in examining it. There should be no drift.

This assesses for lesions in the primary motor cortex (frontal lobe), as well as for deep white matter and brainstem lesions.

6. *Ask the patient to identify which hand is wiggling on the right and left side.* Visual field evaluation is absolutely the most important portion of the examination. Lesions of the occipital lobe will present as visual loss, and the patient will often not realize there is a problem until he or she is examined. To test this, simply have the patient look at your nose, then hold up your hands so you can see them in your peripheral vision. Make sure your hands are equidistant between you and the patient. Then wiggle your fingers on the right and then left and then both sides. Loss of visual field occurs with occipital or parietal lobe damage. The PCA and inferior MCA supply blood to these areas. More sensitive is to have the patient count fingers instead of looking at moving fingers, but acknowledging movement is acceptable.

The examination takes no more than 60 seconds once practiced a few times. It will take longer in sleepy or sedated patients. The examiner occasionally has to be firm with patients to obtain compliance with the examination, and anesthesia can complicate the examination if done early after a procedure. This makes sense, because it is a screen of neurologic function, which is often abnormal in sedated patients. Practice is required to recall the steps and get consistent results, but with only six points, the basic examination is easy to remember. The fill-out form in table format (see Table 90-3) organizes the examination by lobe tested and artery supplied. It is critical to mark what side was abnormal. The form should be filled out and then examined for consistency. For instance, a large right MCA stroke will give left-sided abnormalities on questions 1 to 6. One must remember that the ipsilateral cerebral cortex controls the contralateral body and vice versa. Thus, left-sided weakness and vision loss are due to right-sided brain lesions. Cerebellar lesions are not well screened in this examination. These primarily present as ataxia and clumsiness without weakness. These lesions can be missed by all but experienced neurologists on physical examination. Primary symptoms of cerebellar lesions are vertigo, nausea, vomiting, and ataxia.

SUMMARY

There are many approaches available to treat an acute ischemic stroke that is a complication of angiography, depending on the protocols available at individual institutions. The key is to identify the stroke without delay. The interventionalist will often know the side and artery that has been manipulated, so attention to that side and arterial distribution in the examination is acceptable. In cases where conventional angiography is done, a new stroke can be anywhere in the cerebral cortex and brainstem. Although the full neurologic examination is much more sensitive and specific for new lesions and their localization, the rapid neurologic examination establishes a baseline before the procedure and will help the interventionalist identify a change in the examination. It is important to examine the integrity of the structure of the vessels when performing an angiogram and to examine the function of the parenchyma supplied by the vessels.

- An understanding of basic cerebral vascular anatomy is vital for an interventional radiologist when secondary embolization from a proximal source is possible.

- There is a correlation of vascular anatomy and functional anatomy. A neurologic examination can specifically suggest brain dysfunction and vascular damage.

- The Cincinnati Stroke Scale is an easy-to-use screening implement that is good but nonspecific for location of stroke, and a basic understanding of this evaluation technique is reasonable for nurses and emergency medical technicians but probably too simplistic for interventionalists.

- A reasonable neurologic examination that can be done in 60 seconds will evaluate different functional and vascular territories of the brain.

▶ **SUGGESTED READINGS**

Bendszus M, Koltzenburg M, Burger R, et al. Silent embolism in diagnostic cerebral angiography and neurointerventional procedures: a prospective study. Lancet 1999;354:1594–7.

Bogousslavsky J, Caplan L. Stroke syndromes. 2nd ed. New York: Cambridge University Press; 2001.

Dion, JE, Gates PC, Fox AJ, et al. Clinical events following neuroangiography: a prospective study. Stroke 1987;18:997–1004.

Hankey GJ, Warlow CP, Sellar RJ. Cerebral angiographic risk in mild cerebrovascular disease. Stroke 1990;21:209–22.

The complete reference list is available online at www.expertconsult.com.

CHAPTER 91

Carotid Revascularization

Zinovy M. Katz, Martin G. Radvany, and Mark H. Wholey

Stroke represents the third leading cause of death in the United States, with an incidence of 1.5 deaths per thousand people. Of the more than half-million strokes occurring annually, occlusive disease of the extracranial circulation is responsible for approximately 30%. The traditional standard of care in treating cervical carotid artery occlusive disease has been carotid endarterectomy (CEA), a procedure initially performed in the 1950s and described by Scott, DeBakey, and Cooley. In 1988, the landmark North American Symptomatic Carotid Endarterectomy Trial (NASCET) demonstrated a reduction in stroke and death rates from 26% at 2 years to 9% after endarterectomy.[1] Since that time, additional studies have further validated this approach and demonstrated the benefit of intervening in patients who are asymptomatic from their disease.[2-4]

From a historical standpoint, Mathias, Theron, and Kachel pioneered angioplasty for cervical carotid artery occlusive disease treatment in the early 1980s. With the advent of stent technology, interventional management of carotid artery disease began to develop as a practical technique, as shown by the early work of Diethrich, Roubin, Wholey, and Mathias. Stents provided significant improvements over conventional angioplasty and helped reduce restenosis rates, prevent elastic recoil, and treat dissections. During the pioneering stage of carotid stent placement from 1995 to 1999, especially in the United States, there were primarily only two peripheral stent systems available: the balloon-mounted Palmaz stent (Cordis Corp., Miami Lakes, Fla.) and the Wallstent (Boston Scientific, Natick, Mass.). When nitinol stents became available in 1999 in the United States, many operators had changed or were in the process of changing from balloon-mounted stents to either self-expanding Wallstents or the newer nitinol stents. With rapid technologic advancements in both the stents themselves and distal protection devices, indications for this procedure and its overall application have grown exponentially worldwide.

INDICATIONS

On May 6, 2011, the U.S. Food and Drug Administration (FDA) approved an expanded indication for use of the stent to include all patients with carotid artery stenosis who are at risk for stroke, not just those who are not good candidates for surgery. This decision comes based on the results of the Carotid Revascularization Endarterectomy versus Stenting Trial (CREST). Previously, the Centers for Medicare and Medicaid Services (CMS) decision limited carotid stenting to the "high-risk" surgical subset with 70% stenosis or greater as a service-covered admission with reimbursement for the Medicare population. All other subsets and categories had been excluded from reimbursement unless they had been enrolled in a category B FDA-approved investigational device exemption (IDE) study. This essentially excluded all asymptomatic patients with high-grade preocclusive lesions involving the internal carotid artery (ICA) who did not have appropriate entry criteria for a trial (typically 80% or greater is required for study entry). The ruling also excluded as a service-covered admission stenotic lesions involving the petrosal portion of the internal carotid, base of skull, and cavernous sinus segment. The caveat to the revised criteria is that a postapproval study be conducted that will:

- Follow patients for at least 3 years after treatment.
- Assess how patients older than 80 years of age respond to treatment.
- Evaluate whether treatment success is impacted by operate experience.
- Examine whether asymptomatic and symptomatic patients have different results.

CONTRAINDICATIONS

Currently there are no absolute contraindications for carotid artery stenting (CAS). Relative contraindications to the use of CAS can be divided into anatomic and patient-specific factors. Anatomic factors are physician and trial specific, but general contraindications are similar to those outlined in the CREST trial[5] (asymptomatic lesions < 70% by ultrasound or < 60% by angiography and symptomatic lesions < 70% by ultrasound or < 50% by angiography). Lesion characteristics are also increasingly recognized as being pertinent to the risk of stroke. Lengthy lesions, those with appearance of extensive thrombus (either by conventional angiography or by intravascular ultrasonography), those with globular calcifications, and those with type III and type IV arches are at increased risk and must be approached with caution. Inability to pass the protective filter, and a tortuous vessel in which the angiographer believes he or she is unlikely to pass the stent must be warning flags and must cause the performing physician to have a low threshold for abandoning the procedure. The aortic arch is the "Achilles heel" for carotid stenting, and if the angiographer has difficulty accessing the vessel of interest, with extensive manipulation of the aorta and multiple catheter exchanges, it is best to abandon the procedure and consider alternative methods of treatment.

Other contraindications involve general contraindications to angiography, such as patients with borderline renal function (although this can usually be handled with prehydration, N-acetylcysteine, nonionic contrast, and small contrast volumes), inability to access the femoral arteries (although the brachials or a direct carotid puncture can also be performed), and patients with extensive cervical hardware that will make precise visualization of stent placement difficult. Additional contraindications include:

- Evolving stroke
- Intolerance/resistance to aspirin and/or clopidogrel
- Patient with active bleeding diathesis or absolute contraindication to anticoagulation
- Severe dementia
- Uncontrolled hypertension

Aspirin and clopidogrel are the most common dual platelet therapy in use today. Resistance to antiplatelet agents is not uncommon and can result in in-stent restenosis or thrombosis. Resistance can be assessed by platelet aggregometry. Regarding clopidogrel, some studies have shown that greater than 50%[6] of patients undergoing cerebrovascular stent placement might be low responders, and 0% to 44%[7] may be resistors, which can be related to genetic polymorphisms of cytochrome P450 3A4 and the P2Y12 receptor. Alternatives are available for low responders/resistors and include increasing the clopidogrel dose, ticlopidine, prasugrel, or ticagrelor. Resistance to aspirin is far less common, occurring in approximately 5%[6] of patients undergoing cerebrovascular stent placement.

EQUIPMENT

Endovascular treatment of carotid arterial stenosis was originally performed with equipment that was not specifically designed for this purpose. This initially led to significant complications in the form of periprocedural strokes. The introduction of balloon and stenting systems specifically designed for carotid stenting, along with the introduction of embolic protection devices (EPDs) and greater operator experience, have resulted in a steady decrease in periprocedural stokes.

Endovascular stents come in two designs: balloon-expandable and self-expanding. Balloon-expandable stents, while appropriate for ostial lesions at the aortic arch, should not be used for treatment of cervical carotid arterial lesions, owing to their lack of flexibility or ability to spontaneously reexpand after external compression. Self-expanding stents have essentially two designs: open cell and closed cell. Each design has certain advantages and disadvantages. The open-cell design has more flexibility, which allows for better vessel wall apposition as well as better deliverability through tortuous anatomy. However, open-cell designs have lower radial force, which may result in a weaker scaffold and thus compromise stent expansion due to recoil, especially in heavily calcified lesions. Closed-cell stent designs have more radial force, but they are less flexible and can introduce kinks and stenosis in the blood vessel when used in tortuous anatomy. Data from the Stent-Protected Angioplasty versus Carotid Endarterectomy (SPACE) trial suggest that there is a higher rate of embolic complications with open-cell designs (11%) than with closed-cell carotid stents (5.6%, $P = 0.029$).[8] Several studies have been performed to assess the outcome of incomplete stent apposition; many of these involve intracranial[9] and coronary stenting.[10,11] With respect to carotid stenting, the Wallstent can at times have incomplete apposition at the edges of the stent when deployed at vascular turns.[12] Existence of a segment of incomplete stent apposition has no adverse morphologic or clinical effect.[13]

There are a number of stents available worldwide; those currently available in the United States are:

- Rx Acculink (Abbott Laboratories, Abbott Park, Ill.)
- Xact (Abbott)
- NexStent (Boston Scientific)
- Precise (Cordis)
- ADAPT (Stryker Corp., Kalamazoo, Mich.)
- Zilver (Cook Medical, Bloomington, Ind.)

There are two types of EPDs: (1) those that provide protection distal to the treatment site by blocking flow or filtering flow in the ICA distal to the treatment site, and (2) flow-reversal devices, which occlude inflow to the common carotid artery and external carotid artery causing reversal of flow in the ICA (Fig. 91-1).

Devices that provide occlusion distal to the treatment site may consist of a balloon or, more commonly, a filter attached to a wire. The balloon occlusion concept originally pioneered by Theron has been refined.[14] A balloon is attached to the working wire and advanced distal to the stenosis and inflated (PercuSurge [Medtronic, Minneapolis, Minn.]). After stenting and angioplasty are completed, a catheter is then advanced and used to aspirate debris prior to deflating and recovering the balloon. Disadvantages of the balloon system include occluding the entire flow during all or a majority of the procedure in patients who frequently have a compromised contralateral carotid artery and circle of Willis circulation. In addition, the angiographer cannot evaluate the lesion fluoroscopically while the balloon is inflated in the ICA. There is also a risk of flushing embolic debris retrograde into the common carotid and aorta or into collateral vessels off the external carotid artery, such as the middle meningeal and orbital branches.

With filter-type devices, the filter is attached to the working wire and deployed distal to the stenosis. After the procedure it is recovered, bringing the debris with filter. There are many different filter devices and they are paired with their individual stent platforms; they should not be mixed. The advantage to this type of design is that antegrade flow is maintained unless the filter is full of debris. The various companies in different stages of development and prototypes include:

- AngioGuard (Cordis)
- Accunet (Abbott)
- Emboshield (Abbott)
- Boston Scientific Filter Wire EZ (Boston Scientific)
- Mednova-NeuroShield (Abbott)
- Rubicon (Boston Scientific)
- SpideRX (ev3/Covidien, Minneapolis, Minn.)
- Sci-Pro (SCION, Miami, Fla.)

An operator should become familiar with one or two systems.

Currently there are two flow-reversal devices being tested; they are based on the Parodi design.[15] With a flow-reversal device, a balloon is inflated in the external carotid artery. A second balloon attached to the guiding catheter is inflated in the common carotid artery. Retrograde flow is then created by aspiration or creation of a circuit between the guiding catheter and the venous system to create retrograde flow. Advantages of the proximal occlusion technique include the ability to provide protection in hostile lesions that could not accept conventional distal embolic filters, as well as the potential to provide therapy in stroke management. Disadvantages include the large size of the guiding catheter (10F-11F) and the presence of low-lying superior thyroid arteries that at times can make it difficult to occlude

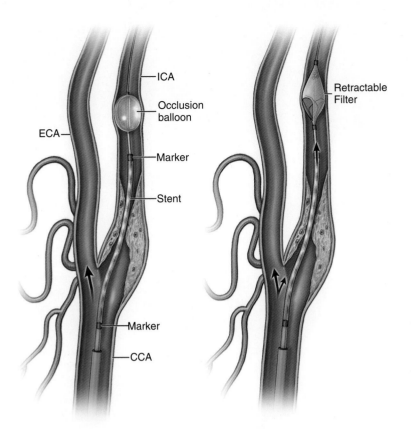

A. Carotid Occlusion

B. Filter Device

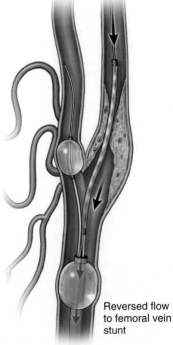

C. Parodi Technique

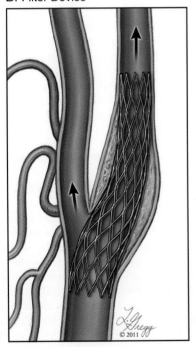

D. Deployed Stent

FIGURE 91-1. **A,** Theron technique. Procedure is performed under flow interruption obtained by inflating a balloon within the internal carotid artery (ICA). After placement of stent (and post dilatation if performed), delivery guide is advanced through the stent and placed immediately below inflated balloon. Blood stagnating below balloon (containing potential plaque debris) is aspirated forcefully. After aspiration, space below balloon is flushed with a bolus of saline solution that chases reminder of dead space content into external carotid artery. **B,** EPD, filter-type. In this technique, filter is advanced through stenosis, using either its built-in wire tip or an over-the-wire technique with a wire selected by operator. Filter is deployed in the ICA and kept open for duration of procedure. At the end, a special recovery catheter is used to retrieve filter and its content. **C,** EPD, flow-reversal type: with this technique, blood flow through lesion is reversed during the procedure, carrying potential debris away from cerebral circulation. Flow reversal is created by inflating two balloons, one in the common carotid artery (CCA) and one in external carotid artery, while blood leaving through the device is reinjected in a femoral vein. **D,** Final result with stent deployed in the ICA, traversing the stenosis into the CCA. (© 2011 lydia Gregg.)

with the balloon system. Early results are promising and the idea of flow reversal quite appealing; however, only those patients with sufficient collateral flow via the circle of Willis will be able to tolerate occlusion of antegrade carotid arterial flow, so this device will not be applicable to all patients.

TECHNIQUE

CAS is conceptually straightforward. Prior to treatment, patients should have a documented neurologic examination, preferably by a neurologist, as well as appropriate premedication with dual antiplatelet therapy. Preprocedure

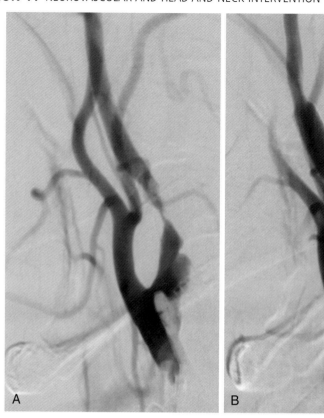

FIGURE 91-2. This 51-year-old man had an occluded right internal carotid artery (ICA) and left subclavian artery and left ICA stenosis. **A,** Before stent placement. Stenosis was predilated with 3 mm × 2 cm balloon. **B,** After stenting with 8 mm × 40 cm stent. Post–stent placement angioplasty was not performed. (© 2011 Martin Radvany.)

imaging with computed tomographic angiography (CTA) or magnetic resonance angiography (MRA) can provide important information on the type of aortic arch as well as anatomic variation that can affect the procedure. If these are not available, an aortic arch arteriogram can be performed. A complete four-vessel cerebral arteriogram should be performed before initiating stenting, to document the cerebral vascular supply.

Once baseline images are obtained (Fig. 91-2, *A*) and the appropriate equipment selected, heparin should be administered to achieve an activated clotting time (ACT) of 250 to 300 seconds. A guiding catheter or a long flexible sheath large enough to support the stent deployment system (6F-7F sheath or 8F-9F guide catheter) is advanced into the common carotid artery over a 0.035-inch guidewire. Avoid excessive manipulation of these catheters within the aortic arch, because this is likely to put the patient at high risk for embolic stroke. In addition, transition dilators should be used with guiding sheaths and guiding catheters to reduce the risk of dissection and embolization (Fig. 91-3).

The stenosis is crossed with a guidewire (0.018-inch or 0.014-inch) and an EPD deployed distal to the stenosis. The safest way to perform this is under roadmap guidance, in which an image of the vessels is overlayed on the live fluoroscopic image. A self-expanding stent that is 1 to 2 mm greater in diameter than the normal vessel and long enough to cover the stenosis is deployed across the stenosis. A follow-up angiogram is performed, and if the stent is adequately expanded, the EPD can be recovered (Fig. 91-2, *B*). If not, angioplasty is performed followed by recovery of the EPD.

Angioplasty prior to EPD placement or stent deployment predilation should only be performed if the EPD and/or stent deployment system cannot be delivered without predilation. Post-stenting angioplasty postdilation is at the operator's discretion. It is important to remember that most embolic events occur during postdilation.[16] If there is good flow with less than 30% residual stenosis, the stent should be allowed to continue to expand on its own, without the additional risk associated with postdilation.[17]

PERIPROCEDURAL MANAGEMENT

Antiplatelet Agents

Antiplatelet agents are essential to good outcomes in CAS. Dual antiplatelet treatment with clopidogrel 75 mg/day and aspirin 325 mg/day is the standard. The patient should be premedicated for at least 3 days prior to the procedure. If a patient cannot tolerate clopidogrel, ticlopidine 250 mg twice daily should be substituted. If a patient cannot tolerate treatment with dual antiplatelet therapy, carotid stenting may have to be reconsidered because the postprocedural stroke risk will be unacceptable. It is essential that patients remain on dual antiplatelet therapy for at least 6 weeks after treatment and continue on daily aspirin for life.

Glycoprotein IIb/IIIa inhibitors are not routinely used in carotid arterial stenting procedures; they have been associated with an increased risk of intracranial hemorrhage during the postprocedural period.[18] Acute thrombus formation during the procedure or in the immediate periprocedural period is an indication for use of these medications. They may be administered intraarterially through the guiding catheter/sheath to treat acute thrombus formation related to stent deployment and angioplasty.

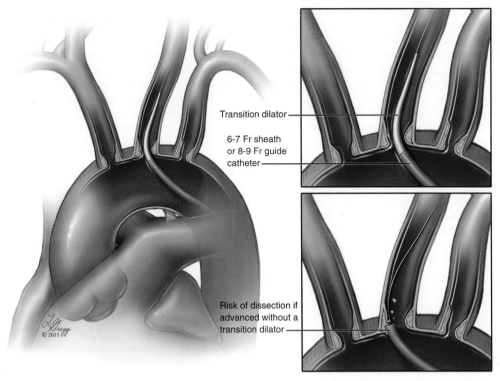

Transition dilator

6-7 Fr sheath
or 8-9 Fr guide
catheter

Risk of dissection if
advanced without a
transition dilator

FIGURE 91-3. If a transition dilator is not used, the guiding catheter or sheath may hang up on a plaque and cause a dissection and/or distal embolization resulting in a stroke. *(© 2011 Lydia Gregg.)*

COMPLICATIONS

Procedural carotid stenting adverse events can be divided into three stages. Stage I (early) complications occur primarily during access of the common carotid artery, including femoral puncture, selection of the common and external carotid arteries, and advancement of the guiding catheter or sheath into the ICA. Complications occur during positioning of the distal protection device (stage II), during predilation and stent deployment, during postdilation, and during recovery of the filter (stage III).

With the advent of distal protection devices, the rate of major strokes and catastrophic events has decreased by about half, but it is still important to know how to recognize and manage any type of complication that can occur. Importantly, the interventionalist must know how to avoid high-risk situations. Complications are directly related to procedure times. Procedures taking an excessively long time increase the risk of dislodging embolic debris from the arch into the targeted carotid or sending the debris to the contralateral carotid or adjacent vertebral arteries, as Jaeger et al. documented in their MRA studies after protected carotid stenting procedures.[19,20]

Periprocedural Neurologic Changes

Adverse events are categorized as neurologic and nonneurologic sequelae. Neurologic complications include transient ischemic attacks (TIAs), minor and major strokes, and consequent deaths. According to the National Institutes of Health Stroke Scale (NIHSS), a TIA is any neurologic deficit that resolves within 24 hours and leaves no residual neurologic damage. Typical TIAs seen during

carotid stent placement have included brief interruptions in vision and speech and transient motor/sensory deficits.

A minor stroke is classified as a new neurologic event that results in slight impairment of neurologic function (speech, motor, or sensory skills) that either completely resolves within 7 days or causes a less than 4 increase in the NIHSS. A new neurologic deficit that persists more than 7 days and increases the NIHSS score by 4 or more is a major stroke. Deaths are usually delineated as procedure related or non–procedure related, with the latter referring to cardiopulmonary and other organ-based causes. Nonneurologic adverse events include groin site complications, retroperitoneal hemorrhages, and infections. Hypotension, cardiac arrhythmias, and bradycardia, which are also major non-neurologic events, can evolve to a neurologic event if left untreated.

When a neurologic event occurs, it is important that the person monitoring the patient recognize the event and report it. Some situations, such as a drug reaction, oversedation, a cardiac event, and contrast encephalopathy, can mimic a neurologic adverse event. The symptoms of contrast-induced neurotoxicity are varied, but the most common manifestation is transient cortical blindness, which can easily masquerade as a stroke.[21] However, it is difficult to differentiate a microembolic stroke from contrast encephalopathy while the patient is on the table. The direct neurotoxic effects of contrast media disrupt the blood-brain barrier, allowing contrast material to enter the brain. Support for this concept has been provided by CT scans that demonstrated blood-brain barrier damage in patients experiencing various acute neurologic sequelae after cerebral angiography.[22] Because of this risk, as well as for the comfort of the patient, the use of nonionic contrast media is generally recommended. Transient blindness usually resolves completely in a few moments but on occasion lasts 48 hours.

Classic signs of a neurologic event relate to the area affected. The patient can present with an abrupt change in mental status and appear agitated and unresponsive to commands. There may be focal motor changes (e.g., dropping the handheld squeaking toy) that are indicative of motor cortex/lenticulostriate arterial involvement. It is vital to have a nurse in constant contact with the patient, who can then respond to repetitive phrases and simple commands without moving excessively during and after the procedure.

Angiographic signs of a neurologic event can vary. It is crucial to have good anteroposterior and lateral views of the intracranial circulation available before stenting, and it is important to note the presence or lack of collateral circulation. Signs of thromboembolic events in the major and distal branches include a cutoff sign in the artery, a filling defect, and delayed capillary and venous return. Another finding is sluggish arterial flow. Other causes such as poor inflow at the common carotid artery and/or the filter must be ruled out first; sluggish flow is a worrisome cause for microembolization, affecting small distal and lenticulostriate vessels.

Management of a Neurologic Event

When a neurologic event does occur, one should have a contingency plan to follow and the necessary equipment and drugs available. The interventionalist must have a good understanding of the intracranial circulation to proceed with a neurologic rescue procedure. Initial steps taken in managing an event include:

- Make sure airway, breathing, and circulation are maintained. General anesthesia should be started to protect the airway and reduce patient movement, including seizure precautions. Systolic blood pressure should be maintained between 100 and 180 mmHg, depending on the clinical condition and the patient's baseline blood pressure.
- Contact auxiliary personnel, such as anesthesia and additional trained nursing staff, if necessary.
- Identify the occlusion angiographically. As stated earlier, findings of thromboembolic occlusions should be compared with previous cerebral angiograms.
- Reestablish perfusion and oxygenation to the brain.
- Decide whether the patient can undergo intraarterial thrombolytic therapy if there has been a recent stroke or evolving stroke. Examine other contraindications to thrombolytic therapy.

Our policy has been to determine clinically whether a TIA or stroke exists. Patients with a TIA or minor stroke and a normal angiogram should be managed medically. We have reduced our general usage of the glycoprotein IIb/IIIa inhibitors except for severe neurologic events, such as poor arterial flow. Patients with minor or major strokes and angiographic evidence of occlusion within the intracranial circulation should undergo thrombolysis. A microcatheter is placed near or in the occluded vessel for intraarterial delivery of thrombolytic agent. We have generally used a bolus of tissue plasminogen activator (2 mg) and an infusion of up to 20 mg over a 1-hour period. Failing these modalities, we would proceed with a mechanical retrieval device.

Angiographic improvement occurs in the majority, but clinical improvement is less assured. These outcomes also compare to patients receiving thrombolytic therapy to manage acute strokes unrelated to carotid stenting. When cerebral infarction does occur from an embolic event, it is important that the ischemic penumbra that exists at the periinfarct site has the potential to be collateralized from the leptomeningeal and lenticulostriate vessels. Disruption at this site can result in hemorrhagic transformation and a mortality that may approach 60%.[6,7]

Hemodynamic Instability

Periprocedural bradycardia can be seen in up to 25% of cases. It occurs most commonly during balloon angioplasty, which may even precipitate hypotension and asystole. This is less common in patients who have previously undergone CEA. Treatment consists of atropine, 0.5 to 1.5 mg intravenously, with cardiac pacing if refractory. Some operators will prophylactically place a transvenous pacer prior to initiating the carotid stenting procedure.

Periprocedural hypotension may accompany bradycardia. Treatment with fluid boluses (colloid and crystalloid) as well as intravenous injection of phenylephrine (Neo-Synephrine) may be required in severe cases. This is thought to be secondary to continued expansion of the stent and pressure on the carotid baroreceptors.

Postprocedural hypertension is seen in up to 35% of patients. The major concern is the development of hyperperfusion syndrome, in which the vessels in the brain are maximally dilated due to poor flow and loss of autoregulation from chronic vasodilation. This can result in vessel rupture and intracranial hemorrhage, with significant morbidity and mortality. Risk factors for this include female gender, a history of hypertension, previous ipsilateral CEA, and intraprocedural hypertension. Treatment consists of intravenous antihypertensive administration with labetalol, hydralazine, nicardipine, or nitroglycerine drip.

Vasospasm of the ICA can be precipitated by guidewire manipulation and EPD placement. It is usually self-limited with removal of the guidewire or EPD. If it is severe and requires treatment, it may be treated with intravenous nitroglycerin or calcium channel blockers.

FOLLOW-UP CARE

Patients should be followed up at regular intervals after CAS. Currently, CMS guidelines require follow-up at 1 month, 3 months, 6 months, and 1 year with ultrasound examination, unless there is contralateral disease, recurrent stenosis, or new symptoms. Follow-up should include a neurologic examination and carotid ultrasound. In-stent restenosis can usually be treated with angioplasty, but repeat stent placement may be required.

Carotid arterial disease is a surrogate marker for coronary artery disease, and patients with atherosclerotic carotid arterial disease should be evaluated for coronary artery disease, as well as other comorbidities such as hypercholesterolemia and hypertension. Treatment with statins should be initiated if appropriate, because they have been shown to be beneficial in long-term treatment of patients with carotid arterial stenosis. Smoking cessation should be strongly emphasized as well.

OUTCOMES

The field of CAS remains among the hotly debated fields in medicine, with surgeons and interventionalists at opposing ends of the debate. Among the controversies are the indications for the procedure (especially inclusion of octogenarians), the definition of the "high-risk" patient, and the increasing application of this technique in the asymptomatic patient. In an effort to compare CAS to CEA, multiple trials were conducted and published.

The Carotid Revascularization using Endarterectomy or Stenting Systems (CaRESS) is a prospective nonrandomized comparative cohort study of a broad risk population of symptomatic and asymptomatic patients with carotid stenosis. This study found no significant differences in a broad-category population. The study did find a 4-year composite endpoint of death/stroke/myocardial infarction that favored CAS (25% CEA vs. 14% CAS) in patients younger than 80 years of age. However, the CAS group had a twofold higher restenosis rate compared to CEA.[13]

The Endarterectomy Versus Stenting in Patients with Symptomatic Severe Carotid Stenosis (EVA-3S) trial was stopped early because of a significantly higher stroke rate in the endovascular arm of the study as compared to the surgical arm (9.6% vs. 3.9%).[23] This study concluded that CAS was as effective as CEA for midterm prevention of ipsilateral stroke, but CAS had a higher periprocedural risk for any stroke. Some of the criticisms of this study are the inclusion of less experienced operators, lack of use of EPDs in 8% of cases, and a 5% failure rate to perform CAS. It is also unclear whether some patients received only a single antiplatelet agent.

During the same time period, the SPACE trial found no difference in the incidence of recurrent ipsilateral ischemic strokes or death between the CAS and CEA groups (6.8% vs. 6.3%). The study was designed to test the hypothesis that CAS is not inferior to CEA, but it failed to prove the non-inferiority of carotid stenting. Weaknesses of the study included lack of EPD use in 73% of patients, variability in the types of stents used, and the fact that the study was underpowered. The study did show a higher incidence of restenosis in the CAS group at 2 years, though restenosis was asymptomatic in most cases.[24]

Most recently, published results of CREST,[5] which enrolled 2502 patients over a median follow-up period of 2.5 years, showed that there was no significant difference in the estimated 4-year rates of the primary endpoint (periprocedural stroke, myocardial infarction, or death and subsequent ipsilateral stroke) between the stenting group and the endarterectomy group (7.2% and 6.8%, respectively; $P = 0.51$). There was no differential treatment effect with regard to the primary endpoint according to symptomatic status ($P = 0.84$) or sex ($P = 0.34$). The 4-year rate of stroke or death was 6.4% with stenting and 4.7% with endarterectomy ($P = 0.03$); the rates among symptomatic patients were 8.0% and 6.4% ($P = 0.14$), and the rates among asymptomatic patients were 4.5% and 2.7% ($P = 0.07$), respectively. Periprocedural rates of individual components of the endpoints differed between the stenting group and the endarterectomy group: no difference in rate of death (0.7% vs. 0.3%, $P = 0.18$), rate of stroke significantly higher in CAS group (4.1% vs. 2.3%, $P = 0.01$), and rate of myocardial infarction significantly higher in CEA group (1.1% vs. 2.3%, $P = 0.03$). After this period, the incidences of ipsilateral stroke with stenting and with endarterectomy were similarly low (2.0% and 2.4%, respectively; $P = 0.85$). An interaction between age and treatment efficacy was detected ($P = 0.02$), with a crossover at 70 years of age; CAS tended to show greater efficacy at younger ages, and CEA at older ages.

CONCLUSIONS

Since the first clinical application of carotid angioplasty as a palliative treatment for inoperable patients with carotid arterial stenosis, technologic improvements have revolutionized endovascular treatment of carotid arterial stenosis and improved patient outcomes. These technologic improvements included the creation of stents and balloons designed specifically for the purpose of treating the cervical carotid arterial system, as well as distal protection devices to decrease the risk of periprocedural complications, including stroke. These technologic improvements have decreased morbidity and mortality associated with the procedure. Current clinical data, particularly CREST, suggest that in experienced centers and with experienced operators, patients and their physicians should be able to individually tailor therapy for stroke prevention by choosing either CAS or CEA. This view is supported by an editorial of the CREST study in which it was concluded "... given the lack of significant difference in the rate of long-term outcomes, the individualization of treatment choices is appropriate."[25]

KEY POINTS

- Carotid artery stenting is a prophylactic procedure designed to prevent stroke in patients who have either had stroke/transient ischemic attack or asymptomatic high-grade stenosis.
- Physicians must be able to perform carotid artery stenting with an approximate 3% and 6% periprocedural stroke and death rate in asymptomatic and symptomatic patients, respectively, to justify the procedure.
- Indications in asymptomatic patients and octogenarians are unclear at this point.

▸ **SUGGESTED READINGS**

Ali OA, Bhindi R, McMahon AC, et al. Distal protection in cardiovascular medicine: current status. Am Heart J 2006;152:207–16.

Bates ER, Babb JD, Casey DE Jr, et al. ACCF/SCAI/SVMB/SIR/ASITN 2007 clinical expert consensus document on carotid stenting: a report of the American College of Cardiology Foundation Task Force on Clinical Expert Consensus Documents (ACCF/SCAI/SVMB/SIR/ASITN Clinical Expert Consensus Document Committee on Carotid Stenting). J Am Coll Cardiol 2007;49:126–70.

Bosiers M, Deloose K, Verbist J, et al. Carotid artery stenting: which stent for which lesion? Vascular 2005;13:205–10.

Bosiers M, Deloose K, Verbist J, et al. Review of stents for the carotid artery. J Cardiovasc Surg (Torino) 2006;47:107–13.

Cunningham EJ, Fiorella D, Masaryk TJ. Neurovascular rescue. Semin Vasc Surg 2005;18:101–9.

Eskandari MK. Cerebral embolic protection. Semin Vasc Surg 2005; 18:95–100.

Faries PL, Chaer RA, Patel S, et al. Current management of extracranial carotid artery disease. Vasc Endovasc Surg 2006;40:165–75.

Macdonald S. The evidence for cerebral protection: an analysis and summary of the literature. Eur J Radiol 2006;60:20–5.

Narins CR, Illig KA. Patient selection for carotid stenting versus endarterectomy: a systematic review. J Vasc Surg 2006;44:661–72.

Wholey MH, Wholey MH. History and current status of endovascular management for the extracranial carotid and supra-aortic vessels. J Endovasc Ther 2004;11(Suppl 2):II43–II61.

CaRESS Steering Committee. J Vasc Surg 2005;42(2):213–9.

The complete reference list is available online at www.expertconsult.com.

CHAPTER 92

Acute Stroke Management

Pierre Y. Gobin and Edward D. Greenberg

Stroke is the leading cause of disability and the third leading cause of death in the United States, with approximately 795,000 patients a year experiencing a stroke, at an annual cost of $40.9 billion.[1] Almost 90% of strokes are ischemic and arise from arterial thrombotic or thromboembolic occlusion. Loss of cerebral blood flow results in cerebral ischemia, which cascades to infarction if brain perfusion is not rapidly restored. The goal of acute ischemic stroke (AIS) intervention is to minimize cerebral damage by restoring blood flow to ischemic brain tissue as efficiently and safely as possible. In 1995, results from the National Institute of Neurological Disorders and Stroke (NINDS) rt-PA Stroke Study Group[2] demonstrated that in carefully selected ischemic stroke patients, significant clinical benefit at 3 months is observed after intravenous (IV) administration of tissue plasminogen activator (tPA) performed within 3 hours of AIS onset. More recent studies have shown that the window for treatment could be extended to 4.5 hours in certain patients.[3,4] Despite the benefits of IV tPA, which resulted in U.S. Food and Drug Administration (FDA) approval for the treatment of AIS, the utility of the drug for the vast majority of AIS patients is limited in actual practice. Because of the limited time window and other stringent exclusion criteria (Table 92-1), only 2% to 6% of stroke patients are administered IV tPA.[5,6] When treated with IV tPA alone, patients with large-vessel ischemic stroke, which carries the highest morbidity and mortality rate, still have overall poor clinical outcomes, most likely because IV tPA fails to recanalize up to 70% of large artery occlusions.[7] Endovascular stroke intervention is aimed at treating these large-vessel strokes and expanding the proportion of the AIS population eligible for acute treatment.

INDICATIONS

Careful patient selection for endovascular acute stroke treatment is paramount to successful clinical outcome. Ideally, at the time of the intervention, the patient should have minimal cerebral infarction, with a large ischemic penumbra that will revitalize once cerebral blood flow is restored. This should ensure maximal clinical benefit and help minimize the principal risk of endovascular AIS therapy, namely intracerebral hemorrhage (ICH). Table 92-2 summarizes the indications, which represent common knowledge within the neuro-interventional community at the time of this writing. It is important to note that mechanical embolectomy using the MERCI and Penumbra devices is not FDA-approved for the specific clinical indication of AIS. Use of these devices is based on single-arm trials sponsored by the respective companies (Concentric Medical and Penumbra), designed to gain 510K clearance from the FDA for the purpose of vessel recanalization and/or thrombus removal. As for intraarterial (IA) thrombolysis, although such treatment is based on the positive results of the

randomized PROACT II trial (Prolyse in Acute Cerebral Thromboembolism),[8] these results were not sufficient to achieve FDA approval.

Patients eligible for interventional stroke therapy include those arriving within 3 hours of stroke onset who have systemic contraindications to IV tPA treatment, as listed in Table 92-1. Endovascular stroke therapy is also indicated for patients arriving after 3 to 8 hours from stroke onset, because mechanical embolectomy and IA thrombolysis theoretically carry a lower risk of ICH than IV tPA after recanalization if performed under the same conditions. The likelihood of postrevascularization ICH depends on both temporal and tissue factors, as well as the extent of the induced coagulopathy. Large tissue infarctions, especially involving the basal ganglia, and prolonged duration of ischemia both elevate the risk of reperfusion hemorrhage. The duration and extent of ischemia determine the degree of neuronal death and cerebral tissue infarction, which progress in a time-dependent fashion.[9] Although these factors are present regardless of treatment, it is the minimalization and even omission of a thrombolytic drug that enables the prolonged time window associated with IA therapy. The upper limit of this time window, however, is not certain. Data from the PROACT II trial, a randomized controlled trial of IA prourokinase, suggest that the upper limit for recanalization should be 8 hours after symptom onset. In the special case of basilar artery occlusion, these time-to-treat guidelines may not apply, and some centers will treat aggressively up to 24 hours after stroke onset, given the dismal 80% to 90% mortality rate associated with untreated acute basilar artery occlusion and the numerous series showing some positive outcomes after late endovascular recanalization.[10] A key concept to consider when treating AIS, besides the time from symptom onset, is the amount of viable brain tissue at risk for infarction (penumbra) and the amount of core infarction present. Most would agree that patients with minimal or no core infarction and a large amount of penumbra are good candidates for endovascular treatment, regardless of the time from symptom onset, whereas patients with a large amount of core infarction (>100 mL) are not considered to be good candidates for endovascular treatment, owing to the higher risk of hemorrhage. Higher risk of hemorrhage may make even patients with greater than 70 mL of core infarction unsuitable candidates for endovascular treatment.

Interventional stroke treatment is limited to patients with significant neurologic deficits, namely patients with National Institutes of Health Stroke Scale (NIHSS) scores greater than 4, except for patients with isolated aphasia or hemianopsia. In addition, patients with fluctuating symptoms and evidence of a large-vessel occlusion, even with little deficit at the time of treatment, may qualify for endovascular therapy. These patients typically have sufficient collateral circulation to maintain adequate cerebral blood flow to minimize neurologic deficits, but this compensation is nearly invariably temporary. IA stroke treatment is also indicated for patients who fail to recanalize after IV tPA administration. Finally, endovascular revascularization requires the angiographically demonstrable arterial occlusion of an accessible artery. Appropriate target vessels include the internal carotid artery (ICA), the first (M1) and second (M2) division of the middle cerebral artery (MCA) (Fig. 92-1), the vertebral artery, the basilar artery, and the first (P1) segment of the posterior cerebral artery.

CONTRAINDICATIONS

Endovascular stroke therapy is contraindicated in patients with ICH, large established infarction (>one third MCA

TABLE 92-1. Exclusion Criteria for Intravenous Administration of Tissue Plasminogen Activator (tPA)

- 3 hours from stroke onset
- Minor or resolving deficits, NIHSS score < 4
- Sustained hypertension (systolic BP > 185 mmHg/diastolic BP > 110 mmHg)
- Seizure at onset
- International normalized ratio > 1.7
- Intravenous heparin with partial thromboplastin time > 40 s or low-molecular-weight heparin in past 48 hours
- Platelet count < 100,000/mm³
- Glucose > 400 mg/dL or < 50 mg/dL
- Stroke, myocardial infarction, or head trauma in past 3 months
- Major gastrointestinal or genitourinary hemorrhage in past 3 weeks
- Major surgery in past 2 weeks
- Noncompressible arterial puncture in past 7 days
- Past intracerebral hemorrhage, subarachnoid hemorrhage, or intraventricular hemorrhage
- CT scan with intracerebral hemorrhage or hypodensity in greater than one third of middle cerebral artery territory

BP, Blood pressure; *CT,* computed tomography; *NIHSS,* National Institutes of Health Stroke Scale.

TABLE 92-2. Indications for Endovascular Acute Stroke Therapy

- Significant neurologic deficit (NIHSS score > 8) or large territory at risk
- Angiographically demonstrable occlusion of an endovascularly accessible vessel*
- No hemorrhage or major infarction on noninvasive imaging
- <3 hours from symptom onset, with contraindications for intravenous tPA
- 3 hours and < 6 hours (chemical) or < 8 hours (mechanical) from symptom onset†
- Failure to significantly recover clinically after intravenous thrombolysis

*Internal carotid artery (including bifurcation, or "T" occlusions), middle cerebral artery (first and second divisions), vertebral artery, basilar artery, or proximal posterior cerebral artery.
†≤12 hours for basilar artery occlusion, although efficacy not proved.
NIHSS, National Institutes of Health Stroke Scale; *tPA,* tissue plasminogen activator.

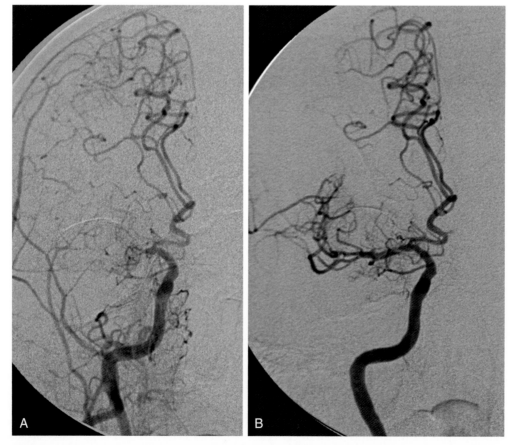

FIGURE 92-1. **A,** Right carotid artery angiogram, intracranial anteroposterior view, demonstrating acute occlusion of proximal M1 segment of right middle cerebral artery (MCA) in a 77-year-old man. **B,** After mechanical embolectomy with the Merci L6 Retriever, right MCA is recanalized. Note dissection flap, seen in proximal M1 segment, that occurred as a consequence of clot retrieval.

TABLE 92-3. Basic Equipment for Acute Stroke Management

Device	Example	Company
Femoral sheath	5F-9F, 11-90 cm*	Cordis Corp., Miami Lakes, Fla.
Diagnostic catheter	TempoVert	Cordis
Guide catheter*	6F Envoy Guider Softip XF guide catheter Shuttle Introducer Balloon Guide Catheter	Cordis Boston Scientific, Natick, Mass. Cook Inc., Bloomington, Ind. Concentric Medical Inc., Mountain View, Calif.
Intermediate catheter	DAC	Concentric Medical
Microcatheter	Excelsior SL10 Excelsior 1018 Prowler Plus	Boston Scientific Boston Scientific Cordis
Microguidewire	Transend-14 Synchro-14	Boston Scientific Boston Scientific
Thrombolytic	tPA Abciximab (ReoPro)	Genentech Inc., San Francisco, Calif. Eli Lilly, Indianapolis, Ind.

*Long 90-cm sheath may be used for support instead of a guide catheter for mechanical embolectomy, intracranial angioplasty, and stenting.

territory computed tomography [CT] hypodensity or magnetic resonance imaging [MRI] diffusion-weighted abnormality), or completed infarction without salvageable territory. CT perfusion, MRI diffusion/perfusion-weighted (DWI-PWI) mismatch, and MRI diffusion-weighted/clinical mismatch are all useful in determining the extent of the latter and aid in patient selection, especially when contemplating late recanalization (>3 hours). A DWI-PWI mismatch may be found in up to 70% of patients imaged within 6 hours from stroke onset,[11] and it is hypothesized that these patients may derive the most clinical benefit from endovascular intervention. Some relative contraindications to IA therapy include rapidly improving neurologic examination, NIHSS over 30, and a history of anaphylaxis to thrombolytic drugs or iodinated contrast material.

EQUIPMENT

Digital biplane angiography with road-mapping capability is optimal for the safe and efficient performance of endovascular acute stroke intervention. General endotracheal anesthesia is required for most procedures, although monitored conscious sedation is at times adequate for cooperative patients. Our experience is that patients with left hemisphere strokes are paradoxically more cooperative than right hemisphere stroke patients. The patient should have an arterial line placed for blood pressure management, which may become crucial after recanalization to prevent reperfusion hemorrhage. In the time before vessel recanalization, it is critical to maintain adequate perfusion pressure by elevating the patient's blood pressure to significantly above the patient's baseline values, particularly during administration of general anesthesia. A recent study comparing outcomes of AIS patients[12] showed that patients placed under general anesthesia during endovascular treatment for anterior circulation had higher rates of poor neurologic outcome and mortality, a difference that could potentially be due to lack of adequate blood pressure support during general anesthesia. Common femoral artery access requires a minimum of a 5F sheath for IA thrombolysis and up to a 9F sheath for the Merci Retrieval System. A 5F diagnostic catheter is used for cerebral angiography to demonstrate and characterize the arterial occlusion. The catheter and sheath are maintained under continuous heparinized saline flush (5000 units heparin per liter normal saline), and nonionic iodinated contrast (Omnipaque [GE Healthcare, Piscataway, N.J.]) is used for angiography. Once an intervention is deemed appropriate, minimal systemic anticoagulation is initiated with 2000 to 3000 units of IV heparin.

A guide catheter is required for device support during thrombolysis and embolectomy. A microcatheter and microwire facilitate navigation past the occlusion, and the microcatheter provides a conduit for IA thrombolytic infusion. More specific details about the basic equipment required for IA treatment are summarized in Table 92-3.

The most commonly used drugs for IA thrombolysis include plasminogen activators such as urokinase, alteplase, reteplase, and prourokinase. Other newer thrombolytics that are not plasminogen dependent include V10153 (Vernalis, Winnersh, U.K.), a recombinant variant of human plasminogen, Microplasmin (ThromboGenics, Heverlee, Belgium), a truncated form of plasmin, Alfimeprase (Nuvelo, San Carlos, Calif.), a truncated form of fibrolase that degrades fibrin directly, and Ancrod, a purified fraction of the venom of the Malayan pit viper, which acts by directly inactivating fibrinogen. Given the prothrombotic activity of fibrinolytics, there is some rationale for adjunctive anticoagulant therapy when administering fibrinolytics in the setting of AIS. Investigations are ongoing involving combinations of fibrinolytics, anticoagulants, and platelet disaggregants for IV, IA, and combined IV/IA AIS therapy, although there is currently no clear evidence to recommend one combination over another. Periprocedural anticoagulation with IV heparin may allow for augmentation of thrombolysis and prevention of arterial reocclusion at the expense of potentially higher rates of ICH. The use of glycoprotein IIb/IIIa antagonists in ischemic stroke remains investigational; only limited data are available, mainly involving IV administration of a glycoprotein IIb/IIIa antagonist in conjunction with IV thrombolysis. A randomized double blinded placebo-controlled study in which 54 ischemic stroke patients were randomly selected to receive IV abciximab did not report a single ICH complication in the group receiving abciximab.[13] The CLEAR trial evaluated the combination of low-dose IV rtPA and eptifibatide, a glycoprotein IIb/IIIa antagonist, in patients with NIHSS scores of less than 5 presenting within 3 hours of stroke onset. The study showed a nonsignificant trend toward increased efficacy with the standard-dose rtPA treatment arm, and there was a non–statistically significant increased incidence on ICH in the eptifibatide group.[14] A small study on the IA administration of glycoprotein IIb/IIIa antagonists as adjunctive therapy in patients with large-vessel occlusion and AIS also suggests that the added risk of ICH is low.[15] However, the AbESTT II trial, a phase III multicenter randomized double-blind placebo-controlled study evaluating the safety and efficacy of IV abciximab in AIS treated within 6 hours after stroke onset or within 3 hours of awakening with stroke symptoms, was stopped early because of high rates of symptomatic ICH in the abciximab-treated patients (5.5% vs. 0.5%, $P = .002$).[16]

Mechanical embolectomy involves the use of devices for mechanical clot extraction or fragmentation. The only two devices currently approved by the FDA for revascularization are the Merci Retriever (Concentric Medical Inc., Mountain View Calif.) and the Penumbra Reperfusion System (Penumbra Inc., San Leandro, Calif.). A myriad of other devices designed for this same purpose have recently become available in this regard, but their usage is off-label and/or investigational. Among these newer devices, the Solitaire and Trevo devices seem to be the most promising. The mechanisms employed by these devices include thrombectomy, thromboaspiration, mechanical disruption, angioplasty, stenting, laser techniques, ultrasound-based methods, flow augmentation, and transvenous retrograde reperfusion. A summary of the devices currently available for IA treatment of AIS is listed in Table 92-4.

TECHNIQUE

Anatomy and Approaches

Specific techniques for endovascular stroke therapy differ depending on whether IA chemical thrombolysis or mechanical embolectomy will be performed in isolation or in combination and on which mechanical device will be deployed. All acute stroke management requires similar equipment (see Table 92-3) and necessitates sufficient guide catheter support from the common femoral artery through the abdominal and thoracic aorta into the ICA for ICA, MCA, or ACA occlusion (Fig. 92-2) and subclavian or vertebral artery access for vertebral artery, basilar artery, and posterior cerebral artery thrombosis (Fig. 92-3). The technical aspects of IA thrombolysis and mechanical embolectomy with the Merci Retriever, the Penumbra Reperfusion System, and the Solitaire FR Revascularization Device are discussed next.

Technical Aspects

Intraarterial Thrombolytic Infusion
Fibrinolytic infusion is best used in conjunction with mechanical embolectomy, especially in the setting of high

TABLE 92-4. Current Mechanical Embolectomy Devices Approved or Under Investigation

Device	Company
Merci Retriever*	Concentric Medical, Mountain View, Calif.
Penumbra System*	Penumbra Inc., San Leandro, Calif.
Solitaire	ev3/Covidien, Irvine, Calif.
Trevo	Concentric Medical
Phenox Clot Retriever and Phenox Clot Retriever CAGE	Phenox, Bochum, Germany
Attracter-18 device	Target Therapeutics, Freemont, Calif.
Alligator Retriever	Chestnut Medical Technologies Inc., Menlo Park, Calif.
EnSnare	InterV, Gainesville, Fla.
AngioJet and NeuroJet	Possis Medical Inc., Minneapolis, Minn.
Oasis Thrombectomy Catheter System	Boston Scientific, Natick, Mass.
Amplatz Thrombectomy Device	Microvena, White Bear Lake, Minn.
Hydrolyzer	Cordis Endovascular, Warren, N.J.
F.A.S.T. Funnel Catheter	Genesis Medical Interventional, Redwood City, Calif.
Microsnare	Microvena
HyperGlide balloon	ev3/Covidien
Gateway angioplasty balloon	Boston Scientific
Enterprise stent	Cordis Corp., Miami Lakes, Fla.
LEO stent	Balt Extrusion, Montmorency, France
Solitaire/Solo stent	ev3/Covidien
Wingspan stent	Boston Scientific
EPAR Laser	Endovasix Inc., San Francisco, Calif.
LaTIS laser device	LaTIS, Minneapolis, Minn.
Locket retrieval	Lazarus Effect, Cambell, Calif.
OmniWave Endovascular System	OmniSonics Medical Technologies, Wilmington, Mass.
EKOS MicroLysUS infusion catheter	EKOS Corporation, Bothel, Wash.
NeuroFlo device	Co-Axia, Maple Grove, Minn.
ReviveFlow System	ReviveFlow, Quincy, Mass.

*510K clearance for recanalization of cerebral arteries.

clot burden (Fig. 92-4). When mechanical embolectomy is not considered, a smaller (6F) guide catheter can be used via a 6F groin sheath. A diagnostic angiogram is performed to identify the branch occlusion(s). The diagnostic catheter can then be exchanged out for the 6F guide catheter. Alternatively, the guide catheter can be navigated directly into the ICA or the vertebral artery and used to perform the initial angiogram in patients with straightforward anatomy. Next, using roadmap technique, the microcatheter is advanced over a microwire into the area of arterial occlusion and then slightly distal to it. A microcatheter

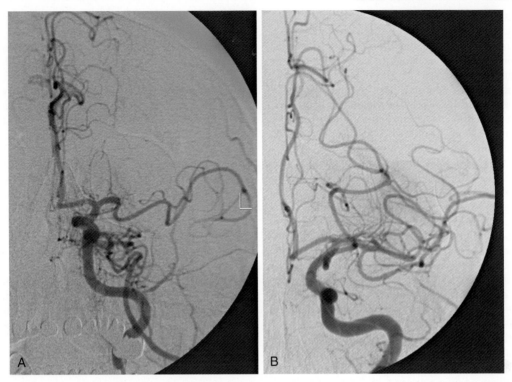

FIGURE 92-2. Left common carotid artery angiogram, intracranial anteroposterior view. **A,** Acute mid-M1 segment left middle cerebral artery (MCA) occlusion in a 65-year-old man with atrial fibrillation. **B,** Complete recanalization was achieved with combination intraarterial tissue plasminogen activator (tPA) infusion and mechanical embolectomy with the Merci L5 Retriever.

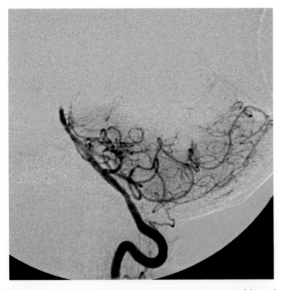

FIGURE 92-3. Left vertebral artery angiogram, intracranial lateral view, shows an acute mid-basilar artery occlusion.

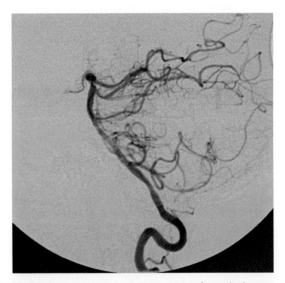

FIGURE 92-4. Same patient as in Figure 92-3. Left vertebral artery angiogram, intracranial lateral view. After mechanical embolectomy, basilar artery is completely recanalized.

angiogram can then delineate the anatomy of the occlusion and the distal vasculature. The microcatheter is then withdrawn into the area of arterial occlusion, and thrombolytic medication is slowly infused. Sequential passes of the microwire through the thrombus increase the surface area for thrombolysis and are typically performed during the infusion. Cerebral angiography through the guide catheter is performed serially (typically every 15 minutes) during the

infusion to assess the progress of recanalization. The procedure is completed when recanalization has been achieved or the maximum dose of medication has been administered. IA thrombolytic infusion is particularly helpful for recanalization of more distal branch occlusions that are inaccessible to mechanical devices, including the treatment of distal branch occlusion after mechanical thrombus extraction of a large proximal occlusion.

The Merci Retriever

After acquisition and interpretation of the diagnostic cerebral angiogram, the femoral sheath used for diagnostic catheterization must be exchanged under fluoroscopic guidance for an 8F or 9F sheath to allow insertion of an 8F or 9F Concentric BGC. Alternatively, the sheath may be exchanged directly for the BGC. The diagnostic catheter is exchanged out for a BGC using an exchange-length hydrophilic 0.035- or 0.038-inch guidewire, or the BGC can be directly navigated into the ICA, subclavian, or vertebral artery over a 0.035- or 0.038-inch wire in patients with straightforward anatomy. If an ICA kink is encountered, the BGC should be kept in the common carotid artery, even though anterograde flow control may be less efficient. In the setting of an ICA stenosis severe enough to inhibit embolus removal, carotid angioplasty and stenting may be performed before embolectomy. For posterior circulation stroke, owing to the small size of the vertebral artery, the BGC should be positioned in the subclavian artery just below the origin of the vertebral artery. At the distal end of the BGC is a 10-mm-diameter soft silicone balloon that is inflated with a 50% contrast-in-saline medium by a 3-mL syringe (0.8 mL maximal inflation volume) at the time of clot retrieval (Fig. 92-5). Once the BGC is in position, the Merci microcatheter (14X for X-series retrievers and 18L for L and V series retrievers) is advanced over a microguidewire under digital roadmap technique into the target artery. The microwire is navigated past the occlusion into a patent large branch (e.g., posterior cerebral artery for basilar artery occlusion), and the microcatheter is coaxially advanced over the microwire. Careful passage of the microwire into the true lumen of the occluded artery is crucial to avoid vessel dissection or perforation. Contrast medium injection through the microcatheter will demonstrate the patency of the branches distal to the occlusion. The microwire is then exchanged for the Merci Retriever device.

The X-series retriever (X5 and X6 devices) is composed of a memory-shaped nitinol wire with five helical loops of tapering diameter at the distal tip (Fig. 92-6). The loops of the L-series retriever (L5 and L6 devices) are arranged at a 90-degree angle to the base wire and are cylindrical. L-series devices additionally have bound suture threads that encircle the helical loops and function to facilitate thrombus capture (Fig. 92-7). The V-series is a hybrid of the X and L series. The Merci device is advanced through the microcatheter and unsheathed past the microcatheter tip. The retriever and microcatheter are withdrawn as a unit into the thrombus. The device will slightly deform once it is in contact with clot (Fig. 92-8). At this point, anterograde blood flow is arrested by inflation of the BGC balloon, and the thrombus-retriever-microcatheter unit is withdrawn into the BGC lumen and removed from the patient under vigorous hand suction with a 60-mL syringe placed at the proximal hub of the BGC (Fig. 92-9). Injection of contrast medium during clot retrieval may demonstrate a thrombus halo, indicating successful thrombus capture (Fig. 92-10). The BGC balloon

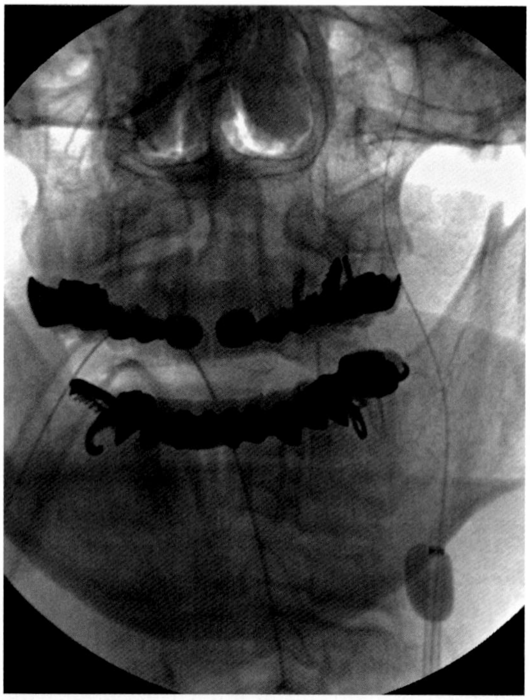

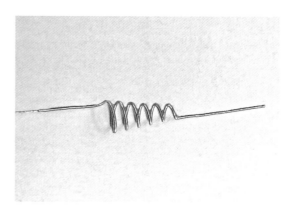

FIGURE 92-6. Photograph of the Merci X-series Retriever with tapered helical loops.

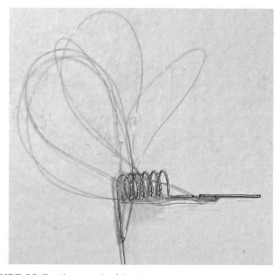

FIGURE 92-7. Photograph of the Merci L-series Retriever with cylindrical helical loops and bound suture thread for enhanced clot capture.

FIGURE 92-5. Unsubtracted anteroposterior view of an inflated Concentric balloon guide catheter used to initiate flow arrest during embolus extraction.

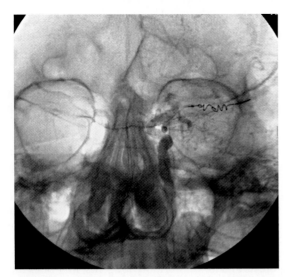

FIGURE 92-8. Unsubtracted anteroposterior view of Merci L5 Retriever in left middle cerebral artery of patient in Figure 92-2. Note deformation of retriever helix as it captures embolus.

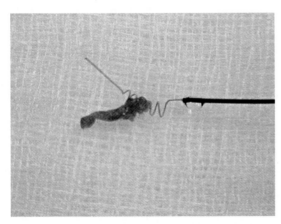

FIGURE 92-9. Photograph of Merci X-series Retriever with ensnared red clot. *(Courtesy Concentric Medical, Mountain View, Calif.)*

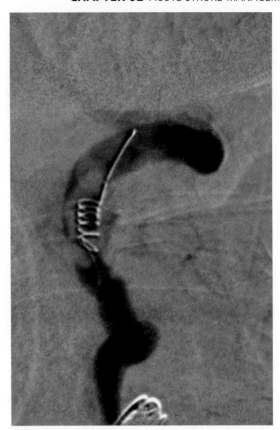

FIGURE 92-10. Left vertebral artery angiogram, intracranial lateral view. Contrast agent injection during flow arrest demonstrates a halo around captured thrombus.

is deflated, and cerebral angiography is then performed to confirm vessel recanalization. Multiple passes with the Merci device may be required to achieve complete vessel recanalization. No more than six passes are recommended by the manufacturer. In our own experience, more than three passes is futile.

The Penumbra Reperfusion System
After performing the initial diagnostic angiogram, the diagnostic catheter is exchanged out for a 6F guide catheter using an exchange-length hydrophilic 0.035- or 0.038-inch guidewire. Alternatively, the 6F guide can be directly navigated into the ICA or vertebral artery over a 0.035- or 0.038-inch wire in patients with straightforward anatomy. Next, using roadmap technique, a Penumbra Reperfusion catheter of appropriate size for use in the target vessel is advanced over a microwire into the area of the vessel just proximal to the occlusion. The 0.54 Reperfusion catheter can be used for vessels larger than 4 mm in caliber (ICA, M1, vertebral, basilar), the 0.41 Reperfusion catheter for

vessels measuring 3 to 4 mm (M1, vertebral, basilar), the 0.32 for vessels measuring 2 to 3 mm (M2, P1), and the 0.26 for vessels smaller than 2 mm, such as M3 branches. The microwire is then exchanged out for an appropriately sized Separator, which is a soft wire with a 6-mm teardrop-shaped enlargement proximal to its tip designed to physically break up the clot and keep the Reperfusion catheter tip from clogging. The RHV of the Reperfusion catheter is then connected to the aspiration pump, which is then turned on to suction, and the baseline aspiration rate is observed. The Separator is then positioned so that the radiopaque marker on it is 4 mm distal to the radioopaque marker on the Reperfusion catheter. The Reperfusion catheter is then advanced until aspiration flow slows or stops signifying that the reperfusion catheter is at the site of the thrombus. The Separator is then gently moved in and out of the Reperfusion catheter to clear it of debris and break up the thrombus. Guide catheter angiograms are performed intermittently to assess progress. Several passes with the device may be required to clear the vessel of thrombus.

Solitaire FR Revascularization Device
After acquisition and interpretation of the diagnostic cerebral angiogram, the femoral sheath used for diagnostic catheterization is exchanged out under fluoroscopic guidance for an 8F Cello Balloon Guide Catheter (ev3/Covidien, Irvine, Calif.), which is placed into the proximal ICA. With the balloon of the guide catheter deflated, a 0.014-inch guidewire (Silverspeed; ev3/Covidien) is advanced over a

Rebar 18 microcatheter (ev3/Covidien) via the guide catheter into the occluded intracranial vessel and navigated distal to the thrombus. The Rebar 18 microcatheter is then advanced over the microwire through the thrombus, and the microwire is removed. The Solitaire FR device is then advanced via the microcatheter and deployed with the distal portion of the stent placed a few millimeters distal to the thrombus. This typically results in immediate flow restoration so long as the stent is longer than the length of the thrombus. A repeat angiogram can be performed at this point to evaluate the potentially reconstituted flow through the previously occluded segment. The stent is kept deployed for a few minutes before its retrieval. The proximal third of the stent is recaptured into the microcatheter, and the balloon on the guide catheter is inflated for flow arrest in the ICA. Then, under continuous proximal aspiration of the guide catheter with a syringe, the stent and microcatheter are gently withdrawn proximally through the guide catheter. Alternatively, in cases with underlying stenosis, the Solitaire Stent can be deployed at the site of occlusion in to help maintain patency of the artery. Several recent reports on the use of the Solitaire Revascularization Device have shown promising revascularization rates of about 90%.[17-20]

CONTROVERSIES

One major controversy in acute stroke management is whether the clinical benefit of reperfusion warrants the risks and cost of the procedures. Currently, no answer to this question exists. However, several studies show relative safety and efficacy and of endovascular stroke therapies in terms of successful vessel recanalization,[11,21,22] and successful recanalization has been shown to be strongly associated with improved patient outcomes.[23] Most interventional acute stroke trials use a time window rather than a tissue window for inclusion and therefore undoubtedly incorporate both patients with salvageable brain tissue and those with completed infarction. This heterogeneity of treated stroke populations makes proof of clinical benefit difficult. As already mentioned, successful clinical outcomes require appropriate patient selection. The concept of patient selection based on the degree of tissue at risk for infarction (tissue window) is being investigated in MR Rescue, a randomized trial of Merci Retriever embolectomy versus standard medical therapy based on the presence or absence of a 20% or more DWI-PWI mismatch. It is hoped that this study will help resolve this controversy.

Another debate is the role of bridging stroke therapy, the concept of administering reduced-dose IV thrombolytic before IA therapy. The IMS I study[24] investigated a bridging tPA protocol in 80 patients with NIHSS scores of 10 or higher. Intravenous tPA (0.6 mg/kg over 30 minutes) was administered within 3 hours of stroke onset and was followed by IA tPA to a total dose of 22 mg over a 2-hour infusion or until complete thrombolysis was achieved. Although this trial was a safety and feasibility study, clinical outcomes were modest, showing a trend toward improved clinical outcome at 30 days (odds ratio [OR]for global test, 1.35; 95% confidence interval [CI] 0.78-2.37) and numerically lower 3-month mortality (16% vs. 21%) compared with historical IV tPA-treated patients from the NINDS tPA stroke trial. The IMS II study differed from the IMS I trial mainly by incorporating the use of the MicroLysUS infusion catheter (EKOS, Bothell, Wash.) to deliver rtPA into the clot and to use ultrasound to augment thrombolysis.[25] The IMS II patients had a lower mortality and better outcomes than NINDS rt-PA–treated subjects, with 3-month mortality in IMS II subjects 16%, compared with a 24% mortality with placebo and 21% mortality in rt-PA–treated subjects in the NINDS rt-PA Stroke Trial. The IMS III study is a 3-hour time window stroke protocol randomizing standard IV tPA (0.9 mg/kg) versus a bridging protocol of IV tPA (0.6 mg/kg) plus IA therapy that uses techniques with proven safety in phase I studies (IMS III). IA treatment may include IA tPA alone (maximum dose 22 mg), ultrasound-enhanced IA tPA with the EKOS microcatheter (demonstrated safety and feasibility in the IMS II Trial), or mechanical embolectomy with the Merci Retriever. Individual technique selection is at the discretion of the operator. These and other bridging strategies, including glycoprotein IIb/IIIa antagonists and newer fibrinolytic agents, may offer thrombolytic synergy and added safety and are currently being investigated.

OUTCOMES

Outcome after endovascular stroke management is measured as both technical success and clinical benefit. Overall, endovascular techniques result in higher rates of recanalization than IV thrombolytic therapy, and these higher rates of recanalization are strongly associated with improved functional outcomes and reduced mortality in AIS patients.[7] A meta-analysis of the most significant trials of IA thrombolysis, including PROACT I and II[8,26] and the Middle Cerebral Artery Embolism Local Fibrinolytic Intervention Trial (MELT),[27] included 204 patients treated with IAT and 130 controls. The analysis showed a lower rate of death or dependency at long-term follow-up with IAT compared with controls.[28] A second, more recent meta-analysis on this topic confirmed these results, concluding that IA fibrinolysis significantly increases recanalization rates and results in improved clinical outcomes in AIS patients.[29] Regarding mechanical embolectomy, in the MERCI trial, arterial recanalization was attained with the X-series Merci Retriever, with and without adjuvant IA thrombolytic therapy, in 57% and 48%, respectively. In the Multi-MERCI trial, a single-arm study of the Merci L5 retriever, the device was deployed in 111 patients, including 30 patients initially treated with IV tPA, and 43 patients were administered adjuvant IA tPA.[22] With other demographics being similar to those of the MERCI trial, revascularization was achieved in 54.1%, increasing to 69.4% when an adjuvant IA thrombolytic agent was used. Clinical outcome also benefited from higher revascularization rates, with lower morbidity (34.3% vs. 27.7% independence at 90 days) and lower mortality (30.6% vs. 43.5%) in Multi-MERCI compared with the MERCI trial. The Penumbra stroke trial is a prospective multicenter single-arm study that included 125 patients with NIHSS scores of 8 or higher presenting with angiographic occlusion of an intracranial vessel within 8 hours of symptom onset. All 125 patients were treated with the Penumbra system with an overall 81.6% recanalization rate, although 28% were found to have intracranial hemorrhage on 24-hour followup CT, and all-cause mortality was 32.8% at 90 days, with 25% of the patients achieving a modified Rankin Scale score of 2 or below.[30] More recent trials involving the Penumbra system have shown even higher recanalization rates and better clinical outcomes.[31] Despite the excellent data from the above studies, there is still an overall lack of controlled clinical outcomes analyses in interventional stroke management. Because clinical outcome is intimately linked with complete vessel recanalization, current device modifications, novel technologies, and newer thrombolytic agents have to be developed to attain improved technical outcomes likely to yield higher rates of clinical success.

COMPLICATIONS

The major complication of endovascular acute stroke management is symptomatic ICH, which is associated with a dismal mortality rate.[32] ICH may be a consequence of reperfusion, where a rapid increase in hydrostatic pressure after revascularization leads to rupture of previously underperfused vessels or hyperperfusion injury. The latter is more common after chronic rather than acute vessel recanalization and is discussed in detail in Chapter 93, Endovascular Management of Chronic Cerebral Ischemia. Reperfusion hemorrhage occurs within infarcted brain tissue, where endothelial integrity is lost, causing small vessels to become friable and easily rupture. Reperfusion hemorrhage typically occurs shortly after recanalization and is significantly affected by hypertension and the volume and location of infarcted tissue. The basal ganglia and posterior cerebral artery territories appear to be at highest risk for reperfusion ICH. Established infarcts greater than one third of the MCA

territory are more likely to bleed once vessel patency is restored. Other risk factors for reperfusion ICH include delayed recanalization, higher pretreatment NIHSS score, inherent or iatrogenic coagulopathy, pretreatment hyperglycemia, and the presence of MRI gradient echo–positive microhemorrhages.[32-34] When similar definitions are used to describe symptomatic ICH in the major interventional stroke trials, the rates of symptomatic ICH are 5% in the MERCI trial,[11] 6.3% in the IMS trial,[24] 9% in the Multi-MERCI trial,[22] and 10% in the PROACT II trial.[8] These rates are of the same order of magnitude as the 6.4% rate of ICH in the NINDS IV tPA trial.[2]

Other complications of endovascular stroke management for the most part have less calamitous prognoses compared with reperfusion ICH. Vessel dissection or perforation may arise from sheath insertion or exchange and from diagnostic catheter, guide catheter, or guidewire manipulation anywhere in the approach to the occluded vessel, including the common femoral artery, aorta, innominate artery, subclavian artery, vertebral artery, and the common carotid or ICA. Consequences of vessel dissection or perforation range from asymptomatic and spontaneously resolving events to stenosis and thrombotic occlusion and pseudoaneurysm formation. Arterial trauma may also involve the occluded intracerebral artery secondary to microguidewire or mechanical embolectomy device manipulation and may result in vessel stenosis, thrombosis, or rupture. Depending on the location and degree of dissection, management options include conservative observation, balloon angioplasty, stent placement, or surgical repair (Fig. 92-11). Failed

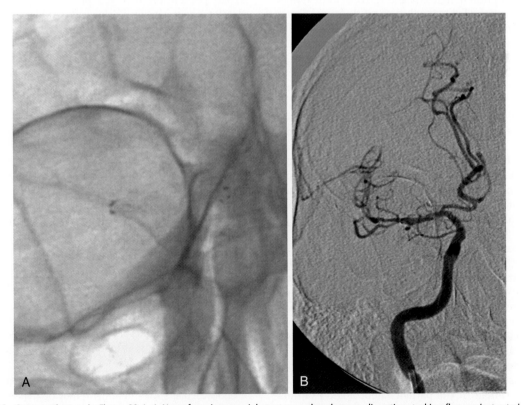

FIGURE 92-11. Same patient as in Figure 92-1. A Neuroform intracranial stent was placed across dissection, tacking flap against arterial wall and thus preventing possible thromboembolic consequences. **A,** Unsubtracted anteroposterior view demonstrating proximal and distal markers of Neuroform stent. **B,** Right internal carotid angiogram, intracranial anteroposterior view, shows complete luminal patency after stent deployment.

common femoral artery hemostasis at the end of the procedure may result in groin hematoma, retroperitoneal hemorrhage, and pseudoaneurysm formation. Occasionally, surgical repair of groin complications is required to restore vessel integrity.

Device fractures and thromboembolic events to uninvolved arterial territories may also occur during endovascular revascularization. Device fractures require removal with foreign-body snare devices. Low-level anticoagulation with IV heparin during the procedure diminishes the risk of catheter- and guidewire-related thromboembolic events. Adverse contrast reaction includes allergy, with potentially fatal consequences if prompt management is not instituted, and renal failure, especially in patients with baseline renal insufficiency. Unfortunately, premedication with *N*-acetylcysteine[35] and prehydration with sodium bicarbonate drip,[36] which have both been shown to diminish the risk of contrast medium-induced nephropathy, is impractical for emergent stroke intervention. Although unproved, intraprocedural and postoperative administration of these agents may help prevent contrast nephropathy even in the absence of preadministration, and should be instituted in patients with renal insufficiency.

POSTPROCEDURAL AND FOLLOW-UP CARE

At the conclusion of an endovascular acute stroke intervention, common femoral artery hemostasis is obtained. Adequate hemostasis is necessary to avoid a groin complication. The nature of these interventions—namely, large groin sheaths and use of thrombolytics and platelet inhibitors—raises the risk of groin hematoma and retroperitoneal hemorrhage. Avoiding the latter involves careful arterial access, specifically avoiding arterial puncture above the inguinal ligament. After an endovascular stroke procedure, hemostasis is best obtained with a closure device (e.g., Angio-Seal Vascular Closure Device [St. Jude Medical Inc., St. Paul, Minn.]). If a closure device is contraindicated (e.g., in a septic patient), the sheath should be kept in place until the thrombolytic coagulopathy is reversed as the infused drugs are metabolized and eliminated. Manual compression is then sufficient for hemostasis.

As soon as revascularization is achieved, elevated blood pressure must be rapidly controlled to avoid reperfusion hemorrhage and hyperperfusion syndrome. Blood pressure can be efficiently managed with IV labetalol or a nicardipine drip. Systolic blood pressure targets of below 140 mmHg is the goal, and lower levels (e.g., 100-120 mmHg) may be required for patients with angiographic evidence of hyperperfusion (e.g., basal ganglia blush) after recanalization. Nicardipine drip is started at 5 mg/h IV infusion and can be titrated to a narrow blood pressure goal at 2.5 mg/h every 5 minutes to a maximum dose up to 15 mg/h. Vasodilating antihypertensives, such as nitroprusside, are best avoided because of their intracranial vasodilatory effects that theoretically can increase cerebral hyperperfusion.

After the procedure, the patient should be examined as quickly as possible to establish clinical improvement, no change, or detriment. If the patient's neurologic examination is worse than before the procedure, or if there is any clinical indication of ICH, such as headache, vomiting, decreased level of consciousness, anisocoria, or Cushing reaction (sudden hypertension and bradycardia associated with brainstem compression from cerebral herniation), an immediate head CT scan should be obtained. If ICH is encountered, procedure-related coagulopathy must be rapidly reversed, blood pressure controlled, and if the hemorrhage is of sufficient size, neurosurgical consultation for intracranial pressure monitoring and hematoma evacuation requested. Reversal of coagulopathy may include any combination of protamine (to reverse intraprocedural heparin), fresh frozen plasma, cryoprecipitate, and platelets, although coagulopathic correction is typically incomplete.

Postoperative observation and management in an intensive care unit, optimally one with specialty in neurologic patients, is obligatory. Within the first 24 hours, patients should have nursing neurologic assessments every hour and immediate head CT scans obtained for any clinical deterioration. Vital signs and blood glucose monitoring are essential for maximizing clinical outcome after stroke intervention. Other poststroke comorbidities must be prevented or managed, including deep vein thrombosis, pulmonary embolus, myocardial infarction, pneumonia, urosepsis, malnutrition, and pressure ulcers. Immediate focus on these issues is the key to maintaining a successful clinical outcome.

The remaining hospitalization is directed at continuing to prevent or manage poststroke complications, obtaining any necessary physical, occupational, or speech therapeutic services, and determining the etiology of the patient's stroke. The extent of the poststroke assessment depends on the supposed etiology of the stroke and patient age, where young patients with cryptogenic stroke and few risk factors generally have the most extensive evaluations. Secondary stroke prevention involves prescribing appropriate antiplatelet agents or warfarin and risk factor modification, including management of chronic hypertension, diabetes mellitus, hyperlipidemia, and counseling for smoking cessation. Key to preventing a second stroke is treatment of symptomatic extracranial carotid artery, vertebral artery, and potentially intracerebral arterial stenosis, the endovascular management of which is discussed in Chapter 93.

KEY POINTS

- The aim of endovascular stroke treatment is rapid restoration of brain perfusion to minimize cerebral tissue loss during an acute ischemic stroke.

- Endovascular stroke interventions include intraarterial thrombolytic infusion and mechanical embolectomy.

- These procedures are indicated for patients with contraindications for systemic tissue plasminogen activator (tPA), or who have failed to recanalize after intravenous tPA, who have accessible arterial occlusions and salvageable brain tissue.

- Devices like the Merci Retriever, the Penumbra Reperfusion System, and stentrievers can restore vessel patency without thrombolytic drugs, extending the time window of stroke treatment.

- Intracerebral hemorrhage, the major adverse consequence of endovascular stroke treatment, may be minimized by careful patient selection, judicious use of thrombolytic drugs, and strict postprocedural blood pressure control.

▶ **SUGGESTED READINGS**

Katz JM, Gobin YP, Segal AZ, Riina HA. Mechanical embolectomy. Neurosurg Clin N Am 2005;16(3):463–74, v.

Nogueira RG, Schwamm LH, Hirsch JA. Endovascular approaches to acute stroke, part 1: Drugs, devices, and data. AJNR Am J Neuroradiol 2009;30(4):649–61.

Nogueira RG, Yoo AJ, Buonanno FS, Hirsch JA. Endovascular approaches to acute stroke, part 2: A comprehensive review of studies and trials. AJNR Am J Neuroradiol 2009;30(5):859–75.

The complete reference list is available online at www.expertconsult.com.

CHAPTER 93

Endovascular Management of Chronic Cerebral Ischemia

Pierre Y. Gobin and Edward D. Greenberg

Chronic cerebral ischemia may be the result of extracranial carotid or vertebral stenosis and/or intracranial arterial stenoses. This chapter is going to focus on intracranial arterial stenoses as well as extracranial vertebral artery stenosis. For an in-depth discussion of extracranial carotid stenosis, please refer to Chapter 91, Carotid Revascularization. Intracranial atherosclerosis is estimated to be the underlying cause of 10% of all ischemic strokes[1,2] and carries a first-year ipsilateral stroke rate of at least 11%.[3] Twenty percent of all ischemic strokes involve the posterior circulation, and the most common area of vascular stenosis or occlusion in the setting of a posterior circulation stroke is the extracranial vertebral artery.[4] Given these strong associations with stroke, intracranial atherosclerotic disease and extracranial vertebral artery atherosclerotic disease have become prime targets for endovascular treatment.

INDICATIONS

The goal of intracerebral artery and extracranial vertebral endovascular revascularization in the setting of atherosclerotic stenosis is ipsilateral stroke prevention. Given the benign nature of asymptomatic intracranial atherosclerotic disease, asymptomatic patients with intracranial atherosclerotic narrowing should not be offered endovascular treatment.[5] Regarding treatment of symptomatic intracranial atherosclerosis, it is generally believed that endovascular treatment should only be considered in patients who remain symptomatic despite maximal medical therapy. The rationale leading up to this conclusion, including the preliminary results of the SAMMPRIS study (Stenting and Aggressive Medical Management for Preventing Recurrent Stroke in Intracranial Stenosis), are discussed in the following paragraphs.

The utility of best medical therapy alone in the treatment of intracranial atherosclerotic disease was evaluated in the Warfarin-Aspirin Symptomatic Intra-cranial Disease Trial (WASID).[3] In this study, patients with a history of stroke or transient ischemic attack (TIA) caused by an angiographically confirmed 50% to 99% intracranial artery stenosis were randomly assigned to receive aspirin (1300 mg; n = 280) or warfarin (target international normalized ratio 2.0 to 3.0; n = 289). The study was prematurely terminated because of higher death, major hemorrhage, and myocardial infarction rates in the warfarin group, without any primary endpoint benefit for either treatment (stroke/brain hemorrhage/vascular death other than stroke, 22.1% for aspirin vs. 21.8% for warfarin). Perhaps most importantly, this study illustrated the high morbidity and lack of effective medical therapy for moderate to severe intracranial atherosclerotic stenosis at that time. The overall 1- and 2-year rates of ischemic stroke in the territory of the stenosed artery were 11% and 14%, respectively. Factors associated with increased stroke risk included stenosis greater than

70%, recent symptoms, and female gender.[6] The risk of a recent index event (TIA or stroke) and the linear increase in stroke risk associated with the degree of stenosis is analogous to the risk stratification observed in cervical carotid artery disease, which is estimated at 22% for severe symptomatic stenosis.

Endovascular stenting is another treatment option that has been studied for the prevention of recurrent stroke or TIA in patients with intracranial atherosclerotic disease. However, evaluation of the efficacy of intracranial angioplasty and stenting is limited by factors such as rapidly evolving technology, the wide variation in endovascular techniques, and the overall lack of controlled data in the literature. Outcome after endovascular treatment for chronic cerebral ischemia is generally measured by technical success, incidence of restenosis, and early and long-term ipsilateral stroke rates. Technical success for intracerebral arterial and extracranial vertebral artery disease, defined as residual stenosis post procedure of less than 50%, is on the order of 95%.[7-10] However, restenosis rates are high, with the Stenting of Symptomatic Atherosclerotic Lesions in the Vertebral or Intracranial Arteries (SSYLVIA) study[8] reporting a 43% restenosis rate over a mean follow-up period of 16 months for extracranial vertebral artery stenting and a 32.4% restenosis rate for intracranial stenting. In estimating the overall risk of stroke and death associated with intracranial angioplasty with or without stenting, a Cochrane systematic review of 79 publications calculated the pooled periprocedural rate of stroke or death at 9.5%.[11]

The SSYLVIA study,[8] a nonrandomized prospective protocol evaluating the feasibility of the Neurolink System (Guidant Corp., Indianapolis, Ind.) for vertebral and intracranial artery stenosis, included patients with 50% or greater stenosis by angiography with a recent history of stroke (60.7%) or TIA (39.3%). Failure of medical therapy before endovascular intervention was not a prerequisite for this study. Of the 61 patients included, 43 underwent treatment for symptomatic intracranial stenosis (15 internal carotid, 5 middle cerebral, 1 posterior cerebral, 17 basilar, 5 vertebral), and 18 underwent treatment for extracranial vertebral artery stenosis (6 ostial lesions and 12 lesions proximal to the posterior inferior cerebellar artery). Successful stenting with residual stenosis of less than 50% was attained in 95% (58/61 patients). However, as noted, restenosis rates were high: 12/37 or 32.4% for the intracranial arteries and 6/14 or 42.9% for the extracranial vertebrals. Among the 18 patients with restenosis, 7 (39%) were symptomatic. Strokes occurred in 6.6% of patients within 30 days and in 7.3% between 30 days and 1 year, and there were no deaths.

In the prospective multicenter Wingspan trial,[7] 45 patients with symptomatic medically refractory intracranial stenosis of more than 50% were treated with angioplasty and Wingspan stent placement (Fig. 93-1). Technical success, defined as residual postprocedure stenosis of less

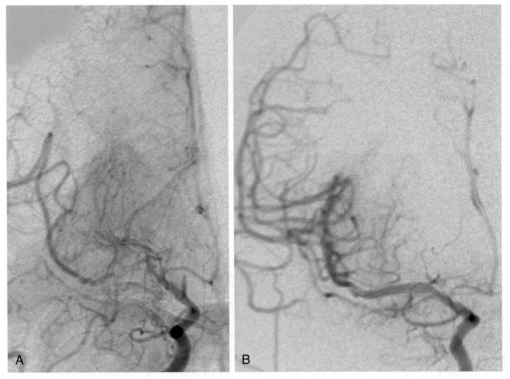

FIGURE 93-1. Intracranial angioplasty and stenting. **A,** Right common carotid artery angiogram, intracranial anteroposterior view, demonstrates a critical right middle cerebral artery (MCA) stenosis in this 57-year-old woman with multiple right MCA distribution infarcts and hypoperfusion on computed tomographic perfusion imaging. **B,** Complete recanalization is achieved after angioplasty with a 2.5-mm Gateway balloon and placement of a 3 × 20 mm Wingspan stent (Boston Scientific, Natick, Mass.).

than 50%, was achieved in 100% of cases. The incidence of restenosis was only 7.5%, much lower than in the SSYLVIA study, and the ipsilateral 30-day and 6-month combined stroke and death rates were 4.4% and 7.1%, respectively.

The only prospective randomized study on the topic of intracranial angioplasty and stenting is the SAMMPRIS trial, which compared aggressive medical management alone to intracranial stenting plus aggressive medical management for the prevention of stroke in patients with symptomatic severe intracranial stenosis (70%-99%) of a major artery (middle cerebral, carotid, vertebral, or basilar arteries). In the context of the study, aggressive medical management consisted of aspirin 325 mg/day for the entire follow-up, clopidogrel 75 mg/day for 90 days after enrollment, intensive management of vascular risk factors (systolic blood pressure < 140 mmHg, [<130 mmHg if diabetic], low-density lipoprotein [LDL] levels below 70 mg/dL), and lifestyle modification programs for all study patients. Recruitment was halted after 451 (59%) of the planned 764 patients were enrolled, owing to the higher risk of stroke and death detected in the stented group (14%) compared to the aggressive medical management alone group (5.8%) in the first 30 days of enrollment.[12] In the period beyond 30 days, the risk of stroke and death appear to be similar in the two groups, although most of the patients have not been followed for 1 year.[12] The preliminary results of the SAMM-PRIS trial illustrate both the significant benefit of aggressive medical management to treat severe symptomatic intracranial stenosis, and the important risks of endovascular treatment in this patient population. In summary, the results of the cited studies support considering endovascular

treatment in patients with intracranial atherosclerotic disease only if they remain symptomatic despite maximal aggressive medical therapy.

Intracranial angioplasty and stenting can also be indicated in a number of conditions besides atherosclerotic disease, although there is an overall paucity of data regarding these entities. Patients with symptomatic vertebral or intracerebral artery traumatic or idiopathic dissection who have failed adequate medical therapy may be considered for angioplasty and stent placement. Additionally, patients with nonatherosclerotic stenosis secondary to Takayasu arteritis, moyamoya disease, and connective tissue diseases such as fibromuscular dysplasia may benefit from angioplasty and possible stenting, although recent evidence in the case of moyamoya disease has shown that although such intervention may temporarily improve brain perfusion, angioplasty/stenting does not appear to provide long-term prevention against ischemic events in these patients.[13] Furthermore, the authors' own experience has shown high restenosis rates when angioplasty and stenting are performed in cases of arteritis.

CONTRAINDICATIONS

Relative clinical contraindications to endovascular management of chronic cerebral ischemia are related to the risk of cerebral angiography and include severe contrast allergy and chronic renal insufficiency. Both of these may be managed with appropriate premedication. Administration of diphenhydramine (50 mg, 1 hour preoperatively) and prednisone (50 mg at 24, 12, and 1 hour preoperatively) is effective contrast allergy prophylaxis. Hydration with intravenous sodium bicarbonate solution and oral administration of *N*-acetylcysteine before and after contrast agent administration has demonstrated efficacy in preventing contrast nephropathy.[14,15] Other relative clinical contraindications are related to the need for combination antiplatelet therapy for at least 4 weeks after stenting. These include allergy or intolerance (excessive bruising) to aspirin and clopidogrel therapy. The requirement for combination antiplatelet therapy, intended to prevent platelet aggregation, embolization, and stent thrombosis until stent endothelialization, also makes the urgent need for a major surgical procedure a relative contraindication for stenting.

Relative anatomic contraindications for stenting procedures are usually manageable by experienced operators when present individually. However, as the number of anatomic difficulties accrues, the procedure becomes significantly higher risk, making medical management preferable to the endovascular approach. Anatomic relative contraindications include severe tortuosity, calcification, or atherosclerotic disease of the aortic arch and origins of the great vessels (Fig. 93-2). These changes make endovascular access difficult and significantly raise the risk of thromboembolic complications. Great-vessel origin stenosis is manageable by angioplasty and stenting concurrently with treatment of the target vessel. Severe tortuosity and acute takeoff of the common carotid artery and severe tortuosity of the internal carotid artery make access for a guide catheter or sheath and delivery of angioplasty balloon and stent challenging. Other anatomic considerations, including tandem stenoses, unruptured intracranial aneurysms, and arteriovenous malformations, are not contraindications to endovascular therapy. Poorly controlled hypertension and a large recent infarct raise the risk of post-revascularization intracerebral hemorrhage from reperfusion injury and hyperperfusion syndrome. Postponing revascularization therapy

(endovascular or surgical) 10 to 14 days after a moderate to large stroke and careful postoperative blood pressure control can effectively minimize these risks. Intensive medical therapy, including combination antiplatelet and high-dose statin therapy, in the first weeks after a stroke may also facilitate plaque stabilization, lowering the thromboembolic risk associated with the endovascular approach.

EQUIPMENT

All stenting procedures necessitate premedication and postmedication with aspirin (325 mg/day) and clopidogrel (75 mg/day; at least 300 mg is required before stent placement). Clopidogrel is continued after the procedure during the period of stent endothelialization to prevent stent thrombosis. Patient monitoring includes cardiac telemetry, pulse oximetry, and continuous arterial blood pressure by radial arterial line. Conscious sedation is preferred for extracranial vertebral artery stenting, whereas general endotracheal anesthesia is preferred for intracranial stenting. All procedures are performed under systemic heparinization to a target activated clotting time of two to three times baseline.

Vascular access is typically with a 6F sheath placed into the common femoral artery. In the setting of severe stenosis or occlusive disease of the aortoiliac vessels or severe aortic arch tortuosity, the transfemoral approach may not be possible. In these circumstances, radial artery access may be required. The transradial approach requires performance of an Allen test (with pulse oximetry) to confirm adequate collateral circulation to the hand from the ulnar artery and a combination of trans–introducer sheath injections, including verapamil (2.5 mg), cardiac lidocaine (2%, 1 mL), and nitroglycerin (0.1 mg) to prevent radial artery vasospasm, and systemic heparinization (80 units/kg) to inhibit thrombosis. The transbrachial approach is a second option, but potential median nerve injury and brachial artery thrombosis make it less favorable. Digital biplane angiography is required for intracranial procedures. Diagnostic catheterization is performed with standard equipment, including a 5F diagnostic catheter (e.g., Torcon Vert [Cook Medical, Bloomington, Ind.]) and a 0.035- or 0.038-inch guidewire (e.g., Glidewire [Terumo Medical Corp., Somerset, N.J.]). Standard nonionic iodinated contrast medium (Omnipaque [GE Healthcare, Piscataway, NJ]) is used for angiography. Angioplasty and stenting requires relatively stiff guide catheter support. For anterior circulation lesions in patients with non-tortuous anatomy, a 6F guide catheter, such as a 6F Envoy Guide Catheter (Cordis Neurovascular, Miami Lakes, Fla.) is usually adequate. In patients with anterior circulation lesions and tortuous anatomy, a 90-cm 6F or 7F sheath (Cordis) or Shuttle Sheath (Cook Medical) may be used in combination with an intermediary catheter such as the Neuron Intracranial Access System (Penumbra Inc., San Leandro, Calif.) or a Distal Access Catheter (DAC) (Concentric Medical, Mountain View, Calif.). For posterior circulation lesions, a 5F or 6F guide catheter, such as an Envoy placed high up in the vertebral artery, provides excellent support. High-pressure angioplasty balloons are inflated with insufflator devices, using a 50% contrast-in-saline solution to achieve nominal filling pressures.

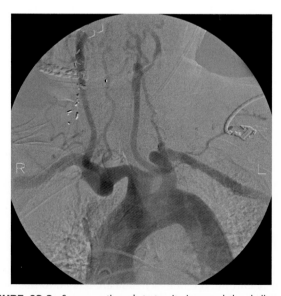

FIGURE 93-2. Severe aortic arch tortuosity increased the challenge of endovascular therapy in this 68-year-old man with symptomatic postirradiation left internal carotid artery stenosis. Note bovine aortic arch and sharp angle made by left common carotid artery as it ascends into neck.

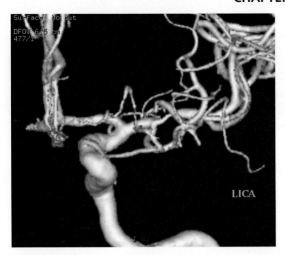

FIGURE 93-3. Computer-generated reconstruction of a left internal carotid artery angiogram in three-dimensional rotational projection demonstrates a short severe stenosis of the mid-M1 segment of the left middle cerebral artery. Arterial lumen diameters generated from these reconstructions enable precise balloon and stent size selection, which is necessary for safe intracranial stenting procedures.

Intracranial angioplasty employs small-diameter (1.5-4 mm) balloons, including the Maverick and Gateway balloons (Boston Scientific, Natick, Mass.), which are navigated coaxially over an exchange-length microguidewire (0.014-inch Transend Floppy exchange wire [Boston Scientific]) that is initially positioned using a microcatheter past the stenosis. Balloon diameter is slightly undersized compared to the normal luminal diameter of the vessel (estimated based on the diameter of the healthy arterial segment distal to the stenosis) to minimize the risk of vessel dissection and rupture. Appropriate size selection is especially crucial to the safety of intracerebral angioplasty, requiring normal luminal diameter measurement on computerized three-dimensional (3D) rotational reconstruction of the diseased artery (Fig. 93-3). Stents may be dichotomized into balloon-expandable stents, including drug-eluting stents, and self-expanding stents that swell to a preset diameter (straight or tapered) and conform to the inherent tortuosity of the cervicocerebral vasculature. Selection of stent diameter is oversized 0.5 to 1 mm compared to the normal diameter of the target vessel. This increases the radial force that implants the stent into the vessel wall, enhancing neo-endothelialization, a process paramount to regeneration of a smooth vessel lumen.[16] The Wingspan stent is a self-expandable stent and is currently the only available stent approved by the U.S. Food and Drug Administration (FDA) for treatment of intracranial stenosis. Balloon-expandable stents may be used for treatment of intracranial atherosclerotic disease as well, but no balloon-expandable stent is currently FDA-approved for this purpose. Such stents are favored for extracranial vertebral artery stenosis because they allow for more precise deployment. Stent restenosis caused by neointimal hyperplasia is a major concern after extracranial vertebral artery stenting. For this reason, drug-eluting stents, including paclitaxel-(Taxus [Boston Scientific]) and sirolimus- (Cypher [Cordis]) eluting stents are often preferred during extracranial vertebral artery revascularization procedures.

TECHNIQUE

Anatomy and Approach

Diagnostic cervicocerebral angiography is performed in the usual fashion from the transfemoral approach through the abdominal and thoracic aorta into the ipsilateral common carotid artery for intracranial internal carotid and middle or anterior cerebral artery stenosis, the ipsilateral subclavian artery for extracranial vertebral origin stenosis, and the ipsilateral vertebral artery for intracranial vertebrobasilar artery stenosis. Cervical as well as intracranial angiography must be performed before intervention to evaluate for tandem stenoses to assess for any baseline distal branch occlusions and gain an understanding of the angioanatomy of the stenosis and the interventional approach. The degree and length of stenosis and the vessel caliber both proximal and distal to the stenotic area are measured. These measurements are more accurately attained during intracranial stenting procedures with the use of 3D rotational angiography.

Technical Aspects

Key equipment is listed in Table 93-1.

A 6F sheath is placed in the femoral artery, and a diagnostic angiogram is performed using a 5F diagnostic catheter. After planning the endovascular approach, a loading dose of intravenous heparin (70 units/kg) is given, and the guide catheter is navigated directly or via exchange technique into the internal carotid, subclavian, or vertebral artery, depending on the location of the stenosis. For intracranial stenosis, the guide catheter is placed as high as possible in the internal carotid or vertebral artery to maximize support during the angioplasty and stenting procedure. The distal cervical portion of the internal carotid artery or the distal V2 segment of the vertebral artery are generally considered excellent guide catheter positions, although in some cases more distal catheterization can be obtained with an intermediary catheter such as a DAC or Neuron. The guide catheter should be positioned proximal to any sharp curves in the vessel to minimize the chance for vessel injury and vasospasm. A good working view is obtained that demonstrates the target stenosis under high magnification and includes the guide catheter in the field of view. A microcatheter is then navigated past the lesion over an exchange-length microwire (Fig. 93-4). The microcatheter is removed, and the angioplasty balloon is advanced over the microwire and positioned across the stenosis. Balloon position is ascertained by the presence of proximal and distal radiopaque markers. The balloon is inflated to nominal pressure using an insufflator and a 50/50 mixture of contrast in heparinized saline to restore the vessel lumen to approximately 80% of its normal caliber (Fig. 93-5). After the angioplasty is completed, the balloon is removed and an angiogram is performed to visualize the angiographic result and determine whether or not stenting will be performed. In this regard, there is great variability in practice; many neurointerventionalists invariably continue on to stenting, while others reserve stenting for cases with significant recoil or dissection. In the case of intracranial angioplasty and stenting, the Wingspan stent, which obtained FDA approval in 2005 as a Humanitarian Device, is typically

TABLE 93-1. Key Equipment for Endovascular Management of Chronic Cerebral Ischemia

Device	Example	Company
Guidewire	Terumo 0.035-inch	Terumo Medical Corp., Somerset, N.J.
Diagnostic catheter	Torcon Vert 5F, 125 cm	Cook Medical, Bloomington, Ind.
Carotid sheath	6F, 90-cm sheath Shuttle Introducer	Cordis Corp., Miami Lakes, Fla. Cook Medical
Guide catheter	Envoy Guide Catheter Guider Softip XF guide catheter	Cordis Neurovascular, Miami Lakes, Fla. Boston Scientific, Natick, Mass.
Intermediary catheters	Neuron Intracranial Access System Distal Access Catheter (DAC)	Penumbra Inc., San Leandro, Calif. Concentric Medical, Mountain View, Calif.
Balloon catheter—ICAS	Gateway PTA balloon	Boston Scientific
Exchange-length microwire	Transend floppy exchange wire 0.014	Boston Scientific
Stent—ICAS	Wingspan	Boston Scientific
Stent—drug eluting	Cypher Taxus	Cordis Boston Scientific

CAS, Carotid artery stent; *ICAS,* intracranial artery stent.

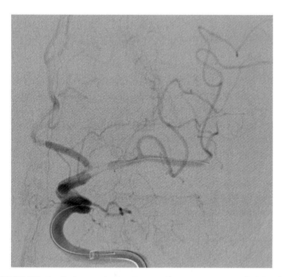

FIGURE 93-4. Endovascular treatment of severe symptomatic left middle cerebral artery stenosis in a 66-year-old woman. Working view shows guide catheter in good position within petrous internal carotid artery. An exchange-length microwire is also present and appropriately placed across area of severe stenosis.

used. The Wingspan stent, made of nitinol, is not radiopaque but instead has four proximal and four distal radiopaque markers that identify its deployed position (Fig. 93-6). The delivery system has four radiopaque indicators representing, from most distal to most proximal, the delivery system tip, compressed distal stent markers, compressed proximal stent markers, and stent stabilizer tip. During deployment, the stent stabilizer is advanced to the proximal stent marker and then held in place as the delivery system sheath is carefully withdrawn, releasing the stent into position. Care must be taken to avoid distal or proximal stent migration during deployment. Subsequent angiography evaluates the accuracy of stent position and degree of residual stenosis. Postprocedural cervical and intracranial angiography can then be used to assess the final degree of revascularization and evaluate for arterial dissection,

catheter-induced vasospasm, and intracranial distal branch occlusion (Fig. 93-7).

CONTROVERSIES

There is much controversy regarding the role of endovascular therapies for extracranial vertebral artery stenosis and intracranial arterial stenosis. No effective surgical option exists for intracranial atherosclerotic stenosis, since the only available operative therapy (i.e., extracranial-intracranial bypass) has been proven ineffective.[17] The risks and benefits of intracranial angioplasty and stenting compared to aggressive medical management have not yet been clearly established. Conflicting data are available from two recent studies,[18,19] as well as the recently discontinued SAMMPRIS trial.[12] For patients with symptomatic intracranial stenosis greater than 50% undergoing percutaneous transluminal angioplasty and stenting with the Gateway-Wingspan stenting system, Fiorella et al. report a perioperative stroke or death rate and ipsilateral stroke rate after 30 days of 13.2% per year.[19] For patients undergoing percutaneous transluminal angioplasty and stenting with the Gateway-Wingspan stenting system for symptomatic intracranial stenosis greater than 70%, Jiang et al. report a perioperative stroke or death rate and ipsilateral stroke rate after 30 days of 5% per year.[18] However, the recent SAMMPRIS trial comparing best medical therapy versus angioplasty and stenting with the Wingspan system plus best medical therapy in patients with symptomatic 70% or more intracranial cerebral artery disease (ICAD) reports a 14% 30-day rate of stroke or death with stenting, compared to 5.8% in the medical arm, a highly significant difference in favor of medical therapy.[12] Given the uncertain risks and efficacy of angioplasty combined with stenting in these patients, the authors of this chapter prefer to treat patients with symptomatic intracranial stenosis of 70% or greater whose neurological deficits are suspected to be related to hypoperfusion, or patients with recurrent symptoms despite optimal medical therapy. Angioplasty alone is performed initially, and stenting is reserved for patients with arterial recoil or dissection. Although angioplasty alone has been shown to result in lower success rates and higher restenosis

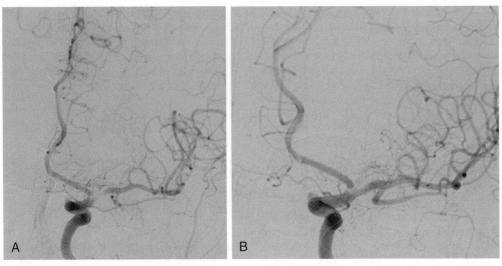

FIGURE 93-5. **A,** Posteroanterior (PA) projection before angioplasty demonstrates severe stenosis of M1 segment of left middle cerebral artery. **B,** PA projection after angioplasty demonstrates marked improvement in vessel caliber.

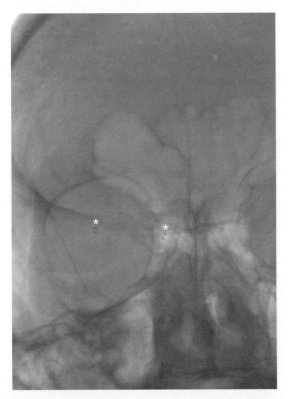

FIGURE 93-6. Unsubtracted anteroposterior view of cranium showing the four proximal and four distal radiopaque markers of the Wingspan stent *(asterisks)*.

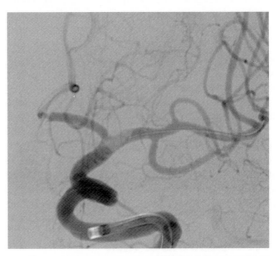

FIGURE 93-7. Posteroanterior projection after left middle cerebral artery stenting using the Wingspan system. Arterial lumen is essentially normal. No evidence of vascular dissection.

rates than angioplasty combined with stenting, the significantly lower rate of procedure-related stroke favors this approach.[20]

Looking to the future, selecting patients who are expected to optimally benefit from intracranial angioplasty and stenting (i.e., patients with distal territory hypoperfusion as opposed to artery-to-artery emboli) has the potential to result in improved patient outcomes.[12] Studies of brain perfusion, such as magnetic resonance (MR) and computed tomographic (CT) perfusion, with or without administration of a vasodilator such as acetazolamide, may be useful in identifying these patients and guiding management of extracranial vertebral artery stenosis and intracranial arterial stenosis by measuring cerebrovascular reserve. However, at the present time, there is a paucity of evidence regarding these techniques, their indications, and their role in management.

COMPLICATIONS

Complications of endovascular treatment of chronic cerebral ischemia are thromboembolic stroke, arterial dissection or perforation, intracranial hemorrhage, reperfusion hemorrhage, cerebral hyperperfusion syndrome, catheter-induced vasospasm, groin hemorrhage, and common femoral artery injury (dissection, pseudoaneurysm formation, perforation, or thrombosis).

Thromboembolic stroke rates during intracranial stenting range from 0% to 20% in several case series,[21] and the 30-day stroke rate was 6.6% in the SSYLVIA trial[8] and 14% in the preliminary results of the SAMMPRIS trial.[12] Reperfusion hemorrhage into a previous cerebral infarct is less common after endovascular management of chronic cerebral ischemia than after acute ischemic stroke intervention and is fully discussed in Chapter 92, Acute Stroke Management. The presence of a large cerebral infarct increases the risk of reperfusion hemorrhage, so in the setting of a large recent stroke, intracranial revascularization should be delayed 10 to 14 days to minimize the risk of reperfusion hemorrhage and maximize the benefit of therapy. Cerebral hyperperfusion syndrome is a rare event, complicating 1.1% of carotid artery stenting procedures.[22] It is caused by impaired autoregulation resulting from chronic hemispheric ischemia distal to a severely narrowed internal carotid artery.[23] The severe form is characterized by headache, seizures, focal neurologic deficits, and intracerebral hemorrhage and may arise several days after revascularization.[22-25] Risk factors include severe bilateral carotid stenosis and periprocedural hypertension.[22] Although most commonly associated with treatment of cervical carotid stenosis, cerebral hyperperfusion syndrome may also complicate intracranial stenting procedures.[26,27] MRI or CT with perfusion-weighted imaging is helpful in the diagnosis of cerebral hyperperfusion and for differentiating this syndrome from thromboembolic stroke, reperfusion hemorrhage, and acute stent thrombosis, which may present with similar clinical manifestations. Early recognition and aggressive blood pressure control are crucial to successful management. In patients deemed at high risk for cerebral hyperperfusion or already symptomatic, inducing hypotension to systolic pressures near 100 mmHg may be required. Medications such as intravenous labetalol and continuous nicardipine infusion are most useful in this regard.

POSTPROCEDURAL AND FOLLOW-UP CARE

The major thrust of postrevascularization management is monitoring for the aforementioned complications during the first 24-hour postoperative period. Patients should be followed with cardiac telemetry and continuous arterial blood pressure monitoring to watch for hemodynamic instability. Frequent neurologic assessments every 1 to 2 hours are necessary to evaluate for cerebral hyperperfusion syndrome and acute stent thrombosis. For intracranial stenting procedures, particularly those patients with multiple medical comorbidities, in-hospital postoperative monitoring may require an observation period of several days. Subsequent to discharge, patients are maintained on aspirin (325 mg daily) and clopidogrel (75 mg daily) for at least 3 months after intracranial stenting. Afterward, the clopidogrel is stopped and the aspirin dose continued or lowered to 81 mg daily indefinitely.

CT angiography and gadolinium-enhanced MR angiography may at some point offer a noninvasive technique for postoperative assessment of poststent intracerebral artery and extracranial vertebral artery evaluation, but catheter angiography is currently the most reliable technique to monitor these patients.

KEY POINTS

- Intracranial atherosclerotic disease has significant morbidity associated with medical therapy, and no beneficial surgical option exists.

- Preliminary results of the SAMMPRIS trial suggest that patients with severe symptomatic intracranial atherosclerotic disease should initially be offered aggressive medical management without endovascular treatment.

- Intracranial stenting can be considered for symptomatic patients refractory to best medical therapy.

▸ **SUGGESTED READINGS**

Bose A, Hartmann M, Henkes H, et al. A novel, self-expanding, nitinol stent in medically refractory intracranial atherosclerotic stenoses: The Wingspan study. Stroke 2007;38(5):1531–7.

Chimowitz MI, Lynn MJ, Howlett-Smith H, et al. Comparison of warfarin and aspirin for symptomatic intracranial arterial stenosis. N Engl J Med 2005;352(13):1305–16.

SSYLVIA Study Investigators. Stenting of symptomatic atherosclerotic lesions in the vertebral or intracranial arteries (SSYLVIA): Study results. Stroke 2004;35(6):1388–92.

Higashida RT, Meyers PM, Connors JJ 3rd, et al. Intracranial angioplasty and stenting for cerebral atherosclerosis: A position statement of the American Society of Interventional and Therapeutic Neuroradiology, Society of Interventional Radiology, and the American Society of Neuroradiology. J Vasc Interv Radiol 2009;20(7 Suppl):S312–6.

The complete reference list is available online at www.expertconsult.com.

CHAPTER 94

Management of Head and Neck Tumors

Todd S. Miller, Elizabeth R. Tang, Randall P. Owen, Jacqueline A. Bello, and Allan L. Brook

The types of masses encountered in the head and neck are diverse, as are their appropriate treatments. Some benign head and neck lesions are treated primarily by surgical means without endovascular intervention. For example, when possible, hemangiomas are commonly excised by laser, and lymphangiomas are sclerosed by direct puncture or surgically resected.[1] Certain highly vascular benign tumors like carotid body paragangliomas and juvenile nasal angiofibromas are frequently treated with preoperative embolization.

Malignancy is treated by surgery whenever possible.[2,3] Often, however, these patients present with the tumor at a high stage. For stage IV squamous cell carcinoma, 5-year survival rates are lower than 25% following surgery and/or radiotherapy.[4] Management of these serious late-stage malignancies is complex, involving substantial teamwork among several disciplines. The interventional radiologist's role on this team is most necessary for advanced tumors or carotid blowout syndrome (CBS) secondary to such tumors and/or complications of treatment. Potential interventions include balloon test occlusion (BTO), preoperative embolization to aid surgery or posttreatment embolization for hemorrhage due to tumor necrosis, emergent treatment of CBS, intraarterial chemotherapy, and image-guided radiofrequency ablation (RFA).[5]

INDICATIONS FOR ENDOVASCULAR THERAPY OF BENIGN HEAD/NECK LESIONS

The two most common endovascularly treated benign lesions of the head and neck are paragangliomas and juvenile nasal angiofibromas (JNAs). Preoperative embolization of other potentially highly vascular head/neck tumors, including angiomyomas (i.e., angioleiomyoma, vascular leiomyoma),[6,7] neurofibromas,[8] schwannomas,[9,10] hemangioendothelioma,[11] and meningioma[1] has been reported. Congenital vascular malformations that have failed to regress or those whose mass effect impinges on vital structures have also been successfully treated with endovascular therapy.[12]

Paragangliomas

Paragangliomas are slow-growing tumors that originate from the neural crest of the autonomic nervous system and can be hereditary in 7% to 9% of cases.[13] Locations in the head and neck include the carotid body (35%), glomus vagale (11%), tympanic and/or jugular regions (almost 50%; jugulotympanic if the tumor is larger and melds together over the two regions), and other locations (6%) including the orbit, nasal cavity, and the rare laryngeal case, 90% of which are supraglottic.[14] The malignant potential of paragangliomas is generally low at around 4%,[15] but it can be up to 10% to 18% for the vagal, carotid, and laryngeal types.[3]

Recommended therapy for paragangliomas is complete surgical excision. Given the high vascularity of these tumors, the role of endovascular management by preoperative angiogram and embolization can be significant. If a paraganglioma is suspected, a diagnostic superselective angiogram should precede any biopsy attempt, lest the attempt lead to arterial rupture. The angiogram should include bilateral exploration,[16] since multicentric paragangliomas occur in up to 80% of familial cases and 10% to 20% of nonfamilial,[17] and bilateral carotid body tumors occur in 5% of sporadic and 33% to 38% of familial lesions.[13] In addition, diagnostic angiography may demonstrate occult lesions not previously demonstrated on computed tomography (CT) or magnetic resonance imaging (MRI).[16] Diagnostic evaluation demonstrates the blood supply and flow dynamics of the tumor. The venous supply can be mapped, allowing the surgeon to preserve the venous drainage, limiting blood loss.

The role of embolization in paraganglioma management depends on the extent of the tumor and the anatomy of its feeding branches.[3,16,17] In jugular or jugulotympanic paragangliomas with more complicated vasculature involvement, preoperative embolization has become a definite part of surgical management and can significantly reduce intraoperative blood loss.[17,18] In most tympanic and laryngeal cases, preoperative embolization is unnecessary.[17,19] Transarterial or direct puncture embolization as an alternative to radiotherapy could be considered as the primary therapy for paragangliomas that are unresectable or where resection would be debilitating.[1,20-22,63]

As for the management of carotid body and vagal paragangliomas, most recommend preoperative embolization, but the role of preoperative embolization is still a matter of debate, especially it seems for carotid body tumors.[14,17,23] Carotid body tumors are potentially the most challenging to resect. This tumor originates in the bifurcation of the common carotid artery (CCA), where it commonly involves the internal carotid artery (ICA) and receives feeding vessels from external carotid branches and muscular branches of the ICA.[24] When small, hemostasis can be controlled during resection through careful preoperative and intraoperative consideration of the ascending pharyngeal artery (Fig. 94-1).[14,13,11]

Finally, if resection of the paraganglioma may require sacrifice of the carotid artery, particularly in the case of

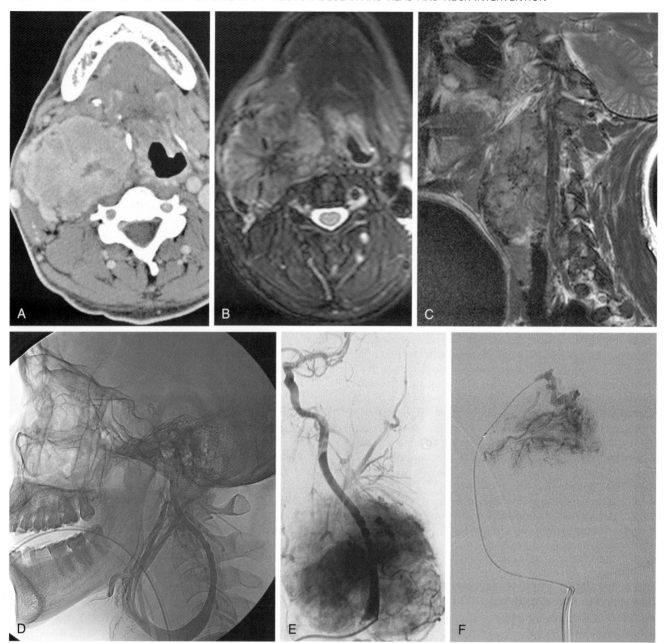

FIGURE 94-1. Carotid body tumor. **A,** Axial contrast-enhanced CT demonstrating large enhancing mass deviating airway. Vessels of carotid sheath are splayed. **B,** Axial Fat Sat T2-weighted fast spin-echo (FSE) magnetic resonance imaging (MRI) demonstrating same findings with flow-related signal voids seen within central tumor. **C,** Sagittal Fat Sat FSE T2-weighted MRI demonstrating flow-related signal voids within mass centered on carotid sheath. **D,** Lateral angiogram demonstrating splayed external and internal carotid arteries. **E,** Capillary phase from same angiogram in anteroposterior view demonstrating diffuse capillary blush. **F,** Lateral angiogram taken with a coaxial microcatheter and guide demonstrating multicompartmental blood supply. This technique was used to deliver polyvinyl alcohol particles 150 to 250 μm in size to each feeding vessel. Immediate surgical resection followed.

large jugulotympanic tumors and larger carotid body tumors, another necessary preoperative endovascular intervention is BTO of the ICA.[24]

Juvenile Nasal Angiofibromas

JNAs are benign, submucosal, unencapsulated, vascular tumors that are most commonly diagnosed in adolescent males between 14 and 25 years old, but can present at any age. The tumor is locally destructive and tends to erode

bone as it spreads.[24] Patients usually present with unilateral nasal obstruction or epistaxis. The majority originate in the sphenopalatine foramen and progress to the pterygo-palatine fossa, infratemporal fossa, sphenoid sinus, and/or other locations within the head/neck.[25,26] Though benign, the risk of bleeding and/or further intracranial extension can be life threatening.[27] Surgical resection is considered one of the best treatment options, in which preoperative embolization plays a significant role to prevent excessive intraoperative blood loss.[28]

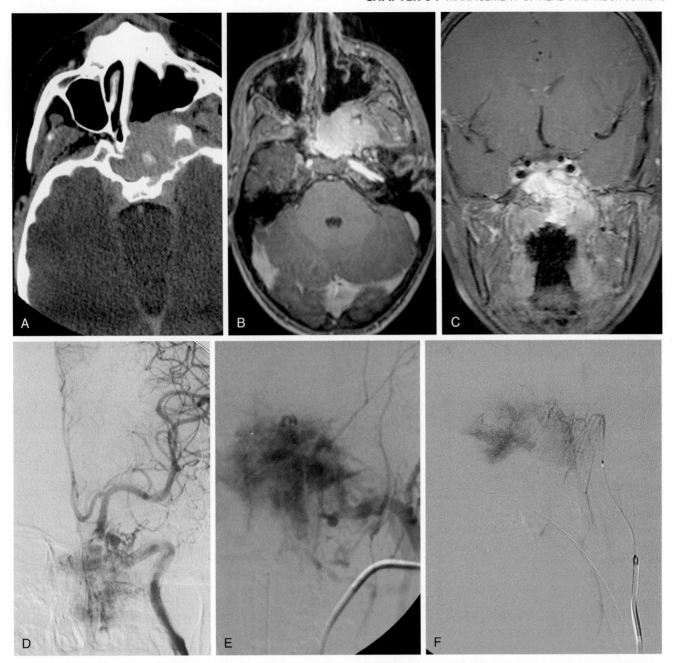

FIGURE 94-2. Juvenile nasopharyngeal angiofibroma. **A,** Axial contrast-enhanced CT demonstrating an enhancing mass expanding pterygopalatine fossa and extending through foramina. Foramina are expanded and bone is eroded. **B,** Axial contrast-enhanced magnetic resonance imaging (MRI) demonstrating similar findings. **C,** Coronal contrast-enhanced MRI with fat suppression demonstrating tumor extent relative to skull base. **D,** Anteroposterior (AP) angiogram demonstrating internal carotid arterial supply and tumor blush. **E,** AP angiogram with a 4F H1 catheter injecting left internal maxillary artery, causing intense tumor blush. **F,** Lateral angiogram demonstrating coaxial microcatheter and guide used to inject ascending pharyngeal artery. This technique was used to deliver 150- to 250-μm polyvinyl alcohol particles to bilateral external carotid artery branches feeding tumor. Immediate surgical resection followed.

Determining the extent of intracranial involvement is crucial to treatment planning for these lesions, as is determining the vascular supply, which may include ipsi- and contralateral, internal and external carotid artery (ECA) systems.[29] Pretherapeutic planning often involves endoscopic biopsy, CT scan, MRI, and diagnostic angiography (Fig. 94-2). In cases where diagnostic angiography shows risk of surgical injury to or potential involvement of the ICA, BTO of the ICA should be used to determine adequacy of collateral blood flow. Because profuse intraoperative bleeding is a hallmark of JNA surgery, preoperative embolization of feeding vessels from the external carotid system is consistently recommended in the ear, nose, and throat literature, although some authors rely on intraoperative ligation of feeding vessels.[25,29,30,31] Decreased blood loss, surgical time and morbidity have been demonstrated with either approach. This consideration is crucial because the relatively lower intravascular blood volume of children

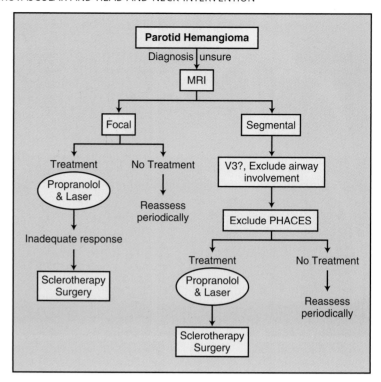

FIGURE 94-3. Decision tree for management of parotid heman-giomas. *(From Weiss I, O TM, Lipari BA, Meyer L, Berenstein A, Waner M. Current treatment of parotid hemangiomas. Laryngoscope 2011;121: 1642–50, Fig. 5.)*

limits their tolerance for blood loss. Direct embolization with Onyx has been performed as part of endoscopic resection as well.[32]

Congenital Vascular Malformations

Congenital vascular malformations are primarily treated with percutaneous therapy, where direct puncture of these lesions allows instillation of sclerosing agents. In some cases, however, endovascular techniques can assist in therapy (Fig. 94-3).

Congenital vascular malformations are categorized as either low- or high-flow lesions. The low-flow group includes telangiectasias, lymphangiomas, and hemangio-mas. Although sclerotherapy is the dominant therapy for this group,[12,33] when hemangiomas present as superficial fungating hemorrhagic lesions large enough to sequester platelets or obstruct vision or vital structures, polyvinyl alcohol (PVA) embolization may be used conservatively.[3,34] To prevent disfigurement or facial nerve injury when hem-angiomas present in the face, surgical excision is usually performed but requires complete resection to minimize the high rate of recurrence. Preoperative embolization assists resection by shrinking the tumor and also helps preserve cosmetic appearance following surgery.[1,35,36]

The high-flow group, in addition to JNAs, includes arte-riovenous fistulas (AVFs)/aneurysms and arteriovenous malformations (AVMs). Kohout et al.'s study (1998), the largest analysis of patients with head/neck AVMs, showed the most success with those lesions treated by a combina-tion of super-selective embolization and aggressive surgical resection.[37,38] Although embolization and surgery lead to a much higher curative rate for head/neck AVMs, the com-plication rate has been reported as almost double that of ethanol sclerotherapy.[39] Thus, Jeong emphasized that

ethanol sclerotherapy should be considered the primary treatment modality, followed by a combination of emboli-zation and surgery if repeated sclerotherapy fails.[39]

INDICATIONS FOR ENDOVASCULAR THERAPY OF MALIGNANT HEAD/NECK CANCER

Surgical resection maintains an important role in the man-agement of head/neck carcinomas; indeed, complete resec-tion of head/neck malignancy with negative histologic margins is the most crucial factor in prognosis.[2] Even in cases of residual or recurrent advanced head/neck carci-noma involving the carotid artery, where prognosis con-tinues to be dim despite resection, surgery can reduce the incidence of life-threatening sequelae like fistula forma-tion, erosion of the pharyngeal wall, or acute tumoral hemorrhage.[40,41]

Carcinoma Involving Carotid Artery

Carotid Occlusion and Tumor Embolization Followed by Resection

Most head/neck malignancies are relatively hypovascular and do not require preoperative embolization for surgical resection,[42] but involvement of the carotid artery by head and neck carcinoma can hinder safe tumor resection. In these cases, preoperative BTO followed by preoperative carotid artery occlusion can greatly reduce neurologic morbidity and assist in planning for resection of tumor involving the carotid artery.

Candidates for surgery with preoperative embolization include those whose carotid arteries are invaded by the less radiosensitive carcinomas (e.g., adenocarcinoma, adenoid cystic carcinoma, melanoma) or any residual or recurrent

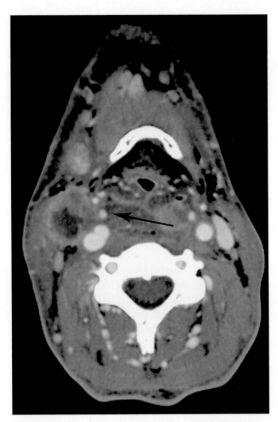

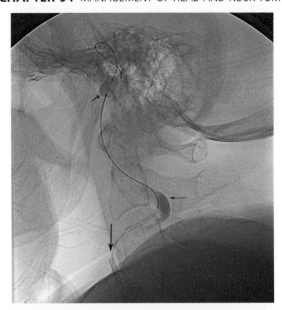

FIGURE 94-5. Balloon test occlusion. Lateral view from angiogram demonstrates occlusive balloon in distal internal carotid artery *(oblique arrow)*. Horizontal arrow indicates stagnant contrast material in carotid bulb. Vertical arrow indicates guiding catheter in distal common carotid artery.

FIGURE 94-4. Axial contrast agent-enhanced computed tomography scan of tumor invading carotid artery. Arrow indicates necrotic tumor surrounding internal carotid artery (right ICA with > 200-degree circumferential involvement). There is high likelihood of carotid invasion by tumor.

head/neck carcinomas including squamous cell.[43] Usually such a patient will present with a fixed neck mass. Clinical presentation, however, has a highly inaccurate (32%-63%) rate of predicting carotid invasion. Circumferential carotid artery involvement of at least 270 degrees should be confirmed by MRI, CT, or ultrasound, which predicts arterial wall invasion with high sensitivity and specificity. In one series, arteriography only identified invasion in 1 of 12 patients[2,44,45] (Fig. 94-4).

Historically, carotid artery ligation can cause up to 45% neurologic morbidity rate and 31% to 41% reported mortality.[2] Stroke can occur either immediately from decreased blood flow or later from a postprocedural thrombus or embolic event.[43] Preoperative BTO with/without single-photon emission computed tomography (SPECT) imaging or induced hypotension can help identify those who would be less neurologically vulnerable to decreased blood flow. Patients whose preocclusion diagnostic evaluation indicates inadequate collateral flow may benefit from a bypass procedure during surgical ligation, though this approach adds morbidity and mortality. For those patients with demonstrated sufficient collateral flow allowing for carotid resection without reconstruction, preoperative coil embolization of the ICA can minimize surgical blood loss as well as minimize postprocedural thromboembolic complications. In particular, coil embolization of the preophthalmic petrous carotid artery with postembolization heparinization has been shown to help prevent distal embolization after surgical resection.[43] After allowing clot formation to

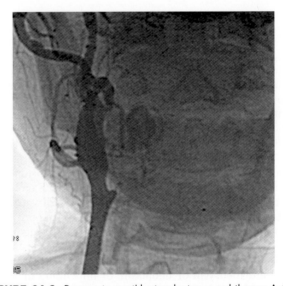

FIGURE 94-6. Damage to carotid artery by tumor and therapy. Anteroposterior angiogram demonstrates severe irregularity of internal and external carotid arteries.

stabilize, surgical ligation can follow 2 to 6 weeks later[42] (Fig. 94-5).

Carotid Blowout Syndrome
Rupture of any branch in the extracranial carotid artery system, known as *carotid blowout*, can follow extravasation, pseudoaneurysm, or AVF from any number of causes and can lead to acute transoral or transcervical hemorrhage. *Carotid blowout syndrome* is a broader term that encompasses carotid blowout as well as the threat of it in cases where the carotid is injured or exposed.[46] Most commonly, the cause leading to carotid blowout is therapy for squamous cell carcinoma (Figs. 94-6 and 94-7). Radiation

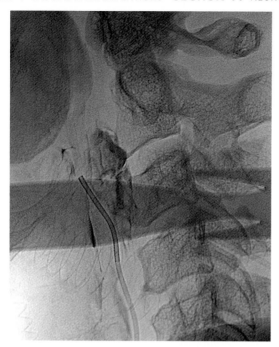

FIGURE 94-7. Carotid blowout syndrome. Lateral angiogram demonstrates contrast material leaking into soft tissue surrounding diseased carotid artery.

weakens the arterial wall and has been associated with a sevenfold increase in the risk of CBS. Other etiologies include other tumors, neck trauma, and functional endoscopic surgery for refractory epistaxis.[47] Historically, treatment of CBS with emergent surgical ligation alone led to a 60% neurologic complication rate and 40% overall mortality.[48,49] With advances in interventional endovascular therapies that include embolization, occlusion, and stenting, morbidity and mortality has been reduced substantially. Attempts should therefore be made to treat CBS endovascularly. A combination of anatomy, severity, and availability of interventional services determines the appropriate endovascular management of CBS. A helpful algorithm has been proposed by Cohen and Rad[47] (Fig. 94-8).

If CBS severity falls under the categories of threatened by pseudoaneurysm or neoplasm, or impending or acute, angiography and CT with contrast should be used to confirm the anatomy and the potential of sentinel hemorrhage.[50] If ICA or CCA involvement is demonstrated by angiography/CT, BTO is indicated to determine extent of collateral flow. If collateral flow is inadequate, stenting is indicated to achieve hemostasis until permanent occlusion with surgical extra-anatomic bypass (i.e., subclavian to carotid) can be performed. Covered stent technologies have advanced to a point where their use in such patients may also be beneficial.[51] ICA/CCA involvement with adequate collateral flow as well as ECA involvement should be managed by distal and proximal occlusion using coils or detachable balloons (currently unavailable in the United States). If the tumor itself is the source of hemorrhage, as indicated by tumor blush on angiography/CT, the entire tumor bed should be embolized. This can be accomplished with PVA particles via superselective transarterial microcatheterization of all arterial supply to the tumor or by

direct-puncture ethanol or cyanoacrylate as a last resort[48] (Table 94-1).

Radplat/Intraarterial Chemotherapy

Surgery and radiotherapy are the primary treatments for head/neck cancer therapy. Yet surgical resection of areas of the larynx, pharynx, and/or tongue can severely diminish quality of life through limits on speech and swallowing.[4] While radiotherapy alone may better preserve organ function, it does not always provide better rates of local control and survival.[52] Chemotherapy is a promising treatment; studies of head/neck squamous cell carcinomas have shown that they may be highly responsive in a dose-related fashion to the drug cisplatin. Systemic delivery of cisplatin, however, can result in side effects like severe nephrotoxicity.

Selective intraarterial chemotherapy may decrease the risk and severity of these systemic effects while permitting high-dose cisplatin delivery directly to the tumor bed by taking advantage of the angiographer's ability to selectively catheterize distal external carotid branches. Intraarterial chemotherapy is often administered in conjunction with radiotherapy, as seen in the most well-known of the intraarterial head/neck regimens, RADPLAT, reported by Robbins et al.[53-55] RADPLAT (radiotherapy and concomitant intraarterial cisplatin) also combines intraarterial chemotherapy with an intravenous systemic infusion of the competitive cisplatin antagonist, sodium thiosulfate, to further protect the rest of the body from cisplatin's systemic toxic effects.[56] In this manner, RADPLAT allows for delivery of high doses of cisplatin to head/neck tumors while limiting systemic exposure. Other applications of intraarterial chemotherapy under investigation include its preoperative use to improve the quality of head/neck tumor resection (neo-RADPLAT), its role in palliative therapy,[57] and its use as a potential prognostic indicator that can guide further management of disease. Patients who completely respond to intraarterial chemoradiation may have a significantly higher overall survival rate than those who have a lesser response.[57,58] Several authors have subsequently reported success with selective intraarterial chemotherapy using direct superficial temporal artery access.[59-62]

CONTRAINDICATIONS

For benign lesions, in the rare event the tumor blood supply extends intradurally (e.g., via anterior inferior cerebellar artery [AICA] or posterior inferior cerebellar artery [PICA]), embolization is contraindicated owing to risks to the intracranial circulation.[63] Specifically, ICA embolization is contraindicated when collateral blood supply is insufficient (Table 94-2), as when a patient fails a BTO or when the contralateral carotid system has previously undergone embolization or ligation. Finally, for congenital vascular malformations other than the cases indicated earlier, percutaneous sclerotherapy may be considered the primary treatment modality rather than embolization and resection.

For malignancy, if involvement of the carotid artery is by a previously untreated case of squamous cell carcinoma, surgical resection with embolization would not be the therapy of choice. Carotid invasion is usually best treated with radiotherapy. Also, if collateral circulation is

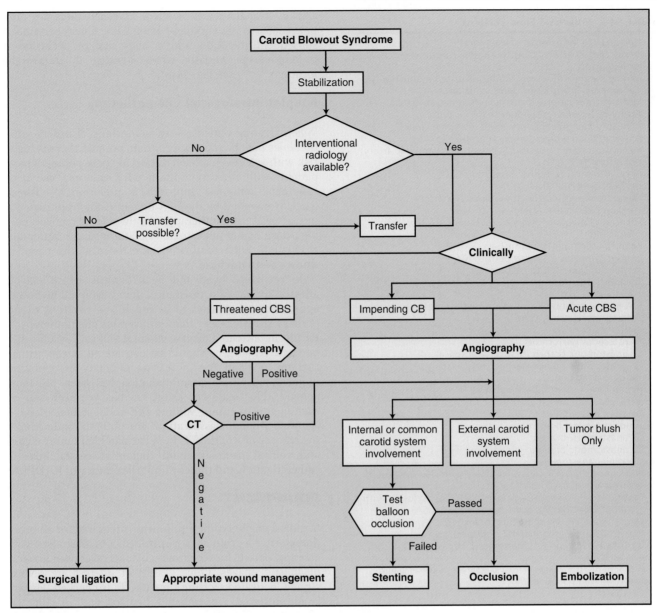

FIGURE 94-8. Management algorithm for carotid blowout syndrome (CBS). Morrissey and colleagues proposed a decision tree for the management CBS. *(From Cohen J, Rad I. Contemporary management of carotid blowout. Curr Opin Otolaryngol Head Neck Surg 2004;12:110–5, after Morrissey DD, Andersen PE, Nesbit GM, et al. Endovascular management of hemorrhage in patients with head and neck cancer. Arch Otolaryngol Head Neck Surg 1997;123:15–9.)*

TABLE 94-1. Balloon Test Occlusion Decision Matrix*: Indications for Bypass from Temporary Balloon Occlusion: Institutional Protocol

Clinical	EEG	SPECT	Hypotension	Intervention
Pass	Pass	Pass	Pass	PO
Pass	Fail	Fail	Fail	PO + low-flow bypass (STA-MCA)
Fail	Fail	Fail	Fail	PO + high-flow bypass (venous/radial artery bypass)
Pass	Pass	Fail	Fail	PO + low-flow bypass (STA-MCA)

*The suggested testing matrix was devised from multiple components of balloon test occlusion and results of surgical management of the carotid artery during tumor resection.
EEG, Electroencephalogram; *PO,* permanent occlusion; *SPECT,* single-photon emission computed tomography; *STA-MCA,* superficial temporal artery to middle cerebral artery.
From Parkinson RJ, Bendok BR, O'Shaughnessy BA, et al. Temporary and permanent occlusion of cervical and cerebral arteries. Neurosurg Clin N Am 2005;16:249–56.

TABLE 94-2. Collateral Flow Patterns

Extracranial to intracranial anastomoses
External carotid artery (ECA) to internal carotid artery (ICA)
Maxillary artery
  Middle meningeal artery (MMA), recurrent meningeal to ethmoidal branches of ophthalmic artery (OA)
  MMA to inferolateral trunk (ILT) (foramen spinosum)
  Artery of foramen rotundum to ILT
  Accessory meningeal artery to ILT (foramen ovale)
  Anterior, middle deep temporal arteries to OA
  Via vidian artery to petrous ICA (anterior tympanic artery)
Facial artery
  Angular branch to orbital branches of OA
Superficial temporal artery (STA)
  Transosseous perforators to anterior falx artery
Ascending pharyngeal artery
  Superior pharyngeal artery to cavernous ICA (foramen lacerum)
  Rami to cavernous ICA branches
  Inferior tympanic artery to petrous ICA
Posterior auricular, OA to petrous ICA
  Stylomastoid artery
Iatrogenic
  STA-middle cerebral artery (MCA) bypass graft
ECA to vertebral artery (VA)
Occipital artery
  Transosseous perforators
  C1 anastomotic branch (first cervical space)
  C2 anastomotic branch (second cervical space)
Ascending pharyngeal
  Hypoglossal (odontoid arterial arch)
  Musculospinal branch
Subclavian artery (SCA) to VA
Ascending cervical branch
  C3 anastomotic branch
  C4 anastomotic branch
Extracranial anastomoses
  Subclavian steal (VA to basilar artery with flow reversal in contralateral VA to distal SCA)
  Carotid steal (common carotid artery [CCA] occlusion with a patent ECA and ICA and flow reversal in ECA)
  Direct VA to VA (via segmental branches)
  ECA to ECA (via contralateral branches)
  Iatrogenic (SCA to CCA anastomosis, bypass graft)

From Osborn AG. Diagnostic cerebral angiography I. Philadelphia: Lippincott Williams & Wilkins; 1999.

inadequate as investigated by diagnostic angiography[16] and BTO with or without SPECT, preoperative embolization is contraindicated. Instead, carotid artery resection with reconstruction, though rarely performed in these cases, can be considered.[43] If carotid artery reconstruction is impossible, palliative chemotherapy or hospice care may be sought.

Carotid Blowout Syndrome

An increasing number of CBS cases are recurrent CBS. In contralateral recurrent cases, if the carotid originally affected by CBS has already been occluded or ligated, contralateral occlusion or ligation is an unavailable option.[48] Endovascular occlusion is also contraindicated in any patient where the contralateral carotid artery is already occluded by atherosclerosis, and in patients who have proven CBS bleeding of the ICA/CCA systems but fail BTO. In cases where occlusion is contraindicated, a self-expandable stent should be placed.[47,51] If using a stent-graft (i.e., covered stent), placement in an uninfected, unexposed

area is strongly recommended. Favorable sites are often unavailable in impending or acute CBS. A near certainty of subsequent infection and a high risk of occlusion or re-hemorrhage persists when stenting in unfavorable locations[51,64,65] (see Fig. 94-8).

Radplat/Intraarterial Chemotherapy

When treating patients with hemostatic disorders, other therapies may be more appropriate because there is higher risk with selective catheterization in these populations. In patients with atherosclerotic femoral anatomy, use of the superficial temporal approach is preferred.[58-62] Tumors partially supplied by the ICA system cannot be treated by intraarterial chemotherapy; this would allow access of high-dose highly neurotoxic cisplatin into the intracranial circulation. Such tumors include those of the paranasal sinuses and skull base.[66]

In recurrent head and neck disease, which may be affected by cisplatin resistance, direct arterial chemotherapy has been reported to be much less effective, though perhaps slightly better than intravenous chemotherapy.[53,55] Finally, in untreated disease where RADPLAT is unlikely to be curative, surgery should be considered as the primary therapy to avoid the increasing difficulty of operations in locations where chemoradiation has been previously applied.[4] No treatment algorithm has yet been set, but such factors as tumor volume and nodal status, as well as age and T-stage classification, are potential indicators of the efficacy of RADPLAT. In particular, high tumor volume and central necrosis could hinder successful selective catheterization and thereby limit the efficacy of RADPLAT.

EQUIPMENT

Standard angiographic equipment is required for all procedures. After a groin sheath is placed, a 4F diagnostic catheter appropriate for cerebrovascular access is used to obtain diagnostic images. Once vessels of interest are demonstrated, activated clotting time (ACT) is checked. Heparin is administered. An exchange Bentson wire or Glidewire is used to safely place a 5F to 8F guiding catheter with an appropriately angled tip. Microcatheters (0.014) and microwire (0.010) are used to obtain selective and superselective images.

Balloon Test Occlusion

For BTO, the HyperForm nondetachable balloon (Micro Therapeutics, Irvine, Calif.) is used after diagnostic angiography demonstrates collateral circulation.[16] Inflation is carefully performed through a thoroughly purged system. Temporary vascular occlusion is performed as distal as is safe to a point just central to the petrous carotid to reduce the noted increased incidence of dissection when working in this carotid segment. Full electroencephalographic (EEG) monitoring is supplied by the neurologist performing the evaluation while circulation is occluded.

Embolization

Embolization procedures may employ particles, acrylate, or coils and are usually performed via a 0.014 microcatheter.

Guglielmi detachable coils (GDCs) may be delivered through this system. PVA particles may also be delivered via this system. Safe and effective particle diameters of the 150 to 250 µm variety offer excellent arteriole occlusion with decreased risk of passing through the capillary bed. Extreme care is used to segregate the embolization equipment from those catheters that may be used for diagnostic image injections after embolization. Onyx or n-butyl cyanoacrylate (NBCA) may also be injected through this system with appropriate catheters.[67,68] Embolization performed by using detachable balloons for managing head/neck cancer–related CBS has been described in depth since it was first reported.[69] However, both permanent balloon occlusion and the requisite temporary BTO may add an additional 15% to 20% delayed and 0.4% immediate occurrence of permanent stroke, respectively.[43,46,70]

Stenting

Stents may be balloon-mounted or self-expandable, uncovered or covered. Stent delivery systems continue to evolve. They frequently come packaged with their own delivery catheters and microwires. Close attention is necessary to ensure the access sheath and guiding wires are compatible with the stent delivery system. Appropriate antiplatelet medications are also necessary.[51]

Selective Catheterization for Intraarterial Chemotherapy

The success of selective arterial catheterization for targeted delivery of cisplatin has been increased with the use of CT scan selective arteriography. Although not widely available, this technique allows for the determination of which branch arteries are feeding tumor masses. A CT machine is attached to the standard fluoroscopy gantry, or cone beam techniques may eventually be used for this purpose. After selective arterial catheterization is performed, injections are made while dynamic CT images are acquired. This method allows the angiographer to elucidate tumor blood supply prior to chemotherapy infusion. Direct superficial temporal artery access requires specifically designed hook catheters.[59-62]

TECHNIQUE

Anatomy and Approaches

Avoidance of postprocedural complications can be helped by paying close attention to collateral ECA-ICA connections during embolization procedures (Figs. 94-9 to 94-13). Emphasis must be placed on the observation that flow dynamics will be altered by embolization, and collateral ECA to ICA connections may be revealed as the embolization proceeds. Specific attention should be paid to direction of ophthalmic artery flow and potential internal maxillary and occipital artery anastomosis to cerebral circulation.

Paragangliomas
Typically the ascending pharyngeal artery and its branches are the rostral-caudal blood supply of paragangliomas. Additional feeding arteries include inferior tympanic for tympanic, neuromeningeal for jugular, and musculospinal

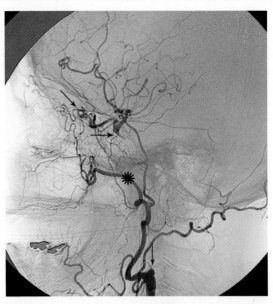

FIGURE 94-9. Collateral flow from ophthalmic artery to internal carotid artery. Lateral angiogram demonstrates common carotid artery injection and blunt occlusion of internal carotid artery *(vertical arrow)*. Enlarged internal maxillary artery *(star)* is feeding sphenopalatine segment and enlarged ophthalmic artery *(oblique arrow)*. Supraclinoid internal carotid artery was reconstituted *(horizontal arrow)*.

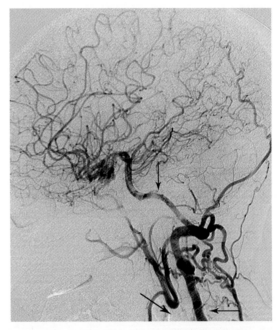

FIGURE 94-10. Collateral flow from vertebral artery to external carotid artery (ECA). Lateral angiogram illustrates vertebral artery injection *(horizontal arrow)*. Vertical arrow points to posterior circulation providing entire cerebral perfusion via posterior communicating arteries. Oblique arrow demonstrates lack of filling of central ECA, proving ECA branches communicate with vertebral artery.

to vagal and carotid body.[16] This can be supplemented by additional feeding vessels such as the internal maxillary artery or superior and inferior laryngeal arteries in their given territories. Contributions from the occipital and posterior auricular arteries, vertebral arteries, or meningeal

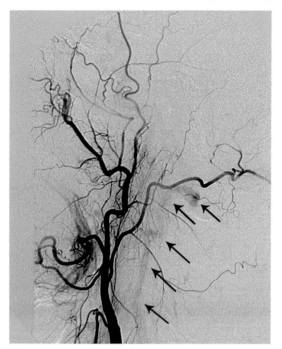

FIGURE 94-11. Collateral flow from external carotid artery to vertebral artery. Lateral view from angiogram demonstrates injection of common carotid artery. Multiple oblique arrows outline vertebral artery shadow, which is reconstituted via muscular branches originating from external carotid artery.

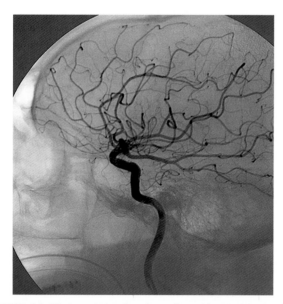

FIGURE 94-12. Lateral view from internal carotid artery injection demonstrating absence of ophthalmic artery filling prior to embolization procedure. This should raise suspicion for aberrant ophthalmic artery supply, which should be confirmed prior to embolic material is injected.

branches of the ICA are also possible and depend on tumor location and extension. Paragangliomas that are solely tympanic are often supplied mainly by the inferior tympanic artery, which eases intraoperative hemostatic control and decreases the need for preoperative embolization. Most (83%) paragangliomas, however, have a "multicompartment" vascular supply; that is, each feeding artery for the

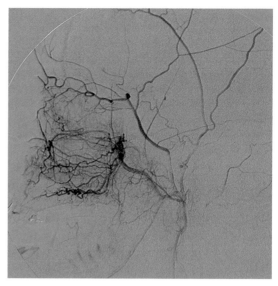

FIGURE 94-13. Angiographic image demonstrating ophthalmic artery supplied by distal internal maxillary artery branch.

tumor supplies only its own respective region of the tumor, as opposed to monocompartment supply, where each artery supplies the entire tumor.[3,13] Angiography should therefore thoroughly investigate the bilateral ascending pharyngeal arteries, as well as the ipsilateral vertebral, internal carotid, distal external carotid, posterior auricular, and occipital arteries.[63]

Juvenile Nasal Angiofibroma
JNAs are supplied by branches of the internal maxillary (sphenopalatine and descending palantine branches) and ascending pharyngeal artery. As tumor spreads, recruitment of other arteries include the ascending pharyngeal/ascending palantine.[66] Ipsilateral/contralateral ICA/ECA involvement has commonly been demonstrated.[29] It is recommended to perform angiography with contralateral injection of the CCA and/or ICA and then ipsilateral injection of the ICA and/or CCA to demonstrate the tumor's extension. In the ECA, attention should be given to anastomoses of the internal maxillary and ascending pharyngeal arteries with the intracranial, intraorbital, and internal carotid arteries.

Carotid Blowout Syndrome
CBS can occur at virtually any portion of the carotid system, but nearly half of cases have been reported at the ICA (43.6%). Other sites include the ECA (23.4%), CCA (11.7%), buccal artery (3.2%), inferior (3.2%) and superior thyroid artery (2.1%), internal mammary artery (2.1%), innominate artery (1.1%), facial artery (1.1%), and aorta (1.1%), as well as rare case reports of the internal maxillary artery.[47] When considering possible CBS sites, it is also necessary to investigate the tumor itself (5.3% of reported cases), as well as the internal jugular vein, which although not technically a part of the carotid artery system is still also a potential source of rupture (Figs. 94-14 to 94-16).

Radplat/Intraarterial Chemotherapy
The physical anatomy of head/neck tumors does not necessarily reflect the vascular anatomy, as shown by Terayama

et al.,[71] who studied the vascular supply of selectively catheterized laryngeal and hypopharyngeal tumors as demonstrated on their CT-visualized enhancement during arteriography. Nearly all ipsilaterally located laryngeal tumors were supplied by the ipsilateral superior thyroid and/or laryngeal arteries, but less than half of ipsilaterally located hypopharyngeal cancers were supplied by ipsilateral vasculature. Almost one quarter of midline-crossing laryngeal tumors, on the other hand, were supplied ipsilaterally. Only 12 of 25 midline-crossing laryngeal tumors were actually supplied by the bilateral superior thyroid arteries. Inclusion of other arterial branches, including the inferior thyroid and lingual arteries, was necessary to completely catalog the arterial supply of the tumors in question (Fig. 94-17). To avoid inadequate distribution of cisplatin, complete investigation of vascular supply is an essential part of treatment planning.

Technical Aspects

General Embolization Procedures in Head and Neck

Standard preoperative precautions are observed. This includes verification of normal renal function and coagulation profile. Some therapeutic agents would produce too much pain in an awake patient, and hemorrhage complicating some procedures often compromises the patient's airway and hemodynamics. For the preceding reasons, these procedures are frequently undertaken with the aid of general anesthesia to increase safety and shorten the procedure. If general anesthesia is planned, appropriate cardiopulmonary evaluation is advised. Frequently general anesthesia is initiated at the beginning of the diagnostic procedure, maintained through the embolization phase of

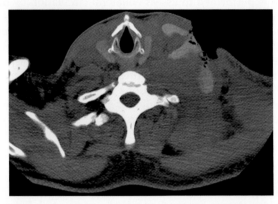

FIGURE 94-14. Blowout. Bleeding was noted after incision and drainage of a supraclavicular abscess. Axial contrast-enhanced computed tomography demonstrates extravasation of contrast material into superficial wound. Pressure dressing was applied immediately, and patient was stabilized.

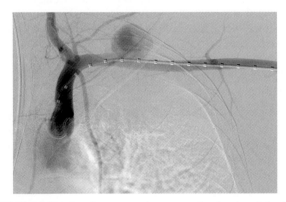

FIGURE 94-15. Pseudoaneurysm. Anteroposterior view from left subclavian angiogram with calibrated catheter demonstrates large subclavian pseudoaneurysm.

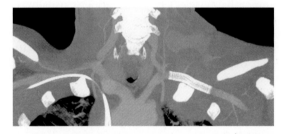

FIGURE 94-16. Stented pseudoaneurysm. Coronal image was reformatted from a computed tomographic angiogram after stenting of subclavian artery.

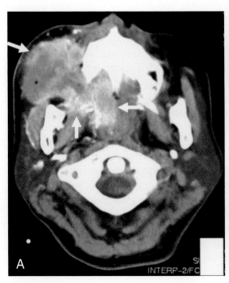
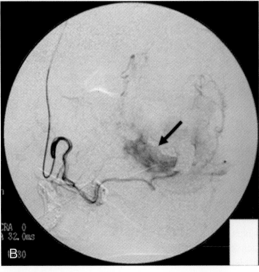

FIGURE 94-17. Computed tomographic angiogram **(A)** and angiographic image **(B)** showing superficial temporal artery access and contrast injection for delineation of tumor blood supply. *(From Mitsudo K, Shigetomi T, Fujimoto Y, et al: Organ preservation with daily concurrent chemoradiotherapy using superselective intra-arterial infusion via a superficial temporal artery for T3 and T4 head and neck cancer. Int J Radiat Oncol Biol Phys 2011;79:1428–35, Fig. 4.)*

the angiogram, and carried into the operative suite. This approach is most useful for the younger patient population affected by JNA.

Endovascular intervention is tailored to the specific disease entity. However, the majority of cases begin in the same fashion. Standard endovascular access techniques are used to obtain safe diagnostic images of the desired circulation. Therapy is usually accomplished through a microcatheter. This may be either a flow-directed-variety catheter over a microwire or a hybrid catheter. These are stabilized by placement of a larger-diameter guide catheter. The diagnostic catheter is exchanged for the guide catheter. To reduce embolic complications, heparin is administered prior to microcatheter deployment. The ACT is monitored with the goal of attaining a safe working range of 1.5 to twice normal. The microcatheter is then used to obtain diagnostic images and deliver various therapeutic agents. This includes Gelfoam, PVA, NBCA, Onyx, alcohol, or coils. Of particular importance, embolic materials should be placed in the ECA in a series of small volumes during the systolic phase; the ECA lacks diastolic forward flow, which would increase the likelihood of material reflux during this phase[63] (Fig. 94-18). Contrast injections demonstrating stagnant flow within the target vessels is considered a technical success.

Care should be taken regarding the ophthalmic artery,[11] since inappropriate occlusion frequently leads to blindness. If a temporalis muscle flap is to be used for reconstruction, it is necessary to communicate this fact to the radiologist so care is taken not to compromise the blood supply to the temporalis muscle.[29] Heparinization is usually recommended during catheterization to prevent clot formation. Corticosteroids are used only with very prolonged procedures or when a significant amount of inflammation is expected, depending on the embolization target and extent of vascular territory involved.[63]

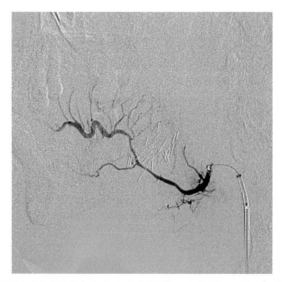

FIGURE 94-18. Polyvinyl alcohol (PVA) embolization of hemorrhagic malignancy. Lateral view from angiogram demonstrates PVA embolization with coaxial guiding catheter and microcatheter. Contrast agent and PVA mixture were injected until a stagnant column of contrast material was demonstrated. Care is taken to avoid extension of contrast column to parent artery, which would signal reflux of PVA particles.

Balloon Test Occlusion

BTO is an exception to the usual approach of general anesthesia. This procedure requires an awake patient because they are frequently monitored via EEG, and their neurologic status is continually monitored throughout the standard 30-minute occlusion session. A standard diagnostic exam is performed to assess collateral circulation by bilateral carotid angiogram. If inadequate collateral vessels are demonstrated, the study is terminated at this point to avoid possible seizure-induced ischemia.[16] If adequate collateral vessels are demonstrated, a balloon is deployed in the proximal ICA via a guide catheter. These patients are heparinized to reduce embolic complications from the stagnant blood column past the balloon. Adjunct methods may be used to increase the sensitivity of the test.[42,72] It is important to note the potential risks associated with prolonged large-diameter balloon inflation in a diseased vessel.

Stenting

Standard diagnostic angiography is performed following contrast CT scan, computed tomographic angiography (CTA), or MRI/MRA with contrast. Once the vessel abnormality is localized, an appropriate stent is chosen predicated on lesion length and parent vessel diameter. Additional considerations include location within the vascular tree and status of the surrounding soft tissue, which may influence the choice of a covered or bare metal stent. This topic is discussed later.

The most significant potential complication is arterial dissection encountered while maneuvering the sheathed stent system across the lesion prior to final deployment. This risk is highest with the larger covered stent systems in narrowed and irregular parent vessels. Patients with atherosclerosis or who have been treated with prior radiation therapy have narrower and more irregular vessels, posing higher dissection risk during stent placement (Figs. 94-19 and 94-20).

Radplat/Intraarterial Chemotherapy

The common intraarterial chemoradiation regimen known as *RADPLAT* consists of four weekly cycles of intraarterial chemotherapy, with radiotherapy during the first week. To administer each cycle of chemotherapy, the carotid anatomy of a well-hydrated patient is assessed by transfemoral digital subtraction angiography. Superselective catheterization of the involved feeding arteries is performed, followed by CT scan. CT concurrent with angiography can help identify feeding arteries. Upon successful catheterization, an intraarterial infusion of cisplatin is rapidly administered (150 mg/m^2 over 3-5 minutes), which is immediately followed by catheter removal to reduce the likelihood of clot formation. CT during the infusion is useful in confirming drug distribution. During the cisplatin infusion, a separate slower intravenous administration of sodium thiosulfate is begun (9 g/m^2 over 15-20 minutes, then 12 g/m^2 over 6 hours). With malignancies that cross the midline, bilateral infusions may be used. Superficial temporal artery access techniques have also been used. Local anesthesia is used for the arterial cutdown. A hooked catheter is placed in the target vessel using standard techniques.

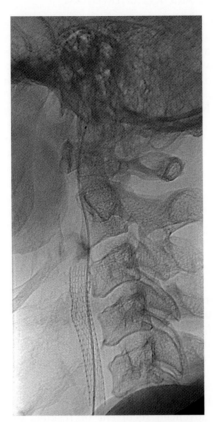

FIGURE 94-19. Lateral angiogram demonstrating an open design nitinol stent used to reduce risk of bleeding from a diseased vessel.

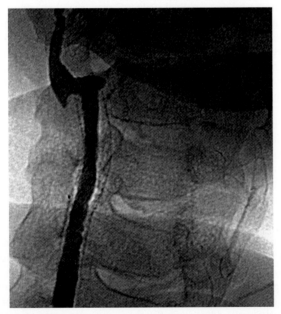

FIGURE 94-20. Anteroposterior angiogram showing stent stabilizing severely diseased common and internal carotid arteries.

CONTROVERSIES

Paraganglioma

Cyanoacrylate Embolization

Direct percutaneous injection of acrylate glue may begin to replace or at least complement intraarterial embolization of

hypervascular tumors. In several studies where embolization therapy involved some component of direct percutaneous acrylate injection, at least some degree of devascularization was observed in over 90% of patients, without any permanent major or minor complications.[21,72,73] Practitioners therefore report increasing use of this technique. In addition to its high success and safety rate, advantages include a greater chance of total devascularization and an "intratumoral casting" of the tumor's vascular bed.[48,74] This "casting" by the colored acrylate glue not only likely aids in achieving complete occlusion but also allows for better distinction of the tumor and its vasculature from surrounding normal tissue during surgery.

Despite this high rate of success, however, drawbacks remain. Clinically, the most significant disadvantage is control of glue migration. In two cases, the acrylate glue has been observed to migrate to the middle cerebral artery,[75] once with no permanent effect but once with subsequent mortality. In the former case, it was attributed to inexperience that led to overinjection of the tumor bed; in the latter, it was related to poor visualization of the vasculature due to a tumor that was already opaque from the procedure. In a third case, glue migration was the cause of blindness when it occluded an ophthalmic artery that was part of the supply to another JNA that had eroded into the orbit. Therefore, great care should be taken during angiographic evaluation of the vasculature, as well as during the subsequent embolization. In cases where the ophthalmic artery is part of the feeding supply, direct glue injection is contraindicated. Other drawbacks are regulatory, technical, and surgical. It has been suggested that intratumoral injection of glue may lead to adherent tumor, making it more difficult to surgically resect; perhaps it should be reserved for larger tumors where endovascular embolization of every feeding artery is difficult to achieve, or where endovascular embolization fails.[11] As we gather more experience with direct percutaneous acrylate injection for hypervascular tumors, its role in embolization therapy will be better understood.[30,67,68]

Carcinoma Involving Carotid Artery

Carotid Occlusion and Tumor Embolization Followed by Resection

Although poor collateral circulation often contraindicates resection of the carotid when invaded by carcinoma, an alternative endovascular/surgical method devised by Nussbaum et al. warrants further investigation.[76] This method involved placement of an endovascular stent in the carotid artery of a patient whose carotid would not tolerate ligation or reconstruction. One month later after the stent formed a complete neoendothelial barrier within the diseased carotid, Nussbaum et al. were able to successfully perform a longitudinal resection and dissection of the tumor surrounding the diseased portion of the carotid. If this method shows continued success, it could be added to the arsenal of endovascular management for head/neck malignancy.[43]

Carotid Blowout Syndrome

Generally, permanent embolic materials have had reported success in controlling CBS hemorrhage; absorbable gelatin particles may also have a similar efficacy, with the added advantage of allowing eventual reestablishment of local circulation to the normal tissue. Kakizawa et al.[70] hypothesize that this absorbability could result in reduced focal necrosis and decreased pain. Furthermore, absorption of the particles could allow for repeat endovascular therapy, especially in the setting of contralateral recurrent carotid disease. A randomized prospective trial comparing permanent embolic materials with the absorbable gelatin particles would be necessary to validate these findings.

Another controversy regarding management of CBS concerns the use of stents. While many advocate the use of therapeutic tumor embolization rather than stenting as the preferred course for CBS treatment, Chaloupka et al. now promote the use of uncovered stents, especially overlapping and in conjunction with coil embolization, as the preferred therapy. The group, possibly one of the most experienced groups in endovascular CBS management, argues that stenting maintains rates of hemostatic control comparable to the rates achieved by embolization and may even reduce the rate of stroke. Also, while the use of uncovered stents alone had a rate of treatment failure similar to the rate for therapeutic embolization alone in one of their series, Chaloupka's group surmises that combining the two techniques may improve on the rates of recurrence, since in the same series, none of the patients under the combined regimen experienced treatment failure. Additional potential advantages of stenting include the immediate ability to treat CBS patients who have inadequate collateral circulation, reinforcement of the damaged arterial wall, and preservation of bilateral carotid artery patency. Maintaining patency could be useful in treating future carotid disease that occurs contralateral to the original site of CBS.[51]

Others argue that the difficulties in managing complications associated with stenting outweigh the advantages. Such complications include infection, rebleeding, and thrombosis. Indeed, reports in the literature concerning stent-grafts (i.e., covered stents) have demonstrated infection-related complications that lead to thrombosis, hemorrhage, stent extrusion, and in one case a brain abscess.[64,65] In a study of stent-graft therapy for CBS by Chang et al., stent-grafts became completely occluded secondary to infection in 3 out of 8 patients.[64]

It is worthwhile to note, however, that the reported incidence of infection associated with covered stents is greater than with uncovered stents. Uncovered stents require smaller-caliber delivery systems and are not as hindered by size limitations as covered stents. Uncovered stents cannot provide an immediate virtual bypass of the affected site as covered stents do. It may be worthwhile to reprioritize the role of stenting in the management of CBS, especially when considering uncovered stents in combination with coil embolization and, perhaps later, stent-grafts if advances in material sciences produce less thrombogenic graft material.

OUTCOMES

Paragangliomas

Eighty percent of preoperatively embolized paragangliomas experience a reduction in tumor size.[13] Often the size reduction is as high as 25%,[16] which reduces surgical blood loss,

intraoperative manipulation of surrounding structures, and the need for intra- or postoperative transfusion. In their surgical management of large paragangliomas (>3 cm) with preoperative embolization, Persky et al.[16] report a mean blood loss of the equivalent of only 1 transfusion unit.

Juvenile Nasal Angiofibromas

Before the common use of endovascular techniques, average blood loss for JNA amounted to approximately 2000 mL per case; that figure has now been reduced to less than 1000 mL.[24] With preoperative embolization, intraoperative time has been significantly reduced, as has tumoral size.[63] This in turn has led to a higher rate of complete surgical resection and thereby a lower rate of recurrence and repeated recurrence.

Carcinoma Involving Carotid Artery

Carotid Occlusion and Tumor Embolization Followed by Resection

In terms of overall survival, resection of carcinoma involving the carotid artery is rarely curative and carries a risk of perioperative mortality. With reconstruction or preoperative embolization, the risk has been reported as less than 5%.[2,40,43] The disease-free survival rate at 1 year following resection has been reported as 60%. The prognosis is worse for advanced recurrent or residual disease. Even with carotid reconstruction, preoperative embolization, or radiotherapy, resection of carcinoma involving the carotid has a 25% to 40% survival at 1 year, with a reported 6.3-month median survival rate. Given the nature of the disease and its prognosis in this patient population, many patients with carotid involvement may not elect for aggressive surgical therapy.

For those patients electing aggressive therapy, resection may provide greater-than-average survival even with residual or recurrent disease.[43] Of those who do undergo resection, endovascular techniques have led to lower rates of morbidity. By using BTO to identify patients who require carotid reconstruction, the 30% risk of stroke from carotid ligation without reconstruction[2,40] has been reduced to 10% to 20% with reconstruction.[42] As for patients who pass BTO, the stroke rate with ligation is favorable compared to that seen in ligation patients who failed BTO.[77] The use of preoperative permanent occlusion has lowered that rate to 10%. Preoperative endovascular occlusion decreases blood loss by precluding the need for intraoperative heparinization of a shunt and minimizes operative time by avoiding reconstruction and the need for well-vascularized coverage of a graft. In addition, by identifying patients who will tolerate ligation without carotid reconstruction, the option of radiotherapy can remain for these patients without worrying about damage to the integrity of a reconstructive graft (Figs. 94-21 and 94-22).

Carotid Blowout Syndrome

Using a variety of methods, endovascular management of CBS has greatly reduced morbidity and mortality. Minor and major neurologic morbidity has been reported to be 10% to 17% and 0% to 7%, respectively; mortality has also been reduced significantly (2%-14%).[48] With endovascular management, however, recurrence of CBS is more

Radplat/Intraarterial Chemotherapy

Early studies of intravenous cisplatin delivery for head and neck malignancies has shown an overall response rate of 40% for previously untreated disease and an average of 28% for recurrent disease.[53] On the other hand, the vast majority of nonrandomized studies pertaining to intraarterial chemotherapy with radiotherapy showed promising rates of complete and partial response—up to 90% and 81%, respectively.[4] In particular, local and regional control has appeared excellent. In a study of 213 patients,[78] only 6% and 3% developed local and regional recurrence, respectively, while 18% were observed to develop distant metastasis. The relatively high rate of metastasis, possibly unmasked by the local therapy, had led to the observation that perhaps a systemic treatment component would be also be necessary. A phase III prospective randomized clinical trial[79-81] comparing intraarterial and intravenous chemoradiation for head/neck cancer was recently completed, with results that appear at odds with previous studies. Preliminary reports of the phase III trial suggest that in 240 patients with stage IV inoperable head and neck cancer, no differences in tumor control, metastasis, or overall survival were observed between intraarterial and intravenous delivery arms. A point of debate has arisen concerning whether the intraarterial treatment was effectively administered based on the anatomy of the treated tumors. Based on preliminary results, the Dutch investigators recommend intravenous chemoradiation as standard therapy.

It should be noted that despite comparable rates of control and survival, systemic complications were observed at a lower rate with intraarterial administration. This appears to confirm the results of earlier nonrandomized studies. The low toxicity profile would not preclude RAD-PLAT's use as a preoperative adjunct to surgery or as a potential prognostic indicator in the management of head/neck tumors. As a preoperative adjunct to surgery (i.e., neo-RADPLAT), RADPLAT has been shown to reduce tumor burden. This has led to a reduction in the extent of subsequent resection, with improved postoperative organ function. It has allowed for surgical removal of otherwise unresectable tumors. Kovacs has reported overall survival rate estimates to be significantly higher for patients who demonstrate complete tumor response to RADPLAT (85%) than those who have poorer responses (33%-64%).[82]

As research continues on intraarterial chemotherapy, another potentially efficacious local therapy being studied is percutaneous image-guided radiofrequency tumor ablation. Given the advantages of local minimally invasive therapy, we should continue to consider all options for our patients.

COMPLICATIONS

General Embolization in Head and Neck

Many postembolization complications are associated with inappropriate occlusion of the vasculature, which can occur either by inadvertent reflux or through ECA-vertebrobasilar or ECA-ICA anastomoses. This has led to stroke, cerebral ischemia, blindness, and cranial nerve (CN) palsies corresponding to affected vasculature (e.g., CN IX-XII, supplied by ascending pharyngeal artery; CN VII, supplied by middle

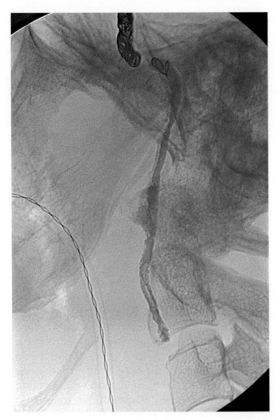

FIGURE 94-21. Endovascular carotid occlusion. Lateral view demonstrates coils, with a proximal glue cast outlining internal carotid artery.

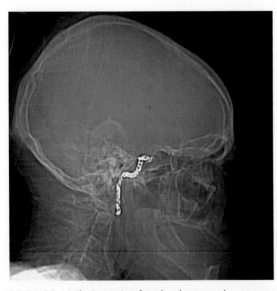

FIGURE 94-22. Coils. Scout view from head computed tomogram shows coils along course of internal carotid artery.

likely and has been reported from 0% to as high as 33%,[70] with 65% resulting from ipsilateral or contralateral progressive disease and 35% from ipsilateral treatment failure. Recurrent CBS can be managed successfully. Chaloupka et al.[72] reported only one of 20 events ending in mortality, and no neurologic or ophthalmologic complications were noted.

meningeal and stylomastoid arteries[13]). Catheterization also increases the risk of stroke and blindness. In general, however, endovascular embolization treatment of head/neck lesions using modern techniques has less than 1% rate of severe neurologic deficit.[24]

Other potential major complications of embolization include necrosis of the mucosa, tongue, and/or skin, ulceration, peripheral neuropathies, and acute muscle ischemia. Muscle is highly sensitive to ischemia, so the latter can result in intense muscular pain. Potential complications more specific to the management of paragangliomas include carotid sinus syndrome and excessive catecholamine secretion, which could be managed with alpha blockade premedication.

Some minor transient complications may include postembolization fever or ear pain due to tumor ischemia.[40] Vasospasm during catheterization can be managed locally by percutaneous nitroglycerin without fear of systemic hypotension.[63]

Carcinoma Involving Carotid Artery

Carotid Occlusion and Tumor Embolization Followed by Resection
Stroke continues to be a concern for patients undergoing this procedure, despite lowered rates with preoperative endovascular occlusion. Other complications may occur during surgical resection. When confronting massive neck malignancy, despite the use of preoperative permanent occlusion, massive hemorrhage and hypotension is still possible during surgical resection.[40] Also, one report of balloon migration during surgical manipulation of the petrous carotid artery resulted in postoperative stroke. In coil-embolized carotid artery systems, dislodging of the clot formation is a theoretical risk of intraoperative manipulation. Detachable balloons are no longer available in the United States.

Carotid Blowout Syndrome
The neurologic morbidity from CBS has been greatly reduced. Reported complications include occasional cases of transient ischemia,[46] Horner syndrome,[47] temporary hemiplegia, or permanent hemiparesis.[70] Occlusion of the facial artery may cause transient facial pain controllable by analgesics.[70] Covered stent placement has been associated with infection, occlusion, and stroke.[83]

Radplat/Intraarterial Chemotherapy

Intraarterial chemotherapy with radiotherapy can result in neurologic sequelae due to catheterization-related injury, chemotoxicity, or general cardiopulmonary effects such as pneumonia. Higher complication rates have been reported at centers with lower case volumes.[4,78,84-88]

POSTPROCEDURE AND FOLLOW-UP CARE

General Embolization in Head and Neck

If significant inflammation is expected, corticosteroid medication may be administered during and following endovascular therapy. Usually, however, postembolization

inflammation is expected to decrease after 1 to 2 days, and follow-up surgery is scheduled accordingly. With paragangliomas, surgical resection is recommended within the period after inflammation has been allowed to decrease (1-2 days postembolization) and before feeding vessels begin to recanalize (no later than 2 weeks postembolization). For JNAs, timely resection within 12 to 48 hours is recommended, before the onset of any postembolization revascularization inflammation and edema; this is particularly important to the preservation of an already tenuous airway in the rare case where angiofibroma involves the larynx (laryngeal angiofibroma).[13,63]

Carcinoma Involving Carotid Artery

Carotid Occlusion and Tumor Embolization Followed by Resection
After preoperative occlusion patients awaiting tumor resection are monitored in the intensive care unit for 3 days of heparinization and fluid dynamic monitoring. Surgical resection of the tumor can be performed 2 to 6 weeks later.[42,43] This equilibration period for the newly embolized arteries helps patients tolerate sudden changes in blood pressure during anesthesia and acute blood loss during surgery. Time interval between carotid occlusion and surgery reduces embolic complications. This may be secondary to clot maturity at the ends of the occluded carotid. Waiting allows coils to stabilize and fix to the vascular wall. For previously untreated carcinomas that have undergone resection, postoperative radiation therapy is indicated.

Carotid Blowout Syndrome
If CBS has been treated by endovascular occlusion, patients should be hemodynamically and neurologically monitored in the intensive care unit, with heparinization for 48 hours and daily aspirin therapy thereafter.[48] In patients with stent treatment, antiplatelet therapy can be administered cautiously. If the patient is at high risk for re-hemorrhage (i.e., in the impending or acute categories of CBS), heparinization should be avoided during and after stent placement.[46] On the other hand, if the patient is in the threatened category or receiving a more thrombogenic stent-graft instead of an uncovered stent, the patient should be immediately placed on clopidogrel with aspirin and maintained following stent-graft placement. Patients receiving stent-grafts should also receive prophylactic antibiotics.[51,64,65] Given the debate over the role of stents in the management of CBS, some follow the emergent stent placement with permanent ligation and vascular bypass surgery. This plan is more strongly advocated if stent placement occurs in a contaminated area. This is also a consideration in patients with stent-grafts, which have a higher occlusion rate.

Radplat/Intraarterial Chemotherapy

After each cycle of chemotherapy, patients should receive intravenous hydration using 1 liter of normal saline with 20 mEq of potassium chloride and 2 g of magnesium sulfate over 6 hours. Patients should also receive 4 mg dexamethasone every 6 hours, either intravenously or orally, until the next morning. Given potential side effects, some patients may require a percutaneous endoscopic gastrostomy (PEG) tube if swallowing problems persist following the completion of RADPLAT, or if hematologic disturbances are observed during therapy. Partial responders with larger nodal malignancies may require selective salvage neck dissection. Complete responders do not need follow-up neck dissection, since their nodes have consistently been found to be negative at neck dissection.[4,53,55]

- Selective arterial catheterization for chemotherapy may be appropriate in some cases.
- Management of complications may require further embolization. Use of covered stents to maintain carotid artery patency instead of endovascular occlusion may help control local complications. This approach may both maintain adequate cerebral perfusion and allow future intervention.

KEY POINTS

- Appropriate therapy for benign tumors of the head and neck may include surgery, endovascular therapy, superficial therapy, or direct puncture. Frequently a combined team approach of experienced physicians offers the best results with the least morbidity.
- Attention to collateral flow from the external carotid artery to the internal carotid artery and the vertebral artery system is crucial to avoid complications from embolic therapy.
- In cases where a paraganglioma is the suspected diagnosis, a preintervention diagnostic bilateral carotid angiogram reduces the likelihood of unforeseen hemorrhagic complications and helps detect bilateral tumors.
- Juvenile nasal angiofibromas are best approached with a preoperative angiogram and possible embolization.
- Late-stage head and neck carcinoma is a complex clinical problem that may require surgery, chemotherapy, radiation therapy, and endovascular intervention.
- Contrast-enhanced computed tomography or magnetic resonance imaging best demonstrates the extent of carotid artery involvement by tumor. It assists in surgical and endovascular treatment planning.
- Diagnostic angiography with balloon test occlusion is the next step when planning treatment for patients with a carotid artery surrounded by malignancy.

▶ **SUGGESTED READINGS**

Ackerstaff AH, Rasch CR, Balm AJ, et al. Five-year quality of life results of the randomized clinical phase III (RADPLAT) trial, comparing concomitant intra-arterial versus intravenous chemoradiotherapy in locally advanced head and neck cancer. Head Neck 2011 Aug 4. doi: 10.1002/hed.21851. [Epub ahead of print]

Chaudhary N, Gemmete JJ, Thompson BG, Pandey AS. Intracranial endovascular balloon test occlusion—indications, methods, and predictive value. Neurosurg Clin N Am 2009;20(3):369–75.

Cherekaev VA, Golbin DA, Kapitanov DN, et al. Advanced craniofacial juvenile nasopharyngeal angiofibroma. Description of surgical series, case report, and review of literature. Acta Neurochir (Wien) 2011; 153(3):499–508. Epub 2011 Jan 28.

Mendenhall WM, Amdur RJ, Vaysberg M, et al. Head and neck paragangliomas. Head Neck 2011;33(10):1530–4. doi: 10.1002/hed.21524. Epub 2010 Nov 4.

Sekhar LN, Biswas A, Hallam D, et al. Neuroendovascular management of tumors and vascular malformations of the head and neck. Neurosurg Clin N Am 2009;20(4):453–85.

Zussman B, Gonzalez LF, Dumont A, et al. Endovascular management of carotid blowout: institutional experience and literature review. World Neurosurg 2011;78:109–14.

The complete reference list is available online at www.expertconsult.com.

CHAPTER 95

Endovascular Management of Epistaxis

Rush H. Chewning, Gerald M. Wyse, Philippe Gailloud, and Kieran P.J. Murphy

CLINICAL RELEVANCE

Nosebleeds so severe they require medical attention are rare. Those severe enough to require transarterial embolization are even rarer. Epistaxis of this type usually occurs in hypertensive elderly individuals with vasculopathy. Serious complications, particularly stroke, can develop quickly during endovascular procedures. It is therefore critical that the physician performing the procedure have both meticulous technique and an understanding of the potentially dangerous anastomoses around the skull base that may allow embolic material to pass from the extracranial circulation into the intracranial circulation. Fortunately, stroke can easily be avoided through knowledge of the vasculature of the head and neck, a well-developed system of preparation for head and neck embolization procedures, and an understanding of microcatheter technique.

TREATMENT OPTIONS

Local conservative treatments are first line in managing epistaxis. A common treatment is insertion of pledgets soaked in an anesthetic vasoconstrictor solution, along with pressure on both sides of the nose.[1] If this or another similar local treatment fails to stop the bleeding, the nose is typically packed, from posterior to anterior, with gauze or a preformed nasal tampon (Merocel or Doyle sponge).

To pack the nose, a catheter is inserted through the nostril and nasopharynx and out the mouth. A gauze pack is then attached to the end of the catheter and positioned in the posterior nasopharynx to seal the region and compress the site of bleeding.[1] Complications of nasal packing procedures include septal hematomas and abscesses from traumatic packing, sinusitis, and pressure necrosis secondary to excessively tight packing. Though rare, major complications such as septicemia, arrhythmia, hypoxia, and death have also been associated with packing.[2,3]

Use of an epistaxis balloon is an alternative method of tamponade. For anterior bleeding, balloons are inserted along the floor of the nasal cavity and inflated slowly with sterile water or air until the bleeding stops. For posterior epistaxis, a double-balloon device is passed into the nasopharynx and seated in the posterior nasal cavity to tamponade the bleeding source. Next, the anterior balloon is inflated in the anterior nasal cavity to prevent retrograde travel of the posterior balloon and subsequent airway obstruction. If a specialized epistaxis balloon is unavailable, a Foley catheter may be substituted using the same general principles. Balloon tamponade is associated with a risk of saline aspiration,[4] pressure necrosis, perforation, infection, and other potential complications of packing.

Persistent bleeding requires endoscopic inspection by an ear, nose, and throat (ENT) specialist to identify the bleeding site. Cautery is first-line management if an anterior source of bleeding has been visualized.[5] However, cautery will not take effect through fluid, so the bleeding point itself cannot be cauterized until hemostasis is achieved. Cautery may cause rhinorrhea and crusting of the mucosa; overzealous use of the technique could lead to ulceration and perforation.[6] For intractable epistaxis, surgical ligation or endoscopic cauterization of the internal maxillary, external carotid, or sphenopalatine artery may be considered. Potential complications of such procedures include excessive blood loss, periorbital infection, and paresthesia. Rare major complications include oculomotor paralysis, oroantral fistulas, and septal perforation.[7]

Angiographic embolization in the case of intractable epistaxis has become an increasingly common management approach. The first successful percutaneous embolization for epistaxis was reported by Sokoloff et al. in 1974.[8] The technique was applied to patients with hereditary hemorrhagic telangiectasia (HHT) by Strother and Newton in 1976, and in 1980, Merland et al. were able to report a 97% success rate in a first series of 54 patients with severe epistaxis.[9,10] The technique has since been widely accepted and its efficacy confirmed.[11] Embolization may be considered a safe and effective therapy for epistaxis.[12] In addition, it is particularly helpful in cases where ENT surgery has failed to stop bleeding, usually after an endoscopic approach.

Although endovascular treatment of epistaxis is safe, serious complications are still possible. Tseng et al. reported 2 cases of stroke in 114 patients treated,[11] Elden et al. noted 1 stroke in 108 patients,[12] and Remonda et al. reported 2 strokes in 47 patients treated endovascularly for severe epistaxis.[13] With the use of calibrated particles, complications such as soft-tissue necrosis and facial paralysis have also been noted.[14] Complications related to coils and Gelfoam include temporofacial pain and headache.[15]

The nasal mucosa receives its blood supply principally from the maxillary artery via the sphenopalatine artery and its branches. Patients with intractable epistaxis commonly show diffuse bilateral mucosal anomalies on catheter angiography (Fig. 95-1). It is therefore not surprising that endovascular management of epistaxis has classically involved bilateral sphenopalatine and sometimes bilateral facial artery angiography, followed by targeted embolization of offending vessel branches with various embolic materials such as calibrated microparticles and Gelfoam pledgets.[15,16] Although the collateral network connecting the sphenopalatine artery and its branches to the facial artery and the anterior and posterior ethmoidal arteries is well recognized,[17] the possibility of mucosal blood supply from branches of the infraorbital artery has not been previously emphasized. In rare cases, the infraorbital artery should be considered a possible source of bleeding and a potential candidate for superselective embolization in patients with intractable epistaxis[18] (Fig. 95-2).

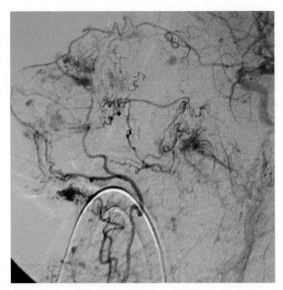

FIGURE 95-1. Digital subtraction angiography. Lateral projection of left common carotid artery demonstrates diffuse hypervascularity of mucosa.

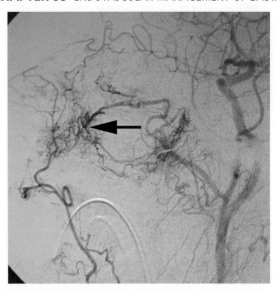

FIGURE 95-3. Digital subtraction angiography. Lateral projection of right common carotid artery demonstrates diffuse hypervascularity of mucosa and dysplastic arteriolar network in right anterior nasal cavity fed by right infraorbital artery *(arrow)*.

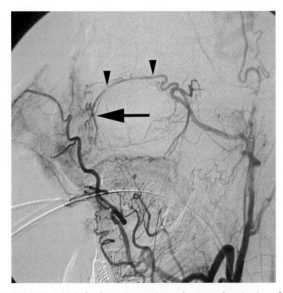

FIGURE 95-2. Digital subtraction angiography. Lateral projection of right external carotid artery demonstrates dysplastic-looking arterial network *(arrow)* in location corresponding to source of bleeding, derived from right infraorbital artery *(arrowheads)*.

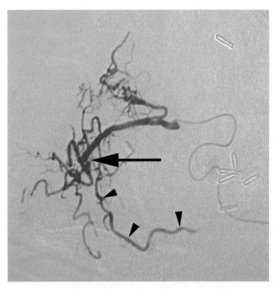

FIGURE 95-4. Digital subtraction angiography. Lateral projection of right infraorbital artery in late stage of n-butyl cyanoacrylate injection shows distribution of glue reaching suspected source of bleeding *(arrow)* and even refluxing into a sphenopalatine artery *(arrowheads)*. Note presence of surgical clips, consistent with history of previous maxillary and ethmoidal ligation.

In addition to diffuse mucosal changes, a focal arterial anomaly can often be detected (Fig. 95-3). The combination of a bleeding source suspected clinically and a focal anomaly seen on angiography allows precise targeting of embolization to a single vessel, despite the presence of widespread mucosal hypervascularity. This strategy, which relies on close collaboration between the otorhinolaryngologist and the interventional neuroradiologist, minimizes the potential for periprocedural complications and recurrent hemorrhage.

The use of n-butyl cyanoacrylate (NBCA) glue as an agent in the treatment of epistaxis has been documented. Merland et al. used Gelfoam occasionally supplemented by NBCA glue at the end of the procedure.[10] Luo et al.

reported using NBCA glue to treat pseudoaneurysms associated with hypervascular tumors of the head and neck.[19] NBCA glue as the primary embolic agent for treatment of severe epistaxis was first documented by Gailloud et al.[18] (Figs. 95-4 and 95-5).

A targeted embolization approach to epistaxis with NBCA glue reduces the duration of the procedure in two ways. First, a selective technique in which only one abnormal vessel is embolized avoids the multiple catheter manipulations necessary for a classic approach involving bilateral

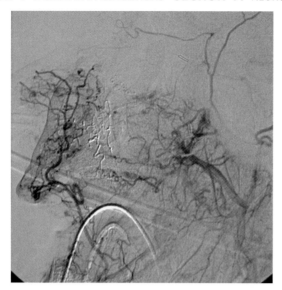

FIGURE 95-5. Digital subtraction angiography. Lateral projection of right external carotid artery shows no opacification of dysplastic network after embolization.

maxillary and facial artery embolization. Second, the use of NBCA glue as the embolic agent is technically faster than embolization with polyvinyl alcohol (PVA) microparticles or Gelfoam. In a population of elderly patients generally manifesting associated cervicocranial atheromatous changes, reducing the complexity and duration of an intervention should help reduce the risk for potential periprocedural complications.

A few technical tricks can be used to optimize embolization of the targeted vessel. Unpacking the nasal cavities in the angiography suite before embolization restores flow in the catheterized vessel and thereby improves both visualization of small focal arterial abnormalities and distal distribution of the NBCA glue. Wedging the microcatheter tip into the targeted vessel and flooding the arterial bed with 5% dextrose before NBCA injection also improves distal progression of the NBCA glue. When a wedged microcatheter tip position cannot be obtained, distal progression of the glue can be optimized by performing a continuous 5% dextrose injection through the guiding catheter simultaneously with microcatheter injection of NBCA.

INDICATIONS

An estimated 60% of the population experiences epistaxis at least once in their lifetime, and about 6% of these patients require treatment.[20] Although the cause of epistaxis is not determined in most cases, possibilities include postsurgical complications, facial trauma, neoplasms, coagulopathy, vascular malformations, arterial hypertension, and HHT.[16] Most cases of epistaxis are managed medically, but such methods are not always effective, especially in patients with a posterior source of bleeding.[15] When conservative management fails, the epistaxis is termed *intractable*.

Patients with intractable epistaxis almost always show diffuse bilateral mucosal anomalies on catheter angiography, with no clearly identifiable source of bleeding. This appearance is often due to nasal packing. Endovascular management of epistaxis has therefore classically involved

bilateral distal internal maxillary artery embolization with calibrated microparticles or Gelfoam pledgets. However, a focal arterial anomaly may be detectable on angiography in addition to diffuse mucosal hypervascularity. A focal angiographic anomaly, when identified, may be selectively embolized with NBCA glue. Angiographic identification of the bleeding source followed by superselective single-vessel embolization with NBCA glue is a successful therapeutic approach to treating intractable epistaxis that reduces the number of endovascular manipulations and duration of the procedure.

Between 1% and 6% of adults experience a large posterior nosebleed. Epistaxis can be due to numerous causes, but usual causes include dry air, nasal oxygen cannulas, hypertension, low platelet count, aspirin use, warfarin (Coumadin) use, and atherosclerosis. Unusual causes of epistaxis include a giant internal carotid artery aneurysm eroding into the sphenoid bone, aneurysmal bone cyst, pseudoaneurysm, HHT, trauma, juvenile angiofibroma, ethmoidal arteriovenous fistula, and cancer of the nose and throat.

CONTRAINDICATIONS

It is critical that a physician performing transarterial embolization have an understanding of the potential dangerous anastomoses around the skull base. These anastomoses may allow embolic material to pass from the extracranial circulation into the intracranial circulation during the embolization and result in a stroke. Relevant anastomoses involve the inferolateral trunk, ethmoidal collaterals, meningohypophyseal arteries, and occipital-vertebral arteries. In addition to being aware of these potentially dangerous anastomoses, use of larger embolic particles can minimize stroke risk. For this reason, it is advisable to never use embolic material smaller than 200 μm during routine embolization for epistaxis.

EQUIPMENT

When selecting a microcatheter, it is important to keep in mind the goal of atraumatic access. The "smaller, softer, and safer principle" applies to all procedures and equipment. Many microcatheters are available. They vary in stiffness, tractability, and inner and outer luminal diameter. Ideally, a catheter that will push and track yet remain stable should be used. Catheter braiding increases axial rigidity and improves stability. Many catheters have a proximal braided shaft with a softer, more flexible distal end.

An appropriately sized microcatheter is selected for each procedure by considering catheter flexibility and stability, the guiding catheter, and devices to be inserted into the microcatheter. The journey traveled by the microcatheter, including the length, morphology, and tortuosity of the anatomy, must also be considered. The technique of steaming a microcatheter is very useful because a shape that conforms to a vessel will give the catheter stability during the procedure. Microcatheters are also available in preshaped form, making steaming unnecessary. A gentle 30- or 45-degree curve is usually sufficient for the procedure. Similarly, a 30- or 45-degree shape on a wire is all that is needed.

Before beginning a procedure, ensure that all equipment sizes are compatible with one another and that everything fits (sizes of wires, coil, etc.). Perform a dry table test if necessary, especially if the equipment is unfamiliar. Choose optimal obliquity. Always remove the slack from the system. Begin slowly and proceed gently. If something is not advancing, understand why. Do not simply push harder!

EMBOLIZATION

Multiple embolic agents are available for use in cases of epistaxis, including PVA, Gelfoam, trisacryl gelatin microspheres, and NBCA glue.

Polyvinyl Alcohol

Because it is both biocompatible and efficient as a permanent embolic agent, PVA has traditionally been the gold-standard embolic particle. However, since it is hydrophobic and irregular in shape, particles tend to cluster and create aggregates of unpredictable size.

Gelfoam

Particles of Gelfoam, made from purified gelatin, may be combined with a mixture of saline and contrast material and then injected into a vessel for embolization. The spongelike material draws in blood via capillary action, and clotting ensues.

Trisacryl Gelatin Microspheres (Embospheres)

These small spheres are composed of a plastic called *trisacryl gelatin.* They are hydrophilic, biocompatible, nonresorbable, and uniformly spherical. These calibrated microspheres are easy to deliver through a microcatheter, and they quickly and reliably reduce blood flow. Their size correlates well with the size of the occluded vessel. They have better sizing and penetration characteristics than PVA, but deaths have been reported from progressive irreversible hypoxemia—especially with smaller microspheres (40-120 μm).

Trufill Liquid Embolic System

This liquid glue system is a combination of NBCA, ethiodized oil, and tantalum powder. It is inserted under fluoroscopic guidance via superselective catheter delivery to obstruct or reduce blood flow. The mixture polymerizes into a solid material on contact with blood or tissue. Higher concentrations of ethiodized oil increase polymerization time, allowing better distal penetration. High concentrations of NBCA result in a faster polymerization rate, which allows proximal embolization. Tantalum powder is added to increase radiopacity and lower viscosity.

TECHNIQUE

Anatomy and Approach

The key to a successful transarterial embolization procedure is proper technique. It is important to keep in mind that the purpose of the procedure is not to devascularize the nose but to allow hemostasis by decreasing arterial inflow pressure to facilitate clotting and epithelial repair. The nose should be packed during the procedure and unpacked at the end of it by an ENT specialist. Of note, procedures should be performed under general anesthesia to protect the patient's airway.

Size 6F guiding catheters should be placed in the external carotid artery, then microcatheters and microwires should be used to access the internal maxillary artery distal to the infraorbital branch. It may be necessary to embolize this vessel bilaterally because it is common for ENT physicians to be unable to identify the source of the bleeding. Occasionally the nasal branches of the facial arteries have to be embolized, particularly in patients with very anterior bleeding, because these branches may supply the anterior aspect of the nose. In patients who have previously been treated by coil embolization, branches may have collateralized more posteriorly and should thus be investigated.

Again, it is imperative that potentially dangerous anastomosis sites be identified by high-quality digital subtraction angiography and careful review. It is also essential to place all embolic materials on a separate table to prevent accidental use of a syringe containing embolic particles for a diagnostic injection or transfer of embolic particles onto a diagnostic catheter or wire, which may cause stroke. Microcatheter injection should be performed with 3-mL syringes. Syringes should be clearly labeled in standard fashion as either saline, contrast material, or particles. Avoid using particles smaller than 200 μm. The best results are achieved with particles in the range of 250 to 350 μm.

Although it may seem counterintuitive in cases of bleeding, administration of heparin (5000-unit bolus, with 1000 units/h thereafter) during the embolization is critical. Prevention of stroke is still the primary concern. Meticulous attention to pressurized catheter flush bags filled with 4 units heparin/mL of normal saline (4000 units of heparin in 1000 mL normal saline) is critical. This ensures that the dead space around the microcatheter is flushed and clot does not accumulate there. Heparin activity should be reversed with protamine at the end of the procedure.

It is crucial to ensure that all guiding catheters are clean and properly flushed. Just one piece of PVA is sufficient to cause a stroke during an injection. Remove all catheters and replace them with new catheters when in doubt; the expense is far less costly than stroke rehabilitation. A cautious approach to embolization is advised because it is never possible to reverse the effects of embolization, especially after devascularization and skin necrosis. Again, staying with midrange particle sizes will help avoid such complications.

Technical Aspects

Though useful, biplane angiography is not required for embolization, but roadmap capability is essential. Two skilled physician operators are needed rather than a scrub nurse and one physician. Size 5F or 6F Cordis Envoy MPC (or comparable) guide catheters should be used. These catheters have 0.057- and 0.067-inch lumens, allowing use of microcatheters and roadmap injections. Use of 0.038-inch-lumen 5F catheters as guiding devices can cause poor vessel visualization and lead to multiple problems. Guiding injections are not possible with this size, and flush will not flow in the dead space, thereby increasing the risk of clotting. Elderly patients with left-sided nosebleeds often need a 6F

Simmons-2 guide catheter or even a shuttle sheath because of a hypertensive arch and challenging left common carotid access. A few such catheters should be kept on hand for this indication.

COMPLICATIONS

Complications of endovascular therapy for epistaxis, though rare, do occur. They include temporofacial pain, headache, soft-tissue necrosis, facial paralysis, and stroke.

POSTPROCEDURAL AND FOLLOW-UP CARE

After the procedure, the nose should be unpacked by an ENT specialist, and heparin activity should be reversed to lower the risk for continued bleeding.

SUMMARY

Transarterial embolization of epistaxis is a safe, cost-effective procedure when performed with adequate technique. During the procedure, an understanding of potential dangerous anastomoses is crucial to avoiding passage of embolic material from the extracranial circulation into the intracranial circulation, which could result in a stroke.

Rapid targeted epistaxis embolization can be performed when clinical suspicion of a bleeding source correlates with a focal arterial anomaly on diagnostic angiography, despite the presence of diffuse bilateral mucosal hypervascularity. Transarterial embolization often follows an unsuccessful attempt at controlling the epistaxis via an endoscopic approach. Communication between the ENT specialist and the interventional neuroradiologist is essential for correlation of the bleeding source with an angiographic anomaly, particularly with respect to lateralization. In certain cases, postembolization endoscopic evaluation may even demonstrate embolic material in the treated vessel. When possible, this therapeutic strategy may avoid long and possibly unwarranted endovascular manipulations that put the patient at higher risk for periprocedural complications. The use of NBCA glue, though not classic in this indication, appears to be ideally suited for rapid targeting of a focal source of arterial bleeding.

The tips and techniques in this chapter are routinely used in a variety of applications, including gunshot wounds to the head and neck, exsanguinating tumors, and preoperative embolization of glomus tumors. The target vessel is the primary difference between the applications.

KEY POINTS

- Intractable epistaxis requiring transarterial embolization is rare.
- Endovascular embolization is a minimally invasive, effective therapy for epistaxis.
- Proper technique and knowledge of anatomy are essential to minimize risks.

▶ **SUGGESTED READINGS**

Elden L, Montanera W, Terbrugge K, et al. Angiographic embolization for the treatment of epistaxis: A review of 108 cases. Otolaryngol Head Neck Surg 1994;111:44–50.

Tseng E, Narducci C, Willing S, Sillers M. Angiographic embolization for epistaxis: a review of 114 cases. Laryngoscope 1998;108:615–9.

The complete reference list is available online at www.expertconsult.com.

CHAPTER 96

Subarachnoid Hemorrhage

Juan Carlos Baez, Rush H. Chewning, Gerald Wyse, and Kieran P.J. Murphy

When a patient has a severe or "thunderclap" headache of sudden onset, subarachnoid hemorrhage (SAH) must be considered and investigated. The most common symptom described by patients with SAH is headache, often the worst they have ever experienced and associated with a sense of doom. Less specific symptoms include stiff neck, change in level of consciousness, vomiting, and focal neurologic deficits, including cranial nerve palsies. Cranial nerve palsies can arise as a result of bleeding, compression from an aneurysm, or ischemia secondary to acute vasoconstriction immediately after aneurysmal rupture. The stereotypic third nerve palsy is manifested as an inferiorly rotated abducted eye with accompanying ptosis and pupil dilation. Patients often describe visual deterioration in the form of diplopia. Onset is sudden, and pain is a common complaint. Third nerve palsy often serves as an indicator of a posterior communicating artery aneurysm, although superior cerebellar and basilar artery aneurysms can less commonly cause the same symptoms.[1]

Ruptured intracranial aneurysms account for approximately 85% of cases of nontraumatic SAH. Although some have suggested familial or genetic causes for the development of intracranial aneurysms, other factors such as smoking, heavy alcohol use, and hypertension play a larger role. Female sex, African American heritage, and hereditary disorders such as autosomal polycystic kidney disease constitute some of the genetic factors also linked to development of these vascular lesions.[2]

Other causes of SAH include cerebral arteriovenous malformation (AVM) and perimesencephalic hemorrhage. AVMs are complex bundles of arteriovenous connections without intervening capillaries. The abnormally high flow commonly results in secondary aneurysms. AVMs are less common than aneurysms as a cause of SAH and will not be discussed further. Perimesencephalic hemorrhage is manifested as blood in the cerebral cisterns, with a predominantly prepontine distribution, and accounts for 10% of all SAH cases. This benign condition is thought to be secondary to rupture of a prepontine vein and poses no threat to the patient.[3]

Multiple grading systems are used for subarachnoid hemorrhage. Two of the more commonly used include the Fisher scale and the Hunt and Hess classification. The Fisher scale scores SAH on computed tomography (CT) appearance and quantification of subarachnoid blood. Patients are in group 1 if no blood is detected. Group 2 consists of those with diffuse deposition of subarachnoid blood, no clots, and no layers of blood greater than 1 mm. Group 3 patients have localized clots or vertical layers of blood 1 mm or greater in thickness, whereas patients in group 4 have intracerebral or intraventricular clots or diffuse subarachnoid blood.[4] The Fisher scale is a radiologic classification and should not be used to predict clinical outcomes.

The Hunt and Hess classification scale grades SAH on a scale from I to V based on clinical manifestations of the patient. A grade of I is given to patients with asymptomatic findings or mild headache. Grade II is assigned for cranial nerve palsies, moderate to severe headache, and nuchal rigidity. Grade III includes mild focal neurologic deficits, lethargy, or confusion. Grade IV consists of stupor, moderate to severe hemiparesis, and early decerebrate rigidity. Grade V is deep coma, decerebrate rigidity, and a moribund appearance.[4] If the patient has a serious systemic disease such as hypertension, diabetes mellitus, or chronic obstructive pulmonary disease or if severe vasospasm occurs during arteriography, the Hunt and Hess grade is increased by one level.[5] The Hunt and Hess system fails to adequately describe the patient's stage of consciousness on admission, which ultimately proves to be the most reliable indicator of recovery. Consequently, interphysician variability exists when using this classification system. In addition to the Hunt and Hess system, use of the Glasgow Coma Scale, which attempts to objectively grade consciousness according to eye opening, verbal ability, and motor function, helps stratify patients and minimize variability among physicians.

INDICATIONS

Outcomes in cases of SAH are poor, with mortality rates ranging from 32% to 67%.[6] Early diagnosis is crucial in minimizing the consequences associated with this condition, because up to 30% of fatalities in individuals with previous SAH result from rebleeding. Among survivors of SAH, 30% will have moderate to severe disability after the event. Unfortunately, between a fourth and half of cases of SAH are missed by the first evaluating physician. Initial evaluation of SAH typically involves the use of noncontrast-enhanced CT in the emergency department. CT scans are fast, readily available, and relatively inexpensive. CT has been demonstrated to have 93% to 95% sensitivity for SAH when conducted within 24 hours of initial bleed.[7] A timely study is critical because 50% of SAH episodes are not visible on CT 1 week after the bleeding.

When clinical suspicion for SAH is high, negative CT findings cannot rule it out. The literature reports a 7% false-negative rate of head CT for the diagnosis of SAH in patients later found to have ruptured aneurysms. Because mortality with untreated SAH is exceedingly high, patients with negative CT findings but clinical suspicion for SAH should undergo additional diagnostic testing. A lumbar puncture (LP) is recommended as the next step in the diagnosis of SAH. Recent work published in the *BMJ* supports modern multislice head CT alone as adequate to exclude SAH if it is performed within 6 hours of ictus.[8] This is being adopted in some emergency departments but not all, and will no doubt be controversial because of cases where LP found CT-negative SAH.

The typical LP involves sequentially drawing four aliquots of cerebrospinal fluid (CSF) from the L4-L5 interspace under local anesthesia of the patient's back. Inspection of CSF for *xanthochromia* (yellowish tint of CSF, indicating hemolyzed blood) provides the best evidence of SAH. A perfectly performed LP in a patient with no SAH yields clear CSF with no red blood cells (RBCs) after violating the L2-L3 interspace. Common parlance refers to this as a "champagne tap," and this result combined with the absence of xanthochromia reliably rules out SAH.[9]

Approximately 10% to 25% of the time, however, LP yields varying amounts of blood. The physician must then decide whether the blood represents SAH or perforation of the epidural venous plexuses and cauda equina vessels during the procedure. The "three-tube test" (named before four tubes became standard) is based on the principle that if the amount of blood present in the aliquots decreases between the first and fourth tubes, the blood is attributed to a traumatic tap. No consensus exists regarding what size decrement of blood indicates a traumatic LP. This results in uncertainty for physicians who must base therapeutic decisions on these results. Although multiple criteria have been used to differentiate between traumatic taps and true SAH, these criteria have been devised on the basis of traditional medical practice and not evidence-based medicine.

A study by Heasley et al., however, showed that a 25% reduction in RBCs between the first and fourth tubes—as one would expect to see in a traumatic tap—does not rule out SAH.[9] Other authors have used different cutoffs for what constitutes a traumatic tap, but these cutoffs have also yielded unacceptably high false-positive and false-negative rates. Heasley's group considers determination of traumatic taps via the three-tube test unreliable and recommend further invasive testing to determine the presence or absence of SAH with certainty if clinical suspicion remains high.

Additional CSF testing for D-dimer, clot formation, and opening pressure have all been studied in an attempt to diagnose SAH with greater accuracy, but the results have been inconclusive; these tests are rarely part of the LP procedure. In cases where a patient is complaining of the worst headache ever experienced, formal evaluation of the cerebral blood vessels is necessary subsequent to any LP that yields blood.

CONTRAINDICATIONS

There are no absolute contraindications to digital subtraction angiography (DSA). Relative contraindications include allergic reactions to contrast material, hypotension, severe hypertension, coagulopathy, renal insufficiency, and congestive heart failure. The patient must also be cooperative and able to remain still during the procedure.

EQUIPMENT

Safe and effective DSA for detection of intracranial aneurysms is ideally performed in an angiography suite with a biplane angiography system staffed by experienced neurointerventionalists. Three-dimensional (3D) DSA requires additional workstations and appropriate software for image reconstruction.

TECHNIQUE

Cerebral DSA is considered the gold standard for finding the aneurysmal source of SAH. This invasive imaging modality relies on manipulation of catheters within the carotid and vertebral arteries to inject radiographic contrast material into the intracranial vessels. DSA provides the best spatial and temporal resolution of aneurysmal sources of SAH, and 3D-DSA further improves aneurysm detection and characterization.

After consent, the patient is brought to the angiography suite and properly draped. Arterial access is gained via a femoral approach, and arterial sheaths and diagnostic catheters are placed within the femoral artery. The sheath is continuously flushed with heparinized saline throughout the procedure. The diagnostic catheter is then advanced to the aortic arch. Imaging of the aortic arch and bilateral vertebral and carotid arteries is performed. Special attention is paid to common locations for aneurysm formation. The three most common sites of aneurysm formation are the anterior communicating artery, posterior communicating artery, and middle cerebral artery. The basilar, posterior inferior cerebellar, and vertebral arteries must also be visualized to clear the angiogram. On DSA, an aneurysm appears as a saccular or irregular dilation of a blood vessel. The interventionalist can use 3D-DSA to better visualize and characterize aneurysms. Special attention should be paid to the neck, shape, size, location, and orientation of the aneurysm because these parameters will help determine therapy.

Both ruptured and unruptured aneurysms should receive immediate treatment by either surgical clipping or endovascular coiling. Once an aneurysm has ruptured, there is a 15% to 20% chance of it rebleeding, with mortality in this scenario exceeding 70%. Studies have shown improvements in mortality and morbidity if treatment of the culprit aneurysm is not delayed.[10] Consequently, quick and accurate diagnosis proves vital for the patient's prognosis.

The high mortality associated with untreated SAH makes diagnosis of it imperative.[11] Any patient with the worst headache ever experienced and a clinical picture consistent with SAH should undergo CT scanning to evaluate for acute bleeding. A negative CT should prompt further invasive testing with LP and possibly DSA. Although improvements in technique and expertise have reduced the risks associated with DSA, a meta-analysis showed that there was a 1.8% chance of complications and less than a 0.2% probability of sustaining permanent neurologic deficits subsequent to DSA.[12] Nevertheless, the benefits of diagnosing an aneurysm causing SAH with DSA far outweigh the risks.

CONTROVERSIES

The increasing popularity of computed tomographic angiography (CTA) and magnetic resonance angiography (MRA) has made prominent the question of whether these noninvasive imaging modalities can replace DSA. DSA is an invasive test that adds time, cost, discomfort, and a small but finite risk to the patient's hospital experience. If noninvasive imaging could match the high sensitivity of DSA for the diagnosis of SAH and localization of an aneurysm, one could minimize the use of DSA.

3D-CTA is increasingly being used for detection and characterization of intracranial aneurysms. In cases of suspected SAH, studies can be conducted immediately after initial noncontrast-enhanced CT scan, because the patient is already on the scanning table. These studies are quick and noninvasive, although contrast agent must be administered through a peripheral intravenous catheter. The sensitivity of 3D-CTA was shown to be 93% in a metaanalysis by Chappell et al.[13] Sensitivity, particularly for small aneurysms, would have to improve for 3D-CTA to fully supplant DSA as the gold standard. Nonetheless, a positive scan proves incredibly useful. Many surgeons now depend solely on 3D-CTA for preoperative evaluation and planning of surgical clipping of aneurysms. As technologic advances in both scanning equipment and software image processing improve, the sensitivity of CT for diagnosing SAH and detecting aneurysms could approach 100%, thereby obviating the need for more invasive tests.

Advances in magnetic resonance imaging (MRI) may allow its use in diagnosing SAH. MRI has been demonstrated to be superior to CT in diagnosing chronic as well as subacute SAH when imaging is performed 5 days after the initial bleed.[14] Although MRI has traditionally been considered less useful than CT for evaluating acute SAH, recent reports indicate that the sensitivity of MRI with fluid-attenuated inversion recovery (FLAIR), proton density–weighted images, or gradient-echo parameters might in fact be equal to if not greater than CT in diagnosing acute SAH.[15,16] Concern about availability of scanners and length of time necessary for scans might limit the utility of MRI in this application. However, acute SAH protocol MRIs can be conducted in as little as 8 minutes without the need for iodinated contrast material or exposure of the patient to radiation.[16] Nevertheless, a hemodynamically unstable sick patient should never undergo MRI. Similar to 3D-CTA, MRI evaluation of SAH adds the benefit of pinpointing the location of an aneurysm, when one is present, without the need for further scans.

CTA and MRA currently have problems detecting small aneurysms, with some studies stating sensitivity as low as 40% for aneurysms smaller than 3 mm. Sensitivity for aneurysms larger than this, however, is significantly higher. Because most aneurysms causing third nerve palsy exceed 5 mm in diameter, CTA and MRA are well positioned to diagnose the culprit aneurysms.[17] Once an aneurysm grows large enough to compress the third nerve, there is a 30% to 60% probability of it causing SAH within the following month. Consequently, presence of a third nerve palsy acts as a herald of potentially catastrophic SAH and should raise multiple red flags in the mind of the physician. Furthermore, a noninvasive imaging modality such as CTA might prove sufficient for diagnosis in this clinical scenario. Nevertheless, until the sensitivity of CTA and MRA improve for aneurysms smaller than 3 mm, DSA will continue being the gold standard in diagnosing intracerebral aneurysms. Whole-head 320-slice CT allows exact aneurysm assessment, and clearly the technology is marching towards a day where catheter angiography will be obsolete (Fig. 96-1).

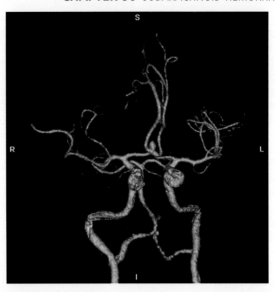

FIGURE 96-1. This 320-slice computed tomographic angiogram demonstrates computed tomography digital subtraction angiographic image of anterior communicating aneurysm filling from right A1-A2 junction, pointing superiorly, with a narrow neck.

OUTCOMES

As noted, DSA is the most definitive method of diagnosing an aneurysm subsequent to SAH, but 10% to 20% of DSA studies performed subsequent to proven SAH will appear normal. In these cases, if the pattern of bleeding appears to be perimesencephalic, the bleeding is attributed to a nonaneurysmal cause, and no further diagnostic evaluation is warranted. These patients go home after observation for 7 to 10 days in the hospital, with no complications and no modifications necessary in their daily lives. If the pattern of blood on CT suggests an aneurysm, but results of DSA appear normal, repeat angiography within 1 to 6 weeks is warranted because the risk of rebleeding is high. Oblique views that fail to visualize the aneurysm, vasospasm, thrombosis of the aneurysm, or saccular obliteration by hematoma have all been posited as reasons why aneurysmal SAH can appear normal on DSA.[18]

If an aneurysm is diagnosed, one must decide whether therapy is to be pursued. Elderly and frail patients in whom the risk of sedation and an interventional procedure exceeds the risk of not treating the aneurysm should undergo observation. Younger and otherwise healthier patients, however, require treatment because the risk of primary or secondary bleeding from an aneurysm accumulates with each passing year. Fifteen years ago, these patients would have undergone neurosurgical clipping of the aneurysm. This technique has been shown to effectively reduce morbidity and mortality when compared with untreated aneurysms.[19] Since the introduction of detachable coils, however, patients can now decide whether they would prefer endovascular therapy.

The morphology and location of an aneurysm, as well as patient status and preference, help determine which therapeutic modality should be used. Coiling selection criteria include anterior circulation aneurysms in patients with Hunt and Hess grade III to V SAH, posterior circulation aneurysms, medical contraindications to surgery, advanced age, and multiple aneurysms. Aneurysms with broad necks (>4 mm) or a fundus-to-neck ratio of less than 2 increase the risk for coil migration and protrusion of the coil into the parent vessel, thereby making clipping clearly favorable in these situations. In terms of location, surgical clipping of anterior circulation aneurysms, particularly anterior communicating artery aneurysms, yields the best results.[20] For all other aneurysms whose morphology and location do not clearly favor one treatment modality over another, controversy still exists regarding optimal therapy.

Two large multicenter studies have attempted to determine whether coiling or clipping provides a better outcome in patients who are equally good candidates for both therapies. The International Subarachnoid Aneurysm Trial (ISAT), a randomized prospective study, showed that coiling yielded significantly better outcomes at 1 year as quantified by Rankin scores, a functional scoring system.[21] Whereas ISAT included patients with ruptured aneurysms, the International Study of Unruptured Intracranial Aneurysms (ISUIA) demonstrated that coiling also yields better outcomes in patients whose aneurysms have not ruptured.[22] Both these studies have drawn criticism from the medical community, but their results, as well as the results of countless smaller studies, suggest that coiling results in reduced morbidity and mortality and decreased use of hospital resources in the short period during which they have been studied. Recent developments in flow-diverting stents are having a remarkable impact on giant aneurysm outcomes. These devices do have side effects, however, including delayed aneurysm rupture and stroke.[23]

COMPLICATIONS

Serious complications from DSA in the hands of experienced interventionalists are rare. Nevertheless, the patient must be informed of the risk of temporary or permanent neurologic deficits. This risk is increased in elderly patients with known histories of extensive atherosclerosis. Additional non-neurologic risks include femoral artery injury, hematoma, allergic reaction to the contrast agent, and nephrotoxicity. Like all invasive procedures, DSA also carries a small but finite risk of death.

POSTPROCEDURAL AND FOLLOW-UP CARE

Patients with aneurysms diagnosed on DSA require treatment unless therapy is contraindicated. If the aneurysm has already led to SAH, the chance of rebleeding is exceedingly high. These patients should undergo either clipping or coiling to reduce SAH morbidity and mortality.

KEY POINTS

- Negative head computed tomography (CT) does not rule out subarachnoid hemorrhage (SAH).
- After a negative head CT, a patient with the worst headache ever experienced should undergo lumbar puncture.
- Digital subtraction angiography remains the gold standard for the diagnosis of aneurysms causing SAH.

► SUGGESTED READINGS

Brisman JL, Song JK, Newell DW. Cerebral aneurysms. N Engl J Med 2006;355:928–39.

Shah KH, Edlow JA. Distinguishing traumatic lumbar puncture from true subarachnoid hemorrhage. J Emerg Med 2002;23:67–74.

van Gijn J, Kerr RS, Rinkel GJ. Subarachnoid haemorrhage. Lancet 2007;369:306–18.

The complete reference list is available online at www.expertconsult.com.

CHAPTER 97

Management of Head and Neck Injuries

M.J. Bernadette Stallmeyer

Traumatic head and neck vascular injuries such as dissections, transections, pseudoaneurysms, arteriovenous fistulas, and large artery occlusions are relatively uncommon but can result in potentially devastating stroke, severe blood loss, and even exsanguination and death. Rapid, early diagnostic imaging followed by effective management of neurovascular injuries can help improve patient outcome by focusing attention on prompt treatment of these lesions.[1,2]

Advances in multidetector computed tomography (CT) technology (Fig. 97-1) have greatly facilitated rapid noninvasive screening of trauma patients with suspected neurovascular injury. Although the use of computed tomographic angiography (CTA) for definitive diagnosis remains somewhat controversial, it can provide sufficient information to "fast-track" a patient with significant vascular injury to definitive surgical or endovascular intervention.[3] Alternatively, CTA may help determine whether a patient with minor injury is better served by delaying angiographic evaluation or treatment in favor of managing concomitant visceral or orthopedic injuries. Angiographic and endovascular resources can thus be directed where they are most appropriate and most needed.

INDICATIONS

- Obvious signs of trauma, including facial fracture; penetrating wounds; epistaxis; hemorrhage from the mouth, orbit, or ears; periorbital ecchymosis, or Battle sign; expanding cervical hematoma or a pulsatile mass, cervical bruising or abrasions; or cervical bruit in a young patient[1,2]
- Fractures in proximity to the internal carotid or vertebral arteries, such as basilar skull fractures, cervical spine fracture-dislocations, or fractures extending into the foramen transversarium[1,2]
- History of significant blunt force injury to the head and neck, especially with a mechanism of injury involving cervical hyperextension-rotation, hyperflexion, or direct blow to the neck
- New focal neurologic deficit or stroke of unexplained cause on head CT in a patient with history of trauma; focal neurologic deficit in the setting of questionable or minimal trauma, especially if the patient was normal at admission[1]
- Pain in the neck, face, scalp, or head in the setting of questionable or minor trauma

CONTRAINDICATIONS

Relative contraindications include:
- Presence of dangerous collaterals or routes of blood flow to the orbit and brain; if these are present and cannot be protected, endovascular therapy may pose a significant risk for stroke.
- Reopening of an acute traumatic vascular occlusion should be done with extreme caution because of the risk of thromboembolic stroke, and should be performed only when essential for cerebral perfusion. In many instances, particularly in patients with an intact circle of Willis and good intracranial collaterals, intentional occlusion of severely injured vessels or coil embolization to secure a traumatic vascular occlusion should be considered among the treatment options.
- Some patients may better be served by medical or surgical therapy.
- Triage issues may dictate the timing or extent of treatment.

EQUIPMENT

- Angiography tray
- Rotating hemostatic valves
- Continuous flush system using heparinized saline (2000-4000 units/L) for sheaths, catheters, and microcatheters) (Fig. e97-1)
- 6F (or larger) access sheath
- 5F to 6F guide catheter
- 6F (or larger) introducer guide sheath, 90 to 100 cm long, for stent delivery
- End-hole microcatheter appropriate for use with chosen embolic agents, and 0.014-inch microwire; exchange length microwire may be needed for some stent delivery systems or tortuous anatomy
- Particulate embolic agents for epistaxis and facial hemorrhage
- Liquid embolic agents (n-butyl cyanoacrylate [NBCA], Onyx) have been used for treatment of life-threatening facial hemorrhage.
- Fibered 0.018-inch push coils and coil pusher for distal arterial injuries
- Fibered 0.035-inch push coils and Benson 0.035-inch wire for proximal arterial injuries
- Detachable 0.020-inch, 0.018-inch, 0.014-inch, 0.012-inch coils for occlusion of pseudoaneurysm sacs
- Stent(s) suitable for delivery into the extracranial internal carotid or vertebral arteries for treatment of cervical arterial dissection or pseudoaneurysm
- Covered stent(s) suitable for delivery into the extracranial internal carotid artery for treatment of cervical arterial lacerations and transections, including arteriovenous and cavernous carotid fistulae (CCF)

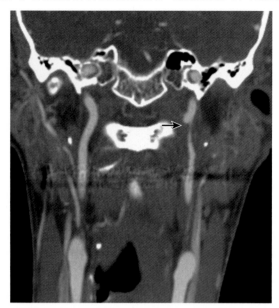

FIGURE 97-1. Computed tomographic angiography coronal multiplanar reconstruction image demonstrates left internal carotid artery (ICA) dissection and pseudoaneurysm *(arrow)*, and normal right ICA.

TECHNIQUE: EPISTAXIS, FACIAL FRACTURES

Anatomy and Approaches

The cervical, facial, and cranial regions are supplied by a rich vascular tree, including the external carotid artery (ECA), internal carotid artery (ICA), vertebral artery (VA), thyrocervical trunk, and costocervical trunk. Branching patterns can be variable, and numerous potential pathways of collateral flow exist between the extracranial and intracranial arteries.[4] Thus, careful vigilance for the presence of these dangerous collaterals is essential in preventing inadvertent embolization of the retina, brain, or cranial nerves.

If time and the patient's condition permit, CTA to evaluate the extent of bony injury and identify potential sites of arterial injury often facilitates delivery of definitive treatment, and is well worth the additional "cost" in examination time, contrast administration, and patient radiation exposure.[3]

In epistaxis and facial smash injuries, the most common culprits amenable to embolization are branches of the facial and internal maxillary arteries. The *facial artery* arises as a proximal branch of the ECA (either directly or as a common trunk with the lingual artery), ascends superficial to the mandible, then courses medially in the superficial soft tissues of the face, giving off branches to the lips, mandible, cheeks, and nasal cavity. The *internal maxillary artery* (IMA) arises as one of the terminal branches of the ECA at the level of the ramus of the mandible. It passes forward almost horizontally, medial to the mandibular ramus, giving off branches to the soft tissues (transverse facial artery), meninges (middle and accessory meningeal arteries) and, as it subsequently courses either deep or superficial to the lateral pterygoid muscle, to the muscles of mastication (masseter, temporalis, mylohyoid, and pterygoids). The

most distal part of the IMA passes through the pterygomaxillary fissure and into the pterygopalatine fossa; this distal segment gives rise to numerous branches that can be injured in facial fractures, particularly LeFort fractures, including the anterior and posterior superior alveolar arteries, descending palatine artery, infraorbital artery, sphenopalatine artery, and branches to the nasal cavity (Fig. 97-2).

Facial and nasal cavity bleeding can also occur as a consequence of injury to intracranial branches of the ICA. Persistent nasal bleeding may arise from the posterior and anterior *ethmoidal arteries*, which arise from the *ophthalmic artery* (OphA) distal to the takeoff of the central retinal artery. The posterior ethmoidal artery courses medially, passing between the medial rectus and superior oblique muscles, and enters the nasal cavity via the posterior ethmoidal canal to supply posterior nasal air cells and the upper nasal septum. The anterior ethmoidal artery also courses medially, passing through the anterior ethmoidal canal, and supplies the anterior and middle ethmoidal air cells, frontal sinus, and anterosuperior aspect of the lateral nasal wall. These ethmoidal branches are generally not amenable to safe direct embolization, and a failure to recognize them prior to ECA branch embolization can result in unilateral vision loss or stroke (Fig. 97-3).

Technical Aspects

In patients with epistaxis or facial injury, it is generally prudent to secure the airway by intubating the patient. The common femoral artery is entered using Seldinger technique, and a 6F or larger sheath inserted. A 5F or 6F guide catheter is then passed over a suitable 0.035- or 0.038-inch guidewire into the aortic arch. The large internal diameter of many available guide catheters is adequate to obtain a good roadmap by injecting around a coaxially placed microcatheter.

There are two general approaches to angiographic protocol: (1) diagnostic angiography of *all* vessels that are potentially a source of bleeding, followed by embolization of relevant arteries, or (2) angiography and embolization of one vessel, then moving on to another. The second approach is recommended only when the source of bleeding is clear on the basis of antecedent clinical or imaging findings. In either case, careful evaluation of the injured vessel and its runoff for possible communication with cerebral collaterals must be performed prior to intervention.

The common carotid artery (CCA) is selected, with care to keep the catheter and wire below any potential site of injury. Digital subtraction angiography (DSA) over the neck, skull base, and head is then performed to evaluate for ICA dissection, pseudoaneurysm, or extravasation arising from the cervical ICA or ECA. Treatment of cervical ICA dissections, pseudoaneurysms, and lacerations is addressed in a separate section later.

Large ECA branch lacerations causing profuse hemorrhage are best treated with particulate embolization followed by coil occlusion. Although the ECA main trunk and proximal portions of ECA branches can be occluded using 0.035-inch fibered push coils (delivered via a 5F catheter) or by 0.018-inch fibered push coils (delivered via microcatheter) alone, the offending ECA branch may continue to fill via retrograde collaterals from the opposite side. Selective roadmap imaging of the ECA, followed by passage of a

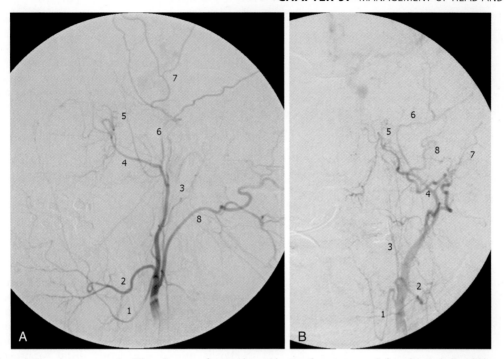

FIGURE 97-2. Lateral **(A)** and anteroposterior **(B)** angiograms of external carotid artery demonstrate main branches, including *(1)* lingual artery, *(2)* facial artery, *(3)* ascending pharyngeal artery, *(4)* internal maxillary artery, *(5)* sphenopalatine artery, *(6)* middle meningeal artery, *(7)* superficial temporal artery, and *(8)* occipital artery.

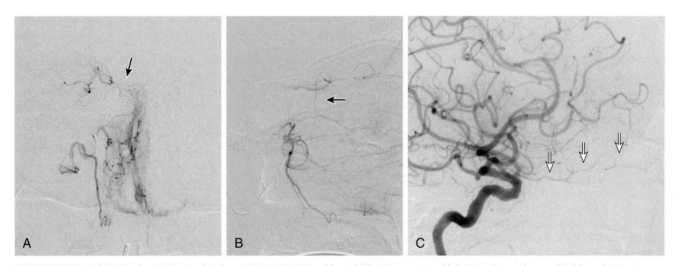

FIGURE 97-3. Left external carotid artery (ECA) anteroposterior **(A)** and lateral **(B)** angiograms, and left internal carotid artery (ICA) lateral **(C)** angiogram reveal anastomosis between distal internal maxillary artery and ophthalmic artery (OphA) *(black arrow)* via posterior ethmoidal artery collaterals. Note retrograde filling of OphA; identical vessel morphology is seen on ICA injection *(open arrows)*.

microwire and microcatheter across (if possible) or closely proximal to the site of extravasation, are performed. Subsequent DSA with microcatheter injection is then done to evaluate for dangerous collaterals. If none are present, small branches that could serve as potential channels for collateral supply are then occluded with polyvinyl alcohol (PVA) particles larger than 250 μm, followed by occlusion of the lacerated branch with 0.018-inch fibered push coils, using either the microwire or a coil pusher for delivery.

In many if not most cases of epistaxis or bleeding due to facial fractures, however, no obvious source of bleeding is evident on the initial CCA angiogram. Often the source of hemorrhage is seen only on selective or superselective angiography. Selective ICA angiography should be performed to rule out laceration of this vessel as a direct source of bleeding into the sphenoid sinus, evaluate ethmoidal branches of the OphA as either direct or collateral sources of hemorrhage, and look for other potential dangerous collaterals. Selective ECA angiography should then be performed to evaluate for arterial truncations (and thus potential lacerations), extravasation, pseudoaneurysms, or regions of unusual vascular blush (Fig. 97-4). The ECA

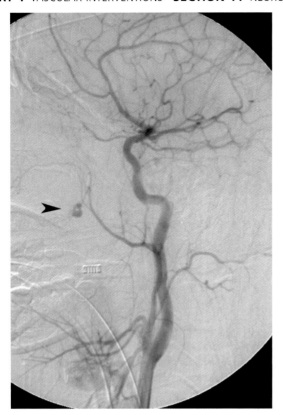

FIGURE 97-4. Lateral external carotid artery angiogram demonstrating a small pseudoaneurysm *(arrowhead)* arising from a branch of internal maxillary artery.

angiogram and any selective branch angiograms should be carefully evaluated for the presence of any branches projecting over the orbit and any collateral branches filling the ICA or OphA prior to performing embolization (see Fig. 97-3).

Therapeutic small-artery occlusion in the setting of epistaxis or trauma is most commonly performed using various preparations of PVA particles, typically 250 to 355 μm in size, suspended in a 1:1 or 2:1 mixture of contrast material to saline. This choice of particulate size effectively controls bleeding but allows small mucosal arteries to remain intact.[5] Particles larger than 250 μm also help avoid inadvertent embolization of perineural vessels and some potentially dangerous collaterals.[4] The concentration of PVA in the suspension should be sufficiently dilute to avoid clumping or clogging of the microcatheter.

Great care should be taken to prevent proximal reflux of particulate material into potential anastomotic branches and the ICA. It is also important to avoid a wedged catheter position, because the resultant increased injection pressure can sometimes open up previously unseen dangerous collateral branches.

If obvious sources of bleeding are seen on the diagnostic angiograms, these vessels are embolized first. If the site of bleeding is occult but clearly unilateral, the ipsilateral IMA and facial arteries may be embolized empirically. When the source of difficult-to-control bleeding is not evident, branches of the IMA are often to blame. In all cases, however, a maximum of three out of the four arteries providing most of the supply to the midline midface (right IMA, left IMA, right facial, left facial) should be embolized.

Internal Maxillary Artery Technique

After obtaining a roadmap image of the ECA, the microcatheter and microwire are passed coaxially through the guide catheter into the IMA. Superselective anteroposterior (AP) and lateral angiography, with hand injection of the microcatheter from a position in the mid-IMA, can be performed prior to embolization to check for dangerous collaterals. If any are seen, great care must be taken to prevent reflux, or embolization of this branch may have to be abandoned. If it appears safe to proceed, the microcatheter is advanced toward the terminal sphenopalatine branch.

Facial Artery Technique

After obtaining roadmap imaging of the ECA, the microcatheter and microwire are passed coaxially into the facial artery, usually just beyond the point where it crosses the mandible. Hand-injection DSA is performed to evaluate for lacerations that may require coil occlusion and for potential dangerous collaterals to the orbit. If embolization is being performed primarily for nasal injury or epistaxis, the catheter is moved sufficiently distal to prevent inadvertent reflux into the main ECA trunk, and even more importantly the ICA.

Internal Maxillary or Facial Artery Technique

A blank roadmap image is obtained. The microcatheter is disconnected from the continuous flush system, and hand injection of particles is performed via a 1-mL syringe, with 0.1- to 0.3-mL aliquots at a time injected under constant direct fluoroscopic visualization. Some operators prefer to inject particulate embolic using a "closed" system: a 3-way stopcock is interposed between the microcatheter hub and 1-mL syringe, with a reservoir syringe containing particulate suspension attached to the 3-way sidearm. Other operators simply draw the embolic suspension from a small medicine cup. Alternating injection of particulate suspension with injection of saline helps prevent clogging of the microcatheter, as does frequent inspection of the microcatheter hub for layering of particles. Embolization should continue until distal branches become "pruned" (Fig. 97-5); nasal blush will decrease concomitantly. Control angiograms via both the microcatheter and guide catheter should be performed intermittently during embolization to assess for additional suspicious vessels and any dangerous collaterals that may open up as small branches are occluded.

Controversies

ECA embolization for control of hemorrhage is safe and effective so long as appropriate care is taken to ensure delivery of embolic agent into target vessels and avoid delivery into intracranial branches and dangerous collaterals.

Outcomes

Technical success is defined as occlusion of the targeted vessels, and in most reported series is greater than 90%.[5] Clinical success is defined in most cases as cessation or control of hemorrhage; this is achieved in the majority of cases.

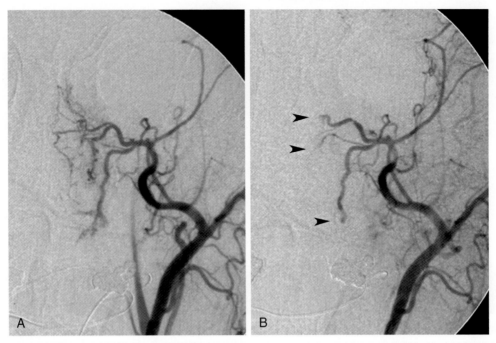

FIGURE 97-5. Lateral external carotid artery (ECA) angiogram before **(A)** and after **(B)** polyvinyl alcohol embolization, demonstrating desired pruning *(arrowheads)* of distal ECA branches.

Complications

Major potential complications include vision loss or cranial nerve palsy (<2%), and neurologic deficit (major permanent deficit in <1%).[5,6] Minor complications include headache and facial or jaw pain. Complications are rare so long as persistent vigilance for dangerous collaterals is maintained. Previously unseen collaterals may open up as distal IMA branches are occluded. If a "new" branch suddenly appears over the orbit or parasellar region, DSA via the microcatheter should be performed after aspiration of microcatheter contents.

TECHNIQUE: CCA, ICA, AND VA DISSECTIONS, PSEUDOANEURYSMS, AND TRANSECTIONS

Anatomy and Approaches

This kind of traumatic injury results from partial or complete disruption of the arterial wall and may occur as a result of either penetrating or blunt trauma. Injury ranges from "minimal intimal injury," in which a small region of endothelium is detached from the underlying media through development of a dissection flap, to perforation of the media or adventitia with pseudoaneurysm, or even complete transection.[7] Arterial occlusion due to expanding hematoma within a false lumen or pressure from extravascular clot may occur. Arteriovenous fistulae occur where transection of an adjacent artery and vein result in communication between the two vessel lumens. Therapy is directed toward two goals: control of hemorrhage and prevention of thromboembolic stroke.

In many institutions, noncontrast CT is the standard exam for initial assessment of head trauma and for both penetrating and blunt neck injuries. CTA is a highly sensitive and specific screening modality when the physical findings or mechanism of injury raise suspicion for neurovascular injury, and a useful precursor to catheter angiography.[3] Because the CCA, ICA, and VA travel for long distances in the neck without giving off large branches, a normal artery maintains a rounded cross-section and a nearly constant caliber; deviations from this appearance should raise concern for injury on CTA.

Many dissections, and even pseudoaneurysms can be managed with medical therapy (heparin, Coumadin, antiplatelets) alone.[2,8] If significant luminal narrowing is present, however, or if a large pseudoaneurysm that may serve as a nidus for thrombus is present, endovascular treatment with stent placement or stent-assisted coiling can be considered. Published criteria for stent placement include impending stroke due to hemodynamically significant luminal compromise, clinical failure of anticoagulation (transient ischemic attack, neurologic deterioration or stroke), or contraindication for anticoagulation because of other injuries.[9] If stent placement is likely and other injuries do not preclude antiplatelet treatment, preloading with aspirin and oral (PO) clopidogrel 300 mg on the day of the procedure, followed by maintenance of 75 mg PO daily for several months post procedure, helps decrease the risk of in-stent occlusion and periprocedural stroke.[10] In cases where the injured artery is occluded on initial exam, coiling of the residual stump may help prevent subsequent thromboembolic stroke.

Technique

In severely injured or uncooperative patients, intubation to secure the airway is generally prudent. It is usually worthwhile to obtain noncontrast head CT within 2 hours prior

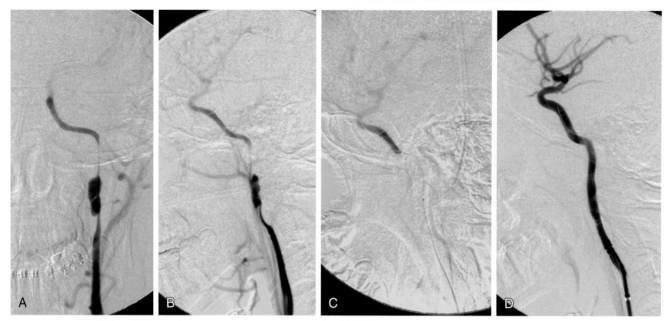

FIGURE 97-6. Lateral common carotid artery angiograms demonstrating endovascular stenting of a long-segment posttraumatic internal carotid artery (ICA) dissection. **A,** Preprocedure angiogram demonstrating severe narrowing of ICA by dissection. **B,** Microcatheter has been negotiated through dissected segment. **C,** Hand injection of contrast material through microcatheter verifies positioning within true lumen. **D,** Appearance of ICA after stent deployment.

to intervention in any patient who cannot be adequately assessed neurologically to exclude a developing stroke. The common femoral artery is entered by means of Seldinger technique, and a 6F or larger sheath placed. Evaluation of the aortic arch and great vessel origins, if necessary, can be performed with a 5F pigtail catheter prior to selective angiography. A 5F or 6F diagnostic catheter (vertebral curve, Berenstein, Headhunter, Vitek, etc.) on a continuous heparinized saline flush line is then passed over a suitable 0.035- or 0.038-inch guidewire, and diagnostic angiography of the neck and head is performed to assess the cervical carotid and vertebral arteries for injury, including intracranial extension. The intracranial collateral circulation must be evaluated prior to intervention. Particular care should be taken not to extend the wire or catheter into any region of suspected injury before it is evaluated with angiography. Additionally, initial injection of all vessels for roadmap images should be performed by gentle hand injection so as not to dislodge any intraluminal clot that may be present. Systemic heparinization with a 2000- to 4000-unit bolus followed by hourly administration of 1000 units should be used if the patient's other injuries permit; efficacy can be measured with serial activated clotting time (ACT).

If stenting of ICA dissection is to be performed, the length of the lesion and diameter of a "normal" segment or diameter of the contralateral artery should be measured to size the stent. Most traumatic ICA dissections involve the distal cervical segment, and some extend above the skull base to involve the very proximal petrous ICA; safe placement of a distal protection device beyond the dissected segment is thus problematic, and in at least some reported series, distal protection was not used.[11,12]

In this location, it is usually easier to deliver self-expanding stents rather than balloon-expandable stents, although the latter have been used successfully. All stents suitable for placement in the carotid or vertebral arteries

can be delivered through a long 6F introducer guide sheath or 7F guide catheter over a 0.014-inch microwire of appropriate length. The microwire is carefully negotiated beyond the dissection, avoiding any resistance. If the residual lumen is very small or tortuous, a microcatheter can be passed over the microwire, and positioning within the true lumen verified by hand injection of the microcatheter (Fig. 97-6). The stent delivery system is flushed with saline according to the manufacturer's directions, taking great care to eliminate all air from the system. The stent delivery system (end-hole or monorail) is then loaded over the microwire, positioned across the injured segment, and deployed according to manufacturer's recommendations. Control angiograms of the cervical and intracranial carotid are then obtained to evaluate for stent patency and intracranial branch occlusions. A delayed control angiogram 10 to 15 minutes after stent deployment should also be performed to assess for further stent expansion and platelet aggregation.

Small pseudoaneurysms will often be obliterated by stent compression alone. With larger pseudoaneurysms, a microcatheter can be positioned through the interstices of the stent into the pseudoaneurysm sac, and the lumen of the sac subsequently occluded with detachable coils (Fig. 97-7).

Vertebral artery dissections can be treated by similar means, although smaller-size stents primarily designed for coronary or intracranial placement will be required in most cases.

With arterial transection or arteriovenous fistulae in the neck, two approaches can be considered to control hemorrhage: placement of a covered stent, essentially identical to delivery of porous stents, or parent vessel sacrifice by occlusion with either detachable or push coils, with coiling technique as described in the previous section on ECA branch injuries. Parent vessel occlusion using the Amplatzer vascular plug has also been reported.[13]

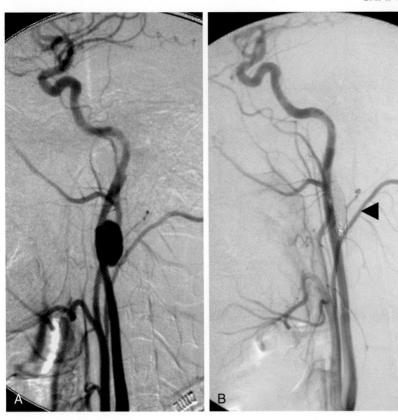

FIGURE 97-7. Lateral common carotid artery angiogram of a patient with traumatic internal carotid artery dissection before **(A)** and after **(B)** stent placement and embolization of residual pseudoaneurysm with detachable coils *(arrowhead)*.

Controversies

Long-term efficacy and durability of stent placement for extracranial carotid and vertebral artery traumatic injury, in comparison with anticoagulation, remains to be determined.[2,14]

Outcomes

Most series report 90% to 95% success in reaching the target lesion and deploying a well-positioned stent across it.[9,14]

Complications

In the short term, occlusion of the parent artery is rare to uncommon (<5%), and the incidence of periprocedural stroke is also low. Concern has been raised, however, about long-term patency rates; a 45% long-term occlusion was reported in one series.[14]

POSTPROCEDURAL AND FOLLOW-UP CARE

All patients should undergo monitoring of vital signs and pulse oximetry during the procedure and in postprocedure recovery.

Depending on the size of the arteriotomy, use of anticoagulant or antiplatelet therapy, and patient-specific disease, the arteriotomy can be closed either by manual pressure or with a closure device. Alternatively the sheath may be left in place temporarily. The puncture site should be periodically monitored for hematoma, and status of the arteries distal to the site of puncture should also be evaluated. If the sheath is left in place, monitoring should be performed by skilled nurses to ensure continuous flushing and patency of the sheath.

The patient should be monitored closely for any signs of postprocedural neurologic deterioration. The operating physician or his/her designee should evaluate the patient's condition immediately after the procedure, and monitoring for delayed neurologic deterioration should continue for at least several hours. When ICA injury has been treated by stenting or coiling of a pseudoaneurysm, the operating physician should be available for continuing care after discharge. Follow-up imaging with CTA or conventional angiography is often appropriate.

KEY POINTS

- Thorough knowledge of cervical and cerebral vascular anatomy, including vascular variants and potentially dangerous collaterals, is essential for safe endovascular management of head and neck traumatic injury.

- The choice of therapy (medical, endovascular, or surgical) is based on the nature and site of injury, but it is heavily influenced by the presence or absence of associated brain, visceral, and orthopedic injuries.

- Noncontrast computed tomography and computed tomographic angiography (CTA) of the head and neck to evaluate the extent of neurovascular injury are useful precursors to angiography in most cases. CTA is often definitive in detecting injury.

► **SUGGESTED READINGS**

Bromberg WJ, Collier BC, Diebel LN, et al. Blunt cerebrovascular injury practice management guidelines: the Eastern Association for the Surgery of Trauma. J Trauma 2010;68(2):471–7.

Burlew CC, Biffl WL. Imaging for blunt carotid and vertebral artery injuries. Surg Clin North Am 2011;91(1):217–31.

Cogbill TH, Cothren CC, Ahearn MK, et al. Management of maxillofacial injuries with severe oronasal hemorrhage: a multicenter perspective. J Trauma 2008;65(5):994–9.

The complete reference list is available online at www.expertconsult.com.

CHAPTER 98

Cervical Artery Dissection

Jennifer Berkeley and Robert Wityk

Cervical artery dissection involving the extracranial carotid and vertebral arteries is an infrequent cause of stroke but accounts for a significant percentage of ischemic strokes in young adults: 20% to 25% of strokes in those younger than 45 years of age can be attributed to cervical artery dissections, whereas only 2% of all strokes overall are believed to be due to dissections.[1] The incidence is equal for men and women and peaks around the age of 40. Reported incidence is 2.5 to 3.0 per 100,000 for carotid dissection and 1.5 to 2.0 per 100,000 for vertebral dissection.[2,3]

Dissections occur when blood accumulates in the vessel wall, usually between the intima and media of the artery, creating an intramural hematoma. The mass effect of the hematoma may result in vessel stenosis or occlusion and affect surrounding structures such as cranial nerves. The underlying etiology of cervical artery dissection is unknown, but two mechanisms have been proposed: (1) an actual tear in the intima allows blood from the lumen into the vessel wall, or (2) rupture of the vasa vasorum in the arterial wall itself leads to intramural hematoma.

CLINICAL PRESENTATION

Carotid dissections may be asymptomatic or present as various combinations of cerebral ischemia (transient ischemic attack [TIA] or stroke), head and neck pain, and cranial neuropathy. Early studies suggested that over 90% of the time they presented as cerebral or retinal ischemia. However, this was likely because they were rarely diagnosed outside the setting of recent TIA or stroke. Currently, some studies suggest that as few as 50% of dissections have associated ischemic manifestations. Furthermore, nearly 80% of those with strokes due to carotid dissections have preceding transient symptoms that include unilateral head, face, orbit, or neck pain; partial Horner syndrome; pulsatile tinnitus; or cranial nerve palsies (with the hypoglossal nerve being the most commonly affected). Ipsilateral Horner syndrome results from injury of sympathetic fibers that travel with the internal carotid artery in the neck on the way to the orbit. Pain typically occurs first. In a carotid dissection, the pain is often over the carotid artery in the neck but can also present as referred pain around the ipsilateral orbit, forehead, or temple. Median time from onset of pain to neurologic symptoms is 4 days.

The presentation of vertebral artery dissections may be more varied. One case series of 49 posterior circulation dissections showed that 44.9% presented with subarachnoid hemorrhage, whereas only 42.8% presented with ischemic stroke.[4] Early signs of vertebral artery dissections include posterior neck pain and occipital headache. Median time from onset of neck pain to ischemic symptoms in these dissections may be up to 2 weeks.[5,6] This delay between actual dissection and onset of neurologic symptoms makes early accurate diagnosis imperative.

The most common locations for cervical artery dissections are in the mobile portions of the vessels. Specifically, dissections in the internal carotid artery typically start 2 to 3 cm above the bifurcation and continue for various lengths up into the petrous portion. The V3 segment of the vertebral arteries is the most common site of posterior circulation dissections. It is also the most common site of bilateral dissections, which account for 12% to 15% of all dissections. Vertebral dissections are much more likely than carotid dissections to extend intracranially, leading to potentially catastrophic subarachnoid hemorrhage. It is also thought that intracranial dissections have a higher likelihood of resulting in ischemic stroke. Thus, those with intracranial dissections have permanent disabling deficits in 44% of cases, versus 14% when the dissection is limited to the cervical portion of the vessel.[7]

Prognosis after a cervical artery dissection is largely dependent on whether the patient presents with a stroke, and on infarct size and location. Although a dissected artery can occlude, patients with good collateral circulation may avoid cerebral ischemia. Strokes are believed to be due to embolization of thrombus that forms at or near the site of dissection, either because of slow blood flow or endothelial disruption. For this reason, the mainstay of treatment has been antithrombotic therapy to prevent embolization (see later discussion). For patients who survive the acute dissection with minimal cerebral ischemia, the prognosis is generally excellent. Recurrent ischemic events are uncommon. Dissecting pseudoaneurysms are discussed later. The lifetime rate of recurrent dissection in another artery is estimated to be between 5% and 10%.[8] Recurrent dissections typically occur within 6 to 12 months.

DIAGNOSTIC TESTING

Angiography is an excellent means for diagnosis, particularly of subtle carotid artery dissections or lesions in the vertebral arteries. Figure 98-1 illustrates several of the characteristic appearances of dissections, such as a flame-shaped tapering of the lumen and a sudden widening of the lumen distal to the dissection. Occasionally, an intimal flap can be seen with a false lumen. Magnetic resonance and computed tomographic angiography (MRA, CTA) can also detect dissections that cause stenosis or occlusion. However, digital subtraction angiography (DSA) may be superior for dissections that occur close to the origin of the vessels in the chest, where MRA or CTA may simply show an absent vessel.

Carotid artery ultrasound may detect a high-resistance flow pattern, but because dissections usually occur distal to the carotid artery bifurcation (typically around the C2

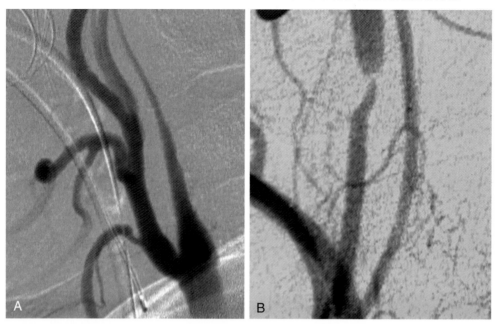

FIGURE 98-1. Angiographic appearance of dissections. **A,** Flame-shaped dissection of right internal carotid artery (ICA) distal to carotid bulb. **B,** Poststenotic dilation distal to right ICA dissection.

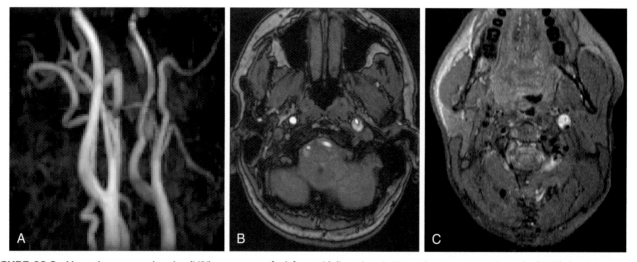

FIGURE 98-2. Magnetic resonance imaging (MRI) appearance of a left carotid dissection. **A,** Magnetic resonance angiography (MRA) showing narrowing of vessel approximately 3 cm above carotid bifurcation. Area of thrombus can be seen adjacent to narrowed vessel lumen. **B,** Axial T1-weighted MRI with gadolinium showing crescent of hemosiderin deposition in wall of a carotid dissection, with narrowing of carotid lumen. **C,** Axial T2-weighted MRI showing a hyperintensity within vessel wall consistent with acute hematoma.

level), the dissection is usually not directly visualized by ultrasound.

Perhaps the gold standard of diagnosis for carotid artery dissection is the use of axial T1- and T2-weighted neck imaging with fat suppression. In acute dissection, the intramural hematoma is visible as a crescent of hyperintense signal in the involved segment of the artery, as shown in Figure 98-2. Visualization of the same process in the vertebral artery is possible but less reliable.

ETIOLOGY

Serious head and neck trauma, as seen with motor vehicle accidents or knife or gunshot wounds, can certainly cause cervical artery dissection. By far the most common presentation, however, is after fairly minor or, at times, almost trivial trauma, such as occurs in turning the head to back up a car or in coughing violently. The remaining dissections are labeled as "spontaneous."

Numerous studies have attempted to elucidate predisposing conditions and risk factors for these spontaneous dissections. Fibromuscular dysplasia may account for 10% to 15% of patients.[5] A minority of patients (1%-5%) have a diagnosable connective tissue disorder, such as Ehlers-Danlos or Marfan disease, whereas a slightly larger percentage (10%-20%) are believed to have an as yet unnamed connective tissue disorder based on subtle ultrastructural changes in collagen, as seen in skin biopsies from patients with dissection.[9] Other associations include hyperhomocysteinemia, α_1-antitrypsin deficiency, migraine, and possibly recent infection.

MANAGEMENT OF ACUTE CERVICAL ARTERY DISSECTION

Management of patients with cervical artery dissection depends on the clinical presentation and time between the dissection and subsequent symptoms. Patients who present within the tissue plasminogen activator (tPA) time window with acute ischemic stroke secondary to dissection have been treated successfully with thrombolytic therapy. Some maintain a theoretical concern that tPA might worsen a dissection by either expanding the intramural hematoma, causing rupture of the vessel, or dislodging a luminal thrombus. A recent meta-analysis of published reports of thrombolysis in patients with strokes secondary to cervical artery dissections suggests that thrombolysis in these patients is safe, and outcomes are similar to those in patients with equivalent strokes of other etiologies. In this analysis, both intravenous and intraarterial tPA were evaluated, and both treatments appeared safe in patients with dissection.[10]

Because of the concern of artery-to-artery embolism, use of antithrombotic therapy (anticoagulation or antiplatelet agents) is currently the standard approach to prevent further strokes, despite the absence of large clinical trials. One small trial showed a nonsignificant benefit of 4.1% for those receiving anticoagulation versus aspirin in terms of preventing recurrent stroke, TIA, or death.[11] A more recent study of 298 patients with spontaneous carotid dissection showed only a 4.7% rate of recurrent ischemic events and no significant difference between those treated with anticoagulants (5.9%) and those treated with aspirin (2.1%).[12]

The suggested duration of antithrombotic therapy is poorly defined, with typical practices ranging between 6 weeks and 6 months. The natural course of a dissection is for recanalization to occur within 3 to 6 months of the initial event.[13,14] Therefore, a common approach to management is to anticoagulate for 3 to 6 months and then to re-image the vessel. When significant healing has occurred, patients are often switched to antiplatelet agents for long-term secondary prevention of stroke, though once again, no

data support this as a necessary therapy. The long-term risk of stroke has been estimated to be 1% or less per year, but it is not known whether this risk diminishes over time.[15]

In several instances, anticoagulation is contraindicated in managing cervical artery dissections; examples are massive trauma with other sites of internal bleeding, and large stroke with mass effect and potential for hemorrhagic transformation. Anticoagulation raises risk when the dissection extends into the intracranial portion of the vessel, not uncommon with distal vertebral artery dissection. When this occurs, it is thought that a higher risk of subarachnoid hemorrhage exists secondary to rupture of the vessel into the subarachnoid space. (Of note, intracranial vertebral artery dissection should be considered in the differential diagnosis of high spinal subarachnoid hemorrhage in the absence of aneurysm.) In cases where anticoagulation is not appropriate, antiplatelet therapy or no therapy is a reasonable option.

Surgery or endovascular therapy is rarely indicated in acute dissection, primarily because of the good outcome most patients have with medical therapy alone. Indications for more aggressive treatment include patients with progressive neurologic deficits from recurrent embolism or worsening vascular occlusion. Surgical treatment, which involves ligation of the artery often combined with an in situ or extracranial-to-intracranial bypass, is associated with a 9% to 12% incidence of death and stroke.[16,17] Good outcomes have been achieved in several cases of acute dissections treated with angioplasty and stenting in patients with fluctuating neurologic symptoms.[18,19]

Another indication for aggressive management is a ruptured aneurysm or enlarging dissecting aneurysm that is at risk for rupture. Figure 98-3 shows images from a patient who presented with a subarachnoid hemorrhage and a Glasgow Coma Scale (GCS) score of 3 and underwent successful coiling of a dissecting vertebral artery aneurysm. Though the vessel had to be sacrificed, the patient went on to have a good functional outcome. Since treatment of these aneurysms in the acute setting is quite rare, no standardized approach has been established. The following is a technical description of the procedure depicted in Figure 98-3.

Under direct fluoroscopic guidance and road mapping, a Boston Scientific SL-10 45-degree microcatheter and a

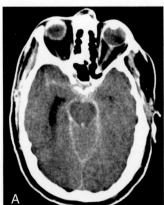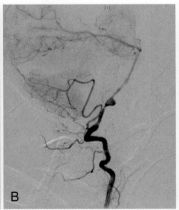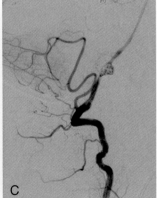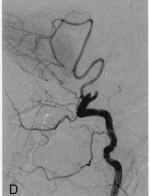

FIGURE 98-3. Interventional management of acutely ruptured vertebral artery dissecting aneurysm that presented as a subarachnoid hemorrhage. **A,** Noncontrast head computed tomography showing diffuse subarachnoid and intraventricular hemorrhage. **B,** Angiographic visualization of right vertebral artery dissecting aneurysm. **C,** Partial filling of aneurysm with coils. **D,** Complete obliteration of aneurysm with occlusion of right vertebral artery.

microfabricated 200-cm Syncro[2] Guidewire (Boston Scientific, Natick, Mass.) were placed into the anatomic region of this aneurysm. A contrast aneurysm study demonstrated the microcatheter to be within the confines of this aneurysm. Using multiple 360-degree Guglielmi detachable coils (GDC 360° Coils [Boston Scientific]), first a 7 mm × 15 cm GDC 360 soft coil was deployed, followed by a 6 mm × 8 cm GDC 360 soft coil, followed by a 5 mm × 9 cm GDC 360 soft coil, followed finally by a GDC 360 4 mm × 8 cm ultrasoft coil. These were placed sequentially within the aneurysm lumen and proximal right vertebral artery at the level of this high-grade stenotic segment and slightly more proximal to that location. Sequential angiographic images demonstrated pronounced stasis of flow within the aneurysm, with ultimate therapeutic occlusion of the right vertebral artery. Angiographic images through the microcatheter demonstrated a patent distal right vertebral artery to the level of the right posterior inferior cerebellar artery. However, angiographic images at the level of the right vertebral artery demonstrated focal tapering at the right vertebral artery just distal to the right posterior inferior cerebral artery takeoff. Approximately 50 µg of intraarterial nitroglycerin was introduced via the guide catheter into the right vertebral artery circulation. Postinfusion angiographic images demonstrated no significant change. The examination demonstrated no filling of the aneurysm and therapeutic occlusion of the pseudoaneurysm and proximal stenotic segment.

Aneurysm recurrence rate in those who are endovascularly treated has become a recent focus of study as this procedure is performed in increasing numbers. A recent series of 111 patients with 119 dissecting vertebrobasilar aneurysms showed a 13% recurrence rate following endovascular treatment. Of the recurrences, 46% presented with rebleeding, and all of these were in patients who had initially presented with hemorrhage.[20]

LONG-TERM MANAGEMENT OF DISSECTING ANEURYSMS AND PERSISTENT STENOSIS

Although rupture of a dissecting aneurysm is occasionally the presenting event for a cervical artery dissection, formation of a "pseudoaneurysm" or "dissecting aneurysm" is more commonly a delayed manifestation. These aneurysms form at the site of the dissection as the intramural hematoma remodels and is reabsorbed. Dissecting aneurysms typically form when the dissection occurs primarily between the media and adventitia. They occur in approximately one fourth (5%-49%) of patients with spontaneous cervical artery dissections and can take two forms: a segmental dilatation (fusiform-type aneurysm) or an extraluminal pouch (a saccular-type aneurysm).[21] Figure 98-4 illustrates the characteristic angiographic presentation of several dissecting aneurysms.

In two large studies on the natural history of dissecting aneurysms, 51 patients with dissecting aneurysms were followed for a mean of more than 3 years.[17,18] During that time, no clinical evidence of rupture or embolization of the aneurysm was observed. Radiographically, 46% to 65% of the aneurysms were unchanged, 18% to 30% decreased in size, and 5% to 36% resolved. Resolution was more common in vertebral artery dissections than in carotid dissections.[21,22] A more recent study of 191 patients with symptomatic but unruptured vertebrobasilar dissecting aneurysms showed good outcomes in all patients who presented with local symptoms (pain without ischemia) and in 90% of patients who presented with ischemic symptoms, regardless of treatment (endovascular procedure vs. antithrombotic treatment with anticoagulation or antiplatelet agents). The unfavorable outcomes resulted from further ischemic events, not from aneurysm rupture, so it would seem that treatment should focus on prevention of further ischemic

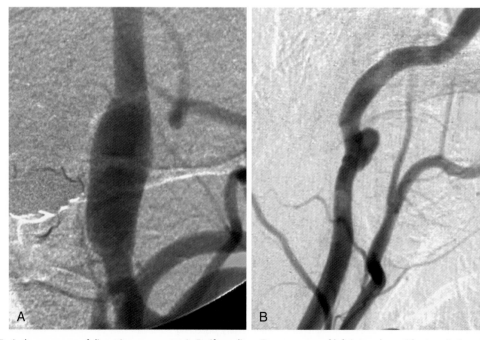

FIGURE 98-4. Typical appearance of dissecting aneurysms. **A,** Fusiform dissecting aneurysm of left internal carotid artery. **B,** Saccular dissecting aneurysm of left internal carotid artery.

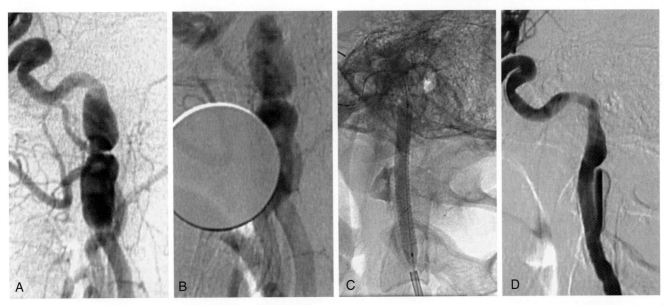

FIGURE 98-5. Interventional management of serial fusiform dissecting aneurysms of right internal carotid artery (ICA). **A,** Angiographic appearance of right ICA dissecting aneurysms. **B,** Coin placed on skin of neck to approximate size of the dissecting aneurysms. **C,** Stent is inflated into proximal dissecting aneurysm. **D,** Contrast agent injection several minutes after stent deployment shows patent flow with decreased filling of dissecting aneurysms.

events rather than concern for rupture of the dissecting aneurysm.[23]

Given that most aneurysms that result from dissections heal spontaneously and the risk of thromboembolic complications from a residual chronic aneurysm is low, it would seem that interventions are unnecessary. However, despite low complication rates, instances of persistent symptoms are attributed to dissecting aneurysms (e.g., recurrent TIAs and strokes) or mass effect and compression from an enlarging aneurysm. Furthermore, antithrombotic therapy to prevent further ischemic events is contraindicated in some instances. In these cases, endovascular treatment may be warranted.

A second long-term complication of cervical artery dissections is persistent stenosis of the dissected vessel. With standard medical management, approximately 90% of stenoses resolve and two thirds of occlusions recanalize in the first 2 to 3 months after the dissection.[24] Even those without complete angiographic resolution rarely have continued complications, likely owing to adequate collateral circulation. However, some patients continue to have hemodynamic symptoms despite anticoagulation and/or antiplatelet therapy.

The literature concerning endovascular management of dissections continues to grow. Appropriately, most of these reports describe interventions limited to patients who have continued to have events despite appropriate medical therapy. For complications due to persistent stenosis, the endovascular approach typically consists of balloon angioplasty followed by deployment of one or multiple stents, resulting in vessel lumen expansion and thrombosis or stabilization of any aneurysm. In some studies, coils have been used to treat dissecting aneurysms, as described earlier. However, even those aneurysms that appear saccular on imaging studies or angiography tend to be fusiform and therefore are often not amenable to coiling.[8] With increasing use of stent-assisted coiling for berry aneurysms, this

approach is also being adopted to treat persistent dissecting aneurysms.

For a technical description of a stenting procedure, we describe a patient treated with carotid stenting for two persistent dissecting aneurysms 2 years after a right carotid dissection (Fig. 98-5). Although this young woman had been medically stable on warfarin, she did not wish to continue on anticoagulation long term because she hoped to become pregnant. She had also had difficulties with anemia and menorrhagia on aspirin therapy. At the beginning of the procedure, the patient received 5000 units of heparin after placement of the sheath. Diagnostic angiography was conducted to confirm the absence of new injuries or collateral vessels. The two dissecting aneurysms were visualized. They extended over a 3.4-cm territory, with the vessel measuring 1.2 mm in diameter. It was deemed impossible to pass a self-expanding stent through this diseased segment. After this diagnostic portion of the procedure, a 6F Envoy guiding catheter was passed through the 6F lumen sheath over a 0.035-inch guidewire into the right internal carotid artery. With a hand injection performed for roadmap guidance, the catheter was advanced into the right internal carotid artery. Using the road map, a 0.014-inch Luge exchange-length wire (Boston Scientific) was passed to the dissecting aneurysms. The first aneurysm had a narrow neck, and the second had a broad neck. The wire was passed into the siphon region. Then, over the Luge wire, a 4-mm-diameter, 2.8-cm-long Guidant Tetra stent (Abbott Vascular, Santa Clara, Calif.) was passed and deployed using an Everest insufflator (Medtronic Inc., Santa Rosa, Calif.) to 10 atm, achieving a 4-mm diameter. The initial angiogram after deflation of the balloon showed that the tip of the stent just entered the petrous segment of the carotid artery, and the inferior aspect of the stent covered the proximal dissecting aneurysm. Further angiography after several minutes showed no branch occlusions and stasis in the dissecting aneurysms. The patient tolerated the procedure well and remained asymptomatic for more than 3 years of follow-up on low-dose aspirin therapy. Figure 98-5 shows images of the dissecting aneurysms before and after deployment of the stent.

SUMMARY

Given the overall success of endovascular management of dissections and dissecting aneurysms, several questions arise. First, could early stenting of uncomplicated dissections improve on the 85% to 90% good outcomes of medical management alone? Second, which patients with dissecting aneurysms are appropriate for endovascular therapy, given the low risk of rupture and the 13% recurrence rate following treatment. These questions cannot be answered without prospective randomized clinical trials. Until such trials are performed, the current standard of care is for initial medical management of uncomplicated dissections and further intervention only in the cases of failure of antithrombotic therapy. For dissecting aneurysms, those who present with rupture should be treated urgently to prevent re-rupture, and those who present with ischemia or pain should be managed conservatively initially and treated only if symptoms recur despite antithrombotic therapy.

KEY POINTS

- Cervical artery dissection is a leading cause of stroke or transient ischemic attack in young adults.
- The underlying etiology of cervical artery dissection is unknown but is hypothesized to be a subtle arteriopathy that predisposes the artery to injury and intramural hematoma formation.

- Stroke from cervical artery dissection may be due to artery-to-artery embolism or hypoperfusion.
- For patients with cervical artery dissection with minor or no neurologic deficits at the time of diagnosis, the prognosis is generally excellent.
- Currently accepted medical therapy is antithrombotic therapy, either with anticoagulation or antiplatelet medications.
- Endovascular therapy is warranted in rare cases, such as patients with ruptured aneurysms or those with recurrent symptoms despite anticoagulation due to persistent stenotic lesions.
- Dissecting aneurysms may form as the dissection heals. These may spontaneously disappear over time. Persistent small dissecting aneurysms are best treated with antiplatelet therapy. Giant dissecting aneurysms can be treated with stenting and/or coiling.

▶ **SUGGESTED READINGS**

Caplan LR, Biousse V. Cervicocranial arterial dissections. J Neuroophthalmol 2004;24:299–305.

Rubenstein SM, Peerdeman SM, van Tulder MW, et al. A systematic review of the risk factors for cervical artery dissection. Stroke 2005;36:1575–80.

Savitz SI, Caplan LR. Vertebrobasilar disease. N Engl J Med 2005;352:2618–26.

Schievink WI. Spontaneous dissection of the carotid and vertebral arteries. N Engl J Med 2001;344:898–906.

Schievink WI. The treatment of spontaneous carotid and vertebral artery dissections. Curr Opin Cardiol 2000;15:316–21.

The complete reference list is available online at www.expertconsult.com.

CHAPTER **99**

Superior Vena Cava Occlusive Disease

Robert F. Dondelinger and John A. Kaufman

Chronic upper extremity (UE) occlusive disease and superior vena cava (SVC) syndrome can be debilitating to the patient and rewarding to treat with endovascular techniques.[1] Chronic UE venous occlusion is more often due to a benign lesion, whereas SVC syndrome is more likely the result of malignant obstruction. The symptoms of chronic UE venous occlusive disease include arm swelling (especially with use or after creation of UE surgical dialysis access.[2] Although the ipsilateral neck may be symptomatic, facial swelling does not occur with obstruction limited to the UE veins. Acute SVC syndrome is considered a medical emergency.[3] Clinical symptoms include headache exacerbated by changes in position, disturbances in consciousness, facial edema, pain in the face and neck, blurred vision, retroorbital pressure, hoarseness, and orthopnea. Edema and pain can involve one or both arms. In patients with slowly progressive obstruction, collateral circulation develops to a variable degree over the chest wall and periscapular region. Acute SVC syndrome may be the first sign of a mediastinal tumor or may be seen later in the course of the disease.[1] Interventional radiologists were early pioneers in the management of these challenging clinical entities.[4,5]

MALIGNANT OBSTRUCTION

Most strictures of the SVC are of malignant origin. Tumors most commonly responsible for compression of the SVC and large mediastinal veins are bronchogenic carcinoma or small cell lung cancer with mediastinal lymph node enlargement caused by metastases from intrathoracic or extrathoracic malignancies, malignant lymphoma or Hodgkin disease, and tracheal malignancies. Other primary mediastinal tumors are less often encountered. The traditional method of treatment of SVC obstruction secondary to malignancy is radiotherapy, chemotherapy, or a combination of both. Such treatment is effective in about 90% of cases, but only after several days and with a recurrence rate of 20% even when the maximum permissible dose of radiation is used.[1]

BENIGN OBSTRUCTION

Approximately 10% of all clinically significant SVC stenoses are due to a benign cause. The main causes of benign stenosis are catheter-related injury, mediastinal

fibrosis, surgery, postanastomotic stenoses, infection, and radiotherapy.[2-3] Conversely, most chronic stenoses or occlusion in the central arm veins are benign in nature and due to venous catheterization, instrumentation, and anatomic compression syndromes.

INDICATIONS FOR INTERVENTION

Patients with acute malignant SVC syndrome that does not respond to radiation, or acute thrombosis of an underlying benign lesion should be considered for catheter-based intervention. Patients with chronic SVC stenosis who present with symptoms consistent with SVC syndrome are good candidates for stent placement. Patients with symptomatic chronic occlusive disease of the central UE veins may benefit from endovascular reconstruction, although anatomic compression syndromes should be surgically corrected first.[6]

CONTRAINDICATIONS

In malignant disease, contraindications to venous stenting include extensive chronic venous thrombosis, anatomic considerations predisposing to severe technical difficulty, and advanced disease in preterminal patients. As a rule, venous access sites should be preserved, and the ostia of large tributaries of the caval system, such as the jugular veins, should not be deliberately covered by a stent to preserve the possibility of further catheterization if necessary. However, the ostium of the azygos vein is routinely covered when stenting the SVC, generally without clinical side effects. Impaired venous flow, such as secondary to limb paralysis, is a relative contraindication to stent placement in the SVC tributaries. Occasionally, transmural venous tumor invasion caused by lymphoma or bronchogenic carcinoma is present. Because uncovered stents may be ineffective in such cases, placement of covered stents is indicated in these infrequent cases.

Patients should be able to cooperate during the procedure. Some patients with severe SVC syndrome may have difficulty lying flat. In these circumstances, the procedure should be undertaken with the patient under general anesthesia. A minority of patients will have simultaneous tracheobronchial narrowing because of malignant compression. Stenting of the airways should precede management of the caval obstruction in such patients.

EQUIPMENT

- Basic angiographic catheters and guidewires are used. A hemostatic valve sheath up to size 10F is placed at the puncture site, depending on the size of the venous stents to be inserted.
- Multipurpose or Cobra-shaped 5F catheters and hydrophilic 0.035-inch guidewires are mainly used to cross the venous obstruction.
- For stent placement, the delivery catheter is pushed over a semi-rigid Amplatz-type guidewire for maximum stability during stent release.

TECHNIQUE

Anatomy and Approach

With regard to the venous anatomy of the upper extremities, brachiocephalic vessels, and SVC, please refer to Chapters 30 and 82.

Stenoses located in the SVC or right innominate vein are most conveniently stented via a right femoral or right jugular approach (Fig. 99-1). Stenoses of the left innominate vein are treated from either a femoral or a left axillary approach. By using a rather unconventional puncture site for catheterization of the axillary vein—namely, at the junction between the axillary and subclavian veins—trauma to the brachial nervous plexus is avoided, particularly when large-diameter catheters are introduced. More direct access to the left innominate vein is also gained with use of this technique. As a general rule, venous stents should be placed sequentially, first in a distal position and then more proximally, in relation to the puncture site. When the confluence of the innominate veins is treated, the technique used depends on the anatomy and type of stents required. Soft and flexible stents can be placed simultaneously in the brachiocephalic vein and left innominate vein, with a parallel course in the SVC (Figs. 99-2 and 99-3). When more rigid stents are used, the SVC and right innominate vein are stented in a line, and stents are placed in the left innominate vein as close as possible to the caval axis. Transesophageal ultrasound can occasionally be helpful in accurate stent placement in the SVC, but it makes an otherwise simple procedure much more complicated.[7,8]

Technical Aspects

Radiographic Technique

Duplex color ultrasound demonstrates stenosis or thrombosis of venous segments accessible to the probe. Loss of cardiac and respiratory variation in the internal jugular veins is suspicious for central obstruction. In most cases, venous-phase helical contrast-enhanced computed tomography (CT) with multiplanar reformatting or magnetic resonance (MR) venography can establish an unequivocal diagnosis of central venous stenosis or obstruction.[9] Both modalities demonstrate the location and extent of disease and also show the collateral network. However, venographic demonstration of the stenosis and collateral pathways remains mandatory immediately before treatment. Venography confirms the location and extent of the stenosis, endoluminal thrombus, or tumor proliferation; the extent of collateral circulation; its hemodynamic significance; and any congenital variants that have to be taken into consideration when planning stent placement. Superior venacavography can be performed by simultaneous bilateral injection of contrast into the basilic or a more peripheral vein in the upper limb or jugular veins.

Crossing the Lesion

Recanalization of the SVC and central venous occlusion sometimes requires a combined femoral-axillary or a bilateral axillary approach. A sequential approach involving increasing stiffness of catheters and guidewires and increased force should be followed for recalcitrant lesions. The back end of a hydrophilic guidewire and even transjugular intrahepatic portosystemic shunt (TIPS) needles can be used for sharp recanalization.[10] Precise localization of the desired reentry point with a contrast-filled intravascular occlusion balloon or cone-beam CT is important to increase the likelihood of success (and decrease the risk of complications). Careful patient monitoring for symptoms suggestive of perforation is important because hemopericardium and hemothorax can result during these interventions.[11] When the guidewire has crossed the occlusion, it can be grasped with a snare, basket, or flexible forceps on the other side and retrieved through the sheath at the second percutaneous entry point. This provides

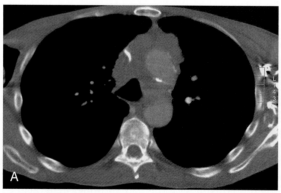
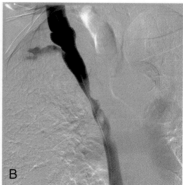
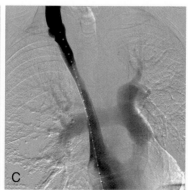

FIGURE 99-1. Superior vena cava (SVC) syndrome in a 55-year-old man. **A,** Contrast-enhanced computed tomography shows large mediastinal mass compressing SVC. Left innominate vein was completely thrombosed. **B,** Superior vena cavography obtained from a right femoral approach confirms tight SVC stenosis. **C,** A Wallstent (10 mm, 7 cm) was placed via femoral approach and expanded immediately. Cavography shows optimal venous flow. Left innominate vein was not treated. Rapid regression of clinical symptoms followed.

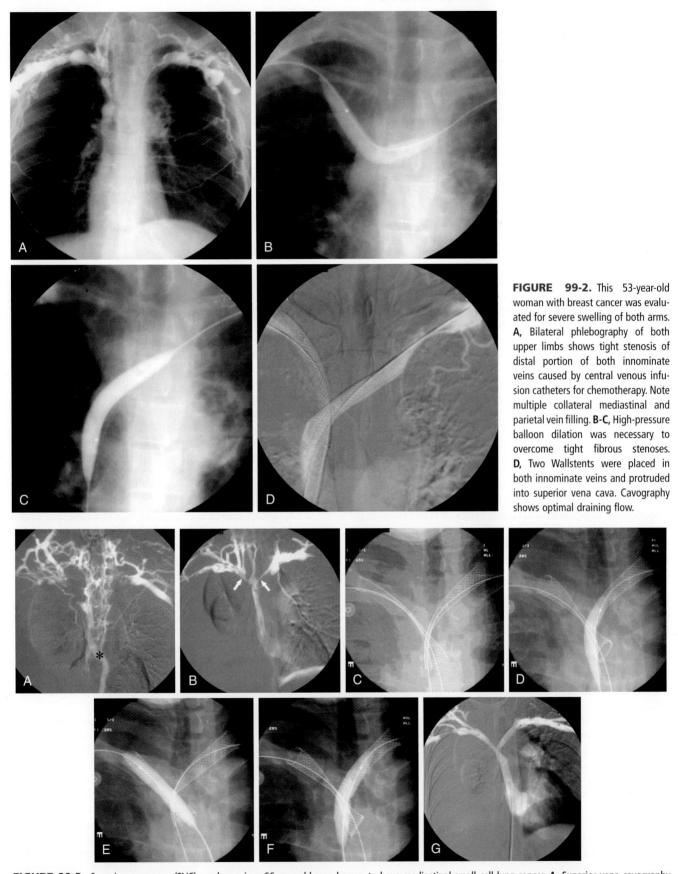

FIGURE 99-2. This 53-year-old woman with breast cancer was evaluated for severe swelling of both arms. **A,** Bilateral phlebography of both upper limbs shows tight stenosis of distal portion of both innominate veins caused by central venous infusion catheters for chemotherapy. Note multiple collateral mediastinal and parietal vein filling. **B-C,** High-pressure balloon dilation was necessary to overcome tight fibrous stenoses. **D,** Two Wallstents were placed in both innominate veins and protruded into superior vena cava. Cavography shows optimal draining flow.

FIGURE 99-3. Superior vena cava (SVC) syndrome in a 66-year-old man known to have mediastinal small cell lung cancer. **A,** Superior vena cavography shows complete obstruction of both innominate veins by mediastinal tumor encasement, a rich venous network, and filling of azygos system *(asterisk)*. **B,** Local infusion of the thrombolytic agent urokinase was started at a rate of 100,000 units/h in both innominate veins. Phlebography obtained 12 hours later shows complete clearing of clots from both innominate veins and unmasked two tight stenoses *(arrows)* at their junction with SVC. **C-F,** Two Wallstents (10 mm, 6 cm) were placed in both innominate veins and protruded into SVC. Balloon dilation inside stents accelerated immediate stent dilation. **G,** Bilateral phlebocavography confirms patency of both stents and optimal venous flow.

through-and-through control of the guidewire ("body floss"), greatly facilitating delivery of devices.

Management of Venous Thrombosis Before Stenting

When venous thrombosis masks the lesion, local thrombolysis or pharmacomechanical thrombectomy should precede stent placement.[1,3,12] A plasminogen activator (tPA, rtPA, urokinase, etc.) is infused directly into the thrombus. Mechanical adjuncts and aspiration thrombectomy accelerate the process.[12] Chronic central venous access catheters may remain in place during thrombolysis but will have to be temporarily displaced during stent placement to avoid entrapment.

The entire length of the thrombus is traversed with a guidewire to detect any underlying stenosis. A stenosis or occlusion that can be traversed with a guidewire can eventually be lysed, so limiting attempts at thrombolysis to such lesions minimizes technical failure. The thrombus is infiltrated with a concentrated bolus of the lytic agent before starting the infusion. The ease with which the guidewire crosses the obstruction is a good predictor of a successful outcome. Percutaneous thrombus aspiration is performed either alone or in combination with local thrombolysis. Similarly, mechanical devices can used with or without thrombolytic agents.

Balloon angioplasty is a very useful adjunct to fragment the clot (especially when there is combined acute and subacute thrombosis), expose a greater surface area to the plasminogen activator, and dilate underlying strictures. Low-dose anticoagulant therapy is given concurrently with local thrombolysis, usually through a peripheral vein.

The endpoint of an uncomplicated thrombolysis is reached when the thrombus has cleared completely or, more often, been reduced sufficiently to unmask the underlying lesion. In patients with malignancy, it is not necessary to achieve the same degree of thrombolysis as when the etiology is benign, and stents are often placed through substantial residual thrombus to restore venous drainage of the head and upper body.

Stent Placement

Stent selection is an important aspect of this procedure. Currently, bare stents are typically used except in special circumstances such as catastrophic venous perforation and recurrent tumor invasion.[13] Large-diameter stents (10-14 mm diameter) are often required. Short focal SVC lesions can be treated with large balloon-expandable stents (Palmaz XL [Cordis Corp., Warren, N.J.]), whereas longer lesions that extend from one venous segment to another are more appropriately managed with self-expanding stents. All guidewires and catheters must be withdrawn from the segment to be stented before release of the stents, except the guidewire contained in the delivery catheter. Pacemaker leads do not have to be removed. Stents across the thoracic outlet should be avoided (see later). For SVC syndrome, restoration of in-line flow from one internal jugular vein to the right atrium is usually sufficient to provide relief of acute symptoms.

Adjuvant Medication

In apprehensive patients, premedication may be helpful. Because placement of an endovascular stent is not painful, only local anesthesia at the puncture site is required.

Percutaneous transluminal angioplasty (PTA) is occasionally painful when the adventitia of the SVC or innominate veins is stretched during full dilation. Dilation of stenoses of peripheral hemodialysis fistulas may also be painful; local infiltration of anesthetic can be helpful. Patients may also briefly experience pain after sudden expansion of a metal stent in the SVC and should be warned of this possibility. If it is anticipated that the stenting procedure will be difficult and prolonged, 5000 IU of heparin should be administered to prevent acute SVC thrombosis during the endoluminal procedure. If SVC stent placement results in immediate and full restoration of flow, there is no need for heparinization after stenting unless the patient had prior underlying thrombosis.

OUTCOMES

Malignant Stenoses

In patients with malignant SVC obstruction, cure of the primary condition is rare. Moreover, because the life expectancy of patients with unresectable mediastinal tumor is limited, the main aim of treatment should be immediate relief from disabling symptoms. PTA alone is rarely effective in such patients. The long-term effects of stent placement are not a major concern. After successful stent deployment, almost immediate complete or partial relief from symptoms is obtained in 68% to 100% of cases and is sustained at follow-up of up to 16 months, without any need for further intervention.[1,3,12,14,15] Patients experience relief of tension in the face and neck almost immediately after stent expansion in the SVC, and the remaining symptoms disappear within a few hours. Edema of the face and neck resolves after 1 to 2 days and in the scapular region and upper limbs in 2 to 3 days. Although the radial force of metal stents is moderate, they expand almost completely within a week. However, long-term patency is not a concern insofar as patients with malignant SVC stenosis generally have limited survival.[12] In patients who do survive, reocclusion occurs in up to 40%.[1] Previous thrombosis and smaller final stent diameters are associated with higher rates of reocclusion.[1,3,12]

Successful long-term results in SVC syndrome are difficult to obtain when stents are placed in more peripheral locations for benign indications, such as the subclavian vein.[2] Reocclusion is common but seems to be reduced by the use of heparin-coated covered stents.[16]

No significant difference in clinical results has been demonstrated after placement of different types of stents. The left innominate vein is particularly prone to tumor encasement because of its long transverse course through the mediastinum. Transmural tumor invasion, however, is a rare event that leads to reobstruction and requires placement of covered stents. In addition, the junction of the left innominate vein and SVC can present an obstacle to stenting. Stent placement should be considered at the onset of clinical symptoms, before the development of a tight stenosis or occlusion involving the SVC bifurcation. Although it may not be necessary to stent both innominate veins to achieve a good clinical result, bilateral stenting helps reestablish optimal flow and limit the number of reinterventions.

Benign Stenoses

Stent placement in the SVC for benign stenosis has excellent overall long-term patency, with almost 100% assisted primary patency at 3 years.[17] However, reintervention is often required for restenosis. These results are significantly better than SVC bypass or reconstruction, with less morbidity.

Like most benign venous stenoses, those occurring in the peripheral arm veins or in the central venous outflow of hemodialysis fistulas respond poorly to PTA alone. In cases of central venous stenoses related to hemodialysis fistulas, a 1-year patency rate of 0% to 35% has been historically been demonstrated, the poorest results being seen with peripheral stenosis[17,18] (Fig. 99-4). The addition of bare metal stents does not significantly improve long-term outcomes but does increase procedural success rates—an important consideration in the chronic dialysis population.[19] In many practices, stents are reserved for patients in whom PTA has failed as a result of recoil or in whom stenosis has recurred. Stents that are flexible and short and have minimal metal surface are probably the most suitable for these lesions. However, the results are not particularly encouraging: a 63% 1-year assisted patency rate. Frequent reinterventions are necessary to maintain patency[19] (Fig. 99-5).

COMPLICATIONS

Complications related to venous stenting are relatively few, occurring in approximately 5% to 7% of procedures.[1] Misplacement or stent migration is the most feared potential complication. Repositioning of a fully opened caval stent that has slipped beyond the stenosis is almost impossible. Stents should be long enough to entirely cover the stenosis. Stents with a too-small diameter are prone to migration even hours after placement.[19] Guidewires or catheters caught inside the mesh of the stent can cause displacement even several weeks after stenting. Stents that have migrated

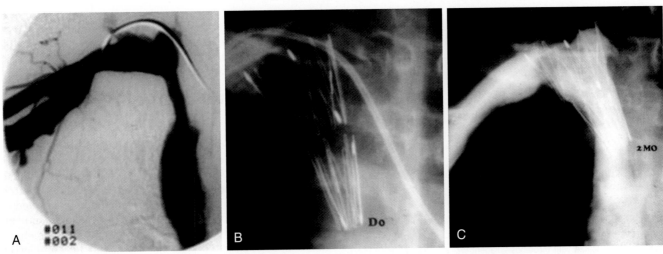

FIGURE 99-4. Impaired function of a hemodialysis shunt in right arm of 73-year-old man undergoing chronic hemodialysis. **A,** Arteriography of right upper limb shows good function of fistula but significant stenosis of right innominate vein. **B,** A 3-cm Gianturco stent with two segments was placed via a right femoral approach and opened correctly immediately after placement. **C,** Phlebography of right upper limb performed 2 months after stenting shows good stent function. Stent remained patent for 11 years until patient's death.

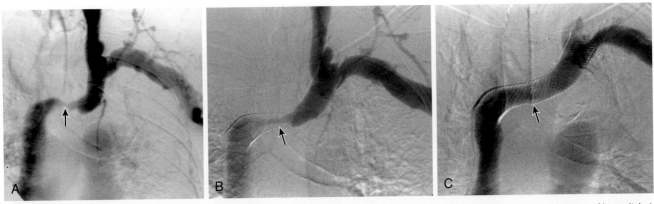

FIGURE 99-5. This 63-year-old woman undergoing hemodialysis experienced pain in her neck and left scapular region during each session of hemodialysis. **A,** Phlebography of left upper limb shows a concentric irregular short-segment stenosis in left innominate vein *(arrow)* and reflux of contrast material in left jugular vein. **B,** Two short 10-mm Wallstents were placed in an overlapping position and produced immediate good flow. Clinical symptoms recurred 1 year later. Phlebography shows regular narrowing *(arrow)* inside stents caused by tissue proliferation. **C,** Stenosis responded well to percutaneous transluminal angioplasty (PTA) *(arrow)*. PTA was again required 1 year later for recurrent intimal hyperplasia.

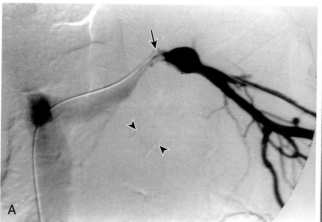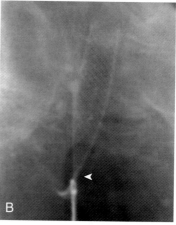

FIGURE 99-6. Extreme thoracic deformity due to ankylosing spondylitis in a 60-year-old man. Patient complained of swelling of both arms. **A,** Phlebography of left upper limb shows compression of left subclavian vein, characteristic of thoracic outlet syndrome *(arrow)*. A Wallstent (10 mm, 3.5 cm) was placed via a left brachial approach. Stent migrated to left pulmonary artery several minutes after release *(arrowheads)*. **B,** Wallstent was grasped and retrieved percutaneously with a gooseneck catheter *(arrowhead)* introduced through a right femoral approach.

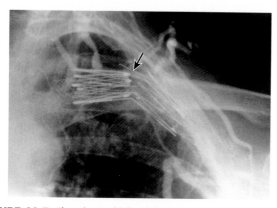

FIGURE 99-7. Thrombosis of left subclavian vein (probably caused by a venous line) in a 69-year-old woman. Phlebography (not shown) of left arm confirmed subclavian vein thrombosis. Patient was treated with local urokinase infusion and placement of a Gianturco stent (1.5 cm, 5 cm) in a subclavian vein stenosis. Stent disintegrated *(arrow)* under external compression by clavicle, and thrombosis recurred. A 10-mm Wallstent was then placed inside Z-stent after repeated local thrombolysis. Phlebography (not shown) performed 9 months later showed obstruction and fragmentation of both stents.

to the heart or pulmonary arteries should be removed with a snare or endovascular forceps if possible to prevent trauma to the cardiac valves and endothelium (Fig. 99-6).[20] A limited venotomy may be necessary for extraction of the stent at the femoral puncture site.

Heparinization during the procedure avoids acute SVC thrombosis. Stent thrombosis caused by external compression and recurrent laryngeal nerve palsy has also been observed.[1] Stent fragmentation can occur when the device crosses the thoracic inlet, because there is continual repetitive compression between the clavicle and first rib (Fig. 99-7).[21] Caval perforation, mediastinal bleeding, and pericardial tamponade are exceptional complications.[1,3,12] Stent infection, bacteremia, septicemia, and shock are potential complications; they should be minimized with the use of strict aseptic technique. Dilation with oversized balloons must be avoided in the SVC, particularly close to the right

atrium, because dysrhythmia or even cardiac arrest is a potential risk. The usual complications that may occur at the venous puncture site are seen: venous thrombosis, arteriovenous fistula, and venous pseudoaneurysm.

POSTPROCEDURAL AND FOLLOW-UP CARE

If SVC stent placement results in immediate and full restoration of flow, there is no need for heparinization after stenting in the absence of thrombus. However, if residual thrombi remain adherent to the stent or vessel wall after local thrombolysis, anticoagulation should be continued if possible.[12] Heparinization is followed by oral anticoagulant therapy and low-dose aspirin for several months, by which time it is anticipated that the stent will be completely covered with neo-endothelium.

If stent thrombosis occurs rapidly after placement, local infusion of a thrombolytic agent can be performed, as described earlier. The cause of the reocclusion must be determined and treated as appropriate, which may include placement of additional stents, redilation, or treatment of another stenosis, the significance of which had previously been underestimated.

KEY POINTS

- Percutaneous management of benign or malignant stenoses of large veins has a high initial success rate.
- Patients with malignant disease should be treated by endoluminal stent placement before full symptoms of superior vena cava (SVC) obstruction develop.
- For acute malignant SVC syndrome due to thrombosis, local treatment thrombolysis/pharmacomechanical thrombectomy should be performed if possible, but primary placement of bare stents provides rapid relief of symptoms.
- In patients with benign disease, frequent reintervention is required to maintain stent patency; SVC stents have better long-term patency than the upper extremity veins.

► **SUGGESTED READINGS**

Reinhold C, Haage P, Hollenbeck M, et al. Multidisciplinary management of vascular access for haemodialysis: from the preparation of the initial access to the treatment of stenosis and thrombosis. Vasa 2011;40: 188–98.

Rowell NP, Gleeson FV. Steroids, radiotherapy, chemotherapy and stents for superior vena caval obstruction in carcinoma of the bronchus. Cochrane Database Syst Rev 2001;(4):CD001316.

Trerotola SO. Interventional radiology in central venous stenosis and occlusion. Semin Intervent Radiol 1994;11:291–304.

Wilson LD, Detterbeck FC, Yahalom J. Clinical practice. Superior vena cava syndrome with malignant causes. N Engl J Med 2007;356: 1862–9.

The complete reference list is available online at www.expertconsult.com.

CHAPTER 100

Percutaneous Management of Chronic Lower Extremity Venous Occlusive Disease

Hyeon Yu and Matthew A. Mauro

Chronic venous insufficiency (CVI) affects millions of people throughout the United States. The higher venous pressure in the lower extremity veins of patients with CVI results in ambulatory venous hypertension. The majority of cases of CVI are due to past deep venous thrombosis of the iliofemoral segments.[1]

CVI is a result of a combination of damaged valves leading to reflux and frank venous obstruction.[2-6] Acute iliofemoral thrombosis is a common problem that is traditionally treated with conventional systemic anticoagulation (heparin followed by warfarin). Despite anticoagulation, chronic changes of the iliac vein with partial or complete obstruction will occur and lead to postthrombotic syndrome (PTS). During the process of chronic obstruction of the iliac vein, inflammatory changes take place and cause vein wall fibrosis that leads to valve dysfunction, reflux, and CVI.[7,8] PTS results in significant morbidity, decreased quality of life, and multiple visits to healthcare providers.[9]

The symptoms of CVI include ulcerations, chronic pain, and swelling.[2] Patients with CVI have traditionally been treated with conservative measures such as medical-grade compression stockings, intermittent compression devices, and wound care in patients with venous stasis ulcers.[10-14] Reestablishment of direct antegrade flow through the iliac venous system can alleviate much of the patient's symptomatology by correcting the obstructive component of CVI.[15,16] The remaining reflux component may be addressed by valvular surgery (valvuloplasty, valve transplantation) or percutaneous valve insertion.[14,17,18]

All patients should have their venous system imaged to determine the adequacy of inflow and outflow. These patients require an initial duplex ultrasound examination of the lower extremity veins to evaluate the patency of venous segments (tibial, popliteal, femoral, and common femoral veins). The pelvic veins and inferior vena cava (IVC) (outflow) are difficult to evaluate with ultrasound, so patients should also undergo either magnetic resonance or computed tomographic venography (MRV, CTV) of the pelvis and abdomen to determine the length of obstruction and adequacy of outflow. Definitive venography will be performed at the time of the intervention.[3,9]

Air plethysmography is a practical, noninvasive, and relatively inexpensive test that provides physiologic quantitative information about the lower leg (excluding the foot) regarding CVI and correlates with ambulatory venous pressure (AVP) measurements.[19-21] The study is performed with an air chamber that surrounds the lower part of the leg and connects to a pressure transducer and recorder. A baseline reading is obtained with the patient in the supine position and the leg elevated to 45 degrees. The patient is then placed in the upright position with all weight on the contralateral limb until the veins are full of blood. This change is the *functional venous volume*. The *venous filling index*

(VFI) can be calculated (90% venous volume divided by the time required for filling to 90% of venous volume). The patient then performs the heel-raise maneuver to displace the venous volume; the volume displaced by this maneuver is the *ejection volume*. The *ejection fraction* (EF) equals ejection volume divided by venous volume. Multiple (10) heel raises are then performed to reach a residual volume plateau. Residual volume divided by venous volume is the *residual volume fraction* (RVF). The VFI is a measure of global reflux, EF is a measure of calf muscle pumping function, and RVF is a reflection of AVP.[9]

INDICATIONS

- Symptomatic patients with partial or complete iliac (unilateral or bilateral) venous obstruction
- Adequate inflow and outflow to ensure continued patency of the reconstructed venous segment

CONTRAINDICATIONS

- Asymptomatic patients
- Occlusion of the common femoral and femoral veins (inadequate inflow)
- Occlusion of the IVC (inadequate outflow) (Occlusion of the infrarenal IVC can be treated by extension of the reconstruction to the level of the renal veins.)

EQUIPMENT

- Ultrasound for initial venous access
- Micropuncture system for venous access
- 6F sheaths (long sheaths may be necessary to provide increased pushability)
- 5F angled catheters (standard plus hydrophilic), along with hydrophilic guidewires for initial recanalization of occluded segments
- Angioplasty balloons for preliminary dilation of venous segments
- 10- to 14-mm nitinol stents (long lengths) to cover the occluded segments
- 16-mm Wallstents

TECHNIQUE

Anatomy and Approach

Knowledge of the normal anatomy and variations of the venous system in the lower extremity, pelvis, and abdomen is required for a safe and successful intervention. A critical review of the preliminary venous studies (ultrasound, MRI, CT) is necessary to determine whether the patient is a candidate for percutaneous intervention, as well as for

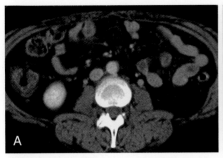 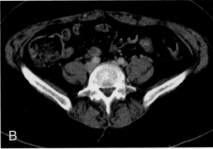 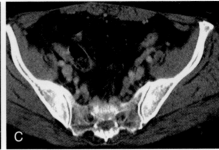

FIGURE 100-1. **A,** Computed tomography (CT) scan of 46-year-old woman with a 16-year history of chronic leg edema and pain after deep venous thrombosis. Lower part of the abdomen shows a patent and normal-appearing inferior vena cava. **B,** CT scan of upper part of pelvis showing normal right common iliac vein and occluded left common iliac vein. **C,** CT of lower part of pelvis shows normal right-sided vein and occluded left external iliac vein.

procedural planning itself (Fig. 100-1). In the popliteal fossa, the vein is often superficial (closer to the posterior skin surface) to the artery, making access more straightforward.[13] Other veins that enter the popliteal vein can also be used for access, including the lesser saphenous vein, soleal vein, and veins draining the gastrocnemius muscle group.[22]

Technical Aspects

Identification of Venous Access Site
Access to the venous system from the popliteal fossa is preferred. This approach allows easy antegrade venography and improved application of directional force to catheters and guidewires while traversing rigid occlusions. The patient is placed prone on the angiographic table. Ultrasound is used for a preliminary review of the venous anatomy of the popliteal fossa. Either the popliteal vein or, preferably, a more superficial vein that drains into the popliteal vein is identified and selected for access. It is preferable (when possible) to avoid direct puncture and subsequent injury to the popliteal vein itself. Access from a more superficial vein will also allow easier hemostasis after the procedure.

Venous Entry
Once identified, the access vein is punctured with a 21-gauge needle under direct ultrasound guidance. The popliteal artery is specifically identified so that it will not be in the course of needle access. Because the vein is collapsible, a brisk sharp thrust may be needed to enter the vein. A tourniquet may be used above the knee to facilitate venous distention. Once the tip of the needle is seen within the vein, insertion of a 0.018-inch guidewire can be performed at this time. If tip placement is uncertain, aspiration of blood and subsequent injection of contrast material may be required to identify an intraluminal position. After insertion of the 0.018-inch guidewire, the micropuncture sheath is inserted, followed by a standard 0.035-inch guidewire. A short 6F sheath is then placed and connected to a heparinized saline infusion via the side arm.

Preliminary Venography
Contrast venography of the popliteal, femoral, and common femoral segments is performed via the sheath (Fig. 100-2, A-C). If satisfactory, a 5F angled multipurpose catheter is advanced into the common femoral vein. Venography of the iliac segment is then performed (Fig. 100-2, D). Multiple

oblique projections will often be required to identify the true course of the occluded iliac venous segment. Because multiple collateral channels will frequently be present, identification of the occluded venous channel is often challenging. Systemic anticoagulation is then initiated.

Iliac Vein Catheterization
The technically challenging portion of the procedure is identification of the native occluded iliac venous channel and traversing it with a catheter-guidewire combination. The catheter tip will have to be wedged into the origin of the occluded segment. If not, guidewires will tend to enter the large and patent collateral channels. Hydrophilic guidewires and catheters are very useful in this situation. Allowing the guidewire to buckle and form a knuckle is helpful (similar to subintimal recanalization techniques). Incremental progress is achieved by advancing the guidewire several centimeters then advancing the catheter. Intermittent injections of contrast material are necessary to ensure an intraluminal catheter position. It is not uncommon to require a long 6F guiding sheath placed at the leading edge of the occlusion to provide increased support and "pushing power," because this chronically occluded and narrow channel is entered. Once the guidewire enters the patent IVC, passage of the guidewire is much easier. The guidewire should be advanced well into the IVC to provide support for catheter advancement. Once the catheter is advanced into the IVC, contrast material is injected to confirm successful traversal of the occluded segment.

Preliminary Balloon Dilation
Once the occluded segment has been successfully traversed, an exchange-length heavy-duty guidewire (Rosen [Cook Medical, Bloomington, Ind.], Amplatz [Boston Scientific, Natick, Mass.]) is placed into the IVC. Incremental balloon dilation is then performed along the entire course of the occluded segment. Size estimates can be obtained by review of the preprocedural CT or MR images of the contralateral iliac vein. Usually, two or three incremental dilations are performed until the final size is reached. The patient is carefully observed for pain during dilation. After the final dilation, the long sheath is advanced into the occluded segment for pull-back injection of contrast material to rule out any vascular perforation (Fig. 100-2, E). If no perforation is identified, the interventionalist can proceed with bare-wire stenting.

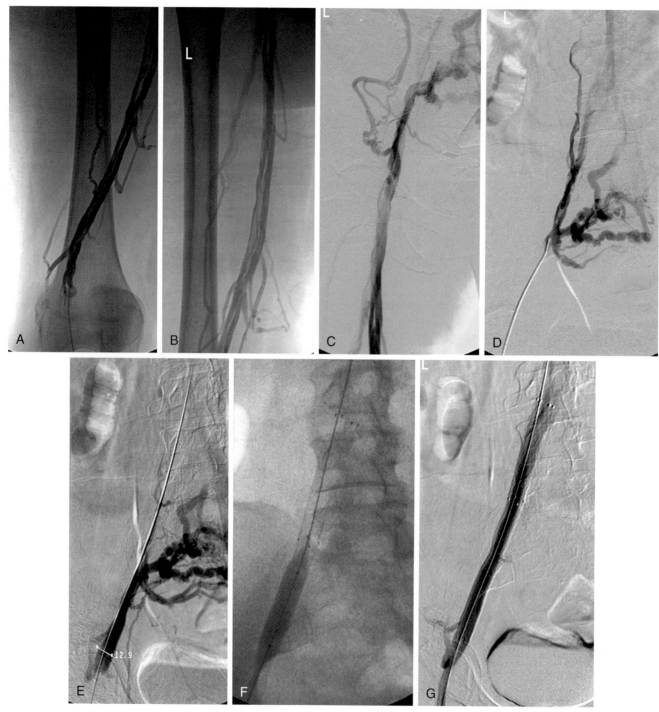

FIGURE 100-2. **A-C,** Contrast venography of left lower extremity shows changes attributable to previous deep venous thrombosis but with continued antegrade flow. Occlusion is apparent at pelvic brim. **D,** Partial recanalization with injection of contrast material opacifies inferior vena cava. Catheter is clearly intraluminal, and recanalization can proceed. **E,** Image after successful traversal of occlusion and predilation. No extravasation of contrast material noted. Stenting can be performed. **F,** Stenting has been completed, and postdilation is being performed. **G,** Final venogram showing brisk antegrade flow in iliac venous system. Patient's symptoms markedly improved.

Venous Stenting

Self-expanding stents are generally preferred for lower tendency of venous perforation during proper fixation, lower risk of migration, longer length, flexibility at the groin, and less susceptibility to permanent deformation.[23,24] Nitinol stents (SMART [Cordis Corp., Miami Lakes, Fla.]) have been increasingly used because of their accuracy in deployment. Stents with diameters of at least 10 to 14 mm will be required. If larger-diameter stents are needed (≥16 mm), Wallstents (Boston Scientific) may be used. If the use of varying diameters is planned, the stents should be telescoped such that the smaller-diameter stents are placed first to ensure adequate apposition of the stents. Long stents should be used to minimize the number of stents deployed. The most central stent should be placed carefully so that flow from the contralateral iliac vein is not impeded. In similar fashion, the most peripheral stent should not interfere with hip motion.

Poststenting Dilation

After deployment of the stents across the entire occluded segment, the region is dilated with the appropriately sized balloons (Fig. 100-2, *F*). Twelve- and 14-mm balloons will require 7F introduction sheaths.

Poststenting Venography

Postdeployment venograms are performed to ensure the entire affected segment is adequately stented and dilated and there is good antegrade flow (Fig. 100-2, *G*). Additional stents and dilations are performed as needed.

Inferior Vena Cava Reconstruction

In some patients, the venous occlusion extends into the infrarenal IVC. Recanalization proceeds through the occluded caval segment into the patent suprarenal IVC. Predilation is performed as described earlier, along with a postdilation sheath venogram to rule out perforation.

Inferior Vena Cava Stenting

Stenting of the IVC is performed in standard fashion. Large Wallstents (Boston Scientific) or Gianturco stents (tracheobronchial stents) (Cook-Z stent [Cook Medical]) may be needed.

Reconstruction of the Caval Bifurcation

If the IVC bifurcation requires reconstruction, bilateral access is obtained. After stenting the IVC proper, access via each iliac vein into the stented IVC is performed. The bifurcation is then reconstructed with simultaneous "kissing" stents beginning in the peripheral portion of the stented IVC and extending into the common iliac veins. Iliac venous stenting can then be completed.

CONTROVERSIES

- Few studies have evaluated the long-term (>5 years) patency of venous stents. Therefore, it has been somewhat controversial to offer this procedure to those with only mild to moderate symptoms.
- Most interventionalists believe that 3 to 6 months of anticoagulation is necessary to allow full reendothelialization. Others think that because of the low-flow venous system, anticoagulation for life is warranted.
- Based on experience with stents in other venous segments, neointimal hyperplasia will develop and eventually cause restenosis. There is value in identifying restenosis before a recurrent thrombosis occurs. Some have advocated more extensive use of physiologic noninvasive monitoring such as air plethysmography.
- Routine use of infrainguinal venous stent placement is currently controversial owing to their poor patency rates. It is recommended to reserve infrainguinal venous stents only for patients with extensive disease and very poor outflow.
- Several investigators have advocated the use of antiplatelet agents.
- The need for a surgically created arteriovenous fistula for the first 3 months to increase flow through the stented area has not been widely endorsed in recent years.

OUTCOMES

Early published series (mid-1990s) from the University of Minnesota and Stanford University reported primary 1-year patency rates for stented iliac venous segments in the 50% to 85% range.[25-27] Secondary patency rates exceeded 90%. In 2002, Raju et al. reviewed results of iliac vein stenting for the relief of iliac vein obstruction (primarily stenoses) in 304 limbs.[16,28] They reported 24-month primary and secondary patency rates of 71% and 90%, respectively. In a more recent study, Neglen et al. published a retrospective evaluation of 870 patients (982 limbs) treated with iliofemorocaval venous stenting.[29] The study showed that at 5 years, primary, assisted-primary, and secondary cumulative patency rates were 79%, 100%, and 100% in nonthrombotic disease and 57%, 80%, and 86% in thrombotic disease, respectively. The authors concluded that venous stenting can be performed with low morbidity and mortality, long-term high patency rate, and a low rate of in-stent restenosis.

Similar to stents in other locations, neointimal hyperplasia may develop. When the hyperplasia leads to flow-limiting stenosis, the patient's symptomatology will probably recur. Many of these patients have become knowledgeable of the symptomatology and will often alert the interventionalist when there is recurrent or a new onset of pain and limb swelling. They require lower extremity duplex ultrasound examination to rule out acute thrombosis. Patients are then scheduled for a venogram and probably a catheter-directed intervention. The venogram will most likely reveal restenosis due to neointimal hyperplasia in the stented segment (Fig. 100-3, *A*). At this stage, the patient is rapidly treated with conventional venoplasty (Fig. 100-3, *B* and *C*) and occasional repeat stenting. If acute thrombus is identified, the patient will require catheter-directed thrombolysis or pharmacomechanical thrombolysis before venoplasty and stenting. This latter group will require lifelong anticoagulation.

COMPLICATIONS

No mortality due to recanalization of chronic iliac/caval occlusions has been reported. Morbidity has been limited to hematomas secondary to perforation of an iliac venous segment, with presumed injury to an adjacent artery. It is important to recognize the importance of staying intraluminal during the recanalization process and being aware of the proximity to the iliac artery. Retroperitoneal bleeding from a high cannulation site has also been reported.[30] Because these procedures are performed during systemic anticoagulation, sheaths traversing the popliteal fossa are often removed while the patient is anticoagulated. This has resulted in self-limited popliteal fossa hematomas.[23]

POSTPROCEDURAL AND FOLLOW-UP CARE

The majority of these procedures are performed on an outpatient basis. Patients are systemically anticoagulated during the procedure. Just before discharge, they receive their first dose of subcutaneous low-molecular-weight heparin (LMWH) and begin oral warfarin therapy the following day. Patients continue LMWH therapy until the international normalized ratio is therapeutic.

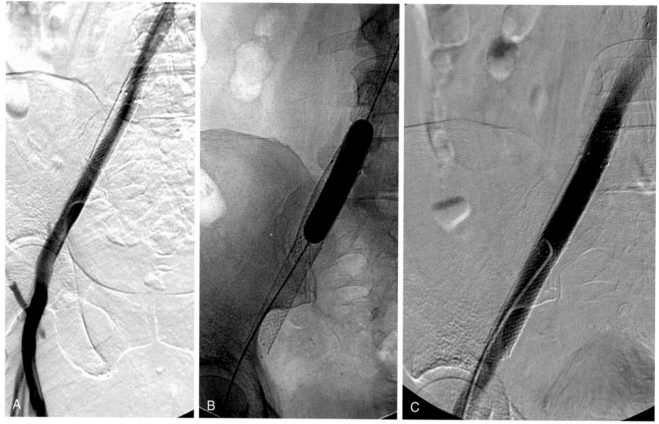

FIGURE 100-3. A, Two-year follow-up of patient in Figure 100-2. Patient experienced increased swelling, and venogram showed stenosis due to neointimal hyperplasia within stent. **B,** Conventional venoplasty performed. **C,** Postvenoplasty venogram shows improved flow. Patient's leg edema resolved. Same group reported on a subset of patients with chronically occluded iliac venous segments in 38 limbs. In nine patients, recanalization extended into inferior vena cava. No morbidity or mortality reported, and 24-month primary, primary assisted, and secondary patency rates were 49%, 62%, and 76%, respectively. Pain and limb swelling were significantly improved. In addition, 62% of patients with venous stasis ulcers/dermatitis showed resolution. Patency rates for long-segment occlusions were clearly lower than those of short-segment stenoses in iliac venous segments.

Anticoagulation is continued for at least 3 to 6 months. Patients with hypercoagulable states or recurrent episodes of venous thrombosis take anticoagulants for life. Patients are monitored clinically, as well as with duplex ultrasonography at 3, 6, and 12 months after the procedure.[23] The follow-up is then often lengthened to 6 to 12 months thereafter. Physiologic follow-up with air plethysmography can also be performed noninvasively.

KEY POINTS

- The two major factors responsible for chronic venous problems are valvular reflux and venous obstruction.

- Chronic iliac venous occlusion is a common result of previous iliofemoral deep venous thrombosis.

- Patients with chronic iliac vein occlusion have chronic leg swelling, pain, limitation of activity, and even venous stasis ulcers.

- Patients with adequate inflow (antegrade flow in the femoral vein) and outflow (patent inferior vena cava) are candidates for iliac vein reconstruction.

- Iliac vein stenting can reestablish antegrade flow and relieve leg swelling and pain.

► **SUGGESTED READINGS**

Hansen E, Razavi M, Semba C, Drake M. Endovascular strategies for inferior vena cava obstruction. Tech Vasc Interv Radiol 2000;3:40–4.

Krishnan S, Nicholls S. Chronic venous insufficiency: clinical assessment and patient selection. Semin Intervent Radiol 2005;22:169–77.

Meissner MH, Moneta G, Burnand K, et al. The hemodynamics and diagnosis of venous disease. J Vasc Surg 2007;46(Suppl S):4S–24S.

Mozes G, Gloviczki P. New discoveries in anatomy and new terminology of leg veins: clinical implications. Vasc Endovasc Surg 2004;38:367–74.

O'Sullivan G. Endovascular management of chronic iliac vein occlusion. Tech Vasc Interv Radiol 2000;3:45–53.

Sharafuddin M, Sun S, Hoballah J, et al. Endovascular management of venous thrombotic and occlusive diseases of the lower extremities. J Vasc Interv Radiol 2003;14:405–23.

The complete reference list is available online at www.expertconsult.com.

CHAPTER 101

Acute Lower Extremity Deep Venous Thrombosis

Haraldur Bjarnason

Early clot lysis may prevent or significantly decrease the incidence and severity of postthrombotic syndrome after acute lower extremity deep vein thrombosis (DVT). Several smaller studies comparing systemic thrombolytic therapy for acute DVT with anticoagulation showed that significant or complete clot lyses can be achieved by giving systemic thrombolysis, but with an unacceptably high rate of bleeding complications.[1,2] Catheter-directed thrombolysis for DVT has proven to be a safe and effective method to remove acute iliofemoral DVT.[3,4] Mechanical thrombectomy has emerged as an alternative or adjunct to pharmacologic thrombolysis.[5]

Population-based studies indicate that the annual incidence of DVT is between 122 and 160 per 100,000.[6] It is thought that approximately 10% of patients with lower extremity DVT will have iliac vein involvement; these patients have an especially high risk of developing severe postthrombotic syndrome, and this may vary significantly. A recently published article from a large tertiary care facility found that 24% of patients diagnosed with DVT did have involvement of the iliac veins.[7] The long-term sequelae of lower extremity DVT are very significant, as has been documented by many authors. Up to two thirds of patients with acute DVT treated according to accepted algorithms will develop postthrombotic syndrome. Patients with iliac vein thrombosis have a much worse prognosis.[8-10]

INDICATIONS

There are no well-established indications for thrombolytic therapy for iliofemoral DVT. The challenge lies in the lack of conclusive randomized studies that document the safety and efficacy of thrombolysis compared to conventional anticoagulation. The decision to offer thrombolytic treatment to a patient with DVT has to be weighed carefully, considering the anticipated clinical outcome of the procedure and potential risks. The decision therefore becomes individualized, taking into account age and comorbid factors such as cancer or bleeding diatheses. Based on several small and large case studies, it is believed that certain indications can be supported on an individual basis.[3,4,11] The Society of Interventional Radiology (SIR) and the Cardiovascular and Interventional Radiology Society of Europe published quality improvement guidelines in 2006 that suggest certain indications. These are listed in Table e101-1.[12,13]

The largest groups of patients currently considered for thrombolytic therapy are patients with acute iliofemoral DVT. These patients are at high risk of developing postthrombotic syndrome and recurrent DVT and are frequently very symptomatic at first presentation. The potential of changing the long-term outcomes for these patients is therefore quite significant. Catheter-directed thrombolysis may be an acceptable alternative treatment and possibly superior to conventional anticoagulation in patients with a long life expectancy and a low risk for bleeding.[14]

A larger group of patients in whom the indications are less studied are patients with acute femoropopliteal DVT. Earlier studies using systemic thrombolysis for femoropopliteal thrombosis did indicate that there was a potential benefit from thrombolysis.[1,2] It has to be borne in mind that many patients with femoropopliteal DVT will become free of symptoms if treated conventionally with anticoagulation and compression garments. Based on this, the threshold for catheter-directed thrombolysis should be higher for femoropopliteal DVT than for iliofemoral DVT. Catheter-directed thrombolysis should be reserved for patients with severe symptoms from femoropopliteal DVT and those who experience progression of thrombosis on anticoagulation.[14]

A limited number of practitioners use thrombolytic therapy in conjunction with iliac vein recanalization in patients with chronic iliac vein thrombosis or subacute thrombosis. This practice is discouraged and probably has very limited benefits in this group of patients.[2,14]

Phlegmasia cerulea dolens, an acute fulminating form of DVT characterized by reactive arterial spasm, pronounced edema, severe cyanosis, petechiae, and purpura, carries a high risk of amputation and significant morbidity and mortality.[15-17] Many patients have significant comorbid factors such that any correctible management—surgical, endovascular, or medical—carries high risk. Several case reports of catheter-directed thrombolysis for phlegmasia cerulea dolens have been published[17,18] describing good short-term clinical improvement. Catheter-directed thrombolysis is found to be justified for most patients with this condition if they do not have a high risk of bleeding. When bleeding risk is believed to be prohibitory for thrombolysis, surgical thrombectomy should be considered. This is regarded as an emergent procedure.[14]

Acute thrombosis of the inferior vena cava is often very symptomatic, leading to bilateral lower extremity leg and genital congestion. If the thrombosis extends above the renal and hepatic veins, renal failure and Budd-Chiari syndrome may result. Filter placement may not be possible to prevent pulmonary emboli. For these reasons, catheter-directed thrombolysis may be justified to prevent or relieve the sequelae mentioned earlier.[14]

Both the American College of Chest Physicians[19] and the American Heart Association[20] have now included catheter-directed thrombolysis as an option for treatment of selected patients with lower extremity deep vein thrombosis.

CONTRAINDICATIONS

Contraindications to venous thrombolysis and mechanical thrombectomy are practically the same as for any other thrombolytic therapy and are listed in Table e101-2.

Contraindications to thrombolysis are often unclear, such as abnormal bleeding parameters in a patient with impaired liver function or in a patient with reduced platelets. Many patients have also undergone surgery on different body parts in the recent past, and it can be difficult to estimate what is a safe time from surgery. For the optimal outcome of thrombolysis, it has to be carried out soon after symptoms first appeared or within 10 to 14 days, which adds to the limitations but still gives some leeway to correct correctable bleeding diatheses.

EQUIPMENT

The equipment needed is the same as that used for arterial thrombolysis. Additional equipment is needed for mechanical thrombectomy. The main items needed are listed in Table e101-3.

Having a good fluoroscopy unit with image-capturing capability for documentation is a necessity. The fluoroscopic unit is used to obtain the necessary venogram and guide placement of the infusion catheters and mechanical thrombectomy. A C-arm fixed to either the floor or ceiling is preferable, and the larger the receptor, the better (40 cm diameter). Mobile fluoroscopic units can be used but should have image-capturing capability. Ultrasound to guide venous access is required, especially when the popliteal vein or posterior tibial vein is used for access. Puncturing the artery inadvertently can have serious consequences when the thrombolytic therapy subsequently starts. For the venous access it is advisable to use a micro-puncture access set. A 20-gauge needle with a 0.018-inch guidewire and 4F coaxial dilator that accepts a 0.035-inch guidewire is available from many vendors. There are many guidewires available, but the basic system is a 0.035-inch guidewire system. A multipurpose guidewire such as the Bentson (Cook Medical, Bloomington, Ind.) can be used, but a glide-coated guidewire such as the Glidewire (Terumo Medical Corp., Somerset, N.J.) may be needed to negotiate the thrombotic veins. To facilitate navigation through the clot, a 5F angiographic catheter, preferably with glide coating, should be used to help direct the guidewire as it is passed through the clotted vein. Contrast medium can be intermittently injected through it to obtain venography as it is advanced. An introducer sheath should be used that is 1F size larger than the infusion catheter so heparin solution can be infused through the side port around the infusion catheter going through it, either for low-dose anticoagulation or to keep the sheath from forming thrombus. There are many brands available, and a 10-cm-long introducer is sufficient. If mechanical thrombectomy is used, a larger introducer is needed, which is then left in place during the following infusion. Selection of an infusion catheter is based on the length of the clot to be treated. There are many different brands offered, but most are available with a 5-, 10-, 20-, 30-, 40-, and 50-cm-long infusion segment and come in 5F diameters, although some are also available in a 4F diameter. Construction of individual catheters differs, but the most important property is equal distribution of the drug throughout the length of the infusion segment.

The large number of mechanical thrombectomy devices available may be an indicator of their shortcomings thus far. They can be divided into so-called wall contact devices and non–wall contact devices (Table e101-4). Many of the

devices have undergone preclinical and clinical evaluation for DVT and have been found to be effective, with very little trauma to the valvular elements, which is one of the main concerns. Concomitant pulmonary emboli have been one of the concerns with mechanical thrombectomy, and placement of an inferior vena caval filter has been recommended with some devices.[21]

TECHNIQUE

Anatomy and Approaches

Anatomic Considerations

The anatomy of the lower extremity, iliac veins, and inferior vena cava is familiar to all interventionists, but the nomenclature of some of the lower extremity veins has recently changed.[22] For example, the superficial femoral vein is now called the *femoral vein*.[23] The following is a short practical review with correlation to the approach for venous thrombolysis. It is important to recognize that the anatomy of the lower leg veins varies.

The three leg veins are paired and travel parallel to the main leg arteries and bear the same names: the *posterior tibial vein, anterior tibial vein*, and *fibular* or *peroneal vein*. The posterior tibial vein pair traverses behind the medial malleoli with the posterior tibial artery. The anatomy here is important because access can be gained into the posterior tibial vein at this level. This access can be used for placement of infusion catheters through which thrombolytic agents can be infused into thrombosed popliteal vein. The deep leg veins communicate with the superficial veins via *perforating veins*. The perforating veins have been used for placement of infusion catheters into thrombosed deep veins.[24] The leg veins will then merge and form the *popliteal vein*. The anatomy in the popliteal fossa is quite variable.[25] The vein is often partially or entirely duplicated.

The *small saphenous vein* (formerly the short saphenous vein) is formed from the dorsal venous arch and travels subcutaneously between the two heads of the gastrocnemius muscle. It then penetrates the fascia to enter the popliteal fossa and joins the popliteal or femoral vein, most commonly above or at the level of the femoral condyles. The small saphenous vein is very useful as an access vein for thrombolysis if the thrombus extends no farther distal than the mid- to distal femoral vein. One has to be aware of variation in the connection of the small saphenous vein, which may join the deep system above the popliteal vein, which will affect the use of this access if thrombus extends caudal to the junction. The sural nerve is just lateral to the vein, and precaution has to be taken not to harm it during puncture.

The *femoral vein* is quite consistent even though it can be duplicated (21.2%) or even have multiple channels (13.8%).[26] Usually only one infusion catheter is placed, so in the case of a split femoral vein, one has to select one channel to infuse into. The femoral vein will then merge with the *profunda femoris vein*, forming the common femoral vein. One major branch drains into it, the *great saphenous vein* (formerly the greater saphenous vein). The transition to the *external iliac vein* is at the inguinal ligament and the deep circumflex iliac vein, which is a tributary and anatomic landmark. As the *internal iliac vein* joins the external iliac vein, the *common iliac vein* is formed. The right and left common iliac veins will subsequently form the *inferior vena cava*, which will ascend to the right and anterior of the spine to the right atrium. A variant that is commonly seen with iliac vein thrombosis is compression of the left common iliac vein by the right common iliac artery crossing it anteriorly. Commonly, a stenosis is present at this point in the left common iliac vein, and the vein is often septate or webbed, which causes partial or complete obstruction with variable collateral formation. It has been estimated that between 14% and 30% of these patients have May-Thurner syndrome.[27]

Access

An access for venous thrombolysis and/or mechanical thrombectomy depends largely on the location and extent of the thrombus. A known history of previous thrombosis (areas of chronic thrombosis) will also play a decisive role in selecting access, because it is difficult to traverse chronically thrombosed vein to get to an acute thrombus for treatment. The main access sites are the right internal jugular vein, common femoral veins, popliteal veins, short saphenous vein, and posterior tibial veins. Other accesses will be mentioned later.

The right internal jugular vein was the access vein of choice during the infancy of the procedure. As interventionists became more experienced, the trend swayed subsequently to popliteal vein access (or small saphenous vein) and the posterior tibial vein.[4,11]

The right internal jugular vein is easily accessed using ultrasound as guidance. The indwelling introducer is reasonably well tolerated by patients, even though it is a rather intimidating proposition to patients to have the jugular vein punctured, not to mention that catheters will be traversing the heart to reach the thrombus. For isolated iliac vein thrombosis it is, as a general rule, easy to traverse the acute thrombus from the jugular vein. Infusion catheters placed from that access will easily span the length of isolated iliac vein thrombus. One of the problems is that during catheter manipulations, there is risk of them looping in the right atrium and even in the right ventricle. Arrhythmias can then occur that almost always are self-limiting after the irritant (looped catheter) has been removed. If an inferior vena cava filter is needed, it can be placed at the same time from the jugular vein. The filter will then be in the path of the infusion system, but this can be overcome by using introducer sheaths that extend beyond the filter. Thrombus sitting even further distal (i.e., in the femoral and even the popliteal vein) causes difficulties if jugular vein access is used. In this case, the valves in the femoral veins have to be traversed retrograde, which is a difficult task because the wire and catheters preferentially sit in the sinus rather than pass through the valve opening.

It was for these reasons practitioners started favoring access from the popliteal vein; popliteal access is easily achieved and well tolerated by the patient. The vein sits superficial to the artery in the popliteal fossa and is usually not very deep. Ultrasound guidance is necessary, and use of a micropuncture access system is recommended.

An alternative to direct popliteal vein access is puncture into the short saphenous vein, which is superficially located in the subcutaneous tissues between the two heads of the gastrocnemius muscle.

Thrombosis of the iliac veins usually carries with it thrombosis of the common femoral vein, but the femoral vein can still be patent. Early on, a contralateral common femoral vein access was sometimes used for treatment of iliofemoral vein thrombosis. This approach has fallen into disfavor because it is poorly tolerated by the patient compared with other used accesses. Second, placing a catheter across the inferior vena caval bifurcation angle to traverse a contralateral iliac vein thrombus was often very difficult.

But what do you do in the case of clot extending into the popliteal vein and distal to that? This is a dilemma many operators have solved by puncturing the posterior tibial vein behind the medial malleoli and placing a second infusion system (in addition to the popliteal vein). This infusion part of the infusion catheter has to be long enough to overlap the infusion catheter from the popliteal vein. Usually a 40- to 50-cm infusion-length system will do that.

Cragg described an alternative technique to accessing the deep calf veins. His method is based on injecting contrast medium into a dorsal superficial foot vein and then using fluoroscopy to guide a needle into the distal posterior tibial vein or, if the posterior tibial vein is not seen, to select a superficial vein and negotiate a catheter via communicating or perforating veins into the deep system. When access is gained to the deep system, preferably via the posterior tibial vein, an introducer sheath is placed and an infusion catheter used as described earlier.[24]

Technical Aspects

The popliteal vein is the preferred access site. Posterior tibial vein access and even jugular vein access are still used occasionally, often in conjunction with popliteal vein access. The jugular vein is only used in rare cases of inferior vena caval thrombosis and isolated iliac vein thrombosis. For the popliteal vein approach, the patient is placed prone (Fig. 101-1) on the procedure table. The vena cava filter can be placed from the jugular vein with the patient supine before turning the patient prone to gain access to the popliteal vein (Fig. 101-2). There have been cases in which filters have been placed from the thrombolysis access in the common femoral vein or even the popliteal vein.

Ultrasound should always be used for guidance during access when thrombolysis is anticipated. Ultrasonography prevents inadvertent puncture of the artery or puncture into a vein that cannot be used for access purposes. These puncture sites may later cause bleeding complications. As soon as access has been gained, an introducer sheath is placed. Usually either a 5F or 6F introducer sheath is used, but if mechanical thrombectomy is to be used, a larger introducer sheath may be needed (Fig. 101-3). When the introducer sheath has been placed, the clot has to be traversed to the most central portion. For this purpose, a glide-coated guidewire and glide-coated angiographic catheter are best fitted. Contrast medium is injected from the introducer to evaluate the distal portion of the thrombus (Fig. 101-4). The guidewire and angiographic catheter are advanced through the clot, and as progress is made, the wire can be intermittently removed and contrast agent injected. This gives an idea of the clot burden.

When the catheter has reached the most proximal or central extent of the thrombus, a venogram should be performed. If the thrombus extends to the upper end of the

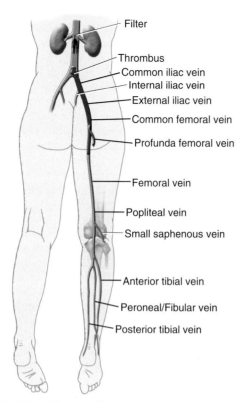

FIGURE 101-1. Diagram of prone patient with thrombosis of right common iliac, external iliac, common femoral and proximal veins. Thrombus extends into inferior vena cava as a "free-floating" thrombus. A filter has been placed infrarenally.

common iliac vein, a good inferior vena cavogram should be obtained through the angiographic catheter, and one might also want to place the catheter into the contralateral iliac vein and obtain a venogram from there (Fig. 101-5). This will verify that the contralateral venous system as well as the inferior vena cava is free of thrombus. At this point, the optimal length of the infusion catheter is selected. An infusion catheter should be selected that has an infusion segment of similar length to the length of the thrombus. The whole thrombus should be covered with infusion holes (infusion segment) (Fig. 101-6; also see Fig. 101-3). An easy way to measure the length is to pass an angiographic catheter through the thrombus to the upper end, and then as the guidewire is removed it is marked at the upper and lower end of the thrombus. Based on this measurement, the length of side hole segment is decided.

Heparin is usually infused through the introducer sheath, and if two accesses are used, the remaining introducer sheath is infused with normal saline with minimal amounts of heparin.

Thrombolysis by itself has been shown to be time consuming, taking between 53 and 75 hours with infusion alone[4,10]; it is expensive, and there is a perceived risk accompanied with thrombolysis. Mechanical thrombectomy has the potential to solve these problems. The thrombus can be either completely removed with mechanical thrombectomy or, as more often is the case, significantly debulked, followed with shorter infusion of the thrombolytic agent. A number of representative mechanical thrombectomy devices are available, as listed in

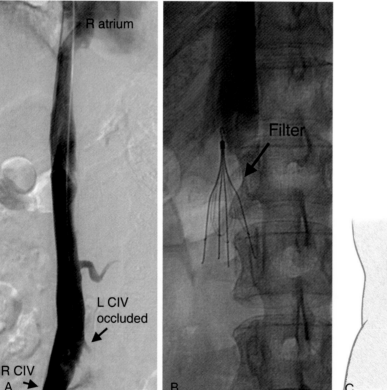

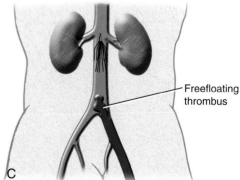

FIGURE 101-2. **A,** This patient has left lower extremity deep vein thrombosis including iliac veins. Inferior vena cavogram was obtained by injecting through a pigtail catheter placed from right internal jugular vein to inferior vena cava bifurcation. There is no reflux into left common iliac vein *(L CIV)*. **B,** Subsequent to inferior vena cavogram in **A,** a Günther Tulip filter (William Cook Europe, Bjaeverskov, Denmark) was placed infrarenally in preparation for mechanical thrombectomy and thrombolysis. **C,** This diagram shows a filter placed above a free-floating thrombus in inferior vena cava.

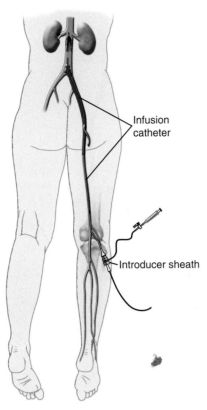

FIGURE 101-3. Diagram showing placement of an introducer sheath into patent popliteal vein. Infusion catheter has been advanced across entire thrombosed segment. Heparin can then be infused through introducer sheath as thrombolytic agent is infused through infusion catheter.

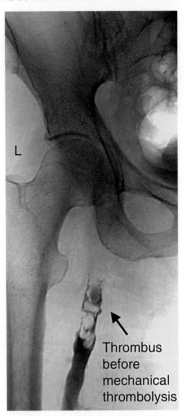

FIGURE 101-4. Patient with left-sided proximal femoral–to–common iliac vein thrombus. Access has been gained into popliteal vein and contrast medium injected from below, showing thrombus filling proximal portion of femoral vein.

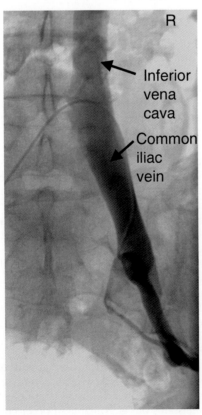

FIGURE 101-5. Catheter is passed through thrombus, and contralateral side as well as upper extent of thrombus are evaluated before any treatment is initiated. Here, catheter has been placed into contralateral right common iliac vein, verifying normal right common iliac vein and inferior vena cava.

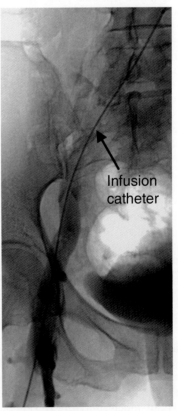

FIGURE 101-6. After mechanical thrombectomy, femoral, common femoral, and external iliac veins are almost cleared of thrombus. Thrombus remained in common iliac vein, and an infusion catheter was left in place and thrombolytic therapy initiated. Infusion catheter covers previously thrombosed segment as well as remaining thrombus.

Table e101-4. The devices can be roughly divided into wall contacting and non–wall contacting devices. Mechanical thrombectomy can usually be performed through the same access site as the thrombolysis, most commonly the popliteal vein. After mechanical thrombectomy, thrombolytic infusion is still needed in most cases.[18] An infusion catheter should be selected with an infusion length that covers the whole previously thrombosed area (see Fig. 101-6).

Not infrequently the thrombus extends beyond the distal femoral vein. Then it is impossible to use mechanical devices or expose the thrombus to the lytic drugs, because the introducer sheath usually covers the popliteal vein and the distal segment of the femoral vein. It has been advocated to actually try to go retrograde from the popliteal vein, which is difficult given that the valves are hard to pass retrograde.[28] An alternative is to either puncture the posterior tibial vein by the medial malleoli or puncture a superficial vein and negotiate through perforators into the deep calf veins. For the posterior tibial vein, a linear ultrasound probe is used (preferably 10 MHz) to identify the posterior tibial vein pair on each side of the artery just behind the medial malleoli. This is done in the same setting as the placement of the popliteal vein access. A 5F or even a 6F introducer sheath can be placed, and usually 5F infusion catheters can be passed up the posterior tibial veins. Occasionally, especially in females, severe spasms will make it difficult to pass the infusion catheters. Subsequently, a Glidewire is passed all the way up to the femoral vein, and finally the infusion catheter is advanced high enough to slightly overlap the one from the popliteal vein. The most distal side hole (closest to the access) should be just above the tip of the introducer sheath. Usually the thrombolytic dose is then evenly split between the two infusion systems.

A separate infusion system is then placed from the popliteal vein, and infusion can then be given from two locations, the posterior tibial vein and the popliteal vein (Fig. 101-7). The thrombolytic dose is then typically split into two even doses.

Infusion is usually continued for 8 to 20 hours or until it is convenient to bring the patient back to the procedure room. One can then inject contrast medium into either the introducer sheath or infusion catheter. At that point, based on the venogram, a decision has to be made whether or not further infusion is needed. It is debated what the endpoint should be. Some authors argue for the so-called open vein concept, which means practically all thrombus has to be removed. That in itself is a good target, especially in the femoral and popliteal veins, where one cannot expect the valvular elements to recover function if there is thrombus burden on them. This has not been proven. This often becomes a question of how long the patient has been infused with the thrombolytic agent, how old the clot is thought to be (and thereby likely to be lysed), and other comorbid factors.

In the iliac veins and even the common femoral veins, one might actually be tempted to stent areas that appear to be resistant to thrombolysis (Fig. 101-8). If in doubt when considering the hemodynamic significance of a venous stenosis, there is not much literature to rely on. If collateral vessels fill around a narrowed vein, that usually indicates that the narrowed segment is hemodynamically significant (see Fig. 101-8, *A* and *B*), but one can also measure

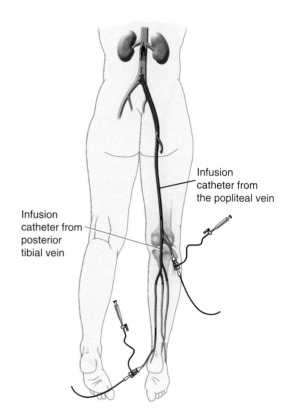

Infusion catheter from the popliteal vein

Infusion catheter from posterior tibial vein

FIGURE 101-7. In this case, thrombus extends distal to femoral and popliteal veins into calf veins. Access has been gained to posterior tibial vein via ankle, and an introducer sheath has been placed there. Infusion catheter has been placed. Infusion catheter should overlap with infusion catheter already in place from popliteal vein.

pressures across the segment. A pressure gradient above 3 mmHg is often cited as a significant pressure gradient in the venous system. Stents are then commonly placed in the iliac veins, typically using 12- to 14-mm-wide self-expanding stents that cover the entire narrowed segment from the inferior vena cava as low as necessary down to the profunda femoral and origin of the great saphenous vein if required. The stents are then dilated to the diameter of the stent using an angioplasty balloon of that diameter. Stent placement and angioplasty can easily be performed from the popliteal vein using the same access as was used for the thrombolysis. The introducer may have to be upsized to accommodate the large diameter of the stent delivery system and balloon shaft size. Angioplasty alone is usually not believed to be adequate for dilation of venous stenosis in the lower extremities and pelvis (Fig. 101-9). Many patients with left-sided iliac vein thrombosis have May-Thurner syndrome, which probably always requires stent placement (see Fig. 101-9).[29-32]

The three agents used for thrombolysis are urokinase (UK, Abbokinase [Abbott Laboratories, Abbott Park, Ill.]), tissue plasminogen activator (tPA, alteplase, Activase [Genentech, South San Francisco, Calif.]), and recombinant tissue plasminogen activator (rtPA, reteplase, Retavase [Centocor, Malvern, Pa.]). Urokinase is no longer available in the United States but is available in other countries and used there. In the United States and many other areas of the world, urokinase was once the drug of choice for

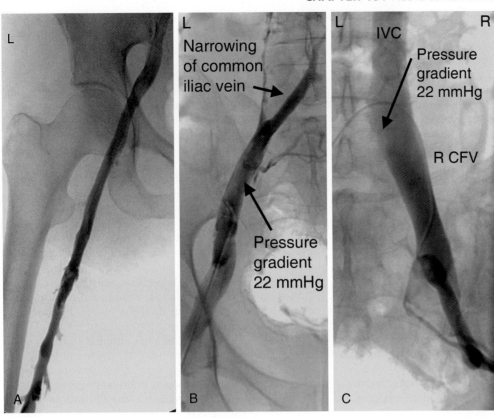

FIGURE 101-8. Venogram obtained after 18 hours of thrombolytic infusion. **A,** Open femoral, common femoral, and external iliac vein, but there is a long segment of common iliac vein narrowing **(B)** that probably is part of May-Thurner syndrome. **C,** Catheter has been passed into contralateral (right) iliac system, and pressure measured there is compared with pressure in left iliac vein peripheral to narrowed segment. Pressure difference (gradient) was 22 mmHg. *IVC,* Inferior vena cava; *R CFV,* right common femoral vein.

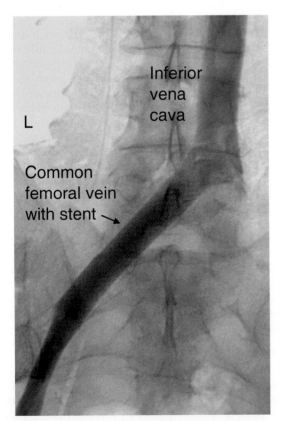

FIGURE 101-9. Narrowed segment shown in Figure 100-8, *B* has now been treated with a 14-mm-wide × 60-mm-long Wallstent (Boston Scientific, Watertown, Mass.) dilated with a 14-mm angioplasty balloon. No measurable residual pressure difference (gradient).

catheter-directed thrombolysis on both the arterial and venous sides, but sales and distribution of urokinase were suspended by the U.S. Food and Drug Administration (FDA). This prompted a search for an alternative in the United States, which led to use of alteplase and reteplase. An advisory panel on catheter-directed thrombolytic therapy published an article in the year 2000 in which alteplase infusion of 0.5 mg/h was recommended.[33] In 2003, Sugimoto et al. published an article comparing alteplase at low dose with that of urokinase. Alteplase infusion was at approximately 0.5 mg/h combined with subtherapeutic heparin infusion, keeping the partial thromboplastin time (PTT) at below 1.5 times baseline. The urokinase dose was 120,000 units/h combined with therapeutic heparin infusion, with a target PTT above 1.5 times baseline values. The study was retrospective, and the basic outcome was 88.9% success rate for alteplase for DVT compared with 85.4% for urokinase thrombolysis. These numbers were not statistically significant, and complication rates were also low and without significant difference.[34]

In 2004, Grunwald et al. published a retrospective evaluation of 74 patients (82 limbs) treated for DVTs. Thrombosed extremities were treated either with urokinase with therapeutic heparin dosing (38 limbs), alteplase with subtherapeutic heparin dosing (32 limbs), or reteplase with subtherapeutic heparin dosing (12 limbs). The authors concluded that in the setting of venous thrombosis, urokinase, alteplase, and reteplase are equally able to resolve thrombi and restore inline flow with a very high success rate (96.9%-100%) and without statistical difference in complication rate.[35]

There have been several infusion regimens published, including pulse-spray,[17,36] but there seems to be a consensus that slow infusion is the method of choice. Pulse-spray infusion fell into disfavor after anecdotal reports of fragmentation of the thrombus and concerns for pulmonary emboli as a direct consequence of the method were raised. Doses can vary significantly. For example, the urokinase infusion has been reported from 60,000 to 370,000 units/h. Doses on a per-kilogram basis have varied between 2000 and 3000 units/kg/h. Similarly, there has been significant variation in the infusion rates of both alteplase and reteplase, but an infusion of less than 1 mg/h of alteplase and 1 unit/h of reteplase seems to be the common theme. When two or even more infusion catheters are used, the infusion is typically split between the infusion systems to make up the aforementioned doses. Streptokinase has been only very rarely used, and the dose has been 50,000 units as a bolus, followed by a dose of 5000 units/h.[37]

Heparin is given concomitantly for all thrombolysis. With urokinase, full anticoagulation was given, with a targeted activated partial thromboplastin time (APTT) of 60 to 80 seconds. However, with the tissue plasminogen activators alteplase and reteplase, the unwritten consensus has been to give low doses of heparin (e.g., 300-500 units/h) and keep the APTT at below 60 seconds. More recently, tenecteplase (TNK [Genentech]) has gained attention as a possible alternative for thrombolytic therapy. Tenecteplase is a tissue plasminogen activator with slightly different properties than either alteplase or reteplase. The typical dose for tenecteplase is 0.25 mg/h and either no heparin or low-dose heparin.[38] Alteplase, reteplase, and urokinase all work through activation of plasminogen.

A thrombolytic agent with significantly different properties, alfimeprase (Nuvelo, San Carlos, Calif.), underwent clinical evaluation but is not yet available for clinical use. Alfimeprase is a direct fibrinolytic metalloproteinase and degrades thrombin directly. It is independent of plasminogen activation and is neutralized in the bloodstream by binding with α_2-macroglobulin, so it does not cause systemic effects. Currently there is no experience with the drug for venous thrombolysis, but it has been evaluated for central venous catheter clearance[39] and has been tested in a phase I trial for peripheral arterial thrombolysis.[40]

CONTROVERSIES

There have been some controversies with regard to what the optimal delivery method for the thrombolytic agents should be. Systemic thrombolysis (i.e., direct intravenous infusion of the agent) for DVT was abandoned many years ago because of high risk for bleeding and lack of studies showing a defined benefit. In the early 1990s, there was considerable interest in so-called flow-directed thrombolysis that was based on infusion of the thrombolytic agent through a dorsal superficial vein in the affected foot, with or without application of tourniquets around the ankle to force the drug into the deep venous system. This method has since fallen into disfavor because of the perceived superiority of catheter-directed thrombolysis. In the venous registry, thrombolysis was found to take significantly longer compared with catheter-directed thrombolysis if this method was used.[4]

Several controversies exist with regard to other aspects of the treatment. The most significant ones have to do with the use of mechanical thrombectomy devices. In the past, many mechanical devices have been developed but few have been used, and reports of the use of even fewer have been publicized. The general feeling is that mechanical devices accelerate the thrombolytic process significantly.

A hotly debated topic is the use of inferior vena caval filters in association with venous thrombolysis. This discussion has taken a turn now in the past few years with introduction of optional filters, filters that can be removed when the perceived need for a filter device has passed. Consensus documents published in the *British Journal of Haematology* on the indications for inferior vena caval filters stated the following: "Thrombolysis is not an indication for filter insertion. A retrievable filter should be used if available."[38] This statement leaves the issue open, indicating on one hand that filters should not be used, but if they are, optional filters should be used. In the venous registry, there were 6 patients (1%) who developed symptomatic pulmonary emboli, 1 of whom died during thrombolysis 16 hours into the infusion therapy.[4]

In Grossman and McPherson's summary article, 49 of 263 patients undergoing thrombolytic treatment had a filter placed (31 of which were optional filters) before the treatment. None of them developed pulmonary emboli.[3]

Of the remaining 214 patients who did not get a filter, there were 2 patients (0.9%) who developed symptomatic pulmonary emboli. Neither patient died.[3] None of the studies looked specifically for pulmonary emboli. The cost of placing a filter is significant, as is that of the removal process, at least in the United States. It still seems logical to place filters given certain circumstances, such as in the case of a free-floating thrombus or reduced cardiopulmonary reserve, where even a small pulmonary embolus could not be tolerated. The other issue is also when the filter should be removed. Some operators recommend that the filter be left in for a few weeks after the procedure before removal. Others take the filter out at the end of the procedure, and the patient is placed on anticoagulant therapy from then on.[41]

It is a myth that patients with acute lower extremity DVT should not be treated with intermittent pneumatic compression because it might cause thrombus dislodgement and pulmonary emboli. Ogawa et al. treated 24 patients with catheter-directed thrombolysis for DVT; 10 were treated with catheter-directed thrombolysis alone, and 14 were treated with intermittent pneumatic compression in addition to the infusion therapy. They found that concomitant application of intermittent pneumatic compression improved the thrombolytic effect and led to better long-term outcomes as well. No pulmonary emboli were observed in either group.[42]

OUTCOMES

Catheter-directed thrombolysis for iliofemoral DVT was first described in 1991 in a report of a single case by Okrent et al.[27] In 1992, Molina et al. described successful treatment in 11 of 12 patients with extensive DVT of the iliofemoral area treated with catheter-directed thrombolysis.[43] Subsequently, several centers acquired considerable experience, resulting in several larger case studies, such as that by

Semba et al. in which 35 patients were treated this way with good outcomes.[44] In 1997, the group from the University of Minnesota expanded on the paper published by Molina et al. by reporting on their experience with 77 patients (87 limbs).[11] Many other smaller reports were published, and at the same time there was a registry (referred to as the *venous registry*) sponsored by Abbott Laboratories that collected and analyzed outcomes from catheter-directed thrombolysis from 63 academic and community hospitals. This was reported by Mewissen et al. in 1999[4] and included 473 patients. Of these, 287 patients had adequate information for meaningful comparison, and that was the group of patients reported on.

The basic results from the University of Minnesota and the venous registry are listed in Table 101-1. Overall technical success was very similar: 79% versus 81%. The outcome was quite similar for the iliac vein alone (86% vs. 83%), but for the femoral veins there was a difference in technical success: 63% versus 79%. The similarity between the two studies was sustained at 1 year, where the primary patency rate was 63% versus 64% for the iliac veins and 40% versus 47% for the femoral veins. The primary patency rate at 1 year was found to be related to the degree of lysis obtained at the end of the thrombolysis procedure. It was also noted that the longer the symptoms had lasted, the less likely there was to be a good procedural outcome. In a similar fashion, a previous history of DVT was predictive for poorer procedural outcome. Stents were placed in 33% of the venous registry patients and were predictive of better long-term outcome. Stents were placed in 45% of the patients' limbs in the University of Minnesota study, with better technical outcome but significantly worse primary patency at 1 year. All or most patients in both of these articles were treated with catheter-directed thrombolysis alone but not mechanical thrombolysis.

At this time, several smaller case studies of venous thrombolysis using catheter delivery were reported. Grossman and McPherson wrote a review article on catheter-directed thrombolysis for lower extremity DVT in 1999 in which they summed up the experience up to that point. This article was written just before Mewissen et al. published the results from the venous registry[4] and contained a meta-analysis from 15 papers with a total of 263 patients, with each study having from 1 to 77 patients.[3] This article is a good review of the status of the procedure to that point.

In 2002, Elsharawy and Elzayat published a small study of 35 patients with iliofemoral DVT who were randomized to either catheter-directed thrombolysis followed by anticoagulation or anticoagulation alone. The thrombolytic agent was streptokinase. There were 18 patients in the thrombolytic arm and 17 patients in the anticoagulation arm of the study. At 1 week, complete lysis of the affected and treated area was seen in none of the patients in the anticoagulation-only group, compared with 61% in the thrombolysis group. At 6 months, 12% had complete lysis in the anticoagulation group, compared with 72% in the thrombolysis group. No lysis was seen in 41% of the anticoagulation group at 6 months, but no patient in the thrombolysis group had no lysis. There were no bleeding complications in either group, but one patient in the anticoagulation group developed symptomatic pulmonary emboli. At 6 months, venous functional studies revealed obstruction or reflux in 88% of the patients in the anticoagulation-only group, compared with 28% of the patients treated with thrombolysis ($P < .001$).[45]

In 2004, Laiho et al. published results from a retrospective evaluation of 32 patients who were treated for iliofemoral DVT either with systemic thrombolysis (16 patients) or catheter-directed thrombolysis (16 patients). This was a nonrandomized review over 1 year at a single institution. All patients were treated with anticoagulation following the thrombolysis. At clinical follow-up 2 to 3 years later, there was a tendency to better CEAP scores (clinical manifestations, etiologic factors, anatomic distribution, pathophysiology)[46] in patients treated with catheter-directed thrombolysis versus systemic thrombolysis, but the clinical disability score was quite similar between the two groups. Valvular competence was found in 44% of the patients undergoing catheter-directed thrombolysis, compared with only 13% of the systemic group ($P = .049$). The deep veins were incompetent in 44% versus 81%, respectively ($P = 03$), and the superficial vein valves were incompetent in 25% versus 63%, respectively ($P = 03$). Major bleeding complications were noted in 2 of 16 (13%) in the catheter-directed group versus 1 of 16 (6%) in the systemic group. There were no intracranial hemorrhages and no reports of pulmonary emboli.[47]

Several smaller series have reported on the use of mechanical thrombectomy and thrombolysis.[21] Vedantham et al. treated 28 limbs with iliofemoral DVT using the HELIX Clot Buster and found that the treatment time was significantly shorter (16.8 hours), compared with previous reports of between 53 and 75 hours.[4,11] They found it necessary to supplement mechanical thrombectomy with thrombolysis.[5]

There are two ongoing large randomized studies comparing catheter-directed thrombolysis to conventional anticoagulation treatment. The first originates from Norway (CaVenT study); published results included 103 patients, 50 of whom were in a catheter-directed thrombolysis group and 53 in an anticoagulation-only group. No mechanical thrombectomy devices were used. The mean duration of infusion ws 2.3 days, with a standard deviation of 1.2 days. In the thrombolysis group, 24 (48%) of the 50 patients had complete lysis, 20 (40%) had 50% to 90% lysis, and two patients had ineffective or failed lysis. At 6-month follow-up (early results), there was a significant gain for the thrombolytic group in terms of iliofemoral patency (based on ultrasound) and functional obstruction (based on air

TABLE 101-1. Comparison of University of Minnesota and Venous Registry Outcomes

	University of Minnesota, 1997[11] N = 77	Venous Registry, 1999[4] N = 287
Initial success	79%	83%
Iliac veins	86%	83%
Femoral veins	63%	79%
Primary patency at 1 year		
Iliac	63%	64%
Femoral veins	40%	47%
Patency at 1 year		
Stented	54%	74%
Not stented	75%	53%

plethysmography), but there was no difference in terms of femoral vein insufficiency (based on Doppler ultrasound). These results demonstrated that thrombolysis did open up the vein, but valvular function did not seem to be affected.[48] The second study, ATTRACT (Acute Venous Thrombosis: Thrombosis Removal with Adjunctive Catheter-Directed Thrombolysis), is a National Institutes of Health (NIH)-funded multicenter study in the United States. This is a randomized study between catheter-directed thrombolysis and anticoagulation, with a targeted enrollment of 700 patients; initial results are not expected for a few years. This study is run out of Washington University in St. Louis by Dr. SureshVedantham.[49]

There are no long-term data available for the clinical or anatomic outcomes of catheter-directed thrombolysis. In an attempt to better understand clinical treatment outcomes, Comerota et al. sent out a health-related quality-of-life questionnaire to 98 patients who had been treated in the preceding 6 to 44 months for iliofemoral DVT. Sixty-eight of the patients had been included in the previously discussed venous registry and had undergone thrombolysis followed by regular anticoagulation. The remaining 30 patients were identified from hospital records and had been treated by standard anticoagulation without thrombolysis.[50] The basic findings were that patients who had undergone thrombolysis reported better overall physical functioning ($P = .046$), less stigma ($P = .033$), less health distress ($P = 022$), and fewer overall symptoms ($P = 006$), compared with patients who were treated with anticoagulation alone. The conclusion drawn from this was that patients with iliofemoral DVT treated with catheter-directed thrombolysis have better functioning and well-being than patients treated with anticoagulation alone. The study also found that patients who underwent thrombolysis that was deemed to have failed had similar outcomes to patients treated with heparin.[50]

COMPLICATIONS

Bleeding complications were the main reason for the cessation of systemic thrombolysis for DVT. Thrombolysis has also traditionally been looked at critically because of the potentially severe complications that can result from thrombolytic therapy. The complications from the University of Minnesota and venous registry studies are listed in Table 101-2.

Major bleeding was seen in 11% of the venous registry patients, the majority of which occurred at and around the introducer sheath (39%); 13% were retroperitoneal, and the remainder came from a variety of other sites. No deaths resulted from bleeding complications. In the University of Minnesota series, the major bleeding incidence was 7%. Pulmonary emboli were not specifically evaluated, so only symptomatic pulmonary emboli were detected. Pulmonary emboli occurred in 1 patient at the University of Minnesota, compared with 6 (1%) in the venous registry. One of the 6 patients died of pulmonary embolism. One patient in the venous registry suffered subdural hematoma, which was surgically managed. In addition to that, 1 patient died of intracranial bleeding. There is not much in the literature on mechanical thrombectomy, but Vedantham et al. did encounter three major bleeding complications in 22 treated patients (14%) who had no intracranial or gastrointestinal bleeding and no pulmonary emboli. With mechanical thrombectomy, hemolysis can be expected, but there are no reports of renal failure associated with the procedure.[5] In the CaVenT study, there were two major complications out of the 49 which did get thrombolytic treatment, one nerve damage and compartment syndrome. There were no major bleeding complications.[4]

POSTPROCEDURAL AND FOLLOW-UP CARE

In general, the postprocedural care for patients after thrombolytic therapy for iliofemoral DVT should be the same as if they had been treated with anticoagulation alone. In other words, the patients should receive anticoagulation according to the DVT management protocol used. Use of elastic stockings is recommended, and follow-up is usually with ultrasonography of the deep veins of the affected limb and pelvic veins, as well as follow-up visits at 3 and 6 months and 1 year. Depending on the clinical situation, annual or biannual follow-up from then on may be all that is needed, including ultrasound evaluation. Patients should be encouraged to be physically active. If stents are placed, many centers advocate antiplatelet therapy for up to 6 weeks, but there is no literature to support this recommendation. A common drug used for this is clopidogrel (Plavix), 75 mg/day for 6 weeks. The rationale is taken from the coronary artery stent literature, which has demonstrated a lower rate of intimal hyperplasia if clopidogrel is given after coronary stent placement.[51]

TABLE 101-2. Comparison of University of Minnesota and Venous Registry Complications Following Venous Thrombolysis

Complication	University of Minnesota, 1997[11] N = 77	Venous Registry, 1999[4] N = 287
Major bleeding	6 (6.5%)	54 (11%)
Intracranial bleeding	0 (0%)	2 (<1%), one death
Pulmonary emboli	1 (1.3%)	6 (1%), one death
Deaths from thrombolysis	0 (0%)	2 (0.4%)

KEY POINTS

- Indications for thrombolysis for lower extremity deep venous thrombosis (DVT) are not established, but patients with iliac and proximal femoral vein thrombosis, especially younger patients and those with thrombosis of short duration (<10 to 14 days), should be seriously considered for thrombolysis. Inferior vena cava thrombosis should fall into the same category.

- Contraindications are the same as for any thrombolysis in general. The main contraindication is a condition that makes the patient especially susceptible to bleeding.

- Several accesses are used for deep vein thrombolysis of the lower extremity, but popliteal vein access is now almost universally used. If the thrombus extends into the popliteal vein and beyond, the posterior tibial vein is also used.

- When administering thrombolysis for lower extremity DVT, infusion catheters should cover the entire thrombus.
- Tissue plasminogen activator (tPA, alteplase) at a dose of 0.5 mg/h is now the primary agent used in the United States. A typical dose for urokinase, where it is available, would be 2000 International Units (IU)/kg/h (140,000 IU/h for a 70-kg person).
- Inferior vena cava filters are not considered indicated for thrombolysis, but in case of loose (free-floating) thrombi or patients with poor cardiopulmonary reserve, filter placement before thrombolysis or mechanical thrombectomy should be strongly considered. Optional or retrievable filters should be considered for this purpose.
- Mechanical thrombectomy may turn out to shorten the treatment time and possibly decrease the risk of complications, but this remains to be proved.
- Endovascular stents are used in 50% of cases or more, and are then almost exclusively used in the iliac veins.

► **SUGGESTED READINGS**

Baglin TP, Brush J, Streiff M. Guidelines on use of vena cava filters. Br J Haematol 2006;134:590–5.

Comerota AJ, Aldridge SC. Thrombolytic therapy for deep venous thrombosis: a clinical review. Can J Surg 1993;36:359–64.

Goldhaber SZ, et al. Pooled analyses of randomized trials of streptokinase and heparin in phlebographically documented acute deep venous thrombosis. Am J Med 1984;76:393–7.

Grossman C, McPherson S. Safety and efficacy of catheter-directed thrombolysis for iliofemoral venous thrombosis. AJR Am J Roentgenol 1999;172:667–72.

Murphy KD. Mechanical thrombectomy for DVT. Tech Vasc Interv Radiol 2004;7:79–85.

Vedantham S, Grassi CJ, Ferral H, et al. Reporting standards for endovascular treatment of lower extremity deep vein thrombosis. J Vasc Interv Radiol 2006;17:417–34.

The complete reference list is available online at www.expertconsult.com.

CHAPTER 102

Acute Upper Extremity Deep Venous Thrombosis

Vineel Kurli, David S. Pryluck, Charan K. Singh, and Timothy W.I. Clark

Upper extremity deep venous thrombosis (UEDVT) most commonly refers to thrombosis involving the axillary, subclavian, or brachiocephalic veins.[1] With an annual incidence of approximately 0.4 to 1 case per 10,000 people, UEDVT has become increasingly more common with higher utilization of long-term central venous access catheters and implanted cardiac devices.[2-5] Current understanding of UEDVT has evolved with recognition of significant potential morbidity and mortality, including thrombophlebitis, postthrombotic syndrome, pulmonary embolism, and rare but devastating phlegmasia cerulea dolens and venous gangrene.[6,7] Pulmonary embolism complicates UEDVT in approximately 5% of cases.[8] Prompt diagnosis and management of UEDVT is therefore important to reduce the short- and long-term consequences of this condition.

To date, there are no prospective randomized controlled trials evaluating treatment of UEDVT. Despite the emergence of different therapeutic strategies, optimal management of acute UEDVT remains controversial and challenging. Catheter-directed thrombolysis after clot debulking with mechanical thrombectomy is becoming more widely adopted as the initial form of therapy, followed by surgery in primary UEDVT and balloon angioplasty in selected secondary causes of UEDVT.

INDICATIONS

Indications for endovascular therapy of UEDVT are guided by the etiology of the thrombosis. UEDVT can be broadly classified into two groups: primary and secondary.

Primary Uedvt: Paget-Schroetter Syndrome

Also referred to as *effort-related thrombosis* or *thoracic outlet syndrome*, this condition more commonly affects otherwise healthy, young, and highly functional individuals, with a male-to-female ratio of approximately 2:1.[2] The inciting event can be any form of excessive or repetitive arm activity, such as weight-lifting, rowing, and swimming,[2] in the presence of one or more compressive elements at the costoclavicular junction. These include hypertrophied or broad insertion of the subclavius and anterior scalene muscles or tendons, cervical ribs, long cervical transverse processes, musculofascial bands, and clavicular or first rib anomalies.[1,9,10] The underlying pathophysiology is thought to be chronic venous stasis secondary to anatomic compression, followed by an acute stress that produces venous intimal damage and inflammation with associated thrombosis.[11] Repeated trauma to the vessel can also result in dense perivascular fibrous scar tissue formation, causing persistent compression.[1] Untreated or inadequately treated patients may suffer from chronic disability due to symptoms of venous obstruction, leading to significant loss of occupational productivity and quality of life.[12]

Conservative treatment involving arm rest, elevation, and anticoagulation is associated with high failure rates and significant long-term disability. Development of intermittent venous distention was reported in 18% of patients in one series, with late symptoms of swelling, pain, and superficial thrombophlebitis in 68% of patients.[13] Treatment is aimed at (1) restoring venous patency, (2) relieving intrinsic venous stenosis, and (3) surgical decompression of the thoracic outlet.[14] Two multidisciplinary strategies are supported in the literature to treat effort-related UEDVT. The first is early thrombolysis followed by surgery and further endovascular interventions, including angioplasty or stenting if residual stenosis develops after surgery. The second strategy is early thrombolysis followed by a short period of anticoagulation and surgical treatment only of symptomatic patients.[15]

Secondary UEDVT

Secondary UEDVT is far more common and accounts for approximately 80% of all UEDVT.[2] It is associated with multiple underlying risk factors, the most common being central venous catheterization and malignancy. Approximately 60% to 70% of cases have a history of central venous catheter placement.[16,17] Endothelial injury at the insertion site or site of chronic vessel wall contact, turbulent or slow flow induced by the catheter, larger catheter sizes, longer duration of use, and a catheter tip position that is too proximal all predispose to thrombosis.[11]

Other risk factors for secondary UEDVT include sepsis, immobility, previous history of venous thrombosis, liver and renal failure, external trauma, coagulation disorders, vasculitis, and treatment with oral contraceptives.[6,18] Screening for hypercoagulable states (e.g., factor V Leiden, prothrombin gene mutation, homocystinemia, antiphospholipid antibody syndrome) should be considered in patients presenting with idiopathic UEDVT, recurrent DVT, or a family history of DVT without evidence of thoracic outlet compression.

CLINICAL PRESENTATION

Patients with true effort-induced thrombosis will almost always be persistently symptomatic.[19] Clinical presentation includes arm swelling, pain and tenderness, vague shoulder or neck discomfort, numbness, or functional impairment of the affected arm.[6,7] Edema is the most common physical sign. Other signs include erythema, tenderness, warmth of the affected arm, distended collateral veins over the shoulder girdle, and limited range of movement.[7,18] A history of repeated exercise or strenuous effort can be elicited from the patients with effort-related thrombosis, with the dominant arm being more commonly affected. If thoracic outlet syndrome is suspected, the supraclavicular fossa should be palpated for brachial plexus tenderness, the hand and arm inspected for atrophy, and provocative tests such as the Adson and Wright maneuvers performed. To perform the Adson test, the examiner extends the patient's arm on the affected side while the patient extends the neck and rotates the head toward the same side. Weakening of the radial pulse with deep inspiration suggests compression of the subclavian artery. The Wright maneuver tests for reproduction of symptoms and weakening of the radial pulse when the patient's shoulder is abducted and the humerus externally rotated.

IMAGING TECHNIQUES

Confirming the clinical diagnosis of UEDVT requires imaging of the axillary/subclavian venous system. Doppler ultrasonography is a rapid, accurate, and noninvasive method of evaluating venous disease in the upper extremities and is currently the screening technique of choice for UEDVT.[20] Sensitivity ranges from 78% to 100%, and specificity ranges from 82% to 100%.[20] Limitations of Doppler ultrasonography include difficulty visualizing the medial segment of the subclavian vein, the brachiocephalic vein, and the confluence with the superior vena cava (SVC) posterior to the clavicle and sternum, potentially resulting in a false-negative study.[20,21]

Venography remains the gold standard for diagnosis of UEDVT and enables diagnosis and initial treatment in a single setting. Although power injectors can be used, hand injections are commonly used and may reduce the risk of contrast agent extravasation.[21] In patients with suspected effort thrombosis, evaluation should also include positional venography, with the arm held in an abducted and externally rotated position to assess the presence and severity of subclavian venous compression.[11] It is important to recognize that venous compression in this region can be seen in normal asymptomatic individuals, and aggressive therapies such as surgical decompression should only be considered in the presence of other symptoms and findings.[11]

Magnetic resonance venography (MRV) is accurate in evaluating the central thoracic veins, including the brachiocephalic veins and SVC. It has been shown to correlate well with conventional contrast venography and to provide better evaluation of central collateral veins.[1,22] More recently, in a prospective study that assessed time-of-flight and gadolinium-enhanced magnetic resonance imaging (MRI) in patients with suspected UEDVT, the calculated sensitivity and specificity were 71% and 89% for time-of-flight and 50% and 80% for gadolinium-enhanced MRI.[23] The utility of MRV in the workup and management of patients with UEDVT is yet to be defined. Similarly, computed tomographic venography continues to have an evolving role in the assessment of UEDVT.[24]

CONTRAINDICATIONS

Contraindications to catheter-directed thrombolysis of UEDVT include:
• Active internal bleeding
• Neurosurgery within the past 2 months
• History of hemorrhagic stroke
• Surgery within the preceding 10 days

• Intraaxial neoplasm and/or metastatic disease
• Known coagulopathy
• Bacterial endocarditis
• Pregnancy
• Hypersensitivity to thrombolytic agent

A contraindication to venous stenting is benign subclavian vein obstruction secondary to compression syndromes (Paget-Schroetter syndrome, effort-related thrombosis, thoracic outlet syndrome). These disorders are not due to an endoluminal abnormality.

Treatment with an endovascular approach without surgery will result in a poor patency rate. Stenting of these segments leads to repetitive compressive trauma to the stent, potentially stent fracture, and reocclusion. Surgical resection of the compressive lever (first rib or the head of the clavicle) is first necessary to treat these patients. Stenting should be reserved for those patients who have previously undergone first rib resection.

EQUIPMENT

• Vascular access: ultrasound- or venographically guided single-wall venous puncture, micropuncture set, vascular sheath (5F-7F) 10 to 30 cm long, able to accommodate thrombolysis catheters and/or thrombectomy catheters
• Crossing the thrombus/occlusion: hydrophilic angle-tip guidewire or soft-tip guidewire (Bentson, Newton), directional catheter (Berenstein, Kumpe, hockey-stick or Cobra), exchange-length working wire (Rosen, Bentson)
• Thrombolysis infusion catheters: multi-sidehole infusion catheters (various vendors) in 5-, 10-, and 20-cm infusion lengths. These infusion systems can be used for "pulse spray" methods as well as continuous infusions. Length is matched to thrombus length.
• Thrombectomy catheters: a variety of rheolytic and maceration mechanical thrombectomy devices have been used for mechanical thrombolysis of UEDVT. These devices may be used alone or be intended for use with a thrombolytic drug (e.g., AngioJet device, Trellis device). When these devices are used off-label, the nature of their use should be discussed with the patient, family, and referring physician. These devices include the AngioJet (Possis Medical Inc., Minneapolis, Minn.), Arrow-Trerotola device (TeleFlex International Inc., Reading, Pa.), and Trellis (Covidien, Mansfield, Mass.), among others.
• Thrombolysis agents: recombinant tissue plasminogen activator (rtPA), urokinase, tenecteplase

TECHNIQUE

Anatomy

The veins of the upper extremity are grouped into a superficial and a deep system. Unlike the lower extremity, the superficial veins of the arm are larger than the deep veins and carry most of the venous return.
  • *Cephalic vein:* forms from the dorsal venous system of the hand and continues on the lateral aspect of the arm to join the axillary vein near the clavicle; it communicates with the basilic vein at the antecubital fossa through the median cubital vein.

• *Basilic vein:* extends from the medial aspect of the distal forearm below the elbow, continues on the medial aspect of arm, and joins the brachial vein to become the axillary vein.

• *Axillary vein:* begins at the lower border of the teres major muscle. At the outer border of first rib it becomes the subclavian vein, which joins the internal jugular vein to become the brachiocephalic vein.

• *Deep veins:* small paired veins that communicate with each other and accompany the arteries of the upper extremity. They drain into the axillary vein but are inconsistently opacified on contrast venography.

Treatment Approaches

• Limb elevation
• Graduated compression arm sleeve
• Anticoagulation:
  • Unfractionated heparin or low-molecular-weight heparin (LMWH) as a "bridge" to warfarin
  • LMWH as monotherapy
• Catheter-directed thrombolysis. The two approaches are antegrade via the arm (preferable) or transfemoral.
• Angioplasty
• Venous stenting
• Surgical thrombectomy
• Thoracic outlet decompression:
  • Surgery
  • Physical therapy
• Superior vena cava filter

Anticoagulation

Anticoagulation is the cornerstone of therapy. It helps maintain patency of venous collaterals and reduces thrombus propagation even if the clot does not completely resolve. LMWH as a bridge may be safe and effective for outpatient treatment or for reducing the duration of hospitalization. Warfarin is typically continued for a minimum of 3 months, with a goal of an International Normalized Ratio (INR) of 2.0 to 3.0. If there is an associated coagulation abnormality, at least 6 months of anticoagulation is recommended.

Thrombolysis

Catheter-directed thrombolysis is now accepted as the initial form of therapy.[12,19,25] Appropriate candidates for thrombolysis are young, otherwise healthy patients with primary UEDVT, patients with symptomatic SVC syndrome, and those who require preservation of a mandatory central venous catheter. Catheter-directed thrombolysis achieves higher rates of clot resolution with lower doses of thrombolytic agent and reduces the risk of serious bleeding compared with systemic thrombolysis. The catheter should be positioned within and along the entire length of thrombus; otherwise, collateral circulation will carry the medication away from the thrombus. Thrombolysis typically works best if used in the acute setting. Studies have shown higher success rates with thrombus less than 2 weeks old.[2,12,26] One retrospective study reported initial treatment success of 84% with thrombolysis.[27] More recently, another retrospective study reported 67% of patients experienced complete thrombolysis with catheter-directed therapy, while 97% of patients had greater than 50% thrombolysis following catheter-directed therapy.[28]

After venography, the thrombus is traversed with a guidewire, and a multi-sidehole catheter is positioned within the thrombus (Fig. 102-1). The thrombolytic agent is infused through the catheter directly into the thrombus. There is no consensus in the literature regarding the dose of the drugs. For urokinase, a loading dose between 200,000 and 250,000 units, followed by an infusion rate ranging between 50,000 and 120,000 units/h and higher has been reported.[12,24,29,30] rtPA is supplied as a sterile lyophilized powder in a 50-mg vial with a 50-mL vial of sterile water. The dose of rtPA is commonly between 0.25 and 1 mg/h. A commonly used regimen is 10 mg of rtPA in 490 mL of 0.9%

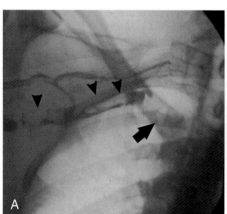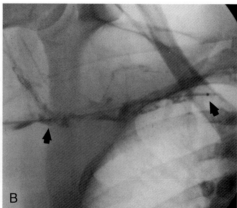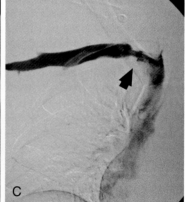

FIGURE 102-1. A, Right upper extremity venogram of a 26-year-old man who developed arm swelling 2 days after a session of strenuous weight training. Thrombus is present in axillary and subclavian veins *(arrowheads),* with occlusion of brachiocephalic vein *(arrow).* **B,** Thrombotic occlusion was traversed with a catheter and guidewire, and a 10-cm infusion-length thrombolysis catheter was placed across occlusion *(infusion length between arrows).* Thrombolysis was initiated with urokinase at 125,000 units/h. **C,** Venogram after 48 hours of thrombolysis showing resolution of thrombus. Note persisting focal stenosis of right subclavian vein at thoracic outlet *(arrow).* Patient was discharged home on low-molecular-weight heparin, then anticoagulated with 6 months of oral warfarin; he has remained asymptomatic and has not required first rib resection.

saline to make a final dilution of 0.02 mg/mL (rate of administration: 1 mg/h or 50 mL/h [titrating dose between 0.25 and 1 mg/h]). Subtherapeutic heparin is given as a 2500-unit bolus followed by 500 units/h through the intravenous site (see Fig. 102-1, C).

Catheter-directed thrombolysis can also be performed using the pulse-spray technique. Pulse-spray thrombolysis consists of brief high-pressure pulsed injections of a lytic agent into the thrombus over a short period of time through a multi-sidehole catheter. The hypothesized advantages of this technique include direct penetration of thrombus to increase its surface area of contact with the thrombolytic agent, higher concentration of the agent within the thrombus to increase the rate of thrombolysis, and minimization of systemic effects because the thrombolytic agent is retained in the thrombus.[26,31]

Mechanical Thrombectomy

Mechanical thrombectomy has been described in recent studies as a safe alternative or useful adjunct to thrombolytic therapy for extensive UEDVT.[32] Thrombus debulking with percutaneous mechanical thrombectomy devices such as the AngioJet may reduce the amount and duration of thrombolytic therapy required, although comparative data are lacking. Mechanical maceration of thrombus may also increase the surface area exposed to the lytic agent.

Mechanical thrombectomy may be used successfully as the only therapy in patients with contraindications to pharmacologic thrombolysis. Moreover, patients presenting with recurrent thrombosis after thoracic outlet decompression surgery may be safely treated with mechanical thrombectomy.[32]

Ultrasound-Enhanced Thrombolysis

The application of ultrasound to enhance catheter-directed thrombolysis represents an emerging technique in the treatment of UEDVT. The EKOS EndoWave Infusion Catheter System (EKOS Corp., Bothell, Wash.) simultaneously delivers low-intensity ultrasound energy and thrombolytic agent to a thrombosed vessel during thrombolysis.[33,34] Ultrasound energy accelerates contact of the lytic agent with plasminogen receptor sites within the thrombus, increases dissemination of the lytic agent throughout the thrombus, and separates fibrin strands to increase surface area for lytic agent activity.[33] In vitro studies have shown ultrasound-assisted thrombolysis to accelerate clot lysis by increasing clot permeability and lytic agent penetration into thrombus.[34,35]

The EKOS EndoWave System was approved by the U.S. Food and Drug Administration (FDA) in 2004 for use in thrombolysis in the peripheral vasculature.[33] Nevertheless, the existing medical literature evaluating its use in thrombolysis—venous or arterial—is limited. In a retrospective study, Parikh et al. evaluated the use of ultrasound-assisted thrombolysis in 47 patients with deep vein thrombosis, 19 of whom had upper extremity thrombosis.[34] Complete lysis was reported in 70% of cases, and median thrombolysis infusion time was 22.0 hours.[34] To date, no study exists that compares use of the EKOS System with standard catheter-directed thrombolysis techniques for venous (upper or lower extremity) or arterial occlusions. Additional research is necessary before this technique can be incorporated into routine clinical practice.

Surgical Decompression

Surgical thoracic outlet decompression as a definitive treatment for effort-related thrombosis after thrombolysis and its timing remains controversial. Many authors advocate surgical decompression for all patients after thrombolysis, which is believed to produce better long-term results.[9,29,30,36,37] Of these, some support immediate surgery during the same hospital admission, while others support a delay in surgery after several weeks to 3 months of anticoagulation. The necessity of every patient needing rib resection has been questioned owing to lack of controlled studies; some authors advocate surgery in only symptomatic patients after thrombolysis and a short course of anticoagulation.[12] Angle et al. compared early and delayed surgical decompression in a small study of 18 patients with UEDVT and demonstrated comparable outcomes between the two study groups, with no significant differences in perioperative morbidity or mortality.[30] In the absence of prospective randomized studies comparing these two treatment strategies, the existing surgical literature appears to support early surgical decompression as being a safe and effective option.[19]

Superior Vena Cava Filters

The incidence if pulmonary embolism with UEDVT has been estimated to be 5.4%.[8] Although the placement of SVC filters may be an appropriate method to prevent pulmonary embolism in selected patients, it constitutes off-label use of these devices, and there are no prospective studies to support their use.[8,38] Indications are similar to placement of inferior vena cava (IVC) filters for lower extremity DVT. Placement of SVC filters can be technically more complex than placement of IVC filters, owing to the small length of vein available for filter deployment. Most authors advocate placement of the filter in the mid-SVC, between the confluence of the brachiocephalic veins and the cavoatrial junction, antegrade to the direction of blood flow as with an IVC filter.

In a comprehensive literature review of the role of SVC filters in patients with UEDVT, Owens et al. identified 21 publications that reported a total of 209 SVC filters, 155 of which were Greenfield filters (Boston Scientific, Natick, Mass.) and 39 of which were TrapEase filters (Cordis Corp., Miami Lakes, Fla.). The remaining 15 SVC filters included 6 Simon Nitinol filters (Nitinol Medical Technologies, Woburn, Mass.), 4 Vena Tech filters (B. Braun, Evanston, Ill.), 2 Gunther Tulip filters (William Cook Europe, Bjaeverskov, Denmark), 1 Bird's Nest filter (Cook Medical, Bloomington, Ind.), 1 Antheor filter (previously sold in Europe by Boston Scientific) and 1 Recovery filter (C.R. Bard, Tempe, Ariz.).[8] The authors reported a major filter-related complication occurring in 8 patients (3.8%), including SVC perforation, cardiac tamponade, aortic perforation, SVC thrombosis, and recurrent pneumothorax.[8] Although no breakthrough pulmonary embolism was reported in any patient, the authors ultimately question the safety and justification of SVC filters and reiterate the need for additional large prospective studies.[8]

Technical Aspects of Thrombolysis

- Venous access is achieved with a micropuncture needle set.
- Venography is performed to define venous anatomy, location, and length of thrombus.

- Placement of a sheath (5F-7F) is highly recommended.
- Thrombus is crossed with a guidewire, preferably one with a hydrophilic coating.
- An infusion catheter is positioned within the entire thrombus burden. Infusion length is matched to catheter (e.g., 10 cm, 20 cm) to length of thrombus.
- Thrombectomy catheter may be applied before lytic infusion while maintaining guidewire access; repeated passes of device may be needed.
- Residual thrombus after thrombectomy may require thrombolysis.
- Repeat catheter injection/venogram in 6 to 12 hours; reposition catheter as appropriate.
- Low-dose heparin is generally given intravenously (400-1000 units/h).
- Fibrinogen levels are monitored for patients receiving longer (>12 hours) infusions.
- Angioplasty is reserved for when the underlying stenosis places the patient at risk of rethrombosis.
- Stents are not used, given the high rates of eventual fracture and restenosis in this location.
- Definitive management after successful thrombolysis/thrombectomy may require surgical decompression of the thoracic outlet.

CONTROVERSIES

The main controversies of endovascular management of acute UEDVT are (1) the role of balloon angioplasty and stents and (2) timing and use of surgical decompression.

Role of Percutaneous Transluminal Angioplasty and Stents

One of the challenges in treating effort thrombosis is managing residual intrinsic venous stenosis within the chronically scarred lumen. Several methods have been suggested, including venolysis, which includes circumferential surgical release of thickened adventitial tissue around the vein, bypass of the stenotic segment, patch angioplasty, and percutaneous balloon angioplasty with or without stent placement.[14] It has been reasonably well established from previous studies that balloon angioplasty is not effective in relieving stenosis before surgical decompression and is not routinely recommended.[14,36] Angioplasty may be more effective after surgical decompression and has been included in several management algorithms for significant stenosis after decompression.[9,12,25,36]

Stent use remains controversial. When placed before decompression, stent deformation and fractures have been reported, particularly with balloon-expandable stents. First rib resection has been recommended after stenting to avoid stent deterioration and improve functional results.[37] Urschel and Patel reported thrombosis of stents in all 22 patients in their series within 6 weeks of placement. They concluded that percutaneous angioplasty and stent use *before* surgery ignores the extrinsic compressive factors in the thoracic outlet and has a high failure rate.[9] An appropriate application for angioplasty and stent placement thus appears limited to treatment of late stenosis after surgical decompression.[2,25,26] The long-term fate of a stent placed in the axillary/subclavian junction in an active individual is also unclear. Additional studies are needed to further define which patients with UEDVT benefit from angioplasty and stenting.

Timing and Use of Surgical Decompression

The timing of surgical decompression remains controversial. Many authors support surgical decompression after thrombolysis, which is believed to produce better long-term patency.[9,29,30,36,37] Some support immediate surgery during the same hospital admission as thrombolysis, whereas others advocate a delay of surgery after an interval (e.g., 3 months) of anticoagulation. The optimal surgical algorithm for treatment of primary UEDVT remains to be established, although early surgical decompression may be as safe and effective as delayed decompression.[19]

COMPLICATIONS

- Complications of vascular access include hematoma, arterial puncture, and median nerve injury.
- Complications of thrombolysis include puncture site oozing/hematoma, bleeding from mucous membranes, and retroperitoneal/intracranial hemorrhage. All patients need continuous hemodynamic monitoring and regular monitoring of neurologic vital signs. Pulmonary embolism may result from manipulations within a thrombosed vein.
- Complications of angioplasty include vascular rupture, dissection, and thrombosis.
- With SVC filter placement, there may be a higher complication rate secondary to intracardiac filter migration or SVC occlusion with SVC filters in comparison to IVC filters.

POSTPROCEDURAL AND FOLLOW-UP CARE

Patients remain in a monitored setting while receiving thrombolytic therapy. Heparin is given concurrently to prevent thrombus formation around the catheter.[1] Heparin infusion is administered at a rate sufficient to maintain the partial thromboplastin time at 2 to 2.5 times normal.[12,29,30]

Serial venograms are done at 12- to 24-hour intervals to assess the effect of thrombolysis. The time to achieve total thrombolysis in UEDVT can take up to 72 hours.[24] Thrombolysis is generally stopped when (1) the desired venous patency is achieved, (2) there are bleeding complications or biochemical evidence of disseminated intravascular coagulation, or (3) when 72 hours of infusion is reached.[12]

The following care is recommended:

- Complete anticoagulation for 3 to 6 months with warfarin instituted after therapy.
- Follow-up examination of the axillary/subclavian region with color Doppler ultrasonography.
- Surgical decompression during the same hospital admission or after 3 months of anticoagulation.

KEY POINTS

- Upper extremity deep venous thrombosis (UEDVT) is frequently underdiagnosed and inadequately managed.
- Catheter-directed thrombolysis (pharmacologic, mechanical, or combined) is an established therapy for patients with primary UEDVT (Paget-Schroetter disease) and for many patients with secondary UEDVT.
- Angioplasty and stenting should be reserved for patients with recurrent stenosis or thrombosis after first rib resection.

▶ **SUGGESTED READINGS**

Adelman MA, Stone DH, Riles TS, et al. A multidisciplinary approach to the treatment of Paget-Schroetter syndrome. Ann Vasc Surg 1997; 11:149–54.

Baarslag HJ, Koopman MM, Reekers JA, van Beek EJ. Diagnosis and management of deep vein thrombosis of the upper extremity: a review. Eur Radiol 2004;14:1263–74.

Illig KA, Doyle AJ. A comprehensive review of Paget-Schroetter syndrome. J Vasc Surg 2010;51:1538–47.

Joffe HV, Goldhaber SZ. Upper-extremity deep vein thrombosis. Circulation 2002;106:1874–80.

Kommareddy A, Zaroukian MH, Hassouna HI. Upper extremity deep venous thrombosis. Semin Thromb Hemost 2002;28:89–99.

Kucher N. Deep-vein thrombosis of the upper extremities. N Engl J Med 2011;364:861–9.

Nemcek AA Jr. Upper extremity deep venous thrombosis: interventional management. Tech Vasc Interv Radiol 2004;7:86–90.

Owens CA, Bui JT, Knuttinen MG, et al. Pulmonary embolism from upper extremity deep vein thrombosis and the role of superior vena cava filters: a review of the literature. J Vasc Interv Radiol 2010;21:779–87.

Rosovsky RP, Kuter DJ. Catheter-related thrombosis in cancer patients: pathophysiology, diagnosis, and management. Hematol Oncol Clin North Am 2005;19:183–202, vii.

Shah MK, Burke DT, Shah SH. Upper-extremity deep vein thrombosis. South Med J 2003;96:669–72.

Sharafuddin MJ, Sun S, Hoballah JJ. Endovascular management of venous thrombotic diseases of the upper torso and extremities. J Vasc Interv Radiol 2002;13:975–90.

The complete reference list is available online at www.expertconsult.com.

CHAPTER 103

Portal-Mesenteric Venous Thrombosis

José I. Bilbao, Pablo D. Domínguez, Isabel Vivas, and Antonio Martínez-Cuesta

The importance of portal vein thrombosis (PVT) lies mainly in the complications of prehepatic portal hypertension, which in the chronic state causes bleeding through varices. Acute PVT is the main cause of prehepatic portal hypertension in the Western world[1] and the primary cause of portal hypertension of any type in noncirrhotic patients in developed countries. PVT accounts for some 8% to 10% of all cases of portal hypertension.

ETIOLOGY

At present, causative factors are detected in most cases, although 8% to 20% are still considered idiopathic.[2,3] In children, up to 50% of cases of PVT are secondary to abdominal infection (chiefly omphalitis), followed by congenital abnormalities of the portal vein (20%), which are generally associated with cardiac and biliary abnormalities (e.g., hypoplasia of the portal vein associated with biliary atresia).[4] In adults, PVT is basically associated with cirrhosis, and its incidence increases as the disease progresses. The prevalence in patients with cirrhosis and hepatocarcinoma is as high as 44%.[3]

Other frequent causes in adults are neoplasm other than hepatocarcinoma, coagulation disorders, and inflammatory-infectious abdominal causes.[2,3,5] When the cause is infectious, septic phlebitis of the portal vein associated with thrombosis may occur, and the process is known as *pylephlebitis.*

Even when local causes of PVT are present, the existence of a prothrombotic predisposition or a latent myeloproliferative disorder should always be ruled out because these are frequent causes of PVT that respond to treatment.[3,6]

CLINICAL PRESENTATION

The acute and chronic forms of PVT are differentiated by the length of time over which they develop. The dividing line between the two has not been defined, and the criteria vary from author to author. Some consider cases diagnosed less than 40 to 60 days from the onset of symptoms to be acute[3,7] in the absence of radiologic findings or complications related to chronic PVT. Others hold that acute cases in noncirrhotic patients must meet three conditions: (1) recent onset of symptoms, (2) no signs of chronic portal hypertension, and (3) absence of portoportal collaterals as shown by computed tomography (CT) or color Doppler ultrasound.[8,9]

The chronic form is diagnosed more frequently because PVT hardly ever produces symptoms or liver function disorders in the acute stage. The absence of acute clinical manifestations is mainly because in most cases, the PVT is not complete and is associated with rapid development of portoportal collaterals (cavernomatosis) and an increase in

hepatic arterial blood supply.[5,10] Consequently, diagnosis in these cases is made in the chronic phase when complications resulting from chronic portal hypertension appear (chiefly variceal bleeding) or abdominal images are taken for some other reason.

At the acute stage, symptoms are generally nonspecific. If the thrombus extends as far as the distal mesenteric branches, it may cause ischemia or infarction of the mesenteric veins, which produces abdominal pain, nausea, vomiting, and slight ascites. The pain is characteristically disproportionate to the findings on clinical exploration of the abdomen.[11] The existence of peritoneal irritation and ascites indicates necrosis of the wall and perforation. In such cases the prognosis is poor,[3,11] and urgent surgery is required, with 13% to 50% mortality being reported.[7] In cases of pylephlebitis, fever, leukocytosis, and abdominal pain are also present.

In the chronic form, complications proper to portal hypertension occur, principally bleeding through varices, splenomegaly, and hypersplenism. The varices are most commonly esophageal (90%-95%), followed by anorectal (80%-90%) and gastric (35%-40%).[4] Portal hypertensive gastropathy is rare in the absence of cirrhosis. In cirrhotic patients, portal hypertension and preexisting poor liver function make PVT and bleeding varices a serious complication that is poorly tolerated.[4] PVT also renders liver transplantation difficult.[12]

In contrast, portal cavernomatosis frequently causes secondary biliary disorders, mainly stenosis and dilation, known by the generic name of *portal biliopathy.* However, only a small proportion of patients with cavernomatosis have clinical manifestations in the form of jaundice, cholangitis, choledocholithiasis, or cholecystitis.[4]

In children, the clinical findings are similar, except that growth is also retarded for reasons not fully understood.[4]

PROGNOSIS

The prognosis for patients with PVT is determined by the pathologic conditions that cause it and, in acute cases, by the degree of mesenteric involvement. The prognosis is good in the absence of malignancy, cirrhosis, sepsis, or thrombosis of the mesenteric vein.[3,5]

Bleeding from varices is the principal complication of PVT, but recent studies have observed no significant changes in survival of these patients as a result of variceal bleeding at diagnosis in the absence of preexisting hepatic pathology,[3] probably because of the efficacy of endoscopic treatment. However, in patients with bleeding from digestive varices in the presence of cirrhosis, mortality is much higher (30%-70% vs. 1%-5%).[2,13] In cases of suppurative pylephlebitis, the prognosis is poor, and mortality may be as high as 80%.[6]

IMAGING

Imaging techniques are essential for the diagnosis of PVT because the clinical manifestations are minor and unspecific. Imaging is also indispensable for planning treatment, be it medical, surgical, or percutaneous. Careful evaluation must be made of the vascular anatomy, size of the thrombus, and the presence or absence of signs of intestinal ischemia and portoportal collaterals (cavernomatosis) or portosystemic collaterals, as well as possible local causes of PVT.

Four anatomic categories related to the extent of PVT[3] have been defined and have clinical relevance for both prognosis and treatment: grade I, thrombus limited to the portal vein that does not reach the splenomesenteric confluence; grade II, thrombus extending to the superior mesenteric vein but with free mesenteric vessels; grade III, thrombus spreading diffusely through the splanchnic venous system but with the presence of large collaterals; and grade IV, thrombus spreading diffusely through the venous system but without large collaterals.

The extent of thrombosis in mesenteric venous branches (grade III-IV) raises the risk for intestinal infarction and consequently the risk for death.[3,14]

Portal Vein Anatomy

The main portal vein is formed by the confluence of the splenic and superior mesenteric veins, and in the absence of anatomic variants, it divides at the porta hepatis into a right and left branch, which lead, respectively, to the right and left hepatic lobes. The left branch is divided into branches for each segment, whereas the right branch is divided into an anterior right branch for segments V and VIII and a posterior branch for segments VI and VII. This normal distribution is present in 65% to 90% of individuals.[15,16]

Anatomic variants usually occur in the right branch, and the most frequent ones are portal trifurcation (absence of the common right branch with direct division of the main portal vein into a left branch and two right branches [Fig. 103-1]), an anterior or posterior right branch originating

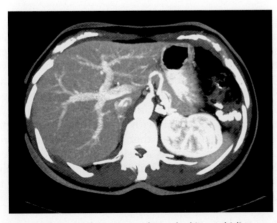

FIGURE 103-1. Axial contrast-enhanced thin multislice computed tomography maximum intensity projection in portal phase depicts portal trifurcation. Surgical metallic clips are present because of left adrenalectomy for renal cell carcinoma metastatic disease.

from the left branch, and a posterior right branch originating from the main portal vein.[11,15,16] The presence of one such variant can have considerable repercussions on surgery and interventional procedures.[15]

Imaging Techniques

Color Doppler Ultrasound

Color Doppler ultrasound is an effective technique for assessing PVT, and it is also fast, economical, and safe. This technique is generally used for detecting and monitoring PVT.[2,8] If ultrasound brings the presence of PVT to light, the investigation must be completed with another technique (CT or magnetic resonance imaging [MRI]) to more accurately evaluate how far it extends into the mesenteric area and detect the presence of signs of intestinal ischemia or abdominal causes of PVT.

The most specific ultrasound finding for PVT on grayscale imaging is the presence of an echogenic thrombus in the lumen of the portal vein, which is present in the case of both chronic thrombi and tumors, but not in acute PVT. An increase in the diameter of the portal vein may also be observed (>15 mm), as may the presence of portoportal collaterals and the absence of an identifiable main portal vein.

At the acute stage, the thrombus may be markedly hypoechoic and pass unnoticed if color Doppler ultrasound is not performed. This study will show an area of absence of flow inside the lumen of the portal vein, with high sensitivity and specificity.[4] Occasionally if portal flow is very slow, it may not be detected in the color Doppler study and might be confused with thrombosis. In such cases, pulsed Doppler imaging may reveal the existence of continuous slow flow.[5,8]

Color Doppler ultrasound also enables the specialist to assess whether arterial flow is present inside the echogenic thrombi. The presence of such arterial flow is highly specific for tumor thrombosis, although its sensitivity is variable.[8]

Regarding the use of intravenous contrast material in ultrasound, several studies have shown better sensitivity in the detection of PVT[17,18] and in the characterization of tumor thrombi[17] than with conventional and color Doppler ultrasound.

Ultrasound assessment may be limited in obese patients, in patients with small livers, or if intestinal gas is present (this affects mainly assessment of the mesenteric branches).[2]

Contrast-Enhanced Computed Tomography

Many authors consider this study to be the technique of choice,[11,14,19] particularly if multislice CT is available. Images obtained with CT offer the advantage of great anatomic detail, which makes them useful for evaluating intraluminal and extraluminal abnormalities, calcification of the portal vein intima, mural thrombosis, existence and distribution of portosystemic collaterals, and any mesenteric edema. Disadvantages include the use of radiation and intravenous iodinated contrast material.

In general, a nonenhanced phase is performed first, followed by injection of 125 to 150 mL of intravenous contrast material at 3 to 5 mL/sec to obtain an arterial and a venous phase (portal, with a delay of 55-70 seconds from the beginning of injection of the contrast material).[11] The initial phase without contrast medium makes it possible to detect

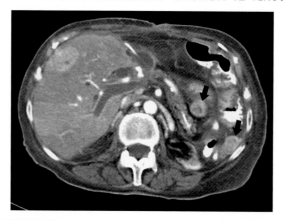

FIGURE 103-2. Mesenteric sarcoma in 75-year-old woman required multiple abdominal surgical interventions, including cephalic duodenopancreatectomy. Contrast-enhanced multislice computed tomography in portal phase shows hypodense thrombus distending portal vein, with portal vein wall enhancement and heterogeneity in enhancement of hepatic parenchyma. Hypervascular hepatic and peritoneal *(arrows)* metastases, pancreatic duct stent, and left renal atrophy are also seen.

very recent thrombi, which are hyperdense, as well as calcifications in the intima of the portal vein, and allows analysis of whether the thrombus enhances after the administration of contrast medium.[1]

After injection of intravenous iodinated contrast medium, the thrombus appears as a persistently hypodense area in the lumen of the portal vein, which is generally associated with peripheral enhancement corresponding to the vein wall (Fig. 103-2).[11,14] If the thrombus is due to a tumor, it may enhance after administration of contrast medium, especially in the arterial phase.[1] Conversely, the coexistence of hypodensity in the superior mesenteric vein, thickening of the wall of bowel loops, and ascites indicates transmural intestinal infarction, and urgent surgery may be necessary.[11]

Another common finding is the presence of heterogeneity in enhancement of the hepatic parenchyma. In general, clearly defined areas of hypodensity are observed and attributable to alterations caused by an irregular decrease in the uptake of contrast medium or the glycogen or fat content. On other occasions, areas of greater enhancement can be seen in the arterial phase because the arterial blood that supplies these areas of decreased portal flow increases more markedly.[1]

Magnetic Resonance Imaging

Magnetic resonance angiography (MRA) is an excellent technique for detecting PVT; its very high sensitivity and specificity (100% and 98%, respectively)[20] are greater than those of CT and color Doppler ultrasound and similar to those of invasive techniques.[20] It involves no ionizing radiation, the intravenous contrast material used is less nephrotoxic, and only in exceptional cases does it trigger allergic reactions. In comparison to CT, spatial resolution is lower, and the technique is less sensitive in detecting calcifications of the portal intima. It may also overestimate the degree of stenosis because the signal is degraded by turbulence, and it is not able to assess the lumen of metal stents. Moreover, much longer exploration time is needed (30-60 minutes),

it is more expensive, and in general it is less widely available.

To assess the portal system, MRA uses ultrafast three-dimensional sequences with digital subtraction angiography (DSA) after administration of paramagnetic intravenous contrast material. The sequences are obtained in the venous phase or in early equilibrium. It offers excellent visualization of the vascular lumen but poor spatial resolution of other structures and should therefore be complemented with conventional spin-echo or gradient-echo sequences.[11] MRA without intravenous contrast material but with time-of-flight or phase-contrast sequences is less sensitive, although the latter can be used to evaluate the direction and speed of flow.[11] MRA has been compared with DSA, and no significant differences were found in the detection of PVT.[20]

In conventional spin-echo and T1-weighted gradient-echo MR sequences, the thrombus is usually hyperintense when it has been developing for less than 6 weeks and isointense in chronic cases. On T2-weighted sequences, it is generally hyperintense.[21]

Invasive Techniques

Invasive techniques are reserved for cases in which other techniques prove inconclusive or a percutaneous therapeutic procedure is to be performed.[4,6,11] Such techniques are limited by the very fact of being invasive, as well as because they depend on flow dynamics and use intravenous iodinated contrast material and ionizing radiation.

Indirect Portography

Indirect portography consists of assessing the venous return time of an injection of contrast medium into the superior mesenteric artery (SMA) or splenic artery. It is the most sensitive procedure for assessing thrombosis in the small mesenteric veins.[19] Signs of thrombosis include the presence of defects in intraluminal repletion, delay in visualization of the venous system, secondary spasm of the mesenteric arteries, and prolonged opacification of the mesenteric arterial arcades.[14] If PVT has developed in the chronic form, portosystemic collaterals will exist and can limit the extent to which the portal tree can be visualized if the contrast medium escapes through them in a hepatofugal direction.

Direct Portography

In direct portography, iodinated contrast medium is directly injected into branches of the portal vein via a transhepatic or transjugular route or through a patent umbilical vein. Less frequently, the transsplenic route or a mesenteric vein after minilaparotomy is used.[22] Direct access to the portal vein has the advantage that the images are not limited by the existence of collaterals with hepatofugal flow, and pressure can be measured and therapeutic procedures carried out. Nonetheless, there is a risk of bleeding through the puncture point, especially if it is transhepatic, and a slight risk of thrombosis or infection of the portal vein also exists.[21]

Carbon Dioxide Wedged Hepatic Venography

In this technique, CO_2 is injected through a catheter with a balloon wedged in a hepatic vein, generally the middle or right vein. The CO_2 spreads backward through the portal

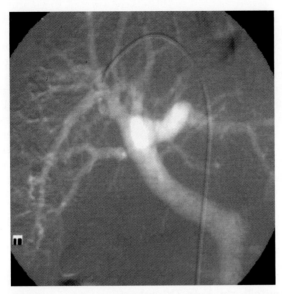

FIGURE 103-3. Wedged CO_2 hepatic venography. Portal venous anatomy is clearly depicted. A double right portal vein is seen, with inferior branch connecting with extrahepatic portal vein.

tree and acts as a negative contrast agent (Fig. 103-3).[23,24] Only one venous puncture is necessary (femoral or jugular), and it is possible to measure free and wedged hepatic pressure and even perform transvenous hepatic biopsy through the same access.

CO_2 is safer than iodinated contrast medium for performing this wedged injection because its lower viscosity means the possibility of capsular rupture due to high pressure is almost ruled out. Moreover, there are no allergic reactions or nephrotoxic effects, cost is low, there is no limit to the dose, and it spreads more easily through smaller vessels, making it possible to more accurately visualize the portal tree.[23,24]

In comparison to direct transjugular portography and indirect arterial portography, this method has been shown to be a safe and effective technique for assessing the portal vein.[23,24] In cases of widespread PVT, it is the best technique for assessing the intrahepatic portal branches.[23] Its drawback is that it does not show portosystemic collaterals as well as other techniques.

TREATMENT

The objective of PVT treatment is to reduce associated morbidity and mortality by reversing the thrombosis, treating its complications (particularly bleeding from varices in the chronic form), and preventing rethrombosis. If possible, the causes of PVT should also be treated.

This section on treatment is divided into two parts: general aspects and a more detailed discussion of percutaneous management.

General Aspects

Acute Portal Vein Thrombosis
At present, the first approach for treating acute PVT is to start anticoagulation with heparin at once.[2,3,14] The dosage and means of administration vary from one study to another.

One article recommends giving 5000 units of heparin in a bolus, followed by perfusion of heparin at the dose needed to maintain the activated partial thromboplastin time (APTT) at twice its normal level in cases of mesenteric thrombosis.[14] Once the thrombosis has resolved, heparin is replaced by oral anticoagulants for 6 months. Anticoagulation alone results in resolution of PVT in up to 80% of cases.[9]

Although no consensus exists because of the lack of randomized studies comparing different treatments, efficacy has been demonstrated for combining systemic fibrinolytic treatment (recombinant tissue plasminogen activator [rtPA] or urokinase) with anticoagulants in patients with acute PVT.[2,3,14]

Several types of percutaneous treatment have been used successfully in these patients, especially in cases of progression or persistence of symptoms despite treatment, as well as from the outset in patients with marked symptoms in whom surgery is not indicated (i.e., had no signs of intestinal infarction).[3,6,7,25,26] Percutaneous techniques include selective pharmacologic fibrinolysis (in the mesenteric artery or directly in the portal vein through a transhepatic or transjugular route) and mechanical thrombectomy or balloon angioplasty (or both), which can be completed by placing a stent in the portal vein and performing embolization of the collaterals with hepatofugal flow.[8,27] It is beneficial to perform a transjugular intrahepatic portosystemic shunt (TIPS) procedure if cirrhosis is present, if the PVT extends to the intrahepatic branches,[8] or if despite correct treatment of PVT and the portosystemic collaterals, portal flow remains slow. In these cases, rethrombosis is more likely to occur because of stagnation of portal blood flow, and it is useful to perform a TIPS procedure because it favors hepatic venous outflow, with a consequent increase in hepatopetal portal flow.[6]

Acute Portal Vein Thrombosis in Noncirrhotic Patients
Anticoagulation alone seems to be effective in the vast majority of cases of acute PVT. In one study it proved efficacious in 25 of 27 patients; in 40%, patency was partial, and in 60% it was complete.[9] Although it is unknown how many of these cases would have resolved spontaneously, estimates are that the treatment is effective in more than 80% of patients. The risk of bleeding from varices did not increase in these patients, and the risk of potentially fatal intestinal infarction was reduced.[2,10,28] For this reason, early treatment with heparin is indicated even in patients undergoing surgery for intestinal infarction.[28] Anticoagulation is generally maintained for 6 months, but if the cause of thrombosis persists, it can be prolonged indefinitely.

In cases of pylephlebitis, broad-spectrum antibiotics should be administered, and an early percutaneous approach may even be considered for insertion of drains, destruction and aspiration of thrombus, and administration of fibrinolytics and antibiotics directly.[6]

Any treatable causal factor should be dealt with to reduce the risk of rethrombosis.[8,10] There is also the possibility that spontaneous resolution of the PVT may occur when the causal factor is removed,[2,8] as has been described in cases secondary to acute pancreatitis. For this reason, some authors think it is better to wait before a more aggressive course is taken in patients who are asymptomatic and have a known cause of PVT that has already been treated.

Percutaneous recanalization is reserved for cases in which anticoagulants and systemic fibrinolysis are not effective, for local application of fibrinolytic agents, and as a first choice in symptomatic patients. Despite the fact that percutaneous techniques such as fibrinolysis, mechanical thrombectomy, and stent placement have been shown to be effective tools for treating PVT, complete patency of the portomesenteric venous system is not always obtained.[29] Possible causes of incomplete resolution or rethrombosis are progression of the thrombosis to the mesenteric veins; existence of damage to the endothelium (e.g., in pylephlebitis or after manipulation), which facilitates rethrombosis because the underlying thrombogenic tissue is exposed; insufficient portal flow; or an underlying hypercoagulability state.[29]

Acute Portal Vein Thrombosis in Cirrhotic Patients

In cirrhotic patients with lower tolerance of PVT, percutaneous recanalization should be considered and a TIPS procedure performed to reduce portal hypertension, the principal cause of PVT in this group of patients.[8]

If PVT is due to a tumor-related thrombus when hepatocarcinoma is present, treating the tumor may reduce the size of the thrombus and resolve the thrombosis.[6] Stents can also be inserted, and a TIPS can be created to palliate complications caused by portal hypertension.[30] Because of the theoretic risk of bleeding or tumor dissemination during the procedure and the limited life expectancy of these patients, the relationship between the risks and benefits of a TIPS procedure in patients with tumor should be assessed with special care. Wallace and Swaim[30] successfully inserted TIPS through tumors in nine patients, four of whom had right PVT, without technical complications. However, they did observe a greater tendency toward early obstruction of the TIPS (33% of patients).

Acute Portal Vein Thrombosis After Liver Transplantation

Liver transplantation was initially contraindicated in patients with PVT, but subsequent improvements in surgical technique made transplantation possible. It was more complex and had a poorer prognosis, mainly owing to a higher incidence of portal rethrombosis after transplantation in these patients. However, recent studies have revealed no significant differences in the follow-up of patients with PVT who underwent transplantation (including surgical thrombectomy) and those with no PVT.[12,21] The exception is massive thrombosis affecting the mesenteric veins, in which the prognosis is worse and mortality is high (33%).[12]

Acute PVT after liver transplantation is a rare complication when PVT is not previously present (1%-2% of liver transplant cases). It occurs mainly during the early postoperative period as a result of stenosis of the surgical anastomosis or stagnation of portal flow when flow is "stolen" by portosystemic collaterals or PVT is present beforehand. It can cause acute failure of the graft and bleeding through varices or ascites and may make retransplantation necessary. It can also prove fatal if associated with simultaneous arterial thrombosis.

Early percutaneous treatment in the form of thrombolysis, angioplasty (to destroy the thrombus and treat stenosis of the surgical anastomosis), insertion of stents,[5,26] and embolization of portosystemic collaterals if they maintain hepatofugal flow have proven to be effective in these patients.[27,31] In selected cases it may be useful to perform a TIPS procedure at the acute stage to temporarily improve outflow, although its usefulness in this context has yet to be determined.

Finally, interventional percutaneous intraoperative procedures have been used successfully in patients with PVT who have undergone orthotopic liver transplant surgery and in whom insufficient portal flow has been observed after surgical thrombectomy.[26,31] Marini et al.[26] successfully performed intraoperative treatment on eight patients with grade III to IV PVT with poor portal flow after eversion thromboendovenectomy or direct portal anastomosis to the splenomesenteric confluence of the recipient. They used the method of recanalization with balloon angioplasty, stent placement, and embolization of portosystemic collaterals and observed no subsequent rethrombosis. Their results are thus extremely promising.

Chronic Portal Vein Thrombosis

Anticoagulation in chronic forms of PVT is more controversial because portosystemic variceal collaterals have developed, which confer a greater risk of bleeding that would be exacerbated by anticoagulation. However, in a recent study in noncirrhotic patients with chronic PVT treated with anticoagulation, no significant differences were observed in either bleeding frequency or survival, and there was a reduction in the number of new episodes of venous thrombosis in any area. It therefore seems anticoagulation can be recommended for chronic PVT in noncirrhotic patients.[3,32]

The most frequent complication of chronic portal hypertension is bleeding from gastroesophageal varices. Initial treatment is endoscopic band ligation of the varices as a first choice or the use of β-blockers. However, in patients with PVT, use of β-blockers is controversial because if flow is reduced still further, the thrombosis may progress.[2,3,33]

Regarding primary and secondary prevention of bleeding in patients with portal hypertension, several authors have failed to find any significant differences between treatment with β-blockers and endoscopic band ligation in both cirrhotic and noncirrhotic patients.[3] However, a recent randomized study revealed that endoscopy was significantly more effective than propranolol in primary prevention of bleeding from severe varices,[34] even though there were no differences in survival. In another study, complete endoscopic eradication of varices in patients with PVT was found to significantly lessen the risk of rebleeding from 0.13% to 0.02% per patient per month, although survival depended on the cause of the PVT rather than on hemorrhage.[33] Nevertheless, in these patients, percutaneous treatments such as thrombectomy, mechanical recanalization, stent placement, embolization of varices, or decompression of the portal venous system by means of TIPS, which is particularly indicated in cirrhotic patients, have also been shown to be effective.[8]

Percutaneous Procedures

Local Fibrinolysis

Prompt administration of anticoagulant therapy and fibrinolytics has been shown to be an effective method for treating acute PVT.[3,7] Selective administration ensures a high concentration of fibrinolytic in the portomesenteric venous system, with lower systemic concentrations, so treatment is more effective and the theoretic risk of systemic complications is lower. The combination of intraportal thrombolysis and mechanical recanalization allows the condition to resolve more rapidly than with systemic thrombolysis.[25]

In view of the high efficacy of anticoagulant treatment in acute PVT[9] and the potential complications with use of local fibrinolysis, the latter should be reserved for cases where the patient's clinical state is deteriorating and symptoms persist despite treatment.[7]

Technique

Local fibrinolysis can be performed through the SMA by placing a catheter from the femoral or radial arteries or directly through the portal vein via a transhepatic or transjugular route. Fibrinolysis through the SMA would seem to be the most advisable method in patients with complete PVT and in cases where the small mesenteric veins are affected (because a fibrinolytic agent administered intraportally fails to reach these distal branches).

If the PVT is located on the splenoportal axis or in the proximal segment of the superior mesenteric vein and if distal veins are patent, a transhepatic portal approach is recommended (which will also allow mechanical thrombectomy to be performed). Although they are less frequently used, transsplenic and transileocolic (through a minilaparotomy) approaches are also feasible.[22]

In general, the transhepatic approach is used most frequently. It is easier than the transjugular route but has a greater risk of bleeding, particularly in patients receiving anticoagulants or in the presence of ascites (or both).[25] Complications can be controlled in these patients with use of ascites drainage and track embolization. If a TIPS is also to be created, the transjugular route allows performing both procedures from a single approach.[6]

Transhepatic puncture of an intrahepatic portal branch is performed with the patient under general anesthesia or moderate sedation, with Chiba needles (21 or 22 gauge),[22,25] and under ultrasound guidance.[7,35] Once access has been secured, the portal thrombus is recanalized with hydrophilic guidewires, and a multiperforated catheter is inserted to perfuse urokinase or rtPA.

If local fibrinolysis is used as an isolated measure, the duration of treatment depends on resolution of the thrombosis. However, it is generally used in association with mechanical thrombectomy,[7,8,25] either before or after fibrinolysis.[8,25] Rossi et al. achieved their best results when the mechanical thrombectomy was performed before fibrinolysis.[36]

If mechanical thrombectomy is to be performed after fibrinolysis, a short infusion of urokinase (e.g., 250,000 international units [IU]/2 h or 1,000,000 IU/6 h) or rtPA (0.25 to 1 mg/h) is given, after which as much of the thrombus as possible is extracted via an 8F or 9F catheter with a large internal lumen.[7,21]

Once patency has been obtained, if hepatofugal flow is detected through portosystemic collaterals, they should be embolized to increase portal inflow. If stenoses are detected, they should be treated. In cirrhotic patients, it is useful to create a TIPS to improve portal flow, and the same is true in the case of certain noncirrhotic patients to provide adequate outflow.

Patients should have their ascites drained if present around the liver. Once the percutaneous procedure is finished, to prevent hemorrhagic complications involving the access, the parenchymatous tract is embolized with coils or gelatin sponge pledgets.[7,25]

Results

Pharmacologic thrombolysis is an effective technique for treating acute PVT. Hollingshead et al.[7] reported a retrospective study of 20 patients with acute or portal mesenteric thrombosis (<40 days from onset of clinical manifestations) treated with systemic anticoagulants as well as local fibrinolysis because of either the severity of symptoms or persistence of the condition despite anticoagulant therapy. They observed a certain degree of lysis in 75% of these patients and clinical improvement in 85%, and in no patient was intestinal resection required. Nonetheless, severe hemorrhagic complications occurred in 60% of cases, so despite their good results, they recommend reserving this technique for severe cases.

Other series have demonstrated that thrombolysis seems more effective than anticoagulation for acute PVT and may be effective in cases where anticoagulation alone failed.[3] The efficacy of fibrinolysis is related to the time over which the thrombus has developed: complete recanalization is possible in thrombi present for less than 14 days, partial results are obtained in thrombi present for 14 to 30 days,[3,8] and only a very slight response can be expected after 40 days.[8]

Complications

Most complications of local fibrinolytic treatment are related to transhepatic puncture, which may cause intraperitoneal bleeding.[8] Systemic fibrinolytic treatment, in contrast, increases the risk for bleeding at any site. Local administration plus combination with other percutaneous techniques makes it possible to reduce the dose of fibrinolytic agent and consequently lessen the complications that result from its use.

Mechanical Percutaneous Thrombectomy and Balloon Angioplasty

Mechanical percutaneous thrombectomy, an alternative to surgical thrombectomy, uses miniature mechanical devices to modify or destroy the thrombus in a minimally invasive manner.[37] This is generally performed in cases of acute PVT. It is especially useful for acute thrombosis in patients with severe symptoms or in those who have a high risk of bleeding; it allows the length of the procedure to be reduced and renders fibrinolytic agents less necessary or even superfluous.[25]

In general, it is performed in conjunction with other treatments to improve the extent to which the thrombosis resolves, such as local administration of fibrinolytics for widespread thrombosis or balloon dilation and stent placement. Balloon dilation with stent placement is the technique of choice for dealing with residual thrombosis after mechanical thrombectomy, when fixed venous stenosis underlies the thrombosis, or when the vein is compressed or invaded by tumors or local inflammatory processes.[6]

Technique

Usual access routes are transjugular (with less risk of bleeding, preferably if a TIPS procedure is to be performed) and transhepatic.[25] In cases of chronic thrombosis, the transhepatic route makes it possible to have more control over thrombus management.

Mechanical recanalization devices can be divided into (1) devices that perform thrombectomy by direct contact (angioplasty balloons, fixed or rotating wire baskets, and pigtail catheters), (2) hydrodynamic thrombectomy devices, and (3) rheolytic thrombectomy devices (based on flow).

The technique of balloon angioplasty fractures and compresses the thrombus against the vessel wall to create a permeable duct. It also allows dilation of fixed stenoses caused by organized thrombi and is therefore useful in cases of chronic PVT. Generally a stent is inserted afterward to maintain vessel patency. An 8- to 10-mm balloon is inserted in the portal vein and inflated repeatedly to fracture and compress the thrombus against the walls of the vein, or the balloon is used to dilate the stenosis and create a permeable central channel into which a stent, usually of the self-expanding type, is then inserted to maintain patency. Before use of the angioplasty balloon, it is possible to try to remove part of the thrombus by aspiration, with fibrinolytic agents, or by other percutaneous mechanical thrombectomy methods.[8]

Other mechanical thrombectomy devices that have been used successfully to treat PVT are the Trerotola nitinol fragmentation basket, the Amplatz thrombectomy device, and the Xpeedier AngioJet thrombectomy device.[37] One other possible technique for fragmenting the thrombus is to rotate the end of a pigtail catheter repeatedly inside the thrombus or to aspirate it.[7]

Results

Mechanical thrombectomy achieves swifter resolution of the thrombosis and is therefore particularly indicated in patients with severe symptoms or in emergencies, such as PVT after liver transplantation. Moreover, it makes it possible to use a lower dose of fibrinolytic agent, thus reducing the associated risk of hemorrhage. Mechanical thrombectomy is very effective for treating fresh thrombi and has been used successfully for PVT,[6] sometimes in combination with various devices. However, it causes damage to the endothelium, which may increase the risk for rethrombosis.

Balloon dilation with stent placement is the method of choice in the presence of organized thrombi or fixed venous stenosis[6] and has been used in cases of PVT caused by portal stenosis after transplantation or tumor-related thrombosis.

Complications

When mechanical thrombectomy devices are used, there is a potential risk of damaging the vessel or its endothelium, which may predispose to rethrombosis, although in published cases, the patency rate at follow-up is acceptable. In a study comparing three direct-contact mechanical thrombectomy devices in thrombosed iliac arteries in dogs, vascular damage occurred and spread to the media in all cases.[37,38]

Use of some of these devices also causes hemolysis secondary to fragmentation of the thrombus, with subsequent hemoglobinemia and hemoglobinuria. Although this has no clinical relevance in itself, in patients who have received transfusions during the procedure it may simulate a posttransfusion immune hemolytic reaction and should not be confused with such reactions.

Transjugular Intrahepatic Portosystemic Shunt

Although the presence of PVT is regarded as a relative contraindication to TIPS because of the greater technical complexity, many articles demonstrate that it can be performed if the specialist is experienced enough,[22,39] even in the presence of portal cavernomatosis[39] or tumor-related PVT.[30]

In cases of portal hypertension with PVT, it is useful to perform TIPS in cirrhotic patients with associated PVT and in cases where slow portal flow persists despite resolution of the thrombosis and adequate flow reaching the portal vein (Fig. 103-4).[6]

In cases of tumor-related PVT or widespread liver tumors, performing a TIPS procedure may actually make it easier for metastases to spread,[8] and these patients' life expectancy is short. However, TIPS can be performed through tumors and tumor-related PVT as a palliative treatment in selected patients.[30]

Technique

Before TIPS, an imaging study (color Doppler ultrasound, CT, or MRI) should be performed to analyze the vascular anatomy and plan the operation. Choosing the correct hepatic vein to use and analyzing its relationship to the portal branches are of enormous importance,[40] as is knowing the position of the hepatic capsule vis-à-vis the portal bifurcation to prevent extracapsular puncture of the portal vein and the subsequent risk of peritoneal bleeding.[13,41] Puncture of a portal branch 2 to 3 cm above the bifurcation is considered safe.[41]

The preferred approach is the internal right jugular vein, and its patency should be tested by ultrasound before the operation commences. The procedure is particularly difficult when the thrombus has extended into the liver occluding the portal vein where access is to be established. The conventional technique of aspiration will not be successful if the portal segment is occluded with thrombus. Other techniques have been used to establish satisfactory portal access in patients with intrahepatic portal vein thrombosis. One technique is to inject small amounts of contrast as the needle is being withdrawn until the occluded vein is identified. Another is to intermittently probe with a hydrophilic guidewire as the needle is withdrawn until it is seen moving along the course of the portal vein. On occasion it may be necessary to complement this approach with a transhepatic access route[6,21,22] to target the portal vein. In this situation, only a small-gauge needle and 0.018-inch guidewire is needed. In these patients, procedures intended to destroy the thrombus[39,40] or embolize collaterals (or both) are also usually performed.[6,8,27,40]

Results

TIPS is an effective treatment for controlling refractory ascites and bleeding from varices in patients with PVT, and the survival rate is similar to that in patients without PVT. Survival rates at 1 year depend on how advanced the underlying liver pathology is and vary from 48% to 90% in

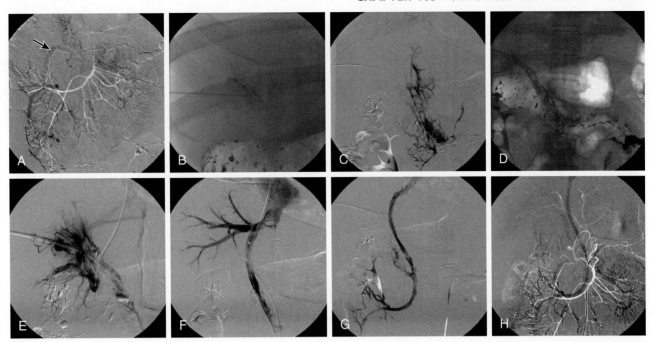

FIGURE 103-4. Abdominal pain in a 55-year-old man. **A,** Superior mesenteric angiography depicts occlusion of superior mesenteric vein and portal vein. A huge right colonic vein is seen *(arrow)*. **B,** Direct transhepatic puncture of portal vein performed under fluoroscopic and ultrasonographic guidance. **C,** Recanalization of portal vein, which was completely occluded with thrombi. **D,** Direct portography after mechanical disruption of thrombi; no flow seen. **E,** Direct transjugular puncture of portal vein. **F,** Prosthesis (transjugular intrahepatic portosystemic shunt [TIPS]) placed from portal vein to right hepatic vein. **G,** Direct portography after TIPS shows good flow within prosthesis. **H,** Indirect portography performed from superior mesenteric artery angiograms 1 month after procedure shows good decompression of superior mesenteric vein area. Patient remained asymptomatic 2 years after procedure, and TIPS was patent.

different series.[42] Various models have been constructed to predict survival (e.g., Model for End-Stage Liver Disease [MELD]); such models make it possible to predict how the condition will develop.[42]

The guidelines developed in 2001 by the Society of Interventional Radiology (SIR) for creating a TIPS to treat portal hypertension indicate that technical success (creation of the shunt and reduction of the hepatic venous pressure gradient to 12 mmHg or less) can be achieved in 95% of patients, and clinical success (resolution of complications of portal hypertension) in 90% of cases.[35]

The clinical success rate is significantly lower when portal cavernomatosis is present, and TIPS should not be performed in these circumstances[21] even though it might prove successful in selected cases.[39]

Complications

The most common complication is dysfunction of the TIPS caused by occlusion or stenosis and, more rarely, by thrombosis. The frequency of stenosis and thrombosis should be significantly reduced by using covered stents.[42] The next most important complication is onset or worsening of hepatic encephalopathy (20%-31% of patients).[42]

The frequency of fatal complications varies from 0.6% to 4.3%,[42] depending on the series, with the mean being 1.7%. Such complications include intraperitoneal hemorrhage, laceration of the hepatic artery or portal vein, and right heart failure.

The use of ultrasound, conventional or intravascular, considerably reduces the frequency of complications such as extracapsular puncture of the portal vein or puncture of

an arterial or biliary branch within the intraparenchymatous tract.[21]

According to SIR guidelines, severe complications should not occur in more than 3% of procedures.[35]

KEY POINTS

- Portal vein thrombosis (PVT) is the leading cause of prehepatic portal hypertension in the Western world and accounts for approximately 8% to 10% of all cases of portal hypertension.

- The diagnosis of PVT is best made by cross-sectional imaging such as color Doppler ultrasound, computed tomographic angiography (CTA), and magnetic resonance angiography (MRA). Invasive techniques are reserved for cases where such modalities are inconclusive or a percutaneous therapeutic procedure is to performed.

- The first approach for treating acute PVT is immediate anticoagulation with heparin, which may be combined with systemic fibrinolytic treatment.

- Percutaneous treatments such as local catheter-directed thrombolysis, mechanical thrombectomy, or balloon angioplasty—which may be completed by stent placement in the portal vein and/or embolization of hepatofugal collaterals—are to be considered in patients who show persistence or progression despite treatment with anticoagulants and systemic fibrinolysis in acute PVT.

- A transjugular intrahepatic portosystemic shunt (TIPS) procedure may be useful in selected cases of acute PVT to improve outflow, particularly in patients with cirrhosis with portofugal collaterals or if PVT extends to the intrahepatic branches.

• In chronic PVT, the main goal is to treat complications of portal hypertension. Bleeding from gastroesophageal varices is the most frequent complication and first-choice treatment is endoscopic band ligation of the varices.

• TIPS is an effective treatment for controlling refractory ascites and bleeding from varices in patients with PVT.

► **SUGGESTED READINGS**

Bilbao JI, Quiroga J, Herrero JI, Benito A. Transjugular intrahepatic portosystemic shunt (TIPS): current status and future possibilities. Cardiovasc Intervent Radiol 2002;25:251–69.

Bilbao JI, Vivas I, Delgado C, et al. Portal thrombosis. In: Rossi P, Ricci P, Broglia L, editors. Portal Hypertension: Diagnostic Imaging and Imaging-Guided Therapy. Berlin: Springer; 2000. p. 233–48.

Bradbury MS, Kavanagh PV, Chen MY, et al. Noninvasive assessment of portomesenteric venous thrombosis: current concepts and imaging strategies. J Comput Assist Tomogr 2002;26:392–404.

Gallego C, Velasco M, Marcuello P, et al. Congenital and acquired anomalies of the portal venous system. Radiographics 2002;22:141–59.

Hidajat N, Stobbe H, Griesshaber V, et al. Imaging and radiological interventions of portal vein thrombosis. Acta Radiol 2005;46:336–43.

Sarin SK, Agarwal SR. Extrahepatic portal vein obstruction. Semin Liver Dis 2002;22:43–58.

Uflacker R. Applications of percutaneous mechanical thrombectomy in transjugular intrahepatic portosystemic shunt and portal vein thrombosis. Tech Vasc Interv Radiol 2003;6:59–69.

Valla DC, Condat B. Portal vein thrombosis in adults: pathophysiology, pathogenesis and management. J Hepatol 2000;32:865–71.

Webster GJ, Burroughs AK, Riordan SM. Review article: portal vein thrombosis—new insights into aetiology and management. Aliment Pharmacol Ther 2005;21:1–9.

The complete reference list is available online at www.expertconsult.com.

CHAPTER 104

Caval Filtration

Christoph A. Binkert

Venous thromboembolism (VTE) is a significant cause of morbidity and mortality. The most feared condition is pulmonary embolism (PE) resulting from blood clot dislodging from the lower extremity or pelvis, and less commonly from the upper extremity, into the lungs. Symptomatic PE is diagnosed in about 355,000 patients per year in the United States and results in 240,000 deaths annually.[1] Anticoagulant medication is the current accepted first-line treatment and prophylaxis for PE.[2] However, in the case of a massive PE, the right side of the heart can become acutely overloaded, leading to right ventricular dysfunction, hemodynamic compromise, and possibly cardiac arrest and death. Anticoagulation alone is often insufficient for these severely ill patients.[3] Thrombolytic therapy[4] or a combined mechanical and fibrinolytic treatment for massive PE has been described, with promising outcomes.[5]

A different and likely more efficient approach is to prevent a symptomatic PE before it happens by capturing the clot on its way to the pulmonary circulation. This idea of PE prevention is more than 100 years old. In 1874, John Hunter described femoral vein ligation to prevent PE.[6] In the mid-1940s, inferior vena cava (IVC) ligation was proposed to include capturing clot coming from the pelvic veins.[7] IVC ligation was effective in preventing PE but associated with a 14% operative mortality rate and a 33% chance of chronic venous stasis.[8] Ligation was therefore replaced by compartmentalization of the IVC with sutures, staples, or clips, which reduced the venous stasis problem, but unfortunately not the operative mortality rate (12%).[8] To reduce operative mortality, the first percutaneous filter, the Mobin-Uddin umbrella, was introduced in 1967.[8] Use of the Mobin-Uddin device, which had the design of a reversed cone, was stopped because of a high IVC occlusion rate of 60%.[8] The cone-shaped Greenfield filter marked the start of the era of permanent IVC filters and is still in use. The first percutaneous placement of a Greenfield filter was reported in 1984.[9] Since then, many different devices designed for percutaneous insertion have been developed. Despite widespread availability and relative ease of use, the frequency of use varies substantially among different countries and even within the United States.

There is little doubt that caval filtration reduces the risk of PE. The only randomized study comparing anticoagulation alone versus anticoagulation with use of an IVC filter showed a significantly lower rate of symptomatic PE in the filter group of 3.4% versus 6.3% without filter at 2 years[10] and 6.2% versus 15.1% at 8 years.[11] The same patient population demonstrated an increased risk of deep venous thrombosis (DVT) at 2 years with 20.8% with a filter in place compared with 11.6% without a filter.[10] This difference continued at 8 years: 35.7% with filter versus 27.5% without.[11] In the same patient population, anticoagulation showed a substantial risk for bleeding, with 3.75% major events at 12 days and 10.3% at 2 years.[10] Because of the lack of good

scientific data, the benefit, risk, and cost of IVC filters compared with standard anticoagulation therapy are assessed rather subjectively, leading to very different usage of IVC filters around the world.

INDICATIONS

The simple idea of an IVC filter is to prevent a PE. The indication for caval filtration has two components: (1) the presence or a high risk of a PE paired with a contraindication, complication, or insufficiency or (2) a high risk of anticoagulation, which is the primary treatment for VTE. One without the other is not enough to place an IVC filter. In an attempt to standardize use of IVC filters, a multidisciplinary consensus conference led by the Society of Interventional Radiology (SIR) described an algorithm for IVC filter placement (Fig. 104-1). Depending on the risk of PE and/or downsides of anticoagulation, the indications for IVC filters can be categorized in three groups: absolute indications, relative indications, or prophylactic indications (Table 104-1). Absolute indications are situations with proven VTE when anticoagulation fails or if anticoagulation led to a bleeding complication or is considered contraindicated. The latter group of patients includes those with an active internal hemorrhage, a hemorrhagic stroke, severe bleeding diathesis, recent major surgery including neurosurgical procedures, or an intracranial neoplasm.

Although there is little controversy about the absolute indications, there are substantial differences about the relative and prophylactic indications. A large free-floating thrombus can look worrisome on imaging, and placement of a filter intuitively seems to be the right thing. However, in a prospective study, no difference in recurrent PE was found between free-floating and occlusive DVT in patients treated with intravenous unfractionated heparin.[12] Other patients with limited cardiopulmonary reserve may not tolerate any further PE and therefore benefit from an IVC filter. The problem in these cases is to define what the critical cardiopulmonary reserve is. The same subjectivity applies for the assessment of increased risks of anticoagulation for patients at higher risk to fall. Besides the medical issues of anticoagulation, patient compliance plays an important role for either oral anticoagulation or subcutaneous low-molecular-weight heparin injection therapy. Therefore, it seems reasonable to place a filter to protect noncompliant patients from PE. Prophylactic IVC filter placement has been proposed for patients with a high risk for VTE undergoing spinal surgery,[13] open gastric bypass surgery with a body mass index greater than 55 kg/m^2, or severe trauma.[14,15] Trauma patients were considered at high risk if they had one of the following injuries: spinal cord injury with neurologic deficit, severe fractures of the pelvis and/or long bone, or severe head injury. Another study showed a benefit of prophylactic filter placement within 48 hours compared with delayed filter placement in the presence of VTE.[16] All these mentioned studies used permanent IVC filters.[13,16]

A new dimension was added to the discussion about prophylactic filter placement by the introduction of optional filters. Optional filters are permanent filters with the option to be removed or converted to a stent if caval filtration is no longer needed. The concept of removing an IVC filter if it is no longer needed is based on the randomized trial by Decousus et al., who showed an early reduction of PE within the filter group with an increased DVT rate after 2 years.[10] The SIR guidelines for optional filters state that "there is no unique new indication for optional filters distinct from permanent IVC filters,"[17] but the option to retrieve a filter and therefore avoid possible long-term complications has somewhat changed the risk/benefit equation of IVC filters. Optional filters are most beneficial if the PE risk and/or the contraindication to anticoagulation is limited to a short time period (see Fig. 104-1). Retrievable filters successfully acted as protection devices and prevented symptomatic PE during catheter-directed thrombolysis in 31 consecutive patients.[18] Because of the potential of preventing a large PE during thrombolysis and a relative low risk of retrievable filters, more and more interventionalists are using retrievable filters during thrombolysis. Optional filters are also increasingly used in trauma patients at high risk of VTE. Retrievable filters have been shown to be safe, prevent fatal PE, and effectively provide a bridge to anticoagulation.[19] However, a critical comment was made that relatively few of these retrievable filters were actually removed.[20] In a retrospective study of a level 1 trauma registry, "only" 35% of filters were retrieved.[20] In a different publication, only 14% of IVC filters with a temporary indication for caval filtration were retrieved.[21] Because of these surprisingly low retrieval rates, specific indications for retrievable IVC filters should be considered cautiously. In addition to medical concerns, there have also been legal issues in the United States around the problem of leaving retrievable filters in place.

Discontinuation of caval filtration is recommended in the following clinical situations. The most important is when the indication for an IVC filter is no longer present and is not anticipated to recur. Retrieval with consecutive placement of another filter should be avoided. The patient's life expectancy should be at least 6 months to benefit from avoiding long-term filter complications. Also, the filter should be reasonably easy to retrieve, and the patient must agree to discontinuation of caval filtration. It is not so unusual that patients want to keep the filter to be protected from PE.

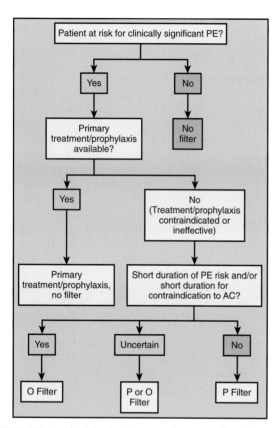

FIGURE 104-1. Algorithm for placement of vena cava filters from Society of Interventional Radiology guidelines. *AC,* Anticoagulation; *O,* optional; *P,* permanent, *PE,* pulmonary embolism. *(From Kaufman JA, Kinney TB, Streiff MB, et al. Guidelines for the use of retrievable and convertible vena cava filters: Report from the Society of Interventional Radiology multidisciplinary consensus conference. J Vasc Interv Radiol 2006;17:449–59.)*

TABLE 104-1. Indications for Inferior Vena Cava Filters

Absolute Indication (Proven VTE)	Relative Indications (Proven VTE)	Prophylactic Indication (No VTE, High Risk for Anticoagulation)
Recurrent VTE despite adequate anticoagulation	Iliocaval DVT	Trauma patient with high risk of VTE
	Large, free-floating thrombus	Surgical procedure in patient at high risk of VTE
Contraindication to anticoagulation	Thrombolysis for iliocaval DVT	Medical condition with high risk of VTE
Complication of anticoagulation	VTE with limited cardiopulmonary reserve	
Inability to achieve/maintain therapeutic anticoagulation	Poor compliance with anticoagulation	
	High risk of complication of anticoagulation (e.g., frequent falls)	

From Kaufman JA, Kinney TB, Streiff MB, et al. Guidelines for the use of retrievable and convertible vena cava filters: Report from the Society of Interventional Radiology multidisciplinary consensus conference. J Vasc Interv Radiol 2006;17:449–59.

CONTRAINDICATIONS

There are very few contraindications for caval filtration. One contraindication for an IVC filter is lack of a location to place the filter. Examples would be occlusion or absence of the IVC. In these conditions, blood returns to the heart through a collateral venous network that consists typically of multiple tortuous and small veins preventing large blood clots from traveling to the pulmonary circulation. However, if a large collateral venous pathway develops over time, placement of a filter into the azygos or hemiazygos vein can be considered.[22] Another contraindication to percutaneous IVC filter placement is lack of access to the IVC in cases when all possible access sites—jugular, subclavian, and femoral veins—are occluded.

Uncontrollable hemostasis is a contraindication for percutaneous procedures in general. However, because of the relatively small insertion profile (as low as 6F), the availability of jugular delivery systems, and the availability of ultrasound-guided venous puncture, IVC filters can be safely placed in almost every patient. Other medical conditions that could interfere with IVC filter placement include allergy to iodinated contrast agents and/or renal insufficiency. Alternative contrast agents (gadolinium or CO_2) can be used in these patients, allowing safe filter placement.[23,24] CO_2 venography before filter placement is safe and accurate in the majority of patients and underestimated IVC diameter in only 3.3% (IVC diameter thought to be below 28 mm when in fact it was above 28 mm).[24] Underestimating IVC diameter can have an impact on certain IVC filters that are approved to a maximal IVC diameter of 28 mm.

EQUIPMENT

The features of all available U.S. Food and Drug Administration (FDA)-approved IVC filters are summarized in Table 104-2. For a more detailed discussion of different filter types and new developments please see Chapter 12.

TECHNIQUE

Anatomy and Approaches

The goal of IVC filtration is to capture clot on the way from the lower extremity and pelvis to the lungs. It is therefore important to know the venous drainage, including congenital anomalies. The embryogenesis of the IVC involves the formation of several anastomoses between three paired embryonic veins.[25] The results are numerous, but rare variations occur in the venous anatomy of the abdomen and pelvis. These include an absent IVC, left-sided or duplicated IVC, and circumaortic or retroaortic left renal veins. In cases of a missing IVC, which occurs in about 0.15% of patients,[26] the blood is drained through the azygos system and is referred to as *azygos continuation*. Because of the absence of the IVC, no IVC filter can be placed. A left IVC is present in about 2% of humans,[27] either as a single left-sided IVC or as duplicated IVCs, in which case the left common iliac vein is typically missing or a left accessory IVC with a left common iliac vein is present (Fig. 104-2). Left-sided IVCs typically drain into the left renal vein, which crosses anterior to the aorta to join the right IVC. It is obvious that in cases of a duplicated IVC, either a suprarenal IVC filter or two IVC filters, one in each IVC, have to be placed for appropriate caval filtration.[28,29] Alternatively, a filter can be placed in the right-sided IVC and the left-sided IVC can be embolized.[30] The most common anomaly is a circumaortic left renal vein (Fig. 104-3), with a frequency of 5.5%.[31] In this anomaly, one left renal vein crosses anterior to the aorta and another crosses posterior to the aorta. IVC filters should be placed below the circumaortic renal vein because if the IVC filter

TABLE 104-2. U.S. FDA-Approved Inferior Vena Cava Filters (2011)

Name	Manufacturer	Retrievability	Access (Delivery Size, French ID)	Material	Maximal IVC Diameter (FDA)
ALN	ALN	Yes	Femoral/ jugular (7F)	Stainless steel	28 mm
Option	Angiotech	Yes	Femoral/ jugular (5F)	Nitinol	30 mm
Recovery G2, G2X	Bard Peripheral	Yes	Femoral (7F), jugular (10F)	Nitinol	28 mm
Simon Nitinol	Bard Peripheral	No	Femoral/ jugular (7 Fr)	Nitinol	28 mm
Greenfield Over-the-Wire SS	Boston Scientific	No	Femoral/ jugular (12F)	316 L stainless steel	28 mm
Greenfield Titanium	Boston Scientific	No	Femoral/ jugular (12F)	Beta III titanium	28 mm
VenaTech LP	B. Braun	No	Femoral/ jugular (7F)	Phynox	28 mm
Vena Tech LGM	B. Braun	No	Femoral/ jugular (10F)	Phynox	28 mm
Bird's Nest	Cook	No	Femoral/ jugular (12F)	Stainless steel	40 mm
Celect	Cook	Yes	Femoral (8.5F), jugular (7F)	Conichrome	30 mm
Günther Tulip	Cook	Yes	Femoral (8.5F), jugular (7F)	Conichrome	30 mm
OptEase	Cordis	Yes	Femoral/ jugular (6F)	Nitinol	30 mm
TrapEase	Cordis	No	Femoral/ jugular (6F)	Nitinol	30 mm
SafeFlo	Rafael Medical Technologies	No (U.S.); Yes (Europe)	Femoral/ jugular (6F)	Nitinol	27 mm

FDA, Food and Drug Administration; *ID,* inner diameter; *U.S.,* United States.

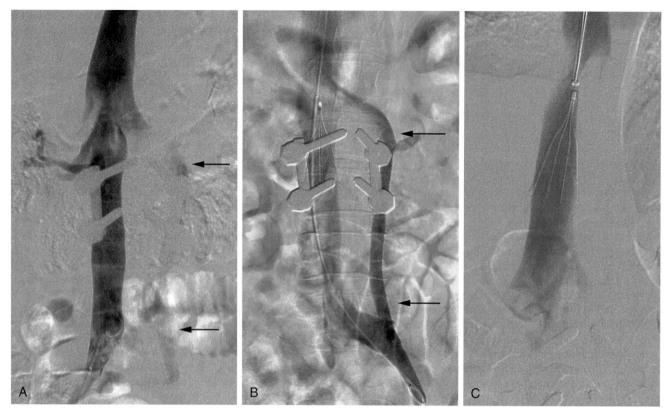

FIGURE 104-2. Inferior vena cava (IVC) anomaly: left accessory IVC. **A,** Initial cavogram showed a faint filling of left accessory IVC partially hidden behind pedicle screws *(arrows)*. Infrarenal Günther Tulip filter was placed because left accessory IVC was not recognized at that time. **B,** On next day's reevaluation, left accessory IVC was clearly visualized *(arrows).* **C,** With infrarenal filter location, thrombus from left lower extremity could bypass filter through left accessory IVC, so filter was moved to suprarenal position. *(Courtesy Dr. John Kaufman, Dotter Institute.)*

is placed between the main left renal vein and the circum-aortic renal vein, a possible conduit exists for clot from the lower extremity to bypass the filter. Retroaortic left renal veins are also quite common (≈4.7%).[31] However, because they do not represent a possible conduit for bypassing an infrarenal IVC filter, they do not impact IVC filter placement.

The vast majority of IVC filter placements today are performed via a percutaneous approach. A more invasive surgical cutdown is no longer needed because of the small profile of today's filters. All FDA-approved IVC filters are available in a jugular or femoral delivery system. For symmetric filters such as the TrapEase (Cordis Corp., Miami Lakes, Fla.), one delivery system can be used for either approach. For nonsymmetric cone-shaped filters, selecting the appropriate delivery system (jugular or femoral) is important to avoid an upside-down placed filter. For superior vena cava (SVC) filter placement, the same filter types can be used, but for a jugular approach a femoral delivery system has to be used. The most commonly used access sites are the right common femoral and right jugular veins because of straight alignment of the delivery system with the IVC. Straight alignment of the sheath with the IVC was found to have the least tilt with Greenfield filters.[32] With newer self-centering devices, tilting seems to be less of a problem even when using the left common femoral vein as an insertion site. The low profile of the delivery systems combined with the high deformability of the mostly nitinol-based filters allow placement even from more peripheral

access sites such as the basilic vein.[33] These peripheral approaches offer easy hemostasis, which can be useful for patients at increased risk of bleeding. For an antecubital approach, it is important to choose a longer insertion sheath, typically 90 cm, to reach the infrarenal IVC.

Technical Aspects

As with any other procedure, good preprocedural assessment is important. The following information should be gathered before IVC filter placement. The anatomy and patency of the IVC should be confirmed. Anomalies have to be depicted to avoid incomplete filtration of the lower extremity and pelvis. In general, IVC filters are placed in an infrarenal position, with the idea to avoid renal vein thrombosis in the case of a filter thrombosis. The infrarenal position for IVC filters is widely accepted, although the suprarenal position does not seem to be associated with significantly increased renal dysfunction.[34,35] One institution reported a higher rate of migration of more than 2 cm with suprarenal filters compared with infrarenal filters: 27.7% versus 3%.[34] For accurate infrarenal placement, the location of the renal veins has to be identified (Fig. 104-4). Placement at the renal veins should be avoided because of the possibility that parts of the filter might engage with a renal vein, causing severe filter tilting. To avoid filter migration, the diameter of the IVC must be measured before placement. There is no minimally required IVC diameter for any device, but there is an upper diameter for each filter.

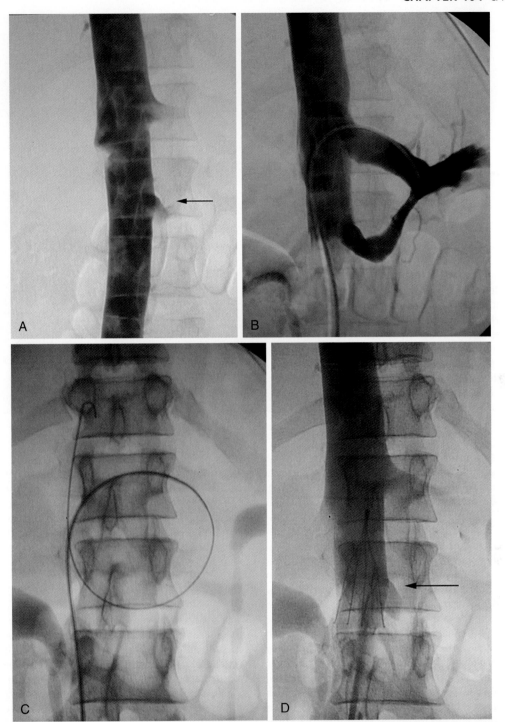

FIGURE 104-3. Inferior vena cava (IVC) anomaly: circumaortic left renal vein. **A,** Initial cavogram revealed a second inflow vein below left main renal vein *(arrow).* **B,** Selective injection into left main renal vein demonstrated a circumaortic renal vein. **C,** Guidewire was advanced through circumaortic vein to illustrate circle shape of vein. **D,** A Günther Tulip filter was placed with legs below inflow of circumaortic left renal vein *(arrow).*

For an IVC larger than 28 mm, only certain devices are approved (see Table 104-2). Also, it is important that possible thrombus in the IVC is detected. Filters should be placed above the most cranial extension of clot for maximal protection against PE. Clot extending beyond the renal veins requires a suprarenal filter placement. It is important to avoid placement of an IVC filter into a thrombus, because the filter may not open properly or does not attach to the IVC wall. In both instances there is an increased risk for filter migration.

The most common guiding modality for IVC filter placement is venography. Venography allows assessing all the just-mentioned factors at once at the time of filter placement (see Fig. 104-4). The main disadvantage is the necessity to transfer the patient to the angiographic suite. Bedside placement with intravascular ultrasound (IVUS) guidance

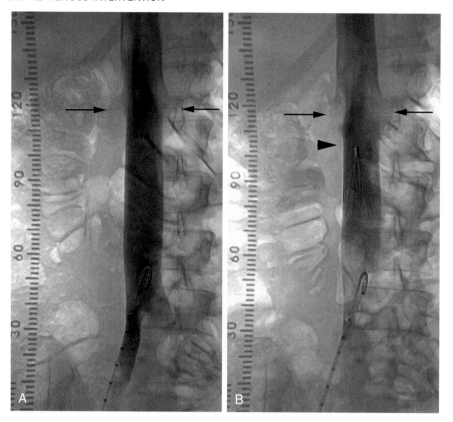

FIGURE 104-4. Technique for inferior vena cava (IVC) filter placement. **A,** Ruler is attached to angiographic table parallel to IVC to estimate IVC diameter and help indicate location of filter placement. Cavogram is injected through a marking pigtail for exact measurement of IVC diameter. Nonopacified inflow from both renal veins allows location of renal veins *(arrows)*. **B,** Recovery G2 was placed with filter tip *(arrowhead)* about 1 cm below renal veins.

followed by an abdominal radiograph to verify filter position has been described to avoid patient transfer for patients who have sustained multiple areas of trauma.[36] A relatively high rate of misplacement of 3.2% was reported, which indicates that IVUS guidance should be reserved for experienced users. A recent report describes the use of contrast-enhanced computed tomography (CT) to analyze the IVC, allowing IVC filter placement with fluoroscopy only.[37] This approach can be helpful to minimize contrast medium administration in patients who must undergo multiple contrast medium administrations. Another way to identify the renal veins without the use of a contrast agent is selective catheterization of the renal veins (Fig. 104-5). This approach can be used to avoid repeat venography in uncooperative patients. Alternatively, CT fluoroscopy has been reported to be successful in two cases.[38] The latter method should, however, be reserved for special instances because of a more difficult device localization, the necessity to use a modern CT scanner, and an increased radiation dose compared with simple fluoroscopy. Magnetic resonance guidance was used successfully for filter placement in an in vitro model.[39] However, it is unlikely that MRI will be used on a regular basis for filter placement because of higher costs without substantial benefits over the existing modalities.

With the new optional filters, the interventionalist is involved not only in placement but also retrieval of IVC filters. Depending on the design of the optional filter, either the hook at the tip or at the bottom (OptEase [Cordis]) is snared for retrieval. The Recovery and Recovery G2 (C.R. Bard, Covington, Ga.) require a dedicated retrieval cone for retrieval (Fig. 104-6).[40] Overall, success rates of filter retrieval are high (71% and 100%).[21,40-43] The most common reasons for retrieval failure are large clots in the

filter[42,43] or a filter tilt preventing snaring of the tip.[21,41,42] Maximum dwell times have not been definitively determined; safe dwell times appear to depend on filter design. Most reported dwell times for the OptEase filter are within a few weeks,[44,45] and for the Günther Tulip up to 3 months.[42,46] No time restriction for retrieval seems to apply for the Recovery filter, owing to its superelastic fixation hooks.[47]

CONTROVERSIES

The main controversy of IVC filters remains the indication for placement, discussed earlier. Technical controversies include differences among filter types, SVC filtration, suprarenal filter placement in women of childbearing age, and exact placement of filter tip in relation to the renal veins.

No studies are available comparing the performance of different IVC filter designs, so no definitive judgment can be made; it is widely assumed there are no differences. However, it was suggested in an in vitro flow model that the design of the TrapEase could lead to increased tendency to trap clot.[48] This laboratory finding is supported by a clinical study that found trapped clot within the TrapEase in a relatively high number of patients: 25.2%.[49] Comparative studies would be desirable to define the strengths and weaknesses of each filter design.

Similar to IVC filtration, the goal of SVC filtration is to prevent significant PE. It is estimated that about 12% of upper extremity DVTs are complicated by PE.[50] Safe and effective placement of SVC filters has been reported,[51] but whether the amount of thrombus located in an upper extremity DVT can be large enough to cause a symptomatic or even fatal PE is controversial. The somewhat unclear

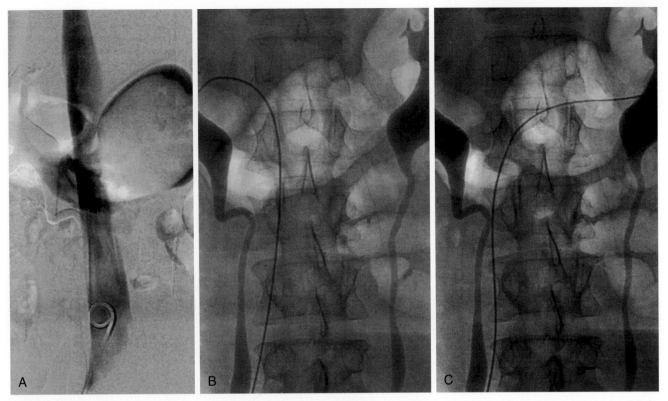

FIGURE 104-5. Localization of renal veins without contrast agent administration. **A,** Initial cavogram does not clearly delineate renal veins. Selective catheterization of right **(B)** and left **(C)** renal veins shows location of both renal veins without additional contrast.

benefit has to be weighed against the possible risk of SVC filter placement, which includes cardiac tamponade.[52] To minimize the risk of a cardiac tamponade by a penetrating leg, the fixation points of the filter should be placed above the pericardial fold.

Suprarenal filter placement was recommended during pregnancy and in women of childbearing age to prevent complications between the fetus and the filter.[53] With the availability of optional filters, many interventionalists place filters in young women at the usual infrarenal position, with the idea of retrieving the filter when it is no longer needed and therefore avoiding all filter-related complications.

Exact placement of the filter tip just at the renal vein is desirable to minimize the space between the filter tip and the inflow of the renal veins. The rationale is to limit the area of stagnant blood in case of a filter thrombosis, which could lead to thrombosis and PE if unprotected by the filter. The proximity of the filter tip to the renal veins can, however, lead to difficulties during filter retrievals. Therefore, placement of the filter tip about 1 cm below the renal veins has become more popular recently with optional filters.

OUTCOMES

The critical outcome measure is prevention of PE. In a meta-analysis, the recurrent PE rate with a filter in place was reported to be 2.8% to 3.8%.[54] In large single-institution series, the recurrent PE rate was 5.6% for different filter types[55] and 7.5% for the TrapEase.[49] In the only randomized trial, IVC filters significantly reduced PE.[11] The cumulative rate of symptomatic PE after 8 years was 6.1% in the filter group compared with 15.1% in the no-filter group. In the same study there was an increased rate of recurrent DVT in the filter group (35.7%) compared with the no-filter group (27.5%).[11] Filters did not affect the rate of postthrombotic syndrome, which was similar for both groups: 70.3% in the filter and 69.7% in the no-filter group.[11] All patients received anticoagulation in the PREPIC study, resulting in major bleeding complications in 15.4% in the filter group and 18.5% in the no-filter group.[11] These bleeding complications could theoretically be avoided if patients were not anticoagulated while having a filter, as is the usual clinical practice in the United States. In a large study of long-term anticoagulation, substantial morbidity and mortality were found: cumulative life-threatening complications and warfarin-related death was 1% at 6 months, 5% at 1 year, and 7% at 2 and 3 years.[56] Avoiding anticoagulation and its possible bleeding complications should be looked at as a secondary benefit of IVC filters in future randomized trials.

COMPLICATIONS

There are two different types of complications: procedure-related complications during filter placement or retrieval and device-related complications that occur during the dwell time of the filter.

Procedure Related

Similar to other interventional procedures, there are general risks to filter placement, including complications related to iodinated contrast (e.g., contrast-induced nephropathy and

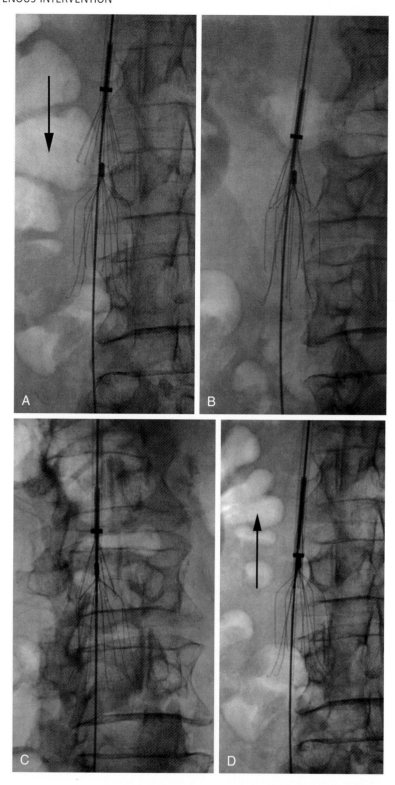

FIGURE 104-6. Retrieval of Recovery G2 with dedicated retrieval cone. **A,** Recovery cone is advanced down over tip of filter. Oblique views are performed (LAO [**B**]) and (RAO [**C**]) to confirm appropriate capturing of filter tip with cone. **D,** Then cone is closed and filter pulled into sheath.

allergy), as well as access site problems, which include bleeding and thrombosis. Groin hematomas were noted in 0.4% with low-profile filters.[49] The main bleeding risk comes from inadvertent arterial puncture.[55] This can be minimized with ultrasound guidance, which is increasingly used, especially for the jugular approach. Access site thrombosis during IVC filter placement is reported to be 2% to 22%,[55,57] but these data were recorded before low-profile introducer systems were available. The newer lower-profile systems likely will decrease the chance of an access site thrombosis. During filter retrieval, there is a risk of caval injury. The chance of an IVC injury seems small, but a mild stenosis was reported after a forceful retrieval of a long-dwelling Günther Tulip filter.[58] However, this stenosis resolved over 3 months.

Device Related

The true number of long-term filter complications is difficult to assess because many complications are asymptomatic. Filter migration, observed in about 6% of cases, is mostly asymptomatic.[57] However, in certain cases, severe complications can occur, such as a cardiac shock from an intracardiac filter migration.[59] Filter fractures are rare and estimated to occur overall in about 1% of cases.[8] The rate of fracture is possibly different among different filter designs. The fracture rate of the TrapEase was observed to be 3%.[49] Fracture of the original Recovery filter was reported as high as 7.5%.[60] Most fractures are asymptomatic, but if a fragment dislodges it can cause a severe problem, including pericardial tamponade.[61] Penetration of filter parts through the IVC is another problem. Penetration of more than 3 mm was observed in 9% of cases.[57] In most cases, small caval penetration is asymptomatic unless the penetrating part interferes with an important adjacent structure. Aortic pseudoaneurysm[62] and duodenal perforation[63] have been reported from penetrating filters. Likely the most commonly discussed complication is caval thrombosis or occlusion. Reported filter thrombosis ranges from 2.7%[55] to 19%[57] to 25.2%.[49] As discussed in the Controversies section, there is a possible relation between design and thrombosis. Other explanations for the observed differences are length and scrutiny of follow-up. The observed rate of caval occlusion varies but is likely higher when imaging is performed, because many caval occlusions happen without clinical symptoms.

A different complication is wire entrapment within an IVC filter. Two cases of Greenfield filter dislodgement during central venous catheter placement have been described.[64] Entrapment particularly occurs with J-tip wires. The chances for wire entrapment differ among different filter types.[65,66] It is important to recognize a wire entrapment to avoid dislodging the filter. Different techniques, either with a special wire torque technique[67] or with use of a myocardial biopsy forceps,[68] have been described to release the entrapped wire from the filter.

POSTPROCEDURAL AND FOLLOW-UP CARE

Before the era of optional filters, no follow-up was usually performed because there was nothing to do after a permanent filter was placed. In the case of optional filters, patients should be reevaluated within the time window of retrievability of a given device if the indication for caval interruption is still present. If the indication for caval filtration no longer exists, discontinuation of caval filtration should be discussed according to the guidelines described in the earlier section on Indications. The decision to leave or retrieve an optional filter should be made in an interdisciplinary approach. The interventionalist as an expert of caval filtration should play a leading role and facilitate coordination among the different clinical specialties. It seems especially important that the interventionalist is actively involved in the follow-up care in order to increase the retrieval rate for optional filters.

KEY POINTS

- The purpose of caval filtration is to prevent pulmonary embolism.
- Caval filtration is generally indicated if there is a high risk for pulmonary embolism combined with a contraindication or high risk for anticoagulation.
- Assessment of the anatomy and the knowledge of an existing deep vein thrombosis is important for accurate filter placement.
- More recently, optional filters were introduced. Optional filters are permanent filters with the option of filter retrieval if the device is no longer needed.

▸ SUGGESTED READINGS

Athanasoulis CA, Kaufman JA, Halpern EF, et al. Inferior vena cava filters: review of 26-year single-center clinical experience. Radiology 2000; 216:54–66.

Binkert CA. The role of optional filters. Endovascular Today 2006; September:50–6.

Decousus H, Leizorovicz A, Parent F, et al. A clinical trial of vena caval filters in the prevention of pulmonary embolism in patients with proximal deep-vein thrombosis. Prevention du Risque d'Embolie Pulmonaire par Interruption Cave Study Group. N Engl J Med 1998;338: 409–15.

Kaufman JA, Kinney TB, Streiff MB, et al. Guidelines for the use of retrievable and convertible vena cava filters: report from the Society of Interventional Radiology multidisciplinary consensus conference. J Vasc Interv Radiol 2006;17:449–59.

Kinney TB. Update on inferior vena cava filters. J Vasc Interv Radiol 2003;14:425–40.

The complete reference list is available online at www.expertconsult.com.

CHAPTER 105

Ambulatory Phlebectomy

Michael D. Darcy

CLINICAL RELEVANCE

Varicose veins are an extremely common problem, affecting over 8 million Americans. Primary management is to treat the underlying reflux, which is most often down the great saphenous vein (GSV), but even after successful GSV ablation, many patients will still have visible varicose veins. Ambulatory phlebectomy (AP) is a simple procedure that can be used to remove these residual varicose veins. AP involves hooking the varicosities through multiple small stab incisions and then pulling the veins out, avulsing them from their attachments. AP was first developed around the time of the Roman Empire by Aulus Cornelius Celsus (56 BC to 30 AD). Although an ancient technique, AP is an integral part of managing varicose veins and should be a part of any modern vein practice.

INDICATIONS

The most common indication for AP is to treat varicose veins that persist despite adequate GSV ablation. Residual varicosities can cause symptoms such as pain or itching, and although GSV ablation may significantly diminish symptoms, it does not always completely eradicate them. Even if ablation relieves all symptoms, some patients will seek further treatment for cosmetic improvement of residual bulging and unsightly varicosities. The timing of AP is slightly controversial and will be discussed later.

There are some reasons to do AP as primary therapy for varicose veins rather than an adjunct to GSV ablation. Local therapy may be preferable when the deep system is compromised and GSV ablation is inadvisable, or if the varicose veins are fed by a focal source of reflux like a perforating vein. In the latter case, doing GSV ablation without addressing the perforator reflux would lead to clinical failure. This is a more common scenario in patients with more severe venous disease, since it has been shown that there is increasing frequency of refluxing perforators as the clinical severity of venous disease increases.[1,2] AP may also be used as palliative treatment to treat local symptoms in a patient who refuses or is medically unable to undergo definitive treatment of the underlying source of reflux.

CONTRAINDICATIONS

There are very few absolute contraindications to AP. Cellulitis in the planned operative field is a firm contraindication. Operating in an infected field may worsen the infection, and poor healing of the AP incisions is likely. The multidisciplinary guidelines on use of AP also list severe peripheral edema, lymphedema, serious illness, inability to follow postoperative instructions, and allergies to local anesthetics as other absolute contraindications.[3] Allergies to local anesthetics may be a contraindication, but switching to a different family of local anesthetics (an ester vs. an amide) can allow safe anesthetic use. Coagulopathy, anticoagulation use, or any other bleeding diatheses are relative contraindications. These abnormalities may increase the risk of bleeding or hematoma. Although these are normally minor complications, greater attention has to be paid to this when doing AP for cosmetic reasons. Even relatively small hematomas or bruising may lead to decreased patient satisfaction if their goal is to improve the cosmetic appearance of the legs. Prior history of deep venous thrombosis is also a relative contraindication, since removal of additional veins may further compromise venous return from the leg. Past episodes of superficial phlebitis or prior attempts at sclerotherapy may not be actual contraindications, but can greatly increase the difficulty of AP if veins are adherent to surrounding tissue. These veins should be approached more cautiously.

ANATOMY

AP can be used to treat a wide variety of veins almost anywhere in the leg. Large truncal varicose veins all the way down to small reticular veins can be removed by phlebectomy. Part of what makes AP suitable for most varicose veins is that these veins are located in the superficial subcutaneous tissue, making them easy to reach with a vein hook. Although incompetent perforating veins that dive deeper can also be treated with AP, it is still the superficial component that is initially hooked.

Although most varicose veins can be treated by AP, complications are more likely for veins on the feet and in the popliteal fossa. Varicose veins on the feet are often small and fragile. This makes it difficult to tease them out, and the extra manipulation of the vein hook plus the higher density of cutaneous nerves in the foot can more frequently lead to paresthesias than in other areas. The popliteal fossa is another risky area. Post-AP hematomas are more common here because it can be difficult to apply a dressing that adequately achieves good postprocedure compression.

EQUIPMENT

Table 105-1 offers a list of necessary equipment for performing the AP procedure.

TECHNIQUE

The initial step is to map the varicose veins to be treated. This is done before the procedure, with the patient standing to distend the veins. The skin over the varices to be removed should be marked on with a marker. If this is not done, the varices may not be visible when the patient is supine (Fig. 105-1).

Local anesthesia alone is generally sufficient. Not only is sedation rarely needed, but it may inhibit early postprocedure ambulation, which is desirable. Tumescent anesthesia is usually recommended, using large volumes of dilute lidocaine. The large volume of anesthetic engorges the perivenous tissue and helps dissect the vein free from the surrounding tissue. The volume of anesthetic also provides some pressure on the veins, which will help decrease postprocedural bleeding.

The tumescent anesthetic solution is formulated by diluting either 25 or 50 mL of 1% lidocaine in 500 mL of saline. This yields 0.05% or 0.1% lidocaine, respectively. To reduce the discomfort of the lidocaine injection, the solution should be buffered by adding 5 mL of 8.4% sodium bicarbonate. It is recommended that the total volume of anesthetic used be limited to 5 mg of lidocaine per kilogram of body weight.[3] Lidocaine with epinephrine can be used to reduce bleeding, but bleeding is rarely severe enough to require it, and skin necrosis has been attributed to epinephrine use in one case report.[4]

For best cosmetic results, incisions should be very small, approximately 1 to 2 mm in length. These small incisions do not require sutures, which facilitates healing without significant scarring. A #11 scalpel blade can be used to make the stab incisions, but care must be taken to avoid advancing the blade in too far, which would lead to a larger incision by virtue of the blade's triangular shape. Placing a clamp on the blade can help limit the depth of penetration (Fig. 105-2). Small stab incisions can also be made with an 18-gauge needle. A Beaver blade (Fig. 105-3) is ideal for phlebectomy; it is a microblade that by virtue of its small size will limit the size of the incision.

It is important to make incisions in the appropriate direction; most (with two exceptions) should be made parallel to the long axis of the leg. Exceptions are around the knee and ankle. Here the incisions should be horizontal to follow the skin lines. Attention to the direction of the incisions will facilitate healing and reduce scar visibility. Incisions should not be made directly over the ink markings used to map out the varicose veins. This can introduce ink under the skin and result in tattooing.

Once the incision is made, the vein has to be snared and delivered up onto the skin surface. The vein hook, which comes in numerous varieties, is the tool used to do this. Some hooks are blunt and used by passing the hook all the way beneath the vein and then lifting the vein up and out. Others have a sharp barb or harpoon at the tip. The barb

---

TABLE 105-1. Necessary Equipment

- Ultrasound and marking pen to map varicose veins and perforators
- Tumescent anesthesia (25 or 50 mL of 1% lidocaine in 500 mL of saline)
- Device for making small stab incisions:
  - Beaver blade
  - #11 scalpel with clamp attached to limit penetration
  - 18-gauge needle
- Phlebectomy hooks: multiple varieties available
  - Alternate option: TriVex powered phlebectomy device (Smith and Nephew, Andover, Mass.)
- Small clamps to grasp vein and help dissect it free
- Dressings: Steri-strips and absorbent gauze dressing
- Class 2 graduated compression stockings (30-40 mmHg of pressure)

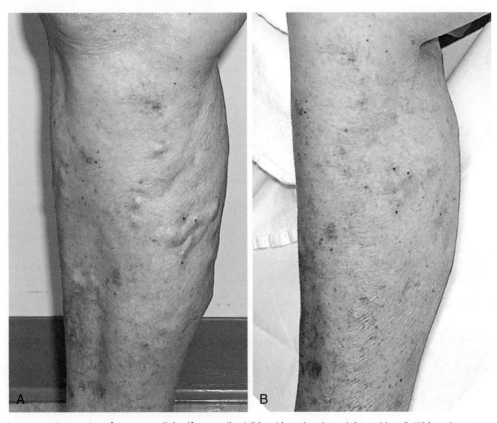

FIGURE 105-1. A, Large varicose veins of posteromedial calf are easily visible with patient in upright position. **B,** With patient now supine, varicose veins are much less visible.

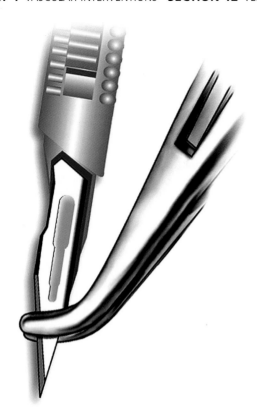

FIGURE 105-2. Use of clamp to limit penetration of #11 blade.

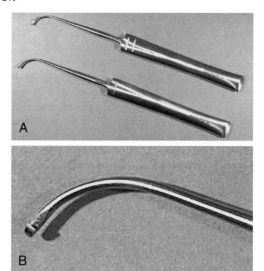

FIGURE 105-4. A, Oesch vein hooks. **B,** Magnified view showing barb used to snag vein adventitia.

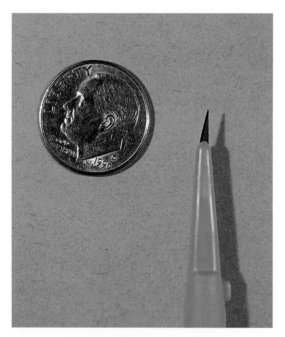

FIGURE 105-3. The Beaver blade.

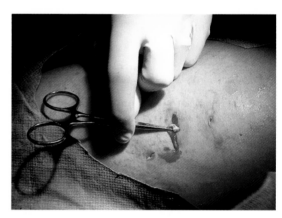

FIGURE 105-5. Varicose vein being wound around clamp as it is slowly pulled out through incision.

snags the venous adventitia and allows the vein to be pulled up without having to pass the hook all the way around the vein. Oesch (Fig. 105-4) and Ramelet hooks are examples of barbed hooks. Choice of a particular hook generally relates to physician preference, but it worth noting that blunt hooks generally require a slightly larger incision and more perivenous dissection. Hooks vary in size to match the size of the veins being treated. They are introduced

through stab incisions and moved in a sweeping motion until the vein is hooked. The hook will generally move through subcutaneous fat without much difficulty, so a greater amount and different type of tension is felt when the vein is hooked. Smooth continuous traction is applied to pull the vein out through the incision.

Additional tools that are useful include fine scissors and several mosquito clamps. These are used for gentle dissection to help dissect the vein from surrounding tissue. Clamps are also used to help extract the vein through the incision. Once the vein is pulled out through the incision, it is grasped close to the skin with the clamps, and traction is applied to pull out more of the vein. As segments of vein are exposed though the incision, the vein is reclamped closer to the incision, and tension is reapplied. This process is repeated in a hand-over-hand fashion until the vein avulses. Alternatively, the vein can be wound around the clamp (Fig. 105-5) with continuous gentle traction. Segments of vein 5 to 10 cm long can be pulled out with gentle technique (Fig. 105-6). If too much tension is applied to the vein too quickly, it will avulse early before much of the vein has been pulled out through the incision.

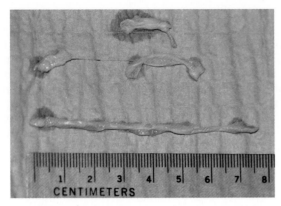

FIGURE 105-6. Vein segments removed by phlebectomy.

Transilluminated powered phlebectomy (TIPP) is a more complex alternative to standard hook phlebectomy. TIPP uses two devices, one of which is a transilluminator and irrigator that provides both infiltration of tumescent anesthesia plus a light source to transilluminate the veins when the device is passed deep to the varicosities. The second device is the powered resector, with a rotating blade that cuts the varicose veins and a suction channel to remove the fragments. These devices, as well as the unit that powers the resector and light source, are marketed as the TriVex system (Smith and Nephew, Andover, Mass.). A recently described hybrid technique involves using external transillumination to help better identify vein and side branches to speed up and increase efficiency of standard AP.[5]

CONTROVERSIES

There has been speculation in recent years that reflux down the major truncal veins may be a secondary effect rather than the reason for development of varicose veins. Based on this idea, some have proposed treating the varicose veins directly. Pittaluga et al.[6] used AP to treated dilated tributaries, with conservation of the dilated GSV. They found that after AP, there were significant reductions in GSV diameter and the degree of reflux down the vessel. Although many showed clinical improvement, 18% had persistent symptoms,

One controversy is whether standard AP with hooks or TIPP is better. TIPP has a number of theoretical advantages. Manual AP is usually a blind technique, since the veins are hooked by feel under the skin through microincisions. On the other hand, the transillumination during TIPP provides visualization of the varicose veins. Another reported benefit of TIPP is that the resector and transilluminator can be moved under the skin in a fanlike distribution, so multiple varicose veins can be removed through a single incision, requiring fewer incisions for TIPP than for standard AP procedures.[7,8] Promotional material from the manufacturer suggests that the TriVex system reduces procedure time, but in one study[7] AP actually took less time than TIPP (45 vs. 56 minutes), and another study[8] yielded only a nonsignificant procedural time reduction for TIPP. A recent meta-analysis showed that although TIPP led to fewer incisions and shorter procedure time (when varicosities were extensive), it was also associated with more hematomas and pain.[9]

TIPP has several disadvantages compared to AP. These include much higher equipment costs and greater anesthesia requirements. TIPP is often done under spinal or general anesthesia, whereas local tumescent anesthesia is generally used for conventional AP.

Most important is the actual outcome. In one randomized trial, Chetter et al. reported that at 6 weeks post procedure, skin bruising and pain were significantly worse after TIPP than after AP.[10] Although not achieving statistical significance, 4 of 29 (13.8%) patients in the TIPP group had a neuropathy, but this occurred in only 1 of 33 (3.0%) AP patients.

The timing of when to do AP is often a matter of personal preference but is a minor source of controversy. Some perform AP immediately after GSV ablation, during the same procedural visit.[11] This can shorten the length of time required to eradicate the patient's varicose veins but may unnecessarily subject patients to an extra procedure. In some patients, varicosities will recede sufficiently after GSV ablation alone. Monahan reported that 42% of above-knee varicose veins and 26% of below-knee varicose veins resolved completely after GSV ablation alone.[12] Similarly, Schanzer found that 58% of extremities required no further treatment after endovenous laser ablation of the truncal veins.[13] A trial that randomized patients to endovenous laser treatment (EVLT) with concomitant AP versus EVLT and delayed AP if needed found that the immediate AP group had better clinical severity scores at 3 months, but by 1 year there was no difference between the groups.[14] Thus a more conservative approach is to assess the patient 1 month after GSV ablation, see if the varicose veins have shrunk or not, and then decide if AP should be performed.

OUTCOMES

Results with AP are quite good, since this procedure actually removes the varicose veins. One study of 30 patients reported 100% eradication of 273 truncal vein segments removed by AP done concurrently with laser ablation of the GSV.[11] This high degree of initial technical success is common, but recurrence of varicose veins is not rare. Sadick[15] reported greater than 90% long-term success for AP, thus 10% recurrence. Others have reported recurrent or residual varicose veins in 9% to 21% of patients.[8,16]

However, in comparison to other therapies, AP seems to fare well. A randomized trial[17] between phlebectomy and compression sclerotherapy reported much lower recurrence rates for AP. The recurrence rates for phlebectomy and sclerotherapy were 3% and 25%, respectively, at 1 year. The 2-year postprocedure recurrence rate for sclerotherapy had increased to 38%, but there was no further increase in recurrence for the AP group. As a gauge of overall success, one might consider the results of patient satisfaction surveys. Patients report being satisfied with the results in 87% to 91% of cases.[8,18]

COMPLICATIONS

Complications are uncommon, but many patients are very focused on the cosmetic result. Thus minor hematoma or discoloration that might be considered inconsequential after other interventions may cause great distress in AP

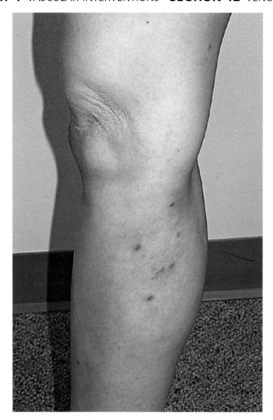

FIGURE 105-7. Hyperpigmented areas beneath phlebectomy incisions. Over time, these faded to near-normal skin color.

patients. Hyperpigmentation (Fig. 105-7) occurs in 5% to 7% of patients, but it usually fades spontaneously within a few months.[11,19] Hematomas are relatively common and are seen more often in areas like the popliteal fossa, where it is difficult to achieve adequate compression with the dressing. In one study,[7] hematoma occurred in 45% of patients after TIPP and in 25% after conventional AP. In another series, as many as 7% of TIPP patients needed a second operation to surgically evacuate hematomas.[18] Transient edema in the surgical region will occur in about 10% of cases.[11] If a segment of vein is not completely removed, the remaining component can become inflamed. This phlebitis can often be managed conservatively with heat and antiinflammatory medications. In severe cases, the inflamed vein segment may be have to be removed by repeat phlebectomy. Wound infection and cellulitis has been reported in 6% and 3.5% of cases, respectively.[16]

Telangiectatic matting is an uncommon complication seen in about 3% to 4% of cases. It consists of clusters of new telangiectasias clustered near the phlebectomy site. The etiology of this process is uncertain. These telangiectasias may disappear spontaneously after several months, so a period of observation is warranted. Sclerotherapy or external laser therapy can be used in those cases that do not resolve spontaneously.

Another uncommon complication, 0.6% incidence in one series,[19] is damage to small cutaneous nerves. This can result in postoperative paresthesias or pain. Even rarer is temporary foot drop, which can be caused by damage to the peroneal nerve when doing AP in the popliteal fossa. There is little that can be done to treat these nerve complications, so prevention is critical. One must pay careful attention to the tissues that are pulled out on the vein hook. Nerves look like fine white threads. An advantage of using dilute tumescent anesthesia is that the patient may feel discomfort if the nerve is pulled by the vein hook, thus alerting you to redirect the hook.

There are other rare complications such as development of a lymphocele in a calf after AP,[20] and necrotizing fasciitis that occured in one case after AP and GSV stripping.[21] A rare complication unique to TIPP is skin perforation by the resector. This has been reported in a few cases[16,18,22] but was successfully treated in all cases by simply suturing the hole closed.

POSTPROCEDURE AND FOLLOW-UP CARE

Since the veins are not usually ligated, hemostasis is achieved by manual compression during the procedure and then by a compressive dressing applied at the end. Because incisions are only 1 to 3 mm in length, no sutures are necessary, and incisions can be closed with simple Steri-strips.

The postprocedure dressing is crucial to a good result. Each incision should be covered with sterile gauze or another form of sterile absorbent padding. The absorbent layer should be taped in place with care to avoid excessive tension on the tape. Tension is not necessary, since the outer elastic layer will hold the inner layers in place and provide the necessary compression. Excessive tension on the tape can cause skin blistering under the tape.

Over the absorbent layer, a compression layer is required to reduce swelling and hematoma formation. Preventing hematomas will not only decrease immediate postoperative pain but also improve the long-term result by decreasing the amount of bruising or pigmentation. Compression can be applied with Ace wraps, but commercial elastic compression stockings are easier to apply correctly and are more likely to maintain appropriate pressure. Stockings should be a class 2 graduated compression stocking that will apply 30 to 40 mmHg of pressure. Since these have to be individually fitted to each patient, it is best to measure legs for stocking size during the initial pre-procedural visit.

Immediate postprocedure instructions are fairly simple. Patients should be encouraged to ambulate, which along with their compression stockings should prevent deep venous thrombosis. Bed rest is not necessary, and return to work is possible the following day. When the patient is at rest, leg elevation can be helpful to reduce swelling. Over-the-counter antiinflammatory medications and analgesics are sufficient, since postoperative pain is generally very mild. Anticoagulation is unnecessary, since the patient remains ambulatory.

The first follow-up visit should be 24 to 48 hours after the procedure. At this visit, the dressings should be removed to allow wound cleansing and inspection. After 2 days, showering over the incisions is permissible, but incisions should not be soaked in a tub, pool, or lake for at least a week. Compression stockings should be worn for another week after AP of typical varicose veins and 2 weeks if very large veins were removed. With careful attention to technique and postoperative care, AP can provide an easy and satisfying solution to some varicose veins.

- Phlebectomy is a well-established technique for removing varicose veins by hooking the varicosities through multiple small stab incisions and then pulling out the veins.
- The tools needed for phlebectomy are simple and inexpensive.
- Phlebectomy can be done as an outpatient procedure under local anesthesia.
- Excellent symptom relief and cosmetic results can be achieved in most patients.

▶ **SUGGESTED READINGS**

Kundu S, Grassi CJ, Khilnani NM, et al. Multi-disciplinary quality improvement guidelines for the treatment of lower extremity superficial venous insufficiency with ambulatory phlebectomy from the Society of Interventional Radiology, Cardiovascular Interventional Radiological Society of Europe, American College of Phlebology and Canadian Interventional Radiology Association. J Vasc Interv Radiol 2010;21(1):1–13.

Pittaluga P, Chastanet S, Locret T, Barbe R. The effect of isolated phlebectomy on reflux and diameter of the great saphenous vein: a prospective study. Eur J Vasc Endovasc Surg 2010;40(1):122–8.

Sadick NS. Advances in the treatment of varicose veins: ambulatory phlebectomy, foam sclerotherapy, endovascular laser, and radiofrequency closure. Dermatol Clin 2005;23(3):443–55

Scavee V. Transilluminated powered phlebectomy: not enough advantages? Review of the literature. Eur J Vasc Endovasc Surg 2006;31(3):316–9.

The complete reference list is available online at www.expertconsult.com

CHAPTER 106

Great Saphenous Vein Ablation

Robert J. Min and Neil M. Khilnani

Chronic venous insufficiency (CVI) is extraordinarily common, with estimates of up to 25% of women and 10% of men suffering from some form of CVI.[1] Most patients with CVI have symptoms that interfere with daily living (e.g., leg aches, fatigue, throbbing, heaviness, night cramps). Severe cases can lead to skin damage resulting from chronic venous hypertension (e.g., eczema, edema, hyperpigmentation, lipodermatosclerosis).

The majority of patients with leg ulceration have superficial venous insufficiency (SVI) as the primary underlying cause, with SVI being the sole factor in 20%.[2]

Initial treatment includes graduated compression and wound care, but long-term control is dependent on the ability to successfully treat the underlying venous disease. Many patients with SVI also seek to rid their legs of spider veins, varicose veins, or other sequelae of SVI, and though not life threatening, the unsightly appearance of CVI can and often does adversely affect quality of life.

Patients with symptoms typical of CVI and clinical signs of CVI require further evaluation with duplex ultrasound (DUS).[3,4] The goal of DUS evaluation is to map out all the incompetent venous pathways responsible for the patient's condition, including the primary or highest points of reflux and the presence of obstruction.[3] Such a map is necessary to determine the best treatment plan.

Over the past 6 years, reports of impressive clinical success and low complication rates have made endovenous laser ablation the treatment of choice for eliminating reflux in incompetent truncal veins.

INDICATIONS

Medical treatment should be contemplated when varicose vein symptoms persist despite conservative methods such as graduated compression and exercise. Other indications may include treatment or prevention of complications arising from chronic venous hypertension, such as bleeding, superficial thrombophlebitis, and skin damage. Patients who are unable or unwilling to tolerate long-term compression or those desiring cosmetic improvement may also be candidates for medical intervention. Indications for endovenous ablation of incompetent truncal veins are similar to those for surgical ligation and stripping.

CONTRAINDICATIONS

Many of the exclusion criteria for sclerotherapy are also relative contraindications to endovenous treatment, including dependency on the saphenous system for venous drainage because of significant deep venous obstruction, active deep venous thrombosis (DVT), nonpalpable pedal pulses, inability to ambulate, general poor health, or women who are pregnant or nursing. Additional relative contraindications to all catheter-based endovenous ablation techniques are nontraversable vein segments as a result of either

thrombosis or extreme tortuosity. Fortunately, these findings are uncommon and should be recognized on pretreatment venous DUS mapping.

EQUIPMENT

Please visit www.expertconsult.com for a listing of the necessary equipment.

TECHNIQUE

Anatomy and Approach

Before treatment, the abnormal venous pathways are mapped with ultrasound guidance, and the veins to be treated are marked on the overlying skin with the patient standing. Additional important landmarks such as the entry point, junctions, aneurysmal segments, and areas of significant blood flow from tributaries or perforators should be noted.

Endovenous ablation of the great saphenous vein (GSV) is performed with the patient in the supine or oblique position and the hip slightly turned to expose the course of the GSV. When the small saphenous vein (SSV) is the target, patients are placed prone with their feet hanging off the end of the table to relax the calf muscle and popliteal fossa. Treating multiple sources of venous reflux may require multiple repositioning and repeat preparation.

In almost all cases, the target vein is entered or access is gained via one of its direct tributaries. Entry through a tributary should be attempted only if the vein is relatively straight and of sufficient diameter, because these veins tend to be more prone to venospasm and can be more difficult to traverse. In general, the vein is punctured at or just peripheral to the lowest level of truncal reflux as determined by DUS. At this point, saphenous vein diameter abruptly decreases, and it regains its competence after escape of the refluxing blood through incompetent varicose tributaries. Saphenous vein incompetence can occur segmentally. Reflux escaping through a tributary vein can reenter the saphenous vein at a lower level. In this case, the lowest incompetent vein segment should be accessed and all refluxing vein segments ablated via one puncture. At times, however, more than one puncture may be necessary.

Technical Aspects

The target vein is entered with either a 19- or 21-gauge needle under real-time ultrasound guidance with a single-wall technique. Using reverse Trendelenburg positioning and keeping the procedure room warm until access is achieved will help minimize shrinkage. Other ancillary procedures advocated by some practitioners to maximize vein size include a heating pad or a small amount of nitroglycerin paste at the access point. Non-GSV segments are especially prone to venospasm, so particular care must be taken when accessing a tributary vein segment or a truncal vein such as the anterior accessory GSV, SSV, or thigh circumflex vein.

A 5F vascular introducer sheath with markings is inserted over a guidewire into the vein and passed through the entire abnormal segment into a more central vein. A bare-tipped laser fiber is inserted into the sheath. The sheath is then pulled back to expose the tip of the fiber, and the fiber is locked in place. Under ultrasound guidance, the introducer sheath and fiber are withdrawn out of the deep veins and positioned within the superficial venous system at the junction, as seen in Figure 106-1. The fiber is left in this position during tumescent anesthetic administration and will be repositioned just before delivery of laser energy. Confirmation of position can be made by direct visualization of the red aiming beam through the skin.

An important part of the procedure is correct delivery of perivenous tumescent anesthesia. Proper use of tumescent anesthesia should make endovenous laser therapy painless, without the need for intravenous sedation or general anesthesia. In fact, it can be argued that sedation adds risk to endovenous laser ablation by blunting patient feedback during the procedure, as well as delaying immediate postprocedure ambulation.

In addition to making the procedure painless, tumescent anesthesia is used to maximize the safety and efficacy of endovenous laser treatment (EVLT). Although venospasm may occur in some veins, proper delivery of tumescent fluid into the perivenous space will ensure compression of the vein around the laser fiber and achieve contact between the vein walls and laser fiber tip. This will allow adequate transfer of laser energy to the target vein walls and result in vein wall damage and subsequent fibrosis. Inadequate vein emptying with too much blood remaining within the vein will lead to suboptimal heating of the vein wall. In this case, the occlusion may be due to thrombosis, which will inevitably result in recanalization.

Many practitioners believe the surrounding cuff of tumescent fluid also serves as a protective barrier to prevent heating of nontarget tissues, including skin, nerves, arteries, and deep veins. Injection of tumescent fluid in the proper plane can be achieved only with DUS guidance. The tumescent fluid should be delivered between the target vein and adjacent nontarget tissues. We prefer to deliver the tumescent anesthetic by hand pressure from a 25-gauge needle attached to a 20-mL syringe. For right-handed operators, the tumescent fluid is injected distally to proximally. Skin punctures are required every 3 to 5 cm until the proper perivenous tissue plane is located. Once this occurs, fluid will track more easily up and around the target vein, and greater distances can be covered with each needle puncture.

To treat a 45-cm segment of vein, approximately 100 to 150 mL of 0.1% lidocaine neutralized with sodium bicarbonate may be required. This mixture can be made by diluting 50 mL of 1% lidocaine in 450 mL of normal saline and adding 5 to 10 mL of 8.4% sodium bicarbonate. If it is anticipated that larger volumes of tumescent anesthetic will be necessary, a concentration of 0.05% lidocaine can be used effectively. These amounts of lidocaine are well within the safe doses of 4.5 mg/kg of lidocaine without epinephrine and 7 mg/kg with epinephrine. Although many practitioners choose to use lidocaine with epinephrine to maximize venospasm and minimize bruising, we achieve adequate and complete vein emptying with plain lidocaine and avoid the risk of toxicity related to epinephrine.

After administration of tumescent anesthesia, ultrasound is used to check for adequacy. A centimeter halo of fluid surrounding the target vein or separating the vein from the overlying skin has been found to be sufficient, as demonstrated in Figure 106-2. Proper delivery of tumescent fluid may be particularly useful for maximizing procedural safety when performing endovenous laser therapy in certain locations such as tributaries close to the skin, the SSV near the saphenopopliteal junction, or the GSV below the knee, owing to the close proximity of nerves or arterial branches. Adequacy of separation of arterial branches from the target vein can be checked with color Doppler ultrasound.

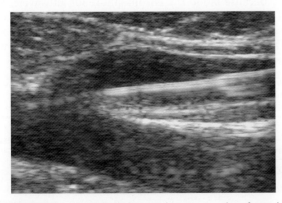

FIGURE 106-1. Longitudinal ultrasound image at saphenofemoral junction during laser fiber positioning. Fiber and sheath are pulled out of femoral vein and positioned within great saphenous vein.

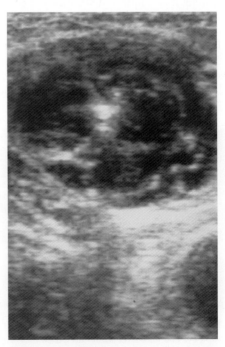

FIGURE 106-2. Transaxial ultrasound image demonstrating a halo of tumescent fluid surrounding saphenous vein compressed onto laser fiber.

Placing the patient in the Trendelenburg position (head down) either before or after the delivery of tumescent anesthesia will facilitate vein emptying. Proper tumescent anesthesia and Trendelenburg position will result in sufficient contact of the laser fiber and vein wall. If additional vein emptying is necessary, other maneuvers can be attempted, including raising the leg, using manual compression, applying suction to the sheath, or cooling the room to induce vasospasm. Because the laser fiber can move during the administration of tumescent anesthesia, the laser fiber is repositioned before delivery of the laser energy. For the GSV, the fiber tip is positioned at or below a competent superficial epigastric vein, or 5 to 10 mm peripheral to the saphenofemoral junction. When treating the SSV, seeing the fiber tip can be difficult because of the acute angle taken by the SSV as it dives to join the popliteal vein. After delivery of tumescent anesthesia and flattening of this angle, the laser fiber tip may be more easily visualized with ultrasound. Accurate preprocedure marking of the saphenopopliteal junction is important, and when used with the red aiming beam will enable precise positioning of the laser fiber. Even in obese patients, this red light can be seen, although dimming the room lights may be necessary. Optimally, the laser fiber tip is placed 10 to 15 mm peripheral to the saphenopopliteal junction where the SSV turns parallel to the skin just below the popliteal fossa.

The marked vascular introducer sheath and fiber are withdrawn together during laser activation, as seen in Figure 106-3. In our practice, 810-nm diode laser energy is delivered in "continuous mode" at 14 W. The amount of laser energy necessary to result in nearly 100% vein closure seems to be at least 70 J/cm throughout the treated segment.[9] The average pullback rate to accomplish such closure is 2 mm/s. Although automatic pullback devices are available, they are an unnecessary expense. Most manufacturers of endovenous laser ablation kits now provide marked vascular sheaths. When used with the elapsed time display of the laser system, it is simple to determine the pullback rate. This combination permits both accurate and standardized delivery of laser energy. Simple manual withdrawal also allows delivery of laser energy to be customized to the particular vein segment being treated, which enhances treatment efficacy and safety. For example, when treating the GSV, higher laser energy is delivered to the most central

portion of the vein, with the first 10 to 15 cm of the vein treated at 140 J/cm, which is achieved by withdrawing the laser fiber at a rate of 1 mm/s. This segment of the GSV is the most prone to treatment failure and the least susceptible to venospasm. Thus, it is necessary to deliver proportionately larger amounts of tumescent anesthesia and more laser energy to adequately treat this important vein segment. Higher laser energy is also delivered in regions of blood inflow, such as near junctions with incompetent tributaries or refluxing perforators. When treating vein segments close to the skin, such as the SSV near the saphenopopliteal junction or the GSV below the knee, faster laser fiber withdrawal rates of approximately 3 mm/s are used to minimize the risk of injury to nontarget tissues. These laser energy parameter guidelines are outlined in Table 106-1.

Class II (30-40 mmHg) graduated compression stockings are placed on the patient immediately after EVLT and worn for a minimum of 2 weeks at all times, except to sleep or shower. The purpose of graduated support stockings is to lower the risk of superficial thrombophlebitis in tributary varices, which will shrink once the underlying saphenous vein reflux is eliminated. Graduated compression stockings, in addition to immediate and frequent ambulation after EVLT, also increases the velocity of blood flow in the deep veins and thus reduces the likelihood of DVT.

CONTROVERSIES

Most treatment failures seem to occur within the first year after treatment, with the majority becoming evident by 6 months. The proximal portions of truncal veins appear to be the most difficult to treat successfully.[10] These vein segments are exposed to the highest central venous pressure and are the least prone to venospasm, so emptying the vein with Trendelenburg positioning, tumescent anesthesia, or other means is especially important. Because transfer of laser energy to the vein walls via direct contact with the laser fiber tip is the predominant mechanism of action of endovenous laser ablation, maximizing this contact will result in sufficient vein wall damage, with eventual fibrosis. It has been postulated by some investigators that absorption of laser energy by blood plays a role in homogeneous distribution of thermal damage to the inner vein wall[11]; however, it is apparent from mathematical calculation that steam formation from blood absorption is grossly inadequate to result in significant vein wall damage.[12] Furthermore, because blood is a chromophore for all wavelengths used for endovenous laser ablation, delivery of laser energy into a blood-filled vein will result in inadequate vein wall damage and nonocclusion or occlusion by thrombosis, with eventual reopening.

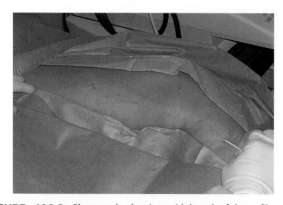

FIGURE 106-3. Photograph showing withdrawal of laser fiber and marked sheath. Fiber and introducer sheath are pulled back at an average rate of 2 mm/s as 14 W of laser energy in continuous mode is delivered from junction to vein entry point.

TABLE 106-1. Laser Energy Parameter Guidelines for 810 nm

Vein Segment	Power (W)	Withdrawal Rate (mm/s)	Energy Delivered (J/cm)
Proximal third	14	1	140
Middle third	14	2	70
Distal third*	14	3	47

*Suggested for vein segments close to skin, nerves, and arteries, below the knee, and so forth.

True recanalization of treated veins can occur but is uncommon. Initial vein diameter is unrelated to procedural success, and there appears to be no upper size limit that cannot be successfully treated by endovenous laser ablation if adequate vein emptying and contact of the laser fiber with the vein wall are achieved. Veins with initial upright diameters in excess of 30 mm have been successfully closed with EVLT by several practitioners.

The complete discussion of controversies surrounding GSV ablation can be found at www.expertconsult.com.

OUTCOMES

Technical success of EVLT is defined as a procedure in which successful access is achieved, the segment to be treated is crossed, the vein is emptied adequately, tumescent anesthesia is administered properly, and sufficient laser energy is delivered to the entire incompetent segment. Clinical success is defined as occlusion of the treated vein segments, with successful elimination of related varicose veins and improvement in the clinical classification of patients.

In many cases, ecchymosis will develop over the treated site because of puncture of the vein during access and administration of tumescent anesthesia. This is of no medical consequence and will resolve within weeks after EVLT. Some patients may experience mild discomfort over the treated vein that begins hours after the procedure and resolves within 24 to 48 hours. Many patients will also note delayed tightness and mild to moderate tenderness over the treated vein, particularly over the distal segment. This sensation, described as a "pulling," will usually start at the end of the first week, reach a peak approximately 7 days after EVLT, and resolve by week 2 or 3. This delayed pain does not correspond to the presence or degree of bruising and is most likely caused by transverse and longitudinal retraction of the vein as the acute inflammation transitions to cicatrization. Most patients feel better with graduated support stockings and ambulation, and nonsteroidal antiinflammatory medications are occasionally required.

In addition to clinical examination, DUS is essential for evaluating treatment success after endovenous laser ablation. Most practitioners perform DUS within 1 week after endovenous laser ablation, at the completion of treatment, and yearly thereafter. DUS criteria for successful treatment are important to recognize. One week after EVLT, DUS imaging will reveal a noncompressible vein that may be decreased in diameter, with echogenic circumferentially thickened walls and no flow seen within the entire treated vein lumen on color Doppler interrogation. Adequate treatment should result in occlusion secondary to vein wall injury, with resultant inflammation. If present, intraluminal thrombus should be minimal and a secondary phenomenon, not the primary cause of occlusion, which would result in recanalization. At 3 to 6 months' follow-up, DUS should demonstrate continued target vein occlusion and a marked reduction in vein diameter. The vein should be absent or only a minimal residual cord visible on DUS imaging 1 year and beyond.[3,4]

The following are results of the first 1000 limbs treated by endovenous laser ablation with an 810-nm diode laser source (Diomed Holdings Inc., Andover, Mass.) for saphenous vein reflux at our center. Successful EVLT, as defined earlier, was seen in 98% (982/1000) of treated limbs at up to 60-month follow-up. Some 99% (457/460) of treated vein segments remained occluded at more than 2-year follow-up. The majority (13/18) of treatment failures occurred before 1 year, and there has been only one failure in more than 500 veins treated at 14 W. All veins treated with at least 70 J/cm of laser energy have remained closed.[15]

Clinical examination correlated well with DUS findings. Subjects demonstrated improvement in visible varicosities, which at times were significant, as shown in Figure 106-4. All subjects with leg pain from SVI noted resolution or substantial improvement in associated symptoms by 6 months.

Several investigators have reported similar success rates of endovenous laser ablation of the GSV.[6-9,15,16] These studies have consistently shown successful nonthrombotic occlusion of the target truncal vein in 90% to 100% of cases, with very rare recanalization of previously occluded vein segments. Clinical improvement was noted in almost all cases after successful truncal vein occlusion. Patient acceptance was high, and adverse reactions were extremely rare, with heat complications such as DVT, paresthesias, or skin burns being virtually nonexistent.

Performing endovenous ablation of the GSV without division of the tributaries at the saphenofemoral junction goes against a cardinal rule in saphenous vein surgery; however, the combined experience with endovenous ablation procedures has shown lower recurrence rates than after surgical ligation and stripping.[17,18] Neovascularization at the groin, often seen after surgical removal of the saphenous vein,[19] has been practically nonexistent after endovenous ablation. It seems that avoiding the trauma of surgery, while preserving venous drainage in normal competent tributaries and removing only the abnormal refluxing segments, does not incite this response.

Published studies comparing catheter-based techniques with one another are limited. One recent investigation by Black et al. demonstrated acceptable results with both procedures at 6 months: 100% (126/126) of veins were closed with endovenous laser ablation and 91.5% (118/129) with radiofrequency ablation. Eight of the radiofrequency failures were retreated with radiofrequency ablation. Interestingly, three veins failing repeat radiofrequency ablation were successfully closed with EVLT.[20] Despite these differences, it is important to emphasize that both these minimally invasive techniques offer advances in both safety and efficacy over traditional surgical treatment of saphenous vein reflux.

COMPLICATIONS

At our institution, nonpuncture site bruising was noted in a quarter of limbs at 1 week, which resolved in all subjects before the 1-month follow-up. The majority of subjects felt a delayed tightness peaking 4 to 7 days after laser treatment and lasting 3 to 10 days. Superficial phlebitis of an associated varicose tributary was noted in approximately 5% of treated limbs after endovenous laser ablation. Most cases of superficial phlebitis required no treatment, although symptomatic patients were encouraged to ambulate, continue to use graduated compression stockings, and take over-the-counter antiinflammatory medications as needed. Two temporary skin paresthesias occurred after treatment

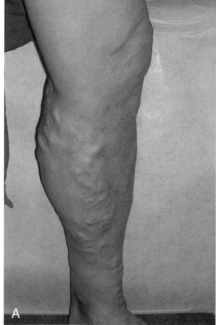
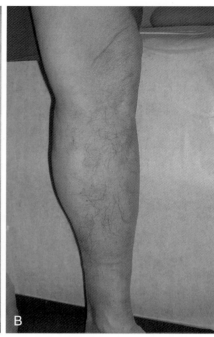

FIGURE 106-4. A, Left lower extremity with large varicose veins due to saphenofemoral junction incompetence and greater saphenous vein (GSV) reflux. **B,** Marked improvement in appearance of leg 1 month after endovenous laser ablation of GSV.

of anterior thigh circumflex segments. No other paresthesias have been noted in other vein segments subjected to endovenous laser therapy. There were no skin burns, DVT, or other adverse reactions in the first 1000 limbs treated at our facility. The procedure was well tolerated by all subjects, with strictly local anesthesia.

When compared with other treatments for saphenous vein reflux such as surgery or other catheter-based procedures, the incidence of adverse reactions after endovenous laser ablation is significantly lower. Complications related to endovenous radiofrequency techniques have included skin paresthesias, skin burns, DVT, and pulmonary emboli. Although liberal use of tumescent anesthesia has helped reduce the incidence of heat-related injury to adjacent nontarget tissues, there has been persistence of paresthesias (13%-15%), clinical phlebitis (2%-20%), thermal skin injury (4%-7%), and DVT (1%-16%) after radiofrequency ablation.[21,22]

POSTPROCEDURAL AND FOLLOW-UP CARE

Most patients will note significant improvement or resolution of symptoms within a month after EVLT but will require additional adjunctive procedures to completely eradicate the visible varicose tributaries and realize the full benefits of treatment. Compression sclerotherapy and ambulatory phlebectomy are the most commonly used techniques to accomplish this goal. The ideal timing of these procedures has been debated. Practitioners who advocate waiting note that most patients will experience a reduction in the size and fullness of associated varices, thus making ancillary treatments easier and more effective. In some cases, the improvement is so dramatic and complete after endovenous laser ablation that additional procedures are not necessary. Proponents of performing adjunctive procedures at the same sitting as endovenous ablation cite the possibility of fewer visits and a lower risk for superficial phlebitis, particularly in large varicose tributaries after elimination of the underlying truncal reflux. Occasionally, treatment of nonsurface tributary veins or persistence of clinically significant perforator reflux will require ultrasound-guided sclerotherapy with foam or strong liquid sclerosants.

Although recanalization of a vein closed by endovenous laser ablation is uncommon, recurrence of varicose veins is not. Even successful endovenous therapy does not eliminate someone's propensity for the development of varicose veins. They can arise from untreated portions of the saphenous vein, incompetent tributaries, perforator reflux, or worsening of veins during pregnancy. Practitioners must counsel patients that venous insufficiency is a chronic condition.

KEY POINTS

- Superficial venous insufficiency is an extremely prevalent condition, but despite its potentially disabling nature and high socioeconomic cost, most patients suffering from SVI are poorly evaluated and often mismanaged.

- Fortunately, advancements in noninvasive examination, in particular DUS, have improved our understanding of SVI by allowing direct visualization and testing of the underlying pathways of venous reflux.

- Making a better diagnosis has led to better treatment. In particular, new and improved minimally invasive techniques for the treatment of incompetent veins now provide practitioners with safe and effective options for managing the whole spectrum of superficial venous disease.

▶ **SUGGESTED READINGS**

Min R, Khilnani N. Endovenous laser ablation of varicose veins. J Cardiovasc Surg 2005;46:395–405.

Min RJ, Khilnani NM, Golia P. Duplex ultrasound of lower extremity venous insufficiency. J Vasc Interv Radiol 2003;14:1233–41.

The complete reference list is available online at www.expertconsult.com

CHAPTER 107

Foreign Body Retrieval

Paul V. Suhocki

INTRODUCTION

Foreign bodies left unattended in the vascular system have been associated with a 71% major complication rate and 24% to 60% mortality rate. Those located within the cardiopulmonary system pose the greatest risk. Foreign objects find their way into the vascular system through trauma, instrumentation, or transmural penetration from adjacent tissues (e.g., ingested foreign bodies). Upon arriving in the heart, wires, stents, inferior vena cava (IVC) filters and filter fragments can cause cardiac arrhythmias, septal or ventricular wall perforation, myocardial infarction, myocarditis, sepsis, pericardial effusion, and pericardial tamponade.[1-6] Continued migration into the pulmonary arteries can result in thromboembolism and sepsis.[7,8]

Percutaneous techniques have dramatically altered the management of foreign bodies over the last several decades. Earliest reports of retrieving misplaced objects were limited to removal of catheter fragments and wires with a Dormia basket, forceps, or a self-made wire loop.[9-13] Unable to be directed over a guidewire, baskets were difficult to manipulate into position. Stiff forceps were prone to traumatizing the vascular media, resulting in spasm, dissection, and perforation. Following reports of the less traumatic self-made wire loop, several improved devices became commercially available. This niche market of retrieval devices has since been driven by the increasing use of stents, filters, coils, and other intravascular devices. Medical literature relating to foreign body retrieval is limited to case reports and short series.[14-19] This chapter will describe the rationale for removing foreign bodies and discuss the various techniques that can be used.

SNARES

The most commonly used retrieval devices today are snares. The Amplatz GooseNeck Snare (ev3/Covidien, Plymouth, Minn.) is constructed of a nitinol cable and a gold-plated tungsten loop.[20] The snare's superelastic construction prevents it from deforming during use. The platinum-iridium radiopaque marker band at the tip of the guiding catheter is highly visible under fluoroscopy. When fully deployed, the snare is oriented at a 90-degree angle with respect to the guiding catheter tip. It is cinched around the foreign body by holding it stationary and advancing the catheter forward. Amplatz GooseNeck Snares are available in 5- to 35-mm diameters.

The Texan Foreign Body Retrieval Device (IDev Technologies, Houston, Tex.) consists of a dual-lumen catheter shaft, a push rod with a handle, and a nitinol wire loop.[21,22] The smaller lumen is used for the loop wire. The larger lumen is used for either a 0.018-inch guidewire or contrast injection. The loop cinches down on the foreign body as the operator pulls back on the push rod. The loop wire opens at a 90-degree angle with respect to the shaft and can be adjusted from 0 to 30 mm in diameter, remaining perpendicular to the shaft throughout deployment. This 90-degree angle being maintained throughout snare deployment accounts for a major difference when compared with the Amplatz GooseNeck Snare, which achieves perpendicular orientation only after it is fully deployed from the catheter tip.

Snares are successful in removing foreign bodies 95% of the time. Objects that are too large or noncompressible for removal through a vascular sheath can be relocated to a less noxious location or moved to a position that is easily accessible through a surgical cutdown.[23]

LOST GUIDEWIRE AND CATHETER FRAGMENTS

A guidewire is usually lost in the vascular system by an inexperienced operator who loses sight of the wire during dilator or catheter exchange while placing a central venous catheter.[24] Catheter fragmentation usually occurs during catheter removal. Catheter shearing may also occur when the catheter is "pinched off" between the clavicle and the anterior portion of the first rib. Peripherally inserted central catheter (PICC) lines usually become torn when the peripheral arm vein goes into spasm during catheter removal.

The interventional radiologist may be called to remove a PICC line while the catheter is still intact but cannot be removed. In this case, a 0.025-inch guidewire is advanced through the PICC line under fluoroscopy until the wire tip exits the catheter. The guidewire and PICC line are then removed by applying traction to both as a unit.

When a catheter of any type has become torn or is found incidentally on imaging or a wire has been lost, use of an endovascular snare becomes necessary.[18] A vascular sheath is placed in either the internal jugular or common femoral vein. A long sheath provides greater support and stability for the snare. The snare is passed through the sheath and advanced or retracted over the fragment tip. The snare is then cinched and drawn out with the fragment through the sheath (Fig. 107-1).

A fragment tip that is caught in a small branch vessel or chronically embedded in the vessel wall must first be freed from the vessel wall in order to be snared. A reverse curve catheter passed through the same sheath or a separate sheath can be used to pull down on the shaft of the foreign body, freeing the tip (Fig. 107-2). A braiding technique can also be used for this purpose.[25] With this method, a pigtail catheter tip is wrapped around the fragment and rotated, braiding itself with the fragment and freeing the tip to allow successful snaring.

The end of a fragment may sometimes extend into the subcutaneous tissues while remaining invisible at the skin

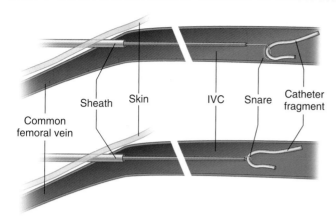

FIGURE 107-1. Catheter fragment has been lost in inferior vena cava *(IVC)*. Amplatz GooseNeck Snare (ev3/Covidien, Plymouth, Minn.) has been passed through a vascular sheath in common femoral vein and used to remove fragment through sheath.

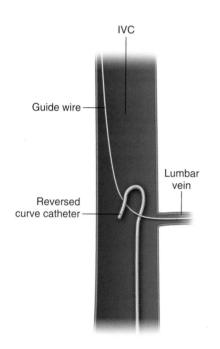

FIGURE 107-2. Tip of a lost wire is in a lumbar vein, preventing its being snared with an Amplatz GooseNeck Snare (ev3/Covidien, Plymouth, Minn.). A reverse curve catheter is used to pull wire tip out of lumbar vein to facilitate wire removal with a snare. *IVC,* Inferior vena cava.

surface. This occurs when the catheter is torn during attempted removal. With the help of fluoroscopy or ultrasound, one can incise the skin and dissect down onto the fragment. The fragment is then secured and extracted along with its intravascular component. An 18- to 20-gauge needle can be formed into a hook on the table for this purpose.[26] If the tip of the foreign body is too deep for a safe or successful cutdown, the intravascular end of the fragment can be snared and removed through a vascular sheath, bringing the soft-tissue component along with it.

Rarely, a catheter will become sutured to the wall of a vein during an operation. Snaring the catheter would risk

tearing the vessel wall. In this setting, two vascular sheaths are placed via femoral and internal jugular access.[27] One snare is passed through each sheath. The catheter is snared on each side of the suture, immediately adjacent to the suture. Steady, equal traction is applied to the catheter fragment from each direction until the fragment is torn into two pieces. Each fragment is subsequently removed through the sheaths. Because of the risks associated with this procedure, anesthesiology and surgery services should first be consulted.

LOST ENDOVASCULAR STENTS

A self-expanding stent can migrate during deployment when the constrained stent is not centered on a stenosis and it "trumpets" or "melon seeds" in either direction during release. A stent can also migrate following a technically successful deployment in a vein as the vessel diameter increases with respirations or Valsalva maneuvers. Using a T-fastener to anchor an IVC stent to the wall of the intrahepatic IVC has been described in this setting.[28] A stent may become irretrievable if left to migrate into the heart chambers, requiring open-heart surgery for its removal.

Maintaining a guidewire through the lumen of a lost stent is key to its successful capture and removal. Keeping the wire in both the superior and inferior vena cavae will prevent the stent from passing into the heart chambers. The vascular sheath is exchanged for one that is wide enough to pull the captured stent through. The snare is cinched around the wire outside of the sheath. The snare and its guiding catheter are passed through the sheath along the guidewire. The snare is opened around the proximal-most end of the lost stent. The snare is then cinched down on the proximal end of the stent, drawing the constrained end of the stent out through the sheath.[29]

A lost stent through which a wire does not pass presents a greater challenge. The snare will tend to get caught on the struts of the stent, constraining only a part of the end of the stent. It will not be possible to pull this stent into the vascular sheath for removal. Passing a wire through the stent before snaring will assist in stent capture. Using a J-tipped wire for this purpose will help avoid passing the wire tip through the side wall of an uncovered stent.

Having successfully passed a wire through the stent, the operator may still find it difficult to avoid hang-up of the snare on the struts at the end of the stent. Use of an angioplasty balloon will provide a transition zone for the snare to approach and slip over the end of the stent. The vascular sheath is first exchanged for an appropriately sized one. An angioplasty balloon 1 to 2 mm greater in diameter than the stent and longer than the stent is selected. A snare is cinched around the balloon catheter shaft outside of the sheath. The balloon/snare combination is passed over the wire just proximal to the stent. The snare is opened. The balloon is advanced into the stent and inflated. The open snare is advanced over the tapered end of the balloon and onto the proximal end of the stent (Fig. 107-3, *A*). The balloon is deflated and pulled out of the stent as the end of the stent is constrained by the snare (Fig. 107-3, *B*). The deflated balloon and captured stent are then drawn out sequentially through the sheath.

Once a stent lies in the right ventricle, the struts may lodge in the chordae tendinae, or access to the stent may

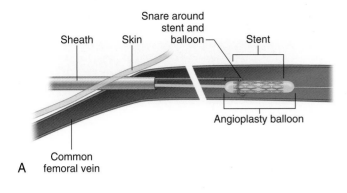

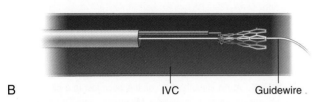

FIGURE 107-3. A, Struts on free end of lost stent have prevented passage of Amplatz GooseNeck Snare (ev3/Covidien, Plymouth, Minn.) around it. An angioplasty balloon is placed inside stent to provide a transition zone for snare to approach and slip over end of stent. **B,** Balloon has been deflated and pulled into sheath. End of stent is constrained by snare as stent is pulled out through sheath. *IVC,* Inferior vena cava.

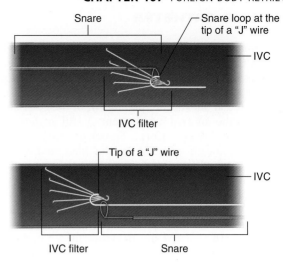

FIGURE 107-4. A, Tip of a J-wire has been caught on an inferior vena cava *(IVC) filter.* A GooseNeck Snare (ev3/Covidien, Plymouth, Minn.) is advanced over J-wire shaft and cinched down on wire near caught end, pushing the wire down to free it from filter. **B,** Alternative method for freeing J-wire from IVC filter involves pulling down on J-wire tip with an Amplatz GooseNeck Snare.

be blocked by the tricuspid valve. Capture is made even more difficult by the moving target created by cardiac motion during fluoroscopy. Changing the angle of approach from femoral vein access to internal jugular vein access (or vice versa) may aid in stent capture. Foreign bodies trapped within the heart pose a greater risk for capture. Attempts at their removal may cause dysrhythmia or damage to the myocardium, chordae tendinae, or tricuspid valve. A defibrillator, code cart, and transvenous pacer should be available for use, and a cardiothoracic surgeon on standby. If all attempts for stent removal become futile, the cardiothoracic surgeon should be consulted for open removal.

Once a stent has traveled through the heart and into the pulmonary arteries, apposition of the stent against the vessel wall may make it impossible to pass a snare around it. If this occurs, an appropriately sized angioplasty balloon can be inflated inside the stent and used to pull the stent from the artery, through the cardiac chambers, and into the vena cavae or iliac veins for snaring through a second vascular sheath.[8]

Once lost stents are snared and constrained, it may not be possible to pull the stent into the sheath. Stent struts or a severely deformed stent may keep the stent from entering the sheath. Three options are available at this point:

1. The stent can be deployed in the iliac vein if it is appropriately sized. If the stent is too small in diameter, a larger and longer self-expanding stent can be deployed within it to trap it in place.
2. A second snare can be used to capture and constrain the other end of the stent from a different approach.
3. The stent can be drawn into the common femoral vein and removed by surgical cutdown.

WIRES CAUGHT ON INFERIOR VENA CAVA FILTERS

J-tipped wires that are used for placement of central lines without imaging guidance are sometimes caught in the apex of an IVC filter. In this setting, a vascular sheath is passed over the caught wire. A snare is passed around the wire and loosely cinched down with its guiding catheter on the end of the J-wire outside the sheath. The snare is advanced over the J-wire and cinched down on the wire near the caught end, pushing the wire down to free it from the filter (Fig. 107-4, *A*).

If the J-wire/catheter combination buckles during attempts to free the wire, a stiffer system can be used. The sheath is replaced by an 8F vascular sheath, and a 6.5F catheter is passed over the caught J-wire. The stiff end of an Amplatz Superstiff guidewire (Boston Scientific, Natick, Mass.) is passed into the 6.5F catheter adjacent to the caught J-wire, being careful not to allow the Amplatz Superstiff guidewire to exit the catheter distally or anywhere along its length. The snare is than drawn over the 6.5F catheter and used to cinch down onto the catheter near the end of the caught wire. Thrusts are made with this stiffer system to free up the tip of the J wire.

If the length of the J-wire is too short to pass a catheter over, a vascular sheath is placed over the wire. A hole is created in the side of a straight 5F catheter 1 cm from its tip. The end of the J-wire is passed through the tip of the catheter and out through the side hole in monorail fashion.[30] The catheter is then advanced over the wire and used to free the wire tip from the catheter. If these methods are not successful in freeing up the tip of the J-wire, a vascular sheath is placed in a vein from an access opposite to that in which the central line wire was placed. A snare is passed through the sheath and used to snare the tip of the J-wire and pull the J-wire away from the filter (Fig. 107-4, *B*).

KNOTTED CATHETER

Knot formation is an uncommon complication of indwelling catheters that may make catheter removal impossible.[31] A double access technique can be used for "untying" a knotted jugular or subclavian vein catheter endovascularly.[32]

Two vascular sheaths are placed. An 8F vascular sheath is placed in the internal jugular vein. A stiff angled Glidewire (Terumo Medical Corp., Somerset, N.J.) is passed through the sheath adjacent to the knot and into the IVC. A second stiff angled Glidewire is then passed into the sheath through a 5F angled catheter. This Glidewire/catheter combination is directed through the knot and into the IVC. The 5F catheter is removed. The sheath is advanced over both wires to exert downward force on the knot. A long 10F vascular sheath is then placed in the right femoral vein. Parallel stiff Glidewires are passed to the level of the knot, one through the knot, one adjacent to it as described earlier, with the help of an angled 5F catheter. The catheter is removed, and the sheath is advanced over the two Glidewires to the knot. This exerts an upward force on the knot. Using the sheaths in concert with each other from both directions, the knot is untied, and the catheter is removed.

A variation on this knot-unraveling approach utilizes one wire and one snare passed through each of the described sheaths. A guidewire is passed through the knot via the right internal jugular vein using an 8F internal jugular vein sheath with the aid of a 5F angled catheter. The catheter is removed. The wire tip is snared via the same sheath. A second guidewire is then passed through the knot with the aid of a 5F catheter via the 10F right femoral vein sheath. The catheter is removed. A snare is used to snare the wire tip via the same femoral sheath. The knot is unraveled by pulling on the wire and snare from each direction.

LOST EMBOLIZATION COILS

Occasionally a coil is deployed in an unintended location during an embolization procedure.[33] This occurs when (1) an undersized coil migrates distal to the intended deployment site, (2) an undersized coil passes through a pulmonary venous malformation to the systemic circulation during pulmonary arteriovenous malformation (AVM) embolization, or (3) the coil is oversized, pushing the catheter tip and the end of the coil back into the parent vessel while it is being deployed. Although the errant coil can cause local thrombosis and ischemia in the unintended location, attempts at retrieving it may cause even more damage to the arterial tree in the form of dissection or vascular occlusion. Therefore, the coil can be left in place if deemed unlikely to cause injury to the patient. If the coil must be removed, anticoagulation should be initiated immediately, and one of several devices chosen for its removal:

- A 3F, 4-mm-diameter Amplatz GooseNeck Microsnare (ev3/Covidien) (Fig. 107-5, *A*)
- An alligator retrieval device (ev3/Covidien) with four interlocking jaws attached to a stainless steel core wire (Fig. 107-5, *B*)
- An EN Snare (Merit Medical, South Jordan, Utah) device with three cabled interlaced kink-resistant nitinol loops

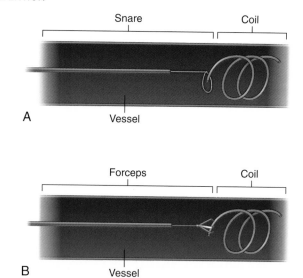

FIGURE 107-5. A, An embolization coil has been lost in a blood vessel. A 3F, 4-mm-diameter Amplatz GooseNeck Microsnare (ev3/Covidien, Plymouth, Minn.) is used to capture end of coil for removal through a vascular sheath. **B,** Alligator retrieval device (ev3/Covidien) with four interlocking jaws is used to capture end of this coil misplaced during embolization procedure.

- A 3F flexible rat-tooth forceps (Cook Urological Inc., Spencer, Ind.).[34]

Following removal of the coil, anticoagulation can be stopped or reversed. If the retrieval procedure has caused intimal damage, long-term anticoagulation should be considered.

LOST NON-RADIOPAQUE FOREIGN BODIES

Non-radiopaque or faintly radiopaque foreign bodies, such as angioplasty balloon fragments or ingested bones/toothpicks that have eroded through the vessel wall, may be seen on computed tomography (CT) or ultrasound but not be visible under fluoroscopy. There are several ways to approach this problem. Using fluoroscopy alone, a large, long vascular sheath can be placed and a snare passed through the sheath.[35] The object is visualized as a negative filling defect while contrast is injected through the sidearm of the sheath. The retrieval process is monitored in this fashion as well. Real-time ultrasound, echocardiography, or intravascular ultrasound (IVUS) can also be used for identification and capture of the foreign body.[36,37]

SUBCLAVIAN ARTERIAL CENTRAL VENOUS CATHETER

Arterial placement of central venous catheters is being seen less frequently as ultrasonographic guidance is increasingly used for their placement. Central venous lines that are found to be intraarterial should not be removed without proper planning. This "pull and hope" technique is inadvisable because the subclavian arterial entry site is posterior to the clavicle and non-compressible. The site of entry may also unknowingly be the brachiocephalic artery or the thoracic aorta. The "pull and hope" approach can result in uncontrollable hemorrhage, hemothorax, pseudoaneurysm, arteriovenous fistula, and death. Surgical removal is difficult and involves partial rib resection, thoracotomy, or sternotomy. Endovascular management provides an attractive alternative. There are three percutaneous methods with which the catheter can be removed in the interventional radiology suite with the least amount of risk to the patient. With all three methods, arteriography of the involved vessel is first performed through a femoral arterial sheath, noting the exact site of catheter entry into the artery. Steep angulation of the image intensifier is usually necessary for proper assessment of the artery. The diameter of the injured artery is measured.

With the balloon occlusion method, a second femoral arterial sheath is placed in the opposite groin. An angioplasty balloon 20% greater in diameter than the injured artery is placed across the access site and hand inflated while the catheter is removed. The balloon is deflated every 15 minutes to reperfuse the limb and reassess the artery for puncture closure with the angiography catheter.

With the covered stent method, proximity of the catheter entry site to the vertebral artery origin must be assessed. If there is a possibility the covered stent will cover the origin of the vertebral artery, a formal cerebral arteriogram is performed to assess vertebral artery dominance. A second femoral arterial sheath is placed in the opposite groin. A self-expanding covered stent 20% greater in diameter than the artery is placed as the catheter is removed. Angiography is repeated to confirm satisfactory stent positioning.

The third method utilizes a percutaneous arteriotomy closure device, which may be used if the catheter is still in situ. The catheter is removed over a guidewire and replaced with the closure device. Perclose (Abbott Laboratories-Vascular Devices, Redwood City, Calif.), Angioseal (St. Jude Medical, St. Paul, Minn.), and VasoSeal (Datascope, Montvale, N.J.) have all been used for this purpose, without or with concomitant balloon occlusion via groin sheath access. Using balloon occlusion along with the closure device, however, does allow for either the balloon occlusion method or the covered stent method to be used in the event the closure device fails.

AIR EMBOLISM

Although one does not typically think of an air embolism as a foreign body, iatrogenic introduction of gas emboli into the vasculature can be fatal. The most common portals for entry of venous air emboli are probably a peel-away sheath used during central venous catheter placement and a catheter stopcock that has been left open. A much rarer portal of entry would be the side holes of a percutaneous biliary drainage catheter, providing a passageway for air from the duodenum into hepatic veins during endoscopy. When venous air embolism is suspected, measures must first be taken to prevent its further entry. The patient is placed in the left lateral decubitus position. Supplemental oxygen should be administered and cardiopulmonary resuscitation initiated if necessary. Removal of air from the right atrium

with a multi-sidehole central venous catheter or a pulmonary artery catheter should be attempted. Hyperbaric oxygen therapy may be necessary in severe cases, particularly if neurologic changes are present and paradoxical embolism is suspected.

Gas emboli can enter the arteries directly through a needle or catheter, through the pulmonary veins (e.g., during CT-guided transthoracic needle biopsy or pulmonary AVM embolization), or via a patent foramen ovale. Gas emboli are particularly serious in the coronary and cerebral circulations. Oxygen should be administered not only to treat hypoxia but also to help eliminate nitrogen in the bubbles through a large diffusion gradient. Cardiopulmonary resuscitation should be started if necessary. Once stable, the patient should be immediately transferred to a hyperbaric chamber.[38] Hyperbaric oxygen therapy decreases the size of gas emboli by raising the ambient pressure and causing hyperoxia. The hyperoxia produces a very large diffusion gradient, driving oxygen into the bubble and nitrogen out. It also greatly increases the amount of oxygen in plasma and oxygen diffusion in tissues.

SUMMARY

In conclusion, the interventional radiologist plays an important role in removing foreign bodies from the vascular system. Leaving such objects unattended can result in fatal consequences. Careful planning and a working knowledge of the tools available will help provide this service in the safest and most expedient manner.

KEY POINTS

- Catheter fragments and lost guidewires that are left in the vascular tree are associated with high morbidity and mortality rates.
- The interventional radiologist plays a key role in removing foreign bodies from the vascular system, using tools readily available on the internet.
- Misplaced stents or coils can be removed or relocated to a safe location if removal is impossible.
- While not often perceived as a foreign body, air embolism is an important cause of morbidity and mortality and must be prevented by using careful catheter technique.

▶ SUGGESTED READINGS
Carroll MI, Ahanchi SS, Kim JH, et al. Endovascular foreign body retrieval. J Vasc Surg 2013;57(2):459–63.
Schechter MA, O'Brien PJ, Cox MW. Retrieval of iatrogenic intravascular foreign bodies. J Vasc Surg 2013;57(1):276–81.

The complete reference list is available online at www.expertconsult.com

CHAPTER 108

Renal Vein Renin Sampling

David W. Trost and Thomas A. Sos

Renal vein renin (RVR) sampling can help determine whether renal artery stenosis is a significant contributor to a patient's hypertension. It can also help determine which patients with renal vascular hypertension (RVH) may benefit from revascularization by percutaneous or surgical methods.

INDICATIONS

• To determine which patients with RVH may benefit from revascularization by percutaneous or surgical methods
• To determine the physiologic significance of an anatomic stenosis that is of indeterminate grade
• To assess whether a tumor secretes renin

CONTRAINDICATIONS

• Patients who are not candidates for revascularization by any means
• Patients without access to the renal veins because of venous occlusion or anatomic abnormalities
• Severe uncorrectable coagulopathy

EQUIPMENT

Catheter

• 4F or 5F Cobra catheter (various vendors) with a side hole close to the distal tip
• Alternatively, a Simmons catheter (various vendors) or other angled catheter may be a better fit for a particular patient's anatomy.
• Rarely a coaxial microcatheter system is necessary to obtain a stable position in a segmental renal vein for segmental sampling (various vendors).

Guidewire

• Bentson (various vendors)
• Rosen (Cook Medical, Bloomington, Ind.)
• Angled Glidewire (Terumo Medical Corp., Somerset, N.J.)
• Wire for microcatheter system (various vendors)

TECHNIQUE

Anatomy and Approach

The renal veins lie ventral to the renal arteries. The left is longer than the right and passes in front of the aorta, just inferior to the origin of the superior mesenteric artery. The renal veins enter the vena cava around the level of L1-L2.

The left renal vein is usually slightly more cephalad than the right. It receives drainage from the left gonadal, left inferior phrenic, and left adrenal veins.

Renal vein anomalies are common. Multiple renal veins can arise from one or both kidneys; there can be circumaortic or retroaortic left renal veins, and rarely the renal veins can arise from the iliac vessels.

Technical Aspects

Patient Preparation

Patients should ideally have all their antihypertensive medications discontinued at least 2 weeks before RVR sampling. This may not be possible, but all β-blockers and angiotensin-converting enzyme (ACE) inhibitors must be discontinued several days before sampling. The predictive value of the test is poor when the patient is taking antihypertensive medications, especially ACE inhibitors.

The accuracy of sampling is increased if it is performed under stimulation. Captopril (1 mg/kg of body weight) is administered orally 60 to 90 minutes before sampling.[1]

Access

Ideal access is via the right common femoral vein, but the left common femoral vein or jugular veins can be used if necessary. The renal veins can be catheterized with a 4F or 5F Cobra 2 catheter with a side hole at the tip.

Right Renal Vein

The catheter should be positioned in the main right renal vein so blood from the whole kidney is sampled.

Left Renal Vein

The catheter should be positioned deep enough into the left renal vein so it is proximal to gonadal vein inflow, which can otherwise dilute the sample and decrease accuracy of the result. The gonadal vein typically enters the left renal vein in the proximal to middle third of the vein. Sometimes a Simmons or other angled catheter will be required to access the renal veins.

The entire vena cava must be surveyed to identify and sample any accessory or aberrant veins. If a branch renal artery a stenosis is suspected to be the cause of RVH, selective segmental sampling should be performed.

IVC

A sample from the IVC below the lowest identified renal vein should be collected after each renal vein sample, or if the patient's heart rate and blood pressure are stable after both selective samples have been obtained. Each selective vein sample should be accompanied by a nonselective vena caval sample. Five milliliters of blood should be discarded before each sample to ensure an uncontaminated sample. All samples should be obtained as rapidly as possible because if the patient's hemodynamic status changes between various samples renin levels can vary spuriously and the renin levels may not represent the true baseline physiologic steady state.

Pitfalls in Renal Vein Renin Sampling

- Patients who are being treated with chronic ACE inhibition or β-blockade and cannot safely discontinue taking these medications may have a suboptimal study.
- Failure to identify multiple renal veins or venous anatomic variants may decrease accuracy of the result.
- Samples obtained from the left renal vein proximal to inflow from the left gonadal vein or samples on the right inadvertently obtained from a low hepatic vein will result in a suboptimal study.

CONTROVERSIES

Renal vein renin sampling may help determine whether a patient with renal artery stenosis will benefit from renal revascularization, but this remains controversial especially in the presence of bilateral renal artery stenosis.[2-7] A review of 143 patients, 20 of whom had RVH, resulted in a sensitivity of 65%, a positive predictive value of 18.6%, and a negative predictive value of 89.3%. The authors concluded that the results were neither sensitive nor specific enough to exclude patients who do not have RVH.[2] Another study[3] of elderly patients (mean age of 60 years) found a very low specificity (21%) and negative predictive value (16%) of RVR analysis, thus limiting its use in this population. This same study also found that performing angioplasty without previous RVR analysis did not significantly affect clinical outcome.

OUTCOMES

Renin-Angiotensin-Aldosterone System

The juxtaglomerular apparatus of the kidney responds to decreased blood pressure and sodium concentration by releasing renin from the macula densa. Renin acts on renin substrate, a glycoprotein manufactured by the liver, to produce angiotensin I. Angiotensin I is inactive and is converted to angiotensin II by an enzyme (ACE) produced in the lung. Angiotensin II is a potent vasoconstrictor, and it stimulates the zona glomerulosa of the adrenal gland to release aldosterone. Aldosterone acts on the kidney to promote sodium and water retention.

Vaughan et al. studied renin release in essential hypertensives and normal individuals. They found that to maintain blood pressure at a steady state, each kidney secreted a 25% increment, for a total increment of 50% over systemic renin levels.[6] Mathematically, this relationship can be expressed as follows:

$$VR - A/A = 25\%; \qquad VL - A/A = 25\%$$

where VR and VL are the renin activity in the right and left renal veins, respectively, and A is systemic arterial renin activity, which in a steady state equals that in the infrarenal inferior vena cava.

Selective Renal Vein Sampling for Renin Assay

Selective sampling of the renal veins and the infrarenal inferior vena cava for renin activity (RVR) permits calculation of the net secretion of renin from each kidney. Hypersecretion of renin from the stenotic kidney ([V − A]/A > 50%) and contralateral suppression of renin release from the normal kidney ([V − A]/A ≈ 0) are hallmarks of potentially curable unilateral RVH. Because the two kidneys normally contribute a 50% increment, (V − A)/A > 50% signifies not only hypersecretion but also decreased renal plasma flow on the involved side. In our experience, use of the Vaughan formula for evaluation of RVR activity has a sensitivity of 75% and a specificity of 100%.[8]

When the same data were analyzed with the simple ratio method, which compares the renin activity of the involved and contralateral kidneys, the result was less accurate. Using a ratio of 1.5 : 1 or greater as abnormal, sensitivity was only 63%, with a specificity of 60%. In patients with bilateral renal artery disease, there is frequently lateralization to the more stenotic side, and this is even more impressive when one side is totally occluded.[8]

Differences between the two kidneys can be accentuated by use of an ACE inhibitor, the "captopril challenge" test.[9]

Pathophysiology of Renovascular Hypertension in Humans

The most frequent cause of RVH is stenosis of the renal artery; however, diffuse parenchymal disease that results in arteriolar obliteration[10] or renal parenchymal compression, as in the "Page kidney" phenomenon,[11] can also produce the changes described at the juxtaglomerular level. In these pathologic states, the involved diseased kidney secretes the entire complement of 50% renin increment, and renin production by the contralateral normal kidney is suppressed. The RVH in patients with unilateral renal artery disease is primarily renin-mediated vasoconstriction produced by angiotensin II. The secondary hyperaldosteronism produced by stimulation of the adrenal cortex is of less significance because the contralateral healthy kidney continues to excrete the retained sodium and water.

The situation is more complex in bilateral renal artery disease or in patients with unilateral renal artery disease but with contralateral parenchymal nephrosclerosis or in uninephric individuals with renal artery stenosis. Initially, renin-mediated vasoconstrictive hypertension occurs, but plasma volume also increases as a result of the secondary hyperaldosteronism and decreased ability of both kidneys to excrete sodium and water. Chronically, renin and aldosterone levels may become normal, but the hypertension persists because of the increased retained plasma volume. In clinical practice, however, even in bilateral renal artery disease, the stenosis on one side is almost invariably more severe, so hypertension tends to remain dependent on renin, angiotensin, and vasoconstriction rather than on volume, although plasma volumes are somewhat higher than in unilateral disease.[12]

If segmental branch stenosis or focal renal infarction is suspected of being the cause of the hypertension, segmental sampling can be performed to determine whether these conditions are significant contributors to the patient's hypertension.[13] Segmental sampling may require use of a coaxial microcatheter system for selection of the desired vein.

COMPLICATIONS

• Damage to the puncture site vein
• Damage to the adjacent artery
• Damage to the vena cava or branch veins
• Nephropathy induced by contrast material
• Allergic reaction to the contrast material

POSTPROCEDURAL AND FOLLOW-UP CARE

Routine post-femoral venipuncture care is all that is needed after RVR sampling.

KEY POINTS

• Renin is a potent regulator of blood pressure via the renin-angiotensin-aldosterone system.

• Renin is produced in the juxtaglomerular apparatus of the kidney and in some tumors.

• Selective renal vein and IVC sampling for renin can help determine whether a renal arterial stenosis is physiologically significant.

▸ **SUGGESTED READINGS**

Trost DW, Sos TA. Percutaneous transluminal angioplasty and stenting in renal artery stenosis. Renal artery thrombolysis. In Pollack HM, McClennan BL, editors. Clinical urography. 2nd ed. Philadelphia: WB Saunders; 2000.

Trost DW, Sos TA. Renal angioplasty and stenting. In Handbook of interventional radiology. 4th ed. Philadelphia: Lippincott Williams & Wilkins; 2011. p. 205–18.

The complete reference list is available online at www.expertconsult.com.

CHAPTER 109

Adrenal Venous Sampling

Kenneth R. Thomson, Jim Koukounaras, and Mark F. Given

In the investigation of adrenocortical function, urine and blood cortisol measurements as well as adrenocorticotropic hormone (ACTH, corticotropin) levels are used. Adrenal venous sampling is almost never required in the investigation of underproduction (Addison disease) or overproduction (Cushing disease) of cortisol. These can be diagnosed by peripheral samples during an ACTH stimulation test. Levels less than 2 µg/dL indicate Addison disease and greater than 22 µg/dL indicate Cushing disease.

Excessive excretion of aldosterone may be primary due to a tumor (Conn syndrome) or hyperactivity of the outer area of the adrenal cortex, or secondary due to nonadrenal conditions that cause a severe imbalance in sodium and potassium. Examples of secondary causes of hyperaldosteronism are congestive heart failure, cirrhosis with ascites, depletion of sodium from diuretics, or toxemia of pregnancy. Plasma renin activity is typically elevated in secondary hyperaldosteronism and reduced in primary aldosteronism. As a result, aldosterone and renin are usually measured together.

Primary aldosteronism is increasingly considered to be a remedial cause of hypertension. Patients with an increased peripheral aldosterone/renin ratio after correction for hypokalemia and removal of interfering medication who also show a positive response to corticosteroid suppression should be considered for adrenal vein sampling to distinguish unilateral from bilateral primary aldosteronism. Because corticosteroid suppression requires sodium loading, it is generally not performed in the elderly or those with severe hypertension. It has been suggested that a saline infusion test is equally reliable, but it is limited in persons with heart failure. In most cases, a prior computed tomography (CT) scan of the adrenal glands will have been performed. If there is evidence of a unilateral enlargement of a portion of the adrenal gland, there is slightly more likelihood of unilateral aldosteronism excess. In about 40% of cases of aldosteronism, however, the CT is unhelpful or even misleading.

INDICATIONS

- Detection of excessive aldosterone excretion (Conn syndrome)
- Differentiation of bilateral hyperplasia, aldosterone-secreting adenoma, and primary adrenal hyperplasia
- Confirmation of unilateral hyperaldosteronism before adrenalectomy

CONTRAINDICATIONS

There are no specific contraindications to sampling. Adrenal venography is of limited value in diagnosis and is most useful for confirming the actual site of the blood sample.

If excessive or wedged injections of contrast agent are used for adrenal venography, there is a risk of rupture of the vein and infarction of the adrenal gland on that side.

EQUIPMENT

- Angiography tray
- 5F access sheath
- 5F Cobra 2 catheter
- 5F Hilal HS1 spinal, RDC, or sidewinder catheter
- Small hole punch
- Nonionic contrast medium (25-50 mL)

TECHNIQUE

Anatomy and Approach

The adrenal gland is a composite retroperitoneal organ with a medulla of ectodermal origin and a cortex of mesodermal origin. The gland shrinks significantly in the first 2 weeks after birth as the fetal cortex degenerates. The adult cortex is fully differentiated by puberty. The cortex forms the main mass (90%) of the gland and is richly supplied by arteries. A single vein emerges from each adrenal gland. The arterial supply is multiple and comes from the aorta directly, the renal artery, and the inferior phrenic artery.

The adrenal glands lie at the anterosuperior aspect of the upper pole of each kidney and are enclosed within the renal fascia but separated from the kidneys by loose fibroareolar tissue (Fig. 109-1). There maybe several small masses of tissue identical with adrenal cortex "cortical bodies" in the neighborhood of the gland.

The right adrenal gland is roughly triangular, with its apex and medial portion of the anterior surface in contact with the posterior aspect of the inferior vena cava (IVC) (Fig. 109-2). The larger lateral portion of the anterior surface is in contact with the bare area of the liver. Medially, the gland is related to the right celiac ganglion and the right inferior phrenic artery. The posterior surface is related above to the diaphragm, and the lower posterior surface and the base of the gland are related to the upper pole or upper medial portion of the right kidney. The right adrenal vein is short and formed from three major tributaries. It emerges from a furrow on the anterior border of the adrenal gland just below the apex to enter the right posterolateral aspect of the IVC above the right renal vein. Occasionally the right adrenal vein drains into a hepatic vein close to the IVC and rarely may drain into the right renal vein. In such cases, a recurved catheter with a longer tip like a Simmons or sidewinder shape may be required.

The left adrenal gland is slightly larger and crescentic, with its concavity applied along the medial border of the upper part of the left kidney. The anterior surface is related

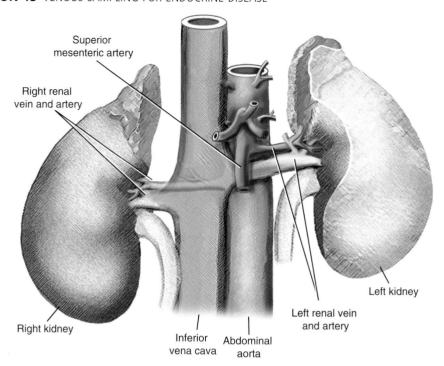

FIGURE 109-1. Diagram of adrenal glands.

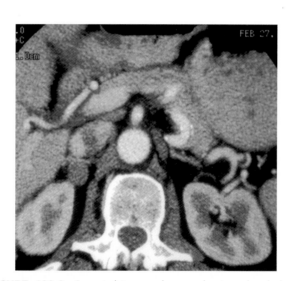

FIGURE 109-2. Computed tomography scan showing adrenal glands. Note focal adenoma in right adrenal gland.

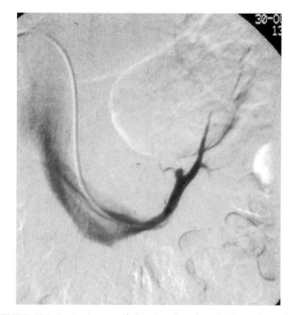

FIGURE 109-3. Angiogram of phrenicoadrenal trunk. Note valve at lower end of left inferior phrenic vein.

to the stomach and spleen above and the pancreas and splenic artery below. The medial portion of the posterior surface is related to the left crus and the lateral portion to the left kidney. The left adrenal vein emerges from the lower portion of the anterior surface and joins the left inferior phrenic vein to form a single trunk that drains into the left renal vein (Fig. 109-3). The left adrenal vein lies lateral to the inferior phrenic vein and, unlike the phrenic vein, it does not contain a valve.

The left adrenal vein is formed from a remnant of the left subcardinal vein, and in cases of left or double IVC it may drain directly into the left portion of the cava.

Technical Aspects

Ideally, all interfering drugs should be stopped for 2 weeks prior to the procedure. In the case of spironolactone, it should be stopped for 6 weeks if possible. The patient should be kept in the supine position from about 10 PM the night before, the logic of this being that approximately one third of aldosterone-producing adenomata are angiotensin sensitive and will respond to the upright position by a rise in aldosterone production. Preferably, the sampling should be done in the morning, since this is when peak aldosterone production occurs. Blood samples should be kept at room

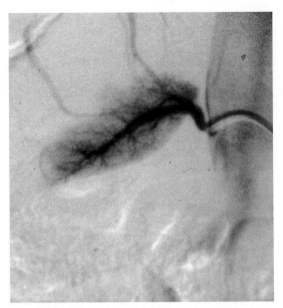

FIGURE 109-4. Right hepatic venogram for comparison with Figure 109-5.

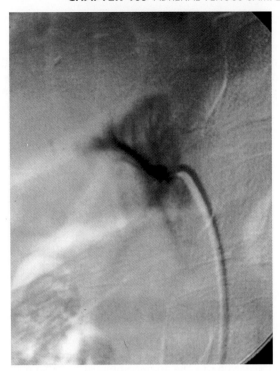

FIGURE 109-5. Normal right adrenal venogram with parenchymal blush.

temperature because the renin precursor prorenin is cryo-activated at −4°C to renin. Each laboratory may have different reference levels for renin and aldosterone.

A small side hole is made as close to the tip of each catheter as possible. If a side hole punch is unavailable, a small V can be made in the tip of the catheter. These reduce the tendency of the catheter to collapse the vein during aspiration of samples.

The IVC is accessed by the Seldinger technique from the right femoral vein. Once the IVC is accessed, a wire guide is not required.

The left renal vein is catheterized with the Cobra 2 catheter, and as the catheter is rotated counterclockwise, it is allowed to withdraw until the tip of the catheter turns upward. The left adrenal vein is usually found near the spinal border, and the catheter will catch in it easily. The catheter is inserted past the confluence of the left phrenic vein. Contrast agent is gently injected by hand with a film run to confirm position. The injection should not totally fill the adrenal veins within the gland until after the blood samples have been taken.

Aspiration is done until blood appears, then a sample of 5 to 8 mL is obtained. A slow and intermittent aspiration is required to avoid vein collapse. If the syringe fills rapidly, the catheter is probably not in the adrenal vein, and the position should be checked fluoroscopically. At the same time, a similar blood sample is taken from the femoral vein access sheath. The left adrenal vein should be accessed easily in all cases because the anatomy is quite constant.

The right adrenal vein is situated just above and posterior to the right renal vein. The biggest problem is finding it and not sampling a hepatic vein instead (Fig. 109-4). A similar side hole is made in the Hilal HS1 catheter. The Cobra catheter does not have enough length of curve at the tip to securely interrogate the wall of the IVC in most adults. Unlike the left adrenal vein, the right adrenal vein is short, and the catheter is more unstable within it. The position is confirmed with a small hand injection of contrast

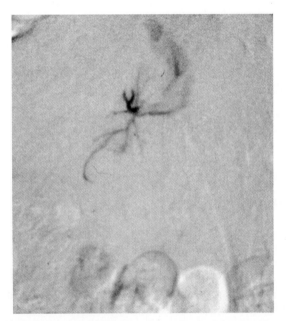

FIGURE 109-6. Right adrenal venogram showing distortion produced by a focal adenoma (same case as Fig. 109-2).

agent and a film run. The appearance of a hepatic vein and the normal right adrenal vein (Fig. 109-5) are quite different. Communication with another large vein indicates a hepatic vein. Although a formal adrenal venogram will show communications with renal capsular and hepatic veins, this is not expected with a small test injection of contrast agent (Fig. 109-6).

It can be difficult to obtain a large enough sample from the right adrenal vein. Most laboratories will make do with

4 to 5 mL, but they may be limited in their ability to perform repeated dilutions and provide exact measurements of aldosterone.

In the few patients in whom the right adrenal gland cannot be found, the alternative is to take IVC samples in the right renal vein and in the IVC between the right renal vein and the right atrium. This method is far less satisfactory because it results in a diluted sample compared with a selective adrenal vein sample. The right renal vein can be imaged on high-quality CT scans after intravenous administration of nonionic dimer contrast media and venous timing. Although this may provide the level of the vein, it does not guarantee a sample at the subsequent catheterization.

Normally, 95% success in achieving bilateral samples is achieved. Measuring the serum cortisol level will confirm that an adrenal sample was obtained. Usually, the adrenal cortisol is at least twice the peripheral level.

CONTROVERSIES

Adrenal venography is not strictly necessary, and it does add to the risk of the procedure, but it removes any debate about the site of the sample, and the samples may be numbered according to the angiographic runs. In some countries, angiography is remunerated but venous sampling is not.

Direct sampling of the adrenal vein will always show a higher level of aldosterone than a peripheral sample, and it is important to ensure that the biochemical workup before the venous sampling is robust and excludes other causes of elevated aldosterone.

OUTCOMES

Venous sampling is the most accurate way of determining what the cause of excessive aldosterone production is, provided patients have been properly selected, and hypokalemia and corticosteroid-induced aldosteronism have been excluded.

COMPLICATIONS

Complications are rare, and if gentle hand injections are used for angiography, adrenal vein damage should not occur.

Rough catheterization of the adrenal veins may cause spasm and result in failure of the procedure or rupture of the vein.

Rupture of an adrenal vein may result in infarction of the gland and loss of function.

POSTPROCEDURAL AND FOLLOW-UP CARE

Damage to the vein and infarction of the gland will cause immediate pain, and there will be biochemical evidence of loss of gland secretions.

Because adrenal vein sampling requires only a venous puncture, observation for 2 hours or so after the procedure is sufficient. If the patient has been sedated, he or she should be accompanied home. Resumption of normal activities is permitted the following day.

Results may take up to several weeks because most analysis laboratories will batch samples.

KEY POINTS

- Understanding the anatomy is the key to successful adrenal vein sampling.
- There is a single draining vein from each gland.
- The results of adrenal venous sampling are highly accurate for aldosteronism.
- Bilateral samples should be achieved in over 95% of attempts.

▶ **SUGGESTED READINGS**

Auchus RJ. Aldo is back: recent advances and unresolved controversies in hyperaldosteronism. Curr Opin Nephrol Hypertens 2003;12:153–8.

Geisinger MA, Zelch MG, Bravo EL, et al. Primary hyperaldosteronism: comparison of CT, adrenal venography, and venous sampling. AJR Am J Roentgenol 1983;141:299–302.

Magill SB, Raff H, Shaker JL, et al. Comparison of adrenal vein sampling and computed tomography in the differentiation of primary aldosteronism. J Clin Endocrinol Metab 2001;86:1066–71.

Mulatero P, Milan A, Fallo F, et al. Comparison of confirmatory tests for the diagnosis of primary aldosteronism. J Clin Endocrinol Metab 2006;91:2618–23.

Rossi GP, Chiesura-Corona M, Tregnaghi A, et al. Imaging of aldosterone-secreting adenomas: a prospective comparison of computed tomography and magnetic resonance imaging in 27 patients with suspected primary aldosteronism. J Hum Hypertens 1993;7:357–63.

Stowasser M, Gordon RD, Gunasekera TG, et al. High rate of detection of primary aldosteronism, including surgically treatable forms, after "non-selective" screening of hypertensive patients. J Hypertens 2003;21:2149–57.

Wheeler MH, Harris DA. Diagnosis and management of primary aldosteronism. World J Surg 2003;27:627–31.

Young WF Jr, Stanson AW, Grant CS, et al. Primary aldosteronism: adrenal venous sampling. Surgery 1996;120:913–9.

Young WF, Stanson AW, Thompson GB, et al. Role for adrenal venous sampling in primary aldosteronism. Surgery 2004;136:1227–35.

CHAPTER 110
Parathyroid Venous Sampling

Jeff Dai-Chee Tam, Mark F. Given, and Kenneth R. Thomson

Hyperparathyroidism is identified by direct assay of the circulating intact parathyroid hormone (iPTH). This leads to loss of regulation of calcium levels and hypercalcemia. Osteoporosis may occur, and if untreated, there is an increased incidence of cancer of the breast, colon, kidney, or prostate. Surgical removal of the hypersecreting gland or glands is the best treatment. In some cases there is diffuse hyperactivity, and in others a single gland is implicated.

Before surgery, enlarged parathyroid glands may be identified by high-resolution ultrasonography, multislice contrast-enhanced computed tomography (CT), magnetic resonance imaging (MRI), and technetium-99m (^{99m}Tc) sestamibi nuclear scanning.

In experienced hands, primary surgical excision is curative in 95% of cases, but only 64% of patients with secondary surgery show success.[1] Recently this outcome has been improved with the use of iPTH assays.[2] When the primary surgery fails, reoperative parathyroidectomy is often difficult and unsuccessful because of scarring and distortion of the tissue planes without localization of the site of excess parathyroid hormone secretion by selective venous sampling (SVS).

In a study of 228 consecutive patients with persistent/recurrent hyperparathyroidism, the single most common site of missed adenoma glands was in the tracheoesophageal groove in the superior compartment of the posterior mediastinum (27%). In this position, the glands may be adherent to the recurrent laryngeal nerve. Other ectopic sites for parathyroid adenomas in this group of patients were thymus (17%), intrathyroidal (10%), undescended glands (8.6%), carotid sheath (3.6%), and retroesophageal space (3.2%). The most sensitive and specific noninvasive imaging test was the ^{99m}Tc-sestamibi subtraction scan, with 67% true-positive and no false-positive results. The rate of true-positive results for ultrasonography, CT, MRI, and technetium thallium scans was approximately 50%.[3]

The accuracy of SVS for localization of the residual adenomas ranges between 75% and 90%[4,5] and is related to the skill and persistence of the operator. It is possible to combine ultrasonography and needle aspiration for parathyroid hormone assay to identify lymph nodes that are the major cause of false-positive scans with ultrasonography, CT, and MRI.[6]

INDICATIONS

- Localization of the site of excess parathyroid hormone secretion by SVS before planned reoperation for parathyroidectomy
- Differentiation of diffuse hyperplasia from a single hyperthyroid adenoma

CONTRAINDICATIONS

Venous sampling should only be used in patients who are planned surgical candidates and not as a triage to decide who should be referred for surgery.

EQUIPMENT

Catheter

A coaxial system is recommended because the normal anatomy is often disrupted by previous surgery, and the guide catheter helps prevent prolapse of the sampling catheter into the right atrium and ventricle. A 7F guide catheter 80 cm in length and an inner catheter of 4F external diameter and 100 cm long is used.

In complicated cases, a variety of catheter shapes tailored to the veins at the time may be required. Alternatively, a microcatheter may be used.

Guidewires

For general venous access, a Teflon-coated J-tip with a 1.5-mm curve radius (0.035-inch) diameter and that is 145 cm long (Cook Medical, Bloomington, Ind.) is used with a standard 0.035-inch angled guidewire (Glidewire, Terumo Medical Corp., Somerset, N.J.).

Deflecting tip wires and torque wires may also be required in difficult cases.

A fine-gauge guidewire (0.018-inch diameter) may be used with a Tuohy-Borst adapter to prevent the 4F catheter tip from obstructing on the vein wall when a sample is obtained from small veins.

Contrast Medium

Iodine, 300 mg/mL, is used. The volume and rate depend on the site of the injection and can be gauged from test injections. Hand injections only are used for filming.

Exposure Sequence

With digital subtraction angiography, two exposures per second for 1 to 2 seconds are obtained. Often this will demonstrate other nearby veins that should also be sampled.

Other Equipment

An ice bucket for the blood samples is required because all samples (usually 20-25) should be placed immediately on ice and transported to the laboratory with a vein diagram (Fig. 110-1) as soon as possible after the procedure.

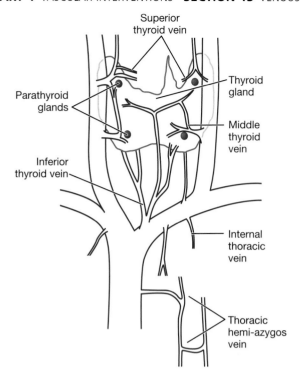

FIGURE 110-1. A diagram such as this one may be copied and used as a standard form when taking parathyroid venous blood samples. One can mark the site of each blood sample and send the marked form along with the blood samples to the laboratory to ensure correct localization.

A urinary catheter may be required for the patient if a long procedure is expected.

TECHNIQUE

Anatomy and Approaches

The inferior parathyroid glands arise from the third branchial cleft along with the thymus, and during development descend with the thymus. This explains why they may be found anywhere from the pericardial sac to the cricoid region. In the mediastinum, they are usually positioned anteriorly. The superior parathyroid glands, which arise from the fourth branchial cleft, are usually more consistent in position posterolateral to the superior pole of the thyroid gland close to the recurrent laryngeal nerve, but when ectopic tend to lie in the superior compartment of the posterior mediastinum.

Technical Aspects

These catheters and guidewire are listed as examples:
- 4F Glidecath, 0.038-inch guidewire compatible, 100 cm long, angle (A) tip shape
- Shapeable Glidewire (Terumo), straight tip, 0.035-inch diameter, 150 cm long, 3 cm flexible tip length
- 7F Pinnacle Destination Guiding Sheath (Terumo) with dilator, 7F inner diameter, 90 cm length, multipurpose curve style, Tuohy-Borst valve
- Progreat O Microcatheter (Terumo), 110 cm length, 2.8F outer diameter distal, 0.027-inch inner diameter, 17-cm tip flexibility, 0.021-inch maximal guidewire,

0.7-mm platinum marker band, 900 psi max pressure, 50-cm coating length, flow rate of 4.7 mL/s
Also needed are:
- Ice bucket and sample tubes. Blood samples must be kept chilled.
- A person to record the site of each sample as it is obtained
- Nonionic contrast medium: iodine, 300 mg/mL

Approach

A standard Seldinger approach from the common femoral vein is used. Sampling the major veins alone is insufficient because the right inferior thyroid vein may drain to the left innominate vein, and mediastinal adenomas may drain to cervical veins and vice versa.

A small venous injection of contrast medium and a short image sequence may be made at the beginning of the procedure to provide a "roadmap" to aid the examination and on which the site of each sample may be recorded. Alternatively, a low-volume venogram can be performed at each sampling site. This site should be marked on a printed diagram and a copy of the diagram sent with the blood samples to ensure correct localization (see Fig. 110-1).

Site of Injection

The best single vein to start the procedure from is the inferior thyroid vein, especially if there is a single inferior thyroid trunk. The middle thyroid veins are usually ligated at the first operation. The anterior jugular veins hardly ever drain parathyroid adenomas and should be avoided.

Samples should be obtained from both inferior thyroid veins because they are the normal drainage route for both the inferior and superior parathyroid glands. The middle thyroid, superior thyroid, vertebral, thymic, and internal mammary veins on each side should be sampled if possible. At surgery, many of these veins are ligated. Most laboratories require 3 to 4 mL of whole blood.

The superior thyroid vein may drain into the facial vein. Samples from midline veins are not usually helpful in localizing adenomas. Samples from the innominate and internal jugular veins are included but are not often helpful in lateralization. Samples should also be taken from the thoracic azygos veins.

A peripheral sample should also be taken from the iliac veins to provide a baseline value at the start and end of the procedure.

A positive sample is defined as a 1.5-fold increase in iPTH concentration compared with the iliac vein sample.

Accurate prediction of the location of a hyperactive parathyroid adenoma in a primary situation (i.e., no previous surgery) is between 75% and 90%. The accuracy in a secondary situation (i.e., persistent postoperative hypercalcemia) decreases because of ligation of the various vessels, resulting in anomalous drainage, which can be via the thyroid venous plexus or to the vertebral or anterior jugular vein.

CONTROVERSIES

In those centers where the cost of investigations is not a consideration, it is not unusual to find that a number of examinations (e.g., nuclear scintiscan, ultrasonography, CT, digital subtraction angiography, and MRI) have been performed in addition to SVS. The question is then in which order should these investigations be performed rather than which is most precise and useful. In our institution, once the diagnosis of hyperparathyroidism is established biochemically, surgery is performed with no further investigations.

Normally, angiography is not necessary, but in those cases in which surgery has been performed more than once or in radical fashion, the venous anatomy may be so disturbed that selective thyroid and internal mammary arteriography should be performed first to outline any anomalous veins. The inferior thyroid artery supplies the cervical spinal cord; proximal large-volume injections in this artery should be avoided.

For mediastinal adenomas, intentional overinjection of the gland with hypertonic contrast medium may result in infarction and cure of the hyperparathyroidism. In one series of 24 patients, the success rate was 83% at 1 month after ablation and 71% at both 5 and 9 years. Ablation was successful in 85% of the patients in whom the catheter could be wedged into the artery feeding the adenoma.[7] This method has not found wide acceptance even though it did not make subsequent surgery more difficult.

With 64-row multidetector CT it may be possible to avoid arteriography, and the delayed phase will provide a basic venous map. Direct aspiration of suspicious lesions with rapid iPTH assay may provide an alternative to lengthy venous sampling procedures.

Intraoperative sampling allows rapid confirmation of adenomas at primary operations but appears to be less useful for second or subsequent operations.

OUTCOMES

Parathyroid venous sampling currently has the highest sensitivity of any localization method for ectopic or overlooked parathyroid adenoma at initial surgery.[8]

COMPLICATIONS

Rupture of veins or extravasation of contrast agent may occur, but generally the examination is without incident.

POSTPROCEDURAL AND FOLLOW-UP CARE

Normal postprocedural care for a 7F femoral venous puncture is rest in the supine position for 2 hours.

KEY POINTS

- Venous sampling requires patience and a meticulous approach.
- It is a precursor to planned reoperative parathyroidectomy.
- Every vein available in the parathyroid region and upper mediastinum should be sampled if possible.
- Baseline peripheral samples are required.
- Samples must be kept chilled on ice as soon as they are taken.

▶ **SUGGESTED READINGS**

Seehofer D, Steinmuller T, Rayes N, et al. Parathyroid hormone venous sampling before reoperative surgery in renal hyperparathyroidism: comparison with noninvasive localization procedures and review of the literature. Arch Surg 2004;139:1331–8.

Winzelberg GG. Parathyroid imaging. Ann Intern Med 1987;107:64–70.

The complete reference list is available online at www.expertconsult.com.

CHAPTER **111**

Arteriography and Arterial Stimulation with Venous Sampling for Localizing Pancreatic Endocrine Tumors

Anthony W. Kam, Bradford J. Wood, and Richard Chang

Pancreatic endocrine tumors are uncommon tumors that belong to the family of amine precursor uptake and decarboxylation (APUD) neoplasms. They are called *functional* if the hormone released is associated with a clinical syndrome and *nonfunctional* if they are not associated with clinical symptoms. The incidence of functional pancreatic endocrine tumors is approximately 4 per million population per year.[1] The most common functional pancreatic endocrine tumors are gastrinomas (20%) and insulinomas (50%).[2] The number of nonfunctional pancreatic endocrine tumors diagnosed annually is 1 to 2 per million population.[3] Pancreatic polypeptide secreting tumors comprise the majority of nonfunctional pancreatic endocrine tumors. Surgical resection is the only treatment that can possibly cure patients with pancreatic endocrine tumors. Preoperative workup includes establishing the diagnosis clinically and biochemically, evaluating for the presence of multiple endocrine neoplasia type 1 (MEN-1), and imaging to determine the location of the primary tumor or tumors and the presence of metastatic disease. The imaging studies needed to localize and stage pancreatic endocrine tumors depend on the tumor type. Because pancreatic endocrine tumors other than gastrinomas and insulinomas are typically large at diagnosis, noninvasive imaging such as somatostatin receptor scintigraphy, computed tomography (CT), and magnetic resonance imaging (MRI) suffices to detect and stage these tumors. In contrast, hormonally active gastrinomas and insulinomas produce dramatic clinical symptoms, so patients come to medical attention when their tumors are small to occult at the time of initial presentation. In fact, 90% of these tumors are detected when 2 cm or less.[2]

This chapter examines the role, technique, and result of arteriography and arterial stimulation with venous sampling (ASVS) in localizing gastrinomas and insulinomas. ASVS involves injecting a secretagogue (secretin or calcium) into selected pancreatic and hepatic arteries and sampling for the appropriate hormone (gastrin or insulin) in hepatic veins.

INDICATIONS

Gastrinoma

Gastrinomas cause the Zollinger-Ellison syndrome (ZES), which is characterized by multiple and unusually located peptic ulcers and diarrhea. In sporadic ZES, the apparent primary gastrinomas are located in the duodenum (40%-50%), pancreas (30%-40%), lymph node (10%-15%), and nonpancreaticoduodenal or nodal sites (≤5%).[1] The percentage of gastrinomas that are malignant, as defined by metastatic disease, is 60% to 90%.[1,3] In contrast to pancreatic gastrinomas, duodenal gastrinomas tend to be small (<1 cm), can be multiple, and are more associated with

lymph node rather than hepatic metastases.[4] About 20% of patients with ZES have MEN-1, which is an autosomal dominant trait characterized by hyperplasia or tumors of the parathyroids, pituitary, and enteropancreatic endocrine system.[1] The tumors in these patients are invariably multiple and typically small; furthermore, the primary tumors are located in the duodenum (70%-95%) and pancreas (10%-25%).[1] For almost all ZES patients, gastric acid hypersecretion can be controlled effectively over the long term with proton pump inhibitors such as omeprazole or lansoprazole. The main limitation on long-term survival in ZES patients is tumor growth.[5] Clinically, there are two forms of gastrinomas. The aggressive form, which involves about 25% of patients with ZES, is more common in females and patients without MEN-1 and is associated with large pancreatic tumors, liver metastases, short disease duration, and a 10-year survival of 30%.[4,5] The nonaggressive form, involving 75% of patients with ZES, is associated more with duodenal gastrinomas, absence of liver metastases, and a 10-year survival of 96%.[4,5]

For patients with sporadic and localized gastrinomas, surgical exploration with intent for a curative resection is the treatment of choice. The cure rate for these patients is 34% at 10 years.[6] In contrast, the role of surgery in patients with ZES and MEN-1 is controversial.[1] Because of multiple tumors in these patients, the cure rate with local resection is less than 10%,[4] and a cure is not possible without a pancreaticoduodenectomy. Pancreaticoduodenectomy is not routinely indicated in patients with ZES, with or without MEN-1, because a survival benefit with this procedure has not been demonstrated, and the procedure itself can have substantial morbidity.[4] However, some surgeons will resect primary tumors larger than 2.5 cm on preoperative imaging in patients with ZES and MEN-1 in an attempt to prevent development of metastatic disease, because development of hepatic metastases correlates with primary tumor size.[1]

The biochemical diagnosis of ZES is established with elevated fasting serum gastrin levels (>200 pg/mL), increased basal gastric acid secretion (≥15 mEq/h), and a positive secretin stimulation test (>110 pg/mL increase in serum gastrin over basal levels after 0.4 μg/kg is given intravenously).[1] The role of preoperative imaging in patients with ZES is to identify the location and number of primary tumors and assess for metastases. The initial imaging study of choice is somatostatin receptor scintigraphy (SRS).[7] Gastrinomas express somatostatin receptors to which the somatostatin analog octreotide binds. SRS is the most sensitive noninvasive imaging modality for detecting primary gastrinomas or liver metastases. It detects approximately 58% of primary tumors and 92% of liver metastases,[8] but sensitivity depends on tumor size. SRS detects 30% of tumors 1.1 cm or less, 64% of tumors between 1.1 and 2 cm, and 96% of tumors larger than 2 cm.[9] SRS misses mainly

816

duodenal gastrinomas, which tend to be small (≤1 cm).[9] Because SRS does not provide information on tumor size and gives only an approximate location, CT or MRI, also performed routinely, are useful for detecting larger primary tumors and distant metastases. Single-photon emission computed tomography (SPECT)-CT hybrid imaging and software fusion of SRS with CT or MRI may help localize areas of increased activity on SRS.

If results of both SRS and CT or MRI are negative, an invasive localization study such as endoscopic ultrasonography (EUS) or arteriography with ASVS using secretin should be considered. The choice depends on local expertise. EUS has a sensitivity of about 85% in detecting pancreatic gastrinomas and about 43% in detecting duodenal gastrinomas.[4,10] Limitations of EUS include low sensitivity for tumors in the duodenal wall, tumors in the pancreatic tail, and small (<0.5 cm) tumors and false-positive results with lymph nodes, splenules, and pancreatic nodules.[10] In patients with sporadic ZES, whether EUS should be a routine preoperative study is controversial.[4,11] In patients with ZES and MEN-1 who are surgical candidates, there is more agreement that EUS should be included in the preoperative workup to identify additional pancreatic endocrine tumors and metastatic lymph nodes.[4] The advantage of ASVS over anatomic imaging is that ASVS is a functional study, so its sensitivity for detecting gastrinomas does not depend on tumor size.

Presently the indications for arteriography with ASVS in patients with ZES are controversial. A relative indication is failure to localize a gastrinoma with noninvasive imaging studies. The sensitivity of all preoperative imaging techniques in detecting duodenal gastrinomas is low. The most sensitive technique for detecting duodenal gastrinomas is intraoperative duodenotomy.[12] A stronger relative indication is to identify the tumor or tumors secreting gastrin in patients with ZES and MEN-1 who are surgical candidates, because these patients typically have multiple pancreatic endocrine tumors.[11,13]

Insulinoma

Insulinomas cause symptoms of hypoglycemia, which can be classified as neurologic or adrenergic. Neurologic symptoms include visual disturbances, confusion, altered consciousness, and less commonly seizures. Adrenergic symptoms include sweating, tremulousness, weakness, and palpitations. Unlike gastrinomas, insulinomas are exclusively found in the pancreas and are distributed evenly throughout the organ. Five to 15% of insulinomas are malignant, as defined by metastatic disease.[1] Most insulinomas are solitary. In the 2% to 10% of patients with multiple insulinomas or pancreatic endocrine tumors, one should evaluate for MEN-1.[1] About 4% of patients with insulinomas have MEN-1.[2] Because of the characteristic symptoms, insulinomas found at surgery are small: 90% less than 2 cm, 66% less than 1.5 cm, and 40% less than 1 cm.[2]

For insulinoma patients without metastases, surgical resection is curative. Preoperative workup includes establishing the diagnosis of insulinoma and obtaining noninvasive imaging. The diagnosis of insulinoma is confirmed by showing inappropriately high serum insulin levels with simultaneous symptomatic hypoglycemia during a supervised 72-hour fast and excluding other causes of hypoglycemia. Patients with insulinoma typically have serum insulin levels 6 μU/mL or higher.[14] The most common definition of hypoglycemia is a blood sugar level less than 45 mg/dL during a fast.[14] Insulinoma patients also should have an elevated plasma C-peptide level (≥200 pmol/L) and no sulfonylurea in the plasma.

There is agreement in using cross-sectional imaging such as CT or MRI to assess for metastatic disease, but the necessity for preoperative imaging to localize insulinomas in cases of presumed benign solitary insulinoma is controversial.[15,16] Because insulinomas are exclusively intrapancreatic, careful exploration and assessment with direct palpation and intraoperative ultrasound allow the surgeon to identify the vast majority of tumors. In fact, the sensitivity of intraoperative ultrasound in localizing insulinomas is 86% to 98% in experienced hands.[14,17], Nevertheless, preoperative localization of insulinomas is useful for several reasons. First, it helps the surgeon decide whether an open or laparoscopic approach is feasible and whether enucleation or resection is required to remove the tumor.[18-21] Second, if surgical exploration fails to localize an insulinoma, blind distal pancreatectomy is no longer recommended.[22] Positive preoperative localization is a requisite for a reoperation for insulinoma. Third, in patients with MEN-1, functional localization with ASVS can identify the tumor or tumors among the multiple pancreatic endocrine tumors responsible for hyperinsulinism. Fourth, because data from ASVS are usually concordant with intraoperative ultrasonography, preoperative data from ASVS can be helpful when expertise with intraoperative ultrasonography is not available or when findings are particularly subtle even to experienced ultrasonographers. Finally, in the differential diagnosis of hypoglycemia with hyperinsulinism, there is an entity called *noninsulinoma pancreatogenous hypoglycemia syndrome* (NIPHS).[23] Histologically, it is characterized by *nesidioblastosis*, which refers to islet cell hypertrophy and neoformation of islet cells from pancreatic exocrine duct cells.[23] Clinically, NIPHS is characterized by postprandial rather than fasting hypoglycemia. In the Mayo Clinic series, NIPHS accounted for 9% of their hyperinsulinemic hypoglycemia patients.[14] ASVS showing an insulin gradient in all pancreatic arterial distributions allows metabolic confirmation of this diagnosis.

Preoperative localization begins with noninvasive imaging such as CT, MRI, and/or transabdominal ultrasonography. The sensitivities of these noninvasive modalities are highly variable in different series but are typically less than 50% to 65%.[14,17] If noninvasive imaging is negative, one should consider invasive modalities such as EUS or arteriography with ASVS using calcium. Again, the choice depends on local expertise. The sensitivity of EUS in localizing insulinomas is about 80%.[10] The sensitivity in the pancreatic tail is lower than that in the pancreatic head.

CONTRAINDICATIONS

Contraindications to abdominal visceral arteriography and ASVS are the same as with any diagnostic arteriography. There is no absolute contraindication to angiography. Relative contraindications include uncontrolled hypertension, uncorrectable coagulopathy, severe allergy to iodinated contrast, severe renal insufficiency, and congestive heart failure.

For secretin ASVS, allergy to secretin and acute pancreatitis are relative contraindications. For calcium ASVS, cardiac glycosides are a relative contraindication. Glycosides and calcium are synergistic in their inotropic and toxic effects. Administration of calcium may induce arrhythmias in patients taking glycosides.

EQUIPMENT

The right hepatic vein is catheterized with a 4F or 5F Simmons-1 catheter from a femoral venous approach. Side holes are cut near the tip of the Simmons-1 catheter to facilitate blood draw by decreasing the possibility of suction against the venous wall. The left hepatic vein may be catheterized with a second Simmons-1 catheter.

Selective visceral arteriography is performed with 4F Cobra-2, SOS Omni, Simmons-1, and/or Simmons-2 catheters from a common femoral arterial approach. For extremely tortuous arteries, a coaxial technique with a microcatheter is helpful. Any microcatheter can be used; the authors prefer the 0.027-inch inner diameter microcatheters such as the Renegade Hi-Flo (Boston Scientific, Natick, Mass.) and Progreat O (Terumo Medical Corp., Somerset, N.J.) because these allow a tighter bolus of secretagogue.

For contrast, a nonionic iodinated agent such as iopamidol (Isovue 300 [Bracco Diagnostics Inc., Princeton, N.J.]) is used. Although there was a shortage of secretin for a period, secretin is now available in synthetic form as SecreFlo (Repligen Corp., Waltham, Mass.). This synthetic secretin has an amino acid sequence identical to porcine secretin. Calcium gluconate 10% is a generic agent (American Pharmaceutical Partners Inc., Schaumburg, Ill.).

TECHNIQUE

Anatomy and Approach

The technique of visceral arteriography for localizing gastrinomas is similar to that for localizing insulinomas. A common femoral arterial approach is most commonly used. The following selective arteriograms are performed: celiac, splenic, common hepatic, gastroduodenal, and superior mesenteric. The order of the selective arteriograms is not important. A celiac arteriogram shows most of the pancreas. In splenic arteriograms, a left anterior oblique projection is occasionally needed in addition to an anteroposterior projection.[13] The part of the pancreas that has a posterior course is seen en face in an anteroposterior projection, and summation of normal pancreatic enhancement in that part sometimes creates an impression of a tumor blush. A left anterior oblique projection lays out the pancreas and can confirm that a questionable blush is a summation effect. The splenic artery gives rise to numerous tiny arteries that supply the body and tail of the pancreas. The gastroduodenal artery gives rise to superior pancreaticoduodenal arteries that supply the head and neck of the pancreas and duodenum. The superior mesenteric artery (SMA) gives rise to an inferior pancreaticoduodenal artery supplying the head and neck of the pancreas and duodenum. In gastrinoma localization, a selective inferior pancreaticoduodenal arteriogram is occasionally needed to demonstrate duodenal primary tumors. In insulinoma

localization, selective dorsal pancreatic, pancreatic magna, and inferior pancreaticoduodenal arteriograms may be needed in addition. Glucagon (0.5-1 mg) can be given intravenously to decrease bowel peristalsis before an arteriogram but should be used with caution in patients with an insulinoma, because it can precipitate hypoglycemia.

Although both gastrinomas and insulinomas are hypervascular tumors, gastrinomas are less vascular than insulinomas.[13] If visualized on arteriography, their blushes appear early in the arterial phase and remain for a variable duration. Figures 111-1 to 111-3 show the typical appearances of a tumor blush in patients with gastrinomas and insulinomas.

Technical Aspects of Arterial Stimulation and Venous Sampling for Gastrinomas

In 1987, Imamura et al. pioneered the technique of ASVS using secretin for localizing gastrinomas in patients with ZES.[24] The technique of ASVS for gastrinomas at the

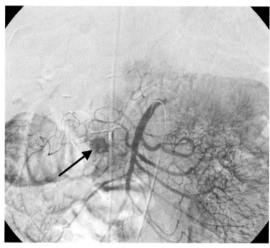

FIGURE 111-1. Selective superior mesenteric arteriogram shows an approximately 1-cm tumor blush at caudal aspect of pancreatic head *(arrow)*, suggesting gastrinoma in patient with Zollinger-Ellison syndrome. Results of secretin arterial stimulation with venous sampling shown in Figure 111-4.

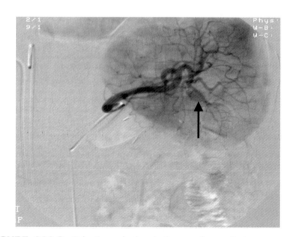

FIGURE 111-2. Selective splenic arteriogram demonstrates an approximately 1-cm tumor blush in tail of pancreas *(arrow)*, consistent with insulinoma in patient with biochemical evidence of insulinoma. Calcium arterial stimulation with venous sampling showed positive insulin gradients from both mid- and proximal splenic artery injections.

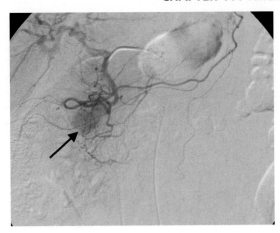

FIGURE 111-3. Selective gastroduodenal arteriogram demonstrates an approximately 3-cm tumor blush in pancreatic head *(arrow)*, suggesting insulinoma in patient with biochemical evidence of insulinoma. Results of calcium arterial stimulation with venous sampling shown in Figure 111-6.

National Institutes of Health (NIH) has evolved since the first report in 1990.[25-27] From a bilateral femoral venous approach, catheters are placed into the right and left hepatic veins. From a femoral arterial approach, standard visceral arteriography is performed with selective injections of contrast agent into the SMA, proximal splenic, proximal gastroduodenal, and proper hepatic arteries. If a tumor blush is visualized, the artery supplying the blush is injected with the secretagogue last. After each selective arteriogram, 4-mL samples are drawn from the right and left hepatic veins for baseline gastrin levels. Then 30 IU of secretin diluted in 5 mL of normal saline is injected into the selected artery as a bolus. The rate of injection should not result in reflux out of the selected artery as determined by a test bolus of contrast agent. Samples from both hepatic veins are obtained 20, 40, and 60 seconds after secretin injection for gastrin assay. Sampling at later times is no longer performed because recirculation can result in nonspecific rises in serum gastrin levels. A *gastrin gradient* is defined as the percent increase in gastrin level above the baseline level obtained before each selective secretin injection. A positive localization requires a gastrin gradient of at least 25% at 20 seconds, 78% at 40 seconds, or 109% at 60 seconds.[26,27] A positive gastrin gradient with injection into the gastroduodenal artery and/or SMA localizes the gastrinoma to the region including the pancreatic head and neck and duodenum (*gastrinoma triangle*). A positive gradient with injection of the splenic artery localizes the gastrinoma to the region of the pancreatic body and tail. A positive gradient with injection of the proper hepatic artery suggests hepatic metastases, but the sensitivity of this test is low.[28]

There are variations to this technique. First, venous sampling can be performed with one hepatic vein. The right hepatic vein is most commonly sampled because it is easier to catheterize. Right and left hepatic veins were sampled during the development of ASVS because of the concern that tumors that drain to the splenic vein may be missed if splenic venous flow preferentially streamed to the left hepatic vein. It has been shown that preferential streaming does not occur for insulinomas in the pancreatic body and tail.[29] Sampling from only the right hepatic vein, however, could further reduce sensitivity in detecting hepatic metastases.

Second, calcium gluconate is an alternative secretagogue to secretin in localizing gastrinomas.[30] Whereas secretin specifically stimulates gastrin release from gastrinomas, a local increase in calcium concentration causes gastrinoma and insulinoma cells to degranulate and secrete their respective hormones. There is a possibility that calcium gluconate is an improvement over secretin. The dose of secretin, 30 IU or 2 nmol per injection, causes a substantial rise in plasma secretin concentration that is on the order of pmol/L; therefore, recirculation is a problem. The doses of calcium used in ASVS do not result in any significant rise in plasma calcium concentration. Because there is only one case report and the experience of the authors in using intra-arterial calcium to localize gastrinomas is preliminary, further evaluation is necessary to determine whether calcium gluconate can replace secretin.

Patients with ZES who are scheduled for ASVS need not stop their proton pump inhibitors. ASVS can be performed with elevated basal gastrin levels.[13]

Technical Aspects of Arterial Stimulation and Venous Sampling for Insulinomas

In 1991, Doppman et al. introduced ASVS using calcium for localizing insulinomas in patients with hyperinsulinemic hypoglycemia.[31] At NIH, the technique of ASVS for insulinomas is similar to that for gastrinomas, with several exceptions. There are selective injections into the mid- and proximal splenic artery in an attempt to localize a tumor to the pancreatic tail or body, respectively. The midsplenic artery is defined as just distal to the origin of the pancreatic magna artery. The secretagogue, 10% calcium gluconate, is diluted to 5 mL with saline and given at a dose of 0.0125 mmol/kg (0.025 mEq/kg). In obese patients, the dose is adjusted to 0.005 mmol/kg. The time between calcium injections should be at least 5 minutes to allow the hepatic venous plasma insulin level to return to its baseline. Then 5-mL samples from the hepatic veins are obtained before and 20, 40, and 60 seconds after calcium injection. The samples are kept in ice until they can be centrifuged, and the resulting plasma is stored at −20°C. Insulin levels are measured by radioimmunoassay. A twofold or more increase in the insulin level (an insulin gradient of at least 100%) from the 20-, 40-, or 60-second sample localizes an insulinoma to the territory of the artery studied. The insulin gradient typically peaks by 60 seconds. A positive insulin gradient in the gastroduodenal artery and/or SMA localizes the insulinoma to the pancreatic head and neck. A positive gradient in the proximal splenic artery localizes the insulinoma to the pancreatic body and tail. Positive gradients in both the proximal and midsplenic artery localize the insulinoma to the pancreatic tail. A positive gradient in the proximal splenic artery and no gradient in the midsplenic artery localize the insulinoma to the pancreatic body.

There are variations to this method. Sometimes only the right hepatic vein is sampled. In patients with occult insulinomas (in whom ASVS is usually performed), hepatic metastases are extremely rare, so the proper hepatic artery injection can be omitted. The arteries that are injected are the SMA, mid- and proximal splenic, and gastroduodenal arteries. There are also variations in the dose of calcium gluconate used for each bolus. Many groups use a dose dependent on body weight. Although 0.0125 mmol/kg is the most common dose, a dose as low as 0.00312 mmol/kg has been reported.[32] Other groups use a fixed dose ranging from 0.23 mmol (1 mL of 10% calcium gluconate) to 0.70 mmol (3 mL of 10% calcium gluconate).[13,33] Some groups obtain two baseline samples separated by 1 minute before calcium injection to ensure the hepatic venous insulin level has returned to baseline.[13] Some groups sample to 180 seconds and define a positive localization as a twofold or more increase in insulin from baseline 30 to 120 seconds after injection.[32] Some groups periodically monitor blood glucose levels during the procedure.[13]

Diazoxide, a nondiuretic benzothiadiazine, is occasionally used to treat insulinoma patients awaiting surgery. It should be suspended before calcium ASVS because it inhibits insulin release.

CONTROVERSIES

Controversies in the indications for secretin and calcium ASVS were discussed under Indications, and variations in the technique for ASVS were discussed under Technical Aspects. The utility of SPECT-CT hybrid imaging with octreotide and software fusion of SRS with CT or MRI in localizing gastrinomas warrants evaluation.

OUTCOMES

Gastrinoma

Angiography is operator dependent. In a 1987 NIH review involving 70 patients with surgically proven gastrinomas, sensitivity of selective angiography was 68% for extrahepatic tumors and 86% for hepatic tumors.[34] In a 1999 NIH review involving 35 surgically proven gastrinoma patients, sensitivity of angiography was 57% on a per-patient basis and 30% on a per-lesion basis.[26] Angiography demonstrated 20% of primary duodenal tumors, 46% of primary pancreatic tumors, and 28% of metastatic nodes.[26]

Figure 111-4 shows the typical results of a secretin ASVS for a patient with a gastrinoma in the pancreatic head.

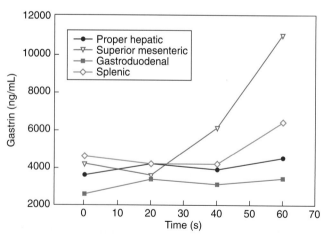

FIGURE 111-4. Secretin arterial stimulation with venous sampling results for patient with sporadic Zollinger-Ellison syndrome with gastrinoma in pancreatic head. Gastrin gradient from a hepatic vein is 162% at 60 seconds after stimulation of superior mesenteric artery and 31% at 20 seconds after stimulation of gastroduodenal artery.

Figure 111-5 illustrates that calcium gluconate can be used as a secretagogue for both insulinomas and gastrinomas. Because ASVS involves catheterizing the main visceral arteries, ASVS is less operator dependent. In a 1992 NIH review of 36 patients with ZES, the sensitivity of ASVS was compared with that of transhepatic portal venous sampling.[27] Portal venous shunting involves a direct access to the right portal vein and selective catheterization of the tributaries of the portal vein. In the review, gastrinomas were found in 33 patients at surgery; sensitivities of secretin ASVS and portal venous shunting were 89% and 60%, respectively.[27] As such, because of its higher complication rate, portal venous shunting is no longer performed in localizing gastrinomas. In the 1999 NIH review of 35 gastrinoma patients, the sensitivity of secretin ASVS was 77%.[26] Secretin ASVS only regionalizes gastrinomas and does not indicate the number of tumors present. Overall,

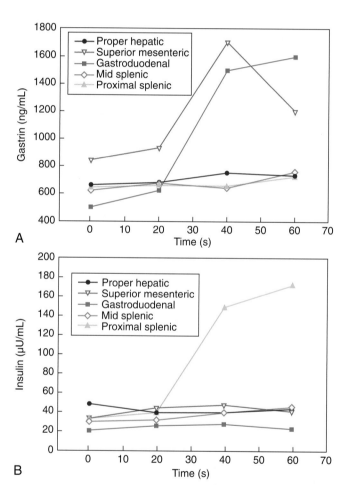

FIGURE 111-5. Calcium arterial stimulation with venous sampling results for patient with multiple endocrine neoplasia type 1 with biochemical evidence of both gastrinoma and insulinoma. **A,** Positive gastrin gradients from stimulation of both superior mesenteric and gastroduodenal arteries localize gastrinomas to pancreatic head and neck and/or duodenum. **B,** Fivefold rise in insulin level from proximal splenic artery stimulation without significant rise in insulin level from stimulation of midsplenic artery localizes insulinomas to body of pancreas. Resection of three duodenal gastrinomas, enucleation of a pancreatic head (due to pancreatic endocrine tumor), and subtotal distal pancreatectomy and splenectomy involving eight pancreatic endocrine tumors and three metastatic nodes resolved hyperinsulinemic hypoglycemia but did not alter hypergastrinemia.

the sensitivity of secretin ASVS is higher than that of SRS in detecting extrahepatic gastrinomas. Unlike other imaging modalities, because it is a functional study, the sensitivity of ASVS is independent of tumor size. The sensitivity of secretin ASVS for detecting hepatic metastases, however, is low at 41%.[28]

Insulinoma

There is considerably more literature on localization of insulinomas with angiography and ASVS. Reported sensitivity of angiography in localizing insulinomas varies widely from 35% to 94%,[16,17,35-39] likely the result of referral bias and operator dependency. In the largest series, the sensitivity of angiography was about 60%.[16,17,35,38]

Figure 111-6 demonstrates a typical sampling result from a patient with an insulinoma in the pancreatic head. The sensitivity of calcium ASVS in localizing insulinomas ranges from 78% to 100%.[17,29,36,37,40,41] In the 1999 NIH review of 39 insulinoma patients, which is the largest published series, the sensitivity of calcium ASVS was 92%.[26] Calcium ASVS has replaced transhepatic portal venous shunting, which has a sensitivity of 55% to 77% in localizing occult insulinomas.[29,35,42]

COMPLICATIONS

Overall, complications of ASVS are uncommon. There is no complication specific to secretin ASVS. For calcium ASVS, there are two reported cases of symptomatic hypoglycemia at a dose of 0.0125 mmol/kg.[17,32] In the first case, the examination was stopped and repeated at a later date at a dose of 0.00312 mmol/kg without complications.[32] In the second case, the hypoglycemic symptoms resolved with an infusion of glucose water.[17] The authors infused dextrose 5% in water into two venous sites during the procedure to prevent hypoglycemia.

Pancreatitis is a potential complication in calcium ASVS. Doppman et al. suggested that injection of calcium into small pancreatic arteries like the dorsal pancreatic and pancreatic magna arteries may cause pancreatitis.[29] In a superselective version of ASVS, Baba et al. injected calcium at a concentration of 0.005 mmol/kg into the dorsal pancreatic arteries of six patients.[41] None developed pancreatitis. Other potential complications are related to the angiography procedure.

POSTPROCEDURAL AND FOLLOW-UP CARE

Postprocedural management is standard postangiographic care. The arterial catheter or sheath is removed, and hemostasis is achieved before removal of the venous catheters. Venous samples are sent to the appropriate laboratory. When results of the hormone levels become available, the radiologist should discuss these results with the endocrine and surgical teams.

KEY POINTS

- Functional pancreatic endocrine tumors such as gastrinomas and insulinomas tend to be small to occult at presentation.
- Visceral arteriography together with arterial stimulation with venous sampling (ASVS) has a high sensitivity in localizing gastrinomas and insulinomas, independent of their size.
- The indications for secretin ASVS are controversial and include failure of noninvasive imaging to localize a gastrinoma and regionalization of the gastrin-secreting tumor when multiple tumors are present.
- The indications for calcium ASVS are controversial and include failure of noninvasive imaging to localize an insulinoma, failure of a surgical exploration to find an insulinoma, regionalization of the insulin-secreting tumor when multiple tumors are present, anticipated difficulty with either intraoperative palpation or ultrasound, and evaluation for noninsulinoma pancreatogenous hypoglycemia syndrome.
- Endoscopic ultrasonography is competitive with ASVS in localizing gastrinomas and insulinomas.
- Calcium gluconate is a secretagogue in ASVS for both insulinomas and gastrinomas.

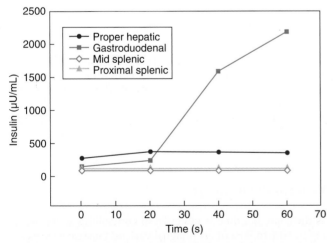

FIGURE 111-6. Calcium arterial stimulation with venous sampling results for hyperinsulinemic patient with insulinoma in pancreatic head. Note 15.5-fold increase in insulin level from a hepatic vein at 60 seconds after stimulation of gastroduodenal artery.

▶ **SUGGESTED READINGS**

Grant CS. Insulinoma. Best Pract Res Clin Gastroenterol 2005;19: 783–98.

Grossman AB, Reznek RH. Commentary: imaging of islet-cell tumours. Best Pract Res Clin Endocrinol Metab 2005;19:241–3.

Jackson JE. Angiography and arterial stimulation venous sampling in the localization of pancreatic neuroendocrine tumours. Best Pract Res Clin Endocrinol Metab 2005;19:229–39.

Norton JA, Jensen RT. Resolved and unresolved controversies in the surgical management of patients with Zollinger-Ellison syndrome. Ann Surg 2004;240:757–73.

The complete reference list is available online at www.expertconsult.com.

CHAPTER **112**

Transjugular Intrahepatic Portosystemic Shunts

Mark Duncan Brooks and Changqing Li

Cirrhosis and its complications are common throughout the world. Hepatitis B and C and alcohol abuse account for about 90% of cases. Autoimmune chronic active hepatitis, primary and secondary biliary cirrhosis, hemochromatosis, Budd-Chiari syndrome, and others make up the remaining 10%. Risk of death comes from variceal bleeding, progressive liver failure, and hepatoma. Key quality-of-life issues include management of ascites and hepatic encephalopathy.

Cirrhosis is an irreversible condition, the only potential cure being liver transplantation. However, liver transplant is an expensive and complex process. There are strict selection criteria and long waiting lists for transplant. The result is a large pool of patients with portal hypertension. Transjugular intrahepatic portosystemic shunt (TIPS) is one of the treatments available to control the complications of portal hypertension.

PATHOPHYSIOLOGY OF PORTAL HYPERTENSION

Venous blood from the gut, spleen, and pancreas drains via the portal venous system into the liver. It reaches the hepatic sinusoids, which drain into the hepatic veins. In cirrhosis, the liver responds to persistent damage by regenerating in nodules of hepatocytes, disrupting normal anatomy. Drainage through the sinusoids is impaired, leading to an increase in the pressure gradient between the portal vein and hepatic veins.

Two additional factors contribute to portal hypertension. Vasoconstriction in intrahepatic vessels elevates sinusoidal resistance further. Vasodilation in splanchnic vessels results in increased intestinal blood flow and a consequent increase in portal venous inflow. When portal pressure is chronically elevated, naturally existing collateral veins enlarge, becoming varices that provide alternative venous drainage from the portal venous system into systemic veins.

Esophageal varices are most common, occurring in 40% of cirrhotic patients at diagnosis and increasing by 6% per year. Gastric varices are seen in about 20% of patients and tend to occur later in the course of cirrhosis. Ectopic varices are less common. Sites include duodenum, jejunum, lienorenal, rectal, and parastomal varices. Although varices close to a mucosal surface are associated with bleeding risk, those distant from the surface are unlikely to bleed. Drainage through these veins helps keep portal pressure down.

Variceal bleeding is a major cause of death in portal hypertension. In patients with varices, the risk of a first hemorrhage is around 4% per year. Risk factors include size of varices, Child-Pugh class B or C, and hepatic vein pressure gradient (HVPG) greater than 12 mmHg. HVPG is measured using a transjugular catheter, comparing pressure when the catheter tip is wedged and free within the vein, and reflects the portal-to-systemic pressure gradient. Esophageal varices account for 70% of bleeding, and most of the remainder are gastric variceal hemorrhages. Mortality within 6 weeks of bleeding is about 30%. It is most often related to uncontrolled bleeding or early rebleeding. Other important causes of death after variceal bleeding are liver failure, multiorgan failure, and sepsis. Without preventive treatment, rebleeding occurs within 2 years in up to 65% of patients, and mortality from rebleeding is 33%.[1]

Ascites in patients with cirrhosis and portal hypertension is a result of multiple factors. Elevated venous pressure in the gut causes low protein fluid transudate into the peritoneal cavity. Elevated sinusoidal pressure causes high protein transudate from the liver surface. Renal effects of cirrhosis result in sodium and water retention. Reduced albumin contributes to extravascular fluid retention. Ascites causes significant impairment of quality of life. Frequent percutaneous drainage procedures may be required. Complications include spontaneous bacterial peritonitis and hepatorenal syndrome. TIPS is most effective in treatment of ascites when the HVPG is high.[2]

TREATMENT OF PORTAL HYPERTENSION

Measures for prevention and treatment of variceal bleeding include endoscopic, interventional, and drug treatments. Endoscopic treatment includes sclerosant injection, band ligation, and cyanoacrylate injection of varices. Interventional treatments include TIPS, transhepatic coil embolization, balloon-occluded retrograde transvenous obliteration (BRTO) and partial splenic embolization.

Drugs that reduce portal pressure include the vasoconstrictor drugs terlipressin and octreotide in acute therapy and propranolol for long-term control. These agents reduce splanchnic blood flow. The vasodilators glyceryl trinitrate and isosorbide mononitrate reduce resistance at the hepatic sinusoidal level.

INDICATIONS

Variceal Hemorrhage

Endoscopic banding is effective in controlling acute bleeding in 80% to 90% of esophageal varices. Gastric varices are more difficult to control but may respond to endoscopic glue injection. Ectopic varices are not treatable endoscopically. Emergency TIPS is indicated when endoscopic therapy fails to control esophageal or gastric variceal bleeding and as a first-line therapy for bleeding ectopic varices. Outcomes are best when TIPS is performed early, ideally within 24 hours of presentation.[3,4]

TIPS is also used for prevention of rebleeding. Recurrence of bleeding after successful endoscopic control is a common problem, with high morbidity, mortality, and cost. Even with preventive medical therapy, rebleeding occurs in 25% to 33% of patients over 18 months.[5] A recent randomized controlled trial identified patients with high risk of rebleed and compared the outcome of endoscopic banding plus TIPS with banding alone. The study demonstrated a marked reduction in rebleeding and improved patient survival at 1 year.[4] The authors identified the timing of TIPS within 72 hours of endoscopy as a critical factor in producing an improved clinical outcome.

Gastric varices have a greater tendency to rebleed acutely after successful TIPS. Rebleeding can occur despite reducing the portal systemic pressure gradient to less than 12 mmHg. For this reason, transvenous embolization and sclerosis of varices should be performed routinely during TIPS for bleeding gastric varices.[6]

Ascites

Transjugular intrahepatic portosystemic shunting is effective in reducing ascites in patients with portal hypertension. In addition to symptomatic control, potential benefits are reduced risk of hepatorenal syndrome and spontaneous bacterial peritonitis. However, its role is limited by the risk of developing the complications of encephalopathy and progressive liver failure. Results of trials and meta-analyses are mixed when assessing benefits to survival and quality of life.[7-11] Improvement in control of ascites can be expected in approximately two thirds of patients. New or worsened encephalopathy is seen in 32%. This can usually be controlled with medication but may require a shunt-reducing stent or shunt occlusion.[12] Six-month mortality is around 36%.[7] Poor outcome is more likely in those with a bilirubin level over 3 mg/dL, creatinine level over 1.5 mg/dL, and age older than 60.[9] Improved ascites control is more likely in those with a higher portosystemic pressure gradient (mean 21 mmHg vs. 15 mmHg).[10]

Because of its potential complications and uncertain effects on life expectancy and quality, TIPS is generally considered to be indicated only in those patients with large-volume ascites that cannot be controlled with medical therapy and requires repeated large-volume paracentesis at less than monthly intervals.

Hepatic hydrothorax, in which ascitic fluid passes through defects in the diaphragm, is similar to ascites in its pathophysiology and responds to TIPS in a similar way.

Budd-Chiari Syndrome

Budd-Chiari syndrome is a rare condition resulting from occlusion of hepatic venous drainage. It can be divided into a classic form, resulting from intrahepatic venous thrombosis, and a suprahepatic form, also known as *membranous occlusion of the vena cava*. Our experience is confined to the classic form. Interventional procedures appear to be important in treating this condition, but its rarity and highly variable prognosis make it difficult to measure improvements in patient outcomes associated with specific

treatments. Presentation is most commonly with subacute disease causing ascites and tender hepatomegaly. Less common is fulminant hepatic failure. A small percentage present with end-stage chronic liver disease. Patients with well-compensated disease, particularly where not all hepatic veins are involved, typically have a good long-term prognosis

Treatment is indicated in patients who are symptomatic or have abnormal liver function tests, suggesting ongoing damage to hepatocytes. Treatments aimed at restoring normal hepatic venous drainage include thrombolysis, angioplasty, and stenting. These may be successful at controlling symptoms in the short term, but in our experience, recurrence due to restenosis is common. If these treatments fail or are not appropriate, TIPS can be used to provide an alternative venous outflow path for the liver. TIPS provides good symptomatic control and improved liver function in both fulminant and subacute Budd-Chiari syndrome. With use of covered stents, long-term TIPS patency can be achieved, but it should be noted that this group has an increased risk of shunt stenosis and thrombosis. Regular long-term follow-up is critical because restenosis is associated with progressive liver damage.

Although no randomized studies have been performed, patients treated with TIPS have a good long-term survival compared with historical series and predicted survival based on biochemical and clinical parameters at presentation.[13,14] Control of symptoms and prevention of disease progression means these patients can delay or avoid the need for liver transplantation.[15]

ALTERNATIVES TO TRANSJUGULAR INTRAHEPATIC PORTOSYSTEMIC SHUNT

With some patients' liver anatomy, it may be feasible or preferred to place percutaneous portosystemic shunts directly from the inferior vena cava (IVC) to the portal vein or potentially between other portal and systemic veins with appropriate anatomy. The direct intrahepatic portosystemic shunt (DIPS) extends from the intrahepatic IVC through a short parenchymal track in the caudate lobe of the liver into the portal vein. Stented to 8 mm with a covered balloon-expandable stent, it provides a short low-resistance shunt with minimal liver trauma and low risk of restenosis.[16]

In patients with predicted poor outcome from TIPS, bleeding can be controlled using alternative interventional techniques, either BRTO[17] or transhepatic transportal injection of sclerosant, with or without coil embolization. Although these techniques are uncommon in Western countries, they are widely practiced in some Japanese and Chinese centers to the point where they are preferred to TIPS, particularly in the treatment of gastric variceal bleeding. Published results suggest these techniques may result in improved survival with lower rates of encephalopathy and rebleeding.

CONTRAINDICATIONS

Relative contraindications to TIPS include:
• Cardiac failure, elevated right-sided heart pressure, and pulmonary hypertension

- Rapidly progressive liver failure
- Severe uncorrectable coagulopathy
- Uncontrolled sepsis
- Unrelieved biliary obstruction
- Extensive primary or metastatic hepatic malignancy
- Clinically significant encephalopathy

Polycystic liver disease has previously been considered a contraindication, but TIPS has been performed safely in these patients with the use of bare metal stents. It is likely to be safe with covered stents, although this remains to be tested.[18] Coagulopathy, shock, and sepsis are relative contraindications, but it may still be appropriate to perform an urgent TIPS procedure while these are being corrected.

A number of anatomic features may make TIPS difficult or impossible. These include absence or thrombosis of the portal vein and distortion of venous anatomy due to liver atrophy. Modified TIPS techniques may be effective in these patients.

Other relative contraindications are predictors of poor prognosis after TIPS. The most accurate prediction of post-TIPS mortality is the Model for End-Stage Liver Disease (MELD) score. The scoring system was developed specifically for use in prediction of post-TIPS outcome.[19] It provides a score based on a weighted mathematical formula including creatinine, bilirubin, and the international normalized ratio (INR):

$$9.6 \times \log e(\text{Creatinine [mg/dL]})$$
$$+ 3.8 \times \log e(\text{Bilirubin [mg/dL]}) + 11.2 \times \log e(\text{INR})$$
$$+ 6.4 \times (\text{etiology: 0 if alcoholic or cholestatic, 1 otherwise})$$

A 30-day mortality of 3.7% (1 in 27) is reported for patients with a MELD score of 1 to 10. Mortality increases to 60% (3 in 5) with a MELD score above 24.[20]

The Child-Pugh score has similar predictive effect on patient outcome after TIPS but may be slightly less accurate.[21] The simplest prognostic measure is the serum bilirubin value alone. A bilirubin value over 3 mg/dL is associated with an increase in 30-day mortality after TIPS.

EQUIPMENT

Equipment required includes a TIPS set, a range of guidewires, angiographic catheters, angioplasty balloons, and stents (Table 112-1). Invasive pressure measuring equipment, appropriate patient monitoring facilities, and high-quality digital subtraction angiographic imaging are essential. Ultrasound imaging is also useful.

The TIPS set we use is the Cook RUPS set (Cook Medical, Bloomington, Ind.). It includes a long 10F sheath, a 10F angle-tipped steel-reinforced cannula, and a 5F catheter with a central pointed trocar. In this set, the steel-reinforced cannula is positioned in the hepatic vein and directed toward the portal vein. Then the 5F catheter/trocar combination is advanced through the liver parenchyma into the portal vein. In other sets, including the Ring (Cook Medical) and Haskal (Cook Medical) sets, the 16-gauge angled steel cannula is the sharp component advanced through the liver. A third design, the Hawkins transjugular access set (Angio-Dynamics, Latham, N.Y.) employs a 68-cm 21-gauge needle introduced through a 14-gauge angled steel cannula. While each different design has its advantages, local availability

TABLE 112-1. Disposable Equipment

TIPS Set
40-cm long, 10F sheath
10F angled introducer with metal stiffener
47-cm, 5F straight catheter with central sharp 0.035-inch trocar wire

Angioplasty Balloons
Predilation balloon: 8 × 40 mm
Postdilation balloons: 10 × 40 mm, 12 × 40 mm

Guidewires
Amplatz Extra Stiff: 0.035 inch, 260 cm
Angled Glidewire: 0.035 inch, 150 cm
Bentson wire: 0.035 inch, 145 cm

Catheters
5F Davis T, 65 cm
5F multipurpose, 65 cm
5F Cobra, 65 cm

Stents
VIATORR. Covered lengths 5 to 8 cm, diameter 10 mm (8 mm and 12 mm also available)

Micropuncture Set
22-gauge Chiba needle
0.021-inch platinum-tipped Mandril wire

Invasive Pressure Measuring Transducer

TIPS, Transjugular intrahepatic portosystemic shunt.

and operator familiarity usually dictate which device is used.

Our preferred TIPS stent is the VIATORR made by W.L. Gore & Associates (Flagstaff, Ariz.). This is a purpose-designed covered TIPS endoprosthesis made from nitinol and expanded polytetrafluoroethylene (ePTFE). Its inner surface is identical to standard vascular grafts, whereas an outer less porous layer is designed to withstand bile intrusion into the lumen. The graft is supported by a nitinol wire skeleton. At its portal end is a highly flexible uncovered segment of nitinol stent that anchors the device in the portal vein without occluding portal flow.

TECHNIQUE

Procedure Planning

In patients referred for treatment of acute upper gastrointestinal bleeding, preprocedural assessment should answer the following questions:

- Is there evidence of portal hypertension?
- Is variceal bleeding the cause of the current presentation? Endoscopy should include a search for other sources of bleeding such as peptic ulcer, sclerotherapy-induced ulcers, and Mallory-Weiss tear.
- Is the patient likely to develop encephalopathy or liver failure as a result of TIPS?
- Have appropriate first-line treatments for variceal bleeding been undertaken?

Review of imaging should ideally include recent contrast-enhanced computed tomography (CT). Points to note are liver size, hepatic vein, and portal vein anatomy.

Approach and Technique

Standard access for TIPS is through the right internal jugular vein (Fig. 112-1). The 40-cm, 10F sheath is advanced into the IVC. A 5F multipurpose shaped catheter is manipulated into the right hepatic vein. The catheter is then exchanged over a stiff wire for the TIPS cannula. The angled metal cannula is positioned 2 cm into the hepatic vein and directed anteriorly and inferiorly toward the right portal vein. The sharp trocar and 5F catheter combination is advanced a few centimeters through liver parenchyma into the right portal vein. The trocar is removed from the catheter. If blood can be freely aspirated, contrast agent is injected to confirm that the catheter has entered a portal vein. Repeated passes of the catheter/trocar combination may be required. For subsequent paths, the catheter is redirected by advancing, withdrawing, rotating, or reshaping the TIPS cannula. Once the portal vein has been entered, the catheter is advanced over an angled hydrophilic guidewire (Radiofocus Guide wire M [Terumo Medical Corp., Somerset, N.J.]) into the main portal vein. The wire is then exchanged for a 260-cm Amplatz Extra Stiff guidewire (Cook Medical). The rest of the TIPS set including the 10F sheath is then advanced over the stiff guidewire into the main portal vein. All components except the sheath and the wire are then removed. The portal pressure is measured through the sheath. The sheath is then pulled back over the stiff wire, and right atrial pressure is measured. An 8-mm angioplasty balloon is inflated across the parenchymal track. The sites of balloon waist formation are good indicators of the portal and hepatic vein ends of the track. A graduated marking catheter is used to determine the length of stent required. Choose a stent with covered segment 1 cm longer than the length measured from portal vein entry site to hepatic vein–IVC junction.

The right hepatic–to–right portal vein approach is preferred, partly for reasons of familiarity. Also it produces a track that remains intrahepatic and does not traverse central anatomic structures such as major ducts or arteries.

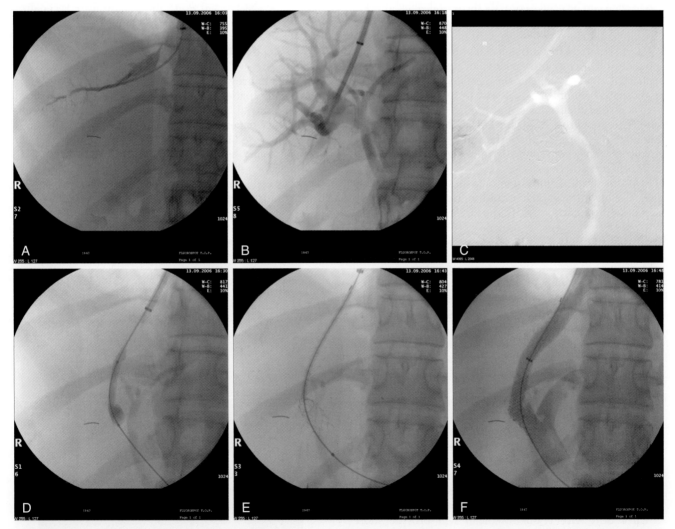

FIGURE 112-1. **A,** Cannulation of right hepatic vein. Note platinum marker already placed beside right portal vein. **B,** Transjugular intrahepatic portosystemic shunt cannula directed anteriorly and inferiorly toward marker to reach right portal vein. **C,** Alternatively, portal vein can be localized by CO_2 wedged hepatic venogram. **D,** Intrahepatic track is dilated with 8-mm, 4-cm balloon. **E,** Bare segment of VIATORR deployed, pulled back to portal vein entry site. **F,** VIATORR fully deployed.

Individual anatomic variation may require the use of alternative vessels. Left hepatic vein to left portal vein, middle hepatic vein to left portal vein, and middle hepatic vein to right portal vein TIPS are also used. Review of CT or magnetic resonance imaging (MRI) before TIPS is useful to plan the ideal access and shunt position. Other pathology such as hepatic or portal vein occlusion requires further variation in technique away from the standard technique. Variations described include right portal vein–to-IVC shunts through the caudate lobe and extrahepatic shunts between the main portal vein to the IVC.[16] When alternative shunt techniques are being considered, thought should be given to future patient management. Some shunt locations may make liver transplant surgery more difficult.

Guidance

The unique component of the TIPS procedure is formation of an intrahepatic track between the hepatic and portal veins. Although this can be achieved using fluoroscopic landmarks, we prefer to use additional techniques to identify the desired portal vein puncture site. Injection of contrast agent or CO_2 through a catheter wedged in a hepatic vein branch can be used to opacify the portal veins. A platinum microcoil or guidewire fragment can be placed under ultrasound guidance beside the right portal vein to act as a target. Alternatively, an intrahepatic portal vein branch can be punctured directly and cannulated. This allows complete angiographic assessment of the portal vein and use of a basket snare, balloon, or a guidewire tip as a target. Imaging in two planes then allows positioning and reshaping of the TIPS cannula so it is directed at the target prior to puncture. The transhepatic portal vein access track can be embolized with gelatin sponge to minimize the risk of intraperitoneal bleeding.

Real-time transabdominal ultrasound guidance is sometimes useful. Intravascular ultrasound guidance has also been described, particularly in the DIPS procedure.

Technical Aspects

TIPS combines a number of endovascular skills practiced more commonly in other interventional procedures:
- Transjugular liver biopsy uses the same skills as the initial steps of TIPS. It provides useful practice to develop and maintain TIPS skills.
- Identify which hepatic vein has been cannulated. The right hepatic vein typically angles posterolaterally from the superior vena cava, and the middle vein angles anterolaterally.
- A cranially angled hepatic vein will be difficult to cannulate with the TIPS cannula. If there is no caudally directed vein, puncture through liver parenchyma may have to be initiated directly from the IVC. This is best performed close to the ostia of the hepatic veins, because the liver is closely adherent to the vena cava at this level.
- If the hepatic vein that is cannulated is very short, a guidewire with a very short soft tip such as an Amplatz Ultra Stiff wire (Cook Medical) will provide more support for the TIPS cannula. (Some operators use the stiff end of an Amplatz Extra Stiff wire.)
- Once portal vein access is achieved, the whole TIPS set including the 10F sheath is advanced into the portal

vein. This maneuver is particularly important to predilate the parenchymal track in tough fibrotic livers. Slightly rotating the device counterclockwise as it advances helps it follow the course of the wire more smoothly.
- If a VIATORR device is used, the sheath must be reintroduced and advanced at least 3 cm beyond the portal vein puncture site. The stent is then positioned with the marker band inside the portal venous system and the sheath withdrawn to allow the uncovered segment to deploy. The stent is gently pulled back until the marker band lies at the portal vein puncture site. The uncovered component remains within the portal vein and maintains alignment of the device with the vein.
- Repeat balloon dilation to 8 mm. Pressure measurements are made in the main portal vein and right atrium. If the gradient remains elevated above 12 mmHg, the stent is redilated using a 9- or 10-mm balloon.
- In patients with acute variceal bleeding, the varices should also be embolized. This can be done most effectively using a sclerosant such as sodium tetradecyl sulfate (STDS) (Fig. 112-2). Coils may be used in combination with sclerosant to slow flow through varices. When coils are used alone, they are prone to recanalization, which may result in rebleeding.

CONTROVERSIES

Early TIPS improves survival in variceal bleeding in Childs-Pugh B and C patients at high risk of rebleeding. The recent randomized trial by Garcia-Pagan et al.[4] showed a significant survival benefit in patients randomized to endoscopic banding followed by TIPS within 72 hours, compared with patients treated by endoscopic banding alone (with TIPS as rescue for rebleeding); 6-week and 12-month survival was 97% versus 67% and 86% versus 61%, respectively, for banding plus early TIPS versus banding plus rescue TIPS

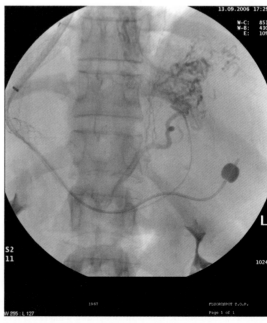

FIGURE 112-2. Flow of sclerosant from varices is controlled with a compliant balloon in splenic vein.

groups. Nevertheless, local Australian experience suggests gastroenterologists continue to use TIPS in small numbers, primarily as a rescue procedure often late in the clinical course.

Role of Surgical Portacaval Shunts

Since the advent of TIPS, the number of surgical shunts performed for acute variceal bleeding has decreased dramatically. A recent study comparing bare metal TIPS with prosthetic mesocaval shunts in acute variceal bleeding showed improved intermediate-term survival and lower rebleeding rates with surgical shunts.[22] A study comparing VIATORR TIPS with prosthetic surgical shunt would be more relevant but is unlikely to be undertaken. A remaining indication for surgical shunting is the small group of patients with frequent symptomatic TIPS restenosis.

OUTCOMES

Procedure Success Rate

Although TIPS is a technically challenging procedure, success should be achieved in about 95% of cases. Increased failure rates can be predicted in patients with additional problems such as portal vein thrombosis. Acute procedural mortality is around 1%.

Clinical Success

Clinical success rate is measured in terms of survival, control of bleeding, or ascites but should also include an assessment of encephalopathy. Survival is related to MELD score and Childs-Pugh class but is worse for patients who are treated for refractory ascites.

Acute Control of Bleeding

Control of bleeding is achieved in approximately 90% of cases.[23,24] Failure to control bleeding should prompt further endoscopic imaging, because nonvariceal bleeding such as a Mallory-Weiss tear or bleeding peptic ulcer may coexist with variceal bleeding.

In patients with HVPG over 12 mmHg at presentation, the acute rebleeding rate in esophageal varices treated with endoscopic sclerosant followed by TIPS is about 12%.[3] This compares with 50% in those treated with endoscopic injection alone.

Acute rebleeding is more common with ectopic varices: 42% when TIPS is performed without embolization and 28% with combined TIPS and embolization.[5]

Late Rebleeding

Late rebleeding is also more common with ectopic varices and is reduced by concurrent embolization and sclerosant injection with TIPS. Late rebleeding appears to have reduced dramatically with widespread introduction of covered stenting, reflecting a much higher long-term primary and secondary patency. Rebleeding with covered devices may be as low as 3% at 12 months and 8% at 2 years.[9,23] This compares with a rebleeding rate of 39% at 2 years for bare stent TIPS.[24] These results fit with

primary patency of 83% to 100% at 1 year for the VIATORR device.

Ascites Control

Improved control of ascites is seen in 60% to 85% of cases. TIPS is significantly better for ascites control than paracentesis. Assessment of survival and quality of life varies between series and meta-analyses.[7-11] The benefits of improved ascites control seem to be balanced by an increase in encephalopathy.

Survival

Two recently published large series of unselected cases with 474 and 523 patients treated with TIPS produced the following respective survival figures[10,25]:
- Early mortality, 27% and 17%
- 1-year survival, 55% and 71%
- 2-year or 3-year survival, 46% and 57%
- 5-year survival, 27% and 49%

In both groups, alcohol was the most common cause of disease, and treatment of variceal bleeding was the most common indication. Percentage of cases with Child-Pugh class C was 53% and 32%, respectively. Survival was related to Child-Pugh class C, age, and ascites as the indication for treatment. Most deaths were due to liver failure and sepsis. In patients treated for ascites, 5-year survival may be as low as 0%.[26]

Encephalopathy occurs in about 30% of patients, and de novo encephalopathy occurs in 12%. It can usually be controlled with medical therapy but may require TIPS reduction or occlusion.

COMPLICATIONS

Major procedural complications are uncommon. Bleeding may occur as a result of perforation of the liver capsule or extrahepatic puncture of the portal vein. Damage to the hepatic artery and bile duct have been reported.[27] Radiation dermatitis and ulceration should be avoided with appropriate radiation technique.

Acute postprocedural complications include liver failure, encephalopathy, and cardiac failure. Failure to control bleeding with TIPS may result from acute TIPS thrombosis, persistent elevation of portal pressure despite TIPS, coagulopathy, or bleeding from a source other than varices. Recurrent or persistent bleeding should be investigated with TIPS venography, portal venography, and pressure measurement. Additional procedures such as embolization and sclerosant injection of varices reduce the risk of acute rebleeding.

Apart from TIPS failure, the main long-term complications are encephalopathy and progressive liver failure. Encephalopathy may be controlled medically, but if it becomes refractory to treatment, TIPS revision or TIPS reversal can be performed. TIPS revision is achieved by partially occluding the shunt using a stent of smaller diameter (Fig. 112-3). No custom-made TIPS-reducing stent is currently available, but a range of techniques has been described using combinations of existing devices.[28] If a TIPS-reducing procedure is unsuccessful, reversal of the TIPS shunt can be performed using embolization coils or other occluding devices (Fig. 112-4). Progressive liver failure

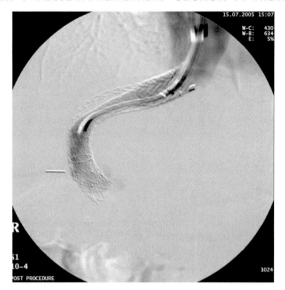

FIGURE 112-3. Transjugular intrahepatic portosystemic shunt reducing stent. Covered balloon-expandable stent has been flared to 10 mm at its ends and 7 mm centrally.

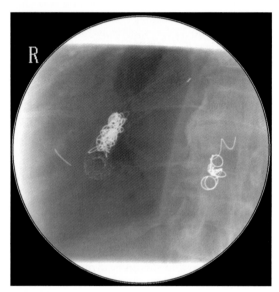

FIGURE 112-4. Transjugular intrahepatic portosystemic shunt occlusion with coils.

may also be responsive to TIPS reversal.[29] Other additional treatment strategies such as partial splenic embolization may complement TIPS reduction.[30]

TIPS infection (so-called endotipsitis) is a rare but recognized complication affecting approximately 1% of cases.[31] Most patients are successfully managed with long-term antibiotic therapy. Cure is possible, but a small percentage of patients die as a result of infection.

POSTPROCEDURAL AND FOLLOW-UP CARE

In the urgent or emergent use of TIPS, early postprocedural management is a continuation of preprocedural resuscitation. One potentially significant hemodynamic change to be considered is the effect of rapid decompression of the portal venous system into the systemic circulation. This is effectively a large-volume transfusion of whole blood and may

lead to elevated central venous pressure. This may lead to cardiac failure. Also, elevated central venous pressure will contribute to elevated portal pressure that may result in acute rebleeding. Once the patient's condition has stabilized, he/she is discharged to chronic liver disease outpatient care. Key issues in clinical follow-up relating to TIPS function are ascites, rebleeding, and encephalopathy.

Doppler ultrasonography is performed before hospital discharge, at 3 months, then every 6 months. Important parameters are flow velocity in the portal end of the shunt, midshunt, and caval end of the shunt, along with flow direction and velocity in the main, left, and right portal veins and the presence of collateral veins. Doppler ultrasound findings suggestive of TIPS restenosis include reduction in flow velocity throughout TIPS, focal increase in flow velocity within TIPS (less common), and change in flow direction in left and right portal veins from hepatofugal to hepatopetal.

TIPS venography and pressure measurement is performed if there is any clinical or imaging evidence of restenosis.

<table>
<tr><td>**KEY POINTS**</td></tr>
</table>

- Transjugular intrahepatic portosystemic shunt (TIPS) is a minimally invasive procedure designed to treat complications of portal hypertension.
- In acute esophageal variceal bleeding, TIPS should be performed when bleeding is not controlled endoscopically or when there is a high risk of rebleeding.
- Survival is improved when TIPS is performed early (within 72 hours of presentation).
- In gastric variceal bleeding, TIPS should be considered alongside endoscopic glue injection and balloon-occluded retrograde transvenous obliteration (BRTO).
- In ectopic variceal bleeding, TIPS is a first-line therapy.
- TIPS is effective in treating ascites that cannot be controlled with medication.
- Covered TIPS endoprostheses provide high long-term patency and have made TIPS a viable long-term treatment for patients who are not suited to transplantation.
- In the management of variceal bleeding, TIPS should be considered as one of a range of treatment strategies, including endoscopic banding of varices, transvenous embolization and sclerosant injection, liver transplantation, and surgical shunts.
- For best patient outcome, TIPS should be combined with best medical management as part of a multidisciplinary approach. Patient selection and timing of TIPS are critical to a good clinical outcome.

▶ **SUGGESTED READINGS**

Garcia-Pagan JC, Caca K, Bureau C, et al. Early use of TIPS in patients with cirrhosis and variceal bleeding. N Engl J Med 2010;362:23970–9.

Rossle M, Grandt D. TIPS: an update. Best Pract Res Clin Gastroenterol 2004;18:99–123.

Zaman A, Chalasani N. Bleeding caused by portal hypertension. Gastroenterol Clin North Am 2005;34:623–42.

The complete reference list is available online at www.expertconsult.com.

CHAPTER 113

Retrograde Balloon Occlusion Variceal Ablation

Hiro Kiyosue and Hiromu Mori

When compared with esophageal variceal bleeding, bleeding from gastric varices is usually more severe and difficult to control. Gastric varices are classified into two types: gastroesophageal varices and isolated varices.[1,2] Gastroesophageal varices located at the cardia are considered part of esophageal varices. Gastroesophageal varices always drain into esophageal varices, and they are usually treated endoscopically (Fig. 113-1). In contrast, isolated varices are usually located at the fundus or at the cardia and fundus and develop independently as part of a large portosystemic shunt that runs through the stomach wall and drains into the left renal vein or inferior vena cava (IVC) (Fig. 113-2).[2] Because of their large size and high flow, endoscopic treatment of isolated gastric varices is difficult.

With recent developments in interventional techniques, the majority of isolated gastric varices can be treated safely with a balloon-occluded retrograde transvenous obliteration (BRTO) technique.[3-5] In BRTO, sclerosant is injected via a balloon catheter positioned at the outlet of the vein draining the gastric varices (gastrorenal or gastrocaval shunt), and the sclerosant fills and stagnates in the varices under balloon occlusion of the shunt (Fig. 113-3). When the sclerosant sufficiently stagnates in the varices, complete thrombosis of the varices can be ensured. Reported success rates of the BRTO technique have ranged from 90% to 100%. Recurrent gastric varices or rebleeding from gastric varices after BRTO occurs rarely.

INDICATIONS

Isolated gastric varices at high risk for rupture or those that have already ruptured are an indication for BRTO. High-risk varices include large varices, those with red spots, and rapidly growing varices. Some authors have performed BRTO for the treatment of portosystemic encephalopathy and ectopic varices such as duodenal varices.[6] However, the long-term efficacy of BRTO for portosystemic encephalopathy has not been confirmed.

CONTRAINDICATIONS

Portal venous pressure will be elevated after BRTO because a large portosystemic shunt is often obliterated concurrently with obliteration of the gastric varices. Therefore, portal venous occlusion or refractory ascites is generally thought to be a contraindication to BRTO. Although a selective infusion technique with a microcatheter may selectively obliterate gastric varices while preserving the portosystemic shunt, it cannot be predicted before treatment whether the shunt will be occluded.[7] Aggravation of esophageal varices is also frequently observed after BRTO[8]; therefore, performance of BRTO for high-risk esophageal varices would increase the risk for bleeding from esophageal varices. In the treatment of patients with both unruptured gastric varices and high-risk esophageal varices, the esophageal varices should be treated by endoscopic techniques before BRTO.

Ethanolamine oleate, commonly used as a sclerosing agent, may induce acute renal failure because of its hemolytic effect.[9] Renal insufficiency (serum creatinine > 1.5 mg/dL) is also a contraindication or should be carefully treated.

EQUIPMENT

Balloon Catheter

A 6F to 7F Simmons-shaped balloon catheter has generally been used for occlusion of gastrorenal shunts (Fig. 113-4). The balloon catheter should have a wide lumen through which a microcatheter can be inserted and should also have a large-diameter balloon (>15 mm) to occlude a large shunt completely. A 5F or 6F C-shaped catheter with a balloon has been used for occlusion of gastrocaval shunts. For the technique of selective BRTO, a 9F/5F coaxial balloon catheter that can easily be advanced proximally to the varices (Fig. 113-5) is used.[10] A microcatheter can be inserted through the 5F coaxial balloon catheter. The 9F guiding balloon is positioned at the outlet of the gastrorenal shunt, and the 5F balloon catheter is introduced coaxially into the proximal portion of the shunt over a microcatheter advanced into the varices. The sclerosing agent is then infused via the microcatheter under balloon occlusion of the shunt at the outlet and proximal portion. Microballoon catheters are recently available, which is useful for selective BRTO in cases with a small and tortuous access route (Fig. 113-6). These catheters come in 3.3F to 3.5F sizes with a 6- to 10-mm balloon (see Fig. 113-5), and they can be introduced through a 6F guiding catheter or 4F sheath over a microguidewire of 0.014 inch.

Sclerosing Agent

For BRTO, 5% ethanolamine oleate iopamidol (EOI), which consists of a mixture of 10% ethanolamine oleate (Oldamin) and the same dose of a contrast agent (iopamidol 300), is commonly used. Because some types of contrast material cannot be mixed with ethanolamine oleate, we used iopamidol 300. Ethanolamine oleate induces hemolysis in blood vessels, and free hemoglobin is released, which may result in renal tubular disturbances and acute renal failure. To prevent renal insufficiency, intravenous administration of 4000 units of haptoglobin, which combines with free hemoglobin, is performed during the procedure. Polidocanol in the form of foam has been recently used as a sclerosing agent alternative to ethanolamine olerate.[11] Foam sclerotherapy using polidocanol may reduce the drug amount and maximize the effect by increasing the contact surface area with the venous wall. However, one should be aware of the

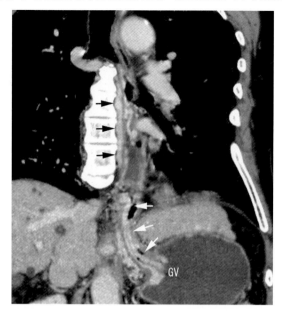

FIGURE 113-1. Gastroesophageal varices. Coronal multiplanar reconstructed computed tomography image shows cardiac gastric varices *(GV)* draining through esophageal varices *(white arrows)* into azygos vein *(black arrows)*.

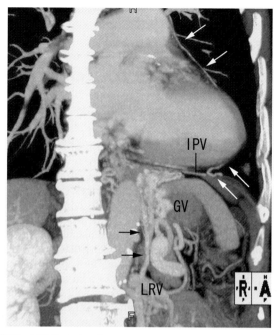

FIGURE 113-2. Isolated gastric varices. Coronal multiplanar reconstructed computed tomography image shows gastric varices *(GV)* draining through left inferior phrenic vein *(IPV)* (gastrorenal shunt *[black arrows]*) into left renal vein *(LRV)*. Note that varices also drain through subdiaphragmatic branch of left inferior phrenic vein into pericardiophrenic vein *(white arrows)*.

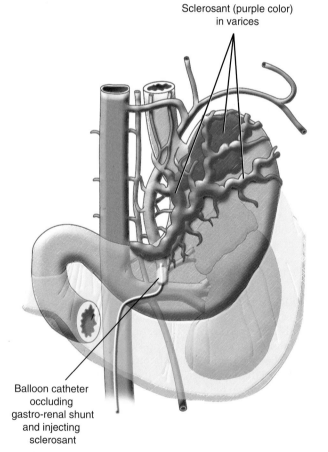

Sclerosant (purple color) in varices

Balloon catheter occluding gastro-renal shunt and injecting sclerosant

FIGURE 113-3. Schematic drawing of standard balloon-occluded retrograde transvenous obliteration technique. Balloon catheter is introduced into outlet of gastrorenal shunt from a femoral venous approach, then sclerosant is slowly injected via balloon catheter, with balloon occlusion of shunt. Sclerosant fills varices.

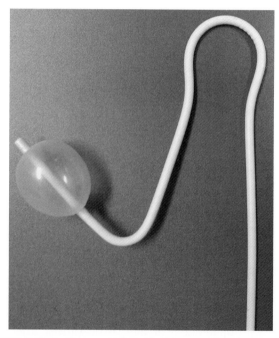

FIGURE 113-4. Photograph of standard Simmons-shaped balloon catheter for balloon-occluded retrograde transvenous obliteration procedure.

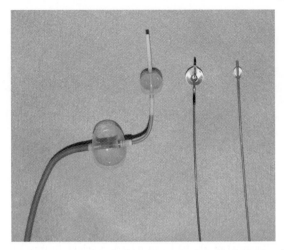

FIGURE 113-5. Photograph of a 9F/5F coaxial double-balloon catheter system *(left)* and microballoons with 3.3F *(middle)* and *(right)* for the selective balloon-occluded retrograde transvenous obliteration technique.

potential risks of air embolism. Some authors used 50% glucose solution, which is infused before injection of EOI to occluded collateral veins or to replace the blood. This technique can reduce the amount of EOI.[12]

Sodium tetradecyl sulfate (STS) is the most commonly used sclerosant within the United States. It is used at the 3% concentration and is often mixed with Ethiodol (for opacity) and air to create a foam solution. A 3:2:1 ratio (air/STS/Ethiodol) has been used successfully by the University of Virginia group. Other ratios have also been used successfully. The added Ethiodol reduces the sclerosing effect to some degree, so there is a balance between opacity and effectiveness.

TECHNIQUE

Anatomy and Approach

Isolated gastric varices are usually located at the fundus or at the cardia and fundus and develop independently as part

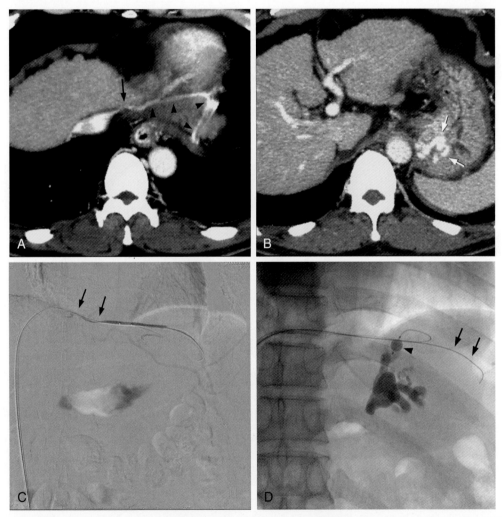

FIGURE 113-6. Gastric varices with gastrocaval shunt treated by selective balloon-occluded retrograde transvenous obliteration (BRTO) with microballoon catheter. **A-B,** Postcontrast computed tomography shows gastric varices *(white arrows)* draining via a small gastrocaval shunt *(arrowheads)* into inferior vena cava. Stenosis *(arrow)* at proximal portion of gastrocaval shunt is noted. **C,** Retrograde venography using a microcatheter shows significant stenosis *(arrows)* at proximal portion of gastrocaval shunt. Multiple collateral drainages are also noted. **D,** A 7F guiding catheter is positioned proximally to stenotic portion of gastrocaval shunt, and a 3.3F microballoon catheter *(arrowhead)* is advanced distally beyond collateral drainage into variceal draining vein. Fluoroscopic image during BRTO shows gastric varices sufficiently opacified with sclerosant. Arrows indicate a guidewire introduced into peripheral branch of inferior phrenic vein to stabilize guiding catheter.

of a large portosystemic shunt that runs through the stomach wall and drains into the left renal vein or IVC.[2] The portosystemic shunt consists of afferent gastric veins and the left inferior phrenic vein, which drains into the left renal vein (gastrorenal shunt; 80%-85%) or directly into the IVC (gastrocaval shunt; 10%-15%) or into both the renal vein and the IVC. The left inferior phrenic vein often communicates with other peridiaphragmatic veins, including the left pericardiophrenic vein, intercostal vein, and azygos vein. These peridiaphragmatic veins, along with the main portosystemic shunt, act as collateral veins draining the gastric varices and would be an obstacle to sufficient filling of sclerosant in the gastric varices during BRTO. Knowledge of potential communications between the gastric varices and peridiaphragmatic veins is very important for successful treatment of gastric varices by BRTO.[4,5,13]

The left inferior phrenic vein often ends in the left renal vein together with the left adrenal vein or passes in front of the esophageal hiatus in the diaphragm and ends in the IVC or left hepatic vein. The proximal portion of the left inferior phrenic vein runs inferior to the diaphragm, and its peripheral branches run superior to the diaphragm. The left inferior phrenic vein potentially communicates with other peridiaphragmatic veins, including the left pericardiophrenic vein, intercostal vein, and anastomotic veins to the right inferior phrenic vein or azygos venous system[14]; consequently, fundic varices can also drain through these potential communications (Fig. 113-7; also see Fig. 113-2). In our experience with portography, balloon-occluded venography, or both in 85 patients with isolated gastric varices, the main drainage routes from the gastric varices were gastrorenal shunts in 52 cases (61.2%), gastrocaval shunts in 3 cases (3.5%), both gastrorenal and gastrocaval shunts in 26 cases (30.6%), and other peridiaphragmatic veins in 4 cases (4.7%). In a portographic study of 20 patients by Chikamori et al., isolated gastric varices drained into a gastrorenal shunt in 85%, a gastrocaval shunt in 10%, and the pericardiophrenic vein in 5%.[2]

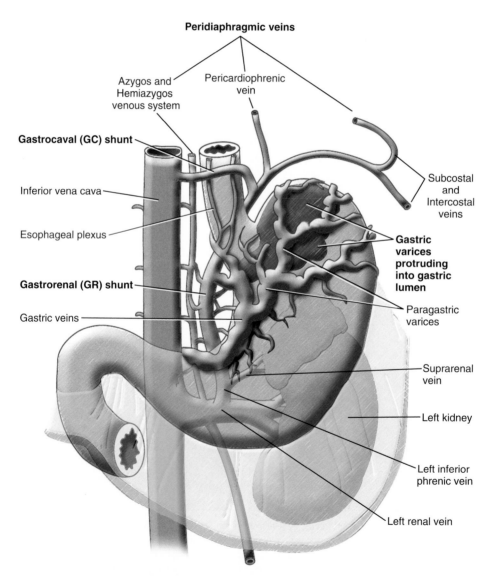

FIGURE 113-7. Schematic drawing of isolated gastric varices draining through various peridiaphragmatic drainage routes. Isolated gastric varices can drain through gastrorenal shunt into left renal vein or through gastrocaval shunt into inferior vena cava or pericardiophrenic vein (or both), intercostal vein, and azygos/hemiazygos vein.

Gastrorenal Shunt

A gastrorenal shunt ends in the left renal vein together with or separately from the left adrenal vein. It often has small retroperitoneal veins communicating with the azygos venous system, and the left adrenal vein and is sometimes associated with other large collaterals through the gastrocaval shunt or left pericardiophrenic vein (see Fig. 113-2).

Gastrocaval Shunt

A gastrocaval shunt ends in the IVC or left hepatic vein (Fig. 113-8). The left inferior phrenic vein runs above the diaphragm peripherally, penetrates the diaphragm near the cardiac apex, and then travels on the inferior surface of the diaphragm. The peripheral portion of the left inferior phrenic vein has many collateral veins, so the majority of gastrocaval shunts are always associated with additional collateral drainage, including the left pericardial vein, veins of the thoracic wall, and an anastomotic vein to the right inferior phrenic vein (see Fig. 113-7). BRTO for this type of gastric variceal drainage is often more difficult than that for varices draining only into the gastrorenal shunt.

Pericardiophrenic Vein

The diaphragmatic branches of the left pericardiophrenic vein anastomose with the supradiaphragmatic portion of the inferior phrenic vein, which ascends parallel to the left cardiac border and drains into the left brachiocephalic vein, the superior intercostal vein, or the internal mammary vein. The vein can function as a collateral pathway in patients with occlusion of the IVC or superior vena cava (SVC) and portal hypertension. Pericardiophrenic venous drainage from varices is usually associated with a gastrocaval or gastrorenal shunt (Fig. 113-9), but it can exist alone. Performance of BRTO through the left pericardiophrenic vein has a potential risk for serious arrhythmia secondary to stimulation by catheter manipulation or sclerosant.

Veins of the Thoracic Wall

Peripheral branches of the left inferior phrenic vein anastomose with the left lower intercostal veins that drain into the hemiazygos vein posteriorly or into the internal mammary vein anteriorly. These thoracic wall veins can also function as drainage veins supplementing the main drainage routes from the gastric varices (Fig. 113-10).

Azygos and Hemiazygos Veins

The azygos vein begins as a continuation of the right ascending lumbar vein, enters the thorax through the aortic hiatus in the diaphragm, ascends along the right side of the vertebral column, and enters the posterior aspect of the SVC. The hemiazygos vein begins in the left ascending lumbar or renal vein, ascends on the left side of the vertebral column,

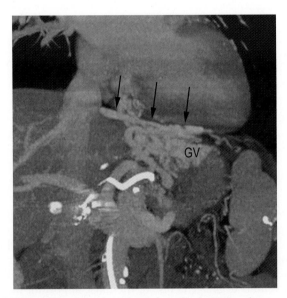

FIGURE 113-8. Coronal maximum intensity projection shows gastric varices *(GV)* draining through gastrocaval shunt *(arrows)* into inferior vena cava.

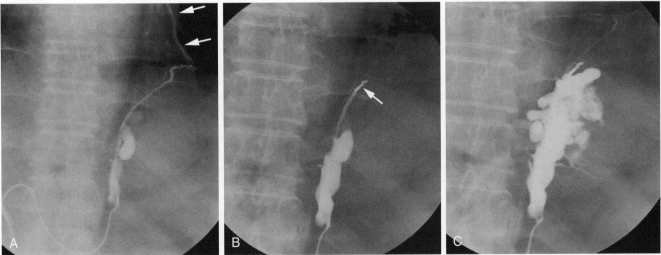

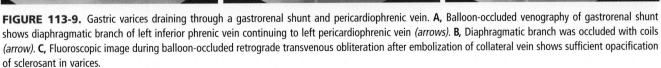

FIGURE 113-9. Gastric varices draining through a gastrorenal shunt and pericardiophrenic vein. **A,** Balloon-occluded venography of gastrorenal shunt shows diaphragmatic branch of left inferior phrenic vein continuing to left pericardiophrenic vein *(arrows)*. **B,** Diaphragmatic branch was occluded with coils *(arrow)*. **C,** Fluoroscopic image during balloon-occluded retrograde transvenous obliteration after embolization of collateral vein shows sufficient opacification of sclerosant in varices.

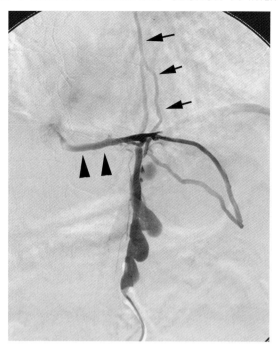

FIGURE 113-10. Balloon-occluded venography of a gastrorenal shunt shows contrast medium draining through diaphragmatic branch of left inferior phrenic vein into inferior vena cava (gastrocaval shunt *[arrowheads]*) and into internal mammary vein *(arrows)*.

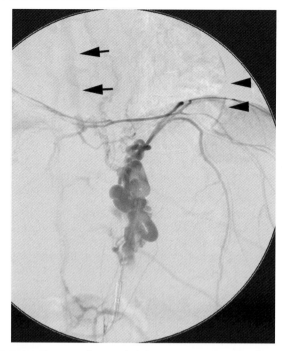

FIGURE 113-11. Balloon-occluded venography of a gastrorenal shunt shows small veins draining to paravertebral plexus and azygos vein *(arrows)*. Note anastomosis with pericardiophrenic vein *(arrowheads)*.

and then joins the azygos vein at the T8-T9 level. The azygos and hemiazygos veins receive the intercostal, pericardial, esophageal, and mediastinal veins. Although the azygos/hemiazygos vein is the most important drainage route from esophageal and gastroesophageal varices that drain directly into the azygos system (see Fig. 113-1), isolated gastric varices less frequently and indirectly drain into the azygos venous system.[2] There are small venous communications between the paravertebral venous plexus and the left inferior phrenic vein. These small anastomotic veins are often observed on balloon-occluded venography of the gastrorenal shunt (Fig. 113-11).

Another important issue regarding the anatomy of gastric varices for BRTO is the existence of a direct shunting vein (paragastric varices).[5,9,13] Gastric varices are located in the submucosal layer and protrude into the gastric lumen. Paragastric varices, which represent variceal shunting veins that connect the afferent gastric veins directly to the draining veins, run around the gastric wall and are sometimes associated with gastric varices. When gastric varices with a large paragastric component are treated by BRTO, sclerosant injected via a balloon catheter may fill the paragastric varices more than the gastric varices.

Technical Aspects

The standard technique of BRTO was introduced by Kanagawa et al.[3] (see Fig. 113-3). According to their description, a balloon catheter is inserted into the outlet of the gastrorenal shunt from a femoral venous approach. After occlusion of the shunt, balloon-occluded venography is performed with the injection of approximately · 8 mL of contrast material (iopamidol 370) via the balloon catheter. Then 5% EOI

is slowly and intermittently injected through the balloon catheter until the gastric varices are completely filled with EOI. After 30 to 50 minutes, EOI is aspirated via the balloon catheter as much as possible. The balloon is then deflated and the balloon catheter withdrawn. The degree of collateral venous drainage is one of the most important factors for a successful procedure. Gastric varices without collateral drainage or with minimum-flow collaterals can easily be treated with the standard BRTO technique because sclerosant infused via the balloon catheter can fill and stagnate in the varices (Fig. 113-12). Some modification in technique is required for the treatment of gastric varices with moderate- or high-flow collateral drainage. We routinely use a 9F/5F coaxial balloon catheter and a microcatheter for selective infusion of sclerosant as mentioned earlier.[10] When the 5F coaxial balloon catheter can be advanced beyond the collateral veins close to the varices, the infused sclerosant can stagnate in the varices under proximal balloon occlusion (Fig. 113-13). For the treatment of cases with moderate- or high-flow collateral drainage, the selective BRTO technique should be attempted first because it requires no further equipment such as coils or an additional balloon (Fig. 113-14). However, in some cases the balloon catheter cannot be advanced beyond the collaterals because of significant tortuosity of the shunt. If proximal balloon occlusion fails, occlusion of these collateral veins is required. Techniques for occlusion of collateral drainage veins, including coil embolization, infusion of liquid occlusive agents such as ethanol or 50% glucose, and balloon occlusion (double-balloon technique), are applied according to the size and ability to catheterize the collateral veins (Figs. 113-15 and 113-16; also see Fig. 113-9). When the collateral drainage vein is large enough that it can be

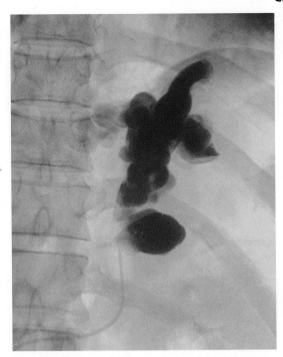

FIGURE 113-12. Gastric varices without collateral venous drainage. Fluoroscopic image during a standard balloon-occluded retrograde transvenous obliteration procedure shows sufficient opacification of sclerosant in varices.

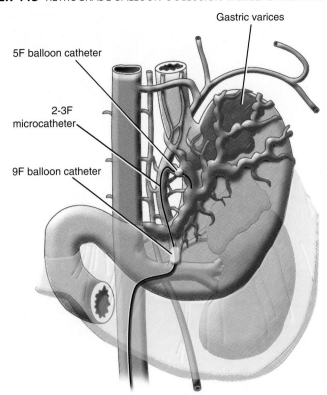

FIGURE 113-13. Schematic drawing of proximal balloon occlusion technique using a coaxial double-balloon catheter system. A 9F balloon catheter is positioned at outlet of gastrorenal shunt, a 5F flexible balloon catheter is coaxially advanced beyond collateral drainage veins, and then a microcatheter is introduced through the 5F catheter into varices. Sclerosant (*purple color*) is slowly injected via microcatheter into varices under balloon occlusion of shunt at both proximal and distal portions.

retrogradely catheterized with a balloon catheter, the double-balloon technique is performed.[5]

Collateral veins with a diameter of 2 to 7 mm can be embolized with coils. Small collateral veins less than 2 mm or those that cannot be catheterized are treated with liquid occlusive agents. Although ethanol can occlude these veins instantly, it is more frequently associated with side effects (e.g., serious arrhythmia) than 50% glucose, so we use 50% glucose for such cases. Treatment strategies related to the size of the collateral drainage vein are summarized in Table 113-1.

Types of afferent veins are another important factor for successful BRTO. Insufficient filling of sclerosant is found in some cases with varices supplied by multiple gastric veins of the left gastric vein, posterior gastric vein, and the short gastric vein, although the systemic drainage from gastric varices is completely blocked by balloon occlusion. Insufficient filling of gastric varices is caused by alternative flow through the gastric varices from a gastric vein to another gastric vein due to pressure gradient under balloon occlusion of systemic drainage. Sclerosant injected retrogradely flows into the gastric vein with lower pressure without filling into the higher pressure part of the gastric varices in such cases (Fig. 113-17). This could result in incomplete thrombosis of the gastric varices after treatment.[15] The addition of afferent venous occlusion with transportal approaches are thought to be useful techniques for ensuring sufficient distribution of sclerosant into complex gastric varices. However, these techniques are associated with periprocedural risks such as peritoneal hemorrhage. Temporary occlusion of the splenic artery during BRTO is a safer and useful technique that can reduce the venous pressure

of the posterior gastric vein and short gastric vein, so altering the pressure gradient in the varices and promoting filling of the entire varices with sclerosant (Fig 113-18).[16]

CONTROVERSIES

In the BRTO technique, there are no significant controversies except for some details. The duration of balloon occlusion varies among physicians.[3-5,9,15] We usually perform BRTO with 30- to 60-minute balloon occlusion times, but several authors have recommended overnight balloon occlusion. In such long-duration balloon occlusion techniques, most physicians perform balloon-occluded venography or contrast-enhanced computed tomography (CT) to evaluate the degree of thrombosis of the varices just before deflation of the balloon. Sclerosant is again injected through the balloon catheter when residual varices are demonstrated by balloon-occluded venography or contrast-enhanced CT. Therefore, the long-duration balloon occlusion technique is more effective for thrombosis of varices than the short-duration balloon occlusion technique. Pulmonary embolism, which can be caused by migration of thrombi formed in the gastric varices and drainage vein, is extremely rare but one of the most serious complications of BRTO. Some physicians believe the risk of

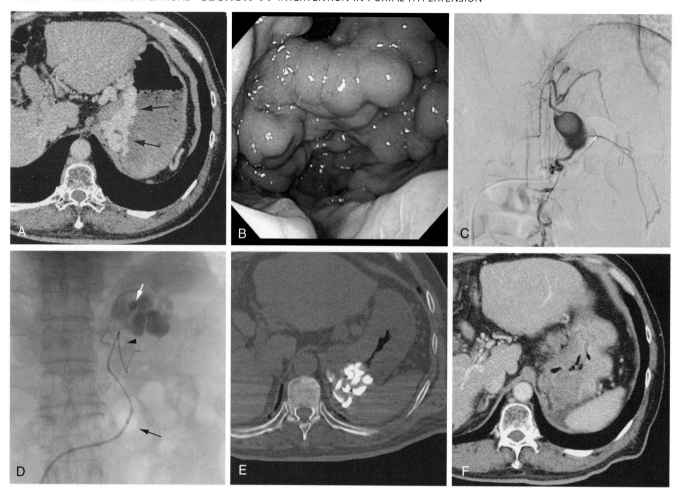

FIGURE 113-14. Gastric varices treated by coaxial double-balloon catheter system. **A,** Computed tomography (CT) after enhancement with contrast material shows large gastric varices *(arrows)* at fundus. **B,** Gastroendoscopy shows large tumorous gastric varices. **C,** Balloon-occluded venography of gastrorenal shunt shows multiple collateral drainage veins. Gastric varices are not opacified. **D,** Fluoroscopic image during balloon-occluded retrograde transvenous obliteration (BRTO) with a coaxial double-balloon catheter system. A 9F balloon catheter *(black arrow)* is positioned at outlet of gastrorenal shunt. A 5F balloon catheter *(arrowhead)* is coaxially advanced beyond collateral drainage, and a microcatheter *(white arrow)* is introduced into varices. Gastric varices are well opacified with sclerosant under double-balloon occlusion of shunt. **E,** CT during a BRTO procedure shows sclerosant sufficiently filling varices. **F,** Follow-up CT 1 week after BRTO shows complete thrombosis of varices. **G,** Gastroendoscopy 1 month after BRTO shows marked regression of gastric varices.

pulmonary embolism after BRTO can be reduced by long-duration balloon occlusion techniques. However, from our data and those reported by other investigators, the results of short-duration balloon occlusion are satisfactory and similar to those of long-duration balloon occlusion techniques in both effectiveness and occurrence of pulmonary embolism.[3,9] Furthermore, the long-duration balloon occlusion technique requires patients to be bedridden for a long period, with the potential risk of malpositioning or thrombogenesis of the balloon catheter. For these reasons we do not recommend the long-duration balloon occlusion technique initially, except for the special case of a very large draining shunt.

For the treatment of collateral drainage, some physicians have infused ethanol via the balloon catheter before infusion of ethanolamine oleate for devascularization of the collaterals. Although infusion of ethanol via the balloon catheter is a simple and effective technique for devascularization of collaterals, it carries a potential risk of minor and major complications such as chest pain, intoxication, and arrhythmia.

Even though the BRTO technique has become the first-line treatment of isolated gastric varices in Japan, it has not yet spread worldwide. Some endoscopists or interventional radiologists recommend endoscopic treatment or a transjugular intrahepatic portosystemic stent shunt (TIPSS) for the treatment of gastric varices.[16-23] TIPSS or endoscopic treatment may be effective for the management of esophageal or gastroesophageal varices that are not associated with a large portosystemic shunt, but these techniques are less effective for isolated varices with a large portosystemic shunt and low portal pressure. Although prospective randomized trials including a large number of cases have not been performed to clarify the efficacy and safety of these three techniques, the reported results of BRTO, including safety and long-term efficacy, are better than those of endoscopic treatment and TIPSS.[3-5,9,18-24,25]

OUTCOMES

Reported technical success rates for BRTO procedures have ranged from 90% to 100%, and regression or disappearance

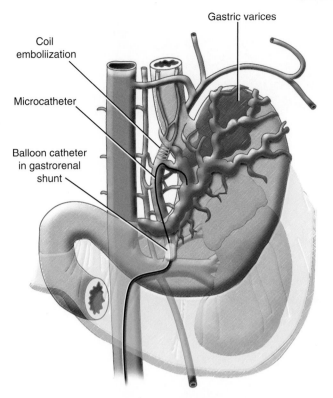

FIGURE 113-15. Schematic drawing of a technique for coil embolization of a collateral vein. A balloon catheter is positioned at outlet of gastrorenal shunt. Collateral drainage veins are occluded with coils, and then a microcatheter is introduced through balloon catheter into gastric varices. Sclerosant *(purple color)* is slowly injected via microcatheter into varices under balloon occlusion of shunt.

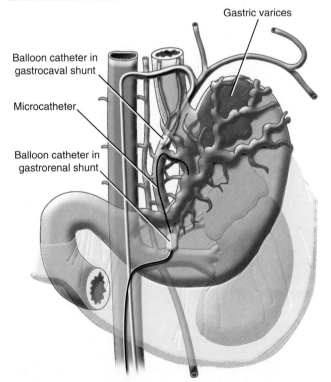

FIGURE 113-16. Schematic drawing of double-balloon catheter technique in a patient with two large portal systemic venous shunts. A balloon catheter is positioned at outlet of gastrorenal shunt, and another balloon catheter is retrogradely introduced into gastrocaval shunt. A microcatheter is then advanced through either catheter into gastric varices, and sclerosant is injected via microcatheter into varices.

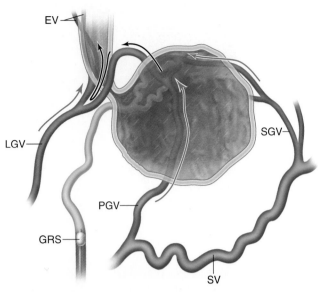

FIGURE 113-17. Schematic drawing of hemodynamic changes occurring in gastric varices supplied by multiple gastric veins after balloon occlusion of drainage shunt. When gastrorenal shunt *(GRS)* is occluded by a balloon, left gastric vein *(LGV)* and (para)esophageal varices *(EV)* can work as a draining vein *(arrows)* because they communicate with systemic vein of azygos venous system, and pressure in LGV would be lower than in other gastric veins. *PGV,* Posterior gastric vein; *SGV,* short gastric vein; *SV,* splenic vein.

TABLE 113-1. Use of BRTO Technique According to Types of Collateral Venous Drainage

Type of Collateral Drainage	Recommended Technique
Collaterals with no or minimum flow	Standard or selective BRTO technique
Collaterals with moderate or high flow	Selective BRTO technique
Small collaterals (<2 mm)	Infusion of liquid embolic material (ethanol, 50% glucose)
Medium collaterals (2-5 mm)	Coil embolization
Large collaterals (gastrocaval shunt > 5 mm)	Double-balloon technique

BRTO, Balloon-occluded retrograde transvenous obliteration.

of gastric varices on endoscopy was achieved in 80% to 100% of patients after BRTO. Some studies with long-term follow-up have shown recurrent gastric varices in 0% to 10% of cases. From our data, including 69 cases monitored over a period of 6 months, recurrence/regrowth of gastric varices was observed in 5 cases (7.2%) on follow-up endoscopy. In all 5 recurrences, partial thrombosis of the gastric varices was noted on follow-up CT 1 or 2 weeks after BRTO. By contrast, in all 58 cases in which complete thrombosis of gastric varices was observed on CT 1 to 2 weeks after BRTO, no recurrences developed. Therefore, CT performed 1 to 2 weeks after BRTO can predict the long-term efficacy of BRTO. Ninoi et al. investigated prognostic factors in 78 patients after BRTO and demonstrated that the presence

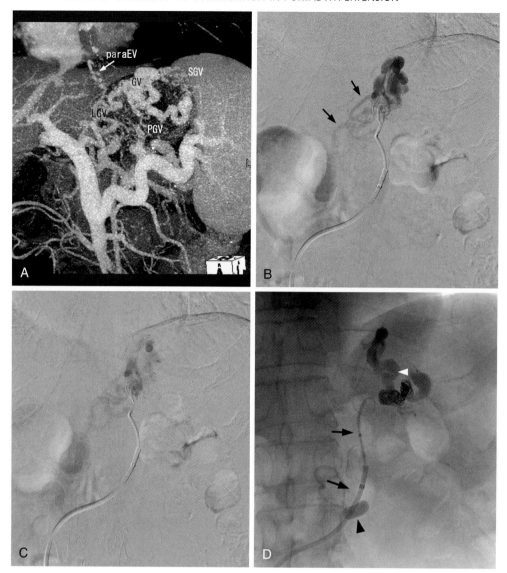

FIGURE 113-18. Gastric varices treated by balloon-occluded retrograde transvenous obliteration (BRTO) combined with temporary balloon occlusion of splenic artery. **A,** Maximum-intensity projection image of enhanced computed tomography shows large gastric varices *(GV)* supplied by multiple gastric veins of posterior gastric vein *(PGV),* left gastric vein *(LGV),* and short gastric vein *(SGV).* LGV continued to paraesophageal varices *(paraEV).* Selective balloon-occluded venography at early **(B)** and delayed **(C)** phases with injection of contrast materials via a microcatheter positioned in gastric varices. Contrast material does not stagnate in varices, which drain into LGV *(arrows)* and paraEV. **D,** Fluoroscopic image during BRTO with temporary occlusion of splenic artery. Sclerosant sufficiently fills and stagnates in gastric varices. Black arrowhead indicates balloon occluding splenic artery. White arrowhead indicates tip of microcatheter introduced into gastric varices. Arrows indicate double coaxial balloon catheter system placed in gastrorenal shunt.

of hepatocellular carcinoma (relative risk [RR] 24.342) and the Child-Pugh classification (RR 5.780) were statistically associated with decreased survival after BRTO.[8] In two studies of BRTO for bleeding gastric varices, rebleeding after BRTO occurred in 0% and 9%.[18,25] Several authors have reported improvement in hepatic function, including serum albumin levels, indocyanine green test, and symptoms of portosystemic encephalopathy after BRTO.[6,26-28] These effects on hepatic function and portosystemic encephalopathy are due to an increase in hepatofugal portal flow as a result of obliteration of a large shunt. Because the majority of patients have hepatic cirrhosis secondary to hepatis B or C and BRTO does not have a direct effect on liver cirrhosis, these improvements in hepatic function and portosystemic

encephalopathy would be transient, and long-term efficacy would depend on the extent of residual hepatic function.

COMPLICATIONS

Hemoglobinuria, abdominal/back pain, and low-grade fever are often observed during and for a few days after BRTO and can be treated conservatively with medication. To prevent renal dysfunction secondary to hemoglobinuria from the hemolytic effect of ethanolamine oleate, intravenous administration of haptoglobin is usually performed during the procedure. We observed one case of acute renal failure (0.5%) in 200 BRTO procedures. Therefore, the dosage of ethanolamine oleate should be decreased as much as possible. We have not encountered any other serious complications, which are extremely rare; however, cardiogenic shock, atrial fibrillation, and pulmonary embolism have been reported.[29] Increased portal venous pressure after BRTO secondary to obliteration of a large portosystemic shunt occurs frequently and would lead to development of ascites and aggravation of esophageal varices. The risk for aggravation of esophageal varices after BRTO was reported to be 27% at 1 year and 58% at 3 years.[8] From our data, aggravation of esophageal varices after BRTO occurred in 45% at 1 year. Therefore, careful follow-up by endoscopy is required. Transient ascites was observed in 15%. Although all such cases could be controlled by medication, it may worsen the condition of patients.

POSTPROCEDURAL AND FOLLOW-UP CARE

Because of the potential risk for acute renal failure secondary to the hemolytic effect of ethanolamine oleate and hepatic injury secondary to migration of the sclerosant into the portal venous system, we routinely check laboratory data, including serum creatinine, blood urea nitrogen, transaminase, and red blood cell and platelet counts on the first, third, and seventh days after BRTO.

CT should be performed within 2 weeks after BRTO for evaluation of the degree of thrombosis of the varices and the development of ascites and for screening for other potential complications. As mentioned earlier, CT performed 1 to 2 weeks after BRTO is useful for predicting the long-term effect.[9] We usually perform gastroendoscopy 1 week, 1 month, and 3 months after BRTO to assess changes in gastric varices, esophageal varices, and portal hypertensive gastropathy. Insufficient regression or regrowth of gastric varices on follow-up gastroendoscopy at 3 months would require repeat treatment. When varices remain or

regrow and drain via a large portosystemic shunt, they can be treated by BRTO again. Other treatment options, including TIPSS and endoscopic treatment, should be performed when an accessible shunt has been already thrombosed by the previous BRTO procedure. Esophageal varices that are exacerbated after BRTO should be treated endoscopically.

KEY POINTS

- Balloon-occluded retrograde transvenous obliteration (BRTO) has become an effective minimally invasive treatment of fundal varices associated with a large portosystemic venous shunt such as a gastrorenal shunt.

- Gastric varices are obliterated by injection of sclerosant via the shunt retrogradely into the varices under balloon occlusion of the shunt.

- Complete obliteration of varices with long-term efficacy can be achieved when sclerosant fills and stagnates in the varices.

- Knowledge of the peridiaphragmatic veins associated with varices is important because the presence of such veins draining gastric varices is well correlated with difficulty performing and reduced efficacy of BRTO.

▸ **SUGGESTED READINGS**

Kiyosue H, Mori H, Matsumoto S, et al. Transcatheter obliteration of gastric varices. Part 1. Anatomic classification. Radiographics 2003;23: 911–20.

Kiyosue H, Mori H, Matsumoto S, et al. Transcatheter obliteration of gastric varices: Part 2. Strategy and techniques based on hemodynamic features. Radiographics 2003;23:921–37.

The complete reference list is available online at www.expertconsult.com.

CHAPTER **114**

Surveillance of Hemodialysis Access

Anne Roberts

Large numbers of patients depend on hemodialysis for their survival. In the United States, approximately 370,000 individuals were receiving hemodialysis for end-stage renal disease (ESRD) through 2009.[1] The increased incidence of diabetes in the U.S. population has led to an increased number of diabetic patients being treated for end-stage renal disease with hemodialysis. Growth in the incident population is particularly marked in the number of patients aged 45 to 64; growth in the population aged 75 and older has grown 12% since 2000.[1] Because older patients are less likely to be candidates for renal transplantation, the number of patients on hemodialysis will increase as the population continues to age. Even patients who are transplant candidates will have a significant period of time on dialysis, because median wait times in the United States are more than 2 years and significantly increasing.[1] In 2009 there were about 83,000 patients listed for transplants.[1] For patients with ESRD either awaiting transplantation or who are not transplant candidates, their hemodialysis access is their "lifeline."

Dialysis access may take the form of dialysis catheters, dialysis grafts, or arteriovenous fistulas (AVFs). The AVF is the preferred access because it provides the greatest chance for long-term function. In the United States, the National Kidney Foundation Disease Outcomes Quality Initiative (NKF KDOQI) guidelines affect all dialysis centers.[2] These guidelines have set a goal of 65% of all patients on hemodialysis having a functional AVF ("Fistula First Initiative") and fewer than 10% of patients having a catheter for permanent dialysis. The rationale behind the encouragement of dialysis fistulas is the fistula's excellent patency and low rate of complications.[2] Synthetic grafts are an alternative to native fistulas, but they do not have the longevity that can be achieved with an endogenous fistula. Primary patency rates at 3 years are reported to be 40% to 60%.[3] Secondary patency rates range from 50% to 90%.[4]

Vascular access function and patency are essential for patients on dialysis. If the access is not functioning properly, the patient will have inadequate dialysis, leading to increased morbidity and mortality.[2] Numerous studies have shown a correlation between delivered dose of hemodialysis and patient mortality and morbidity.[5] Vascular access–related complications account for 15% to 20% of hospitalizations for patients on hemodialysis.[2] Because of the adverse outcomes for dialysis patients, preventing dialysis access dysfunction has become a focus of the KDOQI guidelines.

Dysfunction and failure of AVFs or dialysis grafts are primarily due to development of stenoses in the veins associated with the fistula or graft. These stenoses lead to inadequate dialysis and then, potentially, thrombosis and failure of the access. However, if the stenoses can be detected and treated, such problems can be reduced. Detection of stenoses can often be achieved through a systematic monitoring and surveillance program. It is critical to extend the functional life of each fistula for as long as possible because the sites available for dialysis fistulas are limited, and many patients are dependent on dialysis for survival.

INDICATIONS

All patients who have hemodialysis fistulas or grafts should have periodic surveillance of the dialysis access flows. The KDOQI guidelines recommend an organized monitoring/surveillance approach with regular assessment of clinical parameters of the dialysis access and hemodialysis adequacy. Data from the clinical assessment and hemodialysis measurements should be collected and tracked as part of a quality assurance program. In the KDOQI guidelines, *monitoring* refers to examination and evaluation of the vascular access by means of physical examination to detect physical signs that suggest the presence of dysfunction.[2] *Surveillance* refers to periodic evaluation of the vascular access by using tests that may involve special instrumentation, and for which an abnormal test result suggests the presence of dysfunction.[2] *Diagnostic testing* refers to specialized testing prompted by some abnormality or other medical indication and undertaken to diagnose the cause of the vascular access dysfunction.

Physical examination should be performed on all fistulas and grafts at least monthly to detect dysfunction. Physical examination is useful, reliable, easily performed and inexpensive.[6] A number of techniques may be used for surveillance of grafts. Those preferred include intra-access flow measurements, outlined in Table 114-1 and directly measured or derived from static venous dialysis pressures. In fistulas, recirculation may be measured using a non–urea-based dilutional method.

Abnormal values include a flow rate less than 600 mL/min in grafts and less than 400 to 500 mL/min in fistulas, a venous static pressure ratio greater than 0.5 in grafts or in fistulas, or an arterial segment static pressure ratio greater than 0.75 in grafts. One should not necessarily respond to a single abnormal value, but if a trend is noted, the patient should be referred for diagnosis and treatment.

CONTRAINDICATIONS

There are no contraindications to dialysis access surveillance. Angiographic diagnosis and treatment of the dialysis access may be contraindicated in some patients and would

TABLE 114-1. Methods for Measuring Flow in Dialysis Access

- Duplex Doppler ultrasonography (quantitative color velocity imaging)
- Magnetic resonance angiography
- Variable flow Doppler ultrasonography
- Ultrasound dilution
- Crit-Line III (optodilution by ultrafiltration)
- Crit-Line II (direct transcutaneous)
- Glucose pump infusion technique
- Urea dilution
- Differential conductivity
- In-line dialysance

Based on data from NKF KDOQI Guidelines. Available at http://www.kidney.org/professionals/kdoqi/guidelines.cfm.

include those associated with contrast media, primarily severe allergic reactions. Other contraindications would be systemic infections, particularly in the case of a thrombosed access where the thrombus may be infected.

Early failure is usually due to a technical error in creation of the fistula/graft. Rarely, no underlying anatomic lesion can be identified. These patients may have had excessive postdialysis compression, hypotension, hypovolemia, compression of the graft due to sleeping position, or a hypercoagulable state, any of which may lead to thrombosis.[7]

EQUIPMENT

Surveillance can be performed in a number of ways (see Table 114-1). Flow decreases by less than 20% until the stenosis is 40% to 50%, and then the decrease in flow is rapid as the degree of stenosis increases to 80%.[2] Decreasing flows can be measured by direct flow measurements, most commonly using ultrasound dilution. Graft function can also be evaluated using venous pressure measurements that will slowly increase with the development of stenoses. Recirculation is a very late manifestation of stenosis and a poor predictor of imminent thrombosis, so it is no longer used as a measurement of graft dysfunction in the KDOQI guidelines.[2]

The KDOQI Venous Access Working Group strongly encourages use of physical examination for monitoring dialysis fistulas and grafts.[2] There is a concern that the basic skills of inspection, palpation, and auscultation have been largely abandoned in favor of technology, and the Working Group believes these skills should be taught to all individuals who perform hemodialysis procedures. Physical findings of persistent swelling of the arm, presence of collateral veins, prolonged bleeding after needle withdrawal, or altered characteristics of pulse or thrill in the access suggest the possibility of access dysfunction. Flow through the access can be evaluated by assessing the thrill (vibration) at various points along the access.[8] When there is a stenosis present, a "water-hammer" pulse is felt below the stenosis, and above the stenosis the pulse goes away abruptly.[6] If accessory veins have developed, they may frequently be visible, and the pulse in the main outflow vein decreases above the level of the side branch.[6] Auscultation of the graft, particularly at the region of the venous anastomosis, can be very informative. When a stenosis is present, there is often a high-pitched, harsh, or discontinuous bruit at the affected

site. Because the velocity of flow increases in an area of stenosis, there will be a localized bruit or localized increase in the pitch of the bruit.[6] Marked arm swelling usually indicates the presence of a central venous stenosis. Multiple dilated veins and collaterals are usually apparent in the patient's upper arm and chest, and swelling of the breast may also occur with central venous stenosis.[6] If an abnormality is found on physical examination, about 90% of patients will be found to have an angiographically significant abnormality.[6,9,10]

Duplex Doppler ultrasonography can be used to measure the diameter of the access. The method is operator dependent and subject to error caused by variation in cross-sectional area and the angle of insonation.[2] Duplex Doppler ultrasonography flow measurements do not have good sensitivity and specificity. Duplex ultrasound is much more accurate in performing anatomic assessment and direct evidence for the presence, location, and severity of access stenosis. It is particularly useful to determine reasons for maturation failure of fistulas. Because many fistulas cannot be studied using other surveillance techniques, routine duplex Doppler surveillance of primary fistulas should be considered to identify and refer for correction flow-limiting stenoses that may compromise the long-term patency and use of the fistula.

Magnetic resonance angiography can also be used to evaluate the dialysis access noninvasively and allows anatomic assessment. Its high cost limits its use except in research settings.

A number of indirect methods use some type of dilution technique. The major techniques are ultrasound dilution, timed ultrafiltration method, transcutaneous access flow rate, glucose infusion, differential conductivity, and ionic dialysance.[2] Ultrasound dilution is probably the most common method of measuring access flow. It determines flow by measuring recirculation induced by reversing the blood lines during dialysis. The method detects dilution of blood in the arterial line after injecting saline into the venous line. Glucose pump infusion technology is another way to measure flow. In this method, a glucose solution is infused directly into the access, and the glucose level in a downstream blood sample is compared with a baseline sample.[11] This measures flow with good accuracy when compared with ultrasound dilution measurement.[11]

Access flow is useful for identifying inflow stenosis.[10] However, variations in access flow during dialysis can result from changes in cardiac output, mean arterial pressure, and blood volume.[2] Access flow can increase by up to 11% or decrease by up to 30% from initial values by the end of dialysis, potentially impairing the ability of flow to predict impending vascular access failure.[2] A single abnormal value is thus less valuable than demonstrating a trend over time.[10] When access flow is measured repeatedly, trends of decreasing flow add predictive power for detection of access stenosis or thrombosis.[2]

Access pressures have also been used to evaluate dialysis access function. The pressure required to infuse blood back into the access is recorded as a venous pressure. When a stenosis develops, the pressure increases and the flow decreases. One of the components of the venous pressure is the "static pressure"; when static pressure increases to greater than 50% of the mean arterial pressure, the graft flow commonly has decreased into the thrombosis-prone range of 600 to 800 mL/min, and the presence of a stenosis is likely.[2] Static venous pressure is a better tool for outflow lesions.[10] A mean venous access pressure ratio can be calculated by simultaneous measurement of the static venous access pressure divided by the mean arterial pressure measurement.[12] Although the venous pressure measurement may work relatively well for a graft, in a fistula there may be collateral veins decompressing the fistula, making venous pressures less valuable as a surveillance tool.[2,10] There are situations in which the venous pressure is not accurate, including arterial stenoses or stenosis between the area used for the arterial needle and the area used for the venous needle. In both instances, the venous pressure may be normal or even decrease despite increasing stenosis and decreased flows.[2]

Recirculation, the return of dialyzed blood to the dialyzer, had been used as a measure of dialysis access function, but as noted earlier is no longer recommended by the KDOQI guidelines. It can be a sign of low access blood flow and a marker for stenosis,[2] but it is not recommended as a surveillance test in grafts. This technique may be used in fistulas, although it tends to be a late finding and should have a minor role.[2]

TECHNIQUE

Anatomy and Approaches

In grafts, stenoses tend to develop in the venous outflow, usually within a few centimeters of the graft-vein anastomosis; they are due to neointimal hyperplasia. The cause of intimal hyperplasia is not clear but may be a response to turbulent blood flow, shear stress, endothelial dysfunction, vibratory effects from the placement of the graft,[13] compliance mismatch between the graft material and the vein,[7] or angulation and stretching of the vein.[14] Neointimal hyperplasia includes myointimal proliferation, matrix deposition, infiltration with macrophages, and neovascularization.[15] Venous stenoses increase the amount of recirculation in the graft, increase pressure throughout the graft, and increase the likelihood of thrombosis.

In fistulas, stenoses tend to occur just distal to the arterial anastomosis or in the puncture zone of the vein. There may be ischemic effects[16] as well as injury to the vein resulting from recurrent cannulation and subsequent fibrosis.[2] Stenoses in the fistula have variable effects depending on the anatomy. A stenosis just distal to the arterial anastomosis will cause the fistula to appear flat because blood flow is not going through the outflow vein. A stenosis farther into the outflow vein may increase the pressure in the more proximal vein, or if there are collateral veins, these veins may decompress the fistula and there will be the development of large collateral veins.[6] If side branches are occluded, a venous stenosis will give rise to a situation very similar to a graft, with increased recirculation, increased pressure, and increased risk of thrombosis.

Stenoses can be treated with either angioplasty or surgical revision but are likely to recur, particularly in dialysis grafts, because the conditions that caused the original stenoses are unchanged. These lesions are the most common cause for dialysis graft thrombosis, and the long-term durability of any procedure to improve venous outflow is

constrained by development of such stenoses. Fistula stenoses seem to have a better outcome, although it may take several procedures to get the vein to a suitable caliber.

Technical Aspects

Monitoring (physical examination) and surveillance of the fistula or graft should occur at least monthly. Flow assessment should be performed during the first 1.5 hours of treatment to eliminate error caused by decrease in cardiac output or blood pressure related to the ultrafiltration/hypotension.

Venographic evaluation of a failing dialysis access can be easily performed either before or after dialysis. If performed after dialysis, the dialysis needles can be left in place and a venogram performed. If a stenosis is discovered at the time of the venogram, angioplasty can be performed. Angioplasty should improve the flow through the graft by at least 20%.

CONTROVERSIES

There continues to be controversy regarding the benefit of vascular access surveillance.[15] The KDOQI guidelines recommend diagnostic fistulography if the intragraft blood flow is less than 600 mL/min in a graft, or when the fistula flow has decreased by over 25% (≥33% to avoid potential hemodynamic variation).[17] Fistula referral is recommended when flow is less than 400 to 500 mL/min. It seems there is a relatively good correlation between intragraft blood flow of less than 600 mL/min and development of at least one significant (>50%) stenosis.[18] It is not clear that early detection and treatment of stenoses leads to an improvement in graft patency or longevity.[19] However, one study that evaluated whether prophylactic percutaneous transluminal angioplasty (PTA) of stenosis improved survival in native virgin radiocephalic forearm fistulas suggested that improved fistula survival is the result of increased access flow.[2] PTA was associated with a significant decrease in access-related morbidity, halving the risk for hospitalization, central venous catheterization, and thrombectomy.[2] Many of the studies of surveillance have been nonrandomized, and these studies have shown significant improvement. However, randomized trials show thrombosis rates that are not significantly different between groups.[17] Flow and venous pressure measurements should be combined with clinical monitoring and demonstration of a trend of decrease flow.[17]

OUTCOMES

Stenotic lesions are detected more often by using flow rates of less than 650 mL/min or a 25% to 33% decrease in flow. Early correction of venous stenoses is believed to reduce thrombosis rates, and some studies show a 50% to 90% decrease in thrombosis rate can occur when monitoring is instituted.[12,20,21] Studies also indicate that access viability can be prolonged with surveillance programs.[21,22] Surveillance tends not to decrease the number of angioplasties, but shifts toward a greater proportion of elective PTA vs thrombolysis/thrombectomy with PTA.[12] However, some studies indicate that the rates of graft loss, times to graft loss, and overall thrombosis rates did not differ between patients undergoing elective PTA or those in the control group.[2] A limitation of studies trying to evaluate the interventions in dialysis grafts is the small sample size. Graft survival studies require a sample size of approximately 700 patients to detect an increase in graft survival of 1 year or a 33% difference in survival by 3 years.

COMPLICATIONS

The primary complication of dialysis surveillance is more invasive angiographic study of dialysis grafts and fistulas resulting from a false-positive finding on surveillance. This is why a single measurement should not be used to initiate more invasive studies or treatment. The development of a surveillance abnormality should be correlated with other findings on physical examination and adequacy of hemodialysis. Any abnormality should be confirmed before further referral for duplex Doppler ultrasonography (for stenosis characterization) or angiography.[2]

POSTPROCEDURAL AND FOLLOW-UP CARE

After discovery of an abnormality in a fistula or graft and subsequent treatment, the patient should be placed back into a surveillance program.

▶ **SUGGESTED READINGS**

National Kidney Foundation Disease Outcomes Quality Initiative (NKF KDOQI) Guidelines. Available at http://www.kidney.org/professionals/kdoqi/guidelines.cfm.

U.S. Renal Data System. USRDS 2009 Annual Data Report: Atlas of End-Stage Renal Disease in the United States. Available at http://www.usrds.org.

The complete reference list is available online at www.expertconsult.com.

CHAPTER 115

Management of Failing Hemodialysis Access

Charles T. Burke

The natural history of a vascular access graft or fistula is progressive development of neointimal hyperplastic stenoses that reduces blood flow and compromises performance of the vascular access. If left untreated, these lesions will eventually lead to thrombosis of the vascular access. Early detection and treatment of hemodynamically significant stenosis is a primary tenet of a vascular access management program. Angioplasty remains the most important technique for treating neointimal hyperplastic stenoses associated with hemodialysis grafts and fistulas.

INDICATIONS

The criteria that define failing vascular access and the indications for percutaneous or surgical repair are described in the National Kidney Foundation (NKF) Clinical Practice Guidelines for Vascular Access.[1] These criteria and indications have been incorporated into the Society of Interventional Radiology (SIR) quality improvement guidelines, the American College of Radiology (ACR)-SIR practice guidelines, and the SIR document on standards of reporting.[1-3]

Primary indications for percutaneous intervention of either polytetrafluoroethylene (PTFE) grafts or arteriovenous fistulas (AVFs) include (1) documentation of a clinical or hemodynamic abnormality and (2) a stenosis causing over 50% reduction in luminal diameter. Intervention is not indicated unless the clinical and angiographic findings are both abnormal and correlative. Clinical and hemodynamic abnormalities indicative of significant stenosis include elevated venous pressure, decreased intra-access blood flow, prolonged bleeding after needle removal, and arm swelling.

Several clinical studies have reported that periodic assessment of intra-access blood flow may be the most reliable method for early detection of a developing stenosis.[4-6] Intra-access blood flow is measured during hemodialysis, and if intra-access blood flow is less than 600 mL/min, a fistulogram is recommended to evaluate the entire vascular access circuit.[1]

Over time, there may be degeneration of graft material, resulting in overlying pseudoaneurysms. This is often due to fragmentation of the graft material from repeated cannulation and increased intragraft pressure from venous outflow stenosis.[7] Treatment may be required when the pseudoaneurysm interferes with graft access or there are signs of impending rupture. Indicators for possible graft rupture include skin breakdown over the pseudoaneurysm or rapid pseudoaneurysm expansion. In severe cases or in the setting of graft infection, pseudoaneurysms are treated surgically. In patients with limited surgical options and in whom the anatomy is suitable, endovascular management may be considered.

Early evaluation and intervention may be useful for salvage of nonmaturing fistulas.[8] Recent reports demonstrate that serial dilation of small-diameter veins (balloon maturation) may expedite the maturation process and provide functionality to fistulas that may otherwise have failed.[9-11] Although this indication for percutaneous intervention is not yet fully defined, AVFs that have failed to mature within 3 months of creation should undergo fistulography to determine whether angioplasty or surgical revision would be beneficial. The primary reasons for a fistula that fails to mature include vascular stenosis (outflow vein or arteriovenous anastomosis), competitive outflow veins, or a deep outflow vein that is nonpalpable. Management of vascular stenoses continues to be balloon angioplasty. Small competitive outflow veins can be managed by surgical ligation or endovascular embolization. Deep nonpalpable outflow veins require surgical revision.

Use of stents or stent-grafts for management of failing hemodialysis grafts and fistulas remains controversial. Although angioplasty remains the primary technique for treating neointimal hyperplastic stenosis, stent placement may be indicated in specific situations. The Kidney Disease Outcomes Quality Initiative (KDOQI) guidelines allow for stent use to treat central venous stenoses when there is (1) acute elastic recoil of the vein and over 50% residual stenosis after angioplasty and (2) stenosis that recurs within 3 months after previously successful angioplasty.[1] When treating an aggressive recurring stenosis in a large central vein, a vascular stent may provide better results than angioplasty alone. Another acceptable use of stents is for acute repair of angioplasty-induced venous rupture. Although minor venous injuries can be effectively managed by prolonged inflation of an angioplasty balloon, more substantial injuries with continuing perivascular hemorrhage may require a stent or stent-graft to provide a more durable repair.[12,13]

CONTRAINDICATIONS

The only absolute contraindication to percutaneous intervention is an infected vascular access. Manipulation of an infected graft or fistula may cause intravascular dissemination of microorganisms and thereby elicit acute sepsis or long-term infectious complications such as endocarditis or osteomyelitis. Superficial cellulitis may resolve with appropriate antibiotic treatment, but more extensive infection of a graft or fistula often requires surgical management.

Another important contraindication to percutaneous intervention is allergy to a contrast agent. Patients with a known or suspected allergy should be pretreated according to standardized protocols before fistulography or any interventional procedure requiring use of intravascular contrast material. Alternatively, a noniodinated contrast agent (e.g., CO_2) may be used.[14]

Relative contraindications include intervention on a newly placed graft or fistula; dilation of a new (<30 days) anastomosis may disrupt its integrity. Significant anastomotic stenosis within 30 days after creation of the vascular access suggests a technical or anatomic problem that often requires surgical revision to achieve optimal long-term patency.

Long-segment venous stenoses and occlusions are also relative contraindications to percutaneous management. Compared with treatment of short (<3 cm) lesions, angioplasty of long (>7 cm) venous stenoses and occlusions often results in suboptimal immediate success and reduced long-term patency. Although a stent or stent-graft can be inserted to improve postangioplasty luminal diameter, the long-term durability of such interventions remains questionable. When confronted with long lesions or multiple segments of venous stenosis, the appropriate management decision should include both percutaneous and surgical options.

EQUIPMENT

Though once the domain of hospital-based practices, an increasing number of vascular access–related procedures are being performed in outpatient clinics and freestanding ambulatory surgery centers. Regardless of the setting, the equipment required includes (1) a dedicated procedural room, (2) a digital subtraction angiography system, (3) physiologic monitoring and resuscitation equipment, and (4) procedural supplies such as angiographic catheters, guidewires, and needles.

The extent and type of angiography supplies are dependent on physician preference and the variety of procedures performed. A selection of multipurpose angiographic catheters, guidewires, and vascular sheaths is necessary for basic interventional procedures. High-pressure angioplasty balloons with rated burst pressures of greater than 15 atm are often required for effective treatment of neointimal hyperplastic stenoses. Balloon diameters from 5 to 14 mm are required to treat both peripheral and central stenoses. For very fibrotic and resistant stenoses, a peripheral cutting balloon may be useful.

Although stents and stent-grafts are not frequently used for vascular access–related problems, it is prudent to have several readily available if needed to repair an acute procedure-related complication. Both balloon-expandable and self-expandable stents should be available. Each type has advantages and disadvantages, which should be taken into account when determining appropriate situations for their use.

More advanced procedures may require additional supplies such as microcatheters and microguidewires, embolic agents such as coils, and snares.

TECHNIQUE

Anatomy and Approach

For the relevant venous anatomy, please refer to Chapters 30 and 82.

Physical examination of the vascular access is a reliable method for determining the approximate location of stenoses before fistulography. Information gained from the physical examination should be used to plan an appropriate site for entry into the vascular access. In some instances, particularly with the complicated anatomy of an AVF, a preprocedural ultrasound examination can be useful to locate stenoses and plan the optimal entry site for subsequent interventions.

Assessment of the entire vascular access circuit should be performed before embarking on a reparative procedure. The appropriateness of a percutaneous intervention depends on numerous factors, including the location and length of the lesion, number of lesions, and patency of contiguous and adjacent veins. The complex anatomy of AVFs can present a challenge to novice interventionalists. An understanding of standard fistula configurations is essential for correct interpretation of angiographic images. Evaluation of a nonmaturing fistula can be particularly difficult because of the complexity of the anatomy, the small caliber of the veins, and the multiplicity of problems that can be found during fistulography. It is often useful to review the patient's surgical vascular access records when confronted with unusual or complex vascular anatomy.

Technical Aspects

Fistulography

A diagnostic fistulogram can be performed by inserting a 21-gauge butterfly needle or a Venflon access cannula into the hemodialysis graft or fistula and injecting small aliquots (<5 mL) of radiographic contrast material to opacify the different segments of the vascular access circuit. Some practitioners use a micropuncture vascular access set and insert the 5F dilator into the vascular access for injection of contrast material. The fistulogram is performed to evaluate the hemodialysis graft or fistula and the entire vascular access circuit from the arterial anastomosis to the superior vena cava. For nonmaturing fistulae, ultrasound is often required to identify the primary outflow vein. Occasionally, antegrade micropuncture of the brachial artery is necessary to outline the vascular anatomy. Endovascular interventions would be performed via a subsequent outflow vein access.

The majority of patients referred for fistulography will have at least one significant lesion requiring percutaneous intervention. Ideally the initial entry site into the vascular access should be chosen to provide a favorable route for subsequent interventional procedures. Once identified, the character, extent, and hemodynamic significance of each lesion should be assessed before proceeding with a percutaneous intervention. Multiple angiographic images obtained in different imaging planes are often necessary to thoroughly evaluate a stenosis before proceeding with percutaneous treatment. When measured on a two-dimensional angiographic image, a 50% luminal stenosis corresponds to a 75% to 80% decrease in cross-sectional area and is considered hemodynamically significant.[15] The fistulogram may also demonstrate the presence of venous collateral channels adjacent to a stenosis, a finding indicative of significant obstruction.

The hemodynamic significance of a stenosis can be difficult to determine with angiographic imaging alone.[16] Quantitative measurements can be performed during the procedure, both before and after intervention, to ascertain a lesion's hemodynamic significance. Pullback pressure measurements can be used to measure the transstenotic pressure gradient: a mean pressure gradient above 10 mmHg represents hemodynamically significant stenosis.[17] Intraprocedural measurement of intra-access blood flow using specialized thermodilution catheters can also provide quantitative hemodynamic information.[18] This technique is particularly useful for assessing the functional significance of complicated or multifocal stenoses.

When performing fistulography, it is important to distinguish between fixed stenoses and venous spasm. Venous spasm typically appears as a long, smoothly tapered stenosis in a native vein, often at or near the point of access. Administration of a vasodilator drug (e.g., nitroglycerin) directly into the abnormal venous segment may help differentiate venous spasm from fixed stenosis. Venous spasm will often resolve after vasodilator administration, whereas a true stenosis will persist (Fig. 115-1).

Angioplasty

Percutaneous transluminal angioplasty (PTA) is the most commonly performed percutaneous procedure for treating neointimal hyperplastic stenosis associated with hemodialysis grafts and fistulas. The operator should be prepared to perform angioplasty after completion of the diagnostic fistulogram when an appropriate lesion is identified.

As described earlier, the initial entry site into the vascular access should be planned to allow easy access to stenotic or occluded segments of the vascular access circuit. This may require obtaining new vascular access at a new site or in the opposite direction. Though not mandatory, a vascular sheath can prove advantageous for injection of contrast material and emergency maneuvers in the event of an angioplasty-induced complication. Anticoagulants are not uniformly administered for routine angioplasty procedures.

The first step in performing angioplasty is to cross the lesion with a guidewire. Under fluoroscopy, an angiographic catheter can be used to safely manipulate a guidewire across the stenosis or through the occluded segment. Selection of an appropriate angioplasty balloon should be based on the

diameter of the normal vein adjacent to the stenosis and the length of the stenotic segment. The inflated balloon diameter should be 20% to 30% larger than the diameter of the normal vein adjacent to the stenosis. Typically, 7- and 8-mm-diameter balloons are used to treat vascular access–related stenoses. Lesions close to or across the anastomosis in Cimino shunts may require smaller diameters of 4 to 6 mm. The interventionalist should be aware that overstretching the normal vein may injure the vascular endothelium, possibly inducing rapid restenosis. For this same reason, the length of the angioplasty balloon should be matched as closely as possible to the length of the stenosis, minimizing barotrauma to the adjacent normal vein. Peripheral angioplasty balloons are available in several standardized lengths; balloon lengths of 2 and 4 cm are most commonly used for vascular access–related angioplasty procedures.

The angioplasty balloon catheter is inserted over the guidewire, and the balloon is appropriately positioned across the lesion. Using an inflation device with a pressure gauge, the balloon is slowly inflated with a 1:1 mixture of saline and radiographic contrast material. Dilation of neointimal hyperplastic stenoses often requires use of high-pressure angioplasty balloons with inflation pressures substantially higher than those used to dilate atherosclerotic stenoses.[24] The balloon should remain inflated for 1 to 2 minutes (Fig. 115-2). Balloon inflation may be extremely painful for the patient; subcutaneous infiltration of small amounts of lidocaine (1-2 mL) around the stenotic venous segment may be effective in alleviating pain and allowing the balloon to be fully inflated at high pressure.

If necessary, the balloon can be deflated, repositioned, and reinflated to treat longer lesions. At the end of the procedure, a final fistulogram is performed. Ideally, the guidewire should remain in position across the treated lesion during performance of the final fistulogram. A vascular sheath can be used to inject contrast material

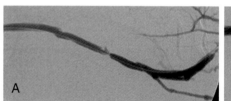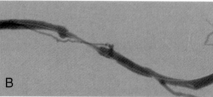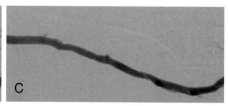

FIGURE 115-1. **A,** Focal stenosis in upper right basilic vein. **B,** Venous spasm after angioplasty. **C,** Resolution of spasm after intravenous nitroglycerin administration.

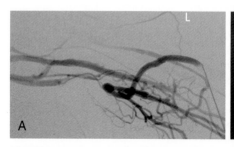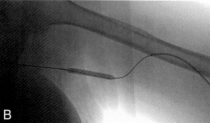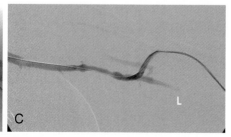

FIGURE 115-2. **A,** Focal outflow vein occlusion with associated collaterals. **B,** Inflation of angioplasty balloon. **C,** Minimal residual narrowing after angioplasty, and significant reduction in venous collaterals.

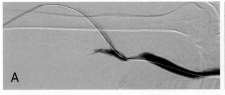 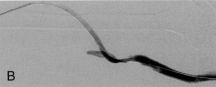 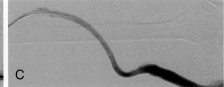

FIGURE 115-3. **A,** Venous anastomotic stenosis. **B,** After angioplasty, there is persistent significant stenosis. **C,** No residual stenosis after insertion of self-expanding stent.

while maintaining position of the guidewire. If the fistulogram reveals an angioplasty-induced complication, the guidewire can be used to immediately perform additional interventions.

Determinants of a successful angioplasty procedure include increased luminal diameter (<30% residual stenosis), resolution of clinical symptoms (i.e., arm swelling), and physical examination revealing the characteristic thrill of a well-functioning vascular access. If a pullback pressure measurement is performed, the transstenotic pressure gradient should be less than 10 mmHg for a successful angioplasty procedure.

Stents
Hemodynamically significant stenoses should initially be treated with angioplasty, which in most instances will be successful, and no additional therapy will be required. If angioplasty fails to improve luminal diameter or if an angioplasty-induced complication occurs, further treatment may be necessary (Fig. 115-3). The decision to proceed with an additional percutaneous intervention or refer the patient for surgical revision is based on the extent and location of the problem and the condition of the adjacent native veins. Use of a stent or stent-graft becomes a viable option when surgical options are limited.

Although a variety of metallic stents and stent-grafts have been used for the management of vascular access–related problems, none of these devices have received approval by the U.S. Food and Drug Administration for use in peripheral veins.

Selection of an appropriate stent is based on the diameter, length, and location of the lesion. Self-expanding stents can be useful for treating both peripheral and central venous stenoses, whereas balloon-expandable stents are more appropriate for treating central venous stenosis. Stent diameter should be the same as or slightly larger than the diameter of the normal vein adjacent to the stenosis. When treating a central venous stenosis, stent diameter should be 20% to 25% larger than the diameter of the normal vein. The central veins expand and contract with respiration, so the stent should be oversized to ensure apposition of the stent against the vein wall and thereby decrease the likelihood of stent migration.[19]

Stent-grafts provide a barrier to the ingrowth of neointimal hyperplastic tissue and are therefore an appealing treatment of aggressive anastomotic stenoses. In addition, a stent-graft can provide a rapid and effective method to repair angioplasty-induced venous rupture and hemodialysis graft pseudoaneurysms.[20]

Before placing a stent, the stenosis should be predilated with standard angioplasty techniques. If a stent or stent-graft is deployed within a stenosis that has not been predilated, the stent may fail to fully expand within the lesion, with no improvement in luminal diameter. Therefore, inability to fully dilate a stenosis via angioplasty is considered a relative contraindication, particularly to placement of a balloon-expandable stent or stent-graft. Self-expanding stents may further expand and dilate a rigid stenosis over time.

Stent insertion and deployment should be performed through a vascular sheath. The nuances of deployment are slightly different for each type of stent delivery catheter, so the manufacturer's instructions for use should be reviewed before proceeding with stent insertion. Although the stenosis should be predilated before the stent insertion procedure, in some instances it may also be beneficial to dilate the stent after deployment to ensure apposition of the stent against the vascular wall and maximize luminal diameter.

A final fistulogram should be performed at the completion of the procedure to reassess the treated segments of the vascular access circuit and identify any procedure-related complications.

Closure Techniques

Use of large-diameter angioplasty balloons, stents, and stent-grafts often necessitates use of large-caliber vascular sheaths. Several different vascular access closure methods have been described for quickly and effectively obtaining hemostasis after removal of the vascular sheath.[21-23] The most popular closure methods use a purse-string suture to close the percutaneous entry site, which has proved useful in both hemodialysis grafts and fistulas.

Although different suture materials can be used, a dissolvable suture works well for this application. A purse-string suture is created by weaving the stitch through the subcutaneous tissue in a circular pattern around the vascular sheath. The stitch is kept superficial in the skin; it is not intended to close the hole in the PTFE graft material. Once the suture has been sewn around the sheath, an assistant places a finger over the skin puncture site and removes the sheath while the purse-string suture is tightened and tied. The suture is pulled taut to cinch the tissue around the puncture site. If the site continues to bleed, lateral tugging on the purse-string suture will effectively control the puncture site until hemostasis is achieved. Of note, a purse-string suture should *not* be used in hemodialysis grafts that are less than 2 months old. The graft must be fully incorporated ("mature") into the surrounding tissue for effective hemostasis with this technique. The stitch is typically removed 2 or 3 days after the endovascular procedure, usually at the time of the next hemodialysis treatment.

CONTROVERSIES

Although angioplasty is a well-accepted initial treatment of vascular access–related stenoses, the use of stents and stent-grafts for the management of angioplasty failures or as a primary treatment strategy remains controversial. Patients with lesions that fail to adequately respond to angioplasty may be referred for surgical revision. The superficial location of most vascular access–related lesions allows easy surgical repair, and long-term results are often superior to those of percutaneous interventions. On the other hand, stents and stent-grafts can effectively salvage angioplasty failures, preserve functionality of the vascular access, and thereby prevent thrombosis and the need for a hemodialysis catheter.

Stents have several advantageous qualities for treating angioplasty failures. A stent can oppose elastic recoil, optimize endoluminal dimensions, and improve blood flow through the vascular access. However, the majority of clinical studies have reported that stents do not provide superior long-term patency and that the results are similar to those obtained with angioplasty alone.[24,25] The neointimal hyperplastic tissue of the underlying stenosis grows unabated through the meshwork of the metallic stent, with gradual redevelopment of the stenotic lesion. Although a stent or stent-graft may allow the interventionalist to salvage an acute angioplasty failure, it may not provide a long-lasting benefit. Furthermore, haphazard deployment of a stent or the use of multiple stents within an outflow vein may interfere with subsequent surgical procedures and necessitate a more extensive revision of the patient's vascular access.

Another controversial subject is early intervention to promote maturation of a nonmaturing fistula. Although most physicians concur that early assessment of a nonmaturing fistula is important for identifying anatomic abnormalities (i.e., small veins), not all would agree that early intervention is necessary or beneficial. Recent clinical studies have reported that percutaneous techniques, such as angioplasty of small-caliber veins and embolization of accessory veins, can accelerate and improve fistula maturation.[10-13] Proponents of these techniques believe that aggressive early intervention can salvage fistulas that would otherwise have failed to mature into a functional vascular access. Alternatively, opponents of early intervention argue that angioplasty is inherently injurious, leads to development of neointimal hyperplasia, and ultimately does more harm than good. This topic continues to be debated in national forums, and long-term clinical studies will be needed to resolve this controversy.

OUTCOMES

The expectations for early and long-term success after vascular access–related interventions are described in the NKF KDOQI guidelines and the SIR quality improvement guidelines.[1,2] These documents defined several parameters for assessment of percutaneous interventions, including anatomic success, hemodynamic success, and clinical success.

Anatomic success, defined as less than 30% residual diameter stenosis, ranges from rates of 80% to 98% after an angioplasty procedure.[26] Hemodynamic success is defined as normalization of hemodynamic parameters such as intra-access blood flow or venous pressure. Hemodynamic success rates range from 70% to 90%, but the value is dependent on the specific parameter being assessed and the measurement method used.[27]

Long-term results after angioplasty of neointimal hyperplastic stenoses are substantially less than those achieved after angioplasty of atherosclerotic stenoses. According to the national guidelines, the expected 6-month primary patency rate is 40% to 50% after angioplasty of a stenosis associated with a failing hemodialysis graft or fistula.[1,2] The reported 12-month primary patency rates range from 23% to 51%.[26]

Inevitably, the treated stenosis will recur or a new stenosis will develop at a second site along the vascular access circuit. Additional angioplasty procedures can be performed to dilate these lesions and maintain functionality of the vascular access. If repeated angioplasty is performed before thrombosis, this extended period of patency is termed *assisted primary patency*. Kanterman et al. reported decreasing assisted primary patency rates with each successive dilation of a venous stenosis.[28] The 6-month primary patency rate for the first angioplasty was 63%, but it decreased to 50% for the second angioplasty and substantially decreased to a 3-month patency rate of 24% after the third angioplasty procedure. In contrast, Beathard reported that repeated dilation of recurrent stenoses provides long-term patency rates equivalent to those of the initial angioplasty procedure.[29]

Angioplasty technology continues to improve. Ultrahigh-pressure angioplasty balloons with rated burst pressures greater than 20 atm and peripheral cutting balloons have proved useful for the treatment of resistant stenoses.[30,31] The peripheral cutting balloon has four atherotomes that score the stenotic lesion during inflation to allow complete dilation of the stenosis at lower inflation pressure. In theory, lower inflation pressure minimizes angioplasty-induced trauma to the normal vascular wall adjacent to the stenosis. Use of the peripheral cutting balloon may also decrease the incidence of elastic recoil, but this potential benefit has not been substantiated. Although ultrahigh-pressure angioplasty balloons and peripheral cutting balloons have improved our ability to treat resistant stenoses, long-term patency rates remain similar to those obtained with conventional angioplasty.[32-35]

Use of stents and stent-grafts has expanded our repertoire of percutaneous interventions for vascular access–related problems. These devices are particularly useful for salvage of angioplasty failures and management of angioplasty-induced venous rupture. However, clinical studies have demonstrated that long-term results after use of these devices is similar to those obtained after a successful angioplasty procedure.[36-38] The expected 6-month primary patency rate is approximately 50% after insertion of a stent.

The use of stent-grafts as a primary treatment strategy for stenoses at the venous anastomosis of a dialysis graft has met with mixed results. In a recent multicenter prospective randomized trial, patients treated with stent-grafts had a 6-month restenosis rate of 28%, compared to 78% for patients treated with balloon angioplasty, resulting in significantly higher patency rates for patients treated with stent-grafts.[39] Despite these promising data, other studies have failed to show this advantage.[40]

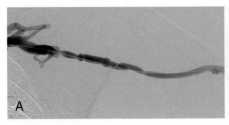 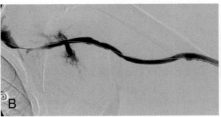 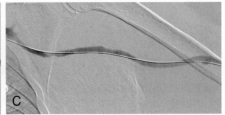

FIGURE 115-4. A, Axillary vein stenosis in patient with left upper extremity dialysis graft. **B,** After angioplasty, there is extravasation from angioplasty site. **C,** No additional extravasation after balloon tamponade.

COMPLICATIONS

The most common complication that occurs during percutaneous treatment of a failing hemodialysis graft or fistula is angioplasty-induced venous rupture, which occurs during 2% to 3% of angioplasty procedures[41] (Fig. 115-4). In many instances, the perivascular hemorrhage can be effectively controlled by manual compression or balloon tamponade. Occasionally the venous injury is more substantial and requires a stent or stent-graft to control bleeding and repair the injury.[12,13,41] Patients with AVFs are prone to develop stenoses within the upper cephalic vein ("cephalic arch"), and these lesions are notorious for angioplasty-induced rupture.[42]

Persistent bleeding from vascular access entry sites is a common minor complication that occurs after completion of an interventional procedure. It may be due to the use of anticoagulants during the procedure. Another cause of access site bleeding is persistence or acute recurrence (i.e., elastic recoil) of a stenosis along the vascular access circuit. A persistent stenosis can increase venous pressure within the vascular access and cause continued bleeding from the percutaneous entry sites. If hemostasis cannot be achieved, a fistulogram may be useful to reassess the outflow veins for significant stenosis.

Embolic complications, peripheral arterial and pulmonary arterial, may be associated with procedures performed on patients with thrombosed vascular access. Endovascular manipulations can dislodge and cause embolization of thrombus fragments, but embolic complications rarely occur during procedures performed on patent but dysfunctional grafts and fistulas.

As with most vascular interventional procedures, administration of intravascular contrast agents or medications for conscious sedation may cause systemic complications. The patient's underlying medical condition and previous history of allergy to contrast agents should be ascertained before the procedure.

POSTPROCEDURE AND FOLLOW-UP CARE

All patients should be monitored by qualified personnel during the immediate postprocedure period. The length of this observation period depends on the level of sedation, complexity of the procedure, occurrence of complications, and overall medical condition of the patient. The vascular access entry sites and distal vasculature should be closely observed for bleeding or other delayed complications. If conscious sedation was administered during the procedure, the patient must be fully recovered before discharge. The

operating physician or qualified designee should evaluate and document the patient's condition before discharge.

It is advantageous for the operating physician to communicate with the patient's hemodialysis treatment center, vascular access coordinator, or nephrologist in timely fashion. The interventionalist should discuss the angiographic findings, outcome of the procedure, and current condition of the patient with other members of the vascular access team. Although this communication does not supplant the requirement for a final written report, this information is beneficial for planning the patient's hemodialysis treatment schedule and formulating a long-term vascular access management plan.

Typically, minimal follow-up care is necessary after the majority of vascular access–related procedures. The condition of the vascular access is routinely examined, and its function is tested at each hemodialysis treatment.

KEY POINTS

- Early identification and repair of a failing hemodialysis graft or fistula improve the quality of hemodialysis treatment and decrease the likelihood of vascular access thrombosis.

- Percutaneous management of failing hemodialysis grafts and fistulas is easier, faster, and less expensive than management of thrombosed grafts and fistulas.

- Angioplasty remains the primary technique for the treatment of neointimal hyperplastic stenoses associated with failing hemodialysis grafts and fistulas.

▶ **SUGGESTED READINGS**

ACR-SIR practice guideline for endovascular management of the thrombosed or dysfunctional dialysis access. Reston, Va: Digest of Council Actions; 2006.

Haskal ZJ, Trerotola S, Dolmatch B, et al. Stent graft versus balloon angioplasty for failing dialysis-access grafts. N Engl J Med 2010;362: 494–503.

Nassar GM. Endovascular management of the "failing to mature" arteriovenous fistula. Tech Vasc Interventional Rad 2008;11:175–80.

National Kidney Foundation, Vascular Access 2006 Work Group. Clinical practice guidelines for vascular access. Am J Kidney Dis 2006;48: S176–247.

Turmel-Rodrigues L, Pengloan J, Bourquelot P. Interventional radiology in hemodialysis fistulae and grafts: a multidisciplinary approach. Cardiovasc Intervent Radiol 2002;25:3–16.

The complete reference list is available online at www.expertconsult.com.

CHAPTER 116

Management of Clotted Hemodialysis Access Grafts
Aalpen A. Patel and Scott Trerotola

Approximately 20 million individuals in the United States have chronic kidney disease, and just as many are at increased risk for development of such disease.[1] In 2004 in the United States alone, 320,000 patients required dialysis (peritoneal dialysis or hemodialysis) for end-stage renal disease.[2] Because many of these patients require hemodialysis, a reliable long-term dialysis access is their lifeline. Although an increase in fistulas is the goal of the National Kidney Foundation Kidney Disease Outcomes Quality Initiative (NKF KDOQI) and the Fistula First Initiative, when a suitable vein is not available, use of an artificial graft is the only option. Regardless of whether it is a graft or fistula, thrombosis is inevitable in time, although evidence suggests that the rate may be lower with fistulas. Clotted access may be managed by open surgery (increasingly rarely) or by various endovascular techniques (including mechanical thrombectomy, pharmacologic thrombolysis, and combination techniques, all with associated angioplasty of the culprit lesions). In the past, surgical thrombectomy was the norm. However, in the last decade, endovascular management has replaced open surgery as the primary method of treatment of a thrombosed dialysis access.[3]

Avoidance of grafts altogether in favor of fistulas will further reduce the need for declotting techniques; a fistula should be created whenever possible. However, grafts will probably always be part of the delivery of hemodialysis in the United States, and thorough familiarity with declotting techniques, results, and complications is essential to any interventionalist. A coordinated effort from a vascular access team consisting of nephrologists, interventionalists, access surgeons, nephrology nurses, and ideally, a vascular access coordinator is critical to achieve optimal outcomes in this population.

In this chapter only the endovascular management of clotted hemodialysis access grafts is discussed.

INDICATIONS

- Clotted hemodialysis access graft

CONTRAINDICATIONS

Absolute

- Hemodialysis access graft infection or overlying cellulitis. Unlike fistulas, in which thrombophlebitis is common, redness, warmth, and swelling at the access site should be considered infection until proven otherwise. Treatment should begin with intravenous antibiotics. Because the infected material in the graft cannot be cleared with antibiotic therapy alone, subsequent surgical intervention is needed, even if the overlying tissue appears to have healed.
- Uncorrectable coagulopathy

Relative

- Severe allergy to contrast material. Because of the current U.S. Food and Drug Administration (FDA) warning on the use of gadolinium in patients with end-stage renal disease (concern over a possible relationship to nephrogenic fibrosing dermopathy), it should not be used until more evidence is gathered and the issue is resolved.[4,5] Pretreatment with prednisone, 40 mg orally 12 and 2 hours before intervention, is usually sufficient for most allergic reactions; some add H_1 and possibly H_2 blockers, but there is little evidence for this.[6]
- Abnormal but correctable coagulation parameters
- Ischemia of the ipsilateral extremity, because restoring flow will worsen the ischemia by exacerbating the steal phenomenon.
- History of a significant right-to-left shunt because of the risk for paradoxical emboli with rare reported strokes from percutaneous declotting.[7,8] However, successful and complication-free thrombectomy in patients with a known patent foramen ovale, even with right-to-left shunting, has been reported.[9]
- Significantly reduced pulmonary reserve (pulmonary hypertension, severe lung disease, right heart failure) because of an inability to tolerate the small pulmonary emboli resulting from virtually any form of declotting. Fatal pulmonary emboli have been reported in this population.[10,11]
- Severe hyperkalemia or acidosis

EQUIPMENT

- Access needle/set (angiocatheter, 19-gauge needle, or a micropuncture set)
- 6F short marker-tip sheath
- 7F short marker-tip sheath
- Two infusion catheters or a mechanical percutaneous thrombectomy device (e.g., Arrow-Trerotola PTD)
- Appropriately sized percutaneous transluminal angioplasty (PTA) balloons
- An inflation device or a 1-mL polycarbonate syringe (preferred), 10-mL syringe, and a flow switch
- Contrast material

TECHNIQUE

Anatomy and Approach

The preferred form of access, arteriovenous fistulas, cannot always be created. When such is the case, 6- to 8-mm or tapered 4- to 7-mm polytetrafluoroethylene (PTFE) grafts or, less commonly, other material such as bovine or porcine xenograft is used to create a dialysis access. Typically, the upper extremities are used and grafts are placed in straight or loop configurations, starting peripherally and moving centrally as grafts fail. Occasionally, more creative approaches in the neck/chest and lower extremities are needed.

Patient Evaluation and Preparation

The importance of clinical evaluation (history, physical examination, and laboratory tests) in the management of a clotted hemodialysis access graft should not be underestimated. It can help the operator prevent futile efforts and avoid complications. The preoperative workup includes a directed history of the dialysis access and previous interventions and a subsequent physical examination.[3,12]

Determining when the access was created, the type of access in place, and when the graft thrombosis occurred is important. If more than two previous interventions have been performed in less than 1 month, the access may require surgical management. It is critical to determine whether there are signs of local (hemodialysis access graft site) infection (warmth, erythema, tenderness) or systemic infection (fever, chills). If along with physical examination it is determined that graft infection is present, access intervention is absolutely contraindicated.[3,12-14] The history should also focus on possible contraindications such as right-to-left shunts and severe pulmonary disease.

Physical examination is just as important. The flow circuit in the extremity should be assessed by palpating and documenting the ipsilateral radial, ulnar, and brachial pulses. Blood supply to the distal part of the extremity must be assessed as well (capillary refill and warmth of the hand/arm). To assess for central venous stenosis or occlusion, chest wall collaterals should be noted with care. If present, it should be determined whether arm swelling was present when the graft was functioning, because swelling may dictate treatment of a central lesion discovered after restoring graft patency.[15] Cardiac and pulmonary examinations are also important to assess for signs of significant fluid overload.[3,12-14] In addition, each graft should be evaluated by physical examination before every intervention. The site should be assessed for warmth, tenderness, and erythema, because these symptoms may indicate graft infection or cellulitis. To choose optimal puncture sites for intervention, one must determine the type of access (straight or loop), direction of inflow and outflow, presence of aneurysmal graft degeneration, and type of anastomosis.[3,12]

Before hemodialysis access graft intervention, coagulation parameters (international normalized ratio [INR] and

platelet count) should be determined and confirmed to be in the normal range. In the authors' practice, the values used are an INR less than 2.0 (<1.5 for central PTA) and a platelet count above 25,000. It is important to have normal or reversible values of the coagulation parameters in case graft or vascular rupture occurs during the intervention.

A few cases of postprocedure septic shock have been reported, and colonization of clotted grafts is very common.[16] Therefore (though not evidence based), most interventionalists give preprocedural prophylactic antibiotics (cefazolin [Ancef], 1 g intravenously). To prevent rethrombosis during the procedure, as well as to blunt any pulmonary vasospastic or bronchospastic response to small pulmonary emboli occurring during declotting, 3000 to 5000 units of heparin should be administered before intervention.

Technical Aspects

Both open surgical and endovascular approaches can be used to declot a thrombosed hemodialysis access graft. Only endovascular approaches (mechanical thrombolysis, pharmacologic thrombolysis, and combination approaches) are addressed in this chapter. Thrombolysis of a hemodialysis access graft has two major steps: clot removal (Fig. 116-1) (including the arterial plug [Fig. 116-2]) and treatment of the underlying anatomic lesion (Fig. 116-3). In the absence of infection, there are usually underlying causes (e.g., stenoses at the venous or arterial anastomoses, outflow veins, or rarely, arteries proximal to the arterial anastomosis) that have to be addressed with PTA. Some common techniques, but not all techniques, are described in this chapter; it is not meant to be a comprehensive review. Many excellent review articles are listed in the Suggested Readings at the end of this chapter.

Graft Access

Access to the graft depends on the configuration of the graft but is the same regardless of declotting technique used. Although there are many individual variations and preferences, the basic crossed-catheter technique has stood the test of time. It should be noted that despite the name, the access sheaths should not actually cross, or flow will be partially obstructed and efforts at declotting will be impeded. In a loop graft, the first puncture is made near the apex, directed toward the venous anastomosis, and the second puncture is made approximately 1 to 2 cm from the venous anastomosis, directed toward the arterial anastomosis. Similarly, for straight grafts, the first puncture in

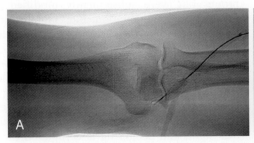
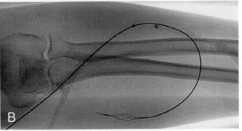

FIGURE 116-1. Mechanical thrombectomy device (Arrow-Trerotola PTD [Teleflex Inc., Limerick, Pa.]) is seen in action while treating venous limb/anastomosis **(A)** and arterial limb **(B)**. It is important that after clot is macerated with mechanical device, it be aspirated thoroughly through both sheaths. If a sheath becomes clotted during this process, it can be removed over a wire and then cleaned outside the body and reinserted.

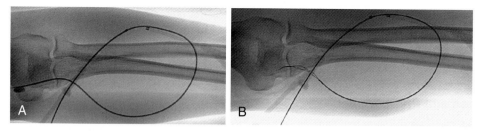

FIGURE 116-2. **A,** Over-the-wire Fogarty method of pulling the plug, which can then be treated with a percutaneous thrombectomy device (PTD). **B,** In contrast, PTD seen here is deformed by plug at arterial anastomosis. Device can be activated at this point to treat plug. If configuration of anastomosis is more complex, an over-the-wire device may be used in same fashion.

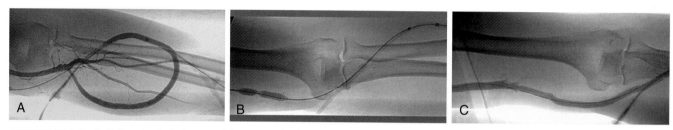

FIGURE 116-3. **A,** Reflux view to look at arterial anastomosis. This is a tapered graft used in a loop configuration. **B,** A "waist" in a balloon at venous anastomosis was noted while performing percutaneous transluminal angioplasty to treat stenosis at this location. **C,** Successful angioplasty with resolution of stenosis.

made near the arterial anastomosis and the second near the venous anastomosis, with each directed toward the other anastomosis. The apex technique[17] deserves mention only because we believe this technique is not suitable for declotting because of the need to repeatedly access both ends of the graft at different times during the procedure.[3,12]

Clot Removal
Mechanical Methods
Mechanical devices for clot fragmentation and removal include those that fragment the clot and those that fragment the clot and aspirate the fragments. Commonly used devices are the Arrow-Trerotola PTD (Teleflex Inc., Limerick, Penn.), AngioJet (Possis Medical Inc., Minneapolis, Minn.), and Helix Clot Buster Thrombectomy devices (ev3/Covidien, Plymouth, Minn.). Although the AngioJet fragmentation/aspiration device is commonly used, published evidence from a randomized trial does not support its use in this setting.[18] Many other devices have been introduced and are infrequently used or have been removed from the market. The reader is directed to several comprehensive reviews on this subject,[19-21] although the proliferation of devices in this field makes even the most recent publication quickly outdated. The reader is cautioned that few of these devices are supported by prospective randomized trials, and it is our firm belief that one's practice should be dictated by evidence wherever possible.

Briefly, the technique is as follows, regardless of the device used. A 7F sheath (preferably with a radiopaque marker and large-bore side arm suitable for aspiration) is directed toward the venous anastomosis, and a 6F sheath is placed at the second puncture site. After negotiating the venous anastomosis, an angled catheter (e.g., Berenstein) is passed into the central veins, and a pullback venogram is performed to evaluate the status of the central veins and

arm veins up to the venous anastomosis (Fig. 116-4). The clotted graft should not be injected, because the resultant increased luminal pressure may give rise to arterial emboli. The thrombus is macerated with a mechanical thrombectomy device and aspirated manually or fragmented and aspirated with a rheolytic device. However, it is important to note that to prevent difficult access as a result of luminal collapse of the graft, the second puncture is made before aspiration of the clot. Similarly, the mechanical device is advanced toward the arterial limb or segment of the graft on the arterial anastomosis side, and a similar mechanical thrombectomy procedure is performed without crossing the arterial anastomosis. Both steps should be repeated until as much of the thrombus can be removed as possible. Intermittent aspiration of the clot should be performed (see Fig. 116-1). (Note: It is the authors' belief, supported by some evidence,[22] that wall contact devices provide more thorough clearance of the luminal clot, especially when used as needed with local massage of the graft.)

Pharmacologic Methods
Infusion methods were the initial pharmacologic techniques but were subsequently modified to incorporate mechanical fragmentation and "mobilization" of the clot to accelerate the procedure and decrease bleeding complications associated with infusion-only techniques; such combined methods were dubbed *pharmacomechanical techniques.* Probably the only remaining indication for infusion thrombolysis in graft declotting is for treatment of a large central clot burden, usually associated with central venous stenosis. In this setting, infusion lysis is performed overnight, and declotting is completed the next day with mechanical or pharmacomechanical techniques. Variations of pharmacomechanical techniques include pulse spray, "lyse and wait," and "lyse and go," to name just a few. Various

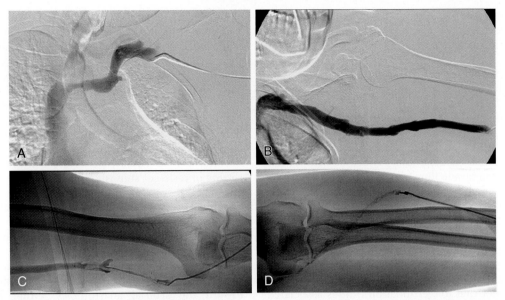

FIGURE 116-4. Pullback venography. **A,** Central venogram. (NOTE: Stenosis in left brachiocephalic vein was not treated because patient did not have a history of arm swelling.) **B-C,** Patent veins centrally, but closer to anastomosis, stenosis is noted. **D,** No contrast material was actually injected into graft, but residual contrast material from catheter pullback outlines thrombus in graft.

thrombolytics, including urokinase, tissue plasminogen activator (tPA), and reteplase, have been used in these methods. In all these techniques, partial thrombolysis is associated with deliberate embolization of the clot (mobilization) to restore flow. Because none has been approved by the FDA for this purpose, the use of pharmacologic agents for declotting is an off-label application. Despite a striking lack of evidence, as well as a randomized trial showing higher complications compared to a mechanical device,[23] the lyse-and-wait technique has become popular. The biggest hurdle with this technique is confirmation of successful graft access, which can be verified by free passage of a guidewire or return of a small amount of blood.

Lyse and Wait (Go)
Urokinase is no longer available in the United States, so it will not be discussed. As a substitute, other lytics such as tPA (2-4 mg) or recombinant (r)tPA (2-3 units) combined with 3000 to 5000 units of heparin are injected into the graft 30 minutes to 2 hours before the patient enters the procedure room. To prevent arterial and central venous emboli (less worrisome), both ends of the graft must be compressed well during the injection. The theory is that during the procedure the clot will undergo partial or full thrombolysis and thus save time in the interventional radiology suite. However, a randomized trial showed no difference in procedure time between a mechanical device and the lyse-and-wait technique.[23] A retrospective nonrandomized study comparing PTD thrombectomy with urokinase-based lyse and wait showed similar immediate and long-term outcomes but higher rupture and stent use rates in the lyse-and-wait group.[24]

Pulse Spray
Again, because urokinase is no longer available in the United States, only off-label use of tPA and rtPA will be discussed. Dosage of tPA varies from 3 to 5 mg to 20 mg.

Two crossing catheters are placed without crossing the anastomosis. Lytic agent and heparin are pulsed into the graft, and then the underlying stenoses are treated.

Non–Device-Associated Mechanical Techniques
Many other techniques for graft declotting have been described but are not in widespread use at present, including deliberate clot embolization, aspiration thrombectomy, and combinations of these techniques.

Arterial Plug
The arterial plug[25] is resistant to pharmacologic thrombolysis, presumably because each layer of lamellated fibrin and red cells protects the next from lysis. Regardless of the method used for treatment of the clot, the arterial plug may require separate treatment. It can be treated with the PTD (the only mechanical device approved by the FDA for treating the arterial plug) or with an over-the-wire occlusion balloon (see Fig. 116-2). For treatment with the PTD, the PTD (either the non–over-the-wire or the over-the-wire version) should be passed beyond the arterial anastomosis into the artery in its constrained state. It should be gently deployed in the artery. The basket should be pulled back until it is seen to deform or indent at the arterial anastomosis (the site of the plug) and then activated to perform mechanical thrombolysis (see Fig. 116-2, *B*). This treats the plug and the arterial segment of the graft and establishes flow in the graft. If incompletely treated as assessed by physical examination, the step may have to be repeated. An additional pass though the venous limb is generally necessary to treat residual thrombus. The sheath may become occluded during these maneuvers; occlusion can be addressed by removing the sheath over a wire, flushing it outside the body while still on the wire, and reinserting it.

For the Fogarty technique, an over-the-wire occlusion balloon should be inflated in the artery and then pulled in the inflated state across the arterial anastomosis to take the plug into the graft (see Fig. 116-2, *A*). It can then be treated by balloon maceration or the PTD and be aspirated or allowed to embolize centrally.

Percutaneous Transluminal Angioplasty

Regardless of the method used, after flow has been established, PTA of the underlying lesions must be performed. Once the graft is determined to have flow on physical examination, and antegrade flow is confirmed with a minute injection of contrast material, diagnostic fistulography should be performed. Fistulography performed without this confirmation of antegrade flow may lead to arterial emboli and is to be avoided, as is flushing of the sheaths (while inside the graft) before flow is restored. Any stenoses identified on diagnostic fistulography should be treated with PTA (see Fig. 116-3). The balloon size should be at least 1 mm larger than the size of the graft; sometimes even larger balloons are needed if there is significant recoil and prolonged dilation fails. At least one paper has shown in a statistically significant manner that longer inflation time is associated with better acute success[26]; a randomized trial comparing 1- versus 3-minute inflations also showed better immediate success with the longer inflation, but 1-, 3-, and 6-month patency were no different.[27] We recommend a 90-second inflation for initial PTA performed in a dialysis access, with prolonged inflation in 5-minute courses as needed to treat elastic lesions. Sometimes a progressive increase in balloon size is needed in addition to prolonged inflation to treat a recoiling lesion.

If all efforts fail to treat a recoiling lesion, consideration should be given to stent placement or surgical revision. At present, the available evidence and KDOQI guidelines suggest that surgical revision is preferable to stent placement, provided the lesion is surgically acceptable. A significant exception to this guideline is PTA-induced rupture not responding to balloon tamponade, because in this setting, surgical revision would be hampered by the surrounding hematoma and would probably be far more extensive (with attendant loss of vein) than otherwise needed. If an elastic lesion is surgically inaccessible, stent placement should be performed. The available evidence suggests that nitinol self-expanding stents may have better patency than Wallstents,[28] but no randomized data support this at present. A prospective randomized trial of a carbon-lined PTFE-encapsulated stent (Bard Peripheral Vascular, Tempe, Ariz.) showed superior patency in comparison to PTA.[29] The device nearly doubled patency in this trial, with the caveat that PTA patency was quite poor. The cost effectiveness of this device versus repeated PTA has not been established. We believe

the best role for this device is in a patient who previously had good response to PTA and is now experiencing diminished patency; it has been our experience one can "reset the patency clock" by placing a covered stent. We also believe that placing any stent, covered or otherwise, out of frustration with repeated short-term PTA failure and/or thrombosis will not yield favorable results and strongly prefer surgical revision or a new access in that setting. As more data emerge concerning the role of covered stents in hemodialysis access circuits, their relative role should become clearer. Finally, stents are contraindicated in the setting of resistant stenosis, and fortunately the problem of resistant stenosis is now rare given the availability of ultrahigh-pressure PTA balloons (Conquest [Bard Peripheral Vascular]).[26,30]

A final postprocedure fistulogram is necessary to evaluate the entire access circuit. The arterial anastomosis is best evaluated while treating the outflow stenosis with PTA (when the outflow is occluded) by injecting the sheath toward the arterial anastomosis. Other less preferred methods include manual compression (increased radiation exposure to the operator's hand) and arterial cannulation.

Endpoint of Treatment

At the end of the procedure, it is imperative that the arteriovenous graft be free of significant lesions on fistulography. Although it makes sense to use objective measures such as pressure gradients to determine the endpoint, the evidence suggests otherwise. The authors reported that postprocedural physical examination findings correlate best with a satisfactory outcome.[31] A uniform thrill without pulsatility is ideal. During this examination, postprocedure pulses should also be assessed to exclude arterial emboli (Fig. 116-5).

Access Hemostasis

Hemostasis may be achieved with manual compression or with purse-string technique variants. If the latter are used, the sutures must be removed before discharge from interventional radiology, or they will probably be forgotten and may well become a nidus for infection or skin breakdown, thereby jeopardizing the graft. Hemostasis has been shown in a randomized trial to take less time with mechanical techniques than with those involving lytic agents.[23]

CONTROVERSIES

There are some controversies in the treatment of a clotted hemodialysis graft, including mechanical versus

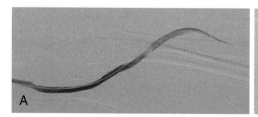
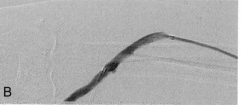

FIGURE 116-5. It is important to treat as much residual clot in graft as possible for optimal patency. **A,** Residual adherent thrombus was treated with percutaneous thrombectomy device (PTD) while massaging area during treatment. **B,** Successful treatment and resolution of clot. Some adherent clots are resistant even to treatment with wall-contact devices such as a PTD. In these rare situations, other devices (e.g., Fogarty Adherent clot catheter) may prove successful.

pharmacologic treatment, covered stent versus surgical revision, prolonged dilation, and dilation of central venous stenosis. These controversies have been addressed in other sections of this chapter. Evidence is building to settle some of them.

OUTCOMES

In most cases, treatment of thrombosed arteriovenous grafts is now performed percutaneously with at least some mechanical means, with or without pharmacologic assistance. Evidence indicates that percutaneous declotting performed by mechanical or pharmacomechanical methods has an approximately 90% initial success rate and a 40% primary patency rate at 3 months. There is little randomized evidence to suggest that one technique provides significantly better long-term patency, with the notable exception of the AngioJet, for which a 15% 3-month patency rate was reported in a randomized trial[18]; it should never be used for dialysis graft declotting in our opinion. We believe strongly, based on several pieces of evidence,[22,32] that removal of wall-adherent clot results in more favorable outcomes and that when eventually compared with non–wall-contact techniques in a randomized fashion, it will prove superior.

COMPLICATIONS

Despite attention to detail and meticulous technique, complications will occur, including arterial emboli, graft or vascular rupture, hand ischemia, and symptomatic pulmonary emboli, among others. The operator must know how to address these problems in an endovascular fashion and recognize when an open approach is needed. Because of space considerations, only the most common complications, arterial emboli and venous rupture, are discussed here.

When an arterial embolus is recognized, the goal is to prevent ischemia. Many emboli are not symptomatic and may be left alone, especially if only partially flow limiting, because they will lyse spontaneously.[33] In contrast, symptomatic emboli should be addressed immediately. First, once an arterial embolus is recognized, the patient should be adequately heparinized to prevent in situ thrombosis and worsening of ischemia. Techniques such as backbleeding, the Fogarty balloon technique, thromboaspiration, or (rarely) surgical embolectomy may be required. Backbleeding is the preferred technique of treating arterial emboli,[34] but for it to work, the graft must be patent and flow established.

Venous rupture, the most common complication of dialysis graft declotting, occurs in up to 5% of procedures. The initial treatment of choice is balloon tamponade, which is at least 70% effective.[35,36] We previously placed uncovered stents when two 5-minute cycles of tamponade failed,[37-39] but we found this to be less effective than placing covered stents.[36] At this time, based upon our experience and the favorable patency for covered stents described earlier, we place covered stents in the small percentage of patients in whom balloon tamponade fails.

POSTPROCEDURE AND FOLLOW-UP CARE

The best "treatment" of a clotted dialysis graft is prevention of access thrombosis. It is well established that surveillance and prophylactic PTA reduce the thrombosis rate in grafts.[40-42] Thus, postthrombectomy monitoring and surveillance are essential components of the overall care of dialysis grafts. Attention to quality assurance and awareness of outcomes at the local level are not just a good idea but are highly likely to be part of Medicare requirements in the near future.

Conflict of Interest Disclosure
Dr. Trerotola receives royalty from, and consults for, Teleflex Inc. (global headquarters: Limerick, Penn.), maker of the Arrow-Trerotola PTD.

KEY POINTS
• Many different methods exist for treating a clotted hemodialysis access graft.
• Prevention of thrombosis is the "best treatment."
• Meticulous technique and attention to details will prevent complications and achieve optimal results.

▶ **SUGGESTED READINGS**

Beathard G. A practioner's resource guide to hemodialysis arteriovenous fistulas. Dallas: ESRD Network of Texas, 2003. Accessed 07 Dec 2011 at http://www.esrdnetwork.org/assets/pdf/fistula-first/BeathardGuidetoAVFs.pdf.

Patel AA, Tuite CM, Trerotola SO. Mechanical thrombectomy of hemodialysis fistulae and grafts. Cardiovasc Intervent Radiol 2005;28:704–13.

Turmel-Rodrigues L, Pengloan J, Baudin S, et al. Treatment of stenosis and thrombosis in haemodialysis fistulas and grafts by interventional radiology. Nephrol Dial Transplant 2000;15:2029–36.

Turmel-Rodrigues L, Pengloan J, Bourquelot P. Interventional radiology in hemodialysis fistulae and grafts: a multidisciplinary approach. Cardiovasc Intervent Radiol 2002;25:3–16.

The complete reference list is available online at www.expertconsult.com.

CHAPTER 117

Percutaneous Management of Thrombosis in Native Hemodialysis Shunts

Dierk Vorwerk

CLINICAL RELEVANCE

Percutaneous procedures for hemodialysis shunts are becoming increasingly important for interventional radiologists. A growing number of patients with renal insufficiency are enrolled in dialysis programs, the majority of them undergoing hemodialysis. In the West, this affects some 150 to 200 persons per million inhabitants. Given the increase in patients' life expectancy, maintaining access to the vascular system continues to be a problem.[1] For example, the number of long-term functioning shunts is estimated to be 15%.[1] Primary patency of hemodialysis shunts is low: approximately 65% of Brescia-Cimino shunts and 50% of polytetrafluoroethylene (PTFE)-covered shunts exhibit primary patency after 1 year, and the numbers sink after 2 and 4 years to 60% and 45% for Brescia-Cimino shunts and to 43% and 10% for PTFE-covered shunts.[1]

In Europe, arteriovenous Brescia-Cimino shunts are the preferred primary shunts, used in conjunction with the radial artery and veins of the lower arm. Autologous veins in the proximal lower arm and elbow region are generally preferred even for renewed shunt application. For percutaneous revascularization, the choice of access site, indications, and interventional technique employed depend on the nature and location of the shunt, site of the lesion, and nature of the obstruction.

Shunt thrombosis of native fistulas is a complication not as frequent as in grafts.[1] Besides an underlying stenosis that is present in almost all cases, cofactors are manifold: clotting abnormalities, thrombocytosis, disturbed fluid balance, hypotension, and aneurysmatic degeneration of the native vein causing low flow may lead to shunt thrombosis. There are, however, different types of shunt thrombosis that require different strategies of percutaneous intervention.

INDICATIONS

Indications for interventional treatment are acute or subacute occlusions in native fistulas that prevent use of the arteriovenous connection for dialysis. Relative indications are occluded fistulae in patients with a functioning renal allograft. Percutaneous intervention is contraindicated in acute infections of the vein or perivenous space. It is, however, worth trying to recanalize even thrombosed immature fistulas because there is a good chance of restoring flow and allowing development of a mature fistula after percutaneous recanalization.[2,3] Natario et al. achieved clinical success in immature fistulas in 97%, with a 1-year primary patency of 51%.[3] Miller et al. achieved 85% technical success in thrombosed immature fistulas, 79% clinical success, and a secondary patency of 90% at 12 months.[2]

Clinical Situation

Clinical examination of the shunt and especially palpation of the venous outflow tract gives an impression of the type of occlusion and its location and is an inevitable part of the clinical checkup prior to an intervention. When in doubt, sonography and duplex sonography may help determine the extent of a thrombosis and its location.

Shunt occlusions in Brescia-Cimino fistulas, especially in the very early phase, may be due to only a very short plug-like thrombus selectively obstructing the arteriovenous anastomosis or a segment of the venous outflow. In those cases, the draining shunt vein is soft and compressible at palpation. If digital manipulation to remove the thrombus fails, this type of obstruction is an ideal candidate for percutaneous transluminal angioplasty (PTA), since the small thrombus can be macerated by balloon inflation alone, and flow can be restored immediately. Treatment, however, should be started soon to avoid propagation of thrombosis.

Palpation also detects those cases where shunt thrombosis is due to an underlying severe stenosis and a subsequent small thrombus formation. If this happens close to the arteriovenous anastomosis, the amount of thrombus is usually small, and balloon dilatation alone may be sufficient for recanalization and treatment of the underlying stenosis.

Long-segment thrombosis of Brescia-Cimino fistulas present with enlarged and incompressible veins that appear rather hard during palpation. PTA alone is mostly insufficient in these cases.

Very rarely, arterial thrombosis or embolism may be a cause for shunt dysfunction. Percutaneous treatment depends on the location and amount of thrombus that has to be removed. It can vary from simple PTA to thrombolysis.

CONTRAINDICATIONS

There are few contraindications to percutaneous thrombectomy from native fistulas. One is definitely a suspected superinfection of the thrombus or vein. This is rare; although thrombosed venosus segments are frequently painful, this does not necessarily indicate infection.

Large amounts of thrombus, especially in large venous aneurysms, are poorer candidates for mechanical thrombectomy, because there is increased risk of pulmonary embolization.

EQUIPMENT

A high-quality angiographic unit with a C-arm, digital pulsed fluoroscopy, and preferably a table that allows lateral

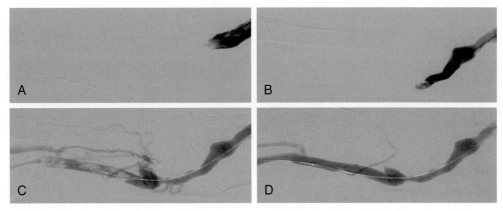

FIGURE 117-1. Distal thrombosis in a Brescia-Cimino (BC) fistula, with a nonthrombosed proximal segment allowing antegrade cannulation. **A,** Complete thrombosis of draining vein in a BC shunt with a proximal nonthrombosed segment. **B,** After aspiration, some thrombus is removed close to elbow region. **C,** By use of a percutaneous thrombectomy device (PTD), larger portions of thrombus have been removed, and flow has been restored. Considerable clots remain in basilic vein. **D,** After continuous application of PTD, remaining clots are removed and free flow obtained.

rotation to position the patient's arm are prerequisites for shunt interventions. For thrombectomy in particular, no special requirements are needed.

TECHNIQUE

Anatomy and Approaches

The anatomy of native hemodialysis fistulas is very individual and may alter due to current arterialized blood stream, pressure, and traumatization. There are some principal forms of fistula that determine which access to the thrombosis is appropriate.

Native Lower Arm Shunts

As a rule, venous access is chosen for Brescia-Cimino shunts. The shunt vein is punctured with the patient wearing a compression bandage. A large-lumen cannula can be employed for the puncture if the vein is large and well palpable, and a regular guidewire (0.035 inch in diameter) can be inserted. However, the micropuncture procedure is recommended if the lumen of the vein is narrow and poorly palpable; in this case, the vein is punctured with a 22-gauge needle and a 0.018-inch wire is inserted. Subsequently, a 16-gauge plastic cannula containing a sharp-pointed needle is inserted into the shunt vein coaxially while being rotated. To prevent it from breaking, imaging must confirm that the thin wire does not suddenly kink. If the position of the plastic cannula is secure, the stylet and guidewire should be replaced by a 0.035-inch wire. A hydrophilically coated wire is well suited.

Retrograde puncture is performed in lesions near anastomoses (i.e., distal venous lesions), stenotic anastomoses, and distal arterial stenoses.

Antegrade transbrachial arterial access as a "backdoor" entrance may be necessary in exceptional cases if the operator does not succeed in probing a stenosis or occlusion near the anastomosis via a venous access. In this case, the brachial artery is punctured in an antegrade manner at the level of the elbow joint, and after thorough probing of the artery supplying the shunt—normally the radial artery—a 4F catheter is inserted. The stenosis is overcome using the wire and

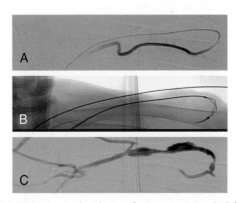

FIGURE 117-2. Proximal occlusion of a Brescia-Cimino (BC) fistula due to extended thrombosis. **A,** Complete thrombosis of a BC shunt from anastomosis onward. Access achieved via basilic vein. **B,** Thrombus is destroyed using a percutaneous thrombectomy device guided via 0.018-inch wire. **C,** Flow has been reestablished.

catheter, and the wire is then guided out via the venous puncture site as a pull-through approach. The intervention is then performed via the venous site to avoid over-enlarging the arterial puncture.

For occlusions in the proximal segments of the draining veins, the shunt vein is punctured antegrade at a peripheral puncture site. If a proximal lesion cannot be probed via the peripheral access, or if probing is prevented by a dissection or perforation, there is still the option of attempting the passage in a retrograde direction via a second access closer to the trunk.

Native Upper Arm Shunts

In lesions near the anastomosis, retrograde puncture of the upper cephalic vein is performed at a position near the trunk. If the lesion is located more centrally, a puncture site is chosen close to the anastomosis (Figs. 117-1 and 117-2). A double access is often advisable in thromboses of upper arm shunts, whereby the puncture can be made in the thrombosed venous portion and thrombectomy first performed on one segment via retrograde access and then the second segment via antegrade access.

Ipsilateral puncture of the internal jugular vein with retrograde probing has been described as an alternative access to the brachiocephalic vein.[4]

Arterial Lesions

For proximal arterial lesions, access can be achieved either retrograde via puncture of the brachial artery or—in the case of the upper arm and synthetic shunts—retrograde transvenously after shunt puncture. If the brachial pulse is weak, the micropuncture technique is occasionally appropriate after the stenosis has been located using a pocket Doppler. Transfemoral arterial access for dilatation is only indicated in the unusual case of arterial stenoses of the proximal brachial artery.

Technical Aspects

Percutaneous Treatment

Published literature describes a number of approaches to treating clotted native fistulas:

- Thrombolysis and spray-lysis
- Mechanical thrombectomy:
- Balloon angioplasty
- Aspiration thrombectomy
- Hydrodynamic thrombectomy
- Mechanical clot dissolution
- Stent placement

Frequently a combination of methods becomes necessary to finalize a case. All methods have been used with success, and interventional radiologists should be familiar with several of them to achieve best possible results.

Thrombolysis

Thrombolysis is (relatively) infrequently described to treat native fistulas. Rajan et al.[5] described their experience in 25 fistulas with 30 episodes of occlusion, including 19 forearm radiocephalic fistulas in 18 patients and 6 upper arm brachiocephalic fistulas in 6 patients. Lytic therapy with urokinase or recombinant tissue plasminogen activator (rtPA) was administered as a bolus into the fistula in 24 cases, with the exception of one case in which a 16-hour infusion of rtPA was initiated. Clinical success was achieved in 73% of cases (22 of 30). All patients were followed for a maximum of 66 months (mean 12 months). Primary patency rates were 36% at 3 months and 24% at 1 year. The assisted primary patency rate was 40% at 3 months and 32% at 6 months. The secondary patency rate stabilized at 3 months was 44%. Patency rates after clot removal were not significantly different between upper and lower arm fistulas.

Schon and Mishler[6] described their experience with 35 procedures in arteriovenous fistulas (AVFs). The technique entailed local instillation of tPA in small doses, together with manual maceration to dissolve clot and balloon angioplasty to correct the underlying stenoses. The procedures were successful in 92% of cases, with an average required tPA dose of 2.3 ± 0.32 mg/procedure. Primary patency was 11.2 months, and secondary patency was 25 months; 55% of fistulas required repeat angioplasty procedures at an average of 3.6-month intervals. In addition, more than half of the fistulas that presented with clotting required repeat interventions for continued patency.

Yehia et al., however, describe failure of thrombolysis in almost 50% of cases[7] and claimed that thrombolysis was considerably inferior to surgery. Poulain et al. in their early paper from 1991, having treated the largest group (55 patients), reported a primary technical success of 59%.[8]

Mechanical Thrombectomy
Balloon Angioplasty

Simple balloon angioplasty is the easiest tool to treat small-segment thrombosis or small thrombus mass complicating a venous stenosis. It is very quick, inexpensive, and effective.[9,10] Its use is limited to native fistulas, since grafts do not show circumscribed thrombosis unless they are treated in a very early stage of thrombus formation.

To avoid propagation of thrombosis, treatment should be performed on an urgent basis after the patient has evidence of circumscribed thrombosis. This should be also executed during evening hours and on weekends.

Access to the shunt depends on thrombus location. In most instances, it is located close to the anastomosis, so retrograde cannulation of the draining vein is most suitable. The arteriovenous anastomosis is then carefully passed by a 5F multipurpose catheter and a hydrophilic guidewire that is advanced into the feeding artery. There is only a minimal risk of arterial thrombus dislodgement during this maneuver. Thereafter, the 5F catheter is exchanged for a 4- to 6-mm balloon catheter that is inflated at the area of thrombosis. This can be repeated until shunt flow is restored. Treatment should not be terminated unless optimal opening of the underlying stenotic area has been achieved.

Combined Surgery and Balloon Angioplasty

Implant grafts may be declotted using Fogarty balloons after surgical cutdown.[11] In native fistulas, however, combining a surgical and percutaneous approach is not a widely used option.

Aspiration Thrombectomy

Clot removal may be also performed using a simple 7F to 9F end-hole aspiration catheter. The technique used is similar to arterial thrombosuction. If a residual flow is present, arterial inflow should be interrupted by digital compression to facilitate aspiration of a clot. It is a simple and cost-effective technique to remove clot effectively.

Turmel-Rodrigues et al.[12] reported on their vast experience with aspiration thrombectomy in native fistulas and grafts with 257 declotting procedures. They recommend application of curved guiding catheters to reach all segments even in enlarged veins. They achieved technical success in 78% to 98% depending on the nature of the shunt connection. Primary patency at 1 year was 50% for native fistulas and 25% for implant grafts. Secondary patency at 1 year was between 80% and 86%.

Technically, besides aspiration, stent placement became necessary in a considerable number of cases.[12] They placed stents in 41% to 45% of declotting cases, including those stents indicated to displace residual clot material. The mean procedure time varied from 119 (grafts) to 134 minutes (forearm fistulas).[12]

Aspiration is also an excellent tool to remove embolized occlusion material from the radial or brachial artery that occurred during declotting procedures, allowing treatment of complications caused by mechanical thrombectomy or lysis.

Hydrodynamic Thrombectomy

Hydrodynamic thrombectomy has been introduced to the treatment of acute thrombosis of arteries, bypass grafts, and hemodialysis fistulas and grafts. Three different devices have been tested for their utility in dialysis connections:

- Hydrolyser (Cordis, Roden, Netherlands), 7F
- Oasis catheter (Boston Scientific, Natick, Mass.), 7F to 8F
- AngioJet catheter (Medrad/Possis Medical, Minneapolis, Minn.), 6F

All work on the same principle: they are double-lumen catheters with retrograde saline injection from a very small supply lumen that is injected in a larger efferent lumen. The resulting pressure gradient between the jet flow and the larger exhaust lumen, known as the *Venturi effect*, causes the injected fluid to instantaneously leave the vessel via the exhaust lumen, thus creating a turbulent flow zone close to the catheter tip and suction. The surrounding thrombus is fragmented by the flow vortex, sucked into the exhaust lumen, and removed as a mixture of saline and thrombus through it. Blood loss is low, and the system is more or less isovolumetric. Saline injection can be performed by conventional angiographic injectors for the Hydrolyser and the Oasis catheter but requires a specially designed power pump for the AngioJet catheter.

Results are available for all three hydrodynamic systems. However, no comparison studies exist, neither comparing other hydrodynamic nor other mechanical devices.

HYDROLYSER Evaluated from 51 procedures,[13] hydrodynamic thrombectomy using the Hydrolyser was completed with 1 to 7 runs (mean 3.2 ± 1.1 runs). Considerable fluid imbalance with overinfusion of 50 to 100 mL to the patient occurred in two cases.

The major amount of thrombus was removed by hydrodynamic thrombectomy in most cases. The estimated amount of residual thrombus was 8% (5%-30% range) on average in grafts and 21% (10%-50% range) in native fistulas. Despite residual thrombus in many cases, arterialized flow was completely established by combining hydrodynamic thrombectomy and PTA in 44 of 51 cases (86%). By additional use of aspiration thrombectomy, stent implantation, or Fogarty embolectomy, overall assisted technical success was therefore 46 of 51 procedures (90%).

Technical failure of combining hydrodynamic thrombectomy and balloon angioplasty occurred in 7 cases. Occlusion time in these cases ranged from 12 to 120 hours (mean 65.2 hours, median 60 hours). In all cases, hydrodynamic thrombectomy was combined with balloon angioplasty and, in two cases, with directional atherectomy for treatment of an additional stenosis or remaining thrombus.

There was one retrograde arterial embolization to the radial artery that was treated by embolectomy using a minibasket, and one case of temporary shortness of breath that might be subsequent to pulmonary embolization of occluding material.

Clinical success was achieved in 39 of 46 technically successful cases (85%) in whom the access was used for hemodialysis again or remained patent for at least 1 week after thrombectomy without hemodialysis (3 patients). Forty-six grafts and fistulas were followed from 1 week to 18 months. Cumulative patency was calculated at 63% after 1 week, 57% after 1 month, 48% after 3 months, 37% after 6 months, and 32% after 12 months.

OASIS CATHETER Barth et al.[14] evaluated the safety and efficacy of a hydrodynamic thrombectomy system in a prospective multicenter randomized comparison with pulse-spray thrombolysis in hemodialysis grafts. Nine centers enrolled 120 adult patients with recently (≤14 days) thrombosed hemodialysis grafts. Clinical success rates were 89% (55 of 62) and 81% (47 of 58).

No particular results have been published for native fistulas.

ANGIOJET CATHETER Vesely et al.[15] compared the clinical effectiveness of the AngioJet F105 rheolytic catheter to that of surgical thrombectomy for treatment of thrombosed hemodialysis grafts. Technical success was 73.2% for the AngioJet group and 78.8% for the surgical thrombectomy group. The AngioJet F105 catheter provides similar clinical results to surgical thrombectomy for treating thrombosed hemodialysis grafts. For this device, no analysis exists for native fistulas.

Endoluminal Clot Dissolution

Other than hydrodynamic thrombectomy that removes the thrombus from the body, endoluminal thrombus dissolution tries to break up thrombus formation into ultrasmall pieces, allowing capillary passage of the fragments. Several different devices are clinically available, but the Amplatz Clot Buster device (Microvena Corp., White Bear Lake, Minn.) and the percutaneous thrombectomy device (PTD) (Arrow-Trerotola PTD with rotating basket [Teleflex Inc., Limerick, Pa.]) are the only devices where clinical data are available for dialysis connections.

Clot Buster

The Clot Buster is a 7F or 8F flexible catheter with no guiding lumen, bearing a housed impeller at its distal end. The impeller is driven by air pressure up to high rotational speed, causing a large vortex around the catheter tip. Thrombus is sucked toward the impeller and fragmented, and its fragments recirculate into the vortex over and over again.

Technical application is similar to hydrodynamic thrombectomy and depends on the type of shunt to be treated. Applicability is easy and quick, since pressured air is available in most angiosuites.

Sometimes guiding problems may occur, since the 8F device cannot be advanced over a wire (however, a 6F over-the-wire version will be available soon) and hemolysis is possible. In large-diameter veins such as the brachial, subclavian, and jugular vein, the Amplatz catheter—in our experience—seems to be more effective than hydrodynamic devices such as the Hydrolyser.

Uflacker et al.[16] reported the final results of the trial comparing the Amplatz thrombectomy device (ATD) with surgical thromboembolectomy to declot thrombosed dialysis access grafts. Patency of the graft (with successful dialysis) at 30 days with the ATD procedure was 79.2% and with surgery was 73.4%. No statistically significant differences were seen.

Haage et al.[10] analyzed technical success of mechanical thrombectomy in acute thrombotic occlusion of native arteriovenous fistulae for hemodialysis. Eighty-one percutaneous procedures were performed in 54 patients presenting with a clotted native dialysis fistula. There were 60 cases of a long-segment thrombosis of the fistula. In 20 cases, a small thrombus usually caused by an underlying severe stenosis was observed. A proximal arterial occlusion was seen in one case. Treatment depended on clot size and included balloon dilation (n = 20), mechanical thrombectomy with various devices including hydrodynamic thrombectomy and the Clot Buster (n = 58), as well as pharmacomechanical thrombolysis (n = 3). Full restoration of flow was established in 72 cases (88.9%). Primary patency rates after a 1-, 3-, 6-, and 12-month period were 74%, 63%, 52%, and 27%, respectively. Overall fistula patency was 75% after 3 months, 65% after 6 months, and 51% after 12 months.

Arrow-Trerotola Percutaneous Thrombectomy Device

The Arrow-Trerotola PTD is a 7F system that carries a nitinol basket which slowly rotates, driven by a small motor. It can be closed and opened by moving an outer protecting catheter. It is an over-the-wire system that accepts a 0.025-inch guidewire.

In dialysis shunts and grafts, some clinical experience has been published. Lazzaro et al.[17] reported on the use of the Arrow-Trerotola PTD as the sole means of mechanical thrombolysis in hemodialysis access grafts. Fifty consecutive patients in whom mechanical thrombolysis of a thrombosed hemodialysis access graft using the PTD was planned were included in the study. Three-month patency using life-table analysis was 42%.

Rocek et al.[18] evaluated the feasibility of using the Arrow-Trerotola PTD in the treatment of thrombosed native fistulas. Ten patients were treated, the technical success rate was 100%, and the clinical success rate was 90%. In all 10 cases, the procedure was associated with angioplasty. The mean time of successful procedures was 126 minutes. The 3- and 6-month primary patency rates were 70% and 60%, respectively; the assisted primary patency rate at 6 months was 80%. Thus, the device could also be safely used in native veins.

Stenting

Another possibility of mechanical "thrombectomy" is use of endoluminal stents to fix the thrombus to the venous wall by compression and flattening.[19] This technique can be especially helpful in large veins where other techniques failed to remove thrombus material. The permanence and cost of stent placement make it an approach not used on a regular basis, but it offers additional possibilities in the event an otherwise desperate situation has to be solved.

Chronic Venous Occlusion

Please visit www.expertconsult.com for more information on chronic venous occlusion.

CONTROVERSIES

There is no real controversy concerning percutaneous treatment of thrombosis in native fistulas. Other than in implant shunts, no good surgical option exists. Frequently surgeons tend to create a new fistula instead of repair, or a new anastomosis is performed. Treatment of thrombosis in the presence of larger venous aneurysms is debatable, and in many of these cases, at least surgical resection of the aneurysm is preferable.

COMPLICATIONS

Complications are mostly benign in the treatment of thrombosis in native fistulas. Turmel-Rodrigues et al.[21] described one case of pulmonary embolism, one subacute pseudoaneurysm, one significant blood loss, and five venous ruptures in 94 cases of thrombectomy of native fistulas (8% including venous rupture, 3% without). Miyayama et al.[22] described minor complications in 20% of 26 patients with thrombosed Brescia-Cimino fistulas, but this included procedural events such as venous rupture in 12% and development of a hematoma in 8%. Liang et al.[23] reported just two cases of venous rupture and two cases of radial arterial emboli in a group of 42 thromboses of Brescia-Cimino fistulas treated by percutaneous means, which counts for a total complication rate of 10% or 5% excluding venous rupture. Rajan and Clark[24] found two complications among 30 treatments for thrombosis of native fistulas: one small hematoma and one small pseudoaneurysm (7% in total).

POSTPROCEDURE AND FOLLOW-UP CARE

Please visit www.expertconsult.com for a full discussion of postprocedure care.

KEY POINTS

- Thrombosis of hemodialysis fistulae and grafts represents a frequent complication of hemodialysis access.
- Nonsurgical treatment using thrombolytic drugs and various mechanical instruments is increasingly applied in native fistulae as a first-line procedure instead of standard surgical thrombectomy.
- At many institutions, surgery is reserved for thrombosed aneurysmal or markedly dilated outflow veins where a large thrombus burden restricts the effectiveness of catheter techniques.

► **SUGGESTED READINGS**

Haage P, Vorwerk D, Wildberger JE, et al. Percutaneous treatment of thrombosed primary arteriovenous hemodialysis access fistulae. Kidney Int 2000;57(3):1169–75.

Turmel-Rodrigues L, Pengloan J, Baudin S, et al. Treatment of stenosis and thrombosis in haemodialysis fistulas and grafts by interventional radiology. Nephrol Dial Transplant 2000;15(12):2029–36.

Uflacker R, Rajagopalan PR, Selby JB, Hannegan C; Investigators of the Clinical Trial Sponsored by Microvena Corporation. Thrombosed dialysis access grafts: randomized comparison of the Amplatz thrombectomy device and surgical thromboembolectomy. Eur Radiol 2004;14(11):2009–14. Epub 2004 Jul 29.

The complete reference list is available online at www.expertconsult.com.

CHAPTER **118**

Peripherally Inserted Central Catheters and Nontunneled Central Venous Catheters

Joseph A. Hughes, Colin P. Cantwell, and Peter N. Waybill

Peripherally inserted central catheters (PICCs) and nontunneled central venous catheters (CVCs) are indispensable in current medical practice, with both serving central venous access needs. They are used for infusion therapy, exchange therapy, and hemodynamic monitoring. The central venous system includes the pulmonary arteries, right heart, superior vena cava (SVC), inferior vena cava (IVC), and brachiocephalic, subclavian, and iliac veins. It should be noted that although these vessels and many other small veins are considered central, they are not necessarily appropriate locations for venous catheter tips. In most cases, the desired position for a CVC tip is in the SVC or right atrium.

Present-day venous access devices are available in a wide variety of sizes, forms, and configurations designed to meet specific needs. It is important to be familiar with the range of venous access devices presently available on the market and the features that affect their selection.

INDICATIONS

There are three main indications for temporary CVC insertion: infusion therapy, exchange therapy, and hemodynamic monitoring. Although many CVCs can be used for phlebotomy, this use alone is rarely an indication for insertion.

PICCs are small-bore catheters placed through a peripheral arm or leg vein into the central veins. Midline catheters are shorter than PICCs and typically terminate in the axillary vein. Nontunneled CVCs are inserted more proximal to the central venous system in the internal jugular (IJ), subclavian, or femoral veins.

Indications for placement of a PICC or nontunneled CVC for infusion therapy include (1) rapid infusion of fluids or blood products to maintain hemodynamic stability, (2) infusion of vesicant solutions such as chemotherapeutic, cytotoxic, or inotropic medications or infusates with pH less than 5 or above 9, more than 500-600 mOsm, more than 10% dextrose, or more than 5% amino acids, (3) total parenteral nutrition, (4) active infection that prevents placement of a more permanent device, and (5) coagulopathy that prevents placement of a more permanent device.[1-3]

Indications for placement of a nontunneled CVC for exchange therapy (hemodialysis and apheresis) include (1) management of acute volume overload not responsive to other medical therapy, (2) management of severe acute electrolyte disorders, (3) management of acute hyperviscosity disorders, (4) short-term apheresis/hemodialysis treatment, (5) stem cell harvesting, (6) active infection that prevents placement of a more permanent device, and (7) coagulopathy that prevents placement of a more permanent device. Owing to small lumen size and low flow rates, current PICC technology does not permit exchange therapy or hemodialysis.

Indications for hemodynamic monitoring are usually encountered in patients in the intensive care unit (ICU). Nontunneled CVCs traditionally serve this function, but PICCs may be used with some limitation based on caliber. These catheters are most commonly inserted at the bedside in the ICU setting.

Catheter choice should be made with expected length of treatment in mind. For short-term access (<2-4 weeks) for infusion, monitoring, or exchange therapy, a PICC or small-bore nontunneled CVC would be indicated. Some studies have reported PICCs functioning for longer than 1 year, and some anecdotal reports have noted functioning PICCs that have been present for longer than 2 years.[4-6] However, such reports represent the exception rather than the rule.

For long-term access (>2-4 weeks) a tunneled catheter or implantable port may be indicated. A selection algorithm for choosing among PICCs, nontunneled CVCs, tunneled CVCs, and ports is provided in Figure 118-1.

PICCs have many advantages. They are safe and easy to place, prevent the need for frequent venipuncture, allow easy care and access for inpatients and outpatients, and they are usually well tolerated by patients. Unlike tunneled catheters and ports that require conscious sedation, PICCs and nontunneled CVCs can be placed without sedation with little patient discomfort. They are also easy to remove or exchange in the event of malfunction or infection.

Bedside ultrasound-guided PICC placement by skilled nurses is becoming the standard at many institutions, saving all but the most challenging of patients the time and cost of a trip to the interventional suite. At our institution, only PICCs that cannot be advanced to the cavoatrial junction or the very difficult-to-access patients come to interventional radiology for placement under fluoroscopic guidance.

Nontunneled CVCs have similar properties to PICCs, with the advantage of accommodating large-bore catheters in the larger IJ, subclavian, and femoral veins. The major disadvantage of nontunneled CVCs is the high rate of catheter-related bloodstream infections. In fact, nontunneled CVCs account for the majority of catheter-related bloodstream infections in the United States.

Indications for pediatric PICCs may include the need for venous access of 6 days or more or the need to administer vesicants or other infusates requiring dilution in the central venous system.[3] Early PICC placement may spare patients numerous venipunctures. Selection criteria for catheter placement in pediatrics are otherwise similar to adults:

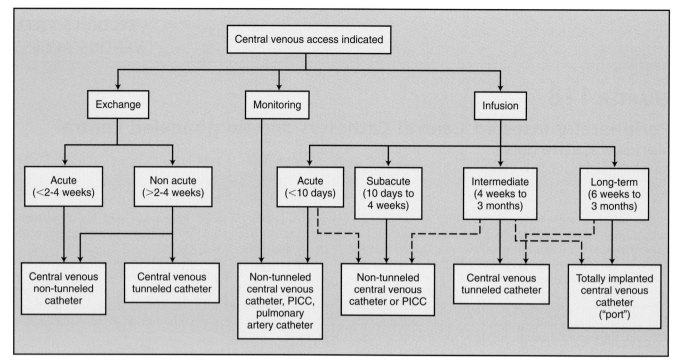

FIGURE 118-1. Clinical algorithm for appropriate catheter selection. *PICC,* Percutaneously inserted central catheter.

- It is important to choose the appropriate type of CVC for the intended use: infusion, exchange, or hemodynamic monitoring.
- PICCs and nontunneled CVCs are appropriate for access needs less than 2-4 weeks.
- Tunneled CVCs and ports are appropriate for access needs longer than 2-4 weeks.

CONTRAINDICATIONS

There are very few strict contraindications to PICC and nontunneled CVC placement. These catheters can usually be placed safely regardless of existing coagulopathy or thrombocytopenia. Unlike with tunneled CVCs and ports, active infection or bacteremia does not contraindicate placement. Allergic reactions to contrast material and elevated serum creatinine are relative contraindications to placement under venographic guidance with iodinated contrast agents. However, ultrasound guidance or use of alternative contrast agents such as carbon dioxide gas or gadolinium negates this contraindication. PICCs should not be placed on the same side as a previous mastectomy or axillary lymph node dissection, in a paretic extremity, or in the location of focal infection, burn, or radiation injury.

PICC placement may be precluded in patients in whom a suitable peripheral vein cannot be identified. Central venous thrombosis or occlusion also poses a relative contraindication. Occasionally a guidewire can be used to traverse the thrombosed vein, or access to the central veins can be achieved through collaterals, thus permitting central venous placement of the catheter tip. When this fails, PICCs may be positioned peripheral to the occluded central veins, thereby resulting in subclavian or axillary placement of the catheter tip. This position may be adequate provided fluids to be administered are not hyperosmolar or vesicant fluids. It has been shown that PICCs placed in a noncentral vein

can provide reliable safe intravenous access for administration of many medications for up to 2 weeks' duration.[7]

Placement of a PICC is contraindicated in any person undergoing hemodialysis or in whom hemodialysis is anticipated, including patients with renal transplants. PICCs are associated with a significant rate of peripheral venous thrombosis.[8] To preserve peripheral veins for future hemodialysis access, the National Kidney Foundation Kidney Disease Outcomes Quality Initiative (NKF KDOQI) advises against placement of PICCs in this patient population.[9,10]

EQUIPMENT

Catheter Types

Multiple catheter designs with varying catheter materials (silicone and polyurethane), catheter diameters, and number of lumina are available commercially. Catheters are made with three basic tip configurations: end hole, staggered tip, and valve tipped:

- End-hole catheters are the most common catheter design, with all lumina opening within close proximity of the catheter tip. These devices may be trimmed at the tip to achieve an appropriate length.
- Staggered-tip dual-lumen catheters are specifically designed for therapies that require simultaneous rapid aspiration and infusion with limited mixing (hemodialysis and apheresis). These devices should not be trimmed, so their staggered-tip configuration is maintained.
- Valve-tipped catheters have a specially designed slitlike two-way valve at the catheter tip that is closed in the resting state. The valve opens inward with aspiration and outward for infusion, with the potential advantage of not requiring routine heparinization to prevent catheter thrombosis. The Groshong catheter (C.R. Bard Access Systems Inc., Salt Lake City, Utah) is a

valve-tipped catheter. Valve-tipped catheters cannot be trimmed at the tip, but they have a removable external connection that allows the back end to be trimmed for adjustment of length. The Vaxcel catheter with pressure activated safety valve (PASV) (Boston Scientific Corp., Natick, Mass.) incorporates a valve into the hub of the catheter, allowing the tip to be trimmed. PASV catheters have a lower recorded rate of infection, thrombosis, and phlebitis compared to distal valve-tipped catheters.[11-13]

Standard PICC technology does not allow for high-pressure power injection, but high-pressure injectable catheters are now available. Typically constructed of polyurethane, they usually allow injection up to a maximum of 300 psi and 5 mL/s. Maximum allowable flow rates may vary for individual catheters. High-pressure injectable catheters are most beneficial to patients requiring power injected contrast enhanced computed tomography (CT) studies.

Procedural Supplies

Required supplies for PICC and nontunneled IJ, subclavian, and femoral CVC placement are listed in Table 118-1.

Ultrasound-guided placement is best performed using a 7.5 to 9 MHz probe. A needle guide attached to the ultrasound probe is optional but makes seeing the needle tip puncture the vessel easier.

When placed at the bedside, tip locator devices increase the accuracy of placement. Some examples of these devices are the Navigator Bionavigation System (Medcomp Inc., Harleysville, Pa.) and Sherlock Tip Positioning System (TPS) (C.R. Bard Access Systems). They use an electronic device external to the patient to detect the catheter tip position or tip direction. These systems are not intended to replace appropriate preinsertion measurements or chest radiographic confirmation of tip location.

Accuracy of bedside placement is also increased using electrocardiogram (ECG)-assisted techniques and is being used in lieu of radiographic tip verification.[14] Traditional bedside ECG monitors can be used, but dedicated systems are now coming to market to emphasize this technique. At our institution, we use the Sapiens Tip Confirmation System (TCS) (C.R. Bard Access Systems) that uses external ECG electrodes to detect intravascular ECG P-wave changes as the catheter approaches the cavoatrial junction.

TECHNIQUE

Anatomy and Approach

The preferred location for PICC placement is in the nondominant arm. Placement above the antecubital fossa is preferred and may lower the risk of phlebitis. The order of preference is the basilic, brachial, cephalic, then median cubital vein. The preferred location for nontunneled CVC placement in order of preference is the right IJ, left IJ, subclavian, then femoral vein. Anatomic reference is provided in Figure 118-2.

Basilic Vein
The basilic vein is the dominant superficial vein of the arm and merges with the axillary vein in the mid- to proximal arm. It is best found in the superficial fat of the medial aspect of the forearm. Approach from the medial part of the arm with the vein interposed between the ultrasound probe and the humerus allows control of the vessel.

TABLE 118-1. Standard Ultrasound-Guided PICC Tray

Cap, mask, sterile gown, and gloves
Ultrasound probe cover, gel, and needle guide
Sterile tourniquet (nonsterile tourniquet can be used outside sterile field)
2% chlorhexidine or povidone iodine
Drapes
Gauze
Lidocaine 1% or 2% with or without epinephrine
10-mL syringe with 25-gauge needle for lidocaine injection
21-gauge needle for vein puncture
0.018-inch guidewire for access
Scalpel with #11 blade
Scissors
Measuring tape
Appropriately selected catheter with guidewire
Appropriately sized peel-away sheath
Saline and 10-mL syringes for aspiration and flushing
Heparin flush (100 IU/mL)
Adhesive securing device
Sharps container

Additional Supplies for Nontunneled CVC Tray

21-gauge needle and 0.018-inch wire including dilator for micropuncture *OR*
18-gauge needle and 0.025- or 0.035-inch wire for puncture
10-mL syringe with attached connecting tubing for aspiration

CVC, central venous catheter; *PICC,* peripherally inserted central catheter.

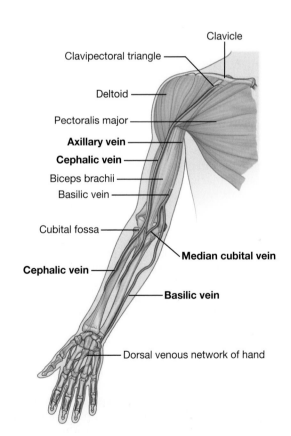

FIGURE 118-2. Upper extremity venous anatomy. *(From Drake RL, Vogl W, Mitchell AWM. Gray's anatomy for students. Philadelphia: Elsevier; 2005, Fig. 7-18.)*

Proximity to the median antebrachial cutaneous nerve may require additional local anesthesia. Care should also be taken to avoid the ulnar nerve located just medial to the vein.

Brachial Vein

The brachial vein is bounded proximally by the teres major muscle, where it continues as the axillary vein. The paired brachial veins parallel the brachial artery. There is increased risk of median nerve injury with brachial venipuncture, and ultrasound-guided placement is preferred to avoid injury to the medially located nerve.

Cephalic Vein

The cephalic vein drains through the clavipectoral fascia into the axillary vein at the shoulder. Approach from the lateral aspect of the arm with the vein interposed between the probe and the humerus allows control of the vessel. Navigation may be difficult in this sometimes tortuous vessel, which often has an acute angular insertion into the axillary vein. Arm abduction may aid passage of the guidewire or PICC through the clavipectoral fascia.

Median Cubital Vein

The median cubital vein drains the superficial forearm and hand and drains into the basilic and cephalic veins. It is often the most prominent vessel in the antecubital fossa, and cannulation can sometimes be made without ultrasound. However, the vein may be occluded if there is a history of frequent cannulation. Numerous venous valves may also make cannulation difficult.

Internal Jugular Vein

The IJ vein is the preferred location for nontunneled CVC placement. A right IJ approach is preferable to a left IJ approach because fewer angulations are encountered. An anterior low-central or posterior approach can be made under ultrasound guidance. The low-central approach between the clavicular and sternal heads of the sternocleidomastoid muscle is the most common. An adequate sonographic window must be identified to exclude the carotid from the direct trajectory of the puncturing needle. An optimal approach creates a catheter entry point into the vein that avoids any acute angulation and the possibility of catheter kinking.

Femoral Vein

At the level of the femoral head, the femoral vein lies medial to the common femoral artery. Palpation of the femoral artery allows the operator to puncture the vein medially over the pubic bone. The catheter tip should lie in the common iliac vein or IVC below the level of the renal veins.

Technical Aspects

Ultrasound-Guided Placement of a Peripherally Inserted Central Catheter

The arm is positioned at 45 to 90 degrees at the patient's side on an arm board with the palm up. An appropriate compressible vein should be identified with a tourniquet applied to the shoulder.

The appropriate length of catheter should be calculated before sterile prep and venipuncture. This is critical in the

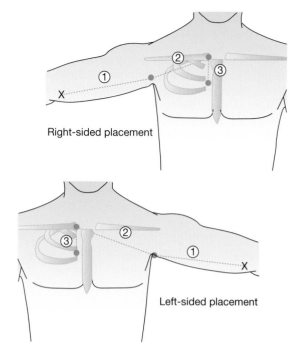

Right-sided placement

Left-sided placement

FIGURE 118-3. Appropriate measurements are taken before placing a PICC. Anatomic landmarks used for estimating PICC length include venipuncture site, ipsilateral axillary crease, right sternoclavicular joint, and right third intercostal space at parasternal border. *(Courtesy Bard Access Systems.)*

absence of fluoroscopy. The desired tip position is in the distal third of the SVC or at the cavoatrial junction. Measurements are taken from the venipuncture site to the ipsilateral axillary crease to the right sternoclavicular joint and inferiorly to the third intercostal space at the right parasternal border (Fig. 118-3). Lower extremity PICCs are measured from the venipuncture site along the course of the vein to the right of the umbilicus to the xiphoid. Adding the estimated depth of subcutaneous fat to the measurement will increase accuracy. When approaching from the left, adding 1 to 2 cm may increase accuracy as well, owing to catheter flexibility as it courses from left to right in the left brachiocephalic vein. Evaluating a chest radiograph prior to measurement may also help judge the tortuosity of the venous system. Lum's CVC Measurement guide provides an estimated catheter length based on patient height (Table 118-2).

Care should be taken in washing hands. The chosen venipuncture site is sterilely prepped and draped. A tourniquet is reapplied. Local anesthetic is administered to a broad tract across the midpoint of the probe or at the heel of the probe. The 21-gauge needle is advanced with or without a guide until it indents the anterior vein wall and then punctures the vessel, and venous return occurs in the needle hub. The 0.018-inch guidewire is then advanced centrally through the needle into the vein. If the guidewire is advanced too far, cardiac ectopy may be observed, and the guidewire should be retracted.

The tourniquet is removed. Additional lidocaine is injected at the venipuncture site. A small incision is made adjacent to the needle with the scalpel, and the 21-gauge needle is removed. A sheath and dilator system appropriately sized for the chosen PICC are inserted over the guidewire. If not already completed, the PICC is trimmed to the

TABLE 118-2. Lum's Central Venous Catheter Measurement Guide

Height (in)	R. PICC (cm)	L. PICC (cm)	R. JC (cm)	L. SC (cm)	R. SC (cm)	Height (cm)
4 ft 8 in	42.5	46.5	13.0	18.0	14.0	143
4 ft 10 in	44.0	48.0	13.5	18.5	14.5	148
5 ft	45.5	49.5	14.0	19.0	15.0	153
5 ft 2 in	47.0	51.0	14.5	19.5	15.5	158
5 ft 4 in	48.5	52.5	15.0	20.0	16.0	163
5 ft 6 in	50.0	54.0	15.5	20.5	16.5	168
5 ft 8 in	51.5	55.5	16.0	21.0	17.0	173
5 ft 10 in	53.0	57.0	16.5	21.5	17.5	178
6 ft	54.5	58.5	17.0	22.0	18.0	183
6 ft 2 in	56.0	60.0	17.5	22.5	18.5	188
6 ft 4 in	57.5	61.5	18.0	23.0	19.0	193

NOTE: Standard insertion site.
For PICC insertion: approximately 2.5 cm below antecubital fossa line.*
For SC insertion: approximately 2.5 cm below midclavicular border (≈2nd anterior rib level).*†
For JC insertion: apex of sternocleidomastoid triangle or cricoids level.*
*Deviation from standard insertion site, CVC length must be adjusted accordingly.
†Pendulous breast must be taped down prior to SC insertion in supine or Trendelenburg position.
CVC, Central venous catheter; JC, jugular catheter; L, left; PICC, peripheral inserted central catheter; R, right; SC, subclavian catheter.
From Lum PL. A new formula-based measurement guide for optimal positioning of central venous catheters. J Assoc Vasc Access 2004;9:80–5. (©Philip Lum, MD Anderson Cancer Center.)

estimated measurement and flushed with sterile saline. The inner stylet of the catheter should not be cut. After removal of the dilator and 0.018-inch guidewire, the trimmed PICC with stylet is advanced. Having the patient turn the head to the side of the catheter helps avoid deflection into the IJ vein.

The catheter should be advanced to the hub unless a tip locator system is being used, in which case the catheter should be advanced until it reaches the estimated lower SVC. The catheter should not be advanced if resistance is met. If advanced too far, cardiac ectopy may be observed, and the catheter should be retracted. If using the ECG-guided technique, the P wave will increase in size as the tip approaches the cavoatrial junction, ultimately peaking and then inverting after it has passed into the atrium. The ideal catheter tip location is when the P wave is half the height of the QRS.[14]

After removal of the peel-away sheath and stylet, aspiration confirms catheter function. Heparin flush is performed to prevent thrombosis in non–valved-tipped catheters. The catheter is secured to the skin with an adhesive device.

Prior to use, a chest radiograph should be done to confirm catheter position in the lower third of the SVC or cavoatrial junction. When catheters are placed using the ECG-guided technique, chest radiographic confirmation may not be required. This is both a time and cost savings for the patient and hospital but not a substitute for good clinical judgment; if there is any question about catheter location, a chest radiograph should be obtained. Bedside ultrasound at the time of placement may also be used to verify the catheter has not deflected into the IJ vein.[14]

Tips
- Do not compress the vein with the ultrasound probe when advancing the needle.
- Withdraw the needle slowly; slow withdrawal may produce a flashback not apparent on advancement because of apposition of the vein walls.

- Failure to advance the PICC may occur secondary to central stenosis or thrombosis. If in doubt, the catheter should be evaluated with fluoroscopy.
- Attempts at arm abduction and adduction may allow passage of the catheter, particularly when inserted into the cephalic vein at the level of the clavipectoral fascia.

Fluoroscopically Guided Placement of a Peripherally Inserted Central Catheter
An intravenous cannula is inserted at the forearm, hand, or antecubital fossa. The arm is positioned at 45 to 90 degrees at the patient's side on an arm board with the palm up, and a tourniquet is placed at the shoulder. Contrast material is injected into the arm veins. The basilic, cephalic, or brachial veins can be identified fluoroscopically, and the skin entry point identified with metal forceps. Local anesthesia is administered. An additional injection of contrast material will allow placement of a 21-gauge needle directly anteroposterior in the center of the imaging intensifier field toward the distended contrast-filled vein. The combination of indentation of the pool of contrast by the puncture needle and observation of return of venous blood will determine appropriate positioning of the needle in the vein.

The 0.018-inch guidewire is placed. The tourniquet is removed. Additional lidocaine is injected at the venipuncture. A small incision is made adjacent to the needle with the scalpel, and the 21-gauge needle is removed. A sheath and dilator system appropriate for the size of the PICC is inserted. A guidewire is advanced centrally under fluoroscopic guidance until the tip is in the right atrium just distal to its junction with the IVC on inspiration, and the wire is marked with a clamp at the skin entry site. The guidewire is removed, and the PICC is trimmed to the measured length. The guidewire is reinserted and appropriately positioned. After removal of the dilator, the PICC is advanced over the guidewire under fluoroscopic guidance to the

SVC/right atrial junction. If there is excessive catheter length external to the percutaneous insertion site, a measurement is taken from the catheter hub to the insertion site, the catheter is removed over the guidewire, excess measured catheter is trimmed, and the catheter is reinserted over the wire. Aspiration confirms catheter function, and a heparin flush in non–valved-tipped catheters is performed to prevent thrombosis. The PICC is secured to the skin with an adhesive device.

Tips

- If primary insertion of the 21-gauge needle is unsuccessful, the tourniquet should be removed, pressure applied at the insertion site for 5 minutes, and the venogram repeated with puncture of an adjacent vein or the same vein at another level.
- If the artery is punctured, compression should be applied for 10 minutes or until no further hemorrhage is noted.
- Failure to advance the PICC may be due to central stenosis or thrombosis. If in doubt, perform a venogram.

Nontunneled Central Venous Catheter Insertion

Nontunneled CVC placement in the IJ, subclavian, and femoral veins is very similar to tunneled catheter and port placement, and the techniques and considerations for insertion are discussed in greater detail in those chapters. We review some key steps and tips here.

Internal Jugular Vein Insertion

Ultrasound should be performed with the patient supine before entering the fluoroscopy room to verify an adequate vein exists on the preferred side and determine whether the patient should perform a Valsalva maneuver or be placed in Trendelenburg position. Distention of the anterior or external jugular vein may also indicate central venous stenosis, right heart failure, or fluid overload. The right IJ vein is preferable to the left. Straightening of the venous system secondary to guidewire stiffness when approaching from the left IJ vein leads to underestimation of the length of catheter needed. Compensate by adding 1 to 2 cm to the length of a catheter from this approach. Suturing the catheter to the skin overlying the clavicle rather than the neck conceals the catheter ports under clothing and enhances patient comfort.

Femoral Vein Insertion

Femoral vein insertion may be performed under ultrasound or fluoroscopic guidance. The femoral vein lies medial to the common femoral artery. The vein is punctured by advancing the needle at 30 degrees of cranial angulation while aspirating. Low-pressure aspiration of the needle helps verify when flow is identified. The tip of the venous catheter placed via the femoral vein should lie at least at the level of the common iliac vein or IVC below the renal veins.

Subclavian Vein Insertion

Subclavian vein puncture may be performed by identifying the subclavian or axillary vein under ultrasound guidance. The vein is entered inferior to the clavicle between its outer and middle thirds. Puncture of the subclavian vein for access should be avoided in any patient who has the potential to become dialysis dependent, because this may lead to thrombosis or stenosis of the subclavian vein and

make future fistula formation difficult from the side of puncture.

PEDIATRIC CONSIDERATIONS

The techniques for venous access in pediatric patients are similar to the adult, with some modifications. Sedation may be required in young patients, which is rarely needed in adults. The utility and effectiveness of topical lidocaine before venipuncture is debated, but in selected patients may be helpful. Swaddling and firmly securing extremities may be required. Choosing the smallest catheter to meet the patient's needs is important. As catheter size decreases, there is an increased risk of catheter occlusion, and catheters smaller than 2F may occlude without continuous infusion. Users should refer to specific catheter manufacturer recommendations for flushing. Some small veins that may be considered for venipuncture in pediatric patients not commonly accessed in adults include the superficial temporal, posterior auricular, greater and lesser saphenous, and popliteal veins (Figs. e118-1 and e118-2).[3]

CONTROVERSIES

Blind versus Ultrasound-Guided Insertion

There is now little controversy that ultrasound-guided insertion of CVCs is preferred over blind placement. Meta-analysis has shown that the use of ultrasound substantially reduces mechanical complications associated with placement of CVCs when compared with the standard landmark placement technique.[15] Procedure time is diminished, and discomfort to the patient is subsequently reduced. The blind or landmark technique, if not initially successful, has a complication rate of up to 20%. Maintenance of the skill of unguided IJ and subclavian vein insertion may be beneficial for emergency situations when ultrasound guidance may not be available.[16]

Catheter Tip Position

There has been much debate about the appropriate tip position of a CVC. Venous perforation has been associated with stiffer catheter material, left-sided catheters, and a perpendicular orientation of the tip to the vein wall. Cardiac tamponade has been reported when the venous catheter tip is positioned in the lower 3 cm of the SVC or right atrium. However, placement of the tip above the pericardial reflection of the SVC has also been reported to be associated with central vein perforation or thrombosis. Most authors believe that tip position at the SVC/right atrial junction or high right atrium is desirable.[17]

Renal Impairment and Dialysis Needs

The NKF has recommended that subclavian vein access and PICC access cease to be used in patients who are seriously ill and may become dialysis dependent at any stage in their life. Their increased risk for thrombosis and stenosis at the level of entry will increase the failure rate of fistula formation in the affected limb.[9,10] When in doubt, use the IJ vein.

Catheter Design

Some evidence suggests use of antimicrobial agents (minocycline or rifampicin) or chlorhexidine- and silver sulfadiazine–impregnated catheters is associated with a lower rate of catheter-related bloodstream infections.[18] However, the primary determinant of catheter-related infection is strict adherence to sterile technique during catheter placement.[19] In relative proportions, the reduction in catheter-related bloodstream infections gained by using impregnated catheters is trivial to the gains made by observing strict sterile technique. Given their relatively greater cost and minimal gain in reduction of infections, most authors do not think use of this type of catheter is mandatory.

OUTCOMES

The technical success rate for elective placement of nontunneled CVCs under fluoroscopic or ultrasound guidance (or both) has been reported to approach 100%, with one large study reporting a mean in-place catheter duration of 109 days.[20,21] The technical success rate for PICC placement under fluoroscopic or ultrasound guidance (or both) has been reported to be 98.2%, with a mean in-place catheter duration of 28.1 days (range 0-288 days).[2]

COMPLICATIONS

Prevention of complications is both desirable and achievable with central venous access and should be emphasized. Strict attention to sterile technique during catheter placement and use of the catheter along with appropriate dressing care and flushing should keep infectious complications to a minimum. Despite the best of preventive measures, complications can and will occur. Complications can be divided into catheter insertion complications and postinsertion complications.

Catheter Insertion Complications

Catheter insertion complications include hemorrhage, arterial puncture, nerve injury, venous valvular damage, air embolism, cardiac arrhythmia, tamponade, catheter malposition, and pneumothorax.

The risk of significant hemorrhage is extremely low (<1%) even in patients with thrombocytopenia or coagulopathy. Inadvertent arterial puncture with a 21-gauge needle is usually of no consequence and can easily be handled by simple manual compression. In many cases, ultrasound guidance can minimize inadvertent arterial puncture.

Nerve injury is extremely rare with nontunneled CVC placement. However, nerve damage may occur with PICC placement, particularly during attempts to catheterize the brachial veins, which run adjacent to the median nerve.

Venous valvular and vessel wall injury can be minimized by avoidance of excessive force during catheter insertion and avoidance of stiff guidewires and stylets during placement.

The risk of air embolism, not infrequent during placement of large-bore CVCs with peel-away sheaths, is relatively low with the use of small-bore catheters.

Cardiac arrhythmia may occur with guidewire and catheter placement in the right atrium or ventricle. This complication can easily be avoided with fluoroscopic guidance. Similarly, most malpositioned catheters can be successfully repositioned under fluoroscopic guidance by manipulation of the guidewire and catheter.

With ultrasound guidance for venous access, the risk of pneumothorax has decreased significantly. However, should pneumothorax occur, it can usually be treated conservatively with oxygen and followed with a short-interval chest radiograph in 4 to 6 hours. If there is enlargement of the pneumothorax or evidence of tension, immediate needle decompression with a 16-gauge or similarly sized needle at the second intercostal space at the midclavicular line will usually alleviate immediate life-threatening complications. Treatment with a small-bore pleural catheter and Heimlich valve if immediately available is nearly always successful for treatment and subsequent monitoring.

Postinsertion Complications

Complications after catheter placement include hematoma, thrombophlebitis, infection, occlusion, dislodgment, malpositioning, and catheter fracture. Infectious and thrombotic complications are by far the most important in the management of CVCs.

Nontunneled CVCs have the highest infection rate of any form of central venous access, with an average infection rate of 5.3 per 1000 catheter-days,[22] although the incidence of infection from elective nontunneled placement of CVCs has been reported to be 1.1 to 3.35 per 1000 catheter-days.[20,23] Infection rates for PICCs are lower than those for nontunneled CVCs and are reported to be 1 to 2 per 1000 catheter-days.[2] These figures compare with a rate of 1.3 per 1000 catheter-days for tunneled infusion catheters and a rate of 0 to 1 per 1000 catheter-days for subcutaneous ports.[23]

Catheter placement site influences the subsequent risk for catheter-related infection and is related to the density of local skin flora. Femoral catheters have demonstrated a relatively high colonization rate when used in adults and should be avoided if possible.[24] Femoral catheters in pediatrics may have a lower infection rate than adults.[3] Subclavian access sites have a lower density of skin flora than jugular sites, so there is a theoretic advantage to placing nontunneled CVCs via a subclavian route. However, no randomized trials have satisfactorily compared infection rates for catheters placed via the IJ versus subclavian site. Other factors, including the risk of subclavian vein stenosis and occlusion associated with subclavian vein insertion, may outweigh the theoretic benefit of reduced infection rates.

Migration of skin organisms at the insertion site into the cutaneous catheter tract, with colonization of the catheter tip, is the most common route of infection for short-term nontunneled catheters and PICCs.[25] Contamination of the catheter hub contributes substantially to intraluminal colonization of both short- and long-term catheters.[26-28] Occasionally, catheters may become hematogenously seeded from another focus of infection. Rarely, contamination of the infusate leads to infection.[29] Coagulase-negative staphylococci account for the majority (37%) of catheter infections. *Enterococcus* is the second most common organism.[30]

Some catheter materials have surface irregularities that enhance the adherence of certain species (e.g., coagulase-negative staphylococci and *Pseudomonas aeruginosa*).[31,32] In vitro studies have demonstrated that catheters made of polyvinyl chloride or polyethylene are less resistant to the adherence of microorganisms than catheters made of Teflon, silicone elastomer, or polyurethane.[33,34] Therefore, the majority of catheters sold in the United States are no longer made of polyvinyl chloride or polyethylene.

Management of infectious complications is best approached by differentiating infections into exit site infections, bacteremia, and catheter sepsis. Management of these complications differs. Exit site infections are managed by local treatment and antibiotics and can frequently be cured without catheter removal. Bacteremia and catheter sepsis often require catheter removal, but when venous access is limited, over-the-wire catheter exchange along with intravenous antibiotics may be attempted.[35]

Thrombosis

CVC-related thrombosis is a common problem and can be divided into two categories: fibrin sheath formation around the catheter tip and central venous thrombosis.

The typical clinical scenario of a fibrin sheath is an inability to withdraw fluids from the catheter but ease of injecting fluids through it. The reason is that the fibrin sheath forms a one-way valve on the tip of the catheter. Frequently a single dose of a thrombolytic agent is sufficient to restore catheter flow; usually 2 to 3 mg of tissue plasminogen activator (tPA). Other techniques for disrupting the sheath include passing a guidewire through the catheter lumen to dislodge the sheath,[36] stripping of the fibrin sheath using a snare from a femoral vein approach, balloon angioplasty disruption of the entire length of the sheath, and catheter exchange.

Although fibrin sheath formation may interfere with therapy, catheter-induced central venous thrombosis is a much more serious problem. Asymptomatic catheter-related venous thrombosis occurs in 28% to 54% of patients,[37-40] whereas symptomatic central venous thrombosis occurs in 2.8% to 16% of patients.[41-43] Almost all symptomatic cases are related to subclavian vein access. Symptomatic central venous thrombosis is rarely reported with IJ access, so despite a higher skin flora colony count, the IJ vein is the preferred route for placement of nontunneled CVCs.

Treatment of asymptomatic venous thrombosis related to CVCs is debated. Many authors believe there is no need to remove the venous access device. Symptomatic venous thrombosis (e.g., arm swelling) will usually resolve with removal of the catheter and anticoagulation therapy alone. The role of thrombolytic therapy in catheter-related central venous thrombosis is limited because the majority of thrombi associated with CVCs have formed over time. Thrombolytics are unsuccessful with clots older than a few days. Even if lysis of acute clot is successful, rethrombosis is not uncommon.

Peripheral venous thrombosis associated with placement is not infrequent, with an overall thrombosis rate of 38%. The incidence of thrombosis by access site has been reported to be 10% for brachial vein access, 14% for basilic vein access, and 57% for cephalic vein access.[8] Dialysis fistula formation requires patent peripheral veins,

especially cephalic veins. Because of the high rate of venous thrombosis associated with PICCs, placement of these catheters is relatively contraindicated in patients undergoing hemodialysis or in whom hemodialysis is potentially anticipated, including patients with renal transplants.

POSTPROCEDURE AND FOLLOW-UP CARE

Documentation of catheter insertion should include the date of insertion, reason for insertion, insertion site, catheter size, catheter length, excess catheter length outside the patient, number of lumina, catheter tip position, complications, and the name of the person who inserted the catheter. For PICC placement, documentation of upper extremity circumference can aid in assessing future complications. Catheter dressing and care should be conducted in strict accordance with hospital and manufacturers' guidelines. Typically, each lumen of a catheter is flushed with 2 to 5 mL of a 10 to 100 IU/mL heparin solution immediately after placement and after each intravenous infusion, or two to three times per week when the catheter is not being used. Valved catheters usually require only weekly saline flushes.

KEY POINTS

- Peripherally inserted central catheters (PICCs) and nontunneled central venous catheters (CVCs) provide short- to intermediate-term venous access, usually less than 2 to 4 weeks.
- In order of preference, PICCs should be placed in the cephalic, brachial, basilic, or median cubital vein.
- In order of preference, nontunneled CVCs should be placed in the right internal jugular (IJ), left IJ, right subclavian, left subclavian, or femoral vein.
- National Kidney Foundation Kidney Disease Outcomes Quality Initiative criteria state that PICCs and subclavian CVCs should be avoided in patients with current or anticipated future hemodialysis needs, owing to an increased risk for venous thrombosis.
- Ultrasound, tip locator systems, and electrocardiogram guidance make bedside PICC placement safer and easier.
- Ideal CVC catheter tip location is debated but should be within the lower third of the superior vena cava, at the cavoatrial junction, or in the upper atrium.
- Smaller catheters in pediatric patients require more rigorous care than in adults to prevent catheter occlusion.

▶ SUGGESTED READINGS

O'Grady NP, Alexander M, Dellinger EP, et al. Guidelines for the prevention of intravascular catheter-related infections. Centers for Disease Control and Prevention. MMWR Recomm Rep 2002;51(RR-10):1–26.

Teichgraber UK, Gebauer B, Benter T, Wagner HJ. Central venous access catheters: radiologic management of complications. Cardiovasc Intervent Radiol 2003;26:321–33.

The complete reference list is available online at www.expertconsult.com.

CHAPTER 119

Tunneled Central Venous Catheters

Peter R. Bream, Jr.

Tunneled central venous catheters (CVCs) fill a vital role in patient treatment, especially with new cancer-fighting regimens. The catheters are durable and fit nicely into interventionalists' armamentarium alongside peripherally inserted central catheter (PICC) lines and chest or arm ports. There are many sizes, lengths, and technologic advancements that allow safe, long-term venous access. These catheters enable the physician to safely administer caustic medications centrally, draw blood for laboratory studies, and even perform pheresis or dialysis multiple times a week. They have become an indispensable tool in the modern-day treatment of patients.

INDICATIONS

One of the keys to successful, safe, long-term central venous access is placement of the most appropriate device at the initiation of therapy. The ordering physician and the proceduralist should maintain an open dialogue regarding the goals and duration of therapy so the device can be individualized for the patient. Generally, cuffed tunneled catheters are suited for intermediate (<6 months) to long (>6 months) use in patients who are not overly debilitated. The design is ideal for patients who need frequent to continuous access and two to three lumina. The ability of the patient (or appropriate caregiver) to care for this device is extremely important and crucial for its long-term success. Cuffed tunneled catheters are ideal for patients receiving continuous therapy, including epoprostenol sodium, dobutamine, and magnesium. The ease of placement and exchange also allows site preservation in these patients, who will need access for many years. These catheters can remain in place long term because of the nature of the tunnel. Tunneling under the skin allows the body's natural defenses to ward off infection and prevents access of pathogens to the venous entry site. The addition of a Dacron cuff or one made of other fiber promotes the ingrowth of fibroblasts and scar tissue, which secures the catheter. Some catheters are designed with an "antimicrobial" cuff (Vitacuff [Vitaphore, Menlo Park, Calif.]) that is used in tandem (closer to the skin exit site) and intended as a temporary barrier until the Dacron cuff is secure.

CONTRAINDICATIONS

Although there are no absolute contraindications to placement of a tunneled CVC, most proceduralists avoid placement in patients with active infection or proven bacteremia. If central venous access is needed in these patients, a nontunneled temporary line can be placed. In our institution, patients must be culture negative for 24 hours before considering placement of a tunneled line. Coagulopathy is a relative contraindication. A tunneled line is an elective procedure in the vast majority of patients, so acute correction of coagulopathy is rarely needed. If necessary, replacement of platelets or administration of fresh frozen plasma can be performed. A total platelet count of greater than 40,000/mm^3 and an international normalized ratio (INR) of less than 1.5 are the standards we adhere to. If the patient is on a regimen of chronic anticoagulation, conversion to either standard or low-molecular-weight heparin (LMWH) is carried out before the procedure. The heparin is discontinued for the appropriate amount of time for each type (1-2 hours for standard heparin and 24 hours for LMWH). Patients taking antiplatelet medication (aspirin, clopidogrel bisulfate) should stop taking it 5 days before the procedure and can resume immediately afterward. Other relative contraindications are lack of a suitable vein for access and severe skin conditions that will not accommodate a tunnel (scleroderma, graft-versus-host disease, or Stevens-Johnson syndrome). Careful evaluation of the venous access needs must be weighed against the risk for infection or bleeding in such patients. Finally, allergy to the material the catheter is made of is rare but can result in replacement with a catheter made of different material.

EQUIPMENT

The history of CVCs dates back to 1733, where an English clergyman, Stephen Hales, inserted a glass tube into the jugular vein of a horse to measure pressure. The first prolonged use of catheters for central venous infusion was reported by B.J. Duffy in 1949, reporting on 72 catheters.[1] The catheter we use most often today was created at the University of Washington by a team including Belding Scribner, John Broviac, and Robert Hickman in 1973.[2] The basic design of the catheter has not changed, although new technologies have allowed different brands to distinguish themselves. Over the past years, valve technology was developed to reduce thrombosis and infection and eliminate the need for heparin packing. Recently, with the advent of faster computed tomography (CT) scanning, power injectibility has been introduced.

Valves have been used on catheters dating back to the Groshong catheter (Bard Access Systems, Salt Lake City, Utah). The Groshong has slits in the sides of the catheter near the tip. The tip is closed with an atraumatic rounded end. The slits are closed except during infusion or aspiration. The company claims this cuts down on infection and occlusion rates. Groshong catheters are flushed with heparin solution.

CT has become an irreplaceable technology for diagnosing all types of diseases. Newer protocols rely on rapid introduction of a bolus of contrast material for CT angiography and evaluation of tissue perfusion. Many patients with chronic disease undergo regularly scheduled CT scans to evaluate the effectiveness of treatment, and these same patients have some form of central venous access for that

869

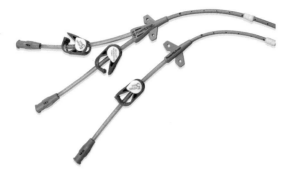

FIGURE 119-1. The POWERHICKMAN single (8F) and dual (9.5F) catheter. Note clear markings of power injection limits on catheter clamps. Bard Access Systems also uses color purple to identify its power injection catheter. *(Courtesy Bard Access Systems, Salt Lake City, Utah.)*

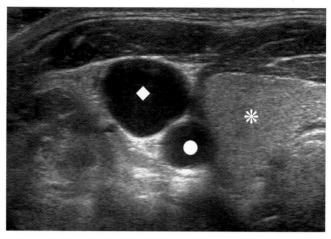

FIGURE 119-2. Normal relationship of right internal jugular vein laterally *(diamond)* to carotid artery medially *(circle)*. Note relationship to thyroid *(asterisk)*, which is medial to carotid and has a distinctive echotexture.

treatment. Rather than start a peripheral intravenous line each time the patient needs a CT scan, it would be desirable to use the patient's existing access. This has been accomplished with newer power-injectable cuffed tunneled catheters. The use of polyurethane for the construction of the catheter has allowed larger inner lumens and faster flow rates. The Power Hickman (Bard Access Systems [Fig 119-1]) was the first such catheter. It is capable of injection rates up to 5 mL/s, which is clearly marked on the catheter's hub. In addition, the catheter has a distinct purple color that has become a universal signal of power injectibility, present on PICC lines and ports from Bard as well as other manufacturers. Although there are many studies[3-6] that have safely shown the use of regular catheters for power injection, these were done off-label, and the readily available power injection safe catheters today render this practice obsolete.

TECHNIQUE

Anatomy and Approach

The right internal jugular (RIJ) vein is the preferred vessel for entry when all other variables are equal. The modern proceduralist will always use ultrasound to guide venous access. When ultrasound is used, the RIJ has been shown to have the lowest rate of complications, including thrombosis, arterial puncture, pneumothorax, and catheter malposition.[7-13] Although some articles have recently settled on the subclavian vein (SCV) as the preferred entry site, this recommendation is for temporary catheters, not tunneled ones. The Kidney Disease Outcomes Quality Initiative (K/DOQI)[14] clearly states that the RIJ is the primary site for dialysis catheters and that tunneled infusion catheters should follow suit. In a retrospective review of subclavian versus IJ tunneled catheters by Trerotola et al. in 2000,[9] there was a 13% incidence of clinically significant central thrombosis when catheters were placed in the SCV (with fluoroscopic guidance) versus 3% when placed in the IJ (with ultrasound guidance). Of note, they did not identify a higher risk for infection in the IJ than in the subclavian site. When the RIJ is not available, the next vein of choice is somewhat controversial. Most interventionalists will proceed to the left internal jugular (LIJ) or resort to the SCV. However, a recent article by Cho et al. proposed that

the right external jugular vein is the preferred second choice. They demonstrated an acceptable success rate and a low complication rate to reach their conclusion. This makes sense because of the tortuous route through the left brachiocephalic vein from an LIJ approach.

A careful history is essential to optimize site selection for each patient. Information such as previous catheters and surgeries and patient preference should be discerned. I have altered the exit or entry site of a catheter based on patient preference. If the patient has undergone a mastectomy or radical node dissection in either the axillary or neck region, that side should be avoided because of the devastating consequence of venous thrombosis on a side that has had the lymphatic system disrupted. After determining the optimal site, a thorough informed consent should be obtained. The consent form should indicate that the risks involved in placing the catheter have been discussed, including bleeding, infection, nerve or lung puncture, air embolism, infection, and cardiac ectopy (see Complications). It is crucial to include the risks associated with conscious sedation if it will be used.

The final step in patient preparation is a preliminary ultrasound scan of the proposed catheter site before the patient is sterilely prepared. The technique for prescanning includes identification of the jugular vein and its relationship to the carotid artery (Fig. 119-2). This is done in the transverse plane and carried down to below the clavicle until the vein cannot be visualized. Test the compressibility of the vein to identify it and exclude acute thrombosis. Note the location of the subclavian artery if it is present and its relationship to the IJ. Finally, look for valves in the jugular bulb. If these valves are moving back and forth with respiration, there is direct communication with the right atrium (RA), which helps assure the operator there is not a significant stenosis in the superior vena cava (SVC).

Hemodynamic monitoring, including noninvasive blood pressure, electrocardiography, and oxygen saturation, is then established. The site is prepared with 1% to 2% chlorhexidine and alcohol, and a full body drape is placed.

The technique for RIJ access (Fig. 119-3) is as follows. Position a linear 7- to 12-MHz transducer that has been placed in a sterile cover parallel to and touching the clavicle.

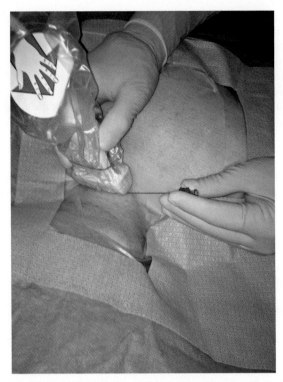

FIGURE 119-3. Proper position of ultrasound probe and needle for internal jugular vein access with use of maximum sterile barriers.

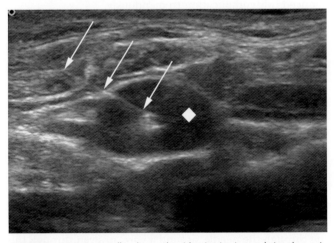

FIGURE 119-4. Needle *(arrows)* with tip in internal jugular vein *(diamond)*.

Identify the RIJ, and palpate the sternal head of the sternocleidomastoid muscle. The puncture site should be just lateral to this muscle, which allows superolateral entry into the RIJ. Use liberal lidocaine with epinephrine and create a wheal. Make the incision appropriate for the catheter size. Use an angled hemostat to dissect the tissues down to the vein and in the direction of the tunnel. With the vein seen in transverse orientation and the needle in longitudinal orientation, advance the needle into the vein until it is seen tenting the wall. Make sure to angle the transducer to visualize the entire subcutaneous course of the needle. When tenting the wall, slowly advance until the wall release and the tip of the needle in the vein are seen (Fig. 119-4). We

use a 21-gauge needle with a 0.018-inch wire for most accesses. If resistance is encountered while advancing the wire from the needle tip, pull the wire back until it is in the needle and then pull the needle back. Readvance the wire until no resistance is met. This maneuver can be repeated until the needle is out of the skin. If at any time resistance is encountered when pulling the wire back into the needle, stop and pull the needle and wire out as a unit. Mandrel-type wire tips can shear off and embolize to the lungs. Once the wire is safely in the vein, advance it several centimeters into the RA while being careful to listen for ectopy, remove the needle, and place a transitional dilator. I prefer the Cope Access Set (Cook Medical, Bloomington, Ind.), which includes a 6.3F dilator with a metal inner stiffener, a 0.018-inch stainless steel Cope mandrel wire, and a 0.035-inch Rosen wire.

It is important to get an accurate measurement from the entry site to the RA as a guide in catheter tip placement. An accurate way to accomplish this is with the wire. After the transitional dilator is placed, advance the stainless steel wire to the middle of the RA. Bend the wire. Place a straight hemostat at the entry site, and pull the wire back under fluoroscopic guidance until the tip lines up with the hemostat. Brace a hand on the sterile field (usually the patient's head), and then clamp the wire with the hemostat at the dilator hub. Pull the bent wire-hemostat unit out, and place a stopcock on the dilator. Save the wire for after tunneling is complete.

Choose an exit site several centimeters from the entry site. Generally, a site in the deltopectoral groove 3 to 4 cm below the clavicle is best. Make sure not to place the exit site in the axilla or too medially. Infiltrate lidocaine and create a wheal. Infiltrate along the expected course of the tunnel. Make an incision corresponding to the size of the catheter. Use the curved hemostats to dissect several centimeters along the tract.

Several different tunnelers come with the various catheters. They can be plastic and blunt tipped or metal and sharp tipped. The metal ones are easier to tunnel but also easier to tunnel too deeply or damage structures. The plastic tunneler is more difficult to get through tissues, but if the tip is rotated back and forth while advancing the tunneler, it will spread the tissues and is a safer device. At the entry site, there is oftentimes a fibrous band preventing the last centimeter of tunneling, especially if sufficient tissue was not dissected when the incision was made. The band may have to be incised with a knife.

Pull the catheter through while making sure it does not come off the tunneler. Pull the cuff through and seesaw it back and forth through the tunnel. This motion roughens the tract and promotes a better scar so the cuff holds better. Leave the cuff 1 to 2 cm from the exit site. Using the wire with the previous measurement, cut the catheter by lining the wire alongside the catheter. Do not stretch the catheter before cutting it. After cutting it, pull the catheter through the tunnel so the cuff is close to the *entry* site. In this manner, the cuff can be pulled back 1 to 2 cm from the exit site, and any kinks along the tunnel straightened out after the catheter is placed.

Catheters are inserted through a special sheath known as a *peel-away sheath*. This sheath temporarily creates a conduit through which the catheter can be placed, and it is then removed from around the catheter once it is in. The

Cope transitional dilator is constructed such that the included Rosen wire will exit a side hole at approximately 45 degrees. This helps direct the wire into the inferior vena cava (IVC). Selecting the IVC is important because it prevents placement into the azygous system. Make sure the wire passes into the IVC below the diaphragm. Also make sure the wire does not engage an IVC filter. Firmly place the peel-away sheath over the wire and into the SVC. To avoid kinking the wire, hold the wire and advance the dilator over the wire. While pausing between advances, move the wire in and out a few centimeters to make sure it runs smoothly. If it does not, the wire is kinked and must be drawn back into the dilator. If it cannot be drawn back, pull the whole unit back until the kink is outside, thread a catheter over the wire, and replace the wire.

Once the peel-away sheath is in place, have the patient perform a maneuver that will temporarily increase intrathoracic pressure to avoid an air embolus (see Complications for ways to prevent air embolism). This can be accomplished by having the patient hold his breath or hum while the operator rapidly removes the wire and dilator. Place the thumb over the hole or pinch the sheath and place the catheter through the peel-away sheath. Once the catheter is in several centimeters, let the patient breathe. Place the catheter and peel the sheath away. Over the past few years, several versions of a valved peel-away sheath have been developed, and many are bundled with the catheters. This valve will reduce the chance for an air embolism, a potentially fatal complication of placement. This is especially helpful if the patient is uncooperative. An alternative strategy in uncooperative patients is to place a longer peel-away sheath at least 30 cm, and advance it so the tip is in the IVC below the diaphragm. This eliminates the negative pressure caused by inspiration in the chest, the cause of air embolism. Once the catheter is in the peel-away and occluding the lumen, the peel-away is removed.

After the peel-away sheath has been removed, pull back on the catheter so the cuff now resides 1 to 2 cm away from the exit site and the tunneled portion of the catheter has been smoothed. Check the position with fluoroscopy while the patient is taking a deep breath. If the initial measurement was with the wire tip in the RA, the deep breath will simulate an upright position and bring the tip up into the SVC/RA junction. Check aspiration and flush the catheter. Use 4-0 Prolene to place a simple suture at the entry site. Place a single stitch adjacent to the exit site and secure it. With the remaining suture, place a roman sandal tie around the catheter four to five times. Cinch the suture down to the exit site, and tie it tight enough to secure it without occluding the lumen. These sutures can be removed once the cuff has grown in, usually 2 to 3 weeks.

COMPLICATIONS

Complications can be divided into two groups: early (periprocedural) and late. Early complications occur at the time of or immediately after placement of the catheter and include failure to gain access, arterial cannulation, pneumothorax, ectopy evolving into atrial or ventricular dysrhythmias, perforation of a vein leading to hemothorax or cardiac tamponade, air embolism, and catheter malposition or kinking. Late complications include infection (bloodstream or tunnel site), thrombosis of the catheter or vein, fibrin

sheath formation, venous stenosis and occlusion, catheter fracture or tip malposition, lymphatic leakage from left-sided placement, and pulmonary thromboembolism.

Most of the immediate complications are avoided with meticulous technique and ultrasound guidance. As image guidance has increasingly been used, the incidence of complications, including arterial puncture, malposition, failure to access, and pneumothorax, is reduced.[15]

Arterial Puncture

Inadvertent arterial puncture most often occurs with blind techniques in the subclavian or IJ veins and is almost always recognized during catheter placement. However, infusion of caustic substances into the carotid artery can lead to thrombosis and stroke if not recognized immediately. Use of micropuncture needles (21 gauge) under direct ultrasound guidance is the best prevention against this complication.

Pneumothorax

Pneumothorax is also a complication that occurs most often with blind techniques in the SCV and less frequently in the jugular vein. Risk factors include an incompetent patient, hyperinflated lungs as in cystic fibrosis and chronic obstructive pulmonary disease, and large body habitus. The preference of interventionalists to use micropuncture technique, ultrasound guidance, and IJ vein cannulation has reduced this complication tremendously.

Air Embolism

During placement of a catheter in the vein, a peel-away sheath is often used to advance the catheter after it has been tunneled. Most catheters now come with a valved peel-away that prevents air aspiration into the SVC during inspiration. This has greatly reduced the incidence of air embolism. However, if a valved peel-away is unavailable, the patient must suspend respiration while the inner dilator is removed and the catheter is placed. If the patient inadvertently takes a breath while the dilator is out, a large amount of air can be drawn into the central veins because of the decrease in intrathoracic pressure, which is a potentially fatal complication. Air can enter during any part of the procedure, including through the needle, around a wire, or even through the catheter after it has been placed. If entry of air is suggested—and oftentimes the proceduralist hears a "sucking" sound during the embolization—fluoroscopy should be performed to look for the site of the air. It is usually seen trapped in the main pulmonary artery. The patient should have a 100% nonrebreathing oxygen masked placed with maximal oxygen infusion. In the majority of cases, such a mask will prevent significant desaturation and is the only therapy to be used. If it is suspected that enough air is present to "lock" the RA, place the patient in the left lateral Trendelenburg position to trap the air in the RA and attempt to suction the air out of the RA with the catheter. Fortunately, this is a rare complication, and prevention is the most effective way to deal with it. Making sure patients understand the instruction for holding their breath or having them hum or perform a Valsalva maneuver is the first step. Some proceduralists advocate pinching off the sheath to prevent any influx of air, but this can damage the peel-away sheath and actually allow more air to enter. Valved peel-away sheaths are the best way to avoid this complication. They have been shown to eliminate the introduction of air during catheter placement.[16] Another method for preventing air embolism is to place a very long (30-45 cm) peel-away sheath all the way into the IVC below the diaphragm. This avoids changes in intrathoracic pressure and allows the catheter to be placed in a patient who is uncooperative with breath holding.

Catheter Malposition or Kinking

Catheter malposition is rarely a problem when proper imaging techniques are used during placement. However, catheters can migrate once the patient assumes an upright position. Therefore, final tip position should be confirmed when the patient has taken a deep breath to simulate an upright position. Large patients and women with pendulous breasts are particularly vulnerable to migration of the tip from its intended SVC/RA junction. Occasionally, this can cause the tip to flip up into the ipsilateral IJ or azygos vein or cross over into the innominate or contralateral jugular vein. Although repositioning with forceful flushing, a wire through the catheter, or even use of a snare from a femoral approach can be done, spontaneous migration in this case points to a catheter that is too short and should be revised. Catheter kinking should also be diagnosed and fixed at the time of placement. The most common cause of kinking is subclavian "pinch." When blind techniques are used to cannulate the SCV, the puncture can cross the costoclavicular ligament and become pinched between the rib and clavicle.[17] Over time, the catheter can become kinked, perforated, or even disrupted. Using the IJ vein or puncturing the SCV more laterally under ultrasound guidance is a way to avoid this complication.

If the catheter breaks off, it most commonly embolizes to the pulmonary arteries and will have to be retrieved with endovascular techniques. Although this problem is rarely serious, the catheter can be a nidus for thrombus formation and infection. Another place for catheter kinking is at the vein entry site in the tunnel. Fibrous bands are commonly present and can kink the catheter as it turns to enter the vein. Careful blunt dissection around the catheter along the tunnel will break up these bands and relieve the pinching. Catheters can also become kinked if the jugular vein is punctured too high and the angle of the tunnel is too acute. This problem is more frequently remedied with the use of stiffer polyurethane catheters rather than the softer silicone.

Infection

Infection is the most common complication that causes a catheter to be removed prematurely. Infection can involve the exit site, subcutaneous tunnel, or bloodstream. Exit site and tunnel infections are typically caused by skin flora, with direct extension from the adjacent skin. *Staphylococcus epidermidis* is the most common organism. The true incidence of infection is difficult to generalize because there are many factors, both dependent and independent, that determine the development of infectious complications. Site and tunnel infections can be treated with systemic antibiotics, with preservation of the site in most cases. Intravenous

vancomycin commonly clears up cellulitis or uncomplicated tract infection, so long as there is no frank suppuration in the tract. An abscess in the tract is treated by prompt removal of the device followed by intravenous antibiotics, presumably guided by culture of the offending organisms. An individual approach to patients is encouraged, especially those with terminal indications for catheter dependence. These patients should be treated like dialysis patients, and every decision regarding removal of catheters should consider future access options. If a patient is running out of such options, conversion of a catheter with a mild tunnel tract infection to a nontunneled catheter plus treatment of the infection may be a viable option. This preserves the access site and allows a new tunnel to be created when the infection clears.

Catheter-related bloodstream infections are a serious, often life-threatening complication of central venous access. The incidence varies considerably depending on type of catheter, frequency of access, and the patient's comorbid conditions. Coagulase-negative staphylococci are the most common hospital-acquired infection, followed by enterococci. An alarming statistic is the increase in vancomycin resistance, determined to be 25.9% in 1999. Although a thorough review of catheter-related bloodstream infections is beyond the scope of this chapter, the Centers for Disease Control and Prevention has issued several general recommendations for the prevention of intravascular catheter-related infections.[18] Readers of this chapter may also want to refer to Miller and O'Grady's article in the *Journal of Vascular and Interventional Radiology*,[19] which summarizes this report with relevance to interventionalists. A brief overview of recommended practice as it relates to cuffed tunneled catheters is included here.

The most common route of infection is migration from the skin into the catheter tract. Use of tunneled catheters or, when appropriate, totally implanted ports reduces this risk. The minimum number of lumina necessary for treatment should be used because contamination from the hub contributes to colonization of the catheter. The site of insertion continues to be a controversial issue, with most authors advocating a subclavian entry site over a jugular or femoral one. Although this has been shown to reduce infections in an intensive care unit setting with temporary catheters, no such advantage has been demonstrated for cuffed tunneled catheters. Site selection must take into account patient factors, as well as the need for future access, because the subclavian site has been shown to increase the risk for central venous thrombosis (see next section).

Maximal sterile barriers, including a hat, mask, gown, and gloves for the operator and large sterile drape for the patient, should be used for insertion of CVCs. A 2% tincture of chlorhexidine gluconate is recommended over tincture of iodine for preparation of skin entry sites.

A combined strategy involving proceduralists and postinsertion caregivers is essential for preventing catheter-related infection.

Thrombosis/Central Stenosis

A variety of patient and catheter factors contribute to catheter-related thrombosis. There are two types of catheter-related thrombosis: extrinsic and intrinsic. *Extrinsic* refers to thrombosis of the vessel in which the catheter

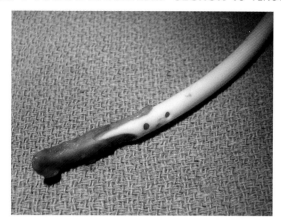

FIGURE 119-5. Catheter tip after removal. Note red fibrin sheath adherent to tip and covering tip and side holes. This is only part of fibrin sheath; rest remains in patient.

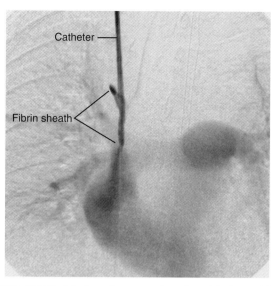

FIGURE 119-6. Injection of contrast through a right internal jugular single-lumen catheter. Contrast fills a fibrin sheath enveloping catheter tip. On this single frame from a digital subtraction venogram, note opacification of right atrium, ventricle, and pulmonary arteries.

resides and includes entry site thrombosis, mural thrombosis, central vein thrombosis, and atrial thrombosis. *Intrinsic thrombosis* relates to the catheter itself and includes intraluminal thrombosis, catheter tip thrombosis, and fibrin sheath formation. Of these complications, the most significant clinically are fibrin sheaths, entry site thrombosis, and central vein thrombosis.

Once a catheter is placed in a vein, thrombus forms at the entry site in response to the presence of the catheter. This thrombus organizes into a cellular and noncellular sheath that contains a mixture of collagen, proliferating smooth muscle cells, and progressive covering by endothelial cells (Fig. 119-5). As the sheath grows down the length of the catheter, bridges form between the sheath and the vein wall, which on histologic evaluation are indistinguishable from each other.[20] Clinically, a fibrin sheath is detected by the ability to flush but not aspirate from the catheter. Radiographically, the sheath is seen as a static column of contrast material beyond the tip of the catheter when it is drawn back over a wire and contrast material is injected. It also can be seen as a column of contrast wider than the tip of the catheter arising from the tip of the catheter and tracking back along the catheter toward the entry site (Fig. 119-6). It is treated with several methods. Once a sheath has been discovered, the catheter can simply be exchanged over a wire or exchanged over a wire with balloon disruption of the sheath, or the sheath can be "stripped" off with a snare from another (usually femoral vein) approach, and the catheter left undisturbed. A recent review of all three methods concluded that each method is effective, and the choice should be up to individual preference and cost considerations.[21] Finally, if the catheter is attached to a totally implanted port, an infusion of recombinant tissue plasminogen activator is effective in dissolving the sheath.

The true incidence of catheter-related central venous thrombosis is difficult to discern because of the low incidence of clinical symptoms. If surveillance is performed to look for thrombosis, the incidence is as high as 74%, but if only clinically symptomatic thrombosis is considered, the incidence is as low as 12%. A recent meta-analysis arrived at a 41% incidence of catheter-related central venous thrombosis, 12% symptomatic and 29% asymptomatic.[22] Factors

that contributed to a higher incidence include catheter tip location not in the distal SVC or SVC/RA junction, left-sided entry site, number of lumina, insertion site not in the jugular vein, insertion without image guidance, and a history of previous catheter placement in the vein.[22]

Entry site thrombosis, like central venous thrombosis, can be largely asymptomatic. This is due in part to well-developed collateralization in the chest wall and neck. Even though it may not produce swelling in the affected extremity, entry site thrombosis, especially in the SCV, can prohibit the development of usable fistulas for hemodialysis or prevent the placement of PICCs, which are becoming a more widely used option for short-term venous access. Trerotola et al. found a 13% incidence of thrombosis of the entry site after subclavian cannulation versus a 3% incidence after jugular cannulation. In addition, the mean time to thrombus formation was 36 days in the SCV versus 142 days in the IJ.[12] There was no difference in the incidence of infection. For this reason, the K/DOQI standards mandate placement of hemodialysis catheters in the IJ over the SCV.[14]

POSTPROCEDURE AND FOLLOW-UP CARE

Tunneled CVCs can be inserted safely as an outpatient procedure with minimal postprocedure care and follow-up. Meticulous sterile technique when accessing the catheter is essential to prevent catheter-related bloodstream infection. Patients should not immerse themselves completely in water and should be instructed in proper bathing techniques. The site sutures should be removed by a medical professional 10 to 14 days after catheter placement, which is usually accomplished by the infusion team. Catheter removal is a bedside procedure that consists of sterile preparation and infiltration of lidocaine around the exit site, blunt dissection of the cuff, freeing it from the fibrin sheath, and removal of the catheter while holding pressure over the catheter entry site until hemostasis is achieved. It is not necessary to check coagulation status in the patient before removal; a recent study showed that this has no significant influence on time to hemostasis following removal of a cuffed catheter.[23] Occasionally, surgical cutdown is required to free the cuff, but this can also be accomplished at the bedside.

KEY POINTS

- Tunneled cuffed central venous catheters are essential to clinical practice for patients who need long-term continuous or frequent access.
- Placement under ultrasound and fluoroscopic guidance yields consistently better-performing catheters with fewer complications.
- Technologic advances such as power injectibility for computed tomography procedures allow patients who have these catheters for therapy to more comfortably chart their progress.
- Infection and central venous thrombosis are the most common complications that limit catheter effectiveness.

▸ **SUGGESTED READINGS**

Miller DL, O'Grady NP. Guidelines for the prevention of intravascular catheter-related infections: recommendations relevant to interventional radiology. J Vasc Interv Radiol 2003;14:133–6.

National Kidney Foundation. Kidney Disease Outcomes Quality Initiative, 2006. Available at http://www.kidney.org/professionals/kdoqi/index.cfm.

O'Grady NP, Alexander M, Dellinger EP, et al. Guidelines for the prevention of intravascular catheter-related infections. Infect Control Hosp Epidemiol 2002;23:759–69.

Pieters P, Tisnado J, Mauro M. Venous Catheters: A Practical Manual. New York: Thieme; 2003.

The complete reference list is available online at www.expertconsult.com.

CHAPTER 120

Subcutaneous Ports

Robert G. Dixon

CLINICAL RELEVANCE

After the introduction of tunneled silicon central venous catheters (CVCs) in the 1970s by Broviac[1] and Hickman,[2] the next decade brought the development of subcutaneous ports.[3] Though originally developed in the surgical arena, subcutaneous port insertion under image guidance soon evolved[4,5] and improved the safety profile of the procedure by essentially eliminating the risk for pneumothorax and arterial puncture.[4,6] Because insertion of subcutaneous ports is a routine part of most busy interventional radiology practices nowadays, familiarity with their insertion and management of related complications is requisite for today's interventionalist.

INDICATIONS

The choice of venous access device is based on the length of therapy and frequency of access required. Patient and physician preferences play a role as well. Insertion of subcutaneous ports is indicated if central venous access is needed intermittently for many months to years. If more frequent (daily) access is needed over a shorter time frame, peripherally inserted central catheters (PICCs) or tunneled CVCs should be considered (see Chapters 118 and 119). The most common indication for long-term central venous access is for chemotherapy administration.[4,7] Additional indications include antibiotic therapy, administration of blood products, and total parenteral nutrition.[4,7] A funnel-shaped subcutaneous port (Cathlink 20 [C.R. Bard Inc., Salt Lake City, Utah]) that accepts an 18-gauge intravenous needle has been used for erythrocytapheresis (red blood cell exchange)[8] and therapeutic plasma exchange.[9] Recently, ports have been developed (Vortex Port System [AngioDynamics, Latham, N.Y.]) through which erythrocytapheresis can be performed with noncoring 16-gauge access needles for patients with sickle cell disease; flow rates of approximately 30 to 60 mL/min have been achieved. However, little data regarding the long-term feasibility of this technology exists, and we have had mixed results at our institution. In many patients, multiple indications for port insertion may exist at any one time.

CONTRAINDICATIONS

Contraindications to the insertion of subcutaneous ports are related to two of the more common complications: infection and hemorrhage. Before inserting an implantable port, patients with active infection or bacteremia should be treated appropriately until the underlying process has resolved. Patients with a coagulopathy or those taking anticoagulants should ideally be corrected until the international normalized ratio (INR) is 1.5 or less. An uncorrectable coagulopathy would prohibit insertion of a port; nontunneled access should be used in this situation until the patient's condition improves. If anticoagulation is of significant import, it may be necessary to convert to enoxaparin (Lovenox) to limit the period during which the degree of anticoagulation is subtherapeutic. Likewise, severe thrombocytopenia could also be prohibitive. Although a platelet count of over 50×10^9/L is traditionally recommended for invasive procedures, there is a paucity of data to support this threshold.[10,11] Preoperative or intraoperative platelet transfusion will usually allow safe insertion in those with platelet counts below 50×10^9/L.[12,13] Insertion of ports should be avoided in severely neutropenic patients. Venous access via the internal jugular (IJ), external jugular, or subclavian routes may be impossible secondary to central venous occlusion and may be severely limited because of anatomic constraints as a result of trauma, recent surgery, or burns. In this situation, access through the femoral vein or inferior vena cava (IVC) via a translumbar or transhepatic route should be considered. Finally, if there is no safe access to the central venous system, a port simply cannot be placed.

EQUIPMENT

Key equipment is listed in Table 120-1.

TECHNIQUE

Anatomy and Approach

The IJ vein begins at the jugular foramen as a direct continuation of the sigmoid sinus and descends in the neck within the carotid sheath along with the carotid artery and the vagus nerve. Posterior to the medial portion of the clavicle, the IJ and subclavian veins join to form the brachiocephalic veins. The IJ vein is directly anterior and lateral to the carotid artery.[6,14] The apex of the bifurcation of the two heads of the sternocleidomastoid muscle is the landmark for locating the distal IJ vein.[14]

The axillary vein begins at the lower border of the teres major as a continuation of the basilic vein and terminates at the lateral border of the first rib, where it continues as the subclavian vein. The subclavian vein ends at the medial border of the anterior scalene muscle, where it joins the IJ vein to form the brachiocephalic vein. Note that the second portion of the subclavian artery is *posterior* to the anterior scalene muscle, whereas the medial portion of the subclavian vein is positioned just anterior to it. The anterior scalene muscle is approximately 10 to 15 mm thick in adults and separates the artery and vein considerably; however, more laterally, the subclavian artery and vein lie much closer together, with the vein anterior and slightly inferior to the artery.[5]

TABLE 120-1. Key Equipment for Insertion of a Subcutaneous Port

Port of choice
Ultrasound with a 5- to 7.5-MHz linear array transducer
Fluoroscopy
1% Lidocaine with epinephrine
Cutdown tray:
  #15 Blade
  #11 Blade
  Knife handle
  Iris forceps, 1 × 2 teeth, straight (4-inch)
  Two-eyed dressing forceps, serrated, straight (4-inch)
  Adson forceps, 1 × 2 (4.75-inch)
  Two tracheal retractors (6-inch)
  Kelly hemostat, straight (5.5-inch)
  Halstead mosquito forceps, curved (5-inch)
  Halstead mosquito forceps, straight (5-inch)
  Ballenger sponge forceps, serrated, straight (7-inch)
  Crile needle holder (6-inch)
  Iris scissors, curved (4.5-inch)
  Iris scissors, straight (4.5-inch)

Technical Aspects

- Review the patient's history and any relevant previous imaging studies.
- Use maximum barrier technique, and maintain sterility at all times.
- Consider preprocedure administration of antibiotics.
- During ultrasound-guided access of the IJ vein, optimize the angle of approach to avoid placing the carotid artery in the path of the needle.
- Intravascular distance is measured with a 0.018-inch mandril wire.
- Create a pocket with a "snug" fit to avoid migration or flipping of the port.
- Plan and construct the tunnel with a gentle curve to prevent a kink from developing in the catheter.
- Avoid air embolism by pinching the sheath or covering the open end of the peel-away sheath (or both) until the catheter is quickly inserted into the sheath.
- Close the port pocket incision in two layers.
- Leave the port accessed if chemotherapy is to be initiated within 3 days.

Initially, surgically placed subcutaneous ports were inserted via a blind percutaneous subclavian vein approach[3] or by cutdown.[15] Although central lines placed by interventional radiologists were also initially placed via the subclavian vein under fluoroscopic guidance,[16] insertion of ports soon evolved from an ultrasound-guided subclavian vein approach[4] to the preferred ultrasound-guided IJ vein approach.[5,6,17] Ultrasound-guided IJ access has become the preferred approach because it allows an easily compressible access (in the rare case of inadvertent arterial puncture), avoids the higher risk for pneumothorax associated with axillary/subclavian vein access,[18] and avoids the "pinch-off syndrome" associated with medially placed subclavian catheters.[19]

Review of the patient's history and any available relevant previous imaging studies is paramount. The goal is to uncover any evidence of central venous stenosis or occlusion. A history of multiple central venous lines or end-stage renal disease should be queried. Access via the subclavian vein should be avoided in dialysis patients in an attempt to preserve patency of the axillary and subclavian veins for any current or future surgical dialysis access (fistulas or shunts). Although it has traditionally been recommended to avoid the ipsilateral approach in patients who have undergone axillary lymph node dissection, it has been shown that the incidence of lymphedema after ipsilateral port placement is no higher than that reported after axillary lymph node dissection alone.[20] In addition, any thoracic malignancy requiring external beam irradiation should be considered and the planned radiation field avoided.

The technique described here is a minor modification of that previously described by Mauro, Jaques, and Morris.[4,5] A routine procedure tray is augmented with a cutdown tray (see Table 120-1 and Fig. e120-1). The neck should be interrogated with ultrasound to confirm patency of the IJ vein, which is supported by easy compressibility of the vein and lack of adjacent collaterals. If ultrasound or previous imaging indicates that the IJ veins are occluded, the subclavian veins are a reasonable alternative. If there is complete central venous occlusion involving the brachiocephalic veins or superior vena cava (SVC), a femoral, translumbar, or transhepatic approach can be considered. Although these approaches are rarely required, they should be part of an interventionalist's armamentarium.

The upper portion of the chest and neck are then prepared and draped in sterile fashion. Povidone-iodine solution has traditionally been used, but many institutions have switched to 2% chlorhexidine gluconate in 70% isopropyl alchohol (Chloraprep).[21] The ultrasound probe is then also draped so it can be used for direct imaging during venous access. The procedure is typically performed with the patient under conscious sedation and continual monitoring of the electrocardiogram and pulse oximetry by a member of the radiology nursing staff. Local anesthesia is achieved at the entry site with 1% lidocaine with epinephrine, and this can be done under ultrasound guidance to plan the path of the access needle and avoid intravascular injection of lidocaine (Fig. 120-1). A small skin incision is made with a #11 blade. Through this small incision, a 21-gauge, 4-cm needle (some obese patients may require a 21-gauge, 7-cm needle) connected to a 20-mL syringe by short connector tubing is advanced in a medial and caudal direction under direct ultrasound guidance (Fig. 120-2). The operator should keep the needle tip visualized throughout the access process. Some operators prefer an 18-gauge needle to eliminate the need for a transition dilator. The operator can often optimize the angle of approach to avoid placing the carotid artery in the path of the trajectory of the needle. Gently "bobbing" the needle may improve localization of the needle tip. Once the tip of the needle "tents" the vein, a short, quick thrust will advance the needle into the vein. A tactile "pop" is often felt as the needle enters the vein. Again, with the aid of ultrasound guidance, care can be taken to avoid going completely through the vein into the carotid artery. Insertion of the tip of the needle within the vein is confirmed by observing the bright tip of the needle within the vein (Fig. 120-3) and by aspiration of blood through the 20-mL syringe. At times, the patient's respirations will intermittently collapse the vein. In such cases, puncturing the vein during expiration will usually allow successful access. A 0.018-inch mandril wire is then advanced into the vein under fluoroscopic guidance so the access needle can be

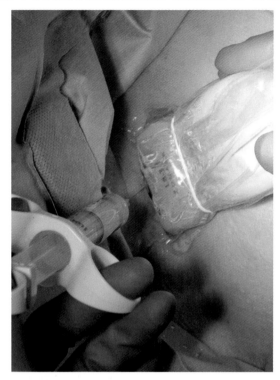

FIGURE 120-1. Local anesthesia can be introduced under ultrasound guidance to plan access needle path and avoid intravascular injection of lidocaine. "Tranverse" relationship between needle and ultrasound probe shown here is the one typically used for access.

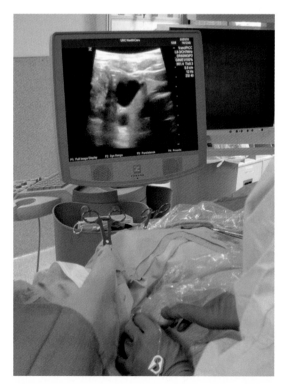

FIGURE 120-2. Ultrasound probe in operator's right hand guides a 21-gauge needle while accessing right internal jugular vein. Operator should keep needle tip visualized throughout access process. *(Courtesy Jaclyn Green, ACNP.)*

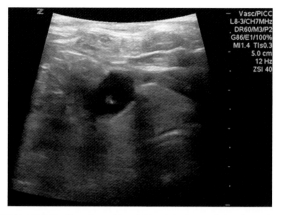

FIGURE 120-3. Tip of needle within right internal jugular vein. One should always confirm position of needle tip with ultrasound before proceeding.

exchanged for a Cope transition dilator (Cook Medical, Bloomington, Ind.). Some operators prefer a micropuncture set (Cook Medical) to make the transition to a 0.035-inch system. The mandril wire is used to measure the distance from the access to the proximal aspect to midportion of the right atrium, and this access is then temporarily capped. The intravascular distance can be measured by placing the tip of the mandril wire in the desired location between the cavoatrial junction and the cephalad aspect of the right atrium, bending the exposed wire as it exits the transition dilator, and then pulling the wire back to the point of access in the vein, which can be visualized under fluoroscopy with a radiopaque marker at the skin. The wire should then be stored in a safe place on the table so it can be used for measurement after the catheter is tunneled to the right neck dermatotomy site.

Next, the tunnel and port pocket are planned. The port pocket should be positioned in the infraclavicular region a few centimeters below the clavicle and medial to the deltopectoral groove. The region of the port pocket and planned tunnel is then anesthetized with 1% lidocaine with epinephrine. The port pocket should allow firm bony support by the underlying ribs and yet avoid mammary tissue. In addition, the tunnel should have a gentle curve so the catheter does not kink. To allow a few minutes for the lidocaine to take effect, the catheter and port can be assembled and secured at this time. The junction of the port and catheter should be tested by accessing the port with a Huber needle, flushing the catheter, and pinching off the distal end of the catheter to challenge the catheter/port junction and confirm the absence of a leak.

An incision is then made with a #15 blade, just long enough to allow insertion of the port. Though originally described as an incision caudal to the port pocket,[4] we now make the insertion incision just cephalad to the pocket. This approach allows easy access to the catheter/port junction and gives some flexibility if last-minute tailoring of catheter length is necessary. However, some practitioners still prefer to use the inferior incision approach. Usually the port pocket can be easily created by blunt dissection with a Kelly hemostat and small tracheal retractors or simply with the operator's finger (Fig. 120-4). This allows any fibrous bands encountered to be freed and gross estimation of the pocket size required (the length of one's distal phalanx is

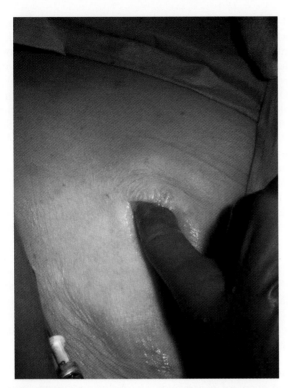

FIGURE 120-4. Blunt dissection can be performed, at least in part, with operator's finger. This allows estimation of pocket size required.

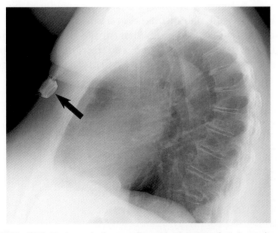

FIGURE 120-5. Lateral chest radiograph showing that 2 weeks after insertion, this port had flipped 180 degrees within pocket. Diaphragm *(arrow)* is identified along deep margin of pocket. This port was manually flipped back into appropriate position (without opening pocket) and successfully accessed thereafter.

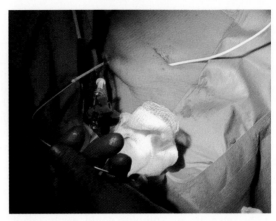

FIGURE 120-6. Tunneler is then brought through neck dermatotomy site. Port will be placed in port pocket and catheter will be cut to length.

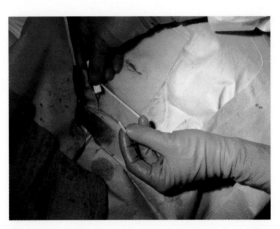

FIGURE 120-7. Operator covers peel-away sheath with right thumb while quickly introducing catheter with left hand.

approximately the depth required for many ports). The pocket should be large enough to allow the port to be inserted easily, the incision to be closed without tension on the skin, and the incision to not overlie the diaphragm of the port. If a snug fit is achieved, anchoring sutures are not usually needed.[22] However, if the port pocket is too large or if the patient is obese, it is prudent to place anchoring sutures to avoid the complication of the port flipping within the pocket and thereby prohibiting access (Fig. 120-5). Usually, two nonabsorbable sutures adequately anchor the port.

Once the port pocket is created, the catheter is tunneled from the infraclavicular incision to the right neck dermatotomy. The metal tunneling device is then shaped with a gentle curve (Fig. e120-2) to facilitate following a cephalad then medial path. The operator should initially tunnel cephalad, then use the curve of the tunneler to turn medially, all the while keeping a finger on the leading point of the tunneler to avoid inadvertent injury to surrounding structures. Attention to the tip of the tunneler is of particular importance when it is passing over the clavicle, to ensure it does in fact pass superficial to the clavicle and avoids an intrathoracic trajectory. Once the catheter is brought through the tunnel (Fig. 120-6), the port is positioned within the pocket. If anchoring sutures are going to be used, they can be placed at this time. The port may be held in place by accessing it with a noncoring Huber needle. The catheter is then cut to length with the previously marked mandril wire used for measuring the distance. The Cope transition dilator is then exchanged over a 0.035-inch wire for a peel-away sheath.

Air embolism can be avoided by pinching the sheath while introducing the catheter into the sheath or by covering the open end of the peel-away sheath (Fig. 120-7) until the catheter is quickly inserted into the sheath. The catheter can then be advanced through the peel-away sheath (Fig. 120-8) and positioned with its tip in the region between the cavoatrial junction and the cephalad aspect of the right atrium. Dialysis catheter manufacturers have developed valved peel-away sheaths to minimize the risk of air embolism and diminish blood loss (AirGuard Valved Introducer [Bard Access Systems, Salt Lake City, Utah]). This technology is now available for the smaller-caliber sheaths used for port insertion. Other maneuvers may be used, such as having patients hold their breath or hum; however, following such simple commands may prove difficult, depending on the degree of sedation at that time. Attention to the patient's respiratory cycle is critical at this step so that occlusion of the sheath is not released at the point of inspiration. The catheter should not be advanced through the peel-away sheath if the patient is agitated, coughing, or crying, because an air embolus could easily result. The length of the catheter should be checked before the entire

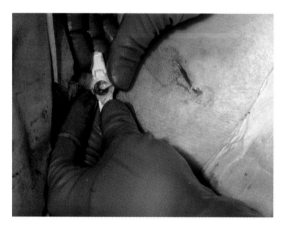

FIGURE 120-8. Catheter advanced into peel-away sheath while sheath is removed.

peel-away sheath is removed. If the catheter is too long or short, this should quickly be remedied at this time. Placement of a new peel-away sheath, which could be temporarily capped while the appropriate alterations are made, may be required.

Once the catheter is in appropriate position, aspiration of blood followed by flushing with normal saline confirms patency. This is followed by 5 mL of dilute heparin flush (100 units/mL) unless the port is a valved port, in which case it can simply be flushed with 20 mL of saline. The Huber needle anchors the port within the pocket while the pocket incision is closed in two layers, usually with subcutaneous 3-0 Vicryl followed by a 4-0 Vicryl running subcuticular suture. Other combinations of two-layer closure may be preferred by individual operators, and some incorporate the use of adhesive strips (Steri-Strips [3M, St. Paul, Minn.]) or liquid skin adhesive (Dermabond [Ethicon, Somerville, N.J.]). Regardless of the precise suturing technique used, two-layer closure is preferred to avoid wound dehiscence. If the patient is to receive chemotherapy within the next 3 days, the port is left accessed. At completion of the procedure, the area is cleaned, and sterile gauze with an occlusive dressing is applied.

Alternative Access

In the event of central venous occlusion, unconventional venous access must be considered.[4,5,7,23] Potential alternative routes include well-developed collaterals, recanalized occluded veins, femoral, translumbar, and transhepatic access.[23] A femoral approach is rarely considered because of the increased risk of infection associated with this site; however, if it is used, maximal sterile barrier technique should be rigorously employed, and the port should be positioned over the ribs to allow a firm backing for access (Fig. 120-9).

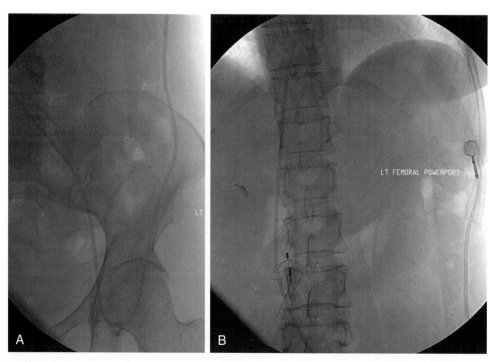

FIGURE 120-9. A, A femoral approach is rarely considered because of increased risk of infection associated with this site; however, if it is used, maximal sterile barrier technique should be rigorously employed. **B,** Port should be positioned over ribs to allow a firm backing for access.

Though more frequently used for dialysis or tunneled catheter access, a translumbar approach should be considered for port insertion if the SVC is occluded. A patent IVC must be confirmed by either venography at the time of the procedure or by review of recent cross-sectional imaging. In addition, the patient must be cooperative and be able to be positioned in a semiprone or decubitus position. The skin should be inspected for any lesions that would prohibit this type of access. After placing a guidewire, snare, or catheter in the IVC from a femoral approach to serve as a target, the catheter or guidewire is secured and the patient placed in the prone or semiprone (right side up) position. After the right flank is prepared and draped, an entry site approximately 7 to 10 cm lateral to the midline and just superior to the right iliac crest is identified, and a local anesthetic is applied. A 21-gauge needle is then advanced medially and superiorly under fluoroscopic guidance by targeting the guidewire or catheter at the L3 level. Angled fluoroscopy and parallax are key components of this procedure. Alternatively, computed tomography (CT) guidance may also be used to confirm access to the IVC.

Once access to the IVC is established, a 0.018-inch mandril wire is advanced into the right atrium. With the use of a transition dilator such as the Cope, the system is upsized to a 0.035-inch system. Oftentimes there is difficulty advancing the catheter through the peel-away sheath at the point of entry into the IVC because of angulation; in such cases, the catheter can be advanced over a stiff hydrophilic guidewire and through the peel-away sheath.[7,23] For port access, the pocket should be created over the lower lateral ribs to provide firm support. A two-stage tunnel may be necessary to allow a gentle curve of the catheter to the entry site.

Translumbar catheter complications are similar to those encountered with other access routes and include infection, catheter tip migration, kinking, fibrin sheath formation, and rarely, caval occlusion.[23] In the pediatric population, interval growth may result in migration of the catheter tip to an extravascular position, so plain radiographs should be obtained intermittently to ensure appropriate tip position.[23]

If both the SVC and IVC are occluded, the transhepatic route is another alternative.[5,7,23] Access to the middle hepatic vein can be achieved with a 21-gauge needle under ultrasound and fluoroscopic guidance. Once access to the hepatic vein is confirmed by injection of contrast material, a mandril guidewire can be advanced into the right atrium to allow the system to be upsized to a 0.035-inch system. The port pocket should be created over the bony support of the rib cage and at a point that is easily accessible. This access is subject to respiratory movement, which may result in migration of the catheter to an extravascular position. Complications of transhepatic catheter placement include intraabdominal hemorrhage (any coagulopathy should be corrected) and hepatic vein thrombosis, although this is uncommon. Again, interval growth is an issue with children, and the catheter tip should be monitored with intermittent plain radiographs.[7,23]

Alternative Port Pocket Locations

Port pocket creation in the midaxillary line at the anterior border of the latissimus muscle has been described.[24] Because this location requires a longer tunnel, it can be difficult to locally anesthetize the entire tunnel, so general anesthesia is preferred.[24] In addition, the long tunnel length may leave the catheter at increased risk of migration. Because of this, the authors recommend strict attention to catheter position at the time of insertion but feel that this location provides a better cosmetic result and have found no increase in complications in this location.[24]

In patients with prior surgery (e.g., bilateral mastectomies), anticipated breast reconstruction, or radiation therapy or burns, alternative pocket locations may be required. The "trapezius port" with the subcutaneous pocket created over the trapezius muscle[25,26] avoids any recent or anticipated treatment fields. A paramedian location or the upper extremities are other potential options as well.[25]

CONTROVERSIES

Although insertion and maintenance of ports are fairly straightforward, there are differences of opinion regarding catheter tip position, port selection, antibiotic prophylaxis, valved ports, and suture fixation.

Tip Position

Perhaps no other topic is more passionately debated in the central venous access arena than the distal catheter tip position. This contentious topic is impacted by operators' experiences, local policies, and conflicting recommendations[27-32] and is further complicated by anatomic misinterpretations.[33,34] At our institution, the catheter tip of a subcutaneous port is considered to be optimally placed if it is in the region between the cavoatrial junction and the cephalad portion of the right atrium (Fig. 120-10). This takes into consideration the expected cephalad migration with the patient in the upright position,[18,28,35,36] and the improved function with the catheter tip in this position.[28,36] However, other authors vehemently recommend that the catheter tip be placed in the SVC[31] no deeper than the cavoatrial junction to avoid potential cardiac complications, including arrhythmias, tricuspid valve injury, and the most dreaded complication, cardiac perforation and tamponade.[37] This is further complicated by the fact that positioning the catheter outside the atrium does not guarantee there will be no vascular perforation.[29,38] Detailed discussion of this debate is beyond the scope of this chapter; the reader is directed to articles that discuss these points in detail.[28,29,32] In addition, review of the anatomy is in order before further contemplating this debate, because the true cavoatrial junction in adolescents and young adults has been identified as more caudally located than commonly believed, and is best estimated by a point approximately two vertebral bodies below the carina.[34]

Port Selection: Material, Size, and Number of Lumina

Most ports are made of either titanium or plastic (Fig. e120-3). Plastic ports cause only minimal if any imaging artifacts, whereas titanium ports cause minimal artifact on CT (Fig. 120-11) and only local artifact on magnetic resonance imaging (MRI). Both materials are MRI compatible. Single- and double-lumen ports are available, with

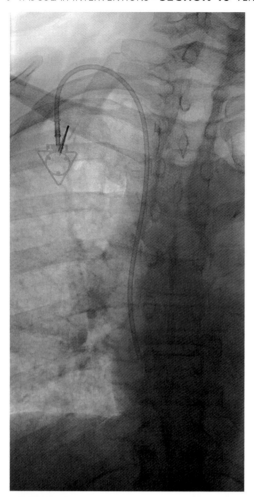

FIGURE 120-10. Single radiograph of a port placed via a right internal jugular approach, with tip at level of cavoatrial junction about two vertebral bodies below carina. Port has been accessed, and radiopaque backing allows identification of port as one that can be injected with a power injector for computed tomography imaging.

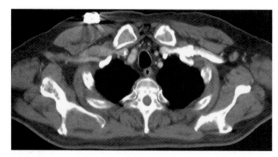

FIGURE 120-11. Titanium port in right anterior chest wall, causing minimal artifact on computed tomography.

single-lumen ports being smaller and less expensive and catheters ranging from 6F to 10F. Dual-lumen ports are larger and more expensive, possibly migrate more,[35] and are attached to larger 10F to 13F catheters. Kowalski et al. showed a significant difference in migration between 10F single-lumen ports and 12F double-lumen ports, possibly because of the larger device settling within the soft tissues of the chest wall and thereby withdrawing the catheter.[35]

Because double-lumen tunneled catheters have been noted to result in more total venous occlusion than is the case with single-lumen catheters,[39] and because catheters smaller than 2.8 mm in outer diameter are associated with few instances of thrombosis,[40] the larger-caliber catheters used in double-lumen ports may also be at increased risk for venous thrombosis. Moreover, one should use central venous devices with the fewest number of lumens necessary to reduce the number of portals for colonization.[41,42] However, dual-lumen ports offer the benefit of being able to administer incompatible medications or concomitantly administer fluids or blood products with chemotherapy. Therefore, double-lumen ports are usually reserved for situations in which incompatible chemotherapeutic agents or concomitant blood product and fluid administration are genuinely anticipated.

The access diaphragm is a compressed silicon disc designed to accept approximately 2000 accesses with a non-coring 20-gauge Huber needle. Catheters are available in both preattached and attachable designs and are made of either silicon or polyurethane because these materials are much less thrombogenic than polyethylene.[40] Polyurethane offers the benefit of greater tensile strength than silicone, thus allowing increased internal diameter (thinner wall) and consequently increased flow rates with diminished overall catheter mass. In addition, the development of segmented polycarbonate-based polyurethanes has led to a more durable polyurethane that is immune to biologically induced stress cracking, which occurs when macrophages attach themselves to the surfaces of ether-based polyurethanes and enzymatically degrade the polymer surface, thereby leading to microcracking and potential failure.[43] Catheter tips have either a simple end-hole design, a staggered tip, or a valved/slit tip (Groshong catheter).

Power-injectable ports are now available from multiple manufacturers and have eliminated the need for additional venous access during the multiple follow-up CT examinations oncology patients undergo. These ports are identifiable with uniquely shaped backing that can be seen on routine radiographs, and personal identification (e.g., card, bracelet, key chain) the patient keeps at all times. In addition, some ports may be identified on physical examination by three raised palpable points along the perimeter of the port diaphragm (Power Port [Bard Access Systems]) (Fig. 120-12).

Antibiotic Prophylaxis

Although no randomized controlled clinical trials have been conducted to validate use of prophylactic antibiotics for insertion of subcutaneous ports, it is widely practiced.[7,17,42,44-46] However, some authors have demonstrated low infection rates without the use of antibiotic prophylaxis.[4] When used, it is best if a broad-spectrum agent (e.g., cefazolin) is administered less than 2 hours before the start of the procedure.[41,47] If antibiotic prophylaxis is given more than 3 hours before the start of the procedure, the incidence of adverse infectious events increases fivefold.[41] It should be noted that antibiotic prophylaxis is no substitute for rigorous adherence to sterile technique by the entire interventional radiology staff.

It is interesting to note that guidelines established by the Centers for Disease Control and Prevention (CDC)

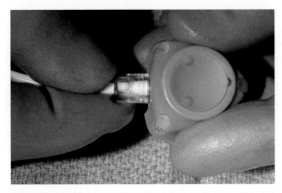

FIGURE 120-12. The Power Port (Bard Access Systems, Salt Lake City, Utah) has a unique shape, and arrangement of three raised palpable points along perimeter of diaphragm of port facilitates identification of diaphragm when port is accessed.

for avoidance of intravascular catheter-related infections emphasize education and training of health care providers who insert and maintain catheters, use of maximal sterile barrier precautions during CVC insertion, 2% chlorhexidine preparation for skin antisepsis, avoidance of routine placement of CVCs, and use of antiseptic- or antibiotic-impregnated short-term CVCs if the rate of infection is high despite adherence to other strategies. However, the guidelines do not recommend prophylactic antibiotics.[48]

Valved versus Nonvalved Ports

A paucity of data exists regarding the benefit and effectiveness of valved ports, which have the potential benefits of allowing blood draws for coagulation studies from the valved port without any concern for contamination (as long as heparin is not inadvertently used), and the use of valved ports in patients with a heparin allergy. One study that evaluated ports with a proximal valve in the port hub showed that an inability to draw blood occurred less frequently in valved ports than in nonvalved ports, and the number of instances where there were difficulties that required additional access time to draw blood were less in the valved port group than in the nonvalved port group.[49] However, Biffi's group looked at valved ports that use a Groshong catheter with a distal valve in the catheter tip versus an open-ended catheter with a nonvalved port.[39] This randomized study of 302 patients did not find valved ports to be superior; in fact, 19 of 152 patients with ports using Groshong catheters experienced more episodes of inability to draw blood samples (12.5%) than those in the nonvalved group (3 of 150 patients [2%]). Because there is not a significant body of work to suggest that valved ports truly outperform nonvalved ports, the decision regarding which type of port to use should be based on local preferences of the patients, nurses, and physicians involved.

Suture Fixation

Fixation of the port using nonabsorbable sutures has traditionally been recommended, but if a small, snug pocket is created, fixation is typically not needed. Some argue that fixation is required to avoid rotation of the port, which precludes access. Others contend that fixation merely adds

to the procedure length at the time of insertion and again at the time of removal.[22] McNutty et al. showed in their retrospective review of over 500 ports, none of which were secured to the pocket, that only one port (0.2%) flipped.[22] Moreover, fixation does not completely eliminate the risk of port rotation, with port rotation reported in up to 0.5% of ports that are fixated.[50-52] The rate of port rotation may be slightly higher without fixation (up to 1.6%); however, this is often early in the authors' experience and secondary to an incorrect pocket size.[53] At our institution, ports are not routinely sutured into place, but if a too-large pocket is inadvertently created, or if the patient is morbidly obese, fixation with nonabsorbable sutures should be considered.

Pediatric Considerations

The tip position of CVCs is also hotly debated in the pediatric literature. The rare, albeit devastating, complication of pericardial effusion and potentially fatal cardiac tamponade exists, particularly in very low-weight premature infants.[54,55] The fine points of the various positions is beyond the scope of this chapter. Suffice it to say that the risk is greatest in very low-birth-weight premature infants,[56,57] where daily radiographic monitoring of lines is paramount.[55] In older children requiring long-term venous access with subcutaneous ports, most authors recommend placing the catheter tip at the cavoatrial junction.[34,58] The important concept to keep in mind is that the cavoatrial junction is best identified with relationship to the carina, and is approximately two vertebral bodies below the carina—a position slightly caudal to what is commonly thought to represent the cavoatrial junction.[34,58]

Most pediatric port insertions are implanted under general anesthesia, with the potential exception being adolescents and teenagers who could conceivably have a port inserted with conscious sedation if the appropriately trained staff is present and local protocol permitted this. The other major concern in pediatric cases is to truly optimize the radiation dose, using only what is needed to accomplish the job at hand.[59]

OUTCOMES

The overall technical success rate for subcutaneous port insertion is 95% to 100%,[4,18,46,60] with the overall incidence of complications similar to or better than that in surgical series.[4,5,18,46] Puncture-related complications for ports and tunneled catheters diminish to essentially zero with ultrasound guidance,[17,44,61] and position-related complications can be avoided with the use of high-quality real-time fluoroscopic equipment and strict attention to guidewire and catheter skills. Specific complications are reviewed in the next section.

COMPLICATIONS

Complications can be divided into early complications (occurring within 30 days of placement) and late complications (occurring after 30 days).[60] Early complications can be further divided into procedure-related complications (occurring at the time of the procedure or within 24 hours of the procedure) and those occurring after that time frame.[60] Early complications include air embolus, pneumothorax, arterial puncture, early migration or malposition, and early infection related to implantation. Multiple studies have shown that access performed under image guidance—in particular, ultrasound guidance—has dramatically reduced the number of procedural complications when compared with blind or landmark-based access.[4,17,44,60-63]

Early Complications

Air Embolism

Air embolism is a rare but potentially lethal complication. The volume of air that can be tolerated in the venous system is not known, but volumes of 100 to 300 mL have proved to be fatal.[64] It has been calculated that with a 5-cm H_2O pressure gradient, 100 mL of air per second can flow through a 14-gauge needle, so a fatal volume of air could easily be aspirated within just a few seconds through most of the peel-away sheaths used for central venous access.[64] The first important point regarding air embolism is to avoid this complication by strict attention to technique during insertion of the catheter through the peel-away sheath. Although some authors recommend Valsalva/breath-holding maneuvers,[46] humming,[18] or the Trendelenburg position, we find that reliance on breath-holding techniques is difficult (especially when the patient is sedated), and we simply avoid the complication by either pinching the sheath[4,5] until a sufficient amount of catheter has been introduced into the peel-away sheath or covering the peel-away sheath with a fingertip until the patient begins to exhale and quickly introducing the catheter before the patient inhales. Attention to the patient's respiratory cycle is mandatory to avoid releasing the pinch or uncovering the peel-away sheath at the moment the patient inhales. Despite these precautions, air embolism may still occur (particularly in the pediatric population) if the patient becomes irritable, coughs, or cries during the critical step of advancing the catheter through the peel-away sheath.[64] Newer peel-away sheaths with an integrated protective valve further limit the risk of air embolism (Airguard [Bard Access Systems]). Finally, it should be kept in mind that air embolism can also occur at the time of catheter removal, because a fibrin sheath may provide a conduit for air to enter the central venous system after the catheter has been removed.[65,66] With this in mind, the optimal patient position for catheter removal is supine or a slight Trendelenburg position (to increase intrathoracic pressure).[65] Catheters should be removed during a Valsalva maneuver, with immediate manual compression of the catheter exit site, followed by the application of an occlusive dressing.[65,66]

The second important point is to promptly recognize the problem if it does occur. This is not usually difficult because it is ushered in by an audible "slurping" sound, and the embolus is often visible with fluoroscopy. When symptomatic, the patient may experience shortness of breath, nausea, light-headedness, substernal pain, or confusion and may exhibit tachypnea, tachycardia, hypoxia, cyanosis, focal neurologic deficits, apnea, and even complete cardiovascular collapse.[18,66] In addition, a "mill wheel" murmur (bruit de moulin) may be heard on auscultation of the chest.[66]

Air embolism should be taken very seriously because the associated mortality rate is 29% to 43%.[66] Traditional treatment recommendations include patient positioning in the left lateral decubitus position (thereby trapping air in the nondependent right atrium)[5,18,65] or with the left side down combined with the Trendelenburg position (Durant position), which should allow air in the pulmonary outflow tract to migrate to the apex of the right ventricle and permit flow of blood into the lungs.[64] However, some authors recommend leaving the patient supine because air has often already passed into the outflow tract of the right ventricle by the time the air embolism is recognized. Moving the patient to a left lateral decubitus position may shift the air embolus into the right pulmonary artery and produce further cardiovascular instability.[5] Oftentimes, supplemental oxygenation and observation are all that is required. If a large embolus is identified and the patient deteriorates despite initial efforts, a steerable catheter and guidewire should promptly be used to gain access to the air embolus and aspirate it immediately. If the patient continues to decompensate, cardiopulmonary resuscitation should ensue.

Pneumothorax

Pneumothorax, previously a complication that occurred approximately 0.69% to 2.4% of the time with a blind subclavian approach[15,67] and diminished to approximately 1% with a fluoroscopically or venographically guided subclavian approach,[4,46] has now virtually been eliminated; it occurs 0% to 1% of the time with the use of ultrasound guidance and the IJ vein approach.[17,44] Lameris et al. demonstrated a decrease in the rate of pneumothorax during subclavian access from 7.5% when done blindly to 0% under ultrasound guidance.[61] However, this complication can occur even with ultrasound guidance, particularly in cachectic patients in whom a subclavian approach is used.[5]

Arterial Puncture

Likewise, arterial puncture is a rare complication in the era of ultrasound guidance, but it can occur, particularly in obese patients with difficult anatomy or in the absence of ultrasound guidance. Very unusual errant passes have occurred during CVC insertion in the absence of image guidance (Fig. 120-13). Hematoma or hemothorax may occur acutely, and rarely, a pseudoaneurysm may develop. Because of these potential puncture-related complications, access with a 21-gauge needle under real-time ultrasound guidance is recommended.

Migration/Malposition

Although early migration or malposition has been reported to occur in 0.6% to 3% of patients[4,46] in both the radiology and surgical literature,[68] attention to detail at the time of implantation should avoid this as an early complication. A malpositioned intravascular catheter can usually be directly repositioned[46] or, if necessary, repositioned from a transfemoral approach[4] (Fig. 120-14). However, if the catheter is of improper length, it is very likely that it will return to its improper position at a later time. Correction of length should therefore be done at the time of insertion to avoid a subsequent delayed malpositioning complication. With high-quality imaging in place (ultrasound, fluoroscopy, and if necessary, venography), early malpositioning should be diminished significantly.[44] However, the position of the catheter tip is dynamic, and significant cephalad migration

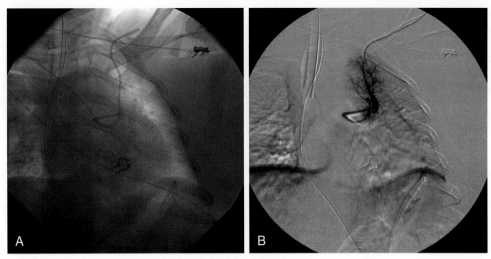

FIGURE 120-13. A, Initial chest radiograph showing an unusual path of attempted subclavian central venous catheterization without image guidance before injection of catheter. **B,** Injection of catheter confirms position of catheter tip within superior segmental branch of left pulmonary artery. Additional computed tomography (CT) views of errant catheter paths **(C-D)** available online.

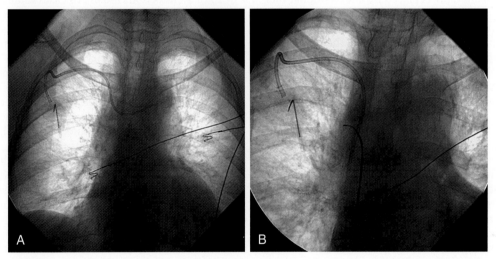

FIGURE 120-14. A, Initial chest radiograph demonstrating that tip of right subclavian port has migrated to left brachiocephalic vein. **B,** With a 25-mm Amplatz Gooseneck snare (Microvena, White Bear Lake, Minn.), catheter was easily repositioned with tip at sinoatrial junction. A 3-month follow-up film (not shown) demonstrated catheter tip to still be at sinoatrial junction.

of the catheter tip (as much as 3-4 cm) can be seen with a change in patient position from supine to upright.[18,35]

The dreaded complication of an extravascular position can be avoided by attention to detail at the time of insertion and intermittent fluoroscopic monitoring of the guidewire, peel-away sheath, and catheter. The peel-away sheath may perforate the brachiocephalic veins or right atrium if it is inadvertently advanced over a kinked guidewire or inserted without the presence of a guidewire.[18] This deadly complication is not unique to port insertion and usually occurs in the absence of fluoroscopy. Unfortunately, it may not be evident until postprocedure imaging is performed[18] and may result in hemothorax, cardiac tamponade, or mediastinal hematoma.

Infection
Infection of the subcutaneous tunnel or pocket within the first week is probably caused by intraoperative contamination[7] but could theoretically also be due to access

complications or simply the presence of a colonizable foreign body.[46] Therefore, strict adherence to sterile technique is of utmost importance. All personnel involved in the procedure should wear surgical masks and caps. In addition, the operator should perform a full surgical scrub and wear a surgical cap, gown, gloves, and mask, and the patient should have the site prepared with Betadine or Chloraprep and then be fully draped. The number of personnel who access the room itself should be limited. Preprocedure administration of antibiotics is controversial, with some practitioners using them and others not (see earlier).

Other Early Complications
Other rare early complications of central venous access include temporary brachial plexopathy,[46] catheter laceration (by a cutting device used for removal of the introducer sheath),[46] catheter embolization requiring retrieval from the pulmonary artery,[15] catheter fracture at the time of

insertion,[69] thoracic duct injury,[70] IVC filter dislodgement,[18,71] and cardiac perforation.[18]

Late Complications

Late complications include infection, venous thrombosis, venous stenosis, catheter dysfunction/fibrin sheath formation, catheter migration (both intravascular and extravascular), and late fracture (pinch-off syndrome).

Infection

Infection remains a leading cause of catheter removal in patients with subcutaneous ports.[17] Delayed infection may be due to hematogenous seeding from a distant site, contiguous spread to the tunnel and endovascular space from the access needle site,[7] from the access site with intraluminal spread of infection,[72] or rarely from contamination of the infusate.[48] The most common pathogens are coagulase-negative staphylococci, *Staphylococcus aureus*, gram-negative bacilli, and *Candida albicans*.[72] Despite early concerns to the contrary, the frequency of infectious complications in implanted ports placed by interventional radiologists is the same or better than the frequency of complications in ports placed by surgeons.[4,44,45] The overall rate of infectious complications reported in the literature in most patient populations ranges from 0% to 22% for subcutaneous port placement,* with many authors reporting rates of less than 6%.† Though somewhat controversial, most authors acknowledge that this rate is considerably lower than that with external tunneled catheters, which have infectious complication rates of up to 38%.[69,75] Groeger's group found that the incidence of infections per device-day was 12 times greater with catheters than with ports.[76] The difference in the infectious morbidity of subcutaneous ports is thought to be secondary to the fact that ports are "irrigated less frequently, require no specific care at home, and are less prone to environmental or cutaneous contamination when they are not accessed."[39,76] Rates of infection increase dramatically in certain populations. For example, Wagner and coauthors reported infectious complications in 15 of 25 (60%) venous ports placed in patients with sickle cell disease in their retrospective study and found a 50% to 100% rate of infectious complications in patients with sickle cell disease on review of the literature.[77]

Treatment of infectious complications often requires removal of the device.[17,45] Port-related infections can be divided into true port pocket infections, less severe localized cutaneous site infection or cellulitis, and device-related bacteremia or fungemia. Frank port pocket infections, characterized by redness, warmth, tenderness, purulent discharge, and culture-positive material aspirated or swabbed from the pocket, are treated by removal of the device, irrigation and packing of the wound, and appropriate antibiotic therapy.[46,76,78] These classic signs of infection may be suppressed or absent in neutropenic patients.[76] At the time of removal, a swab of the port pocket should be sent for culture, with wound checks and packing changes performed until the wound heals and initial empirical antibiotic therapy guided by culture results. A less severe localized cutaneous site infection or cellulitis with erythema,

induration, and tenderness over the port may be treated with antibiotics and the port left in place.[45,76] Removal of the Huber needle is recommended[76] during treatment of the access-site infection. Close follow-up is important, for if the cellulitis progresses to a frank port pocket infection, removal of the port would be indicated. If evidence of concurrent sepsis is noted, the port should be removed and the patient admitted for intravenous antibiotics, supportive care, and close observation. A port should also be removed if it is associated with septic thrombosis or emboli, endocarditis, osteomyelitis, refractory hypotension, or persistent culture positivity without eradication of infection.[72,76,78]

There is conflicting evidence regarding appropriate treatment of device-related bacteremia. Whereas some authors have reported successful port salvage in this situation,[74,76,78] others have not.[17] Groeger et al. were able to salvage 25 of 26 ports associated with device-related bacteremia or fungemia.[76] In addition, later work by this same group found that only 16 of 31 instances of sepsis (52%) and 5 of 15 cases of port-site cellulitis (33%) required port removal.[78] By contrast, Kuizon et al. reported device removal being necessary in 15 of 17 infections (88%) (10 cases of device-related bacteremia, 4 cutaneous site infections, 2 port infections, and 1 unknown infection because this port was removed at an outside hospital).[17] Port salvage failed in two of three attempts in the bacteremia group (n = 10) and in two of three attempts in the cutaneous site infection group (n = 4). Both port pocket infections were treated by immediate port removal. Thus, salvage failed in four of six attempts (67%).

The likelihood of successful catheter salvage depends on the site of infection (exit site infection more likely to respond than tunnel or pocket infection) and the organism (coagulase-negative staphylococci more likely to respond than *S. aureus* and *Pseudomonas aeruginosa*).[72] In addition, most antibiotics are unable to kill microorganisms growing in a biofilm at therapeutic concentrations. Investigators have found that antibiotic concentrations must be 100 to 1000 times greater to kill sessile bacteria growing in a biofilm than to kill planktonic bacteria in solution.[72] These findings are relevant to intraluminal infections and have led to use of the antibiotic lock technique, in which the catheter lumen is filled with pharmacologic concentrations of antibiotics for hours or days. Although more data exist with regard to the use of antibiotic lock therapy for tunneled catheters, antibiotic lock therapy has been shown to improve salvage rates for ports as well.[72]

The conflicting data regarding catheter salvage require that local expertise and clinical assessment of each individual episode guide therapy in cases of device-related bacteremia. As stated in the guidelines from the Infectious Diseases Society of America, the American College of Critical Care Medicine, and the Society for Healthcare Epidemiology of America:

Because the pathogenesis of catheter-related infections is complicated, the virulence of the pathogens is variable, and the host factors have not been well defined, there is notable absence of compelling clinical data to make firm recommendations for an individual patient. Therefore, the recommendations in these guidelines are intended to support, and not replace good clinical judgment.[72]

---

*References 4, 15, 17, 39, 44-46, 67-69, 73, 74.
†References 4, 17, 44-46, 67, 68, 74.

Special note should be made that in the event of documented catheter-related candidemia, the port should be removed and systemic antifungal therapy initiated.[72,79,80] Salvage therapy for port-related candidemia is not recommended as routine therapy because salvage rates for *Candida* species have been on the order of 30%.[72] After removal of the device, systemic antifungal therapy should be instituted because cases of endophthalmitis resulting in blindness have been reported in patients with catheter-related candidemia treated only by device removal.[72] In addition, the decision regarding device removal should be based on the likelihood of the source being the catheter rather than an alternative source such as the gastrointestinal tract.[72] Recent work by Raad et al. showed that in cases of true catheter-related candidemia, removal of the CVC within 72 hours of the onset of candidemia improved the response to antifungal therapy.[80] Care should be taken to identify either microbiologic indicators of true catheter-related candidemia (simultaneous quantitative blood cultures with a ratio of central blood culture colony-forming units [CFUs] to peripheral blood culture CFUs of 5:1 or greater, or time to positivity of central blood culture before simultaneously drawn peripheral blood culture of 2 hours or more) or clinical indicators of catheter-related candidemia (no chemotherapy or steroids within 1 month before onset of the candidemia, no evidence of secondary foci or disseminated candidemia).[72,80] The reader is directed to an extensive review of the literature and detailed outlines of specific treatment guidelines.[72]

Deep Venous Thrombosis/Central
Venous Thrombosis
The incidence of catheter-related venous thrombosis in subcutaneous chest ports varies from 1% to 12%,[40,44] with many series reporting a 3% to 6% incidence.[4,15,45,46,47] However, this risk may be underestimated because the diagnostic criteria vary between studies, and identification of thrombosis is often based on clinical criteria.[40] Via monthly Doppler ultrasound screening, Luciani's group found that catheter-related venous thrombosis developed in 17 of 145 patients (11.7%) within the first 3 months of having a subcutaneous port implanted through a subclavian vein approach.[40] Although this incidence is somewhat higher than in many series, it should be recognized that 13 of these 17 patients (76%) were asymptomatic. Risk factors include the composition, diameter, and position of the catheter.[36,40,81] Polyurethane and silicone catheters are associated with a lower risk of thrombosis than polyethylene or Teflon-coated catheters, and catheters with an outer diameter of less than 2.8 mm are also associated with lower rates of thrombosis.[40] The position of the catheter tip has been found to be a significant risk for the development of thrombosis, with tip positions in the brachiocephalic veins or SVC resulting in higher rates of thrombosis.[36,40,67,81] Caers et al.[67] showed that catheter tips located in the brachiocephalic veins or cranial third of the SVC were associated with a 45% and 19% incidence of thrombosis, respectively, in comparison to the middle or distal thirds of the SVC and the right atrium, in which thrombosis developed in 4.2%, 1.5%, and 5.6%, respectively. Tesselaar's group demonstrated a 2.6-fold increased risk for thrombosis with the catheter tip in the SVC versus the right atrium.[81] These differences are probably related to differences in flow and diameter between the brachiocephalic veins and the sinoatrial junction. In light of this and despite reports of cardiac tamponade associated with catheters positioned in the right atrium,[37] catheter tip position in the cephalad to middle aspect of the right atrium is highly recommended (see Fig. 120-10). Although some investigators have also found increased risk for thrombosis with left-sided versus right-sided catheters,[37,81] others have not been able to confirm this finding.[40] Additional risk factors that have been identified for catheter-related thrombosis include arm ports,[81] elevated homocysteine levels,[81] female gender,[67] lung cancer,[67] and ovarian cancer.[81]

The mechanism of catheter-related thrombus formation is probably multifactorial and involves mechanical trauma (related to catheter insertion, as well as chronic microtrauma caused by movement of the catheter within the venous system), flow abnormalities created by the catheter, local activation of the coagulation process, and irritation of the vessel wall by chemotherapeutic agents.[36,67] The increased dilutional effect in the region of the central SVC and right atrium may be protective.

Treatment of symptomatic catheter-related venous thrombosis initially involves simply anticoagulation. This is usually tried before removal of the device, especially if it is still needed for continued therapy. If anticoagulation fails, port removal should be considered. If the patient still remains symptomatic after port removal and anticoagulation, thrombolytic therapy should be contemplated. It has been shown that low-dose warfarin (Coumadin, 1 mg/day) started 3 days before catheter insertion and continued for 90 days can reduce the incidence of catheter-related thrombosis.[82]

SVC syndrome can occur in this patient population and may be related to the patient's tumor burden, the presence or history of CVCs, and the associated hypercoagulable state of oncology patients. If the patient's device is needed for continued therapy, effort should be made to salvage the port while treating the SVC syndrome (Fig. 120-15).

Port dysfunction secondary to fibrin sheath formation is a relatively common complication of CVCs that is frequently manifested as aspiration failure. Fibrin sheaths form within days[83,84] and are present in the vast majority of CVCs. Two postmortem studies identified fibrin sheaths on all of the catheters studied,[83,85] with sheaths being identified as early as 24 hours after insertion.[83] In addition, fibrin sheaths have been identified in 78% to 100% of venographic studies.[86-88] The fibrin deposition begins at one of two points of intimal injury: the entry point of the catheter into the vein or the tip of the catheter that comes in contact with the intima. Deposition propagates from these points and can encase the entire length of the catheter within 5 to 7 days.[83]

Fortunately, ports are less sensitive than dialysis catheters (which require a high flow rate) to the presence of fibrin sheaths. If a port is not functioning properly, a chest radiograph should be obtained to check the position and course of the catheter and ensure that the port and catheter are in continuity. Two views of the chest or fluoroscopic evaluation in multiple obliquities may be required to identify a kinked or pinched catheter.[84] If one is unable to aspirate from a port but it flushes forward easily, a fibrin sheath is presumed to be the culprit, and the port should be treated with thrombolytics (barring any contraindications to thrombolytics). Instillation of 1 to 2 mg of tissue

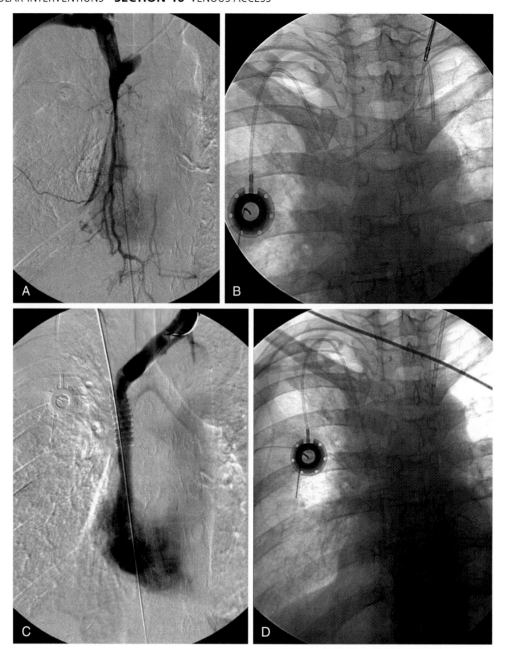

FIGURE 120-15. A, Initial venogram performed from a left internal jugular vein approach demonstrates high-grade stenosis of superior vena cava (SVC) with filling of collaterals and reflux into right subclavian vein. **B,** A 25-mm Amplatz Gooseneck snare (Microvena, White Bear Lake, Minn.) from left internal jugular approach captures port catheter and temporarily retracts catheter into left brachiocephalic vein. **C,** Repeat venogram demonstrates improved flow through newly stented SVC, without filling of collaterals. **D,** Final image of catheter repositioned through stented SVC. Patient's symptoms began to resolve within hours.

plasminogen activator (tPA), which is allowed to dwell for 30 to 60 minutes, is often successful in improving function. This may be repeated once if necessary. For resistant cases, an infusion of tPA (1 mg/h) over a period of a few hours often solves the problem. If tPA does not improve the function, the port should be accessed and evaluated by slowly injecting the port with contrast under fluoroscopy. The operator must be familiar with the varied appearances a fibrin sheath can have. Contrast may track back along the proximal catheter and potentially extravasate into the subcutaneous tissues, or contrast may be confined in the smaller-diameter sheath off the distal tip of the catheter

rather than freely flowing from the catheter tip.[84] If a fibrin sheath is identified, the sheath may be "stripped" from a femoral approach, using a snare to dislodge it. Although stripping may not result in sustained flow in dialysis catheters,[89] it will frequently provide sufficient relief for ports. If all else fails, the port may have to be replaced.

Pinch-Off Syndrome
Pinch-off syndrome is a complication unique to subclavian vein access. Catheters may be compressed in the costoclavicular space, particularly if the catheter enters via a medial access. The costoclavicular space is bounded anteriorly by

the clavicle, subclavius muscle, and costocoracoid ligament; posteriorly by the first rib and the anterior scalene muscle; and medially by the costoclavicular ligament, which joins the clavicle and first rib.[19] Catheters are at greater risk of being compressed and fractured if they enter the costoclavicular space too medially, where they are more susceptible to compression between the clavicle and rib because the costoclavicular space is narrower along its medial aspect. A more lateral approach will allow the catheter to pass through the costoclavicular space within the subclavian vein in a more posterolateral position, where more space is available and the risk of compression diminishes.[19]

The degree of catheter distortion can be graded from 0 to 3, with grade 0 having a smooth, single curved course with no narrowing; grade 1 showing any degree of bending or deviation from a single curved course, but without any luminal narrowing (Fig. 120-16, *A*); grade 2 showing some degree of luminal narrowing while passing beneath the clavicle (Fig. 120-16, *B*); and grade 3 having been completely transected (Fig. 120-17), with embolization of the central segment (Fig. e120-4).[19] The importance of this grading system is to recognize that grade 2 configurations have a high likelihood of transection and embolization. If catheter embolization occurs, an attempt to remove

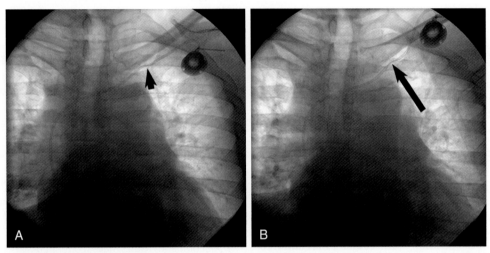

FIGURE 120-16. **A,** Frontal chest radiograph showing a grade 1 pinch-off deformity *(arrowhead)* of catheter of a left subclavian port. **B,** Same patient with arm abducted; a grade 2 deformity *(arrow)* is noted. *(Courtesy David Hayes, M.D.)*

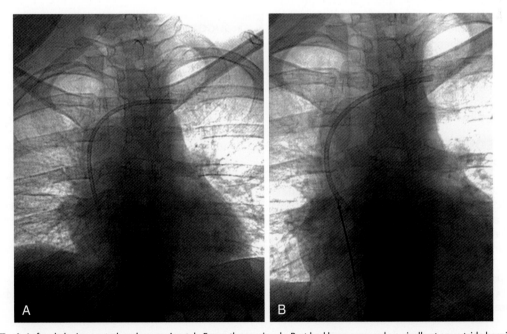

FIGURE 120-17. **A,** Left subclavian port placed approximately 5 months previously. Port had been removed surgically at an outside hospital by the surgeon who placed it, and patient was referred for retrieval of retained catheter fragment shown in this frontal chest radiograph. **B,** Fragment was snared from a femoral vein approach with an 18- to 30-mm En Snare (Medical Device Technologies Inc., Gainesville, Fla.) and removed intact. A follow-up venogram (not shown) showed no injury to left subclavian vein.

the fragment with a snare should be made, and the port should be replaced or removed if it is no longer needed (see Fig. e120-4). Because shoulder position may affect the costoclavicular space and this syndrome often appears within 3 weeks of placement, it has been suggested that CVC placement in the subclavian vein be monitored with an upright arms-at-side chest radiograph immediately after placement, at 1 month, and any time the catheter malfunctions.[19] More importantly, it should also be noted that this syndrome can be avoided altogether by using an IJ vein approach. However, if the IJ veins are occluded, an ultrasound-guided approach to the axillary/subclavian vein will allow a lateral approach that will avoid medial compression of the costoclavicular space.

Rare Complications

Rare complications include cardiac perforation/tamponade, inadvertent puncture of the catheter during suturing, migration to an extravascular position, and catheter fracture and embolization. Although cardiac tamponade resulting in death or anoxic brain injury has been reported in the literature,[37] it is fortunately exceptionally rare with the catheter materials currently available and can be further avoided by maintaining superb catheter and guidewire technique while inserting catheters. One must know where the catheter and guidewire are at all times because cardiac perforation and tamponade can result if poor technique is used (i.e., advancing a catheter, transition dilator, or peel-away sheath over a guidewire without fluoroscopic guidance). In addition, strict attention to suturing technique and complete awareness of the position of the catheter in relation to the suturing needle while closing the port pocket incision and the access site dermatotomy will avoid inadvertent puncture of the catheter. This complication will become evident when the patient complains of pain during any injection of the port. It should be noted that the puncture may be small enough that it might not be evident on injection of contrast material into the port but will be evident when the incision is opened and the port injected while directly visualizing the catheter at the point of discomfort (most often the neck dermatotomy). Catheter migration to an extravascular position[46] and catheter fracture and embolism have been reported,[15] but these complications are fortunately exceptionally rare.

POSTPROCEDURE AND FOLLOW-UP CARE

After the procedure is completed, the residual Betadine or Chloraprep is cleaned off the patient's skin with normal saline and chlorhexidine. The area is then cleaned with Chloraprep once again, and sterile gauze is secured with an occlusive dressing such as Tegaderm (3M Health Care, St. Paul, Minn.) or Mefix (Molynlycke Health Care, Göteborg, Sweden). The patient is given verbal and written instructions outlining care of the port and dressing. If the port is not left accessed, the patient is instructed to keep the

original dressing in place for 2 to 3 days without getting it wet during that time. After 2 to 3 days, the patient is instructed to remove the old dressing, wash the site with warm water and soap, dry the area, and reapply the gauze and occlusive dressing. Dressing changes should be continued daily until the site is healed. If the port is left accessed, the patient is instructed to keep the dressing clean, dry, and intact. The port is usually left accessed if chemotherapy is planned to be initiated within 3 days. The importance of protecting the dressing and access needle until the time of infusion is emphasized to the patient. In addition, information on contacting the interventional radiology department is given to the patient in case there are any questions or concerns. The patient is instructed to contact a physician if any signs of infection are noted.

KEY POINTS

- Subcutaneous ports are ideal for long-term intermittent central venous access, with the most frequent indication being administration of chemotherapy.
- The preferred access is now the internal jugular vein under direct ultrasound guidance. This, in conjunction with high-quality fluoroscopic guidance, has essentially eliminated many of the procedure-related complications (pneumothorax, arterial puncture, and malpositioned catheters).
- Today's interventionalist must be able to identify and manage the acute and chronic complications associated with subcutaneous ports.
- Subcutaneous ports have continued to evolve since their introduction in the 1980s, with the development of improved catheter materials and port designs.

▶ **SUGGESTED READINGS**

Barnacle A, Arthurs OJ, Boebuck D, et al. Malfunctioning central venous catheters in children: a diagnostic approach. Pediatr Radiol 2008;38: 363–78.
Denny DF. Placement and management of long-term central venous access catheters and ports. AJR Am J Roentgenol 1993;161:385–93.
Funaki B. Central venous access: a primer for the diagnostic radiologist. AJR Am J Roentgenol 2002;179:309–18.
Jaques PF, Mauro MA, Keefe B. US guidance for vascular access. Technical note. J Vasc Interv Radiol 1992;3:427–30.
Mauro MA, Jaques PF. Radiologic placement of long-term central venous catheters: a review. J Vasc Interv Radiol 1993;4:127–37.
Mermel LA, Farr BM, Sherertz RJ, et al. Guidelines for the management of intravascular catheter-related infections. Clin Infect Dis 2001;32: 1249–72.
Weeks SM. Unconventional venous access. Tech Vasc Interv Radiol 2002;5:114–20.

The complete reference list is available online at www.expertconsult.com.

CHAPTER 121

Hemodialysis Access: Catheters and Ports

Hyeon Yu, Kyung Rae Kim, and Charles T. Burke

INTRODUCTION

In the United States, the number of patients with end-stage renal disease (ESRD) has been rising each year (often by > 10%), and more than 300,000 individuals undergo hemodialysis treatment.[1] Each of these patients needs some form of vascular access to allow sufficient blood flow to the dialyzer for adequate hemodialysis, which is administered three times weekly. Maintaining vascular access patency and function for these patients is an essential component of their care.

The Clinical Practice Guidelines and Recommendations of the National Kidney Foundation Kidney Disease Outcomes Quality Initiative (NKF KDOQI) state that an ideal vascular access should have the following characteristics: optimum flow rate for adequate hemodialysis, long use-life, and low rate of complications (e.g., infection, stenosis, thrombosis, aneurysm, and limb ischemia).[2] Although no currently available vascular access can perfectly meet these criteria, the surgically created native arteriovenous fistula (AVF) has been reported to have the best patency rates, require the fewest interventions, and have the best results following interventions compared to other types of vascular access.[3-5]

Despite the NKF KDOQI Vascular Access Guidelines that recommend increased placement of AVFs and decreased use of hemodialysis catheters, 10% of total vascular accesses, the patient population with ESRD receiving hemodialysis via catheters has steadily increased from 13% to 25%. This increase of hemodialysis catheters may be partly attributed to advanced patient age, comorbid conditions such as peripheral vascular disease and diabetes, and late referral for creation of an AVF.[6] Hemodialysis catheters still play an important role, not only as a temporary access for patients with acute renal failure but also as a bridge until a more definitive form of vascular access is established.

Currently, there are three different types of hemodialysis catheters available: tunneled cuffed catheters, nontunneled catheters, and ports. This chapter reviews the use of these different types of catheters, techniques of initial placement, and interventional procedures for managing complications associated with hemodialysis catheters.

INDICATIONS

According to the guidelines and recommendations developed by the NKF KDOQI Vascular Access Work Group, one of the goals to improve patients' survival and quality of life is to increase the placement of AVFs. Recently, the target for fistula creation has been reset at 65%.[2]

For patients in whom an AVF cannot be created because of anatomic or technical limitations, an AV graft is the next best option. Typically, a fistula requires approximately 3 months for maturation, and a graft 6 weeks to mature before use. Before fistula or graft creation and during maturation periods, patients may require placement of a dialysis catheter or port.

Patients awaiting renal transplantation or creation of peritoneal access for peritoneal dialysis also have an indication for placement of a hemodialysis catheter or port. Patients who undergo continuous ambulatory peritoneal dialysis may need temporary hemodialysis access via a catheter or port while their peritoneal dialysis access heals or during episodes of peritonitis.

Hemodialysis catheters or ports are also indicated in patients who are not candidates for surgical access. These include patients with anatomic issues such as venous or arterial stenosis or occlusion and patients with severe comorbid conditions that could make the presence of an AV shunt dangerous.

Despite NKF KDOQI recommendations, decreased durability, and a higher rate of complications with catheters, some patients may nonetheless prefer them to AVFs and grafts.[7] One significant difference for the patient is the necessity for needle access to the fistula or graft at two separate skin sites during each dialysis session, versus painless direct connection of the dialysis catheter to the dialysis machine.

CONTRAINDICATIONS

The use of hemodialysis catheters as primary vascular access should be minimized because of the high risk for infection and high malfunction rate. The NKF KDOQI Vascular Access Work Group strongly recommends that catheters be used in less than 10% of hemodialysis patients as their permanent chronic hemodialysis access.[2]

Prolonged presence of a catheter that traverses the central veins may result in central venous stenosis or occlusion. Because the likelihood of this problem increases with the duration of indwelling central access, long-term use of catheters is generally contraindicated in patients with other potential access options.

The preferred site of catheter placement is the right internal jugular (RIJ) vein because of its more direct route to the right atrium than the left-sided venous approach. Catheter placement in the left internal jugular (LIJ) vein may potentially limit permanent access options on the left arm by inducing stenosis or occlusion of the left brachiocephalic vein. It has been reported that catheter placement in the LIJ vein may be associated with decreased blood flow rates and increased risk for stenosis and thrombosis.[8,9]

Catheter placement in the subclavian vein on either side should be avoided because of the risk for stenosis,[10,11] which can significantly reduce the possibility of future upper extremity permanent AVF or graft.

Catheters should not be placed in the vein on the same side as a slowly maturing permanent access. Central venous stenosis due to catheter placement is closely linked to the site of insertion,[12,13] number and duration of catheter uses, and occurrence of infection.[12,14]

Although the common femoral vein may be used for nontunneled temporary access, longer-term access with tunneled catheters and ports is suboptimal and relatively contraindicated because of the higher rate of infection at this site.[15]

EQUIPMENT

A variety of different types of hemodialysis catheters are produced by a number of manufacturers. Although there may be slight differences between them, they are all based on the same principle and are used in the same way. The full discussion of these devices is available at www.expertconsult.com.

TECHNIQUE

Anatomy and Approach

Vascular anatomy is more completely covered elsewhere in the book, so the following will serve only as a brief overview.

The most important approach for all types of hemodialysis catheters and ports is the IJ vein. Accessing the IJ vein at the lowest possible point above the clavicle will help prevent kinking of tunneled catheters. The IJ vein joins with the ipsilateral subclavian vein to form the brachiocephalic vein, which joins with the contralateral brachiocephalic vein to form the superior vena cava (SVC), which conveys blood to the right atrium.

When the IJ vein approach is not available, the external jugular vein may be useful. The external jugular vein sits more lateral and posterior in the neck in relation to the IJ vein and typically empties into the central portion of the ipsilateral subclavian vein.

The subclavian venous approach is rarely used, but one exception is in patients who may no longer have usable arm veins for creation of more permanent access and who also have occlusion of the jugular vein ipsilateral to this arm. In such patients, the ipsilateral subclavian vein may be used if available, because stenosis or occlusion of this vein should not jeopardize the possibility of creation of a future AVF or graft.

Less frequently used approaches include the femoral vein, hepatic vein, translumbar inferior vena cava (IVC), recanalized or collateral veins, and direct approach to the SVC. This is discussed in more detail in the Unconventional Hemodialysis Access section of this chapter.

Technical Aspects

The patient's history and any available relevant prior imaging studies should be thoroughly reviewed to identify any evidence of central venous stenosis or occlusion before planning the procedure. Informed consent for the procedure must be obtained in advance and should include discussion of its risks, benefits, and alternatives. The patient should be allowed to ask questions if desired.

Before sterile preparation, the patient should be examined thoroughly. Frequently, physical examination will reveal important clues about venous anatomy. The presence of chest wall venous collaterals or arm or neck and facial swelling may be a sign of venous occlusion.

Limited ultrasound examination of the planned access site is very useful for quick assessment of the feasibility of an approach. Strict sterile technique should be used, including sterile preparation and draping of the patient. Currently in most institutions, skin is prepared using 2% chlorhexidine gluconate in 70% isopropyl alcohol (Chloraprep).[32] The skin surface should be shaved before sterile preparation if hair is visible. For tunneled catheters placed via the IJ access site, preparation should extend from the upper mid-neck area to the nipple. Full surgical scrubbing is a necessity for all operators, as is the use of surgical caps, masks, and sterile gowns and gloves. Sterile probe covers should be used for ultrasound probes.

For the large majority of patients, a combination of local anesthesia and moderate sedation is well tolerated. Lidocaine 1% with epinephrine is commonly used for local anesthesia, and moderate sedation generally consists of a fast-acting and relatively short-lived benzodiazepine and narcotic combination, such as midazolam and fentanyl. During the entire procedure, the patient should be continuously monitored using electrocardiogram and pulse oximetry by a member of the nursing staff.

Preprocedure antibiotic administration is not required,[33,34] with multiple studies demonstrating low infection rates that are comparable or lower than those documented for surgical placement.[35]

Because the IJ vein is the preferred hemodialysis catheter placement site, discussion will focus on this approach. Real-time ultrasound guidance should be used for IJ venous puncture because it will help guard against complications. The IJ vein should be accessed in the inferior aspect of the neck as close to the superior border of the clavicle as possible. A low puncture will aid in preventing kinking of the catheter as it curves from the subcutaneous tunnel to the venotomy site. After ultrasound is used to select the access site, local anesthesia should be administered. A small, shallow incision or "skin nick" should be made over the access site with a #11 blade (Fig. e121-3). Use of a hemostat to spread the underlying fascia will facilitate subsequent passage of the peel-away sheath and also aid in preventing catheter kinking at the venotomy site. Through the skin incision, the IJ vein is accessed using a 21-gauge needle connected to a 20-mL syringe by a short connecting tubing under ultrasound guidance. Placement of the needle tip within the vein is confirmed by ultrasound and aspiration of blood through the 20-mL syringe (Fig. 121-1). Under fluoroscopic guidance, a 0.018-inch guidewire is advanced through the needle and subsequently exchanged for a Cope transition dilator (Cook Medical, Bloomington, Ind. [Fig. 121-2]). Some operators prefer an 18-gauge needle for venous access to skip the transition from 0.018-inch to 0.035-inch systems. Others prefer a micropuncture set (Cook Medical) to make the transition to a 0.035-inch system.

Fluoroscopy is used to position the wire tip in the upper to mid–right atrium. The wire is then measured to determine the appropriate catheter length for the patient. Two methods of measurement are commonly used, depending on the preference of the operator. One involves marking the wire at the point where it exits the transition dilator

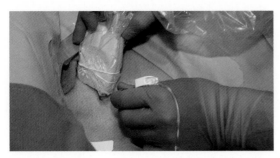

FIGURE 121-1. Under real-time ultrasound guidance, right internal jugular vein is accessed with a micropuncture needle.

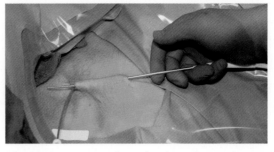

FIGURE 121-4. Using a metal tunneling device that attaches to catheter tip, catheter is pulled through tunnel.

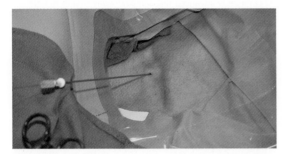

FIGURE 121-2. A 6F Cope transition dilator is placed over 0.018-inch wire through venotomy site and into superior vena cava.

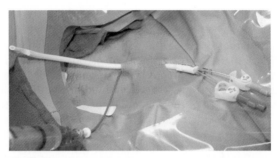

FIGURE 121-5. Catheter is pulled to the point where Dacron cuff is at most cephalad portion of subcutaneous tunnel. This helps facilitate later adjustment of final position of catheter tip.

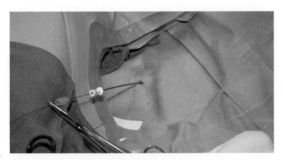

FIGURE 121-3. After placing tip of wire in mid–right atrium under fluoroscopy, hemostat is used to mark wire.

(Fig. 121-3). Then the intravenous portion of the wire can be measured by subtracting the length of the exposed transition dilator from the length of the wire between the tip and the marking. This is the best way to measure the appropriate length for a nontunneled catheter, and many operators also use this measurement to determine the length of a tunneled catheter. However, when placing tunneled catheters, some operators prefer to bend the wire in a curved pathway that simulates the course of the catheter through the tunnel, and mark the wire at a reproducible point intended to be at or near the exit site of the tunnel, such as three fingerbreadths below the clavicle (Fig. e121-4). The distance from this mark to the tip of the wire is the length from the tunnel exit site to the tip of the intravenous portion of the catheter. The wire is subsequently removed from the transition dilator.

For nontunneled catheters, a 0.035-inch wire is placed through the right atrium in the IVC, followed by serial

dilation over the wire to the appropriate French size, and the catheter is placed so its tip lies at or below the junction of the SVC and right atrium. Because commercially available catheters are available in specific lengths and cannot be trimmed, the appropriate catheter length must be chosen from the wire measurement.

For tunneled catheters, the length measurement is used to help determine the length of the subcutaneous tunnel. As with nontunneled catheters, tunneled catheters also come from manufacturers in specified lengths and cannot be trimmed. Flow resistance increases as catheter length increases, so it is best to choose the shortest catheter length that allows a tunnel at least several centimeters long (generally at least three fingerbreadths below the clavicle). The most useful catheter measurement is the distance from the tip to the cuff. Because the catheter cuff must sit inside the tunnel, the distance from the tip to cuff should never exceed the distance between the catheter tip and the tunnel exit site. The tunnel may be created in a parasternal orientation or laterally on the chest wall, and different practitioners have different preferences in this regard. This is discussed in more detail in the Controversies section of this chapter. After an exit site is chosen for the tunnel and the catheter is prepared, a skin dermatotomy is created in much the same way as for the venotomy site (Fig. e121-5). The catheter is pulled through the subcutaneous tunnel from the exit site to the venotomy site (Fig. 121-4), and the cuff is advanced to the most superior portion of the tunnel (Fig. 121-5).

The Cope transition dilator or micropuncture catheter is exchanged over the wire for the peel-away introducer sheath that will be used to place the catheter (Fig. 121-6).

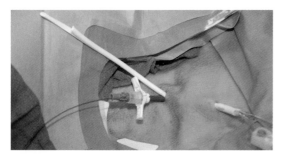

FIGURE 121-6. Peel-away sheath that will be used to introduce tunneled catheter into central veins is placed over wire through venotomy site. Peel-away introducer sheath should be advanced until it is still several centimeters outside venotomy.

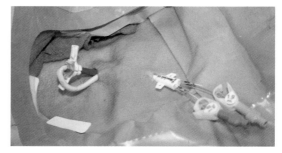

FIGURE 121-7. To prevent air embolism, sheath is usually pinched at venotomy site after removing inner dilator and wire and before advancing tunneled catheter into it. Sheath pictured is packaged with HemoSplit dialysis catheter and has a hemostatic valve that prevents leakage of air into sheath. Tunneled catheter is advanced through peel-away sheath to right atrium.

In most patients, this peel-away sheath is placed after serial dilation, especially in patients who have scar tissue from previous surgery or catheterization. Some operators prefer to advance the peel-away sheath without serial dilation after proper dissection of the subcutaneous tissue at the venotomy site using a hemostat. The peel-away sheath must be passed over the wire under fluoroscopic guidance to ensure that the wire does not kink and that the direction of the sheath conforms to the path of the central veins leading to the SVC. The sheath should be placed so several centimeters of its length is still outside the venotomy (see Fig. 121-6). The wire and inner dilator of the sheath are removed together while the remaining peel-away introducer sheath is pinched just above the venotomy to prevent air embolism. The fact that the sheath is partially outside the venotomy allows both lumina of step-tip design catheters to be placed inside the sheath above the site where it is pinched. This will prevent a size mismatch between the longer lumen alone and the sheath, which could allow leakage of air into the sheath as the operator releases enough pressure to allow the catheter to pass through the sheath. A relatively recent advance was the advent of a valved peel-away sheath, which has a valve that automatically inhibits entry of air into the sheath after the inner dilator is removed. Albeit rare, if symptomatic air embolism does occur, the patient can be placed in the left lateral decubitus and Trendelenburg position to prevent the air from moving into the right ventricle and the veins of the head and neck.

The dialysis catheter is advanced through the sheath (Fig. 121-7). The two halves of the sheath are peeled laterally away from each other. The sheath should be pulled back several millimeters at a time and peeled outside the venotomy (Fig. 121-8). Peeling inside the venotomy could expand the diameter of the venotomy and lead to pericatheter oozing of blood from the jugular vein. Such oozing may be difficult to stop, may require prolonged manual compression, and may even result in hematoma formation, which could cause discomfort and predispose to infection.

Under fluoroscopic guidance, final positioning of the catheter may be performed (Fig. 121-9). During quiet inspiration, the catheter tip should sit approximately in the mid–right atrium. During expiration, the catheter should not touch the inferior portion of the right atrium or the AV valve. During deep inspiration, the catheter tip should sit at or below the junction of the SVC and right atrium.[2] The entire course of the catheter should be evaluated to ensure

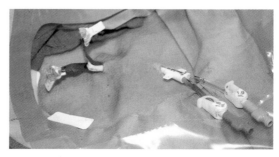

FIGURE 121-8. Two halves of peel-away sheath are separated and pulled laterally and outward from patient to remove it.

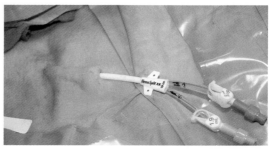

FIGURE 121-9. Tunneled catheter is now in place and ready for final positioning under fluoroscopic guidance.

the absence of kinking (Fig. 121-10). A 20-mL syringe should be used to test for unhindered aspiration and flushing of each lumen. The venotomy site may be closed with absorbable suture or surgical topical skin adhesive (Fig. e121-6). The catheter should be secured to the skin surface at the point where it exits the tunnel. If sutures are tied circumferentially around the catheter, they should be just tight enough to prevent movement, but not so tight that they partially constrict the catheter, because this will decrease flow (Fig. e121-7). A final anteroposterior radiograph of the chest should be obtained to document catheter position.

The catheter lumina should be filled with an optimal volume of heparin (5000 units/mL) when the catheter is not being used for dialysis. Obviously, if the patient is at severe

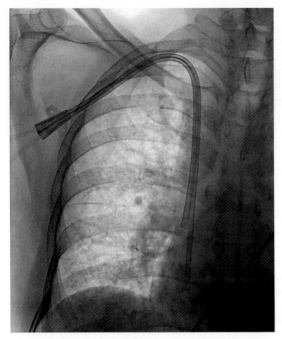

FIGURE 121-10. Anteroposterior chest radiograph demonstrating right internal jugular tunneled dialysis catheter in good position. Note that with patient supine, in expiration, catheter tip should sit within mid- to lower right atrium.

risk for hemorrhage, very dilute heparin or even sterile saline should be used. If the patient has a history of heparin allergy or heparin-induced thrombocytopenia, 1 to 2 mg of tissue plasminogen activator (tPA) may be placed in each lumen and diluted to the proper volume, as generally noted on the hemostatic clamp of each lumen.

Dialysis port placement is somewhat different from tunneled catheter placement and is more similar to placement of venous infusion ports. The LifeSite hemodialysis port system actually consists of two separate reservoirs that are placed in a subcutaneous pocket several centimeters below the clavicle. Each reservoir connects to a catheter that is tunneled and positioned in similar fashion to tunneled hemodialysis catheters. Aside from the subcutaneous reservoirs, the main difference is that the two catheters will be tunneled separately and enter the IJ vein via two separate venotomies. To guard against recirculation, as described earlier, one of the two catheters has to end higher than the other within the right atrium. The chest wall incision is generally closed with subcutaneous and subcuticular layers of absorbable suture. The port reservoirs will then sit completely under the skin surface, with no exposed parts. At dialysis, the skin surface over the reservoirs is prepared in sterile fashion, and the reservoirs are accessed with dialysis needles.[31,36,37]

Unconventional Hemodialysis Access

Because of venous stenosis or occlusion, accessible veins in the neck and chest are eventually depleted as the duration of catheter hemodialysis is prolonged. The next available access sites may include the femoral vein, hepatic vein, translumbar IVC, subclavian vein, a recanalized or collateral vein, and the SVC. These sites require additional technical expertise for placement, and maintenance of catheters at these sites may be somewhat more difficult.

Femoral Vein

Femoral veins are the next best option to jugular veins for long-term catheterization, because they are easily accessed and provide adequate flow for hemodialysis.[38] The femoral veins empty into the ipsilateral iliac veins within the pelvis, with blood subsequently flowing to the IVC and right atrium. To achieve desirable flow rates, the catheter tip should be placed at least into the IVC and, optimally, as close as possible to the right atrium. Although femoral hemodialysis catheters are more susceptible to infection and often require more interventions than thoracic catheters, they may provide alternative permanent tunneled hemodialysis access in patients with difficult central venous access.[39]

Recanalized or Collateral Veins

Using recanalized or collateral veins in the neck and chest for hemodialysis access may preserve other accessible veins for future use. Enlarged peripheral collateral veins including neck, chest wall, and thyrocervical veins may provide suitable access sites for hemodialysis catheter placement. If there are short-segment occlusions in the internal or external jugular veins, recanalization can be achieved with an antegrade approach using a short 5F catheter (e.g., Kumpe catheter) and a 0.035-inch stiff hydrophilic guidewire. If an antegrade approach is not possible, retrograde approach from the femoral vein may be an alternative option for recanalization of the obstructed central or neck veins. For optimal flow rates, recanalized veins should have a straight course without tortuosity to the SVC or right atrium.[38]

Translumbar Inferior Vena Cava

Translumbar catheters are placed through the skin, subcutaneous tissue, and multiple muscle planes of the right side of the back just above the right iliac crest, approximately 7 to 10 cm lateral to the midline at the L3 lumbar level, and enter the IVC directly. A guidewire or pigtail catheter placed in advance through the femoral venous route is used as a marker for direct puncture of the IVC under fluoroscopic guidance.[40] Initial access to the IVC can also be achieved under computed tomography (CT) guidance. The exterior portion of the catheter is tunneled laterally in subcutaneous tissue and exits the skin in the region of the posterior axillary line. The catheter tip should be in the right atrium (Fig. 121-11). Complications associated with translumbar hemodialysis catheters are similar to those for conventional catheter placement and include infection, catheter malfunction, patient discomfort, catheter tip migration, catheter kinking, and fibrin sheath formation. Occlusive thrombosis of the IVC can also occur but is rare.[40]

Hepatic Vein

In patients with an occluded infrarenal IVC, a transhepatic route may provide their final percutaneous access site for hemodialysis catheter placement. The transhepatic approach requires subcostal or intercostal access of a hepatic vein, most commonly the right hepatic vein. The hemodialysis catheter is tunneled subcutaneously along the upper abdominal wall and placed through the liver capsule

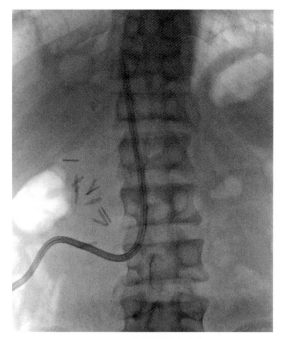

FIGURE 121-11. Anteroposterior abdomen radiograph demonstrating translumbar tunneled dialysis catheter in good position in inferior vena cava.

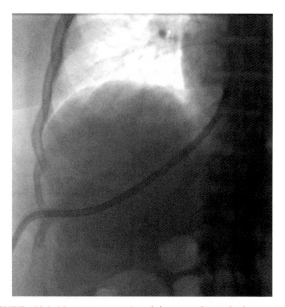

FIGURE 121-12. Anteroposterior abdomen radiograph demonstrating transhepatic tunneled dialysis catheter in good position in right atrium.

into the hepatic vein and the IVC, subsequently ending within the right atrium (Fig. 121-12). Limited data showed that patency of hepatic venous access was poor, and common complications were catheter migration, catheter-related sepsis, and thrombosis.[41,42]

Subclavian Vein
Hemodialysis catheters should be placed via the subclavian veins only in patients who are not candidates for surgical creation of an ipsilateral upper extremity AVF or graft.[2] Access to the subclavian vein and catheter placement result

in central venous stenosis and occlusion that can permanently exclude the possibility of upper extremity fistula or graft.[10,11] The technique for catheter placement in the subclavian vein is similar to that described for jugular catheter placement.

Superior Vena Cava
There has been a report describing percutaneous direct access to the SVC under fluoroscopic guidance in patients with occluded jugular and subclavian veins.[43] Using a femoral venous approach, a 5F catheter is placed in the most superior portion of the SVC, and a venogram is performed to evaluate the location of the SVC in relationship to the right clavicle. With a 5F catheter as a marker, the SVC is then directly accessed from the right supraclavicular area using an 18-gauge needle under fluoroscopic guidance. Once the needle position in the vein is confirmed by aspirating blood, a hemodialysis catheter is inserted in standard fashion. Procedure-related major complications include pneumothorax and hemothorax.

CONTROVERSIES

Location of Tunnel Site

As described previously, as part of tunneled catheter placement, individual practitioners may prefer to create a subcutaneous tunnel to the lateral chest wall, whereas others may prefer to tunnel in a parasternal direction. The lateral tunnel has the advantage of a gentler curve toward the venotomy site, which may limit the incidence of kinking. However, some believe that the catheter tip, which moves somewhat because of chest wall motion as the patient changes position, will move less than with the use of a parasternal tunnel, where the subcutaneous tissue is not as bulky. Although this has not been fully studied, trends suggest that parasternal tunnels may also help prevent infection, probably because they move the catheter exit site farther away from the axilla.

Tunneled versus Nontunneled Catheters

In a patient with newly diagnosed acute renal failure requiring hemodialysis, it may be unclear whether a nontunneled dialysis catheter or a tunneled catheter should be placed. Many patients recover from the various causes of acute renal failure and require only temporary dialysis. Nontunneled dialysis catheter placement is associated with more short-term complications than tunneled access, but some patients will progress to chronic renal failure and require longer-term access, so despite the increased procedural cost and invasiveness of tunneled catheters, they are generally more cost-effective and safer to place when it is unclear how long a patient may require dialysis.[19]

Exchange versus Removal of Catheters

When a dialysis patient has signs of infection and is found to be bacteremic, the tunneled dialysis catheter will often be the source of infection. Medical practitioners unfamiliar with the NKF KDOQI and Centers for Disease Control and Prevention (CDC) guidelines may ask that all such catheters be removed for a "line holiday." Actually, in the setting of bacteremia, most patients can be treated with intravenous antibiotics alone or with a combination of antibiotics and over-the-wire catheter exchange. This has the effect of preserving the access site because venous stenosis from catheterization, if present, may preclude replacement of a new catheter at the same site in the future. Guidewire exchange maintains wire access across any stenosis and is highly unlikely to result in loss of the access site. By contrast, some patients have septic physiology and a hemodialysis catheter as the suspected source. In the setting of sepsis, immediate catheter removal and a line holiday are indicated.[44-47] Blood should be redrawn for culture after the catheter is removed and the septic physiology has resolved. When cultures have been negative for at least 48 to 72 hours, a new tunneled hemodialysis catheter may be placed. If necessary, such patients may be managed by placement of a temporary nontunneled dialysis catheter until cultures clear.

Coated Catheters

Silver-Coated Catheters
Silver-coated catheters were developed in an effort to reduce infection rates; only limited and inconclusive data exist regarding their benefit. In a prospective randomized trial performed by Trerotola et al.,[48] silver-coated catheters showed no significant benefit in infection rate reduction. However, a more recent study by Bambauer et al.[49] showed a significant decrease in bacterial colonization rates in the silver-based antimicrobial catheters compared with uncoated catheters.

Antibiotic-Coated Catheters
Antibiotic-coated catheters are clinically effective and cost saving compared with standard catheters.[50] A meta-analysis of randomized controlled trials have shown that rifampin-impregnated catheters were safe and effective in reducing bacterial colonization rates and catheter-related bacteremia as compared with standard uncoated catheters.[51] According to the 2002 CDC guidelines, antimicrobial-coated catheters should be used in patients with the infection rate exceeding 3.3 per 1000 catheter days.[52]

Antithrombotic-Coated Catheters
Currently at least two types of antithrombotic-coated tunneled hemodialysis catheters are available: (1) the Carmeda BioActive Surface (CBAS) coating on the Spire Biomedical catheter (Spire Biomedical Inc., Bedford, Mass.) and (2) the Trillium Biosurface coating (BioInteractions Ltd., Redding, UK) on the Tal Palindrome Emerald catheter (Covidien, Norwalk, Conn.). As an anticoagulant, heparin bonding is used on the surface of these catheters.[52] Although they may reduce the rates of biofilm and fibrin sheath formation, because of a lack of long-term data, patency and safety of these catheters are yet to be concluded.

OUTCOMES

In skilled and experienced hands, very high technical success rates can be achieved with image guidance for placement of hemodialysis catheters.[35,53] When a combination of review of prior relevant imaging studies, physical examination of the chest wall, arm, and neck veins, and

ultrasound examination of the intended access vein is performed, technical failure from venous stenosis and occlusion can easily be avoided in the large majority of patients.

One of the clinical outcome goals recommended by the NKF KDOQI Work Group is that no more than 5% of tunneled catheters should be unable to achieve a blood flow rate greater than 300 mL/min during the first dialysis session after catheter placement.[2] Again, image guidance is the key because catheter tip position and a catheter course without kinking can be confirmed before conclusion of the placement procedure.

Tunneled catheter longevity after placement is generally limited by two factors: patency and infection. Multiple studies, only a few of which are referenced here, have demonstrated variable catheter survival or median patency, generally varying between 2 and 5 months.[35,54,55]

At 1 year after placement, about 50% of patients who require long-term access remain functional.[18] Infection occurs in up to 54% of catheters over time, and this may be the single most important reason why currently available catheter designs cannot hope to dominate grafts and fistulas for long-term access needs.[34,35,44,56] Studies have shown, however, that infection rates of catheters placed by interventional radiologists in the interventional radiology procedure room do not differ significantly from those in catheters placed in the operating room.[35,44,56]

COMPLICATIONS

Complications of dialysis catheter placement include bleeding, which may be due to either hemorrhage at the venotomy site or internal vascular injury. Risk is minimized by proper use of imaging guidance.[57,58] Because of the close proximity of the carotid artery to the IJ vein, ultrasound-guided puncture should always be performed. As described previously, fluoroscopic guidance should be used to track the course of all devices within the central veins and to be sure no device is placed in an extravascular position. Major vascular injuries are exceedingly rare but can result in hemothorax or hemopericardium and cardiac tamponade, and such injuries may require operative repair.

Air embolism may occur but is rarely clinically significant. If symptomatic, the patient should be placed in the left lateral decubitus and Trendelenburg position, as previously described. Lung injury and pneumothorax are also quite rare, especially with imaging guidance.

The medications used for moderate sedation may cause respiratory depression and increase the risk for aspiration. Patients should be held without oral intake for at least 6 hours before receiving moderate sedation to allow complete emptying of gastric contents into the small bowel. Sedation should be administered by advanced cardiac life support (ACLS)-certified staff, and members of the team should be familiar with the use of pharmacologic antagonists to reverse the effects of sedatives and analgesics in the event it should become necessary.

Rarely, iodinated contrast material may be needed to define the vascular anatomy, especially if stenosis or occlusion is present. For patients who may still have some residual renal function, these agents can be nephrotoxic and hasten the decline of their renal function. In such patients, consideration should be given to an alternative contrast agent such as carbon dioxide. Allergic reaction to contrast material is also a potential risk.

Infection of dialysis catheters can occur at any time from placement onward. It could potentially lead to sepsis and may be life threatening.[35,44,56] Other risks associated with maintenance and use of the catheter include phlebitis and thrombosis, which may result in facial, neck, chest, or arm edema, or any combination of these complications.

It is important to note that all the potential complications of the placement procedure are quite rare and that complication rates of significantly less than 2% can be expected.[35,53]

Infectious complications related to use and maintenance of catheters that occur remote from the time of placement, however, are much more common and increase proportionally with the duration of catheterization, as does the risk for central venous stenosis and occlusion.[11,12,59-61]

POSTPROCEDURAL AND FOLLOW-UP CARE

The full discussion of this topic is available at www.expertconsult.com.

KEY POINTS

- The incidence of end-stage renal disease has been increasing in the United States each year.

- Hemodialysis catheters and ports are intended to be used for temporary dialysis access, optimally while a patient is waiting for creation or maturation of more permanent surgical hemodialysis arteriovenous fistulas, grafts, or peritoneal dialysis access.

- The internal jugular approach is preferred for all types of hemodialysis catheters and ports.

- If accessible veins in the neck and chest are exhausted, unconventional accesses, including femoral vein, hepatic vein, translumbar inferior vena cava, and recanalized or collateral veins, should be considered.

- Imaging guidance enhances both the safety and functionality of dialysis catheter placement.

- Dialysis catheters can be placed in the interventional radiology suite with a high rate of technical success and a very low rate of procedural complications. The risk for central venous stenosis and occlusion rises in proportion to the duration of indwelling hemodialysis catheter access.

- Infection is a frequent long-term complication of hemodialysis catheters, which makes them a source of relatively high morbidity and mortality compared to other types of dialysis access.

- Patients with tunneled catheter-related bacteremia may be treated with antibiotics and over-the-wire catheter exchange, but sepsis should prompt catheter removal and a "line holiday."

▶ **SUGGESTED READINGS**

Agarwal AK, Patel BM, Haddad NJ. Central vein stenosis: a nephrologist's perspective. Semin Dial 2007;20:53–62.

Bagul A, Brook NR, Kaushik M, Nicholson ML. Tunnelled catheters for the haemodialysis patient. Eur J Vasc Endovasc Surg 2007;33: 105–12.

Funaki B, Unconventional Central Access. Catheter insertion in collateral or in recanalized veins. Semin Intervent Radiol 2004;21(2):111–7

Knuttinen MG, Bobra S, Hardman J, et al. A review of evolving dialysis catheter technologies. Semin Intervent Radiol 2009;26:106–14.

Liangos O, Gul A, Madias NE, Jaber BL. Long-term management of the tunneled venous catheter. Semin Dial 2006;19:158–64.

Lok CE. Avoiding trouble down the line: the management and prevention of hemodialysis catheter-related infections. Adv Chronic Kidney Dis 2006;13:225–44.

Moran JE, Prosl F. Totally implantable subcutaneous devices for hemodialysis access. Contrib Nephrol 2004;142:178–92.

NKF KDOQI Clinical Practice Guidelines and Clinical Practice Recommendations for Vascular Access. Update. 2006, Available at http://www.kidney.org/professionals/KDOQI/guideline_upHD_PD_VA/index.htm.

Quarello F, Forneris G, Borca M, Pozzato M. Do central venous catheters have advantages over arteriovenous fistulas or grafts? J Nephrol 2006; 19:265–79.

Rosner MH. Hemodialysis for the non-nephrologist. South Med J 2005; 98:785–91; quiz 792–793.

Saxena AK, Panhotra BR. Prevention of catheter-related bloodstream infections: an appraisal of developments in designing an infection-resistant 'dream dialysis-catheter'. Nephrology (Carlton) 2005;10: 240–8.

Trerotola SO. Hemodialysis catheter placement and management. Radiology 2000;215:651–8.

Work J. Hemodialysis catheters and ports. Semin Nephrol 2002;22: 211–20.

The complete reference list is available online at www.expertconsult.com.

CHAPTER 122
Clinical Manifestations of Lymphatic Disease
Stefan G. Ruehm

The lymphatic system not only plays an important role in maintaining homeostasis of body fluids, it is also a vital component of the immune system. Functions of the lymphatic system include drainage and removal of excess fluids from different body tissues; absorption of fatty acids from the intestine and transportation as *chyle*, a milky substance consisting of milky fluid, lymph, and emulsified fats, to the circulatory system; and production of immune cells such as lymphocytes, mastocytes, and plasma cells. Because of its complexity, imaging the lymphatic system remains challenging. Conventional lymphangiography was once the only imaging modality available, but the technique has been widely abandoned because of its invasiveness, technical difficulties, and potential for side effects. A variety of alternative imaging techniques such as ultrasound, computed tomography (CT), and magnetic resonance imaging (MRI) have taken its place.

LYMPHATIC SYSTEM ANATOMY

Despite various generalized anatomic characteristics of the lymphatic system in the upper and lower extremities, chest (including the axillary region), and pelvis (including the inguinal region), there is a wide variety in shape, size, number, and structure of lymph nodes and vessels. For diagnosis and therapy, knowledge of standard and variant anatomy is important.

In general, the lymphatic system can be described as a one-way or open semicircular transport system for fluid and proteins that begins with lymphatic capillaries, also referred to as *initial lymphatics*. They are located in the interstitial tissue. Several lymphatic capillaries unify to become lymphatic precollectors, which then form lymphatic collectors. In general, *afferent lymphatics*, which carry the lymph toward regional lymph nodes, can be differentiated from *efferent lymphatics*, which exit the nodes and then form several lymphatic trunks. The largest lymphatic trunk is the thoracic duct. It starts in the abdomen, usually with the cisterna chyli, which is typically located anterior to the spine at the L2 level, posterior to the aorta. The thoracic duct takes a course toward the chest through the aortic foramen of the diaphragm and drains into the angulus venosus, the venous junction formed by the left subclavian and left internal jugular veins.[1-3]

LYMPHATIC SYSTEM PHYSIOLOGY

As blood reaches the capillary system, plasma fluid and proteins filter into the interstitial space. This process is influenced by hydrostatic and osmotic pressure gradients. The major portion of the exudate is reabsorbed by postcapillary venules. Because of the osmotic force from proteins in the interstitial space, a small proportion of the capillary filtrate escapes reabsorption and constitutes the lymphatic fluid load. This net ultrafiltrate is conveyed to the interstitial space and initial lymphatics, which are freely permeable to macromolecules. They therefore play an important role in maintaining the balance of hydrostatic and osmotic pressure in the interstitium. The net efflux of fluid or net flow rate of lymph is approximately 100 to 500 times less than the flow rate of blood.[2,4]

The net flow rate in the lymphatic system is influenced by both the formation and propulsion of lymphatic fluid. Lymph flow is generated mainly by contractions of lymph collectors and lymph trunks. Lymph vessels generally contain one-way valves to support lymph propulsion and prevent retrograde flow. The segment of lymph vessels between two valves is called the *lymphangion*. Compared with blood circulation, the lymphatic system lacks a central pump.[5] As opposed to the initial lymphatics, the collecting lymph vessels contain smooth muscle cells that enable phasic contractions to take place and thus aid in lymph transport.[6]

Protein composition in lymphatic fluid is nearly identical to interstitial fluid, which is similar to but usually less concentrated than that in blood plasma. The exception is intestinal lymph, which contains large amounts of fat as a result of direct absorption from the intestine.

In addition to regulation of fluid balance in tissues and organs, the lymphatic vascular system serves as a transport system for immune cells. It may also disseminate tumor cells along with interstitial macromolecules.

Lymphatic fluid has to pass through lymph nodes, which serve as filters and reservoirs and are organized as clusters within the lymphatic network. Lymph nodes also serve as incubators for white blood cells and may allow proliferation of tumor cells in the presence of cancer. Access to systemic blood is established through so-called high endothelial venules within the lymph nodes. Phagocytes in lymph nodes may capture molecules and particles and could thus reduce lymphatic protein concentration. Fluid exchange through the nodal vasculature may also modulate protein concentration.[4,5,7,8]

MANIFESTATIONS OF LYMPHATIC DISEASE

Lymphedema

In the presence of an obstruction of the lymphatic transport system (e.g., due to removal of lymph nodes or interruption of lymph vessels after trauma or surgery), interstitial fluid can accumulate and cause edema. A change in osmotic force in the interstitial space can result in edema as well. In general, *edema* can be characterized as a condition of tissue fluid imbalance. Common causes of *lymphedema* are infection, trauma, burns, surgery, radiation, tissue grafting, and congenital factors.[9-11]

The condition of lymphedema can be characterized by etiology, stage, presence or absence of reflux, and pathogenesis. If the cause of lymphedema is known, it is generally termed *secondary*; if it remains unknown, it is called *primary* or *idiopathic*. Causes of primary lymphedema include aplasia, hypoplasia, hyperplasia, and atresia of lymph vessels, as well as agenesis of lymph nodes and inguinal lymph node fibrosis. Causes of secondary lymphedema include the presence of malignant disease, with lymphangiomatosis, carcinomatosis, or compression of draining lymph structures by tumorous tissue. Iatrogenic causes induced by surgery or radiation therapy, trauma, lymphangitis, infectious diseases (filariasis), artificial self-induced sources (self-mutilation), retroperitoneal fibrosis, and amyloidosis[1,2,12] are regarded as causes of secondary lymphedema as well.

However, this categorization of lymphedema appears to no longer be adequate. Only the etiology of inguinal lymph node fibrosis remains unknown, whereas all other forms of primary lymphedema are due to a variety of known malformations of lymph vessels and nodes.[2,12] The Browse-Stewart classification[13] proposes that primary lymphedema is caused by abnormalities originating in the lymphatic system, whereas secondary lymphedema is caused by an abnormality that does *not* originate in the lymphatic system.

A variety of pathologic conditions can be differentiated on the basis of a correlation between lymph production and transport capacity of the lymph system. In the presence of an excess of lymph fluid that exceeds the transport capacity of the normal lymph system, high-output failure occurs, with resulting edema or fluid accumulation in body cavities. Edema in patients with nephrotic syndrome or ascites in patients with cirrhosis results from high-output lymphatic vascular system failure. However, if there is a decrease in transport capacity of the lymph system below the normal lymphatic load, mainly as a result of a pathologic condition of lymph nodes or vessels, low-output failure is present, and typically an interstitial lymphedema develops. If lymphatic transport capacity decreases but remains higher than the lymph load, a latent stage of lymphedema (stage 0) is present. If transport capacity drops and there is an increase in lymphatic load at the same time, a combined form of lymphedema exists.[3]

Primary lymphedema may be categorized as hereditary or sporadic. In general, the hereditary form has an autosomal dominant pattern of inheritance, typically coupled with incomplete penetrance. Both hereditary and sporadic lymphedema may be present at birth or develop during early childhood. Terms that describe the disease include *congenital lymphedema*, *lymphedema praecox*, and *lymphedema tarda*. The hereditary form is usually called *Milroy disease*, whereas the hereditary praecox form is called *Meige disease*. Primary lymphedema may occur in isolation or in combination with a variety of other abnormalities such as microcephaly, chorioretinal dysplasia, and Turner or Noonan syndromes. Depending on the location of the dysplastic lymphatic structures, primary lymphedema of the lower extremity can be differentiated into high dysplasia when the lumbar lymph trunks or lumbar or iliac lymph nodes are involved. If dysplastic lymph vessels are present in the leg, the term *distal dysplasia* is used.

Even though millions of people worldwide are affected by various forms of lymphatic diseases, understanding of the underlying disease mechanism by medical professionals is often inadequate, and treatment options are limited.[1-3]

Tumors and Lymph Metastases

The lymphatic system is often part of or even the primary route for dissemination of many solid tumors. In particular, tumors of epithelial origin (e.g., breast, colon, lung, prostate cancer) may show dissemination via the lymphatic system. Metastatic spread of cancer is a complex mechanism, with some tumors metastasizing primarily through blood, some through the lymphatic system, and some using both pathways at various stages of the disease process. To date, lymphangiogenesis and the interaction between the tumor and lymphatic system is poorly understood.

Compared with blood circulation, the lymph system may facilitate spread of tumor for several reasons. Lymph fluid is similar to interstitial fluid and may promote cell viability. The smallest lymph vessels are still larger than blood capillaries, and lymph flow velocity is substantially slower. Tumor cells in the bloodstream may experience serum toxicity and mechanical deformation that may contribute to a lower rate of hematogenic versus lymphogenic metastasis. In addition, lymph nodes may serve as incubators with long dwelling times for tumor cells and provide access to the circulatory blood system through high endothelial venules.[14-16] In general, access of tumor cells to the lymphatic system may be more difficult than access to the blood system. However, as soon as tumor cells have invaded lymph vessels, metastatic spread may occur with higher success rates, which explains the focus of research on the pattern of entry of tumor cells into the lymphatic system. According to one theory, tumors may simply invade neighboring lymphatics, such as occurs with melanoma.[17] This theory is supported by the fact that many tumors that preferentially show lymphatic spread commonly have a pattern of aggressive local invasion.[18] However, there is also evidence that carcinomas may directly induce lymphangiogenesis, which may then facilitate tumor spread.[19] The precise mechanism of lymphatic tumor spread remains unclear, and further studies are warranted to understand the interaction between tumor cells and the lymph system to generate a model that describes lymphatic tumor spread comparable to what has been proposed for hematogenous metastasis.[4]

DIAGNOSTIC EVALUATION OF LYMPHATIC DISEASE

Analogous to other medical disciplines, a comprehensive physical examination combined with the medical history of the patient is mandatory as a first step in the process of diagnosing lymphatic diseases.

Physical Examination

Lymphedema of the extremities is usually painless and typically occurs unilaterally; if both extremities are affected, the manifestation is usually asymmetric. Patients may experience pain in tumor-related lymphedema or edema in association with orthopedic or neurologic diseases. In uncomplicated lymphedema, the skin is usually normal in early stages and may show increased pigmentation in later stages, sometimes accompanied by lichenification and keratosis. In addition, swelling of the back of the hands and feet, increased skin folds, and limited mobility of the affected extremities may occur. Lymphedema in conjunction with venous insufficiency may be accompanied by peripheral cyanosis. In patients with advanced lymphostatic elephantiasis, the skin may develop a gray-brown color. Lymph cysts, lymphocutaneous fistulas, and papillomatosis cutis lymphostatica may be associated with the disease process. The *Stemmer sign*[20] describes broadening of the skin folds of the toes or fingers or an inability to lift the skin folds (or both). A positive Stemmer sign suggests the presence of primary lymphedema. It is highly accurate in differentiating primary lymphedema from edema of other causes, except in patients with a descending type of lymphedema. In these patients, swelling reaches the toes last. A descending type of lymphedema may occur in the presence of proximal lymphatic dysplasia or lower abdominal or pelvic masses.[3]

Differential Diagnosis of Lymphedema

Cardiac, hepatic, and renal diseases can lead to lower extremity edema, typically causing bilateral leg swelling. Physical examination and laboratory studies can generally determine the cause of the disease. Several conditions can coincide. Of clinical importance is differentiation of edema due to early-stage venous insufficiency, typically characterized by pitting edema that decreases or disappears during bed rest, and lipedema.

Posttraumatic lymphedema requires differentiation from edema secondary to deep venous thrombosis (DVT) and sympathetic reflex dystrophy syndromes. DVT can be ruled out by duplex sonography, phlebography, contrast-enhanced CT venography, or MR venography. Sympathetic reflex dystrophic syndromes are characterized by persistent burning pain not explained by trauma, hyperpathia, shiny reddish blue discolored skin, and hyperhidrosis. X-ray images of the extremities often show signs of demineralization in the affected extremity. Differentiation between sympathetic reflex dystrophy syndrome and artificial lymphedema induced by the patient can be difficult and may require surveillance of the patient to rule out self-induced strangulation of the extremity.

Lymphostatic elephantiasis (grade III lymphedema) is usually easily diagnosed from the enormous swelling of the affected extremity. It may require differentiation from lipedema, complex angiodysplasia, and other potential causes of elephantiasis such as Recklinghausen disease and lepra tuberosa. In contrast to patients with lymphedema, the dorsa of the feet are not usually swollen in patients with lipedema.[2,3,12] MRI may help in the differential diagnosis of lymphedema, lipedema, and phlebedema.[21]

Swelling of the upper extremity may require differentiation between Paget-von Schroetter syndrome (postthrombotic axillary vein syndrome) and lipedema. Patients with Paget-von Schroetter syndrome typically show spontaneous resolution of the swelling after 4 weeks.[3] Ultrasound, CT, and MRI may be helpful in the assessment of venous patency and can visualize the augmentation of subcutaneous fatty tissue in patients with lipedema.

Imaging Techniques

Morphologic and functional imaging techniques may be used for assessment of the lymphatic system. Direct oily lymphography, an imaging technique commonly used in the past, has been widely abandoned because of its invasiveness, technical challenges, and potential for side effects, including pulmonary embolism and local wound infection.[22] The imaging modalities currently used include lymphangioscintigraphy, indirect lymphography, CT, MRI (Fig. 122-1), ultrasonography, and fluoromicrolymphography. Functional isotope lymphography can be used to assess lymphatic function. Lymphangioscintigraphy and functional isotope lymphography exploit the fact that after interstitial injection, macromolecules are absorbed and transported by the lymphatic system. Both modalities may provide valuable scientific data, but their clinical use is limited.[23]

Indirect lymphography, described in 1984,[24] involves slow-flow infusion of nonionic water-soluble contrast medium into toes or fingers or the backs of the hands or feet via an infusion pump. X-ray images are then used to visualize the precollectors and the initial segments of collector lymphatic pathways. The technique is currently not used in clinical practice but may provide valuable information for research applications.

For both melanoma and breast cancer, sentinel node imaging, typically based on indirect lymphangioscintigraphy, can be performed to identify the first lymph node draining the primary tumor.[25,26]

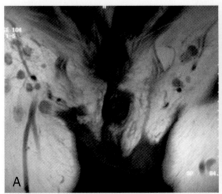 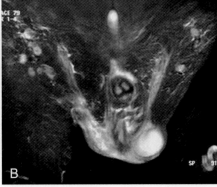 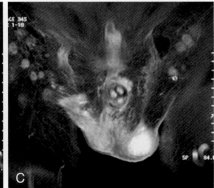

FIGURE 122-1. Noninvasive imaging of inguinal lymph nodes with magnetic resonance imaging shows reactive lymph nodes without evidence of malignancy. **A,** T1-weighted image. **B,** T2-weighted image. **C,** T1-weighted sequence after administration of contrast material.

CT and MRI are currently the imaging modalities of choice for detection of malignant lymphatic disease. In addition, both techniques allow depiction of retroperitoneal fibrosis, which may be a rare cause of secondary lymphedema. High-resolution (duplex) ultrasound may play a role in detection and characterization of lymph node enlargement and, in the presence of lower extremity swelling, allow differentiation between lipedema, lymphedema, and phlebedema as well as MRI.[21,27]

In patients suffering from malignant diseases, therapeutic options and disease prognosis are strongly related to tumor stage.[28] Accurate tumor staging, including detection of malignant involvement of lymph nodes, is of critical importance. However, with currently used cross-sectional imaging modalities, mainly CT and MRI, characterization of lymph node involvement is based largely on the nonspecific criterion of size. Tissue-specific imaging techniques based on newly developed contrast agents such as ultrasmall particles of iron oxide (USPIO), a contrast agent under investigation for MR lymphography, have been proposed to increase accuracy in the diagnosis of lymph node metastases.[29,30]

Ultrasonography

Ultrasound is often used as the first baseline imaging technique for lymph node imaging. Imaging characteristics such as increased size, round shape with loss of the central hilus, and hypoechoic texture are regarded as indicators of malignancy.[31,32] The additional use of power Doppler or color Doppler may contribute to the diagnostic accuracy of ultrasound for detecting lymph node disease. Malignant lymph nodes may show increased vascularity in the periphery of the node, whereas normal or reactive lymph nodes typically show a hilar type of vascularity with a centralized flow pattern.[33] Use of ultrasonographic contrast agents may further increase the accuracy of ultrasound for lymph node imaging,[34] but operator dependence and limited access to deeply located lymph nodes remain critical drawbacks of ultrasound as opposed to CT or MRI.[35]

Magnetic Resonance Imaging

Assessment of lymph nodes with high-resolution MRI can provide valuable information on lymph node morphology. MRI has been used to evaluate axillary lymph nodes, such as in patients with breast cancer. The use of dedicated surface coils appears to be mandatory to obtain sufficient contrast and spatial resolution for diagnostic image quality.[36-38] Indirect MR lymphography (based on interstitial injection of a gadolinium-based contrast agent for the depiction of draining lymph vessels and lymph nodes) has been described in animal experiments and humans[39-41] (Figs. 122-2 and 122-3). The introduction of MR scanners with higher field strengths (3T) and availability of gadolinium-based macromolecular contrast agents may further improve spatial resolution and therefore the diagnostic value of contrast-enhanced MR lymphography techniques.[42] Alternatively, noncontrast-enhanced, heavily T2-weighted sequences may be used to delineate dilated fluid-filled lymph vessels.[43] However, this technique appears to be limited for delineation of normal-sized peripheral lymph vessels in healthy individuals because of limitations

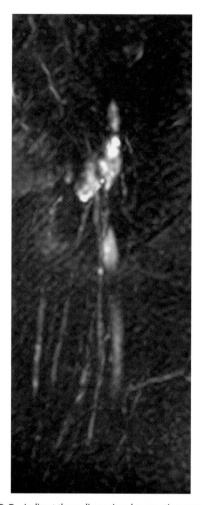

FIGURE 122-2. Indirect three-dimensional magnetic resonance lymphangiogram performed to visualize ascending inguinal lymph vessels and nodes after interstitial administration of gadolinium-based paramagnetic contrast agent in a 28-year-old volunteer.

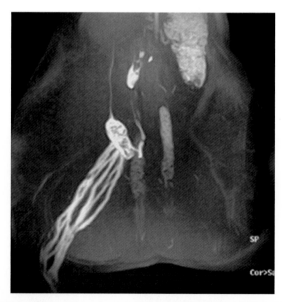

FIGURE 122-3. Contrast-enhanced magnetic resonance (MR) lymphangiogram after interstitial administration of a macromolecular MR contrast agent into dorsum of right foot in a pig model. Note excellent opacification of ascending lymph vessels and inguinal lymph node in right leg.

has been proposed. Studies have shown that after intravenous administration of USPIO, normal lymph nodes show USPIO uptake that results in loss of signal due to iron-induced susceptibility effects. In malignant lymph nodes, cells in the reticuloendothelial system responsible for USPIO uptake are replaced by metastatic tissue. As a result, malignant nodes do not accumulate USPIO and therefore lack signal loss on MRI. This concept allows differentiation of tumor-bearing from reactive lymph nodes, independent of size criteria.[44]

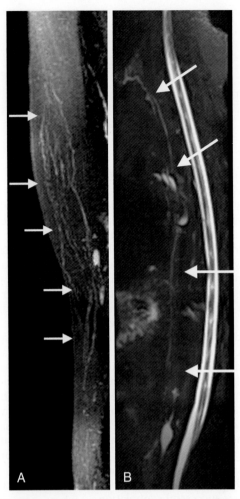

FIGURE 122-4. Depiction of lymph vessels with heavily T2-weighted magnetic resonance (MR) sequence (three-dimensional [3D] turbo spin-echo [TSE] sequence). **A,** Normal superficial lymph vessels *(arrows)* are visualized at medial aspect of calf and thigh. **B,** Sagittal projection of 3D TSE MR lymphangiogram shows course of thoracic duct *(arrows)* anterior to spine. Longitudinal structure on right of image represents spinal fluid, which appears bright as well on T2-weighted MR sequence.

of the signal-to-noise ratio and spatial resolution with currently used MR sequences on standard MRI systems, although high-resolution MR coil technology has shown early promising results (Fig. 122-4).

For differentiating normal from malignant lymph nodes, use of novel MR contrast agents, usually based on USPIO,

---

KEY POINTS

- Knowledge of lymphatic anatomy and physiology is mandatory for a better understanding of the various disease processes affecting the lymphatic system.

- A thorough clinical examination along with the medical history is the first important step in the diagnostic workup of patients with lymphatic diseases.

- Recent advances in imaging techniques, particularly in the field of magnetic resonance imaging and computed tomography, and potentially combined with the development of novel contrast agents, may play an important role in the future, particularly for the staging of lymph node involvement in patients with malignant disease.

- The exact role of the various new imaging modalities has yet to be determined.

- Early promising results from various studies indicate that noninvasive imaging techniques may limit the role of invasive diagnostic procedures (e.g., lymph node biopsy) in routine tumor-staging algorithms.

► **SUGGESTED READINGS**

Földi E. The treatment of lymphedema. Cancer 1998;83:2833–4.
Földi E. Lymphatic vascular diseases. New York: Springer; 2002.
Földi M, Kubik S, editors: Lehrbuch der Lymphologie für Mediziner und Physiotherapeuten. 4th ed. Stuttgart, Germany: Gustav Fischer; 1999.
Ruehm SG, Schroeder T, Debatin JF. Interstitial MR lymphography with gadoterate meglumine: initial experience in humans. Radiology 2001;220:816–21.
Weissleder R, Elizondo G, Josephson L, et al. Experimental lymph node metastases: enhanced detection with MR lymphography. Radiology 1989;171:835–9.

The complete reference list is available online at www.expertconsult.com.

CHAPTER 123

Bipedal Lymphangiography

Linda Kelahan, Denis Primakov, Chad Baarson, Ali Noor, and Anthony C. Venbrux

INTRODUCTION

Lymphangiography is rarely performed today because cross-sectional imaging to evaluate lymph node pathology has replaced it.[1] Years ago, prior to ultrasound (US), computed tomography (CT), and magnetic resonance imaging (MRI), bipedal lymphangiography was used in part to stage malignancies (e.g., lymphomas and metastatic disease to lymph nodes).[2,3]

Injury to the thoracic duct (traumatic, surgical, etc.) may be associated with life-threatening chylous pleural effusions. Surgery to ligate the thoracic duct is associated with significant morbidity and mortality; such patients are frequently severely debilitated.[4-7]

Percutaneous thoracic duct embolization is an alternative technique and in some centers has changed the management of thoracic duct injuries. The key is opacification of the thoracic duct and percutaneous puncture of the duct in the abdomen. Once the thoracic duct has been accessed percutaneously, superselective catheterization of the duct requires use of a microcatheter and guidewire and experience in embolotherapy.[8,9]

The initial step is generally bipedal lymphangiography.[1-3] The technique is briefly outlined here. In some centers, only the lymphatics of the right foot are accessed. Recent developments include ultrasound-guided direct percutaneous puncture of lymph node(s) in the femoral regions. This latter technique may save time, but experience using this approach is anecdotal and limited. In terms of equipment, a lymphangiography injector, once standard equipment in interventional radiology suites, is no longer manufactured. Use of a handheld insufflator (used for angioplasty) will substitute. The goal of this procedure is to opacify the cisterna chyli or other dominant lymphatics in the abdomen.

EQUIPMENT

- Cutdown tray (with scalpels, forceps, hemostats, etc.)
- Adhesive strips (Steri-Strips)
- Lymphangiography needle(s) (Cook Medical, Bloomington, Ind.)
- Angioplasty insufflator(s)
- Lipiodol (Lipiodol Ultra-Fluide [Guerbet, Paris, France])

TECHNIQUE

Although there is some anecdotal evidence that injecting the right pedal lymphatics will provide better opacification of the abdominal lymphatic channels, at our institution the authors typically inject both feet to increase the probability of successful lymphatic opacification.

Initially, 0.1 to 0.2 mL of 1% methylene blue is injected into each interspace between the toes of both feet using a 1-mL syringe (Fig. 123-1). Patients should be warned that their feet may remain blue for days to weeks, and their urine will also develop a blue-green coloration. After waiting approximately 10 minutes to allow the dye to be taken up by the lymphatics, the dorsum of each foot is then anesthetized with 1% lidocaine. A curved blade is then used to make a shallow transverse incision (≈2.5 cm) across the dorsum of each foot, taking care to only cut the epidermis and the topmost layer of the dermis (Fig. 123-2).

The dermis is then carefully spread perpendicular to the incision using a blunt-tipped instrument such as a hemostat. Extreme care must be taken during this step, since lymphatic channels are very thin and easy to tear. Ideally, sufficient dye is taken up by the lymphatics to distend them slightly and give them a light blue–tinted appearance. The process can be helped along by "milking" the tissues upward from the toes toward the incision while simultaneously blocking lymphatic outflow by compressing the dorsum of the foot above the incision. The goal is to identify at least two to three lymphatic channels in each foot to increase the chances of successful cannulation.

Once a lymphatic channel is identified, an approximate 1.5-cm segment is carefully dissected away from surrounding tissues. The authors find it helpful to insert the flat back of small surgical forceps under the lymphatic vessel to assist with exposure, cleaning, and subsequent cannulation. The distal outflow portion of the vessel is secured with a very loose nonocclusive silk suture (e.g., 3-0 silk), which is then slightly tethered up and secured to the skin with Steri-Strips. Gentle traction of the suture will obstruct lymph outflow and ideally distend the vessel (Fig. 123-3). The proximal aspect of the isolated lymphatic is also tethered temporarily with a suture. A third suture is placed and is ready to be tied around the vessel and needle tip once the lymphatic vessel is cannulated. If required, this process may be repeated for each identified lymphatic vessel. Typically only one lymphatic vessel is injected per foot. Given the small size and fragility of peripheral lymphatic vessels and the technical difficulty of cannulation, it is advisable to isolate and prepare 2 or 3 channels per foot to optimize chances of success. Surgical dissection loops may be used to assist the operator during vessel dissection and cannulation.

One lymphatic channel in each foot is then carefully cannulated with a 30-gauge lymphangiogram needle (Cook Medical). The needle is attached to a catheter (cannula) with a hub. A small amount of saline should be injected through the needle to confirm the integrity of the cannulated vessel and appropriate placement of the needle tip within the lumen. If the needle tip is in the lumen, gentle injection of a small amount of saline with a 1-mL syringe

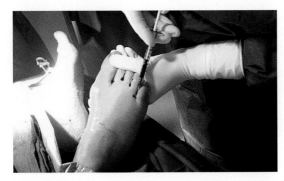

FIGURE 123-1. After sterile preparation of feet, 0.1 to 0.2 mL of 1% methylene blue are injected into each interspace between toes of both feet, using a 1-mL syringe.

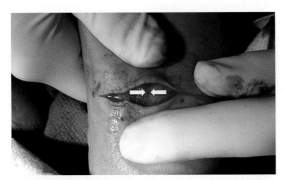

FIGURE 123-2. Transverse incision along dorsum of each foot is used to expose underlying lymphatics *(arrows)*.

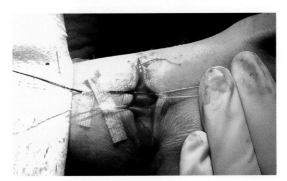

FIGURE 123-3. Lymphatics are elevated and secured with sutures and Steri-Strips.

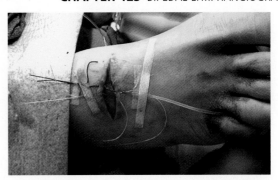

FIGURE 123-4. Lymphatic channel has been cannulated with 30-gauge lymphangiography needle. Suture is tightened around needle to secure it to lymphatic duct, and needle is fixed to skin with Steri-Strips.

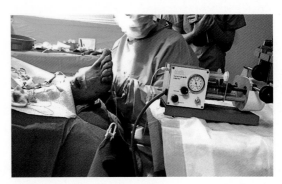

FIGURE 123-5. This image demonstrates completed setup for pedal lymphangiogram portion of procedure, including Cordis Lymphography Injector (Harvard Pump).

will visibly distend the lymphatic vessel. If the lymphatic vessel is disrupted, saline will leak, and the needle should be repositioned or another should be selected. Ideally, one lymphatic vessel per foot will be successfully cannulated. As mentioned earlier, in some centers, injection in only one foot may be sufficient. The suture tethering the distal portion of the duct should then be relaxed, and the knot of a preplaced suture tightened gently around the needle in the lymphatic vessel to hold the two in place (Fig. 123-4). The needle and attached catheter should then be secured to the patient's foot to stabilize it for the next phase of the procedure. We find that simply looping the catheter gently around a toe (e.g., great toe) plus a few adhesive strips (Steri-Strips) will provide sufficient stability.

If a lymphatic vessel in each foot has been successfully cannulated, two syringes with 10 mL of Lipiodol are

attached to the hub ends of the lymphangiography needles. Injection at our institution was initially performed with the aid of a dedicated lymphangiography pump (Harvard Pump) (Fig. 123-5). In addition to providing a slow and steady injection rate, the pump also heats the Lipiodol. As an alternative to the pump, an inflation device such as one used during percutaneous transluminal angioplasty (PTA) may be used. One inflation device should be attached to the end of each catheter hub and inflated to 2 to 4 atmospheres pressure. Pressure must be maintained for the duration of the contrast injection. The progress of Lipiodol up the lymphatics should be monitored with intermittent fluoroscopy (Fig. 123-6).

The cisterna chyli will eventually opacify, followed by the thoracic duct. One may only visualize segments of the thoracic duct in the abdomen as the oily iodinated contrast moves cephalad toward the chest. In the abdomen, the opacified thoracic duct is percutaneously punctured with a skinny needle (e.g., Chiba needle [Cook Medical]). Once the duct has been entered, a fine-caliber guidewire (e.g., 0.018 inches in diameter) is advanced. The needle is removed, and a microcatheter is advanced over the guidewire into the thoracic duct in the chest. If possible, the microcatheter tip is advanced superior to the leak to begin thoracic duct embolization. If the thoracic duct is completely disrupted, it may not be possible to catheterize the duct superior to the injury. If this is the case, begin occlusion at the upper end of the injured duct (see Chapter 124 for additional technical details). In the thorax, the duct may be occluded using a combination of microcoils, tissue adhesive (glue), or

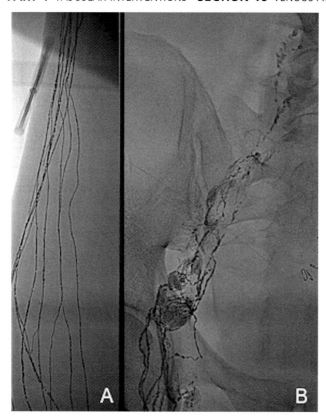

FIGURE 123-6. Lipiodol traveling up upper thigh lymphatics **(A)** and through iliac lymphatic chain **(B)**.

newer copolymer liquid agents (e.g., Onyx, Onyx Liquid Embolic System [Micro Therapeutics Inc./ev3 Neurovascular, Irvine, Calif.]).

The authors wish to thank Ms. Shundra Dinkins for her assistance in the preparation of the manuscript for this chapter.

KEY POINTS

- Massive chylous pleural effusions due to a thoracic duct injury may become life threatening.
- Lymphangiography serves as a means to identify lymphatic leaks and obstruction. In the setting of a thoracic duct leak (injury), the technique is used to opacify the thoracic duct. The thoracic duct may then be occluded using transcatheter embolotherapy techniques.
- Coils, tissue adhesive (i.e., glue), and newer polymers have been used to occlude the thoracic duct.

▸ **SUGGESTED READINGS**

Cerfolio RJ, Allen MS, Deschamps C, et al. Postoperative chylothorax. J Thorac Cardiovasc Surg 1996;112:1361–6.

Cope C, Kaiser LR. Management of unremitting chylothorax by percutaneous embolization and blockage of retroperitoneal lymphatic vessels in 42 patients. J Vasc Interv Radiol 2002;13:1139–48.

The complete reference list is available online at www.expertconsult.com.

CHAPTER 124

Thoracic Duct Embolization for Postoperative Chylothorax

Matthew P. Schenker, Chieh-Min Fan, and Richard A. Baum

The thoracic duct, a primary central common drainage pathway for the lymphatic system of the trunk and lower extremities, exists in close anatomic proximity to the esophagus. Roughly 0.5% to 2.0% of patients undergoing thoracic surgery, especially esophagectomy, will suffer iatrogenic thoracic duct disruption, an injury that can result in intractable high-volume chylous pleural effusions. The thoracic duct carries 2 to 4 liters of lymph daily, the major components of which include proteins, lipids, and lymphocytes. The clinical sequelae of persistent high-volume lymph loss can be severe and life threatening and include respiratory compromise, immune compromise, dehydration, and severe nutritional depletion. Unremitting chylous effusions can be associated with up to 50% mortality.[1] Conservative treatment with parenteral nutrition, cessation of oral intake, and pleural fluid drainage may help resolve some leaks, but these maneuvers are frequently unsuccessful. In one review of 11,315 patients undergoing thoracic surgery, 47 (0.42%) developed postoperative chylothorax, of which only 13 (27.7%) resolved with nonoperative treatment; the remaining 34 (72.3%) required reoperation. In this series, reoperation was associated with a mortality rate of 2.1% and a complication rate of 38.3%.[2] Recently, thoracic duct embolization (TDE) has been described as a minimally invasive treatment for persistent chylous effusions, either by direct thoracic duct cannulation and embolization (type 1) or cisterna chyli maceration (type 2).[3,4]

INDICATIONS

The primary indication for TDE is unremitting true chylous effusion in the clinical setting of suspected thoracic duct injury. Typical predisposing events include pulmonary or esophageal surgery or penetrating thoracic trauma. If lymph production can be minimized by restricting oral and fat intake, thoracic duct leaks with an output of less than 500 mL/day can sometimes heal spontaneously. However, the process can take 2 to 3 weeks, during which the patient may become nutritionally depleted, and many of these effusions may not ultimately resolve. The decision to proceed to intervention in chylous effusions of less than 500 mL/day depends on the clinical status of the patient, duration of the effusion, and daily output trends. Successful nonoperative management of chylous effusions with more than 500 mL/day output is questionable, and with more than 1000 mL/day output, unlikely. Accepted criteria for operative intervention include over 1000 mL chyle output per day for 48 hours, increasing output on conservative management over 5 days, and persistent chylothorax after 2 weeks of conservative management.[5]

Chylous effusions typically have a milky appearance and are categorized as either true chylous effusions or pseudochylous effusions. True chylous effusions can be confirmed by the presence of pleural fluid chylomicrons and/or a pleural fluid triglyceride level above 110 mg/dL. Causes of true chylous effusions include thoracic duct injury and lymphatic disruption by tumor (e.g., lymphoma). Pseudochylous effusions may have a milky appearance, but chemical analysis demonstrates cholesterol to be the dominant lipid component with triglyceride level less than 50 mg/dL and the absence of chylomicrons.[6] The most common causes of pseudochylous effusions include tuberculosis and rheumatoid disease. Pseudochylous effusions do not reflect thoracic duct disruption and are not an indication for TDE.

CONTRAINDICATIONS

Contraindications to TDE include absence of a true chylous effusion, chylothorax that is responding positively to conservative management, allergy to lymphangiographic contrast agents (methylene blue and ethiodized oil), and anatomic unsuitability. Some patients lack a distinct cisterna chyli or suitable upper lumbar lymphatic channel for cannulation. A completely retroaortic position may make the thoracic duct inaccessible to percutaneous cannulation. Prior low ligation of the thoracic duct limits the effectiveness of TDE, although embolization or maceration of the cisterna chyli may still be beneficial. Since passage of the needle and catheter through visceral organs cannot be avoided during TDE, bleeding diatheses and uncorrectable coagulopathies are contraindications as well.

EQUIPMENT

- 21- or 22-gauge 15- to 20-cm Chiba needle (Cook Medical Inc., Bloomington, Ind.)
- Stiff 0.018-inch 150-cm guidewire (V-18 Control Wire [Boston Scientific, Natick, Mass.])
- 4F inner dilator and stiffening cannula from a nonvascular access kit (MAK-NV Introducer System [Merit Medical Systems, South Jordan, Utah])
- Microcatheter (Slip-Cath 3F 80-cm Infusion Catheter [Cook Medical])
- Platinum-fibered microcoils (Nester Embolization Microcoils, 4- to 6-mm, 14-cm [Cook Medical])
- Liquid embolic adhesive (TRUFILL NBCA Liquid Embolic System [Codman & Shurtleff Inc., Raynham, Mass.])

TECHNIQUE

Anatomy and Approaches

The lymphatic system of the lower extremities coalesces in the pelvis with the internal and external iliac lymphatic chains. These in turn join the common iliac lymphatics and coalesce to join the paraaortic and paracaval lymphatic chains. At the level of T12-L2, the paraaortic and paracaval

907

chains join the intestinal trunk to form the cisterna chyli, a fusiform or saclike channel that is distinctly larger than the surrounding lymphatics and visible on lymphography in 80% of patients. In the majority of patients, the cisterna chyli is located to the right posterior aspect of the abdominal aorta. The thoracic duct arises from the cisterna chyli at its cephalad terminus and courses superiorly posterior to the esophagus and slightly right of midline in the lower thorax, crossing to left of midline around T5-T6. It continues cephalad to terminate variably in the region of confluence of the left subclavian and internal jugular veins. The thoracic duct can be a single-channel or multichannel structure, and 10% of patients will have a bilateral duplicated thoracic duct system.[7]

Thoracic duct embolization is a two-phase procedure. In the initial phase, pedal lymphangiography is performed to visualize the cisterna chyli or dominant upper lumbar lymphatics as potential cannulation targets. The cisterna chyli has a predilection for right-sided location in the upper abdomen, and in our experience, for the purposes of TDE, right-sided pedal lymphography results in more efficient and definitive visualization of the cisterna chyli than left-sided lymphography. Alternatively, direct inguinal lymph node injection can be performed to opacify the upper lumbar lymphatics and cisterna chyli. Intranodal lymphangiography allows for very rapid opacification of the lumbar lymphatics, but it requires sonographic guidance for needle placement in a suitable lymph node, which can be challenging in patients with anasarca or obese body habitus. Lastly, retrograde cannulation of the thoracic duct can be achieved by accessing the ostium of the thoracic duct near the left angulus venosus, using a 5F reverse curve or angled catheter and a coaxial microcatheter delivered from a left brachial or basilic vein approach. Of these three methods, the retrograde transvenous approach is the least reliable because of the primary difficulty of locating and seating a catheter in the ostium of the thoracic duct and the secondary difficulty of passing a wire and microcatheter through competent terminal valves.

The second phase of TDE involves cannulation and embolization of the thoracic duct, typically from a right anterior oblique transabdominal approach to avoid the aorta, although a right posterior oblique transhepatic approach is also feasible. If the thoracic duct cannot be cannulated, a secondary strategy of needle maceration and disruption of the cisterna chyli can be performed to divert chyle flow into the retroperitoneum. This results in decompression of the thoracic duct and promotes healing of the breach.

Technical Aspects

Preoperative Evaluation

Preprocedural mapping of the cisterna chyli is achieved with magnetic resonance imaging (MRI) using fat-suppressed, heavily T2-weighted imaging of the thoracolumbar region in coronal and axial planes to localize the cisterna chyli and relative positions of the right renal artery and aorta (Fig. 124-1). The primary objective of MRI is to assess surrounding anatomic structures to guide the needle trajectory. Absence of a distinct cisterna chyli on MRI does not preclude the possibility of visualizing a workable target on lymphangiography. Because thoracic duct access entails

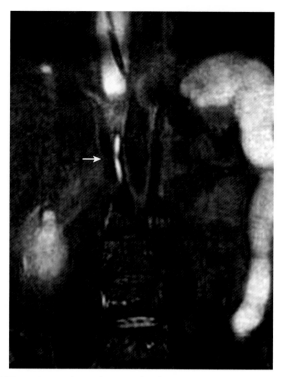

FIGURE 124-1. Coronal T2-weighted magnetic resonance image of abdomen shows periaortic location of a large fusiform cisterna chyli in upper abdomen *(arrow).*

deep retroperitoneal and periaortic penetration with potential transgression of visceral organs and bowel, the patient's coagulation profile should be checked and, if necessary, corrected to within normal limits before proceeding.

Thoracic Duct Access

After sterile prep of the upper abdomen, the cisterna chyli is identified fluoroscopically and accessed with a 21- or 22-gauge needle, usually from a 10- to 20-degree right anterior oblique approach to avoid the aorta (Fig. 124-2, *A*). Use of a "gun site" technique assists in accurate needle guidance into the deep retroperitoneal target (Fig. 124-2, *B*). Once the cisterna chyli has been punctured, a 0.018-inch guidewire is passed into the duct (Fig. 124-2, *C*), and the needle is exchanged for a microcatheter. Predilation with a 4F inner dilator and stiffening cannula from a nonvascular access kit can be employed if the microcatheter fails to track appropriately. Direct hand injection of iodinated contrast medium is performed to locate the site of thoracic duct injury (Fig. 124-3, *A*). The point of chyle extravasation and level of injury relative to the spine should be carefully documented with imaging. In the event the TDE is unsuccessful in resolving the chyle leak, precise localization of the site of duct injury will help guide subsequent surgical en bloc ligation. Given the potential for transintestinal passage of the access system, it is recommended that antibiotics for enteric organisms be administered intraprocedurally and that the access system be kept as small as possible, ideally 3F to 4F.

Embolization Procedure (Type 1 Thoracic Duct Embolization)

The microcatheter is positioned as close to the site of thoracic duct injury as possible, ideally bridging the point of

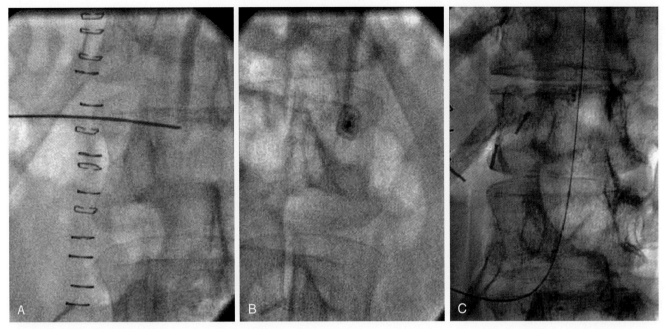

FIGURE 124-2. Radiograph shows step sequence of thoracic duct access. **A,** Right anterior oblique transabdominal approach with 21-gauge needle. **B,** "Gun sight" alignment of needle hub over cisterna chyli. **C,** Wire access into thoracic duct.

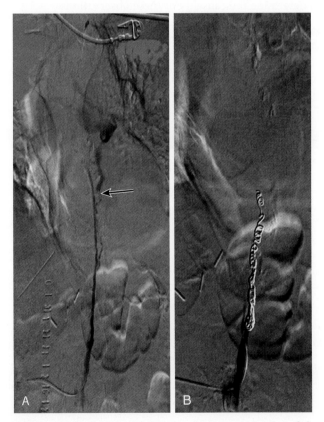

FIGURE 124-3. Thoracic duct injection demonstrates location of duct injury and leakage **(A)** and successful occlusion of leak site with coil embolization **(B).**

extravasation. Coil embolization is then performed using 4- to 6-mm-diameter coils along the entire length of the thoracic duct to within 2 cm of the entry site (see Fig. 124-3, *B*). As the final embolization step, a 2:1 mixture of ethiodized oil and *N*-butyl cyanoacrylate (NBCA) with 0.5

to 1 g of tantalum powder (components included in TRUFILL Liquid Embolic System) is injected to seal off the lower thoracic duct and entry site.

Needle Disruption of Lymphatics (Type 2 Thoracic Duct Embolization)

If the thoracic duct cannot be successfully cannulated, intentional disruption of the cisterna chyli and adjacent lymphatics is performed with serial needle passes. Macerating the cisterna chyli results in decompression of the thoracic duct into the retroperitoneal space (Figs. 124-4 and 124-5), allowing the intrathoracic leak to heal.

CONTROVERSIES

A brief discussion of controversies associated with this procedure is available at www.expertconsult.com.

OUTCOMES

The discussion of postprocedure outcomes can be found at www.expertconsult.com.

COMPLICATIONS

Standard complications of lymphography include permanent tattooing of the foot dermis, Ethiodol-related pulmonary complications including hypoxia and chemical pneumonitis, allergic reaction or anaphylaxis to contrast agents including Ethiodol and methylene blue, wound infection, and persistent lymph leak. As with all embolization procedures, nontarget embolization is a potential complication of TDE, including pulmonary embolism with liquid embolic agent. Although the transabdominal approach likely entails transintestinal or transorgan passage of the cannulation system, to date there are no reports of significant complications directly related to this approach.

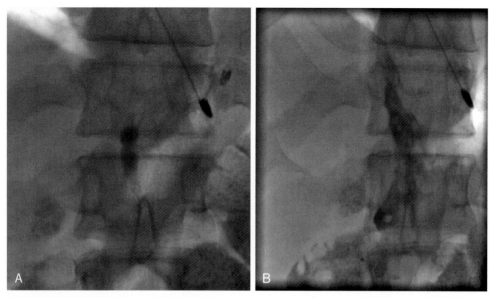

FIGURE 124-4. Radiographs demonstrate appearance of cisterna chyli before needle maceration **(A)** and after needle maceration with extravasation of Ethiodol into retroperitoneum **(B)**.

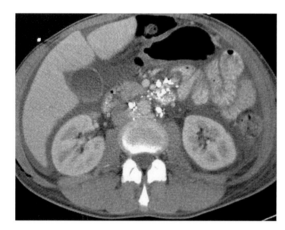

FIGURE 124-5. Axial computed tomography image shows high-density ethiodized oil droplets in retroperitoneum after type 2 thoracic duct embolization.

Delayed complications related to TDE have not been conclusively demonstrated, but the potential exists, given the intentional redistribution of lymphatic flow induced by the procedure. Intractable chylous ascites and peripheral lymphedema are known possible long-term complications of surgical thoracic duct ligation, and protein-losing enteropathy has been induced in dogs after thoracic duct ligation.[10-13] In a contemporary retrospective survey of 169 patients who underwent TDE for symptomatic chylous effusion, several instances of chronic leg swelling, abdominal swelling without evidence of anasarca or ascites, and chronic diarrhea were felt to be "probably related" to the procedure (14.3% overall).[14] A prospective study is needed to determine the causality of these observations.

POSTPROCEDURAL AND FOLLOW-UP CARE

A discussion of postprocedural and follow-up care is available at www.expertconsult.com.

KEY POINTS
• Postoperative high-volume chylothorax is an uncommon but serious complication of thoracic surgery that is associated with high morbidity and high mortality if untreated.
• Percutaneous thoracic duct embolization (TDE) is a minimally invasive method of resolving postoperative chylothorax without reoperation.
• TDE is a safe technique associated with minimal morbidity, despite transabdominal passage of the cannulation system.

▶ SUGGESTED READINGS

Cerfolio RJ, Allen MS, Deschamps C, et al. Postoperative chylothorax. J Thorac Cardiovasc Surg 1996;112:1361–6.

Cope C, Kaiser LR. Management of unremitting chylothorax by percutaneous embolization and blockage of retroperitoneal lymphatic vessels in 42 patients. J Vasc Interv Radiol 2002;13:1139–48.

The complete reference list is available online at www.expertconsult.com.

CHAPTER **125**

Biopsy Devices

Joseph M. Stavas

CLINICAL RELEVANCE

Percutaneous biopsy has become one of the most commonly performed image-guided interventional procedures in radiology practice today. With refinement in imaging guidance, biopsy devices, and techniques, previously inaccessible and difficult-to-biopsy lesions are now routinely diagnosed. Paralleling the advances in image guidance has been the development of histopathologic, cytopathologic, and immunologic stains to further characterize tissue specimens. The minimally invasive nature of current outpatient biopsy techniques allows rapid diagnosis and formulation of treatment plans. Collaboration with cytopathology and histopathology departments is useful to determine the most optimum needle choice for improved tissue adequacy and diagnosis, and can provide valuable quality assurance feedback.

SOFT-TISSUE BIOPSY DEVICES

The various devices used for soft-tissue biopsy of abdominal, thoracic, and other lesions can be classified on the basis of sampling mechanisms and needle tip configurations. Such devices include aspiration needles and small and large cutting core biopsy needles.[1] Selection of biopsy device is based on patient history, location of the lesion, imaging appearance of the mass, intended trajectory of the needle, and importantly, the type of information sought from the pathologic sample. Coagulation status, proximity to vital structures, and expertise of the radiologist also play a role in needle selection. These needles can be used alone or coaxially with guide needles when multiple specimens are needed.

Needle size is typically designated by gauge, whereby the larger the gauge number, the smaller the needle size. An 18-gauge needle is approximately 0.05 inches or 1.27 mm in outside diameter (OD), and a 22-gauge needle is 0.028 inches and 0.77 mm in OD. Histologic diagnosis can be ascertained in most situations with an 18- to 20-gauge biopsy needle.

Aspiration Needles

Aspiration needles are the most frequently used biopsy needles to obtain samples primarily for cytologic analysis.

They are commonly used by both radiologists and clinicians and include the spinal needle and the Chiba needle (Figs. 125-1 and 125-2). These needles are simple smaller-gauge beveled needles that have a noncutting edge.

The Chiba needle is a thin-walled straight needle with a beveled tip angle of 30 degrees as described originally.[2] It is made of stainless steel, has a removable stylet, and is available in 18- to 25-gauge sizes (Cook Medical, Bloomington, Ind.). When compared with Chiba needles, spinal needles have a smaller inner lumen and thicker wall, which makes them easier to control than a comparable gauge Chiba needle. They are also available in multiple sizes. The mechanism of sampling with aspiration needles is rapid to-and-fro movement with simultaneous rotation in the tissue/lesion and the application of suction with a syringe. This motion is continued for a maximum of 10 passes or until blood is obtained in the needle hub. Suction with the syringe is released as the needle is withdrawn to obtain material for cytologic examination. A variety of techniques and devices developed to help aspirate specimens in the needle are available but offer no significant advantage over manual aspiration.[3]

The vanSonnenberg needle set (Cook Medical) has a trocar point introducer needle with a removable hub, an outer cannula, and a 30-degree beveled-tip biopsy needle. A 23-gauge needle with a removable hub is used for a modified coaxial biopsy technique. The needle is useful for biopsy of small (≤2.5 cm) and difficult chest or abdominal lesions near vital structures. After removal of the hub, coaxial insertion of an outer 19-gauge needle is performed. Cutting biopsy or aspirated specimens are obtained coaxially through the 19-gauge needle after the hubless needle is removed. This system allows improved precision for smaller lesions, for which the tandem biopsy technique is not practical.[4]

Cutting Needles

Cutting biopsy needles are specifically designed to provide samples for histologic analysis. These needles remove small pieces of target tissue (0.1-0.4 mm and under) rather than cells. The various cutting mechanisms include end-cutting and side-cutting needles. Side-cutting needles generally work best with soft-tissue masses, whereas end-cutting needles do well in more solid lesions.[1]

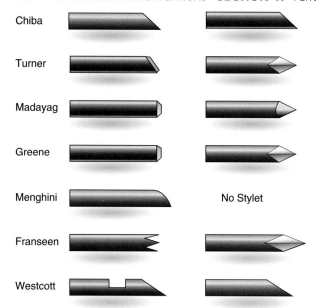

FIGURE 125-1. Biopsy needle tip and stylet configurations.

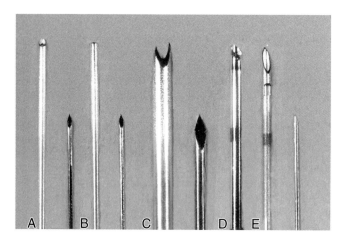

FIGURE 125-2. Biopsy needles with stylets. **A,** Chiba needle. **B,** Greene needle. **C,** Franseen needle. **D,** Menghini needle. **E,** Westcott needle.

End-cutting needles are basically aspiration needles with sharpened cutting tips and varying bevel angles and stylet configurations (see Figs. 125-1 and 125-2). The simplest of these is the Menghini-type needle (Cardinal Health, Woodstock, Ill.), an end-cutting device that has a sharpened beveled convex tip angled at 45 degrees.[5] This configuration cuts out a cylinder of tissue on forward movement of the needle, without any rotation.

The Turner needle (Cook Medical) has a circumferentially sharpened beveled tip with an angle of 45 degrees. When advanced and rotated in conjunction with suction through a syringe, the tip obtains an excellent core of tissue with minimal trauma.[6] The Franseen needle (Cook Medical) is a trocar-point needle with three sharp bevels at the tip that act like cutting teeth once the inner stylet is withdrawn and the needle is rotated.[7]

The Madayag (Popper & Sons, New York, N.Y.) and the Greene (Cook Medical) needles have a sharpened 90-degree

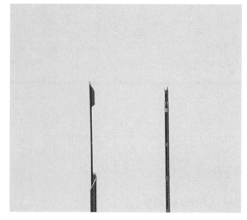

FIGURE 125-3. Side-cutting Tru-Cut biopsy needle *(left)* and end-cutting BioPince biopsy needle *(right)*.

beveled tip with different stylet configurations. The Madayag needle has a conical stylet, whereas the Greene needle has a faceted stylet.[8]

The Westcott needle (Becton-Dickinson, Franklin Lakes, N.J.) is a modified side- and end-cutting needle with a slot measuring 2.2 mm in length located 3 mm from the tip of the needle. The slot creates a cutting edge in addition to the needle tip and enables aspiration of larger amounts of biopsy tissue.[9]

One of the most commonly used needles for core biopsy today is the Tru-Cut needle (Baxter Healthcare, Deerfield, Ill.). It is a side-cutting needle that consists of an outer cutting cannula and an inner slotted stylet (Fig. 125-3). After insertion of the needle tip to the edge of the tissue to be sampled, the inner slotted stylet is advanced and followed by the outer cutting cannula, which slices a piece of the tissue being sampled (Fig. 125-4). The throw of the stylet and slot length (and thus sample size) vary from 17 to 23 mm, depending on various vendors. The needle comes in manual and spring-loaded semiautomated and fully automated configurations (Fig. 125-5). Automated biopsy devices offer a semiautomated or fully automated loading and deployment spring-activated mechanism for side-cutting and end-cutting needles. Automated Tru-Cut–style needles include the ASAP biopsy needle (Medi-Tech/ Boston Scientific, Natick, Mass.) and the Max-Core (C.R. Bard Inc., Tempe, Ariz.). Reusable fully automated side cut-type biopsy devices that are used with disposable needles are also available.

The BioPince full-core biopsy needle (Inter-V, Gainesville, Fla.) is an automated end-cutting needle (see Fig. 125-3). It has a variable throw length of 13, 23, and 33 mm, which yields a specimen length of 9, 19, and 29 mm, respectively. The biopsy specimen obtained is a full cylindrical core, unlike side-cutting devices, which obtain a semi-cylindrical specimen (Figs. 125-6 and 125-7).

COMPARISON OF BIOPSY DEVICES

Several reports comparing cutting and aspiration needles have been published. Before imaging guidance was used for biopsy of lesions, comparisons of different biopsy devices were based on blind techniques, which thus had the potential error of biopsy of a nontarget area. Now, with

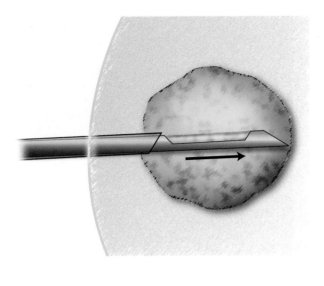

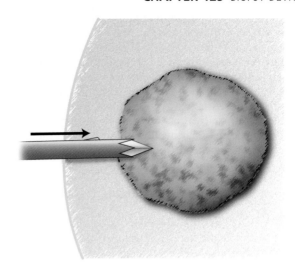

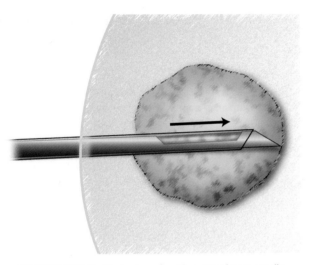

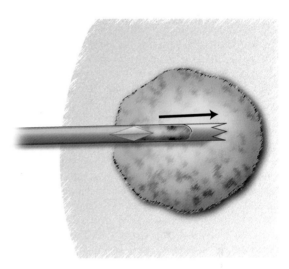

FIGURE 125-4. Mechanism of a side-cutting biopsy needle.

FIGURE 125-6. Mechanism of an automated end-cutting biopsy needle.

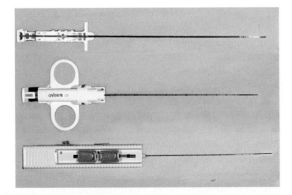

FIGURE 125-5. Side-cutting needles: manual *(top)*, semiautomated *(middle)*, and automated *(bottom)*.

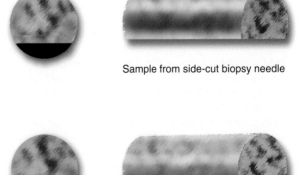

Sample from side-cut biopsy needle

Sample from end-cut biopsy needle

FIGURE 125-7. Comparison of specimens obtained from side-cutting and end-cutting needles.

ultrasound and computed tomography (CT) being used for biopsy of even diffuse disease processes, comparison of various needle types is easier. However, with a variety of new devices being introduced at regular intervals and non-uniform availability of various devices in different parts of the world, a comprehensive comparison of biopsy devices is not feasible. Key biopsy device factors are cost, size, type, and the false-negative rate of samples obtained. Ongoing quality assurance of various organ biopsies in conjunction with the pathology department will allow a radiology practice to decide the most practical biopsy needle inventory.

Aspiration Needle versus Cutting Needle

Selection of a biopsy needle is generally guided by familiarity of the radiologist with the various needle types and the tissue being sampled. The size and design of the needle in addition to the biopsy technique and nature of the tissue are important factors contributing to the amount and quality of tissue retrieved.[10] The thin noncutting aspiration needles are the safest devices available for biopsy, although their use has been associated with complications.[1,11] Cutting needles are generally superior to aspiration needles and offer increased diagnostic accuracy with no significant difference in complication rates.[1,12,13] In general, complication rates with the various biopsy devices have been reduced significantly because of improved imaging localization and procedure techniques and are currently less than 1%.

Fine-needle aspiration biopsy has high cancer-specific diagnostic accuracy, but the accuracy of cancer-negative diagnoses is generally much lower. Moreover, diagnosis of the cancer cell type is also sometimes difficult to assess, such as with poorly differentiated cancer and lymphoma. The advantage of aspiration needles lies in the minimal tissue disruption they cause. They primarily divide tissue planes rather than severing tissue.[14] Increased gauge and decreased bevel angle increase the diagnostic yield, and larger Chiba needles have a higher yield than similar smaller needles.[10,15] With the collaboration of a cytopathologist during biopsy, however, fine-needle aspiration biopsy has diagnostic rates and accuracy comparable to that achieved with larger needles.[16] The smaller-gauge needles can be used to traverse bowel or vessels safely without significantly increasing the risk of complications, but they are more flexible and thus more difficult to control when used for biopsy of deep-seated small lesions. Complications commonly occur when multiple needle passes are made or when used for biopsy of vascular lesions. Bleeding is one of the most frequent complications with larger-gauge needles (≥16 gauge); such needles are associated with greater bleeding than 18-gauge or smaller needles even in patients taking anticoagulants.[14]

Cutting needles have been recommended for biopsy of lesions with an unknown primary, evaluation of suspected benign disease, biopsy of possible second primary cancer, suspected lymphoma, and biopsy after nondiagnostic fine-needle aspiration.[1] Cutting needles with a larger caliber obtain more tissue than smaller needles and are safe to use because fewer passes are required to obtain the same amount of diagnostic tissue.[17] Low overall complication rates are seen with their use in the abdomen, and complication rates are higher with biopsy of the adrenal gland and pancreas than with biopsy of the liver.[18] Under CT

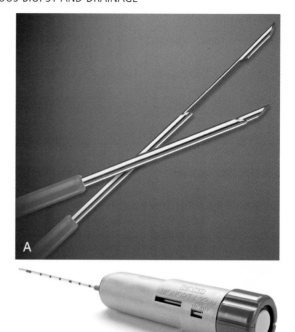

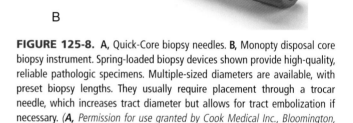

FIGURE 125-8. **A,** Quick-Core biopsy needles. **B,** Monopty disposal core biopsy instrument. Spring-loaded biopsy devices shown provide high-quality, reliable pathologic specimens. Multiple-sized diameters are available, with preset biopsy lengths. They usually require placement through a trocar needle, which increases tract diameter but allows for tract embolization if necessary. (**A,** Permission for use granted by Cook Medical Inc., Bloomington, Ind.; **B** courtesy Bard Biopsy Systems, Tempe, Ariz.)

guidance, the yield of diagnostic tissue is higher with cutting needles, with no significant increase in complication rates over aspiration biopsy needles, even when larger needles are used.[13]

Manual versus Automated Devices

Automated biopsy devices are easy to use and reliable and provide a specimen for histologic analysis that is equal to or better than that obtained with manual needles. Automated biopsy devices are spring levered and require cocking a firing mechanism before use. They provide a simplified and standardized biopsy technique that eliminates operator experience as a variable and provide higher-quality and more intact cores than manual techniques.[19,20] The biopsy motion is quick, with little needle movement during the biopsy. The number of passes and thus procedure time are also shortened. Various cutting trough lengths are available to customize the depth of tissue obtained. Common automated devices currently available are Quick-Core (Cook Medical) and Monopty (C.R. Bard [Fig. 125-8]).

Side-Cutting versus End-Cutting Devices

The side-cutting Tru-Cut needle obtains samples in a side notch on a trocar. In comparison, the automated end-cutting (BioPince) needle has two cannulas, and the sample is obtained with a strong forward stroke of the cutting cannula. Thicker biopsy specimens with a circular cross section are obtained with end-cutting needles, which allows flatter embedding of specimens in paraffin blocks for histopathologic evaluation than is the case with side-cutting needles (see Fig. 125-7). The greater stroke length also provides a longer specimen with higher weight and weight/length ratios.[21] The side-cutting needle is limited in the potential length of the side notch, inasmuch as longer notch and stroke lengths are associated with a risk of the outer cannula hitting the notch when advanced and thus getting stuck in the tissue in the notch. "Zero biopsy" or high failure of the end-cutting device is a major drawback, especially at shorter throw lengths.[21,22] At longer throw lengths, the failure rate is significantly higher than with side-cutting–type needles.[21,22] However, when zero biopsies are excluded, end-cutting biopsy devices obtain a core of tissue of equivalent quality.[23] Fragmentation rates of samples obtained with end-cutting needles are significantly lower, although some authors have found comparable rates for both devices.[22,24]

BREAST BIOPSY DEVICES

Image-guided biopsy of palpable and nonpalpable lesions of the breast has undergone rapid advances in the past decade or so. In fact, percutaneous image-guided breast biopsy has become the standard of care in most communities because it is faster, less invasive, and less expensive than surgical biopsy and can obviate the need for surgery in women, since most biopsies represent benign disease. Rapid development of breast biopsy devices has contributed enormously to this change. A wide array of needles and biopsy devices are now available for breast biopsy under ultrasound or stereotactic guidance. Fine-needle aspiration of solid breast lesions has given way to core biopsies with automated and vacuum-assisted devices at most institutions because of vastly improved sampling with the latter and limitation of fine-needle aspiration to cysts and other fluid collections.[25] Automated large-core coaxial biopsy of the breast with a long-throw (2.3-cm), 14-gauge needle to obtain a minimum of five specimens yields increased diagnostic accuracy, especially for microcalcification clusters.[26,27] Large-core biopsy devices, however, can underestimate disease (e.g., atypical ductal hyperplasia at needle biopsy and carcinoma at open surgery).[25] Directional vacuum-assisted breast biopsy devices and image-guided single-cylinder excision devices (ABBI System, United States Surgical, Norwalk, Conn.) are the most recent innovations in the field of imaging-assisted breast biopsy that provide larger biopsy tissue samples. The more commonly used vacuum-assisted breast biopsy devices include the Mammotome System (Ethicon Endo-surgery, Cincinnati, Ohio) and the ATEC (automated tissue excision and collection) System (Suros Surgical Systems, Indianapolis, Ind.). The Mammotome biopsy needle probe is a single-insertion device that initially draws tissue into an aperture at its distal end with the help of vacuum. A rotating cutter then advances over the tissue and cuts a core from the breast, and continued vacuum suction withdraws the sample without the need to remove the needle probe from the breast. Multiple sequential specimens around the probe can be obtained by rotating the probe 360 degrees. The specimens are larger than those obtained with 14-gauge automated needles, and more

accurate characterization of lesions is possible, with lower underestimation of disease.[25] These devices can be used with ultrasound, stereotactic, and MRI guidance.

MUSCULOSKELETAL BIOPSY DEVICES

The choice of biopsy device for use in musculoskeletal biopsy procedures depends on the location (soft tissue or bone) and type of lesion (osteolytic or osteoblastic). Routinely, these procedures are now performed under CT or fluoroscopic guidance. Trephine needles are commonly used for bone lesions.[28] These large-gauge needles have a serrated or sawtoothed cutting edge and include the Ackermann needle (Becton-Dickinson), Turkel needle (Turkel Instruments, Southfield, Mich.) and the Franseen needle (Cook Medical). An outer cannula with a blunt obturator is introduced through the soft tissue, followed by coaxial introduction of the trephine to harvest biopsy material. Suction is not usually required during biopsy or removal of the needle. For biopsy of lytic lesions with an intact cortex, a window is made in the overlying cortex with a cannula, and an aspiration or cutting needle is coaxially introduced for the biopsy (Bonopty Coaxial Biopsy System [RADI Medical Systems Inc., Wilmington, Mass.], Osteo-Site Bone Biopsy Needle Set [Cook Medical]). The Bonopty bone biopsy system consists of an outer cannula with a stylet and an eccentric drill that is introduced through the cannula, cuts a hole in the intact bone, and helps position the outer cannula. Cutting needles for bone biopsy include the Jamshidi needle (CareFusion Corp., San Diego, Calif.) and the Ostycut (C.R. Bard). The Ostycut needle has a threaded cutting cannula with a trocar point stylet. The needle can be attached to a hand grip. When dense ossification is present, a lightweight hammer or hand drill can be useful to obtain access to the biopsy site. The pathology laboratory should be alerted so a decalcification marrow aspirate is performed. For soft-tissue neoplasms, a 20-gauge or larger side-cutting Tru-Cut biopsy needle (Baxter Health Care) is used. Besides the aforementioned, multiple needle configurations are available, each with its own advantages and disadvantages.[29]

TRANSVENOUS BIOPSY DEVICES

Transvenous biopsy is a commonly performed procedure for evaluation of liver disease when there is a contraindication to direct percutaneous image-guided biopsy (e.g., uncorrectable coagulopathy, ascites, renal failure, obesity). Transvenous biopsy can also be performed for intravenous tumors and evaluation of renal disease. The biopsy is performed under fluoroscopic guidance, preferably from the right internal jugular vein, but the left internal jugular vein can also be used safely. Biopsy devices available include aspiration biopsy needle sets, semiautomated Tru-Cut–type core biopsy needle sets, and biopsy forceps (Fig. 125-9). The Tru-Cut–style devices, Quick-Core (Cook Medical) and Flexcore (Dextera Surgical, Franklin, Ind.) liver access and biopsy sets, consist of 18-gauge, 60-cm-long semiautomated side-cutting needles with a 20-mm throw that is introduced through a 7F introducer sheath and a stiffening directional cannula after accessing the right hepatic vein. With the semiautomated biopsy needle device, the whole procedure is shorter and easier, and fewer passes

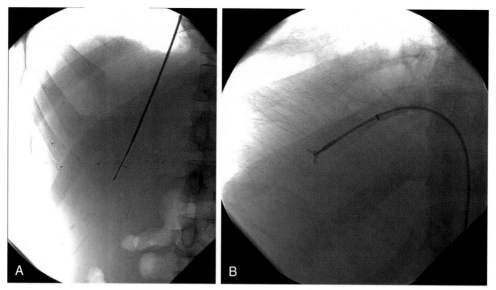

FIGURE 125-9. Transvenous biopsy. **A,** Liver biopsy with a side-cutting needle via internal jugular route. **B,** Forceps biopsy of liver via transfemoral route.

are required to obtain adequate material than is the case with aspiration needle biopsy.[30] The lesser fragmentation of tissue, especially in cirrhotic livers, results in significantly higher rates of definite histologic diagnosis. Sample adequacy, however, and overall complication rates are similar with both needles.[31] Perforation of the liver capsule is the most common complication.[32] Biopsy failure with either device is minimal and usually due to difficult catheterization in patients with an acutely angled hepatic vein as a result of acute angulation with the inferior vena cava or in liver transplant patients.

Transjugular renal biopsy can also be performed in a similar manner with aspiration needle and side-cutting biopsy devices. These biopsies are usually performed in patients with uncontrolled hypertension, bleeding disorders, morbid obesity, and small kidneys. The right vein is anatomically favorable for this manner of biopsy. The Mal transjugular renal biopsy set (Cook Europe, Bjaeverskov, Denmark) has a 16-gauge, 63.8-cm needle with a reverse bevel of 45 degrees. It is a modification of the Colapinto liver biopsy set. The biopsy sample is obtained via the Menghini technique once the catheter is advanced into a peripheral cortical vein of the lower pole of the right kidney. The yield of tissue and the incidence of major complications with this device have been similar to the yield and complications with percutaneous biopsy devices.[33] Potential complications include perforation of the renal capsule, with perirenal hematoma and hematuria. The renal capsule may be thin and the risk of capsular perforation higher than during liver biopsy. Having a pathologist available to stain the specimens may reduce the number of passes if adequate glomeruli are present.

A side-cutting biopsy needle for transjugular renal biopsy, similar to the one used for transjugular liver biopsy, is also available. The renal access and biopsy set (Cook Medical) has a 19-gauge, 70-cm-long Tru-Cut–type semi-automated needle with a blunt tip to prevent perforation of the renal capsule. In addition, the directional cannula has decreased curvature in comparison to the hepatic biopsy set. The needle throw length is 2 cm. The modified set is

associated with a low incidence of capsular penetration and is thus safe to use.[34]

Transvenous biopsy of the liver or biopsy of intravascular tumors can also be performed with flexible endocardial biopsy forceps (Medi-Tech).[35] This device has oval-shaped serrated cutting jaws. Once the position of the introducing sheath is secured, the tip of the biopsy forceps is placed distal to the tip of the sheath, followed by opening of the jaws. The biopsy forceps are then advanced and wedged into the hepatic parenchyma or tumor, and a bite is obtained by closing the jaws. The biopsy forceps are especially useful for liver biopsy in patients with thrombosed internal jugular veins because they are routinely used via the transfemoral route.

PLEURAL BIOPSY DEVICES

The pleural biopsy needles developed initially were used for untargeted or closed biopsy of the parietal pleura in patients with pleural effusion. Such biopsy needles include the Cope and Abrams needles.[36,37] They have a notch near their tips, and the cutting edge of these needles is used to snag the pleura after introduction of the needle assembly. With the advent of image-guided biopsy, there was an increase in the diagnostic yield of pleural biopsy with these devices. Now, automated biopsy devices are routinely used for sampling of focal pleural-based masses under CT or ultrasound guidance. In patients in whom no focal lesion can be identified, biopsy with an Abrams or Cope needle can be performed.[38]

MAGNETIC RESONANCE IMAGING–COMPATIBLE BIOPSY DEVICES

Interventional MRI is a rapidly growing field with a wide array of procedures now being performed with MRI-compatible instruments, albeit at select institutions. As continued experience is gained, there will be growth in MRI-guided procedures. Most of the biopsy devices used in conventional interventional procedures are not compatible for MRI-guided interventions because of safety concerns and degradation of image quality. Theoretically, the ideal material for MRI-guided procedures should have similar magnetic susceptibility as the human body. Unlike stainless steel, nonferromagnetic material such as titanium alloys produce minor local image artifacts, estimated at roughly twice the size of the needle.[39] Titanium alloys are the most commonly used material for manufacturing biopsy needles. The appearance and feel of a titanium needle, however, are different from a stainless steel needle. It is soft and pliable, the products cannot be made sharp enough, and moreover, titanium does not traverse tissue freely. Overall needle performance is not as good as with a normal steel needle.[40]

MRI-assisted biopsy is now gaining popularity, particularly for musculoskeletal, retroperitoneal, breast, and liver lesions that can be detected and visualized only by contrast-enhanced MRI. The choice of MRI-compatible needles includes the Chiba and spinal aspiration biopsy needles (Cook Medical), side-cutting core biopsy needles, and coaxial introducer and bone biopsy sets (Invivo Corp., Pewaukee, Wis., and E-Z-EM, Lake Success, N.Y.), as well as the MRI-compatible vacuum-assisted breast biopsy devices (Mammotome and ATEC Systems).

"TREATED NEEDLES"

Ultrasound-guided needle biopsy has gained widespread popularity because of real-time imaging combined with easy availability, low cost, and lack of ionizing radiation when compared with CT guidance. However, one of the major limitations of ultrasound-guided biopsy has been inadequate visualization of the biopsy needle, especially with small lesions at increased depth. Tissues with increased echogenicity, as well as target lesions with a limited window of access or overlying air or bone, pose additional problems for needle visualization. Poor angle of insonation and smaller gauge also compromise the echogenicity and thus the visualization of needles. Not only does adequate visualization of the biopsy needle during the procedure help in precise placement of the needle in the area of interest, it also serves to avoid small structures such as blood vessels in the needle tract and hence decreases procedure-related complications. Indirect improvement in visibility of the needle tip can be achieved with manual shaking of the needle, pumping air bubbles from the tip of the needle by in-and-out movement of the stylet, or tiny injections of lidocaine or saline that contains microbubbles. Despite needle improvements, a high-quality ultrasound machine is necessary to optimize visualization of the biopsy device.

To circumvent some of the aforementioned issues during ultrasound-guided biopsy, some newer biopsy needle innovations have focused on improving needle visibility. The more common modifications include Teflon-coated, dimpled, and etched-tip needles (Cook Medical), echogenic polymer-coated needles (Echo-Coat [STS Biopolymers Inc., Hernietta, N.Y.]), and the screw-tipped stylet needle (Inrad, Grand Rapids, Mich.). These modifications either create a more reflective surface for the sound waves or trap microbubbles of air, thus improving needle visibility. The etched-tip needle is a low-cost modification with the dimpling limited to the distal 6 mm of the needle. Coated needles, on the other hand, have the whole shaft coated

with Teflon or biopolymer and are usually better seen than etched-tip needles, particularly at small angles of insonation. In dense tissue, in addition to improved echogenicity, there is increased shadowing from the coated needle shaft, which aids visualization.[41] Coated needles, however, do loose their echogenicity significantly with time when compared with uncoated needles, presumably because of resorption of the microbubbles by surrounding fluid when used during biopsy. Of the Teflon-coated and biopolymer-coated needles, subjective visualization of the latter has been described as better. No difference has been observed in the diagnostic yield rates of untreated and treated needles, but better visualization of treated needles during ultrasound-guided biopsy may result in fewer needle passes and thus reduced procedure time and morbidity.[42]

KEY POINTS

- Image-guided biopsy allows safe and rapid diagnosis of disease processes.
- The Chiba needle is one of the safest biopsy needles.
- Biopsy indication may determine needle type and size.
- Collaboration with the pathology department to determine tissue adequacy may impact choice of biopsy needle and assist in practice quality improvement.
- Aspiration needle biopsy has high cancer-specific diagnostic accuracy, but the accuracy of a negative cancer diagnosis is much lower.
- Cutting needles have increased diagnostic accuracy with no significant increase in complication rates over aspiration needles.
- Automated biopsy devices provide a standardized biopsy technique, and specimens for histologic analysis are equal or better in quality than those obtained with manual devices.
- Automated end-cutting needles provide a full cylindrical core specimen with lower fragmentation rates but a higher failure rate than with side-cutting needles.
- Transvenous biopsy devices for liver and renal biopsy have diagnostic accuracy and complication rates similar to percutaneous biopsy devices.
- Magnetic resonance imaging–compatible biopsy devices are made of titanium alloys.

▶ **SUGGESTED READINGS**

Gazelle GS, Haaga JR. Biopsy needle characteristics. Cardiovasc Intervent Radiol 1991;14:13–6.

Gupta S. New techniques in image guided percutaneous biopsy. Cardiovasc Intervent Radiol 2004;27:91–104.

Haaga JR. Image-guided micro procedures: CT and MRI interventional procedures. In: Haaga JR, Lanzieri CF, Gilkeson RC, editors. CT and MR imaging of the whole body. 4th ed. St. Louis: CV Mosby; 2003.

Schulz T, Puccini S, Schneider JP, Kahn T. Interventional and intraoperative MR: review and update of techniques and clinical experience. Eur Radiol 2004;14:2212–27.

The complete reference list is available online at www.expertconsult.com.

CHAPTER 126

Percutaneous Biopsy

Sudhen B. Desai, Robert J. Lewandowski, and Albert A. Nemcek, Jr.

The clinical relevance of biopsy results must be considered before performing a procedure, but numerous patients undergo biopsy before definitive clinical evaluation. Therefore, biopsy results may dramatically alter the future workup of these patients.

Not all radiographic findings merit biopsy. The interventionalist must have awareness and understanding of the radiologic findings of normal variants, "pseudolesions," and insignificant manifestations of pathology (e.g., focal fatty infiltration of the liver, simple renal cysts, hepatic hemangiomas). This avoids unnecessary interventions that are costly and potentially dangerous. It should also be established that less invasive means of establishing a confident diagnosis are unavailable or were previously unsuccessful in establishing a diagnosis, and no other potential biopsy sites that may be safer or easier to access are an option. Finally, there should be a discernible advantage to imaging guidance for accessing the target biopsy site.

INDICATIONS

Indications for percutaneous biopsy are to (1) establish a malignant diagnosis, (2) establish a benign diagnosis, and (3) obtain material for culture or other laboratory studies. Departmental review of patient selection should be undertaken if less than 95% of image-guided percutaneous biopsies are being performed for these three indications.[1] Additionally, it should be requisite that plans for treatment or further investigation will be strongly influenced by the biopsy results.

CONTRAINDICATIONS

Absolute contraindications to biopsy of a lesion include severe uncorrectable coagulopathy and a patient's inability to cooperate.

Relative contraindications to biopsy of a lesion include:
- Coagulopathy (prothrombin time > 15 seconds; platelets < 50,000; patient not withdrawn from anticoagulation for a safe period, e.g., 4 hours for heparin and 7 days for warfarin [Coumadin], clopidogrel [Plavix], and nonsteroidal antiinflammatory drugs [NSAIDs])
- Unsafe target for biopsy (e.g., highly vascular tumor)
- Absence of a safe pathway from the skin to the target site. Consideration should be given to use of other imaging modalities (e.g., ultrasound vs. computed tomography [CT] guidance) or other sites of access (e.g., percutaneous vs. transjugular hepatic biopsy).

Although gross ascites is frequently suggested as a contraindication, there is remarkably little evidence that ascites in the absence of coagulopathy increases the risk related to percutaneous biopsy of abdominal lesions.

TECHNIQUE

Before image-guided biopsy is performed, certain clinical considerations must be entertained. Basic issues such as the initial complaint and site of greatest symptomatology (e.g., pain, palpable mass), allergies to medications, medical comorbidity, surgical history, and a thorough understanding of the procedure must be addressed with the patient. Appropriate laboratory parameters should also be noted, and test results obtained within an acceptable time frame. Many of these questions can easily be answered by referring clinicians and the medical record. However, review of these topics with the patient is mandatory to ensure accuracy of the data.

Review of dedicated imaging of the lesion in question should also have been performed. This enables preprocedural planning, selection of equipment, and targeting of the lesion. It may also change the modality by which the procedure is performed. If preprocedural imaging is not available, time should be set aside for a diagnostic evaluation to be performed with the imaging modality most likely to be used for biopsy.

The choice of which imaging modality to use varies according to a number of parameters. First and foremost is availability. Most institutions now have 24-hour access to ultrasound, fluoroscopy, and CT, but access to magnetic resonance imaging (MRI) remains limited.

Second is operator preference. Many interventionalists are comfortable using ultrasound and CT as guidance for biopsy. Fluoroscopic guidance for percutaneous biopsy is no longer as widespread as it once was, and most interventionalists currently have little experience with MRI guidance (in part because of lack of widespread availability of MRI-compatible devices).

Each imaging modality has relative advantages and disadvantages (Table 126-1), so certain situations may favor the use of specific modalities. Mobile lesions and lesions that require multiple imaging angles, for example, may be better suited to ultrasound-guided biopsy (Fig. 126-1). Deeper lesions that might be obscured by bowel gas or limited by body habitus may be easier to biopsy under CT guidance.

Ultrasound guidance is the preferred modality for percutaneous biopsy at numerous institutions. Most biopsy needles are sonographically visible as long as the scan plane is optimized[2] (Fig. 126-2). Most commonly, nonvisualization of the needle tip is due to misalignment of the needle

TABLE 126-1. Comparison of Imaging Modalities for Biopsy

	Advantages	Disadvantages
CT	Images easy to comprehend Ability to visualize deep structures Images not obscured by bowel gas or bone	Can be time consuming Certain imaging planes (e.g., craniocaudal) may be difficult to obtain. Opportunity and cost (diagnostic evaluations vs. interventions on the scanner) Radiation exposure
Ultrasound	Real-time exposure and imaging No radiation exposure Able to recognize vasculature Patients tend to be more comfortable. Multiplanar/polyplanar imaging Portable Low cost	Inadequate visualization of the target or needle (operator dependent or limited by habitus, bowel gas, fibrous scarring, bony structures, lesion depth)
Fluoroscopy	Minimal cost Real-time imaging Widely available	Radiation exposure Single-dimension imaging Not portable
CT fluoroscopy	Unique cross-sectional imaging visualization	? Impact on time, patient outcomes, radiation exposure
MRI	High contrast resolution Multiplanar imaging Vascular structures can be identified without contrast material. No ionizing radiation (pediatric and obstetric patients)	Expensive MRI-compatible biopsy tools expensive and not in widespread production Opportunity and cost (interventional vs. diagnostic use) Imaging artifacts Imaging time

CT, Computed tomography; *MRI,* magnetic resonance imaging.

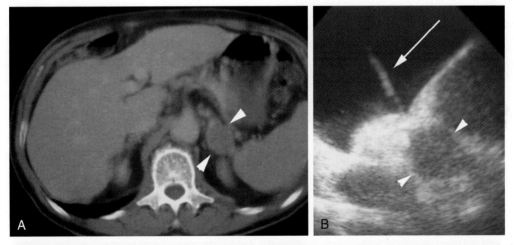

FIGURE 126-1. A, Left adrenal mass *(arrowheads)* noted in patient with history of lung cancer. Biopsy requested to determine whether it represented metastasis. With patient prone, mass is shielded in axial plane by stomach and liver anteriorly, spleen laterally, spine and aorta medially, and lung posteriorly. **B,** Under ultrasound guidance, an acceptable path through left pleural effusion and left hemidiaphragm is chosen. Left adrenal gland *(arrowheads)* is enlarged, and biopsy needle *(arrow)* is apparent.

and the transducer plane. Techniques for enhancing visualization of the needle tip include jiggling the needle tip, the "pump" maneuver,[3] or injection of a small amount of air or saline through the needle tip. Many interventionalists also use commercially available needle guides to perform ultrasound-guided biopsy.

CT guidance may be used in patients who are poor candidates for ultrasound (e.g., because of habitus or previous surgical intervention with resultant scarring). Preliminary scans through the target area allow localization of the lesion in question and assist in planning for the biopsy. Intravenous contrast material may be useful to better visualize the lesion under consideration and the surrounding vascular structures.

Fluoroscopic guidance can be used for lesions (e.g., lung) that may be easier to biopsy under real-time x-ray imaging.

Biopsy needles can be divided into three main groups: small-gauge aspiration needles, small-gauge core biopsy needles, and larger-gauge core biopsy needles. Aspiration needles can provide only cytologic samples, which may occasionally be scant or difficult to interpret. The biggest disadvantage of aspiration, however, is that the architecture of the sampled tissue is not preserved. This technique may also require multiple passes, and it is important that cytopathologic evaluation be undertaken at the time of sampling if aspiration is to be performed. Involvement by on-site pathologists optimizes dissemination of clinical information and ensures that specimens are optimally handled and appropriate samples are taken as required for ancillary investigations (e.g., microbiology or molecular studies).[4]

Small-gauge core biopsy needles are designed to provide small specimens of tissue for histologic analysis. Larger-gauge core biopsy samples provide adequate histologic samples, but the risk of complications may be higher.[5] Core biopsy samples are now commonly required for genetic testing of material.

For fine-needle biopsy, our own preference is to start with a nonaspiration (nonsuction) technique because suction may result in an inordinate amount of blood in the specimen. This technique relies on rapid movement of the needle tip within the target in excursions of approximately

0.5 to 1 cm, generally until the first hint of blood is noted in the needle hub. Tissue enters the lumen of the needle and is expressed with a syringe onto a slide for immediate review by a cytopathologist. The nonaspiration technique may be limited in organs with firm (e.g., heavily fibrotic) tissue, in which case, manual aspiration with a syringe may be undertaken. Suction can also be applied with a number of devices designed for this purpose. A 20- to 25-gauge Chiba-type or cutting needle is generally used for fine-needle biopsies. For core biopsies, the core biopsy device should be placed at the edge of the lesion in question as the needle advances from the tip of the device (Fig. 126-3). Care should be taken to ascertain that the needle throw not extend outside the lesion to be sampled, or if it does, that it will not result in injury to critical structures.

In general, the shortest route from the skin to the lesion should be taken, so long as no vital structures or organs are interposed. In the case of peripheral hepatic lesions, however, a biopsy path that traverses normal liver between the liver capsule and target should be chosen. This can help minimize the risk of intraperitoneal bleeding (particularly for vascular lesions such as hemangiomas) and potentially decreases the likelihood of needle-tract seeding. Certain lesions may merit use of nonstandard technique as well. For instance, a transintestinal approach may be necessary for lesions within the mesentery (Fig. 126-4). Transsplenic biopsy may be necessary for lesions in the upper part of the abdomen that are not approachable even with a craniocaudal trajectory. Retroperitoneal and pelvic biopsy may be more safely approached posteriorly.

Certain organs merit other considerations before biopsy:
1. In patients undergoing adrenal biopsy, potential pheochromocytomas should be handled with caution and may be considered a contraindication to biopsy. Preprocedural α-blockade, urinary metabolic assessment (for catecholamines and vanillylmandelic acid), and evaluation of clinical symptoms will often be enough to avert biopsy-related complications. Potential clinical sequelae of biopsy of pheochromocytomas include paroxysmal hypertension, headache, excessive perspiration, and palpitation. Treatment of

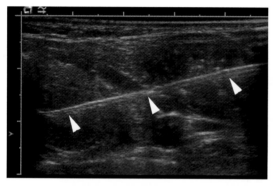

FIGURE 126-2. Biopsy of thyroid lesion under sonographic guidance. Needle *(arrowheads)* is easily visualized within scan plane of transducer and is oriented nearly perpendicular to ultrasound beam.

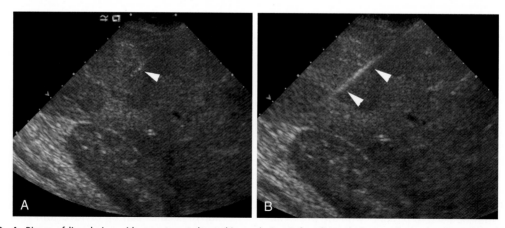

FIGURE 126-3. A, Biopsy of liver lesion with an automated core biopsy device. Before firing device, needle is placed at edge of lesion *(arrowhead)*. **B,** After device activation, needle advances through lesion to opposite edge *(arrowheads)*. Length of throw of device must be taken into account during biopsies with such devices.

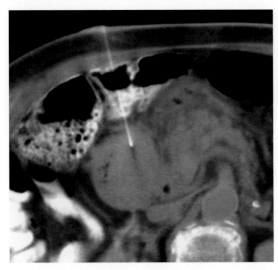

FIGURE 126-4. Biopsy of periduodenal mass. A 20-gauge biopsy needle was passed through colon to lesion. No postbiopsy complications developed.

pheochromocytoma-related complications includes phentolamine (1 mg intravenously) followed by intravenous titration of blood pressure with 5 mg of phentolamine for adults and 1 mg for children. Sodium nitroprusside can also be administered intravenously (50 mg in 500 mL of 5% dextrose in water) for managing hypertensive crisis.[6,7]

2. Patients undergoing pancreatic biopsy are at increased risk for postprocedural pancreatitis. This risk is increased with biopsy of the normal pancreas. There should be no hesitation in obtaining serum amylase and lipase levels after biopsy in any patient in whom abdominal pain, anorexia, or nausea and vomiting develop in short-term follow-up after pancreatic biopsy.

If multiple passes are anticipated, especially in lesions that are difficult to approach anatomically, consideration can be given to using a coaxial or tandem method (Fig. 126-5). In the tandem method, a small-gauge (e.g., 25-gauge) needle is used to work out the appropriate angle of access to the target lesion, followed by a larger-gauge (e.g., 18-gauge core) device placed adjacent and parallel to the first needle. In the coaxial method, a larger-gauge needle is carefully advanced to the target lesion (often in stepwise fashion). Once well positioned, multiple biopsy passes of smaller-gauge needles can be performed to obtain specimens without having to repeatedly traverse a potentially difficult or dangerous biopsy trajectory.

COMPLICATIONS

Complications can be stratified on the basis of outcomes. *Major complications* can be defined as (1) unplanned admission to the hospital for therapy, (2) unplanned increase in the level of care, (3) prolonged hospitalization, (4) permanent adverse sequelae, and (5) death. *Minor complications* can be defined as (1) complications requiring nominal

therapy or (2) complications requiring a short hospital stay for observation.[1]

Complications of percutaneous biopsy are of two types: generic and organ specific. Generic complications are common to all types of biopsy (e.g., bleeding, infection, unintended organ injury). In general, clinically significant bleeding is uncommon, although multiple studies demonstrate increased risk with core renal biopsy.[5,8] Organ-specific complications are those that are only associated (or most commonly associated) with biopsy of a specific organ. For example, pneumothorax is most commonly associated with biopsy of the lung, but it can occur during vertebral, rib, liver, spleen, or other biopsy.

POSTPROCEDURAL AND FOLLOW-UP CARE

Postbiopsy follow-up should include monitored observation with frequent (e.g., every 15 minutes) evaluation of vital signs, depending on the biopsy site, perceived risk associated with the procedure, needle gauge used, and patient reliability. Some sites (e.g., thyroid) rarely require any postprocedural observation. Solid organs such as the liver and kidney may merit 1 to 4 hours of postprocedural observation. In the pediatric populations, a 6-hour period of observation is often undertaken after solid-organ biopsy. Also of note in our practice is that patients who undergo biopsy of their native kidneys are admitted by medical nephrologists for overnight observation and postprocedural laboratory evaluation.

A negative or inconclusive biopsy should be repeated if suspicion of malignancy is high. Repeat biopsy may also be useful for lesions that are incongruent with the radiographic appearance or clinical suspicion. Use of a larger-gauge or core biopsy needle may further increase the sampling yield.

SUMMARY

Use and demand for image-guided procedures have seen a marked increase in recent years; one of the greatest demands is for percutaneous biopsy. Biopsy may be the most common procedure an interventionalist will perform. With appropriate preprocedural planning and postprocedural follow-up, image-guided biopsy is generally a safe and valuable component of patient care.

KEY POINTS

- Percutaneous biopsy plays a key role in the diagnostic evaluation of many lesions detected by imaging studies.
- Choice of imaging modality for biopsy guidance depends on many factors, including physician experience and preference, lesion location, and lesion detectability.
- The interventionalist needs to recognize potential complications and be prepared to initiate appropriate management.
- The presence of on-site cytopathy improves diagnostic yield and enhances patient care.

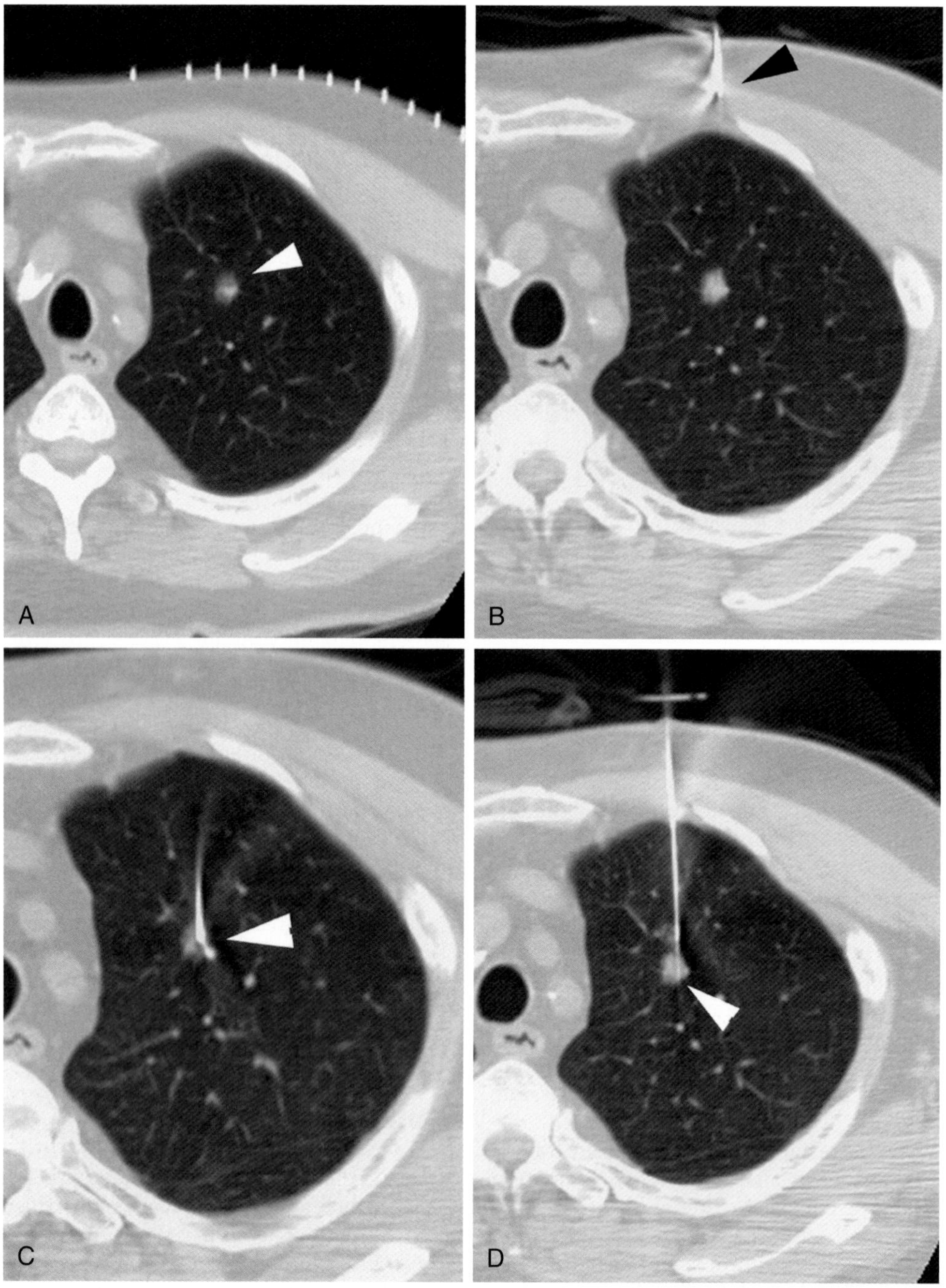

FIGURE 126-5. **A,** Prebiopsy films of 8-mm lung lesion *(arrowhead).* Marker grid is placed on anterior chest wall to help determine optimal entry point. **B,** Initial positioning of 19-gauge guiding needle *(arrowhead).* Direction and position are adjusted before crossing pleural surface. **C,** Guiding needle has been placed within lesion *(arrowhead).* **D,** After pulling back lesion, a 20-gauge coaxial core specimen is obtained through lesion *(arrowhead).* Diagnosis was metastatic melanoma.

▶ **SUGGESTED READINGS**

Ansari NA, Derias NW. Origins of fine needle aspiration cytology. J Clin Pathol 1997;50:541–3.

Dupas B, Frampas E, Leaute F, et al. [Complications of fluoroscopy-, ultrasound-, and CT-guided percutaneous interventional procedures.] J Radiol 2005;86:586–98.

Gupta S. New techniques in image-guided percutaneous biopsy. Cardiovasc Intervent Radiol 2004;27:91–104.

The complete reference list is available online at www.expertconsult.com.

CHAPTER 127

Percutaneous Abscess Drainage Within the Abdomen and Pelvis

Justin J. Campbell and Debra A. Gervais

Since its introduction in the early 1980s, percutaneous abscess drainage (PAD) has become the primary drainage procedure for most infected abdominal fluid collections. Numerous large clinical series have demonstrated the efficacy and safety of this procedure.[1-6] Image-guided drainage allows rapid, minimally invasive drainage of collections that had previously required surgical drainage and necessitated a trip to the operating room, general anesthesia, and was therefore associated with higher morbidity. Benefits of PAD in most cases include avoiding general anesthesia, laparotomy, and prolonged postoperative hospitalization, with a resultant reduction in morbidity, mortality, and hospital costs.

INDICATIONS

As PAD has become more widely used, indications have continued to expand. Currently, the vast majority of infected intraabdominal and pelvic fluid collections are considered amenable to percutaneous drainage. Prerequisites for PAD are presence of a fluid collection and one or more of the following: suspicion the collection is infected, need for fluid analysis, or suspicion the collection is producing symptoms that warrant drainage.[7] PAD may be performed in essentially every organ of the abdomen and pelvis. Liver abscesses, pancreatic abscesses, renal and perirenal abscesses, enteric abscesses, anastomotic abscesses, subphrenic abscesses, splenic abscesses, and pelvic abscesses, as well as subcutaneous abscesses and abscesses within musculature (e.g., psoas muscle) are examples of abscesses that have been successfully drained with percutaneous techniques. The goal of treatment can be complete cure of an infected fluid collection, or PAD may be used as a temporizing measure before definitive surgical treatment. For example, patients with diverticulitis and abscess formation would require, in addition to surgical drainage, a colostomy and subsequent takedown of the colostomy if operated on in the acute period. With PAD, the abscess and any existing or potential acute sepsis are treated first, allowing time for the acute inflammation to subside and ensuring a cleansed bowel at the time of resection so a primary anastomosis can be performed without colostomy. In other instances, PAD can serve as a palliative procedure for patients who are not candidates for curative surgical treatment.

CONTRAINDICATIONS

Contraindications to PAD are relative and should be weighed carefully against the suitable surgical alternative and the alternative of no procedure. Relative contraindications include coagulopathy that cannot be adequately corrected, phlegmons or collections containing a large amount of debris, hemodynamic instability such that the procedure could not be completed, inability of the patient to be positioned or cooperate adequately for the procedure, known adverse reaction to contrast material when administration is deemed necessary for success of the procedure, lack of a safe access route for drainage of a collection, and severely compromised cardiopulmonary status in patients undergoing procedures in which there is risk of further cardiopulmonary compromise inherent in the procedure.[7] In reality, almost all these factors can be mitigated to some degree to allow abscess drainage. For example, most coagulopathies can be corrected to within an acceptable range of risk. In truth, the only absolute contraindication would be absence of a safe percutaneous route to the abscess. However, this is rare with the many options available to the interventional radiologist, such as angling of the computed tomography (CT) gantry, using an angled ultrasound approach, imaging after repositioning the patient, or instilling saline to displace structures at risk. The risks and benefits of PAD must be carefully evaluated in each patient. Decisions regarding whether to pursue abscess drainage in critically ill patients are best made in concert with the surgical and medical teams caring for the patient.

Additionally, imaging facilities should have policies and procedures in place to attempt to identify any pregnant patients before exposing them to ionizing radiation. Pregnant patients undergoing procedures requiring use of ionizing radiation are counseled regarding the risk of radiation exposure to the fetus and the clinical benefit of the procedure. Every attempt should be made to avoid exposing the fetus to radiation in accordance with ALARA (as low as reasonably achievable) principles. This can be accomplished by performing the procedure under ultrasound guidance alone when possible. If CT is required for adequate drainage, exposure factors are minimized to those required to demonstrate the collection and differentiate it from adjacent structures. Likewise, if fluoroscopy is needed to guide wire manipulations, diminished exposure factors and frame rates are advisable.

EQUIPMENT

The primary tool necessary for drainage of an abscess is a drainage catheter. In the early days of PAD, angiography catheters and catheters used by surgeons were the tools available for PAD, but catheters specifically designed for PAD are now available. The majority of catheters are constructed from a proprietary polyurethane material modified for kink resistance. These catheters are designed to be placed by either the Seldinger or trocar method. Standard catheters consist of a pointed metal trocar loaded coaxially through a metal stiffener into the flexible polyurethane catheter. Once the tip is placed in the collection, the catheter is fed off the trocar and stiffener into the collection.

The trocar and stiffener are then removed. Alternatively, the catheter can be placed by the Seldinger method by removing the trocar and placing the catheter and stiffener over a wire. After dilating the tract, the catheter is fed off the stiffener once it has passed through any tissues likely to prevent the catheter from easily following the wire, such as fascial planes and muscle. Catheters are available in sizes ranging from 8F to 16F. Many have a hydrophilic coating to facilitate placement and deployment. Numerous large oblong-shaped holes at the catheter tip facilitate drainage. The majority of catheter tips have a string-locked pigtail configuration for retention, but other internal retention devices, such as balloons and mushroom types, are also available.

Whether using the trocar or Seldinger technique, needle access is generally performed before catheter placement. A variety of needles can be used. Superficial collections are generally amenable to access with spinal needles. Deeper collections can be sampled with 10- to 25-cm Chiba needles. Needle diameters range from 18 to 22 gauge. Fluid sampling is usually possible with 20-gauge needles, but if a viscous collection is suspected, larger-gauge needles can be used. The needle can then be used as a guide for the tandem trocar technique. If the Seldinger technique is performed, the access needle can be used to place the wire over which the drainage catheter will be placed. Several needles designed to accept a 0.038-inch wire can be used to facilitate this technique. Ring sheathed needles (Cook Medical, Bloomington, Ind.) allow direct placement of an 0.038-inch wire, whereas the AccuStick system (MediTech/Boston Scientific, Watertown, Mass.) allows initial placement of an 0.018-inch wire, with upsizing to a 0.038-inch wire via use of a sheath.

When the Seldinger technique is used, the operator may need to redirect a working wire to a specific location for optimal catheter drainage. This is usually achieved by using a directional catheter to guide the wire to a specific target location under fluoroscopic guidance. A number of such catheters exist. We find that a 5.0 Kumpe catheter or cobra catheter is useful for this purpose. These catheters accept 0.038-inch wires. In general, directional catheters measuring 30 to 40 cm in length are preferable to the longer catheters used in vascular interventions, because the distance from the skin puncture to the desired catheter location is usually much shorter than this. A catheter that is too long can make torquing and redirecting the catheter more difficult.

When using the Seldinger technique, tract dilation is often necessary to allow placement of the catheter. This can be achieved with dilators, stiff devices with tapered ends that are placed over the working wire. During tract dilation, care must be taken to not kink the wire. After performing serial dilation, the catheter can then be placed over the wire. Alternatively, the catheter can be placed after dilation with the use of a Peel-Away introducer (Cook Medical). The advantage of the latter is that it provides added stiffness for passing the catheter through tracts that are especially resistant to the softer catheter. This will also require the tract to be dilated 1 to 2 French sizes larger than the nominal drainage catheter size.

Once the catheter has been placed within the collection and secured with the internal retention device, it is usually fixed to the skin to provide additional stability to prevent dislodgment of the catheter from the collection. This can

be performed in a number of different ways. The catheter can be secured with a skin suture, which is then attached directly to the catheter. Alternatively, nonsuture fixation devices can be used. These devices are fixed to the skin with adhesive and lock to the catheter with a plastic locking device designed to accommodate specific catheter sizes. One example is the StatLock system (Venetec, San Diego, Calif.). A hybrid system can be used in which the catheter is sutured to an adhesive ostomy appliance (Hollister Inc., Libertyville, Ill.) that contains a small central opening through which the catheter passes. Finally, a drainage bag is attached to the catheter. A three-way stopcock can be placed between the catheter and bag to facilitate catheter flushing. At our institution, abdominal/pelvic drainage catheters are usually placed under gravity drainage, but some practitioners prefer using suction devices.

TECHNIQUE

Anatomy and Approach

After establishing the presence of a drainable fluid collection, several issues regarding patient preparation must be addressed before performing PAD. First, adequate antibiotic therapy is initiated if there is clinical evidence of infection. In the majority of cases, the team caring for the patient has begun antibiotic therapy before consulting radiology for potential PAD. In the rare instance in which antibiotic therapy has not been initiated, broad-spectrum antibiotics are administered before drainage. Antimicrobial therapy is not withheld for fear of sterilizing cultures; because the interventional manipulation can seed the bloodstream with bacteria, the risk of sepsis is too high.[8] Coagulation factors, including prothrombin time (PT), partial thromboplastin time (PTT), and platelet count, are checked before intervention. Any coagulopathy is then corrected to the degree possible before performing the procedure.

Except for the most superficial abscesses, most abscess drainage procedures cause some intraprocedural pain despite local analgesia, so intravenous (IV) sedation is almost always used. A benzodiazepine and narcotic combination works well. At our institution we use IV fentanyl citrate and midazolam hydrochloride (Versed). Typically, fentanyl (25 μg IV) and midazolam (0.25 to 0.5 mg IV) are administered at 5- to 10-minute intervals until adequate sedation is achieved. IV sedation is administered according to institutional guidelines, and interventional radiologists need to be familiar with their own institution's guidelines.

When planning the drainage route, it is important to consider the most direct route that is free of intervening organs and vital structures such as bowel, solid viscera, vessels, and nerves. Furthermore, every attempt is made to avoid contaminating sterile areas. The catheter is generally placed in the most dependent position possible to facilitate drainage. For example, if the patient will be in the supine position after placing the catheter, a posterior or lateral approach may optimize drainage. Once the route for drainage has been selected, the patient can be placed in the most appropriate position for catheter placement, after which the skin is prepared and draped in the usual sterile fashion, and sedation is initiated.

Initial access to the abscess cavity is obtained under CT or ultrasound guidance. Fluoroscopy can be used in conjunction with either of these two modalities to confirm catheter position or assist with catheter positioning in difficult cases. The decision regarding which imaging modality to use is based on factors that include position of the collection, presence of overlying structures, visibility of the collection and adjacent structures with each modality, availability, and user preference. A limited number of image-guided drainage procedures are performed under magnetic resonance imaging (MRI) guidance, but such techniques are still in the early stages of development and not yet widely used. The decision of which modality to use should be made on a case-by-case basis.

Ultrasound has several advantages. First, it is a real-time imaging modality and for this reason is generally much faster than CT. It is also more widely available and less expensive than CT. The modality is portable, allowing for use at the bedside in critically ill patients not stable enough to travel to the radiology suite. Finally, ultrasound does not expose the patient to ionizing radiation. Unlike CT, however, intervening fat, gas, and bone significantly degrade visualization of collections. Abscesses deep within the abdomen or pelvis can be difficult to visualize. For the same reason, ultrasound can be difficult to use in obese patients with large amounts of subcutaneous fat. Similarly, collections in the retroperitoneum can be difficult to visualize. Limitations of ultrasound also include the need for significant operator experience.

CT is not as operator dependent as ultrasound, and collections deep to bone, gas, or fat are well visualized. Provided the patient's weight does not exceed table limits and his or her size allows placement of the patient with a guiding needle into the gantry, CT-guided drainage is not as limited by obesity as ultrasound-guided drainage. Lastly, both final catheter position and the degree of evacuation of abscess contents are better visualized with CT than with ultrasound. Disadvantages of CT include exposure to ionizing radiation, increased time required for procedures, and lack of portability.

Both CT and ultrasound have limitations in their ability to distinguish solid tissue from drainable fluid collections. CT relies on attenuation measurements to distinguish tissues. The majority of fluid collections have low attenuation, but some drainable fluid collections can contain high-attenuation material such as iodinated contrast material or blood products. Likewise, some nondrainable tissues (e.g., necrotic tissue, certain neoplasms) can be very low in attenuation. Unlike CT, however, ultrasound has particular difficulty visualizing collections that contain gas because of limited sound transmission. Additionally, some hypoechoic through-transmitting tissues (e.g., lymphoma) can be mistaken for fluid. Regardless of which imaging modality is ultimately chosen to guide drainage, a combination of pre-drainage diagnostic imaging modalities can be used to characterize collections and the feasibility of drainage access before attempting PAD.

Technical Aspects

Method
The catheter may be placed by either the trocar or Seldinger technique. Both are viable options and offer advantages and disadvantages in different clinical settings. Although each technique has its proponents and detractors, no randomized trial has been conducted to compare them, and the choice of which to use comes down to operator preference, which itself is usually a function of experience. The trocar technique is generally performed in conjunction with a guiding needle (Fig. 127-1). As discussed earlier, the guiding needle is usually 18 to 22 gauge and variable in length, depending on the depth of the collection. The guiding needle is placed in the collection under CT guidance. Once needle placement within the collection has been confirmed with imaging, the needle acts as a guide for catheter placement. Before placing the catheter, a sample of fluid can be aspirated and sent for laboratory analysis. This initial aspiration can be helpful in charactering the fluid. If no fluid is aspirated, the collection may be very viscous and thus suggest the need for a larger catheter. Alternatively, if the fluid is not grossly purulent and the collection is not thought to be infected, a Gram stain can be performed if the decision of whether to place a catheter will be influenced by these results.

Once the decision to place the catheter has been made, a small nick is made in the skin adjacent to the entrance site of the guiding needle, and the underlying subcutaneous tissue is dissected bluntly. The catheter containing the hollow metal stiffener and inner trocar needle is then advanced into the cavity, adjacent to the guiding needle, to the appropriate predetermined depth. When the catheter tip is within the cavity, the catheter is fed off the trocar needle and metal stiffener. Syringe aspiration can then be performed to help confirm catheter position. Minimal fluid is aspirated at this time because decreasing the size of the target cavity makes subsequent repositioning technically more difficult if required. Catheter position is then confirmed by imaging before securing the device. The guiding needle is removed after satisfactory catheter position is confirmed. The advantage of the trocar method is the speed with which the catheter can be deployed. This can be very helpful when the patient is critically ill or lightly sedated. The main disadvantage of this technique is limited ability to reposition the catheter without removing and reinserting it if initial positioning is suboptimal.

With the Seldinger technique, initial access can be performed with a needle under ultrasound or CT guidance (Fig. 127-2). When needle position within the cavity is confirmed by imaging, a wire is placed through the needle into the cavity. The needle is then removed over the wire, and the tract is serially dilated to the appropriate size to allow placement of the catheter. Two different types of needles can be used for initial access. "One-stick" systems use a 21- to 22-gauge needle that accepts a 0.018-inch wire. A three-component device containing a sheath, dilator, and stiffener is placed over this wire. With removal of the stiffener and dilator, a 0.035- or 0.038-inch working wire can be placed through the sheath. Further dilation can then be performed to place the catheter over this wire into the collection. Alternatively, a larger needle that accepts a 0.035- or 0.038-inch wire, such as a Ring needle, can be placed. The Seldinger technique is helpful when the window to the collection is narrow. This technique offers the further advantage of guiding the catheter into optimal position with the use of directional catheters under fluoroscopic guidance. The disadvantage of this technique is primarily that it can be more time consuming than the trocar technique. This time consideration can be particularly important with

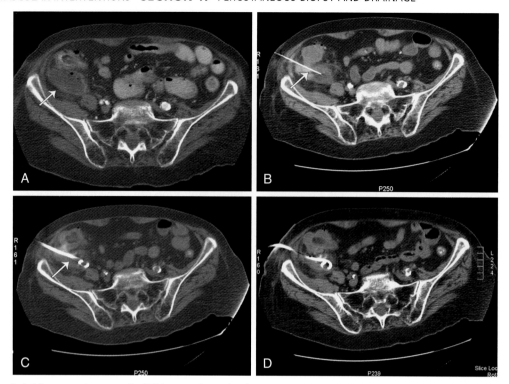

FIGURE 127-1. A, Axial computed tomography (CT) image enhanced with intravenous contrast material shows a gas-containing fluid collection posterior to cecum *(arrow)* in patient with right lower quadrant pain, fever, and leukocytosis. **B,** An 18-gauge needle *(arrow)* is advanced into collection under CT guidance; 2 mL of purulent material was aspirated. **C,** An 8F locking pigtail catheter *(arrow)* is advanced into collection tandem to guiding needle. **D,** Collection is then aspirated and irrigated. Postdrainage image demonstrates decreased size of collection.

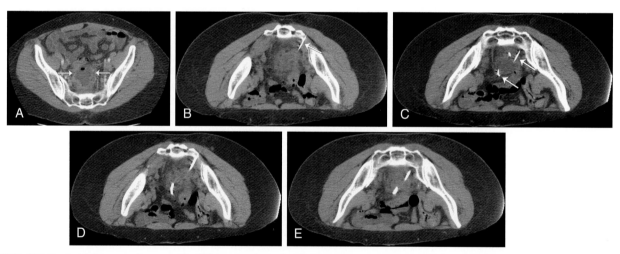

FIGURE 127-2. A, Axial computed tomography (CT) image enhanced with intravenous contrast material demonstrates a gas- and fluid-containing collection *(arrows)* in presacral space in patient with abdominal pain, fever, and leukocytosis. **B,** Using an angled gantry, a 20-gauge needle is advanced through sciatic foramen *(arrow)* into collection, and small amount of purulent material is aspirated. **C,** A 0.018-inch wire *(arrows)* is advanced through needle into collection. **D,** After using "one-stick" system to upsize wire to a 0.035-inch Amplatz wire, a 10F locking pigtail catheter is advanced over wire into collection; 30 mL of purulent material was aspirated. **E,** Postdrainage image shows decreased size of collection.

critically ill patients. Additionally, serial dilation can be painful even in well-sedated patients.

Approach to Challenging Locations
The approach to drainage of abdominal and pelvic abscesses is often straightforward. As discussed, in the majority of cases the most direct route that is free of intervening organs and vital structures is selected. However, specific locations

in the abdomen and pelvis present technical difficulties and merit further discussion, including collections in the subphrenic, posterior epigastric, peripancreatic, and deep pelvic spaces.

Collections in the subphrenic spaces are encountered on both sides. Causes of right-sided collections include abscesses related to hepatic flexure or duodenal pathology, bile leaks, postoperative abscesses, and infected hematomas.

These collections are often seen in postoperative patients after hepatic or biliary surgery or resection of right adrenal masses. Similarly, left-sided collections are frequently seen in the postoperative period after splenectomy and distal pancreatectomy. Drainage can be performed under ultrasound guidance, CT guidance, or a combination of CT or ultrasound with fluoroscopy. When draining these collections, measures to avoid contaminating the pleural space should be taken. A subcostal, transperitoneal lateral, or anterior approach can be used.[9] The catheter can then be angled cranially into the subphrenic space. Access to these collections can be achieved via either the Seldinger or trocar technique. The Seldinger technique is usually preferred because the catheter can be guided into the subphrenic space over a wire (Fig. 127-3). Optimal wire position can be achieved by advancing the wire under fluoroscopy, often with the aid of a directional device such as a Kumpe catheter (Cook Medical). In cases where a subcostal approach is impossible, an intercostal approach can be performed, but the risk of pleural contamination and pneumothorax is increased. Because the pleural reflection is more cranial anteriorly and more caudal posteriorly, consideration of pleural anatomy can guide the location of an intercostal puncture. Anteriorly, the catheter is ideally placed below the seventh rib; laterally, placement of catheter below the tenth rib is generally regarded as safe.

One must remember that there is variation in terms of where the pleural reflection may descend, so the risk of transpleural puncture always exists, even with some posterior subcostal approaches.

Collections in the peripancreatic and posterior epigastric spaces are technically difficult to drain percutaneously because of surrounding vital structures and bones, including organs, vessels, nerves, and spine. Because of the many intervening structures, image guidance for these collections is usually performed with CT. In many cases, these collections lack a safe access route and therefore cannot be drained percutaneously. However, there are a few access routes for draining these collections that should be considered. First, with the patient placed in the lateral decubitus or prone position, a window can be found between the spine and the medial border of the kidney. Similarly, an access route can be present along the lateral border of the kidneys, inferior to the spleen or liver. At times, these collections can be drained via an anterior approach, but overlying bowel (e.g., stomach, transverse colon) usually renders this approach unsafe. In the absence of other safe access routes, catheter placement via a transhepatic approach can be considered (Fig. 127-4). A transhepatic approach can be performed safely by going peripherally through the liver and avoiding the larger vessels and bile ducts of the central portion of the liver. Care is also taken to avoid transgressing

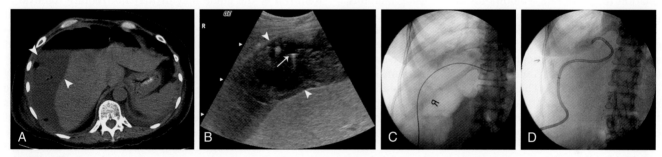

FIGURE 127-3. **A,** Axial computed tomography (CT) image without intravenous contrast enhancement demonstrates large, complex, gas-containing right subphrenic collection *(arrowheads)* in patient after colostomy takedown procedure. **B,** Under ultrasound guidance, a sheathed needle is advanced into collection *(arrowheads)*. Echogenic needle tip is visualized in collection *(arrow)*; 5 mL of thick yellow fluid was aspirated. **C,** Under fluoroscopic guidance, an Amplatz wire is passed through the sheath into subphrenic collection. **D,** A 14F multi-sidehole biliary drainage catheter is advanced over wire into subphrenic collection.

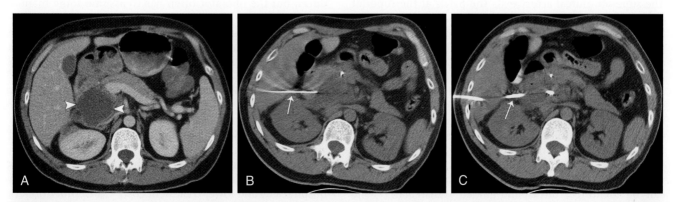

FIGURE 127-4. **A,** Axial computed tomography (CT) image enhanced with intravenous contrast material demonstrates a periduodenal collection *(arrowheads)* in patient in whom fever, abdominal pain, and leukocytosis developed after duodenal perforation from endoscopic retrograde cholangiopancreatography. Access is limited anteriorly by overlying bowel and pancreas. Access posteriorly is limited by spine and kidney. **B,** Under CT guidance, a 20-gauge Chiba needle *(arrow)* is placed into periduodenal collection via transhepatic approach. **C,** A 10F locking pigtail catheter *(arrow)* is then placed into collection using tandem trocar method; 50 mL of purulent material was aspirated.

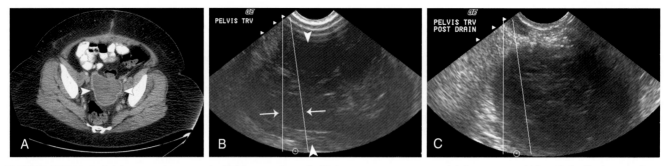

FIGURE 127-5. A, Axial computed tomography (CT) image enhanced with intravenous contrast material demonstrates thick-walled collection superior to vaginal cuff *(arrowheads)*, suggestive of abscess in patient with pelvic pain 1 month after total abdominal hysterectomy and bilateral salpingo-oophorectomy. **B,** Transvaginal ultrasonographic image demonstrating hypoechoic collection in pelvis *(arrowheads)*; 10 mL of bloody fluid was aspirated. Ultrasound software superimposes white lines *(arrows)* over image. Expected needle course lies between these projected lines. **C,** Postaspiration image demonstrates improvement of collection.

any existing hepatic masses or obstructed bile ducts, or both.

Secondary techniques may have to be considered when approaching a seemingly inaccessible collection. Blunt-tipped needles have been used to displace bowel en route to a collection. A curved-needle technique can be used to approach a collection inaccessible with a straight-line approach. Needles should be gently curved, with a guided wire inserted to avoid kinking. Techniques developed for ablation to create safe windows for access using balloons, gas, or fluids can also be employed.

Finally, deep pelvic collections are subject to technical difficulty, also because of intervening vital structures and surrounding bone. Particular care is taken to avoid damage to the urinary bladder and bowel. Decompression of the urinary bladder with a Foley catheter generally reduces the risk of injury to this structure. If time allows, preparing the patient with oral contrast material reduces the risk of confusing unopacified loops of bowel for the target collection.

In addition to the anterior approach, the transgluteal approach should be considered.[10-12] When using a transgluteal approach, in which the catheter is placed through the greater sciatic foramen, care is taken to avoid the sacral and sciatic nerves and the gluteal arteries. This is best achieved by placing the catheter as close to the sacrum as possible. The superior gluteal artery exits the pelvis at the superior aspect of the greater sciatic foramen, which is separated from the lesser sciatic foramen by the sacrospinous ligament. The sciatic nerve and inferior gluteal artery travel along the anterior aspect of the middle third of the piriformis muscle and exit the pelvis immediately below the muscle (see Fig. 127-1). The initial diagnostic CT scans should be studied carefully for safe access to the fluid collection. Modern enhanced scans clearly delineate the location and course of major arteries and nerves to be avoided. If possible, it is preferable not to traverse the piriformis muscle.

In patients in whom no safe percutaneous access route can be identified, ultrasound-guided transrectal[13,14] and transvaginal[15] approaches are viable alternatives for drainage of deep pelvic abscesses. Transvaginal or transrectal drainage under ultrasound guidance can be performed with commercially available needle guides manufactured specifically for each probe and accompanied by appropriate

software demonstrating the expected pathway of the needle on the ultrasound monitor (Fig. 127-5). However, because they are designed for needle placement, most catheters are too large to fit through the guide, so the operator must modify the technique slightly from a simple biopsy. When using the Seldinger technique, drainage can be accomplished by passing a long needle through the guide, passing a wire through the needle, and removing the needle and guide to allow serial dilation and catheter placement. Removal of the guide may or may not require removal of the ultrasound transducer, which can be reinserted without the guide if necessary to monitor the remainder of the procedure. Alternatively, one can use the trocar technique, but this will require that a modified plastic sheath (which sheaths the trocar and metal stiffener components of many commercially available catheters) be used instead of the guide. The diameter of these sheaths generally allows passage of 8F and 10F catheters. In short, the sheath is cut shorter to allow passage of the catheter distal to its tip. The sheath is sliced longitudinally to allow it to be freed from the catheter once the catheter is deployed. Finally, the sheath is placed along the ultrasound transducer along the same side as the guide would go, with the distal ends of the transducer and the sheath aligned. Tight rubber bands are helpful in preventing the sheath from moving and making its angle of entry different from that of the transducer, but the operator often has to assume some manual responsibility for this as well. With the sheath and transducer perfectly aligned and showing the abscess on the monitor, the sheath will guide the catheter into the abscess under direct ultrasound visualization.[16,17]

CONTROVERSIES

Adjunctive use of intracavitary fibrinolytics is a subject of some controversy. The presence of infected hematomas and viscous, thick purulent material has been associated with poor drainage despite proper catheter position. There is some evidence that instillation of fibrinolytics can shorten hospital stay and lower treatment cost.[18] Most practitioners currently use tissue plasminogen activator (tPA). At the authors' institution, 4 to 6 mg of tPA is instilled into the cavity in a volume of up to 50 mL of normal saline. The volume is adjusted according to the size of the cavity. The drainage catheter is then clamped for 30 minutes and subsequently opened to gravity drainage. This process is repeated every 12 hours for 3 days. The cavity is then re-imaged to evaluate the size of the collection.

Another area where there is variation in PAD practice concerns PAD in the setting of coagulopathy. The risk of a bleeding complication increases with the presence of a coagulopathy. Cutoff values for PT and platelet count vary from institution to institution. Although most patients will have recent laboratory values available before PAD, not all practitioners will check values before the procedure. Most institutions use a PT cutoff of 15 to 18, which corresponds to an international normalized ratio (INR) of 1.5 to 2.2. Cutoff values for platelets vary from 50,000 to 70,000. At this time, no scientific trial has established guidelines for practitioners of PAD regarding the necessity to check laboratory values or PT or platelet cutoff values before PAD. Practice also varies concerning performance of PAD in patients being treated with anticoagulation therapies such as aspirin and clopidogrel (Plavix). Additionally, multiple new anticoagulation agents give rise to new challenges regarding whether and when to withhold anticoagulation therapy when performing PAD. In each case, the benefits of PAD must be weighed carefully, as must the risks of a bleeding complication occurring and those related to withholding anticoagulation therapy. These decisions should always be made in concert with other clinicians involved in the patient's care.

Finally, the area of greatest practice variation in PAD concerns use of the trocar and Seldinger techniques. There are proponents of each who closely adhere to one and eschew the other. At this time, no prospective clinical trial has established the supremacy of either technique. As discussed previously, there are situations in which each technique offers advantages and disadvantages. Given the extensive experience with both, the decision of which technique to use depends at present on the preference of a given practitioner in a given situation.

OUTCOMES

Curative drainage of an infected abdominal collection is defined as resolution of the fluid collection and clinical improvement of the patient, without additional operative intervention. *Partial success* in PAD is defined as adequate drainage of a collection before subsequent surgical treatment of the underlying cause of the fluid collection, or PAD that serves as a temporizing measure to stabilize the patient before surgical treatment.[19] There is a spectrum of complexity of collections that are amenable to PAD. As the technical difficulty of the procedure and the complexity of the underlying disease process increase, rates of complication, failure, and recurrence, as well as drainage time, increase. Causes of failure include multiloculated and thick organized collections that communicate with bowel and abscesses in necrotic tissue. Unilocular discrete abscesses are the simplest to drain and are cured in more than 90% of cases.[20] More complicated abscesses, such as those that communicate with the gastrointestinal tract, are cured in 80% to 90% of cases. The most complex abscesses are cured at rates less than 80% and as low as 30%.[21-29]

In addition to the complexity of an abscess, several specific factors should be considered when evaluating the likelihood of success of PAD. Cinat et al.[29] performed a prospective study examining the characteristics of intraabdominal abscesses to predict the success of PAD. Analysis of 96 patients who underwent PAD demonstrated that presence of a postoperative abscess was predictive of success, whereas the presence of yeast and an abscess of pancreatic origin were negative predictors of a successful outcome. Additionally, this analysis demonstrated that PAD requiring more than two attempts was also a negative predictor of success. Gervais et al. examined the incidence and results of repeated abscess drainage. Evaluation of 43 patients requiring secondary abscess drainage also demonstrated that patients with postoperative abscesses were significantly likely to avoid a subsequent surgical procedure, whereas patients with pancreatic abscesses were significantly more likely to require it.[30] An additional retrospective study concerning the technical success of PAD in the setting of Crohn disease demonstrated that success rates are higher in postoperative patients than in those with spontaneous abscesses.[31]

Finally, abscesses that occur in tumors can never be definitively treated with PAD. A septic patient with a tumor abscess may improve substantially after PAD, but because of the underlying tissue pathology, these abscesses almost always recur when the drainage catheter is removed. Many of these patients require surgical resection of the tumor or lifetime catheter drainage. Therefore, before proceeding with PAD in these scenarios, the patient must understand that the catheter will probably remain in place for life, or re-drainage will be required.[26,32]

COMPLICATIONS

Major complications are rare and occur in less than 10% of PAD patients. Published complications include septic shock, bacteremia requiring a significant new intervention, hemorrhage requiring transfusion, superinfection of sterile fluid collections, and bowel or pleural transgression requiring intervention.[4,6]

Hemorrhage requiring transfusion is usually the result of laceration of visceral arteries, the spleen, or the liver. Hemorrhage is more likely in patients with uncorrected coagulopathies, as well as in patients with difficult access routes for drainage. Every attempt is made to correct the underlying coagulopathy to minimize the risk of bleeding, and the safest access route for abscess drainage is selected to avoid organs and vessels. This may involve using different techniques such as transgluteal, transrectal, or transvaginal approaches.

Patients commonly become bacteremic after the procedure and experience a rise in temperature. This is not considered a major complication. The patient will usually defervesce by postprocedure day 2.[4] Septic shock and bacteremia requiring a new intervention are considered major complications. Hypotension and disseminated intravascular coagulation have been reported as a result of sepsis after PAD.[4]

Superinfection of sterile cavities is also considered a major complication. For this reason, sterile technique is used when performing drainage of any fluid collection.[4] Enteric complications include bowel perforation with or without resultant fistula formation or peritonitis. These complications can occur if bowel is transgressed en route to abscess drainage or when a distended loop of bowel is mistaken for a drainable collection. Inadvertent transgression of bowel can result in fistula formation. Management of fistulas is discussed in the section on postprocedural care.

Transgression of the pleura with catheter placement can result in pleural fluid collections, pneumothorax, or both.[33] If clinically significant, these collections and pneumothoraces can be treated by chest tube placement.[34] Similarly, bladder perforation with urinoma formation has been reported. Placement of a Foley catheter before drainage of lower abdominal/pelvic abscesses decompresses the bladder and decreases the risk for bladder perforation. In the event of bladder perforation, a Foley catheter is kept in the bladder for 5 to 7 days to ensure good drainage while the perforation closes. The Foley catheter is then clamped for 4 hours and removed if there is no evidence of urine leak.

POSTPROCEDURAL AND FOLLOW-UP CARE

Immediately after the procedure, imaging is performed to assess the adequacy of cavity drainage and final catheter location. This is generally evaluated with the modality used to place the catheter. Catheters can be hard to visualize with ultrasonography, but a decrease in cavity size can usually be assessed, which suggests correct catheter position. CT offers excellent visualization of both cavity and catheter. Injection of contrast material under fluoroscopy can also be used to confirm catheter position. At the time of initial drainage, care should be taken to inject less volume than the volume of fluid removed from the cavity to minimize the risk for bacteremia and acute sepsis. Because of the viscosity of iodinated contrast material, the injected contrast agent should then be aspirated and the catheter flushed with saline to minimize catheter clogging. Additionally, catheter position can be independently confirmed by flow of appropriate fluid (e.g., pus from an abscess). When satisfactory catheter position is confirmed, the collection is then decompressed with a large aspiration syringe until return of fluid or debris ceases. For large cavities, irrigation of the cavity with small aliquots of sterile saline can be performed until the returning irrigant becomes clear. Irrigation often results in higher volumes of return fluid than the irrigant facilitating drainage. Irrigation must cease immediately if the irrigant volume is not completely returned with aspiration. Failure to achieve complete return indicates that the irrigant is collecting in a location not amenable to aspiration by the catheter, and further irrigant will simply expand this collection.

Irrigation of the cavity must be distinguished from flushing the catheter. *Irrigation* involves instillation of fluid into the cavity for lavage and more complete drainage of the cavity contents. *Flushing* is intended simply to clear the catheter and any associated drainage tubing to prevent catheter occlusion by particulate debris and necrotic tissue.[3,5] Importantly, overzealous irrigation can cause bacteremia and paradoxical worsening of the patient's clinical status. Hence, irrigant volume is always less than the volume of the abscess.

When decompression of the cavity and catheter position have been confirmed, the pigtail is formed when using a pigtail catheter, and the catheter is sutured to the skin. However, this can lead to skin irritation, so a number of retention devices are available that do not require a skin suture. The catheter is then connected to a drainage bag. A three-way stopcock can be placed between the catheter and drainage bag. This device has the advantage of facilitating subsequent catheter flushes but the disadvantage of a narrow lumen that can impede drainage of viscous fluid or collections containing debris. In particular, for catheters larger than 14F, the standard stopcock lumen is narrower than the catheter lumen, although larger-bore stopcocks are available. The catheter is flushed with 10 mL of saline every 8 to 12 hours to prevent drained material from obstructing the catheter lumen. Because the connection tubing to the bag can also become obstructed, this tubing is also flushed.

The major criteria for catheter removal include clinical improvement of the patient, improvement in the patient's laboratory test results, decreased drainage from the catheter, resolution of the cavity, and the absence of a fistula. A collaborative approach with surgical and medical consultants helps maintain a uniform treatment plan. Moreover, because of the wide array of catheters available to different medical specialties, nursing, medical, and surgical staff may be unfamiliar with the types of catheters used in interventional radiology. The interventional radiology service should remain involved to evaluate the need for repositioning, exchange, placement of additional catheters, and removal. On daily rounds, the interventional radiology service can inspect the catheter, assess its connections, and determine the quantity and character of the drainage output, as well as the condition of the patient.[20,35]

It is not unusual for patients to become febrile with transient bacteremia in the first 24 hours, but they usually defervesce by postprocedural day 2. The patient's laboratory test results generally improve over a similar time course and normalize within 48 to 72 hours. If clinical status and laboratory results are not improving, the possibility of undrained collections should be considered.

Catheter output is another useful indicator of when a catheter should be removed. Catheter output must be monitored closely. A nondraining catheter (output of 0 to 20 mL/day) is one of the most common clinical scenarios the team caring for the patient after catheter placement faces. Diagnostic possibilities include obstruction of the drainage catheter, presence of a loculated/fibrinous collection, migration of the catheter out of the abscess, or complete drainage of the collection. When drainage decreases, catheter patency can be evaluated by a simple flush with 3 to 5 mL of sterile saline. Causes of obstruction include stopcock malfunction, internal or external kinking of the catheter, or obstruction of the lumen by debris or blood. Evaluation of the catheter at the bedside includes inspection of the stopcock and external portion of the catheter, as well as gentle flushing of the catheter with saline. If the problem cannot be resolved at the bedside, additional imaging is indicated to evaluate the position of the catheter and the size of the collection. If the catheter is in the correct position and the collection remains, the material within the collection is likely too particulate or fibrinous to drain. Solutions to this problem include exchanging the catheter for a larger one or instilling thrombolytic therapy. If the catheter has moved out of the collection, the catheter can be repositioned or replaced.

If fever persists or drainage increases or remains high (>100 mL/day), it is necessary to re-image with CT or an abscessogram to evaluate for a residual abscess, development of a new abscess, or communication with bowel. Up to 40% of catheters require repositioning or placement of additional drainage catheters.[36]

If output remains persistently high or increases, a fistula should be suspected.[37] Fistulas can be to bowel, bladder, the pancreatic duct, or the bile duct. The most common fistula that occurs after abscess drainage is a gastrointestinal tract fistula; this reflects the cause of many abdominal abscesses. The source of abdominal and pelvic abscesses is often previous bowel surgery or inflammatory conditions of the bowel such as diverticulitis, appendicitis, or inflammatory bowel disease.[31] After pus is aspirated, the purulent drainage usually clears within 48 to 72 hours. The character of the subsequent drainage will generally reflect its source. The presence of a fistula can be confirmed by a fluoroscopically guided injection of iodinated dye via the catheter. The catheter will have to remain in place long enough for the enteric communication to close. Many close within 2 weeks,[20] but it is not unusual for fistulas to close over a period of weeks to months. For such long-term drainage, the patient can be discharged with the catheter in situ and then return for repeat injection in approximately 2 weeks to evaluate the fistula. If no fistula is identified at this time and catheter output has remained low, the catheter may be removed. If a persistent communication is identified, however, the catheter must remain in place until the fistula closes.

An additional cause of fistula formation is communication with the pancreatic duct. This communication can occur in the setting of collections drained in the pancreatic bed or collections occurring in the left upper aspect of the abdomen after procedures such as splenectomy or left nephrectomy.[38,39] If a pancreatic duct fistula is suspected, a sample of fluid can be sent for measurement of the amylase level. An elevated amylase level suggests connection with the pancreatic duct and can be confirmed by fluoroscopic tube injection. Drainage is often then required for an extended period. In severe cases, healing can be facilitated with octreotide, a somatostatin analog, or bowel rest and total parenteral nutrition (or both).

KEY POINTS

- Percutaneous drainage of abscesses is the primary drainage procedure for most infected abdominal and pelvic fluid collections.

- Drainage can be accomplished with either the Seldinger or trocar technique.

- Numerous approaches, including transgluteal, transvaginal, transrectal, and transhepatic techniques, allow the radiologist to drain most collections in the abdomen or pelvis. Careful study of the initial diagnostic imaging studies (ultrasound, computed tomography, magnetic resonance imaging) is critical to planning the most appropriate access route to the collection.

- The success rate of percutaneous drainage decreases with increasing complexity of the collection, as well as in the setting of pancreatic abscess.

▶ SUGGESTED READINGS

Cinat ME, Wilson SE, Din AM. Determinants for successful percutaneous image-guided drainage of intra-abdominal abscess. Arch Surg 2002; 137:845–9.

Gervais DA, Ho CH, O'Neill MJ, et al. Recurrent abdominal and pelvic abscesses: incidence, results of repeated percutaneous drainage, and underlying causes in 956 drainages. AJR Am J Roentgenol 2004;182: 463–6.

Harisinghani MG, Gervais DA, Hahn PF, et al. CT-guided transgluteal drainage of deep pelvic abscesses: Indications, technique, procedure-related complications, and clinical outcome. Radiographics 2002;22: 1353–67.

Maher MM, Gervais DA, Kalra MK, et al. The inaccessible or undrainable abscess: How to drain it. Radiographics 2004;24:717–35.

Maher MM, Kealey S, McNamara A, et al. Management of visceral interventional radiology catheters: A troubleshooting guide for interventional radiologists. Radiographics 2002;22:305–22.

Mueller PR, vanSonnenberg E, Ferrucci Jr JT. Percutaneous drainage of 250 abdominal abscesses and fluid collections. Part II: current procedural concepts. Radiology 1984;151:343–7.

O'Neill MJ, Rafferty EA, Lee SI, et al. Transvaginal interventional procedures: Aspiration, biopsy, and catheter drainage. Radiographics 2001; 21:657–72.

vanSonnenberg E, Ferrucci Jr JT, Mueller PR, et al. Percutaneous drainage of abscesses and fluid collections: Technique, results, and applications. Radiology 1982;142:1–10.

vanSonnenberg E, Mueller PR, Ferrucci Jr JT. Percutaneous drainage of 250 abdominal abscesses and fluid collections. Part I: results, failures, and complications. Radiology 1984;151:337–41.

vanSonnenberg E, Wittich GR, Goodacre BW, et al. Percutaneous abscess drainage: update. World J Surg 2001;25:362–9; discussion 370–2.

The complete reference list is available online at www.expertconsult.com.

CHAPTER 128

Management of Fluid Collections in Acute Pancreatitis

David S. Pryluck, Charan K. Singh, and Timothy W.I. Clark

Sterile and infected fluid collections are common local complications of acute pancreatitis. Initial diagnosis and management of these fluid collections commonly rely on image-guided techniques like fine-needle aspiration and percutaneous catheter drainage. Fine-needle aspiration (often at multiple sites) documents or excludes infection and can be used to guide antimicrobial therapy. Early diagnosis of these conditions can dramatically alter therapy; for example, a diagnosis of infected necrosis may warrant surgery or an aggressive attempt at percutaneous drainage to stabilize such patients.[1,2] Percutaneous catheter drainage can also be used to relieve symptoms caused by sterile fluid collections, such as gastric outlet obstruction or abdominal pain.

Just as acute pancreatitis exists as a spectrum of severity, the fluid collections associated with the disease also exist as a spectrum. After the 1992 International Symposium on Acute Pancreatitis, a classification system describing acute pancreatitis–associated fluid collections was implemented. It defined the terms *acute fluid collection, pancreatic necrosis, acute pseudocyst,* and *pancreatic abscess* based on pathophysiology and prognostic and treatment implications.[3] Ambiguity ensued in the use of these terms in medical literature and clinical practice, as well as difficulty in radiographically distinguishing among them. A revised classification scheme has been proposed that seeks to clarify the nomenclature used to describe acute pancreatitis–associated fluid collections.[4,5] It proposes that acute fluid collections be referred to as *acute peripancreatic fluid collections* (sterile or infected), pancreatic necrosis as *acute postnecrotic pancreatic/peripancreatic fluid collections* (sterile or infected), acute pseudocysts as *pancreatic pseudocysts* (sterile or infected), and pancreatic abscesses as *walled-off pancreatic necrosis* (sterile or infected).[4,5]

Multidetector computed tomography (CT) is the preferred modality used to diagnose and evaluate pancreatitis and associated fluid collections. Dynamic contrast-enhanced CT depicts the distinction between necrotizing and interstitial pancreatitis by demonstrating nonenhancing, nonviable areas of pancreas with necrosis. CT can depict all but the mildest forms of acute pancreatitis, demonstrate most of the major complications, and guide percutaneous needle aspiration and catheter drainage.[6,7] Ultrasonography, endoscopic retrograde cholangiopancreatography (ERCP), and magnetic resonance imaging (MRI) have secondary or adjunctive utility in pancreatitis, for example, in monitoring the size of pseudocysts or defining the relationship between a fluid collection and the pancreatic duct before percutaneous or surgical drainage.

This chapter will review current practices in percutaneous management of fluid collections associated with acute pancreatitis, both diagnosis and treatment. Sterile and infected collections will be considered. Established and new nomenclature will be used as appropriate.

INDICATIONS

Percutaneous therapy for acute pancreatitis can be effectively used to treat complications previously managed only surgically; it can be performed repeatedly and does not preclude any subsequent form of therapy. The decision to drain and the type of drainage are based on the associated CT findings, results of needle aspiration, and the patient's clinical condition.[8-11]

Pancreatic necrosis is defined as diffuse or focal areas of nonviable pancreatic parenchyma, typically associated with peripancreatic fat necrosis. This definition includes both sterile and infected necrosis.[4] Normal nonenhanced pancreas has a CT attenuation of 30 to 50 Hounsfield units (HU) and shows homogeneous enhancement to 100 to 150 HU with contrast material. A focal or well-defined zone of nonenhancing parenchyma larger than 3 cm in diameter or greater than 30% of the pancreas is a reliable CT finding of necrosis. Approximately 30% of patients with necrotizing pancreatitis develop secondary bacterial infection of necrotic debris.[12] The rationale for not using percutaneous drainage is therefore to avoid potentially converting a sterile collection into an infected one. With careful catheter care and judicious use of antimicrobial agents, secondary infection can be avoided and selected patients with sterile necrosis can benefit from percutaneous drainage. Liquefied necrosis that yields a brownish fluid containing debris is amenable to percutaneous drainage. Percutaneous catheter drainage may also decrease morbidity by avoiding surgery, or it can be used to temporize a patient before surgery.

Acute fluid collections (acute peripancreatic fluid collections per revised nomenclature) occur in up to 50% of patients early in the course of acute pancreatitis, usually within the first 48 hours. These collections result from either a rupture of a small branch of the pancreatic duct or from edema associated with parenchymal and/or peripancreatic inflammation.[4] They contain protein-rich fluid, may or may not contain high concentrations of pancreatic enzymes, and resolve spontaneously in about 50% of cases.[4] On CT they are low-attenuation, poorly defined collections of fluid with no recognizable capsule or wall; this radiographically distinguishes them from pseudocysts. Acute peripancreatic fluid collections can be sterile or infected, and intervention is usually unnecessary beyond needle aspiration to rule out infection.[13] The size and location of acute peripancreatic fluid collections can vary; large fluid collections are commonly localized in the lesser sac and anterior pararenal space, left more commonly than right.[14]

Acute pseudocysts (pancreatic pseudocyst per revised nomenclature) are round or oval collections of pancreatic fluid enclosed by a wall of fibrous or granulation tissue that arise at least 4 weeks following acute pancreatitis.[4,15] It is estimated that 30% to 50% of acute peripancreatic fluid collections progress to pseudocyst formation.[4] Although most pseudocysts resolve spontaneously, pseudocysts larger than 5 cm and those increasing in size are less likely to resolve and can be considered for percutaneous drainage. Severe pain and gastrointestinal (GI) or biliary tract obstruction are other indications for percutaneous drainage of noninfected pseudocysts. Approximately 10% of pseudocysts become secondarily infected, presumably from bowel seeding.[4]

Pancreatic abscesses (walled-off pancreatic necrosis per revised nomenclature) are circumscribed intraabdominal collections of pus in proximity to the pancreas. They contain little or no necrosis and usually occur 4 weeks or more after the onset of acute pancreatitis. Differentiation of an abscess from infected necrosis is crucial for appropriate clinical management. Abscesses are infected fluid collections that can be drained percutaneously, whereas infected necrosis develops in relatively solid or incompletely liquefied necrotic tissue and generally requires surgical débridement. Needle aspiration is crucial because visually, the CT appearance of a low-attenuation zone of infected necrosis may be similar to that of an abscess.

Infected necrosis (infected postnecrotic pancreatic/peripancreatic fluid collection [PNPFC] per revised nomenclature), as the name suggests, is infected pancreatic or peripancreatic necrotic tissue. Associated mortality rates range from 15% to 60%, and this is considered the most severe complication of pancreatitis. Traditionally, infected necrosis is an indication for surgical débridement. The rationale against use of percutaneous drainage has been that it is ineffective because necrotic material blocks drainage catheters. Catheter drainage may temporize a patient preoperatively; it does not preclude surgery and may optimize surgical timing. A trend toward minimally invasive organ-preserving therapy with aggressive percutaneous maneuvers is supported by reports of complete success with catheter drainage alone in some cases of liquefied infected necrosis. This approach mandates use of large-bore catheters, with extensive lavage and catheter manipulations performed over multiple sessions.[16-20]

CONTRAINDICATIONS

• Chronic catheterization of sterile pancreatic necrosis
• Drainage of infected pancreatic necrosis without significant liquefaction
• Pseudoaneurysms; all round or oval fluid collections must be adequately imaged to rule out visceral pseudoaneurysms. Pseudoaneurysms are usually managed by transcatheter embolization.

EQUIPMENT

Aspiration

• 20- to 22-gauge Chiba-type needle or 18-gauge sheathed (Yueh) needle

Drainage

• Trocar placement of catheters should be avoided
• Seldinger technique preferable
• 18- to 22-gauge needle for initial access

• A coaxial set may be necessary to convert from a 0.018- to a 0.035/0.038-inch system
• Stiff guidewire
• Fascial dilators
• Large-bore multi-sidehole catheters (14F-16F)
• Drainage bag or suction system

TECHNIQUE

Anatomy and Approach

Drainage catheters are inserted via the Seldinger technique, and this should be preceded by fine-needle aspiration to guide diagnosis. Cultures should be performed routinely, including culture for anaerobes and fungus, since these organisms are known to infect pancreatic collections.

CT or ultrasound guidance can be used for percutaneous drainage. In the majority of instances, CT provides the most information about the extent, number, and location of adjacent neighboring structures. More superficial collections can be drained under ultrasound guidance if a previous localizing CT scan has been performed within the last 72 hours.

Thrombolytic agents may be used to facilitate drainage of loculated or complex collections. A variety of approaches have been described, but no consensus exists on the optimal timing or dose of thrombolytic agents (this also constitutes off-label use). After placement of a percutaneous catheter, the thrombolytic agent is instilled (e.g., tissue plasminogen activator [tPA], 5-10 mg in 20 mL of saline) through the catheter and allowed to dwell for 30 to 60 minutes with the catheter clamped. Drainage is then resumed. This process is repeated two to three times, either on the same day or on consecutive days.

The pancreas lies in the most anterior of the three retroperitoneal compartments, the anterior pararenal space. It is bounded ventrally by the posterior parietal peritoneum and dorsally by the anterior renal or Gerota fascia. Other structures occupying the anterior pararenal space include the duodenal loop and ascending and descending colon. The predominant anterior relationship of the pancreas is the lesser peritoneal sac or omental bursa. The splenic vein courses along the posterior surface of the pancreatic body, and the inferior mesenteric vein may course cephalad, posterior to the body, and join the splenic vein. Other posterior relationships include the left kidney, left renal vessels, left adrenal gland, and the left crus of the diaphragm.

Pancreatic collections contain proteolytic enzymes that facilitate spread of the inflammatory process along established fascial planes. The lesser sac is the site most often involved, followed closely by the left anterior pararenal space. The spleen (which is in close juxtaposition to the intraperitoneal pancreatic tail) and left lobe of the liver (probably by way of the gastrohepatic ligament) are the organs most frequently affected. Intraperitoneal spread through the foramen of Winslow and mediastinal spread along the diaphragmatic crura may also occur.

The incidence and location of pseudoaneurysms occurring in pancreatitis reflect the distribution of pseudocysts and fluid collections seen with the disease. The splenic artery is the vessel most commonly involved, followed by the gastroduodenal, inferior pancreaticoduodenal, and superior pancreaticoduodenal arteries. Additionally, involvement of the superior mesenteric, dorsal pancreatic, hepatic, and gastric arteries has been described. However, any vessel in contiguity with a fluid collection of pancreatic origin may be affected.

Several different approaches to drainage of pancreatic pseudocysts can be taken: surgical, radiologic, and endoscopic. Surgical drainage is accomplished by creating a large anastomosis between the GI tract and the collection; infected collections are drained externally. Radiologically, collections are drained externally with percutaneous transabdominal drainage catheters. Endoscopy facilitates internal drainage with placement of transgastric or transduodenal plastic stents. Most recently, therapeutic endoscopic ultrasound has been used to introduce large stents to provide drainage into the upper GI tract.

A transgastric internal drainage approach for a pseudocyst can be taken to avoid the risk of development of a pancreatic-cutaneous fistula and use of an external catheter. The technique involves using fluoroscopic, ultrasound, or CT guidance (or any combination thereof) to place a needle through the stomach and into the pseudocyst. After dilating the tract, a double-J stent is placed with a pusher catheter to provide communication and drainage of cyst contents into the stomach. All external catheters are then removed.

Drainage of pancreatic necrosis frequently requires large-bore catheters (up to 30F) and multiple catheter exchanges and flushing. Solid debris will often be removed through these large-bore catheters. Nontapered large-bore catheters can be placed percutaneously with aggressive preliminary balloon overdilation of the tract. The drainage catheter is then mounted onto the balloon catheter, which functions as a tapered dilator, and advanced into the collection.

Technical Aspects

- Optimal locations for catheter insertion are sites where fluid collections are largest and in contact with the parietal peritoneum.
- A direct approach that avoids other structures is preferable, except for percutaneous cystogastrostomy.
- A direct approach offers certain advantages: reduced catheter migration, easy catheter exchange when required, daily monitoring of drainage fluid volume and appearance, capability of irrigation, and the ability to detect a fistula with the GI tract or pancreatic duct.
- Relatively small-bore catheters (8F-10F) may be adequate to drain clear fluid collections and noninfected pseudocysts.
- Infected pseudocysts, abscesses, and liquefied necrosis are better drained with large-bore catheters (12F-16F).
- Multiple or complex collections may require more than one catheter.

CONTROVERSIES

Regarding the transgastric approach for a pseudocyst versus the direct percutaneous route, the rationale for performing percutaneous cystogastrostomy is that it avoids the risk of development of a pancreatic-cutaneous fistula, requires no external catheter to maintain, and improves patient comfort. It is debatable whether the risk of a pancreatic-cutaneous fistula is high enough to justify routine use of the

TABLE 128-1. Results of Percutaneous Catheter Drainage for Sterile Pancreatic Pseudocysts

Reference	No. of Patients	Clinical Success Rate (%)
Karlsson et al., 1982[22]	6	100
Gerzof et al., 1984[23]	11	90
Colhoun et al., 1984[24]	10	100
Kuligowska and Olsen, 1985[25]	3	33
Hancke and Henricksen, 1985[26]	18	100
Torres et al., 1986[27]	15	67
Matzinger, et al., 1988[28]	12	67
Grosso et al., 1989[29]	43	76
vanSonnenberg et al., 1989[30]	101	90

technically more challenging transgastric approach; many experts agree that transgastric pseudocyst drainage is unnecessary when no communication exists between the pseudocyst and pancreatic duct. In these patients, percutaneous drainage is sufficient. A detailed description of this technique is beyond the scope of this chapter but can be found in references 21 and 22 and Table 128-1.

OUTCOMES

Percutaneous catheter treatment of noninfected fluid collections and sterile pancreatic pseudocysts is less complicated and more successful than drainage of infected collections. Complete pseudocyst resolution has been reported in over 90% of patients (see Table 128-1). One retrospective study of 92 patients found equal success with surgical and percutaneous drainage of pancreatic pseudocysts.[25] Walser et al. compared needle aspiration and percutaneous catheter drainage of sterile fluid collections in acute pancreatitis. In this retrospective study of 37 patients, there was no apparent clinical benefit for catheter drainage of sterile fluid collections arising in acute pancreatitis in terms of length of hospital stay and mortality. In that study, the authors also reported a greater than 50% rate of bacterial colonization and the need for multiple sinograms and tube changes following catheter drainage.[13]

Series of patients with complicated pancreatitis (i.e., pancreatic abscess, pancreatic and peripancreatic necrosis) who are treated percutaneously are relatively small, but with continued advances in percutaneous drainage techniques, use of large-bore multiple catheters, and appropriate follow-up, a trend toward the percutaneous approach is developing. Reported results indicate a 65% to 90% success rate of percutaneous drainage for pancreatic abscess (Table 128-2) and 40% to 60% for pancreatic necrosis. One study (20 patients with pancreatic necrosis) reported a 100% success rate using large-bore catheters with enlarged side holes, suction catheters, stone baskets, and copious amounts of lavage fluid performed over multiple sessions.[17] In a systematic literature review of 384 patients with necrotizing pancreatitis undergoing percutaneous catheter drainage, van Baal et al. reported a 55.7% success rate, defined as patients surviving without additional surgical necrosectomy.[12]

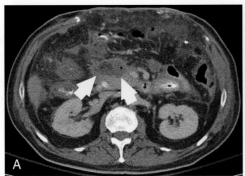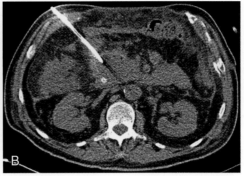

FIGURE 128-1. A, Acute necrotizing pancreatitis in a 71-year-old man after endoscopic retrograde cholangiopancreatography. A peripancreatic fluid collection *(arrows)* was detected 2 weeks after open débridement. Minimal pancreatic necrosis was encountered during surgery. Leukocytosis and a temperature of 102°F developed 48 hours before computed tomography (CT) scan. A narrow percutaneous window for drainage is present from a right subcostal approach. **B,** CT after placement of a 10F drainage catheter yielded pus without debris. Cultures grew *Klebsiella* and *Escherichia coli*. Collection resolved over next 2 weeks with percutaneous drainage.

TABLE 128-2. Results of Percutaneous Drainage For Pancreatic Abscess

Reference	No. of Patients	Successful Results (%)
Karlsson et al., 1982[22]	6	50
Steiner et al., 1988[32]	10	40
Freeny et al., 1988[10]	23	65
Adams et al., 1990[7]	23	79
Lee et al., 1992[6]	30	60
vanSonnenberg et al., 1997[16]	59	86

Percutaneous drainage of appropriate pancreatic fluid collections can be either curative or a valuable adjunct to surgery or endoscopic maneuvers (Fig. 128-1). Strategies for successful percutaneous drainage include choosing safe and uncomplicated catheter routes, permitting adequate time for catheterization and drainage, using more than one large catheter for complex collections, and performing follow-up clinical and imaging studies with appropriate tube adjustments as needed.

COMPLICATIONS

Complications of percutaneous drainage for pancreatitis include organ perforation, secondary infection of a sterile collection, rupture of a pseudocyst, pancreaticocutaneous fistula, and hemorrhage. Insertion of a drainage catheter into a pseudoaneurysm is a rare but potentially lethal complication that can be avoided by ensuring adequate imaging before drainage.

POSTPROCEDURAL AND FOLLOW-UP CARE

- Close monitoring with proper catheter adjustment, revision of catheter size, and repositioning of catheters is often required.
- Daily irrigation with saline until the returning fluid is clear is an important factor. Irrigation is performed three or more times daily. The technique includes first aspirating all the fluid that can be withdrawn, then gentle instillation of 20 mL of saline, usually multiple times. The fluid is withdrawn after each 20-mL infusion and discarded; this process is repeated until the returning fluid is clear.
- Catheterization continues until drainage ceases (usually defined as <20 mL/day for 2 consecutive days).
- Repeat CT or an abscessogram (or both) to document absence of a residual collection may be performed before catheter removal.

KEY POINTS

- Image-guided aspiration of pancreatic necrosis can be used to guide antimicrobial therapy, particularly when polymicrobial or antibiotic-resistant organisms are present.
- Fine-needle aspiration for bacteriology can differentiate between sterile and infected pancreatic necrosis in patients with sepsis syndrome.
- Percutaneous drainage of infected acute peripancreatic fluid collections, pancreatic abscess, and infected pseudocysts can be performed.
- Initial percutaneous drainage plays a limited role in infected pancreatic necrosis because the complex solid tissue elements often require surgical débridement.
- If surgical débridement of infected pancreatic necrosis is incomplete and fluid reaccumulates in the débrided area, percutaneous interventions may be performed.
- Percutaneous drainage may also be used as a temporizing measure in critically ill patients with infected necrosis until operative risk diminishes.
- Inflammatory debris may require large-bore and long-term percutaneous drainage catheters, with additional upsizing and repositioning often needed.
- Small sterile fluid collections can be left alone, or the drainage catheter can be removed at 2 days if 48-hour cultures remain negative.
- Sterile pseudocysts producing a mass effect may be considered for drainage. Pseudocysts may be drained percutaneously or through a cystogastrostomy.

- Thrombolytic agents have an evolving role in difficult fluid collections.
- Large visceral arterial pseudoaneurysms from pancreatitis can masquerade as fluid collections. All fluid collections undergoing percutaneous drainage must be adequately imaged (with computed tomography, ultrasound, or magnetic resonance imaging) to exclude pseudoaneurysm.

▶ SUGGESTED READINGS

Acute Pancreatitis Classification Working Group. Revision of the Atlanta classification of acute pancreatitis 2008; http://pancreasclub.com/wp-content/uploads/2011/11/AtlantaClassification.pdf.

Bollen TL, van Santvoort HC, Besselink MG, et al. The Atlanta Classification of acute pancreatitis revisited. Br J Surg 2008;95:6–21.

Brun A, Agarwal N, Pitchumoni CS. Fluid collections in and around the pancreas in acute pancreatitis. J Clin Gastroenterol 2011;45:614–25.

van Baal MC, van Santvoort HC, Bollen TL, et al. Systematic review of percutaneous catheter drainage as primary treatment for necrotizing pancreatitis. Br J Surg 2011;98:18–27.

vanSonnenberg E, Wittich GR, Chon KS, et al. Percutaneous radiologic drainage of pancreatic abscess. AJR Am J Roentgenol 1997;168:979–84.

The complete reference list is available online at www.expertconsult.com.

CHAPTER **129**

Esophageal Intervention in Malignant and Benign Esophageal Disease

Tarun Sabharwal, Stavros Spiliopoulos, and Andreas Adam

With development and improvement of different technologies and devices, many diseases of the esophagus are now within the scope of minimally invasive interventional radiologic–guided procedures. In this chapter we describe the methods of imaged-guided intervention of benign and malignant conditions of the esophagus. Although endoscopy is helpful in confirming the diagnosis, it is unnecessary in the treatment of esophageal strictures under imaging guidance.

An esophageal stricture is a narrowing of the lumen caused by an abnormality of the esophageal wall. Strictures may be due to esophageal cancer or a range of benign conditions and may be associated with mucosal ulceration and fibrous scarring. Obstruction of the lower esophagus can be also caused by achalasia. The etiology of the stricture is determined by the patient's signs and symptoms, the radiographic and endoscopic appearance of the stricture, esophageal pressure and acidity measurements in patients with suspected functional obstruction, and where appropriate, histologic examination of endoscopic biopsy specimens. Management of the stricture differs among the types.

Dysphagia is the most common symptom associated with esophageal strictures. Patients typically complain of solid-food dysphagia that may progress over time to include liquids. If patients present initially with solid *and* liquid dysphagia, a motility disorder rather than an anatomic abnormality should be suspected. Patients may also report symptoms of regurgitation or aspiration, chest pain, abdominal pain, or weight loss. Analysis of the patient's symptoms can guide the clinician to the correct diagnosis in 80% of dysphagia cases.[1]

The diagnostic evaluation for these patients often begins with a barium esophagogram, which can help direct further endoscopic evaluation and intervention. The location, size, and complexity of the lesion, as well as the presence of associated abnormalities, influence the choice of therapy. If esophagography suggests that the stricture may be malignant, diagnostic endoscopy and biopsy are usually carried out.

Esophageal cancer is the sixth leading cause of death from cancer worldwide.[2,3] Because patients may not experience dysphagia until the luminal diameter has been reduced by 50%, cancer of the esophagus is generally associated with late presentation and poor prognosis. The overall 5-year survival rate is less than 10%, and fewer than 50% of patients are suitable for resection at presentation.[4,5] The aims of palliation are maintenance of oral intake, relief of pain, elimination of reflux and regurgitation, prevention of aspiration, and minimization of hospital stay.[6-8] Current palliative treatment options include thermal ablation,[9] photodynamic therapy,[10] radiotherapy,[11] chemotherapy,[12] chemical injection,[13] argon beam or bipolar electrocoagulation,[14] enteral feeding (nasogastric tube/percutaneous endoscopic gastrostomy),[15] and intubation using either self-expanding metal stents (SEMS) or semirigid plastic tubes.[7,8] Esophageal prostheses have been in use for over a century. Different tubes of the pulsion and traction variety have been described. The earliest device, made of decalcified ivory, was designed by Leroy d'Etiolles in 1845. The first metal esophageal prosthesis was introduced by Charters J. Symonds in 1885.[16] Modern esophageal stenting utilizes either rigid plastic tubes or SEMS.

INDICATIONS

Benign Esophageal Strictures

Benign strictures of the esophagus occur as the result of collagen deposition and fibrous tissue formation stimulated by esophageal injury. Peptic strictures, caused by esophageal exposure to gastric acid, account for 70% to 75% of benign esophageal strictures.[17,18] Other common causes of benign strictures include Schatzki ring, ingestion of corrosive agents (including certain medications), external-beam radiation therapy, sclerotherapy, photodynamic therapy, reaction to a foreign body, infectious esophagitis, and surgical trauma.[19,20]

Corrosive Strictures

Please visit www.expertconsult.com for the discussion of corrosive strictures.

Achalasia

Achalasia is an esophageal motor disorder characterized by increased lower esophageal sphincter (LES) pressure, diminished to absent peristalsis in the distal portion of the esophagus, and lack of a coordinated LES relaxation in response to swallowing.

Primary achalasia is the most common subtype and is associated with loss of ganglion cells in the esophageal myenteric plexus. These important inhibitory neurons induce LES relaxation and coordinate proximal-to-distal peristaltic contraction of the esophagus. LES pressure and relaxation are regulated by excitatory (e.g., acetylcholine, substance P) and inhibitory (e.g., nitric oxide, vasoactive intestinal peptide) neurotransmitters. Patients with achalasia have an imbalance in excitatory and inhibitory neurotransmission. The result is a hypertensive, nonrelaxing esophageal sphincter.

Secondary achalasia, which is relatively uncommon, is caused by conditions other than intrinsic disease of the esophageal myenteric plexus, such as certain malignancies, diabetes mellitus, and Chagas disease.

Please visit www.expertconsult.com for more information on the clinical presentation, diagnosis, and treatment of achalasia.

Epidermolysis Bullosa

Epidermolysis bullosa (EB) is a very rare skin fragility disorder characterized by blister formation following minor mechanical trauma. The clinical subset varies from only mild skin reactions to severe mutilating deformities such as pseudosyndactyly and fatal forms, depending on the genotypic subtype of the disease. In severe types, gastrointestinal, urologic, and corneal abnormalities have been also noted.[23] In general, two major categories are recognized: inherited (IEB) and acquisita (EBA). The inherited type is more common and can be divided into four principal types: EB simplex, dystrophic EB, junctional EB, and Kindler syndrome.[24,25] It is calculated that IEB affects 1 to 3 births in every 100,000 live births; nearly 5000 patients in the United Kingdom suffer from the disease.[26] EBA is an autoimmune primary blistering disease associated with immunoglobulin G (Ig) autoantibodies against type VII collagen, the basal membrane zone (BMZ) of the skin and the malpighian mucosa. Collagen VII is a major component of esophageal epithelium, so high-grade esophageal strictures resulting in severe dysphagia and malnutrition are noted in various EB subtypes. Esophageal involvement is more frequent in the recessive dystrophic EB subtype; almost 70% of these patients will develop at least one esophageal stricture by the age of 25.[27]

A discussion of the diagnosis and treatment of epidermolysis bullosa is available at www.expertconsult.com.

Esophageal Varices

Esophageal varices detected prior to first hemorrhage are usually treated with oral β-adrenergic blocking agents. If varices are of a high endoscopic grade, sclerotherapy or variceal ligation may be performed. In the setting of acute esophageal variceal hemorrhage, control of bleeding can be accomplished endoscopically in 80% to 90% of patients. Radiologic interventions employed in the treatment of esophageal varices include transjugular intrahepatic portocaval shunt, embolization of the varices, or both.

Esophageal Strictures in Children

Esophageal strictures occur in 40% of children after surgical repair of esophageal atresia. The main causes are fibrosis subsequent to natural healing, size difference of the two anastomosed segments, tension, and gastroesophageal reflux. Leaks, as well as use of a two-layer anastomosis and/or silk sutures, increase the likelihood of stricture formation. Dilation is 90% effective, but strictures that do not respond to repeated dilation can be treated with temporary stenting—a technique still under evaluation—or with repeat surgery.

Esophageal atresia is a condition in which the proximal and distal portions of the esophagus do not communicate. The upper segment of the esophagus is a dilated blind-ending pouch with a hypertrophied muscular wall. This pouch typically extends to the level of the second to fourth thoracic vertebrae. The distal esophageal portion has a small diameter and a thin muscular wall; it extends a variable distance above the diaphragm.

Tracheoesophageal fistula is an abnormal communication between the trachea and esophagus. When associated with esophageal atresia, the fistula most commonly occurs between the distal esophageal segment and the trachea, just above the carina.

The frequency and severity of complications after repair of esophageal atresia are related to the extent of the repair required, with primary anastomosis and fistula closure being associated with fewer complications than esophageal replacement. The most common complications are anastomotic leak, recurrent fistula, stricture, and gastroesophageal reflux.

Foreign Body

Prompt treatment of an infant or child with a suspected esophageal foreign body is very important in avoiding severe complications.

Malignant Esophageal Strictures

The main indications for esophageal stenting in malignant disease are:
- Intrinsic esophageal obstruction
- Tracheoesophageal fistula. Spontaneous malignant fistulas between the esophagus and major airways occur as a result of local tumor invasion from the esophagus or tracheobronchial tree (Fig. 129-1) or may be secondary to surgery or esophageal stent placement. Esophageal leaks or perforations are usually iatrogenic following esophageal dilation or surgery, but may also be caused by local tumor invasion. Leaks and fistulas in benign disease should not be stented because leakage occurs around the stent. In many such cases, there is spontaneous healing. However, without definitive treatment, malignant lesions will not heal, and most patients would die of malnutrition and thoracic sepsis within weeks. Until recently, therapy for malignant leaks and fistulas has been unsatisfactory. Attempted surgical repair has a high morbidity and mortality. Parenteral nutrition or feeding via a gastrostomy were often used, but continuing leakage of esophageal contents resulted in mediastinitis in many patients. Attempts to seal the esophageal defect with plastic stents were usually ineffective. Covered self-expanding metallic stents are the treatment of first choice in patients with malignant leaks and fistulas, because the metallic stent expands to the diameter of the esophagus, and the covering material seals the defect.
- Extrinsic esophageal compression by primary or secondary mediastinal tumors
- Esophageal perforation, usually iatrogenic, from direct endoscopic trauma or following stricture dilation
- Symptomatic gastroesophageal anastomotic leaks
- Anastomotic tumor recurrence after surgery

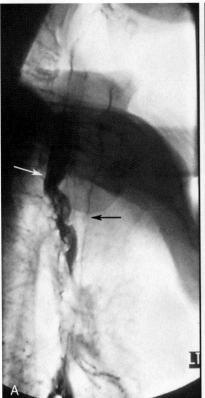 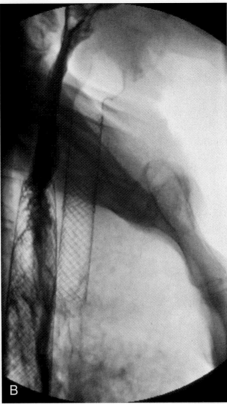

FIGURE 129-1. A, Esophagogram demonstrating large esophago- *(white arrow)* tracheal *(black arrow)* fistula. **B,** Esophagogram demonstrating esophageal and tracheal stents in situ, with no extravasation of contrast agent.

CONTRAINDICATIONS

There are no absolute contraindications for intervention in esophageal disease. Relative contraindications should be considered for both benign and malignant disease:

- Radiotherapy during the previous 6 weeks, which is associated with increased hemorrhage and perforation rates if stents are inserted
- Malignant obstruction of the gastric outlet or small bowel
- Strictures above the level of the cricopharyngeus muscle
- Severe tracheal compression that would be made worse by esophageal intubation
- Severe debility

Particular contraindications for foreign body removal by fluoroscopic balloon catheter removal, esophageal bougienage, and temporization include chest radiographic findings of esophageal edema with airway compromise, esophageal perforation, or pneumomediastinum. Most often, esophageal foreign bodies are retrieved with rigid esophagoscopy. Advantages include a high success rate, direct visualization of the foreign body in the esophagus, and direct visualization of the esophagus after removal of the object.

EQUIPMENT

Materials and Equipment

- Water-soluble nonionic contrast medium
- Tilting fluoroscopic table

- Monitoring equipment (pulse oximeter, blood pressure, and pulse measurement)
- Suction equipment
- Oxygen
- Radiopaque ruler
- Lidocaine spray
- Mouthguard

Catheters and Guidewires

- Biliary manipulation catheter
- Multipurpose 6F, 100-cm catheter
- 0.035-inch Bentson guidewire
- 0.035-inch hydrophilic wire (Terumo Medical Corp., Somerset, N.J.)
- 260-cm, 0.035-inch stiff exchange wire

Balloons

- 14- and 18-mm diameter (Medi-Tech/Boston Scientific, Natick, Mass.), 30- and 40-mm balloons (Rigiflex [Boston Scientific])

Stents

A wide variety of self-expanding metallic or plastic stents are used.

Nitinol Stents

Nitinol is composed of nickel (55%-56%) and titanium (44%-45%), which expands or contracts when its temperature is increased or decreased, respectively. As a result of a "shape memory effect" acquired during heat treatment of the raw material, stents made of nitinol return to a preset shape and size when they reach body temperature.

Esophageal Wallstent

WallFlex stents (Boston Scientific) are fully and partially covered esophageal stents. The Permalume silicone covering encompasses the entire stent in the fully covered type. In both versions, a Teflon-coated polyester removal suture facilitates removal during the initial stent placement procedure. The 18.5F low-profile delivery system helps traverse tight strictures, while the progressive step-flared ends may assist in better stent anchoring.

Ultraflex

The Ultraflex stent (Boston Scientific) is knitted from a highly elastic 0.15-mm-diameter nitinol wire; it is flexible both radially and longitudinally and has a large proximal flare. The stent is stretched and compressed in a low-profile manner and has a suture release mechanism that allows either distal or proximal release. A polyurethane covering is used to counter the problem of tumor ingrowth and enable sealing of the esophageal fistula. The stent is available in 28-mm and 23-mm diameters.

Niti-S Stent

Niti-S stents (Taewoong Medical, Seoul, South Korea) are single- or double-layered polytetrafluoroethylene (PTFE)-covered nitinol stents. The double-layered type consists of an inner PTFE-covered stent and an outer uncovered stent attached to the middle part of the inner covered stent. Its particular design aims to minimize the risk of migration. The single-layer Niti-S stent is constructed of a nitinol monofilament mesh fully or partially covered with polyurethane. It has a thread attached to enable retrieval of the device.

EsophaCoil

The EsophaCoil (Medtronic InStent, Eden Prairie, Minn.) consists of a tightly wound coil of nitinol forming a cylinder that resists tumor ingrowth. It has flared and expanded coils at the proximal and distal ends helping to maintain the stent position. The delivery system allows central, proximal, or distal stent release. The EsophaCoil is available in diameters of 16 and 18 mm, with flanges of 21 and 24 mm.

Memotherm Stent

The Memotherm stent (C.R. Bard Inc., Covington, Ga.) is a single-walled, thermoreactive device covered with PTFE. The particular blend of nitinol used to manufacture the Memotherm stent expands maximally at 35.5°C. Both ends of the stent are slightly flared to minimize the risk of migration. The stent undergoes only minimal foreshortening (3%-4%) on deployment.

Choo Stent

The Choo Stent (Diagmed Healthcare Ltd., Thirsk, North Yorkshire, UK) is made from strands of nitinol wire and is covered with a polyurethane membrane. Several stent segments are interconnected with this membrane to produce stents of 4 to 14 cm. This method of construction increases stent flexibility. The stent has flanges at the proximal and distal ends measuring 24 mm in diameter. There is a

retrieval lasso attached inside the proximal flange to allow retrieval and repositioning of an inappropriately placed stent.

Do Stent

The Do stent is a modified Choo stent with an internal distal antireflux valve made of three polyurethane leaflets.

Stainless Steel Stents

Flamingo Stent

The Flamingo stent (Boston Scientific) is made of a stainless steel mesh with a conical shape, and it has a covering material placed inside the stent. The braiding angle is larger in the upper part of the stent and smaller in the lower part. This feature constitutes an effective antimigration mechanism. The stent is available in 12- and 14-cm lengths and 24-mm and 30-mm maximum diameters.

Gianturco-Rösch Z Stent

The esophageal Z stent (Cook Medical, Bloomington, Ind.) is completely covered by polyurethane. Barbs fix the stent and minimize the risk of migration. The stent is 18 mm in diameter with 25-mm flanges at both ends. It is available in lengths of 10, 12, and 14 cm. A variety of this device is available with a "windsock" valve to prevent gastroesophageal reflux.

Song Stent

The Song stent (Sohoo/Medi-Tech, Seoul, South Korea) has a modified Gianturco design. It is made of stainless steel with a polyurethane covering and is available in a retrievable form. Variations of this stent made of nitinol are available.

FerX-ELLA Stent Family

FerX-ELLA stents are covered and uncovered designs with an optional antireflux valve (ELLA-CS, Hradec Králové, Czech Republic). The Boubela (UK Medical Ltd., Sheffield, UK) stent is a self-expandable covered device made of stainless steel wire covered with two-layer polyurethane foil. The stent can be equipped with an antireflux valve. Both ends of the stent are provided with purse strings that allow retrieval.

Plastic Self-Expanding Stents

The PolyFlex stent (Boston Scientific) is a new type of device made of a polyester mesh and is 100% coated with a silicone membrane that aims to prevent mucosal hyperplasia or tumor ingrowth. This device can be retrieved and may be appropriate for use in benign as well as malignant strictures.

Biodegradable Stent

The ELLA-BD esophageal stent (ELLA-CS) is a biodegradable self-expanding bare stent manufactured of interwoven polydioxanone monofilament, and is currently commercially available in Europe. The stent is designed to disintegrate within 11 to 12 weeks following implantation. The absorption process is accelerated by the reflux of gastric content, and therefore in case of migration it can be left to dissolve in the stomach. It has to be manually loaded on the delivery system. This innovative technology is expected to expand stent indications in the treatment of benign

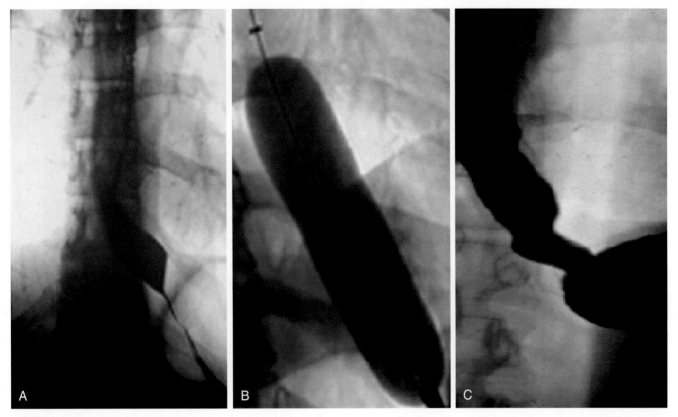

FIGURE 129-2. A, Esophagogram demonstrates patient with achalasia. **B**, Balloon dilation with a 40-mm balloon. **C**, Check esophagogram demonstrates good flow after dilation.

esophageal disease, as well as in the field of neoadjuvant therapy as a bridge to surgery.

TECHNIQUE

Technical Approach for Benign Strictures

After an initial esophagogram (Fig. 129-2) with water-soluble nonionic contrast medium to identify the site and length of the narrow segment, the patient is placed on the fluoroscopic table in the left lateral position. Intravenous sedation is with midazolam, and analgesia is with fentanyl as required. The oropharynx is anesthetized with lidocaine, and a mouthguard is inserted.

A 6.5F biliary manipulation catheter (Cook Medical) is advanced over a Bentson guidewire (Cook Medical) to the level of the gastroesophageal junction. Contrast medium is injected to outline the narrow segment and enable safe manipulation of the catheter and guidewire into the stomach. The catheter is usually advanced into the duodenum because this provides greater stability and allows easier catheter exchange. If the esophagus is grossly dilated and contains food or liquid residue, a large-bore nasogastric tube is inserted, and the contents are aspirated.

A Bentson guidewire is used to cross the stricture, but a hydrophilic wire can be used if the stricture is tortuous or very tight. A stiff exchange wire (Amplatz Super Stiff [Boston Scientific]) is then inserted, over which the balloon catheter is advanced to the cardia.

The balloon is partially inflated until a waist appears (Fig. 129-2, *B*) indicating the position of the muscular ring of the

lower esophageal sphincter. The balloon is always inflated under continuous fluoroscopic guidance, and the position readjusted if it starts to slip. The balloon is inflated by hand pressure using dilute contrast medium (Ultravist 300 [iodine, 300 mg/mL, mixed with equal volume sterile water]).

Elimination of the "waist" is used as an indicator of successful dilation. Immediately after the dilation, water-soluble contrast medium is injected through the catheter to exclude esophageal perforation.

A barium esophagogram is repeated at 4 to 6 hours after the procedure, once the patient has recovered from sedation, to rule out mucosal tear or perforation (Fig. 129-2, *C*). If the imaging studies show no evidence of perforation, the patient is allowed to drink clear fluids and can resume a normal diet the following day.

In patients with esophageal strictures, the choice of balloon diameter is based on severity of the stenosis, length of stricture, and cause or nature of the disease. In patients with fixed strictures, it is common to start with a 12-mm diameter balloon and then use balloons of larger diameters, up to 20 mm. Larger balloons are hardly ever used in this group of patients. In patients with achalasia having balloon dilation for the first time, a 20-mm balloon is used initially. If there is no blood on the balloon or severe pain (pain intolerable despite safe adequate sedation and analgesia) during the dilation, we progress to 30-mm and 35-mm balloons. If blood is seen on the balloon after dilation or the patient experiences severe pain, the procedure is terminated. Balloon inflation is maintained for 1 minute to allow time for disruption of the muscular ring to take place. If the

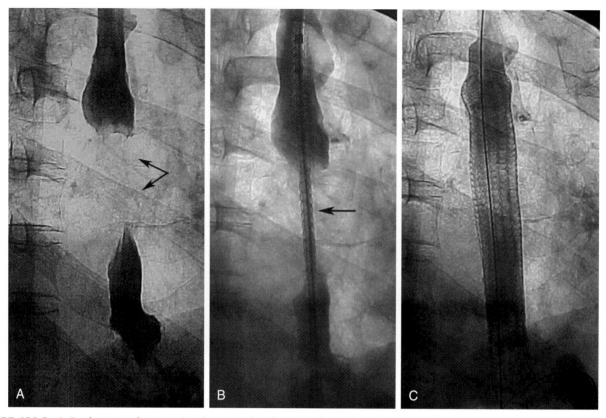

FIGURE 129-3. **A,** Esophagogram demonstrating almost complete obstruction *(arrows)* in mid-esophagus from known cancer. **B,** Ultraflex delivery system in situ *(arrow)* in same patient. **C,** Post-deployment esophagogram shows satisfactory stent position and expansion.

"waist" of the balloon is not eliminated completely during the first inflation, a second or third inflation is carried out.

Balloons larger than 35 mm are not used for patients having their first dilation, even if no blood is seen on the balloon. However, in patients having their second or subsequent dilation, a 40-mm balloon is used if no blood is present on the 35-mm balloon. Many different types of balloon dilators were used in the past, but the Rigiflex balloon (Boston Scientific) is currently the most popular.[30]

Technical Approach for Malignant Strictures

After obtaining an esophagogram to delineate the position and length of the stricture, the patient is placed in the left lateral position. The oropharynx is anesthetized with lidocaine spray, and the catheter is passed orally into the esophagus. The location of the tumor is defined by injecting contrast medium above and below the stricture and by anatomic landmarks.

The stricture is crossed with a variety of angle-tipped catheters and standard or hydrophilic guidewires. A 180- or 260-cm-long stiff guidewire is looped in the stomach or advanced into the proximal duodenum. The stricture may be predilated to 15 mm, because this facilitates introduction of the delivery system, allows rapid expansion of the stent, and enables more accurate placement.

A stent of appropriate size and length is advanced across the stricture on its delivery system and deployed in such a way that slightly more of the stent is above the stricture than below it; this will reduce the likelihood of migration. The stent should cover at least 2 cm of normal esophagus above

and below the stricture. Long strictures may require more than one stent, with one third overlap between the devices. After deployment, contrast medium is injected to confirm correct stent position and exclude esophageal perforation.

Esophagography on the following day is recommended to show that the stent has expanded adequately and remains in a satisfactory position (Fig. 129-3).

Esophageal Atresia and Tracheoesophageal Fistula in Children

Dilation of anastomotic strictures may be performed in a child with 4- to 10-mm angioplasty balloons with the same approach as just described but with the use of general anesthesia.

Foreign-Body Removal

A variety of methods can be used to remove an esophageal foreign body. The chosen strategy depends on the type and location of the foreign body, the length of time it has been in the esophagus, and the relative degree of experience with the different techniques at a given facility.

Current strategies for the removal of retained foreign bodies include endoscopy or surgery; temporization, which allows the foreign body to pass into the stomach on its own; rigid or flexible esophagoscopy; balloon catheter extraction with radiographic guidance; and bougienage or a balloon catheter technique to push the foreign body into the stomach. The last technique is appropriate only when the object is lodged in the distal portion of the esophagus.

Stent Insertion Technique in Esophageal Fistulas

The same technique as described previously for malignant strictures is used for esophageal fistulas. It is usually possible to identify the exact location of the fistula or perforation by injection of contrast medium into the esophagus. Any coexisting stricture should not be predilated with a balloon so as not to risk increasing the size of the esophageal defect. Deployment of a covered stent across a fistula or leak almost always results in prompt and complete closure of the defect. Because most of these patients have malignant strictures, stent insertion not only seals the fistula or leak but also improves the patient's dysphagia.

CONTROVERSIES

Achalasia

Minimally invasive surgery using laparoscopic or thoracoscopic myotomy has shortened hospitalization and decreased morbidity compared with traditional myotomy, without increasing complications.[31] However, no long-term results are available. Medical treatment with anticholinergic agents or calcium antagonists is disappointing, and bougienage produces only transient relief, with a reported 6% incidence of perforation of the esophagus.[32]

Injection of botulinum toxin is an attractive alternative because of its safety and low cost per treatment, but the response is short lasting, and there is a need for repeat injections, leading to higher overall cost compared with pneumatic dilation.[33] Treatment with oral medication or injection of botulinum toxin should be reserved for elderly or infirm patients who are not suitable candidates for pneumatic dilation or surgery. Pneumatic dilation remains the first choice in treatment of esophageal achalasia in many institutions.[34,35]

Some investigators[33] do not consider that routine use of fluoroscopy is necessary for balloon dilations. However, the American Society for Gastrointestinal Endoscopy guidelines state that fluoroscopy is mandatory for placement of a balloon dilator.[36] We think fluoroscopic guidance facilitates the negotiation of tight strictures and enables less traumatic crossing of the cardia, thus helping minimize the risk of perforation due to inappropriate advancement of instruments outside the esophageal lumen. Furthermore, it is not uncommon during inflation for the balloon to slide into the stomach or esophagus. Fluoroscopy enables immediate detection and correction of misplacement; this can be missed during endoscopy, leading to full inflation of a large balloon in the esophagus and consequent perforation, or ineffective inflation within the lumen of the stomach.

OUTCOMES

Corrosive Strictures

Corrosive strictures, especially if long, often lead to severe dysphagia, affecting even liquids, and the lumen may be completely obliterated. The degree of dysphagia is related to the diameter of the residual lumen, but this is not the only factor. The severity of esophagitis is an equally important determinant of dysphagia, and failure of motility is a further contributory factor.

Achalasia

The reported success rate of balloon dilation is high (70%-80%), and complications are relatively infrequent.[33,36,37] This method of treatment is successful in decreasing LES pressure in 60% to 80% of patients, but this change does not always translate into relief or improvement of symptoms. About half of these patients experience recurrent symptoms within 5 years. In most, the disease responds well to repeated dilation therapy.[38] Recently, a 0 to 3 scale has been proposed for quantifying clinical success following balloon dilatation according to patients' symptomatology (weight loss, dysphagia, retrosternal cramps, regurgitation).[39]

Further predictors of outcome include manometric and barium studies. A 50% decrease in LES pressure or reductions to below 10 mmHg are predictors of symptomatic response.[40] Metman et al.[41] found that previous Heller myotomy was not a risk factor for complications after pneumatic dilation. This agrees with our own findings in 76 patients who underwent a total of 110 dilations, in whom no perforations were encountered, including a subgroup of patients who had had previous esophageal surgery.[36] Reported rates of perforation range from 0% to 18%.[29,37,42] Progressive balloon dilations yields excellent results, with balloons larger than 30 mm having to be used in relatively few patients.[33]

The Laplace law, which states that "the tension applied on the wall for a given pressure increases rapidly with the square of the balloon radius" suggests that use of larger balloons is likely to be associated with a substantially higher risk of perforation. However, in a retrospective study evaluating risk factors for esophageal perforation in 218 patients who had 270 pneumatic dilations, Borotto et al.[43] reported that perforation always occurred during the first dilation.

Our policy of not progressing to a balloon of greater size when blood is detected on the balloon being used for the procedure is based on the assumption that tissue damage has occurred in such cases, and that this is a useful marker of success. By terminating the procedure when blood staining of the balloon is observed, we believe we decrease the likelihood of unnecessary further injury to tissues and may reduce the risk of perforation. Rupture of the esophagus after balloon dilation can be treated with fasting, parenteral alimentation, and antibiotics; surgery is rarely needed and is reserved for major perforations.

Accurate positioning of the balloon across the LES and maintaining the position throughout inflation using fluoroscopic guidance is essential to success. Abolition of a balloon "waist" and presence of blood on the balloon are indications of a successful myotomy. Novel trials that tested the use of retrievable partially covered SEMS in achalasia demonstrated satisfactory long-term results. In a prospective study, 75 patients were treated with a custom-made stent that was removed after 4 to 5 days. The reported remission rate was 83.3% after 10 years' follow-up.[44] This strategy could be implied in selective cases in which poor balloon dilatation outcomes are awaited, owing to the presence of various negative predictors. In a recent study, Alderliesten et al.[45] reported that young age at presentation, classic achalasia, high pressure of the LES 3 months after dilatation, and incomplete obliteration of the balloon's waist are the most important predicting factors for clinically driven repeated treatment.

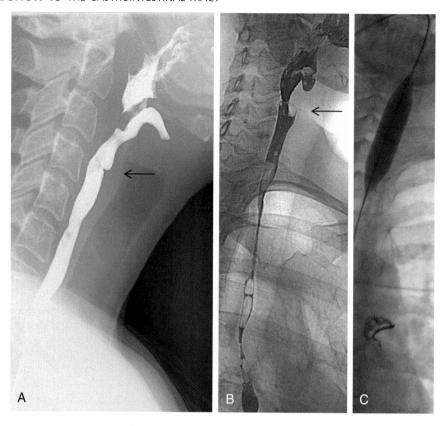

FIGURE 129-4. A, Barium esophagogram demonstrating a characteristic epidermolysis bullosa web stricture at level of cervical esophagus *(arrow)*. **B,** Dilatation of lesion using a 14 × 40 mm balloon. **C,** Check water-soluble esophagogram demonstrating a satisfactory result *(arrow)*. No sign of perforation is noted.

Epidermolysis Bullosa

Data from fluoroscopically guided balloon dilatations for treatment of dysphagia due to EB are scarce because of the rarity of the disease. However, a few case series and case reports have reported that fluoroscopically guided esophageal dilatations are safe and effective. Most of the procedures were performed under general anesthesia. The technical success rate is almost 100%. Complication rates vary from 0% to 14.8% and include perforation, bleeding, and acute dysphagia.[27] The mean intervention-free interval ranges from 10 to 16.5 months, but cases of dilatation-free intervals of almost 5 years have been reported (Figure 129-4).[27,29]

Esophageal Atresia and Tracheoesophageal Fistula

Two recent studies have been published regarding balloon dilation in children. The first study[46] reports the author's experience in three children with achalasia, including one successfully treated with balloon dilation. The second study[47] compares the results and success of balloon dilation of strictures due to caustic ingestion, achalasia, esophagitis, congenital stenosis, and epidermolysis bullosa with those from primary repair of esophageal atresia. Both groups had satisfactory alleviation of symptoms. There were no complications, but the authors noted that patients with chronic diseases such as EB required repeated dilation.

Zhang et al.[48] published their experience with retrievable stents in children with benign esophageal strictures. The devices used in this study were made of nitinol alloy coated with silicon to avoid mucosal ingrowth, and were easy to remove. Most of the patients had developed strictures after ingestion of corrosive agents such as oil of vitriol, hydrochloric acid, sodium hydroxide, and other industrial corrosive substances, which can cause deep esophageal burns, resulting in strictures that do not respond to medical treatment or repeated dilation.

The stents were removed within 1 to 4 weeks (mean, 13.3 days) after placement. There were no serious complications, but all patients experienced chest pain and vomiting caused by visceral tension or gastroesophageal reflux. These symptoms were relieved using oral medications and disappeared after stent removal.

The radial force exerted by stents is uniform, and the rate of stricture recurrence is lower than that associated with balloon dilation. Some authors have suggested that a longer period of stenting might reduce stricture recurrence. In animal studies, stents left in place for 2 weeks caused less stenosis than was observed in control animals without stents. After 3 weeks of stenting, strictures were virtually eliminated, but stent retrieval after 4 weeks can be difficult because of epithelial ingrowth. Gastroesophageal reflux after stenting and the development of squamous cell carcinoma have been reported. Because of these possibilities, long-term follow-up of such patients is required.

Foreign-Body Removal

The success rate for the removal of foreign bodies from the esophagus is 95% to 100% regardless of the technique used. Trained professionals with experience in pediatric resuscitation procedures must be available.

Stent Placement in Esophageal Cancer

The technical success rates of stent placement under fluoroscopy guidance approach 100%. The results of stenting are expressed by means of a dysphagia score with five grades: grade 0, normal diet; grade 1, some solid food; grade 2, semisolids only; grade 3, liquids only; grade 4, complete dysphagia. Dysphagia is relieved in most patients, with an improvement in the dysphagia score of at least one grade in 92% to 98% of patients.[7,8] Although most patients die in the 4 months after stent placement, they experience a substantial improvement in quality of life.[49] Covered metallic stents have a clinical success rate exceeding 95% in the palliation of malignant esophagorespiratory fistulas and perforations.[50,51]

The initial clinical success rate in the use of metallic stents in the treatment of benign strictures resistant to balloon dilation approaches 100%; however, dysphagia due to occlusive tissue hyperplasia almost always recurs in these patients. For this reason, metallic stents should be used in benign disease only as a last resort when the patient's quality of life is unacceptable and the condition cannot be treated by other means. Stenting in this very small group of patients relieves symptoms but requires repeated interventions to maintain patency of the devices. Occlusive epithelial hyperplasia is best treated with balloon dilation or endoscopic laser therapy.

Of note, novel biodegradable stent technology has recently provided new management options for recurrent benign strictures. Initial data are favorable, and more studies are awaited.[52] In addition, experimental studies are in progress testing the safety and feasibility of drug-eluting and radioactive stents for management of esophageal malignant disease.[53]

Stent Placement in Esophageal Fistula

Clinical success, defined as closure of the fistula or leak and relief from symptoms of aspiration, is achieved in 67% to 100% of patients. Recurrent fistulas or leaks occur in 8% to 20% of patients and can usually be treated by insertion of additional stents. In the largest series from our institution, clinical success was achieved in 95% of 39 patients, and recurrent lesions occurred in 10%. Treatment failure occurs with lesions close to the cricopharyngeus and when the esophagus is very dilated, which results in inadequate apposition between the stent and the esophageal wall. Patients in whom treatment fails can be treated with insertion of covered stents into the trachea. Most complications are related to the migration of a covered stent in the lower esophagus.

COMPLICATIONS

Foreign-Body Removal

The most serious complication of balloon catheter removal is transient airway compromise caused by displacement of the foreign body from the esophagus into the airway. Although the reported complication rates with this technique vary, there is a definite risk, and this technique should be used with great care.

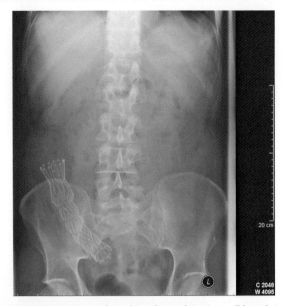

FIGURE 129-5. Migrated esophageal stent lying in small bowel. Patient subsequently required surgery for obstruction.

Malignant Disease

The main procedural complications are perforation, aspiration, hemorrhage, stent migration, and pain. Postprocedural complications include perforation, hemorrhage, stent migration (Fig. 129-5), pain/sensation of a foreign body, tumor ingrowth/overgrowth (Fig. 129-6), stent occlusion due to a bolus of food, reflux esophagitis, mucous membrane ulceration, fistula formation, and sepsis.

Procedure-related complications are lower in patients treated with metallic stents than in those in whom rigid plastic endoprostheses are used. The major complications of stenting are hemorrhage, fistula, perforation, severe pain, migration, and ingrowth/overgrowth. Hemorrhage occurs in 3% to 8%, although it is usually mild and self-limiting. Severe hemorrhage, which is rare, is best managed with arterial embolization. Fistulas and perforation attributable to stent insertion are uncommon. Some chest discomfort is reported by most patients, but in the longer term, chest pain is observed in approximately 13%. Pain is more severe in patients with high strictures and when using large-diameter stents. The incidence of migration of uncovered stents is low (0%-3%) when the lower end of the device is within the esophagus, increasing up to 6% for stents extending into the stomach.

Initial designs of covered stents exhibited a high rate of migration (25% and 32%), especially when positioned across the cardia. Migration is much less common with newer designs of covered stents. New data from a prospective randomized trial investigating the application of the Niti-S double-layered covered stent demonstrated significantly superior results regarding tumor ingrowth and stent migration compared to the single-layer covered control group.[54] Moreover, migration rates as low as 3% following deployment of the double-layer covered Niti-S stents indicate that these stents should be considered as the first choice in cases of malignant disease.[55] Therefore, uncovered stents should only be preferred in cases of extrinsic esophageal compression and very dilated esophagus to avoid food entrapment.

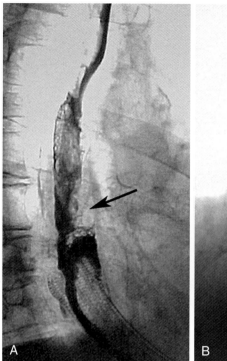 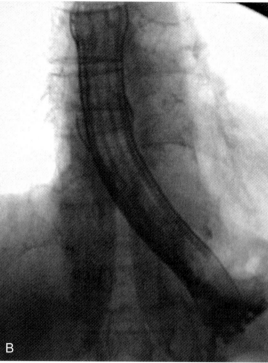

FIGURE 129-6. A, Tumor overgrowth *(arrow)* just above previously stented esophageal stricture. **B,** Second coaxial stent placement to relieve dysphagia from tumor overgrowth.

Partially migrated stents are treated by coaxially inserting another stent that overlaps the upper half of the migrated stent. If there is complete stent migration, the lesion is treated by insertion of a new stent. The asymptomatic patient with a migrated stent in the stomach can be left untreated, but if pain or vomiting occurs, the stent should be removed via a gastrostomy, surgical incision, or endoscopy.

Tumor ingrowth with uncovered stents is reported from 17% to 36% and is very rare with covered stents. Recurrent dysphagia due to tumor overgrowth or ingrowth has been reported in up to 60% of the patients. Ingrowth is much more frequent when uncovered stents are used. Tumor ingrowth or overgrowth can be treated by coaxial stenting. Metallic stent insertion has a very low procedural mortality rate, ranging from 0% to 1.4%.

POSTPROCEDURAL AND FOLLOW-UP CARE

Patients with balloon dilation for benign disease must have a "check swallow" the following day to rule out any perforation and guarantee adequate flow of contrast agent through the esophagus.

In patients with esophageal stent placement, if stent placement is successful and there are no immediate complications, clear fluids are allowed on the same day, and a normal diet can be resumed the following day. However, the patient is advised to avoid large chunks of food. Carbonated drinks with each meal help maintain patency of the stent.[7] Proton pump inhibitors, such as omeprazole, should be used in patients who develop reflux after stent deployment. Antacids may be used prophylactically in all patients in whom nonvalved stents are deployed across the cardia.

KEY POINTS

- Many diseases of the esophagus can be treated with procedures guided by interventional radiology.
- Esophageal strictures can be caused by both benign and malignant diseases and can be appropriately treated by balloon dilation or stent insertion under fluoroscopy guidance.
- Graded balloon dilation in patients with achalasia may help prevent the risk of perforation.
- Esophageal stenting causes rapid relief and palliation of symptoms in patients with malignant esophageal disease.
- Self-expanding metal stents (SEMS) are the most commonly used esophageal stents.

▶ SUGGESTED READINGS

Ferguson DD. Evaluation and management of benign esophageal strictures. Dis Esophagus 2005;18:359–64.

Morgan R, Adam A. Use of metallic stents and balloons in the esophagus and gastrointestinal tract. J Vasc Interv Radiol 2001;12:283–97.

Sabharwal T, Morales JP, Irani FG, Adam A; CIRSE: Cardiovascular and Interventional Radiological Society of Europe. Quality improvement guidelines for placement of esophageal stents. Cardiovasc Intervent Radiol 2005;28:284–8.

Woltman TA, Pellegrini CA, Oelschlager BK. Achalasia. Surg Clin North Am 2005;85:483–93.

The complete reference list is available online at www.expertconsult.com.

CHAPTER 130

Intervention for Gastric Outlet and Duodenal Obstruction

Jin Hyoung Kim, Ho-Young Song, and Chang Jin Yoon

Gastric outlet obstruction is a preterminal complication of advanced malignancies of the pancreas, stomach, and duodenum. Patients with gastric outlet obstruction experience intractable nausea, vomiting, and anorexia, which may in turn cause electrolyte imbalance, dehydration, and malnutrition. Furthermore, these patients are at constant risk for aspiration and pneumonia. The primary goal of treatment is palliation of obstructive symptoms, thereby improving quality of life.[1] Although surgical gastrojejunostomy with or without gastrectomy has been the traditional method of palliative treatment, many patients are unfit for bypass surgery because of poor medical condition at initial evaluation. Moreover, it carries a significant rate of morbidity and mortality and is associated with persistent or delayed relief of symptoms and prolonged hospital stay.[2] Nonsurgical palliation by means of drainage via a nasogastric tube or gastrostomy does little to improve a patient's quality of life. Placement of self-expandable metallic stents is an established treatment option in patients with malignant biliary and esophageal obstruction. Recently, stents have been increasingly used to treat malignant gastroduodenal obstruction, with successful palliation achieved in most patients. Advantages of gastroduodenal stent placement over surgical palliation include more rapid gastric emptying, fewer complications, and improved quality of life.

Causes of benign gastric outlet obstruction include peptic ulcer disease, anastomotic obstruction after gastrectomy, corrosive injury, pyloric dysfunction after esophageal resection and gastric pull-up surgery, and rarely Crohn disease. Traditionally, most of these obstructions were treated surgically. Balloon dilation, as well as placement of metallic stents, has been applied successfully in patients who are not surgical candidates.

INDICATIONS

The main indication for placement of gastroduodenal stents is obstruction of the stomach, duodenum, or proximal jejunum by unresectable malignant tumors. Advanced carcinoma of the pancreatic head is the most common malignancy causing obstruction in these regions. Other malignancies include cholangiocarcinoma, gastric carcinoma, and metastatic disease to the duodenum or proximal jejunum.

Anastomotic malignant obstruction after gastrectomy or esophagectomy is also an indication for stent placement.[3,4] Although stent placement for benign obstruction is still under investigation, it may be a possible alternative treatment when coexisting morbidity involving the cardiopulmonary system limits surgical treatment.[5]

CONTRAINDICATIONS

The only absolute contraindication to stent placement is gastrointestinal (GI) perforation with peritonitis or tension pneumoperitoneum. Multifocal small bowel obstruction has been reported as the main cause of clinical failure after stent placement.[6,7] Therefore, clear evidence of distal small bowel obstruction is also a contraindication to stent placement. Patients with peritoneal carcinomatosis are at high risk for multifocal small bowel obstruction.

EQUIPMENT

Gastroduodenal stents should be flexible enough to allow easy placement along a tortuous GI tract. They should not migrate after deployment and should be conformable in a way that does not permit distortion of the normal anatomy of the upper GI tract. They should have sufficient radial expansile force and diameters large enough to relieve the obstructive symptoms. In addition, such stents should not allow tumor ingrowth and mucosal hyperplasia.

Self-expandable metallic stents have virtually always been used in the stomach and duodenum. Many self-expandable stents composed of a variety of metal alloys with varying structures are available commercially. Although stents made of multiple strands of stainless steel wire have been used frequently, the use of stents woven from a monofilament of nickel-titanium alloy (nitinol) has been increasing recently.

Both covered and bare stents have been used in the stomach and duodenum. Covered stents have the advantage of resisting tumor ingrowth through the stent mesh wire but are prone to migration. They are rigid and require a large delivery system and thus are difficult to deploy at distant locations along a tortuous delivery route. Advantages of bare stents over covered ones include greater flexibility, requirement for a smaller delivery system, and more resistance to migration. When used for long-term palliation of malignant obstruction, they are more prone to obstruction by tumor ingrowth. However, in the majority of cases, tumor ingrowth has not been clinically important because of the limited life expectancy of the patient. Therefore, to date, bare stents have been used much more frequently than covered stents in patients with gastroduodenal obstruction.[7-11]

Until recently, because stents dedicated to GI use were unavailable, interventionalists used stents designed for esophageal or vascular use, including the Wallstent (Boston Scientific, Natick, Mass.), Ultraflex stent (Microinvasive/Boston Scientific), Gianturco Z-stent (Wilson-Cook,

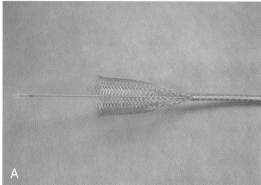
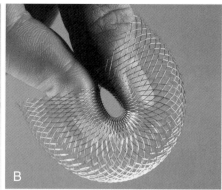

FIGURE 130-1. Enteral Wallstent. **A,** Stent is partially released from a 10F delivery system and can be reconstrained before it has been completely deployed. **B,** Released enteral Wallstent is highly flexible.

Winston-Salem, N.C.), and EsophaCoil (Intra-Therapeutics, Eden Prairie, Minn.).[7-11] The Wallstent endoprosthesis is the most frequently used stent. Vascular Wallstents are very flexible but have a small diameter (16 mm) inadequate for GI use, whereas esophageal Wallstents are sufficiently large (20-25 mm) but relatively rigid. Recently a Wallstent dedicated to GI use has been developed (Fig. 130-1). Available stents range from 18 to 22 mm in diameter and are mounted on 10F delivery systems 230 cm long for endoscopic placement and 160 cm long for peroral fluoroscopic placement. The enteral Wallstent is a bare stent braided from multiple strands of stainless steel wire. Advantages of this stent include high longitudinal flexibility, adequate radial force, and the fact that it uses a small introducer system. Disadvantages of the enteral Wallstent are substantial shortening (≈40%) after deployment, unavailability in a covered version, and potentially traumatic ends of the stent. More recently, a new enteral stent (WallFlex [Boston Scientific]) was introduced that is made of nitinol instead of stainless steel.[12,13] This new stent has been constructed to provide improved flexibility while maintaining lumen integrity, has looped ends to reduce risk of mucosal injury, and has a proximal flared end to minimize risk of stent migration.[12,13] The Ultraflex stent is knitted from nitinol mesh wire, which slowly expands when deployed at body temperature and is available in both covered and bare versions.[14] It has significantly lower radial expansile force than the other stents, but it is highly flexible and thus can be placed across acutely angled stenoses. The stent is available in a 23-mm middle diameter, has a 28-mm funnel-shaped proximal end, and is mounted on a 16F delivery catheter.

The covered version of the stent has a polyurethane external membrane with bare portions at both ends to prevent migration.

The Gianturco Z-stent is available in bare and polyethylene-covered versions. The bare stents are cylindrical or flared at both ends and available in diameters of 15 to 35 mm. The covered esophageal Z-stent is designed with flared ends to prevent migration. The diameter of the stent is 18 mm in its midportion and 25 mm at each end.[15] The stent is delivered through a 28F sheath. The greater inflexibility of these stents limits their use in the GI tract.

In some recent publications from Korea, use of various types of covered enteral stents (Fig. 130-2) has been reported. The Niti-S stent (Taewoong Medical, Ilsan, Korea)

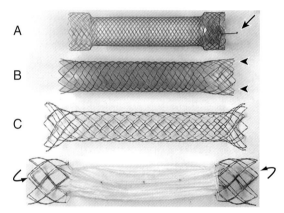

FIGURE 130-2. Various types of covered gastroduodenal stents. **A,** A polyurethane-covered Niti-S stent is woven from nitinol monofilament in an interlacing pattern. Both ends of stent are flared to prevent migration. Note string at proximal (oral side) end of stent *(arrow)* for endoscopic removal. **B,** A HANAROSTENT is woven from a single nitinol wire in an interlocking pattern and covered with silicon membrane. Stent has a bare part at proximal end to prevent migration *(arrowheads)*. **C,** A Dual duodenal stent is composed of a bare stent *(upper)* and a partially covered stent *(lower)*, designed to be placed coaxially. Inner bare stent is knitted from a single nitinol wire, and both its ends are flared. Outer partially covered stent has three parts: a proximal bare nitinol stent *(curved arrow)*, nylon mesh, and a distal bare nitinol stent *(curved arrow)*.

and the HANAROSTENT (M.I.Tech, Pyungtaik, Korea) are woven from a single thread of nitinol wire. The stents are covered with polyurethane (Niti-S) or silicon membrane (HANAROSTENT). The diameters of the body of the stents are 16 or 18 mm, and both ends are flared, which increases the size to 20 to 24 mm. They are mounted on an 18F delivery system.[16] These stents are highly flexible and exert adequate expansile force. Recently, Song et al.[17,18] developed a nylon-covered stent (Dual duodenal stent [S&G Biotech, Sungnam, Korea]) that was designed to be placed coaxially. It is mounted on a very low-profile (3.8 mm) delivery system. Other authors have introduced a new duodenal bare metallic stent (BONASTENT M-Duodenal [Standard Sci-Tech Inc., Seoul, Korea]), through which biliary stent placement is safe and effective for palliative treatment of malignant biliary and duodenal obstruction.[19]

TECHNIQUE

Anatomy and Approach

Before stent placement, upper GI series should be performed to assess the anatomy and evaluate the location, length, and nature of the obstruction. However, such information may not be obtainable with a contrast-enhanced study in cases of complete obstruction, for which nonionic water-soluble contrast material should be used, given that barium will hamper further imaging and intervention. Ionic contrast media may cause pulmonary edema if aspirated. Computed tomography (CT) is the study of choice for diagnosis and staging of the disease. In addition, it may provide important information about the presence of distal obstruction in the small bowel. Although endoscopy with biopsy is desirable before stent placement, it may be difficult to perform in patients with complete gastric outlet obstruction, because such patients have an increased risk of aspiration. Since palliative treatment is usually decided by the time of stent placement, biopsy for tissue diagnosis is not mandatory.

Technical Aspects

Peroral Stent Placement

For peroral placement, stents can be placed under fluoroscopic or combined endoscopic-fluoroscopic guidance. Advantages of endoscopic stent placement over fluoroscopically guided placement include direct visualization of the lesion and greater accessibility to the obstruction by straightening of the access route through the distended stomach. However, technical success rates of fluoroscopic placement have been reported to be similar to those of endoscopic placement.[3-21] In some cases, fluoroscopic stent placement is successful after failed endoscopic placement. The delivery system of a covered stent is too large to place through the endoscope channel. In addition, accurate stent deployment is performed mainly under fluoroscopic monitoring. Therefore, the techniques used often depend on the referral pattern and available local expertise rather than superiority of techniques.

Fluoroscopic Guidance

The procedure can be performed on a conventional fluoroscopic table or within a vascular-interventional suite. Equipment allowing tilting of the table is desirable. Because of prolonged obstruction, the stomach is usually distended and elongated, which may make catheterization of lesions difficult or even impossible. Therefore, decompression of the stomach with a nasogastric tube for 1 to 2 days before the procedure is mandatory. The procedure is generally performed with the patient under conscious sedation and continuous monitoring of vital signs and oxygen saturation. After anesthetizing the pharynx with topical spray, an angiographic catheter with a guidewire is passed perorally into the stomach or duodenum near the obstruction (Fig. 130-3). A curved 100-cm-long angiographic catheter, such as a 5F multipurpose (Terumo Medical Corp., Tokyo, Japan) or Head Hunter catheter (Wilson-Cook), and a 260-cm, 0.035-inch floppy-tipped guidewire (Radiofocus [Terumo]) are most commonly used. A limited amount of iodinated contrast material is injected through the catheter to identify the proximal extent of the stricture. The catheter is manipulated through the obstruction with standard catheter and guidewire techniques. However, when the patient has a markedly distended stomach, manipulating the obstruction may prove difficult because the catheter and guidewire are frequently looped along the greater curvature of the stomach. A guiding sheath may be helpful to prevent looping of the guidewire in these cases.[22] In addition, gastric decompression for several days before the procedure can minimize this problem. After the catheter is advanced as far distally as possible, contrast medium is injected again to demonstrate the distal margin of the obstruction. With the use of a recently developed GI catheter (Song-Lim [S&G Biotech]), the contrast medium can be injected without removing the guidewire from the catheter (Fig. 130-4).[23] The guidewire is exchanged for a long stiff wire (260-cm Amplatz Super Stiff wire [Boston Scientific], Lunderquist Extra Stiff guidewire [Cook Medical, Bloomington, Ind.]). Sometimes the exchange-length guidewire is too short for the procedure because of marked looping of the catheter in the distended stomach. In these cases, use of a 500-cm-long Amplatz Super Stiff wire may solve the problem. Once an exchange stiff wire is placed, looping of the wire is likely to be relieved, and a straight access route can be established.

Present balloon dilation is not usually necessary in most cases. Occasionally, however, gentle balloon dilation (10-15 mm) may facilitate rapid expansion of the stent in the presence of very tight obstruction. Furthermore, balloon dilation may be helpful in determining the exact length and location of the proximal and distal extents of the obstruction when they are not clearly demonstrated by injection of contrast material.

A stent of adequate diameter (at least 16 mm) and length should be chosen to completely cover the obstruction. It is important to place a stent that is at least 2 to 4 cm longer than the site of obstruction so it covers 1 to 2 cm distal and 1 to 2 cm proximal to the obstruction to limit tumor overgrowth. A large-diameter stent (at least 18 mm) is recommended to establish a wide lumen and facilitate passage of food through the stent. The stent delivery system is advanced over the wire across the obstruction. During stent deployment, the distal end of the stent shortens toward the obstruction. The stent delivery system may be pulled back if placed too distally. However, a partially deployed stent should not be advanced. When multiple stents are required, the distal stent should be placed initially, with confirmation that it extends well beyond the lesion. At least 1 to 2 cm of the stents should overlap to prevent migration. It is not generally necessary to dilate the stent after deployment, because most stents will slowly self-expand over time. A postinsertion contrast-enhanced study is performed to assess stent position.

Endoscopic-Fluoroscopic Guidance

Patients should be placed in left lateral decubitus or prone position. With use of intravenous conscious sedation, the esophagus and stomach are intubated with the endoscope. If the endoscope can be passed through the obstruction easily, a 0.035-inch guidewire and a catheter are advanced through the endoscope channel, but it is unnecessary to apply excessive force to the endoscope to make it pass through the obstruction. If the endoscope cannot be passed through the obstruction, a guidewire and catheter are

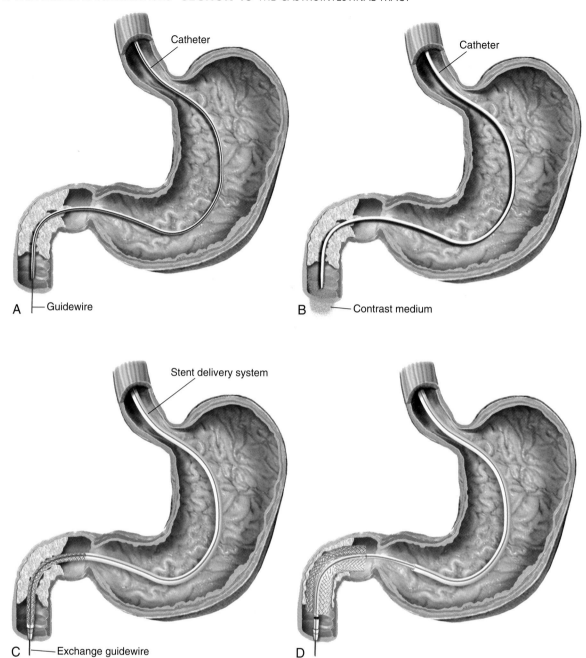

FIGURE 130-3. Diagrams demonstrating gastroduodenal stent placement under fluoroscopic guidance. **A,** Angiographic catheter and guidewire are introduced into stomach and manipulated to pass through obstruction. **B,** Distal end of obstruction is delineated by injection of a limited amount of contrast medium. **C,** Exchange-length stiff guidewire is placed as far distally as possible. Angiographic catheter is removed, and stent delivery system is advanced over stiff guidewire. **D,** Stent is deployed to relieve obstruction. Accurate stent position is confirmed by injection of contrast medium.

advanced to traverse the obstruction under fluoroscopic monitoring, during which the endoscope plays the role of a guiding sheath to provide stability within the distended stomach. Removal of gastric contents by suction may facilitate access to the obstruction and reduce the risk of aspiration. Water-soluble contrast material is injected to identify the length and location of the obstruction. An extralong exchange-length stiff guidewire is placed as far distally as possible.

A stent of adequate diameter (at least 16 mm) and length (at least 2 cm longer than the stricture) should be chosen.

The enteral Wallstent is mounted on a 10F delivery system and can be delivered through the working channel of the endoscope. When a larger stent delivery system is used, the endoscope should be removed. The stent is loaded onto the guidewire and advanced under fluoroscopic monitoring. The endoscope can be reinserted alongside the stent delivery system for endoscopic guidance during stent deployment. The stent is deployed under fluoroscopic monitoring, and the distal end should be located at least 1 to 2 cm beyond the obstruction. The proximal location of the stent can be monitored fluoroscopically and endoscopically.

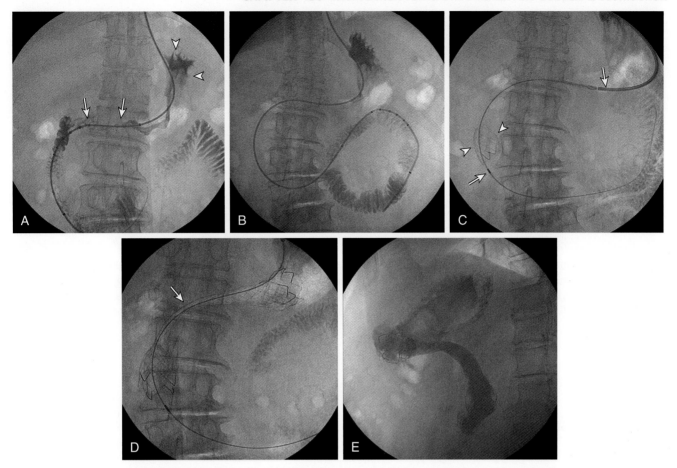

FIGURE 130-4. A 63-year-old patient with gastric cancer. **A,** Radiograph shows a multipurpose catheter crossing obstruction in antrum *(arrows)*. Stomach is adequately decompressed by overnight placement of a Levin tube, which facilitates procedure *(arrowheads)*. **B,** Catheter was advanced into jejunum, and a stiff guidewire is subsequently placed. **C,** Stent delivery system is advanced over stiff guidewire *(arrows)*, and stent is partially deployed *(arrowheads)*. **D,** Radiograph obtained immediately after stent deployment shows a partially expanded stent. Central part of stent is compressed by tumor *(arrow)*. **E,** Upper gastrointestinal series performed 1 day after procedure shows free passage of contrast material through nearly completely expanded stent.

Additional stents can be inserted if necessary. Correct position of the stent is demonstrated by injection of contrast medium after the procedure.

Transgastrostomy Stent Placement

As an alternative to the peroral approach, access to the stomach can be achieved by percutaneous gastrostomy (Fig. 130-5). This access allows placement of a stiff sheath to provide greater catheter and wire control. Consequently, such direct access allows successful catheterization in virtually all cases.[5,16] However, percutaneous gastrostomy is an invasive procedure that has its own associated risks and complications, so it should be reserved as a last option. After placement of the stent by means of the gastrostomy route, a gastrostomy tube is left in place until a mature tract develops, usually 10 days after the procedure. Placement of duodenal and biliary stents from a transhepatic approach has also been reported.[24] This alternative route is useful in patients with complex surgical anastomoses when peroral stent placement is not possible.

Combined Biliary and Duodenal Stent Placement

In patients with duodenal obstruction secondary to pancreatic or ampullary cancer, coexistent biliary obstruction usually precedes gastric outlet obstruction. Late symptomatic duodenal obstruction develops in 7% to 34% of patients with pancreatic cancer and in 23% of patients with ampullary cancer who are treated by surgical biliary bypass.[25]

When biliary obstruction coexists with duodenal obstruction, combined palliation of both lesions is possible in most patients. Endoscopic placement is preferred because it allows simultaneous combined palliation without the need for a separate percutaneous biliary intervention. In patients with a duodenal stent covering the papilla, it is impossible to place a biliary stent through the mesh of the stent endoscopically. A biliary stent should therefore be placed in patients with known or impending biliary obstruction before duodenal stent placement. Kaw et al.[26] treated 18 patients by simultaneous duodenal and biliary stent placement and reported only one technical failure. When biliary obstruction develops after duodenal stent placement, a percutaneous transhepatic approach is required.

Duodenal obstruction may develop after percutaneous[27] or endoscopic[28] placement of metallic biliary stents. It occurs more frequently than after placement of plastic biliary stents. These duodenal obstructions are presumed to be related to mechanical obstruction by the metallic biliary stent, which protrudes into the already

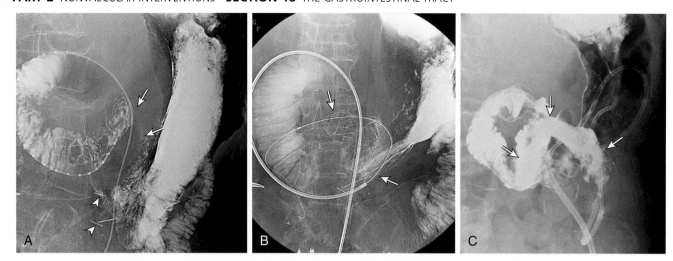

FIGURE 130-5. An 82-year-old patient with pancreatic cancer. Peroral placement of a stent under endoscopic-fluoroscopic guidance failed. **A,** Contrast-enhanced study obtained via percutaneous gastrostomy access shows obstruction at duodenojejunal junction *(arrows).* Note anchoring devices for percutaneous gastrostomy *(arrowheads).* **B,** A partially covered stent is placed via gastrostomy route *(arrows).* Immediately after stent placement, a significant waist is noted in middle part of stent. **C,** Upper gastrointestinal series performed 1 day after stent placement shows free passage of contrast material through expanded stent *(arrows).*

compromised duodenal lumen. These patients can be successfully treated with duodenal stent placement (Fig. 130-6).

CONTROVERSIES

Stent Placement versus Bypass Surgery

Minimal cost and time should be invested in patients with limited life expectancy who are undergoing palliative treatment. Several comparative studies have demonstrated the effectiveness of stent placement and have provided a scientific rationale for the procedure. Yim et al.[29] retrospectively compared the outcome of surgical gastrojejunostomy and endoscopic stent placement in patients with malignant gastric outlet obstruction secondary to metastatic pancreatic cancer. Mean survival was similar in both groups (94 days in the stent group vs. 92 days in the surgery group). However, the stent group had significantly lower median charges ($9921 versus $28,173) and hospital stay (4 vs. 14 days). Five of 12 stent placements were performed on an outpatient basis, whereas all 15 patients in the surgical group underwent surgery in the hospital. Another retrospective comparative study[30] found that the gastrojejunostomy group was more prone to delayed gastric emptying (58.8%) than the stent group (0%). Thirty-day mortality in the gastrojejunostomy group was higher (18%) than that in the stent group (0%). A study by Maetani et al.[30] noted shorter operating time (30 vs. 110 minutes) and more prompt restoration of oral intake (2 vs. 8 days) in the stent group than in the surgery group. A recent prospective randomized trial,[31] however, found that surgical (open or laparoscopic) gastrojejunostomy was associated with better long-term results and lower complication rates despite higher costs and slow initial symptom improvement. Thus, they suggested that surgical gastrojejunostomy may be the treatment of choice in patients with a life expectancy of 2 months or longer, and stent placement may be preferable for patients expected to live less than 2 months, because

stent placement is associated with better short-term outcomes.[31]

Laparoscopy is a less invasive surgical technique that has recently been applied to palliation of gastric outlet obstruction. Initial trials have shown that laparoscopic gastroenterostomy is associated with shorter hospital stay, faster recovery, and less morbidity and mortality than open surgery. However, laparoscopic surgery requires general anesthesia and is contraindicated in patients with malignant ascites. In addition, open conversion may be required in up to 20% of patients. A retrospective study[32] found no differences in technical and clinical success and the incidence of minor and early major complications and survival between a stent placement group (n = 53) and laparoscopic gastrojejunostomy group (n = 42). Food intake improved more rapidly after stent placement than laparoscopic gastrojejunostomy, and hospital stay was also shorter after stent placement. However, the time to late major complications, recurrent obstructive symptoms, and reintervention was significantly shorter after stent placement than laparoscopic gastrojejunostomy in their study. They suggested that stent placement is associated with better short-term outcomes, and laparoscopic gastrojejunostomy with better long-term outcomes.[32]

OUTCOMES

Since reports of four cases of successful stenting for gastroduodenal outlet obstruction in 1992 and 1993, more than 50 case series have been published. In early studies published in the late 1990s, consisting of 6 to 12 patients each, Wallstents designed for vascular or esophageal application were used. Feretis et al.[7] placed 22-mm-diameter esophageal Wallstents under endoscopic-fluoroscopic guidance without passage through the endoscope in 12 patients with pancreatic cancer. Technical success, usually defined as correct placement of the stent in the intended location, with patency confirmed at endoscopy or contrast-enhanced study, was achieved in all patients. Clinical success, defined

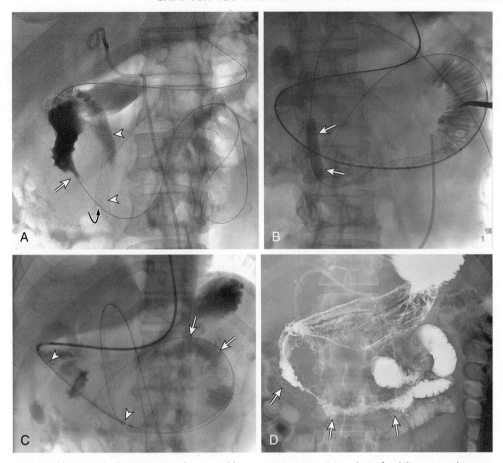

FIGURE 130-6. A 55-year-old man with obstructive jaundice caused by pancreatic cancer. Seven days after biliary stent placement, symptoms of upper gastrointestinal obstruction developed. **A,** Contrast-enhanced study obtained with a perorally inserted catheter shows obstruction at second part of duodenum *(arrow).* Guidewire can be passed through obstruction *(curved arrow)* but only through biliary stent mesh *(arrowheads).* **B,** To avoid passage through biliary stent mesh, a guidewire and catheter are manipulated to cross obstruction during temporary balloon dilation within biliary stent lumen *(arrows).* **C,** After placement of a stiff guidewire into jejunum *(arrows),* stent delivery system *(arrowheads)* is advanced over wire. **D,** Upper gastrointestinal series performed 1 day after duodenal stent placement shows passage of contrast material through a completely expanded stent *(arrows).*

as improvement of the patient's ability to resume oral intake and objective weight gain, was achieved in 11 patients. There was one reobstruction by tumor ingrowth. Only two patients, however, were alive 6 months after stent placement. Binkert et al.[8] placed 16-mm-diameter vascular Wallstents under combined endoscopic-fluoroscopic guidance in nine patients—7 with malignant disease and 2 with chronic ulcer disease. Technical and clinical success was achieved in 8 (89%) and 7 (78%) patients, respectively. During a follow-up period of 1 to 52 weeks, no stent obstruction occurred. De Baere et al.[9] reported on fluoroscopically guided placement of 16-mm-diameter vascular Wallstents without endoscopic assistance in 10 patients; 7 underwent successful peroral placement of the stents. Percutaneous gastrostomy was required in 3. The procedure was clinically successful in 8 of 10 patients. In 2 patients, multiple small bowel obstructions were found after stent placement. Pinto[10] also reported experience with fluoroscopically guided stent placement in 6 patients with malignant gastric outlet obstruction. In 5 of the 6 patients, peroral stent placement was successful, and 1 required a gastrostomy. Vascular or esophageal Wallstents were used, and all patients were relieved of their obstructive symptoms. One

patient died of complications of gastrostomy, and 3 had obstructed stents within 2 months of placement.

Other types of stents, such as the Gianturco Z-stent, the Ultraflex stent, or the EsophaCoil, have been used only occasionally, with scanty reports in the literature. Nevitt et al.[4] used endoscopic-fluoroscopic guidance to place four types of stents (Wallstent, Gianturco Z-stent, Ultraflex, Endocoil) in eight patients with malignant gastroduodenal (three patients) or anastomotic (five patients) obstruction. All stents were deployed successfully. Seven patients had immediate relief of obstructive symptoms, and two had recurrent symptoms as a result of tumor ingrowth. Yates et al.[11] used a variety of stents (Wallstent, Ultraflex, Esopha-Coil) to palliatively treat gastric or proximal jejunal obstruction in 11 patients under combined endoscopic-fluoroscopic guidance. Both technical and clinical success was achieved in 10 of the 11 patients (91%). The single failure was due to severe anastomotic angulation and distal luminal obstruction. Five patients had subsequent stent occlusion due to tumor ingrowth at 3 to 11 weeks after placement. Maetani et al.[33] placed Ultraflex stents (n = 18) and Z-stents (n = 5) as palliation in 23 patients with gastric outlet obstruction. The stents were successfully inserted in all patients with the use of modified techniques consisting of a longer delivery system, grasping forceps, and a home-made sheath. Initial clinical success was achieved in all patients, but three recurrent obstructions developed as a result of tumor ingrowth, mucosal hyperplasia, and stent fracture.

In these early studies, technical failures were relatively common and mainly due to the relatively short and rigid stent delivery systems. Recent advances in the design of stents, with longer and more flexible delivery systems, have significantly improved the technical feasibility of gastroduodenal stents (Table 130-1).[13,18,34-36] At present, the enteral Wallstent, which can be passed through the working channel of an endoscope, is most commonly used. Yim et al.[34] treated 29 patients with enteral Wallstents. Technical success was achieved in 27 patients (93%) with peroral endoscopic-fluoroscopic guidance. Clinical improvement was achieved in 86% and long-term palliation in 79%. In two patients, the stents were obstructed by tumor ingrowth, which was successfully treated with second stents. Van Hooft et al.[13] reported a 98% technical success rate in the endoscopic placement of enteral WallFlex stents (n = 51). Clinical success was achieved in 84% of the patients and World Health Organization performance score improved ($P = .002$) when the score before stenting was compared with the mean score until death.[13] In a series comprising 63 patients,[35] enteral Wallstents and enteral CHOOSTENTs (M.I.Tech) were placed. Technical success was achieved in 60 patients (95%), and an exclusively peroral diet was possible in 58 patients (92%). Complications occurred in 30% of patients, including 13 stent obstructions (12 tumor ingrowth and 1 impaction of the proximal end of the stent in the duodenal bulb), 4 stent migrations, and 2 duodenal perforations.

With the use of dedicated enteral stents, most recent studies report high technical success rates of 93% to 98% (see Table 130-1).[13,18,34-36] In almost all cases in which peroral stent placement fails, the procedure can be successfully performed via gastrostomy access. Initial clinical success has been achieved in 84% to 97% of cases.[13,18,34-36] A clinical failure rate of about 10% is expected despite adequate technical success. The most common causes of clinical failure are associated with distal intestinal obstruction. Other causes include functional gastric outlet obstruction caused by prolonged gastric distention or neural involvement of the celiac axis.[9,11]

Covered self-expandable stents have been used successfully in patients with malignant esophageal obstruction to prevent recurrent obstruction by tumor ingrowth. However, in the gastroduodenal region, they have been used only occasionally because the delivery systems of commercially available covered esophageal stents are too rigid and short to be used routinely in this region. In 2000 and 2001, however, Korean radiologists introduced various types of covered stents dedicated to gastroduodenal use. Park et al.[37] used a polyurethane-covered flexible Z-stent (CHOOSTENT [M.I.Tech]) in 24 patients with malignant gastroduodenal (16 patients) or anastomotic (8 patients) obstruction. They reported a technical success rate of only 75%, mainly attributed to the large and rigid delivery system (6 and 8 mm). There were no procedural complications, but a 24% migration rate was observed. Jung et al.[38] used a polyurethane-covered stent woven from a single thread of nitinol wire. In 18 of the 19 patients, adequate placement

was achieved under fluoroscopic (n = 14) or endoscopic-fluoroscopic (n = 4) guidance. Tumor ingrowth was successfully prevented during a mean follow-up period of 11 weeks, but there were five cases of stent migration (28%), and obstructive jaundice developed in one patient after stent placement covering the duodenal papilla.

Initial experience with covered stents demonstrated two major problems: a high migration rate and technical difficulties caused by the rigid delivery system. Therefore, stent designs have been modified to prevent stent migration, including the use of covered stents placed coaxially inside bare stents,[39] stents with shoulders,[16,37] and partially covered stents.[17,18] To improve technical feasibility, a more flexible stent delivery system with a low profile was developed. Subsequent studies demonstrated improved technical success and stent migration rates. Furthermore, by preventing tumor ingrowth, stent patency rates also improved over those of covered stents. Jung et al.[39] treated 39 patients by placement of a bare stent followed by a coaxial covered stent and reported a 97% technical success rate and a stent migration rate of 8%. Recurrent obstruction was noted in 10 patients, mostly secondary to tumor overgrowth in patients with longer survival times. Lopera et al.[40] performed a prospective study to investigate the use of fully covered, bare, and partially covered stents. Stent migration was observed in 3 of 7 fully covered stents and tumor ingrowth in 2 of 3 bare stents, although no migration or tumor ingrowth was observed in 10 partially covered stents. In a large study comprising 213 patients with malignant gastroduodenal (186 native and 27 postoperative anatomy) obstruction,[18] a partially covered stent and a bare stent were coaxially placed with a 3.8-mm delivery system (Dual duodenal stent [S&G Biotech]). Technical and clinical success rates were 94% and 94%, respectively. Stent migration was observed in only 4% of the patients, and tumor overgrowth in 7% (see Table 130-1).

Benign Gastric Outlet Obstruction

As mentioned earlier, the traditional treatment of benign gastric outlet and gastroduodenal obstruction has been surgery. Balloon dilation is also an effective alternative and can be successful in more than 80% of patients. Recently, balloon dilation combined with antisecretory therapy and removal of the etiologic factors (e.g., *Helicobacter pylori*) was shown to achieve long-term resolution of symptoms in 85% to 100% of patients with peptic ulcer–related gastric outlet obstruction.[41,42] Balloon dilation also led to symptom resolution in 50% to 94% of patients with benign anastomotic obstruction after gastrojejunostomy or gastroduodenostomy.[43-45]

Use of metallic stents for benign gastroduodenal obstruction has been limited because in general, the life expectancy of patients exceeds that of the stent. It is usually attempted in patients at high surgical risk or when other methods, including balloon dilation, have failed. Cowling et al.[46] and Bae et al.[47] demonstrated that stent placement can be an effective form of treatment in patients with postsurgical anastomotic obstruction and pyloric dysfunction when balloon dilation had failed. However, the use of metallic stents for benign gastroduodenal obstruction is still under investigation, and the long-term results are not yet known.

TABLE 130-1. Results from Recent Major Studies

Authors	No. of Patients	Stent Used	Technique	Technical Success	Initial Clinical Success	Recurrent Obstruction	Tumor Ingrowth	Tumor Overgrowth	Complications	Survival Period
Yim et al.[34]	29	Enteral Wallstent	Endoscopic-fluoroscopic	93% (27/29)	85% (23/27)	7% (2/27)	7% (2/27)	—	—	77 days (mean)
van Hooft et al.[13]	51	Enteral WallFlex stent	Endoscopic-fluoroscopic	98% (50/51)	84% (43/51)	24% (12/51)	10% (5/51)	2% (1/51)	Stent migration (1) Cholangitis (3) Bleeding (2) Pain (2)	62 days (median)
Nassif et al.[35]	63	Enteral Wallstent, Enteral CHOOSTENT	Endoscopic-fluoroscopic	95% (60/63)	97% (58/60)	22% (13/60)	20% (12/60)	—	Stent migration (4) Perforation (2)	70 days (mean)
Bessoud et al.[36]	72	Vascular Wallstent (55) Enteral Wallstent (10)	Endoscopic-fluoroscopic	97% (70/72)	93% (65/70)	10% (7/70)	3% (2/70)	7% (5/70)	Stent migration (8) Perforation (1) Stent fracture (1) Death related to general anesthesia (1)	120 days (mean)
Kim et al.[18]	213	Dual nitinol stent	Fluoroscopic	94% (201/213)	94% (196/209)	17% (35/209)		7% (14/209)	Stent migration (8) Stent collapse (9) Food impaction (5) Granulation tissue (2) Bleeding (2) Jaundice (5)	99 days (median)

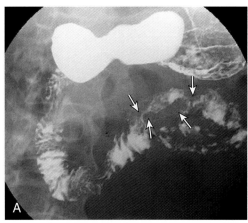
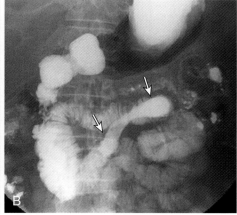

FIGURE 130-7. A 63-year-old man with pancreatic cancer. **A,** An upper gastrointestinal series (UGIS) performed 90 days after placement of a bare stent shows narrowing of stent lumen secondary to tumor ingrowth *(arrows)*. **B,** UGIS performed after placement of a second stent *(arrows)* shows good passage of contrast material into jejunal loops.

Patients should be monitored closely, with reintervention undertaken if complications occur.

COMPLICATIONS

Intraprocedural complications are extremely rare and are related to sedation and complications inherent in endoscopic procedures. To date, only one death related to general anesthesia has been reported.[36] Stent migration or malposition during stent deployment occurs in less than 5% of cases. A distally malpositioned stent can be pulled back to a more desirable location with endoscopic forceps. When this technique fails or is not feasible, the problem can be managed by placing a second stent coaxially.

Late complications include perforation, bleeding, stent migration, and stent obstruction. Major complications, such as perforation and major bleeding, are extremely rare. In a meta-analysis[48] that included 32 recent studies (606 patients), there were 4 duodenal perforations (0.7%) and 3 instances of major bleeding (0.5%). Duodenal perforation after stent placement usually requires emergency surgical treatment. Minimal bleeding and ulceration related to the stent wire are relatively common but usually resolve spontaneously without treatment.

Stent migration rates of bare and covered stents are reported to be 0% to 5% and 21% to 43%, respectively.[6-9,37-39] This complication has been a major problem for covered stents, but with recent advances in stent design, the rate of stent migration is much improved.[17,18,40] Stent migration is related to chemotherapy after stent placement, but not to balloon dilation before or after stent placement.[18] Most patients in whom stent migration has occurred can be managed by placement of a second stent. The migrated stent is eventually expelled through the anus. However, when a migrated stent causes distal bowel obstruction, surgical removal is required.

Stent obstruction is the most common late complication of gastroduodenal stents and is caused by tumor ingrowth or overgrowth, mucosal hyperplasia or prolapse, and food impaction. Stent obstruction secondary to granulation tissue or mucosal hyperplasia has been reported as early as 2 weeks after stent placement. Obstruction due to tumor ingrowth or overgrowth usually develops later. The overall rate of stent obstruction by tumor ingrowth has been reported to be 3% to 25% with bare stents (Fig. 130-7).* This complication can be successfully prevented with use of covered stents,[37-39] but it can still occur rarely when the covering membrane of the stent is disrupted.[34] In patients with long survival times, covered stents can be obstructed by tumor overgrowth, with reported rates of 2% to 5%. Obstruction by tumor ingrowth or overgrowth can be successfully managed by placement of another stent in the majority of cases.

Biliary obstruction is a potential complication when a covered stent is placed over the duodenal papilla.[17,40] Because biliary obstruction has generally occurred before gastric outlet obstruction, external biliary drainage or a biliary stent is usually in place by the time of gastroduodenal stent placement in the majority of cases. When biliary obstruction coexists at the time of duodenal stent placement, simultaneous stenting of both lesions is possible in most patients. Yoon et al.[50] placed a covered stent over the duodenal papilla in 15 patients without biliary obstruction. Obstructive jaundice developed in 3 patients within 7 days after stent placement. In such cases, transhepatic biliary drainage with subsequent biliary stenting should be performed.

In contrast to esophageal stents, gastroduodenal stents do not usually cause pain. If pain does occur, it improves spontaneously in most patients, and significant pain requiring treatment is exceedingly rare. Partial or dynamic obstruction of the stent can be caused by the distal end of the stent abutting against the small bowel wall or the proximal end against the anterior wall of the stomach. This problem can be resolved by placement of another stent. Stent fracture is extremely rare, but one series using a covered Z-stent reported an extraordinarily high rate of 12.5%.[37]

POSTPROCEDURAL AND FOLLOW-UP CARE

The patient should not be allowed any food by mouth overnight. A follow-up upper GI study is usually performed the

*References 6-11, 14, 15, 34, 35, 49.

next day. If the examination shows adequate stent expansion and free passage of contrast medium through the lumen, the patient may resume oral intake and advance from liquids to semisolids. Dietary instructions related to eating habits should be given. A semisolid or pureed diet is generally recommended, and leafy uncooked vegetables and meat should be avoided to minimize episodes of obstruction by solid food boluses.[11]

When a patient with a gastroduodenal stent has recurrent symptoms, an upper GI study, CT, or endoscopy should be performed. Early stent obstruction is usually secondary to stent shortening, stent migration, food impaction, or infrequently, mucosal hyperplasia. Stent obstruction occurring more than 2 weeks after stent placement may be caused by tumor ingrowth or overgrowth.[10]

KEY POINTS

- The most common causes of gastroduodenal obstruction are gastric and pancreatic cancer. Patients with gastroduodenal obstruction suffer from nausea, vomiting, dehydration, jaundice, and pain.

- Curative resection is not possible in 40% of patients with gastric cancer and 80% to 90% of patients with pancreatic cancer. Traditionally, patients with unresectable cancer underwent palliative gastrojejunostomy. This procedure, however, is associated with a relatively high risk of morbidity and mortality, delayed gastric emptying, and prolonged hospital stay.

- Peroral stent placement in the stomach or duodenum has a high technical success rate because of improvement in stent design and its delivery system.

- The main problem associated with bare stents is that progressive tumor ingrowth through the wire filaments can cause recurrent dysphagia. In contrast, the main problems associated with covered stents include disruption of the covering membranes and stent migration.

- A clinical failure rate of about 10% is expected despite adequate technical success. The most common cause of clinical failure is small bowel obstruction secondary to peritoneal seeding.

- Gastroduodenal stent placement seems to be an attractive alternative to palliative gastrojejunostomy in patients with unresectable symptomatic malignant gastroduodenal obstruction with no evidence of small bowel obstruction. It is easy and safe to perform, is effective immediately, and is lower in cost than conventional palliative gastrojejunostomy.

► SUGGESTED READINGS

Baron TH, Harewood GC. Enteral self-expandable stents. Gastrointest Endosc 2003;58:421–33.

Dormann A, Meisner S, Verin N, Wenk Lang A. Self-expanding metal stents for gastroduodenal malignancies: systematic review of their clinical effectiveness. Endoscopy 2004;36:543–50.

Katsanos K, Sabharwal T, Adam A. Stenting of the upper gastrointestinal tract: current status. Cardiovasc Intervent Radiol 2010;33:690–705.

Kim JH, Song HY, Shin JH, et al. Metallic stent placement in the palliative treatment of malignant gastroduodenal obstructions: prospective evaluation of results and factors influencing outcome in 213 patients. Gastrointest Endosc 2007;66:256–64.

Lopera JE, Brazzini A, Gonsales A, Castaneda-Zuniga WR. Gastroduodenal stent placement: current status. Radiographics 2004;24:1561–73.

Mauro MA, Koehler RE, Baron TH. Advances in gastrointestinal interventions: the treatment of gastroduodenal and colorectal obstructions with metallic stent. Radiology 2000;215:659–69.

Zollikofer CL, Jost R, Schoch E, Decurtins M. Stents in gastrointestinal cancer. In: Adam A, Dondelinger RF, Muller PR, editors. Interventional Radiology in Cancer. Berlin: Springer; 2004.

The complete reference list is available online at www.expertconsult.com.

CHAPTER 131

Preoperative and Palliative Colonic Stenting

Christoph L. Zollikofer

Colorectal cancer is the fourth leading cause of cancer death in the United States after lung cancer and carcinoma of the breast and prostate.[1] Close to a million new cases of colorectal cancer are detected each year worldwide, and almost 500,000 deaths are attributed to malignant tumors of the colon and rectum.[2] Up to 30% of these patients experience acute partial or complete obstruction, with up to 75% of colorectal cancers occurring in the left colon.[3] Other, less frequent causes of colorectal obstruction include malignant infiltration from adjacent malignant tumors or metastatic involvement. Benign obstruction such as diverticulitis or other inflammatory bowel diseases and anastomotic or postirradiation strictures are rare.

Colonic cancer causing obstruction tends to be at a more advanced stage when first seen, and a higher proportion of obstructed patients (27%-40%) than unobstructed patients already have liver metastases.[4] Curative surgery is not feasible in up to 30%. The advanced stage is also reflected in the poor 5-year survival rate of less than 20% with obstructive disease.[4]

Acute obstruction of the large bowel usually requires urgent surgical treatment, and these patients generally are high surgical risks because of poor general condition related to dehydration and electrolyte imbalance. Mortality and operative morbidity are in the range of 10% to 20% and 40% to 50%, repectively.[5] If patients can be treated electively, mortality rates drop to 3.5% to 7% and operative morbidity to 2% to 24%.[6,7] Therefore, for many years the standard treatment of acute malignant obstruction of the colon has been a two- or three-stage procedure (Hartmann procedure) consisting of first a decompressing colostomy, including resection of the primary tumor at the same time or in an additional operation, and finally closure of the colostomy.[3] Both approaches result in long hospital stays, and up to 62% of these patients never undergo closure of the colostomy.[4,8]

The best oncologic approach to obstructing carcinoma of the colon is primary resection without colostomy. To facilitate primary anastomosis and avoid colostomy, several techniques such as nasointestinal suction and lavage,[9] colonic decompression with rectal-colonic tubes,[10] lavage during surgery,[10] and tube cecostomy[3] have been used to relieve acute distention of the colon and rectum. However, nasointestinal suction and lavage require several days to become effective, rectal-colonic tubes may be impossible to place in patients with severe tumor stenosis, and tube cecostomy is unreliable because of tube obstruction.[3] Nonsurgical methods such as balloon dilatation[11] and laser recanalization[12] have been used occasionally. Therefore, self-expanding metal stents (SEMS) have been advocated to serve as a bridge to surgery for rapid relief of obstruction and allow the patient to be prepared for elective tumor resection with primary anastomosis. Likewise, stents are used as a method of definitive palliation for colonic obstruction in patients who are not surgical candidates, thereby obviating the need for colostomy.[5]

INDICATIONS

The primary indications for placement of endoluminal colorectal stents are for (1) bridge to surgery in patients with resectable colonic obstruction to allow efficient bowel cleansing and single-stage surgical resection and (2) long-term palliative colonic decompression to avoid colostomy in patients with unresectable obstruction.[5,13-15] Other, less common indications are benign conditions such as preoperative stenting in diverticular disease.[16,17] Rarely, anastomotic, ischemic, and radiation-induced strictures are treated with stents, and finally, colonic fistulas may be handled with covered stents.[18-23]

CONTRAINDICATIONS

Clinical or radiologic evidence of intestinal perforation and distal rectal lesions where a safe landing zone of at least 2 cm above the anal sphincter cannot be obtained are absolute contraindications to stent placement. Colorectal obstruction that is too long or patients with multilevel obstruction should not be stented. Tumors that cannot be passed by a guidewire and stent cannot be treated.[13,14]

EQUIPMENT

In the majority of cases, colonic stenting is performed in an emergency setting requiring an appropriately trained team of interventional radiologists, endoscopists, nursing staff for patient monitoring (including administration of neuroleptanalgesia), and availability of high-quality fluoroscopy.[5] Standard angiographic catheters such as the Cobra or Headhunter type are used in combination with steerable and hydrophilic guidewires (Terumo, Tokyo, Japan) to negotiate the obstruction. Stiff/superstiff guidewires (Amplatz Super Stiff wire, Lunderquist wire [Boston Scientific, Natick, Mass.]) are necessary to advance the stent-bearing instruments. Endoscopic guidance is used at institutions where the procedure is performed by gastroenterologists.

A variety of SEMS specifically designed for colonic use is available today (Table 131-1). They are manufactured from stainless steel, Elgiloy (cobalt-chromium-nickel), or nitinol (nickel-titanium). Postdeployment diameters vary from 18 to 30 mm, and typical unconstraint lengths are 6 to 12 cm (see Table 131-1). Most modern stents are flared at one or even both ends to prevent migration, particularly in covered versions. For many SEMS, the delivery systems are provided for per anus use over the wire (OTW) as well as for through the scope (TTS). Colonic stents should be flexible enough to allow easy placement along acute curves and bends, particularly in the case of an elongated sigmoid

TABLE 131-1. Commercially Available Colonic Stents

Manufacturer/ Model	Material	Deployed Diameter (mm)	Deployed Length (mm)	Features
Boston Scientific Natick, Mass.				
Wallstent Enteral	Stainless steel Uncovered	18, 20, 22	60, 90	Unistep Plus Delivery System 10F OTW and TTS Reconstrainable 39%-49% foreshortening during expansion
Ultraflex Precision Colonic Stent System	Nitinol Uncovered	25, proximal flare 30	57, 87, 117	Proximal suture release Only 22F OTW Not reconstrainable 23% foreshortening during expansion
WallFlex Colonic Stent	Elgiloy (cobalt-chromium-nickel) Uncovered	22 body/25 prox. flare 25 body/30 prox. flare	60, 90, 120	10F Delivery OTW and TTS Reconstrainable 30%-45% foreshortening during expansion
PolyFlex Esophageal Stent (Off-label use for rectosigmoidal benign lesions)	Polyester with silicone coating	16 body/20 proximal flare 18 body/23 proximal flare 21 body/25 proximal flare	90, 120, 150	12-, 13-, 14-mm insertion tube OTW only Repositionable, retrievable
Cook Endoscopy Winston-Salem, N.C.				
Colonic Z-Stent	Stainless steel	25 body/35 flared ends	40, 60, 80, 100, 120	10-mm introducer sheath OTW only
Evolution Colonic	Nitinol	25 body/30 flared ends	60, 90, 120	10F TTS system Reconstrainable 45% foreshortening during expansion
ELLA-CS* Hradec-Králové, Czech Republic				
SX-ELLA Stent Colorectal Enterella	Nitinol Uncovered/Covered	Uncovered: 20, 22, 25, 30 Covered: 22, 25, 30 Uncovered TTS 20	82, 90, 113, 135 75, 82, 90, 113, 136 135	15F (uncovered) and 18F (covered) delivery system; OTW 10F TTS All models are repositionable, retrievable
M.I.Tech* Seoul, South Korea				
HANAROSTENT Colon/Rectum	Nitinol Uncovered Covered	Uncovered: body 20, 22, 24 Flared ends Covered: body 22, 24 Dogbone shape	80, 110, 140 60, 110, 140	10.2F OTW and TTS Partly reconstrainable 8-mm OTW delivery system Retrievable
Taewoong Medical* Seoul, South Korea				
Niti-S Enteral Colonic Stent (D-Type)	Nitinol Uncovered	18, 20, 22, 24, 26, 28 OTW 18, 20, 22, 24 TTS	60, 80, 100, 120 60, 80, 100, 120	16F/18F OTW nonflared ends 10.5F TTS nonflared ends
Niti-S Enteral Colonic Stent Both bare-type 15/15	Nitinol Partly covered (silicone)	18, 20 Dogbone shape 24, 28	40, 60, 80, 100, 120	10.5F TTS, both ends (15 mm) bare Reconstrainable, retrievable
Niti-S Enteral Colonic Stent Both bare type 15/15	Nitinol double layer Partly covered, with PTFE membrane in between	18, 20, 22	60, 80, 100	10.5F TTS Both ends 5/10 or 15/15 bare, nonflared PTFE membrane between two bare nitinol stents

*Not available in the United States.
OTW, Over the wire; *prox.,* proximal; *PTFE,* polytetrafluoroethylene; *TTS,* through the scope.

colon or around the colonic flexures. The Enteral Unistep Colonic Wallstent (Boston Scientific), with a maximum diameter of 22 mm, was most frequently used[13,24-28] until the early 2000s. Recently, more atraumatic and flexible nitinol modifications, such as the Ultraflex Precision Colonic Stent for OTW application[29] and the WallFlex Colonic Stent for both OTW and TTS use (Boston Scientific), have been introduced (Fig. 131-1; see Table 131-1). Because of its atraumatic ends and proximal tulip shape (27/30 mm) to reduce the risk of perforation and migration, and the availability of both OTW and TTS systems, the WallFlex is our standard stent for colonic obstruction and is used at many other institutions.[28,30,31]

The Colonic Z-Stent (Cook Endoscopy, Winston-Salem, N.C.) has a 31F introducer system of only 40-cm in length, limiting its application to distal lesions. Recently a 10F TTS nitinol version has been released (see Table 131-1). Other covered and uncovered stents, such as the HANARO-STENT (M.I.Tech, Seoul, Korea) and Niti-S Colorectal Stent (Taewoong Medical, Seoul, Korea), have either flanges on each side (dogbone) and/or uncovered bare ends, or have an extra outer self-expanding bare nitinol stent body

(Niti-S ComVi [Taewoong Medical]) to prevent migration (see Table 131-1). However, apart from treating malignant fistulae, iatrogenic perforation, or postsurgery leaks, covered stents seem not to have a significant advantage and have not gained wider acceptance in clinical practice in the United States and Europe because of their unavailability.[5,32,33] The SX-ELLA Colorectal-Enterella Stent (ELLA-CS, Hradec Králové, Czech Republic) is repositionable and retrievable, thanks to a plastic loop at the distal end, and may be particularly suited for benign or rectal lesions.[26,34,35] Modern nitinol and Elgiloy SEMS are nonferromagnetic and therefore compatible with magnetic resonance imaging (MRI).

TECHNIQUE

Approach

A radiologic diagnosis of acute colonic obstruction is made by plain film radiography and computed tomography (CT) (Fig. 131-2). Barium enema, colonoscopy, and biopsy can help determine the exact location and nature of the

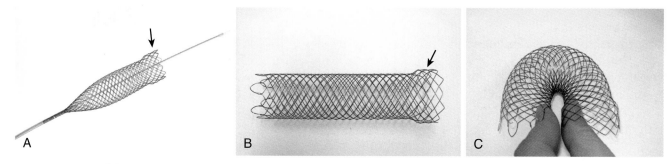

FIGURE 131-1. WallFlex. Note tulip shape at proximal end to prevent migration *(arrow)*. **A,** Stent partly released. **B,** Stent fully expanded. **C,** Demonstration of high flexibility of stent.

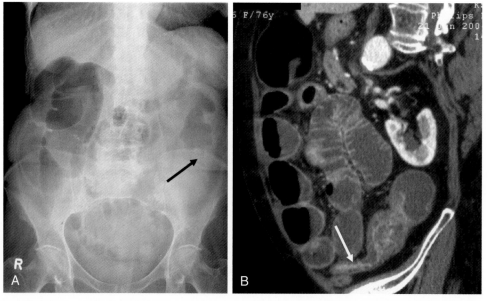

FIGURE 131-2. Acute ileus due to carcinoma of lower descending colon in a 76-year-old patient. **A,** Plain film of abdomen showing a distended large bowel and suggestion of abrupt cessation of air column in descending colon *(arrow)*. **B,** Sagittal reconstruction of computed tomography scan showing tumorous obstruction in lower descending colon area and dilated loops of large bowel with air-fluid levels. Note collapsed bowel loop distal to tumor *(arrow)*.

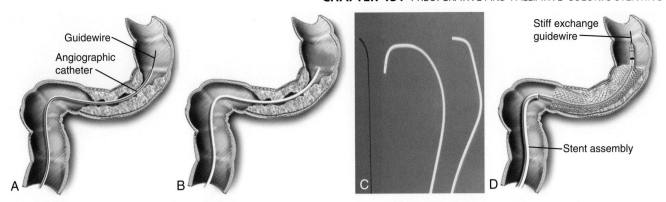

FIGURE 131-3. **A-B,** Schematic drawing of a tumorous lesion in rectosigmoid junction, traversed with a guidewire and catheter. **C,** Terumo Glidewire *(left)* and angiographic catheters *(right)*, Cobra and Headhunter types. **D,** Schematic drawing of stent instrument advanced over superstiff wire, and released stent in place.

obstruction. CT is also the method of choice for staging and may provide important information about the presence of multiple stenoses or concomitant small bowel obstruction in peritoneal carcinosis that have to be ruled out before placement of colonic stents. CT colonography may be of additional value.

The stenosis can be negotiated (1) primarily with radiologic techniques alone, with optional endoscopy reserved for difficult cases,[5,26,29,36,37] (2) with hybrid endoscopic-radiologic methods,[13,17,25,26] and (3) endoscopic stent placement with limited fluoroscopy, probably the preferred method at many institutions where gastroenterologists are in the lead of gastrointestinal stenting.[28,30] Lesions in the proximal portions of the colon are best handled with a combined endoscopic-fluoroscopic approach to overcome the tortuosity of the colonic flexures.[13,17]

Technical Aspects

Fluoroscopic Guidance/Radiologic Technique (OTW)
Patients are best treated under mild sedation and placed in a left lateral position on the fluoroscopy table to start. A high-torque (7F) angiographic catheter (Headhunter or Cobra type) or a guiding catheter is placed in the colon, and the colonic segments are best negotiated with a catheter-guidewire combination (Fig. 131-3, *A-C*). Water-soluble contrast material is used to outline the bowel lumen and the area of the stricture. Conventional or hydrophilic guidewires, or both, may be used. Once the stricture has been passed with the catheter-guidewire assembly, the lesion is best defined by injecting contrast material through a catheter with multiple side holes and rotating the patient to an optimal position for stent insertion. For stent placement, an exchange-length superstiff wire (Amplatz Super Stiff, Lunderquist [Boston Scientific]) is placed well beyond the lesion. After advancing the stent to the desired location under fluoroscopic control, the stent is released (Fig. 131-3, *D*). If acute bends or kinks have to be passed or an elongated rectosigmoidal arch reduces forward pushability, a stiff large-bore guiding catheter (i.e., 11F Mullin sheath [William Cook Europe, Bjaeverskov, Denmark]) may be helpful to advance the stent assembly to the desired location.

Endoscopic-Fluoroscopic Guidance (TTS)
Patients are mildly sedated with midazolam and given pain medication (pethidine chlorhydrate). With the patient in the supine or oblique decubitus position on the fluoroscopy table, the endoscope is advanced to the distal end of the stenosis, and the obstruction is passed with a guidewire under endoscopic and fluoroscopic guidance (Fig. 131-4, *A*). Various types of steerable and hydrophilic guidewires such as the Glidewire (Terumo Medical Corp., Somerset, N.J.), Zebra (Boston Scientific), or endoscopic wires (Wilson-Cook Medical, Winston-Salem, N.C.) may be used to pass the obstruction. After placement of a multi-sidehole endoscopic catheter with its tip passed beyond the obstruction, the extent of the stenosis is visualized with the injection of water-soluble contrast material (Telebrix, Guerbet, France) (Fig. 131-4, *B*). For stent placement, a stiff guidewire at least 400 cm in length (Zebra), with its tip well beyond the obstruction, has to be used to accept any stent delivery system that will fit through the working channel of the endoscope (Fig. 131-4, *C*). The stent is deployed under combined fluoroscopic and endoscopic control such that the middle of the stent covers the stricture, with the stent extending at least 1 to 2 cm on each end of the lesion (Fig. 131-4, *D-F*). If a lesion is not adequately covered, an additional stent must be placed. A plain film is taken 24 to 48 hours after stent placement to confirm adequate position and expansion of the stent, as well as regression of the ileus, and to exclude inadvertant perforation (Fig. 131-4, *G*). Figure 131-4, *H*, shows a resected specimen with the stent in place.

Further Technical Considerations
As a general rule, intraluminal position of guidewires and catheters must be confirmed at all times. The significant shortening of braided stents during release must always be taken into account; stents must have sufficient length to adapt to curves and bends and prevent protrusion of bare stent ends (particularly those of the open-end type, such as the Enteral Wallstent) or obstruction by abutting of the free stent end against the bowel wall. Therefore, placement of the free edges of the stent near sites of bowel angulation should be avoided and treated with additional stents if necessary (Fig. 131-5). Stents placed too close to the anal

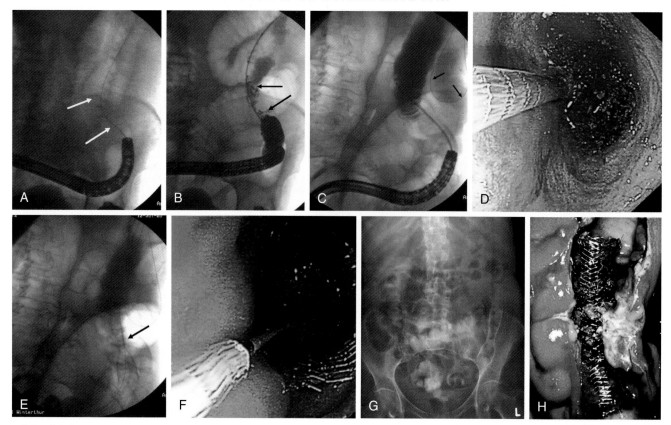

FIGURE 131-4. Same patient as in Figure 131-2. **A,** Guidewire has been passed through obstruction (defect in air-filled column of descending colon *[between arrows]*) via working channel of endoscope. **B,** Injection of contrast material via endoscopic catheter with multiple side holes demonstrates tight and irregular obstruction *(between arrows)*. **C,** Enteral Unistep Wallstent advanced through obstruction via working channel of endoscope. Note how far proximal to obstruction guidewire has been placed for safe stent delivery *(arrows)*. **D,** Endoscopic view and control of stent position before release. **E,** Fluoroscopic view of released stent, showing adequate spontaneous self-expansion at area of tumor *(arrow)*. **F,** Endoscopic view of released stent, confirming perfect positioning. **G,** Plain film of abdomen 24 hours after stent placement, showing further self-expansion of stent and markedly reduced signs of ileus. **H,** Resected specimen with stent in place shows stent in perfect position overlapping tumor ends on both sides by 2 to 3 cm. Patient underwent primary anastomosis without a colostomy. *(**A**, **B**, **D**, and **F**, from Jost RS, Jost R, Schoch E, et al. Colorectal stenting: An effective therapy for preoperative and palliative treatment. Cardiovasc Intervent Radiol 2007;30:433–40.)*

sphincter may cause tenesmus and incontinence[5,18] and carry a higher risk for expulsion.

Balloon dilatation before stent placement should be avoided because of the increased risk for perforation or potential metastatic spread.[5,16,17,28,29] In our experience, additional balloon dilatation to adequately expand the stent is only rarely necessary (see Fig. 131-5, *D* and *E*). Again, this should be done with care to not run the risk of colonic perforation.[5,13,17,28,29]

In cases in which a lesion cannot be passed with the endoscope following the guidewire, or if the stent apparatus used will not fit through an endoscope, a superstiff guidewire has to be placed across the obstruction, then the endoscope must be removed and the stent advanced under fluoroscopy over the superstiff guidewire. For deployment of the stent, the endoscope may be reinserted alongside the stent assembly to monitor correct placement of the stent endoscopically and with simultaneous fluoroscopy. For greater stability around bends and kinks or around the splenic flexure, a large-caliber guiding catheter accepting the stent instrument may be needed to advance the stent assembly (see Fig. 131-5). Some authors mention balloon dilatation of the stricture or even laser ablation to allow

passage of the endoscope.[15] However, we do not recommend this because of the danger of rupture following stent placement.[5,17,28,29]

If a distal (rectosigmoidal) obstruction cannot be passed with the help of either the endoscope or standard angiographic catheter techniques, we have found a rectal tube with balloon occlusion of the anus, as used for barium enemas, to be most helpful in opacifying and distending the rectum and distal part of the colon (Fig. 131-6, *A* and *B*). In this way, by using a coaxial system with a 5F to 7F Cobra or Headhunter catheter passed through a steerable guiding catheter (8F or 9F MPA, Cordis Corp., Miami Lakes, Fla.), difficult and kinked obstructions may be negotiated with a steerable guidewire (Fig. 131-6, *C*). For subsequent positioning of the stent instrument, superstiff exchange wires are mandatory.

Alternative Approaches to the Transanal Route

In cases in which a colonic obstruction cannot be passed via the conventional transanal route, a percutaneous approach by percutaneous cecostomy access may be considered.[38-40] The authors stress the importance of anchoring the colon firmly to the abdominal wall to avoid

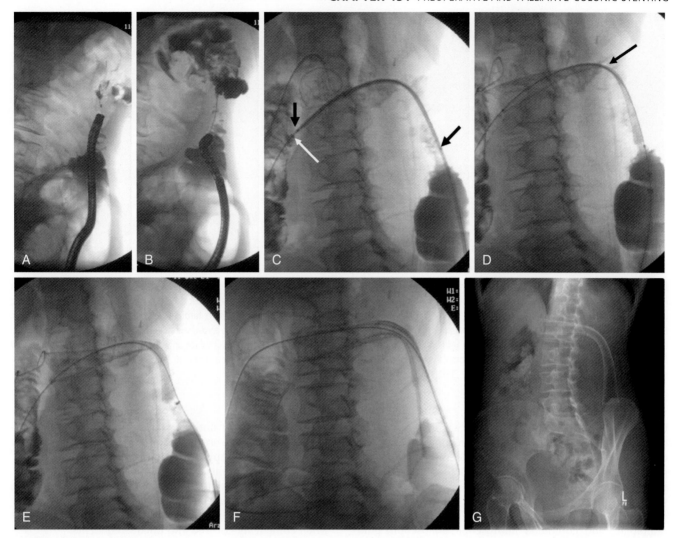

FIGURE 131-5. Carcinoma of stomach and infiltration of left flexure and proximal descending colon in a 55-year-old patient with acute ileus. **A,** Because of a very tortuous and elongated sigmoid colon, only a baby endoscope could be advanced to obstruction. Injection of contrast material shows irregular obstruction. **B,** After manipulation of guidewire through obstruction, injection of contrast material over multi-sidehole catheter shows a long lesion involving entire splenic flexure and parts of descending colon. Endoscope could not be advanced further. **C,** In addition to a superstiff wire, a Mullin sheath *(white arrow marks the tip)* had to be used as an additional stiffening and guiding tool to advance constrained stent *(black arrows)* beyond splenic flexure. **D,** Inadequate self-expansion of a 22/90-mm Enteral Unistep Wallstent after release around splenic flexure *(arrow).* **E,** After dilation with a 12-mm angioplasty balloon, stent lumen is sufficiently expanded, but stent has shortened and does not cover obstruction distally. **F,** Three Enteral Unistep Wallstents had to be placed around splenic flexure through Mullin sheath to cover entire lesion. **G,** One-day follow-up shows good expansion of all three stents, with nice adaptation to splenic flexure.

the danger of complications such as fecaloid peritonitis.[39] Letting the percutaneous tract mature for 6 to 10 days plus good decompression by the stent before removing the percutaneous catheter seems extremely important to avoid the risk of peritonitis or formation of an enterocutaneous fistula.

CONTROVERSIES

Both covered and uncovered stents have been used for colorectal obstruction.* For preoperative stenting, there is no need for a covered stent, since tumor ingrowth is not an issue in the short preoperative interval, but for palliation, covered stents have the potential advantage of preventing

*References 5, 13, 16, 23, 30, 32, 33, 37.

tumor ingrowth that would cause delayed stent obstruction. Covered stents are more rigid and less stable than uncovered versions, however, and seem to have no advantage over uncovered stents.[32] Covered SEMS are beneficial to treat malignant fistulae as well as iatrogenic perforations and postsurgical leaks.[16,21-23]

Colonic cancers located in the rectosigmoid region can be negotiated with interventional catheter techniques alone in the majority of cases. However, we have found the endoscope to be particularly helpful as a stiffening and guiding tool for managing the rectosigmoid curvature, straightening out kinks, dealing with elongation of the bowel, and especially for lesions proximal to the descending colon around the colonic flexures, which may not be managed by radiologic catheter techniques alone. Most interventional radiologists would resort to additional endoscopic

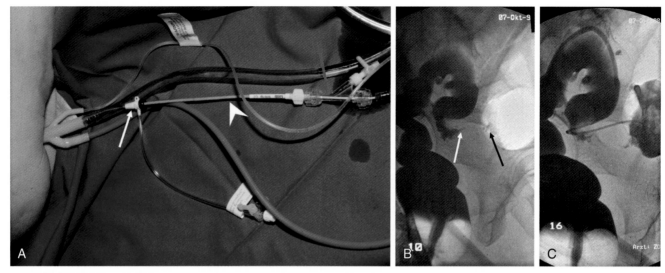

FIGURE 131-6. Metastatic obstruction of sigmoid colon in a 66-year-old patient that could not be passed by endoscopic means. **A,** Balloon-catheter system (Trimline DC [E-Z EM, Westbury, N.Y.]) for a barium enema in situ. Main tube has been punctured, and 8F introducer sheath *(white arrow)* and renal 8F guiding catheter *(arrowhead)* have been introduced. A 5F angiographic Cobra catheter *(red arrow)* has been passed through guiding catheter with a Y-connector. **B,** Barium enema with distal colon and rectum extended shows distal end of tumorous obstruction *(white arrow)* and air-filled sigmoid delineating proximal end of obstruction *(black arrow)*. **C,** Obstruction has been passed with a steerable hydrophilic guidewire over which angiographic catheter could be advanced for injection of contrast material to delineate length of lesion for final stent placement after exchange for a superstiff wire. *(**A** and **B** from Zollikofer CL. Gastroduodenal and colonic stents. Semin Interv Radiol 2001;18:265–80.)*

techniques in such cases.[17,26,31] A further potential advantage of endoscopy is the ability to obtain biopsies at the time of the procedure. Yet another consideration to favor a hybrid procedure might be the radiation dose. De Gregorio et al.[26] found a significant 12.5% reduction in radiation dose with a combined endoscopic-fluoroscopic technique.

Though there are no direct comparisons of endoscopic, radiologic, and combined fluoroscopic-endoscopic guidance, they seem to have similar technical success rates and procedure times,[13,14,26] with marginally lower success for purely radiologic methods in one pooled study.[41]

OUTCOMES

Technical success is defined as successful deployment of the SEMS across the obstruction, with at least 1 to 2.5 cm of normal colon bridged by both ends of the stent and stent patency. Clinical success is defined as significant improvement of radiologic signs of obstruction and clinical signs at 24 to 48 hours after stent placement.[5,17,26]

Despite little high-level data, colorectal stenting has gained widespread acceptance.[5,15,33] In large pooled and systematic overview studies,[13,16,25,33,41] as well as large single-center studies,[26,28,31] the results of preoperative and palliative stenting via endoscopic, radiologic, or combined methods showed high overall technical success rates of 92% to 98%. The main reasons for failures were inability to cross the obstruction with a guidewire and iatrogenic colonic perforation.[26] Clinical improvement was seen in 88% to 99%, with a rate of recurrent obstruction of 7.3% to 12%,[5,15] mainly in cases of palliative stenting. Primary reasons for early clinical failure were paralytic ileus and perforation.[13,16,25,26,28]

Major complications other than stent obstruction were reported in an average of 8% to 24.4% and consisted mostly of stent migration (3.0%-11.8%) and perforation

(0%-4.5%).[5,23,26,31] Of note is an up to threefold risk of perforation in patients receiving chemotherapy, particularly bevacizumab therapy following palliative stenting.[5,28,42] Stent-related mortality is less than 1%.[5] No significant differences between different uncovered stent designs (no detailed analysis available) were found, and only minor differences were reported for technical and clinical success when comparing covered and uncovered stents.[32,33]

Preoperative Stenting

Preoperative stenting is intended as a bridge to one-stage surgery to lower morbidity and mortality rates, shorten hospital stay, and reduce costs.

In two recent large pooled studies, two single-center studies, and two registries, the technical and clinical success rates were 90% to 98% (range 66%-100%), with a 72% to 94% chance for one-stage surgery with primary anastomosis.[26,28,31,33,41] The majority of patients (where specified) were treated with Wallstents (Enteral Wallstent Unistep, Ultraflex Precision, and WallFlex). The mean time to surgery after stent placement was 7 to 11 days.[26,29,33] In these studies, lower rates of colostomies and serious adverse events and shorter hospital stays were shown. This is in line with the most recent meta-analysis of some 600 patients by Zhang et al.,[43] where 38.6% underwent preoperative stent placement, versus 61.4% having emergency surgery. Fewer patients needed intensive care ($P = 0.03$) and stoma creation ($P = 0.04$). The primary anastomosis rate was higher ($P = 0.001$) and the overall complications reduced by stent placement ($P = 0.004$). There was no adverse effect on mortality or long-term survival in the stent group. The overall complication rate in the two multinational registries (182 patients) was only 7.8%, including 3% perforation, 1.2% stent migration, and 1.8% persistent colonic obstruction.[31]

At this time, there are few published prospective randomized trials. Two recent multicenter randomized trials by Pirlet et al.[44] and van Hooft et al.[45] failed to show any advantage of preoperative stenting over emergency surgery. In both studies, low technical success rates of 53%[44] and 70%[45] and high perforation rates of 33% (7% procedure, 26% stent related)[44] and 13% (4% procedure, 8% stent related)[45] were noted. The unexpected high rates of adverse effects and high rate of technical failures led to cessation of the studies. These disappointing results may be attributed to the large number of participating centers (9 and 25) for only 30 and 47 stented patients, so that a sufficient threshold for highest proficiency in colonic stenting at all centers may be questioned. As Song and Baron state in their commentary,[46] preoperative stenting should be best done in selected centers where a team of highly experienced interventional radiologists and endoscopists cooperate. This concurs with the recommendation (level B) of a recent consensus conference of the World Society of Emergency Surgery (WSES).[47]

Stenting of Benign Lesions (Diverticulitis)

Because it is not always possible to distinguish between malignant and benign obstruction caused by diverticulitis in the acute stage, even with endoscopy, stent placement may be necessary for immediate relief of obstruction before the results of biopsy are available. The experience with stenting of obstruction in inflammatory stenosis secondary to diverticulitis is limited, with small numbers reported in the recent literature.[16-19,25,48] Results are encouraging, and prompt relief of obstruction was achieved in most patients. However, because of a relatively high risk of complications (38%-43%), particularly perforation in inflammatory lesions, patients should be operated on as soon as clinical decompression allows elective one-stage surgery if a diagnosis of diverticulitis is confirmed.[17,18] Delayed surgery or palliation in acute diverticular disease carry an increased risk of perforation.[17-19] Stenting should therefore only be used in patients unfit for emergency surgery as a bridge to resection.[17-19]

Palliative Stenting

Technical and immediate clinical success rates in large retrospective studies,[26,33] as well as two prospective studies,[29,49] were in the range of 90% to 100% and 86% to 99%, respectively. Major complications including perforation, stent migration, and reobstruction were in the range of 11% to 28%. Recurrent symptoms due to fecal impaction and tumor and/or overgrowth ranged from 5% to 16%, and secondary clinical success at 6 months was 77% to 86%.[19,26,29,49] The median rate for reintervention in the review by Watt et al.[33] was 20%. The median survival was 205 days (range 87-327 days). Median stent patency was 157 days (range 106-204 days). Stent patency until death was a reported 89.5%, and median stent patency at 6 months ranged from 53% to 77% (mean 66%).[19,26,29,33,49] In all these studies, the need for stoma creation was rare.

Comparative data are scarce. The only randomized trial for either surgery or palliation by endoscopic stenting in advanced stage IV colorectal cancer had to be stopped prematurely because of an excessive number perforations,[42] but this study had important limitations.[30]

Overall, the available data confirm that SEMS for palliation of malignant colorectal obstruction is safe and effective if an experienced team of specialists is available. In comparison to surgery, SEMS placement has positive outcomes, including shorter hospitalization time, lower rate of serious complications, and similar postprocedure mortality rates. The WSES recommended in their guidelines for palliative decompression for nonresectable colorectal malignancies that SEMS should be preferred to colostomy.[47] However, caution is advised if additional treatment with specific chemotherapeutic drugs is planned, which may predispose to perforation.[28,50]

In addition, in our experience the length of the stenosis is an important determination of long-term patency. Stenting of long (>5 cm) metastatic lesions that required more than one stent gave rather disappointing results.[17] The higher tendency for dysfunction is probably related to a disturbance in propulsive peristalsis, which leads to stool impaction. Therefore, we are currently reluctant to stent lesions that require more than one stent of 90 mm in length. However, if stent dysfunction occurs, this may be relieved by colorectal tubes, which can easily be advanced through an obstructed stent, thereby still allowing decompression of obstructed bowel before palliative surgery.

Palliative, Midterm, and Long-Term Stenting of Benign Obstruction (Non-diverticulitis)

Little data on SEMS in benign non-diverticular colorectal obstruction exists.[16,18,19] Anastomotic obstruction and other rare causes (ischemic, radiation) have been treated with balloon dilatation or surgery when neccessary.[18,19] Keränen et al.[18] have treated 10 patients with anastomotic strictures (two Crohn disease) and one radiogenic stricture; 9 of the 11 patients were treated with covered stents, and 6 patients had mid- to long-term stenting (4 weeks to 63 months) without requiring surgery. Stents spontaneously discharged (two cases) or were electively removed (three cases). In one patient with Crohn disease, the surgery could be postponed by 1 month; in the other, an ileostoma had to be performed because of perforation after 53 months. The results of Keränen et al. and Small et al.[18,19] suggest that stenting could be a valid alternative in non-diverticular strictures and patients who are unfit for surgery. The devices of choice are probably retrievable covered stents that allow temporary stenting to minimize complications (e.g., SX-ELLA stent [ELLA-CS] or PolyFlex stent [Boston Scientific]).[34]

Restenosis Secondary to Tumor Progression

An overall rate of recurrent obstruction of 7.3% to 11.8% has been reported.[5] Tumor ingrowth has been reported in 2% to 20%.* Although tumor ingrowth is not a problem in patients in whom stents are applied for short-term decompression before surgery, for palliative treatment of obstruction, restenosis secondary to tumor ingrowth may well be problematic. Therefore, covered stents were developed to address this problem in the late 1990s.[23,51] Because of the limited length and bulkiness of the delivery catheter, only distal lesions of the rectosigmoid region could be treated. In addition, these cylindrical types of covered stents had a high migration rate.[23,32,51] Therefore, new designs of covered

*References 23, 26, 28, 29, 33, 49.

stents with a dogbone shape and uncovered flanged ends and more flexible delivery systems, including TTS, were developed to address this problem.[32,33,52,53] However, no significant advantages could be demonstrated with the improved designs. In their recent prospective study comparing covered and uncovered stents, Lee et al.[32] reported an identical clinical efficacy until 7 days. In the palliative group treated with covered stents, the symptoms of obstruction became more frequent beyond 7 days (60% vs. 18.8%). Late stent migration occurred only in the covered stent group. There was an 18.8% tumor ingrowth rate (treated with additional stents) in the uncovered stent group, and 12.5% of the covered stent group experienced fecal impaction and 6% tumor overgrowth, treated with endoscopic lavage or additional stents, respectively. Covered stents provided no advantage in either the bridge to surgery or palliative group and did not prevent reobstruction from tumor overgrowth or fecal impaction.

When restenosis secondary to tumor ingrowth does occur, a new stent can be placed coaxially within the first stent. Likewise, tumor overgrowth above or below the stent can be treated by placing a second stent. Fecal impaction and mucosal prolapse can usually be treated with endoscopic cleansing and/or balloon dilatation.[17]

Therefore, at this time it seems that the additional costs of a covered stent are not warranted. The obvious exceptions are, as mentioned previously, colovesical and colointestinal fistulas (see later).

Cost-Effectiveness

Cost-effectiveness and evidence-based treatment are major issues today and naturally also apply to colonic stenting. In two retrospective cost analysis studies,[54,55] the total costs generated for a group of patients with preoperative stent placement and follow-up surgery were compared with those of a control group undergoing only surgical treatment at the same hospital. The average cost savings in the group who underwent preoperative stenting versus the control group was 19.7% and 21.9%, respectively. The cost savings were mainly due to shorter hospitalization time (26.1 vs. 31.7 days), fewer days in the intensive care unit (0.4 vs. 4.9 days), and lower surgical fees ($23,669 vs. $31,120). Eighty-six percent of the patients treated by surgery after stent placement underwent primary anastomosis, and only 14% needed a temporary colostomy.

In two other studies addressing the cost differences between stenting and stoma creation[56] and analyzing three competing strategies[57]—preoperative stenting with elective resective surgery, emergent surgery with either primary reanastomosis or protective colostomy, and emergent colostomy followed by elective resection—the cost savings with preoperative SEMS were only marginal, but a significantly better quality of life and reduced rate of permanent or temporary stomas were achieved. Therefore, preoperative stenting should be strongly considered as a first-line bridge to surgery management and should also be offered in selected patients for palliation.

Stenting for Colonic Fistulas

Several cases of successful treatment of coloenteric or colovesical fistulas and anastomotic leakage with covered stents have been reported.[18,20-23,51,58] Various designs such as esophageal covered nitinol Ultraflex stents, covered esophageal Wallstents, and the polyester PolyFlex stent (Boston Scientific) were used in the United States and Europe,[20-23,58] whereas Choo et al. used their own design.[51] Dedicated covered colonic stents such as the SX-ELLA, Niti-S, and HANAROSTENT, which all have been used for colorectal obstruction,[26,30,52,53] are available outside the United States and are advocated for treatment of rectocolic fistulas (see Table 131-1).

COMPLICATIONS

Perforation, stent migration, and inadequate bowel decompression are the major procedure-related complications encountered with colonic stent placement. The mean rate of severe complications in the recent literature covering perforation with sepsis and stent migration ranges from 7%-15.5%. It is usually less than 10% in experienced hands.[†] Anal hemorrhage and tenesmus are usually self-limited and considered minor complications.

Perforation of the colon is a potentially serious complication that was reported in 0% to 4.5% in large pooled[5,31,33] and single and multicenter studies.[26,29,49] In their large retrospective study, Small et al.[28] reported 9% perforations, but this was negatively influenced by prior stricture dilatation up to 14 mm before stent placement, the experience of the endoscopist, and bevacizumab therapy following stent insertion. Early perforation caused by guidewire manipulation can usually be managed conservatively without sequelae.[5,13,54] Symptomatic perforations, which may be provoked by excessive guidewire manipulation and diverticular disease,[36] require vigilant treatment in 70% with emergency surgery, because of the 10% mortality risk.[16,41] The risk of perforation also increases two- to threefold with balloon dilatation before or after stent placement.[16,28,43] Therefore, we never use balloon dilatation before stent placement and only rarely after implantation if the stent does not expand adequately (see Fig. 131-5). In general, however, early symptomatic procedure-related perforation is rare.

Late perforations are usually stent related and may be caused by the sharp free ends of metal filaments (i.e., of enteral Unistep Wallstents).[13,28] Stents should be long enough to adapt around bends and acute angles, preventing the stent end from protruding into the bowel wall. Steroids, radiation therapy, and chemotherapy, which may enhance the fragility of the bowel wall, are further risk factors.[5,28] Bevacizumab therapy may result in an up to threefold risk of perforation.[28,42,50]

Stent migration of uncovered colonic stents in pooled and large single-center studies has been reported in the 7% to 12% range.[5,26,28,33] In a multinational registry using 22/25-mm and 25/30-mm WallFlex stents[39] and a prospective multicenter study using 25/30-mm Ultraflex precision stents,[29] the rates were only 1.2% and 2%, respectively. This supports the findings that stents with larger diameters (22-25 mm) and flared ends, longitudinal flexibility, and at least 6 cm in length reduce stent migration.[‡] Apart from stent type and size, the degree of obstruction and location influences fixation of the stent. Therefore, tumor debulking (laser ablation), balloon dilatation, and prophylactic

---

[†]References 5, 15, 26, 28, 31-33, 49.
[‡]References 5, 13, 16, 28, 49, 54.

stenting for subileus with incomplete obstruction or noncircular lesions is not recommended. Stents in the distal descending and rectosigmoid region are more likely to migrate because of the greater mobility and curvature, as well as the vigorous propulsive peristaltic activity in the rectum.[26,29] Chemo- and radiotherapy may be a cause of delayed migration.[15,29] Most stents migrate distally and may be spontaneously expelled through the anus. If patients become symptomatic following stent dislocation, the endoprosthesis may be removed by endoscopic or combined radiologic-endoscopic techniques, although in some cases migrated stents may have to be removed surgically.[15] Recurrent obstruction after stent dislocation/migration may be treated in many cases with a further stent insertion.[17,27]

Covered stents are more prone to migrate; rates as high as 30% to 50% have been reported, particularly for fully covered stents.[51] Dumbbell configurations (Niti-S stent) showed reduced migration rates (19%).[32] A dual design consisting of an outer covered and an inner bare stent (S&G Biotech, Seongnam, Korea) used by Song et al.[52] and Kim et al.[53] had a migration rate of 4% to 10% and up to 11% perforations. However, 7% of the patients required predilatation to pass the 4.5-mm-diameter stent assembly, and 48% needed additional balloon dilatation (15-20 mm) to achieve adequate stent expansion. Therefore, these stents do not seem to have any significant advantage for colorectal tumor stenting.

Inadequate bowel decompression is usually related to stent malpositioning, incomplete expansion,[17] stent migration,[5,13,25,33,54] or valve mechanisms if the stent end is abutting the bowel wall. In our own experience with stenting of long-segment stenosis (>7 cm), particularly in patients with extensive metastatic disease, early dysfunction secondary to fecal impaction or inadequate peristaltic propulsion (or both) was not infrequent (27%). Furthermore, the presence of multiple obstructions undetected before stent placement must be considered if decompression is delayed despite stent patency. Thus, to rule out synchronous lesions that might prevent clinical success, particularly in metastatic disease, abdominal CT with special attention to additional sites of small/large bowel obstruction should be performed before stent deployment. If recurrent fecal impaction, inadequate peristalsis, or both lead to stent dysfunction, placement of a large bowel tube through the stented segment has proved to be an effective method of bowel cleansing and preparation for elective palliative surgery.[13,17] In cases of valve mechanisms with the stent end abutting the bowel wall, which can result from stent shortening with progressive stent expansion, placement of an additional stent usually solves the problem (Fig. 131-7). Stent fracture in the colon and rectum seems to be a very rare event.[59]

Other potential complications such as severe hemorrhage or excessive pain are rarely encountered.[15,26,35] In general, minor rectal bleeding and tenesmus can be treated

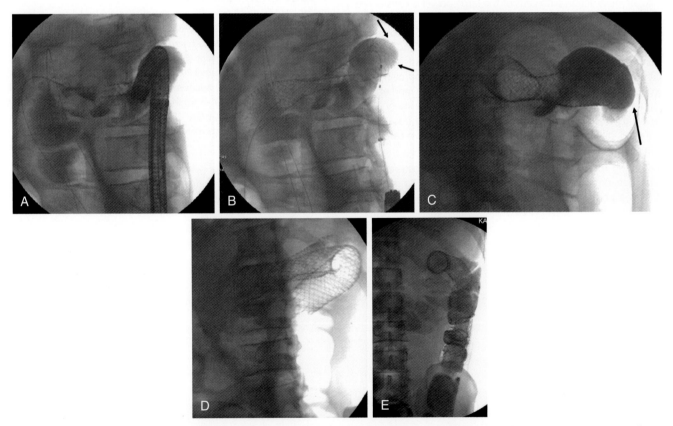

FIGURE 131-7. Infiltrating pancreatic carcinoma in a 37-year-old patient referred for palliative stenting of a colonic obstruction proximal to splenic flexure. **A,** Injection of contrast material through a multi-sidehole catheter placed endoscopically shows long irregular stenosis close to splenic flexure. **B,** Adequate expansion of a 25/90-mm WallFlex. Note that distal end is very close to lateral wall of descending colon *(arrows)*. **C,** Three days later, patient had inadequate bowel movements. Distal stent end is abutting descending wall at splenic flexure *(arrow)*, causing partial obstruction. **D,** A second 25/90-mm WallFlex has been placed coaxially to extend first stent around flexure. **E,** Plain film after computed tomography examination 1 month after placement of second stent shows good function and no signs of obstruction proximal to stent. The two stents adapt well to curvature of left colonic flexure.

medically. Stents within 5 cm of the anal verge may cause severe tenesmus and pain and seem more prone to migration and expulsion.[35] Retrievable stents such as the covered PolyFlex (Boston Scientific) and SX-ELLA (ELLA-CS) seem valid choices in low rectal obstruction.[35]

POSTPROCEDURAL AND FOLLOW-UP CARE

Immediate postprocedural care consists of monitoring vital signs, treatment of electrolyte imbalance, and intravenous administration of fluids. Patients are kept fasting for a 12-hour period. Plain films of the abdomen are usually obtained after 24 to 48 hours to assess adequate position and expansion of the stent and resolution of the radiologic signs of ileus. Patients stented for bridge-to-surgery are prepared with bowel cleansing for elective surgery, which is best performed after a period of 3 to 7 days.[5,27] Patients should be warned about potential complications such as early or late stent migration, perforation, bleeding, tenesmus, and fecal impaction of the stents. To avoid the last, patients in whom stents are placed for palliation without subsequent surgery should be kept on a low-residue diet and stool softeners, including phosphate enemas.[15]

obstruction is short, and elective surgery after treatment with antibiotics is performed in due course.

- In patients with nonresectable malignant disease, stenting may provide adequate long-term palliation obviating colostomy, but long-segment stenoses have a relatively high risk of reocclusion due to stool impaction or mucosal prolapse. Tumor ingrowth or overgrowth may be of further concern in patients with prolonged survival, but covered stents do not seem to provide significantly better long-term patency. Caution is advised if treatment with specific chemotherapeutic drugs is planned, which may predispose to late perforation.
- Covered stents may be indicated in treating fistulas of the rectosigmoid colon. Retrievable stents may be advisable for palliative stenting of nonmalignant strictures or rectal stents.
- Stents may be placed with a combined endoscopic-radiologic approach as far proximally as the right colon, whereas with radiologic guidance alone, stent placement is generally limited to the left colon distal to the splenic flexure. If both facilities and the expertise of fully trained interventional radiologists and gastroenterologists are available, a hybrid approach would seem optimal for treating obstructing lesions throughout the colon.

KEY POINTS

- Acute obstruction with ileus of the large bowel is considered an emergency, and rapid treatment is required. Bridge-to-surgery use of self-expanding metal stents (SEMS) in obstructive colorectal cancer, particularly of the descending and sigmoid colon, is a cost-effective, minimally invasive alternative to emergency surgery. It buys time for improving the patient's overall condition, staging of the disease, and appropriate bowel cleansing for elective one-stage surgery. Cost savings of up to 22% can be achieved, mainly because of shorter hospital stay, fewer days in the intensive care unit, and fewer surgical procedures.
- Stenting for diverticulitis with severe colonic obstruction in patients unfit for emergency surgery as a bridge to resection can be performed safely, provided the inflammatory tumor

▶ **SUGGESTED READINGS**

Baron TH. Minimizing endoscopic complications: endoluminal stents. Gastrointest Endosc Clin N Am 2007;17:83–104.

De Gregorio MA, Laborda A, Tejero E, et al. Ten-year retrospective study of treatment of malignant colonic obstructions with self-expandable stents. J Vasc Interv Radiol 2011;22:870–8.

Katsanos K, Sabharwal T, Adam A. Stenting of the lower gastrointestinal tract: Current status. Cardiovasc Intervent Radiol 2011;34:462–73.

Watt AM, Faragher IG, Griffin TT, et al. Self-expanding metallic stents for relieving malignant colorectal obstruction. Ann Surg 2007;246(1):24–30.

The complete reference list is available online at www.expertconsult.com.

CHAPTER 132

Gastrostomy and Gastrojejunostomy

Sarah Power and Michael J. Lee

Traditionally, enteral feeding tubes were placed by surgical or endoscopic techniques, but the interventional radiologist now plays a central role in providing patient enteral nutrition by placing gastrostomy and gastrojejunostomy tubes. The first successful placement of a percutaneous endoscopic gastrostomy (PEG) was described in 1979 by Gauderer and Ponsky.[1] This was followed 2 years later by the first percutaneous radiologic gastrostomy (PRG) performed under fluoroscopic guidance by Preshaw.[2] PRG is a well-tolerated procedure that provides nutritional support where required. The procedure is associated with low morbidity and mortality,[3] with recent technical advances improving the long-term patency of enteral catheters.[4] The advantage of PRG is the relative simplicity of the technique, facilitating enteral feeding in either the hospital or home environment.

INDICATIONS

PRG is indicated in a wide range of patients who cannot maintain their nutrition orally. The most common patient subgroups are those with neurologic impairment resulting in absent gag reflex or disorders of swallowing, and esophageal or head and neck malignancy.[3-6] Indeed, PRG is particularly advantageous in these patient subgroups, since it can be performed with minimal sedation, thereby decreasing the risk of aspiration,[7,8] and avoidance of endoscopy, which is often precluded by upper tract stenosis in the case of malignancy.[9] Other patient groups who benefit from gastrostomy placement and enteral feeding include those with intestinal malabsorption secondary to small bowel pathology such as Crohn disease, radiation enteritis, and scleroderma; patients who require supplementary enteral support, such as those with cystic fibrosis or significant burns; and patients with psychological ailments such as eating disorders or profound depression.[10,11]

Less commonly, gastrostomy is placed for decompression of gastrointestinal (GI) obstruction.[3,11-13] Patients with diabetes-related gastroparesis can benefit from dual-lumen cannulation[13]; one lumen decompresses the stomach while a distal limb is placed beyond the ligament of Treitz for feeding. When not feeding during the day, the two loops are attached, obviating the need for a drainage bag.[10]

CONTRAINDICATIONS

There are few contraindications to PRG placement. As with most interventional procedures, the patient's coagulation status should be evaluated, and any abnormality corrected prior to the procedure. In our unit, an international normalized ratio (INR) of 1.5 or less and a platelet count in excess of 80,000/mm^3 are considered acceptable.

Difficulties with percutaneous access to the stomach, such as interposition of the colon between the stomach and anterior abdominal wall, or a large/low-lying liver are considered relative contraindications. In the case of colonic interposition, an infracolic approach is possible.[14,15] Previously it was thought that gastric fixation (gastropexy) should not be performed with this approach, owing to the increased potential for complications including colonic obstruction. However, more recently an infracolic approach with gastropexy has been described with no additional complications.[14] In the presence of a low-lying or large liver, computed tomography (CT) and/or ultrasound can facilitate gastric cannulation.[11] PRG placement can be challenging in patients with a high-lying stomach, often seen in patients with amyotrophic lateral sclerosis and due to diaphragmatic weakness; an intercostal approach may be required.[7]

Previous surgery (e.g., Billroth II gastroenterostomy, partial gastrectomy, or gastric pull-through surgery) is considered a relative contraindication owing to anatomic distortion.[16] Balloon distension of the stomach remnant and/or CT-guided placement of the gastrostomy tube may render the procedure possible.[17-19]

In head and neck or esophageal malignancy, significant stenosis of the upper GI tract may preclude placement of the nasogastric tube required for gaseous distension of the stomach. In such cases, a small-diameter catheter and hydrophilic guidewire may be used to cross the stenosis[9]; alternatively, the stomach can be punctured under ultrasound[20] or CT guidance.[21]

The presence of ascites is no longer considered an absolute contraindication to PRG placement,[21] and most interventional radiologists will perform the procedure in the presence of mild ascites. In the case of significant ascites, preprocedural paracentesis and gastropexy is mandatory to reduce the risk of catheter looping in the peritoneal cavity, tube dislodgement, and peritubal leakage.[11] It is also necessary to prevent reaccumulation of ascites post procedure, since the weight of fluid can result in separation of the stomach from the anterior abdominal wall despite gastropexy.[22] Sonographic follow-up and repeated paracentesis should therefore be performed as required. Patients undergoing peritoneal dialysis require similar consideration.

The presence of gastric varices, as in portal hypertension, remains one of the only absolute contraindications to PRG because of the associated risk of significant hemorrhage.[11,12]

EQUIPMENT

The required equipment for PRG insertion is detailed in Table 132-1.

TABLE 132-1. List of Equipment Required for Standard Gastrostomy Tube Insertion

Equipment	Comments
Nasogastric tube and air insufflation balloon	Placed prior to procedure
200 mL of dilute barium suspension	Optional; colonic air usually visible fluoroscopically
Noninvasive monitoring equipment	To monitor HR, BP, oxygen saturation
Paralytic agents	Hyoscine-*N*-butylbromide or glucagon hydrochloride
Local anesthetic	1% lignocaine
Medications for conscious sedation	Fentanyl citrate, midazolam
T-fasteners, slotted needle, and stylet	For gastropexy
10-mL syringe with 5-mL sterile saline	For gastropexy and gastric puncture
18-gauge needle	For gastric puncture
0.035-inch Amplatz Super Stiff guidewire	
Serial fascial dilators or tapered dilator	
Gastrostomy catheter of choice	
Peel-away sheath	If balloon retention type catheter used
Contrast medium	To confirm placement

BP, Blood pressure; *HR*, heart rate.

GASTROSTOMY

Patient Preparation

The procedure and potential complications are discussed with the patient, and informed consent is obtained. A coagulation study is performed and any abnormalities corrected. The patient is required to fast from the evening prior to the procedure, and a nasogastric tube (NG) placed. Approximately 200 mL of dilute barium suspension can be administered (orally or via NG) 12 hours prior to the procedure to help identify the colon so it can be avoided during PRG. However, similar to other investigators,[23,24] we have discontinued routine use of barium in our unit because we find gas in the colon is usually a sufficient marker when lateral screening is used. If there is insufficient gas in the colon, a small amount of air can be insufflated per rectum. Although advocated by some, particularly in head and neck cancer patients,[25] antibiotic prophylaxis is not routinely administered in our unit unless a hybrid PEG/PRG procedure is planned, as described later.

Noninvasive monitoring equipment is applied. The patient's heart rate, blood pressure, and oxygen saturation are monitored throughout the procedure. When appropriate, intravenous midazolam and fentanyl citrate are used in combination for sedation and analgesia. We routinely start with 1 mg midazolam and 50 µg fentanyl, giving further increments as required. The abdominal skin is cleansed with an appropriate solution, and sterile drapes placed.

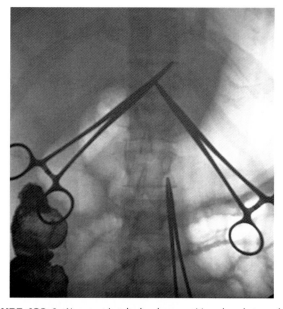

FIGURE 132-1. Nasogastric tube has been positioned, and stomach has been distended with air. Two forceps outline costochondral junctions. A pair of scissors overlies proposed site of gastrostomy tube insertion. In this case, barium was administered to outline colon.

One of the key factors to a successful outcome is maintaining adequate gastric distension. The stomach is insufflated with air via the indwelling NG tube and the degree of gastric distension monitored fluoroscopically. Hyoscine-*N*-butylbromide (Buscopan) or glucagon hydrochloride (GlucaGen) is administered intravenously to facilitate gastroparesis. This is of particular importance in cases where the stomach is suboptimally distended due to poor air retention.

Technique

The following is a description of the technique for placing a standard gastrostomy tube with gastropexy under fluoroscopic guidance. Figures 132-1 through 132-6 illustrate various aspects of the insertion technique. Certain tube types, such as low-profile gastrostomies, require some modification of technique, and this is addressed later in the chapter with the discussion on tube types.

An appropriate puncture site for gastrostomy is chosen using fluoroscopy and anatomic landmarks; we do not routinely use ultrasound to delineate the liver edge. The optimum insertion site is usually to the left of midline overlying the antrum or mid- to distal body of the stomach, equidistant from the greater and lesser curves to avoid gastric and gastroepiploic vessels, and lateral to the rectus muscle to avoid the inferior epigastric vessels.[12,21] A curved artery forceps is placed over the planned puncture site under fluoroscopy to confirm the proposed gastropexy position (Fig. 132-1).

Local anesthetic (5-10 mL 1% lignocaine) is infiltrated at the four corners of a 2-cm square surrounding the planned puncture site (Fig. 132-2, *A*), and the gastropexy is formed using four T-fasteners, one at each corner of the gastropexy square (Fig. 132-2, *B*). Traditional T-fasteners (Boston Scientific, Natick, Mass.) (Fig. 132-3, *A*) consist of a nylon

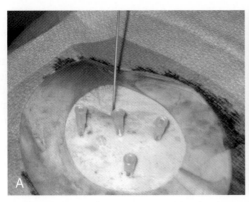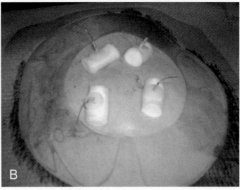

FIGURE 132-2. A, Local anesthetic is infiltrated at four corners of a 2-cm square surrounding planned puncture site. **B,** Four T-fasteners (Boston Scientific, Natick, Mass.) have been inserted into stomach before gastrostomy tube placement.

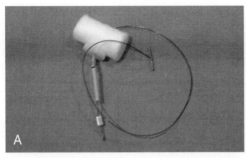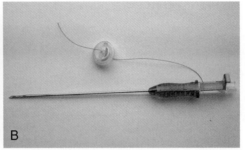

FIGURE 132-3. A, T-fasteners from Boston Scientific (Natick, Mass.) consist of a nylon suture with a metal T-bar, cotton pledget, two metal cylinders, and a plastic washer, and are inserted into distended stomach using a slotted 18-gauge needle. **B,** Gastropexy sutures (Saf-T-Pexy T-fasteners) from Kimberley Clark (Draper, Utah) are preloaded safety needles that contain a monofilament absorbable suture (3-0 Biosyn), eliminating need for suture removal. They also contain a polyurethane suture lock that secures suture connection and maintains tension.

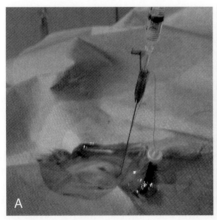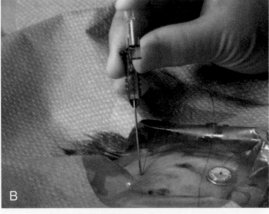

FIGURE 132-4. Insertion of Saf-T-Pexy T-fasteners from Kimberley Clark (Draper, Utah). **A,** Syringe containing sterile saline is attached to preloaded safety needle, which is inserted into stomach with a single sharp thrust. Intragastric position is confirmed by aspiration of air into syringe. **B,** Once intragastric position is confirmed, syringe is removed. T-fasteners are deployed by releasing suture strand, bending locking tabs on needle hub, and pushing inner hub to outer hub as shown. Following this, needle is withdrawn, T-bar is pulled flush against gastric wall, suture lock is slid down to abdominal wall, and suture is temporarily clamped with hemostat. Once all T-fasteners are in place, gentle traction is placed on sutures to appose stomach to anterior abdominal wall, and suture lock is closed with hemostat until an audible click is heard.

suture with a metal T-bar, cotton pledget, two metal cylinders, and a plastic washer, and are inserted into the distended stomach using a slotted 18-gauge needle. A syringe containing sterile saline is attached to the slotted needle, and an intragastric position confirmed by aspiration of air into the syringe. A stylet is then passed through the slotted needle to deploy the T-fastener. Stylet and needle are subsequently removed, and the stomach is approximated to the anterior abdominal wall by gentle traction on the T-fastener suture. T-fasteners are then secured in position by crimping the small metal cylinders at the base of the nylon suture. Such T-fasteners require removal post procedure. More

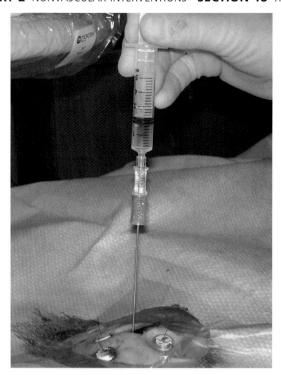

FIGURE 132-5. Sterile syringe is attached to 18-gauge introducer needle, which is then inserted into stomach through incision made in center of gastropexy square. Aspiration of air confirms intragastric location.

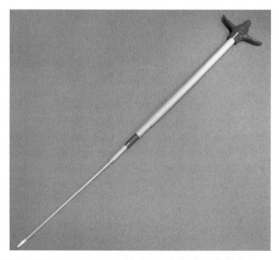

FIGURE 132-6. Gastrostomy kit from Kimberley Clark (Draper, Utah) contains a serial telescoping dilator with integrated peel-away sheath, eliminating need for multiple dilators and separate peel-away sheath.

recently we have switched to using T-fasteners with an absorbable suture (Saf-T-Pexy T-fasteners, Kimberley Clark, Draper, Utah) (Fig. 132-3, *B*) that do not require postprocedure removal. Their insertion technique is described in Figure 132-4, *A* and *B*.

Following gastropexy, the center of the square is anesthetized, an incision is made using a #11 blade, and the subcutaneous tissue dissected. An 18-gauge needle is inserted through the incision and into the stomach (Fig. 132-5). Usually the puncture needle is directed vertically

downward or slightly toward the fundus, but if conversion to a gastrojejunostomy procedure is anticipated, the needle should be directed toward the pylorus.[12] Again, aspiration of air confirms an intragastric position, and a 0.035-inch Amplatz Super Stiff guidewire (Boston Scientific) is introduced through the needle and coiled within the gastric lumen. The percutaneous tract is then dilated to a size 2F larger than the selected catheter, and each dilatation is monitored fluoroscopically. Previously we used a series of fascial dilators for tract dilatation. More recently we have switched to using a gastrostomy kit from Kimberley Clark that contains a serial telescoping dilator with an integrated peel-away sheath (Fig. 132-6). This eliminates the need for multiple dilators and a separate peel-away sheath and is available in a variety of sizes dependent on the French size of the gastrostomy tube. Alternatively, an angioplasty balloon can be used to dilate the tract.[4,26]

Finally, a 14F to 18F gastrostomy catheter is placed into the stomach, either through a peel-away sheath if a soft balloon retention catheter is used, or directly over the guidewire if a pigtail retention-type catheter is used. Depending on tube type, normal saline is then instilled into the balloon, or the pigtail formed. At the end of the procedure, contrast material is injected through the gastrostomy to confirm an intraluminal position.

For gastrostomy catheter exchange in mature tracts, the old tube can be removed over a wire and a new tube placed. In immature tracts where the gastrostomy tube is no longer in place, a small hockey stick catheter can be used to probe the tract and gain access to the stomach under fluoroscopic guidance.

Postprocedural and Follow-up Care

The patient remains fasting for 12 hours after the procedure, and the gastrostomy tube is not used. Following review by the interventional radiology team the next morning, a decision is made as to whether enteral feeding can commence. The tube should be flushed after each use to prevent occlusion. Should an occlusion occur, gentle flushing with saline or a carbonated beverage usually unblocks the tube. If these measures fail, a guidewire placed through the tube can facilitate clearance. If unsuccessful, the tube may have to be replaced.

As noted earlier, if the T-fasteners used do not have an absorbable suture, they are removed 48 hours after tube placement. This is performed at the bedside by gently lifting each T-fastener away from the abdominal wall and cutting the suture, allowing the metal T-bar to fall into the gastric lumen. Traditionally, the recommended time for removal of T-fasteners was 7 to 12 days, but we advocate early removal of T-fasteners. In a study conducted in our unit, early removal of T-fasteners resulted in reduced postprocedural pain and superficial skin infection.[27]

Once the patient is discharged, regular review by trained personnel (e.g., public health nurse or dietician) should be performed. Skin excoriation due to peritubal leakage of gastric juices can be problematic to deal with, and neutralization of acid with standard antacids may be beneficial, along with local skin cleansing. Local superficial infections can be treated with topical antibiotic ointments, but systemic antibiotics are required should signs such as fever or raised white cell count develop.[11] Potential complications of gastrostomy placement are discussed later in the chapter. Any complications relating to the gastrostomy placement should be referred to the interventional radiologist who performed the procedure.

Gastrostomy Tube Types

Please visit www.expertconsult.com for a discussion of the full range of gastrostomy catheters available.

Controversies

Some controversy has surrounded gastropexy since the origins of PRG. From the literature, most interventionalists would advocate gastropexy for tubes that are pushed through the abdominal wall.[28,29] Gastropexy results in close apposition of the stomach and anterior abdominal wall, preventing the stomach being pushed away during tract dilatation[33] and theoretically allowing placement of larger-bore catheters.[34] In a prospective randomized trial performed by Thornton et al., gastropexy was shown to reduce the risk of intraperitoneal tube placement.[33] Other cited advantages of gastropexy include rapid maturation of the gastrocutaneous tract, reduced intraperitoneal leakage of gastric contents with peritonitis, and tract access in case of inadvertent early tube removal.[9,21,34] There is also the theoretical benefit of reducing the risk of hemorrhage owing to the tamponade effect,[21] although the possibility that hemorrhagic risk may be increased due to the increased number of punctures has also been suggested.[35] While T-fasteners have themselves been associated with pain and skin excoriation, these are minor complications that resolve on their removal.[7,27] As already noted, the recommended time for removal of T-fasteners was traditionally 7 to 12 days, but we advocate early removal at 48 hours after the procedure, since this results in reduced postprocedural pain and superficial skin infection, without increased complication.[27]

Tract dilatation exerts a large amount of force, and gastropexy is generally performed using multiple (typically four) anchors. Gastropexy with a single anchor has been performed with conflicting results.[36-38] Shin et al. reported a single-anchor technique to be feasible, safe, and effective, with low complication rates,[36] but other authors have shown increased complication rates, including peritonitis and bleeding, when only one T-fastener was used.[37,38]

Both PEG and PRG are widely used as a minimally invasive means of placing gastrostomy tubes. Debate remains over which is the better procedure. PEG has been shown to have lower success rates than PRG, largely due to failure of transillumination in obese patients or those with a high-lying stomach.[3,7] Silas et al. showed PRG was associated with more early complications than PEG, but there was no difference in late complications.[5] A meta-analysis performed by Wollman et al. showed PRG had significantly fewer major complications than PEG,[3] whereas other groups have reported comparable complication rates for the two procedures.[39] There is evidence to suggest that PRG is safer in certain patient subgroups. These include patients with amyotrophic lateral sclerosis, since it can be performed with minimal sedation and avoidance of the endoscopic route, thereby decreasing the risk of aspiration.[7,8] PEG may not be possible in some patient groups, such as those with

obstructing head and neck or esophageal malignancy.[9,20] Furthermore, stomal metastases are a rare but possible complication of upper GI tract passage.[40] The incidence of tube replacement is greater with PRG than PEG, owing to the difference in retaining mechanisms,[7] already discussed.

Complications

Major complications related to PRG can be broadly defined as those resulting in an unplanned increase in level of care, prolonged hospitalization, permanent adverse sequelae, or death,[4,23,28] and include deep stomal infection, peritonitis, septicemia, aspiration, GI perforation, and hemorrhage requiring transfusion. From the literature, recorded rates of major complications vary from 0% to 8%,[4,24,25,28,41] whereas a meta-analysis performed by Wollman et al. reported a major complication rate of 5.9%.

Minor complications are those resulting in no sequelae and requiring only nominal therapy or observation.[4,23,28] Peristomal leakage, tube dislodgment without peritonitis, and superficial wound infection are all minor complications associated with gastrostomy placement. From the literature, other minor complications include postprocedural pain, minor abdominal wall hematoma, ileus, decreased consciousness requiring reversal of sedation, and hypotension.[5,23,25] Pneumoperitoneum, once uncomplicated, is considered to be a normal finding after gastrostomy.[25,42,43] Reported minor complication rates vary widely from 3.2%[21] to 36%,[6] although many authors quote rates of 14% to 24%.[5,23,24,27,37] A meta-analysis performed by Wollman et al. quotes a minor complication rate of 7.8%. Some authors have included tube-related complications such as blockage and balloon rupture as minor complications,[5,9] which may in part account for the wide variation. Ideally, such issues should be reported separately, since they are related to tube failure and do not directly reflect the efficacy of the procedure.[3,11] Tube-related complications vary with the type of tube placed, as already discussed. For example, Funaki et al. reported a tube complication rate of 68% for balloon-retained gastrostomies, compared with a rate of 3.6% for mushroom-retained tubes.[28] Mushroom-retained tubes do, however, have their own complication in the form of "buried bumper syndrome," where excessive traction, either from a too tight tube or manipulation, can cause the internal bumper to migrate into the abdominal wall and become overgrown by gastric mucosa.[43] This can be managed by tube manipulation without the need for tube replacement,[23] but occasionally endoscopic assistance or surgical removal may be required.[43]

Outcomes

Many studies have shown the safety and efficacy of PRG, and most series report a high technical success rate of between 98% and 100%.[7,9,21,36,37] Equally high success rates have been reported for de novo insertion of both balloon- and mushroom-retained gastrostomy buttons,[4,23,24] as well as hybrid PEG/PRG tubes.[28,29,41]

Reported 30-day mortality rates vary widely, with rates ranging from 3.1% to 19%.* This likely reflects the wide

*References 5, 21, 23, 36, 37, 41.

variety of indications for PRG, which is often performed in an ill patient population.

GASTROJEJUNOSTOMY

Gastrojejunostomy can be performed as an initial feeding tube placement (primary PRGJ) or as a conversion procedure from an existing gastrostomy (conversion PRGJ). Primary gastrojejunal tube placement remains controversial. It is postulated that catheter placement distal to the ligament of Treitz reduces the incidence of aspiration pneumonia,[11] and some advocate primary PRGJ placement in patients with a history of gastroesophageal reflux or aspiration.[34,44] In one series, primary PRGJ was predominantly performed in cases of recurrent aspiration pneumonia or to prevent gastroesophageal reflux in cases of a disrupted upper GI tract (e.g., esophageal or gastric perforation).[44] PRGJ, however, offers no protection against aspiration of oropharyngeal secretions, a problem common to a significant number of patients requiring gastrostomy.[11] Some authors favor routine PRGJ placement[13,34] and believe the absence of clinically significant aspiration in their series to be due to this routine placement,[13] but continued gastroesophageal reflux has been demonstrated in predisposed patients despite gastrojejunal catheter placement.[45,46]

Conversion PRGJ can be considered where patients with prior gastrostomy show signs of gastroesophageal reflux or aspiration[44] or where there are large gastric residuals.[12] Conversion PRGJ has also been performed to bypass a duodenal obstruction and to alleviate the gastrostomy-related complication of food oozing at the skin insertion site.[44]

Gastrojejunostomy catheters are longer and tend to be of narrower caliber than those placed for gastrostomy. As a result, they may be more prone to occlusion, and early catheter blockage has been reported.[13] In our experience, PRGJ procedures can require longer table times than gastrostomy, particularly if difficulty is experienced cannulating the pylorus. This may have resource implications when access to the interventional suite is limited.

The technique of primary gastrojejunostomy placement is similar to that described for percutaneous gastrostomy, however, the stomach puncture is directed toward the pylorus to facilitate cannulation. The pylorus is cannulated using a 5F torquable catheter and a 0.035-inch hydrophilic guidewire (Terumo Medical Corp.). The 5F catheter is advanced to the proximal jejunum, and the hydrophilic guidewire exchanged for a 0.035-inch Amplatz Super Stiff guidewire (Boston Scientific). After tract dilation, a gastrojejunal catheter is placed (Fig. 132-7). Our catheter of choice is a low-profile skin-level gastrojejunostomy catheter (MICKEY G).

Conversion procedures from gastrostomy to gastrojejunostomy may be technically challenging, since the initial angle of entry for the gastrostomy tube is directed to the fundus of the stomach, rendering intubation of the pylorus difficult. When pyloric catheterization is difficult to achieve, there have been reports of using fascial dilators to stabilize the guidewire and aid cannulation[13,44]; rigid sheaths can also be used to facilitate redirection of the tract.

Success rates for primary PRGJ placement are high,[13,34,44] with some authors reporting up to 100% successful placement.[44] Success rates for conversion PRGJ are also high, particularly in a mature tract.[13] Bell et al. reported 9 out of

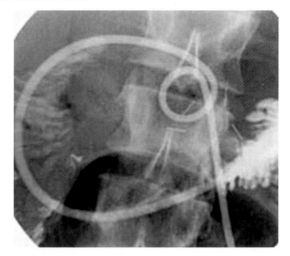

FIGURE 132-7. Gastrojejunal catheter with pigtail retention device has been inserted; contrast instilled to confirm position.

12 procedures to be successful,[13] whereas Shin et al. have reported a 100% success rate.[44]

Direct Percutaneous Jejunostomy

Radiologically guided direct percutaneous jejunostomy (PRJ) may be considered when prolonged enteral feeding is required in patients whose stomach is inaccessible for gastrostomy placement, or who have undergone previous gastrectomy. Less common indications include small bowel decompression for obstruction and biliary tree recanalization after biliary-enteric anastomosis.[47-50] Particular care must be taken to avoid any overlying loops of colon, and large-bowel decompression may be required before the procedure.

The technique for PRJ is as follows. As with gastrostomy, the patient fasts from the evening prior to the procedure, and informed consent is obtained. Intravenous midazolam and fentanyl citrate can be used in combination for sedation and analgesia as already described. A 5F vascular catheter in combination with a 0.035-inch hydrophilic guidewire is introduced through the nose, directed through the esophagus and stomach, and into the jejunum under fluoroscopic guidance. Dilation of jejunal loops is achieved by slow instillation of warm saline solution. Puncture of the distended jejunum is then performed under ultrasound guidance. Van Overhagen et al. describe the use of a 17-gauge needle preloaded with a Cope suture anchor (Cook Medical) to puncture the jejunum.[48] The Cope anchor is displaced from the needle tip using a 0.035-inch Amplatz Super Stiff guidewire. The guidewire is then positioned in the lumen of the jejunum, and the tract dilated. During tract dilation, traction is maintained on the suture to stabilize the jejunum. A 10F hydrophilic pigtail catheter (Cook Medical) is then introduced over the guidewire, and its position confirmed by injection of contrast medium. The catheter is secured to the skin surface and allowed to drain for 24 hours after insertion. A trial infusion of saline is performed initially. If no pain is experienced by the patient, feeding is begun. The Cope anchor suture is then cut on day 10.

Technical success rates for PRJ range between 85% and 95%.[47,48,50,51] Reasons for failure include difficulty in puncturing the jejunum or displacement of the jejunum during anchor or catheter insertion. The most serious complication is intraperitoneal leak. The cumulative procedure mortality rate from three published trials is 2.4%.[47-50]

catheters. Interventional radiologists can therefore offer a wide range of service to referring physicians.

- Disadvantages of percutaneous radiologic gastrostomy include the cosmetic appearance of the gastrostomy tube, the potential for tube occlusion, and inadvertent tube displacement or removal.

KEY POINTS

- The interventional radiologist plays a central role in the provision of enteral nutrition through placement of gastrostomy/gastrojejunostomy tubes.

- The perceived advantages of image-guided placement of enteral feeding tubes include high rates of successful insertion and low morbidity and mortality rates.

- Percutaneous radiologically guided catheters may be placed in patients where gastrostomy insertion by other routes is technically difficult or impossible, such as patients with malignancy of the head and neck or esophagus.

- Technical advances in radiologic gastrostomy include peroral placement of percutaneous endoscopic gastrostomy (PEG) tubes and primary placement of gastrostomy button

▶ SUGGESTED READINGS

Given MF, Hanson JJ, Lee MJ. Interventional radiology techniques for provision of enteral feeding. Cardiovasc Intervent Radiol 2005;28: 692–703.

Laasch HU, Martin DF. Radiologic gastrostomy. Endoscopy 2007;39: 247–55.

Shin JH, Park AW. Updates on percutaneous radiologic gastrostomy/gastrojejunostomy and jejunostomy. Gut and Liver 2010;4(Suppl 1): S25–31.

The complete reference list is available online at www.expertconsult.com.

CHAPTER 133

Pediatric Gastrostomy and Gastrojejunostomy

Bairbre Connolly

INTRODUCTION

Nutrition is vitally important for children's growth and development. Ensuring adequate nutrition in the at-risk child (because of disease or disability) is a challenge. If oral feeding is not possible, adequate, or safe, alternative methods are required. Nasogastric (NG) or nasojejunal (NJ) tubes are suitable for temporary feeding requirements (<3 months). Longer-term requirements can be achieved through tubes placed surgically (open, laparoscopic), endoscopically (percutaneous endoscopic gastrostomy [PEG]) or radiologically (antegrade, retrograde).[1-5] There are a wide variety of tube types, each with inherent advantages, disadvantages, complications, and required maintenance procedures.[1,2,3,6,7] This chapter describes an approach to enterostomy access in children, focusing on those aspects most pertinent to the pediatric age group and emphasizing how they differ from adults.

INDICATIONS

Children referred for gastrostomy (G) or gastrojejunostomy (GJ) frequently require lifelong feeding support. Growth, development, and maturation are important factors to take into consideration when deciding to place a G/GJ tube in a child.[8,9] The underlying diagnoses most commonly encountered include (1) neurologic impairment such as congenital, developmental, or acquired brain abnormalities (e.g., cerebral palsy), (2) gastrointestinal problems (e.g., severe gastroesophageal reflux, absorptive problems), (3) generalized problems (e.g., genetic/chromosomal abnormalities or "syndromes"), and (4) organ-specific conditions (e.g., severe complex cardiac diseases, end-stage renal failure, cystic fibrosis, high metabolic states, catabolic states such as oncologic diseases with severe mucositis/esophagitis, etc.).[8,10-14] Achieving specific weight or growth milestones is a prerequisite to undergoing certain surgeries or transplant; enteral nutrition is a means to promote this growth. Within any of these diagnostic categories, individual patients may have more than one clinical indication for their G/GJ, such as failure to thrive, recurrent aspiration, inadequate caloric intake, gastroesophageal reflux disease, swallowing dysfunction, special dietary requirements, or medications (e.g., human immunodeficiency virus [HIV]-infected patients receiving highly active antiretroviral therapy [HAART]).[15,16]

A child with any of the above indications/diagnoses and associated severe gastroesophageal reflux disease is unlikely to tolerate G feeds. A surgical antireflux procedure combined with gastrostomy is one approach.[17,18] In the medically fragile child with significant comorbidities, a GJ tube may be a more suitable option. Referral preferences depend on institutional practices, local expertise, and the like. There is a major difference for families between maintaining a child on G feeds (bolus feeds, shorter feeding hours) compared to GJ feeds (more continuous feeds, longer hours), so it is often worthwhile to try G feeds initially, despite reflux. Removal of the NG tube alone may alleviate reflux and facilitate tolerance of G feeds. If, however, gastroesophageal reflux remains problematic, the radiologic G tube can be readily converted to a GJ tube.[19,20] A GJ tube does not provide protection against aspiration of oropharyngeal secretions from above or gastric secretions from below. GJ tubes are also indicated in children with duodenal or gastric outlet issues (e.g., superior mesenteric artery syndrome, duodenal trauma, etc.).

CONTRAINDICATIONS

There are few absolute contraindications to placing a G or GJ tube. They include uncorrectable severe coagulopathy, unfavorable abnormal anatomy where there is no safe percutaneous route to the stomach (such as may occur in severe scoliosis) post congenital diaphragmatic hernia repair or anterior abdominal wall defect surgery (e.g., omphalocele).[21] Intestinal obstruction is a contraindication unless placed for decompression (e.g., severe motility disorders).

Relative contraindications include coagulopathy requiring correction, clinical instability, or critical comorbidities. Ascites may require interim drainage until the G-tube tract is healed. Neonates with esophageal atresia without a tracheoesophageal fistula (i.e., a gasless abdomen) can undergo a radiologic G tube, but it requires sonographically guided needle puncture of the stomach to inflate the stomach with air, since an NG tube cannot be passed from above.[22] Dilated gas-filled colon anterior to the stomach can be deflated by aspirating the luminal gas using a 27G needle, T-piece and Luer-Lok syringe.[5,23] Placing a G tube in the presence of a ventriculoperitoneal (VP) shunt may be associated with a risk of ascending ventriculitis.[24-26] Temporally distancing the G tube insertion as much as possible from the VP shunt insertion (>1 month), and physically separating it from the shunt tubing in the abdominal wall and the peritoneum may help to reduce this chance of infection.[24-27]

ASSESSMENT

In children, there are significant psychosocial factors that have to be addressed a priori because they have major impact on parents/caregivers in their relationship with the child and acceptance of a feeding tube.[9,28,29] The importance of these factors should not be underestimated, and parental expectations must be realistic and informed.[7,28,30] Assessment requires a comprehensive multidisciplinary approach to ensure that a G/GJ tube is medically indicated and that the parents support the decision, are in agreement to proceed, and are thoroughly educated regarding what caring for a child with a G tube entails (i.e., site care and tube maintenance).[7,28,30] This involves discussions among the patient's family, referring physician, an expert in gastrostomies (specialist pediatrician or nurse practitioner), a dietitian, an occupational therapist, and interventional radiology (IR).

TECHNIQUE

General Aspects of Pediatric Interventional Radiology Procedures

There are important differences between interventional procedures in children and adults.[31] Dosages of drugs and intravenous (IV) fluids must be calculated tightly on a per kilogram basis. Temperature preservation and monitoring is crucial in the small child who is prone to hypothermia; body warmers such as Bair Huggers (Arizant Healthcare Inc., Eden Prairie, Minn.), plastic coverings, chemical blankets, and hats are required.[31,32] The IR suite must be equipped with different sizes of pediatric devices (e.g., BP cuffs, endotracheal tubes, pediatric resuscitation cart, etc.). Sedation should be performed either by anesthesiologists or persons trained in pediatric sedation and airway rescue (Pediatric Advanced Life Support [PALS] certification). Radiation protection is especially important in children. Dose-reduction strategies include low pulse rate fluoroscopy (e.g., 4 or 7 pulses/s), limited use of magnification and alternate use of postprocessing zoom, removal of the grid (vendor specific in children < 20 kg), last image hold techniques, and so forth.[33-35] Protection of the operator is also important, given patients' small size, the operator's proximity to the beam, and potential hand exposure.[36]

Preprocedure

The process of obtaining informed consent from parents/substitute decision maker is time consuming. Ideally it is obtained after family education and prior to the day of the procedure, rather on entry to the IR suites. Procedural risks include bleeding, injury to bowel or abdominal viscera, and inability to reach the stomach (≈1%). Postprocedural risks include infection/peritonitis (≈2%-3%), tube dislodgement, retention anchor suture (RAS) problems, any specific problems secondary to their comorbidities or underlying diagnosis, and common site and maintenance issues.[7,37,38] Procedural mortality is rare.

For fasting, a commonly used rule of thumb in children is the "2-4-6-8 rule" (2 hours for clear fluids, 4 hours for breast milk, 6 hours for formula, and 8 hours for solids). Avoidance of prolonged fasting and hydration with IV or oral (PO) clear fluids containing dextrose is important to avoid hypoglycemia. Adult guidelines suggest checking full blood cell count and coagulation prior to gastrostomy, but this is not routine in pediatric practices.[39]

Procedure Techniques

The technique described here is the percutaneous retrograde method we currently practice. A preprocedural time out (±the aid of checklist) is conducted, including need for and dose of antibiotics, glucagon, and dextrose-containing IV fluids; date of last menstrual period (where applicable);

radiation protection strategies; any additional procedures to be performed; and any patient-specific precautions (e.g., metabolic issues, allergies, medications, skin issues, etc.).[40,41]

Most frequently, G and GJ tubes are placed under IV sedation or anesthesia, although placement is possible using local anesthetic only. The inferior margin of the liver, spleen, and left costal margin are identified with ultrasound and marked on the skin with a safe skin marker. The lateral edge of the rectus muscle and the position of the superior epigastric artery may also be outlined. Dilute barium may be infused rectally to outline the transverse colon. The abdomen is then prepped and draped in the usual fashion. Prophylactic antibiotics are given (30 mg/kg IV cephazolin). Glucagon IV (0.2-0.5 mg) may be given to achieve gastric atony and pyloric constriction.[42,43] An NG tube is inserted and secured.

Gastrostomy

A combination of ultrasound and fluoroscopy is used. Air is introduced into the stomach through the NG tube. Once tense, a site is chosen, ideally lateral to the rectus muscle and 2 cm or more from the lower costal margin to allow for growth. Alternatively, the puncture can be in the midline or perhaps (least favored by the author) through the rectus muscle and sheath. Local anesthetic (Xylocaine 1%, 0.5 mL/kg; or bupivacaine 0.25%, 1 mL/kg) is infiltrated down to the peritoneum. A small skin incision is made. The stomach is punctured using an 18G needle preloaded with a single pediatric RAS (Cook Medical, Bloomington, Ind.), using a short, sharp, fairly vertical stab, and confirmed with contrast. The RAS is deployed into the stomach with a 0.035-inch straight short guidewire. It is our practice currently to use only one RAS; others may choose to use any number from none to four. The needle is removed over the wire, and slight tension is maintained on the end of the thread with a small forceps for gastropexy. The tract is dilated over the wire using the appropriate-sized dilator and holding additional tension on the RAS thread. The dilator is then exchanged for a pigtail catheter. The position is confirmed with contrast injection (±additional air in stomach via NG) in posteroanterior, lateral, and various oblique projections to document that it is intragastric (gastric rugae outlined with contrast, rotation of the pigtail freely in the gastric lumen, movement of the NG) and clear of other bowel loops (steep craniocaudal x-ray projection showing tube separate from colon). The thread of the RAS is wound around a small roll of gauze until it is gently taut and secured. The NG tube and G tube are secured and put to gravity drainage. Colonic barium is drained via the rectal tube, which is then removed.

Gastrojejunostomy

When placing a GJ tube, some interventionalists may omit the use of barium and glucagon. However, both can be used without interfering with the safe and successful insertion of a GJ tube. The initial steps are as outlined for gastrostomy. The RAS is deployed with a long 0.035-inch floppy-tipped wire (e.g., Bentson [Cook Medical]) and the needle removed. Using a directional catheter (e.g., 5F JB1 [Cook Medical]) advanced directly over the wire, it is directed to the pylorus and negotiated through the duodenum and into the upper jejunum. The catheter is then removed, the tract dilated to the required size, and the GJ then placed over the wire. The retention mechanism is secured, the GJ position confirmed with contrast, the NG put to straight drainage, and the GJ tube is capped off.

Antegrade Gastrostomy Tube Placement

This "push-pull" method is favored by some centers; insertion is more complicated but has the advantage of greater tube security and less risk of dislodgement.[44,45] Access to the stomach is obtained through the mouth with a wire and snare. The esophagus must be patent. The stomach is punctured from outside, aiming for the open snare in the stomach. The wire is snared and exteriorized through the mouth. The G tube is pulled down through the esophagus using a loop mechanism that draws the tube and its bumper into the stomach and out the abdominal wall antegradely. The external bumper is then advanced snug to the abdominal wall. The tube is trimmed to length.[44-46]

Jejunostomy

Experience with radiologically placed direct primary percutaneous jejunostomy tubes is limited worldwide and is not discussed here.[47,48] Surgically placed jejunostomies, on the other hand, are more common in pediatrics. The ongoing maintenance of jejunostomy tubes is usually performed by IR.

Choice of Tubes

Gastrostomy

The initial G tube is usually an 8F, 10F, or 12F pigtail catheter. Choice of product and size is operator/institution dependent. In our practice, an 8F pigtail is generally suitable for a neonate or small infant, a 10F pigtail for a child over 10 kg, and 12F for children over 30 kg. Other institutions will place a larger tube (e.g., 16F) even in small children. New devices with a series of graduated dilators are available for primary placement of low-profile balloon button tubes, rather than a pigtail.

Gastrojejunostomy

There are many varieties of tubes available in different lengths, French sizes, retention mechanisms (loop, balloon, Malecot), straight and pigtail, weighted and nonweighted, and single or dual lumens (feeding J, venting G). There is no one ideal GJ tube for children; each has advantages and disadvantages. Gastric loops can leak feedings at the point of the thread in the retaining gastric coil; Malecot/mushrooms easily become dislodged because of the small size of their gastric retention mechanism; balloons perish with time and gastric acidity; pigtail distal ends are associated with intussusceptions; small jejunal components occlude easily.[30,38,49,50] For children requiring feeding and venting, as an alternative to a dual-lumen tube we frequently place a second tube through an entirely separate puncture—one for the venting G and one for the GJ.

POSTPROCEDURE CARE

Post procedure, the patient is kept fasting for 12 hours. Isotonic IV fluids containing glucose are given. We check blood sugar if glucagon has been used because of the risk of rebound hypoglycemia. Morphine 0.05 mg/kg IV may be

required on day 1; subsequently, acetaminophen (15 mg/kg PO or rectally) is usually adequate. After 12 hours, if active bowel sounds are heard, clear fluids are commenced via the G tube, advancing gradually over the next 48 hours to full feeds. The NG tube is then removed. Because barium is constipating, a stool softener may be required on day 2 or 3. Patients are usually discharged by day 3. At day 14, the RAS thread is cut, and the metallic portion passes per rectum. The tract is considered mature by 6 weeks.

TECHNICAL ASPECTS SPECIFIC TO CHILDREN

Technical aspects related to the pediatric procedure itself include:

- *Choice of site.* Options are limited on the abdominal wall in a young child. Avoid proximity to the ribs.
- *Access.* Frequently the stomach is covered by the inferior margin of the left lobe of the liver. However, after gastric inflation, reevaluation of the liver with ultrasound frequently shows the liver has been pushed up and out of the way, creating a safe access route for tube placement.
- *Pylorus.* Be aware of placing the G tube where it abuts the pylorus because it may cause gagging and intolerance of feeds.
- *Depth.* Use of a short needle for puncture (e.g., 4 cm) will avoid inadvertently puncturing the posterior wall of the stomach with a longer needle (e.g., 7 cm).
- *Loss of access.* In a small patient, when steering to the pylorus for a GJ, it is important not to withdraw the directional catheter so close to the puncture site that one looses access altogether.
- *Compromise.* If placement if a GJ proves very difficult, in the interest of patient safety, a G tube can be placed instead and later converted to a GJ.
- *Nasojejunal tubes.* If a patient with complex anatomy has an NJ tube in place, leaving it in situ may be helpful as a guide to the pylorus.
- *Fragility.* The younger the child, the more fragile the tissues; dilatation and traversing the duodenum must be done gently to avoid tearing of tissues or the duodenum.
- *Ultrasound.* In children use of real-time ultrasound is invaluable for safe needle guidance between viscera.

Technical aspects related to the child's normal growth and development include:

- *Costal margin.* With growth, the child's thoracic cage elongates, and the ribs may encroach on the G tube site, causing severe irritation, pain, and distortion of the ribs. Ideally one should leave more than a finger's breadth (≈2cm) between the ribs and the puncture site to allow for this growth. Occasionally a child's G tube may have to be re-sited because of this issue.
- *Upsizing.* As the child grows, the tube is upsized to accommodate their nutritional needs.
- *Reassessment.* Nutritional needs, feeding ability, and reflux change with growth (see later).

COMPLICATIONS

Complication rates for G and GJ tubes vary widely in the literature, since definitions and descriptions are not standardized. Where pediatric data are unavailable, we rely on adult data.[1] Major complications are on the order of 5%.[2] Minor complication rates depend on definitions used and methods of tracking, with rates as high as 73% reported.[5,7,38]

Procedural

Procedural complications are not limited to technical problems but also include sedation or anesthesia issues, temperature control, and others:

- *Organ puncture.* Using real-time ultrasound in conjunction with fluoroscopy has helped prevent inadvertent puncture of other viscera (small or large bowel, liver).
- *RAS.* The RAS thread will snap with excessive tension. If this occurs, one may leave the G tube without any RAS, or alternatively puncture again alongside the pigtail and place a new RAS. The RAS can be deployed incorrectly (e.g., posteriorly [in lesser sac or posterior gastric wall] or anteriorly [in the tube tract, peritoneum]).
- *Peritoneal placement.* After successful puncture of the stomach, the dilator can fail to advance through the gastric wall but invaginate the anterior gastric wall, resulting in the pigtail forming in the peritoneum. Careful fluoroscopy during dilatation or a stiffer wire may help avoid this. Re-puncture is usually required.
- *Pneumoperitoneum.* A small pneumoperitoneum occurs frequently and will absorb. If large, it is our practice to aspirate the air to reduce the air gap (midline puncture using a 27G needle, a 20-mL Luer-Lok syringe on an extension piece, lateral fluoroscopy).
- *Bleeding.* Uncommon. In patients with portal hypertension who require endoscopy (e.g., in cystic fibrosis), it has been helpful to coordinate the scope and the G tube together, keeping the scope in situ while we puncture the stomach, and assisting in directing the puncture away from varices.
- *Temperature.* Hypothermia is a risk, especially in the neonate/young infant. Bair Huggers, plastic covers, hats, and so forth are important measures to avoid this complication.
- *Mortality.* Procedural mortality is rare unless from comorbidities.
- *Anesthesia/sedation.* These children are medically fragile and at high risk for aspiration and airway problems.

Postprocedural

Early

- *Blood sugar.* Hyperglycemia follows stressful interventions.[51] When glucagon is used, this peak is accentuated and may be followed by a rebound hypoglycemia that can be precipitous, causing irritability, seizures, and even cardiac arrest. Use of dextrose-containing IV fluids and monitoring the child's blood sugar post glucagon will avoid this.
- *Pain.* Unusual focal site pain may be due to irritation from the RAS, necessitating early cutting of the thread to enable the T-piece to pass.
- *Peritonitis.* Signs of peritonitis (pain, fever, vomiting) occur in 2% to 3% of patients secondary to a small leak of gastric contents into the peritoneum. A G-tube contrast check is frequently negative for peritoneal spill. Conservative treatment with antibiotics, G and NG to drainage, and

withholding feeds is indicated. Symptoms usually resolve after 48 hours. If a large pneumoperitoneum has developed, aspiration of the air is indicated. Peritoneal fluid collections rarely require drainage.
- *Dislodgement.* Tube dislodgement is not uncommon.[7,38] If dislodgement occurs before the RAS is cut, one can regain access by unwinding the thread of the RAS, passing a dilator or angiocatheter over the thread, and advancing a wire through the angiocatheter to regain gastric access.

Late

- *RAS.* Persistence of the metallic RAS at the G-tube site may be a source of pain, site infections, or extrusion out through the tract, and require manual removal with a forceps. The metal may cause image artifact/degradation on magnetic resonance imaging (MRI), and potentially movement of the RAS in the magnet can occur. Review of available imaging before an MRI may confirm the RAS has passed.
- *Intussusception.* This occurs around the jejunal limb of a GJ tube, either at the tip of the tube or along its length, especially in the younger child with non-silicone pigtail tubes.[38,49,50] It can be reduced by exchanging the tube over a wire, thereby releasing the mucosa from the tube tip, and the centrifugal force of the wire undoing the intussusception. Replacement with a shorter tube without a distal pigtail usually suffices. Confirmation of reduction by ultrasound is important. Ischemia of the intussusception is rare.[52]
- *Site issues.* These are common and include granulation tissue, purulent discharge, and recurrent infection, even up to 30%.[1,5,30,38] Keeping the site clean and dry is important, using saline soaks and air drying. Granulation tissue (treated with topical silver nitrate) must be distinguished from everted gastric mucosa (may require surgical removal/closure).[4] Gaping of the stoma may occur, resulting in gastric fluid leakage and skin excoriation. Tube upsizing usually results in further enlargement of the stoma. Removing the tube entirely for a few days allows the stoma to shrink down quickly, and a new tube can be reinserted.
- *Reflux.* New or worsening reflux can occur post surgical or radiologic G-tube insertion.

OUTCOMES AND FOLLOW-UP

The discussion of outcomes, follow-up, tube maintenance, and new developments in methods and materials is available at www.expertconsult.com.

KEY POINTS

- The majority of children requiring tube feeding are neurologically impaired.
- For many, tube feeding is a lifelong requirement.
- Pediatric-appropriate equipment is required to undertake the intervention safely.
- Placement requires awareness of the size and depth of the child.
- Fragile tissues in the young child require gentle handling.

- Hypothermia and hypoglycemia occur, especially in the young child.
- Repeat reevaluation is necessary to assess a child's ongoing need for tube feeding.
- Tube and site maintenance issues are common.

▶ SUGGESTED READINGS

Friedman JN. Enterostomy tube feeding: The ins and outs. Paediatr Child Health Dec 2004;9(10):695–9.

Itkin M, DeLegge MH, Fang JC, et al. Multidisciplinary practical guidelines for gastrointestinal access for enteral nutrition and decompression from the Society of Interventional Radiology and American Gastroenterological Association (AGA) Institute, with endorsement by Canadian Interventional Radiological Association (CIRA) and Cardiovascular and Interventional Radiological Society of Europe (CIRSE). J Vasc Interv Radiol 2011;22(8):1089–106.

Wollman B, D'Agostino HB, Walus-Wigle JR, et al. Radiologic, endoscopic, and surgical gastrostomy: an institutional evaluation and meta-analysis of the literature. Radiology 1995;197(3):699–704.

The complete reference list is available online at www.expertconsult.com.

CHAPTER **134**

Management of Malignant Biliary Tract Obstruction

Raymond H. Thornton and Anne M. Covey

Malignant bile duct obstruction (MBDO) occurs when tumor within or adjacent to bile ducts impedes the normal passage of bile from the liver to the intestinal tract. Tumors of pancreobiliary origin, such as cholangiocarcinoma and gallbladder and pancreas cancer, are the most common causes of MBDO. Other etiologies include lymphoma and metastases from any primary neoplasm. Many benign conditions may also cause biliary obstruction. Differentiation of benign and malignant causes of bile duct obstruction is essential because treatments are different.

Obstruction of the biliary tree blocks the normal pathway for bile excretion, resulting in cholestasis (Greek *chole*, "bile," + *stasis*, "standing still"). This leads to measurable biochemical derangements including elevation in serum bilirubin (conjugated hyperbilirubinemia), γ-glutamyl transpeptidase, and alkaline phosphatase. Physical signs and symptoms are often present, and many are explained by the absence of bile in the intestinal tract or the appearance of bilirubin and bile salts in the serum. The presence of one or more of these signs and symptoms of obstructive jaundice usually prompts referral for biliary drainage.

Jaundice, a yellowish discoloration of tissues caused by the deposition of bilirubin, may be first detected as scleral icterus when the total serum bilirubin level exceeds 2 to 3 mg/dL. Darkening of the urine *(bilirubinuria)* occurs with renal excretion of conjugated bilirubin. Light-colored, *acholic stool* is observed because of the absence of pigmented bilirubin breakdown products in the intestinal tract. *Pruritus*, a well-known but poorly understood symptom of cholestasis, is thought to be mediated by bile salt retention. Patients with jaundice may also experience constitutional symptoms including anorexia, nausea, and fatigue. Infection of obstructed bile ducts, termed *cholangitis*, is a clinical syndrome of broad spectrum ranging from low-grade fever to septic shock. Charcot described the triad of right upper quadrant pain, fever, and jaundice for diagnosis of cholangitis. To these, Reynolds added mental status changes and sepsis, for a total of five clinical findings suggestive of the diagnosis. Although cholangitis is relatively uncommon in MBDO when there has been no prior intervention to contaminate the biliary tree, it remains an important diagnostic consideration whenever a patient with biliary obstruction has fever.

Modern imaging capabilities permit robust noninvasive evaluation of the obstructed biliary tree. Regardless of which imaging modality is employed, certain observations about the pattern of biliary obstruction must be made. Chief among these observations is description of the point (or points) of biliary obstruction in anatomic terms. This can be accomplished by tracing dilated bile ducts as they pass from the periphery of the liver to the liver hilus and subsequently to the intestine, recognizing points of obstruction as sites where there is interruption or narrowing of dilated bile ducts. This is important because it facilitates preprocedural prediction of the cholangiogram so an optimal drainage procedure can be planned. Another key observation is evaluation of the patency of the portal vein and its intrahepatic branches. This is important because portal vein occlusion leads to atrophy of liver parenchyma, and drainage of atrophic liver segments will not result in recovery of liver function.

Sonographic examination is a common starting point in the imaging assessment, although overlying bowel gas can limit evaluation of the extrahepatic bile duct. Computed tomography (CT) and magnetic resonance imaging (MRI), including magnetic resonance cholangiopancreatography (MRCP), offer powerful cross-sectional and multiplanar anatomic methods to evaluate the biliary tree and surrounding structures. With this armamentarium of noninvasive imaging tests, it is now unusual to require diagnostic percutaneous cholangiography (PTC) for evaluation of MBDO.

Endoscopic retrograde cholangiopancreatography (ERCP) and biliary drainage (ERBD) are often preferred over percutaneous approaches in centers where skilled endoscopists offer this service. For patients with low bile duct obstruction (obstruction of the common bile duct or common hepatic duct not involving the biliary confluence), endoscopic techniques permit diagnosis and therapy without the need for percutaneous approaches or exteriorized drainage catheters. High bile duct obstruction (obstruction proximal to or involving the confluence of left and right hepatic ducts) is more often managed percutaneously by interventional radiologists, as are patients for whom ERBD is either not possible or unsuccessful. Interventional radiologic procedures used in the management of MBDO include PTC, percutaneous transhepatic biliary drainage (PTBD) and stent placement, and bile duct biopsy.

INDICATIONS

The indication for biliary intervention typically includes imaging evidence of biliary obstruction plus the need for diagnosis or treatment of one or more of the clinical manifestations associated with MBDO.

981

Percutaneous Transhepatic Cholangiography

- As the initial step in PTBD
- For anatomic depiction of the pattern and extent of biliary obstruction when attempts to obtain this information noninvasively have either failed or been inconclusive

Percutaneous Transhepatic Biliary Drainage

In the presence of MBDO when ERBD cannot be performed, PTBD is indicated:
- For treatment of cholangitis. Hydration and antibiotic therapy are successful initial interventions for 80% to 85% of patients with cholangitis.[1] Those with ongoing sepsis despite these therapies require urgent biliary decompression, and those who do respond to initial medical therapies frequently require subsequent biliary drainage.
- To relieve pruritus. Medical therapies including the bile acid–binding resins cholestyramine and colestipol, antihistamines, naloxone, and rifampin are variably effective treatments for pruritus related to cholestasis. Biliary drainage is an effective treatment[2,3] when results of these medications are suboptimal, even when only one or two segments of the liver can be effectively drained. Following biliary drainage for this indication, symptomatic improvement is often observed within 24 hours.
- To relieve symptoms of jaundice. Symptoms such as nausea and anorexia may improve with delivery of bile salts to the intestine.
- To reduce serum bilirubin to facilitate administration of chemotherapy. Some chemotherapeutic agents require intact mechanisms of bile excretion for safe use, and others require dose modification when the serum bilirubin is elevated. To receive optimal chemotherapy at full dose, some patients may require biliary drainage to lower serum bilirubin.[4]
- Prior to surgery. Preoperative biliary drainage is highly controversial; many studies have shown it increases complication rates.[5-8] One meta-analysis suggested neither positive nor negative outcomes in association with preoperative biliary drainage.[9] Others have suggested improved postoperative results following internal drainage.[10-12]
- In association with other percutaneous biliary procedures such as bile duct biopsy and placement of biliary stents or brachytherapy catheters

Biliary Stent Placement

- For palliation of symptomatic MBDO in patients unable to undergo endoscopic or surgical treatment

CONTRAINDICATIONS

Percutaneous Transhepatic Cholangiography

Relative contraindications include:
- Coagulopathy. Every effort should be made to correct or improve coagulopathy prior to biliary drainage procedures.

- Allergy to iodinated contrast agents. Patients with history of allergy to iodinated contrast material should be appropriately premedicated because contrast material may be introduced into the vascular system or absorbed during biliary drainage. Typical premedication regimens include administration of both an antihistamine and a corticosteroid.
- Ascites. Large ascites may complicate transhepatic biliary access and intervention, and leakage of ascites around biliary catheters may occur. Consider paracentesis in such instances. Left-side biliary access may provide an access window away from ascites.

Percutaneous Transhepatic Biliary Drainage

- All contraindications to PTC
- Segmental or subsegmental high bile duct obstruction depending on the indication for drainage. Drainage of a biliary tree with multiple isolations is unlikely to provide palliation and may introduce further complications. This should generally be avoided.

Biliary Stent Placement

- All contraindications to PTBD
- Sepsis. PTBD with minimal manipulation is indicated for patients with sepsis and bile duct obstruction. If appropriate, stent placement can be considered after sepsis has resolved.
- Potential surgical candidate. Because determination of resectability presupposes knowledge of the diagnosis, metallic stents are not placed when the diagnosis is not known. Historically, biliary drainage catheters rather than biliary stents have been placed for preoperative patients. There is a trend in recent literature to suggest that stents can be safely used in preoperative patients with low bile duct obstruction.[13-16] Because this represents a substantial change in approach, local surgical preferences should be sought and considered.
- Benign disease. Metallic stents are generally not used for treatment of benign causes of biliary obstruction.

EQUIPMENT

Either moderate sedation or anesthesia services can be used for performance of PTC, PTBD, and biliary stent placement. In either case, patient monitoring equipment including pulse oximetry and electrocardiographic monitors are required.

Owing to the length of biliary cases and proximity of the operator to the x-ray beam, modern fluoroscopic equipment capable of recording radiation dose should be used. Ceiling-mounted translucent leaded shields or leaded eyeglasses can be used as protective barriers in addition to leaded gowns.

Example equipment needs include:
- Water-soluble, nonionic radiographic contrast material
- Local anesthetic
- #11 blade or other suitable blade for dermatotomy creation

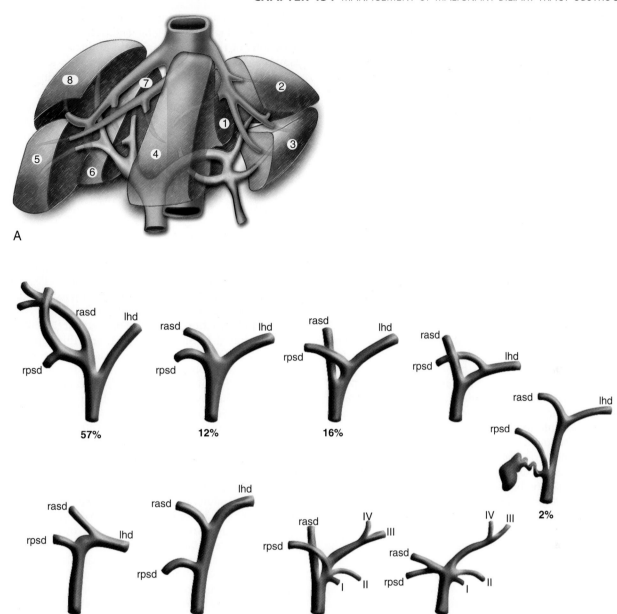

FIGURE 134-1. Couinaud anatomy. **A,** Segmental anatomy of the liver. Portal venous supply to each segment is shown schematically. **B,** Common anatomic variants in confluence of segmental ducts at level of liver hilum. Incidence of each variant is shown. *lhd,* Left hepatic duct; *rasd,* right anterior sectoral duct; *rpsd,* right posterior sectoral duct.

- 21-gauge needle with stylet, capable of accepting a 0.018-inch guidewire
- A coaxial introducer system including an innermost component tapered to accept a 0.018-inch guidewire and an outer 4F or 5F sheath. Examples include the Neff Percutaneous Access Set (Cook Medical, Bloomington, Ind.) and the GrebSet (Vascular Solutions, Minneapolis, Minn.).
- 4F or 5F catheters (e.g., Berenstein, C2)
- Guidewires, including a torquable 0.035-inch hydrophilic wire and a 0.035-inch Amplatz Super Stiff guidewire (Boston Scientific, Natick, Mass.)
- 6- to 10-mm inflatable balloon catheters
- 8F and 10F biliary drainage catheters

TECHNIQUE

Anatomy and Approach

Understanding the segmental anatomy of the liver is essential for interventional radiologists who perform biliary interventions. The Couinaud classification of liver anatomy (Fig. 134-1, *A*) is most useful in this regard. The liver is divided right from left by the plane that includes the middle hepatic vein and gallbladder fossa.

Left Hepatic Lobe
The caudate lobe is segment 1. The lateral segment of the left hepatic lobe comprises segments 2 and 3. Segment 2 is

more superior and posterior, and segment 3 is more anterior and inferior. Therefore, left-sided biliary drainages often use segment 3 for access because it is ordinarily the most superficial and inferior portion of the lateral sector under the skin of the epigastrium. The medial segment of the left hepatic lobe, segment 4, is separated from the lateral segment by the umbilical fissure and falciform ligament.

The left hepatic duct is formed by the confluence of tributary bile ducts from segments 1 through 4. The lateral sector ducts (segments 2 and 3) have a typical appearance, joining to create an acute angle to form a single duct that subsequently receives the segment 4 and segment 1 branches, forming the left hepatic duct. The left hepatic duct is characteristically longer than the right. This anatomic fact is functionally important when MBDO is centered at or above the hilus, because progression of disease will usually involve second-order and higher biliary confluences on the right side before the same thing occurs on the left. In such a context, left-sided biliary drainage may be preferred.

Right Hepatic Lobe

The right hemiliver is separated into anterior and posterior segments by the plane of the right hepatic vein, and into superior and inferior segments by the plane of the portal vein. The posterior sector is composed of segment 6 (the posterior inferior segment) and segment 7 (the posterior superior segment). The anterior sector is formed by segment 5 (the anterior inferior segment) and segment 8 (the anterior superior segment).

The right posterior sector bile duct is formed by the union of the ducts from segment 6 and segment 7, and the right anterior sector bile duct is formed by the union of the ducts from segment 5 and segment 8. The right hepatic duct is formed by the union of the right posterior and right anterior sectoral ducts.

The confluence of the right and left hepatic ducts (the primary biliary confluence) forms the common hepatic duct. The common hepatic duct receives the cystic duct to form the common bile duct. The common bile duct receives the pancreatic duct close to the ampulla of Vater.

Important common variants of biliary anatomy must be understood (Fig. 134-1, *B*). Several of these involve variant insertions of the right-sided sectoral ducts. One common example occurs when the right posterior sectoral duct drains to the left hepatic duct instead of joining the right anterior duct. In certain hilar occlusions where this anatomic variant is present, drainage of the right posterior sector may confer drainage of 6 liver segments (segments 1-4, 6, and 7), whereas drainage of the anterior sector would accomplish drainage of only 2 segments (segments 5 and 8) in such instances. Therefore, careful study of preprocedure imaging and real-time scrutiny of the procedural cholangiogram for the presence of variant biliary anatomy is essential.

Pathologic Anatomy

As obstructed bile ducts pass from peripheral to central, they become larger in caliber, and this appearance can be appreciated by ultrasound, CT, MRI, and PTC. Sudden decrease in the caliber of a bile duct as it passes centrally is a clue to a point of biliary obstruction.

Biliary obstruction may cause one part of the biliary tree to be separated from another part, and this separation is termed *isolation*. The extent or degree of isolation may be characterized as complete or incomplete. In *complete isolation*, there is no obvious remaining connection between the segments of biliary tree that have been separated by the obstruction (Fig. 134-2). Contrast material injected into the bile duct during cholangiography stops at the point of obstruction, and catheter-guidewire manipulations are required to find the obliterated connection between completely isolated segments of bile duct. *Incomplete isolation*, on the other hand, occurs when disease has pathologically narrowed segments of bile duct that still remain in communication. This is depicted by passage of injected contrast material through areas of bile duct narrowing into other portions of the biliary tree (Fig. 134-3). Some refer to incomplete isolation as *impending isolation* to convey the likelihood that with time, disease progression will transform incomplete isolation into complete isolation (Fig. 134-4). Clinically, incomplete isolation is important because

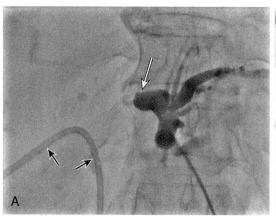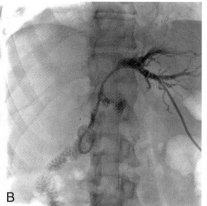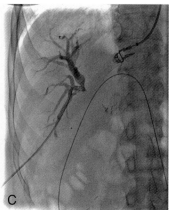

FIGURE 134-2. A, Cholangiogram obtained during left biliary drainage shows that contrast injected into segments 2 and 3 (left lateral sector) *(white arrow)* does not pass into left hepatic duct or right-side ducts, already drained by a catheter *(black arrows)*. Lateral sector is completely isolated from rest of liver. **B,** In this patient who has undergone hepaticojejunostomy, contrast injected into left biliary drain does not opacify right-side bile ducts. Opacified ducts are completely isolated from rest of liver. **C,** In this oblique image, a guidewire is in place via left bile ducts. Right biliary tree has been opacified. There is complete isolation between right-side bile ducts and left bile ducts.

it is functionally equivalent to partial obstruction; when it is present, there are poorly drained segments of the biliary tree that are substrates for infection. Instrumentation or injection can contaminate such ducts with bacteria, leading to cholangitis.

The Bismuth-Corlette classification of hilar cholangiocarcinoma provides a useful scheme for describing high bile duct obstructions (Fig. 134-5). Type 1 obstructions involve the common hepatic duct but do not extend into the confluence. This pattern is functionally equivalent to a low bile duct obstruction in that it can be treated with a single catheter or stent from either a right- or left-sided approach. Type 2 obstructions isolate the right and left hepatic ducts from each other. Complete drainage of such obstructions can be accomplished by placement of a right-to-left (or left-to-right) external biliary drainage catheter, placement of bilateral internal-external biliary drainage catheters, or

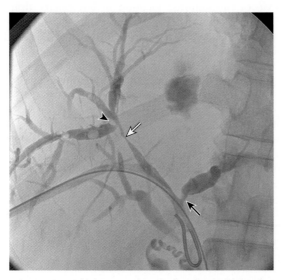

FIGURE 134-3. Multiple areas of incomplete (impending) isolation are present: left hepatic duct *(black arrow)*, segment 8 duct *(white arrow)*, and subsegment 8 ducts *(arrowhead)*. Filling defects are injected gas bubbles.

placement of metallic stents in either a Y or T configuration. In type 3 obstructions, disease extends into either the left or right hepatic duct, producing sectoral or segmental isolations. Complete drainage of either the left (type 3A) or right (type 3B) hemiliver can be accomplished using a single catheter or stent; drainage of more liver parenchyma would require additional drains or stents. Type 4 obstructions extend into both left and right hepatic ducts and/or into segmental bile ducts, creating multiple intrahepatic biliary isolations. For patients with this type of obstruction, the appropriateness and type of biliary drainage should be carefully considered on a case-by-case basis in view of the indication, likelihood of success in achieving the desired clinical endpoint, and potential attendant complications. Complete biliary drainage cannot usually be obtained for patients with such advanced disease.

Evaluation of Preprocedural Imaging Studies

In MBDO, preprocedural imaging studies must be carefully studied to predict the procedural cholangiogram. This is important so as to plan a biliary drainage that will provide maximal drainage with as few catheters/stents as possible. Important considerations include prediction of cholangiographic findings, review of prior biliary interventions, recognition of variant biliary ductal anatomy, parenchymal atrophy, portal vein status, and ascites.

Prediction of Cholangiographic Findings
During review of preprocedural imaging, bile ducts should be followed from liver segments centrally using an orderly search pattern that confirms which ducts communicate and which ducts are isolated from each other (Fig. 134-6). By doing this, the interventional radiologist can construct a mental model of the biliary tree and plan the intervention to accomplish maximal biliary drainage.

Review of Prior Biliary Interventions
In the setting of high bile duct obstruction, it is important to review the patient's imaging history for evidence of prior biliary interventions. This information is critical when a

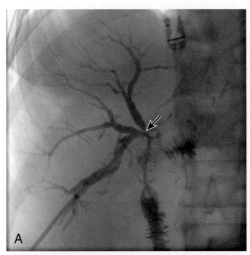
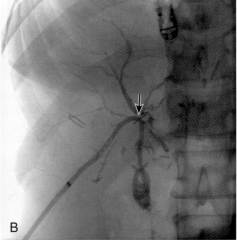

FIGURE 134-4. A, Impending/incomplete isolation (tube cholangiogram). Note narrowing of segment 8 bile duct where it joins central biliary tree. **B,** Although contrast material can be injected into duct, its drainage is impaired by narrowing.

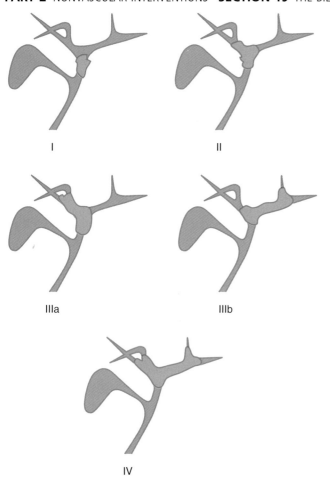

FIGURE 134-5. Bismuth-Corlette classification system for perihilar cholangiocarcinoma. *(From Dalrymple N, Leyendecker J, Oliphant M. Problem solving in abdominal imaging. Philadelphia: Mosby; 2009, Fig 10-31.)*

patient with high bile duct obstruction presents with cholangitis. When such patients have a history of endoscopic or percutaneous intervention, it is important to identify what parts of the liver have been previously contaminated by contrast injection and/or stent placement. This information provides a rational basis for deciding what portion of the biliary tree is most likely to be infected, and therefore what portion of the biliary tree should be targeted for drainage.

Recognition of Variant Biliary Ductal Anatomy
Recognition of common biliary anatomic variants on cross-sectional imaging is important, as previously discussed.

Parenchymal Atrophy
Long-standing biliary and/or portal venous obstruction causes atrophy of the affected liver segments. Atrophic liver parenchyma has a characteristic appearance, with dilated bile ducts that are crowded together due to regression of intervening liver parenchyma (Fig. 134-7). Drainage of dilated bile ducts in atrophic liver segments is unlikely to provide benefit in terms of recovered liver function, so it is important to recognize and avoid them.

Portal Vein Status
Similarly, it is important to evaluate and verify patency of the portal vein on preprocedural imaging. Normal liver

parenchyma derives up to 80% of its blood supply from the portal vein. Therefore, if recovery of liver function is the intended goal of drainage, only liver segments with patent portal venous supply should be targeted during biliary drainage.

Ascites
Ascites is a common occurrence in many advanced cancers, and for several reasons, its presence should be considered when planning biliary interventions. Large amounts of ascites may displace the liver from the abdominal wall, increasing the distance of target bile ducts from the skin. This can increase the technical difficulty of the procedure. After placement of a biliary drainage catheter, pericatheter leakage of ascites may occur, causing substantial discomfort and distress to the patient. Preprocedure paracentesis is an effective immediate solution. If ascites is predominantly dependent in the abdomen, a left-sided approach to biliary drainage may help avoid pericatheter leakage of ascites because of the anterior location of left biliary drains. If ascites leaks around a biliary drainage catheter despite these efforts, an ostomy device can be placed around the catheter exit site to capture the leaking fluid. Ascites refractory to medical management may be palliated by placement of a tunneled peritoneal ascites drainage catheter, peritoneal-venous shunt, or transhepatic portosystemic shunt.

Technique

Antibiotic Prophylaxis
Administration of antibiotics before biliary drainage is routinely recommended, but there is no consensus on a first-choice agent. Common choices include intravenous ceftriaxone, ampicillin/sulbactam, cefotetan and mezlocillin, ampicillin and gentamicin, or for penicillin-allergic patients, vancomycin or clindamycin and an aminoglycoside.[17]

Right Side Biliary Drainage
A low intercostal approach is selected near the midaxillary line. However, the position and anatomy of the liver (or liver remnant) will occasionally dictate a different approach. Fluoroscopic evaluation of the location of the costophrenic sulcus should be made to avoid pleural transgression. Needle entry that projects at or below the superior margin of the 11th rib during anteroposterior fluoroscopy will usually prevent this complication. Following site selection and sterile skin preparation, local anesthesia is obtained by lidocaine injection. Creation of a small dermatotomy facilitates needle passage and subsequent sheath and catheter exchanges. A 10-mL syringe attached to connector tubing is filled with contrast and purged of air. A 21-gauge styleted (noncoring) needle is advanced into the liver toward the midclavicular line during fluoroscopic observation. The stylet is removed from the needle, and the contrast-filled syringe/connector tubing assembly is attached to the needle. During continuous fluoroscopic observation, contrast is gently injected as the needle is slowly withdrawn. Care must be taken not to intravasate contrast material into liver parenchyma, since this causes parenchymal stains that subsequently degrade visualization.

A variety of tubular structures may be encountered as the needle is withdrawn, and it is important to recognize

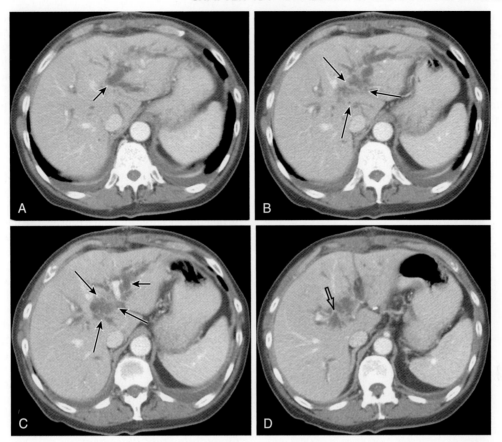

FIGURE 134-6. **A,** Converging ducts from segment 2 abruptly taper *(arrow),* indicating a point of obstruction. **B,** Ill-defined low-attenuation mass in central liver is the cause of high bile duct obstruction *(arrows).* **C,** Segment 3 duct, dilated in liver periphery *(arrows, same as on B),* abruptly tapers *(short black arrow)* and does not appear to join segment 2 duct. **D,** Similarly, groups of right-side bile ducts abruptly taper *(open arrow)* in proximity to central liver lesion. These findings suggest Bismuth-Corlette type IV high bile duct obstruction.

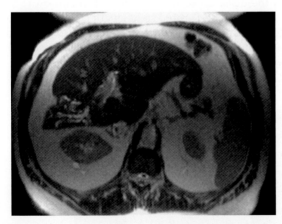

FIGURE 134-7. Axial magnetic resonance cholangiopancreatography image shows atrophy of right hepatic lobe with dilated right bile ducts.

the appearance of hepatic arteries, hepatic veins, portal veins, and lymphatics opacified in this manner so as to distinguish these from bile ducts. In general, hepatic arteries are recognized by pulsatile flow toward the liver periphery, hepatic veins by nonpulsatile flow directed cranially, portal veins by nonpulsatile peripheral flow into branches with multiple characteristic right-angle tributaries, and lymphatics by slow flow through tortuous beaded channels

draining toward the liver hilus. Bile ducts are recognized by nonpulsatile slow gravitational filling of tubular structures.

Once a bile duct has been opacified, the decision must be made whether the site of puncture is acceptable for catheter access. In general, third-order or higher bile ducts are selected for catheter placement (Fig. 134-8). This is both to avoid injury to larger central vascular structures and to ensure an adequate length of bile duct proximal to occlusions for adequate drainage or working room during biliary stent placements. When the initial puncture is judged too central or suboptimal for some other reason (Fig. 134-9, *A*), a second needle is used to target a more suitable peripheral duct (Fig. 134-9, *B*) that has been opacified by injection of the first needle. Once a suitable duct has been accessed, a 0.018-inch guidewire is inserted through the needle into the biliary tree (Fig. 134-10). Over this wire, a coaxial transition set such as the Neff Introducer can be advanced into the biliary tree. The inner components of such a set consist of a metallic stiffener and a 3F cannula tapered to the 0.018 wire. Once in place, the inner components are removed, leaving the outer 5F sheath in place. Through this sheath, a 4F or 5F catheter and guidewire can be advanced into the biliary tree. Alternately, a 0.035-inch guidewire can be placed through it, and it can be exchanged for a 6F or 7F sidearm sheath to permit drainage of bile during subsequent catheter manipulations.

Contrast injections can be performed through the sheath or catheter to depict bile duct anatomy above the obstruction. Next, a catheter and guidewire are used to cross the obstruction. Once past the obstruction, another contrast injection is performed to depict the length of the bile duct occlusion. Over the wire, the catheter is then positioned into the duodenum (or jejunum in the case of prior biliary bypass). Contrast injection into the intestine is performed to verify intraluminal position and assess intestinal outflow for obstruction (Fig. 134-11).

A 0.035-inch Amplatz Super Stiff guidewire is then placed through the catheter. Over this wire, an 8F or 10F

biliary drainage catheter is advanced. A peel-away sheath can be used to facilitate catheter introduction. The drainage catheter's locking loop is formed in the intestine, and side holes are always positioned proximal to the level of bile duct occlusion (Fig. 134-12). Adequacy of catheter position is then assessed by injection and aspiration of contrast material. Catheter maintenance typically includes twice-daily forward flushes of 10 mL of normal saline and exchange every 3 months.

Left Side Biliary Drainage

Dilated left-side bile ducts are readily visualized with ultrasound, facilitating ultrasound-guided bile duct access using a 21-gauge needle with an echogenic tip (Fig. 134-13). When fluoroscopic guidance is used, the needle is advanced into the liver and angled approximately 30 to 45 degrees posteriorly and superiorly. Subsequent procedural steps are identical to those for right-side access.

Placement of Metallic Biliary Stents

Biliary stenting may be performed either at the time of biliary drainage or after a period of catheter drainage. Immediate stent placement should be considered for (1) nonsurgical, noncholangitic patients with MBDO who have low bile duct obstruction, (2) patients with ascites who might otherwise suffer pericatheter leakage of peritoneal fluid, and (3) patients with high bile duct obstruction when biliary access permits drainage of the intended volume of liver.

Immediate Stent Placement

Once wire access to the duodenum has been achieved and a contrast injection has been performed, a sidearm sheath large enough to accommodate the selected stent is placed. Stents 10 mm in diameter are usually selected for the common bile duct, and 8 mm stents are usually selected when the diseased segment extends into either the left or right hepatic duct. Desired stent length can be estimated by comparing the length of duct to be treated to the height of an adjacent lumbar vertebral body, which is ordinarily about 3 to 3.5 cm.

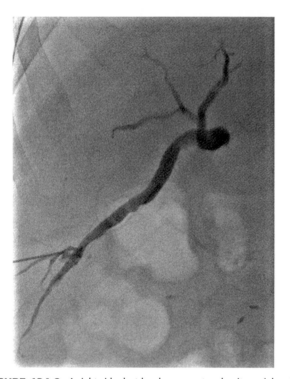

FIGURE 134-8. A right side duct has been punctured quite peripherally.

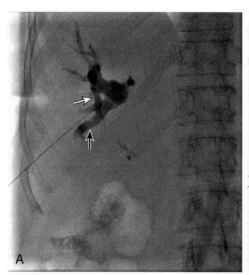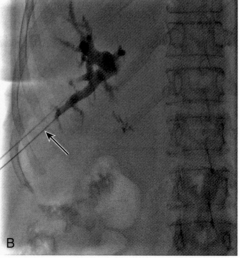

FIGURE 134-9. Two-needle drainage. **A,** Initial biliary puncture was into an up-going radical *(white arrow)*. More inferior duct *(black arrow)* had fewer angles and was judged more favorable for catheter access. **B,** A second needle *(arrow)* was therefore used to puncture the more inferior duct.

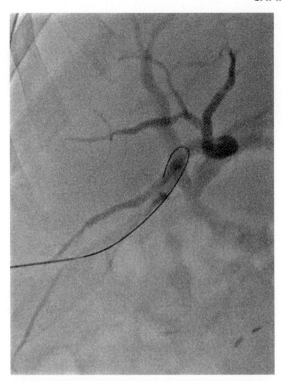

FIGURE 134-10. Following puncture of a suitable bile duct, 0.018-inch guidewire is inserted into biliary tree through needle.

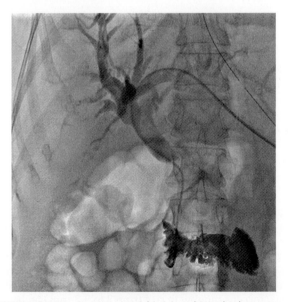

FIGURE 134-11. Contrast material is injected into duodenum to verify that intestinal outflow is not obstructed.

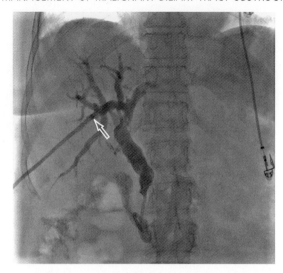

FIGURE 134-12. Appearance following placement of internal-external biliary drain. Position of the most proximal sidehole is indicated by radiopaque marker *(arrow)* on this biliary drain. Side holes have been positioned well above distal common bile duct obstruction.

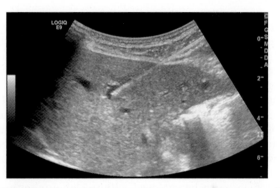

FIGURE 134-13. Needle placement into a segment 3 duct is visualized with ultrasound in this longitudinal image of left hemiliver.

The stent is then advanced through the sheath, over the wire, and positioned distal to its intended final position. Stents intended to be positioned across the ampulla of Vater ideally project about 10 mm into the duodenal lumen. Stents not intended to cross the ampulla of Vater are ideally positioned no closer than 2 cm to it so as not to cause ampullary spasm. Several centimeters distal to its intended final position, stent deployment is started. After several centimeters of the stent are exposed, the catheter-stent delivery system can be pulled back to place the distal aspect of the stent in its intended position. Subsequently, the stent is released (Fig. 134-14, *A*), and the result is assessed by injection of contrast material through the sheath's sidearm port. If required, an additional coaxial stent can be placed to modify the result.

Balloon dilation of self-expanding stents is usually not necessary because they are engineered to expand to their nominal diameter over time. Predilation of biliary stenoses prior to stent placement is also usually not necessary in such instances; in addition to adding expense and causing pain, predilation of malignant obstructions can cause hemobilia, leading to poor stent function. When completion cholangiography shows antegrade passage of injected contrast material through the stent into the intestinal outflow, a decision must be made about whether or not percutaneous access to the biliary tree has to be preserved. If the stent is patent and the biliary tree does not contain blood clots that might block it, percutaneous access can be immediately abandoned by placing a Gelfoam pledget through the access sheath at the site of bile duct puncture. Short-term continued access to the biliary tree may be

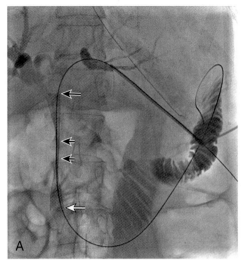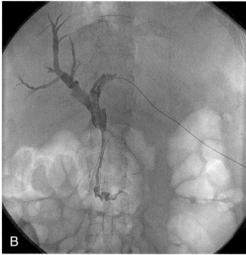

FIGURE 134-14. **A,** From a segment 3 bile duct puncture, a 10 mm × 68 mm Wallstent has been positioned across an occlusion of mid–common duct. Note that flaring of stent both proximally *(long black arrow)* and distally *(white arrow)* provides immediate confirmation that both cranial and caudal aspects of stent are above and below obstruction, respectively. Waist in stent *(short arrows)* indicates segment of biliary obstruction. As radial forces of stent cause it to open, it will shorten slightly. **B,** Contrast material injected through an angiographic catheter passes down stent and into intestine, confirming patency.

desired when procedural hemobilia has occurred or when there are doubts regarding the adequacy of stent function. In such cases, a 4F or 5F angiographic catheter can be placed over wire into the biliary tree to preserve access. If the stent has been placed across the ampulla of Vater, this catheter can be placed into the duodenum. If the stent has been placed above the ampulla of Vater, the catheter should be placed within the stent but not through the ampulla, so as not to cause ampullary spasm. When there is need to provide ongoing external drainage, an 8F external drain can be positioned at the proximal aspect of the stent. Size 4F or 5F catheters can be removed within 24 hours, either on clinical grounds or following contrast injection that verifies adequate stent function (Fig. 134-14, *B*). Larger drainage catheters can be removed in 7 to 10 days following formation of a tract, as a safeguard against peritoneal leakage of bile.

Delayed Stent Placement
Patients with biliary drainage catheters may be referred for internalization of drainage with a metallic stent after resolution of cholangitis, after determination of nonsurgical status has been made, or when another desired clinical endpoint (e.g., adequate bilirubin reduction for chemotherapy) has been attained following catheter drainage. The indwelling biliary catheter is removed over wire, a sidearm sheath is placed, and cholangiograms are obtained to depict the proximal and distal extent of the biliary occlusion, permitting selection of an appropriate stent. The remainder of the procedure is as previously described.

Bile Duct Biopsy
Benign and malignant strictures often are indistinguishable by cholangiographic appearance alone. For this reason, bile duct biopsy may be indicated. Sampling of the bile duct can be achieved by both endoluminal and percutaneous approaches. Tumors that grow within the duct, including cholangiocarcinoma and intraductal metastases, may be

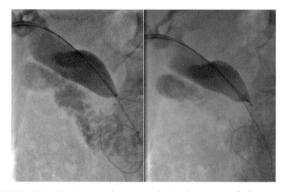

FIGURE 134-15. Forceps biopsy is obtained at point of obstruction in common bile duct.

diagnosed by brush or forceps biopsy. To obtain a sample with brush biopsy, a 3-mm brush at the end of a braided wire is advanced through a sheath to the level of stricture. The sheath is withdrawn to expose the brush, and the brush is manipulated at the site. The brush is removed from the patient and sent for cytologic analysis. Alternatively, alligator jaw forceps ranging in size from 2 to 3.7 mm can be used to grasp a specimen from the stricture (Fig. 134-15). Sensitivity with these techniques is approximately 60%; higher for intraluminal lesions and lower for extraluminal. Specificity is very high, approaching 98%.[18]

Another technique to sample a biliary stricture is percutaneous biopsy. At the time of percutaneous drainage or through an existing biliary drainage catheter, the bile ducts are opacified with contrast to delineate the area of bile duct stenosis. A biopsy needle is then advanced to the stricture under fluoroscopic guidance, and a specimen is obtained. A combination of movement of the bile duct by the biopsy needle and oblique images confirm accurate needle position.

Drainage Systems

Internal-External Biliary Drains

The internal-external biliary drain (IEBD) is a drainage catheter with a locking loop and multiple side holes. The IEBD is positioned such that its locking loop is in the intestine (typically the duodenum), and its side holes are positioned so that some are above (proximal to) the level of the biliary obstruction (Fig. 134-16). Because the catheter's side holes extend from above the level of bile duct obstruction and distally along its length where it terminates in the intestine, the exteriorized portion of the catheter can be capped to force internal drainage of bile. Alternately, the exteriorized portion of the catheter can be attached to a drainage

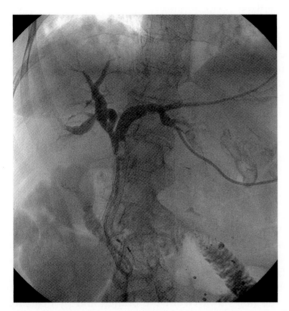

FIGURE 134-16. An internal-external biliary drain has been placed through an occluded metallic stent. Note that obstruction approaches primary biliary confluence, but right and left hepatic ducts still communicate.

bag for external drainage. The ability to provide either internal or external biliary drainage using such a device yields the name *internal-external biliary drain*. Advantages include the versatility of drainage options (internal or external), relative catheter stability compared to external biliary drains because of the position of the locking loop in the intestine, and the option to force internal drainage that delivers bile to the intestinal tract, simulating normal physiology. Presence of an exteriorized catheter limb, however, can be an inconvenience for patients, limiting lifestyle. When used for external drainage, substantial fluid losses from the intestinal limb can occur, so drainage outputs must be monitored.

Scenarios in which IEBDs might be selected for the drainage device in MBDO include: (1) for initial drainage of obstructed bile ducts when the diagnosis is unknown, (2) when a clinical endpoint such as a particular bilirubin value is required prior to internalization of an incompletely drained biliary tree, (3) when the intent was to place a metallic stent immediately, but procedural hemobilia precluded this, (4) for preoperative drainages when metallic stents are specifically not requested, (5) in cases where duodenal disease is likely to preclude metallic stent function, but a stable catheter is desired, and (6) to rescue occluded metallic common duct stents placed by either percutaneous or endoscopic techniques (see Fig. 134-16). IEBDs typically require routine exchange every 3 months.

External Biliary Drains

The external biliary drain (EBD) is a catheter that terminates in a bile duct, not in the intestine (Fig. 134-17). By definition, it provides external biliary drainage and cannot be capped in the setting of bile duct obstruction. Although most drains used for this purpose include some retention device, an external biliary drain is inherently less stable and more prone to dislodge than an IEBD. A variety of scenarios may prompt placement of an EBD. Common examples include (1) when the biliary obstruction cannot be crossed or attempts to cross result in perforation of the biliary tree, (2) when there is a desire to drain two portions of the biliary tree separated by an obstruction using a single catheter (this

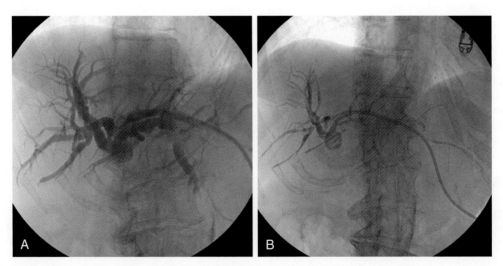

FIGURE 134-17 A, Image from a routine catheter exchange in a patient with common hepatic duct occlusion whose obstruction could not be catheterized; an external biliary drain has been maintained. **B,** External biliary drain imaged after aspiration of injected contrast material.

usually requires making extra side holes in the catheter to span the segments to be drained), (3) in septic patients in whom minimal manipulation is desired, and (4) to preserve transhepatic drainage following placement of a metallic stent. In general, the clinical intent will be to eventually exchange an EBD for a more stable drainage device (IEBD or metallic stent) when this is possible. Otherwise, routine catheter exchanges should be planned about every 3 months.

Metallic Stents

A variety of self-expanding and balloon-expandable stents are available for use in the biliary system. Deploying a metallic stent across a biliary obstruction recreates anatomic internal drainage. Although an exteriorized catheter may be maintained for a variable number of days following metallic stent placement to verify stent patency and adequate patient response, it is eventually removed so that the patient has internal biliary drainage with no external device. This minimizes the impact on patient lifestyle when compared to IEBDs and EBDs. Although percutaneous biliary access is abandoned following metallic stent placement, any needed revisions can often be accomplished endoscopically. Metallic stent placement is a good choice for MBDO when the patient has unresectable biliary obstruction, the target volume of liver would be drained by the stent, or when ascites is present and pericatheter leakage is anticipated. Median stent patency is 6 to 9 months.

Other Special Circumstances

Patients with biliary obstruction can present with one or more symptomatic intrahepatic bilomas. These are recognized as new low-attenuation collections in the liver. Ultrasound- or CT-guided biloma drainage can be effective in such instances. After acute symptoms have resolved, the catheter can be injected with contrast material, often demonstrating connection of the cavity to the obstructed bile ducts. The ducts opacified in this manner can then be fluoroscopically targeted for biliary drainage.

It is useful to remember that in patients with low bile duct obstruction, drainage of the gallbladder may provide external drainage of the biliary tree, provided the cystic duct is patent and inserts above the point of obstruction. Under similar anatomic circumstances, the biliary tree can be opacified by injection of the gallbladder through a needle or a preexisting cholecystostomy tube.

Percutaneous brachytherapy can be delivered to biliary obstructions caused by malignancy. Initially a metallic stent is placed across the diseased segment of duct. A special brachytherapy catheter is then positioned across the stented area for dose delivery by radiation oncology.

OUTCOMES

Successful access to dilated bile ducts approaches 100%. Nondilated bile ducts, which are uncommon in MBDO, are more difficult to access, and Society of Interventional Radiology Quality Improvement Guidelines suggest that success rates greater than 70% are anticipated in this setting.[19]

The clinical outcomes of biliary drainage vary widely depending on the indication and patient selection factors. Cholangitis and pruritus are effectively treated by biliary drainage. The likelihood of success in reducing serum bilirubin to levels appropriate for administration of chemotherapy has been shown to be associated with lower pre-drainage bilirubin levels and anatomy suitable for complete or near-complete biliary drainage. Metallic stents placed in the biliary tree have a median patency of 6 to 9 months, which often coincides with the life expectancy of patients with MBDO.

COMPLICATIONS

Major complications of biliary drainage include sepsis, hemorrhage, pleural transgression, and death. The reported rate for both sepsis and hemorrhage, the most common major complications, is 2.5%. Use of appropriate preprocedure antibiotics, permitting bile to drain from the obstructed biliary tree prior to contrast injection, minimizing the volume of contrast injected, and minimizing manipulation of the biliary tree are techniques to decrease the risk of sepsis related to biliary drainage.

Transcatheter bleeding (bloody bile draining through the catheter) has several potential explanations. Some hemobilia is often present in the immediate postprocedural setting, but catheter output typically clears to non-bloody bile within 12 to 24 hours. When transcatheter bleeding persists, other explanations should be sought. Such bleeding may be due to the presence of catheter side holes near a portal or hepatic venous branch that has been transgressed by the access trajectory. This diagnosis can be made by catheter injection or by over-the-wire, pull-back sheath cholangiogram, permitting visualization of the culprit vascular structure. Venous causes can be treated by repositioning side holes away from the branch and by upsizing the drainage catheter to provide better tamponade. If bleeding persists or is associated with pericatheter bleeding (bleeding around the catheter) and/or a drop in hemoglobin, a hepatic arterial injury should be suspected. Angiography with coil embolization is effective for treatment of arterial injuries related to biliary drainage. Such injuries should be sought angiographically where the drainage catheter crosses or is in close proximity to a hepatic artery branch at the bile duct puncture site. If the injury is not observed with the biliary catheter in place, angiography can be repeated following removal of the drainage catheter over a wire. As with any arterial injury, angiographic findings can be diverse, including pseudoaneurysm, focal arterial spasm, arterial-biliary and arterial-venous fistulas.

KEY POINTS

- Careful review of recent imaging studies is essential prior to percutaneous biliary drainage procedures. This permits the interventional radiologist to predict the procedural cholangiogram, make wise choices regarding what part of the liver should be targeted for drainage, and counsel the patient and referring physician regarding the likelihood the procedure will accomplish the desired clinical endpoint.

- Patients with malignant bile duct obstruction often have a relatively short life expectancy, so when clinically possible, plan the procedure to provide both optimal treatment and optimal palliation. Place an immediate metallic stent instead of a drainage catheter (or actively facilitate timely transition to a metallic stent after a drainage catheter has been placed), and avoid approaches likely to be complicated by pericatheter leakage of ascites (or anticipate this problem and offer solutions).

► **SUGGESTED READINGS**

Covey AM, Brown KT. Palliative percutaneous drainage in malignant biliary obstruction. Part 1: indications and preprocedure evaluation. J Support Oncol 2006;4:269–73.

Hii MW, Gibson RN. Role of radiology in the treatment of malignant hilar biliary strictures 1: review of the literature. Australas Radiol 2004; 48:3–13.

The complete reference list is available online at www.expertconsult.com.

CHAPTER 135

Management of Benign Biliary Strictures

Wael E.A. Saad

INTRODUCTION

Management of benign biliary strictures (whether surgical, percutaneous-transhepatic, or by endoscopic means) is difficult.[1-4] These lesions are formed of cicatricial fibrosis and are recalcitrant to many minimally invasive techniques.[1-3] They can be a contributing factor to recurrent cholangitis, hepatic segmental atrophy, hepatic graft dysfunction (in cases of transplanted livers), and in the long-run, obstructive biliary cirrhosis.[2-4]

Benign biliary strictures are a heterogenous group of lesions that differ in demographics (patient types), locations within the biliary tract, etiology, and disease process (pathology). Firstly, there are pediatric transplant recipients, adult transplant recipients, and adult non-transplant patients with native livers. Pediatric transplant recipients have smaller ducts than adults (transplanted or native livers), and transplant recipients (pediatric or adults) have transplanted livers that have a relatively compromised arterial supply compared to most patients with native livers (see Outcomes for relevance). Secondly, they vary in morphology and location (Fig. 135-1). Thirdly, they vary in etiology and pathogenesis, including inflammatory processes, infectious processes, inflammatory-ischemic processes, thermal injuries from laparoscopic complications, surgical-technical complications at surgical anastomoses (scarring), and (less commonly) radiation injury.[1,5-11] Many key studies amalgamate disease processes, and/or transplant versus non-transplants, and/or stricture locations (peripheral vs. anastomotic), and/or types of anastomoses (duct-to-duct vs. biliary-enteric anastomoses (see Fig. 135-1).[4,12-13] As a result, it is difficult to discuss anatomic and functional (clinical) outcomes specific to a uniform population or a particular pathologic-anatomic biliary stricture.

The types and locations of benign biliary strictures that are encountered vary depending on the referral pattern and expertise of the institution. However, overall, the vast majority of benign biliary strictures are either (1) peripheral intrahepatic (the ones that are solitary and treatable), commonly related to liver transplantation, and/or (2) anastomotic biliary strictures (whether in transplanted or native livers). For the purpose of this chapter (with its limited scope), these two lesions will be discussed. Non-anastomotic central (hilar or common hepatic bile duct) lesions are treated similarly to anastomotic benign biliary strictures, and they will be discussed as one entity.

INDICATIONS

Peripheral Intrahepatic Benign Biliary Strictures

The limited indications for managing peripheral intrahepatic benign biliary strictures are confined to cholangitis with or without biliary stones. The primary issue when contemplating the management of peripheral intrahepatic benign biliary strictures is to make sure this is not a diffuse hepatobiliary process that will develop multiple lesions. Diffuse hepatobiliary processes include primary sclerosing cholangitis and diffuse hepatic graft ischemia. Percutaneous transhepatic biliary management of multiple lesions is futile and probably requires several transhepatic biliary drains. The risks versus benefit of managing multiple lesions tilts heavily toward the risks. Furthermore, treat the patient and not the lesion. If the patient is asymptomatic and has no cholangitis, leave the biliary stricture alone, which will probably cause segmental atrophy of the hepatic segment being drained by the constricted biliary duct segment, with compensatory hypertrophy of adjacent hepatic segments. The only exception is an undersized hepatic graft (usually a pediatric recipient) with involvement of a relatively large hepatic segment. In this case, the involved hepatic segment may not be dispensable.

Central Benign Biliary Strictures (Anastomotic and Nonanastomotic)

Indications include cholangitis with or without biliary stones, biliary stones, cholestasis with pruritus, abnormal liver function tests with concern for developing biliary cirrhosis, and hepatic graft dysfunction. The most definitive treatment of central strictures is a hepaticojejunostomy.[4,14-16] However, redo hepaticojejunostomies have a lower clinical success rate.[4,17] Difficult hepaticojejunostomy candidates (candidates for percutaneous or endoscopic management) include poor surgical candidates owing to comorbidities, patients refusing surgery, numerous adhesions and inflammatory process in the porta hepatis, and short biliary stumps in patients with preexisting hepaticojejunostomies.[4]

CONTRAINDICATIONS

Peripheral Intrahepatic Benign Biliary Strictures

Non-candidacy includes asymptomatic patients and/or patients with diffuse hepatobiliary processes with multiple lesions (see earlier). General contraindications include active sepsis, uncorrected coagulopathy, hemobilia, and possibly ascites. Ascites may have a higher risk for bleeding and may cause leakage of ascitic fluid around the internal-external percutaneous transhepatic biliary drain (PTBD) (high morbidity). However, it is not an absolute contraindication in the author's opinion.

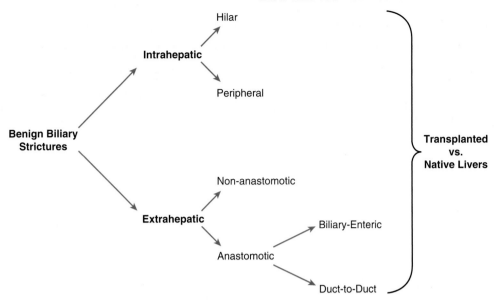

FIGURE 135-1. Flow chart demonstrating classification of benign biliary strictures based on transplant vs. native livers and based on lesion location. Another dimension of variation not included in flow chart is etiology of benign stricture. Non-anastomotic extrahepatic lesions are in common hepatic duct. Hilar intrahepatic lesions are lesions at confluence of main right and main left biliary ducts or in main right or left biliary ducts. Only exception is if a surgical anastomosis is right at the confluence (almost no biliary stump). In this case, we would consider it anastomotic (extrahepatic).

Central Benign Biliary Strictures (Anastomotic and Non-anastomotic)

General contraindications include active sepsis, uncorrected coagulopathy, hemobilia, and possibly ascites (see earlier). In addition, an active biliary leak from the surgical anastomosis is a contraindication to transhepatic balloon dilation, which may increase the leak or rupture the surgical anastomosis.

EQUIPMENT

Peripheral Intrahepatic Benign Biliary Strictures

This includes standard internal-external as well as external PTBDs to establish and maintain percutaneous transhepatic access to the biliary tract. Small-caliber, high-pressure (>12 atm), noncompliant balloons are used. The balloon is sized 100% to 110% of the target biliary duct and probably does not exceed 5 to 6 mm.[2-3,13] Remember that right or left main bile duct (hilar) strictures are included in central benign biliary strictures (see later).

Central Benign Biliary Strictures (Anastomotic and Non-anastomotic)

This includes standard internal-external as well as external PTBDs to establish and maintain percutaneous transhepatic access to the biliary tract. High-pressure (>12 atm) noncompliant balloons are used. The balloon is sized 100% to 125% of the target biliary duct and usually ranges from 6 to 15 mm (Table 135-1).[2-3,13,18] Pediatric and adult split-graft transplant recipients usually require smaller balloons (6-10 mm) compared to whole grafts or native livers (7-15 mm).[2]

Unconventional balloons that have been used include the cutting balloon (Boston Scientific, Natick, Mass.). This

is a noncompliant balloon with four microsurgical blades (atherotomes) mounted longitudinally along the outer surface of the balloon. The atherotomes are 1.5 to 2.0 centimeters in length and are 0.127 in depth for all balloon sizes.[3] The cutting balloon comes in diameters from 5 to 8 mm and requires use of a coaxial 0.018-inch wire. The 7- and 8-mm diameters require a 7F introducer sheath.[3] A drawback is that available diameters of this balloon are limited; 40% of lesions have been found to require balloon sizes greater than 8 mm, which are not available for cutting balloons.[3] The PolarCath (for cryoplasty) from Boston Scientific has been mentioned as a potential tool for managing benign biliary strictures,[2-3] but to the best of our knowledge, its use has not been published.

Covered stents (stent-grafts) can also be used.[19] There are two commercially available stent-grafts that can be placed percutaneously or endoscopically but are mostly removed by endoscopic means. However, they can be removed transhepatically, but not by design. These two stents-grafts are the VIABIL (W.L. Gore & Associates, Flagstaff, Ariz.) and the WallFlex (Boston Scientific).

TECHNIQUE

The primary step of percutaneous transhepatic management of benign biliary strictures is establishing transhepatic access by an initial percutaneous transhepatic cholangiogram (PTC) followed by PTBD placement.[20] The details of the procedure(s) required for access will not be discussed in this chapter. Only the focus of transhepatic management is described.

There are two schools of managing benign biliary stricture. The traditional/historical school is to chronically place a large-bore (14F-16F) internal-external biliary drain to "splinter" (author's term) the stricture and keep it opened/stented for an extended period of time that usually requires a PTBD in place for months (4-12 months). Occasionally

TABLE-135-1 Technical Features and Results of Four Transhepatic Balloon Dilation Protocols for Percutaneous Management of Benign Biliary Strictures

Study and Year		Zajko, 1995[13]	Saad, 2005[18]	Saad, 2006[3]	Cantwell, 2008[4]
Sample Size		**N = 56**	**N = 38**	**N = 22**	**N = 85**
Balloon Features	Type	Conventional	Conventional	Conv + cutting	Conventional
	Max pressure (atm)	10-12	>12-15	>12-15	N/M
	Max diameters (mm) (mean)	7-15 (N/M)	6-14 (8.0)	7-12 (9.1)	8-12 (N/M)
	Cumulative duration of inflation per session (min)	20-30	1-5	10-20	3-15
Regimen/ Treatment*	Dilation session per treatment (mean)	1-6 (3.0)	1-3 (1.2)	1-3 (1.8)	1-4 (1.4)
	Balloon inflations per session	2-3	1	2-3	3-5
	Duration of regimen (weeks)	1-2	0-12	0-4.3	0-12[†]
Technical Results	Overall technical success (%)	<89%[‡]	85	93	100
	Major traumatic complications (%)	<5.6%[‡]	3.8	0.0	2.0

*Terminology may differ.
[†]Estimate.
[‡]Overall technical success rate and complication rates by Zajko et al. amalgamated intrahepatic peripheral lesion dilation and extrahepatic anastomotic dilations.
atm, Atmosphere; *Conv,* conventional; *Max,* maximum; *min,* minutes; *mm,* millimeters; *(N/M),* not mentioned.
Modified from Saad WEA. Percutaneous management of postoperative anastomotic biliary strictures. Tech Vasc Interv Radiol 2008;11:143–53.

balloon dilation can also be an adjunct to chronic drain placement. The second school relies on a relatively "fast-track" sequential balloon dilation (see later) and ridding the patient of the PTBD sooner rather than later. There are no studies (randomized controlled or retrospective) comparing the effectiveness of these two approaches to managing benign biliary strictures.

The traditional school has an admirable thought process, but it has two problems. The first is the high patient morbidity (patient discomfort) of a chronically indwelling large drain in patients who are otherwise healthy and active.[2-4,18] This is particularly true in liver transplant recipients who are generally younger and less tolerant of percutaneous drains.[21] The second problem is a mathematical size problem. On review of the literature, one can glean the diameters of the central bile ducts from the balloon sizes that are used, with a balloon oversize of 110% to 125%.[2-4,13,18] The balloon diameters shown in Table 135-1 place the diameters of central extrahepatic bile ducts at 5.6 to 10 mm, with an average diameter of 8 mm. A drain that truly occupies and splinters these diameters would range from 17F to 30F, with an average of 24F.[2-4,13,18] Even proponents of this method do not place percutaneous biliary drains of this size because it is unacceptable to most patients even when using soft Silastic drains. Ideally, multiple drains should be placed to reach the total occupying diameters required to truly splinter the biliary stricture. This is not feasible percutaneously, but is feasible by endoscopy (Fig. 135-2). Some operators try to maximize the biliary drain diameter to 22F while keeping the transhepatic drain diameter to 14F by placing an 8F drain (partly coaxially) through a 14F drain, where the 8F drain exits the 14F drain through a side hole within the biliary system (Fig. 135-3).

Peripheral Intrahepatic Benign Biliary Strictures

This author adopts the traditional school of benign biliary stricture management for peripheral intrahepatic benign biliary strictures, because most can be splintered appropriately (occupied completely) by a 12F internal-external biliary drain. The key issue, obviously, is to access the

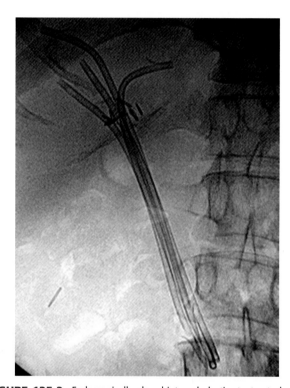

FIGURE 135-2. Endoscopically placed internal plastic stents, stacked to occupy or stretch benign biliary stricture.

peripheral biliary radicals that *lead to* the target benign biliary stricture. Balloon dilation can be used as an adjunct, especially in intrahepatic peripheral biliary strictures that are close to the porta hepatis.

Central Benign Biliary Strictures (Anastomotic and Non-anastomotic)

For left-lobe split-graft recipients (infants and small children), benign biliary stricture management is again our preferred approach because most central/anastomotic biliary strictures can also be splintered appropriately (occupied completely) by a 12F internal-external biliary drain. In addition, sequential balloon dilation protocol is used (see later).[2,3] In adults (native or transplanted livers), sequential balloon dilation protocol is preferred.[3,4,12,13,18]

Sequential Transhepatic Balloon Dilation Protocol

There are enumerable variations to the sequential balloon dilation technique, varying from one institution to another.[2] Certain institutions do not necessarily wait after establishing transhepatic access (fresh after a de novo PTC) to start dilations.[4] Others (this author included) wait for transhepatic tract maturity (≈4 weeks).[2,3] The overall theme is that transhepatic dilations are performed in multiple dilation sessions (a dilation session is any balloon dilation occurring within a procedure day) whereby the patient returns for a repeat dilation session with a maximum of 3 to 6 sessions for each treatment (dilation regimen), depending on the institution.[2-4,13,18] For clarification, a dilation treatment (or regimen) consists of 1 to 6 dilations sessions over 1 to 6 procedural visits (Fig. 135-4).[2-4,13,18] The time lapse between each dilation session also varies greatly between institutions (range, 1-22 days), making the entire treatment regimen last between 0 and 3 months (see Table 135-1).[2-4,13,18] In our practice, the treatment/regimen consists of 2 to 3 dilation sessions 5 to 10 days apart, making the maximum treatment duration 20 or 21 days. Other experienced institutions (University of Pittsburgh) perform 3 dilation sessions 1 to 2 days apart and are typically confined to 1 week (Monday-Wednesday-Friday regimen).[2]

An additional variable in the sequential transhepatic dilation protocol is the type of balloon used. Most institutions use conventional high-pressure balloons (maximum pressure > 12-15 atm). In our practice, we follow a combined cutting-conventional balloon protocol wherein the cutting balloon is routinely used first then followed by a high-pressure conventional balloon of the same size or greater (Fig. 135-5).[3] Other institutions and operators only use cutting balloons (due to their added expense) for benign biliary strictures that are refractory to conventional balloon dilation (type-II and type-III failures [Fig. 135-6]).[2] The duration of inflations range from 1 to 30 minutes.[2-4,13,18] Some operators keep the balloon inflated for 1 to 5 minutes,[18] others inflate the balloons cumulatively for 20 to 30 minutes.[2,13] We keep balloons inflated for 15 to 20 minutes (see Table 135-1).[3]

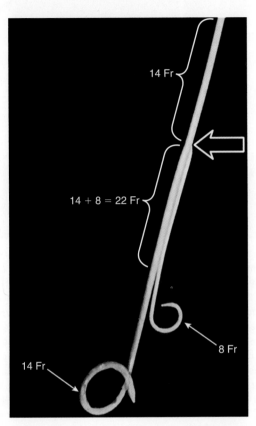

FIGURE 135-3. This is a set-up/technique to maximize biliary drain diameter internally inside biliary tract (22F, 7.3 mm) while minimizing size of drain through transhepatic tract (14F). It is achieved by passing an 8F drain through a 14F drain; 8F drain exits 14F biliary drain within biliary tract through a side hole *(open arrow)* in 14F biliary drain.

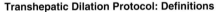

Transhepatic Dilation Protocol: Definitions

Dilation regimen
1 to 3 circuits

Dilation session

(x3)

<30% residual   >30% residual

End of successful
treatment regimen

A

Transhepatic Dilation Protocol: Technical Failure

No improvement after
single dilation session

Dilation session

(>3)

<30% residual   >30% residual

End of successful   End of failed
treatment regimen   treatment regimen

B

FIGURE 135-4. Schematic for balloon dilation protocol. **A,** A dilation treatment regimen *(shaded)* is composed of multiple dilation sessions. Patient returns for more dilation sessions for a maximum of 3 to 6 sessions (in this case, 3) until residual stenosis is less than 30%. **B,** After set maximum number of dilation sessions (in this example, 3) and residual stenosis still more than 30%, treatment is deemed a failure. No improvement whatsoever after any dilation session is considered a technical failure (defined as failure to resolve stricture to < 30%). For clarification, a failed dilation session (inability to improve an anastomotic stricture by any degree) translates to a failed dilation regimen. *(From Saad WEA. Percutaneous management of postoperative anastomotic biliary strictures. Tech Vasc Interv Radiol 2008;11:143–53.)*

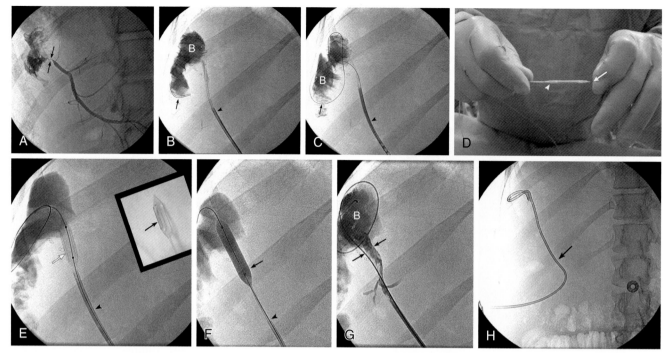

FIGURE 135-5. Cutting balloon dilation of hepaticojejunostomy (biliary-enteric) anastomosis in pediatric left hepatic lobe liver transplant recipient. **A,** Fluoroscopic image from initial percutaneous transhepatic cholangiogram (PTC) demonstrating significant stenosis at biliary-enteric anastomosis *(arrows)*. **B,** Fluoroscopic image during exchange of 0.035-inch wire for 0.018-inch wire. Kumpe catheter *(arrow)* is used for exchange. It is passed into bowel via a 7F sheath *(arrowhead)*. Kumpe catheter sits where a 0.035-inch wire lay. Next, the 0.018-inch wire is to be placed (cutting balloons require 0.018-inch wire). *B,* Bowel. **C,** Fluoroscopic image after exchange of 0.035-inch wire for 0.018-inch wire *(arrow)*. Kumpe catheter has been removed. The 7F sheath *(arrowhead)* is full of contrast. *B,* Bowel. **D,** Photograph of cutting balloon *(arrowhead)* being mounted on 0.018-inch wire *(arrow)*. **E,** Fluoroscopic image after a 7-mm cutting balloon *(open arrow)* has been placed across stenosis via sheath *(arrowhead)*. Inset is a photograph of balloon outside body. Black arrow points to one of four microsurgical blades (atherotomes) of balloon. Inset is oriented and sized to be comparable with its en vivo fluoroscopic image. Cutting balloon is a noncompliant balloon with four atherotomes mounted longitudinally on its outer surface. Atherotomes are 2 cm long and 0.127 mm (0.005 inch) in height/depth for all balloon sizes. **F,** Fluoroscopic image after exchanging 7-mm cutting balloon for 7-mm conventional balloon *(arrow)*, which is placed across stenosis via sheath *(arrowhead)*. **G,** Fluoroscopic image of postdilation transhepatic cholangiogram (performed through sheath), demonstrating resolution of significant stenosis at biliary-enteric anastomosis *(arrows)*. Compare with **A.** *B,* Bowel. **H,** Fluoroscopic image of 8F internal-external drain *(arrow)* placed after dilation. Sheath, wire, and balloon have been removed. Patient is instructed to keep drain to gravity drainage (internal *and* external drainage) for 24 hours after dilation session, then instructed to cap drain after 24 hours (if no fevers) so that biliary system is drained internally (anatomically) only. *(From Saad WEA. Percutaneous management of postoperative anastomotic biliary strictures. Tech Vasc Interv Radiol 2008;11:143–53.)*

A detailed step-by-step dilation session using a combined cutting balloon and subsequent conventional balloon protocol is shown in Figure 135-5.[2,3]

OUTCOMES

Peripheral Intrahepatic Benign Biliary Strictures

Transhepatic balloon dilation with and without mid- to long-term internal-external transhepatic biliary drain placement is a relatively successful technique both technically and anatomically (patency). In fact, peripheral intrahepatic benign biliary strictures respond better to balloon dilation than central/anastomotic benign biliary strictures, where each have a 6- to 12-month patency of 90% to 94% and 70% to 77%, respectively.[13]

Central Benign Biliary Strictures (Anastomotic and Non-anastomotic)

The technical success rate for transhepatic conventional balloon dilation of newcomers (first time treatment) with central/anastomotic benign biliary strictures ranges from 85% to 100% (see Table 135-1).[2-4,13,18] Recurrent anastomotic biliary strictures have been found to be more refractory (2.5-fold more resistant) to conventional balloon dilation than newcomers, with a technical failure rate of 27% and 11%, respectively.[18] Technical failures have been classified by Saad into three types (see Fig. 135-6).[2] A more aggressive combined cutting-conventional balloon protocol (Figs. 135-7 and 135-8) has been found to be more technically successful than conventional balloon dilation only (100% vs. 89%, respectively, for newcomers; 90% vs. 73%, respectively, for recurrent lesions), without an increase in complications.[3]

Patency of central/anastomotic biliary strictures after transhepatic balloon dilation depends on definitions and methodology. Proof of patency based on laboratory values and clinical follow-up would be expected to be higher than patency based on imaging (cholangiography, to be specific). This is because restenosis can occur without being clinically evident or evident by laboratory values (serum bilirubin, alkaline phosphatase, and γ-glutamyl transferase).[2,3] Furthermore, two key studies did not include

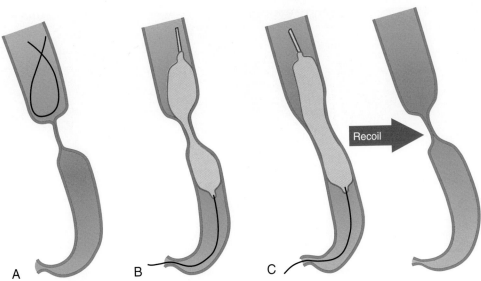

FIGURE 135-6. Types (causes) of technical failures. **A,** Line drawing of a critical stricture at choledochocholedochal anastomosis. Failure to cross anastomotic stricture with a wire, catheter, or balloon is considered by the author's institution a type 1 failure, which is uncommon and occurs in less than 5% of cases. **B,** Line drawing of balloon dilation of significant stricture at choledochocholedochal anastomosis. Balloon has a waist that is not effaced despite applying an atmospheric pressure of more than 15 atm. Failure to efface balloon waist at atmospheres above 15 is considered by the author's institution a type 2 failure. This is a rare type of failure and is due to tough fibrotic tissue at anastomosis. **C,** Line drawing of balloon dilation of significant stricture at choledochocholedochal anastomosis. Balloon is inflated fully (effaced waist), but lesions return immediately (recoil) after balloon deflation. Immediate intraprocedural recoil of an anastomotic lesion is considered by the author's institution a type 3 failure, the most common type (>95% of failures) and due to recoil of elastic fibrotic tissue at anastomosis. *(From Saad WEA. Percutaneous management of postoperative anastomotic biliary strictures. Tech Vasc Interv Radiol 2008;11:143–53.)*

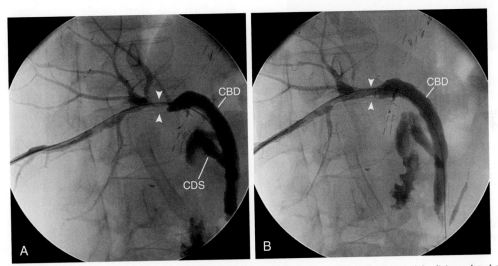

FIGURE 135-7. Cutting balloon dilation of a hepaticocholedochostomy anastomosis in an adult right hepatic lobe living related transplant recipient. **A,** Fluoroscopic image of critical stenosis at bile duct–to–bile duct anastomosis *(arrowheads)*. *CBD,* Common bile duct; *CDS,* cystic duct stump. **B,** Fluoroscopic image after dilation. Patient underwent 7-mm cutting balloon dilation followed by 7-mm conventional balloon dilation. Anastomotic stricture has resolved *(arrowheads)*. *CBD,* Common bile duct of recipient. *(From Saad WEA. Percutaneous management of postoperative anastomotic biliary strictures. Tech Vasc Interv Radiol 2008;11:143–53.)*

an intent-to-treat analysis, but only evaluated patency for technically successful cases and cases with "adequate" follow-up.[4,13] Amalgamation of lesion types, etiology, and locations also adds to the confusion. Overall, the 1- to 3-year intent-to-treat patency ranges from 38% to 73%, based on cholangiography and/or clinical follow-up.[2,4,13,18,22-25] The 5- to 6-year patency of technically successful procedures by clinical/laboratory follow-up is 52% to

66%.[4,13] The only study comparing the patency of duct-to-duct anastomoses with biliary-enteric (hepaticojejunostomies) was by Saad et al., who showed there was no statistical difference ($P = 0.1$) between the 1-year primary unassisted patency (by cholangiography) of either method: 43% and 48%, respectively.[18] This study also showed that liver transplants with patent hepatic arteries had far better 1-year patency results compared to liver transplants with

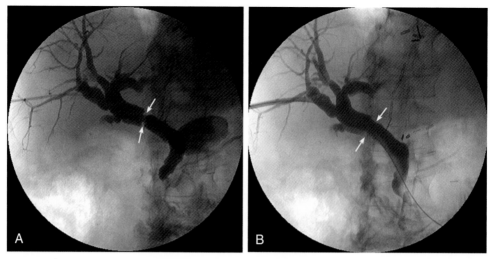

FIGURE 135-8. Cutting balloon dilation of a choledochocholedochostomy anastomosis in an adult cadaveric liver transplant recipient. **A,** Fluoroscopic image of significant stenosis at bile duct–to–bile duct anastomosis *(arrows).* **B,** Fluoroscopic image after dilation. Patient underwent 8-mm cutting balloon dilation followed by 10- and 12-mm conventional balloon dilation. Anastomotic stricture has resolved *(arrows). (From Saad WEA. Percutaneous management of postoperative anastomotic biliary strictures. Tech Vasc Interv Radiol 2008;11:143–53.)*

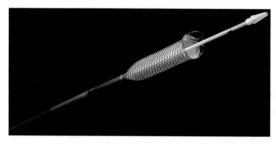

FIGURE 135-9. Photograph of partly deployed WallFlex stent (Boston Scientific, Natick, Mass.). "Bucket handle" (retrievable loop) can be seen at tip of delivery platform from percutaneous transhepatic approach. *(Image courtesy Boston Scientific; © 2012 Boston Scientific Corporation or its affiliates. All rights reserved.)*

stenosed or thrombosed hepatic arteries: 55% versus 0%, respectively.[18]

Retrievable Stents for Central Benign Biliary Strictures

The experience of placing and removing retrievable covered stents (removable stent-grafts) from a percutaneous transhepatic approach is limited compared to endoscopically placed stent-grafts.[2,19] Nevertheless, in the United States, the two most common commercially available stent-grafts used for subsequent transhepatic removals are the most commonly placed and removed stents from an endoscopic approach. These are the VIABIL (W.L. Gore) and the WallFlex (Boston Scientific) stent-grafts. The VIABIL is has expanded polytetrafluoroethylene (e-PTFE) covering a nitinol frame, and the WallFlex has a platinum-cored nitinol (Platinol) braid design covered on the inside with silicone (Permalume). The WallFlex has a retrievable loop ("bucket handle" [author's term]) only on the bowel side (caudad), not on the transhepatic side (cephalad) (Fig. 135-9). In other words, it is currently designed primarily to be removed by

endoscopic means. Transhepatically, the WallFlex can be deployed through a 9F sheath. Both the VIABIL and Wall-Flex come in fully covered and partly covered stent-grafts.

Essentially, retrievable stent-graft placement belongs to the school of prolonged dilation or splintering (see earlier) in which the stent dwells across the benign central/anastomotic biliary stricture, stretching it for months and remodeling the biliary stricture during this dwell period.[2] The issue is how long to keep the covered stent in place to allow remodeling and prevent restenosis. Theoretically, if the stent-graft is removed before a certain dwell time (time x) the stricture will restenose as if it was a dilation, and the only time "bought" would be the dwell time of the stent (Fig. 135-10).[2] However, beyond a certain dwell time (time x) where enough remodeling has occurred, the actual patency of the benign biliary stricture will be improved (stay open longer). This particular dwell time (time x), if this hypothesis is correct, is still to be determined and is the subject of current investigation, primarily in Europe.[2]

COMPLICATIONS

The overall risk of major and minor complications is 4% to 12%.[2-4,13,18] Major complications can be classified into traumatic complications or postprocedural infectious complications (cholangitis with or without sepsis). Hemobilia not requiring blood transfusion is considered a minor complication and has been described in up to 10% of cases.[3] Major traumatic complications occur in 0% to 5.6% of cases (see Table 135-1),[2-4,13,18] and these include anastomotic rupture/biliary leak (0%-1.9%), hemobilia requiring transfusion (0%-1.9%), and pseudoaneurysm formation (0%-0.5%).[3,4,18] Postdilation cholangitis with or without sepsis is actually rarely mentioned.[2-4,13,18] This author does not believe transhepatic balloon dilation of benign biliary strictures adds to the risk of cholangitis or sepsis after a routine biliary drain cholangiogram and biliary drain exchange, which has a cholangitis rate and a sepsis rate of 2.1% and 0.4%, respectively.[21]

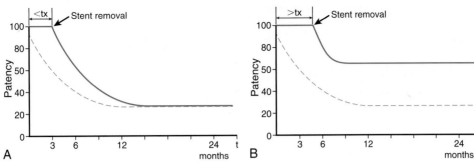

FIGURE 135-10. Graphs depicting hypothetical response of biliary anastomotic patency after stent removal, depending on dwell time of covered stents in biliary tract. **A,** Graph depicting hypothetical response of biliary anastomotic patency after covered stents have dwelled in biliary tract for less than time x (<tx). *Time x* refers to a hypothetical time period before which, if stents were removed (removed prematurely), there will be no increase in patency of biliary anastomoses. **B,** Graph depicting hypothetical response of biliary anastomotic patency after covered stents have dwelled in biliary tract for more than or equal to time x (>tx). Hypothetically, a particular dwell time for covered stent is required to achieve desired effect of improved patency after stent removal. Premature stent removal (<tx) before this particular dwell time does not lead to improved patency, but stent retrieval after this particular dwell time (>tx) may lead to improved patency. This particular dwell time, if the theory is correct, is to be determined and is the subject of current investigation. *(From Saad WEA. Percutaneous management of postoperative anastomotic biliary strictures. Tech Vasc Interv Radiol 2008;11:143–53.)*

Covered stents (stent-grafts) have two main complications: migration (up to 25% of cases) and potential occlusion.

POSTPROCEDURAL AND FOLLOW-UP CARE

After each over-the-wire biliary dilation session, the balloon is removed and replaced with an internal-external PTBD.[2-4,13,18] Removal of the catheter depends on the "school of management" (see earlier). If prolonged splintering of the stricture is the preferred approach, the drain is removed 4 to 12 months after the dilation. If fast-track balloon dilation is preferred (and if there is residual stenosis < 20%-30%), the transhepatic biliary drain is externalized (pigtail placed above the level of the target stricture) and capped for up to 1 to 2 weeks. If the patient tolerates capping and the cholangiogram continues to show adequate biliary patency, the external biliary drain is removed.

- Two schools/approaches exist: (1) chronic percutaneous biliary drainage ± balloon dilations and (2) sequential balloon dilation.
- Aggressive balloon dilation (e.g., cutting balloons) have improved technical results.
- The 1- to 3-year patency of transhepatic balloon dilation of benign biliary strictures ranges 33% to 67%.
- Removable stent-grafts may be a better management option, but well-designed studies are needed to verify this assertion.

▶ SUGGESTED READINGS

Cantwell CP, Pena CS, Gervais DA, et al. Thirty years' experience with balloon dilation of benign postoperative biliary strictures: Long-term outcomes. Radiology 2008;249:1050–7.

Saad WE, Saad NE, Davies MG, et al. Transhepatic balloon dilation of anastomotic biliary strictures in liver transplant recipients: The significance of a patent hepatic artery. J Vasc Interv Radiol 2005;16:1221–8.

Saad WE. Percutaneous management of postoperative anastomotic biliary strictures. Tech Vasc Interv Radiol 2008;11:143–53.

The complete reference list is available online at www.expertconsult.com.

KEY POINTS

- Benign biliary strictures are difficult to manage, probably because of the cicatricial fibrotic nature of the lesions.
- There are numerous variables in etiology, pathology, locations, and management techniques for benign biliary strictures.

CHAPTER 136

Management of Biliary Leaks

Rupert H. Portugaller and Klaus A. Hausegger

Biliary leakage is defined as diversion of bile via a defect in the ductal wall leading to the formation of bilomas, fistulas, or free spillage into the peritoneal cavity. It is a common complication after liver and biliary surgery. With emerging laparoscopic techniques and transplantation, the rate of bile leakage is reported to range from 0.8% to 12%.[1-4] Massive hepatic trauma with subsequent biliary leakage has also been reported.[5] Leaks can originate from biliary-enteric anastomoses, choledochocholedochostomy, bile or cystic duct stumps, cystohepatic ducts, blind-ending aberrant bile ducts (*ducts of Luschka*),[6] intraoperative bile duct injury, or ablation of the surface of the liver, or they may be due to loose or dislocated T-tube drainage.[7] Biliary anastomotic or T-tube exit site leaks attract early attention, whereas symptoms from bile duct necrosis occur relatively late[3] (Fig. 136-1).

Small leaks can be managed conservatively with antibiotics and maintenance of perioperatively placed drains,[8] but massive biliary extravasation can result in bilomas, fistulas, or biliary peritonitis, with subsequent abscess formation and sepsis. Patients usually have localized or diffuse abdominal pain and tenderness and fever and chills. Jaundice is indicative of concomitant biliary strictures. Leukocytosis and elevated C-reactive protein levels are signs of active inflammation. Older patients, however, may lack typical symptoms. Because biliary leakage can provoke a life-threatening condition, early diagnosis and therapy are crucial. Intravenous administration of broad-spectrum antibiotics is mandatory. When bile or blood cultures are available, specific antibiotic therapy is initiated. Bilomas should be diverted percutaneously under ultrasound or computed tomography (CT) guidance or with perioperatively placed drains. Irrigation and low-pressure suction prevent stasis of fluid in a closed space and thus decrease the likelihood of infection.[9,10]

INDICATIONS

- Major biliary leakage unlikely to resolve spontaneously (ongoing abdominal drainage of a significant amount of bilious fluid)
- Surgical therapy not necessary (definitive healing of the leakage expected after endoluminal decompression alone)
- Surgical therapy impossible because of extensive tissue adhesions (previous operations)
- Poor patient condition, with high anesthesiology risk
- Endoscopic management not possible because of
  - Enteric Roux-en-Y anastomosis
  - Recent duodenotomy (air insufflation can cause rupture of the suture)

- Inability to probe the duodenal papilla or the common/hepatic bile duct
- Inability to negotiate an additional biliary stricture retrogradely

In patients with massive biliary peritonitis, surgical revision and peritoneal lavage are usually necessary. Bile duct transection or disruption requires surgical therapy as well. In contrast to the blind-ending ducts of Luschka, the cystohepatic ducts drain liver parenchyma. Thus, injuries to the cystohepatic ducts must be treated by either surgical biliary reconstruction or diversion to the jejunum.[6]

If surgical treatment is not necessary or impossible, endoluminal biliary drainage is indicated for persistent biliary leakage. The principle of healing a bile leak is to create a low-pressure system along the biliary tract by means of internal or external drainage. Endoscopic therapy with nasobiliary drainage, sphincterotomy, or placement of an endoprosthesis has been reported to result in a high closure rate of up to 82%.[11-13] Because percutaneous transhepatic access is more invasive, endoscopic retrograde cholangiopancreatography (ERCP) is recommended as the first option. However, when the duodenum or the common bile duct cannot be cannulated, percutaneous transhepatic biliary drainage (PTBD) is the only endoluminal treatment option. PTBD serves to decompress the biliary system and redirect bile flow from the defect into the bile ducts. This may lead to sufficient healing of the leakage that additional surgery is not necessary (see Fig. 136-1). In critically ill patients, PTBD may allow the patient's condition to improve before subsequent definitive surgery (Fig. 136-2).

CONTRAINDICATIONS

- Coagulopathy that cannot be corrected. Because the risk of uncontrollable hemorrhage from the liver is high in patients with coagulopathy, every effort should be made to correct or improve coagulation status before the procedure.[14]
- History of allergies to contrast material. During hepatic puncture for PTBD, contrast material is likely to be injected into blood vessels before a bile duct is opacified. If a patient is known to be allergic to contrast agents, cortisone and antihistamine should be used prophylactically.

EQUIPMENT

A modern C-arm unit with pulsed fluoroscopy is desirable because fluoroscopy times can be extensive when probing nondilated bile ducts. Apart from the anesthesiology

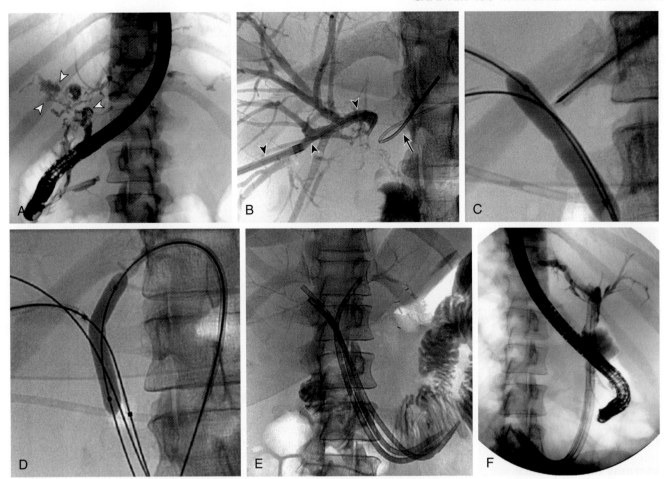

FIGURE 136-1. This 29-year-old woman underwent surgical resection of retropancreatic teratoma. Intraoperative injury to portal vessels resulted in massive hemorrhage with subsequent multiorgan failure. Pancreas and spleen had to be resected, and a venous bypass was performed to bridge iatrogenic occlusion of celiac trunk. Eight months later, patient had jaundice. **A,** Endoscopic retrograde cholangiopancreatography (ERCP) demonstrated a complex central biliary lesion with leakage *(arrowheads)* that was probably due to bile duct ischemia. **B,** Percutaneous transhepatic puncture of right *(arrowheads)* and left *(arrow)* biliary tract was performed. **C,** Because occlusion of left hepatic duct could not be negotiated with a guidewire, balloon-targeted needle passage was successfully performed. **D,** Left hepatic duct was predilated with a balloon. **E,** Finally, biliary system was drained internally by three percutaneously implanted plastic stents. **F,** One year later, because ERCP demonstrated no further biliary leakage and patent bile ducts, plastic stents were removed endoscopically.

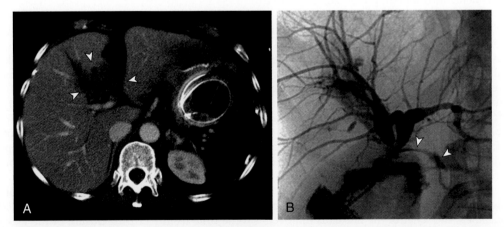

FIGURE 136-2. This 64-year-old woman with pancreatic carcinoma underwent duodenopancreatectomy (Whipple technique). Persistent bilious effluence from abdominal drain and signs of bilious peritonitis occurred. **A,** Abdominal computed tomography study revealed free fluid at porta hepatis *(arrowheads)*. Because postoperative course was complicated by cardiac insufficiency, no repeated laparotomy was performed. **B,** Percutaneous transhepatic cholangiography on postoperative day 8 showed leakage at bilioenteric anastomosis *(arrowheads)*, with free spillage of contrast material into abdominal cavity. Right and left hepatic ducts were narrowed at site of anastomosis, probably because of edema.

equipment, in our unit the following material is at the interventionist's disposal:

- 5- and 10-mL syringes; sterile swabs
- Nonionic water-soluble contrast agent (300-370 mg iodine/mL)
- Local anesthetic: 5 to 10 mL of 2% lidocaine; injection needles
- Single-puncture technique: Neff Percutaneous Access Set (William Cook Europe, Bjaeverskov, Denmark):
  - Small-gauge stainless steel access needle with an inner stylet
  - 0.018-inch guidewire
  - Coaxial introducer system consisting of three parts: an outer sheath, an inner tapered introducer, and an innermost metal stiffening cannula
- 0.035-inch hydrophilic Radiofocus guidewire M (Terumo Medical Corp., Tokyo, Japan)
- 5F Angled Taper Glidecath (Terumo)
- 0.035-inch Amplatz Extra Stiff guidewire (William Cook Europe)
- 8.3F ring, Lunderquist biliary drainage catheter
- 3-0 cutaneous suture
- 10F and 12F Munich drainage catheters (Peter Pflugbeil GmbH, Zorneding, Germany): perforated bile duct drainage with a special flange (perforation distance, 7.5, 10, or 15 cm), connecting tube, sealing cap, and adapter
- Bandage material

TECHNIQUE

Anatomy and Approach

Biliary leakage is suspected when persistent bilious-looking effluent from the abdominal drain is noted. Injection of contrast material through the drain may result in opacification of a bile duct.[15] Before PTBD, contrast-enhanced CT or magnetic resonance imaging (MRI) yields important anatomic information. Bilomas or fistulas, as well as abscesses, are especially well visualized with magnetic resonance cholangiopancreatography (MRCP),[16] and the site of the bile leak may be tentatively established. Though more investigator dependent, ultrasonography is an alternative preinterventional imaging method.[8]

Generally, PTBD for biliary leakage is performed in similar fashion as for biliary obstruction. However, in 88% to 100% of cases, the intrahepatic bile ducts are not dilated or only minimally dilated, and hence more difficult to cannulate.[5,8,15,17] The percutaneous access site is chosen according to the estimated site of leakage, because the biliary drainage catheter should finally be able to cross the injured portion of the bile duct.

A single-puncture technique is acceptable for nondilated bile ducts.[16] This technique requires that the initial puncture be appropriate for definitive catheter placement (Fig. 136-3). After hepatic puncture, the access needle is slowly withdrawn while contrast material is gently injected. When a bile duct is opacified, the stylet of the needle is removed and a 0.018-inch guidewire is advanced into the biliary system. After removal of the cannula, the locked coaxial introducer system is pushed over the guidewire into the bile duct. The metal stiffener is unlocked from the catheter, and only the catheter with its dilator is advanced. After

the 0.018-inch guidewire, tapered dilator, and metal stiffener are pulled out, a 0.035-inch hydrophilic steerable guidewire is advanced into the bowel lumen. Once the intestine has been entered, the hydrophilic guidewire is exchanged for a 0.035-inch extrastiff guidewire (Amplatz type). After dilation of the hepatic puncture tract, an 8.3F self-retaining loop catheter (Lunderquist biliary drainage catheter) is introduced for external/internal biliary drainage. Catheter side holes must be located on both sides of the bile leak to keep intraluminal resistance as low as possible.

Technical Aspects

Sometimes the initial puncture site reveals a bile duct too central for definitive drainage because of the presence of major vessels. In such cases, cholangiography can be performed over the puncture needle. Then, with the double-puncture technique, a proper bile duct is targeted and punctured again with the access needle under fluoroscopic guidance.

If biliary ascites is present, leakage of acidic fluid along the percutaneous puncture route often causes skin irritation. Additional drainage of peritoneal fluid helps minimize puncture tract extravasation.

CONTROVERSIES

There is controversy about when to remove the biliary drainage catheter. Whereas some authors remove the catheter when cholangiography shows that the leak has healed without residual stenosis,[15,17] others keep the tubes in place for a certain period after it has been proved that the leak has sealed.[10] Because no randomized studies have compared early and late catheter removal, no definitive advice can be given for catheter dwell time. Ernst et al. encountered residual stenoses in 4 of 16 patients after PTBD. They suggested that use of a large drainage catheter (12F) and drainage for at least 7 to 8 weeks might prevent secondary biliary stenosis after closure of the leak.[15]

OUTCOMES

Technical success of PTBD is defined as placement of the tube to provide continuous drainage of bile. The Society of Interventional Radiology has established a success threshold of 70% for percutaneous cannulation of nondilated bile ducts.[14] In a series of 130 patients with nondilated bile ducts, a technical success rate of 90% has been reported.[16] In case of biliary leakage, procedural success means either closure of a biliary leak with sole percutaneous biliary drainage or improvement of the patient's condition such that definitive surgical repair is possible. Table 136-1 presents the outcomes reported by several authors.*

For biliary leakage, PTBD has been reported to be effective in 50% to 100% of patients without additional surgery. The time from PTBD to closure of the leak ranged from 7 to 150 days (mean, 10-80 days), and the time to catheter removal ranged from 7 to 274 days. Reasons for extended catheter dwell time after closure of the leak were

*References 5, 7, 8, 10, 12, 15, 17-20.

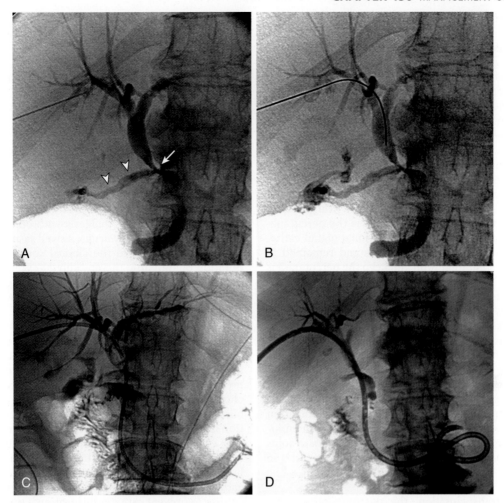

FIGURE 136-3. This 88-year-old-woman with contained perforation of an inflamed gallbladder underwent open cholecystectomy. Operation was complicated by extensive inflammatory tissue alterations. **A,** Postoperatively, percutaneous single puncture of a right intrahepatic bile duct revealed biliary extravasation from cystic duct stump *(arrowheads)* and stricture in common hepatic/common bile duct *(arrow)*. After probing biliary system with 0.018-inch guidewire **(B),** an 8.3F catheter was placed for internal/external drainage **(C). D,** Two weeks later, inflammatory markers had decreased, and only cystic duct stump without further bile extravasation was seen. A 12F Munich drainage catheter was placed and kept on internal drainage.

TABLE 136-1. Outcomes of Percutaneous Transhepatic Biliary Drainage for Biliary Leakage

	n	Technical Success	Leak Healing	Procedural Success	Closure Time (days)	Catheter Dwell Time (days)	Complications	Follow-up (months)
Ernst et al.[15]	16	16 (100%)	13 (81%)	13 (81%)	78 (30-150)	n.s.	2 (12%)	38 (11-76)
Kaufman et al.[5]	12	12 (100%)	6 (50%)	6 (50%)	27 (9-61)	140 (61-274)	3 (25%)	n.s.
Zhang et al.[7]	4	4 (100%)	2 (50%)	3 (75%)	14-21	n.s.	0 (0%)	n.s.
de Castro et al.[8]	11	11 (100%)	9 (90%)	9 (90%)	n.s.	n.s.	0 (0%)	n.s.
Vaccaro et al.[10]	3	3 (100%)	3 (100%)	3 (100%)	25-75	46-70	0 (0%)	36
Tsukamoto et al.[12]	3	3 (100%)	2 (100%)	2 (100%)	14	14	0 (0%)	72
Chen et al.[18]	2	2 (100%)	2 (100%)	2 (100%)	14	n.s.	0 (0%)	n.s.
Civelli et al.[20]	8	8 (100%)	5 (62%)	5 (62%)	80	n.s.	0 (0%)	18
Righi et al.[19]	22	22 (100%)	21 (91%)	21 (91%)	10 (7-41)	15 (7-74)	0 (0%)	36
Stampfl et al.[17]	30	30 (100%)	22 (73%)	22 (73%)	55 (15-116)	55 (15-116)	2 (7%)	n.s.

n.s., Not specified.

concomitant strictures or calculi that were also treated percutaneously.

If PTBD fails to seal a biliary leak, bile duct necrosis, complete duct disruption, or extensive laceration is frequently responsible. Typical signs of procedural failures include persistent septic states and continuous outflow of bile-stained fluid from abdominal drains.

Gwon et al. used retrievable covered stents (Song retrievable stent [Taewoong Medical, Kimpo, Korea]) in complex biliary leakages.[21] Eleven patients with major bile leaks (>500 mL drained bile/24 h) or leaks with concomitant biliary strictures untreatable by endoscopic means or refractory bile leaks despite more than 10 days of external/internal drainage were included in their study. In all patients, the covered stents could be introduced via the percutaneous transhepatic puncture tracts. Additional pigtail catheters were placed coaxially in the stents and remained in place to prevent stent migration and keep the percutaneous puncture tracts patent until stent retrieval. Via the PTBD tracts, all covered stents were removed successfully after a mean of 31 days (range, 14-64 days). In all patients, sealing of the bile leaks without biliary stenosis was proven by cholangiography. The PTBD catheters were extracted after a mean indwelling period of 41 days (range, 20-80 days). No recurrent biliary leakages were noted after a mean follow-up of 366 days (range, 215-730 days).

Endoscopic stent placement has been reported to be effective in sealing biliary leaks in 71% of cases. Cannulation of the bile duct could not be achieved in 4%.[11] With endoscopically placed retrievable covered stents, 100% resolutions were achieved after a mean stent dwell time of 156 days (range, 67-493 days) in 11 patients with complex bile leaks.[22]

After liver transplantation, the outcome of patients with anastomotic bile leaks or leaks from bile duct necrosis is relatively poor. Even after surgical revision, a death rate of 32% has been reported in a series of 34 patients. All deaths were associated with uncontrollable sepsis.[3]

COMPLICATIONS

Because bile ducts are often nondilated in patients with biliary leakage, the complication rate of PTBD for this indication may exceed that of PTBD for biliary obstructive disease. The frequency of complications is shown in Table 136-1 and ranged from 0% to 25%.[5,15] Most authors did not differentiate minor from major complications. There is one report of PTBD in 130 patients with nondilated bile ducts performed for different indications, not just for biliary leakage. Major procedure-related complications occurred in 4%.[16] Hemobilia secondary to arterial injury has been reported, as well as arterial bleeding after catheter removal. If bleeding does not stop spontaneously, selective arterial embolization is the treatment of choice. In another study, subcapsular hepatic hematoma developed in a patient with necrotizing pancreatitis after PTBD and was treated by laparotomy. However, the patient died of recurrent bleeding.[15] Lethal gastrointestinal hemorrhage from duodenal ulcer has also been reported.[5] Residual biliary stenosis occurred in up to 31% and was managed successfully by balloon dilation or stent insertion.[15] Metabolic acidosis

secondary to continuous bile loss from external drainage was treated successfully by fluid replacement and administration of bicarbonate.[5] Intermittent fever with chills after catheter exchange is a minor complication that can be prevented by prophylactic single-dose administration of antibiotics.

POSTPROCEDURAL AND FOLLOW-UP CARE

Immediately after PTBD, patients are kept in a recovery room under cardiovascular monitoring. Depending on their general condition, they return to a normal ward or to an intensive care unit. Analgesia with opioids and nonsteroidal antiinflammatory drugs, as well as antibiotic therapy, continues according to the clinical course. Generally, the duration of antibiotic therapy should exceed the decline in clinical symptoms and inflammation by a few days. Patient monitoring plus replacement of bile losses with intravenous fluid and electrolytes is necessary during external biliary drainage.[5]

The percutaneous biliary drainage catheter can be irrigated during the first postinterventional days, but irrigation must be performed gently to prevent any intraductal overpressure that may keep the leak patent. Frequent catheter cholangiograms are performed during the patient's hospitalization. When a significant reduction in biliary extravasation is noted, drainage is internalized. Before discharge, the 8.3F catheter is exchanged for a larger softer catheter. For instance, a 10F or 12F Munich catheter with various sidehole configurations can be introduced. The outer end of this catheter has the form of a flat hat with holes for placing sutures to prevent catheter dislocation. Using a special connection tube, additional external drainage or irrigation is possible. Regular sterile cleaning and bandaging of the catheter access site must be performed by an instructed relative, a nurse, or the family doctor to prevent access-related infections. Patients should not take baths or go swimming. They can take showers, with the tubes protected by plastic covering that is impervious to water.

The time needed to heal a biliary leak extends beyond that required for drainage of an associated biloma.[9] Prolonged biliary drainage for several weeks to months may be necessary. Catheters are usually exchanged every 2 months on an outpatient basis.[5] If abdominal pain and signs of infection recur, the patient should immediately go to the interventional unit for testing of tube patency and eventual catheter exchange.

If no further biliary leak is demonstrated on repeated cholangiograms and the patient is doing well, the drainage catheter is exchanged for a catheter of smaller diameter that has no side holes and therefore no draining function. This tube is left in place to preserve biliary access and let the hepatic puncture tract gradually contract. After a test period of about 4 weeks, the catheter can be removed, provided the bile ducts are normal and the patient is free of complaints.

Associated biliary strictures can be treated percutaneously[23] (Fig. 136-4). However, complete sealing of the biliary defect is advocated before cholangioplasty is performed at the site of the former leak. Otherwise, repeated rupture may occur when the duct wall is stressed.

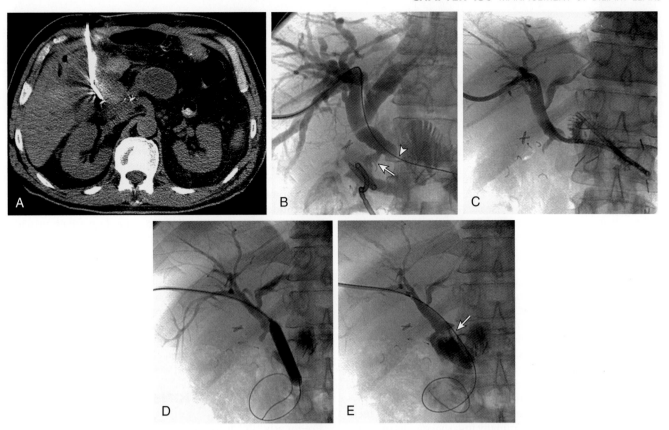

FIGURE 136-4. Carcinoma of duodenal papilla in a 55-year-old man. After duodenopancreatectomy (Whipple technique) and cholecystectomy, patient was evaluated for jaundice and persistent biliary effluence from abdominal drain. **A,** Under computed tomography guidance, a subhepatic fluid collection was drained percutaneously. **B,** Percutaneous transhepatic cholangiography revealed extravasation of bile from cystic duct stump *(arrow)* as well as stricture at biliodigestive anastomosis *(arrowhead).* **C,** Three weeks after percutaneous transhepatic biliary drainage (PTBD), no further bile extravasation was noted. Repeat dilation of biliodigestive anastomosis with a 10/40-mm balloon catheter **(D)** finally resulted in bile flow into jejunum **(E)** *(arrow).* Percutaneous access was discontinued 5 months after initiation of PTBD.

KEY POINTS

- Elderly patients can lack clinical symptoms of biliary leakage.
- Whereas small bile leaks may be managed conservatively, ongoing biliary leakage has to be treated by endoscopic or percutaneous biliary decompression or surgical repair.
- Because percutaneous biliary drainage (PTBD) is more invasive, it should be performed only when endoscopic relief is not possible.
- In biliary leakage, the bile ducts are frequently not dilated.
- In complex lesions, a biliary drainage catheter should cross the injured part of the bile duct with its side holes above and below the leak.
- Prolonged dwell time of the drainage catheter is recommended after bile leak closure.
- Retrievable covered stents can be used to treat complex biliary leaks.

► **SUGGESTED READINGS**

Vecchio R, MacFadyen BV, Ricardo AE. Bile duct injury: management options during and after gallbladder surgery. Semin Laparosc Surg 1998;5:135–44.

The complete reference list is available online at www.expertconsult.com.

CHAPTER 137

Percutaneous Cholecystostomy

Thomas M. Fahrbach, Gerald M. Wyse, Leo P. Lawler, and Hyun S. Kim

CLINICAL RELEVANCE

Acute cholecystitis (AC) is a prevalent condition that carries significant risks of morbidity and mortality.[1] AC may present with a spectrum of disease stages ranging from a mild self-limited illness to a fulminant potentially life-threatening illness.[2] Laparoscopic or open surgical removal of the inflamed gallbladder remains the gold-standard therapy when the patient is a surgical candidate.[3,4] However, because surgery requires general anesthesia, incisions, and postoperative recuperation, percutaneous cholecystostomy (PC) has served to largely replace surgery in patients who have significant comorbidities or anatomic variations that may preclude or delay surgical therapy.[5-8] This minimally invasive nonsurgical approach has in fact been suggested as definitive therapy in critically ill and elderly patients,[9] as well as to provide a bridge to surgery.[10,11] The overall goal of PC is gallbladder decompression and drainage for prevention of gallbladder perforation and sepsis.[12-16] The technique of PC also offers a minimally invasive means of access to the biliary system for other interventions such as stent placement and stone retrieval.[17-20]

INDICATIONS

As just noted, there are primarily two clinical reasons patients are referred for cholecystostomy: (1) to decompress the gallbladder for management of cholecystitis[21] or (2) to provide a portal of access to the biliary tract for therapeutic purposes.[22]

A multidisciplinary approach to determine whether to proceed with PC is ideal and should be guided by clinical symptomatology, laboratory data, and supporting imaging evidence.[22] The clinical manifestations of cholecystitis include fever, elevated white blood cell count, right upper quadrant pain, and Murphy sign. Patients may suffer from either calculous or acalculous cholecystitis (Figs. 137-1 to 137-4).[23,24] Those with calculous cholecystitis have gallstones and possibly sludge causing mechanical obstruction of the cystic duct. The exact pathogenesis of acalculous cholecystitis is unclear but tends to occur in the critically ill, debilitated, or intensive care patients. Associations with diabetes, malignant disease, vasculitis, and congestive heart failure also exist,[25] as well as being secondary to mechanical obstruction of the cystic duct from biliary stent placement in the common bile duct. Empirical cholecystostomy may be indicated in patients with fever of unknown origin or other clinical evidence of sepsis where there is no apparent source other than classic imaging features of cholecystitis.

Sonographic, computed tomography (CT), or magnetic resonance imaging (MRI) findings of uncomplicated cholecystitis include gallbladder wall thickening, pericholecystic fluid/stranding, gallbladder distension, sonographic Murphy sign (right upper quadrant pain with probe pressure), or a gallstone impacted in the neck of the gallbladder or cystic duct.[26,27] Findings of complicated cholecystitis such as pericholecystic abscess, intraluminal membranes, and/or gas suggest a gangrenous or perforated gallbladder.[28] Hepatobiliary nuclear scintigraphy with technetium (Tc)-99m iminodiacetic acid derivatives provides highly specific diagnostic confirmation, with nonvisualization of the gallbladder at 4 hours suggesting cystic duct obstruction and cholecystitis.[29]

Cholecystostomy may also be employed as a means to access the biliary system when transhepatic or endoscopic routes are not feasible or contraindicated. This portal to the biliary system provides a pathway for a variety of therapeutic interventions, including internal/external biliary drain placement, metallic stent placement, gallstone extraction, dissolution, lithotripsy, and even gallbladder ablation.

CONTRAINDICATIONS

Frequently, PC is performed in gravely ill and high-risk patients, and there are few absolute contraindications. Interposed bowel (e.g., as in Chilaiditi syndrome) may preclude safe access to the gallbladder. Coagulopathy is a relative contraindication, and a severe bleeding diathesis may not allow transhepatic access. Other relative contraindications include gallbladder tumor that may be seeded by percutaneous access, or a gallbladder greatly distended by calculi that prevent drainage tube formation and locking (Fig. 137-5). Finally, it may be difficult or impossible to place a PC tube in a perforated decompressed gallbladder.

EQUIPMENT

Percutaneous access to the gallbladder can be achieved via direct image guidance with ultrasound, fluoroscopy, or CT. The preferred method of ultrasound guidance is normally performed with a midrange frequency 2- to 8-Hz curvilinear array sector probe. The procedure may be performed at the bedside when necessary,[16,30] but catheter insertion is best performed in a fluoroscopy suite. Axial noncontrast CT may be used, and CT fluoroscopy tools are rarely necessary but may be helpful when a significantly diseased or calcular gallbladder limits sonographic visualization of the lumen.[31] Standard sterile technique should always be used.

Local anesthesia and moderate sedation with subcutaneous lidocaine 2% and intravenous (IV) midazolam and fentanyl is sufficient for the vast majority of patients, although critical care support is needed in critically ill patients. IV antibiotics with gram-negative coverage is administered.

The gallbladder is usually accessed with an 18G percutaneous entry needle or trocar needle, with length dependent on the distance measured to the gallbladder. A 21G micropuncture or 22G Chiba needle with a 0.018-inch wire may be employed with a wire guide exchange set that allows

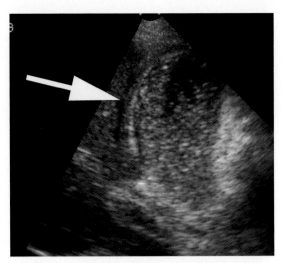

FIGURE 137-1. Ultrasound of acalculous cholecystitis showing a sludge-filled gallbladder with gallbladder wall thickening and pericholecystic fluid *(arrow)*.

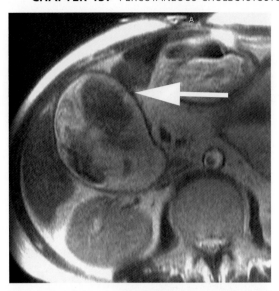

FIGURE 137-4. Axial T2-weighted magnetic resonance imaging shows a distended gallbladder with mixed signal within it *(arrow)*, consistent with blood products and hemorrhagic cholecystitis.

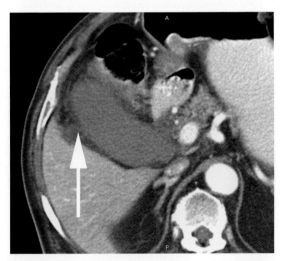

FIGURE 137-2. Axial contrast-enhanced computed tomography shows a distended gallbladder and stranding of pericholecystic fat *(arrow)*.

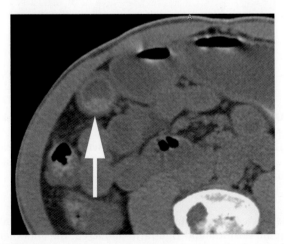

FIGURE 137-3. Axial noncontrast computed tomography shows multiple gallstones, increased attenuation in gallbladder mucosa, and edema of gallbladder wall *(arrow)*.

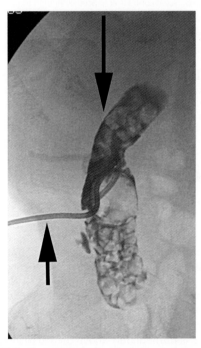

FIGURE 137-5. Contrast study through cholecystostomy catheter *(short black arrow)* shows a gallbladder packed with stones *(long black arrow)*. Note absence of cystic duct filling.

transition to a 0.035-inch system; 8F and 10F tissue dilators may be required. The biliary system is opacified with iodinated contrast such as Hypaque (diatrizoate sodium and diatrizoate meglumine [Nycomed Inc., Princeton, N.J.]). A 0.035-inch Rosen (Cook Medical, Bloomington, Ind.) or short Amplatz Super Stiff wire (Boston Scientific, Natick, Mass.) have the necessary stiffness to support drainage tube placement and may also be partly looped within the gallbladder. A self-retaining all-purpose drain with distal side holes (e.g., Flexima [Boston Scientific]) is used for gravity drainage and connected to a bag. A variety of

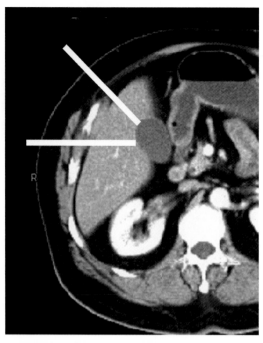

FIGURE 137-6. Axial contrast-enhanced computed tomography showing potential intercostal access routes *(white lines)* for transhepatic cholecystostomy.

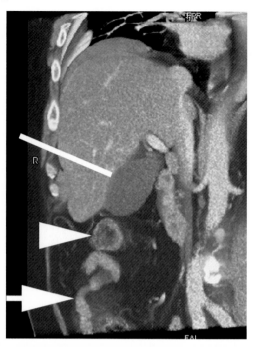

FIGURE 137-7. Coronal contrast-enhanced computed tomography shows an intercostal transhepatic route to gallbladder *(white line)*. Note close relationship of colon *(arrowhead)* and small bowel *(arrow)*.

cholangioplasty balloons, snares, and lithotripsy may be employed when gallstone extraction is contemplated. The gallbladder and biliary system may be directly visualized with a 15F choledochoscope, which will require an 18F tract.

TECHNIQUE

Anatomy and Approach

The gallbladder may be approached via one of two basic methods: transhepatic or transperitoneal. In general, the transhepatic route involves an arc from the right midaxillary line to the midclavicular line (Fig. 137-6), and hypothetically traverses the bare area of the gallbladder (superior third portion of the gallbladder).[31] A track is chosen below the diaphragm, which may or may not be intercostal. Intercostal access is immediately above the rib to avoid the neurovascular bundle (Fig. 137-7). It is important to exclude any ascending colon or hepatic flexure interposed between the liver and abdominal wall along the anticipated track. The transhepatic approach generally traverses segments 5 or 6 and enters the gallbladder through the gallbladder fossa (see Fig. 137-7). The transperitoneal approach is generally anterior or anterolateral, and similarly, interposed bowel must be excluded (Fig. 137-8).[21]

Technical Aspects

Fully informed consent is obtained. Prothrombin time or international normalized ratio (INR), partial thromboplastin time (PTT), and platelet count are checked, and any coagulopathy is corrected. Available imaging is reviewed

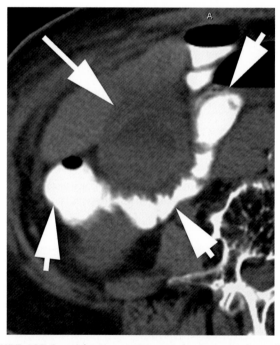

FIGURE 137-8. Axial noncontrast computed tomography shows sludge within gallbladder, a thickened gallbladder wall, and pericholecystic fluid *(long arrow)* in a patient with acalculous cholecystitis. Note close relationship of transverse colon *(short arrows)* along potential anterior or posterior approaches.

to assess a safe percutaneous window. With the patient in a supine position and right arm abducted, the abdomen is sonographically evaluated for determination of access site and the transhepatic/transperitoneal route to the gallbladder. Depth is measured for needle length selection. Under fluoroscopy, the level of the diaphragm and the planned level of access is marked, and a scout image is taken to avoid a transpulmonary or transpleural approach. Lidocaine 2% local anesthetic is applied, and a small nick is made at the needle puncture site. If necessary, the subcutaneous fat and muscle may be bluntly dissected with a curved forceps.

There are two methods for catheter placement when performing PC: the Seldinger technique or the trocar technique.[16] The Seldinger technique is better suited for difficult access or a small gallbladder and uses an 18G to 22G needle, which is advanced into the gallbladder under image guidance with visualization of the needle tip at all times. Upon aspiration of bile, contrast can be injected for cholecystography/cholangiography and to fluoroscopically confirm intraluminal placement within the gallbladder. A guidewire is then advanced through the needle and coiled within the gallbladder, taking care not to overdistend or stretch the inflamed gallbladder. An 8F to 10F self-retaining/locking all-purpose drain is then advanced into the gallbladder and fed off its stiffener to form it. Prior soft-tissue tract dilation may be required. The trocar technique is better suited to those with a large distended gallbladder that can be easily visualized with a clear percutaneous window. With the trocar technique, the needle tip is placed within the all-purpose drain, and the entire system is advanced into the gallbladder. This technique also has the advantage of a single step and access to the gallbladder with no exchanges over a wire. With either technique, the placed drain is formed, locked, and injected with a small amount of contrast (3-5 mL) to confirm position (Fig. 137-9). It is sutured to the skin and attached to a gravity bag. A sample of bile is sent for culture and Gram stain.[21]

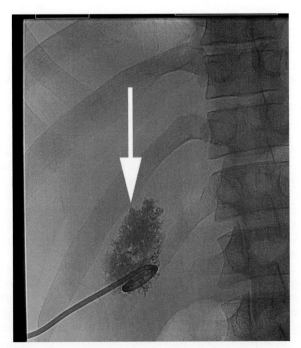

FIGURE 137-9. Contrast injection through cholecystostomy catheter shows irregular filling of gallbladder, characteristic of mucosal inflammation. Note absent cystic duct filling *(arrow)*.

EQUIPMENT

- Imaging:
  - 2- to 8-Hz ultrasound curvilinear array probe
  - Fluoroscopic systems: full angiographic suite, mobile C-arm
  - CT, with or without CT fluoroscopy
- Medications and contrast:
  - Gram-negative antibiotic coverage
  - Lidocaine 2%
  - Moderate sedation: midazolam, fentanyl
  - Contrast (e.g., Hypaque [diatrizoate sodium and diatrizoate meglumine])
- Access:
  - 18G percutaneous entry needle or trocar needle with 0.035-inch wire
  Or
  - 21G micropuncture or 22G Chiba with 0.018-inch wire and a transitional wire guide exchange set
  - 8F to 10F tissue tract dilators
- Wires:
  - 0.035-inch, 145-cm Rosen (Cook Medical, Bloomington, Ind.)
  Or
  - Short 0.035-inch, 75-cm Amplatz Super Stiff wire (Boston Scientific)
- Drain:
  - Self-retaining all-purpose drain (e.g., Flexima [Boston Scientific])
  - Drainage bag
  - 2-0 Prolene suture

CONTROVERSIES

The transhepatic approach for cholecystostomy drain placement is generally preferred. Advantages include a theoretical decreased risk of intraperitoneal bile leakage, more rapid tract maturation, and greater catheter stability as the decompressed gallbladder collapses toward the tube, thus preventing bile leak. If the bare area of the gallbladder was successfully targeted, any bile leak that does occur should be extraperitoneal. The transhepatic access is also more stable, because the less mobile point of access is better suited for exchanges or interventional procedures through the tract, especially in the setting of ascites. Decreased risks of bleeding and liver contamination with infected bile have been postulated with the transperitoneal approach, but concerns remain for an increased risk of bile spillage and subsequent peritonitis due to longer tract maturation time. The transperitoneal approach has also been associated with an increased risk of colon perforation, portal vessel injury, and displacement of the catheter after decompression of the gallbladder as the decompressing gallbladder recedes away from the catheter tip.[32] However, satisfactory results have been reported for the transperitoneal approach, and it may be considered favorable in patients with liver disease or coagulopathy. Its advocates note that the inflamed gallbladder is thickened and distended, so it is thus relatively immobile for ease of puncture.

Simple bile aspiration without drain placement for decompression of the gallbladder may suffice, and there are limited studies in support of this.[33] However, if aspiration fails to initially resolve the acute inflammation, the patient bears the risk, pain, and cost of a repeat procedure. The lack of definitive tube placement also prevents subsequent tube cholangiograms and biliary access.

OUTCOMES

The technique of cholecystostomy tube placement is relatively straightforward, and as such it has enjoyed good technical success in 95% to 100% of patients.[14,15,34-36] Technical failures occur with thick bilious aspirate not amenable for drainage, decompressed gallbladders, porcelain gallbladders, and pronounced gallbladder wall thickening. The results of clinical success are more varied with efficacy from 60 to over 90%.* This is in large measure due to the wide variation in patient clinical status and patient selection. Frequently a PC is requested in patients too sick for a definitive surgery, and frequently—despite successful cholecystostomy placement—they succumb to the other comorbidities, which are difficult to discriminate from the failure of biliary decompression.[1] Outcomes after PC for AC are better when the disease is primary and not precipitated by concurrent illness.[38] The best clinical results are in those with good clinical and imaging evidence of cholecystitis, and the response is rapid within 72 hours of placement.[15,16]

COMPLICATIONS

Major complications of PC are rare, and similar to most minimally invasive procedures, PC is considered low risk. Intraprocedural major complications include sepsis, peritonitis, abscess, hemorrhage, or transgression of adjacent structures, all of which are reported to occur in less than 3% of cases.[22] A recent critical review of peer-reviewed articles reports an intraprocedural death rate of 1.7%.[22]

The most common complication of PC is biliary leak, which may occur during placement or removal of catheters (Fig. 137-10).[34,39] The acutely inflamed gallbladder wall is friable and may perforate with wire or catheter manipulation. Upon catheter removal, major and minor bile leaks have been reported in 3% of patients.[39] Leakage may be self-limited and managed conservatively. Development of a biloma may require placement of an additional subhepatic drain. Large-volume contrast injections into the gallbladder may precipitate rigors and sepsis.

Without diligent evaluation of preprocedural imaging, transgression of surrounding structures may occur, with breaching of the pleural space or bowel, resulting in pneumothorax, bowel perforation, and fistula formation. Transpleural tubes must be removed and replaced because they can result in bile tracking into the pleural space, resulting in pleural reaction and effusion. Transpulmonary tubes will likely result in pneumothorax. If injury to bowel is questioned during the procedure, it may be confirmed by placing a sheath over the wire and injecting while pulling back. One may withdraw the wire or catheter immediately and replace or allow the tract to mature, creating a controlled fistula that may resolve with time if surgery is not an option. Alternately, some will primarily repair such

*References 12-14, 16, 21, 23, 34, 35, 37.

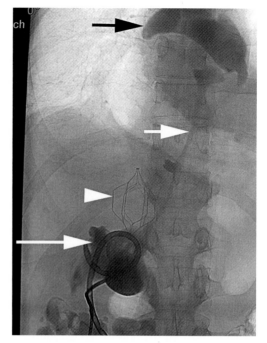

FIGURE 137-10. Contrast study through cholecystostomy catheter *(long white arrow)* shows a bile leak *(short white arrow)* tracting superiorly, with formation of a biloma within mediastinum *(black arrow)*. Arrowhead points to inferior vena cava filter.

injuries by surgery if clinically indicated. Hemorrhage may result from hepatic arterial, venous, or portal venous injury via transhepatic placement and may necessitate vascular intervention and embolization if hemodynamically significant. Most hemobilia is self-limited and responds well to tamponade by catheter upsizing.[21,40]

POSTPROCEDURE AND FOLLOW-UP CARE

Watchful monitoring of postprocedure vital signs and symptoms should occur initially at short intervals for the first 2 hours, and then every subsequent 2 to 4 hours. Antibiotic coverage should be adjusted based on the results of Gram stain and culture. The cholecystostomy catheter should be attached to external bag drainage to gravity and should be flushed with 5 to 10 mL normal saline twice daily. The tube should remain to external drainage and not be capped. Early cholecystograms are not required unless they will effect a management change. The tract is left to mature for 3 to 6 weeks; early removal after as little 14 days can be safe, but tract maturation may be prolonged in immunocompromised or critically ill patients.

Determination of tube removal depends on the initial intention-to-treat and clinical goals.[1] For acalculous cholecystitis, PC may be the definitive treatment, and the tube may be removed once the episode has passed. A tube cholangiogram is performed in anticipation of tube removal or subsequent cholecystectomy[11] to exclude cystic duct obstruction or extrahepatic biliary tract stones (Fig. 137-11).[19,20] Prior to tube removal, a clinical trial may be initiated by capping the drain for 48 hours to exclude recurrent cholecystitis. For calculous cholecystitis, the tube usually remains in place until cholecystectomy. Nonsurgical options of percutaneous stone removal require tract dilatation up to 18F or larger for stone extraction or lithotripsy using fluoroscopic or choledochoscope guidance (Fig. 137-12).[19,20]

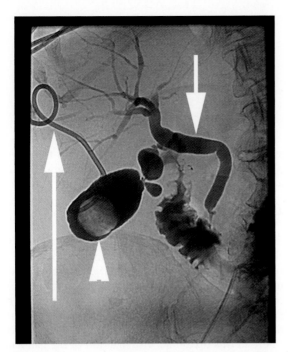

FIGURE 137-11. Contrast study through cholecystostomy catheter *(long arrow)* shows a large stone in gallbladder fundus *(arrowhead)*, with a patent cystic duct filling a stone-free common bile duct *(short arrow)*.

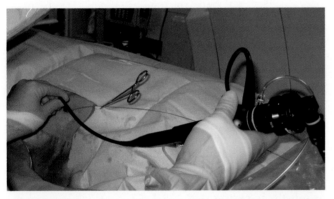

FIGURE 137-12. Photograph of a 15F cholangioscope being passed into biliary system for stone retrieval. Safety wire maintains biliary system access.

KEY POINTS

- Acute cholecystitis (AC) is a prevalent condition that may present with a spectrum of disease stages ranging from a mild self-limited illness to a fulminant potentially life-threatening illness.

- Percutaneous cholecystostomy is a minimally invasive non-surgical treatment proven to be a safe and effective first-line therapy for AC.

- Cholecystostomy offers an alternate interventional access to the biliary system for other biliary procedures.

► **SUGGESTED READINGS**

Ginat D, Saad WE. Cholecystostomy and transcholecystic biliary access. Tech Vasc Interv Radiol 2008;11(1):2–13. Review. PubMed PMID: 18725137.

Joseph T, Unver K, Hwang GL, et al. Percutaneous cholecystostomy for acute cholecystitis: ten-year experience. J Vasc Interv Radiol 2012;23(1):83–8.e1. Epub 2011 Nov 30. PubMed PMID: 22133709.

Pomerantz BJ. Biliary tract interventions.Tech Vasc Interv Radiol 2009;12(2):162–70. Review. PubMed PMID: 19853234.

Saad WE, Wallace MJ, Wojak JC, et al. Quality improvement guidelines for percutaneous transhepatic cholangiography, biliary drainage, and percutaneous cholecystostomy. J Vasc Interv Radiol 2010;21(6):789–95. Epub 2010 Mar 21. PubMed PMID: 20307987.

The complete reference list is available online at www.expertconsult.com.

CHAPTER 138

Management of Biliary Calculi

Daniel B. Brown and Daniel D. Picus

CLINICAL RELEVANCE

Symptomatic gallstones affect 260,000 Americans every year.[1] The majority of patients are treated definitively with surgery, and with the advent of laparoscopic cholecystectomy, surgeons can treat patients less invasively and allow for a quicker recovery. Even in the setting of laparoscopic cholecystectomy, significant medical comorbidities will make some patients unsuitable candidates for surgery. This group can greatly benefit from percutaneous drainage and staged stone extraction. Patients with symptomatic gallstones often simultaneously have calculi in the intrahepatic or extrahepatic bile ducts. Endoscopic retrograde cholangiopancreatography (ERCP) is the principle technique to clear these stones in the majority of patients.[2] However, in patients with challenging anatomy (duodenal diverticulum, impacted stones > 15 mm), endoscopic techniques are more prone to failure. Finally, patients who have undergone previous biliary reconstruction as part of a Billroth II or Roux-en-Y anastomosis may be inaccessible via endoscopy, and intrahepatic calculi in these patients may require percutaneous removal.

INDICATIONS

Indications for percutaneous biliary stone management are relatively straightforward. The principal indication for gallstone extraction is treatment of symptomatic calculi in patients who are not candidates for surgery. The majority of patients with retained biliary duct stones following surgery will be referred following failed ERCP. If hepatolithiasis is diagnosed shortly after surgery and the patient still has a surgical T-tube in place, some surgeons will primarily refer these patients for interventional radiologic management. Peripheral to the hilum of the liver, intraductal calculi are beyond the reach of virtually all endoscopists, and percutaneous management plays a larger role.

CONTRAINDICATIONS

The primary absolute contraindication is the presence of an uncorrectable coagulopathy; bleeding complications are a significant source of morbidity when using large-bore percutaneous transhepatic tracts. Relative contraindications include a nondistensible gallbladder and the presence of active infection. Gallstone extraction can be challenging if not impossible in a chronically diseased, contracted gallbladder. Lack of distensibility can limit needle access and tract dilation. In patients with active infection related to stone disease, appropriate drainage catheter(s) must be placed, with a "cooling off" period to limit septicemia during or following stone extraction. One author has reported successful treatment of a patient with unrelenting fevers secondary to an infected stone burden.[3] Only clearance of the stones allowed this patient's fever to clear. In the majority of patients, drainage and appropriate antibiotics for 24 to 48 hours will allow recovery to perform stone extraction.

EQUIPMENT

Much of the equipment used for percutaneous stone extraction is familiar to trained interventional radiologists. Procedures are staged so initially patients will undergo drainage of the gallbladder with either a locking loop retention catheter or placement of an external or (preferably) internal-external biliary drainage catheter. Details of these initial drainage procedures and required equipment are described elsewhere in this textbook. Visualization of the gallbladder and biliary ducts is performed with injections of ionic contrast material unless the patient has a significant contrast allergy, in which case the patient is premedicated with corticosteroids, and nonionic contrast material is used.

To perform stone removal, we use a 15F flexible choledochoscope (model CHF-4B [Olympus, New Hyde Park, N.Y.]) (Fig. 138-1, *A*). The scope contains a working channel that allows use of standard instruments measuring up to 5F in diameter, including graspers and baskets. The existing tube tract is dilated to 18F with a series of Teflon dilators (Cook Medical, Bloomington, Ind.) (Fig. 138-1, *B*). The outer Teflon sheath allows easy passage of the choledochoscope into the biliary tree, providing a large-bore access to flush out stone debris during the procedure. The scope is connected to continuous normal saline irrigation during use. A principal advantage of the choledochoscope is that it allows the operator to characterize filling defects identified at cholangiography as stones, mucus, air bubbles, clots, or soft-tissue masses (Fig. 138-1, *C*).

For stones that are too large to dislodge and fragment with baskets or other tools, we perform intracorporeal electrohydraulic lithotripsy (EHL). The principle of intracorporeal EHL is similar to extracorporeal EHL. A spark from the electrode generates a shockwave in the fluid medium of the gallbladder or bile duct, which then fragments the stone. We use a foot pedal–controlled EHL shockwave generator (EL-115 [American ACMI, Stamford, Conn.]) with 70- to 80-watt power output. The EHL electrode (Northgate, Chicago, Ill.) is 3F and passes through the working channel to allow direct visualization during activation.

Others have described use of an 11F choledochoscope (URF type P2 [Olympus]). Potential advantages of the smaller device are that it requires a smaller percutaneous access (14F) to use and may pass more easily beyond strictures within the intrahepatic biliary ducts. The working channel of this scope is 3F. Authors using it described use of a coumarin green pulsed dye laser (MDL-1 LaserTripter [Candela Laser, Wayland, Mass.]) to fracture resistant stones. The laser operates at a wavelength of 504 nm, and power output is between 40 and 100 mJ. A downside of this

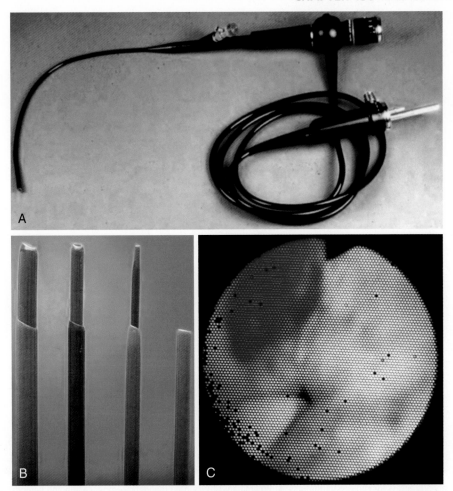

FIGURE 138-1. Equipment used for percutaneous choledochoscopy. **A,** 15F choledochoscope. **B,** Telescoping Teflon dilators used to create a tract large enough to place endoscope. **C,** Narrowing of duct around guidewire is identified. Biopsy of this unsuspected mass was positive for cholangiocarcinoma.

device is a smaller working channel to pass baskets and other tools. Additionally, the laser-based equipment is more costly than EHL. Use of ultrasound lithotripters has been described, but the access required for application is prohibitively large (24F) for most operators and has a small field of view.[4]

TECHNIQUE

Percutaneous Cholecystolithotomy

This procedure has three components: (1) percutaneous cholecystostomy, (2) tract dilation and stone removal, and (3) tract evaluation and tube removal.

Patients are sedated and given intravenous antibiotics (3.375 g of piperacillin/tazobactam or 3 g ampicillin/sulbactam) prior to the procedure. Some operators may prefer administration of atropine (0.6-1 mg) to limit the potential of a vagal response secondary to gallbladder dilation. Initial access may be either transhepatic or transperitoneal, although the latter approach is more commonly associated with acute pain during catheter placement. The gallbladder may be targeted with any combination of fluoroscopic, computed tomographic (CT), or ultrasonic guidance. Optimally the route of entry will be at the end of the

gallbladder fundus to simplify reaching calculi with the EHL probe and to ease clearance of the entire lumen of calculi with baskets. Via the Seldinger technique, a 10F to 14F retention loop catheter is placed (Fig. 138-2).

In patients with chronic cholecystitis, tract dilation and stone extraction is performed the following day. Patients who have drains placed for acute cholecystitis should recover from their presenting symptoms prior to stone removal. A safety wire is left in the gallbladder lumen outside the 18F working access. In cases where tract dilation is difficult, removable T-tac fasteners are available.[5]

Stones too large to remove via the sheath and resistant to basket fragmentation can be broken up with the EHL probe. Important factors to consider when using EHL are that the probe has to be 1 to 2 mm beyond the tip of the scope to avoid damaging the choledochoscope (Fig. 138-3). The probe has to be in direct contact with the stone and not the gallbladder wall. Activation of the EHL probe while in contact with the biliary endothelium can lead to bleeding or bile leakage that will make visualization difficult for the remainder of the case. When the operator believes all stones have been removed, final choledochoscopy is performed to ensure no residual stones remain. Contrast cholangiography is performed to evaluate the cystic and biliary ducts. Calculi are identified in cystic and biliary ducts 28% and 24% of the time, respectively.[6] Stones in these structures are

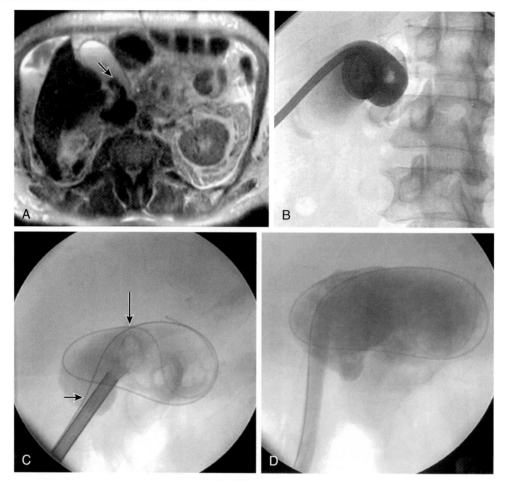

FIGURE 138-2. Percutaneous access for cholecystolithotomy. **A,** Preliminary T2-weighted magnetic resonance imaging demonstrates gallstones *(arrow)* in a nonsurgical candidate. **B,** A 14F Cope loop catheter is placed and left to gravity drainage overnight. **C,** Next morning, tract was dilated to 18F, and a basket was advanced. Note stone ensnared in basket *(long arrow)* and safety wire outside access sheath *(short arrow).* **D,** Final cholangiography demonstrates clearance of stones. Tube was removed 4 weeks later.

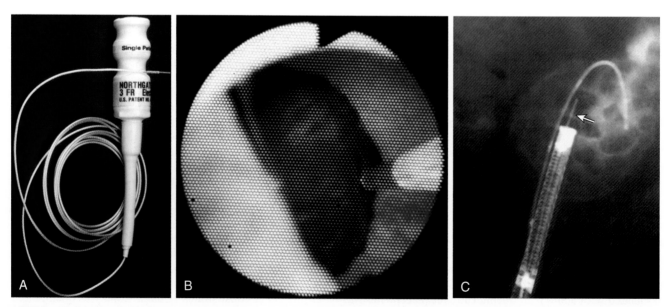

FIGURE 138-3. Electrohydraulic lithotripsy (EHL) probe. **A,** Prior to being advanced through working channel of choledochoscope. **B,** Directly impacting calculus and avoiding contact with biliary endothelium. **C,** Fluoroscopic image demonstrating EHL probe appropriately positioned beyond end of choledochoscope *(arrow).*

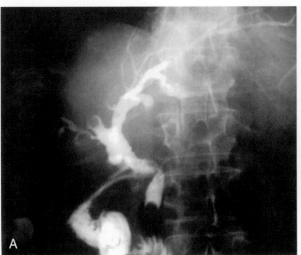
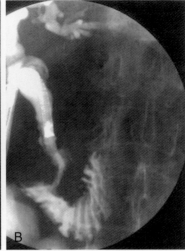

FIGURE 138-4. Percutaneous hepatolithotomy via a T-tube tract. **A,** Cholangiography via T-tube demonstrates calculus at sphincter of Oddi and at entry to right main hepatic duct. **B,** Cholangiography after electrohydraulic lithotripsy demonstrates clearance of common duct calculus.

removed via the gallbladder access if possible or by ERCP if necessary. Calculi in the cystic duct are often impossible to ensnare in a basket or treat with EHL. We have found that leaving an internal-external biliary drain through the gallbladder and cystic duct into the common bile duct and duodenum will usually passively fragment the stones and allow them to pass into the duodenum or out the cholecystostomy catheter. At the end of the procedure, a retention loop catheter is again left in the gallbladder (14F-16F). A large-bore catheter is left in place to tamponade the tract used for endoscopy and allow drainage of any residual "gravel" from calculus fragmentation. The catheter is left to gravity drainage.

Percutaneous Hepatolithotomy

Planning Route of Access

The route of access for these patients is variable and depends upon the timing of presentation. Patients with retained calculi following cholecystectomy may present shortly after surgery with a surgical T-tube in place. These tubes usually form a mature tract quickly and can be used for definitive access approximately 2 weeks after surgery. For patients who present in a delayed fashion following cholecystectomy or those with stones related to primary abnormalities of the biliary ducts or bilioenteric anastomosis, access is usually similar to that used for percutaneous biliary drainage. Approximately half of patients with biliary stones will have multiple calculi, and a careful search for additional stones must be performed during percutaneous cholangiography. If all intrahepatic calculi are located in one lobe of the liver, many operators prefer to access the opposite side to limit any acute angles that may be needed to enter the stone-bearing ducts. Preprocedural noninvasive imaging can be useful to determine stone burden and distribution when planning access. Magnetic resonance cholangiopancreatography has been shown superior to standard CT.[7] Compared with ERCP, it has a 96% sensitivity, 100% specificity, 100% positive predictive value, and 96% negative predictive value.

Accessing the Ducts

If a T-tube tract is to be used, we perform an initial cholangiogram through the existing catheter. Preprocedure sedation and antibiotic prophylaxis is performed similarly to cholecystolithotomy. The T-tube is removed over a guidewire. Depending on the treatment plan (see later), either a vascular sheath can be placed, or telescoping Teflon dilators can be placed to allow scope placement (Fig. 138-4).

If de novo transhepatic access is used, the left, right, or both ducts are accessed in a fashion described in the chapters covering biliary obstruction. Similar to the staged procedure described for cholecystolithotomy, we place an internal-external catheter at the initial visit. If the patient is scheduled electively and is not acutely ill, tract dilation and lithotomy can be performed the next day (Fig. 138-5). If the patient presents acutely, a "cooling-off" period may be required prior to stone removal. If the patient presents with septicemia and the stones are impacted in the common bile duct, it is wise to leave an external drain in place rather than risk septic shock by manipulating through the calculi into the bowel.

Stone Extraction

There are two principal and complementary methods to treat/remove ductal calculi:

1. Balloon dilation of the ampulla followed by use of balloons to dislodge and push calculi into the bowel. This technique works best for smaller, non-impacted stones.
2. Basket/EHL fragmentation similar to that used for cholecystolithotomy. This method is important to treat larger calculi.

Balloon Manipulation

The main advantage of this technique is that the procedure can be performed via a smaller access than is needed for choledochoscope use. Whether via a T-tube tract or percutaneous access, the procedure is performed similarly. For the purposes of this discussion, we will focus on access via a T-tube tract, since the variables are slightly more involved. After removing the T-tube over a guidewire, a sheath is placed in the hepatic ducts. A safety wire is then coiled in

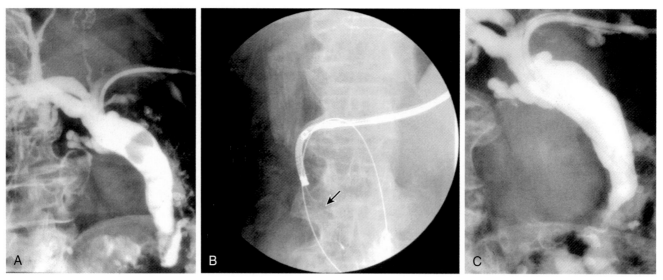

FIGURE 138-5. Percutaneous hepatolithotomy via left duct access in a patient drained for cholangitis. **A,** Cholangiography demonstrates calculus in common bile duct. **B,** After placing a safety wire in duodenum, a basket *(arrow)* is advanced through working port of choledochoscope. **C,** Follow-up cholangiography reveals clearance of stone.

the small bowel. Cholangiography confirms the location of the stone(s). A 10- or 12-mm balloon is then inflated across the ampulla of Vater for 45 to 90 seconds over one or two inflations to facilitate stone passage. A balloon approximating the size of the largest calculus is then used to fragment the stone. Authors advocating this approach have limited maximal balloon size to 12 mm.[8,9] The balloon is then deflated and carefully withdrawn above the stone, reinflated, and used to push the debris into the small bowel.

If the calculi are peripheral to the insertion site of the T-tube, standard catheter and guidewire techniques are used to negotiate past the stones into the respective duct(s), and the stones are pulled into the common bile duct with a Fogarty balloon. The calculi are then fragmented and pushed into the small bowel as described earlier. This technique is generally successful for smaller stones. As calculi exceed 15 mm in diameter, adjunctive techniques become necessary, including basket fragmentation and EHL. After cholangiography and/or endoscopy confirm that all calculi have been treated, an internal-external biliary drain is placed across the ampulla and into the small bowel. The catheter is left to gravity drainage overnight and capped in the morning if the patient is afebrile and otherwise asymptomatic.

The decision whether to routinely perform intrahepatic choledochoscopy is mildly controversial. Preferences are likely related to expertise in choledochoscope manipulation. Although it requires a larger access, EHL via the 15F scope can successfully treat calculi as large as 4 cm in the central bile ducts.[10] A principal advantage of the choledochoscope is that it allows characterization of filling defects in the bile ducts as residual calculi, mucus, blood clots, or soft tissue. Diagnosis and biopsy of unsuspected ductal tumors has been described during cholangioscopy. These tumors may have been diagnosed much later without use of the choledochoscope. Biliary endoscopy by a skilled operator likely cuts down procedure time in complex cases with large or impacted calculi. Operators may elect to use the smaller (11F) scope. This device may pass more easily

past impacted intrahepatic calculi in smaller ducts that are not dislodged by balloon techniques.

OUTCOMES

Percutaneous Cholecystolithotomy

Complete stone removal can be achieved in over 90% of patients.[11,12] A common cause of failure to remove all calculi is missing small fragments discovered at follow-up ultrasound imaging. This factor reinforces the need for careful and thorough inspection of the entire gallbladder lumen with the choledochoscope prior to the end of the extraction procedure, along with critical review of postprocedure cholangiograms. One group found that switching from a rigid to a flexible scope helped them find more residual fragments because it facilitated inspection of the entire gallbladder lumen.[11]

At a mean follow-up of 33 months, Courtois found that eight out of 65 patients (12%) had recurrent symptoms.[6] During follow-up, 30 patients had follow-up ultrasounds, and recurrent stones were found in 12 (40%). Interestingly, only half of these patients had recurrent symptoms. Overall recurrence rates for gallstones in patients undergoing percutaneous cholecystolithotomy are uncertain. Estimates range anywhere from 40% to 70% at 3 to 4 years following the procedure.[11,13-15] Even though not all patients with recurrent stones get recurrent cholecystitis, these long-term outcomes dictate that removal of the diseased gallbladder when feasible remains the best option.

Percutaneous Hepatolithotomy

Success can be achieved in over 90% of cases.[4,8-10,16] Most patients are completely cleared of calculi in one treatment session. An increase in the number of sessions is likely directly related to stone burden. Approximately half of patients will have more than one stone. The majority of calculi are located in the extrahepatic bile duct. On average,

10% to 30% of calculi will be located in the intrahepatic biliary system. In contrast to the frequency of recurrence with percutaneous cholecystolithotomy, successful outcomes with intraductal biliary calculi are typically far more durable, with one report describing no recurrences in 100 patients after a mean of 55 months.[9] Patients presenting with ductal stones related to cholecystitis will be most likely to mirror these outcomes, whereas those with diseases centered in the intrahepatic ducts will be more likely to have recurrence. One study focusing on treatment in the intrahepatic ducts found a relatively lower success rate (70.3%) than in other studies. This same group found a significant rate of recurrent sepsis in their patients (26%-42% depending on whether or not the patient had associated biliary strictures).[17]

COMPLICATIONS

Percutaneous Cholecystolithotomy

Major complications occur in approximately 6% of patients.[4] Most reported complications are related to bile leakage, ranging from simple loculated bilomas to severe bile peritonitis. Thirty-day mortality is approximately 3%.[12] This value is in keeping with the very ill patient population undergoing this procedure. As a reference point, in one study, over 20% of treated patients expired of unrelated causes within 18 months of the procedure.[11] The most important step to avoid complications related to bile leakage is to leave the tube in place long enough to allow a mature tract to form and perform an over-the-wire "tractogram" prior to removing the catheter. Doing so has diminished this specific complication in our practice. Given the prohibitive morbidity and mortality that would be associated with this patient group with surgical intervention, the outcomes with percutaneous cholecystolithotomy are very reasonable.

Percutaneous Hepatolithotomy

Similar to cholecystolithotomy, complications with hepatolithotomy have decreased with time and operator experience. In an early report, Stokes et al. had a 17% major complication rate, with 4% mortality within 30 days.[18] Another operator directed a 20F metal introducer into the biliary tree to perform choledochoscopy.[19] This group had an 8% 30-day mortality and 12% incidence of major hemobilia. Bower et al. reported only one major complication in 68 patients.[10] Harris reported no bleeding complications with use of a smaller scope. However, this patient group had a 24% rate of symptomatic bacteremia following endoscopy.[3] Their group involved a number of patients with intrahepatic stones secondary to vascular compromise in transplanted livers, and they recommend aggressive antibiotic coverage in this setting based upon their results. Groups who have focused on use of balloons and pushing stone fragments into the small bowel have not avoided hemobilia.[8,9,16] Pushing stones into the small bowel is associated with a small but definite risk of pancreatitis. Some operators think that use of octreotide can limit the risk of pancreatitis.[9] It should be remembered that although ERCP is a useful adjunct to manage hepatolithiasis, it is not without adverse events. Complications occur in 8% to 12% of patients, and mortality is 0.5% to 1%.[20,21] Additionally, some operators believe balloon cholangioplasty of the sphincter of Oddi is less traumatic over the long term than formal sphincterotomy performed at ERCP.[8,9]

POSTPROCEDURE AND FOLLOW-UP CARE

Percutaneous Cholecystolithotomy

In approximately 2 weeks, the patient is brought back for an outpatient catheter injection. If no residual stones are identified and the gallbladder drains appropriately into the central bile ducts, the catheter is capped to simulate internal drainage. Once the patient tolerates internal drainage for 2 weeks, the catheter is injected over a guidewire to ensure a mature cholecystocutaneous tract is present. Once the tract is mature, the catheter may be removed. Patients are typically seen in the interventional radiology clinic in follow-up on an as-needed basis. Given that many patients with recurrent calculi are asymptomatic, we do not schedule routine follow-up imaging to evaluate for stone recurrence, and rely on patient findings.

Percutaneous Hepatolithotomy

Patients are similarly allowed to develop a mature tract, and the catheter is removed upon confirmation of the clearance of all calculi. Given the lack of recurrence for the majority of patients, we do not routinely follow patients with stones secondary to cholecystitis. Patients with more complex scenarios are managed conjointly with the referring surgeon or gastroenterologist.

KEY POINTS

- Percutaneous biliary stone management involves two groups of patients:
  - Patients with symptomatic gallstones but not eligible for cholecystectomy
  - Patients with calculi in the extra- or intrahepatic biliary ductal system who are not treatable by endoscopic means. This group will often have recently undergone cholecystectomy.
- With experience and a variety of equipment, operators can remove all calculi in over 90% of patients.
- Patients with symptomatic gallstones are much more likely than patients with hepatolithiasis to have recurrence, because the diseased gallbladder remains in place.

▶ **SUGGESTED READINGS**

Akiyama H, Okazaki T, Takashima I, et al. Percutaneous treatments for biliary diseases. Radiology 1990;176:25–30.

Burhenne HJ. Percutaneous extraction of retained biliary tract stones: 661 patients. AJR Am J Roentgenol 1980;134:888–98.

Fache JS. Interventional radiology of the biliary tract. Transcholecystic intervention. Radiol Clin North Am 1990;28:1157–69.

Malone DE. Interventional radiologic alternatives to cholecystectomy. Radiol Clin North Am 1990;28:1145–56.

Picus D. Intracorporeal biliary lithotripsy. Radiol Clin North Am 1990;28:1241–9.

The complete reference list is available online at www.expertconsult.com.

CHAPTER 139

Biliary Complications Associated with Liver Transplantation

Robert K. Kerlan, Jr. and Jeanne M. LaBerge

Orthotopic liver transplantation (OLT) is a critical therapeutic alternative for managing patients with progressive liver failure and selected patients with hepatocellular carcinoma. Refinements in surgical technique, improved immunosuppressive agents, and the evolution of minimally invasive image-guided procedures have allowed 5-year survival rates to approach 85%.[1-3]

The most common source of a replacement organ is a deceased donor. Usually the whole liver is used as the allograft, but the donor organ can be split, with the right lobe or right lobe and medial segment of the left lobe donated to an adult and the left lateral segment given to a child.[4-6] Unfortunately, there remains a critical shortage of donor organs when compared with the number of patients on the liver transplant waiting list. This shortage of organs stimulated the development of using right and left hepatic lobes from living donors with matching ABO blood types for urgent transplantation. Despite the use of living donors, the availability of organs falls well short of the demand, and up to 50% of potential recipients die while awaiting transplantation.[7,8]

As with any complex surgical procedure, complications after orthotopic liver transplantation are not infrequent and occur in both the acute postoperative period and months to years later. The most common source of significant complications in a liver transplant patient is the biliary tract.[9-12] To understand the types of complications that occur, thorough comprehension of the surgical anatomy is essential.

SURGICAL ANATOMY OF THE BILIARY ANASTOMOSIS

The type of biliary anastomosis created depends on several factors,[13,14] including whether a whole cadaveric liver or a split liver has been used, the condition of the recipient's bile duct, and whether it is an adult or pediatric patient receiving the allograft.

Whole Liver

For whole-liver transplantation, two types of biliary anastomosis are constructed: (1) choledochocholedochostomy (CDCD) and (2) biliodigestive choledochojejunostomy (CDJ) or hepaticojejunostomy (HJ).

CDCD is an anastomosis of the donor common bile duct to the recipient common bile duct. CDCD is the preferred biliary anastomosis, because sphincteric function is preserved, bowel surgery in a patient who will be immunosuppressed is avoided, and retrograde cholangiography with appropriate endoscopic interventions can be performed postoperatively.

The CDCD anastomosis may be performed over a T-tube. If a T-tube is placed, postoperative bile production

can be monitored and the biliary tree can be investigated easily by T-tube cholangiography. Moreover, the presence of the T-tube may make the anastomosis technically easier to create. However, because of complications associated with T-tube placement, as well as biliary leakage after tube removal, many centers have abandoned routine T-tube placement during creation of a CDCD anastomosis.[15-17] A recent meta-analysis suggests that biliary complications may not be increased by T-tube insertion, however, and suggests the incidence of biliary strictures may be reduced.[18]

In some clinical situations, a CDCD anastomosis should not be created. Such circumstances arise when the native recipient extrahepatic bile duct is unsuitable as a conduit, as commonly encountered in patients with primary sclerosing cholangitis and all pediatric patients with biliary atresia. Moreover, if there is a substantial donor/recipient duct size mismatch, a CDCD anastomosis may not be the most attractive option.

When a CDCD anastomosis is not the optimal surgical option, a CDJ or hepaticojejunostomy is constructed.[19,20] These anastomoses are created by attaching the end or obliquely cut side (to create a larger channel) of the common bile duct or common hepatic duct to the side of a loop of jejunum pulled up to the region of the porta hepatis in a Roux-en-Y configuration. This maneuver requires surgical closure of the free end of the jejunal loop adjacent to the biliary anastomosis, as well as distal jejunojejunostomy to maintain continuity of the alimentary tract.

Split Liver

The biliary anastomosis in split-liver transplantation can be more technically challenging than in whole-liver transplantation. This is particularly true with living donor transplantation, because not causing harm to the donor is of paramount importance. When harvesting a lobe from a living donor, the biliary duct is severed at a safe distance from the common hepatic duct to avoid stricture formation. This maneuver often results in only a short segment of donor right (or left) hepatic duct being available to anastomose to the recipient duct, making creation of a tension-free anastomosis difficult. Moreover, variations in donor biliary anatomy may necessitate the creation of more than one biliary anastomosis.

Numerous variations in biliary anatomy exist, with so-called normal anatomy being present in only 57% of patients.[20] "Normal" anatomy is considered to be a common hepatic duct bifurcating into left and right hepatic ducts, and the right duct subsequently bifurcating into anterior and posterior segmental ducts. A trifurcation of the common hepatic duct into left, right anterior segmental, and right posterior segmental ducts is observed in 12%. Other common variations include origin of the right anterior or posterior segmental ducts from either the common hepatic duct or the left hepatic duct. Rarely, the right posterior or anterior segmental duct joins the cystic duct prior to its entry into the extrahepatic bile duct.

When variant biliary anatomy is present in the right lobe of the donor organ and it is desirable to create anastomoses to the recipient bile duct, unconventional anastomoses may be required, including the donor segmental right hepatic duct anastomosed to the recipient's left hepatic duct or cystic duct.[21,22] As an alternative, separate biliary-enteric anastomoses to a Roux-en-Y loop can be created. In some cases, the segmental duct is ligated, and that segment of the liver subsequently atrophies.

When living donor transplantation is being considered, presurgical evaluation of the potential donor is performed so that the biliary and vascular anatomy can be delineated prior to transplantation. Accurate assessment of the biliary anatomy is critical in living donor transplantation because a biliary injury potentially has great significance. Complications related to the biliary tree are encountered in 4.4% of donor hepatectomies.[23]

The optimal method for preoperative anatomic evaluation of potential living hepatic donors remains to be defined. The ideal technique would clearly delineate the hepatic arteries, portal veins, hepatic veins, bile ducts, and hepatic parenchyma without requiring contrast media or ionizing radiation. Although magnetic resonance imaging (MRI) and MR angiography (MRA) potentially fulfill some of these requirements, delineation of small hepatic arteries and diminutive biliary radicles can be problematic.[24] Three-dimensional reconstruction renderings will usually provide adequate information for surgical planning. A more detailed biliary evaluation would be advantageous, but the risks associated with retrograde cholangiography are considered excessive for routine evaluation of a healthy living donor.

BILIARY COMPLICATIONS

The surgical anastomosis between the donor biliary tract and the recipient may be technically difficult to create. Moreover, the biliary system is sensitive to ischemia and may be damaged either by prolonged preservation before transplantation or by problems with either hepatic arterial and possibly portal venous flow.[25]

Despite refinements in surgical technique, biliary complications continue to be a common source of morbidity in the transplant patient. In a systematic review of 14,359 transplants, biliary complications were observed in 12% of deceased donor recipients and 19% of live donor grafts.[11] Two major types of complications related to the biliary tract are observed: bile leak and biliary obstruction.

Bile Leak

Bile leaks usually occur early in the postoperative period and originate from three sources: the T-tube entry site (in patients who have had T-tubes placed), the biliary anastomosis, or the cut surface of the liver (in patients with split or reduced-size allografts).

In a patient with a CDCD anastomosis performed over a T-tube, seepage through the T-tube choledochostomy is the most common cause of a bile leak.[26] This type of leak is usually identified on routine postoperative T-tube cholangiography. Initial treatment consists of opening the T-tube to gravity drainage, which is curative in up to 60% of patients.[27] If this is unsuccessful, endoscopic sphincterotomy may be useful.

Bile leaks may also develop when the T-tube is removed 3 to 6 months after the transplant operation. Immunosuppression often prevents formation of a connective tissue tract to allow bile to drain freely into the peritoneal cavity. Retrograde stent placement or percutaneous transhepatic drainage coupled with percutaneous drainage of the biloma controls the leak in most patients. However, up to a third of these patients require operative intervention with surgical revision for closure.[28]

Because of the aforementioned problems related to T-tubes, some centers have elected to perform the CDCD anastomosis without T-tube insertion. In a study by Randall et al.,[29] a group of 59 patients who had T-tubes placed were compared with 51 patients who underwent CDCD anastomoses without T-tubes. This comparison revealed no difference in biliary complication rates or survival.

Bile leaks that occur at the anastomotic site (Fig. 139-1) may be difficult to manage conservatively. The principles of nonoperative management of bile leaks include (1) exclusion of hepatic artery thrombosis or stenosis, (2) drainage of any associated bilomas or abscesses, (3) diversion of bile flow, (4) eradication of any coexistent infection, and (5) optimization of the nutritional status of the patient.

Patency of the hepatic artery should be confirmed in all patients with a bilious postoperative collection. This is usually accomplished with duplex ultrasound though MRA, or CTA may be used when the ultrasound examination is inconclusive. When hepatic artery thrombosis (HAT) is detected, retransplantation may be required. Kaplan et al.[30] reported percutaneous drainage in 15 patients with hepatic artery occlusion; 11 required retransplantation, and 4 were managed for more than 30 months with indwelling drainage catheters.

Drainage of infected or uninfected bilomas is critical to percutaneous management. Healing requires the area of dehiscence to be invested with healthy connective tissue to provide blood flow as well as structural support. Evacuation of infected fluid promotes ingrowth of healthy tissue.

Management of bilomas in a transplant patient is identical to that in a nontransplant patient, and consists of image-guided percutaneous drainage for accessible collections in the majority of patients. The most common area in which a biloma develops is adjacent to the extrahepatic biliary system in the subhepatic space. However, the bile may track and accumulate some distance from the site of leakage. The right subphrenic space is not an uncommon site, particularly if the size of the allograft is poorly matched to the configuration of the right subphrenic space. The right subphrenic space offers unique challenges for percutaneous drainage because of its location. Frequently a choice must be made between a transhepatic approach, which can potentially lead to damage to the allograft, and a transpleural approach, which may potentially contaminate the pleural space. Overall, percutaneous drainage of postoperative bile collections in a liver transplant patient carries high success and low complication rates.[31]

After drainage of any associated bilomas, bile flow should be diverted. In so doing, the amount of bile effluent through

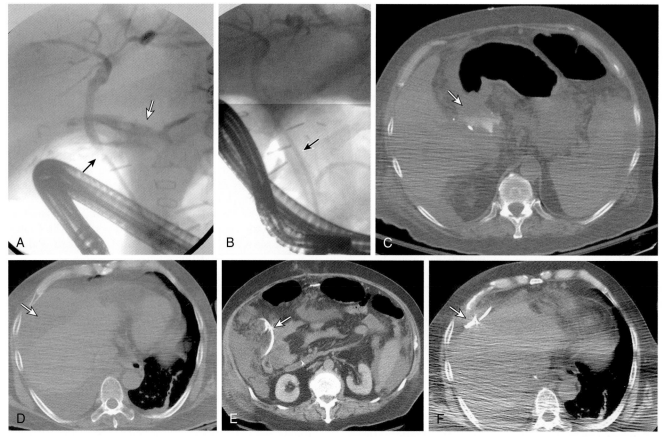

FIGURE 139-1. This 60-year-old man with cryptogenic cirrhosis underwent orthotopic liver transplantation. Two weeks after surgery, his alkaline phosphatase level was elevated, and he underwent endoscopic retrograde cholangiopancreatography (ERCP) for biliary tract evaluation. **A,** Endoscopic injection of contrast material into common bile duct demonstrates a duct-to-duct anastomotic leak. Note duct-to-duct anastomosis *(black arrow)* and collection of contrast material in subhepatic space *(white arrow)*. **B,** Patient was treated by placement of an endoscopic stent *(arrow)* across anastomosis to facilitate drainage. **C,** Computed tomography (CT) performed after ERCP demonstrated extravasation of ERCP contrast material into subhepatic space *(arrow)*. **D,** Also noted on CT were large subphrenic *(arrow)* and subhepatic fluid collections. **E,** Percutaneous drainage of bilomas was accomplished with CT guidance and placement of two 10F pigtail drains. One drain was inserted into subhepatic space *(arrow)*. **F,** Another drain was placed in subphrenic space *(arrow)*.

the defect can be diminished, thereby improving the chance of spontaneous closure. Diversion of bile flow can be accomplished by either placement of an endoscopically guided retrograde stent (if a CDCD anastomosis has been created) or by percutaneous transhepatic biliary drainage (PTBD). Retrograde endoscopic drainage via retrograde stent placement has the major advantage of not requiring a transhepatic puncture and an external drainage tube. PTBD has two advantages over endoscopically guided internal stent placement: the ability to provide both internal and external drainage and the ease with which cholangiography can be repeated.

The ability to provide external drainage allows more efficient evacuation of bile. Both character and amount of bile output can be easily monitored. However, if internal drainage is deemed appropriate, it can be accomplished by merely capping the internal-external drainage tube, provided that the catheter has been positioned across the area of leakage into the bowel. The tube is not usually capped until a cholangiogram no longer demonstrates the presence of a leak. Moreover, monitoring the healing process by tube cholangiography avoids the necessity of sedation and an endoscopic procedure. Unfortunately,

performance of transhepatic biliary drainage requires the risk and discomfort of a transhepatic puncture and may be technically challenging in patients with nondilated intrahepatic ducts. For these reasons, the endoscopic retrograde approach is favored in many centers for patients with CDCD anastomoses to achieve biliary drainage. Patients with CDJ anastomoses require PTBD because it is usually impossible to reach the biliary anastomosis with an endoscope.

Whatever method of biliary diversion is selected, the final two principles in the management of anastomotic leaks have to be followed: eradication of infection and maintenance of nutrition. The former can be accomplished by adequate drainage and appropriate antibiotic therapy. The latter may require enteral or parenteral hyperalimentation to maintain a positive nitrogen balance.

With these principles, it may be possible to treat anastomotic leaks nonoperatively. Osorio et al.[15] reported successful healing of 14 of 17 CDCD anastomotic leaks; 3 of 17 CDCD anastomoses that were entirely dehiscent required operative revision. In this same series, only 3 of 9 bile leaks originating from CDJ anastomoses healed with conservative therapy.

This resistance to healing with conservative therapy may in part be a reflection of the immunosuppressive corticosteroids these patients are taking, which inhibits the healing response. In our institution, a short trial of either PTBD or retrograde stent placement is often attempted, but surgical revision is performed if the perforation does not seal rapidly. That said, many patients have comorbid conditions that make reoperation an unattractive therapeutic option.

Patients with split-liver transplants (either deceased or living donor) deserve special consideration.[32-34] The technical aspects of creating a biliary anastomosis are more challenging in this group. Cadaveric split livers generally contain an ample amount of extrahepatic bile duct when the right lobe is harvested. To prevent a bile leak, care must be taken to ligate the left hepatic duct origin at the point where it is divided from the confluence of the hepatic ducts. The left lobe from the same donor may be used for pediatric transplantation, with anastomosis of the left hepatic duct to a Roux-en-Y loop. The technical demands of creating a biliary anastomosis to the right hepatic duct in patients receiving an allograft from a living donor are even greater because of the short length of right hepatic duct available for creation of the anastomosis. These anastomoses may be created under tension, which can lead to focal necrosis and development of a bile leak. Because of these anatomic restrictions, biliary complications are more frequent after living donor right lobe transplantation, with bile leakage being observed in 4.7% to 18.2% of patients.[35-37]

Because of the presence of the biliary anastomosis cephalically within the porta hepatis, these patients are extremely difficult to surgically revise. When anastomotic leaks occur, an extensive trial of nonoperative therapy before surgical revision is usually attempted.

When transhepatic cholangiography and biliary drainage are performed on patients who are recipients of a right lobe from a split-liver transplant, detailed knowledge of the postoperative anatomy is required. Because of the variable segmental ductal anatomy of the right hepatic ducts, it is sometimes necessary to ligate a substantial-sized duct such as the right anterior or right posterior segmental duct. When this is performed in a sterile environment, the ducts dilate and the parenchyma atrophies. However, if these ducts are punctured and a tube is placed, it is not usually possible to reconnect to a biliary system that has been anastomosed to the recipient's native duct (in the case of a duct-to-duct anastomosis) or to the jejunum (in the case of a hepaticojejunal anastomosis). The punctured ligated duct may leak if the needle is removed. Alternatively, if a tube is placed, it is likely that the external drainage tube must remain indefinitely, probably for the remainder of the patient's life. Therefore, the operative report must be carefully scrutinized and all previous imaging studies reviewed before attempting a diagnostic or therapeutic intervention on a biliary system that has been anastomosed to the recipient. MR cholangiography may be very useful before percutaneous interventions to delineate the appearance of both the ligated and anastomosed systems when a donor system has been intentionally occluded.

Split-liver allografts may also leak from the cut edge of the liver (Fig. 139-2). Because surgical division of the right and left lobe occurs along the plane of the middle hepatic vein, small ductal radicles are divided, ligated, and cauterized in the course of the dissection. Occlusion of these radicles is sometimes incomplete, so bile leakage may occur from this cut surface. In a series of 72 patients reported by Wojcicki et al.,[38] bile leakage from the hepatic parenchyma was the most common biliary complication, observed in 11% of patients. Leaks from the cut edge of the liver often resolve spontaneously with simple drainage of the leak. If the leak continues, drainage of the biliary tract from either an antegrade or retrograde approach may be required. In rare circumstances, it may be necessary to occlude the offending radicle. This can be accomplished with fluoroscopically guided catheter techniques and 2,3-isobutyl cyanoacrylate as the occlusive agent.

Biliary Obstruction

Biliary obstruction represents the other major complication related to the biliary tract after orthotopic liver transplantation. This complication is detected to a varying degree in 10% to 20% of patients.[11,39] The most common problem is a stricture at the biliary anastomosis (Fig. 139-3).

Clinical manifestations of biliary obstruction may be nonspecific. Liver transplant recipients have many potential causes of fever, abnormal liver function tests, and leukocytosis. Biliary obstruction is often just one of the potential explanations. Noninvasive evaluation for biliary obstruction with ultrasound, CT, and MRI may be difficult because patients may not have ductal dilation.[40] Therefore, direct cholangiography may be necessary to exclude or confirm the diagnosis. In a patient with a CDCD anastomosis, endoscopic retrograde cholangiography is usually performed. In a patient with a CDJ anastomosis, percutaneous transhepatic cholangiography is the appropriate examination.[41]

When stenosis of a CDCD anastomosis is identified in the early postoperative period, it may merely represent edema or an inflammatory reaction (or both) at the anastomotic site. In this circumstance, a short period (2-6 weeks) of endoscopic stenting may be curative.[42] If endoscopic cannulation cannot be achieved, a transhepatic internal-external biliary drainage tube should be placed. However, if the stenosis persists or recurs, surgical revision to a CDJ is often the most efficient and durable solution.

As an alternative to surgical reconstruction, balloon dilation via the endoscopic retrograde approach may be attempted, followed by a variable period of retrograde stenting. With this strategy, success rates ranging from 64% to 90% have been reported.[43-45]

When retrograde access to the biliary tree cannot be achieved, percutaneous transhepatic dilation may be attempted (Fig. 139-4). This is accomplished technically by using a standard transhepatic approach to gain access to the intrahepatic biliary system. A sheath large enough to allow passage of the appropriate-sized balloon is inserted. Using a small curved catheter and a probing guidewire, the stenotic anastomosis is crossed. The guidewire is advanced into the duodenum for patients with a CDCD anastomosis or into the Roux-en-Y loop for a patient with a CDJ. A balloon size is selected that exceeds the normal ductal caliber by approximately 10%. This balloon is inflated across the anastomosis for a variable period. Some investigators recommend prolonged balloon inflation (for periods of up to 20 minutes) and repeating the procedure two to three times within 2 weeks to achieve a durable result. Using this technique with balloons ranging from 7 to 14 mm in

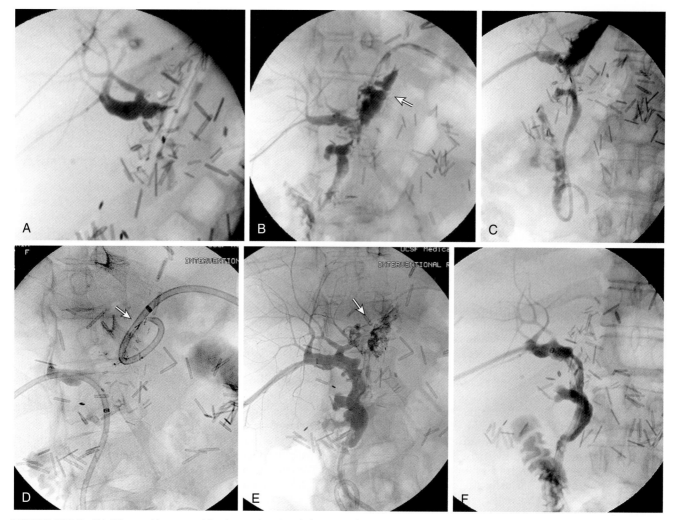

FIGURE 139-2. This 20-year-old woman with primary sclerosing cholangitis underwent liver transplantation with a split liver (she received right lobe and medial segment of left). Postoperatively, abdominal pain and fever developed. **A,** Initial percutaneous transhepatic cholangiography demonstrates mild biliary ductal dilation. **B,** After placement of a drainage catheter into bile duct, injection of contrast material reveals leak at cut edge of liver, with extravasated contrast material filling a small biloma cavity *(arrow)*. Note presence of an operative drain in region of leak. **C,** A percutaneous internal-external biliary drain was inserted into biliary tree. **D,** Surgical drain was then exchanged for a percutaneous pigtail drain *(arrow)*. **E,** After several weeks of percutaneous drainage, biloma drain was removed. A small residual leak was noted at cut edge of liver *(arrow)*. **F,** Three months after transplantation, leak was healed. Injection of biliary drain did not demonstrate a leak, and biliary drainage catheter was removed.

diameter, Zajko et al.[46] reported a 73% success rate at 2 years and a 66% success rate at 6 years in a series of 56 patients with anastomotic strictures.

However, use of conventional dilation balloons for treatment of anastomotic strictures has not been uniformly successful. For this reason, some practitioners[47] have advocated using a cutting balloon (Boston Scientific, Natick, Mass.). This device has four surgical blades embedded in the dilating balloon. During balloon inflation, the blades incise the dense fibrous tissue of the stricture in the hope of preventing elastic recoil and achieving a more durable result of the dilation. Frequently, a cutting balloon smaller than the anticipated necessary diameter is selected to achieve complete dilation, and a conventional balloon is then used to enlarge the lumen to the desired size. Using this technique, Saad et al.[47] treated 22 patients with posttransplant anastomotic strictures during 49 cutting balloon sessions, usually combined with conventional balloon dilation. A technical

success rate of 93% was achieved without incurring a major complication. Long-term durability of this strategy in comparison to conventional balloon dilation has not been assessed.

Before the advent of the cutting balloon, when conventional dilation of an anastomotic stricture failed in a patient who was considered to be a poor surgical risk, metallic stent placement was occasionally performed.[48] Unfortunately, the rate of recurrent stenosis and formation of obstructing debris in the biliary tree was extremely high, and most centers have abandoned this therapeutic alternative. Moreover, it should be noted that stent placement can potentially preclude or complicate definitive surgical repair. To circumvent this problem, the concept of retrievable stent-graft placement was put forth by Petersen et al.[49] In this series, Gianturco-Rosch Z-stents were covered with expanded polytetrafluoroethylene (ePTFE) and inserted for a period of 2 to 9 months. All patients had the stents successfully

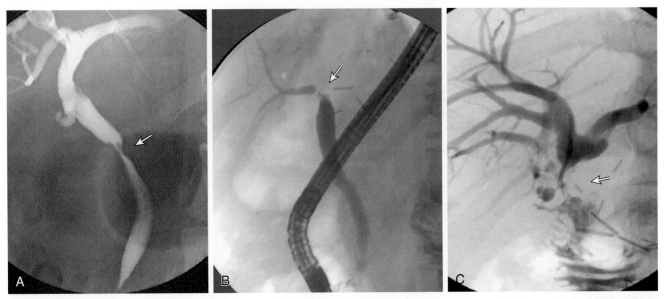

FIGURE 139-3. Biliary strictures after liver transplantation. **A,** Duct-to-duct anastomotic stricture *(arrow)*. Such strictures are often treated by operative repair with a Roux anastomosis. Nonoperative candidates can be treated by balloon dilation. **B,** In right lobe living donor or split-liver transplants, a high stricture can develop in hilum at operative site *(arrow)*. **C,** Stricture can develop at enteric anastomosis *(arrow)* in patients who receive a Roux-en-Y. These strictures are often treated by balloon dilation because reoperation is difficult.

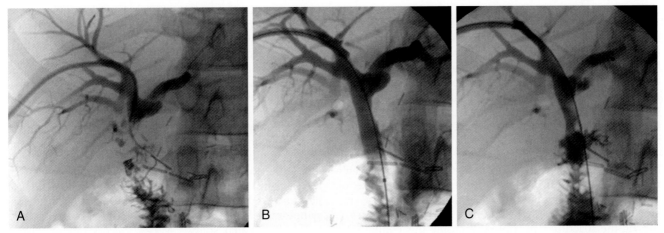

FIGURE 139-4. Stricture at hepaticojejunal anastomosis developed in this 38-year-old man who underwent orthotopic liver transplantation for sclerosing cholangitis. **A,** Tube cholangiogram reveals high-grade narrowing at surgical anastomosis. **B,** A 10 mm × 4 cm dilation balloon is inflated across anastomosis. **C,** Repeat cholangiogram after dilation shows good cosmetic result.

retrieved. Five of six patients with anastomotic strictures (2 CDCD, 4 CDJ) had successful outcomes during the 6- to 20-month follow-up period. Unfortunately, since no commercial devices have been created for this technique, there have been no further reports in over a decade.

Special consideration must be given to patients with biliary obstruction who are recipients of split-liver transplants. Left duct anastomoses in pediatric patients receiving a left lobe transplant tend to not pose a technical problem, because the length of the left hepatic duct is longer and thus allows a relatively straightforward anastomosis, usually to a Roux-en-Y loop. Right lobe transplantation is not problematic when a cadaveric organ is used, because the extrahepatic bile duct is also harvested. However, when a living donor is used, the procedure is considerably more difficult because of the short length of

the right hepatic duct that is available. Not only is the duct small, but the arterial supply may be compromised during the donation right hepatectomy.[50] It is not surprising that biliary obstructions complicate 8.3% to 31.7% of right lobe transplants.[51]

Multiple types of biliary anastomoses can be created with a donated right lobe. A direct anastomosis to the recipient's common hepatic duct or right hepatic duct is usually performed if a single right donor duct drains both the anterior and posterior segments. If the donor biliary anatomy has the posterior and anterior segments draining into variant locations, such as the left hepatic duct, separate anastomoses may be required. If a Roux-en-Y loop is constructed, it is generally straightforward to anastomose each segmental duct into the loop. However, if a duct-to-duct anastomosis is desired, the ducts may be anastomosed to

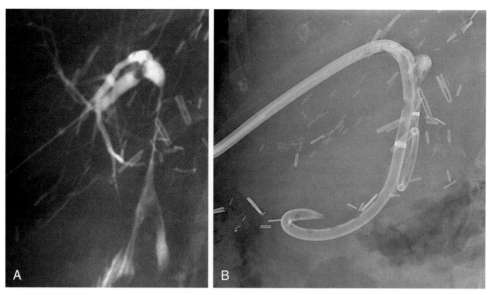

FIGURE 139-5. Stricture of proximal common hepatic duct following right lobe liver transplant. **A,** Tube cholangiogram reveals diffuse narrowing of hepaticojejunostomy. **B,** A 14F catheter with a coaxial 8F catheter exiting a proximal side hole bridges stenotic duct.

the recipient's right and left hepatic ducts or even to the recipient's right or common hepatic duct and cystic duct stump.

Strictures that occur in living donor recipients are managed in a similar fashion to patients with cadaveric liver transplants. If the anastomosis is created to the recipient's bile duct, retrograde cholangiography and therapy is generally performed. When the anastomosis is created to a Roux-en-Y loop, the percutaneous transhepatic route is required. Conventional balloon dilatation and cutting balloons followed by a variable period of transhepatic internal-external stenting is usually performed.

An innovative method of transhepatic management of biliary strictures following living donor transplant has been recommended by Gwon et al.[52] These investigators use a 14F biliary drainage tube through which an 8F catheter is coaxially inserted, exiting a side hole proximally and traversing the stricture (Fig. 139-5). By using this configuration, a 22F channel is created across the strictured area. With this technique, primary patency rates of 96%, 92%, and 91% were reported at 1, 2, and 3 years, respectively, in a series of 79 patients.[46]

An additional novel technique in managing biliary strictures was reported by Itoi et al.[53] These authors inserted a samarium-cobalt magnet from a transhepatic approach with an additional magnet inserted from the retrograde endoscopic approach. The compressive force created through the magnetic attraction eradicated the stricture and created a new anastomosis that remained patent following removal of the magnets.

In some circumstances, segmental ductal systems may be intentionally divided and ligated, which leads to gradual segmental atrophy. If postoperative obstruction develops in such patients, retrograde cholangiography may be performed in the usual manner, and the ligated system will not be opacified. However, if a percutaneous cholangiogram and drainage are necessary, it is crucial to be aware of the ligated system before embarking on the procedure. If a tube is inadvertently placed into a ligated system, the patient may

require an external drainage tube for the remainder of life or a major surgical procedure to rectify the situation. It is prudent to obtain an MR or CT cholangiogram before percutaneous interventions on these patients so that intentionally ligated systems can be avoided during percutaneous interventions.

Biliary strictures unrelated to the surgical anastomosis may also develop.[54] Nonanastomotic strictures related to hepatic artery thrombosis, prolonged cold preservation times, acute or chronic rejection, and cytomegalovirus infection may be encountered. In addition, recurrent intrahepatic biliary strictures develop in 5% to 20% of patients undergoing transplantation for primary sclerosing cholangitis.[55] Because there are no surgical options other than retransplantation for this group of patients, balloon dilation has formed the mainstay of clinical management when symptoms related to such narrowing develop. In the previously cited Zajko study,[46] a 94% success rate at 2 years and 84% at 5 years was reported with the use of balloon dilation in a group of 16 patients with non-anastomotic strictures.

As with anastomotic strictures, metallic stents have also been used rarely in the management of non-anastomotic strictures that fail to respond to balloon dilation. Before placement of a metallic stent, a trial of cutting balloon cholangioplasty should be considered. Although the immediate result of metallic stent placement is often gratifying, there is a tendency for these stents to serve as a nidus for stone and debris formation. The long-term durability of stents in these patients has not been thoroughly evaluated, and such stents should be considered only when other therapeutic alternatives, including prolonged tube drainage, have been exhausted.

In a patient who has had the biliary anastomosis performed with placement of a T-tube, the tube may become occluded with debris or the limb displaced, with subsequent biliary obstruction. It is often possible to rectify T-tube problems via interventional radiologic techniques. However, because transplant patients form mature tracts at a much slower rate than patients who are not immunosuppressed, simple replacement is sometimes not possible. If access is lost during attempted revision of a T-tube, it may be necessary to perform an additional transhepatic or retrograde procedure to ensure adequate biliary drainage.

Mucocele of the donor cystic duct remnant is an unusual but well-recognized cause of biliary obstruction.[56] Although percutaneous aspiration of a cystic duct mucocele may provide temporary relief of obstruction,[57] surgical revision is usually required for definitive therapy. Dysfunction of the sphincter of Oddi in a patient with a CDCD anastomosis can also inhibit bile flow.[58] Even though the cause of this disorder is not clearly defined, its occurrence is well recognized. Endoscopically guided sphincterotomy is curative.

Obstruction of the bile duct by stones, sludge, or necrotic debris may also be encountered. Although stones may develop in any patient with biliary obstruction, the presence of necrotic debris usually indicates a prolonged cold preservation injury, rejection, or hepatic arterial insufficiency. Stones and debris can generally be treated with percutaneous transhepatic or endoscopic retrograde techniques, including basket retrieval and balloon sweeping.[59] However, unless the underlying cause is addressed, recurrent obstruction from newly formed material is likely to occur.

KEY POINTS

- The most common complications after orthotopic liver transplantation are related to the biliary tract. These complications can be divided into two major groups: leak and obstruction.

- Bile leaks develop in the early postoperative period and can often be managed by draining the associated biloma in conjunction with controlling the drainage of bile from the liver with either a retrograde stent or a percutaneous transhepatic biliary drainage tube.

- Biliary obstruction usually develops more than 1 month after transplant surgery and can be managed in many cases by balloon dilatation and stenting.

- Special challenges are posed in patients receiving split organs, with right lobe transplants being most common in the adult population.

▶ SUGGESTED READINGS

Akamatsu N, Sugawara Y, Hashimoto D. Biliary reconstruction, its complications and management of biliary complications after adult transplantation: a systematic review of the incidence, risk factors and outcome. Transpl Int 2011;24:379–92.

Gwon DI, Ko GY, Sung KB, et al. A novel double stent system for palliative treatment of malignant extrahepatic biliary obstructions: a pilot study. AJR Am J Roentgenol 2011;197(5):W942–7.

Perrakis A, Fortsch T, Schellerer V, et al. Biliary tract complications after orthotopic liver transplantation: still the "Achilles heel"? Transpl Proc 2010;10:4154–7.

Piardi T, Greget M, Audet M, et al. Biliary strictures after liver transplantation: is percutaneous treatment indicated? Ann Transplant 2011;16: 5–13.

The complete reference list is available online at www.expertconsult.com.

CHAPTER **140**

Image-Guided Thermal Tumor Ablation: Basic Science and Combination Therapies

Muneeb Ahmed and S. Nahum Goldberg

UNDERSTANDING TUMOR ABLATION: AN OVERVIEW

Image-guided tumor ablation is a minimally invasive strategy to treat focal tumors by inducing irreversible cellular injury through application of thermal and, more recently, nonthermal energy or chemical injection. This approach has become a widely accepted technique, incorporated into the treatment of a range of clinical circumstances, including treatment of focal tumors in the liver, lung, kidney, bone, and adrenal glands.[1-4] Benefits of minimally invasive therapies compared to surgical resection include lesser mortality and morbidity, lower cost, and the ability to perform procedures on outpatients who are not good candidates for surgery.[5] However, additional work is required to improve outcomes and overcome limitations in ablative efficacy, including persistent growth of residual tumor at the ablation margin, the inability to effectively treat larger tumors, and variability in complete treatment based upon tumor location.[1]

Given the multiplicity of treatment types and potential complexity of paradigms in oncology and the wider application of thermal ablation techniques, a thorough understanding of the basic principles and recent advances in thermal ablation is a necessary prerequisite for their effective clinical use. These key concepts related to tumor ablation can be broadly divided into (1) those that relate to performing a clinical ablation, such as understanding the goals of therapy and mechanisms of tissue heating or tumor destruction, and (2) understanding the proper role of tumor ablation and the strategies being pursued to improve overall ablation outcome. These latter concepts include a systematic approach to technologic development, understanding and using the biophysiologic environment to maximize ablation outcome, combining tumor ablation with adjuvant therapies to synergistically increase tumor destruction, and improving tumor visualization and targeting through image navigation and fusion technology. Given that the greatest experimental and clinical experience exists for radiofrequency (RF)-based ablation, this will be the representative model used to discuss many of these concepts. However, many of these principles also apply when using alternative ablative modalities.

Goals of Minimally Invasive Therapy

The overall goal of minimally invasive focal tumor ablation encompasses several specific aims. First and foremost, a successful ablation completely treats all malignant cells within the target. This includes both achieving homogenous ablation within the tumor (so no focal areas of viable tumor remain) and adequately treating a rim of apparently "normal" tissue around the tumor, which often contains microscopic invasion of malignant cells at the tumor periphery. Thus, based upon examinations of tumor progression in patients undergoing surgical resection and the demonstration of viable malignant cells beyond visible tumor boundaries, in most cases (or except when otherwise indicated) tumor ablation therapies attempt to include at least a 0.5- to 1-cm "ablative margin" of seemingly normal tissue for liver and lung, though less may be needed for some tumors in the kidney.[6,7]

A secondary goal is to ensure accuracy of therapy to minimize the damage to nontarget normal tissue surrounding the ablative zone. As such, one significant advantage of percutaneous ablative therapies over conventional standard surgical resection is the potential to remove or destroy only a minimal amount of normal tissue. This is critical in clinical situations where the functional state of the background organ parenchyma is as important in determining patient outcome as the primary tumor. Examples of clinical situations where this is relevant include focal hepatic tumors in patients with underlying cirrhosis and limited hepatic reserve, patients with von Hippel-Lindau syndrome who have limited renal function and require treatment of multiple renal tumors, and patients with primary lung tumors with extensive underlying emphysema and limited lung function.[8-10] Many of these patients are not surgical candidates owing to limited native organ functional reserve, placing them at a higher risk for postoperative complications or organ failure. Other clinical circumstances in which high specificity and accuracy of targeting have proven useful include providing symptomatic relief for patients with symptomatic osseous metastases or hormonally active neuroendocrine tumors, and in using percutaneous therapies to improve focal interstitial drug delivery.[2,11,12]

Finally, maximizing ablation efficiency is an additional consideration. For example, appropriate and complete tumor destruction only occurs when the entire target tumor is exposed to appropriate temperatures, and therefore determined by the pattern of tissue heating in the target tumor. For larger tumors (usually defined as > 3-5 cm in diameter), a single ablation treatment may not be sufficient to entirely encompass the target volume.[13] In these cases, multiple overlapping ablations or simultaneous use of multiple applicators may be required to successfully treat the entire tumor and achieve an ablative margin, though accurate targeting and probe placement can often be technically

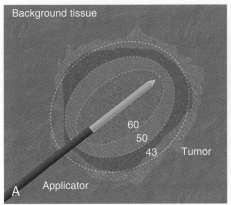
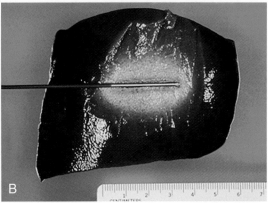

FIGURE 140-1. Schematic **(A)** and pictorial **(B)** representation of focal thermal ablation therapy. Electrode applicators are positioned either with image guidance or direct visualization within target tumor, and thermal energy is applied via electrode. This creates a central zone of high temperatures in tissue immediately around electrode (can exceed 100°C), surrounded by more peripheral zones of sublethal tissue heating (<50°C) and background liver parenchyma. *(From Ahmed M, Brace CL, Lee FT Jr, Goldberg SN. Principles of and advances in percutaneous ablation. Radiology 2011;258:351–69.)*

challenging.[14] Tumor biology can also affect ablation efficiency. Growth patterns of the tumor itself can influence overall treatment outcomes, with slow-growing tumors more amenable to multiple treatment sessions over longer periods of time. Optimizing ablation efficiency is applicable to a wide range of ablative technologies, including both thermal and nonthermal strategies.

PRINCIPLES OF TISSUE HEATING IN THERMAL ABLATION

Ablative tissue heating occurs though two specific mechanisms. First, an applicator placed within the center of the target tumor delivers energy that interacts with tissue to generate focal heat immediately around it. This approach is similar for all thermal ablation strategies regardless of the type of energy source used, though specific mechanisms of heat induction are energy specific (as discussed later in this chapter).[1] The second mechanism of tissue heating in thermal ablation uses thermal tissue conduction.[15] Heat generated around the electrode diffuses through the tumor and results in additional high-temperature heating separate from the direct energy/tissue interactions that occur around the electrode. The contribution of thermal conduction to overall tissue ablation is determined by several factors. Tissue heating patterns vary based upon the specific energy source used; for example, microwave-based systems induce tissue heating at a much faster rate than RF-based systems, so thermal conduction contributes less to overall tissue heating.[15] Tumor and tissue characteristics also affect thermal conduction. As an example, primary hepatic tumors (hepatocellular carcinoma) transmit heat better than the surrounding cirrhotic hepatic parenchyma.[13,16]

Regardless of the energy source used, the endpoint of thermal ablation is adequate tissue heating so as to induce coagulative necrosis throughout the defined target area. Relatively mild increases in tissue temperature above baseline (40°C-42°C) can be tolerated by normal cellular homeostatic mechanisms.[17] Low-temperature hyperthermia (42°C-45°C) results in reversible cellular injury, though

this can increase cellular susceptibility to additional adjuvant therapies such as chemotherapy and radiation.[18,19] Irreversible cellular injury occurs when cells are heated to 46°C to 48°C for 55 to 60 minutes and occurs more rapidly as the temperature rises, so most cell types die in a few minutes when heated at 50°C (Fig. 140-1).[20] Immediate cellular damage centers on protein coagulation of cytosolic and mitochondrial enzymes and nucleic acid–histone protein complexes, which triggers cellular death over the course of several days.[21] *Heat fixation* or *coagulation necrosis* is used to describe this thermal damage, even though ultimate manifestations of cell death may not fulfill strict histopathologic criteria of coagulative necrosis.[22] This has implications with regard to clinical practice because percutaneous biopsy and standard histopathologic interpretation may not be a reliable measure of adequate ablation.[22] Therefore, optimal temperatures for ablation range likely exceed 50°C. On the other end of the temperature spectrum, tissue vaporization occurs at temperatures above 110°C, which in turn limits further current deposition in RF-based systems (e.g., compared to microwave systems, which do not have this limitation).

The exact temperature at which cell death occurs is multifactorial and tissue specific. Based on prior studies demonstrating that tissue coagulation can be induced by focal tissue heating to 50°C for 4 to 6 minutes,[23] this has become the standard surrogate endpoint for thermal ablation therapies in both experimental studies and current clinical paradigms. However, studies have shown that depending on heating time, rate of heat increase, and the tissue being heated, maximum temperatures at the edge of ablation are variable. For example, maximum temperatures at the edge of the ablation zone, known as the *critical temperature*, have been shown to range from 30°C to 77°C for normal tissues and from 41°C to 64°C for tumor models (a 23°C difference).[24,25] Likewise, the total amount of heat administered for a given time, known as the *thermal dose*, varies significantly between different tissues.[24,25] Thus, the threshold target temperature of 50°C should be used only as a general guideline. This conceptual framework is also clearly applicable in determining optimal energy delivery paradigms for nonthermal energy sources.[26]

Different Thermal Ablation Modalities

Thermal ablation strategies attempt to destroy tumor tissue in a minimally invasive manner by increasing or decreasing temperatures sufficiently to induce irreversible cellular injury. RF energy–based systems remain the most clinically ubiquitous technology to date, but alternative energy sources for high-temperature thermal ablation include microwave, laser, and high-intensity focused ultrasound (HIFU). Extreme cooling using cryoablation technologies is also being used for focal thermal tumor ablation. Most recently, an additional ablation technology, irreversible electroporation (IRE), is also being developed as an alternative to thermal technologies.

Radiofrequency

By far, the most well-studied and clinically ubiquitous and relevant percutaneous ablation source to date has been radiofrequency energy. During radiofrequency ablation (RFA), electric current from the generator oscillates between electrodes through ion channels present in most biological tissues. In this way, the RFA setup can be thought of as a simple electrical circuit where the current loop comprises a generator, cabling, electrodes, and tissue as the resistive element. Tissues are imperfect conductors of electricity (i.e., they have electrical impedance), so current flow leads to frictional agitation at the ionic level and heat generation, known as the *Joule effect*. Heating occurs most rapidly in areas of high current density; tissues nearest to an electrode are heated most effectively, whereas more peripheral areas receive heat by thermal conduction.[27] Excessive ablative heating (to temperatures > 100°C) leads to tissue dehydration and water vaporization, which cause dramatic increases in circuit impedance, and ultimately limits further heating.[28] When these effects begin to inhibit current flow from a generator, alternative methods (described later) to decrease circuit impedance, such as expanding the electrode surface area, pulsing the input power, and injections of saline, can be used to augment RF current flow.[29,30]

Microwave

Microwaves are a second thermal energy source used for percutaneous image-guided tumor ablation. In contrast to RFA, where the inserted electrode functions as the active source, in microwave ablation (MWA) the inserted applicators (usually 14-17 gauge) function as antennae for externally applied energy at 1000 to 2450 MHz.[31] The microwave energy applied to tissues results in rotation of polar molecules, which is opposed by frictional forces. As a result, there is conversion of rotational energy into heat.[32] There are several potential advantages of MWA for tissue ablation.[33,34] Microwaves readily penetrate through biological materials, including those with low electrical conductivity (e.g., lung, bone) and dehydrated or charred tissue. Consequently, microwave power can be continually applied to produce very high temperatures (>150°C), improving ablation efficacy by increasing thermal conduction into surrounding tissue.[35] Microwaves also heat tissue more efficiently than RF energy in tissue, do not require ground pads, and multiple antennas can be operated simultaneously.[36] The superposition of microwaves may even be exploited to augment performance.[136-137]

On the other hand, microwave energy is inherently more difficult to distribute than RF energy. Microwaves must be carried in waveguides (e.g., coaxial cable) that are typically more cumbersome than the small wires used to feed energy to RF electrodes, and prone to heating when carrying large amounts of power. It is well known that higher microwave powers increase ablation zone size, but excessive power in the antenna shaft can lead to unintended injuries to other tissues such as the skin.[33,37] Recent investigations have shown that adding a cooling jacket around the antenna can reduce cable heating and eliminate skin burns while effectively increasing the amount of power that can safely be delivered to the tumor.[38]

In clinical practice, MWA has been utilized most in Japan and China, where several systems have been described.[39,40] Most of these systems operate at 2.45 GHz and use monopole, dipole, or slotted coaxial antennas to deliver up to 60 W. Recently, 915 MHz and water-cooled systems have been described that appear to deliver up to 80 W and create larger ablations than previous generation systems.[41] Recently a number of U.S. Food and Drug Administration (FDA)-approved MWA devices have become available for commercial use. Complete clinical characterization of each of these devices is currently ongoing.

Laser

Laser ablation or laser photocoagulation is another method for inducing thermally mediated coagulation necrosis that has been employed for percutaneous tumor ablation. For this procedure, flexible thin optic fibers are inserted into the target through percutaneously placed needles, using imaging guidance. The laser provides sufficient energy to allow for significant heat deposition surrounding the fiber tip, inducing protein denaturation and cellular death. As with RF systems, thermal profiles have been demonstrated to correlate well with the extent of coagulation necrosis observed histopathologically,[42,43] as well as with ultrasound[43,44] and T1-weighted magnetic resonance (MR) images.[45,46] Most devices use a standard laser source (Nd:YAG, erbium, holmium, etc.) that produces precise wavelengths. Additional device modifications have been developed to increase the size of the heated volume, including: (1) type of laser fiber (flexible/glass dome), (2) modifications to the tip (i.e., flexible diffuser tip or scattering dome), (3) length of applicator and diameter of the optic fiber, and (4) the number of laser applicators used (i.e., single vs. multiple applicators).[47] Similar to RF technologies, additional device modifications such as pulsing algorithms and internal cooling of the applicator have also been reported.[48]

Ultrasound

High-intensity focused ultrasound (HIFU) is a transcutaneous technique that has recently been studied for minimally invasive treatment of localized malignancy.[49,50] HIFU uses a parabolic transducer to focus the ultrasound energy at a distance, creating a focused beam of energy with very high peak intensity. This focusing of energy has been likened to using a magnifying glass to focus sunlight.[51] The focused energy is transmitted transcutaneously into the targeted tissue without requiring percutaneous insertion of an electrode or transducer. The ultrasound energy absorbed by tissue is converted to heat, which ablates tissue via

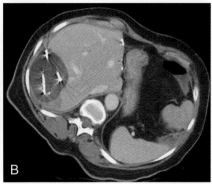

FIGURE 140-2. Cryoablation. **A,** Schematic illustration of tip of a cryoprobe with surrounding iceball formation. **B,** Axial contrast-enhanced computed tomography image demonstrates multiple cryoprobes placed and iceball formation during cryoablation of tumor in right lobe of liver. *(From Ahmed M, Brace CL, Lee FT Jr, Goldberg SN. Principles of and advances in percutaneous ablation. Radiology 2011;258:351–69.)*

coagulation necrosis. Since insertion of a percutaneous applicator is not required, HIFU can be considered the least invasive of the "minimally invasive" therapies. However, limitations in time and coverage, especially given respiratory motion, have limited most clinical investigations to benign conditions in static organs such as the breast,[52] uterus,[53] and prostate.[54]

Cryoablation

Cryoablation induces focal tissue injury using alternating sessions of freezing and tissue thawing[55-59] (Fig. 140-2). Minimally invasive cryoablation is performed using a closed specially constructed cryoprobe that is placed on or inside a tumor. In the past, cryoablation had to be performed in the setting of an open procedure owing to the large caliber of available probes; however, technologic developments have led to smaller probes that can be placed percutaneously under MR or computed tomography (CT) guidance. Liquid forms of inert gases are cycled through the hollow probes, resulting in tissue cooling. The two main types of systems use gas or liquid nitrogen, or argon gas. Many of the systems that use argon gas base their freezing on the Joule-Thompson effect.[60-62] More recent work has involved probes that use "super-critical" nitrogen to cool faster and deeper into tissue.[63]

Cryoablation induces direct cellular injury through multiple mechanisms including tissue cooling.[64] At low cooling rates, freezing primarily propagates extracellularly, which draws water from the cell and results in osmotic dehydration.[65] The intracellular high solute concentration that develops leads to damaged enzymatic systems, protein damage, and injury to the cell membrane.[66,67] At higher cooling rates, water is trapped within the cell, intracellular ice formation occurs, and organelle and membrane injury results.[65,68] A second hypothesized mechanism of cryoablative tissue destruction centers on vascular injury consisting of mechanical injury to the vessel wall, direct injury to cells lining the vessel, and post-thaw injury from reperfusion.[64] Mechanical injury to the vessel wall from intravascular ice formation results in increased vessel porosity, reduced plasma oncotic pressure, and perivascular edema.[69] Endothelial injury further results from the exposure of underlying connective tissue to the vessel lumen and subsequent thrombus formation.[70] Damage to endothelial cells occurs in a fashion similar to the direct cellular injury described

earlier. Reperfusion injury results from the release of vasoactive factors after the tissue thaws, which leads to vasodilation and increased blood flow to treated areas. Subsequent high oxygen delivery[71] and neutrophil migration[72] into the damaged area results in increased free radical formation, and through the peroxidation of membrane lipids, further endothelial damage.

The degree to which each mechanism of cellular and tissue injury described determines overall tissue destruction is governed by characteristics of the administration algorithm, including freezing and thawing rate, the minimum (i.e., coldest) temperature reached, and the duration that temperature was maintained.[64] However, for current commonly used systems, argon provides a heat sink of about 9 kJ and can generate temperatures as low as −140°C inside the iceball, which expands by thermal conduction.[73] Finally, the fact that the lethal isotherm (−20°C to −40°C) rests several millimeters inside the iceball boundary must be considered when using imaging to assess cryoablation treatment efficacy.[74]

Irreversible Electroporation

Percutaneous irreversible electroporation (IRE) is new ablation technology and is most notable because it is presumed to be inherently nonthermal (i.e., no heat is produced to cause cell death). Rather, cells are eradicated using several microsecond- to millisecond-long pulses of electric current. The pulses generate electrical fields up to 3 kV/cm that cause irreversible damage to the cell membrane, thereby inducing apoptosis.[75,76] Since IRE is predominantly nonthermal, heat sinks, such as large vessels, should have a much smaller influence on the ablation zone than with thermal treatments. IRE also appears to limit damage to more collagenous tissues and nerves, which if verified in larger trials will make it an attractive option for thermally sensitive areas (e.g., in the prostate, near large blood vessels, or the renal cortex).[77]

IRE electrodes consist of insulated 19-gauge (1.1 mm diameter) or larger needles with an exposed active portion of 1 to 4 cm. For most applications, multiple electrodes are required and spaced 1 to 3 cm apart to provide sufficient electrical field strengths for irreversible cell damage. A single-needle bipolar electrode is also available for more localized treatments. Initial studies required very high-voltage pulses, but recent reports have shown that lower-voltage pulses can be used when repeated several hundred times.[78] Current IRE devices do have notable drawbacks, including generation of potentially dangerous electrical harmonics that can stimulate muscle contraction or cardiac arrhythmias. These techniques require general anesthesia and paralytic induction and have treatment times on the order of seconds that prevent treatment monitoring or adjustment. There is also a requirement for accurate placement of several needles to achieve moderate-sized ablations (≈3-4 cm), and a lack of coagulation around needle insertion sites, which theoretically could elevate bleeding complication risks. Ongoing research aims to minimize these complications.

ADVANCES IN RADIOFREQUENCY ABLATION: A MODEL FOR TECHNOLOGIC EVOLUTION

The full discussion of technologic advances that have been and continue to be made in RFA is available at www.expertconsult.com.

Practical Application of Technologic Developments: Choosing an Ablation Device

Several different commercially available RFA devices are commonly used, and vary based on their power application algorithms and electrode designs.

Selecting a Radiofrequency Ablation System: Is One System Better Than Another?

Zones of adequate thermal ablation can achieved with most commercially available RFA devices when properly used as described in the instructions for use. Though the specific size of the ablation zone and the time required to achieve adequate ablation will likely vary between different manufacturers and devices, a recent study by Lin et al. compared four separate and commonly used devices in over 100 patients with primary and secondary hepatic tumors, and found little difference in ablation time and local tumor progression.[101] Thus, it is important for operators to be completely familiar with their device of choice, including electrode shapes and deployment techniques, power-input algorithms, and common trouble-shooting issues, so as to permit thorough treatment planning and maximize optimal clinical outcomes. Ultimately, good operator technique and careful patient selection contributes at least as much to treatment success as does the specific electrode choice.

Understanding the Principles or Algorithm of the Selected Device

Several commonly used RF devices use different power application algorithms based upon current flow, impedance, or time to deliver RF energy. Current electrode designs are paired to specific devices and companies, and RF power algorithms are also commonly tailored to specific electrode designs (such that operators can not interchange electrodes from one device to another, and the greatest efficiencies in use are likely found by following company-recommended application protocols). Several specific electrode designs are available, most commonly divided into those that are needle-like versus multi-tined expandable. Specifically, practitioners should be familiar with the shape of the coagulation zone each system generates. For example, needle-like electrodes induce a more oval ablation zone *parallel* to the axis of the electrode, whereas expandable electrodes generate ablation zones that are oval shaped *perpendicular* to the shaft of the electrode.

Examples of several commercially available systems (limited to the most common FDA-approved devices) are illustrated in Figure 140-3. The Cool-Tip RF electrode system (Valleylab Inc., Boulder, Colo.) uses a pulsed application applied over a 12-minute time period that inputs high amounts of current, alternating frequently with "off-periods" triggered by rises in impedance, to reduce tissue overheating around the electrode. The Cool-Tip RF system uses 17-gauge needle-like electrodes as single, cluster, or multiple single electrodes that are internally cooled with icewater (to a temperature of < 10°C). Electrode switching technology (described earlier) is currently only available with the Cool-Tip RF system. In contrast, the Boston Scientific RF 3000 ablation system (Boston Scientific, Natick, Mass.) employs two rounds of slowly increasing power to achieve tissue heating, which occurs until tissue impedance starts to rise (thereby limiting further current input) to threshold levels, colloquially termed *roll-off*. The RF 3000 system uses umbrella-shaped expandable electrodes with multiple (10-12) tines extending out from the needle shaft. Finally, the RITA system (AngioDynamics, Queensbury, N.Y.), another commonly used device, administers RF energy to set temperature endpoints (usually 105°C as measured by sensors within the electrode tips) combined with incremental extension of an expandable electrode system.

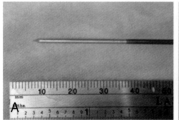
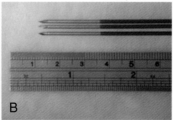
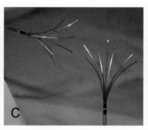
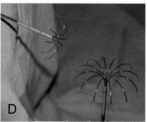

FIGURE 140-3. Commonly used and commercially available electrode designs. **A,** A single internally cooled electrode with a 3-cm active tip (Cool-Tip system [Valleylab, Boulder, Colo.]). **B,** A cluster internally cooled electrode system with three 2.5-cm active tips (Cluster electrode system [Valleylab]). **C-D,** Two variations of an expandable electrode system: **C,** Starburst (RITA Medical Systems, Mountain View, Calif.) and, **D,** LeVeen (Boston Scientific, Natick, Mass.). *(From Ahmed M, Brace CL, Lee FT Jr, Goldberg SN. Principles of and advances in percutaneous ablation. Radiology 2011;258:351–69.)*

The RITA system uses an expandable electrode system paired with slow saline drip infusion.

MODIFICATION OF THE BIOPHYSIOLOGIC ENVIRONMENT

Although larger coagulation zones have been created by modifying electrode design in ablative procedures, limitations due to the tumor physiology itself have to be considered. Recent investigations have centered on altering underlying tumor physiology as a means to improving thermal ablation. Current studies have focused on the effects of tissue characteristics in the setting of temperature-based therapies such as tissue perfusion, thermal conductivity, and system-specific characteristics such as electrical conductivity for RFA.

Tissue Perfusion

The leading factor constraining thermal ablation coagulation size in tumors continues to be tissue blood flow, which has two effects: a large-vessel heat sink effect and a microvascular perfusion-mediated tissue cooling effect. Firstly, larger-diameter blood vessels with higher flow act as heat sinks, drawing away heat from the ablative area. Lu et al. show this in an in vivo porcine model by examining the effect of hepatic vessel diameter on RFA outcome. Using CT and histopathologic analysis, more complete thermal heating and a reduced heat sink effect is seen when the heating zone was less than 3 mm in diameter.[102] In contrast, vessels over 3 mm in diameter had higher patency rates, less endothelial injury, and greater viability of surrounding hepatocytes after RFA. Studies confirm the effect of hepatic blood flow on RF-induced coagulation, in which increased coagulation volumes were obtained with decreased hepatic blood flow either by embolotherapy, angiographic balloon occlusion, coil embolization, or the Pringle maneuver (total portal inflow occlusion).[103,104]

The second effect of tissue vasculature is due to perfusion-mediated tissue cooling (capillary vascular flow), which also functions as a heat sink. By drawing heat from the treatment zone, this effect reduces the volume of tissue that receives the required minimal thermal dose for coagulation. Targeted microvascular perfusion by using pharmacologic alteration of blood flow can also improve overall RFA efficacy. Goldberg et al. modulated hepatic blood flow using intraarterial vasopressin and high-dose halothane in conjunction with RFA in in vivo porcine liver.[105] Horkan et al. modulated the use of arsenic trioxide, showing reduced blood flow and increased tumor destruction.[106] More recently, another antiangiogenic drug, sorafenib, has been combined with RFA to increase overall tumor coagulation in small-animal models.[107] In this regard, newer nonthermal energy sources (e.g., IRE) have been shown to be less affected by these effects and will likely provide an alternative in clinical situations where perfusion-mediated cooling impacts ablation outcome.[108]

Thermal Conductivity

Initial clinical studies using RFA for hepatocellular carcinoma in the setting of underlying cirrhosis noted an "oven" effect (i.e., increased heating efficacy for tumors surrounded by cirrhotic liver or fat, such as exophytic renal cell carcinomas) or altered thermal transmission at the junction of tumor tissue and surrounding tissue.[13] Subsequent experimental studies in ex vivo agar phantoms and bovine liver have confirmed the effects of varying tumor and surrounding tissue thermal conductivity on effective heat transmission during RFA, and further demonstrated the role of "optimal" thermal conductivity characteristics on ablation outcome.[16,109] For example, very poor tumor thermal conductivity limits heat transmission centrifugally away from the electrode, with marked heating in the central portion of the tumor and limited, potentially incomplete, heating in peripheral portions of the tumor. In contrast, increased thermal conductivity (e.g., in cystic lesions) results in fast heat transmission (i.e., heat dissipation), with potentially incomplete and heterogeneous tumor heating. Furthermore, in agar phantom and computer modeling studies, Liu et al. demonstrated that differences in thermal conductivity between the tumor and surrounding background tissue (specifically, decreased thermal conductivity from increased fat content of surrounding tissue) results in increased temperatures at the tumor margin. However, heating was limited in the surrounding medium, making a 1-cm "ablative margin" more difficult to achieve.[16,109] Understanding the role of thermal conductivity and tissue and tumor-specific characteristics on tissue heating may be useful when trying to predict ablation outcome in varying clinical settings (e.g., in exophytic renal cell carcinomas surrounded by perirenal fat, lung tumors surrounded by aerated normal parenchyma, or osseous metastases surrounded by cortical bone).[16]

Electrical Conductivity

The power deposition in RF-induced tissue heating is strongly dependent on local electrical conductivity; its effect can be divided into two main categories. First, altering the electrical activity environment immediately around the RF electrode with ionic agents can increase electrical conductivity prior to or during RFA. High local saline concentration increases the area of the active surface electrode, allowing greater energy deposition, thereby increasing the extent of coagulation necrosis.[110] Saline may be beneficial when ablating cavitary lesions that might not have a sufficient current path. However, it should be noted that saline infusion is not always a predictable process, since fluid can migrate to unintended locations and cause complications if not used properly.[111] Second, different electrical conductivities between the tumor and surrounding background organ can affect tissue heating at the tumor margin. Several studies show increases in tissue heating at the tumor/organ interface when the surrounding medium is characterized by reduced lower electrical conductivity.[109] In certain clinical settings, such as treating focal tumors in either lung or bone, marked differences in electrical conductivity may result in variable heating at the tumor/organ interface and, indeed, limit heating in the surrounding organ and make obtaining a 1-cm ablative margin difficult. Lastly, electrical conductivity must be taken into account when using techniques such as hydrodissection to protect adjacent organs. Nonionic fluids can be used to protect tissues adjacent to the ablation zone (e.g., diaphragm, bowel) from thermal injury. For this application, fluids with low ion content, such as 5% dextrose in water (D_5W) should be used, since they have been proven to electrically force RF current away from the protected organ, decrease the size and incidence of burns on the diaphragm and bowel, and reduce pain scores in patients treated with D_5W when compared to ionic solutions such as saline.[82,83] Ionic solutions like 0.9% saline should *not* be used for hydrodissection since, as noted, they actually increase RF current flow.[112]

Tissue Fluid Content

Microwave-based systems use electromagnetic energy to forcibly align molecules with an intrinsic dipole moment (e.g., water) to the externally applied magnetic field, which generates kinetic energy and results in local tissue heating. Therefore, higher tissue water content influences the rates and maximum amounts of achievable tissue heating in these systems.[35] Incorporating tissue internal water content into computer modeling of tumor ablation to more accurately predict tissue heating has also been proposed.[113] In addition, Brace et al. have demonstrated that greater dehydration (and resultant contraction of the ablation zone) occurs with MWA compared to RFA systems.[114] Optimization of microwave heating by modulating the tissue fluid content is also being investigated.[115]

RATIONALE FOR COMBINING THERMAL ABLATION WITH OTHER THERAPIES

Substantial efforts have been made in modifying ablation systems and the biological environment to improve the clinical utility of percutaneous ablation, but limitations in clinical efficacy persist. For example, with further long-term follow-up of patients undergoing ablation therapy, there has been an increased incidence of detection of progressive local tumor growth for all tumor types and sizes, despite initial indications of adequate therapy, suggesting there are residual foci of viable untreated disease in a substantial but unknown number of cases.[13] The ability to achieve complete and uniform eradication of all malignant cells remains a key barrier to clinical success, so strategies that can increase the completeness of RF tumor destruction, even for small lesions, are needed.

Several studies have demonstrated that tumor death can be enhanced when combining RF thermal therapy with adjuvant chemo- or radiosensitizers. The goal of this combined approach is to increase tumor destruction occurring within the sizable peripheral zone of sublethal temperatures (i.e., largely reversible cell damage induced by mildly elevating tissue temperatures to 41°C-45°C) surrounding the heat-induced coagulation.[116] Modeling studies demonstrate that were the threshold for cell death to be decreased by as few as 5°C, tumor coagulation could be increased up to 1.5 cm (up to a 59% increase in spherical volume of the ablation zone).[109] Improved tumor cytotoxicity is also likely to reduce the local recurrence rate at the treatment site. Although there is high temperature heating throughout the zone of RFA, heterogeneity of thermal diffusion (especially in the presence of vascularity) retards uniform and complete ablation.[117] Since local control requires complete tumor destruction, ablation may be inadequate even if large

zones of ablation that encompass the entire tumor are created. By killing tumor cells at lower temperatures, this combined paradigm will not only increase necrosis volume but may also create a more complete area of tumor destruction by filling in untreated gaps within the ablation zone.[118] Combined treatment also has the potential to achieve equivalent tumor destruction with a concomitant reduction of the duration or course of therapy (a process that currently takes hours to treat larger tumors, with many protocols requiring repeat sessions). A reduction in the time required to completely ablate a given tumor volume would permit patients with larger or greater numbers of tumors to be treated. Shorter heating time could also potentially improve their quality of life by reducing the number of patient visits and the substantial costs of prolonged procedures that require image guidance.

Combined Radiofrequency Ablation and Transarterial Chemoembolization

Independently, RFA and transarterial chemoembolization (TACE) are both commonly used modalities for locoregional treatment of liver tumors such as hepatocellular carcinoma (HCC), but several limitations to their optimal outcomes persist. RFA is less effective in larger tumors and difficult to use in specific locations or near larger blood vessels. TACE can be used for larger tumors, but rates of tumor necrosis are lower (30%-90% compared to > 90% for RFA). Therefore, several experimental and clinical studies have investigated administering them in a combined manner.

The rationale for combined RF/TACE is based upon several potential advantages. This includes combined two-hit cytotoxic effects of exposure to nonlethal low-level hyperthermia in peri-ablational tumor and adjuvant chemotherapy. Alterations in tumor perfusion can potentiate the effects of either RFA through pre-ablation embolization of tumor vasculature, or TACE with postablation peripheral hyperemia increasing blood flow for TACE. Finally, performing TACE first can improve tumor visualization (through intratumoral iodized oil deposition) for RFA.

RFA and TACE can be administered in varying paradigms based upon the sequence and time between therapies. Mostafa et al. demonstrated in VX2 tumors implanted in rabbit liver that the largest treatment volumes were obtained when TACE preceded RFA, compared with RF before TACE or either therapy alone.[104] Ahrar et al. investigated the effects of high-temperature heating on commonly used TACE agents (doxorubicin, mitomycin-C, and cisplatin) and found minimal change in the cytotoxic activity of the agents when exposed to clinically relevant durations of heating (>100°C for < 20 minutes).[119] For HCC tumors invisible on ultrasound and unenhanced CT, Lee et al. reported that 71% of tumors could be adequately visualized for subsequent RFA.[120] Based upon this, the optimal strategy for administration is likely performing TACE first, followed by RFA. This is confirmed in a recent randomized controlled study by Morimoto et al. comparing TACE-RF (on the same day) to RF alone for intermediate-sized HCC (3.1-5 cm diameter), where TACE-RF resulted in lower rates of local tumor progression at 3 years.[121]

Another approach in combination therapy is to primarily treat the target tumor with a single modality (either TACE

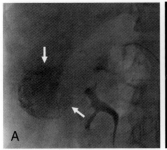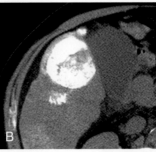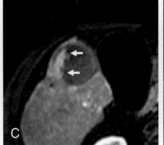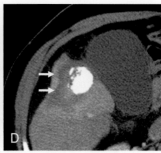

FIGURE 140-4. Combining transarterial chemoembolization (TACE) with radiofrequency ablation (RFA) in a 45-year-old man with a 4.2-cm focal hepatocellular carcinoma. Initially, Lipiodol-based TACE was performed, with good Lipiodol tumor staining on immediate fluoroscopic images **(A)** and follow-up non-contrast axial computed tomography (CT) images **(B)**. **C,** On 1-month follow-up contrast-enhanced T1-weighted axial magnetic resonance imaging, however, a residual focus of arterial enhancement can be seen along lateral aspect of tumor. This was successfully treated with percutaneous RFA using a single 3-cm internally cooled electrode. **D,** Follow-up contrast-enhanced axial CT image demonstrates complete treatment (determined by lack of residual contrast enhancement in ablated tumor).

or RF) followed by additional adjuvant treatments using either one or both modalities for residual disease. For example, RFA can be performed for an initial presentation of limited disease, followed by TACE performed at a later date for residual peripheral tumor, satellite nodules, or new foci. Likewise, TACE can be performed initially to control more extensive disease, with subsequent RF directed at small foci of local recurrence or new small nodules (Fig. 140-4).

Several studies using combination therapy have reported increases in ablation size and increased treatment efficacy with combination RF-TACE, particularly as the primary treatment of large (>5 cm) unresectable tumors. For example, Yang et al. treated 103 patients with recurrent unresectable HCC after hepatectomy and reported lower intrahepatic recurrence and longer 3-year survival compared to either therapy alone.[122] The potential benefit of combining RF with TACE for small (<3 cm) tumors remains less clear. A recent meta-analysis of randomized controlled studies reported no significant survival benefit for combination RF-TACE over RF alone.[123] Finally, tailoring treatment to each individual case remains important because each modality can be adjuvantly used to "mop-up" residual disease after primary therapy.

Combining Thermal Ablation with Adjuvant Chemotherapy

Several investigators have combined RF thermal ablation with adjuvant chemotherapy, most commonly using doxorubicin.[116,124] In an initial study, Goldberg et al. performed RFA in conjunction with percutaneous intratumoral injection of free doxorubicin, demonstrating a significant increase when treated with both RF and intratumoral doxorubicin (11.4 mm) compared to RF alone (6.7 mm).[124] However, many difficulties have been encountered in the clinical setting with image-guided direct intratumoral injection, including non-uniform drug diffusion and limited control of drug distribution. Systemic intravenous injection of free chemotherapy is also associated with dose-limiting side effects. Therefore, the use of doxorubicin encapsulated within a liposome as an adjuvant to RFA has also been advanced. Advantages of using liposome nanoparticles as a

delivery vehicle are prolonged circulation time, selective agent delivery through the leaky tumor endothelium (an enhanced permeability and retention effect), and reduced toxicity profiles. Therefore, liposomal doxorubicin has proved beneficial in the clinical setting.

Several studies have focused on combining RFA with a commercially available preparation of liposomal doxorubicin (Doxil) or thermosensitive (preparations designed to release their contents when exposed to specific temperatures, e.g., 37°C-41°C) liposomal doxorubicin[125-127] (Fig. 140-5). Initial animal experiments demonstrated large ablation zones, increased intratumoral drug accumulation, and longer survival times (with correlative reduced tumor growth rates) for combination RF and intravenous liposomal doxorubicin compared to RF alone. A pilot study was conducted combining RFA (using internally cooled electrodes) with adjuvant Doxil therapy in 10 patients who were randomized into two treatment groups of RFA alone and RFA with pretreatment Doxil (24 hours pre-RFA)[118] (Fig. 140-6). Patients receiving Doxil therapy with RFA showed a 25% increase in coagulation volume 4 weeks post ablation, compared to a decrease of 76% to 88% for tumors treated with RFA alone. Additional clinically beneficial findings were observed only in the combination therapy group, including increased diameter of the treatment effect for multiple tumor types, improved completeness of tumor destruction (particularly adjacent to intratumoral vessels), and increased treatment effect including the peritumoral liver parenchyma (suggesting a contribution to achieving an adequate ablative margin).

Additional studies on this combination therapy demonstrated greatest coagulation effect when given post RF, pointing to a potential two-hit effect, with initial reversible cell injury inflicted by sublethal doses of heat in the more peripheral ablation zone, followed by irreversible injury by doxorubicin on already susceptible cells. More recent mechanistic studies have identified upregulation of cellular stress pathways with combination therapy, including increased expression of markers of apoptosis, and nitrative and oxidative stress. Strategies to potentiate this tumor cell injury even further by using additional pro-apoptotic and anti–heat shock protein agents in liposomes are also being actively investigated.

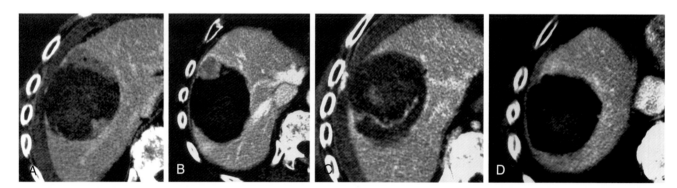

FIGURE 140-5. Method for combining thermal ablation with targeted drug delivery. *Left,* Drugs are brought to tumor site as part of normal circulation. *Middle,* Temperature elevations inside ablation zone facilitate local drug release, which then accumulates in sublethal region at periphery of ablation zone. *Right,* Net result is a larger zone of ablation than possible with ablation alone. (© 2008 by the Board of Regents of the University of Wisconsin System.)

FIGURE 140-6. Increased tumor destruction with combined RF and liposomal doxorubicin in an 82-year-old male with an 8.2-cm vascular hepatoma. **A,** Computed tomography (CT) image obtained immediately following radiofrequency ablation (RFA) shows persistent regions of residual untreated tumor (black zone = ablated region). **B,** Two weeks following therapy, there is interval increase in coagulation; 1.5-cm inferior region of residual tumor and 1.2-cm anteromedial portion of tumor no longer enhance. A persistent nodule of viable tumor is identified. This was successfully treated with a course of RFA. **C,** CT image obtained immediately following RFA demonstrates persistence of a large vessel coursing through nonenhancing ablated lesion. **D,** Two weeks post therapy, there is no enhancement throughout this region, and no vessel was seen on any of three phases of contrast enhancement. No evidence of local tumor recurrence was identified at 48-month follow-up. *(From Goldberg SN, Kamel IR, Kruskal JB, et al. Radiofrequency ablation of hepatic tumors: Increased tumor destruction with adjuvant liposomal doxorubicin therapy. AJR Am J Roentgenol 2002;179:93–101.)*

Combining Thermal Ablation with Adjuvant Radiation

Several studies have reported early investigation into combination RFA and radiation therapy, with promising results.[3,128-130] There are known synergistic effects of combined external beam radiation therapy and low-temperature hyperthermia.[52] Experimental animal studies have demonstrated increased tumor necrosis, reduced tumor growth, and improved survival with combined external beam radiation and RFA, compared to either therapy alone.[130,131] For example, in a rat breast adenocarcinoma model, Horkan et al. demonstrated significantly longer mean endpoint survival for animals treated with combination RFA and 20-Gy external beam radiation (94 days) compared to either radiation (40 days) or RFA (20 days) alone. Preliminary clinical studies in primary lung malignancies confirm the synergistic effects of these therapies.[3] Potential causes for the synergy include sensitization of the tumor to subsequent radiation due to the increased oxygenation resulting from hyperthermia-induced increased blood flow to the tumor.[132]

Another possible mechanism, which has been seen in animal tumor models, is an inhibition of radiation-induced repair and recovery and increased free radical formation.[133] Future work is needed to identify the optimal temperature for ablation and optimal radiation dose, as well as the most effective method of administering radiation therapy (external beam radiation therapy, brachytherapy, or yttrium microspheres), on an organ-by-organ basis.

IMPROVING IMAGE GUIDANCE AND TUMOR TARGETING

For a discussion of some of the major challenges posed by thermal ablation and advances in overcoming them, please visit www.expertconsult.com.

CONCLUSIONS

Several different percutaneous and minimally invasive therapies have been well described for use in treating focal malignancies. Investigators have characterized many of the basic principles underlying the tumor ablative features of these treatments. We have provided an overview of the basic principles of each of these strategies and described the recent technologic modifications that have been developed to further improve clinical success of these therapies. Future directions of research are now looking to combination therapies, such as combining chemotherapy and/or radiation therapy with thermal ablation, as the next step to better understand how thermal energy interacts with tissue to further improve predictability and clinical effectiveness of percutaneous thermal tumor ablations.

KEY POINTS

- Focal thermal tumor ablation is a viable alternative for the treatment of many solid focal malignancies, especially in nonsurgical candidates.
- Benefits of thermal ablation include low morbidity and mortality, low cost, nonsurgical patient inclusion, and same-day discharge.

- Successful treatment is a balance between complete tumor destruction and minimizing damage to surrounding normal parenchyma and adjacent structures.
- Widespread adoption of radiofrequency ablation will rely upon improving and increasing tumor ablation volume. Adjuvant therapies such as antiangiogenic agents, chemotherapeutics, and radiation in this capacity hold great promise.

▶ SUGGESTED READINGS

Goldberg SN, Grassi CJ, Cardella JF, et al. for the Society of Interventional Radiology Technology Assessment Committee and the International Working Group on Image-Guided Tumor Ablation. Image-guided tumor ablation: standardization of terminology and reporting criteria. J Vasc Interv Radiol 2009;20(7 Suppl):S377–90.

The complete reference list is available online at www.expertconsult.com.

CHAPTER 141

Energy-Based Ablation of Hepatocellular Cancer

Riccardo Lencioni, Elena Bozzi, Laura Crocetti, and Carlo Bartolozzi

Hepatocellular carcinoma (HCC) is the fifth most common cause of cancer, and its incidence is increasing worldwide because of the dissemination of hepatitis B and C virus infection.[1,2] Patients with cirrhosis are at the highest risk of developing HCC and should be monitored every 6 months to diagnose the tumor at an asymptomatic stage.[2]

If diagnosed at an early stage, patients should be considered for any of the available options that may provide a high rate of complete response. These include surgical resection, liver transplantation, and percutaneous techniques of tumor ablation.[3] Indication for surgical resection is currently restricted to patients with single asymptomatic HCC and extremely well-preserved liver function who have neither clinically significant portal hypertension nor abnormal bilirubin.[4,5] Cadaveric liver transplantation is limited by the shortage of donors, and living donor liver transplantation is still at an early stage of clinical application.[4,5] As a result, percutaneous ablation plays a key role in therapeutic management of HCC.

PRETREATMENT EVALUATION

Imaging Assessment

In the setting of a patient with known hepatitis B or cirrhosis of other etiology, a solid nodular lesion found during surveillance has a high likelihood of being HCC. However, it has been shown by pathologic studies that many small nodules detected in cirrhotic livers do not correspond to HCC.[6]

Current guidelines recommend further investigation of nodules detected during surveillance with dynamic imaging techniques, including contrast-enhanced multidetector computed tomography (MDCT) and contrast-enhanced magnetic resonance imaging (MRI).[4] In fact, one of the key pathologic factors for differential diagnosis that is reflected in dynamic imaging studies is the vascular supply to the lesion. Through the progression from regenerative nodule, to low-grade dysplastic nodule (DN), to high-grade DN, to frank HCC, one sees loss of visualization of portal tracts and development of new arterial vessels, termed *nontriadal arteries*, which become the dominant blood supply in overt HCC lesions.[6] It is this neovascularity that allows HCC to be diagnosed and is the key for imaging cirrhotic patients.

A rational diagnostic protocol should be structured according to the actual risk of malignancy and the possibility of achieving a reliable diagnosis. Since the prevalence of HCC among ultrasound-detected nodules is strongly related to the size of the lesion, the diagnostic workup depends on lesion size. Lesions smaller than 1 cm in diameter have a low likelihood of being HCC, but minute hepatic nodules detected by ultrasound may become malignant over time. Therefore, these nodules should be followed up to detect growth suggestive of malignant transformation. A reasonable protocol is to repeat ultrasound every 3 months until the lesion grows to more than 1 cm, at which point additional diagnostic techniques are applied.[4] It has to be emphasized, however, that the absence of growth during the follow-up period does not rule out the malignant nature of the nodule, because even an early HCC may take more than 1 year to increase in size.[4] When the nodule exceeds 1 cm in size, the lesion is more likely to be HCC, and diagnostic confirmation should be pursued. Current guidelines recommend that the diagnosis of HCC can be made noninvasively without biopsy in a nodule larger than 1 cm that shows the characteristic vascular features of HCC (i.e., arterial hypervascularization with washout in the portal venous or delayed phase) even in patients with normal α-fetoprotein values. Such lesions should be treated as HCC, since the positive predictive value of the clinical and radiologic findings exceeds 95%, provided that examinations are conducted by using state-of-the-art equipment and interpreted by radiologists with extensive expertise in liver imaging.[7] For lesions above 1 cm without a characteristic vascular profile, a second dynamic study is required. If definitive diagnosis is not reached with these techniques, biopsy is recommended.[4]

It has to be pointed out that noninvasive criteria based on imaging findings can be applied only in patients with established cirrhosis.[4] For nodules detected in noncirrhotic livers, as well as for those showing atypical vascular patterns, biopsy is recommended. Ultrasound is widely accepted for HCC surveillance, but multidetector CT or dynamic MRI are required for intrahepatic staging of the disease; these examinations provide a comprehensive assessment of the liver parenchyma and can identify additional tumor foci.

Clinical Staging

In most solid malignancies, tumor stage at presentation determines prognosis and treatment management. Most patients with HCC, however, have two diseases—liver cirrhosis and HCC—and complex interactions between the two have major implications for prognosis and treatment choice.[8] Therefore, the TNM system has limited usefulness in the clinical decision-making process because it does not take into account hepatic functional status. Several scoring systems have been developed in the past few years in attempts to stratify patients according to expected survival.

However, the only system that links staging with treatment modalities is the Barcelona Clinic Liver Cancer (BCLC) staging system.[9,10]

The BCLC includes variables related to tumor stage, liver functional status, physical status, and cancer-related symptoms and provides an estimation of life expectancy that is based on published response rates to the various treatments. In the BCLC system, early-stage HCC includes patients with World Health Organization (WHO) performance status of 0, preserved liver function (Child-Pugh class A or B), and solitary tumor or up to 3 nodules smaller than 3 cm each, in the absence of macroscopic vascular invasion and extrahepatic spread. If the patient has Child-Pugh class A cirrhosis and a solitary tumor smaller than 2 cm, the stage may be defined as very early. Patients with multinodular HCC with neither vascular invasion nor extrahepatic spread are classified as intermediate-stage according to the BCLC staging system, provided they have a performance status of 0 and Child-Pugh class A or B cirrhosis.[11] Patients with portal vein invasion or extrahepatic disease are classified as advanced stage. The terminal stage includes patients who have either severe hepatic decompensation (Child-Pugh class C) or performance status greater than 2.

TREATMENT OF EARLY-STAGE HEPATOCELLULAR CARCINOMA

Patients with early-stage HCC can benefit from curative therapies including surgical resection, liver transplantation, and percutaneous ablation, and have the possibility of long-term cure, with 5-year survival figures ranging from 50% to 75%.[10] However, there is no firm evidence to establish the optimal first-line treatment for early-stage HCC because of the lack of randomized controlled trials (RCTs) comparing radical therapies. Patients should be evaluated in referral centers by multidisciplinary teams involving hepatologists, oncologists, interventional radiologists, surgeons, and pathologists to guarantee careful selection of candidates for each treatment option and ensure expert application of these treatments.[10]

Surgical Resection

Resection is the treatment of choice for HCC in noncirrhotic patients, who account for about 5% of the cases in Western countries. However, in patients with cirrhosis, candidates for resection have to be carefully selected to reduce the risk of postoperative liver failure. It has been shown that a normal bilirubin concentration and the absence of clinically significant portal hypertension are the best predictors of excellent outcomes after surgery.[12] In experienced hands, such patients have treatment-related mortality of less than 1% to 3% and may achieve 5-year survival higher than 70%.[12-14] In contrast, survival drops to less than 50% at 5 years in patients with significant portal hypertension, and to less than 30% at 5 years in those with both adverse factors (portal hypertension and elevated bilirubin).[12] Most groups restrict the indication for resection to patients with a single tumor in a suitable location. Anatomic resections guided by intraoperative ultrasound techniques are preferred to wedge resections, because they

include any microsatellite lesions possibly located in the same hepatic segment as the main tumor. In fact, it is known that neoplastic dissemination occurs at very early stages in HCC via the invasion of small peripheral portal vein branches.[6] After resection, tumor recurrence rate exceeds 70% at 5 years, including recurrence due to dissemination and de novo tumors developing in the remnant cirrhotic liver. The most powerful predictors of recurrence are the presence of microvascular invasion and/or additional tumor sites besides the primary lesion.[12]

Liver Transplantation

Liver transplantation is the only option that provides cure of both the tumor and the underlying chronic liver disease. It is recognized as the best treatment for patients with solitary HCC smaller than 5 cm in the setting of decompensated cirrhosis and for those with early multifocal disease (up to 3 lesions, none larger than 3 cm).[4] However, for patients with a solitary small tumor in well-compensated cirrhosis, the optimal treatment strategy is still under debate.[15] The reported outcomes of patients who actually underwent transplantation are better than those of patients submitted to resection, especially if the substantially lower rates of tumor recurrence (<10%-20% at 5 years) are considered.[15] Overall survival, however, decreases from an intention-to-treat perspective.[12,15-17] In fact, because of the lack of sufficient liver donation, there is always a waiting period between listing and transplantation during which the tumor may grow and develop contraindications to transplantation (vascular invasion, extrahepatic spread). The rate of dropouts may be as high as 25% if the waiting list is longer than 12 months.[18] Most groups perform interventional treatments, including transarterial chemoembolization (TACE) and percutaneous ablation, to achieve local control of the tumor during the waiting period. Living donor liver transplantation is a viable option to expand the number of available livers, but it requires a highly skilled group of senior liver surgeons, increases surgery-related morbidity, and carries the risk of donor mortality. In addition, the applicability of the technique is low, and only about one fourth of potential recipients eventually undergo the procedure.[15]

Image-Guided Ablation

Image-guided percutaneous ablation is currently accepted as the best therapeutic choice for nonsurgical patients with early-stage HCC.[4] Over the past 2 decades, several methods for percutaneous chemical ablation or energy-based tumor destruction through localized heating, freezing, or energy delivery have been developed and clinically tested (Table 141-1).

The seminal technique used for local ablation of HCC is percutaneous ethanol injection (PEI). Ethanol induces coagulation necrosis of the lesion as a result of cellular dehydration, protein denaturation, and chemical occlusion of small tumor vessels. PEI is a well-established technique for the treatment of nodular-type HCC. HCC nodules have a soft consistency and are surrounded by a firm cirrhotic liver. Consequently, injected ethanol diffuses within them easily and selectively, leading to complete necrosis of about 70% of small lesions.[19] Although there have been no RCTs

TABLE 141-1. Percutaneous Methods for Ablation of Hepatocellular Carcinoma

Chemical Ablation
Ethanol injection
Acetic acid injection

Energy-Based Ablation
Radiofrequency ablation
Microwave ablation
Laser ablation
Cryoablation
Irreversible electroporation

comparing PEI and best supportive care or PEI and surgical resection, several retrospective studies have provided indirect evidence that PEI improves the natural history of HCC. The long-term outcomes of patients with small tumors who were treated with PEI were similar to those reported in surgical series, with 5-year survival rates ranging from 41% to 60% in Child A patients.[19-24] Of importance, two cohort studies and one retrospective case-control study comparing surgical resection and PEI failed to identify any difference in survival, despite patients in PEI groups having poorer liver function.[25-27]

The major limitation of PEI is the high local recurrence rate, which may reach 33% in lesions smaller than 3 cm and 43% in lesions exceeding 3 cm.[28,29] The injected ethanol does not always accomplish complete tumor necrosis because of its inhomogeneous distribution within the lesion—especially in presence of intratumoral septa—and the limited effect on extracapsular cancerous spread. Moreover, PEI is unable to create a safety margin of ablation in the liver parenchyma surrounding the nodule, and therefore may not destroy tiny satellite lesions that even in small tumors may be located in close proximity to the main nodule.

TECHNICAL ASPECTS

Thermal Ablation

Application of localized heating or freezing enables in situ destruction of malignant liver tumors, preserving normal liver parenchyma. The energy-based ablative therapies involved in clinical practice can be classified as either hepatic hyperthermic treatments—including radiofrequency ablation (RFA), microwave ablation (MWA), and laser ablation (LA)—or hepatic cryotherapy. Hepatic hyperthermic treatments are mostly performed via a percutaneous approach, while an open or laparoscopic approach has been widely adopted until recently for hepatic cryotherapy. This chapter is focused on percutaneous hyperthermic treatments, particularly RFA, which has been by far the most widely used thermal ablative modality in HCC.

The thermal damage caused by heating is dependent on both the tissue temperature achieved and the duration of heating. Heating of tissue at 50°C to 55°C for 4 to 6 minutes produces irreversible cellular damage. At temperatures between 60°C and 100°C, near-immediate coagulation of tissue is induced, with irreversible damage to mitochondrial

and cytosolic enzymes of the cells. At more than 100°C to 110°C, tissue vaporizes and carbonizes.[30] For adequate destruction of tumor tissue, the entire target volume must be subjected to cytotoxic temperatures. Different physical mechanisms are involved in the hepatic hyperthermic treatments to generate a lethal temperature. A common important factor that affects the success of thermal ablation is the ability to ablate all viable tumor tissue and possibly an adequate tumor-free margin. Ideally, a 360-degree, 0.5- to 1-cm-thick ablative margin should be produced around the tumor.[30] This cuff would ensure that microscopic invasions around the periphery of a tumor have been eradicated. Thus, the target diameter of an ablation, or of overlapping ablations, must be larger than the diameter of the tumor that undergoes treatment.[31]

Thermal ablation is usually performed under intravenous sedation with standard cardiac, pressure, and oxygen monitoring. Targeting of the lesion can be performed with ultrasound, CT, or MR imaging. The guidance system is chosen largely on the basis of operator preference and local availability of dedicated equipment such as CT fluoroscopy or open MR systems. Real-time ultrasound/CT (or ultrasound/MRI) fusion imaging systems recently developed can substantially improve the ability to guide and monitor liver tumor ablation procedures. Current virtual navigation systems help define the extent of liver tumor burden, plan and simulate needle insertion, and predict the amount of induced necrosis. During the procedure, important aspects to be monitored include how well the tumor is being covered and whether any adjacent normal structures are being affected at the same time. Although the transient hyperechoic zone seen at ultrasound within and surrounding a tumor during and immediately after RFA can be used as a rough guide to the extent of tumor destruction, MR is currently the only imaging modality with validated techniques for real-time temperature monitoring. To control an image-guided ablation procedure, the operator can use the image-based information obtained during monitoring or automated systems that terminates the ablation at a critical point in the procedure. At the end of the procedure, most systems allow ablation of the needle track, which is aimed at preventing any tumor cell dissemination. Contrast-enhanced ultrasound performed after the end of the procedure may allow an initial evaluation of treatment effects (Fig. 141-1). However, CT or MRI are recognized as the standard modalities to assess treatment outcome, showing, in cases of successful ablation, a nonenhancing area with or without a peripheral enhancing rim. The enhancing rim that may be observed along the periphery of the ablation zone appears as a relatively concentric, symmetric, and uniform process in an area with smooth inner margins. This is a transient finding that represents a benign physiologic response to thermal injury (initially, reactive hyperemia; subsequently, fibrosis and giant cell reaction). Benign periablational enhancement has to be differentiated from irregular peripheral enhancement due to residual tumor that occurs at the treatment margin. In contrast to benign periablational enhancement, residual unablated tumor often grows in scattered, nodular, or eccentric patterns.[32] Later follow-up imaging studies should be aimed at detecting recurrence of the treated lesion (i.e., local tumor progression), development of new hepatic lesions, or emergence of extrahepatic disease.

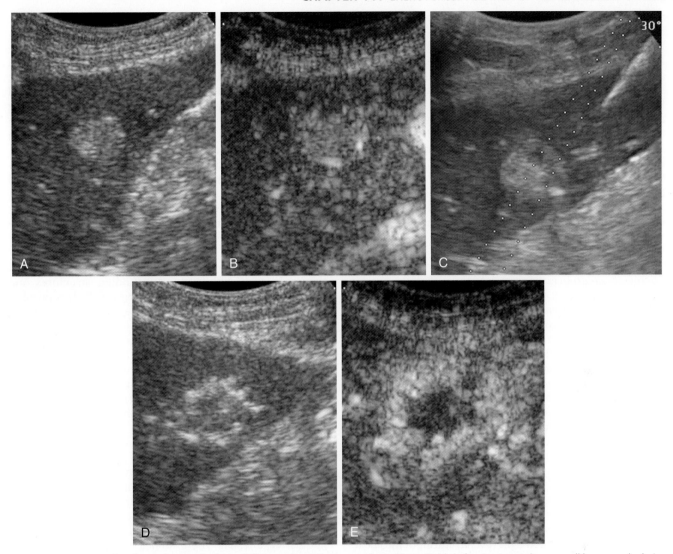

FIGURE 141-1. **A-B,** Baseline and contrast-enhanced ultrasound examinations performed immediately before treatment show a small hypervascular lesion on left liver lobe. **C,** Under ultrasound guidance, a radiofrequency needle is inserted into lesion. **D-E,** Contrast-enhanced ultrasound repeated at end of the procedure allows initial evaluation of treatment effects, showing a hypoechoic area surrounded by a homogeneous hypervascular rim due to hyperemia.

Radiofrequency Ablation

The goal of RFA is to induce thermal injury to tissue through electromagnetic energy deposition. The patient is part of a closed-loop circuit that includes an RF generator, an electrode needle, and a large dispersive electrode (ground pads). An alternating electric field is created within patient's tissue. Because of the relatively high electrical resistance of tissue in comparison with the metal electrodes, there is marked agitation of the ions present in the target tissue that surrounds the electrode, since the tissue ions attempt to follow the changes in direction of alternating electric current. The agitation results in frictional heat around the electrode. The discrepancy between the small surface area of the needle electrode and the large area of the ground pads causes the generated heat to be focused and concentrated around the needle electrode.

Several electrode types are available for clinical RFA, including internally cooled electrodes and multi-tined expandable electrodes with or without perfusion.[32] Cooled-tip electrodes consist of dual-lumen needles with

uninsulated active tips in which internal cooling is obtained by continuous perfusion with chilled saline. Needle cooling is aimed at preventing overheating of tissues nearest to the electrode, which may cause charring, thereby limiting the propagation of RF waves. They are available in either single-needle or cluster array with three needles spaced 0.5 cm apart. Expandable needles have an active surface that can be substantially expanded by hooks deployed laterally from the tip. The number of hooks and length of hook deployment may vary according to the desired volume of necrosis. These techniques enabled a substantial and reproducible enlargement of the volume of thermal necrosis produced with a single-needle insertion and prompted the start of clinical application of RFA.

RFA of HCC is associated with very low mortality rates and acceptable morbidity. Recently, three separate multicenter surveys have reported mortality rates ranging from 0.1% to 0.5%, major complication rates ranging from 2.2% to 3.1%, and minor complication rates ranging from 5% to 8.9%.[33] The most common causes of death were sepsis, hepatic failure, colon perforation, and portal vein thrombosis, while the most common complications were intraperitoneal bleeding, hepatic abscess, bile duct injury, hepatic decompensation, and grounding pad burns.[34-36] Minor complications and side effects were usually transient and self-limiting. An uncommon late complication of RFA is tumor seeding along the needle track. In patients with HCC, tumor seeding occurred in 8 (0.5%) of 1610 cases in a multicenter survey[34] and in 1 (0.5%) of 187 cases in a single-institution series.[37] Lesions with subcapsular location and an invasive tumoral pattern, as shown by a poor differentiation degree, seem to be at higher risk for such a complication.[38] These data indicate that RFA is a relatively safe procedure, but a careful assessment of the risks and benefits associated with the treatment has to be made in each individual patient by a multidisciplinary team (Fig. 141-2).

Microwave Ablation

Microwave ablation is the term used for all electromagnetic methods of inducing tumor destruction by using devices with frequencies greater than or equal to 900 kHz. The passage of MWA into cells or other materials containing water results in the rotation of individual molecules. This rapid molecular rotation generates and uniformly distributes heat, which is instantaneous and continuous until the radiation is stopped. MW irradiation creates an ablation area around the needle in a column or round shape, depending on the type of needle used and the generating power.[39] The potential benefits of MW technology include higher intratumoral temperatures, larger tumor ablation volumes and shorter ablation times.[40,41] In addition, MWA does not require placement of grounding pads (Fig. 141-3).

Laser Ablation

The term *laser ablation* refers to thermal tissue destruction by conversion of absorbed light (usually infrared) into heat. Light is delivered via 300- to 600-μm-diameter flexible quartz fibers directly inserted into the tissue. A great variety in laser sources and wavelength are available. In addition, different types of laser fibers, modified tips, and single or multiple laser applicators can be used. From a single bare 400-μm laser fiber, a spherical volume of coagulative necrosis up to 2 cm in diameter can be produced. The use of higher power results in charring and vaporization around the fiber tip. Two methods have been developed for producing larger volumes of necrosis. The first consists of firing multiple bare fibers arrayed at 2-cm spacing throughout a target lesion, and the second uses cooled-tip diffuser fibers that can deposit up to 30 W over a large surface area, thus diminishing local overheating.[42] LA appears to be relatively safe, with a major complication rate less than 2%.[43] The major drawback of current laser technology appears to be the small volume of ablation that can be created with a single-probe insertion. Insertion of multiple fibers is technically cumbersome and may not be feasible in lesions that are not conveniently located. New devices could overcome this limitation.

Irreversible Electroporation

Electroporation is a technique that increases the permeability of cell membranes by changing the transmembrane potential and subsequently disrupting the lipid bilayer integrity. Irreversible electroporation (IRE) is obtained by applying a greater amount of energy that is able to disintegrate cell membranes permanently, causing leakage of intracellular ions followed by collapse of the homeostatic conditions inside the cell, resulting in cell death. Repeated electric pulses of up to 1 kV of energy cause destabilizing electrical potentials across cell membranes, without an additional thermal effect. The energy is discharged via mono- or bipolar probes with an active tip of a few centimeters, and tissue death is obtained in micro- to millisecond ranges of treatment time compared to conventional ablation techniques, which require several minutes.

During treatment, general anesthesia with complete muscle blockade is mandatory to avoid generalized muscle contractions, as is electrocardiograph-gated delivery of the high voltage pulses to avoid serious cardiac arrhythmias.[44] IRE created a sharp margin between treated and untreated tissues in vivo, preserving surrounding structures and maintaining blood flow in adjacent vessels.[45] This peculiar property is useful for local treatment of lesions located in very crucial anatomic structures, such as in close proximity to the bowel, biliary ducts, neural, and vascular structures.

Moreover, unlike established thermal ablation techniques, IRE creates tissue death by changing the permeability of the cell membrane without thermal energy. Therefore, it will not be affected by the "heat sink effect" as in RFA.

CONTRAINDICATIONS

To be considered eligible for local treatment, patients must meet some general requirements. First, disease should be ideally confined to the liver, without evidence of vascular invasion or extrahepatic metastases.[46] In addition, the tumor to be treated by thermal ablation must be a focal nodular-type lesion. The presence of a clear and easy-to-detect target for needle placement is crucial to treatment outcome.

Tumor size is of utmost importance to determine the outcome of ablation. It has to be taken into account that ablation of appropriate margins beyond the borders of the tumor is necessary to achieve complete tumor destruction.

With particular focus on RFA, which produces in vivo ablation spheres of 5.5 to 5.6 cm in diameter, the tumor should not exceed 3.5 cm in longest axis to obtain a safety margin of 1 cm all around the lesion.[47] In addition, RFA treatment of lesions adjacent to the gallbladder or hepatic hilum is at risk for thermal injury of the biliary tract. Nevertheless, in experienced hands, RFA of tumors adjacent to the gallbladder was shown to be feasible, although associated in most cases with self-limited iatrogenic cholecystitis.[48] Lesions located along the surface of the liver can be considered for RFA, although their treatment requires experienced hands and may be associated with a higher risk of complications. Percutaneous treatment of superficial lesions adjacent to any part of the gastrointestinal tract must be avoided because of the risk of thermal injury of the gastric or bowel wall.[49] The colon appears to be at greater risk than the stomach or small bowel for thermally mediated perforation.[50] Gastric complications are rare, likely owing to the relatively greater wall thickness of the stomach

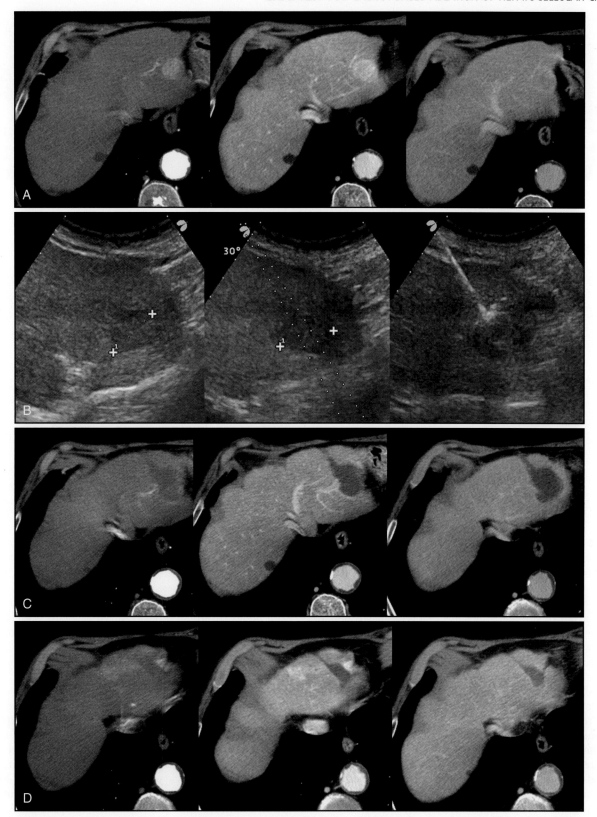

FIGURE 141-2. Complete response of small hepatocellular carcinoma treated with radiofrequency ablation. **A,** Pretreatment computed tomography (CT) shows hypervascular tumor. **B,** Expandable multi-tined electrode is placed into lesion under ultrasound guidance. Follow-up CT after 1 month **(C)** and 3 months **(D)** show complete tumor ablation with progressive lesion shrinkage.

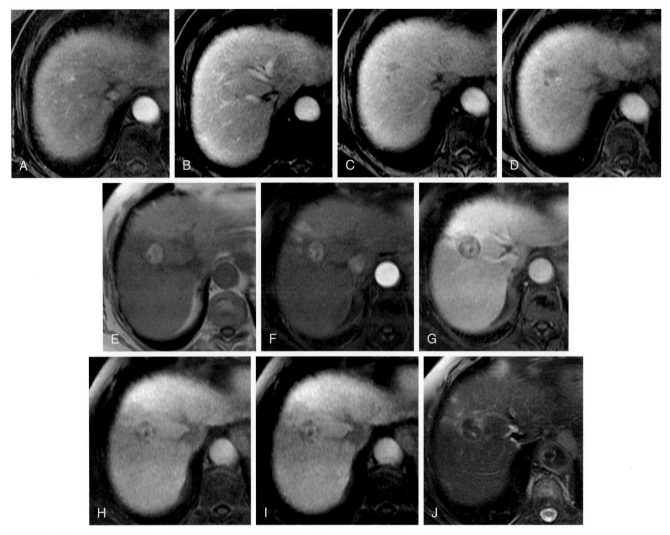

FIGURE 141-3. Complete response of small hepatocellular carcinoma treated with microwave ablation. **A-D,** Pretreatment magnetic resonance imaging (MRI) shows a typical hypervascular tumor on hepatic dome. **E-J,** One-month MRI follow-up shows an area of coagulative necrosis including treated lesion, without signs of viable tumor. Triangle-shaped subcapsular area visible in arterial phase (**F**) is due to presence of intraparenchymal shunts.

or the rarity of surgical adhesions along the gastrohepatic ligament. The mobility of the small bowel may also provide the bowel with greater protection, compared with the relatively fixed colon. The potential risk of thermal damage to adjacent structures should be weighed against benefits on a case-by-case basis. A laparoscopy approach can also be considered in such instances, since the bowel may be lifted away from the tumor.[50]

A multicenter study conducted retrospectively to assess complications of LA for the treatment of HCC indicate that the rate of bile duct damage due to treatment of a lesion located near the liver hilum is lower than that reported for RFA and PEI (0.3% vs. 2.0% and 3.3%, respectively.[51]

In contrast, RF treatment of lesions located in the vicinity of hepatic vessels is possible because flowing blood usually "refrigerates" the vascular wall, protecting it from thermal injury. In these cases, however, the risk of incomplete ablation of the neoplastic tissue adjacent to the vessel may increase because of the heat loss caused by the vessel itself. On the contrary, MWA technique is not influenced by the presence of a large vessel near the target lesion because of the minimal heat sink effect. In fact, it is shown

in a hepatic porcine model that large blood vessels in the resection specimens did not create typical ablation zone distortion because of the minimal heat sink effect.[52]

OUTCOMES

RFA has been the most widely assessed alternative to PEI for local ablation of HCC.[53] Histologic data from explanted liver specimens in patients who underwent RFA showed that tumor size and presence of large (3 mm or more) abutting vessels significantly affect local treatment effect. Complete tumor necrosis was pathologically shown in 83% of tumors less than 3 cm and 88% of tumors in nonperivascular locations.[54] Three RCTs compared RFA versus PEI for the treatment of early-stage HCC[55-57] (Table 141-2). All three investigations showed that RFA had higher local anticancer effect than PEI, leading to better local control of the disease. Therefore, RFA appears to be the preferred percutaneous treatment for patients with early-stage HCC on the basis of more consistent local tumor control.

Recently, the long-term survival outcomes of RFA-treated patients were reported (Table 141-3). In the first

TABLE 141-2. Randomized Studies Comparing Radiofrequency Ablation and Percutaneous Ethanol Injection in the Treatment of Early-Stage Hepatocellular Carcinoma

Author, Year	Complete Response	2-Year Local Progression	Survival Rates		P
			2-Year	3-Year	
Lencioni et al., 2003[38]					
PEI (n = 50)	82%	38%*	88	NA	
RFA (n = 52)	95%	4%*	96	NA	NS
Lin et al., 2004[39]					
PEI, low dose (n = 52)	88%	45%	61	50	
PEI, high dose (n = 53)	92%	33%	63	55	
RFA (n = 52)	96%	18%	82	74	<.05
Shiina et al., 2005[40]					
PEI (n = 114)	100%	11%	82	63	
RFA (n = 118)	100%	2%	90	80	<.05

*2-year local recurrence-free survival: PEI 62%, RF ablation 96%.
NA, Not available; NS, not significant; PEI, percutaneous ethanol injection; RFA, radiofrequency ablation.

TABLE 141-3. Studies Reporting Long-Term Survival Outcomes of Patients with Early-Stage Hepatocellular Carcinoma Who Underwent Percutaneous Radiofrequency Ablation

Author, Year	No. Patients	Survival Rates (%)		
		1-Year	3-Year	5-Year
Lencioni et al., 2005[41]				
Child A, 1 HCC < 5 cm or 3 < 3 cm	144	100	76	51
1 HCC < 5 cm	116	100	89	61
Child B, 1 HCC < 5 cm or 3 < 3 cm	43	89	46	31
Tateishi et al., 2005[42]				
Naive patients*	319	95	78	54
Non-naive patients†	345	92	62	38
Cabassa et al., 2006[43]	59	94	65	43
Choi et al., 2007[44]				
Child A, 1 HCC < 5 cm or 3 < 3 cm	359	NA	78	64
Child B, 1 HCC < 5 cm or 3 < 3 cm	160	NA	49	38

*Patients who received radiofrequency ablation as primary treatment.
†Patients who received radiofrequency ablation for recurrent tumor after previous treatment including resection, ethanol injection, microwave ablation, and transarterial embolization.
HCC, Hepatocellular carcinoma; NA, not available.

published report, 206 patients with early-stage HCC who were not candidates for resection or transplantation were enrolled in a prospective intention-to-treat clinical trial.[58] RFA was considered the first-line nonsurgical treatment and was actually performed in 187 (91%) of 206 patients. Nineteen (9%) of 206 patients had to be excluded from RF treatment because of the unfavorable location of the tumor. In patients who underwent RFA, survival depended on the severity of the underlying cirrhosis and the tumor multiplicity. Patients in Child class A with solitary HCC had a 5-year survival rate of 61%. Three other studies confirmed that survival of naive patients with well-compensated cirrhosis bearing early-stage HCC ranges from 43% to 64%.[59-61] Of interest, in a randomized trial of RFA versus surgical resection in patients with solitary HCC less than 5 cm in diameter, no differences in overall survival rates and cumulative recurrence-free survival rates were observed.[62]

Despite the many published reports, some questions concerning image-guided RFA in HCC treatment are still unanswered. Some authors have reported that RFA may be a safe and effective bridge to liver transplantation.[63-66] However, randomized studies would be needed to

determine advantages and disadvantages of RFA with respect to TACE for HCC patients awaiting transplantation. Recent studies have reported encouraging results in the treatment of intermediate-size HCC lesions with a combination of RFA and TACE.[67-69] However, further clinical trials are warranted to determine the survival benefit associated with this approach.

With regard to MWA, the local effect of treatment in HCC was assessed by examining the histologic changes of the tumor after ablation.[70,71] In one study, 89% of 18 small tumors were ablated completely.[72] Coagulative necrosis with faded nuclei and eosinophilic cytoplasm were the predominant findings in the ablated areas. There were also areas in which the tumors maintained their native morphologic features as if the area was fixed, but their cellular activity was destroyed, as demonstrated by succinic dehydrogenase stain. One study compared MWA and PEI in a retrospective evaluation of 90 patients with small HCC.[73] The overall 5-year survival rates for patients with well-differentiated HCC treated with MWA and PEI were not significantly different. However, among the patients with moderately or poorly differentiated HCC, overall survival with MWA was significantly better than with PEI. In a large series including 234 patients, the 3- and 5-year survival rates were 73% and 57%, respectively.[74] At a multivariate analysis, tumor size, number of nodules, and Child-Pugh classification had significant effects on survival.[75] Only one randomized trial compared the effectiveness of MWA with that of RFA.[76] Seventy-two patients with 94 HCC nodules were randomly assigned to RFA and MWA groups. Unfortunately, in this study the data were analyzed with respect to lesions and not to patients. Although no statistically significant differences were observed with respect to the efficacy of the two procedures, a tendency favoring RFA was recognized with respect to local recurrences and complication rates.

To date, few data are available concerning the clinical efficacy of LA. No randomized trials to compare LA with any other treatment have been published thus far. In one study including 74 patients with early-stage HCC, overall survival rates were 68% at 3 years and 15% at 5 years, respectively.[77] The same authors reported long-term survival rates of 89%, 52% and 27% for 1, 3 and 5 years, respectively, in a series of 169 sub–40-mm lesions in 148 patients (144 biopsy-proven HCC) treated with 239 sessions, with an overall 82% complete lesion ablation rate.[78]

POSTPROCEDURE AND FOLLOW-UP CARE

A careful posttreatment protocol is to be recommended following percutaneous ablation. The patient is kept under close medical observation and re-scanned with ultrasound 1 to 2 hours after the procedure. An overnight hospital stay is scheduled. Contrast-enhanced ultrasound performed shortly after the procedure may allow an initial evaluation of tumor response by showing disappearance of intratumoral signals, surrounded by an enhancing rim. The thin peripheral enhancing rim—which is due to the inflammatory reaction surrounding the area of necrosis—should not be misinterpreted as tumor persistence. Since the enhancing rim tends to disappear over time, dynamic multidetector CT or MRI at 1 month are considered the most reliable methods to evaluate treatment outcome. If there is imaging evidence of residual tumor, the patient can be considered for repeated treatment, provided requirements for treatment are still met. Follow-up is usually scheduled at 3- or 6-month intervals.

KEY POINTS

- Percutaneous ablation is considered the best treatment option for patients with early-stage hepatocellular cancer who are not candidates for surgical resection or liver transplantation.

- Percutaneous ethanol injection has been the most widely used technique. The major limitation of this technique is a high local recurrence rate, which may reach 33% in lesions smaller than 3 cm and 43% in lesions exceeding 3 cm.

- Several new methods of heat ablation have been developed more recently, including thermal ablation with radiofrequency, laser, microwave energy, and irreversible electroporation.

▸ **SUGGESTED READINGS**

Gervais DA, Arellano RS. Percutaneous tumor ablation for hepatocellular carcinoma. Am J Roentgenol 2011;197(4):789–94.

Lu MD, Chen JW, Xie XY, et al. Hepatocellular carcinoma: US-guided percutaneous microwave coagulation therapy. Radiology 2001;221:167–72.

Meza-Junco J, Montano-Loza AJ, Liu DM, et al. Locoregional radiological treatment for hepatocellular carcinoma; Which, when and how? Cancer Treat Rev 2012;38:54–62.

Rempp H, Boss A, Helmberger T, et al. The current role of minimally invasive therapies in the management of liver tumors. Abdom Imaging 2011;36:635–47.

The complete reference list is available online at www.expertconsult.com.

CHAPTER 142

Energy-Based Ablation of Other Liver Lesions
Luigi Solbiati

Metastatic liver disease is a very common issue in oncology practice. Currently, multiple treatment options are available, including hepatic resection, chemoembolization, intraarterial and systemic chemotherapy, cryotherapy, laser therapy, and radiofrequency ablation (RFA).[1,2]

Over the last few years, advances in diagnostic imaging modalities such as contrast-enhanced ultrasound, single- and multidetector helical computed tomography (CT), and magnetic resonance imaging (MRI) with hepatobiliary and reticuloendothelial-specific contrast agents have allowed early detection and accurate quantification of liver metastatic involvement.[3-10] As a result, correct selection of patients for different treatment options is usually possible.

When feasible, surgical resection of hepatic metastases is the accepted standard therapeutic approach in patients with colorectal cancer and offers potential for cure in selected patients with other primary tumors.[2,11-28]

RFA remains the most commonly used method of thermal ablation. Radiofrequency waves operate in the 30 kHz to 1 MHz range. Microwave ablation is also being performed with increasing popularity. Microwaves operate in the 1000 to 3000 MHz range. Microwave ablation can produce heat at a much faster rate than RFA, yielding shorter ablation times. In addition, the relatively rapid heat production with microwaves may minimize the impact of heat loss when lesions are in close proximity to large vessels. Microwave ablation is now being used frequently within the liver but may have particular advantages within the lung and bone, owing to relatively poor electrical conductivity within those tissues.

High-intensity focused ultrasound (HIFU) is yet another method of creating tumoricidal heat production. In the United States, HIFU is currently approved for treatment of uterine fibroids. Areas of investigation include prostate cancer, liver cancer, and brain cancers. The HIFU unit is coupled to and guided with MRI. Irreversible electroporation (IRE) is a method of rapidly increasing the sizes of pores within cell membranes, causing instantaneous cell death. Cell death is not based on thermal heating. IRE can interfere with the conduction system of the heart and is often performed with electrocardiographic gating.

Percutaneous (or laparoscopic) RFA is an established therapeutic option for liver metastases that may obviate the need for major surgery and result in prolonged survival and chance for cure. Extensive operator experience and technical advances provide larger coagulation volumes and therefore allow safe and effective treatment of medium and occasionally even large metastases. Results of RFA in terms of global and disease-free survival currently approach those reported for surgical metastasectomy. In published series, this technique has demonstrated significant advantages:

- Feasibility of treatment in previously resected patients and nonsurgical candidates because of the number or intrahepatic location of metastatic deposits, age, and comorbidity
- Repeatability of treatment when incomplete and in the event of local recurrence or development of metachronous lesions
- Combination with systemic or regional chemotherapy
- Minimal invasiveness with a limited complication rate and preservation of liver function
- Limited hospital stay and procedure cost[29-42]

INDICATIONS

Colorectal Metastases

Patients with new metastases or local recurrence after previous hepatic resection, patients with multiple bilobar liver metastases, and those refusing or ineligible for surgery because of general health reasons are all candidates for RFA. Recently increased awareness among referring oncologists, satisfactory long-term survival reported in the scientific literature, and minimal invasiveness of RFA versus surgery have contributed to the widely accepted status of RFA as a valid therapeutic option for local treatment of patients with limited metastatic liver disease.

RFA is applicable to patients with one to five metachronous liver metastases measuring up to 3.5 to 4 cm in largest diameter (but preferably not > 3 cm) from previous radically treated colorectal cancer in whom surgery cannot be performed either because it is contraindicated or because it was simply refused.

Some patients with large lesions or more than five nodules may undergo RFA after successful tumor debulking by means of chemotherapy (neoadjuvant).

Noncolorectal Metastases

In our experience, RFA is a useful treatment in patients with metastases from previously treated malignancies, provided local control of liver disease may be beneficial from an oncologic perspective in terms of improved survival or quality of life. At our institution, patients with liver metastases from neuroendocrine, gastric, pancreatic, renal, pulmonary, uterine, or ovarian cancer and melanoma have been successfully treated with RFA.

Under these conditions, RFA has to be considered a less invasive therapeutic alternative to surgery. Indications for RFA of liver metastases from other primary cancers may follow those of surgical resection. Hepatectomy for liver metastases appears to be favorable in patients with gynecologic, gastric, and testicular primary tumors, with survival rates higher than 20%; unfortunately, no definite selection criteria have been reported in the literature.[22,26,27]

Particular considerations are reserved for patients with neuroendocrine tumors, which commonly metastasize to the liver. The frequency of metastatic disease, the hormone production, and the protracted clinical course make metastases from neuroendocrine tumors responsive to multiple therapeutic modalities, including surgical resection, hepatic artery embolization, cryotherapy, and RFA. Specific indications for RFA include patients who need intraoperative ablation as an adjunct to resection, who have limited hepatic disease but are not operative candidates, or who are inoperable and unresponsive to embolization treatments or experience recurrence after resection.

RFA can be applied to liver metastases from breast cancer when the liver is the only location of metastases, when extrahepatic metastases are demonstrated to be stable or in regression as a result of other treatment modalities, or when liver involvement is limited (one to five lesions, each 4 cm or less in maximum diameter) and systemic chemotherapy has been partially or completely unsuccessful.

Indications for ablation of hepatic metastases are summarized in Table 142-1.

CONTRAINDICATIONS

Percutaneous RFA is a minimally invasive procedure, so there are few absolute contraindications to its use. Exclusion criteria include the presence of severe coagulopathy, renal or liver failure, portal vein neoplastic thrombosis, and obstructive jaundice. Active extrahepatic disease is a contraindication to RFA, with the exception of bone or lung metastases in breast cancer patients whose disease is responding or is unchanged with systemic chemotherapy.[30]

Contraindications to general anesthesia can be considered relative because the procedure can be performed under conscious sedation if necessary. Conscious sedation

is not applicable if extended breath-holding is necessary during the procedure, depending on the position of the lesion within the liver.

Caution has to be exercised to not damage adjacent structures. Liver lesions adjacent to the hepatic hilum, gallbladder, stomach, and colon are potential candidates for ablation but require precise and careful planning. Adjacent vascular structures do not represent an obstacle alone; high blood flow in major hepatic vessels allows prompt dissipation of the warming effect secondary to RFA (heat sink effect), but the biliary system is vulnerable, especially if harboring bacteria. Proximity of the gastric wall or bowel loops to the area of treatment may be a critical safety issue when selecting candidates for treatment. Perforation of bowel loops by heating may occur many hours after ablation and could be clinically misleading in that it is usually less painful than perforation secondary to inflammatory diseases.

Relatively simple practical measures such as patient positioning, selection of a safe path to the target, and intraperitoneal injection of 500 mL of dextrose (to create "artificial ascites") can provide adequate distance to avoid injury to critical structures.

EQUIPMENT

In most centers, thermal ablation of liver metastases is performed with radiofrequency energy (using both cooled-tip and multihooked needles), but cryoprobes can also be used. Microwaves are under investigation as an ablative modality and will soon become available commercially.

Single or cluster (three needles mounted on one handle) 16-gauge internally cooled electrodes are connected to a 200-W, 480-kHz RF generator system (Radionics, Burlington, Mass.). Ablation is impedance guided with an automated pulsed-RF algorithm. The choice of electrodes is based on the size of the target nodule. For lesions smaller than 2 cm, single insertion of a 3-cm exposed-tip single electrode is sufficient. Lesions 2 to 3 cm in size can be treated by single insertion of a cluster electrode or multiple insertions of a 3-cm exposed-tip electrode. Lesions exceeding 3 cm can be treated with only one to two insertions of a cluster electrode and one to two single-electrode insertions.[43,44]

The applied energy is variable and usually reaches 1600 to 1800 mA for single electrodes and 1800 to 2000 mA for cluster electrodes.[45,46] Each application of energy lasts 8 to 12 minutes, and total procedure time ranges from 12 to 15 minutes for small solitary lesions to 45 to 60 minutes for large or multiple ablations.[47-49]

As an alternative, four to eight hooked 14-gauge electrodes (RITA-AngioDynamics, Mountain View, Calif.; Boston Scientific, Natick, Mass.) connected to 100- to 200-W generators can be used. Temperature monitoring for each hook is available. Each application of energy lasts 10 to 15 minutes. For treatment of large lesions, 60- or 90-degree rotations of the electrode and multiple insertions are required, with a total treatment time of 50 to 60 minutes.

Cooled-tip and multihooked electrodes can achieve comparable volumes of necrosis. In general, ablation with cooled-tip electrodes is faster and technically easier, whereas multihooked electrodes allow accurate real-time monitoring of temperature at the periphery of treated targets.

TABLE 142-1. Indications for Radiofrequency Ablation Treatment of Patients with Liver Metastases

Primary tumor (most frequently colorectal or breast cancer) previously treated radically with surgery and radiotherapy but without adjuvant chemotherapy

No evidence of active extrahepatic disease, with the possible exception of breast cancer metastases in the lung or bone showing regression or stability over time with hormonal therapy or chemotherapy

Liver metastasis (cytologically/histologically confirmed, compatible with the primary tumor), *or*

Residual tumor after previous RFA or other treatment, *or*

Local recurrence after surgical resection, RFA, or other treatment, *or*

Metachronous new metastasis after previous resection, RFA, or other treatment

Up to 4 to 5 lesions, each ≤ 4 cm in maximum diameter; lesions > 4 cm may be treated after debulking by systemic or regional chemotherapy.

Metastases identified with B-mode and/or contrast-enhanced ultrasound

Feasible and safe percutaneous access (not abutting hepatic hilum, gallbladder, or colon)

Adequate coagulation and hepatic and renal function

Informed consent obtained

RFA, Radiofrequency ablation.

Because of the unfeasibility of real-time monitoring of the exact location of each hook, particularly with respect to "risky" anatomic structures, use of multihooked electrodes is technically more challenging than that of cooled-tip needles.

TECHNIQUE

Technical Aspects

Patient enrollment in the treatment process requires evaluation by an anesthesiologist. Laboratory tests include a complete blood cell count (CBC), coagulation screen, urea, electrolytes, liver function tests, and tumor markers.

International guidelines recommend a dedicated operating room in which general anesthesia, endotracheal intubation, and mechanical ventilation can be optimally performed if needed. Standard surgical asepsis rules must be strictly observed by the operating team. Patients receive antibiotic prophylaxis (i.e., ceftriaxone) before treatment and antiemetic and analgesic drugs as needed postoperatively.

In our department, RFA sessions are carried out in a dedicated operating room. Conscious sedation is used in most patients. General anesthesia with endotracheal intubation and mechanical ventilation may be applied only for the treatment of lesions adjacent to the Glisson capsule (usually painful) or for risky anatomic structures.

RFA can be guided either by sonography or by fluoroscopy with CT. Sonography is used in most centers because of some favorable advantages: real-time control, low cost, and no use of ionizing radiation. CT guidance is used when sonographic targeting is not possible, but procedure time is significantly increased.

When sonography is used as the guidance modality, contrast-enhanced ultrasound is particularly useful for pretreatment planning, targeting of lesions undetectable in basal studies, and immediate evaluation of the early results of treatment.

B-mode and color/power Doppler ultrasound is unreliable in assessing the size and completeness of induced coagulation necrosis at the end of the application of energy. Furthermore, additional repositioning of the electrode is usually made difficult by the hyperechogenic "cloud" appearing around the distal probe. Therefore, we routinely perform contrast-enhanced ultrasound at the presumed end of the treatment session to enable rapid assessment of the extent of tissue ablation and detect viable tumor requiring additional immediate treatment.[50]

Keeping a "safety peripheral margin," as in surgical treatment of tumor lesions, is crucial in the long-term outcome. A minimum margin of 0.5 cm is necessary; enlarging the target area by a 1-cm margin when feasible is highly recommended (Fig. 142-1).

Real-time ultrasound/CT fusion imaging technology allows targeting of lesions visible only with CT (Fig. 142-2), real-time calculation of the volume to be treated before treatment is undertaken, and guidance of further electrode insertion into the same target, which is often completely obscured for sonography by the gas formed during RFA.

In our experience, patients are hospitalized for 24 hours after treatment, with discharge following documentation of necrosis and exclusion of complications via a contrast-enhanced CT scan.

CONTROVERSIES

The liver is the first, most common, and often unique site of metastasis from colorectal cancer. Recurrent disease involving the liver develops in approximately 50% of colorectal cancer patients during the course of their disease.

If cure is the therapeutic goal, hepatic resection remains the most effective treatment option for liver metastases of colorectal origin, but metastatic liver involvement is often multifocal, with only 20% to 25% of patients having resectable disease. Moreover, surgery may be excluded because of old age and associated pathologic conditions that increase

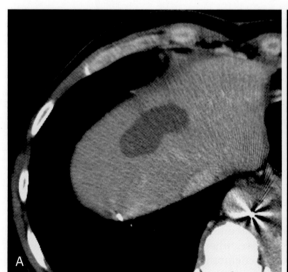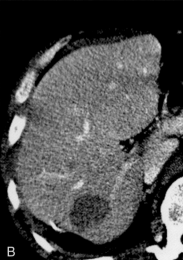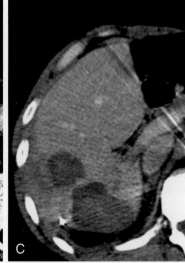

FIGURE 142-1. This 39-year-old man with history of colon carcinoma had prior wedge resection and radiofrequency ablation (RFA) of liver metastases (in **A**, resulting necrotic area caused by thermal ablation). **B**, Two adjacent new metastases were found 20 months later in segments VII and V (respectively 2.7 cm and 0.8 cm in size). **C**, Percutaneous ultrasound-guided RFA was performed, and contrast-enhanced computed tomography scans acquired 1 month later showed complete necrosis with sufficiently large safety margins at periphery of treated lesions.

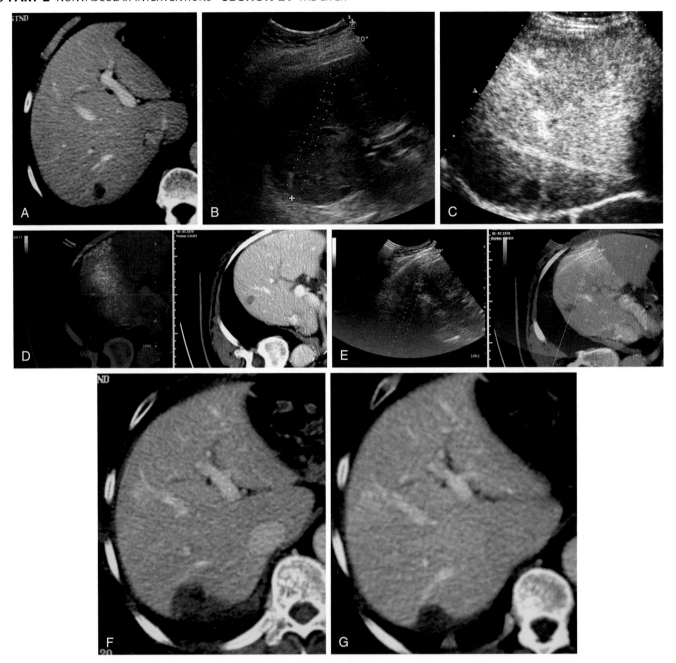

FIGURE 142-2. A 14-mm single metachronous metastasis in segment VII from colon carcinoma, detected on computed tomography (CT) **(A)**, but not on ultrasound **(B)**. **C**, Contrast-enhanced ultra sonography (CEUS) showed lesion as a hypovascular nodule in portal phase. **D-E,** Consequently, percutaneous radiofrequency ablation was guided using CT-CEUS fusion imaging. **F,** A 24-hour contrast-enhanced CT (CECT) showed lesion had been correctly targeted and necrotic area achieved was sufficiently large. **G,** CECT at 1 year showed partial shrinkage of necrotic area and no evidence of local recurrence.

the risk related to anesthesia, and it is associated with prolonged hospital stay, significant perioperative morbidity, and a 2% to 8% mortality rate.

The 5-year overall survival rate after hepatic surgical resection has been reported to range between 25% and 40%,[51-53] but recurrence in the liver or extrahepatic sites can develop in many successfully resected patients, and repeated resection can be performed in only a minority of these patients.[11-20] Prognostic factors include stage of the primary tumor, biological factors (carcinoembryonic antigen [CEA] level, differentiation, cellular ploidy), number of hepatic lesions and size of the dominant lesion, and infiltration of resection margins.

Regional therapies such as RFA can be offered to patients with limited but unresectable liver metastases and no extrahepatic disease, whereas chemoembolization and hepatic intraarterial chemotherapy are applicable to patients with extensive liver involvement unsuitable for ablation.[12,18]

In patients with liver recurrence after hepatectomy, RFA increases the possibility of curative treatment from 17% to 26% and is preferred over repeated surgery because it is less invasive (see Fig. 142-1).[54]

TABLE 142-2. Local Control and Long-Term Survival After Radiofrequency Ablation for Colorectal Cancer Liver Metastases: Literature Review

Author	Patients (N)	Metastases (N)	Size (cm)	Technique	Follow-up (mo)	Local Control	Survival
Solbiati L, 2012[61]	128	261	0.5-6.6; mean, 2.0	Percutaneous	3-126	83.1%	3 yr: 62% 5 yr: 39.5%
Berber E, 2005[63]	135	432	1.2-10.2	Laparoscopic	12-52		3 yr: 28% Median: 28.9%
Gillams AR, 2004[64]	167	354	1-12; mean, 39	Percutaneous	0-89; mean, 17	74.9%	5 yr: 26%
Veltri A, 2005[65]	98	163	0.5-8.0; mean, 2.7	Percutaneous intraoperative (21)	12-108	59%	3 yr: 48% 5 yr: 30%
Jakobs TF, 2006[66]	68	183	0.5-5.0; mean, 2.2	Percutaneous	8-38; mean, 21	82%	3 yr: 68%
Tumor RFA Italian Network (Lencioni R), 2005[67]	423	543	0.5-5.0; mean, 2.7	Percutaneous	1-78; mean, 19	85.4%	3 yr: 47% 5 yr: 24%
Sorensen et al., 2007[68]	102	332		Percutaneous	1-92; mean, 23-6		3 yr: 64% 5 yr: 44%

The results of cryoablation or microwave ablation reported in the literature are very limited thus far, and no conclusion can be drawn regarding the possible role of these ablative modalities as an alternative to RFA.

OUTCOMES

Colorectal Metastases

Several published series have reported promising results of RFA for liver metastases, but these early reports had only short-term follow-up and included patients with both primary and metastatic liver tumors.[37-41]

Currently, survival rates 5 years after RFA for liver metastases from colorectal cancer (Table 142-2) are comparable to those reported for surgical resection.

In the most recent (still unpublished) long-term follow-up study at our institution, 128 patients have been treated by RFA over a period of 7 years; 12% had previously undergone surgery for neoplastic involvement of the liver, and repeated resection was considered unfeasible or too invasive. One to five metastases (mean, 2.28) were ablated in each patient for a total of 261 treated lesions. Of the treated lesions, 87.5% were 3 cm or less in size, with the remaining 12.5% larger than 3 cm.

In our series, local tumor control was achieved in 83.1% of lesions, whereas local recurrence occurred in the remaining 16.9% (77.2% of these recurring metastases were > 3 cm). In a study reported by DeBaere et al., a percutaneous approach allowed local control of 90% of treated lesions after 1 year of follow-up, but the mean diameter of these lesions was significantly smaller than those in our series.[47]

In our experience, the time interval from treatment to recurrence was related to the size of the lesion; local relapse occurred in virtually all cases during the first 12-month period. The median time to local recurrence was 9.3 months. Repeat RFA was carried out in 37.6% of metastases with progressive local tumor growth (Fig. 142-3).

Distant metachronous metastases had developed at follow-up in 36% of our patients (Fig. 142-4). The estimated

median time until detection of new metastases was 12.3 months in our experience.

Kaplan-Meier analysis of the overall survival rates at 1, 3, and 5 years in our series was 96.2%, 62.0%, and 39.5%, respectively, with an estimated median survival time of 51 months.

The overlapping long-term outcome of both surgical resection and RFA will allow future randomized studies to compare RFA with surgery for resectable metastatic liver tumors and enable proper evaluation of the impact of RFA. RFA should not replace hepatic resection whenever applicable, especially for large metastases (>6 cm) because of the higher risk of local recurrence as a result of residual viable tumor tissue within the necrotic area. The precise role of RFA in currently adopted therapeutic regimens has yet to be defined.[55]

RFA performed after previous chemotherapy regimens is still associated with worse survival because of extensive liver disease stage, chemotherapy-refractory tumor, or diffuse extrahepatic disease. A comparison by Machi et al.[56] of RFA used as first- or second-line treatment or in the salvage setting showed greater survival benefit when used as a first-line therapeutic option. Randomized controlled trials to evaluate the value of combined adjuvant systemic chemotherapy are urgently required in the short term.

Not so long ago, the "test-of-time" approach was proposed by surgeons to delay resection of liver metastases so additional, still undetected lesions could develop and become identifiable, thus limiting the number of resections carried out in patients in whom more metastases may ultimately develop. On the one hand, RFA applied in this setting can significantly decrease the number of potential resections, resulting in complete tumor control in some of these patients and avoiding major surgery. Furthermore, offering cancer patients a treatment option such as RFA rather than a "wait-and-see" approach is favorable for the patient. In a recent study using RFA as a "test of time" before resection in a group of 88 potentially operable patients with 134 metastases from colorectal carcinoma monitored for a period of 18 to 75 months, RFA was successful in 60.2% of the patients, 43.4% of whom were

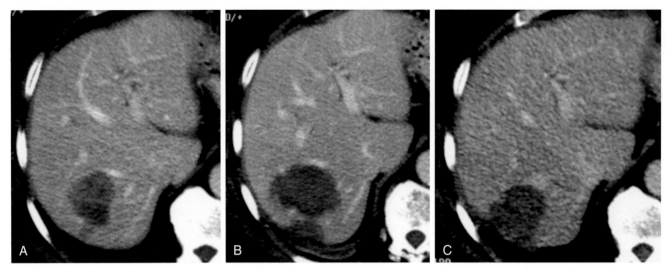

FIGURE 142-3. A 72-year-old man with history of colon carcinoma and prior radiofrequency ablation of three metachronous liver metastases. **A,** The 9-month follow-up computed tomography (CT) study showed a small (12 mm) local recurrence along posterior margin of treated metastasis in segment VII. Percutaneous ultrasound-guided local re-treatment of recurrence was performed; 24-hour **(B)** and 2-year **(C)** CT scans showed complete local control of metastasis.

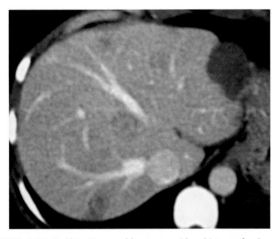

FIGURE 142-4. This 48-year-old woman with a history of colon carcinoma underwent percutaneous ultrasound-guided radiofrequency ablation (RFA) of three metachronous liver metastases. One year after RFA, computed tomography showed complete local control of treated lesions (one necrotic area is seen in segment II in subcapsular location) but also development of multiple new metastases that cannot undergo local treatment.

disease free during the course of the study. In the remaining patients (56.6%), new untreatable intrahepatic or extrahepatic metastases developed. RFA was unsuccessful in 39.8% of the patients; 57.1% of them underwent resection, and new untreatable metastases developed in the remaining 42.9%. No patients became untreatable because of the growth of incompletely ablated lesions. In summary, 50% of patients were spared surgery that would have been noncurative, whereas an additional 26.1% of patients avoided resection because of the curative result of RFA.[57]

Noncolorectal Metastases

Although the vast majority of RFA procedures address liver metastases of colorectal origin, a significant subset of secondary hepatic tumors occurs in patients with breast cancer.[30] Metastatic breast cancer has traditionally been considered a manifestation of systemic disease requiring chemotherapy; however, liver-only metastatic disease occurs in 5% to 12% of breast cancer patients and may be suitable for surgical metastasectomy. Early reports demonstrated improved survival rates (18%-24% at 5 years' follow-up) in patients undergoing resection of limited hepatic metastases from breast cancer.[21-23] More recent reports have yielded even superior survival rates (51% with disease-free interval and stage of the primary as prognostic factors).[24] Therefore, surgery may allow long-lasting benefit and be potentially curative; resected patients with the liver as the first and sole site of relapse have a threefold greater median survival than patients treated with standard nonsurgical treatment.

On this background, we used percutaneous RFA to achieve local control of liver metastases in patients with breast cancer; 24 patients with 64 liver metastases were treated, and in 92% of lesions, complete necrosis was achieved with a single treatment session (Fig. 142-5). Interestingly, the rate of complete necrosis was superior to that obtained with colorectal metastases of comparable size (96% for lesions < 3 cm and 75% for 3- to 5-cm lesions); these figures suggest that occult microangioinvasion of surrounding liver tissue may be absent or less pronounced in metastatic breast tumors.[30]

In more than half the patients (58%), new metastases developed during follow-up, but 63% of 16 patients with liver-only metastatic breast cancer were free of disease 4 to 44 months after the treatment. In view of the natural history of the disease and its minimal invasiveness, RFA is an effective local therapeutic alternative to surgical resection of liver metastases in breast cancer patients. Furthermore, RFA may be extremely useful for tumor recurrence after hepatectomy, because in more than half of these cases the liver is the only involved site of relapse. Combination treatment with hormonal therapy and systemic or intraarterial infusion chemotherapy is required.

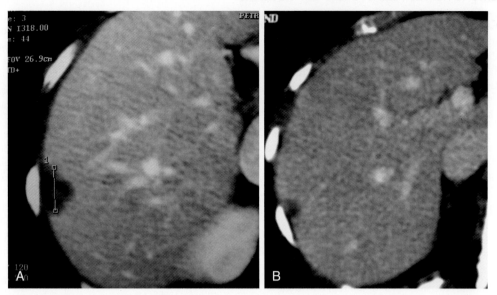

FIGURE 142-5. A, A 1.9-cm subcapsular liver metastasis in segment V from breast carcinoma treated with percutaneous ultrasound-guided radiofrequency ablation after unsuccessful chemotherapy. **B,** Three-year follow-up contrast-enhanced computed tomography scan showed complete local control and marked shrinkage of necrotic area.

Liver metastasectomy from an endocrine primary tumor is followed by long survival in a substantial proportion of patients, with 56% to 74% 5-year survival rates.[22,25-27] Interesting results have been reported with RFA used alone or in combination with surgery for local control of metastases from neuroendocrine tumors.[28] Eradication of disease was achieved in 28.5% of patients treated with curative intent.[29]

COMPLICATIONS

Major complications such as hemorrhage, cholecystitis, and gastric or bowel wall involvement occur in a small percentage of cases (range, 0.7% to 2.6%). Reported mortality rates are usually lower than 0.5%.

In our experience, patients usually experience mild to moderate pain in the right side of the abdomen that lasts for 2 to 5 days; the pain may become severe in patients with subcapsular lesions, but pericapsular injection of a long-acting anesthetic (ropivacaine) immediately after the procedure for postoperative pain control can obviate this problem. Fever may be present for the first 2 or 3 days after treatment and recedes with antipyretic drugs (acetaminophen). No impairment in liver function test results has been observed. Minimal pleural effusion may be documented by CT performed at 24 hours and usually resolves within a week.

POSTPROCEDURAL AND FOLLOW-UP CARE

Antiemetic therapy and analgesia are offered on demand. Laboratory tests include CBC, coagulation parameters, and a liver function test the day after the procedure.

RFA is considered successful when complete coagulative necrosis of the lesion and a safety margin are obtained.

Initial cross-sectional examination is crucial to assess the completeness of treatment, exclude complications, and provide baseline imaging for follow-up purposes. Spiral contrast-enhanced CT (or MRI) at 24 hours is the most widely used technique in follow-up schemes. Other methods, especially diffusion-weighted MRI combined with contrast-enhanced MRI, are being performed with the goal of increasing sensitivity in the evaluation of necrotic tissue. Recent studies have demonstrated diffusion-weighted imaging to be accurate in distinguishing between viable tumor tissue and necrosis.[58,59]

Patients continue to undergo contrast-enhanced multi-detector CT or MRI on a routine basis in the long-term assessment of response to therapy to allow prompt identification of new lesions. Cross-sectional imaging studies obtained at 3- to 4-month intervals must be integrated with liver function tests and serum CEA levels to detect local or distant recurrence. In our experience, contrast-enhanced ultrasonography has also proved valuable in the follow-up setting to confirm local recurrences/new metastases and plan further treatment.[48]

Nevertheless, although effort is continually being expended to increase the resolution and accuracy of imaging techniques, residual peripheral microscopic foci of malignancy or foci within the treated lesion may go undetected and give rise to local recurrence in the short term. Fluorodeoxyglucose (FDG)-labeled positron emission tomography (PET) is a complementary imaging modality in the event of uncertain treatment response when applied after a reasonable time interval.[60] Areas of abnormal FDG uptake after ablative procedures have been reported to represent disease relapse or residual viable tumor after ablation with a high degree of sensitivity.[50,51] In some institutions, it may be proposed as a whole-body surveillance technique in treated patients. When diffusion-weighted MRI is readily available and routinely performed, it has become a valuable diagnostic option.[62]

- Because thermal ablation is a local treatment, metastases that can undergo ablation are those originating from tumors that mostly (if not even exclusively) metastasize to the liver (e.g., colorectal malignancies) or slow-growing metastases from tumors treated by chemotherapy with incomplete local control of the disease (e.g., endocrine and breast malignancies).

- Accurate selection of patients and lesions to be treated and use of state-of-the-art technology for guiding and performing ablation are of crucial importance for achieving good results.

- In experienced hands, thermal ablation can achieve local control of liver metastases in up to 85% to 90% of treated lesions. Repeated thermal ablation for either local recurrence or new metastases is technically feasible and very often performed.

- In long-term studies, survival rates of patients who have undergone thermal ablation can equal those of patients who have undergone surgical resection.

- Adverse effects, cost, and duration of hospitalization after thermal ablation are usually lower than after surgical resection.

► **SUGGESTED READINGS**

Atwell TD, Charboneau JW, Nagorney DM, Que FG. Radiofrequency ablation of neuroendocrine metastases. In: vanSonnenberg E, McMullen W, Solbiati L, editors. Tumor Ablation. Principles and Practice. New York: Springer; 2005. p. 332–41.

Cheung L, Livraghi T, Solbiati L, et al. Complications of tumor ablation. In: vanSonnenberg E, McMullen W, Solbiati L, editors. Tumor Ablation. Principles and Practice. New York: Springer; 2005. p. 440–58.

Fahy BN, Jarnagin WR. Evolving techniques in the treatment of liver colorectal metastases: role of laparoscopy, radiofrequency ablation, microwave coagulation, hepatic arterial chemotherapy, indications and contraindications for resection, role of transplantation, and timing of chemotherapy. Surg Clin North Am 2006;86(4):1005–22.

Solbiati L, Ierace T, Tonolini M, Cova L. Ablation of liver metastases. In: vanSonnenberg E, McMullen W, Solbiati L, editors. Tumor Ablation. Principles and Practice. New York: Springer; 2005. p. 311–21.

Solbiati L, Ahmed M, Cova L, et al. Small liver colorectal metastases treated with percutaneous radiofrequency ablation: local response rate and long-term survival with up to 10-year follow-up. Radiology 2012;265(3):958–68.

The complete reference list is available online at www.expertconsult.com.

CHAPTER 143

Cryoablation of Liver Tumors

Mark D. Mamlouk, Eric vanSonnenberg, Stuart G. Silverman, Paul R. Morrison, Charles D. Crum, and Kemal Tuncali

With the development and maturity of ablation techniques, radiologists now can treat a wide variety of solid tumors. There are several options when deciding which technique to use. Radiofrequency, microwave, laser, ethanol, and cryoablation all have been shown to destroy tumor tissue effectively.[1-5] Although the choice of ablation strategy is usually based on institutional expertise and availability, these techniques (and other nonradiologic methods—i.e., surgery, chemotherapy, and radiation therapy) occasionally can be combined for a given patient, depending on the location and specifics of the target. This chapter focuses on the use of cryoablation to treat neoplasms that involve the liver.

INDICATIONS

Cryoablation can be used to treat primary malignant liver lesions such as hepatocellular carcinoma (HCC), as well as benign lesions such as symptomatic hemangiomas and liver adenomas.[10,11] Nonetheless, the most common use of ablation in the liver in the United States is for metastatic disease from colon, breast, and neuroendocrine primaries (Fig. 143-1). Because fewer than 15% of patients with metastatic liver tumors are candidates for curative surgical resection, percutaneous tumor ablation is a viable alternative. Likewise, a minority of patients with primary HCC are candidates for curative surgical resection. Tumors often are deemed surgically unresectable because too much liver parenchyma would be sacrificed, or the tumor lies too close to major biliary or vascular structures such that adequate margins cannot be obtained. Another restriction for surgery is various comorbid conditions, such as cardiopulmonary disease or nutritional status. A percutaneous approach allows treatment of these problematic tumors for surgery because the tissue destruction can be targeted precisely at the tumor and the immediately surrounding adjacent liver parenchyma, with preservation of a greater percentage of normal parenchyma.[10] Likewise, cryoablation also may be able to induce tumor necrosis when vascular or biliary structures are challenging for the surgeon because of proximity of the tumor to vital structures in the hepatic hilum (although radiologists too must exercise great caution in these same anatomic regions).

Cryoablation is indicated in patients who have pathologically proven metastatic lesions in which surgical cure is not an option. Surgery may not be feasible because of bilobar disease, limited hepatic reserve, or cardiopulmonary compromise. Cryoablation generally is used for one to five lesions that are confined to the liver and measure up to 5 cm in diameter. Most institutions consider the presence of metastatic disease outside the liver to be a relative contraindication to cryoablation, with the possible exception of lung or bone metastases in patients with breast cancer. Cryoablation is indicated for the treatment of residual

tumor or local recurrence in patients who have previously undergone treatment with surgery or ablation, as well as new metachronous lesions after primary treatment.

Cryoablation also has been used to treat primary liver neoplasms, most commonly HCC. Indications for cryoablation of primary HCC are different from those for metastatic disease because of the underlying pathology. HCC is caused by underlying chronic liver disease that is usually secondary to hepatitis or alcoholic liver disease. Because of the underlying disease, the only definitive treatment of HCC is liver transplantation. As a result of the limited availability of donated livers and the high cost of transplantation, only a very small percentage of patients can undergo this option. Surgery can offer complete resection of the first HCC and any satellite lesions, but a second or more lesions may have already developed or will develop in the overwhelming majority of patients. If surgical resection was chosen to treat the primary lesion, only a fraction will be able to undergo a second resection.[12] Ablation affords the possibility of complete destruction of the first and subsequent lesions, without significant loss of functioning liver parenchyma. We have treated patients up to five times percutaneously for secondarily diagnosed lesions. Strategically, patients undergo surveillance, and as new lesions appear, they too can undergo ablation.

Cryoablation also has been used to treat benign liver lesions, specifically hemangiomas and adenomas.[10,11] Adenomas are seen predominantly in younger women taking oral contraceptives; the tumors occasionally cause abdominal pain. Cessation of oral contraceptives is first-line therapy, but with persistent problems (especially pain), more invasive treatment may be necessary. Cryoablation is a valuable alternative because of the amount of liver that can be preserved and the low risks involved in the ablation procedure. Symptomatic focal nodular hyperplasia can be treated as well.

CONTRAINDICATIONS

Percutaneous cryoablation is a relatively safe procedure, so there are few absolute contraindications to its use. As with most invasive procedures, the only absolute contraindications are an uncorrectable coagulopathy or an uncooperative patient. Contraindications to general anesthesia can be considered relative because the procedure can be done under intravenous conscious sedation if needed. However, intravenous conscious sedation is suboptimal if extended breath-holds will be necessary and the patient is unable to be completely cooperative.

When cryoablation is used to treat liver masses, there are several hazardous areas where special care has to be taken to avoid damage to adjacent structures. Ablating liver lesions that are adjacent to the hepatic hilum, gallbladder,

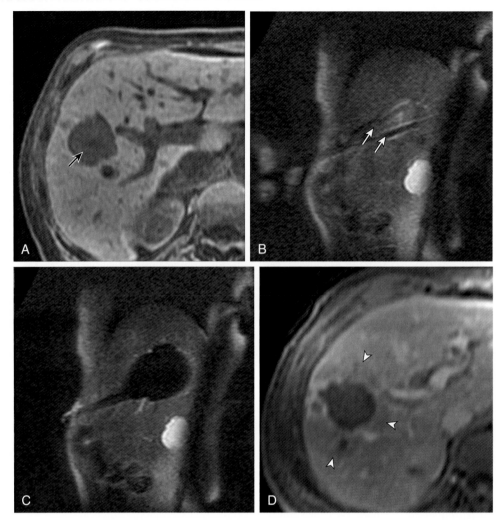

FIGURE 143-1. **A,** Axial contrast-enhanced magnetic resonance imaging (MRI) shows a large minimally enhancing liver metastasis *(arrow)* from a primary breast cancer. **B,** T2 oblique sagittal image shows intraprocedural MRI-guided placement of multiple cryoprobes *(arrows)* into hyperintense tumor. **C,** T2 oblique sagittal image shows a hypointense iceball after 15 minutes of freezing. **D,** Axial contrast-enhanced MRI shows treated tumor surrounded by a nonenhancing margin of ablated normal tissue *(arrowheads)* 24 hours after procedure.

stomach, kidney, pancreas, and colon can be accomplished, but careful planning and execution are essential. Vascular structures are relatively resistant to cryoablation because of the warming effects of flowing blood. However, the biliary system is vulnerable, especially if harboring bacteria. If the lesion to be ablated is juxtaposed to major branches of the biliary system, warm fluid can be circulated through the system via a catheter placed percutaneously or by the endoscopic route. Care also must be taken not to cause damage to structures outside the liver, such as adjacent stomach or bowel.

Sometimes patient positioning (i.e., prone versus supine) can provide adequate distance to avoid injury to critical structures. If positioning of the patient does not provide adequate safety of adjacent structures, sterile water, dextrose, or a normal saline barrier can be interposed (Fig. 143-2). This is accomplished percutaneously by injecting sterile fluid through a fine needle between the lesion and the bowel to be displaced, termed *hydrodissection*.[13,14] Overall, when care is taken in both planning and execution of cryoablation, it is a relatively safe procedure.

EQUIPMENT

During the early days of cryosurgery, the probes were cooled with liquid nitrogen. Because these LN_2 probes were relatively large (3- to 8-mm in outer diameter), for years cryoablation was practical only in a surgical setting.[15] Because the size of the probe was less than optimal, a complicated Seldinger technique was used that required several minutes to position and reposition the probes. Even though these probes were effective in causing tissue destruction, the probe size and handling of the liquid nitrogen were negative features in light of the now contemporary gas-based systems.

The argon gas–based systems that were developed in the 1990s have virtually replaced liquid nitrogen devices. Argon systems work on the Joule-Thompson principle, in which low temperatures are achieved by the rapid expansion of a high-pressure gas through a thin aperture.[15] Because of the low viscosity of argon gas, it can be circulated rapidly within the probe tip. This allows faster cooling at the probe tip, which hastens removal and repositioning (if necessary) of

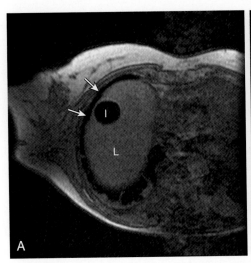 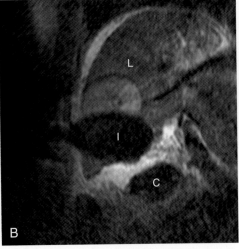

FIGURE 143-2. Image-guided control demonstrated in two separate ablation procedures. **A,** Intraprocedural axial T1 magnetic resonance imaging (MRI) shows critical relationships several minutes into a multiprobe freeze of a liver metastasis in dome of liver. Iceball *(I)* within liver *(L)* is observed as its lateral edge approaches adjacent lung *(arrows)*. Such clear visualization of field allows radiologist to adjust rate of freezing to protect normal tissues. **B,** Intraprocedural coronal T2 MRI provides guidance to protect adjacent structures by additional interventional techniques. Multiprobe freezing of a metastasis is conducted in liver *(L)*. Colon *(C)* is protected from iceball *(I)* because it has been distanced by injection of saline through additional percutaneous needles (not seen in image plane). Saline is seen here as hyperintense region between ice *(I)* and colon *(C)*.

the cryoprobes. After the freezing phase is complete, high-pressure helium gas can then be circulated through the probe tip to cause rapid thawing. Helium provides an effect opposite to that of argon gas under the Joule-Thompson principle, causing a warming of the probe to allow rapid thawing for probe removal from the frozen tissue or repositioning.

There are currently two major manufacturers of cryoablation equipment: Galil Medical (Yokneam, Israel) and EndoCare Inc. (Endo Pharmaceuticals, Chadds Ford, Pa.). Both companies use an argon/helium-based system to cool and thaw the probe tip, respectively, and have stand-alone consoles that are connected to gas tanks. Both systems have a similar computer-based interface that demonstrates the vital statistics of the different probes and their respective temperatures (Fig. e143-1). Currently, Galil Medical is the only company to offer a system that is MRI compatible. Galil Medical and EndoCare cryoprobes for percutaneous ablation are needle-like, 17-gauge in size. The Galil system can accommodate up to 25 probes; the EndoCare system up to 8 probes.

All three main cross-sectional imaging techniques can be used to guide percutaneous placement of cryoprobes for ablation. Ultrasound, CT, and MRI each has advantages and disadvantages. Ultrasound was first used in the early 1980s; its utility has since expanded to guide percutaneous cryoablation. Ultrasound allows real-time imaging during probe placement, and therefore major structures such as the gallbladder, large bile ducts, and larger hepatic vessels are well visualized and can be avoided.

The iceball created during cryoablation is intensely echogenic on ultrasound; this allows real-time monitoring as the iceball forms and propagates. Therefore, damage to the surrounding normal liver parenchyma is limited. The main drawback of ultrasound is the distal acoustic shadow produced by the iceball. Because of the echogenicity of the iceball, ultrasound cannot penetrate beyond it, and

structures distal to the iceball are not visualized because of acoustic shadowing. This can be problematic when trying to avoid critical structures that are deep to the tumor being ablated. Reverberation artifact and the critical angle effect are also troublesome when ultrasound guidance is used. The critical angle effect can cause the iceball to appear speciously larger, whereas reverberation causes apparent echoes within the iceball.[16] The critical angle effect is due to variation in the speed of sound as it travels through soft tissue versus ice, and is more apparent when using a vector transducer than a linear transducer.

CT has many attributes that make it an appealing imaging choice for ablation. CT is widely available and is often primarily used to detect and monitor lesions that have been ablated. CT also shows the anatomy of the liver and adjacent structures well. This allows identification of adjacent structures that may need to be avoided, such as major vessels, the gallbladder, and bowel. In soft tissue, such as liver parenchyma and solid tumors, the iceball is generally well seen as a hypodense region (Fig. 143-3). The margins of cell death and the visible iceball also correlate well when using CT.[17-19] One drawback of the use of CT for image-guided ablation is exposure of the patient and personnel to ionizing radiation. In a retrospective study of 20 CT-guided percutaneous liver tumor cryoablations, the total effective dose for the procedure was 72 ± 18 mSv.[20] Although that report does suggest ways to reduce such exposures, it calls attention to an added risk with CT guidance. Of course, the uncertain risk due to the radiation is weighed against the imminent health risks associated with the disease state for which the ablation is being utilized.

One technological assist to identifying a tumor location in unenhanced CT images is to "register" (map; overlay) preprocedural MRI images with an intraprocedural CT scan. Contemporary efforts use a technique of nonrigid registration to elastically morph the MRI into fitting the CT scan. The resulting information-rich MRI-CT can improve

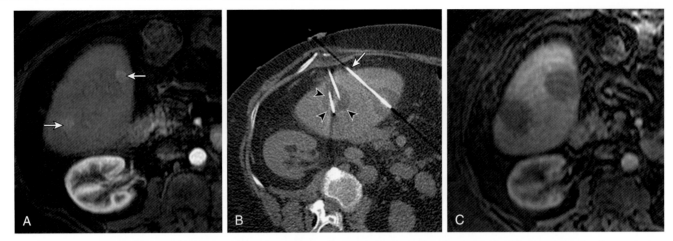

FIGURE 143-3. Image-guided cryoablation. **A,** Axial contrast-enhanced magnetic resonance imaging (MRI) identifies two enhancing liver metastases *(arrows)*. **B,** Unenhanced axial computed tomography (CT) shows cryoprobes *(arrow)* placed under CT guidance. Iceball appears as a hypodense rounded shape *(arrowheads)* around probes. **C,** Axial contrast-enhanced postprocedure MRI at 24 hours shows corresponding nonenhancing regions of ablation covering tumors.

tumor visualization during interventional planning, targeting, and monitoring.[21,22]

In recent years, MRI has been used for a variety of interventional procedures and ablations.[10,23] In one institution's experience of over 300 cryoablation procedures, two thirds were MRI guided.[9] MRI has a distinct advantage over CT in that the tumor is nearly always distinguishable from normal liver parenchyma, without the aid of intravenous contrast agents.[24] The multiplanar capability of MRI is another advantage. The cryoprobes can be accurately placed and verified in all three planes—axial, sagittal, and coronal. Cryoablation can be performed in traditional MRI scanners with the development of MRI-compatible probes; however, with open or wide-bore systems, the radiologist has sufficient access to the patient and can guide the position of the probes during cryoablation.[10,25] This allows nearly real-time imaging during ablation and greater accuracy in controlling the developing iceball.[10,26] Another benefit of MRI is assessing temperature within the iceball and tissues because of T1-weighted imaging characteristics.[27,28] Like ultrasound and CT, the visible iceball on MRI corresponds well to the actual ablative zone size.[29,30] However, MRI demonstrates the demarcations from iceball to tumor to normal parenchyma without any interference or artifact, unlike ultrasound and CT.

For information on the use of PET and PET-CT in cryoablation and radiofrequency ablation, please visit www.expertconsult.com.

TECHNIQUE

Anatomy and Preprocedural Care

Thorough knowledge of hepatic anatomy is essential to safely ablate primary and metastatic hepatic neoplasms. Hepatobiliary surgeons have used the Couinaud system since the 1950s.[32] This system is used to divide the liver into eight segments that are supplied by the portal triad and drained by the hepatic veins. The plane that divides the inferior vena cava (IVC) and the middle hepatic vein separates the left lobe from the right lobe of the liver and is

known as *Cantlie's line.* The left lobe of the liver is divided into segments II, III, and IV, with the umbilical fissure dividing segments II and III from IV. The right lobe of the liver is divided into segments V, VI, VII, and VIII. The plane formed by the IVC and the right hepatic vein separates the anterior segments V and VIII from the posterior segments VI and VII. The portal veins divide the liver into upper and lower segments. The caudate lobe is considered segment I and receives portal flow from both the right and left sides. This knowledge allows the radiologist to communicate with surgeons more appropriately about available options when considering surgery or ablation. Hepatic resection varies from single or double segmentectomies (II and III, IV and V, or VI and VII) to extended lobectomies or trisegmentectomies that include parenchyma from both lobes of the liver.

One of the most important principles in all of interventional radiology is to define a safe access route before beginning the procedure. This requires the identification of all key structures before commencing liver ablation. First, care must be taken to avoid any bowel that may be interposed between the liver and the abdominal wall, the so-called Chilaiditi variant. The liver also has an intimate relationship with the diaphragm. Care must be taken to avoid the diaphragm and not cause a pneumothorax, diaphragmatic injury, or other intrathoracic complications. Planning should also include identification and avoidance of the larger vascular structures (IVC, portal and hepatic veins), porta hepatis, and central biliary ducts.

With regard to antibiotic prophylaxis, we administer 1 g of cefazolin sodium (Ancef [SmithKline Beecham Pharmaceuticals, Philadelphia, Pa.]) intravenously before each procedure, and every 8 hours thereafter for a total of three doses after the procedure.[33] However, there are different views regarding the need for routine antibiotic usage with ablation, and without clear consensus.

Technical Aspects

Before starting an ablation procedure, appropriate imaging (CT, ultrasound, or MRI) is performed to identify the target

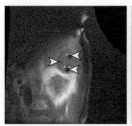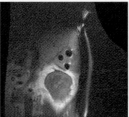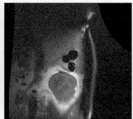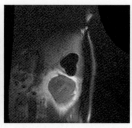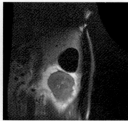

FIGURE 143-4. Monitoring ablation over time. That cryoablation is a dynamic process is evident in coronal T2 magnetic resonance imaging (MRI) acquired in oblique sagittal plane during treatment of a liver metastasis. First image shows three cryoprobes *(arrowheads)* in cross-section situated within tumor. Probes are spaced so individual iceball from each probe can work synergistically to form one large, hypointense iceball *(last image)* to cover target. Images between show same image plane at intervals of approximately 2 to 4 minutes. Although MRI and computed tomography do not provide images in real time, it is possible to scan on a time frame that delineates rate of iceball growth.

and define the safest access route. A small, 22- to 25-gauge needle is used for biopsy if not previously done. Another needle is left in the proper location in the tumor to be ablated as a marker, and the cryoprobe is inserted into the neoplasm by using the tandem technique adjacent to the marker. Alternatively, a modified Seldinger technique can be used. Additional cryoprobes can be placed for adequate coverage of larger lesions. One advantage of multiple small cryoprobes is a more uniform and predictable freeze, with improved control of the iceball.[15] After proper placement of the cryoprobes, two 15-minute freezes separated by a 10-minute thaw are completed to achieve sufficient necrosis of the lesion. The freeze cycle routinely reaches temperatures between −110°C and −120°C, whereas the thaw cycle temperature rises to approximately 40°C. Imaging can be continued throughout the procedure to monitor iceball growth (Fig. 143-4). After successful ablation of the lesion and complete thawing, the probe(s) is removed. Postprocedural imaging is performed to document the adequacy of ablation and whether additional freeze/thaw cycles are needed.

OUTCOMES

Many metrics are used to measure success when evaluating an innovative approach to the care of a patient with cancer. The gold standard by which all treatments are measured is the 5-year survival rate. In a study of 420 patients with unresectable HCC, comparisons were made with a subset that had transarterial chemoembolization (TACE) plus cryoablation, while another group had cryoablation alone. The 5-year survival rates were 39% in the combined group versus 23% in the cryoablation-alone group.[34] In another study of percutaneous ablation of 20 patients with HCC less than 3 cm in diameter, complete response was achieved in 65%, 20% partial response, and 15% stable disease.[35]

The initial measure of ablation is assessed on immediate postablation scans as the percentage of tumor destroyed. In two studies, the initial success of hepatic tumor cryoablation was 60% to 85%.[34,36] Tumor size is a key factor in adequacy of therapy. In the first study, HCCs were ablated with the aid of percutaneous ethanol,[34] whereas in the latter study,[36] all unresectable hepatic malignancies were ablated without any adjunctive therapy. Local recurrence at follow-up ranges from 3% to 53%.[37]

There is evidence in the surgical literature that open or laparoscopic cryoablation does not increase the 2- or 5-year

survival rate in metastatic colon cancer over standard surgical treatment, even though local recurrence is reduced and a greater amount of normal liver parenchyma is preserved with cryoablation alone.[38] Several studies also have evaluated surgical cryoablation of neuroendocrine metastases to the liver; the endpoint for success was relief of symptoms after ablation and reduction of serum markers.[39,40]

COMPLICATIONS

The mortality rate with surgical cryoablation ranges from 1.2% to 7.5%, with the major complication rate from 5.9% to 45%.[41-43] There is a strong correlation between the volume of liver ablated and major complications. Studies have demonstrated that when approximately 30% to 35% of the liver volume or more is ablated, a dramatic increase in complications occurs.[41-43] Ablation of tumors larger than 5 cm, or an area of liver 30 cm^2 or greater, also increases the major complication rate.[44-46]

Major complications include parenchymal fracture, coagulopathy, acute renal failure secondary to myoglobinuria, and cryoshock. Cryoablation hemorrhage is attributed mainly to fracture of the hepatic parenchyma and capsule, whereas coagulopathy plays a minor role. Hemorrhage results from parenchymal fracture that extends from the center of the iceball through the hepatic vessels, either arterial or venous, to the liver capsule. Limiting the torque or movement of cryoprobes during freezing and thawing cycles can minimize this complication. This is extremely important when the freeze cycle is near its end and the liver is coldest. Care also must be taken to allow complete thawing of the iceball before removal of the probe when the liver is most vulnerable to cracking, which was a risk with cryosurgery.

The least understood cause of cryoablation-related mortality has been described as *cryoshock*. This is a constellation of acute respiratory distress syndrome, thrombocytopenia, disseminated intravascular coagulation (DIC), hypotension, and multiorgan failure.[47] Cryoshock has been likened to septic shock without an identifiable infectious source. This syndrome was seen in 21 of 2173 patients following cryosurgery; 6 of these 21 died postprocedurally.[43] This phenomenon appears to be mostly specific to cryoablation, but a recent study has shown that a moderate systemic inflammatory response can occur with RFA.[48] Cryoshock has occurred after ablation of both primary liver tumors and metastases. Cryoshock is related to the volume of liver or tumor ablated (or both) and the number of freeze/thaw cycles.

Minor complications may occur after cryoablation. Patients routinely experience mild to moderate right upper quadrant pain that is treated with narcotic analgesics. Most minor complications from ablation are similar to those that occur with biopsy of tumors: bleeding, diaphragmatic injury, pneumothorax, hepatic abscess (sometimes delayed), and subcapsular hematoma.[36,42,49,50] Injury to the biliary system can occur during cryoablation. The smaller blood vessels of the liver are warmed by blood, but bile ducts do not have this protection. Therefore, specific care must be taken to avoid injury to the biliary system. Warm saline, sterile water, or 5% dextrose in water can be circulated through a catheter placed in the bile ducts percutaneously or endoscopically to protect the main bile ducts.[51] Hypothermia can also be associated with cryoablation; it can be avoided with routine use of the Bair Hugger heating blanket (Arizant Healthcare, Prairie, Minn.) throughout the procedure; this problem is more likely to occur in small children.[14]

Of concern during cryoablation in the liver is the production of myoglobin. Myoglobinemia may develop but usually is transient, and uncommonly severe enough to require prophylactic treatment.[33] Rarely, myoglobinemia can progress to acute tubular necrosis and renal failure from myoglobinuria.[41,52] Ensuring proper hydration before the procedure, as well as use of mannitol diuresis and alkalinization of urine if myoglobinuria develops, can help protect the kidneys from this complication. Lastly, self-limited biochemical and hematologic changes commonly occur after percutaneous cryoablation of liver tumors and are usually milder than those reported after liver cryosurgery.[33] However, as has been suggested following cryosurgery, percutaneous cryoablation can cause thrombocytopenia and even DIC. The amount of decrease in the platelet count correlates with the amount of normal parenchyma sacrificed and included in the ablation. Necrosis of normal parenchyma is associated with a rise in aspartate aminotransferase (AST) and alanine aminotransferase (ALT) and may be a harbinger of thrombocytopenia.[33] Because of this phenomenon, we have often considered other ablative agents, such as RFA, when planning the ablation of multiple tumors in which large amounts of normal liver parenchyma are expected to be included in the ablation zones.

Several other causes of mortality seen after cryoablation are not specific to this method: postablation myocardial infarction, pulmonary embolism, sepsis, colonic perforation, and hepatic insufficiency. There also have been reports of hepatorenal syndrome, portal vein thrombosis, strangulated bowel, variceal hemorrhage, and rupture of the ablated area into the abdominal cavity, resulting in postablation death.*

CRYOABLATION VERSUS RADIOFREQUENCY ABLATION

 For a discussion of this topic, please visit www.expertconsult.com.

*References 36, 39, 40, 44, 47, 53.

POSTPROCEDURAL AND FOLLOW-UP CARE

Immediately after the cryoablation procedure, we perform contrast-enhanced CT or MRI to assess the effectiveness of ablation. Patients are subsequently sent to the postprocedure unit for 2 hours to recover from the effects of general anesthesia. They are then transferred to a regular floor for overnight observation. During this time, blood is drawn for follow-up laboratory studies, including hemoglobin and hematocrit, white blood cell count, platelet count, AST and ALT, coagulation profile, creatinine, and myoglobin. Follow-up imaging is arranged for 3 months after the ablation procedure. If the postablation course is uneventful, most patients are discharged from the hospital the day after the procedure.

After discharge, contact by telephone is maintained for a few days. The patient is seen as an outpatient 1 week after the procedure. Three-month imaging follow-up—CT, MRI, PET-CT, or any combination—is performed and the results compared with preprocedure images to further document the results of the ablation and regression or progression of disease. The latter may require another ablative procedure.

KEY POINTS

- Percutaneous cryoablation is an effective method for tumor destruction in the liver and has been used for both primary and metastatic lesions.
- With proper planning and care, most tumors in the liver can safely undergo cryoablation as an alternative to liver resection.
- Computed tomography, ultrasound, and magnetic resonance imaging all have been used to guide placement of cryoprobes to monitor intraprocedural iceball formation and for postprocedural follow-up.

▶ SUGGESTED READINGS

Atwell TD, Charboneau JW, Que FG, et al. Treatment of neuroendocrine cancer metastatic to the liver: the role of ablative techniques. Cardiovasc Intervent Radiol 2005;28:409–21.

Jain S, Sacchi M, Vrachnos P, et al. Recent advances in the treatment of colorectal liver metastases. Hepatogastroenterology 2005;52:1567–84.

Jansen MC, van Hillegersberg R, Chamuleau RA, et al. Outcome of regional and local ablative therapies for hepatocellular carcinoma: a collective review. Eur J Surg Oncol 2005;31:331–47.

vanSonnenberg E, McMullen W, Solbiati L. Tumor Ablation: Principles and Practice. New York: Springer; 2005.

Weber SM, Lee FT Jr. Expanded treatment of hepatic tumors with radiofrequency ablation and cryoablation. Oncology 2005;19(11 Suppl 4):27–32.

The complete reference list is available online at www.expertconsult.com.

CHAPTER 144
Chemical Ablation of Liver Lesions

Joshua L. Weintraub, Thomas J. Ward, and John H. Rundback

The presentation of a patient with a liver lesion ranges from the patient with an incidentally discovered and asymptomatic simple liver cyst to the patient with multifocal primary or metastatic liver tumors. The interventions used to treat this wide range of lesions is equally as varied, with percutaneous chemical ablation having a continually evolving role.

CHEMICAL ABLATION OF BENIGN LIVER LESIONS

Simple Liver Cysts

Liver cysts are common, with a prevalence of approximately 2.5% in the general population and a female predominance.[1] A majority of these cysts are incidentally discovered by ultrasound or computed tomography (CT) and are clinically insignificant, so no further evaluation or treatment is necessary. For a minority of patients, larger cysts can produce symptoms that range from abdominal discomfort and nausea to compression of the biliary tree or inferior vena cava, intraperitoneal rupture, hemorrhage, torsion, or infection.[2-6] The majority of symptomatic cysts occur in females older than 50, with a 9:1 female-to-male ratio and a predisposition for the right hepatic lobe.[7]

Previous attempts at percutaneous treatment of the symptomatic cyst focused on cyst aspiration. This strategy produced suboptimal results due to high rates of cyst recurrence, with reported recurrence rates between 78% and 100%.[8,9] Advances in percutaneous treatment of liver cysts occurred with the introduction of ablative agents that treat the underlying pathology of the process. True simple hepatic cysts have an epithelial lining and are the result of congenitally aberrant bile ducts that are separated from the remainder of the intrahepatic biliary tract. The columnar or cuboidal epithelial cells that line the cyst produce fluid that reaccumulates after simple aspiration.

With newer techniques, after cyst aspiration a variety of chemical agents (e.g., tetracycline hydrochloride, doxycycline, minocycline hydrochloride, hypertonic saline) have been injected into the cyst in an attempt to decrease previously observed recurrence rates by damaging the fluid-producing cells.[10-13] The most studied chemical agent administered for this purpose is ethanol, which produces epithelial cell damage that prevents fluid secretion and results in subsequent cyst destruction.

The topics Percutaneous Ethanol Sclerotherapy (PES) and Puncture, Aspiration, Injection, and Reaspiration of Cystic Echinococcosis (PAIR of CE) are discussed in full at www.expertconsult.com.

CHEMICAL ABLATION OF MALIGNANT LIVER LESIONS

Unresectable hepatic malignancies, whether primary or metastatic, represent one of the more difficult challenges in the care of patients with cancer. Hepatocellular carcinoma (HCC) is the most common primary liver cancer worldwide, with over 500,000 new cases diagnosed annually. HCC is an extremely malignant tumor that generally occurs in the setting of chronic hepatic cirrhosis. Its association with hepatitis B and C infection is expected to increase its incidence. Treatment options for HCC are limited, with less than half of all patients being candidates for surgical resection. In these patients, median survival from time of diagnosis is approximately 6 to 20 months, despite aggressive therapy.

Colorectal carcinoma accounts for 148,000 new cases of cancer a year and is the second most common cause of cancer death in the United States. Of the 55,000 deaths annually, over 50% are due to liver metastases after the primary lesion has been resected. Surgical resection of the hepatic metastases has been demonstrated to improve survival. In patients who are not resection candidates, regional therapy may show a benefit.

Some other rare tumors (e.g., neuroendocrine, carcinoid, and islet cell tumors; ocular melanoma) have a unique propensity to metastasize exclusively to the liver. Systemic chemotherapies have been shown to be largely ineffective. Because of this, regional cancer therapy and hepatic artery embolization have been employed to control symptoms and attempt to improve overall survival.

Percutaneous chemical ablation is an established technique of regional therapy for small (<3 cm) hepatocellular malignancies, and it continues to have a role despite the emergence and proliferation of newer technologies such as radiofrequency ablation (RFA), cryoablation, and laser interstitial ablation. Diffusion of ablative agents such as ethanol or acetic acid is more favorable in HCC because it is a "soft" tumor in a "hard" (fibrotic, cirrhotic) liver. In contrast, chemical ablation is less effective in treating metastatic lesions such as colorectal carcinoma because the consistency of such lesions is that of a "hard" tumor in a "soft" liver.

Chemical ablation offers many distinct advantages over other regional therapies, in part due to its relative simplicity, low cost, and safety. Chemical ablation techniques with either acetic acid or ethanol, when compared with RFA, have the advantage of not requiring dedicated instrumentation and may allow ablation of tumors difficult to treat with RFA because of proximity to other organs or pronounced heat sink effect from adjacent vascular structures.

Percutaneous Ethanol Injection

Indications

Current indications for percutaneous ethanol injection (PEI) are generally limited to HCC. Most investigators have used PEI for HCC less than 3 cm in greatest diameter, because ethanol may not diffuse evenly through larger tumors, and thus some areas could be left untreated. This shortcoming can be overcome by inserting multiple needles, injecting ethanol into various parts of the lesion through each needle. Our current size limit for use of ethanol injection is 5 cm or less in diameter. Patients are treated in a staged approach, with up to 4 sessions over a 4-week period. Again, PEI is generally reserved for patients with HCC rather than metastasis because hepatic metastases, unlike HCCs, tend to become fibrotic and resistant to diffusion of ethanol the longer the treatment protocol takes to complete. In addition, metastases are often set in a noncirrhotic liver, which allows greater diffusion of ethanol into nondiseased tissue surrounding a more fibrotic tumor.[38] In comparison, HCC is a soft tumor encapsulated by a fibrous capsule that helps contain the ethanol within the tumor.

For ethanol to effectively act on neoplastic cells remote from the point of injection, it must readily distribute through the interstitial compartment of the tumor. Because of its low molecular weight and the high interstitial diffusion coefficient of neoplastic interstitium, as well as the large amount of tissue convection, ethanol can efficiently diffuse through the tumor interstitium. As ethanol distributes through the interstitium, its cytotoxic mechanisms are exerted through a combination of cytoplasmic dehydration, denaturation of cellular proteins, and small-vessel thrombosis. These processes effectively result in coagulation necrosis of the tumor.[39]

The number of lesions treated also varies between investigators. Although most interventional radiologists have used PEI on patients with three or fewer lesions, some investigators have recently widened the indication for this treatment for up to five lesions. The more lesions treated, the more treatment sessions required, which becomes impractical at a certain point. We currently limit PEI use to patients with four or fewer lesions.

Contraindications

Contraindications to percutaneous ethanol injection include extrahepatic metastatic disease as the predominant clinical problem and irreversible coagulopathy as previously defined.

Equipment

The equipment necessary to perform PEI is minimal. By far the most important tool is excellent imaging guidance, which can usually be accomplished with ultrasound via a 3- to 5-MHz curved-array transducer. Occasionally we will supplement this with CT scanning for difficult lesions. A 20- to 22-gauge end-hole or conical-tip multi-sidehole needle is used for delivery of an appropriate volume of 98% ethanol. Other required equipment includes a sterile tray, sterile sheets, local anesthetic, and imaging guidance.

Techniques

Percutaneous ethanol ablation is usually performed with real-time ultrasound guidance. In cases where lesions are

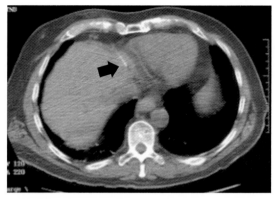

FIGURE 144-1. Chemical ablation of hepatocellular carcinoma (HCC) at dome of liver. Computed tomography showing insertion tract of infusion needle *(arrow)* in patient with small (1.5 cm) HCC in dome of liver. Proximity of lesion to heart and diaphragm made thermal ablative techniques higher risk in this patient, and patient's hepatic synthetic function was inadequate for transcatheter arterial chemoembolization. After two treatment sessions, patient had stable disease that was sustained another 18 months before HCC developed in new locations in right lobe of liver.

near the dome of the liver, CT or MRI guidance may be preferred for better visualization (Fig. 144-1). A 20- to 22-gauge end-hole or conical-tip multi-sidehole needle is used. With MRI guidance, titanium needles are preferred to reduce magnetic susceptibility artifact. Prophylactic antibiotics are not routinely administered. The infusion needle may be placed with either a freehand technique or a needle guide by using a 3.5- or 5-MHz curved-array transducer. For small lesions (<2 cm), the needle is inserted to the margin of the tumor farthest from the ultrasound transducer. Larger lesions may necessitate insertion of the needle at more than one site or insertion of more than one needle. Infusion is performed slowly in 0.1- to 0.2-mL aliquots with continuous ultrasound monitoring. When the area of the tumor has been rendered echogenic, the needle is withdrawn into the area of the tumor closer to the transducer and infusion resumed. Care must be taken to not allow air into the system, because this produces unwanted acoustic shadowing. It must be remembered that the spread of ethanol is often overestimated with ultrasound. When filling of a bile duct, portal vein, hepatic vein, or hepatic artery branch is seen, the infusion is stopped and the needle withdrawn and repositioned. The procedure should be terminated if gallbladder filling is seen during infusion; this has been associated with development of hemobilia. When injection is being performed with CT or MRI guidance, real-time monitoring for filling of nontarget structures is not possible. In this setting, many operators obtain one or two images during the injection procedure to assess distribution of the agent (Fig. 144-2). When the tumor has been rendered completely echogenic or the target volume has been reached, the needle is left in place for 1 to 2 minutes and then withdrawn under aspiration.

Most investigators use a final target volume based on tumor volume and a surgical margin of 1 cm beyond the periphery of the lesion. This volume is calculated as:

$$V = 4/3\pi(r + 0.5)^3$$

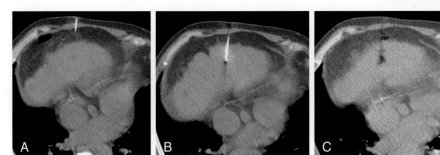

FIGURE 144-2. Chemical ablation of hepatocellular carcinoma (HCC). **A-C,** Computed tomography guidance was used during insertion of infusion needle in this 69-year-old patient with HCC. His initial α-fetoprotein (AFP) level was 600 ng/mL. **D,** Three-month follow-up imaging demonstrates a necrotic area in region of percutaneous ethanol injection therapy. AFP had decreased to 5 ng/mL.

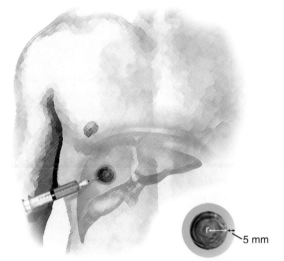

Volume of infusion=$4/3\pi(r + 0.5)^3$

FIGURE 144-3. Final target volume for percutaneous ethanol injection therapy.

where V is the target volume of ethanol, r the radius of the lesion (in centimeters), and 0.5 is the correction for the additional surgical margin (Fig. 144-3).

Cases of HCC recurrence after PEI are usually seen at the periphery of the lesion, which implies that this area is frequently undertreated. For these reasons, many interventional radiologists regard this volume equation as a guideline and have the patient return for additional treatment sessions if areas of viable tumor are seen at follow-up imaging.

In an attempt to circumvent the need for multiple treatment sessions, Livraghi et al. described a "one-shot" technique in which the amount of ethanol injected was higher than the intended final target volume, and lesions larger than 3 cm can be treated.[40] This technique requires an intravenous infusion of 1,6-diphosphate (FDP) and glutathione to be given immediately prior to the procedure to increase the rate of hepatic oxidation of ethanol. This technique is more painful than standard ethanol ablation and is therefore performed under general anesthesia. Glutathione and FDP are unavailable in the United States.

Controversies

Although PEI for HCC is a safe procedure with a complication rate less than 2%, controversy has arisen concerning its efficacy in comparison to RFA, as well as its use in tumors larger than 3 cm in diameter.

When compared to PEI, RFA requires fewer treatment sessions to achieve comparable antitumor effects. Complete response rates were 96% to 100% for RFA versus 86% to 89% for PEI.[41] However, the main drawback of RFA is a higher rate of adverse events than with PEI. The mortality rate ranged from 0.1% to 0.5%, the major complication rate ranged from 2.2% to 3.1%, and the minor complication rate ranged from 5% to 8.9%. The most common cause of death were sepsis and hepatic failure, and the most common complications were intraperitoneal bleeding, hepatic abscess, bile duct injury, hepatic decompensation, and grounding pad burns.[42] Therefore, because deaths have been associated with RFA, there has been controversy regarding the decision to use either RFA or PEI as first-line treatment for ablation of HCC.

There has also been controversy surrounding the use of PEI as first-line therapy for tumors larger than 3 cm in diameter. Studies show that PEI achieves complete responses in more than 80% of tumors smaller than 3 cm in diameter, but only 50% of tumors 3 to 5 cm in size.[43] A retrospective study comparing 39 patients treated with PEI and 58 patients who underwent surgical resection for small HCC (<3 cm each and three or fewer in number) reported no difference in 1-, 3-, and 5-year recurrence-free survival and overall survival.[44] In contrast, another large retrospective study of patients with HCC less than 5 cm in diameter enrolled in the Liver Cancer Study Group of Japan found that patients who underwent liver resection (n = 8010) had better survival than those treated by PEI (n = 4037) or transarterial chemoembolization (TACE; n = 841).[45]

Outcomes

Survival after PEI for HCC is dependent on histologic grade, Child-Pugh score, and size and number of lesions. In patients with Child-Pugh class A cirrhosis and solitary lesions 3 cm or smaller in diameter, 3-year survival rates of 60% to 70% and 5-year survival rates of 30% to 50% have been reported.[46] A recent cohort study found no difference in the 5-year survival rate between patients with three or fewer HCCs 3 cm in diameter or smaller who underwent

PEI or surgical resection.[47] The 5-year survival rate was 59% in the PEI group and 61% in the resection group.

The overall survival using the one-shot technique at 3 years was 74%. The 3-year survival rate for patients with a single HCC with a diameter of 5 cm or less was 82%.[48]

Complications

Conventional PEI is usually well tolerated, with minor complications of local pain, transient fever, and intoxication being easily managed. Major complications are rare, with an overall complication rate less than 2%. Complications include intraperitoneal hemorrhage, pleural effusion, hemobilia, hepatic abscess, hepatic necrosis, cholangitis, esophageal hemorrhage, and hypotension. These are secondary to either the local effects of the ethanol or inadvertent injection into the vascular or biliary system. Hypotension is thought to be related to systemic absorption and subsequent pulmonary artery constriction.[49] It is of critical importance to maintain vascular access throughout PEI procedures with frequent blood pressure monitoring to allow for rapid response to unexpected changes in the patient's vital signs.

Follow-up Imaging

Currently the most widely used modality for measuring treatment response is contrast-enhanced triple-phase CT scanning. MRI is believed to be better at distinguishing viable tumor from fluid and blood products, but early studies did not demonstrate MRI to be a reliable indicator of tumor viability.[50] More recent literature has suggested that MRI is comparable. As functional techniques evolve (diffusion imaging, spectroscopy, etc.), MRI will be increasingly utilized. Currently, positron emission tomography (PET) has not shown to be useful for imaging of hepatocellular carcinoma. Nagoaka et al. demonstrated that the detection rate of PET was 56% for intrahepatic HCC lesions.[51]

The presence of early arterial enhancement is an indicator of residual viable tissue. Necrotic nonviable tissue does not enhance. We currently use the "Modified Response Evaluation Criteria in Solid Tumors" (mRECIST) to evaluate tumor response, using the concept of viable tumor as depicted by arterial phase imaging as recommended by the American Association for the Study of Liver Disease (AASLD).[52] Power Doppler ultrasound has been found to aid in detecting local recurrence. Although tumor arterial Doppler signal could be detected in only a third of HCC nodules, when arterial signal could be detected, correlation of posttreatment arterial signal was predictive of local recurrence. Patients with residual arterial signal had an odds of local recurrence nearly 50 times that of patients without residual arterial power Doppler signal after ethanol ablation during the 25-month follow-up.[53] We routinely perform follow-up on our patients at 3-month intervals after successful ablation for the first year and then lengthen the follow-up imaging period to every 6 months.

Percutaneous Acetic Acid Injection

Indications

Indications for the use of acetic acid are quite similar to PEI. Patients must have unresectable hepatic malignancies. Our experience has suggested that septated or fibrotic tumors show better response with acetic acid than with PEI because of acetic acid's unique diffusion characteristics.[54]

Acetic acid ablation exhibits the same advantages of ethanol ablation, including ease of diffusion, denaturation of cellular proteins, and cellular dehydration. In addition, it also has the ability to dissolve the cellular basement membranes and interstitial collagen, essentially destroying septa within the tumor. As a result, there is more homogeneous diffusion and distribution of effect after acetic acid injection than after intrahepatic injection of absolute ethanol. This in effect allows the entire tumor rather than a small segment to be exposed to the necrotic effects of the drug, thereby potentially reducing the volume needed for treatment. In contradistinction, absolute ethanol denatures proteins only within a particular tumor segment, without septal destruction, thus limiting the chemical diffusion and regional necrotic effect. As a result, the extent of coagulative necrosis is increased, although the histologic appearance is indistinguishable from that achieved with ethanol.[54]

Contraindications

Contraindications to percutaneous acetic acid injection include extrahepatic metastatic disease as the predominant clinical problem and irreversible coagulopathy as defined previously.

Equipment

A 20- to 22-gauge end-hole or conical-tip multi-sidehole needle is used for delivery of an appropriate volume of 50% ascetic acid. Some operators have used an 18-gauge multi-pronged needle with 27-gauge needle array system (Quadra-Fuse [Rex Medical, Radnor, Pa.]) for delivery. This allows for single-needle distribution into a spherical array.[55] Other required equipment includes a sterile tray, sterile sheets, local anesthetic, and imaging guidance.

Technique

A 50% acetic acid solution is injected with a 20- or 22-gauge multi-sidehole needle under real-time ultrasound or CT guidance. Estimation of the volume required for treatment has evolved empirically because acetic acid penetrates the tumor tissue more readily than ethanol. One such formula to determine the injected volume (in mL) for each tumor is to add 1 mL to the largest tumor diameter (i.e., a tumor with a 3-cm diameter would require 4 mL) (Fig. 144-4). Tumor diameter is measured as the greatest transverse diameter of enhancing tumor. Smaller volumes are injected if resistance is encountered, complete lesion filling is observed on real-time ultrasound, or intravasation occurs. In cases of intravasation, the needle should be repositioned before resuming the injection. The total injected volume for each treatment session should not exceed 10 mL because of the risk for renal injury or metabolic acidosis.

Given the high incidence of hemolysis (approximately 30%), pretreatment with *N*-acetylcysteine (600 mg orally twice daily for 3 days beginning 1 day before the procedure) and sodium bicarbonate (100 mEq/L infused at 150 mL/h) is recommended before ablation and continued afterwards for at least 2 hours or until microscopic hematuria resolves. Because the injection is painful, intravenous conscious sedation is recommended with bolus dosing immediately prior to administration of the acetic acid.

The needle is advanced to near the distal wall of the lesion, and slow injection of an ablation agent performed as the needle is slowly retracted. Diffusion of acid through the tumor is evident by confluent areas of echogenicity (Fig 144-5). The target volume may be injected during the initial session. More commonly, the session is terminated when the entire lesion has been rendered echogenic and further injection produces echoes refluxing into hepatic or portal veins (or both). After injection, the needle is removed. If the tumor under treatment was located adjacent to the surface of the liver, occlusion of the needle tract by injection of surgical Gelfoam, thrombin, collagen, or any combination of these agents through the needle can be performed at the discretion of the operator. The patient is monitored for at least 4 hours for possible complications. Injections are done once or twice a week with a minimum 2-day interval until therapy is completed or residual tumor is not amenable to further acetic acid therapy.

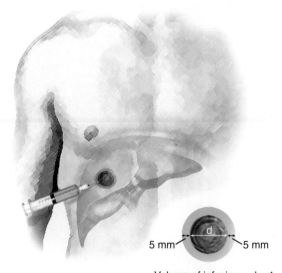

FIGURE 144-4. Final target volume for acetic acid therapy.

Controversies

When percutaneous acetic acid injection was performed for larger HCC nodules measuring 3 to 5 cm in diameter, eight of nine HCC nodules showed complete necrosis on contrast-enhanced CT, and the 3-year local recurrence rate was relatively low (20%).[56] With respect to adverse effects, no serious complications requiring intensive care were observed during or after injection, despite the stronger killing effect of acetic acid. However, although both acetic acid and ethanol treatments provide good results in larger tumors (3-5 cm), studies show they are unable to achieve response rates and outcomes comparable to those of surgical treatment, even when applied as the first option.[57] Therefore, even though surgical treatment is associated with a higher risk for serious complications, there is debate surrounding the decision to initially attempt percutaneous interventions for tumors larger than 3 cm in diameter.

Outcomes

Compared to ethanol, acetic acid is associated with fewer treatment sessions and a smaller total volume injected for all sessions. A significant and substantial difference was observed in cancer-free and overall survival. One-year and 2-year cancer-free survival rates were 83% and 63% in the acetic acid group and 59% and 33% in the ethanol group. One-year and 2-year survival rates were 100% and 92% in the acetic acid group and 83% and 63% in the ethanol group. A randomized controlled trial suggested that acetic acid ablation is more effective than ethanol ablation in patients with HCC smaller than 3 cm. In addition, direct comparisons of ethanol and acetic acid in ex vivo animal and human studies has shown acetic acid to produce larger zones of tissue coagulation, thereby resulting in fewer necessary treatments for complete ablation of a given target tissue volume.[58,59]

Complications

Adverse events of the procedure were the same as for routine percutaneous needle biopsies and injection of absolute ethanol into tumors. These adverse events include hemolysis and hemoglobinuria, intraabdominal bleeding,

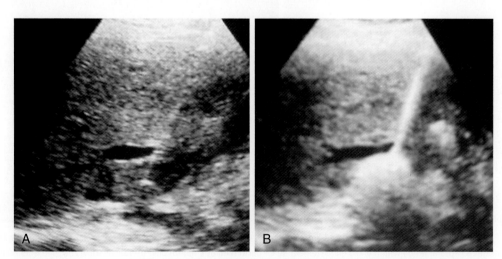

FIGURE 144-5. Ultrasound-guided acetic acid ablation in a 59-year-old with hepatitis B and hepatocellular carcinoma. **A,** Real-time ultrasound guidance was used for insertion of infusion needle into a mass posterior to portal vein. **B,** Diffusion of acetic acid seen as confluent areas of echogenicity. Distal portions of mass are no longer visible.

mild to moderate pain, pneumothorax, perforation of the intraabdominal organs, peritonitis, acute renal failure, transient increase in body temperature, and facial flushing.[60] The acute renal failure is a result of direct renal toxicity of acetic acid or secondary to hemolysis. Hemolysis and hemoglobinuria are common complications of ascetic acid injection and clear within several urinary voidings; the serum creatinine level is not affected.[61] Pretreatment of patients with sodium bicarbonate and *N*-acetylcysteine is recommended to decrease the incidence of hemolysis. Urine pH can be monitored and the bicarbonate infusion adjusted or continued until the pH is consistently above 5.0.

Postprocedural and Follow-up Care

Completion of therapy is determined on a postcontrast CT showing the lesion to be hypoattenuated (low density) and nonenhancing. Postprocedure follow-up is similar to that for PEI (Fig. 144-6). In addition, the α-fetoprotein (AFP)

level is closely monitored. Transient hepatic heterogeneity or peripheral perfusion defects may be observed and are presumably due to intravasation during treatment; in most cases, these findings spontaneously improve during serial imaging. To facilitate identification of the extent of diffusion, small volumes of iodinated contrast may be mixed with the acetic acid during injection (1:9 contrast agent/acetic acid ratio). In these cases, ex vivo diffusion mapping has shown that the distribution of acetic acid is slightly greater than the observed distribution of the contrast agent.

Chemical Ablation and Transarterial Chemoembolization

For lesions larger than 3 cm, the effect of ethanol can be augmented when ablation is performed after TACE, because the pathologic changes that occur after chemoembolization

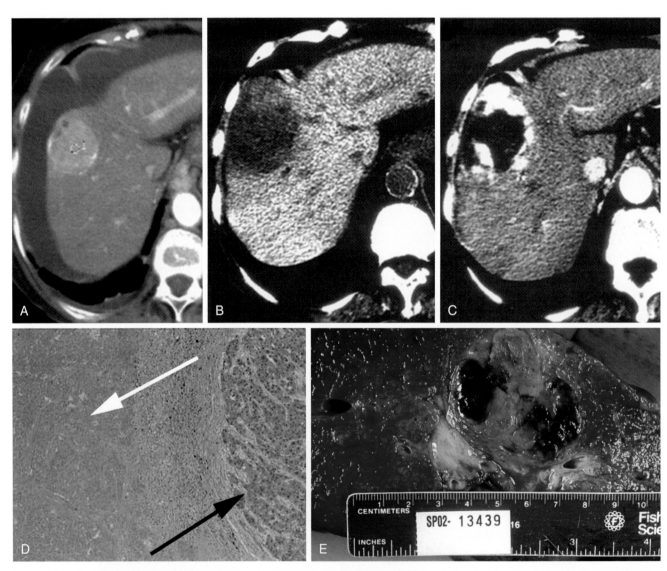

FIGURE 144-6. Follow-up computed tomography (CT) and gross specimen after acetic acid ablation for hepatocellular carcinoma in a 76-year-old woman. **A,** Initial CT demonstrates a capsular lesion with marked enhancement. **B,** CT performed at 1 month post treatment shows no area of enhancement, consistent with complete necrosis. **C,** At 9 months, nodular contrast enhancement is present along periphery. This may be secondary to dilutional effect, with acetic acid being less effective as it diffuses out from central injection region. Microscopic **(D)** and gross **(E)** pathology on a hepatic explant demonstrates viable residual tumor *(black arrow)* and necrotic tissue *(white arrow).*

may increase the diffusion of ethanol through the tumor. Results of a randomized Italian study showed that the survival rate with a single session of TACE combined with ethanol ablation was equivalent to that with two to five sessions of TACE alone for large (3-8 cm) HCCs.[62] The utility of combination therapy for small HCCs was evaluated by Koda et al. Their study demonstrated that fewer PEI treatment sessions were required in patients treated with TACE-PEI than in those treated with PEI alone. A significantly higher local recurrence rate was seen at 2 years in the PEI group than in the TACE-PEI group (65% vs. 35%, respectively). When patients with HCCs smaller than 2 cm were analyzed separately, a significant benefit in 3-year survival was seen (100% with TACE-PEI vs. 62% with PEI alone).[63]

A meta-analysis of 4 randomized trials comparing TACE to TACE-PEI demonstrated increased 2- and 3-year survival with combination therapy for large tumors with odds ratios of 4.33 and 6.79, respectively—both statistically significant.[64]

Chemical Ablation with Radiofrequency Ablation

Anatomic considerations with some HCC lesions (i.e., proximity to vessels, with a resultant heat sink effect) can make them difficult to destroy with RFA. In this setting, chemical ablation can be performed as a first-line therapy or as an adjunctive procedure during follow-up if residual HCC is detected.

A randomized control trial of 133 patients with HCC treated with either RFA alone or RFA-PEI demonstrated statistically significant improved 3- and 5-year survival rates and decreased recurrence rates with combination therapy. RFA-PEI 3- and 5-year survival rates were 75.8% and 49.3%, compared to 58.4% and 35.9% for RFA alone. When subgroup analysis was performed, however, survival benefit was only demonstrated in patients with tumors between 3.1 and 5 cm.[65]

Ahmed et al. studied the effects of combined acetic acid therapy and RFA and showed the combination resulted in greater coagulation than with either therapy alone. In addition, they showed that RFA combined with ethanol produced less coagulation than RFA/acetic acid ablation.[66]

Patients with HCC near the dome of the liver who are not candidates for laparoscopic or surgical RFA represent a unique challenge for percutaneous RFA. In such patients, chemical ablation as first-line therapy may be especially helpful.

▶ **SUGGESTED READINGS**

Brunetti E, Kern P, Vuitton DA. Writing Panel for the WHO-IWGE. Expert consensus for the diagnosis and treatment of cystic and alveolar echinococcosis in humans. Acta Trop 2010;114:1.

Clark TW, Soulen MC. Chemical ablation of hepatocellular carcinoma. J Vasc Interv Radiol 2002;13:S245–252.

Cormier JN, Thomas KT, Chari RS, Pinson CW. Management of hepatocellular carcinoma. J Gastrointest Surg 2006;10:761–80.

Goldberg SN, Ahmed M. Minimally invasive image-guided therapies for hepatocellular carcinoma. J Clin Gastroenterol 2002;35:S115–129.

Lin SM, Lin CJ, Lin CC, et al. Randomized controlled trial comparing percutaneous radiofrequency thermal ablation, percutaneous ethanol injection, and percutaneous acetic acid injection to treat hepatocellular carcinoma of 3 cm or less. Gut 2005;54:1151–6.

Shields A, Reddy KR. Hepatocellular carcinoma: current treatment strategies. Curr Treat Options Gastroenterol 2005;8:457–66.

Tikkakoski T, Makela JT, Leinonen S, et al. Treatment of symptomatic congenital hepatic cysts with single-session percutaneous drainage and ethanol sclerosis: technique and outcome. J Vasc Interv Radiol 1996;7:235–9.

Wright AS, Mahvi DM, Haemmerich DG, Lee Jr FT. Minimally invasive approaches in management of hepatic tumors. Surg Technol Int 2003;11:144–53.

The complete reference list is available online at www.expertconsult.com.

CHAPTER **145**

Urodynamics
Sally E. Mitchell

Causes of nonobstructive dilatation of the renal collecting system include vesicoureteral reflux, urinary tract infection, previous obstruction, congenital malformations, and a noncompliant bladder. Distinguishing between obstructive hydronephrosis and nonobstructive dilatation presents a problem in a number of clinical scenarios. Anatomic evaluation by means such as ultrasonography measures the degree of dilatation but does not delineate the degree of obstruction. Often, this differentiation can be made using radiologic tests such as diuretic renography and intravenous urography, as well as retrograde pyelography. However, these tests sometimes fail to conclusively determine whether an anatomic obstruction exists. It is in such cases that urodynamics can prove most useful.[1]

The renal collecting system and ureters are components of a dynamic system, and it is the resistance within this system that must be taken into account in determining whether an obstruction exists. Poiseuille's equation, which originally characterized the flow of fluid through rigid tubes, has been adapted to physiologic systems. This law describes the relationship between resistance, flow, and pressure. Specifically, resistance through any conduit is directly proportional to pressure and indirectly proportionate to flow. Urodynamic studies, therefore, serve an optimal role in the evaluation of the renal collecting system and ureters because they deal directly with both the pressure and flow of fluid through these systems.

INDICATIONS

- Congenital megaureter—obstructed or nonobstructed?[2,3]
- Congenital megacalyces[4]
- Congenital ureteropelvic junction obstruction—severe enough to require surgical repair?[5,6]
- Any congenital hydronephrosis requiring assessment for obstruction (Fig. 145-1)
- Postoperative ureteropelvic junction repair. Is the urine draining well antegrade through the repair? This is often difficult to assess because the renal pelvis will remain large and baggy owing to the previous chronic obstruction.[7,8]
- Postoperative distal ureteral reimplantation. This also may be difficult to assess if the upper collecting systems remain large or dilated from previous obstruction.
- Postoperative balloon dilatation of urinary stricture
- Assessment of ureteral strictures after injury, either traumatic or surgical (Fig. 145-2)
- Assessment of malignant obstruction resolution after chemotherapy or irradiation

- Transplant kidneys with question of obstruction (Fig. 145-3)[9-11]
- Equivocal results from less invasive tests[12]
- Suspected obstruction in presence of poor ipsilateral renal function[12]
- Continued loin pain with upper urinary tract dilatation and a nonobstructive diuresis renogram[12]
- Unexplained loin pain that might be due to intermittent obstruction at high urine flow rates[12]
- Definitive investigation of the grossly dilated upper urinary tract where there is concern about the implications of an obstructive diuresis renogram with minimal symptoms[12]

In adults, hydronephrosis is often the result of obstruction due to a ureteropelvic junction obstruction, calculus, postoperative scarring, or malignancy. Such pathology is evaluated adequately with ultrasonography, intravenous pyelography, or cross-sectional imaging such as computed tomography (CT), and further examinations are usually unnecessary. In the absence of an obvious obstructing lesion, the Whitaker test can be considered the gold standard test to determine whether a dilated collecting system is obstructed. A common use of the Whitaker test in adults is in patients with hydronephrosis with suspected postoperative obstruction. As urologic diversion procedures and renal transplantation become more common, the Whitaker test is often used to evaluate a dilated renal collecting system in these settings. It is, however, an invasive test, and is therefore reserved for instances in which the results of less invasive examinations, such as CT, ultrasonography, and diuretic renography, are equivocal.

Hydronephrosis is being diagnosed with greater frequency among children, owing to the widespread use of prenatal and perinatal ultrasonography; the distinction between obstructive and nonobstructive causes has particularly immense therapeutic value in this age group. The most common cause of pediatric hydronephrosis is ureteropelvic junction obstruction. As in adults, the Whitaker test can help determine the presence or absence of a functional obstruction. Other causes of pediatric hydronephrosis include vesicoureteral reflux, posterior urethral valves, prune-belly syndrome, and primary megaureter.

The Whitaker test can also be useful in assessing the results of percutaneous treatment (see Fig. 145-3). For example, a ureteral stricture can be assessed by a Whitaker test for significance. If the Whitaker test is positive, the stricture can be dilated and a nephroureteral stent placed for several weeks for healing. The stent is then changed for a nephrostomy tube, which is clamped for a clinical trial. During this time of clinical trial, the patient needs

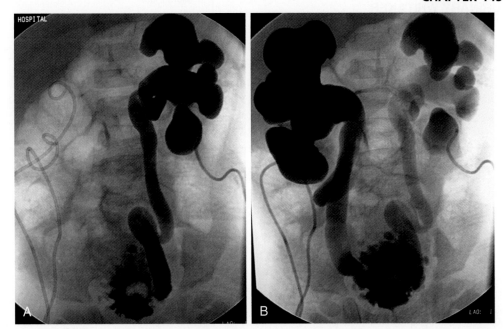

FIGURE 145-1. This 2-year-old boy presented with bilateral hydronephrosis. Despite bilateral nephrostomies (including two placed in different calyces on the right) and a Foley catheter, his ureters remained very dilated. To assess the ureterovesical junction for obstruction, a urinary Whitaker test was requested. **A,** Supine view of left collecting system during left urinary Whitaker test. Note hydronephrosis on left, dilated ureter, and trabeculated bladder. **B,** Supine view of right collecting system during right urinary Whitaker test. Note hydronephrosis on right, dilated and very tortuous right ureter, and more filled view of extremely trabeculated bladder.

instruction to unclamp the tube if he or she experiences pain, fever, or leaking around the nephrostomy due to high intrarenal pressures. An alternative is to have the patient monitor residuals. This is especially useful in children. For residuals, the nephrostomy tube is unclamped every 2 hours, and the amount of urine that drains is measured. These results are called into the physician's office at the end of each day for instructions on how long to keep the tube clamped the following day. If the amount is low, the following day the residuals are measured every 4 hours, and so on, until the tube remains clamped for 12 to 24 hours with a low residual. In this way, the kidney is protected from potential high intrarenal pressures during the initial clamping. After a few days of acceptable residuals, the nephrostomy can remain clamped. The urinary Whitaker test is then performed after this 2-week clinical trial. If the Whitaker test is negative at that time, the percutaneous access is removed.

CONTRAINDICATIONS

- Uncorrectable coagulopathy
- Urinary tract infection

EQUIPMENT

- Normal saline
- Iodinated contrast medium (50%-60% dilution)
- Power injector or Harvard pump
- Disposable manometer × 2
- Simms connector
- Ureteral connecting tubing × 2
- Pressure lines × 2
- Three-way stopcocks × 2
- Sterile hole punch
- Micropuncture set, 5F sheath, or Huey needle/sheath set

TECHNIQUE

If the patient undergoing the Whitaker test arrives with an indwelling nephrostomy, the Whitaker technique is easy. Those patients without an indwelling catheter require access to the renal collecting system for contrast injection and pressure recording. An appropriately sized urinary catheter should be inserted into the bladder using sterile technique. The nephrostomy tube or flank region for collecting system access should be prepped and draped using standard sterile technique. The patient can be supine if he or she has an indwelling nephrostomy tube, but usually the prone position is used for insertion of a needle or tube or if any work through the nephrostomy access site is anticipated.

In the classic two-needle technique using continuous pressure monitoring with the urodynamic recorders, a small 21- to 23-gauge needle was inserted posteriorly into the renal pelvis for contrast injection. A larger 18- to 20-gauge needle was placed via a flank approach into the renal pelvis via a posterior infundibulum approach. Thus, continuous monitoring of the pressure changes occurring during contrast medium injection could be done.

We have adapted the study to be done through a single access site, using an existing nephrostomy tube without additional access, or by placing a small multi-sidehole straight catheter from the usual nephrostomy flank approach. We use a micropuncture sheath with extra side holes created near the tip using a sterile hole punch. (One

PEDIATRIC URINARY WHITAKER

Patient Plate

Date of procedure _____

Weight ___10.9___ Kg   OR 10.4

Length ___82___ cm

Body Surface Area ___.55___ m2

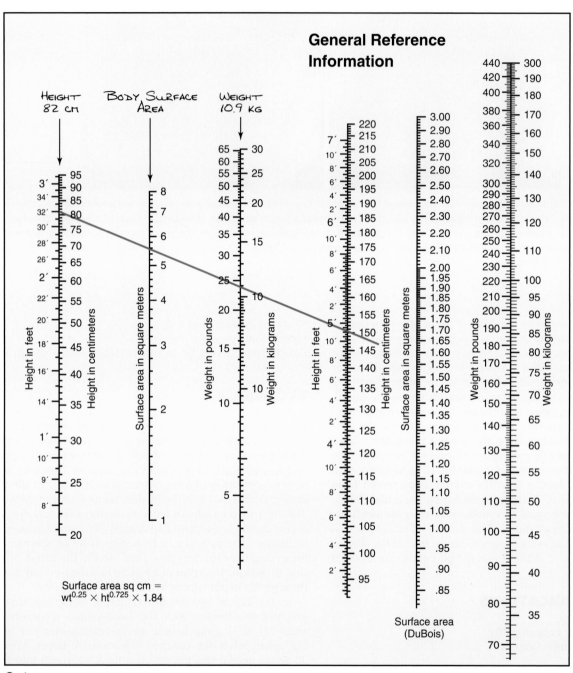

General Reference Information

HEIGHT 82 cm

BODY SURFACE AREA

WEIGHT 10.9 KG

Surface area sq cm = wt$^{0.25}$ × ht$^{0.725}$ × 1.84

Surface area (DuBois)

Cp1

FIGURE 145-1, cont'd. C, Pediatric urinary Whitaker test form filled out for this patient's height (length) of 82 cm and weight of 10.9 kg. By using the DuBois chart for finding body surface area, a straight edge is placed between patient's height and weight to cross the surface area, which can be read off the nomogram. A standard glomerular filtration rate (GFR) can be chosen by patient's age. These numbers are then used to calculate patient's maximal physiologic urine output per kidney in milliliters per minute. This is the rate at which urinary Whitaker test should be infused to match the rate at which kidney produces urine. In this patient, we had estimated 5 mL/min. Using the form, his rate calculated to be 4 mL/min. (In actuality, his rate of infusion should probably have been even lower because his creatinine value was 0.8 owing to chronic renal obstruction. Using the Schwartz formula, his estimated GFR was only 56.1. Using this GFR in the calculation would have calculated his maximal physiologic urine output per kidney to be 1.8 mL/min! However, keep in mind that the point of this pediatric form is to avoid infusing the adult rate of 10 mL/min in small children to avoid infusing renal pelvis above patient's physiologic rate, which could result in collecting system rupture if there is obstruction.) Pressure results and nephroureterograms demonstrate that this patient had no ureteral obstruction but had a very trabeculated bladder with a low capacity, consistent with previously undiagnosed posterior urethral valves.

Date _____ Patient _____ History Number _____

Glomerular filtration rate (ml min^{-1} 1.73m^{-1} SA, inulin clearance)[16]		
Age	GFR	
	Mean	Range (± 2 SD)
Premature	47	29–65
2–8 days	38	29–60
4–28 days	48	28–68
35–95 days	58	30–86
1–5.9 months	77	41–103
6–11.9 months	103	49–157
12–18 months	127	63–191
2–12 years	127	89–165
Adult male	131	88–174
Adult female	117	87–147

$$X = \frac{.55 \times 127 \times .2}{1.73 \times 2} = \frac{13.97}{3.46} = 4$$

Maximum physiological urine output per kidney (ml. per minute)	=	Surface area (m.²) ×	Age adjusted GFR (ml. per minute per 1.73 m.²) ×	20% For total urine output
		1.73 m.² ×	Number of kidneys.	

GFR ___127___

Max physiological urine output per kidney ___4___ ml/min. <u>Infuse at this rate, maximum rate of 10ml/min.</u>

	Flow Rate/min ml/min 5	Injected Volume ml	Total Volume Infused ml	Pressure in Kidney cm H2O	Pressure in Bladder cm H2O	Differential pressure cm H2O
LEFT	Baseline Pressures	0	0	6	2	4
		15	15	10	7	3
		15	30	15	12	3
		15	45	20	14	6
	POST DRAIN			11	0	11
RIGHT		0	0	4	0	4
		15	15	6	1	5
		15	30	8	3	5
		15	45	10	4	6
		15	60	11.5	4	7.5
		15	75	13.5	4	9.5
		15	90	14	4	10
		15	105	15	5	10
		15	130	16	5	11
		15	155	18	Assume 0 in 6	12
	Pressures after emptying Bladder			10	bladder if empty 0	10

Normal = 0 – 12 cm H2O
Indeterminate = 12 – 18 cm H2O
Abnormal = <18 cm H2O

Cp2

FIGURE 145-1, cont'd

could use any 4F or 5F sheath for this so long as multiple side holes are created or already in the tip of the sheath for accurate pressure monitoring.) The posterior and usually the inferior infundibulum is accessed peripherally with the micropuncture needle. The 0.018-inch guidewire is advanced into the renal pelvis, followed by the modified micropuncture sheath. (Note that some adults will require a longer sheath.) With this technique, pressure measurements are more accurate, the risk of hemorrhage is diminished due to access along the avascular plane of the kidney, and one can easily convert the sheath for the Whitaker test to a nephrostomy or to any interventional catheters that may be needed.

The setup for the Whitaker test is diagrammed in Figure 145-4, *A*. Photographs of components of the setup are shown in Figure 145-4, *B* to *E*.

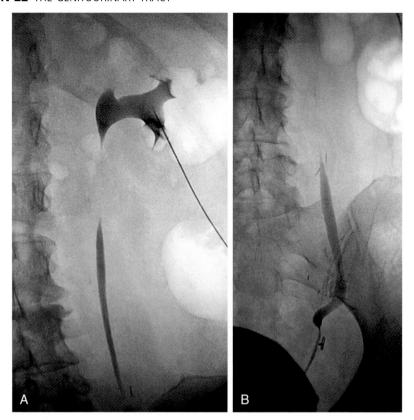

FIGURE 145-2. This 52-year-old woman presented with a history of right ureteral injury 8 years earlier after a hysterectomy. Obstruction was managed with nephrostomies, attempted nonsurgical management, and repair. Eventually, patient underwent ureteral reimplant but developed right flank pain again and had a new hydronephrosis managed by a stent. She improved clinically, but her intravenous pyelogram showed a narrowing in the mid- to distal ureter. She was referred from an outside hospital for evaluation and a urinary Whitaker test. **A,** Prone image of right renal collecting system accessed with a 21-gauge needle from flank approach into lower pole posterior calyx. Note nondilated collecting system and rapid filling of ureter. Needle was exchanged over 0.018-inch guidewire for inner sheath of a Jeffrey set (5F) with multiple side holes punched near end of sheath for good pressure measurements. If a nephrostomy or nephroureteral stent or any ureteral interventions were needed, this access would be excellent for proceeding with definitive management. **B,** Prone image of right renal collecting system during urinary Whitaker test. Note tightly narrowed distal ureter with slight dilation above, and bladder filled with contrast medium.

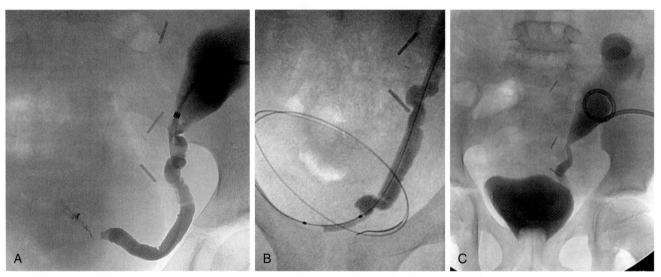

FIGURE 145-3. **A,** Transplant ureteral stricture in 10-year-old boy with history of autosomal-recessive polycystic kidney disease and living related kidney transplant 3 weeks previously. **B,** After crossing stricture, it was carefully dilated with a 2-mm and then a 4-mm balloon to allow placement of an 8F nephroureteral stent. **C,** After stenting stricture for 6 weeks, then changing stent to a nephrostomy tube in renal pelvis, patient went home for 2 weeks of a clinical trial. This image taken during urinary Whitaker procedure done after clinical trial. Pressure in renal pelvis for this image is 23 cm H_2O, with bladder pressure of 11 cm H_2O, for a differential pressure of 12 cm H_2O. Note good flow of contrast medium into bladder.

The catheter in the renal pelvis is connected using sterile tubing to a three-way stopcock on a manometer placed at the level of the kidney, which is connected on the other side of the stopcock to the power injector (see Fig. 145-4, *B* and *C*). Another manometer is placed at the level of the bladder and connected to the Foley catheter using a three-way stop-cock that is also connected to a drainage bag (see Fig. 145-4, *D*).

The power injector is filled with 50% contrast/50% saline, and the injector is set to 700 psi. The fluid levels are read in both manometers and recorded in centimeters of water as the baseline opening pressures. The manometer stopcock

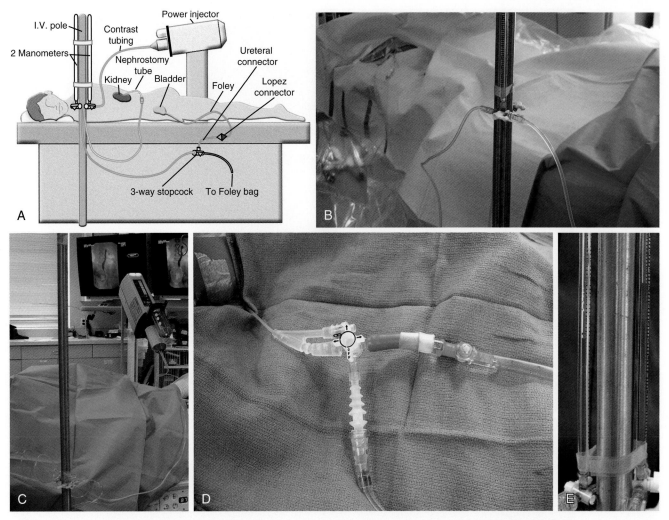

FIGURE 145-4. A, Diagram of setup for urinary Whitaker. Manometers are connected to nephrostomy tube and to Foley catheter and positioned at same height as renal pelvis and bladder. We connect the injector to nephrostomy manometer and a Foley bag to bladder system via three-way stopcocks. This allows stopcock to be turned to injector while infusing dilute contrast medium into renal pelvis, and then turned to pressure after each 25 mL injected, to assess Whitaker pressures. For Foley catheter, this three-way stopcock should always be on pressure until bladder is full and study is completed. At that time, stopcock should be turned to bag drainage. As bladder is drained, renal pelvis pressure should decrease. These pressures are then recorded as final pressures after bladder is emptied. **B,** Manometer connected to patient's left nephrostomy tube. Three-way stopcock is turned off to injector and open to nephrostomy tube to record pressure in kidney. **C,** Manometer system during a urinary Whitaker test. There are two manometers taped to IV pole, with yellow three-way stopcocks at bottoms of manometers. Injector is connected to manometer via yellow three-way stopcock behind and partially hidden by IV pole. This stopcock is open to injector, and other side is open to nephrostomy tube (not shown). The more visible yellow three-way stopcock on front of IV pole is open to pressure from bladder. **D,** Urinary Foley catheter connection. Catheter is taped to patient's leg and connected via a white three-way stopcock to drainage bag to right and to pressure manometer below. This catheter is opened to bag drainage at end of Whitaker procedure. **E,** Appearance of manometers as pressures are measured in renal pelvis *(to the right)* and in urinary bladder *(to the left)*. Note that renal pelvis pressure is 2 to 3 cm H_2O higher than bladder pressure, a normal differential pressure.

at the nephrostomy tube is turned "off" to pressure, and the injection is begun. The bladder manometer remains open to the manometer pressure continuously during the Whitaker test. The pressures are measured for both renal pelvis and bladder at several points throughout the Whitaker. The difference between the renal pelvis pressure and the bladder pressure is called the *differential pressure* (see Fig. 145-4, *E*).

OUTCOMES

Upper tract urodynamic studies, also known as *pressure-flow studies*, have been referred to by some as a "urologic stress test." As fluid is infused at varying rates, pressures within the renal pelvis and urinary bladder are measured. A range of flow rates has been determined in attempts to appropriately challenge the collecting system. With regard to pressure measurements, upper limits have also been established to delineate physiologically appropriate increases versus excessively elevated renal pelvis pressures.

Flow of urine through the upper urinary tract varies greatly depending on physiologic conditions. The normal renal collecting system and ureter should accommodate this normal range of flow rates without excessive change in pressure. However, a collecting system with increased

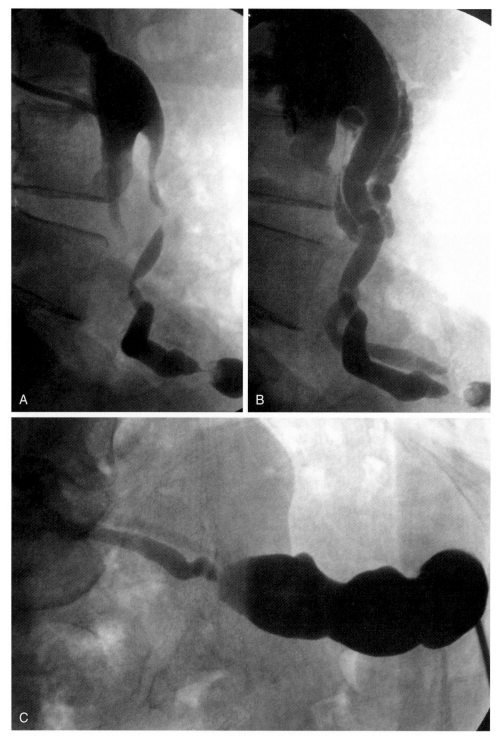

FIGURE 145-5. This 43-year-old woman with an ileal loop diversion presented after multiple urologic surgeries for interstitial cystitis. Because of a recurrent urinary tract infection, she underwent computed tomography that showed bilateral hydroureter (right > left). Loopogram demonstrated bilaterally dilated collecting systems (right > left) and a possible ureteral stricture on right. However, a DTPA renal scan with furosemide showed good flow on both right and left, with no obstruction on either side. She was therefore referred for a urinary Whitaker test. **A,** Lateral view demonstrates a nephrostomy placed into collecting system. Contrast injection during test demonstrates a distal ureteral/ileal loop anastomotic stenosis, but with contrast medium coursing into ileal loop. **B,** After only 125-mL infusion, renal pressure suddenly increased from 15 to 24 cm H_2O. Extravasation of contrast agent around right renal collecting system was noted at this time, resulting from high intrarenal pressure. Whitaker study was stopped at this point. Note that patent left ureter fills by reflux from ileal loop. **C,** Injection of contrast medium into ileal loop to define anatomy of loop and confirm good position of Foley catheter, because loop pressure was 0 cm H_2O during test.

resistance—that is, an obstructed collecting system—responds by increasing pressure when the flow rate surpasses its ability to conduct fluid. According to the Poiseuille equation, the elevation in pressure within an obstructed collecting system is directly proportional to the resistance, or degree of obstruction, as well as the rate of flow. Even a normal unobstructed collecting system may be overstressed by an excessive flow rate and thereby develop increased pressures. Thus, it is important to choose flow rates that are in fact within physiologic ranges.

The original Whitaker test described a standard infusion rate of 10 mL/min for adults (Fig. e145-1 is a printable copy of the adult Whitaker test form), with decreased rates of 5 mL/min or 2 mL/min for small children. Since then, studies have been performed in attempts to determine a child's maximal physiologic urine output, and three patient parameters have been used: (1) body surface area, (2) age-adjusted 90th percentile glomerular filtration rate (GFR), and (3) the maximum percentage of the GFR one can physiologically diurese.[13] Surface area and age-adjusted 90th percentile GFR can be acquired from standard nomograms and tables.[14-16] We have adapted these nomograms into a pediatric Whitaker form for calculation of flow rates for children so that the accuracy of the Whitaker is improved for the pediatric patient (Fig. e145-2 is a printable copy of the pediatric Whitaker test form; also see Fig. 145-1).

In assessing 145 Whitaker studies, Lupton and George[12] found accuracy in its prediction of outcome in 77% of cases. The Whitaker test determined or contributed to the clinical management in 84%. Veenboer and de Jong[17] evaluated 16 patients with a follow-up of 12 years (range 3.5-17.5 years) and found that the 7 patients who were not treated surgically due to low differential pressures did not need reintervention later on during follow-up, indicating the Whitaker test to have a high negative predictive value.

The Whitaker test is considered the gold standard for evaluation of urinary obstruction. While less invasive tests can be most useful in evaluating patients and in follow-up, when questions arise and management issues are dependent on accurate evaluation, the Whitaker test allows precise determination of the urinary physiology as well as anatomy.

COMPLICATIONS

- Bleeding if newly accessing the collecting system
- Infection if there is urinary tract infection in the presence of increasing the pressure in the collecting system with contrast infusions. One may see pyelovenous backflow of contrast medium with elevated intrarenal pressures. This is an indication to stop the infusion.

- Rupture of the collecting system may occur if the intrarenal pressure is allowed to increase above 20 to 25 cm H_2O (Fig. 145-5).

POSTPROCEDURAL AND FOLLOW-UP CARE

Depending on the age of the patient and the underlying urinary tract status, we may admit the patient overnight for intravenous antibiotic therapy. When the Whitaker test is normal, there is less risk for the patient to develop infection after the procedure.

After the test, the bladder catheter is monitored acutely for any hematuria. If the urine is clear, we remove the Foley catheter. If there is any hematuria, the catheter is left in place until the urine clears.

KEY POINTS

- The urinary Whitaker test is named after Robert Whitaker, who first demonstrated the importance of combining radiographic and urodynamic information in assessing the dilated urinary collecting system.[18]
- This technique measures the renal pelvis pressure compared with the bladder pressure during infusion of dilute contrast in the renal pelvis to determine the presence and degree of obstruction between the two.
- The infusion rate into the renal pelvis should be adjusted for the pediatric patient.
- The combination of pressure measurements and the imaging of the urinary collecting system is the gold standard for assessing the presence or absence of obstruction.

▶ **SUGGESTED READINGS**

Aruny JE. The Whitaker test. In: Kandarpa K, Aruny JE, editors. Handbook of Interventional Radiologic Procedures. 3rd ed. Philadelphia: Lippincott Williams & Wilkins; 2002. p. 738–41.

Fung LCT, Lakshmanan Y. Assessment of renal obstructive disorders: urodynamics of the upper tract. In: Docimo SG, Canning DA, Khoury AE, editors. Clinical Pediatric Urology. 5th ed. London: Martin Dunitz; 2006.

Lee MJ. Percutaneous genitourinary intervention. In: Kaufman JA, Lee MJ, editors. Vascular and Interventional Radiology: The Requisites. Philadelphia: Elsevier; 2004. p. 602–35.

The complete reference list is available online at www.expertconsult.com.

CHAPTER 146

Percutaneous Nephrostomy, Cystostomy, and Nephroureteral Stenting

LeAnn S. Stokes and Steven G. Meranze

PERCUTANEOUS NEPHROSTOMY AND NEPHROURETERAL STENTING

Since the original description of percutaneous access of a hydronephrotic kidney using a trocar technique and fluoroscopic guidance in 1955,[1] percutaneous nephrostomy (PCN) has become the cornerstone of a wide variety of diagnostic and therapeutic endourologic procedures. Percutaneous access to the renal collecting system plays a vital role in the treatment of both adult and pediatric patients with complex urologic problems ranging from malignant obstruction to stone disease to congenital obstruction of the ureteropelvic junction (UPJ). High technical success and low complication rates for PCN make it a valuable tool in the management of urologic disease.

Indications

Indications for PCN may be grouped into the following general categories: relief of urinary obstruction, urinary diversion, and access for diagnostic and therapeutic procedures (Table 146-1).

Urinary obstruction is most frequently caused by pelvic malignancy or renal stone disease (Table 146-2). PCN is performed for rapid decompression of an obstructed renal collecting system when retrograde drainage is not feasible, and may be life saving in patients with urosepsis or acute renal failure. PCN may even be preferred over retrograde stenting in patients with obvious infection, because it accomplishes more rapid drainage.[2] In patients who have hypotension and leukocytosis, mortality from urosepsis may be reduced from 40% to 8% with emergency PCN.[3]

Placement of a PCN for urinary diversion may be indicated in several different clinical situations. A urine leak may occur as the result of a traumatic or iatrogenic injury to the renal collecting system, or a leak may arise at a surgical anastomotic site. A urinary fistula may develop in patients with a pelvic malignancy, a pelvic inflammatory process, or a history of irradiation of the pelvis. Another indication for emergency PCN for urinary diversion is the presence of severe refractory hemorrhagic cystitis, which is most commonly due to intravesical chemotherapy or external beam radiation and has a mortality rate of up to 4%.[4] In all these scenarios, placement of a PCN alone may not accomplish sufficient urinary diversion to allow healing of the underlying process, and ureteral occlusion may ultimately be necessary.[5]

Although PCN may still be performed for a wide variety of diagnostic purposes, antegrade pyelography has been replaced in most instances by noninvasive imaging. In a recent series of patients with renal impairment from ureteral obstruction, non–contrast-enhanced computed tomography (CT) was determined to be the best imaging modality for evaluating calculus disease, and magnetic resonance (MR) urography was thought to be optimal for identifying noncalculous causes of obtstruction.[6] In cases in which noninvasive imaging is inconclusive, antegrade pyelography can help determine the severity of an obstruction and can provide very detailed information about stenoses, particularly those at ureteroenteric anastomoses. The access established for antegrade pyelography can also be used for further diagnostic testing, such as brush biopsy of urothelial lesions.

Diagnostic PCN can be definitive in other situations in which noninvasive imaging is unreliable. In the setting of chronic obstruction, the finding of mild to moderate cortical atrophy on CT or ultrasound cannot be used to predict whether renal function will recover after decompression, so PCN should be performed before functional testing. If a kidney contributes greater than 20% of overall renal function after percutaneous drainage, it is generally considered worth salvaging. It may also be impossible to determine whether hydronephrosis is due to functional or mechanical obstruction with noninvasive imaging. The Whitaker test, which measures the pressure gradient between the renal pelvis and the bladder, was devised to answer this question (Fig. 146-1).[7] This test is most commonly performed either before or after pyeloplasty in patients with UPJ obstruction to determine whether surgical or endourologic treatment is indicated or to determine whether it was successful (Table 146-3).

Finally, PCN is frequently performed prior to other interventional procedures, especially in centers with active endourologic surgeons. A wide variety of procedures may be performed via percutaneous access of the kidney, including stone removal, dilation or stenting of a ureteral stricture, endopyelotomy, and foreign body retrieval. Among these procedures, access for treatment of stone disease with percutaneous nephrostolithotomy (PCNL) is by far the most common (Fig. 146-2).[2]

Contraindications

The strongest contraindication to PCN is severe coagulopathy, with most authors in agreement that an international normalized ratio (INR) less than 1.5 and a platelet count greater than 50,000 should be achieved before the procedure.[8-10] Severe hyperkalemia (potassium level > 7 mEq/L) should be corrected with dialysis before the procedure,[9] and systolic blood pressure less than 180 mmHg is desirable. If the PCN is elective, antiplatelet agents or anticoagulants should be withheld for 5 days before the procedure when feasible.[10] Patients who are allergic to contrast media should receive premedication with either oral or

TABLE 146-1. Indications for Percutaneous Nephrostomy

Relief of Urinary Obstruction

Urosepsis or suspected infection
Acute renal failure
Intractable pain

Urinary Diversion

Hemorrhagic cystitis
Traumatic or iatrogenic ureteral injury
Inflammatory or malignant urinary fistula

Diagnostic Testing

Antegrade pyelography
Ureteral perfusion (i.e., Whitaker test)
Biopsy of a urothelial lesion

Access for Endourologic Procedures

Stone removal
Dilation or stenting of a ureteral stricture
Endopyelotomy
Foreign body retrieval
Ureteral occlusion for urinary fistula
Fungus ball removal or direct infusion of antifungal agents

TABLE 146-2. Causes of Urinary Obstruction

		Benign	Malignant
Intrinsic		Stone	Urothelial tumor
		Clot	
		Sequestered papilla	
		Fungus ball	
Extrinsic		Postoperative scar tissue	Pelvic tumor
		Surgical ligature	Adenopathy
		Crossing vessel	
		Retroperitoneal fibrosis	

TABLE 146-3. Whitaker Test

Pressure Gradient	Result
<15 cm H$_2$O	Normal
15-22 cm H$_2$O	Indeterminate
>22 cm H$_2$O	Positive for upper urinary tract obstruction

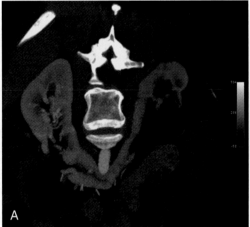
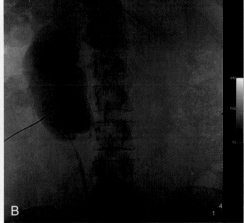

FIGURE 146-1. Whitaker test in a patient after pyeloplasty of left ureteropelvic junction. **A,** Curved maximum intensity projection of abdomen demonstrates a horseshoe kidney with hydronephrosis and cortical thinning of left moiety. Furosemide (Lasix) renogram was consistent with obstruction on left, and a Whitaker test was requested. **B,** Despite marked dilation of left renal collecting system, there was no pressure gradient between left renal pelvis and bladder.

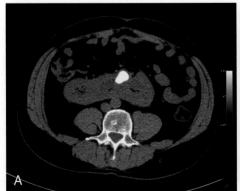
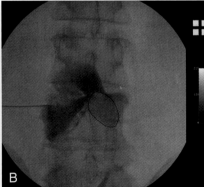
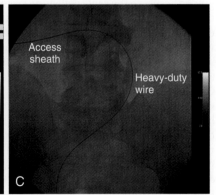

FIGURE 146-2. Access for percutaneous nephrolithotomy (PCNL) in a patient with a large obstructing stone in a horseshoe kidney. **A,** Axial image from a non–contrast-enhanced computed tomography scan demonstrates stone. **B,** Sonographic and fluoroscopic guidance was used to access collecting system from a left posterior approach. Contrast material is seen surrounding stone *(outline)* lodged at ureteropelvic junction. **C,** A 6F coaxial access sheath is in renal pelvis, and a heavy-duty wire has been advanced through sheath into bladder. A 5F Kumpe catheter was advanced over the wire into bladder and left in place to provide access for PCNL, which followed.

TABLE 146-4. Contraindications to Percutaneous Nephrostomy

Absolute
Severe uncorrectable coagulopathy
Percutaneous approach to kidney that crosses colon, spleen, or liver

Relative
Severe hyperkalemia or other metabolic imbalance
Uncontrolled hypertension
Ongoing use of antiplatelet agents or anticoagulants
Extremely short life expectancy because of underlying terminal illness

TABLE 146-5. Key Equipment for Percutaneous Nephrostomy

Basic Equipment
21- or 22-gauge needle with stylet
0.018-inch mandril wire
6F coaxial introducer
0.038-inch heavy-duty J-tipped wire
Fascial dilators
Locking pigtail drain

Additional Equipment
0.018-inch nitinol wire
0.035-inch stiff glidewire
0.035-inch stiff Amplatz wire
5F Kumpe catheter
Peel-away sheath

intravenous (IV) steroids. Rarely, patients will have an anatomic variant such as a retrorenal colon that precludes safe percutaneous access to the kidney (Table 146-4).

Equipment

Equipment for PCN is listed in Table 146-5. Image guidance for PCN may be accomplished with ultrasound, CT, fluoroscopy, or some combination of these modalities, most commonly ultrasound and fluoroscopy. For ultrasound-guided access to the renal collecting system, a low-frequency transducer, usually 3.5 MHz, is necessary for sufficient penetration of the retroperitoneal soft tissues to allow good visualization of the kidney. Any multislice CT scanner should provide adequate imaging to identify an appropriate access site and guide needle placement, and combined CT-fluoroscopy can provide real-time guidance for placement of the PCN. If CT-fluoroscopy is not available, it may be necessary to establish needle access to the kidney and then transfer the patient to a fluoroscopy unit for the remainder of the procedure. In the fluoroscopy suite, a rotating image intensifier is extremely helpful because oblique positioning of the tube allows real-time visualization of wire and catheter manipulations while keeping the operator's hands outside the field of view.

Ultrasound-guided access is often performed with a freehand technique, but needle guides are available and may be useful, especially for less experienced operators. A sterile cover is necessary for the transducer and cord. It may also be helpful to place a clear plastic drape over the ultrasound control panel to allow the operator to make adjustments to the settings.

If fluoroscopic guidance alone is used, IV administration of contrast material may be necessary to aid in visualization of the collecting system, especially if it is not dilated. Depending on the patient's size, an initial injection of 75 to 100 mL of 68% ioversol (Optiray 320) is typically given, and an additional bolus can be administered if needed.

Several different sets are available for percutaneous access to the kidney. The Neff Percutaneous Access Set (Cook Medical, Bloomington, Ind.) and the AccuStick II Introducer System (Boston Scientific, Natick, Mass.) include a 21- or 22-gauge needle with a stylet, a 6F coaxial introducer with a locking cannula, a 0.018-inch mandril wire, and a heavy-duty 0.038-inch J-tipped guidewire (150 cm).

A few other tools may be helpful in certain situations. An 80-cm, 0.018-inch nitinol wire (ev3/Covidien, Plymouth, Minn.) is easier to advance through the access needle into the collecting system than the standard 0.018-inch mandril wire and may be extremely useful when the collecting system is not very dilated. If the patient is obese or has scar tissue in the retroperitoneum, an 18-gauge needle with a stylet is sturdier and less likely to be deflected during initial access, and a stiffer wire like a 0.035-inch Amplatz wire (Boston Scientific) may greatly facilitate dilation of the tract for placement of the drainage catheter.

If placement of a nephroureteral stent or internal double-J ureteral stent is planned, a 5F Kumpe catheter (Cook Medical) and 0.035-inch stiff or regular glidewire (Boston Scientific) will facilitate access into the ureter and bladder. In the presence of a tight ureteral stricture, a 4F Glide catheter (Boston Scientific) or 6.3F or 8F van Andel catheters (Cook Medical), which taper to 3F or 5F, respectively, may be useful to cross the stricture. Occasionally, balloon dilation of a stricture is necessary before placement of a ureteral stent, in which case a noncompliant balloon should be used. Side-port sheaths may also aid in crossing a stricture, and peel-away sheaths are useful for placement of internal ureteral stents.

Nephrostomy, nephroureteral, or double-J ureteral drains are available in many different varieties. Most of the nephrostomy tubes placed by interventional radiologists are 8F, 10F, or 12F all-purpose locking pigtail drains, although mini-pigtail drains may be placed when the renal pelvis is not capacious enough to allow a standard pigtail to form. Nephroureteral drains have a loop in the bladder and a locking pigtail in the renal pelvis and are available in different diameters, usually 8F and 10F, and lengths, typically 20 to 28 cm. Internal double-J ureteral drains are available in essentially the same sizes as nephroureteral drains.

Technique

Anatomy and Approach

Planning the approach for access is the most crucial step in performing successful uncomplicated PCN placement. Before the procedure, any prior studies or cross-sectional imaging should be reviewed to evaluate the anatomy, location, and orientation of the target kidney. Malrotation or malposition of the kidney, duplication of the collecting system, and any cysts, diverticula, tumor, or stones should be noted.[11] The location of the lung, liver, spleen, and colon relative to the kidney should be considered, as well as body habitus, such as morbid obesity or spina bifida.

For routine PCN, the patient should be placed in a prone or prone oblique position with the ipsilateral side elevated 20 to 30 degrees. If ultrasound guidance is planned for access, it is often helpful to scan the patient before sterile preparation to optimize positioning. In some patients, placement of a roll or pillow beneath the lower abdomen will reverse the normal lordotic curvature of the lumbar spine and improve sonographic visualization of the approach.

The ideal entry site to the kidney is through a relatively avascular plane known as the *Brödel line* that lies at an angle of about 30 to 45 degrees from midline when the patient is prone. The collecting system should be accessed peripherally via the tip of the calyx to decrease the likelihood of significant bleeding, and a posterior calyx should be chosen to facilitate placement of a nephrostomy tube or any additional endourologic procedures.

The ideal skin entry site is approximately 10 cm lateral to the midline but not beyond the posterior axillary line. If the entry site is too medial, the PCN will cross the paraspinal musculature and make dilation of the tract more difficult and the tube more painful for the patient, and an entry site that is too lateral increases the risk of colonic perforation. The tract should avoid the inferior margin of the rib to decrease the risk of injury to an intercostal artery. If a supracostal approach is necessary for treatment of an upper pole stone, the risk of injury to lung, liver, or spleen is significantly less in the T11-T12 interspace than in the T10-T11 interspace.[12]

Technical Aspects
Numerous techniques for image-guided PCN placement have been described. The renal collecting system can be accessed using a single-stick or double-stick method with ultrasound, fluoroscopy, or CT, alone or in combination. The single-stick method is more likely to be possible in patients with moderate to severe hydronephrosis, because it facilitates visualization of a calyx for direct access. A double-stick method is useful when the collecting system is not dilated, making it initially more difficult to access a calyx. In this technique, the first needle is used to access and opacify the collecting system so a more appropriate site for definitive access can be targeted (Fig. 146-3). There is reportedly no difference in technical success and complication rates for a single- versus double-stick technique.[3,13]

If ultrasound is used for guidance, the probe should be oriented along the long axis of the kidney, and the needle tip should be visualized from the skin entry site to the point of entry in the calyx. If fluoroscopic guidance alone is used, the site for access can be chosen on the basis of anatomic landmarks, by targeting a stone, or by opacification of the collecting system with IV contrast material. The C-arm should be rotated initially so that the needle is viewed end on as it is advanced toward the appropriate calyx, then the C-arm can be rotated to the orthogonal view to determine the depth.

CT guidance for PCN may be required when the patient has variant anatomy. In addition, CT guidance can allow the procedure to be performed with the patient in a supine oblique position when the patient is unable to lie prone. In CT-guided cases, it is important to select the calyx that can be approached most easily in the horizontal plane.

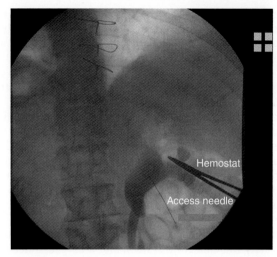

FIGURE 146-3. Double-stick technique for percutaneous nephrostomy. After direct access of left renal pelvis with a 21-gauge needle, contrast material and air were injected to identify appropriate site for placement of nephrostomy drain. A posterior calyx is seen outlined by air and is marked with hemostat for access with a second 21-gauge needle.

Routine Percutaneous Nephrostomy Placement
Once the access site has been chosen, the skin and subcutaneous tissues along the expected path for the nephrostomy are infiltrated with a local anesthetic, and a small dermatotomy is made with a scalpel. After needle access is achieved, a small amount of urine should be aspirated for culture, then a small amount of contrast material should be injected to determine the precise point of entry.

If the needle entry site is not appropriate, the first needle can be used to further opacify the collecting system with contrast material and air if necessary so a more appropriate site can be targeted for entry with a second needle. When opacified, the posterior calyces are typically seen end on, whereas the anterior calyces project more laterally in the anteroposterior projection; however, injection of a small amount of air or CO_2, which will fill the nondependent posterior calyces in a prone patient, may be necessary for confirmation. Care should be taken to aspirate a larger volume of urine than the amount of contrast material injected to avoid overdistention and possible sepsis.

If the needle entry site is appropriate, the 0.018-inch wire is advanced through the needle and coiled in the renal collecting system. If the system is not very dilated, a 0.018-inch nitinol wire may be much easier to manipulate into the renal pelvis. More stable access is obtained when the wire is advanced into the ureter. Fluoroscopic guidance is very helpful to ensure that the wire is in good position and does not become kinked during the subsequent steps of the procedure.

Once the 0.018-inch wire is in appropriate position, the access needle is exchanged over the wire for the 6F coaxial sheath, and the 0.018-inch wire and inner stiffeners are removed. A heavy-duty J-tipped 0.038-inch wire is advanced into the renal collecting system, and serial dilation of the tract is performed over the wire. The percutaneous drainage catheter, usually a locking pigtail drain, is advanced over the wire, and the wire and inner stiffener are removed. The pigtail is formed and locked. All the urine should be aspirated from the collecting system if there is any suspicion of infection, and a small amount of contrast material can then be injected to confirm appropriate position of the drain. The drain should be flushed and secured to the skin with either suture or an adhesive retention device.

Percutaneous Nephrostomy Placement in a Nondilated Collecting System

Occasionally, PCN will be necessary in a patient who has a nondilated system, which can be seen in the setting of a ureteral leak or fistula, hemorrhagic cystitis, or nondilated obstruction. The pathophysiology of obstruction without hydronephrosis is not well understood, but reversal of acute renal failure after PCN in a nondilated system has been well documented.[14] A double-stick technique for fluoroscopically guided access to a nondilated system has been described.[15] Intravenous contrast material is administered to opacify the collecting system, and a 22-gauge needle is quickly advanced directly into the renal pelvis. This needle can be used to distend the collecting system with a small amount of contrast material and air, then PCN can be performed as described previously. If the patient is in renal failure and IV contrast material cannot be given, ultrasound guidance can be used to access the renal pelvis as well.

Nephroureteral Drain Placement

Additional endourologic manipulations should not be performed at the time of the initial PCN if there is any possibility of infection or if there is significant bleeding after PCN. If neither of these conditions is present and the patient would benefit from a ureteral stent, placement of an internal-external nephroureteral stent or an internal double-J ureteral stent can be attempted. Placement of a double-J internal ureteral stent is the ultimate goal in patients who are candidates for this type of stent because it is much more comfortable and convenient for them. Cystoscopic retrograde exchange of the double-J stent must be possible, or an internal stent should not be placed. Other contraindications to placement of either type of ureteral stent include bladder outlet obstruction, irritable or neurogenic bladder, incontinence, and bladder tumors.[3]

A 5F Kumpe catheter and a 0.035-inch stiff glidewire is usually a good combination for traversal of the ureter into the bladder or an ileal conduit. If a stricture that cannot be crossed easily is present, several options are available. If the wire crosses the lesion but the catheter does not, a 4F Glide catheter or a van Andel catheter that tapers from 6.3F to 3F may work. If these catheters do not work alone, placement of a long side-arm 7F sheath that extends into the ureter will provide extra support while pushing the catheter over the wire.[16] Successful use of a microwire and microcatheter to cross a tight ureteral stricture has also been described.[17]

If the lesion is difficult to cross with the catheter, balloon dilation of the stricture will probably be necessary before placement of the nephroureteral stent. Once the catheter is advanced into the bladder or conduit, the guidewire should be exchanged for a stiffer wire (e.g., 0.035-inch Amplatz wire) to facilitate advancement of the balloon across the lesion. Dilation with a 4-mm balloon should allow placement of an 8F nephroureteral stent. If these steps fail initially, the collecting system should be allowed to decompress via a PCN for 24 to 48 hours and then a repeat attempt made. The second attempt is often successful because the edema surrounding the stricture has resolved. If the

TABLE 146-6. Ureteral Stent Length Based on Patient Height

Patient Height	Ureteral Stent Length
<5'10″	22 cm
5'10″ to 6'4″	24 cm
>6'4″	26 cm

ureteral stricture still proves impassible, sharp recanalization with a transjugular intrahepatic portosystemic shunt or transseptal needle has been described, or a rendezvous procedure with both antegrade and retrograde access to the stricture may be helpful.[3,18,19]

Selection of the length of the nephroureteral stent can be based on the height of the patient, which is a very reliable method, or on a measurement made with the wire, which tends to overestimate the length of the ureter (Table 146-6). When the stent is placed into the bladder, the distal pigtail should extend far enough beyond the ureterovesical junction (UVJ) that it will not retract into the ureter, but not so far that an excess amount of catheter is present in the bladder. The nephroureteral stent is advanced over the wire until the distal pigtail is beyond the ureteral orifice and the side holes for the proximal pigtail are just beyond the UPJ. The wire and inner stiffener are pulled back to allow first the distal loop and then the proximal pigtail to form. If the proximal pigtail is going to be in appropriate position in the renal pelvis, the wire and stiffener are removed and the catheter is locked. If the proximal pigtail is not in good position, the wire and stiffener can be used to reposition the stent before they are removed.

Double-J Internal Ureteral Stent Placement

Placement of a double-J internal ureteral stent is the same as placement of a nephroureteral stent up until the point at which a stiff guidewire is coiled in the bladder, but it may be a bit trickier thereafter. A 9F peel-away sheath is advanced over the wire until the tip of the sheath is at the UPJ or just in the proximal part of the ureter. The double-J stent system (Boston Scientific, Cook Medical) consists of an inner plastic cannula, a pusher, and the stent. A nylon suture is attached to the proximal end of the stent, and there is a radiopaque marker on the distal end of the pusher. The pusher typically comes loaded on the inner plastic cannula. The stent is loaded over the plastic cannula while making sure the suture does not become tangled and that the proximal end of the stent does not overlap the pusher; the whole assembly is advanced over the wire until the marker on the pusher is in the renal pelvis. The wire and inner plastic cannula are removed, leaving the pusher and the stent through the peel-away sheath. The distal loop forms automatically when the wire and stiffener are removed, and the proximal loop is formed by pulling on the nylon suture while applying pressure with the pusher. Once the proximal loop is formed, the suture is cut and the pusher is removed, leaving the peel-away sheath. A safety PCN can be advanced through the peel-away before its removal (Fig. 146-4).

A safety PCN that is capped is typically left in the renal pelvis for 24 to 48 hours after placement of an internal ureteral stent to ensure the patient will tolerate internal

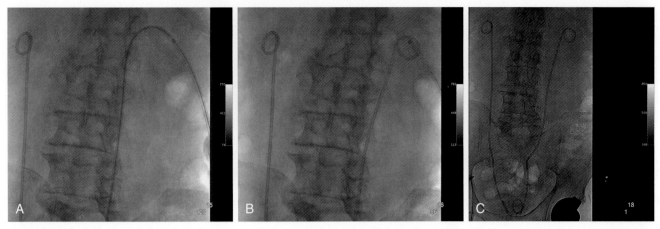

FIGURE 146-4. Conversion of bilateral nephroureteral stents to double-J internal ureteral stents in a patient with extrinsic malignant ureteral obstruction. **A,** Right nephroureteral stent has been removed over a 0.035-inch stiff guidewire, and 8F 26-cm double-J stent has been advanced over wire through a 9F peel-away sheath. Radiopaque tip of pusher is visible in renal pelvis. **B,** Wire and plastic inner stiffener have been removed, and pusher has been used to help form proximal pigtail. **C,** Final fluoroscopic image demonstrates both stents in good position. A safety percutaneous nephrostomy was not placed on either side because exchanges were atraumatic and patient had tolerated capping of both nephroureteral stents for several weeks before procedure.

drainage. An antegrade nephrostogram can be performed via the PCN to confirm that the internal stent is functioning before removal. If a locking pigtail drain is used, fluoroscopic visualization during removal is recommended to avoid dislodging the ureteral stent with the pigtail, but this potential problem can be avoided by using a nonlocking pigtail drain as the safety PCN. The need for a safety PCN at all may be debatable because primary placement of an internal ureteral stent alone was successful in 83% of carefully selected patients in a recent study.[20]

Retrograde Nephroureteral Stent Placement

Placement of a ureteral stent across a ureteroenteric anastomosis into an ileostomy may be accomplished via either an antegrade or retrograde approach. If an internal ureteral stent was placed at the time of surgical anastomosis, the stent may not have an end hole for over-the-wire exchange or repositioning, but it is usually possible to advance a 0.035-inch glidewire alongside the existing stent. After wire access into the renal pelvis is achieved, the existing stent can be removed, and a 7F 70-cm pigtail drain, called a *urinary diversion soft stent* (Boston Scientific), can be placed over the wire.

If a ureteroenteric stent is not present, the anastomosis may be difficult to locate from a retrograde approach through the ostomy, and antegrade access via a PCN may become necessary. A routine PCN can be performed with the patient in the prone position, but after the guidewire is manipulated across the anastomosis and into the ostomy, it is helpful to have the patient in a lateral decubitus position so that both the flank and ostomy can be accessed.

Once in the ostomy, the wire can usually be retrieved with hemostats, although snare retrieval may occasionally be required to establish through-and-through access (Fig. 146-5). After through-and-through access is achieved, the 7F 70-cm pigtail drain can be advanced retrogradely over the wire and formed in the renal pelvis. The drain can be shortened as needed but should be left long enough to extend into the ostomy bag to facilitate exchange of the drain.

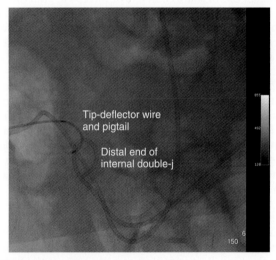

Tip-deflector wire and pigtail

Distal end of internal double-j

FIGURE 146-5. Retrograde exchange of bilateral double-J internal ureteral stents placed across ileoureteral anastomosis in a patient after ileal urinary diversion for severe radiation-induced cystitis. Distal end of double-J stent had retracted into ileal conduit and could not be grasped through stoma. A pigtail catheter and tip deflector wire were used to pull stent out through ostomy so it could be exchanged.

Removal of an Encrusted Percutaneous Nephrostomy

Encrustation of the tube can make it extremely difficult to remove, and it may be impossible to exchange the tube over a guidewire. A hydrophilic wire can be advanced in the existing tract alongside the PCN to maintain access to the collecting system when the tube is removed. Removal of a pigtail that does not completely release when the catheter is cut may result in laceration of the renal parenchyma, and it may be necessary to advance a peel-away sheath over the tube to straighten the pigtail for safe removal.

Removal of Internal Double-J Stents

Antegrade access may be used for percutaneous retrieval of double-J ureteral stents that have fractured or become

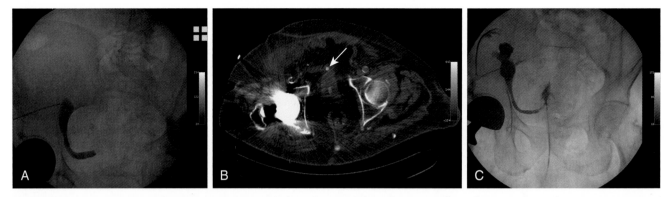

FIGURE 146-6. Percutaneous nephrostomy in a patient with hydronephrosis and elevated creatinine after cadaveric renal transplantation. **A,** An antegrade nephrostogram via a 5F Kumpe catheter demonstrates a rounded filling defect at ureterovesical junction, consistent with a stone. **B,** Axial image from a non–contrast-enhanced CT scan confirms presence of stone *(arrow)*. **C,** Patient's nephrostomy drain was inadvertently dislodged, and a 5F Kumpe catheter was manipulated along existing tract to reestablish access into collecting system. A repeat nephrostogram demonstrated a residual stricture in distal part of ureter after passage of stone. Patient later underwent antegrade ureteroscopy with holmium laser ablation of a calcified stricture in distal end of ureter.

dislodged or can no longer be accessed from a retrograde approach. Use of snare catheters or forceps to grab the stent and use of balloon catheters inflated alongside to pull or push a stent into better position for snaring have been described, with technical success rates of 95% and 100% in two series.[21,22]

Replacement of a Dislodged Percutaneous Nephrostomy

Catheter dislodgement within the first week of placement usually requires creation of a new tract, but mature tracts can frequently be reaccessed under fluoroscopic guidance. Gentle injection of a small amount of contrast material at the exit site will often help delineate the tract, which can then be traversed with a 5F Kumpe catheter and a 0.035-inch stiff glidewire.

Ureteral Occlusion

Ureteral occlusion may be necessary in addition to urinary diversion in patients with a urine leak or fistula, urinary incontinence, or intractable hemorrhagic cystitis. Numerous methods for ureteral occlusion have been described, including antegrade placement of coils, Gelfoam, tissue adhesive, and detachable balloons, as well as retrograde injection of glutaraldehyde cross-linked collagen in the submucosa at the ureteral orifice.[4,5] One technique with durable success was described by Farrell et al. and involves the use of Gianturco steel coils (Cook Medical) with or without Gelfoam. Gianturco coils ranging in size from 5 mm × 5 cm to 12 mm × 5 cm were packed in the distal part of the ureter. Placement of larger coils at both the proximal and distal ends of the nest was suggested to help avoid migration of smaller coils into the renal pelvis, and occlusion of the distal ureter was recommended to reduce the risk for a uretero–iliac artery fistula or infection related to a sort of "blind-loop" syndrome.[5]

Percutaneous Nephrostomy Placement in a Transplant Kidney

In patients with posttransplant complications, an antegrade nephrostogram is performed first to establish the diagnosis and is followed by placement of a PCN or nephroureteral drain, with dilation of strictures if indicated. A severely narrowed, tapered, aperistaltic ureter should be considered to be partially obstructed in these patients.[23] An anterolateral calyx should be targeted, and a transperitoneal puncture, which increases the risk of complications, should be avoided by access of a mid- to upper-pole calyx from a lateral approach (Fig. 146-6). The remainder of the procedure is the same as in the native kidney, although short nephroureteral stents with 8 or 10 cm between the pigtails (Cook Medical) are available for use in renal transplant patients (Fig. 146-7). A biliary drain (Cook Medical) may also be the right length for use as an internal-external nephroureteral drain in a transplant kidney.

Percutaneous Nephrostomy Placement in Pregnancy

Relief of urinary obstruction may be accomplished by either a retrograde or antegrade approach in pregnant patients. The advantages of PCN are that it provides more rapid decompression of the obstructed kidney, avoids the potential for bladder irritability, facilitates routine drain exchanges, and provides access for definitive stone management after delivery. The challenges of PCN include difficulty positioning a patient who is often unable to lie prone, administering sedation that is safe for the fetus as well as the mother, and keeping the radiation dose to the absolute minimum required for accurate PCN placement. Although it may be possible to perform the entire procedure with ultrasound guidance, the potential need for fluoroscopy and the risk of radiation exposure to the fetus should be discussed with the patient when informed consent is obtained.

Percutaneous Nephrostomy Placement in Pediatric Patients

PCN in infants and newborns is often performed for temporary urinary drainage until definitive management is possible for conditions such as bilateral UPJ obstruction, UPJ obstruction with a single functional kidney, obstruction after pyeloplasty, UVJ obstruction, posterior urethral valves, and primary obstructing megaureter. In addition to the issues of appropriate sedation and monitoring for these patients, the procedure may be technically challenging even when the collecting system is extremely dilated. In infants, the kidney is so small that even with severe hydronephrosis,

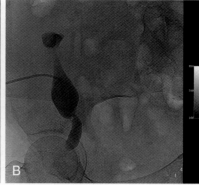

FIGURE 146-7. Percutaneous nephrostomy in a patient with hydronephrosis and elevated creatinine after revision of a right renal transplant ureteral anastomosis with a ureteroureterostomy. **A,** Sagittal ultrasound image obtained during access to right pelvic transplant kidney with a 21-gauge micropuncture needle, which is easily visible entering an anterior calyx. **B,** Antegrade nephrostogram after placement of an 8F locking pigtail drain demonstrates distal ureteral obstruction that is probably ischemic in nature.

TABLE 146-7. Technical Success Rates for Percutaneous Nephrostomy

Obstructed dilated system without stones	98%
Obstructed system in renal transplant	98%
Nondilated system (with or without stones)	85%
Complex stone disease, staghorn calculi	85%

Modified from Ramchandani P, Cardella JF, Grassi CJ, et al. Quality improvement guidelines for percutaneous nephrostomy. J Vasc Interv Radiol 2003;14:S277–81.

the total volume of urine is actually minimal, and it may be difficult to coil a guidewire within the collecting system, a problem that is magnified when UPJ obstruction prevents passage of the wire down the ureter. In addition, the renal parenchyma is often thin and offers little resistance to leakage of urine, and there is less support from the retroperitoneal soft tissues, so the kidney is quite mobile and readily displaced during attempts at dilation of the tract.

Difficulty with PCN placement via a standard micropuncture technique in patients younger than 14 weeks with severe dilation led Koral et al. to describe a modified technique. Access to the collecting system with a 0.018-inch system was replaced by access with a 19-gauge needle followed by a 0.035-inch wire and a 6F Navarre drain (C.R. Bard Inc., Covington, Ga.) to minimize the need for exchanges that allow urine to leak out of the collecting system. The Navarre drain was favored because its taper allows primary placement without dilation, and it coils easily in a small renal pelvis. The modified technique was thought to provide a greater level of success in infants and newborns, particularly those with UPJ obstruction.[24]

Outcomes

Outcomes for PCN are shown in Table 146-7. A PCN can be successfully placed in 98% to 99% of obstructed dilated kidneys. Success rates drop to 85% in patients with nondilated collecting systems, complex stone disease, or staghorn calculi.[9] Success rates are also lower (≈91%-92%) when ultrasound guidance alone is used for the procedure.[25] One

analysis of emergency PCN outcomes reported that fluoroscopy and overall procedure times were significantly less for experienced operators than for inexperienced operators, and that 20% to 33% of procedures performed by inexperienced operators were repeated the next day because of catheter dislodgement or malposition.[26] A simple technique for producing a gelatin-based phantom for use as a training simulator for ultrasound-guided PCN has been described and may improve outcomes for inexperienced operators.[27]

Antegrade ureteral stenting is technically successful in 88% to 96% of cases, and 80% of obstructed ureters can be stented primarily.[20,28] If stenting is not possible initially, a repeat attempt after decompression is often successful. The clinical success of ureteral stenting depends on the cause of the ureteral stricture, with higher long-term success rates being reported in patients with intrinsic disease rather than extrinsic obstruction.[29]

Several studies have evaluated the results of balloon dilation of both benign and malignant strictures and consistently report the most durable success when treating benign strictures that are short and not associated with ischemia.[30,31] In one study comparing the results of a single dilation followed by 3 weeks of internal ureteral stenting, benign strictures showed a patency rate of 67% and 57% at 12- and 36-month follow-up, versus 18% and 14% for malignant strictures.[30] Another study found a 90% patency rate at 2 years after balloon dilation of benign strictures with no evidence of vascular compromise, but the study also came to the conclusion that endopyelotomy or endoureterotomy is indicated for treatment of all other benign strictures.[31] Finally, a recent report on the use of a cutting balloon for treatment of benign ureteroenteric anastomotic strictures described a 3-year patency rate of 62% regardless of whether the stricture was ischemic in nature.[32]

In patients with malignant obstruction, plastic internal stents have a major complication rate of 34% and a failure rate of 36% over a mean indwelling time of 95 days.[33] Unfortunately, metallic stents are little if any better. One review of standard vascular metal stents used to treat 90 patients with malignant ureteral obstruction reported primary patency in 51% but failed to discuss the outcomes in detail.[34] Use of a 6F metallic double-J stent (Resonance [Cook Medical]) has been reported in a series of 40 patients treated with 76 stents, with somewhat positive results. At follow-up, 6 of the 40 patients had been able to avoid nephrostomy because of the metallic stent.[33]

Complications

The overall complication rate for PCN is approximately 10% (Table 146-8).[9] The most commonly occurring complications are sepsis and bleeding, both of which have a wide range of severity. The reported rate of sepsis requiring a major increase in the level of care is 1% to 3%, whereas the reported rate of hemorrhage requiring transfusion is 1% to 4%. Other complications that are reported to occur in less than 1% of patients include vascular injury requiring embolization or nephrectomy, bowel perforation, pleural complications, and injury to the renal pelvis (Fig. 146-8).[9,35] As would be expected, there is evidence that complication rates are higher for inexperienced operators than for experienced ones.[26]

Other problems with PCN tubes that are frequent but not universally considered complications include catheter dislodgement and blockage. Catheter dislodgement occurs in 1% to 2% of patients within the first 30 days of placement but may occur in up to 11% to 30% of patients who are monitored long term.[37] Reported success rates for reinsertion were significantly higher for catheters with a longer indwelling time (93% when in place > 3 months) and for those with a shorter interval between dislodgement and reinsertion (91% within 24 hours).[36] PCN blockage is reported to occur in approximately 1% of patients and is more likely in those with very crystalline urine and in patients who are noncompliant.[37]

The most common problem associated with nephroureteral and double-J ureteral stents is obstruction related to encrustation of the stent (Fig. 146-9).[20] Other common complications include bladder irritative symptoms and flank pain that may occasionally be severe enough to warrant removal of the stent, mild hematuria, ascending urinary tract infection (UTI), and malpositioning.[3]

Finally, a rare complication of ureteral stents is erosion of the stent, either through the renal pelvis, with resultant urinoma, bleeding from vessels in the renal hilum, or retroperitoneal abscess; or into the iliac artery, with resultant intermittent or massive hematuria. Extensive pelvic surgery and pelvic irradiation are risk factors for the formation of a fistula between the ureter and iliac artery, which can be difficult to diagnose.[20]

Patient Care

Patient preparation for PCN placement includes correction of any significant coagulopathy, premedication for contrast allergy, and treatment of hyperkalemia. Patients should be given prophylactic antibiotics, which have been shown to be beneficial in decreasing the incidence of sepsis both in high-risk patients, including those with stones, bacteriuria, ureteroenteric conduits, indwelling catheters, and diabetes, and in those who are at low risk.[38] If the patient is considered to be at low risk for a septic complication, IV administration of a single dose of a first-generation cephalosporin

TABLE 146-8. Complication Rates for Percutaneous Nephrostomy

Septic shock with major increase in level of care	1%-3%
Septic shock in setting of pyonephrosis	7%-9%
Hemorrhage requiring transfusion	1%-4%
Vascular injury requiring embolization or nephrectomy	0.1%-1%
Bowel transgression	0.2%
Pleural complications	0.1%-0.2%
Catheter dislodgement within 30 days	1%-2%

Modified from Ramchandani P, Cardella JF, Grassi CJ, et al. Quality improvement guidelines for percutaneous nephrostomy. J Vasc Interv Radiol 2003;14:S277–81; and Millward SF. Percutaneous nephrostomy: a practical approach. J Vasc Interv Radiol 2000;11:955–64.

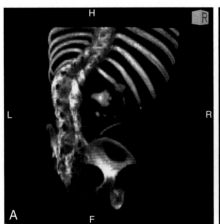
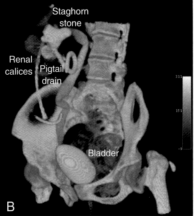
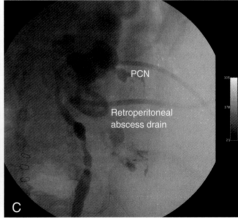

FIGURE 146-8. Young patient with spina bifida, renal and bladder stones, and fever. **A,** Posterior view from coronal maximum intensity projection reconstruction demonstrates spina bifida and a right staghorn stone. **B,** After percutaneous access of right renal collecting system, pigtail drain was very difficult to position because of size of staghorn stone. An attempt to place a nephroureteral drain instead was complicated by perforation of renal pelvis by wire. Volume-rendered image obtained 1 day after percutaneous nephrostomy (PCN) demonstrates pigtail outside renal pelvis. **C,** Retroperitoneal abscess developed and required placement of a drainage catheter. Nephrostomy drain had been repositioned into renal pelvis, but pigtail remained poorly formed. PCN was ultimately converted to a more stable nephroureteral stent, and retroperitoneal abscess resolved with percutaneous drainage.

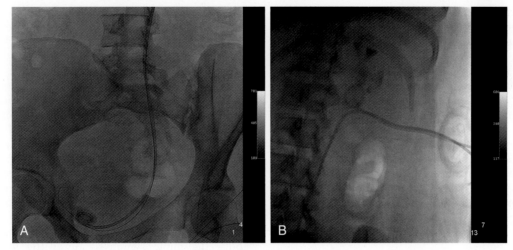

FIGURE 146-9. Noncompliant patient with a right renal stone, fever, and flank pain during pregnancy. A percutaneous nephrostomy drain was placed initially but was later converted to a nephroureteral stent because nephrostomy drain kept coming out. Patient was lost to follow-up and returned several months after delivery with fever and flank pain. **A,** Distal pigtail of nephroureteral stent is completely encrusted, and a wire could not be advanced through stent. A 0.035-inch stiff guidewire was advanced along stent into bladder. **B,** A locking pigtail drain was placed over guidewire and positioned in renal pelvis for decompression until patient could undergo cystoscopic lithotripsy.

within 2 hours of the start of the procedure should be sufficient. If the patient is considered to be at high risk, broad antibiotic coverage against the organisms that typically infect the genitourinary tract, including gram-negative rods such as *Escherichia coli*, *Proteus*, *Klebsiella*, and *Enterococcus*, should be chosen.[38] UTIs in the urology patient population demonstrate higher resistance rates than community UTIs, and significant increases in resistance to ampicillin and trimethoprim have been shown[39]; however, antibiotic susceptibilities vary by region and patient population, and the patient's medical record should be reviewed for any prior urine culture sensitivities to aid in selection of the most appropriate antibiotic. Antibiotics should be continued for 48 to 72 hours or longer if necessary in high-risk groups.

Conscious sedation is often administered during PCN, typically as a combination of short-acting agents such as fentanyl and midazolam. Regardless of whether conscious sedation is used, continuous physiologic monitoring of the heart rate, blood pressure, and oxygen saturation should be performed throughout the procedure by dedicated nursing personnel. The patient should have stable IV access, both for administering periprocedural medications and for resuscitation in the event of sepsis, and should receive oxygen via nasal cannula.

Immediately after the procedure, the patient should be transferred to a recovery area where frequent monitoring of vital signs can be continued at intervals of 15 or 30 minutes for at least 4 hours. Output from the nephrostomy should be recorded to ensure that it is draining well and that hematuria, if present, is clearing. Antibiotic therapy should be continued as appropriate. Because patients with urosepsis before the procedure are at increased risk for septic complications, it may be prudent to monitor these patients in an intensive care setting where intubation and aggressive fluid resuscitation can be performed rapidly if needed.[37]

PCN may be performed safely as an outpatient procedure in a carefully selected group of patients.[40] Outpatient PCN should not be considered for patients who are elderly,

debilitated, or live alone or for those who are at increased risk for complications because of conditions such as staghorn calculi, severe hypertension, diabetes, or ongoing use of antiplatelet or anticoagulant agents.

After initial placement, PCN drains should be left to external gravity drainage, which should be continued until the underlying problem has been treated or has resolved. Some patients, especially those with malignancies, may require long-term drainage, and patient education is the key to successful management. Patients should be given written instructions that describe how to care for the drain and what to do if the tube becomes blocked or displaced. Patients should understand when and how to contact the interventional radiology department in the event of a problem. Drains should be flushed twice daily, or patients instructed to remain well hydrated, or both, to prevent encrustation. Finally, routine PCN exchanges should be scheduled at 2- to 3-month intervals.

If a nephroureteral drain is placed, external drainage should continue until any hematuria has resolved, then the drain can be capped to promote internal drainage. If the patient tolerates capping of a nephroureteral drain, the drain can be exchanged for either a PCN or an internal double-J with a safety PCN, depending on the clinical situation. If the patient continues to drain well internally, the PCN can be removed. The capping trial should last at least 24 to 48 hours to ensure that the internal drainage is adequate. The drain should be returned to external gravity drainage if the patient experiences fever, chills, flank pain, or leakage around the drain at any time while it is capped.

SUPRAPUBIC CYSTOSTOMY

Indications

Percutaneous suprapubic cystostomy is indicated for the treatment of acute urinary retention when transurethral catheterization of the bladder is not possible or is contraindicated. The most common underlying problems in patients requiring suprapubic cystostomy are bladder outlet obstruction secondary to benign prostatic hypertrophy or prostatic cancer and neurogenic bladder dysfunction, but the procedure may also be beneficial in patients with urethral trauma, radiation-induced cystitis, vesicocolonic or vesicovaginal fistulas, and urinary incontinence.[41]

Contraindications

Relative contraindications to percutaneous cystostomy include coagulopathy, multiple previous abdominal and pelvic surgeries with extensive scar tissue, bladder tumor, morbid obesity, and inability to adequately distend the bladder to displace overlying small-bowel loops.

Equipment

The sonographic and fluoroscopic equipment used for placement of a suprapubic cystostomy is the same as that for PCN. Access into the bladder can be achieved with a 19-gauge needle, which is exchanged over a 0.035-inch stiff Amplatz wire (Boston Scientific) for sequential fascial dilators. If a small-bore drainage catheter is desired, an 8F or 10F locking pigtail drain should be placed. If a large-bore catheter is required for long-term drainage, a 16F, 18F, or 20F Foley catheter should be placed through a peel-away sheath that is 2 French sizes larger than the Foley catheter (Table 146-9). A Stamey percutaneous suprapubic catheter

set (Cook Medical) is also available in 8F to 16F for placement of a suprapubic cystostomy via a trocar technique (Fig. 146-10).

Technique

The preprocedural workup should include correction of any coagulation abnormalities, administration of prophylactic antibiotics, and placement of a transurethral Foley catheter if possible. The procedure is usually performed with the patient under conscious sedation, so appropriately trained personnel must be present to monitor the patient during and after the procedure. Percutaneous suprapubic cystostomy may be performed on an outpatient basis in selected patients.

The bladder should be accessed approximately 2 to 3 cm above the pubic symphysis or at the junction of the

TABLE 146-9. Key Equipment for Percutaneous Suprapubic Cystostomy

18- or 19-gauge needle
0.035-inch stiff Amplatz wire
Fascial dilators or balloon catheter
Drainage catheter:
    10F or 12F locking pigtail drain
    16F to 20F Foley catheter (requires a peel-away sheath)

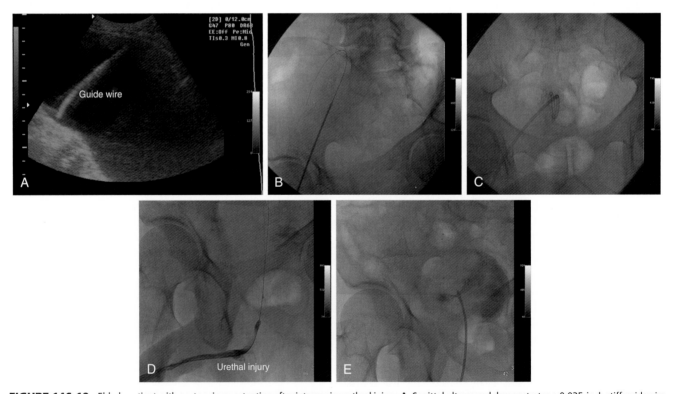

FIGURE 146-10. Elderly patient with acute urinary retention after iatrogenic urethral injury. **A,** Sagittal ultrasound demonstrates a 0.035-inch stiff guidewire that was advanced through a 19-gauge access needle. **B,** After fascial dilation, a 10F locking pigtail drain was advanced over the wire. **C,** Appearance of pigtail drain after aspiration of 1000 mL of urine. **D,** Three days after placement, suprapubic drain became dislodged and tract could not be identified again. Bladder was not distended, and a decision was made to attempt retrograde placement of a transurethral Foley catheter. A 5F Kumpe catheter and a 0.035-inch stiff guidewire were manipulated across urethral injury into bladder, and a 16F Foley catheter was placed over the wire. **E,** Injection of contrast material demonstrated appropriate position of Foley catheter.

mid- and lower thirds of the anterior bladder wall. The area of the trigone should be spared to avoid bladder spasm.[42] A vertical midline or slight paramedian approach will avoid injury to the inferior epigastric artery, which lies along the lateral edge of the rectus sheath.

If the bladder is fully distended or can be adequately distended with a transurethral Foley catheter, percutaneous suprapubic cystostomy may be performed under ultrasound guidance alone via a trocar technique.[43] Otherwise, a combination of sonographic and fluoroscopic guidance can be used for placement of a suprapubic cystostomy via a modified Seldinger technique.[41] If the bladder is not well distended initially, a 19-gauge needle should be advanced into the bladder under direct sonographic guidance to ensure that no bowel loops are traversed, and this needle can then be used to distend the bladder to capacity, usually with 150 to 500 mL of dilute contrast medium, before catheter placement. Once the bladder is fully distended, a 0.035-inch stiff Amplatz wire is advanced through the needle and coiled within the urinary bladder under fluoroscopic guidance. The tract can be dilated with sequential fascial dilators or a balloon catheter. A peel-away sheath that is 2 French sizes larger than the Foley catheter to be placed is advanced over the wire. An end hole is created in the tip of the Foley, and it is advanced over the wire through the peel-away sheath. The wire and peel-away sheath are removed, the Foley balloon is inflated with sterile saline and pulled up against the anterior wall of the bladder, and the Foley catheter is connected to a gravity drainage bag. Retention sutures are avoided because they can cause local skin irritation and typically are not necessary.

Whereas placement of a small-bore catheter (e.g., 10F or 12F locking pigtail drain) is usually adequate for urgent decompression of the bladder, placement of a Foley catheter that is at least 16F in diameter is required for effective long-term bladder drainage. Placement of a large catheter may be difficult in patients with extensive scar tissue related to previous surgeries or in patients who are obese, in which case a two-step procedure may be necessary, with initial placement of a small pigtail drain that can be upsized after the tract has formed.[41]

Creation of a suprapubic cystostomy may enable placement of a transurethral Foley catheter in patients who have suffered a traumatic or iatrogenic injury to the urethra. After bladder access is achieved, a 5F Kumpe catheter and a 0.035-inch stiff guidewire can be used to probe for the urethra. It may be possible to advance the catheter and wire in antegrade fashion across the urethra to establish through-and-through access over which a transurethral Foley catheter can be placed from a retrograde approach.

Outcomes

The reported success rates for placement of a percutaneous suprapubic cystostomy are essentially 100%.[41,43] Although initial placement of a large-bore drainage catheter may not be possible in patients who are obese or have extensive scarring that prevents adequate dilation of the tract, it is almost always successful with a two-step procedure. In two series with follow-up of up to 18 and 36 months, all catheters were well tolerated and remained functional until they were no longer needed.[41,42]

Complications

Potential complications associated with the procedure include hematuria (which is usually transient), sepsis, and injury to the bowel. Chronically indwelling catheters are associated with an increased risk for infection and stone formation, and as with other types of drainage catheters, suprapubic cystostomy tubes can become blocked or dislodged.

Postprocedural and Follow-up Care

All patients should be monitored by checking vital signs at 15- to 30-minute intervals for 4 hours after the procedure. Patients or caregivers should be educated about routine maintenance of the drainage catheter and should be given detailed information about whom to contact in the event the drain stops working, starts leaking, or becomes dislodged. Because long-term bladder catheters are associated with an increased risk for stone formation and infection, patients should be maintained on low-dose trimethoprim-sulfamethoxazole, and routine catheter exchanges should be scheduled every 2 to 3 months. Once the tract has matured, the catheter can be safely exchanged at the bedside.

KEY POINTS

- Review of the patient's medical history and any prior imaging studies should always be performed prior to percutaneous nephrostomy (PCN) or suprapubic cystostomy.

- Emergency PCN can be life saving in patients with urinary obstruction and urosepsis or acute renal failure.

- Treatment of renal stone disease is the most common indication for PCN, but PCN can also be extremely valuable in the management of ureteral injuries or strictures, urine leaks, and hemorrhagic cystitis.

- When PCN is performed for access prior to a urologic procedure such as percutaneous nephrostolithotomy, discussion with the referring urologist to plan the approach is essential to a successful outcome.

- Technical success rates for PCN range from 85% in patients with nondilated collecting systems or complex stone disease to 99% in patients with obstructed dilated kidneys.

- Percutaneous suprapubic cystostomy can provide rapid relief of acute urinary retention when transurethral catheterization of the bladder is not possible.

▶ **SUGGESTED READINGS**

Adamo R, Saad WEA, Brown DB. Percutaneous ureteral interventions. Tech Vasc Interv Radiol 2009;3(12):205–15.

American College of Radiology (ACR) practice guideline for the performance of percutaneous nephrostomy. ACR Practice Guideline; Amended 2004 (Res.25), p. 463–71.

Barnacle AM, Wilkinson AG, Roebuck DJ. Paediatric interventional uroradiology. Cardiovasc Intervent Radiol 2011;2(34):227–40.

Funaki B, Tepper JA. Percutaneous nephrostomy. Semin Intervent Radiol 2006;23(2):205–8.

Hausegger KA. Percutaneous nephrostomy and antegrade ureteral stenting: technique-indications-complications. Eur Radiol 2006;16: 2016–30.

Millward SF. Percutaneous nephrostomy: a practical approach. J Vasc Interv Radiol 2000;11:955–64.

Ramchandani P, Cardella JF, Grassi CJ, et al. Quality improvement guidelines for percutaneous nephrostomy. J Vasc Interv Radiol 2003;14: S277–81.

Saad WEA, Moorthy M, Ginat D. Percutaneous nephrostomy: native and transplanted kidneys. Tech Vasc Interv Radiol 2009;3(12):172–92.

Uppot RN. Emergent nephrostomy tube placement for acute urinary obstruction. Tech Vasc Interv Radiol 2009;2(12):154–61.

The complete reference list is available online at www.expertconsult.com.

CHAPTER 147

Renal and Perirenal Fluid Collection Drainage

Justin J. Campbell and Debra A. Gervais

Percutaneous image-guided drainage is a useful technique for managing many fluid collections involving the upper genitourinary tract. For infected collections in the peritoneal cavity, percutaneous abscess drainage (PAD) has become the primary drainage procedure since its introduction in the early 1980s. This procedure's safety and efficacy has been demonstrated in numerous large clinical trials.[1-5] The logical extension of the technique to collections in the kidney and perirenal space has gained acceptance and in many cases obviated the need for urologic surgery. Benefits of percutaneous drainage of fluid collections in most cases include avoiding general anesthesia, laparotomy, and prolonged postoperative hospitalization, with resultant reduction in morbidity, mortality, and hospital costs. In this chapter, we address techniques for percutaneously draining renal and perirenal abscesses as well as other fluid collections such as hematomas and urinomas. Percutaneous nephrostomy techniques and ureteral stenting are addressed in other chapters.

INDICATIONS

Percutaneous fluid drainage is a therapeutic option that lies between medical and surgical management. In general, the prerequisites for percutaneous renal and perirenal fluid collection drainage are identical to the indications for fluid collection drainage elsewhere in the abdomen—presence of a fluid collection and one or more of the following: suspicion the collection is infected, need for fluid characterization, or suspicion the collection is producing symptoms that warrant drainage.[6] A few caveats should be added in the setting of suspected urinomas. The majority of small urinomas will resolve spontaneously, but if a small urinoma fails to resolve in several days or if a large urinoma is discovered, percutaneous drainage should be considered. Regardless of the collection size, if there is any suspicion a urinoma is infected, drainage should be pursued. The goal of drainage can be complete cure of a collection, or drainage may be employed as a temporizing measure before definitive surgical treatment. For example, in a critically ill patient with a suspected abscess in a nonfunctioning kidney, PAD can be performed to stabilize the patient before performing a definitive urologic procedure like nephrectomy. Similarly, treatment of urinomas caused by obstruction mandate not only drainage of the urinoma but also correction of the underlying leak and/or obstruction and reestablishment of urine flow to the bladder or to the outside for successful treatment of the urinoma.

CONTRAINDICATIONS

Contraindications to percutaneous fluid collection drainage are relative and should be weighed carefully against the suitable medical and surgical alternatives. According to the American College of Radiology (ACR) guidelines, the relative contraindications include coagulopathy that cannot be adequately corrected, hemodynamic instability that precludes completion of the procedure, inability of the patient to be positioned or cooperate adequately for the procedure, known adverse reaction to contrast medium when its administration is deemed necessary for success of the procedure, lack of a safe access route for drainage of a collection, and severely compromised cardiopulmonary status in patients undergoing procedures where risk or further cardiopulmonary compromise are inherent to the procedure.[6] In each case, the risks of the procedure must be carefully assessed. The decision regarding management of renal and perirenal fluid collections is best made in concert with the surgical and medical teams caring for the patient. Lastly, every attempt is made to identify pregnant patients before their exposure to ionizing radiation. Pregnant patients undergoing procedures requiring use of ionizing radiation are counseled regarding the risk to the fetus of radiation exposure, as well as the clinical benefit of the procedure. Every attempt is made to avoid exposing the fetus to radiation in accordance with ALARA (as low as reasonably achievable) principles. Efforts to reduce radiation exposure for these patients include ultrasound guidance whenever possible. If computed tomography (CT) is required for a procedure, imaging is limited to only those areas of the body required to perform the procedure.

EQUIPMENT

As with abscess drainage in the peritoneal cavity, the primary tool necessary for abscess drainage is the drainage catheter. A large number of catheters are designed for fluid collection drainage. The majority are constructed from a kink-resistant polyurethane material. Catheters can be placed by either the Seldinger or trocar method. The trocar method consists of placing a flexible polyurethane catheter loaded with a metal stiffener and pointed metal trocar directly into a collection. Once the tip is placed into the collection, the catheter is fed off the trocar and stiffener into the collection. The trocar and stiffener are then removed. Alternatively, the catheter can be placed by the Seldinger method, which consists of placing the catheter into a collection over a wire. After placing a wire into a collection, the tract is dilated using serial dilators over the wire. The catheter containing the metal stiffener is placed over the wire and fed off the stiffener once it has passed through any tissues likely to prevent the catheter from easily following the wire (e.g., fascial planes, muscle). Many catheters are available with a hydrophilic coating that facilitates placement and deployment. Catheters are available in sizes ranging from 8F to 16F. Numerous large, "oblong-shaped" holes at the catheter tip facilitate drainage. The majority of catheter tips have a string-locked pigtail configuration for retention, but other internal retention devices such as balloons and mushroom types are also available.

Needle access is generally performed before catheter placement. A variety of needles can be used. Superficial collections are generally amenable to access with spinal needles. Deeper collections can be sampled using 10- to 25-cm Chiba needles. Needle diameters range from 18 to 22 gauge. Sampling of fluid is usually possible with 20-gauge needles, but if there is suspicion that the collection is viscous, larger-gauge needles can be employed. This needle can then be used as a guide for the tandem trocar technique. If the Seldinger technique is employed, the access needle can be used to place the wire over which the drainage catheter will be placed. Several needles designed to accept a 0.038-inch wire can be used to facilitate this technique. At our institution, Ring (Cook Medical, Bloomington, Ind.) and AccuStick (MediTech/Boston Scientific, Natick, Mass.) are used in this setting.

When the Seldinger technique is used, one may have to redirect a working wire to a specific location for ultimate catheter deployment. This is usually achieved with a directional catheter to guide the wire to a specific target location under fluoroscopic guidance. A number of such catheters have been developed for vascular radiology. A 5F Kumpe catheter or Cobra catheter are useful for this purpose. These catheters accept 0.038-inch wires. In general, directional catheters measuring 40 to 65 cm in length are used in the nonvascular interventional radiology setting.

When using the Seldinger technique, tract dilation is often necessary to allow catheter placement. This can be achieved using dilators, stiff devices with tapered ends that are placed over the working wire. When dilating the tract, care must be taken to not kink the wire. After performing serial dilation, the catheter can then be placed over the wire. Alternatively, the catheter can be placed after dilation with a Peel-Away introducer (Cook Medical).

TECHNIQUE

Anatomy and Approaches

Pus, urine, blood, and even pancreatic fluid can accumulate in the renal parenchyma and surrounding tissues. An understanding of distribution of the fluid in the renal and perirenal spaces must be founded on an understanding of the fascial planes that compose this area. The fascia that surrounds the kidneys envelops the perirenal spaces that contain the adrenal glands, proximal ureters, and fat that surrounds the kidneys. This perirenal fascia forms a long, tapered cone that reflects the embryologic ascent of the kidneys from the pelvis into their adult position in the retroperitoneum. The eponymous names of the anterior and posterior layers of the renal fascia are the *Gerota fascia* and *Zuckerkandl fascia*, respectively, but the name *Gerota fascia* is frequently used in the medical literature to describe both the anterior and posterior layers of renal fascia.[7] The anterior and posterior layers fuse laterally to join the lateral conal fascia. Although there is no consensus on the strength or completeness of the inferior fascia, published reports suggest that inferior patency exists in some patients, allowing bidirectional flow of fluid between the perirenal and pelvic compartments.[8-10] Similarly, although there is some controversy about the medial boundaries of the perirenal spaces, there is published evidence that patency between the right and left perirenal spaces across the midline exists at and below the level of the lower poles of the kidneys.[9] The lower abdominal aorta and inferior vena cava are within this midline communication between the two perirenal spaces.

Posterior to the perirenal space is the posterior pararenal space, which contains only a variable amount of properitoneal fat. This space is bounded posteriorly by the transversalis fascia and anteriorly by the perirenal fascia. Because this space contains only fat, it is rarely the primary site of a pathologic process. The perirenal fascia fuses at its posterior and lateral aspects to the surface of the pro-peritoneal fat. The fused surfaces of the posterior perirenal fascia and anterior surface of the posterior pararenal space create a potential space, the posterior interfascial or retrorenal plane, which may be filled from fluid arising in either of the compartments it bounds.[11] Anterior to the perirenal space lies the anterior pararenal space that contains the ascending and descending colon, pancreas, and portions of the duodenum. As with the fusion of the posterior perirenal fascia and anterior surface of the posterior pararenal space, the fusion of the anterior perirenal fascia creates an additional potential space, the anterior interfascial plane or retromesenteric fusion plane, which can also be filled with fluid arising from the compartment it bounds.[11] On the left, lateral in relation to the anterior renal fascia, the dorsal mesocolon fuses with the surface of the posterior pararenal fat to form the lateral conal fascia. Similarly, on the right, lateral in relation to the anterior pararenal fascia, the mesentery of the ascending colon fuses with the posterior renal fat to form the lateral conal fascia. Potential spaces are created with the formation of these interfascial planes as well. The retromesenteric anterior interfascial space, retrorenal posterior interfascial space, and lateral conal plane communicate at the fascial trifurcation.[11]

Within the perirenal space, the perinephric fat is divided by numerous thin fibrous lamellae into multiple smaller compartments that may or may not communicate. These fibrous structures are continuous with and interconnect the renal capsule and anterior and posterior renal fascia planes. These connections allow for bidirectional spread of blood, fluid, or edema from the perirenal fascial planes into the perinephric space.[11]

The majority of abscesses in the kidney and perirenal space are the result of pyelonephritis. Other processes that can result in renal and perirenal abscesses include direct extension of infection from an adjacent compartment, superinfection of collections in the perirenal space, and rare processes such as a dropped gallstone. Before discussing drainage of these collections, it is important to clarify terminology. The literature regarding imaging and treatment of acute bacterial renal infections is plagued with inconsistency and ambiguity. The terms *acute pyelonephritis*, *acute bacterial nephritis*, and *lobar nephronia* are frequently used, but there is no consensus among radiologists, urologists, pathologists, nephrologists, and infectious disease experts on the meaning of these terms.

The terms *bacterial nephritis*[12] and *lobar nephronia*[13] were initially introduced to identify a subset of patients with acute pyelonephritis who had severe regional or generalized parenchymal abnormalities without abscess, a protracted clinical course, and eventual atrophy of the affected parenchyma. The majority of these patients were diabetic or immunocompromised. The goal of identifying this group of patients was to distinguish them from patients with uncomplicated acute pyelonephritis who responded rapidly to antibiotics, as well as from patients with renal and/or extrarenal abscesses. The term *lobar nephronia* was used to describe a lobar distribution of pathology. For the most part, infections of the renal parenchyma are the result of ascending spread of pathogens from the lower tract or hematogenous seeding of the renal parenchyma.[14] In experimental models of acute ascending nonobstructive renal infection, vesicoureteral and intrarenal reflux have been demonstrated to carry bacteria to the pyelocaliceal system and papillary ducts and tubules, where an inflammatory response is initiated.[15] Inflammation then radiates centrifugally from the papilla to the cortex along medullary rays in a lobar or sublobar distribution. The configuration of the duct openings at the papilla in part determines which papilla will allow reflux of urine and which will not.[16] It was this proposed lobar distribution that gave rise to the term *lobar nephronia*.[13]

Bacterial nephritis was an additional term used for those patients who did not have lobar distribution of infection but who were likely to have a severe disease process with a protracted clinical course. Both of these terms have shortcomings. First, the literature now clearly demonstrates that otherwise healthy children and adults can have severe infections of the renal parenchyma that prolong treatment and result in parenchymal loss.[17,18] Second, extensive experience with CT has now demonstrated that renal infections frequently do not correspond to a renal lobe. Although most renal infections are thought to be the result of an ascending infection, the extent to which reflux of urine is responsible for inoculation is unclear; acute pyelonephritis occurs in both adults and children, without evidence of reflux. One model used to explain this phenomenon is the ability of certain strains of virulent *Escherichia coli* to ascend the ureter against the flow of urine by the expression of surface adhesins. The bacteria then colonize the upper tract and penetrate parenchyma via collecting ducts and tubules.[14] Furthermore, although less common, hematogenous spread of infection also accounts for many cases of renal infection. In animal models, bacteria reaching the renal parenchyma by this route begin in the cortex and involve the medulla within 24 to 48 hours. These lesions are typically multiple and rounded and have a nonlobar distribution throughout the periphery of the kidney. After 48 hours, however, distinguishing the two patterns is often not possible because spreading inflammation obscures the initial underlying pattern.[19]

To escape this nosologic quagmire in a way that reflects the underlying pathophysiologic process, takes into account the continuous nature of the spectrum of focal or diffuse renal infections, and allows the radiologist to convey an accurate, easily understood report of the process involving the kidney that will help guide therapeutic decisions, the Society of Uroradiology proposes a simplified nomenclature based on the term *acute pyelonephritis*.[19] For CT imaging of patients clinically diagnosed with acute pyelonephritis, the society recommends that all regions of hypoattenuation visualized in the kidney be considered

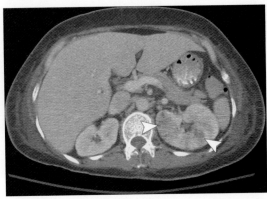

FIGURE 147-1. Axial computed tomography image with intravenous contrast enhancement demonstrates slight enlargement of left kidney relative to right. Note areas of heterogeneous enhancement *(arrowheads)* without a discrete area of hypoattenuation with a discrete wall to suggest abscess formation. These findings are most consistent with acute pyelonephritis in this patient with fever, left flank pain, and leukocytosis.

evidence of acute pyelonephritis (Fig. 147-1). The report should then further characterize the process as (1) focal (uni- or multi-) or diffuse, (2) unilateral or bilateral, (3) with or without focal or diffuse enlargement of the kidney, and (4) complicated (renal or extrarenal abscess, obstruction, gas formation) or not.[19]

If treated too late or inadequately, severe bacterial renal infections may progress to form an abscess. Initially, microabscesses will form that can then coalesce to form macroabscesses. Historically, pathologists and surgeons have used the term *renal carbuncle* to describe multiple coalescent hematogenously seeded renal abscesses. Over time, the term came to be used to describe any renal abscess. Although there is a distinctive macroscopic appearance to this entity, no corresponding imaging features have been described, so the term should be avoided by radiologists. A mature abscess will have a well-defined wall and on CT imaging will appear as an area of nonenhancement within renal parenchyma, with a peripheral rim of enhancement (Fig. 147-2). Before forming a mature abscess, however, there is an initial liquefaction of renal parenchyma in regions of inflammation. On CT, this can appear as an area of low attenuation measuring near water density that does not enhance. Importantly, this lesion may not yet be a drainable collection. When CT findings are indeterminate, needle aspiration can be performed. If less than 1 mL of fluid is aspirated, it is likely this lesion is not drainable and will heal with long-term antibiotic therapy.[19]

Abscesses in the perirenal space most commonly result from rupture of a renal abscess into the perinephric fat. Additional causes of perirenal abscesses include extension of abscesses from adjacent compartments into the perirenal space and superinfection of collections in the perirenal space (e.g., urinomas, hematomas). Continuous leak of urine into the perinephric fat will result in a collection of urine. These collections are most commonly referred to as *urinomas*, but other names have been used in the medical literature, including *uriniferous perirenal pseudocyst*.[20] Urinomas are most commonly the result of forniceal rupture in the setting of obstructive uropathy. Other causes include both iatrogenic and noniatrogenic trauma (Fig. 147-3).

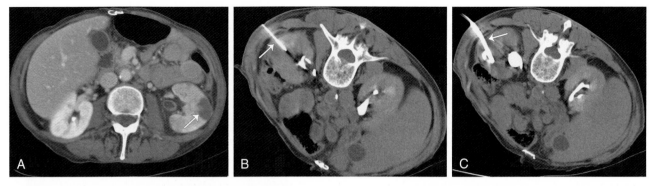

FIGURE 147-2. A, Axial computed tomography (CT) image with intravenous contrast enhancement demonstrates slight enlargement of left kidney relative to right. Note areas of heterogeneous enhancement with a discrete area of hypoattenuation with a perceptible wall in interpolar region of left kidney *(arrow)*. These findings are most consistent with acute pyelonephritis and abscess in this patient with fever, left flank pain, and leukocytosis. **B,** Under CT guidance, a 20-gauge Chiba needle *(arrow)* was placed into area of discrete hypoattenuation; 2 mL of purulent material was aspirated. **C,** A 12F locking pigtail catheter *(arrow)* was then placed into collection using tandem trocar method; 10 mL of purulent material was aspirated.

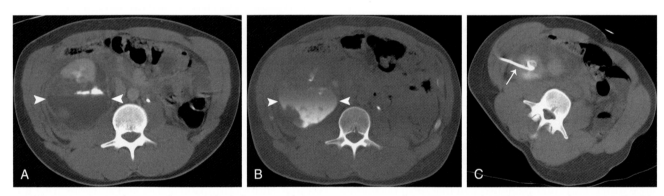

FIGURE 147-3. A, Axial computed tomography (CT) image with intravenous contrast enhancement in pyelographic phase in this patient after blunt abdominal trauma demonstrates fractured right kidney. A large low-attenuation collection is visualized adjacent to lower pole of kidney *(arrowheads)*. A small amount of high-density excreted contrast is visualized within this low-attenuation collection. **B,** Delayed image demonstrates filling of this large low-attenuation collection with excreted contrast *(arrowheads)* consistent with a large urinoma. **C,** A 10F pigtail catheter *(arrow)* was placed into this collection by trocar method under CT guidance. Urinoma resolved without need for additional urinary diversion.

Hematomas in the perirenal space have numerous causes. Abdominal trauma with resultant renal contusion, laceration, or fracture can cause a perinephric hematoma. Additionally, rupture of an aortic aneurysm can lead to a hematoma confined to the perirenal space.[21] Spontaneous perirenal hematomas raise concern for an underlying neoplasm such as renal cell carcinoma or angiomyelolipoma.[22] The underlying lesion may be small and can be obscured by the hematoma in the acute setting. Therefore, management of a completely spontaneous perirenal hematoma or a perirenal hematoma arising in the setting of minimal trauma always includes follow-up imaging until the hematoma has resorbed or another cause for the hemorrhage has been identified.

Collections in the anterior pararenal space are more common on the left than on the right. Collections in the left anterior pararenal space are most frequently associated with inflammatory disease involving the tail of the pancreas (Fig. 147-4). Collections in the right anterior pararenal space can also be associated with inflammatory disease of the pancreas, but duodenal injury or perforation can also cause collections in this compartment (Fig. 147-5). Because the posterior pararenal space contains only fat, collections rarely originate from this compartment and are usually the result of extension of fluid from an adjacent compartment (Fig. 147-6). The most common cause of a collection arising from the posterior pararenal space is a hematoma. These hematomas can occur in the setting of anticoagulation or a bleeding diathesis. Because of the intimate association of the anterior interfascial and lateral conal planes to the retroperitoneal ascending colon on the right and descending colon on the left, edema and inflammatory change associated with diverticulitis, ischemia, infectious colitis, and retrocecal appendicitis can cause fluid collections that spread into these planes.[11]

Technical Aspects

Patient Preparation

Before draining a renal or perirenal fluid collection, several issues regarding patient preparation must be addressed. Coagulation factors including prothrombin time (PT), partial thromboplastin time (PTT), and platelet count are usually checked before intervention. Any coagulopathy is then corrected to the degree possible before performing the procedure. Second, adequate antibiotic therapy is initiated if there is clinical evidence of infection. In the majority of cases, the team caring for the patient has begun antibiotic

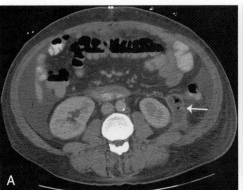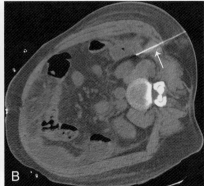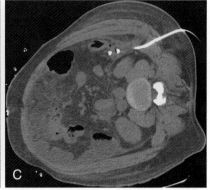

FIGURE 147-4. A, Axial computed tomography (CT) image with intravenous contrast enhancement demonstrates a gas- and fluid-containing collection in left anterior pararenal space *(arrow)* most consistent with an abscess in this patient with pancreatitis. **B,** Under CT guidance, a 20-gauge Chiba needle *(arrow)* was placed into collection. **C,** A 10F locking pigtail catheter was then placed into collection using tandem trocar method; 15 mL of purulent material was aspirated.

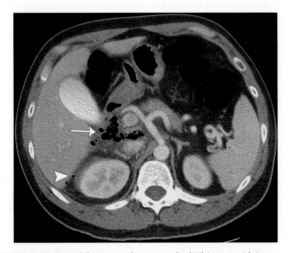

FIGURE 147-5. Axial computed tomography (CT) image with intravenous contrast enhancement demonstrates gas-containing periduodenal collection *(arrow)* with gas tracking into right anterior pararenal space *(arrowhead)* in patient who developed fever, abdominal pain, and leukocytosis after duodenal perforation from endoscopic retrograde cholangiopancreatography. Patient ultimately underwent successful transhepatic percutaneous drainage of collection.

therapy before consulting radiology for potential PAD. In the rare instance in which antibiotic therapy has not been initiated, broad-spectrum antibiotics are given before drainage. Antimicrobial therapy is not withheld for fear of sterilizing cultures; because the interventional manipulation can seed the bloodstream with bacteria, the risk of sepsis is high.[23]

Because most patients will experience some intraprocedural pain despite local anesthesia, intravenous (IV) sedation is almost always employed; a benzodiazepine and narcotic combination works well. At our institution, we use intravenously administered fentanyl and midazolam (Versed). Typically, fentanyl (25 μg IV) and midazolam (0.25-0.5 mg IV) are administered at 5- to 10-minute intervals until adequate sedation is achieved. IV sedation is administered according to institutional guidelines, and interventional radiologists should be familiar with their own institution's guidelines.

Placing the Catheter

There are several important considerations when planning the route for abscess drainage. The primary consideration is identifying the most direct route from skin to collection that is free of intervening organs and vital structures such as bowel, solid viscera, vessels, and nerves. Additionally, every attempt is made to avoid contaminating sterile areas. In the case of renal and perirenal fluid collection drainage, particular attention is given to the possibility of pleural transgression, but avoidance of the pleural space is not possible in all cases. Lastly, the catheter is generally placed in the most dependent position possible to facilitate drainage. For example, if the patient will be in the supine position after the catheter is placed, a posterior or lateral approach may optimize drainage. When the route for drainage has been selected, the patient can be positioned in the most appropriate position for catheter placement. When the patient is properly positioned, the skin is prepped and draped in the usual sterile fashion, and sedation is initiated.

Whether employing the Seldinger or trocar technique, initial access to the abscess cavity is obtained under CT or ultrasound guidance. Fluoroscopy can be used in conjunction with either of these two modalities to confirm catheter position or assist with optimal catheter positioning in difficult cases. The decision regarding which imaging modality to employ is made on the basis of several factors, including position of the collection, presence of overlying structures, and visibility of the collection and adjacent structures with each modality. Availability and user preference also play a role in this decision. Ultrasonography has a number of advantages. The first is speed. Because ultrasonography is a real-time imaging modality, it is generally much faster than CT. Additionally, ultrasonography is also generally more widely available and less expensive than CT. The modality is portable, which allows for use at the bedside in critically ill patients whose condition is not stable enough to allow travel to the radiology suite. Lastly, ultrasound does not expose the patient to ionizing radiation. Unlike CT, however, intervening fat, gas, and bone significantly degrade visualization of collections. Abscesses deep within the abdomen or pelvis can be difficult to visualize. For the same reason, ultrasonography can be difficult to use in obese

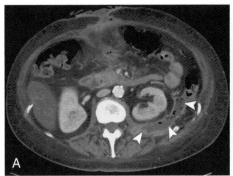 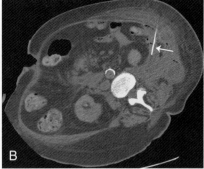 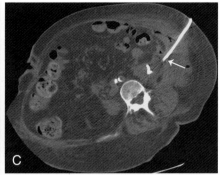

FIGURE 147-6. A, Axial computed tomography (CT) image with intravenous contrast enhancement demonstrates gas- and fluid-containing collection in left posterior pararenal space *(arrowheads)* in patient with severe necrotizing pancreatitis. **B,** Under CT guidance, a 20-gauge Chiba needle *(arrow)* was placed into collection. **C,** A 12F locking pigtail catheter *(arrow)* was then placed into collection using tandem trocar method; 130 mL of purulent material was aspirated.

patients with large amounts of subcutaneous fat. Similarly, some collections in the retroperitoneum can be difficult to visualize. Limitations of ultrasonography also include the need for significant operator experience.

CT is not as operator dependent as ultrasonography. Furthermore, deep collections and collections with overlying bone, gas, or fat are easily visualized. Provided the patient's weight does not exceed table limits, and patient size allows placement of both the patient and a guiding needle into the gantry, CT-guided drainage is not limited by obesity to the same degree as ultrasound. Finally, both final catheter position and degree of evacuation of abscess contents are better visualized with CT than ultrasound. Disadvantages of CT include the use of ionizing radiation, increased time required for procedures, and lack of portability.

Both CT and ultrasound have limitations in their ability to distinguish solid tissue from drainable fluid collections. CT relies on attenuation measurements to distinguish tissues. The majority of fluid collections are low attenuation, but some drainable fluid collections can contain high-attenuation materials like iodinated contrast medium or blood products. Likewise, some nondrainable tissues (e.g., necrotic tissues, certain neoplasms) can be very low in attenuation. Unlike CT, however, ultrasound has particular difficulty visualizing collections that contain gas, secondary to limited sound transmission. Additionally, some hypoechoic through-transmitting tissues (e.g., lymphoma) can be mistaken for fluid. Regardless of which imaging modality is ultimately chosen to guide drainage, a combination of pre-drainage diagnostic imaging modalities can be used to characterize collections and assess feasibility of drainage before attempting percutaneous drainage.

The catheter may be placed using either a trocar or Seldinger technique. Both techniques are viable options and offer advantages and disadvantages in different clinical settings. Although each technique has its proponents and detractors, no randomized trial exists to compare them, and the choice of which to employ comes down to operator preference, which itself is usually a function of experience. The trocar technique is generally performed in tandem to a guiding needle. As discussed earlier, the guiding needle is usually 18 to 22 gauge and variable in length, depending on the depth of the collection. The guiding needle is placed

into the collection under CT guidance. Once needle placement within the collection has been confirmed with imaging, the needle acts as a guide for catheter placement. Before placing the catheter, a sample of fluid can be aspirated and sent for laboratory analysis. This initial aspiration can be helpful in characterizing the fluid. If no fluid is aspirated, the collection may be very viscous, suggesting the need for a larger catheter. Alternatively, if the fluid is not grossly purulent and there is a suspicion the collection is not infected, a Gram stain can be performed if the decision of whether to place a catheter will be influenced by these results.

Once the decision to place the catheter has been made, a small nick is made in the skin adjacent to the guiding needle entrance site, and the underlying subcutaneous tissue is bluntly dissected. The catheter containing the hollow metal stiffener and inner trocar needle is then advanced into the cavity adjacent to the guiding needle to the appropriate predetermined depth. When the catheter tip is within the cavity, the catheter is fed off the trocar needle and metal stiffener. Syringe aspiration can then be performed to help confirm catheter position. Minimal fluid is aspirated at this time because decreasing the size of the target cavity makes subsequent repositioning technically more difficult if repositioning is required. The catheter position is then confirmed with imaging before securing the device. The guiding needle is removed after satisfactory catheter position is confirmed. The advantage of the trocar method is the speed with which the catheter can be deployed. This can be very helpful when the patient is critically ill or lightly sedated. The main disadvantage of this technique is limited ability to reposition the catheter without removing and reinserting it if initial positioning is suboptimal.

Using the Seldinger technique, the initial access can be performed with a needle under ultrasound or CT guidance. When the needle position within the cavity is confirmed with imaging, a wire is placed through the needle into the cavity. The needle is then removed over the wire, and the tract is serially dilated to the appropriate size to allow catheter placement. Two different types of needles can be used for initial access. "One-stick" systems use a 21- to 22-gauge needle that accepts a 0.018-inch wire. A three-component device containing a sheath, dilator, and stiffener is placed over this wire. With removal of the stiffener and dilator, a 0.035- or 0.038-inch working wire can be placed through the sheath. Further dilation can then be performed to place the catheter over this wire into the collection. Alternatively, a larger needle such as a Ring needle (Cook Medical) can be placed that accepts a 0.035- or 0.038-inch wire. The Seldinger technique is helpful when the window to the collection is narrow. Furthermore, this technique offers the advantage of guiding the catheter into optimal position with the use of directional catheters under fluoroscopic guidance. The disadvantage of this technique is primarily that it can be more time consuming than the trocar technique, which can be a particularly important consideration in critically ill patients. Additionally, serial dilation can be painful even in well-sedated patients.

After Placing the Catheter
Immediately after the procedure, imaging is performed to assess adequacy of cavity drainage and final catheter location. This is generally evaluated with the modality used to place the catheter. The catheter can be hard to visualize with ultrasound, but decrease in cavity size can usually be assessed that suggests the correct catheter position. CT offers excellent visualization of both the cavity and catheter. Injection of contrast medium under fluoroscopy can also be used to confirm catheter position. At the time of initial drainage, care is exercised to be sure to inject less volume than the volume of fluid removed from the cavity so as to minimize the risk of bacteremia and acute sepsis. Because of the viscosity of iodinated contrast, the injected contrast medium is then aspirated and the catheter flushed with saline to minimize catheter clogging. Additionally, catheter position can be independently confirmed by flow of appropriate fluid (e.g., pus from an abscess). When satisfactory catheter position is confirmed, the collection is then decompressed with a large aspiration syringe until return of fluid or debris ceases. For large cavities, irrigation of the cavity with small aliquots of sterile saline can be performed until the return of the irrigant turns clear. Irrigation will often result in higher volumes of return fluid than the irrigant facilitating drainage. Irrigation must cease immediately if the irrigant volume is not completely returned with aspiration. Failure to achieve complete return indicates that the irrigant is collecting in a location not amenable to aspiration by the catheter, and further irrigant will simply expand this collection. Irrigation of the cavity must be distinguished from flushing the catheter. *Irrigation* involves instillation of fluid into the cavity for lavage and more complete drainage of cavity contents. *Flushing* is simply to clear the catheter and any associated drainage tubing to prevent occlusion of the catheter by particulate debris and necrotic tissue.[24,25] Importantly, overzealous irrigation can cause bacteremia and paradoxical worsening of the patient's clinical status.

When decompression of the cavity and catheter position have been confirmed, the pigtail is formed (when using pigtail catheter), and the catheter is secured to the skin. The catheter can be sutured to the skin, but this can lead to irritation. For this reason, a number of retention devices are available that do not require a skin suture. The catheter is then connected to a drainage bag. A three-way stopcock can be placed between the catheter and drainage bag. This device has the advantage of facilitating subsequent catheter flushes, but has the disadvantage of a narrow lumen that can impede drainage with viscous fluid or collections containing debris. In particular, for catheters larger than 14F, the standard stopcock lumen is narrower than the catheter lumen, although larger-bore stopcocks are available. The catheter is flushed with 10 mL of saline every 8 to 12 hours to prevent drained material from obstructing the catheter lumen. Additionally, the connection tubing to the bag is flushed because this tubing can also become obstructed.

CONTROVERSIES

Areas of variation in the practice of percutaneous drainage of renal and perirenal collections include the use of intracavitary fibrinolytics, drainage in the setting of coagulopathies or anticoagulation therapy, and use of the Seldinger or trocar technique. The presence of infected hematomas and viscous purulent material have been associated with poor drainage despite proper catheter position. There is some evidence that instillation of fibrinolytics can shorten hospital stays and lower treatment costs, but to date no large clinical trials have been performed to establish definitive guidelines concerning the use of intracavitary fibrinolytics for the practitioner for renal and perirenal fluid collection drainage. The decision regarding intracavitary fibrinolytic use is made by the radiologist together with the other members of the team caring for the patient.

Similarly, there is variation in the practice of percutaneous renal and perirenal fluid collection drainage in the setting of coagulopathies. The risk of a bleeding complication increases with the presence of a coagulopathy, but the cutoff values for PT and platelet count vary from institution to institution. Although most patients will have recent laboratory values available before percutaneous drainage, not all practitioners will check values before the procedure. Most institutions will use a cutoff for PT of 15 to 18 seconds, corresponding to an international normalized ratio of 1.5 to 2.2. Cutoff values for platelets vary from 50,000 to 70,000/mm^3. At this time, no scientific trial has established guidelines for practitioners of percutaneous drainage concerning either the necessity of checking laboratory values before percutaneous drainage or for cutoff values of PT or platelets. Practice also varies concerning percutaneous drainage in the setting of patients receiving anticoagulation therapies such as aspirin and clopidogrel (Plavix). Multiple new anticoagulation agents give rise to new challenges concerning if and when to withhold anticoagulation therapy when performing percutaneous drainage. In each case, the benefits of percutaneous drainage must be weighed carefully along with the risks of a bleeding complication, as well as the risks of withholding anticoagulation therapy. These decisions are always made in concert with the other clinicians involved in the patient's care.

Lastly, the area of greatest practice variation in percutaneous drainage concerns use of the trocar or Seldinger technique. Proponents of each may closely adhere to one and eschew the other, but at this time, no prospective clinical trial has established the supremacy of either technique. As discussed previously, there are situations in which each technique offers advantages and disadvantages. Given the extensive experience with both, at this time the decision of which technique to employ comes down to the preference of a given practitioner in a given situation.

OUTCOMES

The efficacy of percutaneous renal and perirenal abscess drainage with the use of antibiotics has been well documented. Rives et al. found that treatment of renal and perirenal abscesses with antibiotics alone is not effective in the majority of cases.[26] In 1981, Elyaderani reported successful treatment of a renal abscess with percutaneous drainage in a patient too ill to undergo surgery.[27] Several small series subsequently demonstrated variable success with percutaneous drainage of renal abscesses.[28-31] In 1988, Sacks et al. reported a series of 18 patients who underwent percutaneous treatment of infected renal and perirenal collections; 61% required no surgical intervention, and the remaining 39% underwent subsequent surgery after being "cooled off" with percutaneous drainage. These patients experienced a reduced rate of surgical morbidity.[32] The results were echoed in the 1990 report of a series of 30 patients with renal or perirenal abscesses reported by Deyoe et al.[33] In this series, patients who did not improve clinically with antibiotics alone underwent percutaneous drainage; the treatment was curative in 67% of cases. The remaining patients required additional surgical intervention. In the same year, Lang reported a series of 33 patients with percutaneously drained renal and perirenal abscesses. In this series, 90% of the abscesses were eradicated without surgical intervention. All patients required some repositioning of catheter subsequent to the initial drainage, and 11 patients required additional catheter placement to break up loculations.[34]

Causes of failure in these series include complex collections with multiple loculations, renal stones, osteomyelitis, necrotic renal tissue, and tumor. As with percutaneous drainage of collections elsewhere in the abdomen, there is an inverse relationship between the complexity of a renal or perirenal collection and the success of percutaneous drainage. As complexity increases, efficacy of percutaneous drainage generally decreases. As demonstrated by Lang, this can be offset by aggressive catheter repositioning, as well as placement of additional catheters to break up loculations. In the setting of an infected renal cyst, renal stones can serve as a nidus of infection and therefore decrease the success of percutaneous drainage. When possible, an attempt is made to remove such stones percutaneously at the time of drainage. Similarly, if bone adjacent to a perirenal infection has become colonized, the success of percutaneous abscess drainage decreases. Definitive surgical treatment of infected bone is usually required to eradicate a perirenal abscess. Lastly, colonization of necrotic tissue or tumor by bacteria can give rise to abscesses. These collections are almost never successfully eradicated with percutaneous drainage and require surgical intervention. Percutaneous drainage can be used as a temporizing measure in this setting before definitive surgical treatment. In rare cases, a drain may be placed in a tumor abscess as a palliative measure in a patient who is not a surgical candidate. Before placement, the patient is made aware that the drain will have to remain in place for the life of the patient.

COMPLICATIONS

Major complications resulting from percutaneous renal and perirenal collections are rare. Published complications include sepsis requiring intervention, hemorrhage requiring transfusion, superinfection of sterile fluid collections, bowel transgression requiring intervention, and pleural transgression requiring intervention.[32-34] Hemorrhage requiring transfusion usually is the result of laceration of visceral arteries, spleen, or liver. Hemorrhage is more likely in patients with uncorrected coagulopathies and patients with difficult access routes for drainage. Every attempt should be made to correct any underlying coagulopathy to minimize bleeding risks. Additionally, the safest access route for collection drainage is selected to avoid organs and vessels.

Patients commonly become bacteremic after the procedure and develop a fever.[34] This is not considered a major complication and occurs with relative frequency. Four of 33 patients in the series published by Lang experienced transient febrile episodes.[34] The patient should defervesce by postprocedure day 2.[35] Septic shock and bacteremia requiring new intervention are considered major complications. Superinfection of sterile cavities is also considered a major complication. For this reason, sterile technique is employed when performing drainage of any fluid collection.[35]

Enteric complications include bowel perforation with resultant fistula formation and/or peritonitis. These complications can occur if bowel is transgressed en route to abscess drainage or when a catheter erodes into adjacent bowel.[32] In either case, if the catheter tip is placed within the bowel, the catheter is left in place, and a second catheter is placed into the abscess cavity. The catheter is then left within the bowel to allow an epithelialized tract to form, which takes between 10 and 15 days. The catheter can then be safely removed, and the tract will close spontaneously. Transgression of the pleura with catheter placement can result in pleural fluid collections and/or pneumothorax.[34,36] If clinically significant, these collections and pneumothoraces can be treated with chest tube placement.[37]

POSTPROCEDURAL AND FOLLOW-UP CARE

After the catheter has been placed in a renal or perirenal collection, the interventional radiology service should play an active role in catheter management. A collaborative approach with surgical and medical consultants helps maintain a uniform treatment plan. Moreover, because of the wide array of catheters available to different medical specialties, nursing, medical, and surgical staff may not be familiar with the types of catheters employed by interventional radiologists. Therefore, staying involved to evaluate the need for repositioning, exchange, placement of additional catheters, and removal is an important part of interventional radiology follow-up. On daily rounds, the radiologist can inspect the catheter, assess its connections, and determine the quantity and character of the drainage output as well as condition of the patient.[38,39]

The major criteria for catheter removal include clinical improvement of the patient, improvement in the patient's laboratory tests, decreased drainage from the catheter, resolution of the cavity, and absence of a fistula. As already noted, it is not unusual for patients to become febrile in the first 24 hours with transient bacteremia, but they should defervesce by postprocedural day 2. Additionally, a patient's laboratory tests should improve over a similar time course and normalize within 48 to 72 hours. If clinical status and laboratory tests are not improving, the possibility of undrained collections should be considered.

Catheter outputs are another useful indicator of when a catheter should be removed. Catheter outputs must be followed closely. The nondraining catheter (outputs of 0 to 20 mL/day) is one of the most common clinical scenarios to face the team caring for the patient after catheter placement. Diagnostic possibilities include obstruction of the drainage catheter, presence of a loculated/fibrinous collection, catheter migration out of the abscess, or complete drainage of the collection. When drainage decreases, catheter patency is evaluated by a simple flush with 3 to 5 mL of sterile saline. Causes of obstruction include stopcock malfunction, internal or external kinking of the catheter, or obstruction of the lumen by debris or blood. Evaluation of the catheter at the bedside includes inspection of the stopcock and external portion of the catheter as well as gentle flushing of the catheter with saline. If the problem cannot be resolved at the bedside, additional imaging is indicated to evaluate catheter position and collection size. If the catheter is in the correct position and the collection remains, it is likely the material within the collection is too particulate or fibrinous to drain. Solutions to this problem include exchanging the catheter for a larger catheter or instilling thrombolytic therapy. If the catheter has moved out of the collection, the catheter can be repositioned or replaced.

In the setting of an infected collection, if fever persists or drainage increases or remains high (>100 mL/day), it is necessary to re-image with CT or an abscessogram to evaluate for a residual abscess or development of new abscesses or communication with the bowel. Up to 40% of catheters require repositioning or placement of additional drainage catheters.[40] In the series published by Lang et al., which reported the highest success curative rate for percutaneous renal/perirenal abscess drainage, catheter repositioning was performed in all 33 cases, and additional catheters were added in 11 patients. Fistulas can be to the bladder, pancreatic duct, or bile duct, but the most common fistula to occur after abscess drainage is to the bowel.[41] The presence of a fistula can be confirmed with a fluoroscopically guided catheter injection using iodinated dye. The catheter should remain in place long enough for enteric communication to close. Many of these communications close within 2 weeks,[39] but it is not unusual for fistulas to close over weeks to months.

In the case of a urinoma, although there is no absolute quantity of output from a drainage catheter that indicates the presence of a continuous urine leak, outputs are expected to decrease daily. Similarly, on follow-up imaging, the urinoma should decrease in size. If outputs from the catheter do not decrease, or if the urinoma does not demonstrate evidence of resolution on follow-up imaging despite an appropriately placed urinoma drainage catheter, diversion of urine to allow healing of the defect in the collecting system should be considered. This can be achieved with a percutaneous nephrostomy catheter in addition to the percutaneous urinoma drainage catheter to decompress the collecting system and facilitate urinary drainage. In some cases, however, a nephrostomy catheter alone may not be sufficient to divert enough urine to allow for healing of the defect in the collecting system. In these cases, it is necessary to place a nephrostomy catheter in combination with placement of a ureteral stent or nephro-ureteral catheter. The combination of a percutaneous drainage catheter with either a nephrostomy catheter and a ureteral stent or with a nephroureteral catheter can allow for greater diversion of urine away from the area of the leak and promote healing of the collecting system.[42-44]

KEY POINTS

- Percutaneous drainage is an effective technique for treating many infected renal and perirenal collections.
- The technique can be employed as a curative procedure or as a temporizing measure before definitive surgical treatment.
- Urinomas are frequently amenable to treatment with percutaneous drainage alone or percutaneous drainage in combination with urinary diversion techniques.

► **SUGGESTED READINGS**

Bernardino ME, Baumgartner BR. Abscess drainage in the genitourinary tract. Radiol Clin North Am 1986;24:539–49.

Deyoe LA, Cronan JJ, Lambiase RE, Dorfman GS. Percutaneous drainage of renal and perirenal abscesses: Results in 30 patients. AJR Am J Roentgenol 1990;155:81–3.

Gore RM, Balfe DM, Aizenstein RI, Silverman PM. The great escape: interfascial decompression planes of the retroperitoneum. AJR Am J Roentgenol 2000;175:363–70.

Lambiase RE, Deyoe L, Cronan JJ, Dorfman GS. Percutaneous drainage of 335 consecutive abscesses: results of primary drainage with 1-year follow-up. Radiology 1992;184:167–79.

Lang EK. Renal, perirenal, and pararenal abscesses: percutaneous drainage. Radiology 1990;174:109–13.

Lang EK, Glorioso 3rd L. Management of urinomas by percutaneous drainage procedures. Radiol Clin North Am 1986;24:551–9.

Sacks D, Banner MP, Meranze SG, et al. Renal and related retroperitoneal abscesses: Percutaneous drainage. Radiology 1988;167:447–51.

Talner LB, Davidson AJ, Lebowitz RL, et al. Acute pyelonephritis: Can we agree on terminology? Radiology 1994;192:297–305.

Titton RL, Gervais DA, Hahn PF, et al. Urine leaks and urinomas: diagnosis and imaging-guided intervention. Radiographics 2003;23:1133–47.

vanSonnenberg E, Wittich GR, Goodacre BW, et al. Percutaneous abscess drainage: update. World J Surg 2001;25:362–9; discussion 370–72.

The complete reference list is available online at www.expertconsult.com.

CHAPTER 148

Thermal Ablation of Renal Cell Carcinoma

Kamran Ahrar, Surena F. Matin, and Michael J. Wallace

In 2013, over 65,150 new cases of kidney cancer were diagnosed in the United States, resulting in over 13,680 deaths.[1] Renal parenchymal tumors (i.e., renal cell carcinoma [RCC]) account for the majority (85%) of kidney cancers.[2] Urothelial cancers of the renal pelvis (i.e., transitional cell carcinoma [TCC]) account for most of the remaining cases. The incidence of RCC has increased on average 2% to 3% a year for the past 3 decades.[3] At present, over 50% of RCCs are detected incidentally during imaging studies prompted by nonurologic complaints.[4,5] Tumors detected incidentally are smaller (stage I [Table 148-1]) at diagnosis and are often asymptomatic.[3] Partial nephrectomy is the standard of care for small RCCs and provides excellent results. Recurrence-free survival, cancer-specific survival, and overall survival rates for open or laparoscopic partial nephrectomy have been reported as better than 95%, 97%, and 89%, respectively.[6] Other alternative treatment options advocated by the American Urological Association (AUA) include active surveillance and thermal ablative therapies.[6]

Thermal ablative therapies destroy tumors by using thermal energy—either heat (e.g., radiofrequency [RF], laser, microwave, or focused ultrasound) or cold (e.g., cryoablation).[7] The technologies most widely used in clinical practice for ablation of renal tumors are RF ablation (RFA) (Figs. 148-1 to 148-4) and cryoablation (Figs 148-5 and 148-6). Laser, microwave, and high-intensity focused ultrasound technologies are in various stages of experimental or early clinical application but have not been utilized to any substantial degree in clinical practice for treating renal tumors. With either cryoablation or RFA, once the tumor is ablated, it is left in situ. This is a departure from the basic oncologic surgical principle of excision with clear margins. For ablation technology to be considered a clinically acceptable alternative to extirpation, it must be reliable and completely destroy all viable tumor. There must also be a means of imaging and monitoring the area of ablation to preserve and protect surrounding vital structures while ensuring complete tumor destruction. Thermal ablation of renal tumors can be performed either intraoperatively or percutaneously. Historically, RFA has been used most commonly for percutaneous image-guided ablation, whereas cryoablation has been used most commonly in open or laparoscopic approaches.[8] More recently, small-diameter cryoprobes have become available for percutaneous use, resulting in an increasing number of percutaneous cryoablation procedures. At the same time, more urologic surgeons have adopted intraoperative RFA over cryoablation, resulting in an increasing number of laparoscopic RFA procedures.

The basic principles of thermal ablation are discussed elsewhere in this volume. In this chapter, we briefly discuss specific ablation devices that are commonly used to treat RCC. Our main focus is a review of indications, contraindications, technique, complications, follow-up care, and outcomes of percutaneous thermal ablation of RCC.

ABLATION DEVICES

Radiofrequency Ablation

Currently, three RFA devices have been approved by the U.S. Food and Drug Administration (FDA) and are commercially available in the United States. Each of these uses a generator to deliver alternating electric current via an electrode, causing ionic agitation and frictional heating within the target tissue. Each of these ablation systems uses a different strategy to obtain the largest possible zone of ablation. The maximum attainable in vivo ablation zone varies by applicator size and design and is consistently less than the ex vivo maximum,[9] in part owing to the presence of adjacent flowing blood or large fluid-filled structures that produce a cooling or heat sink effect.

RF applicators range in size from 17 to 14 gauge and vary in design. The RITA StarBurst probe (AngioDynamics, Latham, N.Y.) and the LeVeen electrode (Boston Scientific, Natick, Mass.) are both multi-tined applicators with an expandable array design that allows for a scalable teardrop-shaped or spherical ablation zone. The Covidien system (Covidien, Mansfield, Mass.) uses a straight probe design with a central channel that allows for circulation of chilled fluid as the basis for an internally cooled electrode. The cooling of the electrode tip and the pulsed delivery of energy help prevent tissue charring or excess gas formation. This strategy is expected to maximize the potential zone of ablation. The Cool-tip electrodes (Covidien) are available as either a single configuration or a cluster configuration in which three closely spaced (<1 cm) straight electrodes in a triangle configuration are used to create a larger zone of ablation.

Cryoablation

The two cryoablation systems currently available in the United States for percutaneous image-guided ablation are the SeedNet System (Galil Medical, Arden Hills, Minn.) and Endocare (HealthTronics, Austin, Tex.). In both systems, highly compressed argon gas is allowed to expand in a Joules-Thompson chamber in the distal end of the cryoprobe, resulting in intense cooling that creates an ice ball within the target tissue. Helium is used in a similar fashion to actively thaw the ice ball. Cryoprobes used in percutaneous ablation range in size from 17 gauge to 2.4 mm in diameter. The critical temperature required to achieve tissue necrosis is −19.4°C in normal renal tissue[10] and −40°C in cancer cells.[11] This temperature must be transmitted throughout the entire tumor. There is a rapid drop in temperature at the edge of the ice ball, so to achieve the required temperature for cell death throughout the entire tumor, the ice ball must extend at least 3.1 mm beyond the tumor margin.[12]

TABLE 148-1. American Joint Committee on Cancer TNM Staging of Renal Cell Carcinoma

	Primary Tumor*	Node	Metastasis
Stage I	T1	N0	M0
Stage II	T2	N0	M0
Stage III	T1 or T2	N1	M0
	T3	N0 or N1	M0
Stage IV	T4	Any N	M0
	Any T	Any N	M1

From Edge SB, Byrd DR, Compton CC, et al, editors. AJCC Cancer Staging Manual. 7th ed. New York: Springer; 2009.
*Primary Tumor:
T1: Tumor is 7 cm or less in greatest dimension and is limited to the kidney.
T1a: Tumor is 4 cm or less.
T1b: Tumor is greater than 4 cm but less than 7 cm.
T2: Tumor is more than 7 cm in greatest dimension and is limited to the kidney.
T3: Tumor extends into major veins or invades the adrenal gland, sinus fat, or perinephric fat, but does not extend beyond Gerota fascia.
T3a: Tumor invades the adrenal gland.
T3b: Tumor grossly extends into the renal vein or vena cava below the diaphragm.
T3c: Tumor grossly extends into the vena cava above the diaphragm.
T4: Tumor invades beyond Gerota fascia.

INDICATIONS

The technical and clinical success rates of thermal ablation procedures are highly dependent on the appropriate selection of cases. Both patient factors and tumor factors must be carefully considered.

Patient Selection

Thermal ablation is an alternative to partial nephrectomy in patients who may not be good surgical candidates, have multiple RCCs, have limited renal function, or refuse surgical intervention.[13] The majority of incidentally detected small renal tumors are diagnosed in older patients who may have other medical comorbidities (e.g., cardiovascular or respiratory conditions) that result in an unacceptably high operative risk (see Fig. 148-1). In patients with renal insufficiency and those with only one anatomic or functioning kidney, preservation of renal function is of utmost importance.[14] Thermal ablative therapies are superior to partial nephrectomy in preserving renal function, so ablative therapy should be considered for patients with limited renal function, because it may help minimize the need for dialysis in the future. When residual or recurrent disease is identified after nephron-sparing surgery or ablation, thermal ablation should be considered as the least invasive therapy.

Patients with von Hippel-Lindau disease, hereditary papillary cell carcinoma, or hereditary clear cell carcinoma have a genetic predisposition for RCC. Many of these patients will ultimately require nephrectomy, but ablative therapy may prolong the time to resection.[15] Patients with multiple synchronous RCCs (sporadic or genetic) may be treated with surgical resection of the larger lesions and ablation of the smaller lesions (see Fig. 148-3).

Proximity of the RCC to the central collecting system, bowel, pancreas, adrenal glands, liver, or gallbladder may be a relative contraindication to percutaneous thermal ablation or may necessitate additional measures to avoid thermal injury to these structures during the procedure.

For the most part, thermal ablation of renal tumors is indicated for patients with tumors confined to the kidney. As such, metastatic disease, local invasion, nodal involvement, and extension into the renal vein or inferior vena cava are relative contraindications to ablative therapy. On the other hand, when isolated metastases are amenable to surgical or ablative therapy, ablation of the primary tumor can provide durable local control.[16]

When RCC causes hematuria, embolization should be considered first-line therapy; however, utilizing RFA for palliation of intractable hematuria has also been reported.[17,18]

Tumor Selection

Tumor size and location should be carefully considered prior to choosing ablation therapy. Most published series indicate that complete ablation can be more easily achieved for smaller tumors. In general, an ideal tumor for percutaneous RFA is smaller than 4 cm.[19,20] As the tumor size increases, the technical success rate decreases. In a study of 125 RCCs, for each 1-cm increase in tumor diameter beyond 3.6 cm, the likelihood of tumor-free survival decreased by a factor of 2.19.[20] Furthermore, when RCC grows outward and does not abut or invade the collecting system, thermal ablation can be more easily achieved.[19,21] Gervais et al. described a classification scheme for renal tumors with respect to their location.[22] In their system, tumors with at least 25% of their volume extending beyond the renal contour, with no tumor extending into or adjacent to the renal sinus, are classified as *exophytic*. RCCs that are entirely confined to the cortex without any contact with or invasion of the renal sinus are classified as *intraparenchymal*. Tumors that grow internally into the renal sinus are classified as *central*. And finally, when tumors have both exophytic and central components, they are classified as *mixed tumors*. From a practical standpoint, the exophytic and intraparenchymal tumors can be considered "noncentral" tumors, and similarly, the central and mixed tumors can be considered "central" tumors. Satisfactory short-term results have been reported with ablation of large tumors (>4 cm) and central tumors, but more than one ablation session may be necessary, and hemorrhagic complications may be more common in these cases.[19,21,23]

Close proximity of the tumor to other vital structures such as bowel or pancreas should be considered. Adjuvant techniques may have to be used to isolate the kidney and separate the tumor from other structures that may be damaged by thermal energy.

CONTRAINDICATIONS

The only absolute contraindication to ablation therapy is uncorrectable coagulopathy. The majority of other "relative" contraindications, such as systemic illness or sepsis, usually can be treated before the ablation procedure. An additional contraindication to percutaneous ablation is when adjacent vital structures such as bowel cannot be separated from the zone of ablation by accepted techniques and thus cannot be protected from the effects of thermal energy.

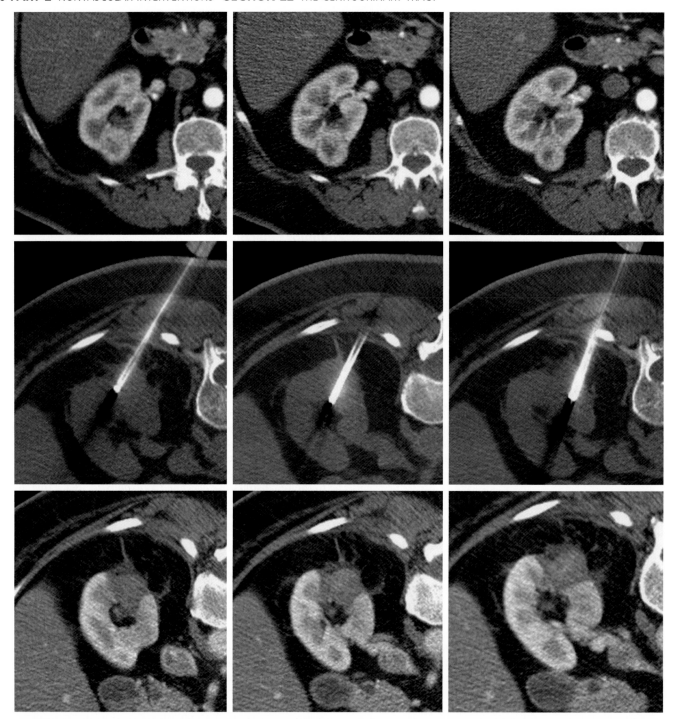

FIGURE 148-1. *Top row,* This 70-year-old woman with multiple medical comorbid conditions was found to have a 3-cm solid, enhancing mass involving posterior aspect of right kidney. *Middle row,* She was treated with computed tomography (CT)-guided percutaneous radiofrequency ablation. Three overlapping ablations were performed. *Bottom row,* Immediately after ablation, axial contrast-enhanced CT images demonstrate high-density changes within tumor, lack of enhancement indicating margin of ablation zone, and a general reduction in size of exophytic tumor. *(Copyright Kamran Arhar, MD.)*

TECHNIQUE

Patient Assessment

All patients should undergo a preprocedural assessment that includes serum creatinine level, estimated glomerular filtration rate (GFR), platelet count, and a coagulation profile. Patients with proven RCC should have chest imaging (e.g., chest radiograph) and a metabolic profile. These are standard basic tests for surveillance of metastatic disease, the incidence of which is very low but still possible for small tumors. Patients also should be assessed for their ability to tolerate intravenous sedation and should meet institutional criteria. Local institutional factors and physician preferences determine whether intravenous sedation[19] or general anesthesia[24,25] is used during ablation therapy. General

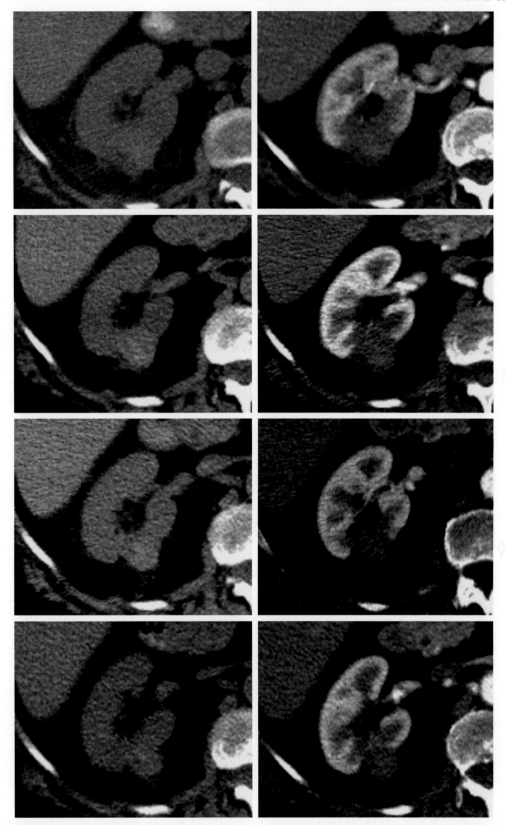

FIGURE 148-2. Follow-up unenhanced *(left)* and contrast-enhanced *(right)* axial computed tomography images of patient in Figure 148-1 at 1, 6, 12, and 24 months demonstrate evolution of postablation changes: persistent high-density material in ablation zone, lack of enhancement, and a thin halo of soft tissue density in perinephric fat. *(Copyright Kamran Arhar, MD.)*

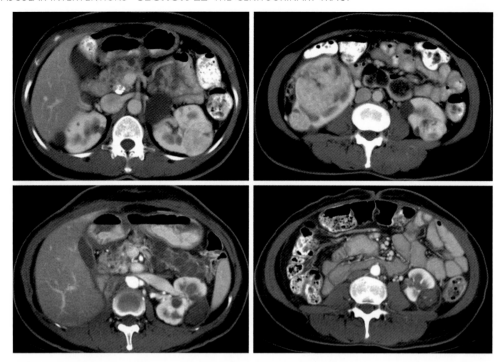

FIGURE 148-3. *Top,* This 42-year-old woman was diagnosed with bilateral solid, enhancing renal tumors. She also had bilateral renal cysts and multiple pancreatic cysts. A genetic workup confirmed diagnosis of von Hippel-Lindau disease. She required right nephrectomy for a large renal cell carcinoma that had replaced most of right kidney. Two separate tumors in left kidney were treated with percutaneous radiofrequency ablation. *Bottom,* Axial computed tomography images at 2 years demonstrate no enhancement in ablation zones in left kidney. *(Copyright Kamran Arhar, MD.)*

anesthesia optimizes patient tolerance, allows greater control of respiratory motion when the applicators are being placed, and may facilitate accurate tumor targeting.

A percutaneous biopsy is recommended prior to ablation of renal tumors.[26] The differential diagnosis of a small enhancing renal mass includes benign entities such as lipid-poor angiomyolipoma, oncocytoma, papillary adenoma, and metanephric adenoma. As the size of a renal mass decreases, the likelihood of a benign diagnosis increases. Approximately 25% of renal tumors smaller than 4 cm are benign, but when tumors smaller than 1 cm were resected, over 40% were benign.[27] About 5% of angiomyolipomas are indistinguishable from small RCCs on cross-sectional imaging.[28] Tuncali et al. reviewed biopsy and imaging data of 27 patients referred for cryoablation of a small renal mass.[29] Ten lesions (37%) smaller than 2 cm were deemed benign.

The "diagnostic accuracy" of renal biopsy has improved over the years, particularly with the addition of routine core biopsies, and is better than 95% in most contemporary series. Sensitivity for detection of malignancy ranges from 84% to 100% in studies of renal masses published after 2006.[30] When percutaneous biopsy establishes a diagnosis (e.g., lymphoma or angiomyolipoma) other than RCC, ablation is not indicated. A positive result with diagnosis of RCC provides details about tumor subtype and grade, information that may become relevant during follow-up visits, insurance claims, or should the patient ever develop metastatic disease requiring systemic therapy. A positive result is also important for the validation of ablation therapy and defining the standard of care for small renal masses in the future. On the other hand, concerns over false-negative biopsy results remain; some clinicians recommend

proceeding with therapy when a negative histologic result conflicts with imaging findings.[31,32] Ideally, the biopsy should be performed during a separate encounter so sufficient time is given for a complete histologic evaluation.

For large tumors (>4 cm), consideration may be given to selective embolization prior to ablation. Embolization may help improve the effectiveness of ablation by reducing perfusion-mediated cooling (the "heat sink effect" during RFA) or heating (during cryoablation) and may help reduce the risk of hemorrhagic complications.[33-35]

Imaging Modalities

Ultrasonography, computed tomography (CT), and magnetic resonance imaging (MRI) have been used to guide renal ablation proceures.[25,36-38] Ultrasonography provides valuable real-time multiplanar imaging for initial tumor targeting and placement of the applicators. Some investigators have reported favorable outcomes for ultrasound-guided RFA compared with other imaging modalities.[39] However, inability to visualize the tumor, gas bubbles during RFA, and large tumor size limit the effectiveness of ultrasonography.[40] During cryoablation procedures, the edge of the ice ball creates intense acoustic shadowing that precludes assessment of the leading edge of the ablation zone.[41-43] Ultrasonography is not optimal for assessment of nearby loops of bowel, and images may become degraded by perinephric hematoma that may develop during the procedure.

Currently, CT is the imaging modality most widely used for percutaneous image-guided renal ablation.[19,24,25] It provides guidance for precise probe placement and is not affected by gas formation during RFA. CT is ideal for

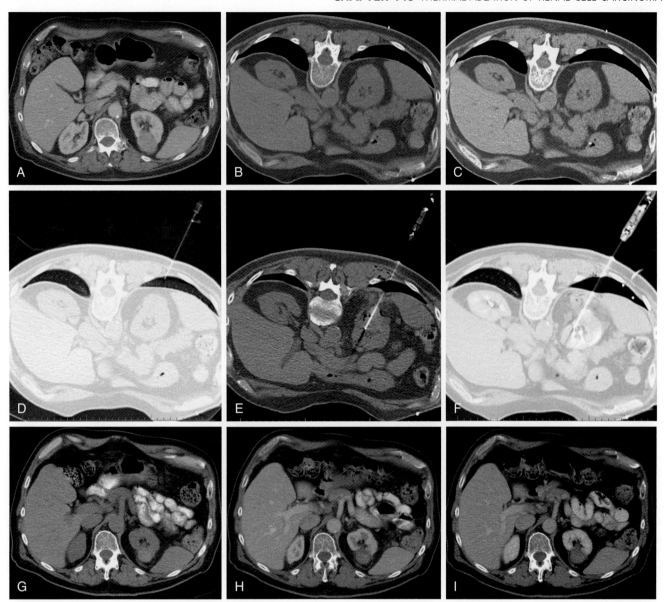

FIGURE 148-4. A, This 70-year-old man with multiple medical comorbid conditions was found to have a 4-cm mass involving upper pole of left kidney. **B-C,** He was referred for percutaneous radiofrequency ablation. Axial computed tomography (CT) images obtained with patient prone demonstrate interposition of lung parenchyma between chest wall and renal tumor. **D,** A blunt-tipped needle was placed in pleural space, and air was injected to separate parietal and visceral pleura, creating a controlled pneumothorax. **E-F,** Axial CT images demonstrate transpleural course of radiofrequency ablation electrode without puncturing visceral pleura. A pneumothorax evacuation tube was placed under CT guidance before termination of procedure. Tube was removed the next morning. **G-I,** Follow-up axial CT images at 6 months taken before contrast, in arterial phase, and in late phase demonstrate stable high-density changes with no evidence of enhancement (CT Hounsfield units measured 64, 60, and 59, respectively). *(Copyright Kamran Arhar, MD.)*

monitoring other vital structures (e.g., bowel) that may come in contact with the tumor. During cryoablation, the location and size of the ice ball can be visualized rather clearly on CT (see Fig. 148-6),[44] whereas in RFA the ablation zone is less clearly visualized, and the boundary between treated and untreated tissue is not precisely demarcated. To overcome this problem, a contrast-enhanced postablation CT examination is typically performed just before completing the RFA (see Fig. 148-1).[24,25] CT fluoroscopy enables real-time visualization of the applicator tip as it is being placed and facilitates precise targeting of the tumor. The main disadvantage of CT or CT fluoroscopy is patient and operator exposure to ionizing radiation. For this reason,

some researchers advocate using a combination of ultrasonography and CT. Ultrasonography can be used for initial placement of the applicators, and CT can be used for any additional imaging during the procedure, including repositioning the electrodes, monitoring adjacent loops of bowel, assessing the size and margins of the ice ball, and performing a contrast-enhanced study to confirm complete tumor ablation.

MRI is an ideal imaging modality for ablation guidance and monitoring because it provides excellent soft-tissue contrast and spatial resolution compared with CT and ultrasound.[37,38,45] In addition to providing multiplanar and near real-time imaging, MRI also allows for monitoring of

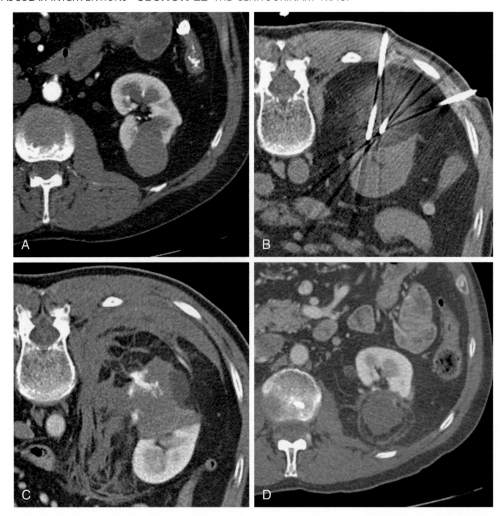

FIGURE 148-5. **A,** This 53-year-old man with history of esophageal cancer was found to have a 3.6 cm left renal tumor. Biopsy showed renal cell carcinoma, papillary type 1. **B,** Axial computed tomography (CT) image of kidney during cryoablation shows three of the four cryoprobes engulfed in a low-density ice ball. **C,** Immediately after two freeze/thaw cycles, contrast-enhanced CT showed active extravasation and associated retroperitoneal hematoma. Selective embolization (not shown) was promptly performed because of dropping blood pressure. **D,** Contrast-enhanced follow-up CT image at 12 months shows zone of ablation with no evidence of residual disease. *(Copyright Kamran Arhar, MD.)*

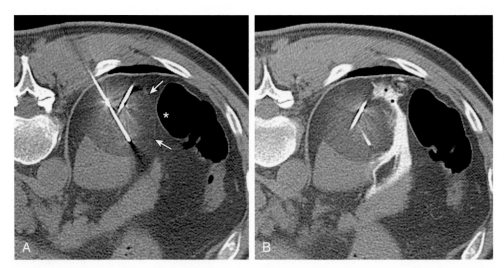

FIGURE 148-6. **A,** Axial computed tomography image of kidney during cryoablation of a left upper pole tumor shows close proximity of growing ice ball *(arrows)* to colon *(star)*. **B,** Hydrodissection was performed by injection of 180 mL of sterile fluid with a small amount of iodinated contrast to separate colon from ice ball. *(Copyright Kamran Arhar, MD.)*

tissue coagulation and treatment results,[37] which CT does not. Also, the lack of ionizing radiation is a significant advantage over CT. Unfortunately, current challenges in producing special MRI-compatible equipment and the lack of availability of interventional MRI units have limited its use in daily clinical practice.

Ablation Procedure

Optimal patient positioning is determined during the planning phase when cross-sectional images are reviewed to assess the feasibility and safety of access to the target tumor. In a typical ablation procedure, the patient is placed in the prone position. During CT-guided procedures, it is helpful to move the arms away from the body in an abducted and extended position and place them next to the patient's head ("the superman position"). This reduces streak artifact and facilitates tumor visualization. When patients are under general anesthesia, care must be taken to not overextend the arms and to provide adequate padding to avoid brachial plexus injury.[46] An ipsilateral decubitus position can help reduce the risk of pneumothorax, although it may limit access to the tumor for insertion of the applicators. A contralateral decubitus position can help separate loops of bowel from a tumor in the anterior or lateral aspect of the kidney. In rare instances, anteriorly or laterally located tumors may be treated with the patient in the supine position. An ablation margin of 5 to 10 mm around the tumor is desirable.[12] The size of the ablation zone depends on the size and vascularity of the lesion, the lesion's proximity to vascular structures, the ablation modality used, and the number, size, and configuration of the applicators. Care must be taken to avoid adjacent vital structures such as bowel and large vessels, and consideration must be given to both the potential applicator path and the projected zone of ablation. When vital structures are detected in the path of the applicator or are contiguous with the expected ablation zone, simple and noninvasive measures may suffice to render the procedure safe. These maneuvers include changing the patient's position or levering the applicator against the skin to lift the tumor off the bowel or vascular structure. Torquing the applicator can potentially increase the distance from the tumor to the bowel by 3 or 4 mm.[47] Ideally, a safe margin between the probe tines and the nearest adjacent bowel is 1 to 2 cm.[48]

To protect nearby structures such as bowel, nerves, or muscles, gas insufflation or hydrodissection (see Fig. 148-6) can be used to create a barrier for heat transmission.[19,49,50] During RFA procedures, nonionic sterile fluid may be instilled using a small-gauge needle placed between the tumor and the bowel under CT or MRI guidance. With injection of 135 to 150 mL of fluid, one can displace the adjacent bowel loop by 2.1 to 2.5 cm.[50] Often, additional hydrodissection attempts are necessary because the fluid spills into the paracolic gutters or Morrison pouch.[50] Alternatively, gas can be insufflated into the peritoneal cavity or perinephric space to prevent thermal damage to adjacent vital structures. Gas has a tendency to dissipate throughout the peritoneal space; thus, larger volumes of gas are required compared with fluid. When injected into the peritoneum, a gas volume of 1200 mL yields 1.5 cm of bowel displacement.[51] When injected into the perirenal space, 15 to 20 mL of gas may be sufficient to achieve a similar degree of bowel separation.[52] Adequacy of insufflation is best monitored with CT because gas can obscure the view of the tumor when MRI or ultrasonography is used.[51]

If hydrodissection does not create the desired effect, large angioplasty or esophageal dilation balloons may be inserted between the tumor and the structure at risk.[48] More than one balloon may be necessary to create an adequate separation between the ablation zone and adjacent structures. Each balloon may be placed in coaxial fashion through an introducer sheath. Initially, a needle is inserted into the desired space. Over a guidewire, an introducer sheath is advanced into the desired position. The balloon is then placed into the sheath but not beyond it. With the balloon in position, the sheath is withdrawn. Balloon expansion is completed once the optimal position has been obtained.

Peripheral thermosensors can be placed to ensure adequate ablation and to prevent thermal injury to normal renal parenchyma and adjacent structures (e.g., periureteric tissue). Carey et al. reported 100% primary effectiveness for RFA of 37 tumors that were 3-5 cm in diameter in which real-time temperature feedback of the ablation zone was used to determine the appropriate treatment endpoint.[53] Ablation was continued until both deep and peripheral thermosensors recorded temperatures of at least 60°C. These independent real-time thermosensors can also be used to determine whether and where an electrode has to be redeployed.

Thermal damage to the ureter or ureteropelvic junction (UPJ) can lead to stricture formation. To reduce this risk during RFA of an adjacent renal mass, retrograde pyeloperfusion with a cooled nonionic solution can be performed.[54-56] In this technique, a 5F to 6F ureteral catheter is placed in retrograde fashion for infusion of cooled fluid into the renal pelvis. A 14F to 16F Foley catheter is placed in the bladder for drainage. Cantwell et al. described infusion of 1.5 to 2.0 L of 5% dextrose in water cooled overnight to 2° to 6°C at a pressure of 80 cm H_2O.[56] The ureteral catheter and the Foley catheter are removed at the end of the procedure.

Froemming et al. described a probe retraction technique used to protect the ureter during cryoablation.[57] After the cryoprobe is positioned, its proximity to important structures is assessed using CT. Activation of the cryoprobe creates an initial small ice ball that fixes the cryoprobe in relation to the tumor and also acts as a point of fixation for manipulation. By manipulating the applicators, one can retract the tumor and kidney away from structures to be avoided (e.g., the ureter). Cryoablation can then be resumed with standard freeze/thaw cycles.

Renal tumors involving the upper pole of the kidney pose a risk of pneumothorax. To minimize this risk, triangulation and oblique trajectories may be considered, avoiding the lung base. Placing the patient in the ipsilateral decubitus position elevates the lung base on that side and thus reduces the plane of contact between the tumor and overlying lung. However, access to the tumor may be more limited in this position. In order to access tumors in the upper pole of the kidney, an iatrogenic pneumothorax may be created such that the electrodes would not traverse the visceral pleura or lung parenchyma (see Fig. 148-4).[58] This procedure involves placing an 18- or 20-gauge needle and injecting gas (e.g., air) into the pleural space. After ablation is completed, the pneumothorax is treated with simple aspiration or placement of a small-bore (8F-10F) chest catheter under CT guidance. Alternatively, one can create an iatrogenic pleural effusion by injecting nonionic fluid instead of gas. This technique allows for precise placement and repositioning of the RFA electrodes under CT guidance, without repeated puncture of the visceral pleura.

For RFA with unipolar devices, two to four dispersive electrodes are applied to the upper thighs. During prolonged ablations, the thighs should be checked periodically to assess for potential skin burns around the dispersive electrodes. Multi-tined RFA electrodes can be used for ablation of renal tumors, but care must be taken to avoid puncturing the collecting system, renal vasculature, or adjacent structures with the tines. Cool-tip RFA electrodes are needle-like in design and easier to place than multi-tined electrodes. Using a single electrode, overlapping ablations are often required to create a zone of ablation large enough to cover the entire tumor and a tumor-free margin. As many as three Cool-tip RFA electrodes can be inserted simultaneously. A switch box allows delivery of power to each electrode sequentially to achieve large areas of ablation.

Cryoprobes used for percutaneous ablation are small in diameter (17 gauge to 2.4 mm) and create ice balls with cytotoxic isotherms that are often too small to completely ablate most renal tumors.[59] For this reason, multiple cryoprobes are often placed at the onset to take advantage of the synergy between the probes. Cryoprobes are placed 1 to 2 cm apart and no more than 1 cm from the tumor margin.[60] High technical success rates can be achieved even in large tumors (>4 cm), but hemorrhagic complication rates may be higher with insertion of multiple cryoprobes.[23]

Immediately after ablation, contrast-enhanced CT or MRI should be performed to assess the ablation zone, confirm complete ablation of the tumor, and rule out any complications. This is particularly relevant to RFA, during which treatment efficacy is difficult to assess. Immediately after RFA, contrast-enhanced CT shows a mild diffuse enhancement within the ablation zone. This should not be mistaken for residual tumor. The ablation zone can be better appreciated by identifying the relatively low-density, sharply demarcated margins and comparing these with the preablation imaging findings.[61] Additional imaging findings include perinephric fat stranding, thickening of the perirenal fascia, locules of gas in the surrounding tissue, perinephric or subcapsular hemorrhage, and fluid in the adjacent tissues or paracolic gutters that may relate to hydrodissection.[62] At some institutions, renal ablation procedures are performed on an outpatient basis,[20] whereas other institutions routinely admit patients[24] for overnight observation.

COMPLICATIONS

The incidence of complications after thermal ablation of RCC has been reported as 3% to 12%.[19,20,63,64] In a multicenter study of 271 ablation procedures,[63] a total of 30 complications (11.1%) were reported. Procedures included both RFA and cryoablation that were performed either percutaneously or intraoperatively. There were 5 major complications (1.8%), 25 minor complications (9.2%), and 1 death (0.4%). Major and minor complication rates were 1.4% and 12.2% for cryoablation and 2.2% and 6% for RFA,

respectively. Minor complications associated with the percutaneous approach included probe site pain or paresthesia, wound infection, hematuria, and (rarely) infarction.

Complications may arise from probe insertion or may be due to application of thermal energy. In most series, hemorrhage accounts for most of the major complications; it usually arises from direct mechanical injury to a vessel by the applicator. Tumors that are centrally located have an increased risk of hemorrhage, which may lead to hematuria and/or perinephric hematoma. In most cases, hemorrhage is self-limited and does not require treatment. Up to 2% of cases treated with RFA may require blood transfusion.[19] The risk of hemorrhage may be higher with cryoablation, particularly when large and central tumors are ablated (see Fig. 148-5). In a retrospective review of 108 lesions that were larger than 3 cm and treated with percutaneous cryoablation, Schmit et al. reported an 8% major complication rate.[65] Significant hemorrhage following removal of the cryoprobes from the ablated tumor occurred in four of the six patients who sustained a major complication. Fracture of the ice ball with associated parenchymal injury is a recognized complication of cryoablation that can result in significant hemorrhage.[66] Potential risk factors include use of larger-diameter or multiple cryoablation probes, initiation of a second adjacent ice ball after the primary ice ball has already been formed, and removal of the cryoablation probes before the ice ball has completely thawed.[66,67] If bleeding persists despite conservative measures and blood transfusion, transarterial embolization may be required. Massive hemorrhage due to an arteriovenous fistula is rare but has been described.[68]

When tumors are located in the upper pole of the kidney, the applicators may traverse the parietal pleura. In most cases, the visceral pleura remains intact and a pneumothorax is not encountered. The incidence of pneumothorax following ablation has been reported in up to 2% of cases.[20] The majority of cases can be managed conservatively. Moderate to severe pneumothorax or pneumothorax associated with new respiratory symptoms may require aspiration or chest tube placement. Seeding of the needle tract is another potential but rare complication of ablation therapy.[69]

Structures that are at greatest risk of thermal injury are the ureter, nerves, and adjacent bowel. During RFA of central tumors, the UPJ is at risk of thermal injury resulting in stricture and UPJ obstruction.[70] Some investigators think that compared to RFA, cryoablation has a higher safety profile with respect to the urothelium.[71] In a review of 129 CT-guided percutaneous cryoablation cases, the radiographic ice ball involved the sinus, with 41 ice balls overlapping the renal sinus by 6 mm or more. There were no cases of collecting system injuries in this series.[71] More inferiorly, thermal injury to the ureter has been reported at a rate of 1% to 2%,[19,20] and tumors in the medial aspect of the lower pole are at greatest risk of injury because of their close proximity to the ureter. The risk of ureteral stricture is higher when the distance between the tumor and ureter is less than 2 cm.[21] Retrograde pyeloperfusion can reduce the risk of thermal injury to the UPJ and ureter during ablation.[54-56] These injuries can manifest radiologically as ureteral wall thickening, periureteral fat stranding, hydronephrosis, or urinoma. If not promptly identified and treated, acute renal failure can ensue, leading to loss of the renal unit.[70] When the ablation zone involves the psoas muscle or posterior abdominal wall, nerve injuries may cause pain, paresthesia, or abdominal wall laxity.[72,73] A distance of less than 5 mm between the tumor and bowel is associated with increased risk of thermal injury to the bowel; this is most commonly encountered with lower-pole and posterior tumors.[48] Shortly after ablation, CT may demonstrate bowel wall thickening. In the weeks after the procedure, the bowel may adhere to the kidney, which may lead to a fistula.[74] Long-term serious sequelae include stricture, obstruction, and perforation. As discussed earlier, hydrodissection, injection of gas, and probe manipulation render ablation safer when bowel loops are in close proximity to the ablation zone.

FOLLOW-UP CARE

The technical success for ablation of renal tumors is determined by follow-up imaging consisting of CT or MRI studies. Detection of subtle abnormalities, which may be the only sign of residual or recurrent tumor, heavily depends on the quality of imaging studies. Renal protocol CT algorithms at most institutions consist of images that are obtained prior to contrast administration, in the corticomedullary phase of contrast enhancement, and in the excretory phase. Similarly, MRI studies are obtained before and after contrast administration. Persistent enhancing nodules in the ablation zone up to 3 months post treatment can indicate residual disease.[62] Recurrent disease is suspected if the ablation zone is enlarging on serial scans or if nodular contrast enhancement that was not present on the initial postablation study is identified.[62] In a multicenter study by Matin et al., 70% of all incomplete treatments were detected in the first 3 months after ablation, and over 90% were detected within 12 months of ablation.[75] Based on these observations, three to four imaging studies are recommended in the first year after ablative therapy, at 1, 3, 6 (optional), and 12 months (see Fig. 148-2).[75] In addition to evaluation of the ablation zone, the renal vein and inferior vena cava are evaluated for evidence of enlargement or abnormal enhancement. A search for a new primary tumor and metastatic disease is performed.

The RFA zone on follow-up CT studies appears as an area of nonenhancing soft tissue surrounded by normal enhancing renal parenchyma, giving it a "bull's-eye" appearance.[62] Over time, a thin band of soft tissue density forms, which engulfs the ablated tumor and the perinephric fat that was involved in the ablation zone. This "halo sign" develops in 75% of the cases.[76]

On MRI studies, the RFA zone is hypointense on T2-weighted sequences compared with normal renal parenchyma and can have variable intensity on T1-weighted sequences.[77,78] Subtraction of postgadolinium and noncontrast T1-weighted data may enhance detection of subtle foci of residual or recurrent disease.[77] Hemorrhage can artificially increase the size of the ablation zone on the immediate postprocedure scan, but the lesion should slowly involute to preablation size on serial scans.[79]

After cryotherapy, the zone of ablation is typically nonenhancing on CT and MRI surveillance studies, but residual contrast enhancement has been reported despite complete tumor ablation.[80-82] In a review of 32 lesions treated with laparoscopic cryoablation, Stein et al. identified persistent ablation zone enhancement in 15.6% (5/32) at 3 months; 3

of these lesions displayed enhancement at 6 months, and 1 displayed enhancement at 9 months.[80] The latter underwent partial nephrectomy that did not confirm recurrent cancer.[80] The ablation zone is frequently isointense on T1-weighted sequences and hypointense on T2-weighted sequences relative to the renal parenchyma. Involution of the tumor mass on surveillance studies is more prominent following cryoablation than RFA because of tissue resorption. After RFA, the lesion is replaced by scar tissue.[62] Gill et al. reported that tumor size decreased by an average of 75% 3 years after ablation, and an additional 38% of cryoablated tumors were not detectable by MRI at 3 years.[83]

With an increasing number of patients undergoing ablation, management and outcome of tumor recurrence after ablative therapy has received some attention in recent years. For recurrent tumors, further management options include active surveillance, repeat ablation, and surgical extirpation. Given that the median annual growth rate of small renal masses (<3.5 cm) is estimated at less than 0.28 cm, surveillance is acceptable.[84] Enhancement may be related to postprocedure inflammation, which often resolves with time. The majority of recurrences are managed with repeat ablation. Between 7.4% and 8.5% of all lesions treated with RFA and between 0.9% and 1.3% of all lesions treated with cryoablation are reablated.[8,85] In a review of 337 patients who underwent cryoablation and 283 patients who underwent RFA, Long et al. reported reablation rates of 2.5% for those who underwent percutaneous cryoablation, 8.8% for those who underwent percutaneous RFA, and 0% for those who underwent laparoscopic RFA or cryoablation.[85] The inferior results observed with RFA may relate to the inability to precisely monitor treatment efficacy during the procedure compared with cryoablation, and perhaps a lower threshold to repeat the percutaneous ablation in the presence of suspicious imaging results. Repeat ablation may be performed laparoscopically or percutaneously, although a second laparoscopic intervention is more difficult. Matin et al. reported a 4.2% incidence of local disease progression after repeat ablation at 2-year follow-up.[75] Salvage nephrectomy is reserved for patients for whom reablation failed or for patients whose tumor is too large for reablation. Partial nephrectomy is challenging but feasible,[86] and in our experience is much more facile after percutaneous ablation than after laparoscopic ablation. To preserve renal function, partial nephrectomy is preferred over total nephrectomy. Surgical resection is technically feasible, but intraoperative and postoperative complications are greater than with a first-time partial nephrectomy.

Patients with confirmed stage T1 RCC have a low but quantifiable risk of recurrence. Although there are no standardized guidelines based on prospective studies, most experts recommend an annual history and physical, chest imaging, and complete metabolic profiles in the first 5 years after treatment, with additional testing based on any abnormalities found.[87,88]

OUTCOMES

Assessment of outcomes after percutaneous ablative therapies for RCC has been very challenging for several reasons. The strongest criticisms of ablation therapy are the lack of pretreatment biopsies confirming the presence of malignancy, as well as lack of histologic evidence to confirm

TABLE 148-2. Long-Term Outcomes of Radiofrequency Ablation for Treatment of Renal Cell Carcinoma

Author, Year	Pts	No. of Tumors	Tumor Size	Pathology	Follow-up Period	Local Recurrence-Free Survival	Metastasis-Free Survival	Cancer-Specific Survival	Overall Survival
McDougal, 2005[95]	16	20	3.2 Mean (1.1-7.1)	100% RCC	55.2 (48-60)	93%	100%	100%	68.8%
Levinson, 2008[94]	31	31	2 Median (1-4)	Entire cohort	61.6 Median (41-80)	89.2%*	100%*	100%*	62%*
				16/31 (52%) RCC	57.4 Mean (41-80)	79.9%*	100%*	100%*	58%*
Tracy, 2010[96]	208	243	2.4 Mean (1-5.4)	Entire cohort	27 Mean (1.5-90)	93%†	NR	NR	85%†
				160/208 (76.9%) RCC	27 Mean (1.5-90)	90%†	95%†	99%†	NR
Zagoria, 2011[97]	41	48	2.6 Median (0.7-8.2)	100% RCC	56 Median (36-64)	88%	83%	97%	66%

Copyright Kamran Ahrar, MD.
*Eighty-month actuarial survival rates.
†Five-year actuarial survival rates.
NR, Not reported; *Pts,* patients; *RCC,* renal cell carcinoma.

eradication of the cancer from the kidney. Imaging with contrast-enhanced CT or MRI has been used as a surrogate for technical success after ablation of renal tumors. Successful complete ablation is defined as the absence of contrast enhancement on CT or MRI and is based on earlier radiologic-pathologic studies in RFA of the liver performed by Goldberg et al.[89] But the strategy of using imaging studies to define complete ablation is not free of pitfalls; both false-positive and false-negative results have been reported.[90,91]

Another criticism is that outcome data from many studies include lesions for which no histologic confirmation of malignancy was obtained prior to ablation. In a meta-analysis of studies performed prior to 2008, approximately 40% of lesions treated with percutaneous RFA were of unknown pathology.[8] Considering that 20% to 40% of small solid renal masses are benign or indolent cancers that would have done well without any treatment,[27,92] survival outcomes of ablation therapy may be overestimated, and an argument can be made in favor of active surveillance for some indolent tumors.

Finally, the lack of uniform reporting criteria has led to significant confusion when comparing different studies and different treatment options. For example, urologists performing laparoscopic cryoablation aim at eradicating the tumor in one session; therefore, in the urology literature any unablated tumor beyond the first attempt of ablation is considered a treatment failure. On the other hand, some radiologists have advocated that a single tumor may be ablated in more than one session, and thus residual tumor after a single ablation session should not be considered a treatment failure.[93]

The impact of these seemingly simple academic discrepancies is immense. In a meta-analysis that led to the development of "Guidelines for Management of the Clinical Stage I Renal Mass," the AUA defined a tumor as incompletely ablated if it required more than one ablation session to achieve elimination by radiographic criteria.[6] As such, when ablation studies were compared based only on the technique, percutaneous studies had significantly higher incomplete ablation rates than laparoscopic studies (13.9%

vs. 2.1%), and ablative studies were less optimal compared with surgical excision. Nevertheless, long-term data are now emerging in support of ablative therapy as a durable treatment option for patients with clinical stage I RCC, both in terms of oncologic efficacy and preservation of renal function.

Since the initial feasibility reports of RFA in the late 1990s, follow-up periods have increased progressively (Table 148-2).[94-97] Gervais et al. reported their single-institution experience over 6 years in which 100 tumors were ablated.[19,21] The rate of complete tumor ablation by imaging criteria was 90%, with tumors ranging from 1.1 to 5.5 cm in diameter (mean, 2.9 cm). Lesions 3 cm or smaller (n = 52), between 3 cm and 5 cm, and larger than 5 cm yielded complete ablation rates of 100%, 92%, and 25%, respectively. Ninety-two percent of all tumors 4 cm in diameter or smaller were completely ablated in the first session, and 8% required a second session for complete ablation. The mean follow-up period was 2.3 years (range, 3.5 months to 6 years). In a selected group of patients (n = 80) without multifocal/metastatic RCC or von Hippel-Lindau disease, Gervais et al. reported only one local recurrence during follow-up. McDougal et al. reported a 91% recurrence-free survival rate following RFA, with a mean follow-up of 54 months in 11 patients.[95] There were no reports of metastatic disease. Levinson et al. demonstrated an initial RFA success rate of 97%, a recurrence-free survival rate of 90.3%, and a metastasis-free survival rate of 100% in 34 patients with a mean follow-up of 62.4 months.[94] Tracy et al. reviewed outcomes of 208 patients with 243 renal masses who underwent RFA, with a mean follow-up of 27 months.[96] Of these patients, 93% underwent preablation biopsy, and 79% of the masses were confirmed as RCC. The initial treatment success rate was 97%. The 5-year recurrence-free survival rate of the 160 patients with biopsy-proven RCC was 90%. Three patients developed metastatic disease, and one patient died of RCC. The 5-year actuarial metastasis-free and cancer-specific survival rates were 95% and 99%, respectively.[96] Zagoria et al. reported long-term outcomes after percutaneous RFA of 48 RCC in

TABLE 148-3. Outcomes of Cryoablation for Treatment of Renal Cell Carcinoma

Author, Year	Pts	No. of Tumors	Tumor Size	Pathology	Follow-up Period	Local Recurrence-Free Survival	Metastasis-Free Survival	Cancer-Specific Survival	Overall Survival
Shingleton, 2001[82]	20	22	3 Mean (1.8-7)	NR	9.1 (3-14)	100%	NR	NR	NR
Silverman, 2005[38]	23	26	2.6 Mean (1-4.6)	24/26 (92%)	14 (4-30)	92%	NR	NR	NR
Gupta, 2006[44]	12	16	2.5 Mean (1-4.6)	12/16 (75%) RCC	5.9 (1.2-10.3)	94%	NR	NR	NR
Littrup, 2007[60]	48	49	3.3 Mean (1.7-7.2)	33/48 (69%) RCC	13.2 (0.2-45.6)	92%	NR	NR	88%
Atwell, 2010[59]	91	93	3.4 Mean (1.5-7.3)	44/93 (47%) RCC	26 (5-61)	95%	NR	NR	85%

Copyright Kamran Ahrar, MD.
NR, Not reported; *Pts,* patients; *RCC,* renal cell carcinoma.

41 patients.[97] Recurrent tumor was identified after a single ablation session in 5 (12%) tumors. The median size of RCC for this group was 5.2 cm. For tumors smaller than 4 cm, there were no recurrences. Local recurrence-free, disease-free, and overall 5-year survival after initial RFA was 88%, 83%, and 66%, respectively.

Traditionally, cryoablation has been performed by laparoscopic approach more frequently. Using this approach, Aron et al. reported a 5-year disease-free survival rate of 81% and a 10-year disease-free survival rate of 78% in 55 patients with biopsy-proven RCC at a median follow-up of 93 months (range, 60-132 months).[98]

The experience with percutaneous cryoablation is less mature than that with RFA, but several investigators have reported promising short-term results (Table 148-3).[38,44,59,60,82] Three small series reported the use of percutaneous cryoablation under guidance of CT[44] or MRI.[38,82] Gupta et al. reported technical success (i.e., the ice ball exceeded the dimensions of the tumor in all three planes) in all 27 lesions treated with cryoablation.[44] In this series, 16 tumors (12 patients) were available for imaging follow-up (mean, 5.9 months). Tumor size decreased in 13 of the 16 lesions and increased slightly in 3 lesions. The apparent increases in size were attributed to difficulty in interpreting the boundaries of the tumor, and these three lesions were not considered treatment failures because of the lack of enhancement on follow-up imaging.[44]

More recently, Atwell et al. reported their experience with 92 percutaneous cryoablations in 91 patients with 93 tumors.[59] The mean tumor diameter was 3.4 cm (range, 1.5-7.3 cm), and the mean follow-up was 26 months (range, 5-61 months). Technically successful ablation was performed in 89 of 93 tumors (96%), and overall local control was achieved in 88 of 93 tumors (95%).

In a meta-analysis of the published literature, Long et al. reviewed 42 studies in which 1447 tumors were treated by either surgical approach (n = 28) or percutaneous cryoablation (n = 14).[99] The surgical and percutaneous cryoablation groups contained similar patients, and there were no significant differences in the rates of unknown pathology, residual tumor, or recurrent tumor between the two groups. Long et al.[96] concluded that surgical and percutaneous cryoablation procedures have similar oncologic outcomes.

Both percutaneous cryoablation and RFA technologies are widely available and used by different investigators for ablation of renal tumors. The overall outcomes from single-arm studies for both technologies are comparable. There is no randomized study comparing the two techniques. Pirasteh et al. compared recurrence rates after percutaneous RFA (n = 41) to those of percutaneous cryoablation (n = 70) at two major academic centers. There was no difference between rates of imaging recurrence between the two groups.[100] Some investigators believe that cryoablation potentially has lower risk of injury to the urothelium of the UPJ or ureter.[101] Other advantages of cryoablation include less intraprocedural pain and more accurate monitoring of treatment efficacy during the procedure.[59,102] The ice ball is well delineated with both CT and MRI, and the size of the ablation zone correlates well with the width of the ice ball. The ablation zone with RFA is predictable, but no imaging modality can accurately monitor treatment efficacy during RFA. On the other hand, RFA has a cauterizing effect and achieves hemostasis, whereas ice ball fracture may lead to hemorrhagic complications with cryoablation.[67]

One of the most appealing aspects of ablative therapies is that they can be safely applied to patients with limited renal reserve. Several groups have reported the safety of ablation in patients with solitary kidneys. Jacobsohn et al. demonstrated the safety of ablation in patients with a solitary kidney, with an average of 9.1% decline in the creatinine clearance after RFA.[103] None of the patients in this group required dialysis. In a multicenter study of 89 patients with 98 renal tumors in a solitary kidney, 47 patients were treated by RFA and 42 underwent open partial nephrectomy.[104] Patients in the ablation group were older, had higher American Society of Anesthesiologists (ASA) scores, and had lower preablation GFR levels. The tumor size was larger in the partial nephrectomy group. Compared with RFA, patients who had partial nephrectomy had a greater decline in GFR (28.6% vs. 11.4% at last follow-up; $P < 0.001$). For patients with a preablation GFR above 60 or over 30 mL/min/1.73 m^2, there was a new onset of decline in GFR of less than 60 and less than 30 mL/min/1.73m^2 in 0% and 7% of patients after RFA and in 35% and 17% after open partial nephrectomy.[104] Lucas et al. examined the impact of RFA, partial nephrectomy, and radical nephrectomy on renal function in patients with small renal masses (<4 cm).[105]

The mean pretreatment GFRs were 73.4, 70.9, and 74.8 mL/min/1.73 m^2, respectively, in the RFA, partial nephrectomy, and radical nephrectomy groups. Following intervention, the 3-year rates of freedom from stage III chronic kidney disease were 95.2% for RFA, 70.7% for partial nephrectomy, and 39.9% for radical nephrectomy ($P < 0.001$). Patients who underwent radical and partial nephrectomy were 34.3 ($P = 0.001$) and 10.9 ($P = 0.024$) times more likely to develop stage III chronic kidney disease compared with their counterparts who underwent RFA.

KEY POINTS

- The discovery of incidental early-stage renal tumors has increased owing to the liberal use of noninvasive abdominal imaging.
- Current thermal technologies commercially available for percutaneous ablation of renal tumors include radiofrequency ablation and cryoablation.
- Image-guided thermal ablation is an excellent treatment option for patients who are not surgical candidates.
- Technical success rates have been reported in excess of 90% for small tumors (<4 cm in diameter), but the use of imaging for assessment of success has limitations.
- Histologic determination of malignancy should be considered prior to therapy.
- Percutaneous thermal ablation is a safe procedure with complication rates ranging from 3% to 12%.

▶ SUGGESTED READINGS

Atwell TD, Callstrom MR, Farrell MA, et al. Percutaneous renal cryoablation: local control at mean 26 months of followup. J Urol 2010; 184(4):1291–5.

Campbell SC, Krishnamurthi V, Chow G, et al. Renal cryosurgery: experimental evaluation of treatment parameters. Urology 1998;52(1):29–33; discussion 33–24.

Gervais DA, Arellano RS, McGovern FJ, et al. Radiofrequency ablation of renal cell carcinoma: part 2. Lessons learned with ablation of 100 tumors. AJR Am J Roentgenol 2005;185(1):72–80.

Guideline for management of the clinical stage 1 renal mass http://www.auanet.org/content/guidelines-and-quality-care/clinical-guidelines.cfm.

Matin SF, Ahrar K, Wood CG, et al. Patterns of intervention for renal lesions in von Hippel-Lindau disease. BJU Int 2008;102(8):940–5.

Tracy CR, Raman JD, Donnally C, et al. Durable oncologic outcomes after radiofrequency ablation: experience from treating 243 small renal masses over 7.5 years. Cancer 2010;116(13):3135–42.

Zagoria RJ, Pettus JA, Rogers M, et al. Long-term outcomes after percutaneous radiofrequency ablation for renal cell carcinoma. Urology 2011;77(6):1393–7.

The complete reference list is available online at www.expertconsult.com.

CHAPTER 149

Magnetic Resonance–Guided Focused Ultrasound Treatment of Uterine Leiomyomas

Marc H. Schiffman, Stephen B. Solomon, and Neil M. Khilnani

Uterine leiomyomas, also called *fibroids*, are gonadal steroid-dependent benign smooth-muscle tumors arising from uterine muscle tissue. Fibroids are estimated to occur in 20% to 50% of women of reproductive age,[1] representing the most common female pelvic tumor. The incidence of uterine fibroids is two to three times higher in African American women, who also present at a younger age and with more symptomatic cases.[2] Treatment of fibroids is reserved for symptomatic myomas and those thought to contribute to difficulties with fertility.

Significant symptoms related to these tumors occur in up to 25% of women and include menorrhagia and pressure-related symptoms such as pelvic fullness, urinary urgency and frequency, and dyspareunia. It is thought that a reduction of fibroid size strongly correlates with a reduction in pelvic symptoms.[3]

Currently there are several treatment options available for symptomatic fibroids. Hysterectomy is the definitive treatment for uterine leiomyomas, with surgical removal of the uterus resulting in 100% relief of all fibroid-related symptoms. However, it does eliminate the possibility of future childbearing, requires general anesthesia, and typically includes a 4-day in-hospital stay and a 4- to 6-week outpatient recovery before returning to usual levels of activity and work. In addition, there are several anatomic and psychological side effects of hysterectomy that many women wish to avoid. As a result, patients often pursue less invasive and uterine-sparing alternatives.

Surgical myomectomy has been used as a uterine-sparing procedure to palliate fibroid-related problems and as the treatment for fibroids interfering with fertility. It is usually performed with laparotomy and requires general anesthesia; recovery time can be as long as after hysterectomy. In addition, the number, size, and location of fibroids may limit its applicability.

Laparoscopic and hysteroscopic myomectomies are minimally invasive options performed when the patient wants to preserve fertility through selective resection of the fibroids while leaving the uterus behind. Unfortunately, these treatment options can only be performed in selected cases, depending on size and location of the myomas.[4] Robot-assisted laparoscopic myomectomy represents the most recent surgical advance in uterine-sparing surgery, but safe application of this technique is also limited, depending on the number and size of the fibroids and condition of the uterus.[5]

Uterine fibroid embolization is another alternative that is good for treating a wide range of fibroid locations and sizes. However, the procedure leads to amenorrhea in 1% to 2% of women younger than 45 and 15% of women older than 45, and may be associated with postembolization syndrome (postprocedural pain and fatigue), which results on average in an 8- to 10-day recovery.[6]

Magnetic resonance–guided high-intensity focused ultrasound (MRgFUS) represents the least invasive tool in the treatment of symptomatic fibroids, and preliminary results are encouraging in selected patients. It represents the only truly noninvasive procedure among the uterine-sparing therapeutic options. Focused ultrasound ablation is generally performed with magnetic resonance imaging (MRI) guidance, allowing for precise target definition as well as temperature monitoring during the entire procedure.

INDICATIONS

Ultrasound-induced thermal coagulative necrosis is a thermoablative technique that has been studied for over 60 years and was first used in 1942.[7] However, clinical applications were hampered by the inability to accurately target the focus and control temperature during the procedure. Recent advances in MRI have overcome these limitations. In the case of fibroids, MRI has excellent anatomic resolution for targeting, high sensitivity for localizing tumors, and enables real-time monitoring of temperature changes induced by ultrasound sonications during the procedure in the targeted tissues.[8] This last feature provides necessary feedback for intraprocedural monitoring of MRgFUS therapy.

Focused ultrasound has been applied in the treatment of a variety of clinical conditions, including prostate hyperplasia and cancer, kidney tumors, and breast lesions.[9] In October 2004, MRgFUS for fibroid treatment received approval by the U.S. Food and Drug Administration (FDA), representing the first commercially available method of treating patients with focused ultrasound in the United States (ExAblate 2000 [InSightec, Haifa, Israel]).

Initial eligibility criteria for enrollment for MRgFUS treatment of fibroids were defined by the FDA commercial guideline labeling. Patients had to be older than 18 and premenopausal (there have been no documented adverse effects on fertility or pregnancy to date, but those restrictions were recommended until data substantiating safety have been collected). Uterine size should be less than a 24-week pregnancy, and the targeted fibroid must be smaller than 12 cm, because this is the amount of tissue that can currently be treated in two 3-hour treatment sessions. The FDA originally specified that the targeted ablation volume must be no more than 33% of the volume of each fibroid, and no sonication should be closer than 15 mm to the endometrium or serosal surface of the uterus. Subsequently, treatment guidelines have been relaxed, first permitting the percentage of ablation to increase to 50%, and very recently allowing for 100% tumor volume ablation, with no minimum distance from the endometrium or maximum fibroid size, only prohibiting ablation within 10 mm of the uterine serosa. One additional treatment session to completely treat the fibroids is permitted within a 2-week period. Previous guidelines stated that "patients *must* have completed child bearing," but the current FDA label states that "patients *should* have completed child bearing."

CONTRAINDICATIONS

Patients with other pelvic diseases (i.e., endometriosis or dermoids) may not be suitable for MRgFUS. Other exclusions include pregnancy, calcified fibroids, and surgical clips or intrauterine devices (IUDs), which could reflect focused ultrasound energy to other locations. Women who are not candidates for MRI, such as those with cardiac pacemakers, should not receive this treatment. Several recent articles on MRgFUS of adenomyosis have demonstrated promise for this modality in treating this entity, initially felt to be a relative contraindication.[10] Previous experience has shown that abdominal scars have higher ultrasound absorption compared to regular tissue and when in the ultrasound beam path may lead to pain and thermal skin damage; therefore, patients with cutaneous scars in the proposed beam path may have to be excluded.[11] The fibroid(s) to be treated must be accessible, and its center can be no more than 12 cm from the skin surface, which is no more than 20 cm from the focused ultrasound transducer using existing technology. Homogeneously dark fibroids on T2-weighted spin-echo MRI respond well to MRgFUS. Fibroid tissue that is bright on T2-weighted spin-echo sequences has been thought by several investigators to respond less well to standard sonications and has previously been considered a relative contraindication. However, a recent publication showed no statistically significant correlation between T2 appearance and 12-month clinical and imaging outcome so long as sufficiently high energies are used to treat these fibroids.[12]

EQUIPMENT

The first FDA-approved clinical MRgFUS system (ExAblate 2000) was developed by InSightec Inc. (Haifa, Israel). It is built into a modified MRI table that docks with a compatible 1.5T or 3T GE MR scanner.[13] The ultrasound transducer is located in a water tank within the ExAblate table and covered by a thin plastic membrane, which allows the ultrasound beam to propagate through to the patient from the table.[7]

TECHNIQUE

Anatomy and Approaches

The patient lies in a prone position with the anterior abdominal wall over the water tank, using a gel pad to enhance acoustic coupling. The transducer can be moved along three axes to allow correct localization of the focal spot within the desired target. The transducer can also be pitched to allow angled sonications to avoid or minimize heating of near and far field structures.

Some anatomic issues must be considered. When performing the treatment, it is of great importance to check the far field of the ultrasound beam. In the series by Stewart et al.,[14] the most serious complication after MRgFUS was development of sciatic nerve palsy, which resolved by the 12-month follow-up visit. In this case, the fibroid was posteriorly located and, reviewing all treatment images, the nerve was not directly sonicated, but heat transfer from the adjacent pelvic bones led to indirect injury of the nerve. Furthermore, it is also essential to check the proximal field before treatment, because critical structures interposed in the treatment field may be harmed. Air-filled viscera such as the small intestine can interfere in the treatment, reflecting the ultrasound beam, injuring the intestine, and reducing the overall effectiveness.

Technical Aspects

The topics Principles of Focused Ultrasound Imaging and Principles of Magnetic Resonance Thermometry are available at www.expertconsult.com.

Patient Preparation

Because conscious sedation is used, the patient must fast for 6 hours before the procedure. A Foley catheter is placed to drain and keep the bladder empty. Otherwise, as the bladder fills during a procedure, it can displace the uterus and hamper the ability to correctly and safely target the fibroid. Hair must be carefully shaved from the lower abdominal wall to the level of the pubic symphysis because it can trap small air bubbles that can reflect ultrasound energy and lead to skin burns. Similarly, when positioning the patient on the table, care must be taken to avoid any air between the coupling membrane, the thin layer of water on top of it, and the patient's skin. Air bubbles can be identified on the preliminary localizing images and if present must be removed before proceeding. Light conscious sedation is used for anxiolysis and to minimize motion while allowing the patient to remain awake to provide constant feedback about any pain or sensation she may feel during the procedure.

Treatment Planning

T2-weighted, nonenhanced MR images in three orthogonal dimensions are acquired for treatment planning. The physician reviews the images then uses planning software to target the parts of the fibroids to be treated. As mentioned, current FDA-approved commercial guidelines allow for 100% treatment of the fibroid volume, with none of the sonications closer than 10 mm to the serosal surface of the uterus. The software on commercially available units allows the treating physician to graphically view the beam path to each targeted sonication as well as the entire treatment volume. It then allows the operator to manually manipulate parameters of each sonication to ensure safety, including altering the beam path or intensity or eliminating spots that could generate sufficient heat to injure nearby critical structures. The parameters at the physician's control include craniocaudal and mediolateral tilting of the transducer (pitch and roll), frequency, power, and size of the focal spot. Newer recently evaluated software incorporates safety controls that allow the physician during the setup to identify vulnerable nontargeted structures such as bowel and nerve roots in front of the spine. After preliminary treatment planning, the software will then alert the physician to sonications that may result in nontarget injury (Fig. 149-1).

Sonications

Before treatment, a representative target volume is defined within the planned treatment volume. Then a low-dose geometric verification sonication is performed and monitored by an MR thermal map. Any correction of the targeting of the transducer is made then verified. Subsequently, a therapeutic dose is delivered to the same spot to see if an appropriate temperature is developed to result in successful tissue

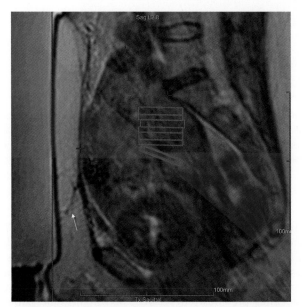

FIGURE 149-1. Sagittal T2-weighted image taken with patient prone on focused ultrasound table, demonstrating use of angled sonication, employed in this case to (1) eliminate nerve root irritation due to heating beyond fibroid by acoustic energy and (2) avoid scar on anterior abdominal wall *(white arrow)*. Green box delineates focal spot; blue shadow anterior and posterior to box represents ultrasound beam's path. Red boxes are planned sonications where a calculation has shown that without altering sonication, nerve root irritation is likely. Tilting the beam was necessary to complete these sonications.

destruction. This ensures the energy is correctly targeting the desired tissue, no errant heating is occurring, and the fibroid is responsive to the selected settings. As an example, if the targeted fibroid tissue has any calcification, the acoustic energy may be reflected and tissue heating may occur anterior to the target.

The treatment itself consists of multiple sonications desired to produce a single larger area of ablated tissue within the previously defined target volume. Temperature elevations within the patient during sonications are monitored by obtaining temperature-sensitive MR images in coronal, axial, or sagittal planes. The operator carefully inspects the thermal images to ensure adequate target heating without any significant heating outside the target (Fig. 149-2). This includes periodic observation of the skin and nerve roots, particularly if the patient describes any excessive skin warmth or neurologic stimulation. The images are also evaluated to identify any potential patient motion; fiducial markers placed on the reference images are carried over to the thermal images, helping the operator recognize significant movement. Most sonication parameters can be optimized during the treatment in response to the thermal maps being created.

The entire procedure, including preprocedural imaging planning and treatment, is guided by a physician and limited by commercial guidelines to approximately 3 hours. In clinical practice, the procedure may be repeated another day to treat more fibroid volume. In the clinical trials, two 3-hour treatments were allowed for each patient. Fibroids that are more vascular (less dark on T2-weighted spin-echo images) or have greater treatable volume may require more treatment time.

Treatment Effect Verification

After all the planned sonications are delivered, the patient remains in the same position for posttreatment T1-weighted spin-echo contrast-enhanced MR sequences to confirm treatment success by detecting a nonperfused area in the location of the target (Fig. 149-3). The abdominal wall is clinically examined to ensure no skin injury is

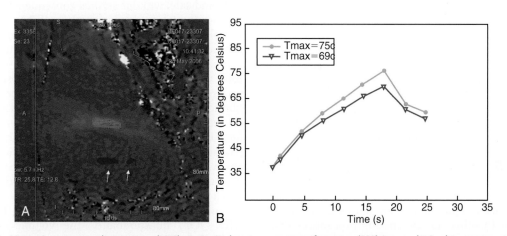

FIGURE 149-2. Magnetic resonance thermometry (MRT). **A,** Sagittal proton resonance frequency (PRF) image obtained to measure temperature in the plane of sonication. Increased signal intensity seen in fibroid on this image indicates temperature elevation. *Green* region around rectangle is acquired thermal dose in most recent sonication, which targeted tissue in rectangle. *Blue* areas are accumulated thermal dose from prior sonications *(white arrows)*. **B,** Thermal curves: graph of temperature over time, depicting temperature elevation during sonication length. Reported temperature is for hottest area in imaging plane *(rectangle in A)*. Green curve shows average temperature in the area; orange curve represents maximum temperature in that region. Temperatures above 54°C for more than 1 second are thought to cause tissue necrosis.

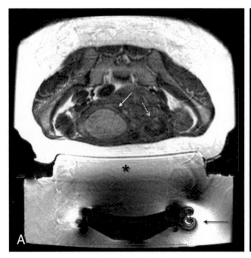
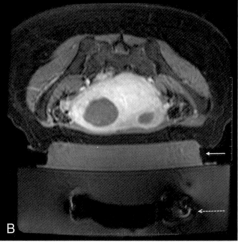

FIGURE 149-3. Treatment effect verification. **A,** Pretreatment axial T2-weighted magnetic resonance imaging (MRI) of patient in prone position reveals a bright fibroid on left *(solid white arrow)* and a smaller, darker fibroid on right *(dashed white arrow)*. Note position of ultrasound transducer in table *(black arrow)* and acoustic gel pad above table *(black star)*. **B,** Contrast-enhanced axial T1-weighted MRI demonstrates nonperfused segments within fibroids, corresponding well to administered sonications. Again note position of ultrasound transducer in table *(dashed white arrow)* and gel pad *(solid white arrow)*.

evident, and the patient stays for a short period of observation before being discharged. Patients usually return to work the next day with minor uterine cramping medicated with nonsteroidal antiinflammatory drugs (NSAIDs). Some minor vaginal bleeding also may occur for a few days.

In clinical practice, the nonperfused volume (hypovascular area) on MRI after ablation is generally larger than the thermal dose volume created during the therapy. This is hypothesized as being the result of the thermal volume occluding small vessels that create an ischemic necrosis beyond the direct thermal-induced necrosis.

Follow-up imaging has been performed every 6 months as part of the clinical trials evaluating this technique. Limited data on volumetric reductions and durability of treatment are currently available. Anecdotally, the nonperfused area seen on immediate posttreatment imaging usually becomes smaller on follow-up scans, with an overall size reduction in fibroid volume consistent with shrinkage of the postablation nonperfused volume. In most cases, viable fibroid tissue remains in the untreated portion of the fibroid.

CONTROVERSIES

The discussion of controversies surrounding this treatment is available at www.expertconsult.com.

OUTCOMES

Data on risks and benefits of MRgFUS for treating uterine fibroids have been reported by few authors. No direct comparisons with other uterine-sparing procedures (e.g., uterine fibroid embolization) have been completed to date.

An initial study conducted by Tempany et al.[23] was performed to evaluate the technical feasibility of performing focused ultrasound therapy with MR guidance and temperature monitoring for uterine fibroids. This study enrolled nine patients with symptomatic fibroids who underwent

subsequent hysterectomy after MRgFUS treatment. The study objective was not to completely treat the myoma but to correlate the surgical specimen with the MR images of post-MRgFUS therapy. Eligibility criteria, patient preparation, sonications, and posttreatment analysis followed the guidelines previously described. Six of the nine patients completed the entire MRgFUS treatment; in four, both MRI-calculated nonenhancing volumes and pathologic volumes were larger than the planned treated volumes. On average, the targeted treatment volume was 14.1 mL, the nonperfused volume on posttreatment MRI was 30 mL, and the pathologic confirmed lesion volume was 18.8 mL. One potential explanation for these results is that the focused ultrasound beam caused coagulation of blood vessels and resulted in downstream necrosis. The authors concluded that MRgFUS therapy for uterine fibroids is feasible and safe, without serious consequences.

The pivotal study designed for FDA approval of the ExAblate 2000 device was described by Hindley et al.[24] and subsequently by InSightec[25]; in the latter, there was also a comparison with a group of 83 patients who underwent total abdominal hysterectomy. The purpose of this study was to explore the hypothesis that treatment of uterine fibroids with MRgFUS therapy would lead to a significant decrease in symptoms and an improvement in quality of life. This was a multicenter clinical trial in which 109 patients were treated in 7 different sites. Suitable patients answered a Symptom Severity Score (SSS) questionnaire before and 6 months after treatment. The primary endpoint was a reduction of 10 points or more from baseline on the SSS of the Uterine Fibroid Symptom and Quality of Life (UFS-QOL) questionnaire. The volume of the fibroid treated was limited by safety restrictions imposed by regulatory authorities. Treatment was limited to four or fewer fibroids, 33% or less of the total volume of a fibroid, and less than 100 or 150 cm³ total treated volume for single or multiple fibroids, respectively. Of note, as mentioned earlier, this is less than the FDA currently allows for its commercial use. The primary endpoint of 10-point or greater SSS improvement at 6 months was achieved by 71% of treated patients, and treatment satisfaction was reported by 76% within the same period. Also, at 6 months, the mean reduction in leiomyoma volume was 13.5%. The better improvement in symptoms was noted during the first 3 months. There were fewer complications compared to hysterectomy, and patients could resume normal activity 1 day after the procedure. At 12 months, however, 21% of the InSightec study patients underwent further procedures to treat their symptoms (repeated MRgFUS session or hysterectomy), owing to SSS worsening. One possible explanation has been that limitations on the permissible size of the treated volume led to only partial treatment of some fibroids, and there was a potential for tumor regrowth. Subsequently, Stewart et al.[14] described follow-up results for the same patients initially observed by Hindley's group.[24] Of the 109 patients studied at 6 months, 82 were evaluated at 12 months, and the primary endpoint of 10-point reduction in the SSS, which was achieved by 71% of patients at 6 months, was reduced to 51% at the end of 1 year.

More recent multicenter data analyzed 359 women completing 24 months of follow-up after MRgFUS. These results showed durable symptom relief as measured by the SSS at 24 months. This multicenter cohort of patients included both early patients who had smaller volumes treated and more recent patients with larger portions of their fibroids treated. Results have shown significantly better results in patients with larger portions of their fibroids ablated.[26] LeBlang et al. described treatment of 147 symptomatic leiomyomas in 80 women, and with the relaxed guidelines approved several years ago were able to achieve average nonperfused volume ratios (NPV) of 55% ± 25% for the fibroid mass immediately after the procedure. The group showed that fibroid volume shrinkage at 6-month follow-up correlated with NPVs at the end of the procedure. They also found a statistically significant difference between patients in whom less than 50% NPV (and less fibroid shrinkage) was obtained and those in whom 50% to 75% and 75% to 100% NPVs were obtained.[27]

Funaki et al. reported 24-month follow-up of 91 women and described type 1 and type 2 myoma patients (type 1, very low intensity on T2-weighted images; type 2, image intensity lower than that of myometrium and higher than that of skeletal muscle) who had mean volume decreases at 24 months of 39.5%, mean drops in SSS from 35.1 ± 21.0 to a mean of 15.0, and mean reintervention rates of 14%. Type 3 myoma patients (T2 image intensity ≥ myometrium) demonstrated less size decrease and had a higher reintervention rate at 24 months (21.6%), but this was a smaller subgroup (n = 11) of patients, limiting more definitive conclusions.[28]

Gorny et al. recently reported 12-month outcomes of 130 MRgFUS patients. In phone interviews, 86%, 93%, and 88% of patients reported relief of symptoms at 3, 6, and 12 months, respectively. Although several authors have suggested that fibroids that demonstrate low T2 signal intensity respond best to sonication, and some have even suggested excluding fibroids with high T2 signal intensity from this treatment, this group found no statistical significance in terms of a correlation between T2-weighted appearance and outcome. Higher sonication energies were needed in the bright T2 group to achieve desired temperatures.[12]

COMPLICATIONS

Complications observed during treatment were rare, with the most significant being skin burns and sacral or lumbar nerve root injuries leading to transient neuropathic pain.[24] There was one episode of a temporary footdrop in the reported experience that resolved completely over the ensuing weeks. The nerve injury was most likely the result of the sound waves heating bone and injuring a nearby nerve. Recognition of these phenomena led to recommendations to cease sonications if a patient described *any* nerve-type symptoms. Software modifications incorporated safeguards that would allow the operator to be warned that a treatment prescription might lead to excessive nerve warming. Such treatment strategies have essentially eliminated this complication, but concern for nerve injury still limits accessibility to some fibroids.

Skin burns probably result from an air bubble interfering with ultrasound penetration and causing excessive skin energy deposition, or at a skin scar with its diminished blood flow and ability to clear accumulated energy. With careful examination of the abdominal wall, hair shaving before the treatment, and exclusion of patients with skin scars that cannot be avoided by the beam path, the skin burn rate has decreased significantly. During the treatment, it is also important to routinely check the thermal images in both the near field and far field to identify any heating of nontarget structures that may lead to injury.

Vaginal expulsion of uterine myomas, an event described after uterine fibroid embolization, has recently been reported after treatment of an intracavitary submucosal fibroid. Spontaneous vaginal expulsion occurred 3.5 months after treatment completion.[29]

POSTPROCEDURAL AND FOLLOW-UP CARE

The patient stays for a short observation period before being discharged, primarily because of the use of moderate sedation and a Foley catheter. They may return to usual activities when they feel ready, typically the next day. Patients may have some pelvic cramping and vaginal bleeding for a few days; the cramping is easily managed with NSAIDs. Some patients complain of musculoskeletal discomfort related to the positioning for the procedure, which is almost always self-limited. Imaging follow-up as previously described is not mandated by labeling but is certainly recommended for patients with ineffective response or recurrent symptoms.

SUMMARY

Focused ultrasound therapy has thus far been shown to be relatively safe and feasible in the treatment of symptomatic uterine fibroids in selected cases. MRT is a powerful adjunctive tool, assuring effective thermal coagulation of the target lesion while avoiding damage to surrounding structures. Currently there are limited short-term data in the literature to compare this treatment for uterine fibroids with its alternatives, and available data do not demonstrate clinical or anatomic features that would necessarily predict

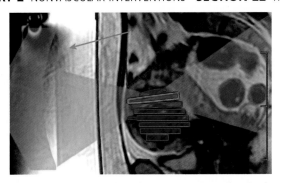

FIGURE 149-4. Future technical improvements under development include features such as beam shaping, which enables shaping ultrasound beam by closing elements in transducer *(red arrow)* to overcome obstacles, allowing wider patient selection and greater treatment volume.

success. Finally, we do not know how much fibroid and uterine volumetric reduction to anticipate in any given patient.

MRgFUS therapy may be an attractive option for those women who are anatomic candidates who wish to avoid invasive therapies and desire an outpatient procedure to palliate their fibroid-related symptoms. It offers potential advantages over surgical treatments, with potential benefits of a shorter recovery period and fewer complications, but multiple sessions may be required.

Modifications from early protocols seem to be leading to better and more durable results. Future technical improvements including robotic transducers, software modifications to allow parallel operations to be performed simultaneously, and enhanced treatment strategies will hopefully reduce the treatment times and result in decreased costs in scanner time (Fig. 149-4). Long-term follow-up and comparative studies are needed to precisely evaluate the efficacy of this noninvasive therapeutic option.

The experience with MRgFUS of uterine fibroids serves to demonstrate the potential of noninvasive thermoablation for other pathologic processes. Application of this technique to lesions of the prostate, bone, breast, liver, kidney, and brain is currently being investigated.

- *Uterine leiomyomas*, also called *fibroids*, are gonadal steroid-dependent benign smooth-muscle tumors arising from uterine muscle tissue.
- Fibroids are estimated to occur in 20% to 50% of women of reproductive age.
- Significant symptoms related to these tumors occur in up to 25% of the women who have them.
- Magnetic resonance–guided focused ultrasound (MRgFUS) represents a new tool in the treatment of symptomatic fibroids.
- MRgFUS allows for precise target definition as well as temperature monitoring during the entire ablation procedure.
- Magnetic resonance thermometry (MRT) is a powerful adjunctive tool, ensuring effective thermal coagulation of the target lesion while avoiding damage to surrounding structures.
- MRgFUS has been applied clinically with promising results, but more data are necessary to determine its optimal clinical application, and head-to-head comparative trials with other fibroid therapies will have to be performed.

► **SUGGESTED READINGS**

Bachmann G. Expanding treatment options for women with symptomatic uterine leiomyomas: timely medical breakthroughs. Fertil Steril 2006;85:46–7; discussion 48–50.

Fennessy FM, Tempany CM. MRI-guided focused ultrasound surgery of uterine leiomyomas. Acad Radiol 2005;12:1158–66.

Hindley J, Gedroyc WM, Regan L, et al. MRI guidance of focused ultrasound therapy of uterine fibroids: early results. AJR Am J Roentgenol 2004;183:1713–19.

Kennedy JE, Ter Haar GR, Cranston D. High intensity focused ultrasound: surgery of the future? Br J Radiol 2003;76:590–9.

Stewart EA, Gostout B, Rabinovici J, et al. Sustaining relief of leiomyoma symptoms by using focused ultrasound surgery. Obstet Gynecol 2007;110:279–87.

The complete reference list is available online at www.expertconsult.com.

CHAPTER 150

Fallopian Tube Interventions

Lee D. Hall and Mark F. Brodie

Image-guided interventions of the fallopian tubes can be divided into recanalization and embolization. Although the earliest reports of both procedures appeared in the literature in 1849,[1,2] the current techniques for fallopian tube recanalization (FTR) were described in the mid-1980s[3-5] and for fluoroscopic-guided fallopian tube embolization (FTE) in 2005.[6]

FALLOPIAN TUBE RECANALIZATION

An estimated 15% of Western couples seek treatment for infertility at some point in their reproductive years.[7] Selective salpingography and FTR are performed as part of the evaluation and treatment for female infertility and subfertility.[4,8] Definitions of fertility are arbitrary and confusing. In reproductive medicine, *subfertility* refers to at least 1 year of unprotected intercourse without achieving conception, and *infertility* is synonymous with sterility or absolute inability to conceive.[9,10] Most couples who have difficulty conceiving are not truly infertile but have decreased fertility (i.e., subfertile). Since the terms *infertility* and *subfertility* are commonly interchanged, we will consider them synonymous for the purpose of this discussion.

Female subfertility can result from one or more factors and varies from one geographic and social area to another. Most developed countries have a similar distribution of causes, with tubal factors responsible for 36%, ovulatory disorders 33%, endometriosis 6%, and indeterminate causes 30%.[9,10] Tubal pathology is usually secondary to pelvic inflammatory disease (PID), with *Chlamydia* and (less often) *Neisseria gonorrhoeae* the most common pathogens. The proximal (interstitial) and/or distal (fimbriated) ends of the tube are usually involved. Distal disease is best treated with laparoscopic or open microsurgery or with in vitro fertilization (IVF),[10] whereas proximal tubal obstruction (PTO) is treated endoscopically or surgically. PTO can be due to a number of processes, including salpingitis isthmica nodosa, fibrosis, adhesions, amorphous debris, mucus plugs, endometriosis, polyps, and spasm.[11-13]

Endoscopic recanalization of PTO can be performed using a variety of methods (falloposcopy, hysteroscopy, laparoscopy, sonography, and fluoroscopy),[12] but most often fluoroscopic guidance is used. The first successful transcervical fluoroscopic recanalization of a PTO was reported by Platia and Krudy in 1985.[3] Thurmond and coworkers described the currently used technique in 1987 in a series of patients who underwent selective salpingography to differentiate spasm from true tubal obstruction and recanalization to treat PTO.[4]

Indications

When a diagnostic hysterosalpingogram (HSG) reveals obstruction of one or both fallopian tubes, the American Society for Reproductive Medicine recommends selective salpingography as the next step in evaluating infertility.[14] An FTR procedure is indicated for a woman with bilateral PTO after initial HSG performed during an evaluation for infertility. At the time of the FTR procedure, repeat HSG is performed to reassess the fallopian tubes and exclude transient tubal obstruction or cornual spasm at the time of the initial HSG. Selective salpingography is performed in an attempt to clear any tubal blockage. If the PTO persists, an FTR is then attempted. If a patient has a unilateral patent tube discovered at the time of the FTR procedure, it is recommended that any PTO of the contralateral tube be treated with FTR to give the patient her best chance at conception.[15,16]

Contraindications

The two main contraindications to performing selective salpingography/FTR are pregnancy and active pelvic infection at the time of the procedure. A urine pregnancy test should be performed on the day of procedure; if this test is positive, it is then confirmed with a serum β-human chorionic gonadotropin (β-hCG) level. Before the FTR procedure, the patient should have a pelvic examination by her gynecologist, with negative gonorrhea and *Chlamydia* cultures documented. FTR should not be performed in cases of known distal tubal blockage (Fig. 150-1) or if both fallopian tubes are patent on HSG or selective salpingography performed immediately before FTR. If one fallopian tube demonstrates tubal patency with free intraperitoneal spillage of contrast on initial diagnostic HSG, the contralateral blocked proximal tube should be treated, especially when the patent tube has an underlying intrinsic abnormality (e.g., salpingitis isthmica nodosa, tubal polyp, or synechiae).

Equipment

The optimal setup for performing fluoroscopy-guided FTR includes an all-purpose fluoroscopy room with a rotating C-arm and lithotomy stirrups. Foam padding beneath the pelvis allows for more room to manipulate the speculum, and padding behind the knees adds to patient comfort. A kit for sterilely preparing the perineum and vagina and draping the legs and abdomen is necessary. Either a resterilizable metal or a disposable plastic speculum can be used to access the cervix. A transcervical catheter is used (e.g., 12F Cook balloon cervical cannula with a 5F inner diameter and a side arm) for injecting contrast medium and saline. A sterile cervical tenaculum for traction and a sterile set of disposable cervical dilators should be available if needed. Long-handled sponge forceps are useful to keep the vaginal vault dry during and after the procedure. Iodinated contrast is used to perform the initial HSG with selective salpingography if necessary. The contrast is diluted with equal volumes of normal saline to improve visualization of the catheter and guidewire. A 40-cm angled-tip 4F or 5F catheter is preferred for selective salpingography. Both 0.018-inch and 0.035-inch hydrophilic angled-tip guidewires (Terumo Medical Corp., Somerset, N.J.) may be used to traverse the obstructed fallopian tube. A 3F microcatheter is useful to provide column strength for the microguidewire and additionally can be used for injections of contrast medium to better evaluate the distal tube.

Technique

Anatomy and Approach

The fallopian tube provides a conduit from the ovary to the uterus and is made up primarily of circular and longitudinal

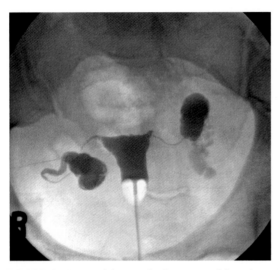

FIGURE 150-1. Hysterosalpingography demonstrates bilateral ampullary/infundibular blockages with hydrosalpinges. This patient gave birth after successful in vitro fertilization.

smooth muscle fibers with multiple epithelial folds. The smooth muscle layers become thinner as the tube tracks from the uterus to the ovary; the diameter of the tube also increases correspondingly. The average fallopian tube measures 11 cm (range 7-16 cm) in length and is divided into four segments (Fig. 150-2): intramural (interstitial), isthmic, ampullary, and infundibular.

The intramural segment is contained in the wall of the uterus beginning at the uterotubal ostium (UTO) and ending at the uterotubal junction (UTJ). It measures 1.5 to 2.5 cm in length, with a lumen of 0.8 to 1.4 mm in diameter observed in vivo specimens.[17] The narrowest point of the fallopian tube is at the UTJ. The isthmus begins at the UTJ and ends at the ampullary-isthmic junction. Its length ranges from 2 to 3 cm, and its diameter is 1 to 2 mm, making it the narrowest extrauterine segment. The ampullary segment is the most variable; it ranges from 5 to 8 cm in length, with a diameter of 1.5 mm at the ampullary-isthmic junction to 10 mm at the ampullary-infundibular junction. The infundibular segment contains the fimbria and the opening to the peritoneal cavity.

The preprocedure workup includes documentation of a recent pelvic examination with a normal Papanicolaou smear and negative gonorrhea and *Chlamydia* cultures. The procedure is performed in the follicular phase of the patient's menstrual cycle. Oral doxycycline is given for periprocedural antibiotic prophylaxis: 100 mg twice daily for 5 days, starting 2 days before the procedure. A negative pregnancy test is confirmed on the day of the procedure. The procedure can be performed with local anesthetic in the form of a paracervical block, but intravenous conscious sedation with midazolam and fentanyl is suggested for the procedure to ensure maximum patient comfort and relaxation. Unless contraindicated, 30 mg of intravenous or intramuscular ketorolac can be prophylactically administered before the procedure for abdominal and pelvic cramping. The patient is positioned, prepped, and sterilely draped as described earlier. The same equipment and techniques

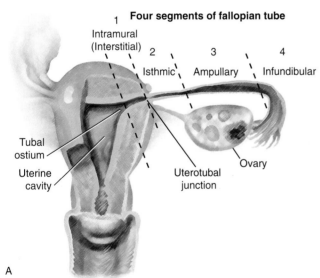

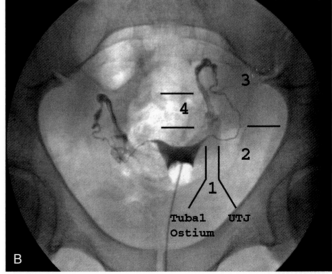

FIGURE 150-2. Drawing **(A)** and hysterosalpingogram **(B)** demonstrate relevant uterotubal anatomy. Labeled segments of fallopian tube include *(1)* intramural (interstitial), *(2)* isthmic, *(3)* ampullary, and *(4)* infundibular. Note uterotubal junction (UTJ), the narrowest portion of fallopian tube. UTJ should be spanned with coil to effectively occlude tube.

already described are used for cervical cannulation, HSG, and selective salpingography.

HSG is first performed as a routine part of the FTR procedure to evaluate the uterus and fallopian tubes; bilateral normal patent tubes can be present in up to 20% of patients referred for an FTR. Selective salpingography through the 4F or 5F angled-tip catheter is performed for any persisting tubal blockage or suboptimal opacification of the tube (Fig. 150-3). If a PTO is present after selective salpingography, FTR can be performed with a hydrophilic 0.035-inch or 0.018-inch guidewire (with or without a microcatheter) (Fig. 150-4). A repeat selective salpingogram is performed after the FTR to document tubal patency. Endpoints for FTR are a patent tube with free intraperitoneal contrast spillage, a patent proximal tube with a distal blockage, or inability to successfully recanalize the tube.

Controversies

The use of water- and oil-soluble contrast agents for HSG and FTR has been extensively debated. The subsequent live birth rate after use of these agents during the procedure is the most important consideration, with the pregnancy rate second. Pinto et al. retrospectively reviewed their cases of FTR, comparing pregnancy rates for patients who underwent successful FTR.[18] The two groups included use of water-soluble contrast medium only and use of water-soluble contrast medium plus addition of an oil-soluble contrast agent after confirmation of tubal patency. In 93 patients, there was no significant difference in pregnancy rates between the two groups, but the mean time to conception was 3.3 months less for the group who underwent the addition of oil-soluble contrast. However, a larger number of patients in the water-soluble-only group were lost to follow-up, with possible skewing of the data. Thus far, Pinto's work is the only study dealing with FTR. A Cochrane review in 2005[19] found two randomized controlled trials for HSG using the same study groups as Pinto et al., but these demonstrated no significant benefit in pregnancy rates. Trials with other combinations of oil- versus water-soluble contrast media have shown increased pregnancy and live birth rates using oil-based contrast agents. Pinto's work

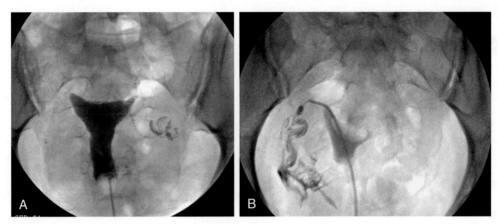

FIGURE 150-3. **A,** Hysterosalpingogram demonstrates nonvisualization of right tube and filling of left tube, with no free spill of contrast. **B,** Selective salpingogram of right tube demonstrates a patent tube with free intraperitoneal contrast medium.

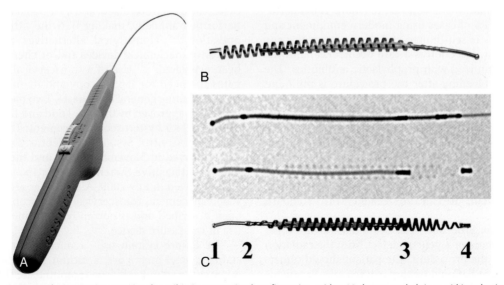

FIGURE 150-4. **A,** Essure device. Device contains the coil in its constrained configuration, with a 10-degree angled tip to aid in selecting out tubal ostium for placement. Outer diameter of device shaft is 4.3F. **B,** Detailed view of Essure coil. **C,** *(top to bottom),* Fluoroscopic images of Essure device and a deployed coil, with a photograph of a deployed coil. Radiopaque markers are labeled *1* to *4*. Third marker is ideally placed at tubal ostium. *(A and B images courtesy Conceptus Inc., Mountain View, Calif.)*

holds the most relevance because it was based on FTR using standard clinical practices. A prospective randomized trial will be useful in determining the role of oil-soluble contrast in FTR.

Tubal perfusion pressure (TPP) has received new attention in the field of female infertility. TPP is measured as the resistance encountered when injecting contrast agent during a selective salpingography. Work by Papaioannou et al.[20] relates poor TPP (>500 mmHg) to significantly lower pregnancy rates than a good TPP (<300 mmHg). Improved fertility was noted in women who had poor TPP at baseline and then underwent successful FTR, with TPP reduction. The concept of TPP for measuring tubal function is intriguing but has not received any attention in the radiology literature. There have been no controlled randomized trials to date to support its routine use in clinical practice.

Outcomes

About 30% of HSGs will demonstrate bilateral PTO. Selective salpingography alone can restore tubal patency in about one third of these previously blocked tubes. For the remaining PTO after selective salpingography, FTR will be technically successful in 80% to 90% of attempts. Reported pregnancy rates after successful FTR vary between 10% and 60% depending on the individual studies' primary patient populations.[21] Overall, an average unassisted conception rate after successful FTR can be expected in the 30% to 35% range. Patients with patent normal tubes after selective salpingography/FTR have a 50% to 60% chance of tubal blockage recurring within the first year after the FTR procedure.[22,23]

Complications

No major complications resulting from an FTR procedure have been reported. Minor complications are uncommon, and the majority of these can be managed conservatively. Complications include tubal perforation, infection, bleeding, ectopic pregnancy, and contrast reaction. Tubal perforation occurs in 2% of cases using modern equipment and techniques.[23] This is self-limited and does not require any further treatment. Infection is a rare occurrence, and the risks can be minimized with prophylactic antibiotics. The vast majority of bleeding after the procedure is mild and can last 2 to 3 days after the procedure. The risk of an ectopic pregnancy is higher for patients who have undergone FTR, but this is thought to be primarily due to underlying tubal abnormalities rather than the procedure itself. Normal monitoring for pregnancy should be performed after FTR. The possibility of a reaction to the contrast agent during the procedure exists but has not been reported. If this does occur, it can be treated with standard medications.

One risk of the procedure that bears discussion is that of developing cancer or a genetic defect from the radiation exposure during the procedure. The patient should understand there is no radiation dose that is 100% safe. Papaioannou et al.[24] reviewed 366 cases of selective salpingography/FTR and retrospectively calculated the median effective dose for the various combinations of procedures performed during an FTR. This dose ranged from 0.087 millisieverts

(mSv) for a unilateral selective salpingogram to 0.271 mSv for bilateral salpingography and FTR. From these doses, the excess risks of cancer and genetic defects were calculated and reported as the number of cases occurring per 1 million procedures performed. These risks ranged from 4.3 to 13.5 for cancer and from 1.9 to 5.9 for genetic defects. They concluded that the overall risks associated with the radiation doses observed in selective salpingography/FTR are low.

Postprocedural and Follow-up Care

Discussion of this topic is available at www.expertconsult.com.

KEY POINTS: FALLOPIAN TUBE RECANALIZATION

- Infertility causes an estimated 10% to 15% of Western couples to seek medical attention.
- Fallopian tube disease causes 10% to 35% of female infertility.
- Fallopian tube recanalization (FTR) is a safe and effective treatment for proximal tubal obstruction.
- Absolute contraindications to FTR include pregnancy and active pelvic infection.
- FTR has a technical success rate of 80% to 90%.
- About one third of patients who undergo a successful FTR will conceive spontaneously.
- The complication rate for FTR is low, and no major complications have been reported.

FALLOPIAN TUBE EMBOLIZATION

Bilateral tubal sterilization (BTS) is one of the most common methods of contraception, used by one third of women worldwide. An estimated 10.3 million women in the United States have been sterilized, and over 650,000 procedures are performed annually, making BTS the fifth most common operation.[25,26] Nonsurgical alternatives to BTS using a variety of mechanical devices and/or chemical agents have been evaluated.[27-35] Use of a transcervical approach eliminates the need for laparoscopy and its inherent operative risks, including general anesthesia. Two mechanical devices have been approved by the U.S. Food and Drug Administration (FDA) for hysteroscopic placement. The Essure Permanent Birth Control System (Conceptus, San Carlos, Calif.) was approved in November 2002, and the Adiana Permanent Contraceptive System (Hologic Inc., Bedford, Mass.) was approved in July 2009. Although approved for hysteroscopic placement, transcervical fluoroscopic placement has been described and is currently performed as an off-label use of the Essure device.[36,37]

The Essure system uses a microinsert consisting of a stainless steel inert core, a nitinol expanding superelastic outer coil, and polyethylene terephthalate (PET)-imbedded fibers (Fig. 150-5). The insert is placed in the interstitial portion of the fallopian tube such that the third (radiopaque) marker is at the level of the tubal ostium. After deployment, the outer coil expands up to 2 mm to anchor

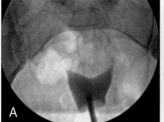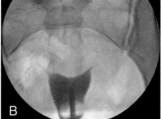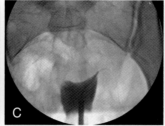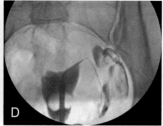

FIGURE 150-5. **A,** Hysterosalpingogram demonstrates nonfilling of bilateral tubes. **B,** Selective salpingogram of left tube demonstrates proximal tubal blockage. **C,** A 0.035-inch hydrophilic guidewire was advanced beyond level of occlusion. **D,** Repeat selective salpingogram demonstrates left tubal patency, with intraperitoneal contrast agent outlining small bowel loops.

the device. The PET fibers incite tissue ingrowth to produce occlusion over the next few weeks.[38,39]

The Adiana system uses a combination of controlled radiofrequency thermal damage to the epithelial lining of the fallopian tube, followed by insertion of a nonabsorbable silicone elastomer matrix. A special catheter is used to deliver radiofrequency energy to the intramural portion of the fallopian tube for 60 seconds, creating a superficial (0.5 mm) injury. The 3.5-mm silicone matrix is then deployed as the catheter is withdrawn. Fibrous tissue ingrowth into the matrix over the next few weeks provides permanent occlusion.[39-41]

Both embolization systems require alternative methods of birth control for 3 months until occlusion is confirmed on a follow-up HSG. The HSG protocol includes a minimum of 6 radiographs: scout, minimal fill of the uterine cavity, partial fill of the uterine cavity, total fill of the uterine cavity, and bilateral oblique magnification views of the uterine cornua. Coil placement (for the Essure device) and tubal occlusion are assessed. Unequivocal total occlusion must be confirmed for the patient to discontinue alternative methods of birth control. Equivocal results require another HSG 3 months later while the patient continues alternate birth control measures. If total occlusion is not demonstrated, the patient should seek another form of birth control.

Indications

Tubal sterilization is indicated when a woman does not want or cannot tolerate a pregnancy; included are multiparous women not yet at menopause and women whose medical conditions are aggravated by or whose lives may be at risk during a pregnancy. The typical patient is a woman who is older than 30 years of age, with two or more children and no plans for future childbearing. A patient should be screened carefully to determine whether permanent sterilization is the best form of birth control for her particular situation. If she is concerned about protection against sexually transmitted diseases and human immunodeficiency virus infection or regulating her menstrual cycle, permanent tubal sterilization may not be the best choice.

Contraindications

The foremost contraindications to tubal sterilization are a desire to maintain childbearing potential or any uncertainty about permanent sterility. Other contraindications include

pregnancy, recent or current pelvic infection, prior tubal ligation, known contrast allergy, immunosuppression, intrauterine pathology that would prevent access to either tubal ostium or the intramural portion of either fallopian tube (e.g., large submucosal fibroid, uterine adhesions, apparent unilateral or bilateral proximal tubal occlusion, suspected unicornuate uterus, etc.), and delivery or termination of pregnancy within 6 weeks (Essure) or 3 months (Adiana).[38-40] Patients with a nickel allergy may still be candidates for the Essure device but should be counseled regarding the risks and benefits of the procedure even though the possibility of an adverse reaction is extremely low (<1 : 5000).[42] Nickel hypersensitivity with intravascular stents and orthopedic prostheses has been addressed in the literature.[43-45] The possibility of early restenosis with nitinol intravascular stents in patients who exhibit nickel hypersensitivity has been debated.[44,45]

Equipment

The optimal setup for performing fluoroscopy-guided transcervical tubal sterilization includes all the equipment described in the FTR section, with the exception of the microguidewire and microcatheter used for recanalization.

Although both the Essure and Adiana systems are FDA approved for hysteroscopic transcervical BTS, our experience with fluoroscopic guidance is limited to the Essure device, so most of the following discussion refers to this product.

Technique

Preprocedural workup includes documentation of a recent pelvic examination with a normal Papanicolaou smear and negative gonorrhea and *Chlamydia* cultures. FTE should be performed in the follicular phase (day 7-14) of the patient's menstrual cycle to limit the chance of a luteal-phase pregnancy. A qualitative urine β-hCG test is performed on the day of the procedure and the negative result documented before the start of the procedure. Patients are given 30 mg of ketorolac and 1 gm of ceftriaxone intravenously before the procedure. With radiologic procedures such as HSG and FTR, periprocedural administration of antibiotics (e.g., doxycycline) is widely practiced but not universal. Antibiotics are given for all our fallopian tube interventions. No preoperative antibiotics were given during the Essure pivotal trial with 507 attempted hysteroscopic device placement procedures, and there were no reported cases of infection.[46]

This procedure can be performed under intravenous conscious sedation (e.g., midazolam and fentanyl) or with local anesthetic using paracervical block anesthesia. If a paracervical block without intravenous conscious sedation is used for pain control during placement, several anatomic factors should be considered. The uterovaginal plexus lies predominantly lateral and posterior to the junction of uterus and cervix. The cardinal ligaments transmit uterine nerves at the 3 and 9 o'clock positions and, similarly, the uterosacral ligaments transmit nerves at the 5 and 7 o'clock positions. Although injections of 1% lidocaine at the 3, 5, 7, and 9 o'clock positions at the cervicovaginal junction place the local anesthetic adjacent to the appropriate nerves, the injections at the 3 and 9 o'clock positions along the cervix risk entering the uterine arteries or veins that are present in the neurovascular bundles. Lidocaine injections with 3 to 5 mL at the 4 and 8 o'clock or 5 and 7 o'clock positions are recommended to maximize anesthesia and minimize risk to adjacent vessels.

The procedure begins with the patient in the lithotomy stirrups on the angiography table. Foam padding under the knees and pelvis aids in patient comfort, and pelvic elevation allows for more room to manipulate the speculum. The vulvar and perineal areas are sterilely prepped with an iodine-based solution, then sterile drapes are placed over the legs and abdomen. A sterile speculum is placed in the vaginal vault, and the cervix is identified. Both the vaginal vault and cervix are prepped with iodine solution. A 12F balloon cannula is used to access the uterine cavity transcervically. The internal balloon is inflated to seal against leakage of the contrast agent. A cervical tenaculum can be used if needed for traction on the uterus. HSG is performed with injection of the contrast medium through the cannula side arm. If neither or only one of the fallopian tubes is identified on the HSG, a 4F or 5F angled-tip catheter is used for selective salpingogram(s). Both fallopian tubes should be clearly seen in their entirety before placing the device. After identification of the fallopian tubes, the tube that appears to offer more of a challenge to correct device placement should be selected for initial placement. This is based on the recommendation by Conceptus that if bilateral microcoils cannot be placed, the procedure should be aborted.[38] We have identified several factors that correlate with a more difficult device placement: a smaller-caliber tube, a more tortuous tube, and a more acute angle at the UTJ.

The Essure device has a 4.3F outer diameter; it is placed through the cervical cannula 5F working port. Using fluoroscopy, the device is engaged into the tubal ostium. The device is then advanced into the fallopian tube until the third radiopaque marker is at the level of the tubal ostium (Fig. 150-6). The coil is deployed, and the placement process is then repeated with another Essure device to occlude the contralateral fallopian tube (Fig. 150-7). The internal balloon is deflated, and the cervical cannula is then removed from the patient. The long-handled sponge forceps are used if needed to clean the vaginal vault of contrast agent and/or blood. The patient is taken to the periprocedural holding room for recovery and monitoring by a nurse after the procedure.

The patient is instructed to use another form of contraception until correct coil position and tubal occlusion can be documented by HSG at the 3-month follow-up

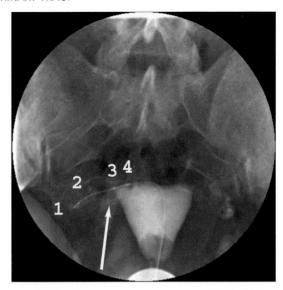

FIGURE 150-6. Placement of the Essure device into right fallopian tube, with radiopaque markers labeled *1* to *4*. Device has been advanced to place third marker at tubal ostium *(arrow)*. After satisfactory positioning, coil is deployed.

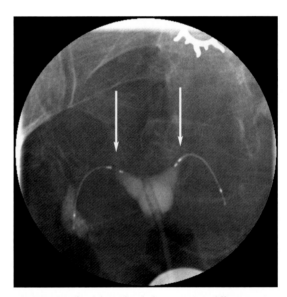

FIGURE 150-7. After bilateral coil placement in a different patient. Note approximation of third radiopaque markers to tubal ostia *(arrows)*.

appointment. Alternate forms of birth control do not include a condom alone (it must be used in combination with another method) or an intrauterine method (e.g., intrauterine device or intrauterine system, which may cause problems with the coils).

The 3-month follow-up HSG is performed in a fashion similar to the FTE procedure previously described in the technique section, with the following exceptions: no conscious sedation or local anesthesia is used, and a 3F balloon transcervical catheter is used for uterine cavity access. Conceptus has a prescribed protocol for the HSG, with a minimum of six radiographs: scout, minimal fill of the uterine cavity, partial fill of the uterine cavity, total fill of the uterine cavity, and bilateral oblique magnification views of

TABLE 150-1. Criteria for Hysterosalpingography for Grading Coil Placement and Tubal Occlusion

Grade	Coil Placement	Tubal Occlusion
I	Expulsion of coil, or >50% of the coil inner length trails into uterine cavity	Tube occluded at the cornua
II	<50% of the inner coil length trails into uterine cavity, or proximal end of inner coil is <30 mm into the tube from the tubal ostium	Contrast within the tube but not past any portion of the coil
III	Coil inner length proximal end is > 30 mm distal to the tubal ostium, or coil is within peritoneal cavity	Contrast past the coil or in peritoneal cavity

To rely on the coils for the sole method of birth control, the coil placement must be grade II and tubal occlusion must be grade I or II. The *coil inner length* is defined as the coil between the first (distal end) and third (proximal end) radiopaque markers.

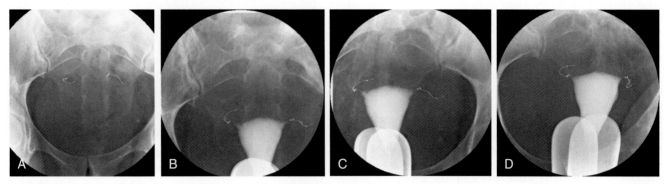

FIGURE 150-8. Three-month follow-up hysterosalpingogram after Essure coil placement. **A,** Scout film. **B,** Film showing total fill of uterine cavity. **C,** Oblique view of left cornua. **D,** Oblique view of right cornua. Minimal and partial fill images are not included.

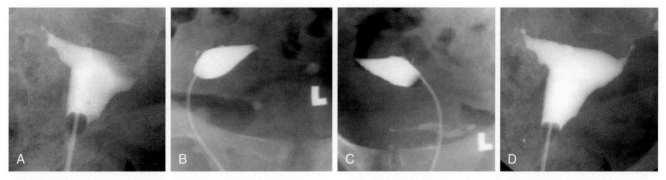

FIGURE 150-9. Follow-up hysterosalpingogram after Adiana placement with **(A)** partial fill, **(B)** left oblique, **(C)** right oblique, and **(D)** total fill shows unequivocal bilateral tubal occlusion.

the uterine cornua (Fig. 150-8). The coil placement and tubal occlusion are assessed and graded (Table 150-1).

The Adiana device is not radiopaque and will not be visible on HSG, but the 3-month follow-up HSG protocol is similar to the Essure protocol. Bilateral tubal occlusion is the unequivocal sign of successful placement (Fig. 150-9).

Technical Aspects

Although the procedure is not technically difficult in most cases, there are situations that can be challenging. In the case of a flexed uterus, the device can have problems tracking into the tubal ostium. Use of a cervical tenaculum to straighten the angles of the cervix and uterus is invaluable in allowing the device tip to engage the tubal ostium. Once the device has engaged the tubal ostium, there is a high likelihood the device will track across the UTJ without difficulty.

In our series, two patients had the device tip engage the tubal ostium and advance into the intramural tube segment, but it would not progress past the UTJ. A selective tubal ostium injection of 100 µg of nitroglycerin in a normal saline solution (concentration 100 µg/mL) permitted advancement of the device distally past the UTJ for successful device deployment.

In the intramural and isthmic segments, the largest portion of the tubal wall consists of smooth muscle cells. Ekerhovd et al.[47] documented the effects of nitric oxide donors on the contractility of the isthmic segment of human fallopian tubes. Nitroglycerin had a concentration-dependent inhibition of the smooth muscle contraction of fallopian tubes. Although our evidence is anecdotal, we think that the use of intratubal nitroglycerin has a physiologic basis for use during the procedure to relieve tubal spasm, with few inherent risks.

The Adiana device requires shorter tubal penetrance and may be successful in patients where the Essure system cannot be fully advanced into the fallopian tube to the third marker.[48]

Controversies

The patient undergoes radiation exposure during fluoroscopic placement, which she would not normally experience had she elected for hysteroscopic placement. The radiation dose for the follow-up HSG is equivalent for both placement methods. Hedgpeth et al.[49] reported their dose for FTR patients as an estimated mean ovarian dose of 8.5 mGy. We reported our initial results for device placement with a similar estimated dose of 8.5 mGy, based on the fluoroscopy time and spot radiographs.[36] This dose is believed to represent a minimal risk to the ovaries.

The necessity of the 3-month follow-up HSG is mandated by the FDA, but this requirement is undesirable for most patients. Other methods to assess coil location at 3 months after the procedure, including pelvic radiographs or ultrasonography, have been described in the literature[50,51] and are in clinical use in Europe and Australia. Follow-up with radiographs is limited to patients in whom the initial placement was judged satisfactory by the physician performing the procedure. A pelvic radiograph is obtained 3 months after the procedure, and bilateral coil retention and location are confirmed. In the absence of abnormal positioning of the coils, tubal occlusion is assumed. HSG is only performed if the placement is believed to be suboptimal or there is an abnormality on the radiograph at 3 months. Using the guidelines described earlier, Heredia et al.[50] followed a series of 78 patients from October 2001 to early 2004; 65 (83%) underwent only pelvic radiographic follow-up, whereas 17% underwent HSG due to perceived suboptimal placement at the time of the procedure. No pregnancies were reported in this patient population. This algorithm is used to limit the patients' discomfort, added cost, and inconvenience from HSG.

Ultrasonography is used in a similar fashion,[51] with or without contrast media to detect tubal patency; the Essure coils are highly echogenic and easily visible (Fig. 150-10). Although these methods may eventually replace HSG, they are not currently approved by the FDA and should not be considered as alternatives to HSG in the United States.

Outcomes

Data from the Essure phase II and pivotal trial[46,52] using hysteroscopic placement included attempted placements in 745 patients (n = 227 and n = 518, respectively). The bilateral placement rates were 88% (phase II) and 90% (pivotal). The reliance rate (i.e., number of women able to rely on the coils for birth control/number of women with bilateral coil placement × 100) was 97% for both trials. The efficacy rate for the device in preventing pregnancy is 99.8%, effectively equal to bilateral tubal ligation and vasectomy.

We have performed 35 fluoroscopic placement procedures on 34 patients[36]; 31 completed follow-up HSG, and 3 patients were lost to follow-up. The three lost to follow-up all underwent bilateral coil placement that appeared to be adequate at the time of procedure. Because the placement cannot be judged as adequate without follow-up HSG,

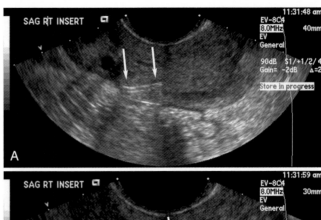

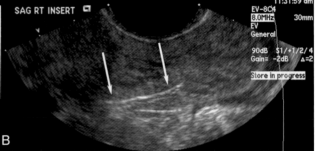

FIGURE 150-10. A-B, Endovaginal ultrasonography. Echogenic outer nitinol coils *(arrows)* are easily distinguishable from surrounding uterus and fallopian tube.

these patients are not counted as successful placements. One patient treated early in our experience underwent an initial unsuccessful placement procedure; she subsequently returned for another placement procedure that resulted in bilateral coil placement. Our placement rate after an initial placement procedure was 88% (30/34). Including the second placement procedure, the rate rises to 91% (31/34), which is comparable to hysteroscopic placement rates. All 31 patients who underwent subsequent HSG were able to use the coils as their primary birth control.

Experience with the Adiana device is limited, but the data from the Evaluation of the Adiana System for Transcervical Sterilization Using Electrothermal Energy (EASE) international phase II trial showed a bilateral successful placement rate of 95%, a 6-month bilateral occlusion rate of 88%, and a 12-month effectiveness rate of 98.9%.[53] These numbers compare favorably with the Essure system and bilateral tubal ligation.[52]

Palmer compared the Essure and Adiana devices and found both systems had high patient satisfaction, low procedural discomfort, and favorable cost profiles compared to laparoscopic tubal ligation.[39]

Complications

In the pivotal trial for the Essure device,[46] the most common complications for hysteroscopic placement included coil expulsion (2.9%) and perforation (1.1%). Pelvic cramping and/or pain and vaginal spotting occurred in the majority of patients and should be considered expected events after coil placement.

No method of birth control is 100% effective. The possibility of pregnancy, including a high risk for an ectopic location, exists after a patient begins to rely on the coils for her primary birth control. For all methods of tubal sterilization, the probability of pregnancy after 10 years with tubal sterilization is 1.3%, with 32.9% of these pregnancies occurring in ectopic locations.[54] As of October 2005, there have been 40,568 hysteroscopic Essure placements worldwide; 52 pregnancies have been reported in these patients.[55] No device failures have been documented in the 52 cases. The most common cause (57%) of pregnancy in these patients is noncompliance with postplacement procedure protocol (physicians and patients). This includes failure to undergo follow-up HSG and failure to prescribe alternative contraception after device placement. Also contributing to these pregnancies were probable pregnancy before coil placement (16%) and failure to adequately interpret the follow-up HSG (16%).

Our known complication rate thus far with fluoroscopic placement is 1 of 35 placements. This placement was in a patient who had an extensive prior history of pelvic pain that was exacerbated by the procedure. Her pain returned to baseline 1 week after the procedure with pain control using a nonsteroidal antiinflammatory drug (NSAID). None of our patients to our knowledge have had a documented positive hCG pregnancy test, although these data are skewed because our patients were followed retrospectively and not prospectively. However, we believe if there is adequate coil placement and tubal occlusion on the follow-up HSG, there should be no difference in the efficacy of the coils compared with that experienced with hysteroscopic placement. Although we have not experienced the breadth of complications reported from the Essure trials, this may be due to our small patient population size.

Postprocedural and Follow-up Care

Discussion of this topic is available at www.expertconsult.com.

KEY POINTS: FALLOPIAN TUBE EMBOLIZATION

- The FDA-approved devices for transcervical sterilization using hysteroscopic placement are the Essure Permanent Birth Control System approved in November 2002 and the Adiana Permanent Contraceptive System approved in July 2009.
- The procedure is indicated for women who wish to permanently end their fertility.
- The Essure microinsert and the Adiana silicone matrix are inert and do not affect the patient's hormonal levels.
- There have been more than 40,000 hysteroscopic placements worldwide, with a 99.8% efficacy rate.
- Off-label fluoroscopic placement of the Essure device has been performed but has not been validated by a long-term prospective trial.
- The procedure uses techniques similar to those for fallopian tube recanalization.
- Patients must return 3 months after placement for a follow-up hysterosalpingogram (HSG) and use another form of birth control in the interim.
- Once tubal occlusion and proper coil placement have been documented by HSG, the patient is able to use the coils as her primary birth control method.

▶ **SUGGESTED READINGS**

Abbott J. Transcervical sterilization. Best Pract Res Clin Obstet Gynecol 2005;19:743–56.
Kodaman PH, Arici A, Seli E. Evidence-based diagnosis and management of tubal factor infertility. Curr Opin Obstet Gynecol 2004;16:221–9.
Magos A, Chapman L. Hysteroscopic tubal sterilization. Obstet Gynecol Clin North Am 2004;31:705–19.
Maubon AJ, Graef M, Boncoeur MP, et al. Interventional radiology in infertility: technique and role. Eur Radiol 2001;11:771–8.
Papaioannou S, Afnan M, Sharif K. The role of selective salpingography and tubal catheterization in the management of the infertile couple. Curr Opin Obstet Gynecol 2004;16:325–9.
Papaioannou S, Bourdrez P, Varma R, et al. Tubal evaluation in the investigation of subfertility: a structured comparison of tests. Br J Obstet Gynaecol 2004;111:1313–21.
Peterson HB, Curtis KM. Long-acting methods of contraception. N Engl J Med 2005;353:2169–75.
Pollock A. ACOG practice bulletin: Benefits and risks of sterilization. Obstet Gynecol 2003;102:647–58.
Thurmond AS, Machan LS, Maubon AJ, et al. A review of selective salpingography and fallopian tube catheterization. Radiographics 2000;20:1759–68.
World Health Organization. Selected Practice Recommendations for Contraceptive Use. 2nd ed. Geneva: World Health Organization; 2004.

The complete reference list is available online at www.expertconsult.com.

CHAPTER **151**

Thermal Ablation of the Adrenal Gland

Deepak Sudheendra and Bradford J. Wood

The primary treatment for adrenal gland tumors has traditionally been open or laparoscopic surgical resection. It has been suggested in a few small series that aggressive local surgical resection may improve outcomes in selected patients with isolated metastatic disease limited to one adrenal gland from nonadrenal primary tumors. Although controversial, this has been especially postulated for patients with solitary adrenal metastases and favorable tumor biology, long disease-free intervals, symptomatic disease, or specific histologic findings such as adenocarcinoma, lung carcinoma, renal cell carcinoma, colorectal carcinoma, or melanoma.[1-3]

In patients with adrenocortical carcinoma (ACC), there is stronger historical evidence that an aggressive surgical approach for recurrent and metastatic disease can improve survival.[4] However, despite such measures, the 5-year survival rate in different series ranged between 16% and 38%, and recurrence rates of 35% to 85% after complete resection yield a poor prognosis.[4-6] Adjunct therapy with mitotane, a synthetic derivative of the insecticide dichlorodiphenyltrichloroethane (DDT), has shown limited efficacy on the natural course of this disease.[7,8] Newer therapies with cytotoxic chemotherapy are limited and under investigation.[6]

Besides the high morbidity associated with repeat surgical resections, which must be weighed against the benefits of such procedures, successive surgeries are further complicated by adhesions. However, image-guided radiofrequency ablation (RFA) may provide an alternative minimally invasive treatment option for patients who are not operative candidates and have multiple comorbid conditions, an aggressive tumor focus, and/or no other treatment options for local control of tumor. In addition to malignant adrenal disease, including pheochromocytomas, benign functioning lesions seen in patients with primary hyperaldosteronism secondary to an adrenal aldosteronoma may benefit from RFA, with its lower morbidity, shorter hospitalization, and less expense than open surgery.[9]

INDICATIONS

RFA can be performed for the treatment of primary and metastatic adrenal neoplasms, including ACCs, pheochromocytomas, adenomas, extraadrenal metastases from adrenal neoplasms, and palliation in selected cases. Surgical indications for adrenalectomy from solitary metastases can be found for specific histologic findings, including adenocarcinoma, lung carcinoma, renal cell carcinoma, colorectal carcinoma, or melanoma.[1-3] Extrapolation to indications for RFA assumes that it is an alternate method for nonsurgical tissue destruction. Image-guided ablation can provide a safe treatment alternative for patients with painful lesions or symptoms related to catecholamine-producing neuroendocrine tumors.[10] Tumor debulking by ablation can subsequently play a palliative role by the resultant decrease in catecholamine release.

In addition, RFA has also been described in the treatment of primary hyperaldosteronism and metastatic pheochromocytoma.[11,12] RFA can be used to treat lesions 5 cm in diameter or smaller. Larger lesions can be treated by overlapping ablations, but the success rate markedly diminishes as the size increases. Nonoperative candidates—those with high surgical risk, several comorbid conditions, unresectable tumors, multiple prior recurrent surgeries, and an aggressively growing tumor—can benefit from RFA in the appropriate clinical scenario. Patients with bilateral adrenal metastases may be well served by RFA for palliative purposes and in some cases may be treated for bilateral disease in a single sitting.[13]

CONTRAINDICATIONS

Uncorrectable coagulopathies and bleeding diatheses are relative contraindications for RFA. Blood product support may be given as per typical surgical procedures. The procedure should not be performed in those patients who are acutely ill and/or septic. Comorbid conditions such as chronic obstructive pulmonary disease and congestive heart failure are not contraindications to RFA, but multiple comorbid conditions may increase the risk profile. Prior hypertensive crisis or elevated levels of catecholamines raise the risks but are not absolute contraindications.

EQUIPMENT

- 200-W, 460- to 480-kHz alternating current RF generator
- RF electrodes (single or cluster electrode)
- 2 to 4 grounding pads or dispersive electrodes
- Chilled saline
- Computed tomography (CT) and/or ultrasound guidance (microwave, cryoablation, high-intensity focused ultrasound equipment may also be used, although there is less historical experience)

TECHNIQUE

Anatomy and Approaches

Thermal ablation of the adrenal gland can be performed from several approaches. When deciding which approach

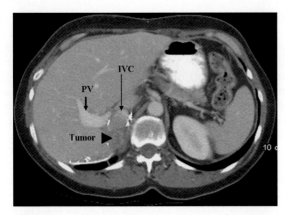

FIGURE 151-1. Before radiofrequency ablation, enhanced computed tomography scan shows right adrenal tumor in close proximity to liver, portal vein *(PV)*, and inferior vena cava *(IVC)*.

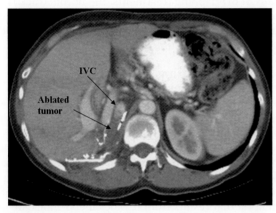

FIGURE 151-2. Enhanced computed tomography scan showing pericaval necrosis of adrenal tumor with patent inferior vena cava *(IVC)* 2.5 years after ablation.

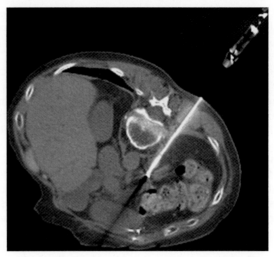

FIGURE 151-3. Radiofrequency ablation of adrenal tumor near aorta and bowel, with patient in prone position.

Technical Aspects

The following technical points must be considered:
- Take into account organ shift when positioning the patient.
- Always be aware of surrounding organ structures to prevent inadvertent thermal injury; consider a fluid blanket to protect bowel, pancreas, lung, kidney, diaphragm, chest wall (including intercostals nerves), and other adjacent structures
- If hypertension develops during adrenal, renal, or lower liver thermal ablation, consider adrenal irritation or catecholamine release as a possible cause.
- Ensure patient has received adequate premedication to prevent hypertensive crises during ablation of pheochromocytomas and other functional neoplasms.
- Cauterize needle track to prevent tumor seeding and bleeding.

Patients may be treated in the interventional or CT scan suite under conscious sedation or general anesthesia, often with additional real-time feedback from ultrasound guidance. When positioning the patient for the procedure, one should keep in mind the location of the lesion, surrounding structures, and overall safety of the patient. Adrenal ablation can be performed from a posterior, lateral, or anterior approach. Organ shift that may occur from supine to decubitus positioning should also be considered when deciding which approach to use.

Although cranial angulation can avoid pleural transgression, one should use caution so as not to injure bowel wall, regardless of the procedural approach, because the consequences of bowel injury can lead to significant morbidity and mortality. For adrenal lesions on the right, transgression through the kidney and liver may provide a window to the target during an anterior or lateral approach. Risk of renal and hepatic thermal injury is usually inconsequential, and a transhepatic or transrenal access route is often ideal. However, care should also be taken to avoid traversing the pleural space and causing a pneumothorax. Left-sided adrenal lesions may rarely mandate transsplenic access, which carries a higher risk of bleeding and thus should be

to use, the location of nearby organs, vessels, and nerves should be considered. Figures 151-1 and 151-2 show the intimate relationship of a right-sided adrenal tumor with the liver, portal vein, and inferior vena cava. In this instance, the close proximity of the tumor to a major vessel should warrant concern as to whether thermal ablation can be done successfully, owing to the large heat sink effect that may occur and result in inadequate treatment.

Adrenal tumors are most readily accessible via a posterior or lateral approach with the patient in an ipsilateral decubitus position.[14] Although the risk of ipsilateral lung injury and pneumothorax is minimized in the decubitus position, one must also take into account the organ shift that occurs with positioning. In Figure 151-3, the adrenal tumor of a patient in the prone position is near the abdominal aorta and loops of bowel. An appropriate treatment window must be selected to allow placement of the electrode without interference of the ribs and to prevent thermal injury to the nearby aorta and large bowel. Thorough planning and preprocedural imaging with multiphase contrast-enhanced CT or magnetic resonance imaging (MRI) with gadolinium can help with tumor staging and avoid intraprocedural complications.

concluded with aggressive ablation of splenic tissue on needle removal, sometimes as long as 12 to 15 minutes.

Access sites very close to the edge of moving targets may add risk of organ laceration (Figs. 151-4 and 151-5). This can occur at the edge of the liver, kidney, or spleen because they move with breathing. It is better to go through the organ and then aggressively cauterize on the way out, rather than traverse a mobile narrow window, lacerate an organ, and not have needle access at the exact bleeding point. Real-time feedback with ultrasound or CT fluoroscopy is vital for narrow windows, as often occurs with adrenal RFA. The stomach may present added risk if in proximity or abutting tumor. Although it is fairly thick walled, injury to the stomach may cause catastrophic perforation. We have given properistaltic drugs, performed orogastric iced saline lavage, and instilled 5% dextrose percutaneously between tumor and stomach to protect the stomach from thermal injury. The last of these may be the easiest and most effective. Although 5% dextrose may be safer than saline due to conduction differences, one should be aware of possible hyponatremia that can ensue from irrigation with hypotonic solutions.[15]

Once the patient has been positioned, two to four grounding pads are placed on the patient's thighs. Using a combination of ultrasound and/or CT guidance (Figs. 151-6 and 151-7), the appropriate electrode is placed into the tumor, often with the help of a radiopaque skin grid placed on the patient before the CT surview. Generally, nondeployable electrodes (Cool-tip [Covidien/Valleylab, Boulder, Colo.]) are easier to pierce small or mobile targets, because inserting and deploying arrays may add technical difficulty for monitoring in three dimensions. An estimation of the treatment zone is made on the ultrasound or CT as a mental treatment plan is formulated. After confirming that the patient is hemodynamically stable, the RF generator is turned on gradually, starting at 0.1 A and then increasing in 0.1-A increments as tolerated. If at any time the patient's mean arterial pressure increases 10 to 20 mmHg above baseline, a 10- to 60-second pause without current is applied while a nitroprusside drip is equilibrated.[16] During the procedure, repeat scanning during 50-mL miniboluses of contrast in between needle repositioning may define target tissue geometry. On completion, which is typically 12 to 16 minutes of overlapping treatments, the needle track is cauterized to prevent needle track seeding and bleeding. A contrast-enhanced CT scan may then be performed to ensure that the entire tumor has been ablated.

Special Considerations

If a pheochromocytoma is being ablated, extreme care must be taken to prevent the possibility of a hypertensive crisis (Figs. 151-8 and 151-9). Several weeks before the procedure, the patient should receive α-adrenergic blockade (with phenoxybenzamine) with or without β-adrenergic blockade to help prevent a hypertensive crisis during the procedure. Often β-blockade must be added because of the tachycardia that results from α-blockade. β-Blockade must only be administered *after* adequate α-blockade because unopposed α-adrenergic receptor stimulation can also precipitate a hypertensive crisis.[17] In our institution, the tyrosine hydroxylase inhibitor metyrosine (Demser [Merck Sharp & Dohme Corp., West Point, Pa.]) is combined with α-blockade because this regimen may provide better blood pressure control and require less intraoperative fluid replacement than the traditional method of single-agent α-adrenergic blockade.[18,19] Since cases of hypertensive

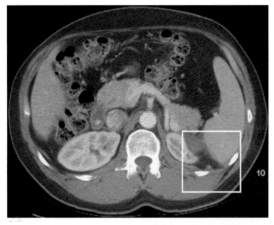

FIGURE 151-4. Enhanced computed tomography scan of recurrent left suprarenal lesion with narrow window *(box)* for electrode placement.

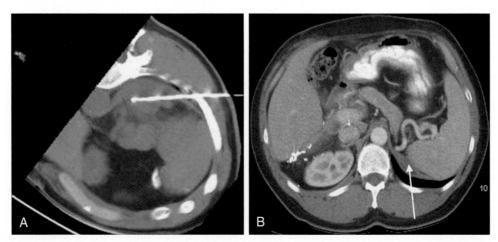

FIGURE 151-5. A, Oblique multiplanar reconstruction of radiofrequency electrode in tumor. **B,** Enhanced computed tomography scan 6 years after radiofrequency ablation shows long-term success. One tumor has disappeared, and one thermal scar *(arrow)* remains.

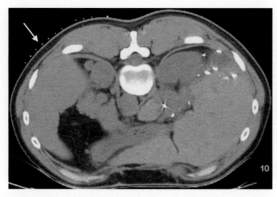

FIGURE 151-6. Computed tomography surview with skin grid *(arrow)* on patient to assist with skin insertion site of electrode.

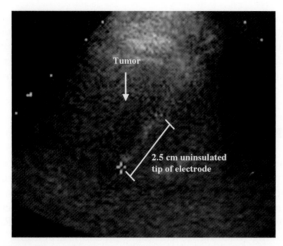

FIGURE 151-7. Ultrasound image showing measurement of uninsulated portion of electrode within tumor *(arrow)*.

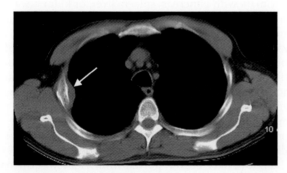

FIGURE 151-8. Preablation computed tomography scan of metastatic pheochromocytoma *(arrow)* to right rib.

crisis, including those leading to temporary cardiac arrest, have been reported during ablation of both pheochromocytomas and adrenal metastases, it may be prudent to premedicate all patients with α-adrenergic blockade prior to any adrenal ablation, although no formal recommendations are yet available.[20,21]

Cryoablation and microwave ablation are other forms of thermal ablation with limited experience in the adrenal

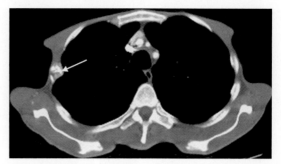

FIGURE 151-9. Enhanced computed tomography scan of metastatic pheochromocytoma *(arrow)* 29 months after ablation.

gland. A retrospective review by Welch et al. analyzed the hemodynamic changes during cryoablation of the adrenal gland in 12 patients. Local control was achieved in 92% of the 12 tumors ablated. Furthermore, it was found that like RFA, patients premedicated with α-adrenergic blockade had a reduced risk of hypertensive crisis. Of notable interest is the fact that the hypertensive crises occurred during the thaw phase, after the active cryoablation treatment.[22] This raises the possibility that cryoablation is less titratable than RFA. RFA can incrementally be turned higher and higher, with pauses to allow the operator to tightly control the catecholamine release. The thawing phase of cryoablation may result in larger bursts of catecholamine release, although this is speculative. Preliminary results of CT-guided microwave ablation has been studied by Li et al. and shows promising results.[23]

With so few cases of thermal ablation of the adrenal gland performed, a prospective study to evaluate various premedication protocols to prevent hypertensive crises would be difficult to conduct. However, in our experience we suggest that appropriate premedication be considered for all patients with nonfunctional and functional adrenal tumors to prevent hypertensive crises.

CONTROVERSIES

Although clinically isolated adrenal metastasis is unusual, the role of surgical resection and its effect on long-term survival is controversial. Kim et al. retrospectively studied 37 patients who had undergone adrenalectomy for isolated adrenal metastasis and found that the overall actuarial 5-year survival was 24% with a median of 21 months.[2] However, the incidence of complications was 19%, of which 12% were major complications. Median length of stay was 8 days.

Because few cases of isolated adrenal metastasis are seen, a randomized prospective trial of surgery versus RFA is highly unlikely. However, given the invasiveness and potential morbidity associated with surgery, RFA may prove to be an alternative minimally invasive treatment modality that could provide similar benefits and survival rates, with fewer complications, shorter hospital stay, and decreased cost.

OUTCOMES

Further studies are needed to determine the long-term efficacy and survival impact of RFA on ablation of adrenal

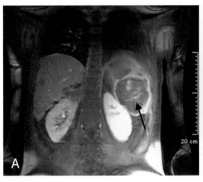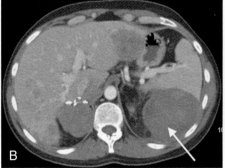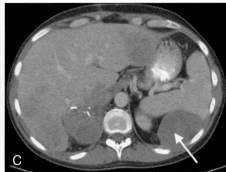

FIGURE 151-10. **A,** Coronal magnetic resonance image of large left adrenal tumor *(arrow)* before ablation. **B,** Preablation enhanced computed tomography (CT) scan of 9.9 × 8.2 cm left adrenal tumor *(arrow)*. **C,** Postablation enhanced CT scan of necrotic left adrenal tumor measuring 6.7 × 5.2 cm *(arrow)* 20 weeks after ablation.

neoplasms. Evidence-based data from hypothesis-driven studies are lacking owing to small numbers and low incidence, but extrapolation from the surgical literature provides a rational approach, with admittedly some major assumptions. RFA may offer a safe and effective treatment option for local tumor control. In our early experience treating 8 patients with 15 ACC recurrences or metastases, 57% of the tumors decreased in size or lost enhancement, and 27% showed no change in size. Tumors smaller than 5 cm achieved better results, with 67% of such tumors completely ablated. One patient subsequently developed a delayed abscess 11 weeks after his third RFA session, which was treated successfully with antibiotics.[24] More recent updates of our institutional experience with thermal ablation of 27 adrenocortical tumors in 16 patients (unpublished data) imply that ACC histology may confer a sensitivity to heat or, alternatively, may conduct radiofrequency current better than surrounding tissue or other tumor histologies. Anecdotally, larger ACC tumors than one would otherwise think possible may be successfully treated with thermal ablation, perhaps due to this speculative hypothesis (Fig. 151-10).

Dupuy et al. ablated 13 adrenal lesions in 12 patients.[25] Eleven of the lesions, including one pheochromocytoma and one patient with bilateral adrenal metastases, were treated successfully. One patient developed a small retroperitoneal hematoma that did not require transfusion, and another patient developed shortness of breath that resolved with diuresis. In these two studies, the mean follow-up ranged from 10.3 to 11.2 months. While the early results are preliminary, these studies also highlight the importance of local tumor control.

Although systemic therapies for metastatic disease remain the foundation of medical oncology, local and regional cancer therapies are playing an ever-increasing role. Hellman and Weichselbaum[26] comment that local tumor control is an important element of treatment strategy in four instances: (1) before tumors metastasize, (2) when combined with adjuvant chemotherapy for occult metastatic disease, (3) to treat oligometastases, and (4) to eliminate residual metastatic disease after effective systemic therapy. Debulking for local tumor control is becoming an increasingly more accepted approach in the oncology community, with the rationale that this could strengthen systemic therapies, which then have less tumor volume to

eradicate or potentially more tumor targets exposed. The ablation process may also elicit a tumor-specific systemic immune response, which may be combined with immunotherapy in the future.[27-29] RFA can be done safely and may be effective for local control of small primary and metastatic adrenal tumors.

COMPLICATIONS

Although the complications associated with RFA are rare when performed by experienced physicians, the adrenal gland may present special considerations and specific risks. Many of the myriad of general complications associated with RFA may also occur in the setting of adrenal RFA, including bleeding, discomfort, infection, grounding pad burns, and tumor seeding. More specific organ-related injuries include bowel perforation, pneumothorax, pancreatitis, and fistula and depend on the exact location and proximity of the tumor from other organs. When tumors are intimate with pancreas, spleen, liver, or kidney, we have seen thermal damage to these organs without clinical sequelae. The spleen has an increased risk of bleeding, and the pancreas a risk of fistula; the kidney and liver can often be burned to excess to ensure complete tumor treatment. Instillation of 5% dextrose water adjacent to the target tumor should be considered in cases in which the tumor is intimate with bowel or pancreas.[30] This should only be performed when absolutely necessary; long-term data are incomplete about whether fluid instillation affects tumor seeding. At least three instances of hypertensive crises in the literature have been reported while right lower hepatic or adrenal RFA was being performed.[21,31] Likewise, we have observed one instance of hypertensive crisis during RFA of pheochromocytoma that was safely managed with premedication, a nitroprusside drip, and careful anesthesia and pharmacologic support.

Hematoma, infarct, urinoma, cutaneous fistula, ureteral stricture, retroperitoneal bleeding, and injuries to the spleen, kidney, or pancreas are also possible complications.[32] Renal, splenic, and hepatic thermal damage is usually well tolerated. However, thermal injury to the bowel is probably the most significant complication that may occur and, if not noticed, may lead to immediate or delayed bowel perforation, peritonitis, and possible death. Although rare, damage to subcostal, ilioinguinal, iliohypogastric, or genitofemoral nerves may occur during ablation of lesions growing caudal or medial onto the psoas muscle.[32] Instillation of 5% dextrose may be protective in this setting. If there is a chance of adrenal insufficiency from the procedure, proper medical replacement therapy should be administered before the procedure to avoid adrenal crises. A postablation syndrome consisting of flulike symptoms may be seen after the procedure and lasts for about 1 week.[33]

POSTPROCEDURAL AND FOLLOW-UP CARE

Contrast-enhanced CT may be done immediately after ablation to evaluate treatment response. A lack of enhancement in the tumor bed or periphery usually indicates adequately ablated tumor. Residual enhancement of the tumor or postablation tumor growth indicates incomplete treatment or tumor recurrence. The primary goal of long-term diagnostic imaging follow-up after RFA is to identify possible recurrences of tumor when they are small and easily treatable. Exact frequency of imaging surveillance is dependent on the overall disease, natural history, and other patient-specific issues and should be determined in conjunction with a multidisciplinary team.

▶ **SUGGESTED READINGS**

Brown DB. Concepts, considerations, and concerns on the cutting edge of radiofrequency ablation. J Vasc Interv Radiol 2005;16:597–613.
Dupuy DE, Goldberg SN. Image-guided radiofrequency tumor ablation: challenges and opportunities: II. J Vasc Interv Radiol 2001;12:1135–48.
Goldberg SN, Grassi CJ, Cardella JF, et al. Image-guided tumor ablation: standardization of terminology and reporting criteria. Radiology 2005;235:728–39.
Ng L, Libertino JM. Adrenocortical carcinoma: diagnosis, evaluation and treatment. J Urol 2003;169:5–11.

The complete reference list is available online at www.expertconsult.com.

CHAPTER 152

Percutaneous Biopsy of the Lung, Mediastinum, and Pleura

Mark F. Given, Alison Corr, Kenneth R. Thomson, and Stuart M. Lyon

Percutaneous biopsy of chest lesions is performed for evaluation of focal lung lesions, mediastinal or hilar masses, and pleural or chest wall lesions. This procedure has become an essential part of staging of pulmonary and extrathoracic tumors.[1]

In the case of lung carcinoma, aspiration biopsy results in a positive diagnosis in 80% to 90% of cases. If a cutting needle is used, a positive diagnosis is expected in up to 95% to 98% of patients unless the lesion is necrotic.[2-5] A cutting needle (Fig. 152-1) is generally required for benign lesions, because more material is required to allow use of the special stains necessary for the pathologist to make a definitive diagnosis. The presence of a cytopathologist at the time of biopsy reduces the number of passes needed for diagnosis and avoids the unfortunate necessity for repeat examinations because of an inadequate sample.

With computed tomography (CT) guidance, it is possible to perform a biopsy on almost any portion of the chest with a high degree of safety and minimal morbidity because of the ability to plan a needle path such that major vascular structures are avoided (Fig. 152-2). The smallest needle suitable for the biopsy should be used to reduce complications.[6]

When there is a suspicious mass in a subcarinal location, endoscopic ultrasound-guided biopsy is a useful and safe technique. It is also associated with a lower risk for pneumothorax than percutaneous biopsy and may be indicated in patients with severe emphysema and a mediastinal mass. Needle biopsy has led to far less frequent use of mediastinoscopy for staging than in the past.

INDICATIONS

- Staging of bronchial carcinoma
- Diagnosis of focal lung lesions (nodules or consolidation)
- Diagnosis of metastatic lung lesions
- Evaluation of chronic infectious diseases when bronchoscopy is unsuccessful
- Diagnosis of mediastinal masses or lymphadenopathy
- Diagnosis of focal or diffuse pleural thickening

CONTRAINDICATIONS

- Severe emphysema. Patients with severe emphysema may not have sufficient lung capacity in the event of pneumothorax and have a higher risk for bronchopleural fistula (forced expiratory volume in 1 second [FEV_1] < 1.0 L).
- Insufficient lung capacity in the case of unilateral pneumothorax. Patients with extensive fibrosis or other causes of restricted lung capacity may not tolerate

pneumothorax. Patients who have undergone pneumonectomy should have an intercostal tube placed before the biopsy.
- Bleeding diathesis (international normalized ratio [INR] > 1.5 or platelets < 50,000/mm³). This is a relative risk, and the bleeding tendency should be corrected unless an urgent biopsy is imperative.
- Uncooperative patients, including those with an intractable cough. In these patients, development of pneumothorax is a certainty, and a diagnostic specimen may be impossible to obtain.
- Positive pressure ventilation, which increases the risk for pneumothorax and bronchopleural fistula.
- Pulmonary arterial hypertension when a central biopsy is contemplated. There is an increased risk for fatal hemorrhage if a major central artery is punctured.
- Suspected hydatid cyst. Diagnosis of a hydatid cyst is usually made on the preliminary CT scan. There is a possible risk for anaphylaxis if the cyst is intact, but if it has already ruptured, this is debatable.

EQUIPMENT

- An appropriate imaging modality (usually a CT scanner but may be a fixed fluoroscopy unit or ultrasound)
- Informed consent
- Intravenous access
- Equipment suitable for resuscitation
- Aspiration needle (Chiba or Westcott, 20-25 gauge)
- Fragment/aspiration needle (20-22 gauge)
- Coaxial needle system (19-gauge outer, 22-gauge inner)
- Core cutting needle (spring activated, 18-20 gauge)
- Cytologist to assess the sample immediately
- Microscope, slides, stains, and specimen pots (air and formalin)
- Percutaneous pneumothorax drainage system

TECHNIQUE

Anatomy and Approach

The shortest possible path to the lesion should be chosen that will avoid vital structures such as pulmonary arteries and major bronchii.

Biopsy of the mediastinum should be undertaken only when adequate imaging of the mediastinal structures is available and there is a safe path for the needle. In cases in which a subcarinal mass requires biopsy, transesophageal ultrasound-guided biopsy may be the method of choice.

Biopsy of a pleural mass almost always requires a cutting needle and a sample for histologic rather than cytopathologic analysis. If special stains are to be used, multiple samples will be required, and provision should be made using a coaxial technique.

Biopsy of the ribs generally requires special bone biopsy needles, even when it appears on the imaging that little bone is present. Unless the lesion is large or a tangential approach can be taken, it is difficult to use a cutting needle for rib lesions.

When it is possible to biopsy a lung lesion percutaneously, a direct vertical approach is preferred, with the skin entry site upright. After the biopsy, the patient is turned so that the punctured side is lowermost to reduce ventilation of that lung and, one hopes, the incidence of pneumothorax. One study comparing conventional treatment with side-down treatment found a reduction in both the pneumothorax rate (41.6% reduced to 12.9%) and the incidence of chest tube requirements (18% reduced to 2.7%).[7]

Technical Aspects

- Informed consent, including discussion of the risk for hemoptysis and pneumothorax, must be obtained. Ensure the patient is cooperative enough and can make an effort to not cough after the biopsy.
- Anticoagulants, including aspirin, should be discontinued for 3 to 5 days before biopsy. A clotting profile should be obtained in the 24 hours before biopsy. If it is abnormal,

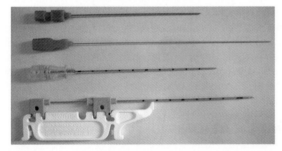

FIGURE 152-1. Biopsy needles suitable for use in the thorax. Sizes range from 22 to 18 gauge and aspiration to cutting type *(lowermost).*

fresh frozen plasma, platelets, or vitamin K should be administered as indicated.
- If CT is used for guidance, it is helpful to place markers on the skin and obtain scans at a phase of respiration easy for the patient to reproduce. Make sure the display on the screen is being projected in the same-side aspect the patient is being viewed.
- If fluoroscopy is used for guidance, the lesion must be visible in two views.
- Preferably, plan to approach the target by crossing as little aerated lung as possible.
- If malignancy is suspected, aspiration biopsy is probably all that is required. For benign lesions in which multiple passes may be required, a coaxial technique is preferred unless a core-cutting biopsy is to be performed.
- After antiseptic skin preparation and draping, infiltrate down to the pleura with local anesthetic while taking care to not cross the pleura. The British Thoracic Society guidelines state that percutaneous lung biopsies should be performed without administration of sedation in most cases.[8]
- Insert the needle along the planned trajectory to the target. When CT is used, perform a series of thin slices around the expected point of the needle to confirm placement within the lesion. When fluoroscopy is used, passage of the needle into the lesion should be visible.
- Perform the biopsy. With aspiration, the stylet is removed from the needle and the needle gently jiggled while the needle is aspirated with a 10-mL syringe. Avoid filling the syringe with blood, and release the suction before the needle is withdrawn. With a cutting needle, remember to allow for the "throw" of the device when positioning the needle.
- When CT is used, ensure the final tip position of the needle is imaged before a biopsy is performed. If a long needle is used, it may impact the CT gantry in some positions.
- Check with the cytologist that the sample is adequate, and if necessary, repeat the biopsy until the sample is pronounced adequate. Percutaneous lung biopsy is preferably performed in the presence of an onsite pathologist to avoid unnecessary recall of patients with inconclusive tissue sampling. If a core-cutting biopsy is performed and

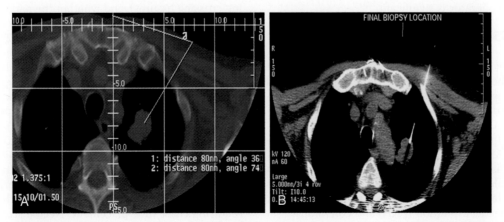

FIGURE 152-2. Computed tomography (CT)-guided biopsy. Planning approach with CT allows assessment of the "throw" of a cutting needle. **A,** Planning image. **B,** Needle in position within mass.

the needle tip has been shown to be within the lesion, one pass of the needle is usually sufficient.
• Place an occlusive patch over the puncture site and turn the patient so the point of puncture is dependent to reduce the incidence of pneumothorax.

CONTROVERSIES

The major controversy regarding biopsy of the lung is who should perform the biopsy. If the lesion is accessible by bronchoscopy, most thoracic physicians will attempt to obtain a cellular diagnosis before referring the patient for percutaneous biopsy. The advent of endoscopic ultrasound-guided biopsy has added another method for thoracic physicians to obtain tissue, with further advances in the introduction of endobronchial ultrasound approaches. Endobronchial ultrasound (EBUS)-guided sampling of mediastinal lymph nodes has been shown to have favorable specificity (100%) and sensitivity (88%) rates over CT-guided approaches.[9] Some limitations in EBUS assessment of mediastinal adenopathy exist, with blind spots including the aortopulmonary window, paraaortic station, paraesophageal stations, and the inferior pulmonary ligament.[9] Combination EBUS and esophageal ultrasound techniques will increase the accessibility of mediastinal nodes, further avoiding mediastinoscopy. More peripheral lesions are less successfully biopsied using an endobronchial approach and should be referred for percutaneous sampling.

Video-assisted thoracoscopic surgery (VATS) is generally indicated when there is a pleural-based mass or a more diffuse lung lesion such as fibrosis of unknown origin. VATS has almost completely replaced percutaneous drainage of empyema and infected bullae and remains the optimal approach for pleural sampling in patients who are deemed fit.

Widespread use of positron emission tomography (PET) in combination with percutaneous biopsy has almost completely obviated the need for mediastinoscopy, because the biopsy establishes the cellular diagnosis, and the PET scan demonstrates metastasis.

Presence of a cytopathologist at the biopsy significantly increases the yield of aspiration biopsy, but it is debatable whether value is added when a cutting-needle biopsy is performed and the sample is returned in formalin.

Use of CT fluoroscopy has declined because although there is some time savings, the increase in radiation dose to the patient and operator is significant.[10,11]

OUTCOMES

There is a low (1 in 5000) incidence of death after needle biopsy of the thorax. Causes of death have been pericardial tamponade, tension pneumothorax, air embolism, and pulmonary hemorrhage.[12,13] With good technique and a cooperative patient, these risks can be minimized.

Provided sufficient tissue is obtained, a definitive diagnosis is usual. Although it has been assumed that the complication rate is higher with cutting needles than with aspiration needles, a study of 182 sequential lung biopsies showed no difference in the incidence of pneumothorax between fine-needle aspiration (FNA) and core biopsy.[14]

Regarding the diagnosis of small cell lung cancer (SCLC) and non–small cell lung cancer (NSCLC), the accuracy of

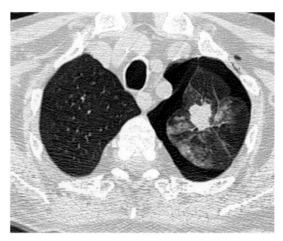

FIGURE 152-3. Pneumothorax after biopsy is always easily seen on computed tomography. Note increase in density of mass, indicative of hemorrhage.

FNA versus core biopsy is comparable, and complications are equal. However, to further subtype the carcinoma—which is becoming progressively more important with the advent of individualized chemotherapeutic approaches—FNA is inferior to larger-core biopsy and cutting-needle samples. It is becoming more important to acquire sufficient tissue to perform molecular analysis, and core biopsy should be considered in any patient being considered for nonsurgical therapeutic options.[15]

With CT-guided cutting-needle biopsy, overall accuracy is reported to be 95%, with a sensitivity of 93%, specificity of 98%, false-positive rate of 0.7%, and false-negative rate of 15%. Failure to obtain a diagnostic sample is more likely in benign lesions, those smaller than 1.5 cm, and large lesions (>5 cm) with central necrosis.[5] Core biopsy should always be the first consideration (over FNA) in a likely benign lesion.[16]

COMPLICATIONS

The most common complication is pneumothorax (Fig. 152-3). Its incidence is generally quoted in the range of 12% to 30%, with most not requiring drainage. In our experience, the incidence is related to the "dwell time" of the needle, the number of holes in the pleural surfaces (including crossing fissures), and whether the patient coughs a lot. In a recent study of 117 consecutive cases, Yeow et al.[17] found that pneumothorax occurred in 12% (14 of 117). Lesion depth ($P = .0097$), measured from the pleural puncture site to the edge of the intrapulmonary lesion along the needle path, was the single significant predictor of pneumothorax. The highest risk for pneumothorax occurred with subpleural lesions 2 cm or shorter in depth (this represented 33% of lung lesions but caused 71% of all cases of pneumothorax; odds ratio [OR], 7.1; 95% confidence interval [CI], 1.3-50.8). Most are visible on initial postbiopsy imaging, but only 30% require treatment. In their series of 283 biopsy procedures, Yamagami et al.[14] performed aspiration of pneumothorax on 52 patients, with only 9 (8.7%) requiring chest tube placement. Needle size (18-22 gauge) has been shown to not significantly affect pneumothorax rates.[18]

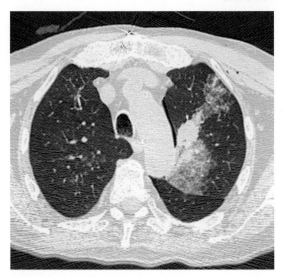

FIGURE 152-4. Pulmonary hemorrhage after biopsy. Despite extensive parenchymal hemorrhage outlining border of upper lobe at oblique fissure after biopsy, there was no evidence of hemoptysis.

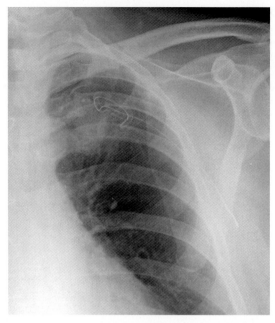

FIGURE 152-5. Percutaneous drainage of pneumothorax with 6F drainage catheter (Safe-T-Centesis kit [Cardinal Health, Dublin, Ohio]).

Hemoptysis may occur and at times may appear significant, but it almost always stops, although deaths have been reported. If there is time, angiography may show a bleeding site, and embolization is possible. Most often the bleeding site is indicated by a severed vessel. Some hemorrhage around the lesion and along the needle tract is common, especially on CT imaging (Fig. 152-4). Yeow et al.[17] reported bleeding manifested as lung parenchyma hemorrhage in 30 patients (26%). Hemoptysis occurred in four patients (3%). Univariate analysis identified lesion depth ($P < .0001$), lesion size ($P < .015$), and pathology type ($P = .007$) as risk factors for bleeding. Multivariate logistic regression analysis identified lesion depth as the most important risk factor, with the highest bleeding risk noted for lesions deeper than 2 cm (14% of lesions caused 46% of all bleeding; OR, 17.3; 95% CI, 3.3-121.4).

Biopsy of the mediastinum when a large vessel or the pericardium is in the target area requires notification of the time of the biopsy to a cardiothoracic surgeon. Because the pericardial reflection reaches well above the aortic valve, pericardial tamponade may occur if the aorta or great vessels are punctured within the pericardial sac. This is more likely to occur with a cutting needle.

POSTPROCEDURAL AND FOLLOW-UP CARE

- Always image the chest at the end of the biopsy procedure. Most significant pneumothoraces develop within 1 hour or less after the biopsy.
- Ask the patient to breathe quietly, and keep the patient resting for 2 to 3 hours. A chest radiograph should then be performed to exclude pneumothorax. An outpatient may be discharged if there is no pneumothorax.[14]
- In cases of tension pneumothorax, an intravenous cannula (Introcan Safety [B. Braun, Bethlehem, Pa.]) can be used to reduce the pressure, and the pneumothorax can be aspirated completely.

- If the pneumothorax is significant (>25%), it should be drained either with an intravenous cannula and a syringe or with a catheter and a one-way valve (Heimlich) or underwater drain (Fig. 152-5). Once the pneumothorax disappears and the lung has reexpanded, the drain can be removed.
- If hemoptysis does occur, it is important to reassure the patient that it will stop. If there is significant bleeding, an urgent angiogram may help but in most circumstances is unnecessary.
- Ensure the sample is labeled correctly and the patient's identification is correct. The laboratory may refuse to process an unidentified sample.

KEY POINTS

- Percutaneous biopsy is a rapid and efficient method of obtaining a cytologic and histologic diagnosis.
- Diagnostic results are highest for malignant lesions.
- Benign lesions usually require core biopsy rather than aspiration biopsy.
- Computed tomography (CT)-guided biopsy is now the preferred method of percutaneous lung and pleural biopsy because of its higher yield. While CT-guided biopsy is favored for most mediastinal adenopathy, subcarinal nodes may be more amenable to biopsy under endobronchial ultrasound guidance.
- Preferably, a cytopathologist should be present at the time of biopsy to indicate whether more material is required.
- Use of a coaxial needle reduces the number of pleural punctures and decreases the risk for pneumothorax.
- Pneumothorax resulting from lung or pleural biopsy can usually be managed by the interventional radiologist.
- Turning the patient onto the side of the biopsy afterward will reduce the incidence of pneumothorax.

► **SUGGESTED READINGS**

Anderson JM, Murchison J, Patel D. CT-guided lung biopsy: factors influencing diagnostic yield and complication rate. Clin Radiol 2003; 58:791–7.

Heck SL, Blom P, Berstad A. Accuracy and complications in computed tomography fluoroscopy-guided needle biopsies of lung masses. Eur Radiol 2006;16:1387–92.

House AJS. Biopsy techniques in the investigation of diseases of the lung, mediastinum and chest wall. Radiol Clin North Am 1979;17: 393–412.

The complete reference list is available online at www.expertconsult.com.

CHAPTER 153

Treatment of Effusions and Abscesses

Robert J. Lewandowski, Sudhen B. Desai, and Albert A. Nemcek, Jr.

Percutaneous management of thoracic and abdominal fluid collections, including pleural effusions and abscesses, has become standard of care in many clinical scenarios.[1] This shift from operative management has been facilitated by advances in quality and rapidity of cross-sectional imaging and interventional radiology technology. Percutaneous management of effusions and abscesses is cost-effective and decreases both morbidity and mortality compared with alternative treatments.[2-8] To be truly effective, the interventional radiologist must participate in the clinical care of the patient and coordinate care with referring medical and surgical colleagues.

INDICATIONS

Most patients undergoing percutaneous management of effusions or abscesses are symptomatic and have had recent imaging studies performed. In fact, these symptoms have typically led to the imaging examination (i.e., most effusions or abscesses are not found incidentally). If the patient is asymptomatic, percutaneous drainage may not be needed as an adjunct to antibiotic or other medical therapy, although diagnostic sampling may be necessary. The patient's symptoms help categorize the urgency of draining an effusion or abscess. Patients with symptoms of pain, low-grade fever, and a mildly elevated white blood cell (WBC) count do not require urgent attention. However, patients with hypotension, tachycardia, high-grade fever or fever spikes, or a markedly elevated WBC count require decompression as soon as possible.

When percutaneous management of an effusion or abscess is clearly indicated, a decision regarding fluid aspiration versus catheter placement should be made. In general, drainage catheters are placed unless a fluid collection is small, not walled off, or known to be sterile. If aspirated fluid appears purulent, a drainage catheter is generally placed.

CONTRAINDICATIONS

There are few contraindications to percutaneous management of effusions or abscesses. Two are lack of a safe route for catheter insertion and uncorrectable coagulopathy, issues that often become evident when reviewing the patient's imaging studies and laboratory results. Any apparent contraindication should be discussed with the referring service to ascertain the risks versus potential benefits.

To allow percutaneous therapy, the abnormal fluid collection must be clearly visualized on imaging, and there must be an acceptable path from a skin entry site to the abnormality. Although it is often necessary and acceptable to place a needle or catheter through normal organ parenchyma when managing an intraparenchymal abscess, it is often unacceptable to traverse an uninvolved organ or normal bowel. However, some have argued for the benefits of transgastric drainage, and normal hepatic parenchyma may be transgressed if it is the only route to the fluid collection.[9] It is sometimes possible to create a more direct and safer access route to the target fluid by injecting saline, lidocaine, or CO_2 into the intervening tissues.[10,11] This may displace potential obstacles out of the way, but it also may make the target less conspicuous on imaging. Manual compression of tissues with the ultrasound probe may help displace intervening bowel loops, and alternative patient positioning may help clear a potential passageway. It should be noted that a referring surgeon may accept traversal of diseased bowel if an operation is impending.

All patients being considered for percutaneous intervention should have their coagulation profile evaluated, including platelet counts, prothrombin time, international normalized ratio (INR), and partial thromboplastin time. Although it is difficult to give strict coagulation parameters, the platelet count should be greater than 50,000 and the INR should be 1.5 or lower.[12] All abnormalities are best corrected in conjunction with the referring service. Some patients will need platelet transfusion, fresh frozen plasma, vitamin K, protamine, or other strategies to make the procedure safer.[13] The medication administration record should also be reviewed. Specifically, drugs such as aspirin, heparin, subcutaneous heparin, and clopidogrel (Plavix) should be sought because they may increase the risk for a hemorrhagic complication without significantly altering the patient's coagulation profile. Ideally these medications are stopped for a defined period (aspirin and Plavix, 1 week; subcutaneous heparin, 12 hours; intravenous heparin, 2 hours) before percutaneous intervention,[14] but each case must be considered individually.

EQUIPMENT

Image-guided procedures are facilitated by ultrasound, fluoroscopy, computed tomography (CT), or a combination of these modalities. Factors that influence which modality is most appropriate include target location, target size, and operator preference. At our institution, percutaneous drainage procedures are typically performed with a combination of ultrasound and fluoroscopy. Ultrasound is used to place a needle into the effusion or abscess, whereas fluoroscopy is used to visualize placement of a drainage catheter. Ultrasound is frequently our preferred modality to access an abnormal fluid collection because it is fast and readily available, produces no ionizing radiation, and allows real-time visualization of needle placement. However, it is operator dependent, and smaller, deeper fluid collections may not be readily seen. Patient body habitus and intervening bowel gas are further detriments to optimal visualization with ultrasonography. Fluoroscopy may be the sole imaging modality if a few criteria are met: the effusion or abscess must be diagnosed on previous cross-sectional imaging, and there must be a previously determined safe passage to this abnormal fluid collection. A recognizable collection of air (air/fluid level) is helpful in ensuring proper needle placement. In our practice, CT is usually reserved for lesions not visible sonographically or fluoroscopically. Abscesses that are deeply located, retroperitoneal, or small in size frequently require CT localization.

Once an imaging modality is selected, the interventionalist must decide on an access needle, guidewire, dilators, and drainage catheter. The preferred access needle is at least a few centimeters longer than needed to reach the fluid collection and allows passage of a 0.035- to 0.038-inch guidewire. The guidewire enables progressive dilation and subsequent catheter placement. Dilators should be chosen to at least the size of the drainage catheter. Some advocate dilating to 2 French sizes larger than the catheter. Various types of drainage catheters are available. A locking 10F pigtail catheter is a reasonable standard catheter. If the fluid collection is small, an 8F drain can be used, and if the aspirated fluid appears viscous, a 12F or larger catheter may be placed. Large-bore tunneled catheters are being placed with greater frequency for longer-term home drainage.

TECHNIQUE

Anatomy and Approach

The most crucial aspect of percutaneous drainage is determining an access route. The safest and shortest distance between the skin access site and target fluid collection should be sought. Review of available imaging studies and knowledge of anatomic landmarks and the expected location of blood vessels, nerves, and other tissues facilitate avoidance of these structures. Once chosen, the access site is marked, prepared, and draped in sterile fashion. The skin access site is then infiltrated with a local anesthetic, a small incision is made with a scalpel, and the tissues are locally dissected to aid subsequent catheter placement. At this point, either the Seldinger or trocar technique is used to place the drainage catheter. With the *Seldinger technique*, an access needle is placed into the fluid collection. A wire is passed through the access needle and coiled in the collection. Serial dilation over the wire precedes placement of the catheter over the wire. The catheter is then advanced without a stylet (a metal or plastic stiffener is used instead). The wire is removed, and the catheter is secured in place. The *trocar technique* does not make use of an access wire. Instead, a sharp stylet passed through the catheter aids its advancement. The *tandem trocar approach* makes use of a reference needle placed into the fluid collection under imaging guidance. The drainage catheter is then advanced via the trocar technique into the cavity adjacent to the reference needle in the same direction as the reference needle until the fluid collection is entered. The *direct trocar approach* does not make use of a reference needle. The drainage catheter is simply advanced into the fluid collection based on previous imaging studies. This technique is generally reserved for large superficial collections.

Technical Aspects

Thoracic
Pleural Effusions
Pleural effusions have many causes and can usually be aspirated (thoracentesis) for symptom relief. Malignant pleural effusions tend to recur rapidly, however, and some special strategies are used to deal with these. A reasonable management plan is to place a tunneled drainage catheter (e.g., Denver Pleurx catheter [Denver Biomaterials, Golden, Colo.]) and monitor the patient on an outpatient basis. Autopleurodesis has been shown to occur in 40% to 50% of these patients.[15] If pleurodesis does not occur, a sclerosing agent may be used to scar the parietal and visceral pleural layers together. Such agents include talc, bleomycin, and tetracycline/doxycycline.[16,17]

Empyema
Infected pleural fluid collections typically result from pneumonia or are posttraumatic in nature (Fig. 153-1). They can often be successfully managed percutaneously with drains. Infusion of thrombolytic agents into these drains has been used to eradicate the fibrinous components of the inflammatory process.[18,19]

Lung Abscess
Lung abscesses are typically secondary to aspiration, hematogenous spread of infection, or spread from an adjacent inflammatory process. More than 80% of lung abscesses respond to the traditional therapy of antibiotics and bronchial lavage. In patients who fail such therapy, percutaneous management may be an alternative to thoracotomy.[7,20] A risk of placing a percutaneous drain in the lung is creation of a bronchopleural fistula. Minimizing drainage catheter size and avoiding traversal of normal lung help minimize this risk.

Pericardial Effusions
Interventional radiologists may be asked to drain pericardial fluid. In our experience, this is best approached with ultrasound guidance. Percutaneous creation of a pericardial window with an angioplasty balloon is a safe therapeutic option, particularly in patients with symptomatic malignant effusions.[21]

Abdominal
Hepatic
Pyogenic hepatic abscesses are most frequently sequelae of previous hepatic or biliary surgery, but they may also result from trauma, an infectious process elsewhere in the abdomen (e.g., diverticulitis), or an existing hepatic malignancy (Fig. 153-2). Percutaneous management of these abscesses is quite effective for both pyogenic and amebic hepatic abscesses.[22,23] A subcostal approach is preferred because it is less painful and there is less chance of crossing the pleural space and causing empyema. The intercostal approach is reserved for instances where a subcostal approach is not possible. It should be noted that although drainage of hydatid (echinococcal) hepatic cysts was once considered a contraindication because of the risk of sepsis, the literature now supports percutaneous management. Hypertonic saline can be injected into the cystic cavities as a scolicidal agent.[24]

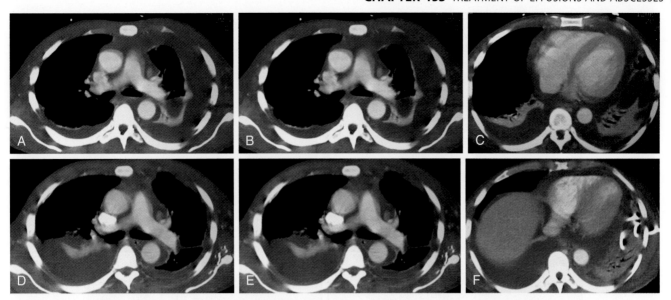

FIGURE 153-1. A-C, Loculated left pleural fluid collection complicating a case of pneumonia. **D-F,** Correlative images after drain placement via interventional radiology and management with thrombolytic therapy; note marked improvement in left fluid collection.

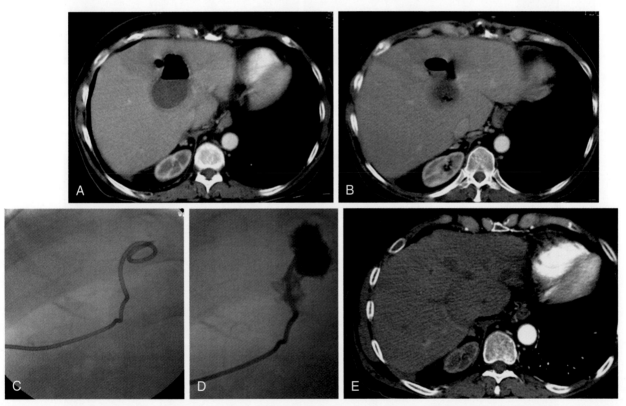

FIGURE 153-2. A-B, Hepatic abscess in segments 4 and 8 post liver transplantation complicated by hepatic artery occlusion. **C,** Fluoroscopic spot image of percutaneously placed drain via interventional radiology. **D,** Tube check of that drain demonstrates small, irregular, persistent cavity without a fistula to biliary tree. **E,** Follow-up computed tomography image demonstrating resolution of abscess and removal of drain.

Renal

Renal abscesses result from hematogenous spread of infection or from pyelonephritis (Fig. 153-3). The infectious process may extend into the perinephric space. Percutaneous management is typically reserved for large parenchymal abscesses, those with a perinephric component, or small intrarenal abscesses that do not respond to appropriate antibiotic therapy. These fluid collections often contain an inflammatory component that may not respond to percutaneous drainage. A retroperitoneal approach through the avascular plane of Brödel is recommended.[25,26]

Splenic

Splenic abscesses result from hematogenous spread of infection, direct extension from an adjacent infectious process, or previous trauma (Figs. 153-4 and 153-5).

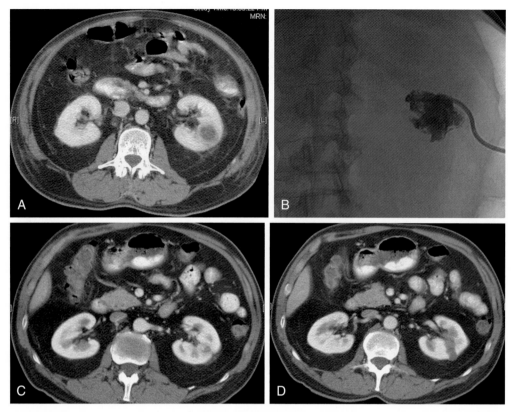

FIGURE 153-3. A, Computed tomography (CT) scan demonstrating left renal abscess complicating a case of pyelonephritis that failed to resolve with intravenous antibiotic therapy. **B,** Fluoroscopic image after percutaneous intrarenal drain placement and manual injection of contrast material; note irregular cavity without a fistula to renal collecting system. **C-D,** CT images after drain removal demonstrate resolution of left renal abscess.

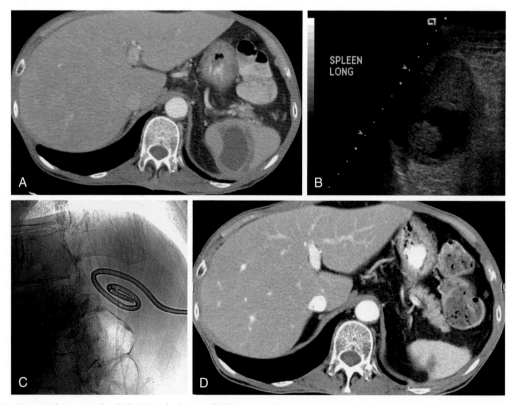

FIGURE 153-4. Computed tomography (CT) **(A)** and ultrasound **(B)** images demonstrating splenic abscess in human immunodeficiency virus–positive patient who complained of fevers and chills on return from trip to Thailand. **C,** Fluoroscopic image after interventional radiology placement of percutaneous drain. **D,** CT image after drain removal demonstrating resolution of abscess.

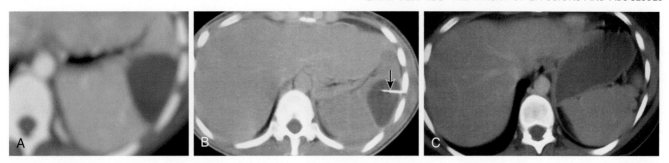

FIGURE 153-5. A, Computed tomography (CT) image demonstrating splenic abscess in patient with mycotic pseudoaneurysm of femoral artery. **B,** CT image during needle placement *(arrow)* into splenic abscess. **C,** CT image taken after completion of abscess management demonstrates resolution of infective process.

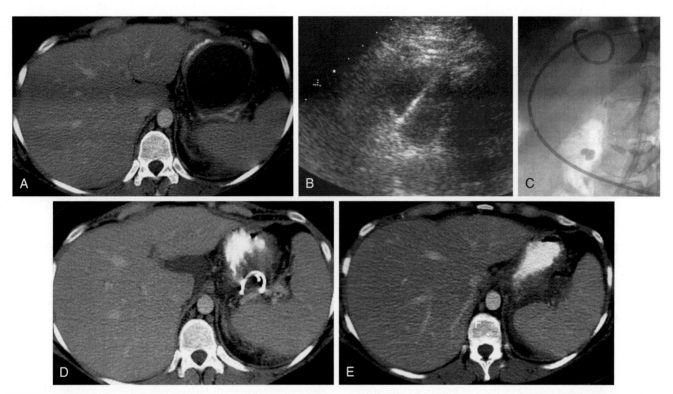

FIGURE 153-6. A, Computed tomography (CT) image depicting large fluid collection in lesser sac complicating a case of pancreatitis. **B,** Ultrasound image during drain placement. **C,** Fluoroscopic image taken after drain placement via interventional radiology. **D-E,** CT images after drain placement and removal demonstrate resolution of fluid collection.

Percutaneous management of these abscesses has historically been avoided because of the risk for significant hemorrhage, but percutaneous drainage techniques have proved to be safe and effective.[27] To minimize bleeding risk, a small (8F or 10F) catheter is typically used, and the catheter is placed such that it traverses the least possible amount of normal splenic parenchyma. Transpleural catheter placement is best avoided to prevent direct spread of infection to the pleural space.

Pancreatic
Management of pancreatic abscesses can be medical, operative, endoscopic, or percutaneous (Fig. 153-6). The role of the interventional radiologist in percutaneous management is evolving. The presence of tissue fragments and saponified fat often makes percutaneous drainage difficult,

and surgical débridement may be needed. Fluid aspiration or sampling is often useful in differentiating sterile from infected fluid collections and helps refine antibiotic therapy. Percutaneous abscess drainage may result in cure or can make future operative management less technically demanding.[28,29]

Enteric
Enteric abscesses typically complicate disease processes such as appendicitis, diverticulitis, or inflammatory bowel disease (Fig. 153-7). The goal of percutaneous abscess drainage in these cases is to facilitate an elective one-stage operation at a time remote from the initial evaluation. Operating on these patients often initially results in multistage procedures and can result in significant morbidity. Drainage catheters may be left in place for several weeks

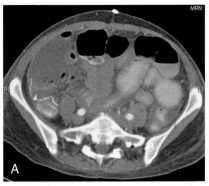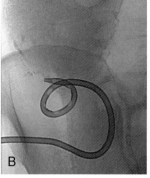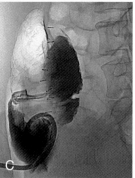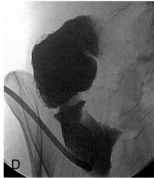

FIGURE 153-7. A, Computed tomography image from woman with fever 5 days after right hemicolectomy for cecal volvulus; note large abscess in right lower quadrant adjacent to surgical anastomosis. **B,** Fluoroscopic image taken after percutaneous drain placement via interventional radiology. **C-D,** Fluoroscopic images taken during routine tube check. A fistula to colon, representing a hole at surgical anastomosis, was detected. Patient had continued to have high drain output for several months.

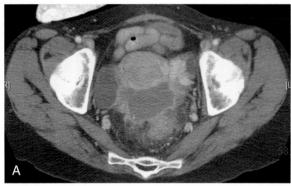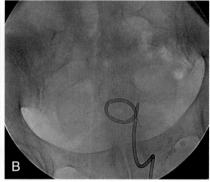

FIGURE 153-8. A, Computed tomography image of woman with Crohn disease; note abscess in pelvic cul-de-sac posterior to vagina. **B,** Fluoroscopic image taken after drain placement via interventional radiology; drain was placed from transvaginal approach.

because it is not uncommon for an abscess-fistula complex to be present.[30-33]

Pelvic

Pelvic abscesses are often challenging to access because of the surrounding bony pelvis (Fig. 153-8). An anterior transperitoneal approach cannot be used in many circumstances because of overlying structures, most notably bowel and bladder. Alternative routes include transgluteal, transrectal, and transvaginal approaches.[34-36] Although the transgluteal route has been used for deep pelvic abscesses, this method is frequently quite painful and not well tolerated by patients. The catheter should be directed near the sacrum if possible to avoid the sciatic nerve as it exits through the greater sciatic foramen.

Subphrenic

Subphrenic abscesses are most often postoperative complications (Fig. 153-9). They may be technically challenging to access because of their location under the diaphragm, bordered by the rib cage. Although an extrapleural route is advised because of the risk of pleural contamination, an intercostal approach may be necessary.[37]

OUTCOMES

The efficacy of percutaneous management of abscesses and effusions has been demonstrated in multiple series.[2-8]

However, it should be stated that success of percutaneous drainage depends on more than just drainage technique and patient management. Comorbid conditions and complexity of fluid collections can also affect success rates.

The Society of Interventional Radiology (SIR) has published a quality initiative for percutaneous drainage of abscesses.[38] Successful diagnostic fluid aspiration is defined as aspiration of sufficient material for diagnosis. Per these guidelines, success should be achieved 95% of the time. Regarding drainage of infected fluid collections, results are defined in terms of success (complete or partial success) or failure (including recurrence). Complete resolution of infection implies that no further intervention is needed, whereas partial success means either that drainage of the abscess was adequate and surgery was subsequently performed to repair an underlying problem, or that the drainage was a temporizing measure before surgery. By SIR guidelines, curative drainage should occur in more than 80% of cases, whereas partial success occurs in 5% to 10%. The SIR set a threshold of 85% for successful drainage (curative and partial success). Failure and recurrence both occur in 5% to 10% of patients.

COMPLICATIONS

The SIR Standards of Practice Committee has published criteria for complications by outcome. Minor complications are defined as those that require no therapy (A) and those

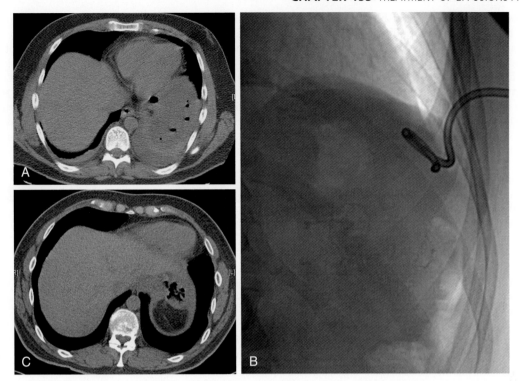

FIGURE 153-9. A, Computed tomography (CT) image from young man complaining of fever and left upper quadrant pain after resection of a desmoid tumor; large subphrenic abscess is present. **B,** Fluoroscopic image taken after percutaneous drain placement via interventional radiology. **C,** CT image after drain removal demonstrates resolution of subphrenic abscess.

that require nominal therapy or admission for overnight observation (B). Major complications include those that require major therapy and hospitalization for less than 48 hours (C) or those that require major therapy, an increased level of patient care, and prolonged hospitalization for more than 48 hours (D). Permanent adverse sequelae (E) and death (F) are other classifications of major complications. According to the SIR, the overall procedure threshold in adults for all major complications resulting from percutaneous drainage of abscesses and fluid is 10%.[38]

Major complications of percutaneous procedures may include bleeding, infection, and inadvertent injury to bowel or viscera. Hemorrhage is often avoided by correcting any coagulopathy before the procedure. Hemorrhage is suspected in the setting of increasing postprocedural pain accompanied by tachycardia or hypotension. Occasionally blood is seen draining from the catheter. If hemorrhage is suspected, the drain should be left in place and the coagulation profile repeated. A CT scan should be obtained urgently because this study can verify hemorrhage and assess its cause and extent. If clinically stable, the patient can be observed closely and serial complete blood cell counts obtained. If the patient appears unstable, angiography with potential embolization of a bleeding vessel could be performed (if CT demonstrates bleeding from an intraabdominal visceral source).

Infection or sepsis is best avoided by ensuring the patient is on an appropriate antibiotic regimen before the procedure. If the patient is not taking preprocedure antibiotics, broad-spectrum coverage should be provided before catheter placement. Sepsis risk can also be decreased by minimizing catheter manipulation during the procedure.

Irrigation of the abscess cavity should be gentle. If contrast material is to be injected, a minimal amount should be used.

Inadvertent injury to bowel or viscera is best avoided by optimizing the access route and directly visualizing catheter advancement under real-time imaging. If a catheter mistakenly perforates a solid organ, bleeding may result. This should be managed as described earlier. If a catheter is mistakenly placed into a loop of bowel, the catheter should remain in place until a mature tract develops. The tract will close spontaneously. If the bladder is mistakenly perforated by a drainage catheter, the catheter should be removed and a Foley catheter placed in the bladder. The Foley catheter should remain in place for approximately 1 week to allow the perforation to heal.

POSTPROCEDURAL AND FOLLOW-UP CARE

After insertion of the catheter and aspiration of fluid, the catheter must be secured to the patient's skin to prevent inadvertent removal or displacement. There are many methods of catheter fixation involving commercially available fixation devices or suturing techniques. A collection bag is connected to the catheter and placed for dependent gravity drainage. Thoracic collections or those with particulate matter or highly viscous fluid may be placed under continuous low wall suction. Drain output should be monitored and recorded at routine intervals. Abscess drains are often irrigated with 5 to 10 mL of normal saline every 8 hours to facilitate tube patency.

The catheter and external fixation device must be inspected daily on ward rounds. Signs of catheter dislodgment or malfunction should be sought. The fluid draining into the collecting bag should also be evaluated; changes in character or quality provide clinical insight. For example, catheter output that does not decrease over time or increases after a few days of drainage probably indicates a fistulous communication. If a fistula is suspected, a catheter sinogram is performed. Otherwise, there is no definitive rule when it comes to repeat imaging after percutaneous drainage. Certainly, if the patient does not respond clinically to percutaneous drainage, cross-sectional imaging may divulge new or inadequately drained fluid collections.

There is some controversy in the published literature regarding the best methods of draining complex fluid collections and abscesses. Specifically, the role of adjunctive fibrinolytic therapy is debated. These agents have been shown to decrease viscosity of the fluid collection, making its removal theoretically easier.[39] In vitro studies with urokinase have demonstrated promising results in decreasing the draining fluid's viscosity.[40] However, a recent *New England Journal of Medicine* article reported no improvement in the treatment of pleural infections treated with streptokinase in nonselected patients.[41]

The endpoint of percutaneous drainage is multifactorial. It is crucial to discuss catheter plans with the referring medical or surgical service before catheter removal to avoid the necessity of replacing the catheter. Major criteria before catheter removal are clinical improvement (fever, pain, appetite), normalization of laboratory parameters (WBC count), decreasing catheter output (≤10 mL/day), resolution of cavity size (either repeat imaging or catheter sonogram), and absence of a fistulous communication. Some advocate exchanging the pigtail catheter for a straight catheter and gradually withdrawing the drain over a period of a few days, a surgical approach to drain management. This theoretically prevents reaccumulation of fluid secondary to premature closure of the drainage tract.[42] However, because catheter removal is typically delayed until drainage is minimal and a mature tract has formed, this process is no longer routinely advocated.[4] After catheter removal, a clean dressing should be applied. It is not unusual to observe a small amount of drainage from the catheter insertion site after catheter removal.

KEY POINTS

- Percutaneous management of abscesses and effusions is safe and effective.
- The role of percutaneous management is evolving.
- Percutaneous management of disease processes should be performed in conjunction with referring physicians.

► **SUGGESTED READINGS**

Mueller PR, vanSonnenberg E, Ferrucci JT Jr. Percutaneous drainage of 250 abdominal abscesses and fluid collections. Part II: current procedural concepts. Radiology 1984;151:343–7.

vanSonnenberg E, Mueller PR, Ferrucci JT Jr. Percutaneous drainage of 250 abdominal abscesses and fluid collections. Part I: results, failures, and complications. Radiology 1984;151:337–41.

The complete reference list is available online at www.expertconsult.com.

CHAPTER 154

Lung Ablation

Jeffrey P. Guenette and Damian E. Dupuy

Lung cancer is the most common primary cancer, with over 220,000 new cases in 2010, and is the most common cause of cancer death, with nearly 160,000 deaths per year.[1,2] Surgery is the mainstay of treatment for primary lung cancer, but it is estimated that over 15% of all patients and 30% of patients over age 75 with stage I or II non–small cell lung cancer (NSCLC) are medically inoperable.[3] Moreover, local therapy with external beam radiation has shown a best 2-year overall survival of only 51%,[4] with newer stereotactic body radiotherapy techniques (i.e., stereotactic body radiation therapy [SBRT]) showing 3-year survival rates of 42% to 60% for early-stage, medically inoperable NSCLC.[5,6]

Pulmonary metastatic disease is generally an indicator of wide disease dissemination requiring systemic therapy, but when a finite number of metastatic deposits exist in the lung, resection may improve prognosis for certain pathologies, including primary sarcoma, renal cell carcinoma, colorectal carcinoma, and breast carcinoma.[7-12] In the case of colorectal carcinoma with isolated pulmonary metastases, 5-year survival rates can exceed 50%.[12] Again, as with primary lung cancer, pulmonary metastases are often inoperable owing to patients' poor cardiopulmonary function, advanced age, and other medical comorbidities.

Image-guided thermal ablation is an increasingly studied and used treatment for both cure and palliation of primary and secondary lung cancer. The technique has been used for a little over a decade and has been shown to be safe and effective in treating a variety of solid tumors including many in the lung, liver, kidney, breast, bone, and adrenal gland. It may be used in conjunction with radiotherapy and systemic chemotherapy and is relatively low cost. Thermal ablation modalities include radiofrequency, microwave, laser, and cryotherapy. Randomized controlled clinical trials have not yet been conducted to establish efficacy of thermal ablation alone, in combination with, or relative to other established treatments of lung neoplasms. However, an increasing number of single and multicenter cohort studies have consistently established the safety and suggest efficacy for medically inoperable disease. The remainder of this chapter highlights the basic biophysics underlying thermal ablation modalities, specifically within the unique anatomy and physiology of the lung, the understood safety and efficacy of thermal lung ablation given our experience to date, newly introduced advances in thermal lung ablation techniques, and the current role of thermal ablation in the treatment of lung cancer.

BASIC BIOPHYSICS OF LUNG ABLATION

Electromagnetic (EM) energy takes form as oscillating perpendicular waves of electrical and magnetic fields traveling at the speed of light. EM wave frequencies range from 10 Hz (waves per second) to 10^{24} Hz, with radio waves having frequencies as low as 10^4 Hz, followed by microwaves, infrared waves, visible light, ultraviolet waves, x-rays, and gamma rays in increasing order of wave frequency.[13,14] Three of the four thermal ablation modalities utilize waves along this spectrum.

Radiofrequency Ablation

Radiofrequency ablation (RFA) is the most widely used ablation modality for the treatment of solid tumors; its safety has been firmly established in solid malignancies of the lung (Fig. 154-1 and Table 154-1), liver, bone, breast, kidney, and adrenals.[15] With this technique, an active RF electrode (applicator) is placed in the tumor under imaging guidance, and a grounding pad (reference electrode) is applied to the chest wall opposite the applicator or on the thigh. Most clinical RFA electrodes emit radio waves in the range of 375 to 500 kHz, generating electrical field lines between the applicator and reference electrode that oscillate with the alternating current. These fields result in collision of electrons with molecules adjacent to the applicator, generating frictional heat.[16] Temperatures exceeding 60°C, regardless of the heating source, induce cell cytotoxicity via thermolabile protein denaturation,[17] and this temperature is generally considered the baseline for inducing immediate coagulative necrosis. Care is taken to keep the electrode tip temperature below 100°C to avoid charring and vaporization, which occur at 110°C, because these processes increase electrical impedance and inhibit heat dissipation to surrounding tissue.[18] The goal is to ablate an appropriate circumferential margin: 95% of microscopic neoplastic extension is within a margin of 8 mm from the tumor border for adenocarcinoma and 6 mm for squamous cell carcinoma.[19]

Three RFA systems are currently commercially available in the United States. The LeVeen system (Boston Scientific/RadioTherapeutics, Watertown, Mass.]) consists of an array of electrode tines that are deployed through a 14- to 17-gauge needle and curve backward toward the device handle. The device measures impedance. The RITA system (RITA Medical Systems Inc., Mountain View, Calif.) is also composed of an array of electrode tines that are deployed through a 14- to 17-gauge needle, but these tines course forward and laterally. The RITA system measures temperature through multiple peripheral thermocouples and includes perfusion electrodes that infuse saline into the tissue to enhance energy distribution. The Cool-tip system (Covidien, Boulder, Colo.) consists of either a single electrode or a triple "cluster" of three electrodes spaced 5 mm apart. The Cool-tip electrodes are perfused with cold saline or water to minimize charring and include a thermocouple at the tip for temperature measurement. There have been no head-to-head comparisons of safety or efficacy between these devices in the lung.

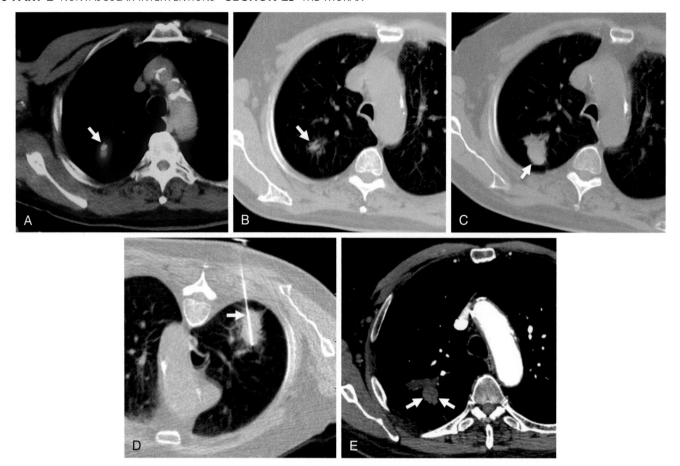

FIGURE 154-1. Biopsy-proven right upper lobe non–small cell carcinoma in a 64-year-old man who was referred for lung ablation. **A,** Axial positron emission tomography (PET)/computed tomography (CT) image shows focally intense metabolic activity *(arrow)* in right upper lobe. **B,** Axial nonenhanced CT image shows initial lesion *(arrow)*. **C,** Axial nonenhanced CT image shows new tumor growth *(arrow)* following initial ablation. **D,** Prone axial CT image obtained during repeat radiofrequency ablation shows electrode *(arrow)* appropriately placed in mass. **E,** Axial contrast-enhanced 6-month follow-up CT scan shows residual thermal scar *(arrow)* in right upper lobe, without evidence of growth or enhancement.

The lung presents unique considerations for RFA because of the large quantities of air between thin layers of parenchyma, continuous air flow, and high volume of pulmonary vascular flow. Air acts as an insulator, so RF energy is concentrated in the tumor. However, the air exchange and vascular flow dissipate heat from normal surrounding parenchyma,[20,21] creating difficulty in establishing a therapeutic ablation margin. Compared to solid organs, the lung has less water per unit volume of tissue,[22] so the infusion of saline may be warranted to help promote conduction of electric current.[23]

Microwave Ablation

Microwave ablation (MWA) has been established as a treatment option for many tumors of the lung (Fig. 154-2; also see Table 154-1), liver, kidney, and bone. Most MWA antennae (applicators) available for clinical use emit microwaves in the range of 900 to 2450 MHz.[24] Unlike RF waves, which generate heat via the friction induced by an electric current, microwaves generate heat by increasing the kinetic energy of water molecules: water molecules in the tissue adjacent to a microwave antenna function as electrical dipoles that repeatedly rotate to align with the applied oscillating

electromagnetic field, thus raising the heat of the tissue.[25] Microwave energy is transferred to a much larger area, up to 2 cm surrounding the antenna, than RF wave energy, so MWA creates a larger zone of active heating.[26]

Six MWA systems are currently available in the United States. Three systems use a 915-MHz generator (Evident [Covidien, Boulder, Colo.], AveCure [MedWaves, San Diego, Calif.], MicroTherm X [BSD Medical, Salt Lake City, Utah]), and three systems use a 2450-MHz generator (Certus 140 [NeuWave Medical, Madison, Wis.], Amica [Hospital Service, Rome, Italy], Acculis MTA [Microsulis Medical Ltd., Hampshire, United Kingdom]), and all use straight antennas. Two of the systems (MicroTherm X, Certus 140) allow synchronous delivery of MW energy in three antennas simultaneously. One system (AveCure) does not require shaft cooling to protect the skin. The other five manufacturers use antennae that are perfused with room-temperature fluid or carbon dioxide gas (Certus 140) to reduce heating of the nonactive proximal portion of the applicator and prevent damage to the skin and other proximal tissues.

Microwaves behave differently than RF waves in the lung. Microwave propagation is not insulated by air and not hindered by the limited water content of lung parenchyma.[25] In theory, MWA may have some advantages over RFA in

TABLE 154-1. Outcomes from Leading and Supportive Studies Conducted on Various Lung Ablation Modalities

Author	Year	No. Patients	No. Tumors	Notable Findings
Radiofrequency Ablation				
Hiraki et al.[49]	2011	50	52 primary	Overall survival 94% at 1 year, 86% at 2 years, 74% at 3 years, 67% at 4 years, 61% at 5 years Stage IA survival 95% at 1 year, 89% at 2 years, 83% at 3 years, 73% at 4 years, 66% at 5 years Stage IB survival 92% at 1 year, 75% at 2 years, 50% at 3 years, 50% at 4 years, 50% at 5 years Cancer-specific survival 100% at 1 year, 93% at 2 years, 80% at 3 years, 80% at 4 years, 74% at 5 years Disease-free survival 82% at 1 year, 64% at 2 years, 53% at 3 years, 46% at 4 years, 46% at 5 years Median and mean disease-free survival 42 months
Palussiere et al.[39]	2010	127	210	Probability of survival 72% at 2 years, 60% at 3 years, 51% at 5 years
Zemlyak et al.[50]	2010	64 25 resection 12 RFA 27 cryo		Overall survival at 3 years for resection (wedge or segmentectomy) 87.1%, for RFA 87.5%, for cryo 77%, with no statistically significant difference Cancer-specific survival at 3 years for resection 90.6%, for RFA 87.5%, for cryo 90.2%, with no statistically significant difference Length of hospital stay significantly shorter for RFA/cryo than resection
Huang et al.[35]	2010	329 237 primary 92 mets		Median progression-free interval 21.6 months Overall survival 68.2% at 1 year, 35.3% at 2 years, 20.1% at 5 years NSCLC survival 80.1% at 1 year, 45.8% at 2 years, 24.3% at 5 years Pulmonary mets survival 50.6% at 1 year, 30.1% at 2 years, 17.3% at 5 years Local progression in 78 (23.7%) during follow-up, most likely related to incomplete ablation due to technical issues or tumor size >4 cm
Beland et al.[51]	2010	79	79 primary	Median disease-free survival 23 months Recurrence in 43% at mean follow-up of 17 months Larger tumor sizes associated with larger risk of recurrence, suggesting initial volume of ablation not adequate
Lanuti et al.[52]	2009	31	34 primary	Overall survival 78% at 2 years, 47% at 3 years Median overall survival 30 months, median disease-free survival 25.5 months Disease-free survival 57% at 2 years, 39% at 3 years Mean progression-free survival 33 ± 3.8 months Local progression in 31.5%, tumors >3 cm had greatest recurrence rate, tumors <2 cm had lowest recurrence rate
Lencioni et al.[53]	2008	106	183 33 primary 150 mets	Local control 88% at 1 year Primary lung cancer overall survival 70% at 1 year, 48% at 2 years Colorectal pulmonary mets overall survival 89% at 1 year, 60% at 2 years
Pennathur et al.[54]	2007	19		Local control 58% Overall survival 95% at 1 year
Simon et al.[55]	2007	153	189 116 primary 73 mets	Local control 83% at 1 year, 64% at 2 years, 57% at 3 years, 47% at 4 years, and 47% at 5 years for tumors ≤3 cm Local control 45% at 1 year, 25% at 2 years, 25% at 3 years, 25% at 4 years, and 25% at 5 years for tumors >3 cm Stage I NSCLC overall survival 78% at 1 year, 57% at 2 years, 36% at 3 years, 27% at 4 years, and 27% at 5 years Colorectal pulmonary mets overall survival 87% at 1 year, 78% at 2 years, 57% at 3 years, 57% at 4 years, and 57% at 5 years
de Baere et al.[56]	2006	60	100	Local control 93% at 18 months Overall survival 71% at 18 months Lung disease free 34% at 18 months
Dupuy et al.[57]	2006	24		Local control 92% Stage IA cumulative survival 92% at 12 months, 62% at 24 months, and 46% at 56 months Stage IB cumulative survival 73% at 12 months, 42% at 24 months, and 31% at 60 months
Thanos et al.[58]	2006	22	22 14 primary 8 mets	Primary lung cancer overall survival 14% at 3 years Pulmonary mets overall survival 42% at 3 years
Yan et al.[59]	2006	55	55 mets	Overall median survival 33 months, despite 30/55 with previously resected liver mets Actuarial survival 85% at 1 year, 64% at 2 years, and 46% at 3 years Univariate analysis: lesion size, location, repeat RFA predictive of survival Multivariate analysis: only lesion size remained predictive

Continued

TABLE 154-1. Outcomes from Leading and Supportive Studies Conducted on Various Lung Ablation Modalities—cont'd

Author	Year	No. Patients	No. Tumors	Notable Findings
Fernando et al.[60]	2005	18 5 primary 13 mets	33	Only 13 patients treated percutaneously Disease progression seen in 8 nodules (38%) in 6 patients (33%) Overall mean survival 20.97 months, median survival not reached Stage I mean progression-free interval 17.6 months Other stages progression-free interval 14.98 months
Akeboshi et al.[61]	2004	31	54 13 primary 41 mets	Complete tumor necrosis 69% in 36 lesions <3 cm Complete tumor necrosis 39% in 18 lesions >3 cm
Kang et al.[62]	2004	50 23 primary 27 mets	120	Complete tumor necrosis in tumors >3.5 cm In tumors >3.5 cm, complete tumor necrosis area within 3.5 cm diameter PET-demonstrated tumor destruction in 70% of cases
Lee et al.[63]	2004	30	32 27 NSCLC 5 mets	Complete tumor necrosis in tumors <3 cm In tumors >3 cm, 23% complete ablation In 20 lesions with incomplete necrosis, 50% necrosis In 8/12 cases of complete necrosis, 5-mm well-demarcated nonenhancing zone of ground-glass opacity surrounding ablated lesion No local tumor recurrence at 22.2 months
Yasui et al.[64]	2004	35	99 3 primary 96 mets	Complete tumor necrosis 91%, mean diameter of 1.9 cm
Herrera[65]	2003	18	33	Complete response 6% Partial response 44% Stable response 33% Progression 17%
Microwave Ablation				
Wolf et al.[66]	2008	50		Primary local control 74% at median follow-up of 10 months Additional 6% secondary local control for total 80% local control rate Actuarial survival 65% at 1 year, 55% at 2 years, and 45% at 3 years
Feng[67]	2002	20	28 8 primary 20 mets	Local response rate 57%
Laser Ablation				
Rosenberg et al.[29]	2009	64	108 mets	Primary local control rate 78% Secondary local control rate of 72% Survival rate 81% at 1 year, 59% at 2 years, 44% at 3 years, 44% at 4 years, 27% at 5 years
Cryoablation				
Zemlyak et al.[50]	2010	64 25 resection 12 RFA 27 cryo		Overall survival at 3 years for resection (wedge or segmentectomy) 87.1%, for RFA 87.5%, for cryo 77%, with no statistically significant difference Cancer-specific survival at 3 years for resection 90.6%, for RFA 87.5%, for cryo 90.2%, with no statistically significant difference Length of hospital stay significantly shorter for RFA/cryo than resection
Kawamura et al.[68]	2006	20	35 mets	Local control rate 80% Survival rate 90% at 1 year
Wang et al.[69]	2005	187	234 196 primary 38 mets	Mean Karnofsky performance score increased from 75.2 ± 1.3 before ablation to 82.6 ± 1.4 1 week post ablation

cryo, Cryoablation; *mets*, metastases; *NSCLC*, non–small cell lung cancer; *PET*, positron emission tomography; *RFA*, radiofrequency ablation.

the lung, including a greater convection profile, resistance to heat sinks, lack of charring and related impedance limitations, and the ability to more rapidly create larger ablative volumes by using multiple applicators simultaneously.[25,27] Such advantages could theoretically improve ablation of the tumor margin and thus reduce recurrence rates. A literature search reveals only one study of MWA versus RFA in the lung. This study examined MWA and RFA in normal porcine lung parenchyma and revealed MWA lesion diameters were larger and more circular than those created by RFA.[27]

Laser Ablation

Laser ablation utilizes electromagnetic waves whose frequencies fall in the infrared spectrum and are of a monochromic wavelength (generally 1064 nm) generated by an Nd:YAG source and transmitted through fiberoptic cables. Lasers generate heat via molecular photon absorption.[28] Only one laser system (Biotex Inc., Houston, Tex.) is currently available commercially in the United States, and that system has not yet been applied to primary lung tumors. European studies (see Table 154-1) have shown laser

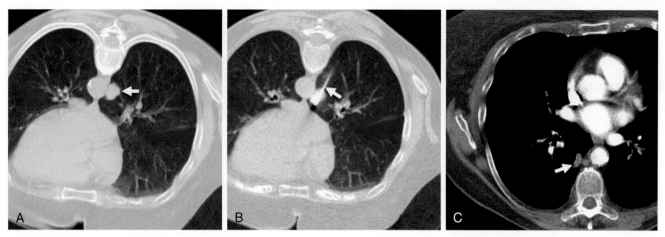

FIGURE 154-2. Biopsy-proven right lower lobe carcinoid tumor in a 79-year-old woman who was referred for lung ablation. **A,** Prone axial computed tomography (CT) image obtained immediately prior to microwave ablation (MWA) shows periaortic mass *(arrow)*. **B,** Prone axial CT image obtained during MWA shows antenna *(arrow)* appropriately placed in mass. **C,** Axial contrast-enhanced 1-year follow-up CT scan shows residual thermal scar *(arrow)* in right lower lobe, without evidence of growth or enhancement.

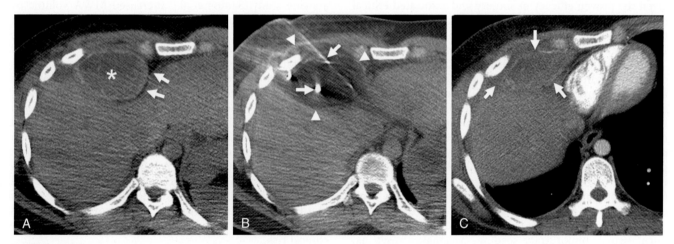

FIGURE 154-3. Biopsy-proven right lower lobe osteosarcoma metastasis in a 22-year-old man who was referred for tumor ablation. **A,** Axial computed tomography (CT) image obtained immediately prior to cryoablation shows 6.8 cm × 5.4 cm mass *(star)* with internal mineralization adjacent to pericardium *(arrows)* and diaphragm. **B,** Axial CT image obtained after fourth freeze cycle shows cryoprobes *(arrows)* in ice ball *(arrowheads)*, which extends to pericardium. **C,** Axial contrast-enhanced 2-month follow-up CT scan shows consolidated nonenhancing region *(arrows)* consistent with tumor necrosis.

ablation of secondary tumors in the lung to be safe and suggest that laser ablation has the potential for improving long-term survival.[29]

Cryoablation

Cryoablation does not utilize the electromagnetic spectrum, but relies on applicators perfused with either liquid nitrogen or pressurized argon gas. Liquid nitrogen has been used in the operating room setting to treat liver tumors for over 3 decades,[30] but the more recent development of pressurized argon gas systems has significantly decreased applicator diameters and made percutaneous cryoablation of other tissues, including the lung (Fig. 154-3; also see Table 154-1), more feasible. Pressurized argon gas can cool to −140°C owing to the Joule-Thomson effect. Temperatures below −40°C induce direct cell destruction primarily through ice crystal formation, which leads to osmotic shifts in intracellular and extracellular water. In addition, as the

tissue thaws, endothelial damage via the same mechanism results in increased capillary permeability, edema, aggregation of platelets, and thrombosis, eliminating the blood supply to the tumor. Necrosis is generally seen in the central part of the lesion closest to the applicator, and apoptosis is seen in the peripheral part of the lesion.[31,32] A freeze/thaw/freeze cycle is typically used as the second freeze/thaw produces faster and more extensive cooling and thereby extends certain tissue destruction closer to the outer limit of the frozen volume.[32]

Two systems, CryoHit (Galil Medical, Plymouth Meeting, Pa.) and Cryocare (Endocare Inc., Irvine, Calif.), are currently available for clinical use in the United States. Both systems allow simultaneous placement of and treatment with up to 15 probes of 1.5 to 2.4 mm diameter.

In the lung, the airways do not appear to affect the size of the ablation zone.[33] As with cryoablation in other tissues, the ice ball may be visualized under computed tomography (CT) or magnetic resonance imaging (MRI), allowing direct comparison of ablative volume borders to tumor margins, increasing operator confidence in measuring cytotoxic margins and managing treatments near critical structures.[34]

EXPERIENCE TO DATE

The majority of lung ablation literature has focused on RFA and is in the form of single-institution case series and retrospective cohort studies. These studies have shown the safety and efficacy of thermal ablation as a palliative and potentially curative treatment option for medically inoperable NSCLC and pulmonary metastases. The outcomes from the major leading and supporting thermal lung ablation studies are summarized in Table 154-1.

There have been no prospective trials directly comparing thermal ablation methods to one another, to radiation therapy, or to chemotherapy. Neither have there been significant series studying the efficacy of thermal ablation for medically operable lung disease or comparing thermal ablation to surgery. Such studies are unlikely in the near future, given the proven efficacy of surgery and associated ethical concerns. A prospective pilot trial looking at the 2-year post-RFA survival and local control in patients with stage IA medically inoperable NSCLC is currently in progress.

Complications related to thermal ablation have been well documented. In a series of 329 RFA ablations, Huang et al.[35] experienced pneumothorax (19.1%), pneumonia (4.5%), hemoptysis (4.2%), hemothorax (3.0%), and pericardial tamponade (0.9%). Additional documented complications of lung ablation include chronic obstructive pulmonary disease exacerbation (0%-6%), pulmonary abscess (0%-6%), pleural effusion requiring drainage (0%-4%), acute respiratory distress syndrome (0%-3%), parenchymal hemorrhage (0%-1%), phrenic nerve injury (0%-1%), death (0%-1%), and case reports of acute renal failure, vocal cord paralysis, atrial fibrillation, pulmonary embolus, third-degree skin burn, stroke, tumor tract seeding, pacemaker resetting, hypertonic saline-induced lobar necrosis, and prolonged bronchopleural fistula.[36]

Immunohistologic analysis by Schneider et al.[37] confirmed RFA-induced cell death in a series of 32 tumors treated intraoperatively prior to curative resection. Incomplete ablation was associated with vascular structures within the tumor tissue and in the marginal zones of the tumor tissue. In addition, scattered vital tumor tissue was identified in 50% of the ablations. A similar study was performed by Jaskolka et al.[38] on tumors ablated percutaneously 2 to 4 weeks prior to scheduled resection. This study confirmed coagulative necrosis by hematoxylin and eosin (H&E) staining and loss of proliferating cell nuclear antigen (PCNA) protein staining but retention of MIB-1 staining. Given the complete necrosis identified by Jaskolka, it is possible that the scattered vital tissues found by Schneider may have been due to the very short period between ablation and resection, but emphasizes the need for close periprocedural management of temperature and impedance and suggests utility in further histologic studies of ablated lung tissues.

In general, ablation success is assessed on imaging follow-up. In a study of 350 tumors treated with RFA, Palussiere et al.[39] found four patterns of evolution at 1 year post procedure: fibrosis (50.5%), nodules (44.8%), cavitation (2.4%), and atelectasis (1.4%). The nodular pattern was most frequently associated with local tumor progression, but the pattern was not indicative of outcome, and thus no pattern warrants discontinuation of follow-up. Imaging features associated with local recurrence following RFA are outlined in a review by Eradat et al.[40]: contrast enhancement on CT at 3 months should never exceed that of the original tumor, but benign peripheral enhancement can be expected to persist for up to 6 months, while nodular or central enhancement of 10 to 15 Hounsfield units suggests incomplete ablation, progression, or recurrence.

NEWLY INTRODUCED ADVANCES IN THERMAL LUNG ABLATION

Several recent studies have revealed new techniques that may improve thermal ablation efficacy and have shown potential in aggressively treating patients who have not been included in the more conservative typical cohorts studied to date. Healey et al.[41] have described a technique for securing lung tumors during RF electrode insertion. In a swine study, Santos et al.[42] increased MWA volume by occluding the bronchus prior to ablation to reduce heat dissipation via air exchange. In a series of six patients, de Baere et al.[43] successfully performed complete ablations of metastatic tumors adjacent to large pulmonary arteries by temporarily occluding the arteries with a percutaneous balloon catheter to reduce heat dissipation via perfusion, but with complications of long-lasting vascular occlusion and atelectasis. Chan et al.[44] have proposed RFA followed by single-fraction high-dose-rate (HDR) radiotherapy, with a promising small case series, and Leung et al.[45] have shown thermal ablation (RFA, MWA, and cryoablation) to be a potential alternative to re-irradiation. Two separate small studies by Hess et al.[46] and Sofocleous et al.[47] have shown that thermal ablation can provide local control in patients with a single lung, despite a potentially high postprocedure clinical risk.

CURRENT ROLE OF THERMAL ABLATION THERAPY IN LUNG CANCER

Given that sublobar resection can achieve 89% 5-year survival for tumors smaller than 2 cm,[48] resection remains the standard of treatment, and ethical concerns prohibit comparison of resection to other modes of treatment, including thermal ablation and radiation. However, with an estimated 15% to 30% of stage I and II NSCLC considered medically inoperable, there is a considerable role for these second-line therapies in both palliative and curative capacities. Significant improvement in overall survival following RFA over the last several years appears to have brought the efficacy of RFA parallel to that of SBRT. Moreover, it is a much cheaper mode of therapy with less theoretical risk of long-term therapy-related morbidity.

Patients with NSCLC and pulmonary metastases with limited treatment options are already benefiting from image-guided thermal ablation therapy while the technology and associated techniques continue to improve. Although rapid advances and the variety of thermal sources and devices employed make it difficult to study thermal ablation treatment on a large and long-term scale, prospective comparisons of the technologies and with SBRT are necessary to solidify the role of thermal ablation in oncology treatment algorithms and regimens.

KEY POINTS

- Thermal ablation modalities include radiofrequency, microwave, laser, and cryotherapy.

- Randomized controlled clinical trials have not yet been conducted to compare thermal ablation modalities with one another or with SBRT or surgery, but an increasing number of single and multicenter cohort studies continue to consistently establish the safety and efficacy of thermal ablation for inoperable lung lesions.

- The majority of lung ablation literature has focused on RFA and, despite the lack of randomized comparison trials, with an estimated 15% to 30% of Stage I and II NSCLC considered inoperable there is already a considerable role for RFA of NSCLC and, for similar reasons, for RFA of pulmonary metastases.

► **SUGGESTED READINGS**

Dupuy DE. Image-guided thermal ablation of lung malignancies. Radiology 2011;260(3):633–55.

Dupuy DE, Goldberg SN. Image-guided radiofrequency tumor ablation: challenges and opportunities–part II. J Vasc Interv Radiol 2001;12(10): 1135–48.

Todd TR. The surgical treatment of pulmonary metastases. Chest 1997; 112(4 Suppl):287S–90S.

Vogl TJ, Naguib NN, Lehnert T, Nour-Eldin NE. Radiofrequency, microwave and laser ablation of pulmonary neoplasms: clinical studies and technical considerations–review article. Eur J Radiol 2011;77(2): 346–57.

The complete reference list is available online at www.expertconsult.com.

CHAPTER 155

Minimally Invasive Image-Guided Breast Biopsy and Ablation

Jessica Torrente and Rachel F. Brem

INTRODUCTION

Screening mammography has been shown to decrease the incidence of mortality associated with breast cancer.[1] Since the initial implementation of widespread screening mammography programs, breast imaging has evolved to include full-field digital mammography (FFDM), ultrasound (US), magnetic resonance imaging (MRI), and more recently, molecular imaging techniques including breast-specific gamma imaging (BSGI) and positron emission mammography (PEM) to aid in the evaluation of breast pathology. The ultimate goal of these technologic advances is to allow for the detection of small and early-stage breast cancer, thus providing patients with the best chance of cure and the least amount of treatment-associated morbidity. However, with the detection of smaller lesions comes the challenge of developing methods to arrive at a pathologic diagnosis in an accurate, cost-effective, and safe manner. Wire-guided surgical breast biopsy was the gold standard for the diagnosis of nonpalpable radiographically detected breast lesions, but given that 80% of indeterminate breast lesions that undergo biopsy are subsequently found to be benign, development of less invasive, more cost-effective techniques was needed.[2]

Breast imaging and intervention has undergone great changes over the past several decades because of the development of many image-guided minimally invasive technologies allowing for accurate and cost-effective diagnosis of breast cancer and high-risk lesions. Such techniques are now available utilizing all traditional forms of breast imaging, including mammography (stereotactic), US, MRI, and now most recently, more novel approaches such as nuclear medicine guidance for molecular breast imaging techniques. As methods for pathologic diagnosis of breast cancer have trended toward minimally invasive techniques, so have potential options for treatment. Various methods of image-guided ablation of small focal breast cancers are now under investigation, with promising initial results. This chapter will review available methods for minimally invasive breast biopsy, including the various modalities of imaging guidance and equipment, and provide an algorithm for clinicians to best tailor their biopsy approach. A brief review of new ablative treatment techniques, specifically radiofrequency ablation (RFA) and cryoablation, will be provided.

STEREOTACTIC INTERVENTIONS

Targeting mammographically detected lesions for minimally invasive biopsy employs stereotactic guidance. The most common type of suspicious mammographic abnormality targeted for biopsy via this method are microcalcifications, although any suspicious abnormality seen solely or best with mammography, including masses or asymmetries, can be targeted and biopsied via stereotaxis. In a large multicenter trial performed in 2003, investigators found that 70% of stereotactic vacuum-assisted biopsy (VAB) was performed for lesions containing suspicious microcalcifications.[3]

For a stereotactic breast biopsy, either a dedicated table is needed or an attachment to a digital mammography unit and a special chair to allow for proper patient positioning. If a dedicated table is used, the patient is prone with the breast positioned dependently through an aperture in the table (Fig. 155-1). Attached to the underside of the table is a mammography unit on an articulating arm, which can be moved such that +15-degree and −15-degree images are obtained. These angles are used by the computer to determine the coordinates of the targeted lesions to within 1 mm of accuracy. If a standard mammography unit with an attachment allowing stereotactic guidance is used, a chair can be positioned to optimally target the lesion. The advantages of a dedicated stereotactic table include greater comfort for the patient and physician and no risk of a vasovagal reaction. However, it requires a dedicated room and space. A mammography unit allows for more efficient use of space and equipment because it can be used for routine imaging when not being used for biopsy. This latter solution may be best suited for practices with lower volumes where use of a mammography unit for biopsy will not impact workflow of screening and diagnostic mammography.

The position used to approach the lesion is decided preprocedurally by examining the patient's diagnostic mammogram. The decision as to approach should be based on the projection in which the lesion is best visualized, not necessarily the shortest distance, as well as considerations for ease of patient positioning. Images of the lesion are obtained at stereotactic angles, typically 15 or 20 degrees, and computer-generated x, y, and z coordinates are obtained. These coordinates place the targeted lesion in the center of the biopsy chamber of the probe. The biopsy probe is then loaded onto a base that is mobilized to the determined x and y coordinates. To minimize bleeding during the procedure, care should to be taken to ensure there is no (or minimal) blood vessel overlying the lesion and that the depth coordinate (z) is neither too superficial nor too deep. A too-superficial depth runs the risk of including skin within the biopsy specimen, and a depth too deep may make it impossible to sample the lesion without compromising the equipment if the biopsy probe should contact the image detector, potentially resulting in misalignment of the equipment. However, there are certainly strategies to overcome these challenges. For a superficial lesion, the probe can be advanced to a position where the entire biopsy chamber is just beyond the skin. This will allow for inclusion of the targeted lesion, even though the z coordinate will be deeper than determined. For a depth that is too deep, the patient can be repositioned.

The overlying skin is prepped in a sterile fashion, followed by injection of topical anesthetic into the skin and subcutaneous and parenchymal tissue.[4] A 3-mm incision is made with a scalpel, and the biopsy probe is advanced through this incision to the predetermined depth. Typically, 6 to 12 samples are obtained. Following biopsy, the device is removed, and a titanium marker is placed through the biopsy probe to denote the area of biopsy. A postprocedure mammogram is critical to confirm the targeted lesion was indeed biopsied, determine clip placement, and have a new baseline; an image of the entire breast rather than the small field of view of the stereotactic device is paramount (Fig. 155-2).

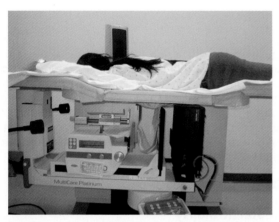

FIGURE 155-1. Patient lying in prone position on a dedicated stereotactic biopsy table.

ULTRASOUND-GUIDED INTERVENTIONS

US is an indispensable tool in the breast imager's armamentarium. This technology not only allows for differentiation of cystic versus solid lesions but can also provide more detailed characterization of solid lesions into probably benign, indeterminate, or suspicious categories.[5-14] This detailed evaluation has largely been made possible by the introduction of high-frequency 7.5- to 10-MHz linear array transducers in the mid-1990s. The ability to carefully evaluate a mass sonographically has proven extremely useful clinically and can improve the specificity of mammographically detected abnormalities. Findings at sonography can also serve to help tailor interventional procedures.

US allows for accurate diagnosis of a mammographic or palpable mass as a simple cyst, a benign lesion. Specific criteria have been developed to allow for classification of a breast lesion as a cyst. When all criteria for a simple cyst are strictly adhered to, the accuracy of US is 96% to 100%.[15] These criteria are demonstration of an imperceptible wall, through transmission of sound, and lack of internal echoes (anechoic). Cysts are typically round or oval in shape and can vary in size from several millimeters to several centimeters. Once a lesion has been diagnosed as a simple cyst, intervention may occur for one of several reasons. Most commonly, the patient may be complaining of a palpable lump or pain and tenderness related to the cyst, and aspiration may alleviate these symptoms.[16] However, it is important to relate to the patient that recurrence of a cyst after aspiration is very common. A second reason to aspirate a benign cyst is very large size, which may obscure a significant portion of the breast and thereby limit mammographic interpretation. In this case, the cyst is aspirated and the mammogram is repeated to allow adequate evaluation.

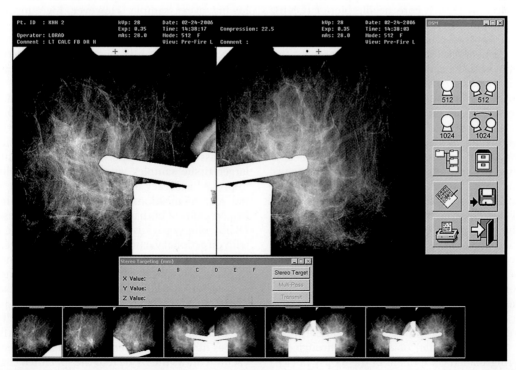

FIGURE 155-2. Images acquired stepwise through a stereotactic biopsy, including scout image, stereo pairs, and pre- and postfire images.

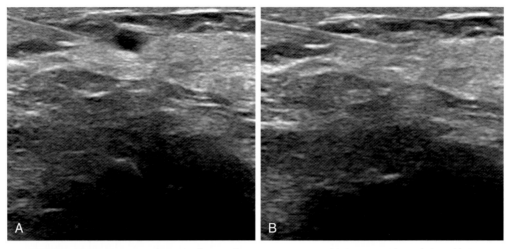

FIGURE 155-3. **A,** Pre– and, **B,** post–fine-needle aspiration sonographic images, with resolution of lesion.

A cyst is typically aspirated under sonographic guidance (Fig. 155-3). The lesion is first localized, and a skin entry site is chosen. The skin is then prepped with alcohol, and intradermal and subcutaneous local anesthesia is injected. Under direct sonographic visualization, a 22- to 25-gauge needle is advanced into the lesion, and the fluid contained within the cyst is aspirated through sterile tubing into a syringe. At many facilities, the aspirated fluid may be discarded if it is clear, straw-colored, green, milky or "motor-oil" colored, since these are compatible with benign cystic fluid. If the cyst contains bloody fluid, even if the sonographic criteria of a simple cyst were met, the fluid should be sent for cytologic evaluation.

Once the possibility that a mass is a simple cyst has been excluded sonographically, the possibility of a solid or complex cystic/solid lesion must be entertained. These are lesions for which biopsy is considered. Options include fine-needle aspiration (FNA), core needle biopsy (CNB), or vacuum-assisted biopsy (VAB).

Regardless of the type of needle chosen, all US-guided interventional procedures follow a similar protocol. The patient lies supine on the sonography table, with the ipsilateral arm raised up and over the head. For a lesion in the lateral portion of the breast, particularly in women with pendulous breasts, positioning the patient at an oblique angle with the shoulder on a bolster or pillow may aid in the biopsy. First the area is prepped and draped using sterile technique. The lesion is then localized sonographically. Lidocaine is used to anesthetize the skin and subcutaneous and intraparenchymal tissues. This is also done with sonographic guidance. Following this, a small (3-mm) skin incision is made 1 to 2 cm from the edge of the US probe. The distance of the skin insertion site to the lesion should include considerations of the amount of purchase needed as well as needle angle. Deeper lesions generally require more purchase, and the incision should be farther from the lesion. Additionally, a very steep needle angle hinders visualization of the needle with US. Through this incision, the biopsy device is advanced to the edge of the lesion. The needle is then either advanced into the lesion manually (e.g., with a 22- to 25-gauge needle) or advanced through the lesion via a spring-loaded component of the biopsy device. It may be optimal to include the transition of the breast parenchyma and the lesion in at least one of the samples, because this may facilitate radiologic/pathologic correlation of a mass lesion. In general, a minimum of three samples are collected, and a biopsy clip may be deployed at the site of biopsy. Care should be taken that the biopsy needle remains parallel to the chest wall throughout the procedure to eliminate the possibility of a pneumothorax or injury to the pectoralis muscle.

BIOPSY DEVICES

Stereotactic Biopsy

Through the years, the stereotactic biopsy needle has undergone many developments. Initial stereotactic biopsy efforts were focused on FNA or biopsy with a spring loaded-device, which required removal from the breast following every sample. However, high insufficiency rates (10%-38%)[17,18] plus the inability to determine invasion from ductal carcinoma in situ (DCIS) were significant limitations to FNA, and substantial undersampling, particularly of calcifications with a spring-loaded device, resulted in important modifications to this original technique. Gradually the gauge of biopsy needles increased to the now used 11-, 9-, 8-, and even 7-gauge probes. Further development followed the introduction of VAB to actively draw tissue into the biopsy chamber, as opposed to sampling that tissue which was passively in the specimen chamber. This resulted in larger tissue samples with decreased sampling error and improved accuracy of diagnosis.[19-24] Because of the potential for calcifications to be histologically heterogeneous (e.g., regions of both atypical ductal hyperplasia [ADH] and DCIS), biopsy performed with a larger-gauge needle, along with directional vacuum assistance, has proved very helpful in obtaining larger samples and decreasing underestimation rates.[25-28] Overall, in comparison to CNB, underestimation drops about 1.8-fold when using vacuum-assisted devices.[29] Therefore, directional VAB is now used to biopsy lesions with mammographically detected microcalcifications.

An additional advantage of the use of a VAB probe is that it does not have to be removed and reinserted. Instead, the vacuum draws the tissue into the specimen chamber, cuts it, and transports the specimen into a collection chamber at the other end of the device. The result is that multiple samples can be obtained while the needle remains in the breast. The vacuum device has been shown to produce tissue samples larger in size and heavier in weight.[29-32] Acquisition of larger tissue samples significantly increases the accuracy of diagnosis of ADH and DCIS.[33] The reported rates of upgrade for ADH lesions average 44% for 14-gauge spring-loaded stereotactic core biopsy, 24% for 14-gauge directional vacuum-assisted breast biopsy, and 19% for 11-gauge vacuum-assisted breast biopsy needles (range, 0%-58%). The diagnosis of ADH following percutaneous biopsy is an indication for surgical excision to exclude the diagnosis of breast carcinoma. A diagnosis of lobular atypia at minimally invasive biopsy remains controversial, with some institutions not recommending surgical excision at all. Increasingly, the recommendations are for surgical excision of all lobular neoplasia diagnosed at minimally invasive biopsy, or the excision of pleomorphic lobular carcinoma in situ.[34,35]

Ultrasound-Guided Biopsy

FNA may be performed on cystic, solid, or mixed solid lesions. A 22- to 25-gauge needle is used, and the technique is similar to the aforementioned description of cyst aspiration. Typically, several passes are made with the needle through different parts of the lesion with a back and forth motion while aspirating with a syringe (Fig. 155-4). Benefits of FNA include decreased cost of procedure and decreased likelihood of hematoma. However, as stated earlier, there are significant and well-established limitations to FNA. The success of FNA is operator dependent, with the best results achieved when performed by an experienced operator. Insufficiency rates have been found to improve with the presence of a cytopathologist during the procedure.[36] Another disadvantage of FNA is its inability to differentiate between DCIS and invasive cancer when malignant ductal cells are identified due to the lack of tissue architecture. Therefore, lesions chosen for biopsy with FNA should be selected based on the sonographic appearance, with less suspicious lesions favored for biopsy with this method, to lessen the likelihood of re-biopsy with a larger gauge needle to establish a diagnosis, or in clinical situations where a core biopsy is more challenging, such as when a lesion is immediately abutting an implant or large vessel. Radiologic-pathologic concordance is paramount when performing FNA.

US-guided CNB has been shown to be a reliable alternative to surgical excision.[37,38] The procedure is cost-effective and well tolerated by patients and has become a mainstay in clinical practice. US-guided CNB enables accurate diagnosis of malignancy and allows for improved surgical planning for treatment. Even lesions that are considered highly suspicious for malignancy should undergo biopsy prior to definitive surgical procedure; this will alleviate the need for a second surgical procedure for nodal sampling. Estrogen and progesterone receptor status, as well as Her-2 status, can be ascertained on a CNB and are generally performed on the biopsy obtained at minimally invasive biopsy. Such assessment can assist with patient counseling and treatment options prior to surgery and can result in a less traumatic and more complete discussion of surgical options. Studies have shown that when a diagnosis of cancer is known prior to lumpectomy/partial mastectomy, the likelihood of negative margins is higher as the surgical excision is more extensive.[39] Additionally, it can reduce the need for repeat surgeries to evaluate and/or treat the axilla in the case of a diagnosis of invasive versus in situ disease. These procedures can be performed utilizing automated or vacuum-assisted devices.

Automated CNB devices are typically spring loaded. Once the skin has been prepped and anesthetized and the CNB device has been advanced under US guidance, it should be placed 1 to 3 cm proximal to the edge of the lesion. The device is fired into the lesion, resulting in a core biopsy specimen that maintains the architecture of the lesion, thereby allowing for a surgical-quality specimen (Fig. 155-5). Real-time documentation of the needle within

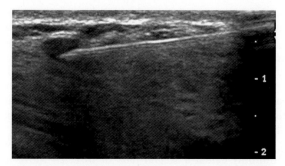

FIGURE 155-4. Sonographic image depicting fine-needle aspiration with needle in persistent lesion.

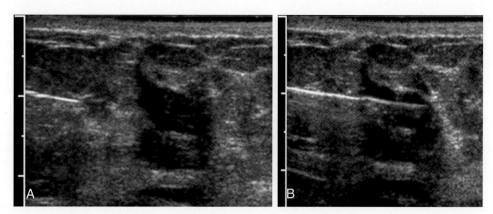

FIGURE 155-5. **A,** Pre- and, **B,** postfire sonographic images obtained during ultrasound-guided core needle biopsy of a hypoechoic mass.

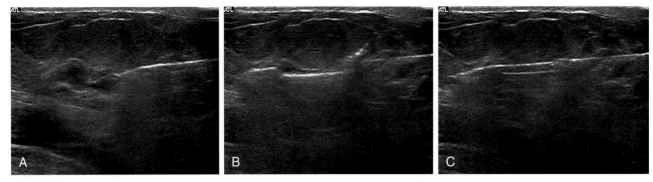

FIGURE 155-6. A, Pre-, **B,** post- (aperture open), and, **C,** post- (aperture closed) sonographic images obtained during ultrasound-guided vacuum-assisted biopsy of an intraductal papilloma.

the lesion is critical to confirm sampling of the targeted lesion. The "throw" of the needle varies with the manufacturer, as does the gauge of the needle and chamber size. It has been noted in the literature that one disadvantage of this US-guided CNB using a spring-loaded device is the need for multiple reinsertions of the needle through the skin incision. Typically, three to five passes are made through various aspects of the lesion, thereby sampling all quadrants of the lesion and decreasing sampling error. There has been debate in the literature as to the number of specimens needed to achieve a reliable histologic diagnosis, with some groups reporting the greatest accuracy achieved with three passes,[40] and over 90% accuracy in the first pass.[41]

A more recent development for US-guided percutaneous breast biopsy is the availability of VAB probes. These are larger-gauge needles[9,11] and allow for procurement of larger cores under real-time imaging (Fig. 155-6). These devices obtain a larger amount of tissue to further increase accuracy of diagnosis, similar to stereotactic-guided vacuum-assisted devices. Additionally, these are typically single-insertion devices, eliminating the need for multiple reentries into the breast. These VAB probes may be useful when a lesion is sonographically visible but also contains microcalcifications, and therefore inherently contain the issues of heterogeneity and underestimation of disease associated with microcalcifications, as previously discussed. The use of sonographically guided VAB is increasingly being used to excise biopsy-proven benign masses, such as fibroadenomas, when excision is desired but surgery is not. This requires additional time, but with the acquisition of sequential samples, the sonographically visible lesion can be excised. Of course, this does not ensure complete pathologic excision.

Most lesions biopsied under sonographic guidance are masses.[42] If the mass is sufficiently small that there is concern that the entire lesion is removed, or if there is a possibility of neoadjuvant chemotherapy with subsequent disappearance of the lesion, a metallic marker should be placed immediately following biopsy to identify the lesion's precise location. In our practice, all lesions that undergo biopsy have a metallic clip placed to ensure accurate localization of the lesion that underwent biopsy.

Most masses are adequately sampled with a spring-loaded device, usually 12 to 14 gauge. However, in certain clinical situations, such as with intraluminal lesions where there is the possibility of a papillary lesion, use of

sonographically guided VAB may be helpful. In the specific case of papillomas, it was found in a recent study that the sensitivity and specificity at automated CNB was 28% and 100%, respectively. For vacuum-assisted CNB, both sensitivity and specificity were found to be 100%.[43] Therefore, use of sonographically guided VAB if the diagnosis of a papilloma is favored may be preferential.

LESION RETRIEVAL AND RADIOLOGIC-PATHOLOGIC CONCORDANCE

The full discussion of this topic is available at www.expertconsult.com.

Magnetic Resonance Imaging

Breast MRI has emerged as valuable adjunct to more traditional methods of breast imaging such as mammography and US. Although the sensitivity of MRI has been shown to be high for detection of cancer, the specificity is quite variable.[48] MRI has been shown to be most useful for screening high-risk women and evaluating the extent of disease in a patient with a diagnosis of cancer, particularly in detecting malignancy that is occult on both mammography and US.

It has become standard clinical practice to perform what is commonly called a *second-look* or *directed ultrasound*, which is a focused sonographic evaluation of the lesion in question to evaluate an abnormal focus of enhancement on MRI that may be suspicious for malignancy. This is performed even if the patient already had US evaluation of the breast, because the directed approach uses a lower threshold to identify the lesion and often can identify a lesion that might not have been appreciated on initial sonographic evaluation. If the lesion is not visualized with directed US, an MRI-guided biopsy can be performed. A recent study by DeMartini et al. demonstrated that just under half of the lesions identified with MRI for which directed second-look US was performed (46%) demonstrated sonographic correlates. These sonographically depicted lesions were more likely to be masses (50%) than non-masslike areas of enhancement (32%) and foci (18%).[49] Therefore, techniques have been developed to percutaneously biopsy lesions that can only be seen on MRI.

In experienced hands, the approximate time to perform an MRI-guided biopsy of a single lesion is approximately 30 to 35 minutes. The patient is placed in a prone position on the MR table in an MRI biopsy coil, which includes a grid for lesion localization. Initial scout images are obtained. Following intravenous injection of gadolinium, the lesion is again identified and correlated with the previous MRI. The literature reports an approximately 4% to 13% nonvisualization rate of lesions recommended for biopsy.[50-52] The majority of these have been found in premenopausal women and are thought to represent variability due to hormonal enhancement. Scheduling surveillance MRI in high-risk women at midcycle (i.e., week 2 or 3) may minimize the likelihood of these false positives.[53] One technique used to "bring out" a potentially nonvisualized lesion is loosening of breast compression, which might be a consequence of blood flow restriction due to tight compression in the biopsy coil.[54] If following this technique, the lesion remains invisible, a second dose of contrast may be used, and finally, a short-interval follow-up MRI is scheduled when the lesion initially recommended for biopsy is no longer visualized. The literature underscores the importance of short-term follow-up for nonvisualized lesions that were recommended for biopsy at initial MRI examination. In a study of 29 lesions recommended for MRI-guided biopsy, 2 (7%) were not visualized on the day of biopsy but were identified at short-interval follow-up.[55]

Once the lesion of interest is identified, with the aid of various software packages and a grid localizing system placed either laterally or medially over the surface of the breast, x, y, and z coordinates of the lesion are calculated, and the skin entry site is chosen. The technique for calculating coordinates varies with the coil and software used. The skin is then prepped in sterile fashion, and lidocaine is injected in the skin and along the biopsy tract. Components of the introducer set include a needle guide, a coaxial introducer sheath, a sharp nonferrous inner stylet, and a plastic localizing obturator (Fig. 155-7). The sterile plastic coaxial sheath is inserted into the breast via the inner sharp nonferrous metallic stylet to the calculated depth. Occasionally, new coordinates are required after administration of lidocaine, owing to movement of the lesion. The stylet is then removed, and the plastic obturator is placed. A scan is performed to ensure placement of the distal tip of the obturator within the lesion. The obturator is then removed, a VAB device is advanced into the breast, and samples (generally 6-12) are obtained. The biopsy device is removed, and a localizing titanium clip is placed through the sheath after sequences confirm biopsy of the targeted lesion (Fig. 155-8). A postbiopsy scan is then performed to document proper deployment of the clip and removal or decrease in size of

the lesion. Technical success rates reported in the literature range from 96% to 100%, with a positive predictive value for carcinoma of 22% to 37%.[52]

Nuclear Medicine–Guided Biopsy: Gamma and Positron Emission Mammography

Molecular breast imaging techniques like BSGI and PEM are increasing in use. Similar to MRI, both provide physiologic breast imaging but do not pose many of the challenges associated with gadolinium administration and use of magnetic fields for image acquisition. Therefore, patients with poor renal function, pacemakers and other metallic implants, or large body habitus can undergo physiologic imaging with BSGI or PEM. Common indications are similar to those for MRI and include surveillance in the high-risk population, preoperative staging, and diagnostic problem solving for cases in which mammography and US are equivocal.

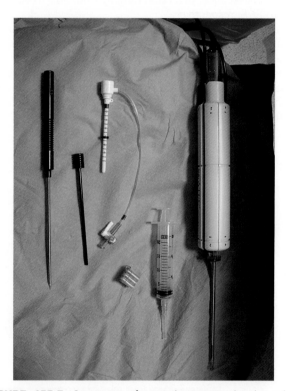

FIGURE 155-7. Components of magnetic resonance imaging–guided biopsy: (from left to right) nonferrous stylet, obturator, introducer sheath, localizing cube, syringe for local anesthesia, and nonferrous vacuum-assisted biopsy device.

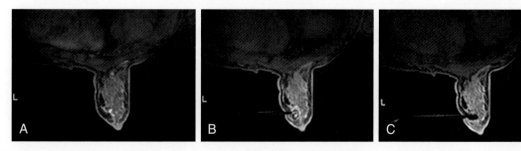

FIGURE 155-8. Images obtained at various stages during magnetic resonance imaging–guided biopsy. **A,** Image of enhancing target lesion. **B,** With obturator in place, following specimen acquisition (small hematoma). **C,** Following clip placement.

BSGI utilizes a high-resolution, small field-of-view gamma camera and technetium (Tc)99m-sestamibi, which is administered intravenously into a peripheral vein immediately prior to image acquisition. Images are acquired with patients in light compression, and four to six images are obtained in positions comparable to mammography. Similar to other nuclear medicine imaging modalities, a suspicious lesion on BSGI is manifested by focal increased radiotracer uptake. Studies have demonstrated sensitivities for breast cancer detection ranging from 100% to 89% (similar to MRI) and specificity from 59.5% to 87%.[56-61] Importantly, these results are not affected by breast density.[56] Similarly, PEM uses fluorine-18 fluorodeoxyglucose (^{18}F-FDG) administered intravenously 60 to 90 minutes prior to imaging. PEM produces 12-slice images of the breasts in analogous mammographic positions.[62] An abnormality is manifested as focally increased radiotracer uptake. For PEM, studies have shown favorable sensitivity and specificity for breast cancer detection ranging from 90% to 96% and 84% to 86%, respectively.[61-63]

Lack of a practical biopsy system was once a limitation for more widespread use of these molecular breast imaging techniques, but vacuum-assisted nuclear medicine breast biopsy techniques have recently gained approval and been introduced into the cadre of image-guided breast biopsy methods. The two systems that have been developed are gamma guidance for BSGI and PET guidance for PEM, using images generated by either BSGI or PEM to target a lesion. Only BSGI biopsy has an accreditation program by the American College of Radiology.

For BSGI, the newly approved system consists of an accessory component that can be added to existing devices for the purpose of biopsy and uses a stereotactic localization method very similar to mammographically guided biopsy. A specialized collimator generates images −20 and +20 degrees to the lesion, and lesion depth and location are clearly generated into a "centered view," which is used for pre- and postfire images. Once the preverification centered view has been generated, a unique software package and grid localizing system similar to MRI are used to choose the skin location. This area is sterilized in the usual fashion, and local anesthesia is administered into the skin and subcutaneous and parenchymal tissues. A skin nick is made, and a cesium-containing obturator in a disposable sleeve is inserted into the area. Postverification centered images are then obtained, the cesium localizing probe is removed, and a handheld vacuum-assisted device is inserted to the determined depth (Fig. 155-9). Several samples are obtained, and postprocedure images are generated; successful lesion removal is demonstrated by lack of increased radiotracer uptake in the area of interest and confirmatory imaging of the specimen, which should demonstrate increased activity (Fig. 155-10). A localizing marker is placed through the biopsy probe, and a postprocedure

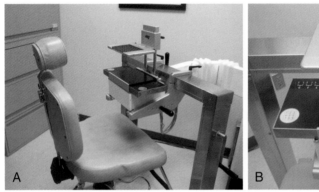
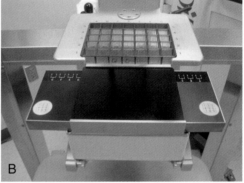

FIGURE 155-9. **A,** Breast-specific gamma imaging with chair and overlying biopsy attachment. **B,** Close-up of biopsy attachment.

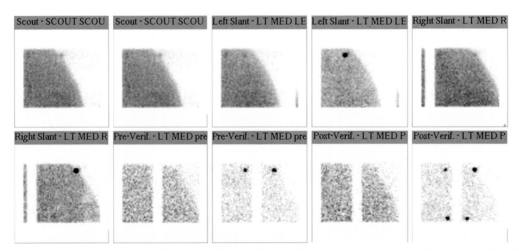

FIGURE 155-10. Multiple images depicting steps of breast-specific gamma imaging biopsy: scout images, stereo pairs, and pre- and postbiopsy verification images.

mammogram is obtained to confirm the location of the metallic marker.

The PEM-guided biopsy method is similar. Using gentle craniocaudal breast compression with the patient in a seated position, the breast is positioned against a support plate, with the fenestrated plate positioned so as to minimize the distance from the skin to the lesion. The initial scan to identify the lesion is generated with a limited field of view. Software is then used to calculate the shortest distance from the skin to the lesion. After sterile preparation of overlying skin and administration of local lidocaine, the biopsy cannula/trocar is introduced via a medial or lateral approach, the inner trocar is removed, and a weak radioactive (1 µCi, germanium-68) sterile stylet is inserted. An alignment scan to confirm the x,y plane is performed. Following validation, the radioactive stylet is removed, and the biopsy device is advanced through the cannula. A pre-biopsy scan is performed with the needle in place to confirm z depth. The biopsy is then performed, with retrieval of a minimum of six samples recommended. A postbiopsy scan is performed to evaluate for lesion removal or modification in appearance. The biopsy device is removed, and a biopsy clip is deployed to denote the area biopsied. Specimens are then scanned and a postprocedural mammogram is performed to evaluate clip placement. A recent study has shown a median time of 32 minutes to complete a PEM-guided biopsy (from initial pre-biopsy scan to insertion of postbiopsy clip).[64]

POSTBIOPSY CARE, CONTRAINDICATIONS, COMPLICATIONS, PRACTICAL APPROACHES TO BIOPSY, AND PROCEDURE DISCUSSION WITH PATIENT

Available at www.expertconsult.com.

ABLATION TECHNIQUES

Ablation techniques for the treatment of small focal breast cancers and some biopsy-proven benign tumors are receiving increasing attention, paralleling the trend of minimally invasive biopsy methods in the breast. Of the various techniques, two of the more promising and well-studied include RFA and cryoablation.

RFA has been previously used for the treatment of other solid tumors, such as liver metastases, primary hepatocellular carcinoma, pulmonary malignancy, and renal cell carcinoma. This technique is performed by placing electrode tips within the lesion and creating a high-frequency alternating current. This causes heating of the tissue, resulting in destruction through thermal coagulation and protein denaturation. The probes are typically placed in the lesion through sonographic guidance, and the procedure is performed under real-time sonographic visualization. Treatment is completed once the tumor reaches a specific predetermined temperature.

Multiple clinical trials have yielded promising results in the treatment of early-stage (stage I-II) invasive breast cancers. An early trial by Jeffrey et al.[68] in 1999 demonstrated RFA was effective at causing breast cancer cell death in five patients. Later studies showed the procedure was well tolerated, with the most common complication being skin burn overlying the treatment area.[69,70] More recently, studies have focused on using MRI to assess response to treatment with RFA. In a protocol by Manenti et al. in 2009,[71] tumor viability following RFA was assessed with pretreatment and sequential posttreatment MRI. Investigators looked for resolution of contrast enhancement of the cancers to be consistent with successful RFA. Definitive surgical excision of the tumor was performed 4 weeks post RFA. In this study, 34 patients with unifocal biopsy-proven invasive breast carcinoma measuring 2 cm or less, visible on both US and MRI, and at least 1 cm from the skin and chest wall underwent RFA. MRI was performed at 1 week and 4 weeks post ablation. On hematoxylin and eosin staining of the surgical specimens, complete changes were found in 94% (32/34) of tumors. In addition, NADH-diaphorase revealed cell death in 97% (33/34) of the tumors. One week after ablation, MRI showed no residual suspicious enhancement in all but three lesions. A similar study was conducted by Vilar et al. in 2012, yielding 100% agreement in 14 cases between post-RFA breast MRI results and histopathology after surgery.[72]

Cryoablation uses the opposite end of the thermal spectrum—freezing—to destroy tumors. In this technique, a percutaneous cryoprobe is inserted into the tumor under sonographic guidance via a trocar, and nitrogen or argon gas flow is initiated into the probe tip via a computer system. The gas undergoes chemical changes and causes a local freezing reaction termed an *ice ball*. The ice ball creates an even ablation field, allowing for homogeneity of tissue destruction. Tumors are destroyed by direct cell injury and death due to vasoconstriction. This process can be halted by application of a second gas, usually helium, or by passive thawing by discontinuation of the flow of argon or nitrogen. At least two freeze/thaw cycles are required to complete treatment, with cycle length based on tumor diameter.

There are multiple studies evaluating the efficacy of cryoablation for the treatment of both benign and malignant tumors. In several studies by Kaufman et al.[73-75] from 2004-2005, researchers examined efficacy, safety, and cost-effectiveness of cryoablation of fibroadenomata. The endpoints of the studies were elimination of the palpability of the mass and patient and physician satisfaction with the procedure. Their most recent report in 2005 was performed for 32 fibroadenomata in 29 patients, with an average follow-up period of 2.6 years. The study demonstrated resolution of palpability of the treated masses from 84% to 16% and with a median volume reduction of the tumor of 99%. The technique has also been shown effective in treating solitary small invasive breast cancers (≤2 cm). Sabel et al.[76] showed in a phase I clinical study that 27/29 (85%) of treated patients had no viable invasive cancer on surgical pathology following cryoablation. Of the 11 patients with tumors smaller than 1 cm, 100% had complete ablation of their tumors. In a more recent publication, Manenti et al. assessed the effectiveness of cryoablation in solitary invasive breast cancers less than 1 cm in size, and compared the accuracy of postablation MRI to detect residual tumor versus delayed surgical excision.[77] Their results yielded 100% correlation between posttreatment MRI and findings at surgical pathology. In 14/15 patients, results demonstrated complete necrosis, and 1/15 had evidence of residual enhancing tumor on MRI, all of which were corroborated at pathology.

CONCLUSIONS

Over 2 million minimally invasive breast biopsies will be performed in the United States this year. It is now the standard of care for tissue acquisition of indeterminate breast lesions and is a safe and accurate approach to the pathologic examination of indeterminate breast lesions. In many practices, as in ours, virtually every breast lesion undergoes biopsy with minimally invasive approaches and not surgical excision. There are numerous imaging approaches to the biopsy of breast lesions, including mammography, US, MRI, BSGI, and other nuclear medicine approaches. Additionally, there is an entire array of biopsy devices, ranging from a 25-gauge needle to a 7-gauge probe.

Each individual lesion should be assessed for optimal approach. Minimally invasive breast biopsy should be performed by a physician adept at all the various techniques, such that the best approach is chosen for the patient.

The accuracy of minimally invasive breast biopsy is 98%. Therefore, in our practice and many others, minimally invasive breast biopsies yielding benign findings undergo short-term follow-up. If there is interval growth, the lesion is either re-biopsied or surgically excised to detect the 2% of lesions missed at initial biopsy. Only well-circumscribed, oval, parallel masses determined to be fibroadenomata may not require short-interval follow-up. However, in our practice, we follow all lesions at 6 months for stability assurance.

The field of minimally invasive tissue acquisition is ever expanding, and now with the detection of smaller breast cancers and more accurate cancer targeting, as well as the ability to ablate lesions, the field is moving from tissue sampling to therapeutic approaches for breast cancer. It is an exciting field that will undoubtedly continue to expand and identify additional approaches to tissue acquisition and treatment.

KEY POINTS

- Image-guided minimally invasive procedures are currently the preferred method for biopsy of indeterminate breast lesions.
- Vacuum-assisted stereotactic biopsy is the preferred method to sample lesions predominantly composed of indeterminate calcifications.
- Core needle biopsy is the method of choice for acquisition of breast tissue from a mass lesion.

- Suspicious lesions seen exclusively on magnetic resonance imaging (MRI) warrant MRI-guided biopsy.
- Breast-specific gamma imaging (BSGI) and positron emission mammography (PEM) are novel physiologic imaging techniques comparable to MRI that also have biopsy capability.
- Ablative techniques, either radiofrequency ablation or cryoablation, are currently under investigation, with promising initial results.

▶ **SUGGESTED READINGS**

Berg WA. Image-guided breast biopsy and management of high-risk lesions. Radiol Clin North Am 2004;42:935–46.

Brem RF, Schoonjans JM, Gatewood OMB. Local anesthesia in stereotactic breast biopsy. Breast J 2001;7:72–3.

Jackman RJ, Marzoni FA. Stereotactic histologic biopsy with patients prone: technical feasibility in 98% of mammographically detected lesions. AJR Am J Roentgenol 2003;180:785–94.

Langer SA, Horst KC, Ikeda DM, et al. Pathologic correlates of false positive breast magnetic resonance imaging findings: which lesions warrant biopsy? Am J Surg 2005;190:633–40.

Liberman L. Percutaneous image-guided core breast biopsy. Radiol Clin North Am 2002;40:483–500.

Liberman L, Cody HS. Percutaneous biopsy and sentinel lymphadenectomy: minimally invasive diagnosis and treatment of nonpalpable breast cancer. AJR Am J Roentgenol 2001;177:887–91.

Liberman L, Drofman M, Morris EA, et al. Imaging-histologic discordance at percutaneous breast biopsy an indicator of missed cancer. Cancer 2000;89:2538–46.

Liberman L, Lalrenta LR, Dershaw DD, et al. Impact of core biopsy on the surgical management of impalpable breast cancer. AJR Am J Roentgenol 1997;168:495–9.

Nasuti JF, Gupta PK, Baloch ZW. Diagnostic value and cost-effectiveness of on-site evaluation of fine needle aspiration specimens: review of 5688 cases. Diagn Cytopathol 2001;27:1–3.

Pisano ED, Fajardo LL, Tsimikas J, et al. Rate of insufficient samples for fine needle aspiration for nonpalpable breast lesions in a multi-center clinical trial. Cancer 1998;82:679–88.

Tardivan AA, Guinebretiere JM, Dromain C, et al. Histological findings in surgical specimens after core biopsy of the breast. Eur J Radiol 2002;42:40–51.

The complete reference list is available online at www.expertconsult.com.

CHAPTER 156

Tracheobronchial Interventions

Ji Hoon Shin, Auh Whan Park, John F. Angle, and Alan H. Matsumoto

Central airway obstruction represents a great challenge to physicians from all subspecialties. Narrowing of the main tracheobronchial airways and proximal branches can cause significant and distressing symptoms for the patient and can be life threatening. Signs and symptoms of large-airway compromise include breathlessness, wheezing, stridor, and recurrent infections.[1] Treatment for airway obstruction varies depending upon the length of the lesion, etiology of the obstruction, and age and overall prognosis for the patient.

Malignancy is the most frequent cause of tracheobronchial obstruction in the adult population. Of the approximately 200,000 new cases of lung cancer diagnosed yearly in the United States, 20% to 30% will develop associated complications related to airway obstruction that can cause significant clinical problems such as resting and exertional dyspnea, atelectasis, postobstructive pneumonia, and hemoptysis.[2-4]

Resection of the pathology and reconstructive airway surgery provide the most definitive therapy, but many of these patients are not amenable to curative or corrective surgery. External beam irradiation and endobronchial brachytherapy, laser therapy, argon plasma coagulation, cryotherapy, photodynamic therapy, and electrocautery have been used in this setting. Most of these treatment options only provide temporary relief of symptoms because of the rapid regrowth of residual tumor.[5-7]

The majority of benign strictures of the trachea and major bronchi are due to iatrogenic causes, but prior infections, sarcoidosis, amyloid disease, vascular rings, trauma, or disease processes that affect the integrity of the cartilaginous rings of the trachea can also lead to airway stenosis. Short, circumscribed, benign lesions of the cervical trachea are usually best treated by surgical resection and reanastomosis. Long strictures (>5-7 cm in length) are more difficult to treat, but can occasionally be treated by very experienced thoracic surgeons.

Surgical options, although rarely feasible, should always be explored first for both malignant and benign lesions, but a large number of patients with symptomatic and life-threatening airway pathology are not candidates for definitive surgical correction because of the extent of the disease or comorbidities. A multidisciplinary approach to obstructing malignancies, with bronchoscopic debulking or removal of the obstructing lesion, balloon dilation of the airway, stenting of the airway, or a combination of techniques, has proven to be highly effective in reestablishing functional airway patency and palliating patient symptoms.[1] Benign lesions have been treated with a variety of endoscopic and fluoroscopic techniques. These therapeutic modalities usually provide immediate improvement and occasional long-term successes, but recurrences are the general rule.[1,5,6] The etiology for the obstruction will determine the need for bronchoscopic tumor debulking, airway stenting (covered or uncovered), balloon dilation, or a combination of these techniques. Central airway obstruction can be divided into four main categories: intraluminal, extraluminal or extrinsic, dynamic (due to loss of airway integrity and dynamic collapse causing obstruction), or mixed. Although intraluminal obstruction typically requires tumor debulking prior to stent placement, pure extraluminal or extrinsic compression and dynamic airway collapse will mainly benefit from airway stenting, with or without prior bronchoscopic balloon dilation.[1] On occasion, intraluminal benign scar tissue (e.g., lung transplant anastomosis or postinflammatory synechiae) can be treated with balloon dilation alone, but often stenting will be necessary.[8-11]

There are three major indications for airway stenting (Table 156-1). Two of these are for (1) enhancing airway patency by stenting an obstructed bronchus or trachea and creating a barrier for further tumor ingrowth (by using a covered stent) and (2) preventing extrinsic compression or dynamic obstruction by serving as a scaffold or supporting weakened airway walls (due to chondromalacia) and preventing airway collapse related to the static and dynamic behaviors of the stent.[12,13] A third indication for using stents in the airway is for sealing airway dehiscences and fistulas.

There have been no recent major advances in airway stent technology. The ideal stent should have limited migration, be easily removed if necessary, demonstrate long-term luminal patency without causing ischemia, be nonallergic, not erode into adjacent structures, induce minimal granulation tissue, be easy to accurately position, allow patency of bronchial branches, be durable, and allow for continued functioning of the mucociliary system. However, such an ideal stent is not yet available. A variety of stents are available from many different manufacturers (Table 156-2). Tracheobronchial stents can be divided into two main categories according to materials used in their construction: silicone and metallic-based stents. Hybrid stents result from the combination of these two major categories.[13]

In 1965, Montgomery described the use of a T-shaped silicone tube designed to be used both as a tracheal stent and as a tracheostomy tube. The tube is positioned in the trachea, with the sidearm of the T projecting through the tracheostomy. The sidearm prevents tube migration and provides access for clearance of secretions.[14] In 1990, Dumon developed the first silicone stent that could be inserted with a bronchoscope and did not require a tracheostomy. It was designed with no external components and could be inserted using a rigid bronchoscope. The outside surface of this stent had rounded studs protruding from its surface. The studs are designed to prevent the stent from sliding or turning. The Dumon stent is available in several sizes for both tracheal and bronchial applications. Different types or designs of silicone stents are also available.[15]

Silicone stents are fairly well tolerated and have been shown to be effective in relieving respiratory symptoms; they have the advantage of being easily removed and exchanged when necessary. The most frequent problems associated with silicone stents are migration and mucous plugging of the stents.[15] Migration is most likely to occur in short conical stenoses with intact smooth mucosa, or in the presence of tracheobronchomalacia. In both situations, the underlying anatomy does not permit firm anchorage of the stent. The mucosa under most silicone stents undergoes a metaplastic alteration, reducing the effectiveness of the mucociliary clearance mechanism, leading to recurrent stent plugging. In most cases, migration or mucous plugging of the stent can be managed by frequent endoscopic repositioning or replacement of the silicone stent.[16]

Metallic tracheobronchial devices have been in use since the early 1950s, but were refined when metallic stents were developed for use in the vascular system. Metallic stents offer several potential advantages over silicone stents for treatment of complex airway obstruction. Metallic stents have a small profile and are fairly easy to insert; the open lattice design allows treatment of more peripheral bronchi with less fear of causing obstructive pneumonia and/or atelectasis. Following placement of a metallic stent, the normal respiratory epithelium can protrude through the open lattice, and metaplastic squamous epithelium overgrows and incorporates the stent into the wall of the airway. The neoepithelium overlying the stent also appears to maintain some rudimentary ciliary function (Fig. 156-1).[16,17] However, granulation tissue and tumor can grow through the open lattice of these stents and lead to recurrence of airway obstruction. In addition, once metallic stents become incorporated into the wall of the airway, they are very difficult to remove without surgery. Covered stents are used to prevent intraluminal tumor ingrowth or when a fistula has to be excluded or sealed. Covered stents also have the advantage of relatively easy removal or exchange compared with uncovered stents (Table 156-3). However, covered stents may prevent neoepithelialization and compromise the mucociliary clearance mechanism of the airway.

Balloon dilation has been proposed for management of benign stenoses of the airways. The noncompliant balloon dilates the stenotic trachea or bronchus by stretching, tearing, and expanding scar tissue and the airway wall. Balloon dilation is associated with little morbidity and mortality,[18] but this technique is of little value in the treatment of malacic segments or airway narrowing secondary to tumor ingrowth or extrinsic compression. In addition, balloon dilation has failed to be of durable benefit for lung-transplant anastomotic strictures.[11]

Increased availability and ease of delivery of metallic balloon-expandable or self-expanding stents has resulted in a lower threshold for considering placement of airway stents. However, other therapeutic modalities and possible long-term complications inherent with the use of a metallic stent should be considered, because these patients will likely require lifelong management and revision. Indeed, an increasing number of adverse events reported in association with use of metallic stents for treatment of patients with benign airway disease led the U.S. Food and Drug Administration (FDA) to publish an advisory in 2005 on their use.[19] These were the recommendations:

* Appropriate patient selection is crucial.
* Use metallic tracheal stents in patients with benign airway disorders *only* after thoroughly exploring all other treatment options (e.g., tracheal surgical procedures or placement of silicone stents).
* Using metallic tracheal stents as a bridging therapy is *not* recommended, because removal of the metallic stent can result in serious complications.

TABLE 156-1. Specific Indications for Tracheobronchial Stent Placement

Malignant

Bronchogenic carcinoma
Primary airway tumor such as adenoid cystic carcinoma
Extraluminal malignancy such as esophageal or thyroid cancer
Metastases from renal cell or colon cancer
Esophagorespiratory fistula

Benign

Post–lung transplant strictures
Postintubation or posttracheostomy tracheal stenosis
Postoperative anastomotic stenosis
Inflammatory obstructive pathology such as tuberculosis
Tracheobronchomalacia
Prolonged radiation therapy
Compression by esophageal stent
Postinflammatory (prior infection [not TB]) stricture
Congenital

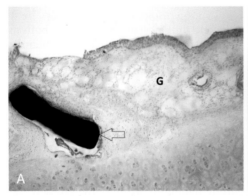
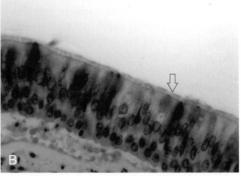

FIGURE 156-1. **A,** Microscopic section of autopsy specimen from patient with endobronchial Palmaz stent in place for 27 months shows stent strut *(arrow)* with overlying granulation tissue *(G)*. **B,** Further magnification of specimen reveals ciliated neoepithelium *(arrow)* along luminal surface of airway. *(Photos courtesy Maria I. Almira-Suarez, MD.)*

TABLE 156-2. Types of Stents

Device	Company Name	Construction/Materials Used	Shape	Expansion Mechanism	Introducer Size (F)	Delivery Catheter Endhole Size (inches)	Stent Diameter (mm)	Stent Length (mm)	FDA Approval
Gianturco-Z	Cook Endoscopy, Winston-Salem, N.C.	Zigzag stainless steel	Straight	Self-expanding	14-16	0.035	15-35	50	Yes
Palmaz	Cordis Endovascular/ Johnson & Johnson, Warren, N.J.	316L Slotted stainless steel tube	Straight	Balloon-expandable	Dependent on balloon catheter	Dependent on balloon catheter	4-12	10-30	Yes
Strecker	Boston Scientific, Natick, Mass.	Single-strand tantalum mesh	Straight	Balloon-expandable	Dependent on balloon catheter	Dependent on balloon catheter	8-11	20-40	Yes
Uncovered Wallstent	Boston Scientific	Woven cobalt-chrome alloy (Elgiloy) monofilaments	Straight	Self-expanding	6-12	0.035	5-24	20-94	Yes
Covered Wallstent	Boston Scientific	Woven cobalt-chrome alloy (Elgiloy) monofilaments with outer-layer Permalume partial covering and both ends bare	Straight	Self-expanding	7.5-11	0.035	8-14	20-80	Yes
Uncovered Ultraflex	Boston Scientific	Single-strand woven nickel-titanium alloy (nitinol)	Straight	Self-expanding	15-22	0.035	8-20	20-80	Yes
Covered Ultraflex	Boston Scientific	Single-strand woven nickel-titanium alloy (nitinol) with outer-layer polyurethane partial covering and both ends bare	Straight	Self-expanding	16-22	0.035	10-20	30-80	Yes
Alveolus	Merit Medical Systems Inc., South Jordan, Utah	Nitinol with inner- and outer-layer full polyurethane covering	Straight	Self-expanding	16-22	0.035	10-20	20-80	Yes
Hercules	S&G Biotech, Seongnam, Korea	Nitinol with outer-layer silicone covering	Straight	Self-expanding	14-21	0.035	8-24	40-90	No
Wallgraft	Boston Scientific	Woven cobalt-chrome alloy (Elgiloy) monofilaments with polyester	Straight	Self-expanding	9-12	0.035	6-14	27-104	Yes
iCAST	Atrium Medical Corp., Hudson, N.H.	316L Stainless steel encapsulated with ePTFE	Straight	Balloon-expandable	6-7	0.035	5-12	16-59	Yes
Viabahn	W.L. Gore & Associates, Flagstaff, Ariz.	Nitinol with external ePTFE layer	Straight	Self-expanding	6-7/9-12	0.014-0.018/0.035	5-8/9-13	25-150/25-150	Yes
Fluency Plus	Bard Peripheral Vascular Inc., Tempe, Ariz.	Nitinol with internal and external ePTFE layers	Straight	Self-expanding	8-9	0.035	6-10	40-80	Yes

ePTFE, Expanded polytetrafluoroethylene; *FDA*, U.S. Food and Drug Administration.

TABLE 156-3. Comparison Between Silicone and Metallic-Based Stents

	Silicone	Metallic
Bronchoscopy	Rigid	Rigid or flexible
Flexibility	No	Easily conform to the anatomy
Secretions	Mucous plugging	Less epithelial/cilia ingrowth
Migration	More frequent	Less frequent
Tumor ingrowth	No	Possible
Granulation tissue formation	Little	Profound
Mucociliary function	Impaired	Preserved
Removal/adjustment	Easy	Difficult

* If a metallic tracheal stent is the only option for a patient, insertion should be done by a physician trained or experienced in metallic tracheal stent procedures.
* Should removal be necessary, the procedure should be performed by a physician trained or experienced in removing metallic tracheal stents.
* Always review the indications for use, warnings, and precautions.
* Be aware of the guidelines from professional organizations regarding recommended provider skills and competency for these procedures (i.e., training requirements and clinical experience).

TRACHEOBRONCHIAL BALLOON DILATION

Indications and Contraindications

The primary indication for using balloon dilation is for treatment of benign tracheobronchial strictures. Postintubation tracheal stenosis, postoperative anastomotic stenosis, chemical aspiration–induced scarring, granulation tissue due to granulomatous disease (tuberculosis, sarcoidosis, histoplasmosis), postinflammatory stricture, and stenosis induced by radiation therapy are the principal etiologies for benign airway stenosis.[20-24] Balloon dilation can also be used either before or after stent placement to optimize airway patency.[20,21] Presence of an active inflammatory process or infection of the tracheobronchial tree is a relative contraindication to balloon dilation, owing to the potential for aggravating the underlying process.

Outcomes of Balloon Dilation

Small case series and limited reports in which balloon dilation was the only treatment used for benign tracheobronchial stenoses have shown a high initial technical success rate, but recurrence of symptoms necessitated further treatment with repeat dilation, stenting, or laser therapy in 71% to 80% of patients.[25,26] Ipsilateral bronchial stenosis is found in 7% to 15% of lung transplantation recipients,[27] and ischemic damage (which often affects the bronchial anastomosis), rejection, and infection have been considered as individual and/or concomitant predisposing causes.[28] In

one retrospective study of lung-transplant bronchial stenoses, bronchoscopic balloon dilation showed effective results in only 50% (5 of 10 bronchial stenosis) after an average of four balloon dilation procedures, suggesting that single or multiple sessions of balloon dilation could be used as a possible approach to management of bronchial stenoses after lung transplantation.[22,27] In cases of bronchial stenosis refractory to repeated sessions of balloon dilation, stent placement was often employed.[22,29]

For treatment of benign bronchial strictures resistant to conventional balloon dilation, use of a cutting balloon has shown some preliminary promise.[30] Kim et al. reported successful use of the cutting balloon, no major complications, and a demonstrated clinical benefit of approximately 60% (11 patients) at 2 years (Fig. 156-2).

Endobronchial brachytherapy has also been used to treat benign bronchial strictures resistant to conventional balloon dilation or as an adjuvant treatment to treat granulation tissue formation after airway restoration.[24,31]

EQUIPMENT

The optimal setup for performing fluoroscopic-guided tracheobronchial balloon dilation includes an all-purpose fluoroscopy room with a rotating C-arm. Flexible standard bronchoscopes with an outer diameter of 4.9 to 5.9 mm at the distal tip and a working channel of 2- to 2.8-mm diameter are usually available. Devices used include any standard 5F 65-cm multipurpose shaped catheter (Cook Medical, Bloomington, Ind.; Boston Scientific, Natick, Mass.; Cordis Endovascular, Warrenton, N.J.; AngioDynamics, Glen Falls, N.Y.) and either a steerable nonhydrophilic 0.035-inch guidewire that comes with a locking wire extension component (Wholey wire [Mallinckrodt, Hazelwood, Mo.]), a 0.035-inch J nonhydrophilic guidewire (Cook Medical, AngioDynamics), or Magic Torque guidewire (Boston Scientific) and the appropriate-diameter balloon catheter. A hydrophilic guidewire should *not* be used, since it may inadvertently pass too peripherally and cause a pneumothorax, and is too slippery to adequately control during catheter exchanges. In adults, 8-mm to 12-mm-diameter balloon catheters are used in the bronchi, and 14-mm to 28-mm-diameter balloon catheters are used in the trachea. The diameter of the balloon is chosen to be closest to that of the lumen measured at the proximal-region normal airway, which is determined based upon a pretreatment computed tomography (CT) scan. It is helpful to partner with a pulmonologist to allow bronchoscopy to be combined with the fluoroscopic procedure to provide additional guidance and assessment of the stenosis before and after balloon dilation.

Technique

Before balloon dilation, stenosis severity, proximal and distal extent of the lesion, tapering in size of the airways, and location of the stricture relative to the vocal cords and branch airways should be evaluated by conventional radiography, pretreatment CT scans, including three-dimensional (3D) and multiplanar reconstructions, and/or bronchoscopy. The presence of malignancy or a benign tumor should have already been excluded, even if a bronchoscopic biopsy is necessary.

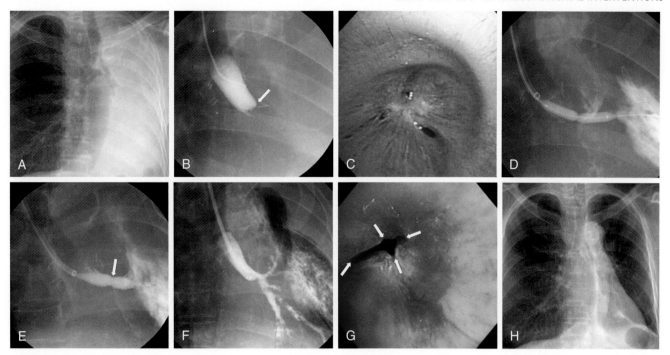

FIGURE 156-2. Images from 71-year-old man with anastomotic bronchial stricture detected 4 months after left lower lobectomy. **A,** Chest radiograph shows total collapse of left lung. **B,** Selective bronchogram shows complete occlusion of left mainstem bronchus at bronchial anastomosis *(arrow)*. Stricture could be negotiated with TIPS dilator with a stiff guidewire (not shown). **C,** Bronchoscopic image shows hard scar tissue. **D,** Using a conventional balloon, lesion could not be dilated. **E,** An 8-mm cutting balloon catheter was successfully used *(arrow)*. Then a conventional balloon (10 mm) was used without difficulty (not shown). **F,** Final bronchogram shows recanalization of anastomotic stricture. **G,** Bronchoscopic image just after cutting balloon dilation shows four directions of laceration *(arrows)* corresponding to the four microtomes on cutting balloon catheter. **H,** Four months later, chest radiograph shows complete left lung aeration.

The pharynx and larynx are topically anesthetized with lidocaine aerosol spray 3 to 5 minutes before the procedure. Patients are sedated using intravenous administration of midazolam and fentanyl while their oxygen saturation, electrocardiogram, blood pressure, and pulse are monitored throughout the procedure. General anesthesia is rarely indicated for simple balloon dilation. Bronchoscopy is first performed to localize the airway obstruction and assess for the presence of a secondary infection. A guidewire is inserted through the working channel of the bronchoscope and is passed through the obstruction. With the guidewire held in place, the bronchoscope is withdrawn, and a sizing catheter (Accu-Vu Sizing Catheter [AngioDynamics, Latham, N.Y.]) is passed over the guidewire to the distal part of the stricture to measure the lesion length, although this calculation can often be performed based upon measurements from the CT scan and the virtual bronchoscopic reconstructions. Alternatively, use of a calibrated guidewire (Magic Torque wire [Boston Scientific]) can be used as an internal reference for calibration. The degree and length of the stricture can be further evaluated in detail by selective tracheobronchography by injecting approximately 5 mL of water-soluble nonionic contrast medium (Visipaque 270 [GE Healthcare, Milwaukee, Wis.]) mixed 1:1 with lidocaine through the sizing catheter while the catheter is pulled back proximal to the lesion, without withdrawing the catheter through the vocal cords. Fluoroscopy is performed, and digital spot images are obtained without moving the image intensifier. This maneuver may cause the patient to cough, and it will also necessitate passage of the

guidewire through the lesion again. However, the tracheobronchogram can be used as a reference such that radiopaque markers can be placed on the surface of the patient's skin to allow fluoroscopic identification of the proximal and distal limits of the stricture.[21,32] Again, to minimize misregistration of the reference image due to parallax, the image intensifier and patient should not be moved. Tracheobronchography could be skipped in cases where exact position of the balloon dilation catheter is not critical or the location of the stricture is seen with simple fluoroscopy. An angioplasty balloon catheter is then passed over the guidewire under fluoroscopic guidance, correctly positioned across the stenosis, and inflated with diluted water-soluble contrast medium at inflation pressures as high as 20 atm. Use of a noncompliant balloon (e.g., Dorado [Bard Peripheral Vascular, Tempe, Ariz.] or Ultrathin Diamond [Boston Scientific]) is recommended to optimize translation of the dilating forces to the lesion.

If the stenosis is too narrow to allow passage of a balloon catheter of 10 mm or more in diameter (which is extremely rare), a 6-mm-diameter balloon catheter can be used first to provide a passage for the larger balloon catheter. Two to three serial balloon inflations are performed for 60 to 120 seconds during balloon bronchoplasty until the balloon waist formed by the stenosis disappears, or until the patient cannot tolerate further inflations. For a tracheal stenosis, balloon inflation and deflation should be very quick (e.g., <20 seconds) because patients cannot tolerate longer inflations within the trachea. As the balloon catheter is being deflated, it is very helpful to push the balloon catheter

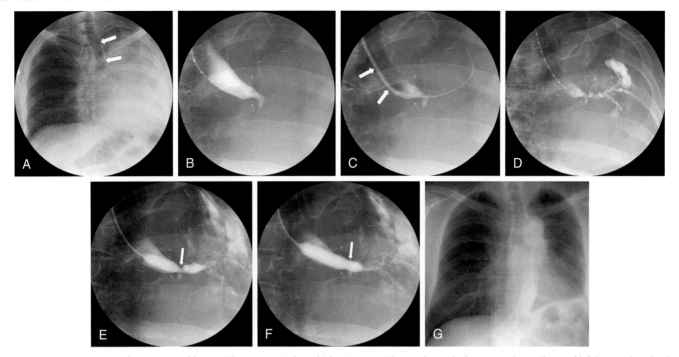

FIGURE 156-3. Images from 60-year-old man with anastomotic bronchial stricture. **A,** Chest radiograph shows complete collapse of left lung and tracheal deviation *(arrows)* toward left lung. **B,** Attempts at negotiating an opening using a graduated sizing catheter and guidewire resulted in guidewire twisting on itself. **C,** Using a TIPS dilator *(arrows)*, guidewire was introduced beyond stricture. **D,** Selective bronchogram shows very short and tight stricture. **E-F,** Subsequently, balloon dilation was successfully performed, with widening of stricture *(arrows)*. **G,** One day after procedure, chest radiograph shows good left lung aeration.

distally to allow improved air flow at the stenotic area. After the procedure, repeat bronchoscopy is performed to evaluate procedure results and assess for complications such as bleeding or a mucosal laceration.

When catheterization with a guidewire and conventional vascular catheter is not successful because a bronchial stricture is tight or complete, catheterization with an angled-tip introducer set (Flexor Check Flo Introducer Set [Cook Medical]) could be very effective to negotiate the guidewire into the stricture (Fig. 156-3; also see Fig. 156-2).[23] The inner dilator has a suitable angle to allow passage of the tapered end of the dilator into the bronchus.

On occasion, some patients do not tolerate balloon dilation of the trachea and/or bronchial segment. In these situations, it may be necessary to employ general anesthesia for the procedure. It is helpful to use a #8 endotracheal tube, which is large enough to allow continued ventilation during flexible bronchoscopy. It is also helpful to use an adapter on the back end of the endotracheal tube through which the bronchoscope can be inserted without having the anesthetic gases leak. During the catheter-based endotracheal/bronchial intervention, a 14F 11-cm vascular sheath can be inserted into the port of the endotracheal tube adapter to minimize back-leakage of the anesthesia gases.

Complications

Although balloon dilation of the airway is a very safe procedure, complications can occur and include coughing during tracheobronchography or balloon dilation, chest pain during the dilation, bronchospasm, atelectasis after dilation, superficial or deep mucosal laceration, pneumothorax, pneumomediastinum, mediastinitis, and/or massive bleeding.[18,25,33,34] In one large series, bronchial lacerations occurred during 64 of 124 (52%) tracheobronchial balloon dilation procedures, but none of these progressed to a transmural laceration.[18] Among them, superficial laceration (defined as 2 mm or less in depth on bronchoscopy) was much more common than deep laceration. The median cumulative airway patency period was significantly longer in patients with a laceration than in those without lacerations (24 months vs. 4 months), indicating that laceration secondary to balloon dilation may improve patency outcomes.[18] In addition, complications can occur during the course of the bronchoscopic examinations.

Postprocedure and Follow-up Care

Postprocedure care generally follows that of standard postbronchoscopy care. The patient is appropriately recovered as per the standard post–conscious sedation or postanesthesia protocols. Patients are also evaluated with a clinical examination, chest radiograph, and bronchoscopy (if symptomatic) within the first week. Additional follow-up evaluation will occur at 1 month, 3 months, and then every 3 months thereafter. Patients are instructed to contact a physician as soon as they notice any worsening of symptoms. They are seen within 24 to 48 hours of notification and further evaluated. The evaluation is tailored to the patient (e.g., lung transplant patient vs. patient with history of postinflammatory stricture), which might also include bronchoscopy to evaluate for lesion recurrence. Pulmonary function testing with flow loops to assess for large-airway obstruction is often obtained before and after balloon dilation to provide objective physiologic data with regard to lesion severity and worsening or improvement.

TRACHEOBRONCHIAL METALLIC STENT PLACEMENT

Up to 30% of patients with lung cancer have been reported to develop central airway obstruction secondary to intraluminal disease or external compression by a hilar tumor or bulky lymphadenopathy.[35] Recent technologic advances have increased the popularity of tracheobronchial stents, particularly because stenting can be effective at alleviating airway obstruction for both extrinsic compressive and intraluminal lesions.

Before stent placement, the airway anatomy should be fully evaluated with detailed CT evaluation, conventional radiography, and/or bronchoscopy. A chest CT with intravenous contrast material is also often useful to evaluate the vascularity of the lesion and detect the presence of metastatic disease. In addition, based upon the CT, the length of the obstruction, diameter of the airway to be stented, and adjacency of the vocal cords or airway branching points can be determined in anticipation of tracheobronchial stent placement.[36]

Indications and Contraindications

Stent placement is indicated for patients with submucosal and extraluminal (extrinsic) pathology or intraluminal (intrinsic) pathology causing airway compromise that cannot be addressed with surgical options, radiation therapy, or chemotherapy. In addition, some patients with tracheobronchomalacia causing severe collapse of the airway during expiration may benefit from metallic stent placement (Table 156-3).

Intraluminal obstruction is most often caused by invasive bronchogenic or metastatic carcinoma (e.g., renal cell). Malignant intraluminal lesions growing into the airway lumen are best managed with initial tumor debulking using transbronchoscopic laser or electrocautery tissue ablation techniques prior to stent placement. However, advanced malignancy with the expectation of extremely limited patient longevity may dictate that stent placement alone without tumor debulking is adequate for palliation, while avoiding the risks of bleeding and perforation.[36] In general, use of a covered stent is preferred for exclusion and displacement of intraluminal tumors.

Extrinsic compression by an extraluminal process can result from malignancies but also from benign conditions such as congenital or acquired vascular abnormalities (e.g., vascular slings or aneurysms) or mediastinal lymphadenopathy or fibrosis due to histoplasmosis. Whenever possible, benign or malignant pathology causing airway obstruction should be addressed with medical and/or surgical therapy. However, if surgical therapy is not a consideration, medical therapy will require too much time to address the acute situation. If there is no other viable treatment option, tracheobronchial stenting may be necessary to stabilize a threatened airway to allow treatment of the extraluminal tumor with radiation or chemotherapy or as the primary therapy. Because of suboptimal primary patency rates, tracheobronchial stenting for benign disease, particularly in young patients, should only be undertaken after careful risk and benefit analysis. Retrievable or absorbable tracheobronchial stents have a definite theoretic advantage in these patients, with the assumption that the stent will no longer be needed after treatment of the underlying process.[20,36,37]

Contraindications to tracheobronchial stenting include uncontrolled hemorrhage, uncorrected coagulopathy, and the presence of an active inflammatory process of the airways. Anatomic contraindications to stent placement include high tracheal lesions where placement would result in the upper end of the stent being within 1 cm of the vocal cords, and absence of a patent distal landing site.[38] Attention should be paid when the tracheobronchial airway bifurcation or the bronchial branches are involved by the primary obstructing process. When tracheobronchial stenting at the mainstem bronchus and more distal obstruction are being considered for stenting, preprocedure planning should involve the issue of whether patency of side branches can be maintained. This planning process is particularly important when placement of a covered stent is being contemplated.[36,39]

For catheter-based or endoscopic/bronchoscopic treatment of an esophagorespiratory fistula, the following treatment algorithm has been proposed[40]: (1) tracheobronchial stent placement if the patient has no or only a very mild stricture in the esophagus and has a moderate to severe stricture in the airways (Fig. 156-4), (2) esophageal stent placement if the patient has a stricture in the esophagus with no or a very mild airway stricture, or (3) both airway and esophageal stent placement when there is a moderate to severe stricture involving both the airway and esophagus.

The only definitive contraindication for placement of a tracheobronchial stent is in a patient with external compression of the airways by an artery (i.e., innominate artery). Stent placement in these patients is associated with an unacceptably high rate of erosion of the stent through the airway into the adjacent compressing artery, leading to an arterial-tracheal fistula, massive hemoptysis, and death.[35]

Outcomes of Tracheobronchial Stenting Using Metallic Stents

For benign tracheobronchial stenoses, technical success rates associated with metallic stent use have been reported to be 100%. However, long-term patency rates vary depending on underlying diseases and stent type used. In one of the largest series by Thornton et al.,[10] 40 patients underwent uncovered metallic stent implantations for benign stenosis related to lung transplantation (n = 13), tracheal tube injury (n = 10), or inflammation/infection (n = 9). Survival rates at 1, 2, 3, 4, 5, and 6 years were 79%, 76%, 51%, 47%, 38%, and 23%, respectively. Loss of primary patency was most rapid during the first year. With repeat intervention, assisted patency rates were 90% at 6.8 years, suggesting that good long-term patency rates can be achieved with secondary interventions. In two representative studies using uncovered or retrievable covered stents for bronchial strictures and/or bronchomalacia secondary to lung transplantation complications,[22,29] significant improvement in pulmonary function tests could be achieved. However, long-term patency of the uncovered stents in this patient population was plagued by abundant

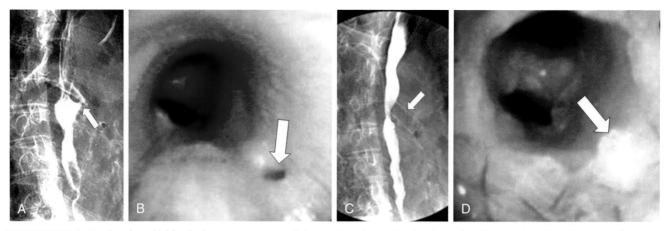

FIGURE 156-4. Esophagobronchial fistula due to pressure necrosis by esophageal stent that had been placed for esophageal carcinoma. Esophagogram (A) and bronchoscopy (B) after esophageal stent removal show a definite fistula *(arrows)* at proximal end of stent site. Esophagogram (C) and bronchoscopy (D) after bronchial stent placement *(arrows)* show successful closure of fistula.

granulation tissue formation (in up to 20% of patients) and stent migration in cases where covered stents were used.

In another study, 30 covered retrievable self-expanding metallic stents were placed in 24 patients with benign airway stenoses, resulting in technical and short-term clinical success rates of 100% (Fig. 156-5).[37] All stents were successfully removed electively, either 2 (n = 12) or 6 (n = 12) months after placement or when complications occurred (n = 6). The group of patients who underwent stent removal at 6 months showed a lower rate of recurrent symptoms (41.7% vs. 83.3%; *P* = 0.045) and a better mean duration of airway patency (39.7 ± 7.8 months vs. 9.4 ± 5.4 months; *P* = 0.001) than the patients whose stents were removed after only 2 months. Although stent migration and granulation tissue formation at either end of the stent was observed in 13% and 37% of these patients, respectively, stent removal was easy and safe.

Postintubation tracheal stenosis is caused by either cuff-induced ischemic damage to the trachea and/or stomal injury from a tracheostomy, and is primarily managed with surgical resection and reconstruction. However, balloon dilation or other bronchoscopic treatment options have been used in selected patients with severe comorbidities and very debilitated health status, or for stenoses less than 2 cm in length.[41] When a stenosis is greater than 2 cm in length or is associated with tracheomalacia, a covered stent could also be used as the primary treatment, but migration, compromise of the mucociliary clearance mechanism, and formation of granulation tissue at the stent ends can occur. Silicone stents have been used as a bridge to curative surgery or as definitive treatment, but migration and mucous plugging occur with these devices when left in place for long periods.[42] Uncovered metallic stents should be avoided in patients who are potential candidates for resection, because these are highly likely to cause additional granulation tissue formation and may make a potentially short-segment surgical repair more difficult or inoperable.[41,42]

Four representative studies of metallic stent placement, two with uncovered and two with covered stents, in 269 patients with malignant tracheobronchial obstructions showed technical success rates of 100% and initial clinical success rates of 82% to 100%.[39,43-45] Since the restoration of airway patency in malignant strictures is a palliative rather than curative procedure, median survival of patients in most studies remains poor, between 3 and 4 months.[43-45]

In another study comparing imaging and clinical outcomes with special reference to tumor involvement pattern after stent placement for malignant bronchial obstructions,[46] involvement of the lower-lobe segmental bronchus has been associated with significantly lower rates of imaging (33% vs. 92%) and clinical (63% vs. 96%) improvement following stent placement. Temporary airway stenting with concurrent radiation therapy and/or chemotherapy may have greater potential for improving a patient's quality of life by reducing stent-related complications when compared with use of a permanent metallic stent for treatment of inoperable malignant tracheobronchial strictures (Fig. 156-6).[47]

In infants and children, use of uncovered or covered metallic stents as well as silicone stents has been reported to be effective in relieving respiratory obstruction in 85% to 100% of patients.[48-50] In cases where uncovered stents were used, stent removal was arduous at best and associated with a high risk of significant complications,[49,50] whereas stent removal was much easier in patients in whom retrievable covered stents were employed (Fig. 156-7).[48]

Equipment

Fluoroscopy equipment and flexible standard bronchoscopes are the same as for balloon dilation procedures. In general, since precise stent placement is required, the procedure is performed while the patient is under general anesthesia to minimize the cough reflex and patient movement. Again, a #8 or larger endotracheal tube with an adapter on the back end of the endotracheal tube should be used to allow the operator to work through the endotracheal tube while maintaining continuous ventilatory support.

As previously discussed, silicone and metallic stents are the two major classes of commercially available tracheobronchial stents (Fig. 156-8). There is an ever-increasing variety of balloon-expandable, self-expanding, and covered metallic stents, but none of these available stents is ideal.

Silicone stents range in size from 8 to 20 mm in outer diameter, and their lengths vary from 2 to 8 cm. The longer-length devices are generally used in the trachea, whereas

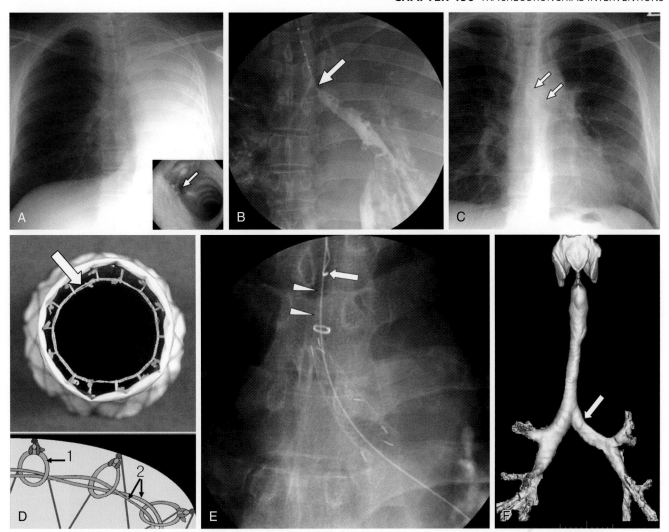

FIGURE 156-5. Images from 36-year-old man with left mainstem bronchial obstruction due to endobronchial tuberculosis. **A,** Chest radiograph shows total left lung collapse and total occlusion of left mainstem bronchus. Bronchoscopy shows complete occlusion *(arrow)* of left mainstem bronchus *(inset).* **B,** Selective bronchogram shows very tight stenosis *(arrow)* of left mainstem bronchus orifice. **C,** Radiograph after left bronchial stent *(arrows)* placement shows complete left lung aeration. Stent was in place for 6 months. **D,** To make stent removable, two drawstrings *(arrows, 2)* and nylon loops *(1)* were attached to its proximal end. **E,** Radiograph shows stent removal, with its proximal end collapsed while drawstrings were grasped by a hookwire *(arrow)* and withdrawn into sheath *(arrowhead).* **F,** Three-dimensional reconstruction computed tomography image 1 year after stent removal shows good patency of left mainstem bronchus *(arrow).*

the shorter lengths are employed as bronchial stents. A limited number of Y-shaped silicone stents are commercially available for placement at the carina, with the limbs positioned in the mainstem bronchi. An advantage of silicone stents is their ability to be repositioned or removed as many times as necessary—especially important for benign tracheobronchial stenoses, slowly growing tumors, and a stenosis that frequently recurs.[35] Disadvantages of silicone stents are high rates of migration, impairment of the mucociliary clearance mechanism and consequent problems with secretions, and unfavorable inner/outer-diameter ratios. General anesthesia and use of a rigid bronchoscope are mandatory for placement and removal of silicone stents.

Both balloon-expandable and self-expanding metallic stents have relatively low profiles, can be delivered to the airways much easier than a silicone stent, and can also be accurately positioned with fluoroscopic guidance. Balloon-expandable stents typically have greater hoop strength than self-expanding stents, but balloon-expandable stents are rigid and do not expand or contract with the airways during normal breathing. Balloon-expandable stents also demonstrate characteristics of plastic deformation—that is, they can be permanently deformed if traumatized during a bronchoscopic procedure. Because the airways are very dynamic, expanding and contracting during inspiration and expiration, respectively, self-expanding metallic stents may be better suited for and better tolerated in the airways. Additional advantages of uncovered balloon-expandable metallic stents (Palmaz [Cordis Endovascular]) and uncovered self-expanding metallic stents (Gianturco Z [Cook Medical], Ultraflex [Boston Scientific], and Polyflex [Boston Scientific]) are their lower rates of migration (if sized appropriately) and less interference with the mucociliary clearance mechanism. Among their disadvantages is their difficult removal due to incorporation of these bare metallic stents into the airway wall from the neoepithelialization that

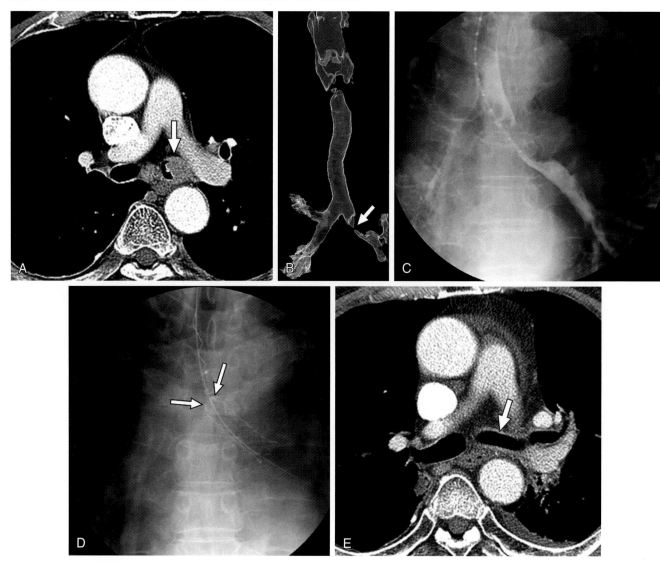

FIGURE 156-6. Images from 67-year-old man with a left mainstem bronchial stricture caused by non–small cell lung cancer. Axial computed tomography (CT) scan **(A)** and three-dimensional surface-rendered reconstruction CT images **(B)** obtained 3 days before stent placement show severe left mainstem bronchial stricture *(arrows)*. **C,** Selective bronchogram shows very tight stricture. Stent was deployed and had been in place for 2 months (not shown). **D,** Radiograph shows stent removal after completion of radiation therapy and chemotherapy. Collapse of proximal end of stent *(arrows)* is seen while a hookwire was withdrawn into sheath. **E,** Axial CT scan obtained 6 months after stent removal shows marked improvement of stricture *(arrow)*.

occurs within 3 weeks of device implantation. Bare metallic stents also have the potential for tumor or granulation tissue ingrowth through the open lattice of the stent, leading to reobstruction of the airway.

Whereas uncovered self-expanding metallic stents cannot be removed or exchanged easily, covered self-expanding metallic stents, such as the Ultraflex (Boston Scientific), Wallstent (Boston Scientific), or Alveolus (Alveolus Inc., Charlotte, N.C.), can be removed or exchanged relatively easily. Specifically designed to be retrievable, a covered self-expanding metallic stent (Hercules stent [S&G Biotech, Seongnam, Korea]) has been used successfully and safely in many different clinical settings.[51] Therefore, retrievable covered self-expanding metallic stents may be the best device to use to treat benign airway strictures, as well as to treat malignant airway strictures, especially when used in combination with radiation therapy and/or chemotherapy.[37,47] In addition, covered self-expanding metallic stents

are reserved for situations such as esophagorespiratory fistula. A retrievable covered metallic stent with barbs has recently been introduced and has shown particularly low migration rates.[52] A balloon-expandable covered stent is also FDA-approved for use in the tracheobronchial system (iCAST [Atrium Medical, Hudson, N.H.]), but its rigidity makes it difficult to remove once it has been placed. In cases of airway stenosis distal to the mainstem bronchi, the problem of preserving or obliterating branch airways is the primary concern. To maximize air flow, especially in severely dyspneic patients, use of uncovered stents is preferred if the stent must be positioned across the ostia of side branches.[36]

Technique

Although silicone stent placement procedures have been performed under general anesthesia using an endotracheal

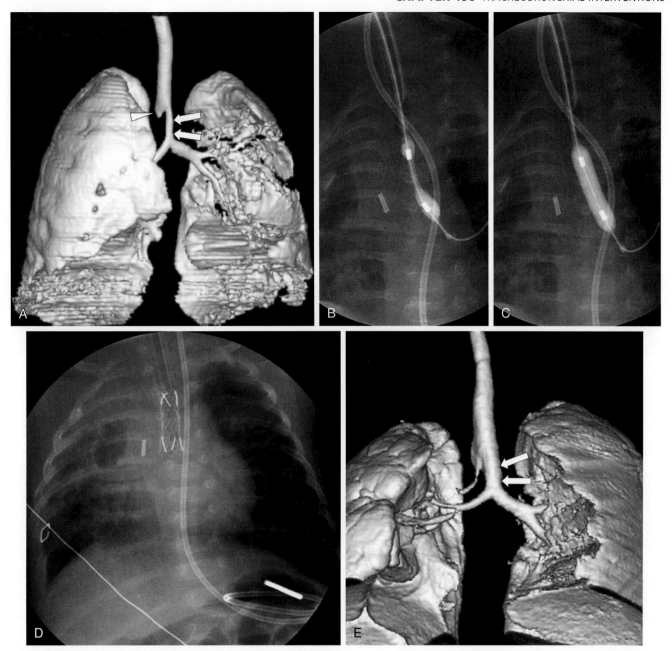

FIGURE 156-7. Images from 2-month-old boy with congenital tracheal stenosis. **A,** Three-dimensional (3D) reconstruction computed tomography (CT) image shows a 13-mm segment of severe narrowing *(arrows)* of lower trachea from below tracheal bronchus *(arrowhead)* to carina. **B,** During balloon dilation, formation of waist on balloon was seen initially during fluoroscopy. Surgical clip from a prior right upper lobectomy is seen. **C,** Balloon was able to be expanded to its full diameter (6 mm). **D,** Stent was then deployed using endotracheal tube as conduit. Stent was left in place for 5 months and then removed. **E,** 3D reconstruction CT image obtained 4 years after stent removal shows an 8-mm patent lumen *(arrows)* of lower trachea.

tube, metallic stents have been placed with fluoroscopic guidance using only conscious sedation and topical anesthesia. However, in most instances, these cases were performed outside the United States. Every case must be tailored to the interventionalist's experience and the patient's desires and ability to cooperate. A collaborative effort with a pulmonologist or thoracic surgeon is generally recommended so immediate bronchoscopic evaluation of the adequacy of the stent procedure can follow. Moreover, it is relatively easy to insert a guidewire across the stricture into the distal portion of the trachea or bronchus through

the working channel of the bronchoscope during fluoroscopic visualization.

Techniques for providing topical anesthesia, introducing the guidewire and catheter into the tracheobronchial tree, obtaining selective tracheobronchography, and placing radiopaque markers on the patient's skin are the same as previously described for balloon dilation. With the patient in a supine position and the neck fully extended, the delivery system is passed over the guidewire into the trachea and is advanced until the distal tip reaches beyond the stricture. When the stricture is severe (i.e., more than two thirds of

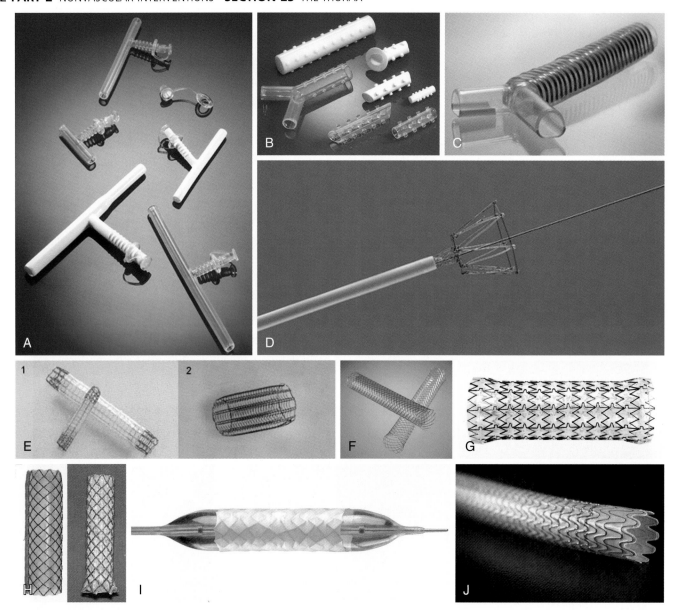

FIGURE 156-8. Various silicone and metallic stents. **A,** Montgomery silicone stent (Boston Medical Products, Westborough, Mass.). **B,** Dumon stent (Novatech S.A., La Ciotat, France). **C,** Dynamic stent (Boston Scientific, Natick, Mass.). **D,** Gianturco Z stent (Cook Medical, Bloomington, Ind.). **E,** Covered and uncovered Ultraflex (Boston Scientific). **F,** Covered and uncovered Wallstent (Boston Scientific). **G,** Alveolus stent (NVSS Corp., Charlotte, N.C.). **H,** Hercules airway stent (S&G Biotech Inc., Gyeonggi-Do, Republic of Korea). **I,** iCAST tracheobronchial covered stent (Atrium Medical, a Maquet Getinge Company, Hudson, N.H.). **J,** Viabahn stent (Gore Medical, Flagstaff, Ariz.). *(Permission for use of **D** granted by Cook Medical Inc., Bloomington, Ind. All other photos courtesy of the respective manufacturers.)*

the lumen is narrowed), the stenosis is predilated with a balloon about 2 mm smaller than the normal airway to allow easier passage of the stent delivery system. The stent should extend at least 5 to 10 mm proximal and distal to the stricture. Fluoroscopy, the tracheobronchography, and the metal markers on the chest are used to monitor stent positioning. Following stent placement and any supplemental balloon dilation, bronchoscopy is performed to check for satisfactory stent placement and adequacy of the airway lumen, assess for any bleeding or mucosal injury, and allow removal of any secretions, retained contrast, or blood. If the stent is not fully expanded, it is further dilated utilizing a balloon catheter inserted over the retained guidewire.[38] It is important to avoid inexact stent deployment that results

in partial obstruction of a bronchial orifice or incomplete coverage of a tumor stenosis. If the stent's position is not optimal, it can often be repositioned in this acute setting using bronchoscopic biopsy forceps. If it is difficult to reposition, it may be easier to remove the stent and place a new one at a more appropriate location.[39]

Lesions involving the carina or other branch points in the main airways present special problems. Three stents could be utilized to have the proximal ends of bilateral bronchial stents cover the most proximal parts of the mainstem bronchi, and to have the distal end of a tracheal stent cover the most distal part of the trachea, much like treating the aortic bifurcation with kissing stents and an aortic stent.[38] Upside-down Y-shaped stents have been devised to completely cover the carina, but these devices are not widely available.[53]

Use of metallic stents in the airways of infants and children is challenging because the stents cannot grow to keep pace with the children's growth. Therefore, a covered stent should be placed temporarily because use of an uncovered stent will make its removal difficult and traumatic. In this regard, there is one small series in which six retrievable covered metallic stents were placed and successfully removed in five infants or children (see Fig. 156-7).[48]

Complications Associated with Use of Metallic Stents

Complications related to the use of metallic stents in the airway are different between uncovered and covered stents, as well as between the treatments of benign versus malignant pathologies.

In benign pathologies, granulation tissue formation and stent fracture are fairly common occurrences in cases where uncovered stents were used. Sputum retention and stent migration occur more frequently with the use of covered stents.[10,22,37,54]

In four representative studies of stent placement in patients with malignant tracheobronchial stenoses,[39,43-45] covered metallic stents were associated with much higher rates of stent migration and sputum retention than uncovered metallic stents. In contrast, tumor ingrowth into the stent lumen occurred more often with uncovered than with covered metallic stents.

Complications related to stent placement may affect a patient's quality of life. More severe complications, including pneumonia or hemoptysis caused by stent placement, may reduce a patient's survival period. In one study,[39] survival of patients who died of pneumonia or hemoptysis was significantly shorter than that of patients who died of disease progression after stent placement (4.47 vs. 13.94 weeks; $P < 0.01$). Therefore, eliminating potential stent-related complications may improve a patient's quality of life and period of survival.

In summary, uncovered stents rarely migrate or impede mucociliary clearance, yet their use is complicated by granulation tissue or tumor ingrowth. Once restenosis occurs, intraluminal treatment with laser or electrocautery to ablate the obstructing tissue or restenting can be performed. Often, management of restenosis becomes a lifelong process, which significantly limits use of uncovered stents in patients with benign disease.[36]

Postprocedure and Follow-up Care

Postprocedure care and follow-up protocols are the same as for balloon dilation patients. To address a complication related to stenting of the airways, bronchoscopic evaluation and intraluminal treatment are performed primarily, then interventional procedures such as stent removal, stent repositioning, or restenting can follow as necessary. To assess for stent fracture, plain films of the chest are easiest and most cost-effective.

KEY POINTS

- Therapeutic strategies for patients with chronic airway obstruction are best developed and managed within a multidisciplinary team inclusive of a pulmonologist, interventional radiologist, thoracic surgeon, oncologist (if malignancy is the underlying problem), and anesthesiologist.

- Tracheobronchial resection and reconstruction should be the first consideration for benign or malignant obstructive lesions, but immediate improvement of respiratory symptoms can be achieved with tracheobronchial stenting to serve as a bridge to more definitive therapy. In patients for whom there is no surgical or medical option, tracheobronchial stenting can provide some palliation and improve quality of life.

- Tracheobronchial stenting is a valuable adjunct to other therapeutic bronchoscopic techniques to relieve airway obstruction and has become a common palliative treatment for both malignant and benign diseases.

- Clinical key factors, such as likelihood of tumor growth or recurrence despite treatment, overall patient prognosis, and the patient's ability to tolerate the procedure, should be considered before placement of a stent is undertaken.

- It is important to understand the inherent properties and outcomes associated with use of the different types of stents, recognizing the advantages and disadvantages of each device.

- For benign lesions, placement of an uncovered metallic stent should be done, recognizing that ingrowth of granulation tissue will likely occur, and removing an uncovered stent is fraught with significant complications.

- Frequently, multiple stent and endoscopic procedures will be necessary to maintain a satisfactory airway, especially for benign disease.

▶ SUGGESTED READINGS

Shin JH, Song HY, Ko GY, et al. Esophagorespiratory fistula: long-term results of palliative treatment with covered expandable metallic stents in 61 patients. Radiology 2004;232:252–9.

Shin JH. Interventional management of tracheobronchial strictures. World J Radiol 2010;2:323–8.

Thornton RH, Gordon RL, Kerlan RK, et al. Outcomes of tracheobronchial stent placement for benign disease. Radiology 2006;240:273–82.

Walser EM. Stent placement for tracheobronchial disease. Eur J Radiol 2005;55:321–30.

The complete reference list is available online at www.expertconsult.com.

CHAPTER **157**

Image-Guided Percutaneous Biopsy of Musculoskeletal Lesions

Yung-Hsin Chen, John A. Carrino, and Laura M. Fayad

Image-guided percutaneous needle biopsy (PNB) has emerged as a safe, effective, and accurate tool for the diagnosis of musculoskeletal lesions.[1-5] Information obtained from percutaneous biopsy helps determine appropriate therapy and disease prognosis. Whether a lesion is benign or malignant and its specific histologic type and grade (in the case of malignant lesions) is vital knowledge for treatment planning. Because diagnostic accuracy may be greatly influenced by the biopsy method used and location of sampling, a well-planned and well-executed percutaneous biopsy is essential for providing an accurate diagnosis and facilitating treatment. When a biopsy is performed poorly, the outcome may be disastrous from a number of standpoints. If an incorrect diagnosis is obtained, a delay in treatment may result, and complications may ensue. In addition, when the percutaneous route taken is badly planned, treatment options can become limited, thus endangering potential limb preservation surgery and creating a significant negative impact on ultimate survival.[6-10]

Traditionally, open incisional biopsy was considered the gold standard for ensuring that adequate tissue was obtained from a musculoskeletal lesion for proper diagnosis. In conjunction with clinical and imaging characteristics, the final histologic diagnosis would then be made. However, open biopsies have a complication rate of 16%, and 8.2% of all patients who have undergone biopsy have their treatment plan affected by these complications.[8] In addition, 1.2% of patients who have had a biopsy undergo unnecessary amputations because of diagnostic errors that are based on the results of an open biopsy.[8]

Historically it was believed that needle biopsy was ineffective for the diagnosis of some lesions, specifically primary mesenchymal musculoskeletal tumors, because such tumors are among the most difficult of pathologies to accurately diagnose. As such, in a survey of practices in the early 1980s, only 9% of patients reportedly underwent needle biopsy,[11] whereas approximately 40% of patients underwent needle biopsy in the late 1990s.[12] Today, PNB is thought to be the initial procedure of choice for establishing the diagnosis of a musculoskeletal lesion.[12,13]

Well-established, consistently good results for core needle biopsy (CNB) have been reported.[14-19] Welker et al. found no significant deleterious effects on patient outcome when diagnostic errors occurred after needle biopsy.[12] Needle track seeding has not been a relevant clinical issue, since en bloc resection of the biopsy track and local field radiation is commonly practiced. The reported accuracy of a needle biopsy procedure in distinguishing benign from malignant lesions, the exact grade, and the exact pathology was 92.4%, 88.6%, and 72.7%, respectively, with a major diagnostic error rate of 1.1%, none of which ultimately had an impact on patient outcome.[12] More recently, PNB was established as a highly accurate and clinically useful technique for characterizing musculoskeletal lesions, with often higher accuracy in soft-tissue masses than with bone lesions. Certain histologies such as lymphoma and histiocytosis may require a second biopsy for final diagnosis.[19]

In addition to having good diagnostic accuracy, additional benefits of PNB include a three- to fivefold increase in cost-effectiveness over traditional open biopsy,[20-22] minimal limitation of activity after the procedure, rapid recovery time, quicker initiation of patient treatment, and assistance with operative planning.[7-9,16,23] Contrary to open biopsy, PNB does not significantly alter the strength of weight-bearing areas, thus avoiding the need for immobilization.[6,9,24]

INDICATIONS

- Establish whether a musculoskeletal lesion is benign or malignant
- Obtain material for microbiologic analysis in patients with known or suspected infection
- Stage patients with known or suspected malignancy when local spread or distant metastasis is suspected
- Determine the nature and extent of systemic diseases (e.g., connective tissue diseases)

Histopathologic studies are often needed in patients with musculoskeletal lesions to establish a definitive diagnosis of tumor, infection, or systemic process. A lytic or blastic lesion may occur in a patient without a history of cancer and may appear malignant or indeterminate; PNB in this setting is requested for clarification. More commonly, however, a lytic or blastic bone lesion or soft-tissue mass appears in a patient with a history of malignancy. PNB is needed to establish the diagnosis of metastasis for staging and initiation of radiation or adjuvant therapy. In addition, in a patient with known cancer and a lesion developing more than 10 years after the initial diagnosis, PNB is needed to distinguish whether the lesion is the same histology as the original tumor or a new neoplasm. Another common indication for PNB is a bone or soft-tissue lesion in a patient whose history, physical examination, laboratory values, and imaging point to infection. Treatment in such a case relies on determining the cause of infection, and biopsy allows identification of the organism in question. The rarest indication for PNB is a systemic disease such as a connective tissue disorder; PNB is performed to exclude other more insidious processes.

CONTRAINDICATIONS

There is no absolute contraindication to PNB, but several factors can be considered relative contraindications because they render PNB unsafe to perform:

- Known coagulopathy that cannot be corrected adequately
- Inability of the patient to cooperate or be positioned for the procedure
- Known adverse reaction to potential medication given during the procedure
- Hemodynamic instability
- Lack of a safe pathway to the lesion
- Pregnancy

Biopsy should be delayed until critical parameters are satisfied, including coagulopathy, infection, and hemodynamic instability. Technical considerations such as lack of a safe pathway to the lesion, adverse reaction to potential medications given during the procedure, and inability of the patient to cooperate or be positioned for the procedure, as well as pregnancy, have to be addressed before initiating or proceeding with PNB. Careful review of imaging and clinical correlation are critical to avoid unnecessary biopsy of a classic "do-not-touch" lesion such as traumatic avulsion of an apophysis in young patients, evolving myositis ossificans, and subchondral geodes that may appear histologically aggressive and confuse clinical management.

EQUIPMENT

Percutaneous needle biopsy may be performed under fluoroscopic,[25-27] ultrasound,[25-28] computed tomography (CT),[3,25-26] or magnetic resonance imaging (MRI) guidance.[29-31] The imaging choice is primarily dependent on the location and imaging characteristics of a lesion and, to a lesser degree, on the available imaging modalities and patient positioning.

For a superficial soft-tissue lesion or a lesion with cortical disruption that allows an acoustic window for passage of a needle, ultrasound may be used (Figs. 157-1 and 157-2). Ultrasound provides real-time visualization, minimal patient and preprocedure preparation, and no radiation exposure to the patient. Obviously, poor sound penetration or a hard surface precludes the use of ultrasound for deep medullary bone lesions. Moreover, deep soft-tissue lesions also preclude ultrasound use because poor sound penetration may lead to unknowing disruption of critical soft-tissue compartments.

For a radiographically identifiable lesion that does not require careful negotiation of neurovascular structures, fluoroscopy allows fast multidirectional real-time visualization with ease of use and less cost than CT or MRI (Fig. 157-3). However, low soft-tissue contrast makes fluoroscopy less ideal for lesions with large cystic or necrotic areas.

For a deep lesion or a lesion adjacent to neurovascular bundles, CT and MRI are ideal for creating high-resolution

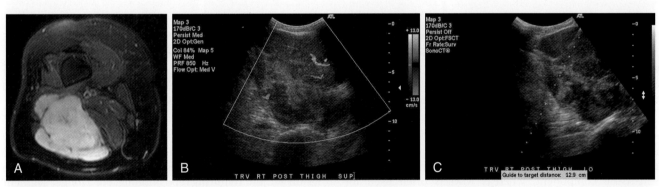

FIGURE 157-1. A, This 64-year-old woman noticed fullness and discrepancy in her thigh diameters, right being larger than left for several months. Magnetic resonance imaging axial short tau inversion recovery shows hyperintense lobular lesion. **B,** Ultrasound shows heterogeneous echogenic 10.5 × 16.7 × 10.5 cm posterior thigh mass with areas of color Doppler flow. **C,** One of four sequential biopsies with 18-gauge core biopsy needle. High-grade myxoid liposarcoma was found on pathologic examination.

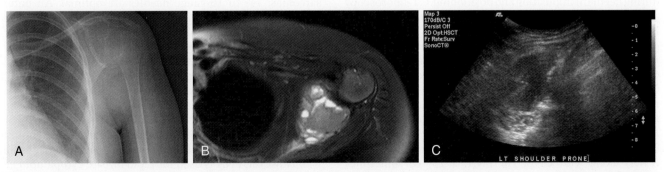

FIGURE 157-2. A, This 12-year-old girl experienced increasing left arm pain over the period of 1 year. Increasing weakness and inability to perform overhand activities with left arm appeared a few months prior to imaging. Radiograph of left shoulder demonstrates expansile radiolucent lesion in left glenoid. **B,** Magnetic resonance imaging shows numerous cystic components with fluid-fluid levels on T2-weighted image. **C,** Ultrasound-guided biopsy was performed with 18-gauge core biopsy needle. Pathologic evaluation confirmed aneurysmal bone cyst.

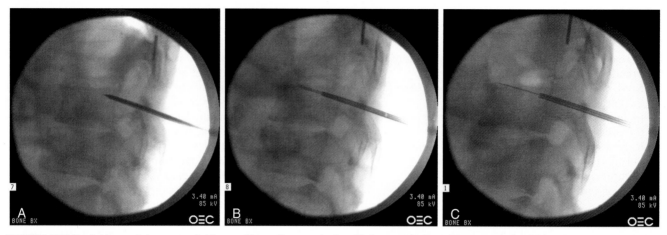

FIGURE 157-3. **A,** Metastatic lung cancer in 78-year-old man; fluoroscopically guided transpedicular L1 biopsy was performed. **B,** Intravertebral core biopsy. **C,** Fine-needle aspiration with 25-gauge needle.

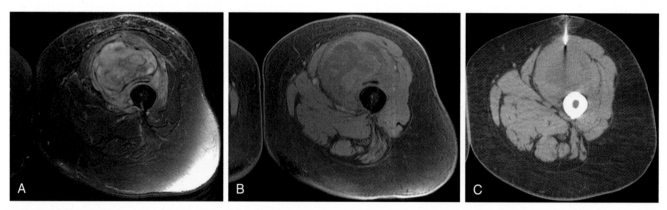

FIGURE 157-4. **A,** Large mass in anterior thigh of 61-year-old woman. T2-weighted magnetic resonance imaging shows heterogeneous signal in anterior compartment soft tissue. **B,** After administration of gadolinium contrast agent, lesion demonstrates some internal lobular enhancement. **C,** Anterior computed tomography–guided biopsy performed with 18-gauge biopsy device. Pathologic examination demonstrated high-grade malignant fibrous histiocytoma.

road maps of compartmental anatomy. In practice, CT is routinely used for lytic or blastic lesions with or without a soft-tissue component, whereas MRI is often used for lesions that are not identified on other imaging modalities and for targeting a focal marrow abnormality (Figs. 157-4 and 157-5). However, conventional CT can occasionally be a slow, arduous modality because of the lack of real-time visualization and the requirement for repeated scanning during needle manipulation and positioning. CT-fluoroscopy allows the combined convenience of real-time guidance and instantaneous cross-sectional anatomy. Although MRI guidance requires MRI-compatible (high nickel content) needles (E-Z-EM Inc., Westbury, N.Y.; Somatex, Berlin, Germany; MD Tech, Gainesville, Fla.; InVivo, Berlin, Germany), imaging with frequency encoding parallel to the needle path reduces susceptibility artifact, and specialized monitor devices and platforms are being developed for MRI-guided procedures[32,33] (Figs. 157-6 and 157-7).

Sampling should be performed by fine-needle aspiration (FNA) along with CNB. For FNA, a 25- or sometimes 22-gauge needle is typically used. For CNB, options depend on whether the lesion is composed of soft tissue or bone. For bone lesions, 11- to 15-gauge trephine needles are typically used. These needles consist of a coaxial system with

an outer trocar that remains fixed in the cortex and an inner trephine needle that makes multiple passes through the lesion without requiring repositioning. For a longer segment of bone, a drill-based trephine needle can be used.

For soft-tissue lesions, biopsy can be performed with cutting needles or core biopsy devices such as automated core biopsy guns and vacuum-assisted needles. Needle sizes range from 14 to 22 gauge, although for the diagnosis of sarcomas, 14- to 16-gauge needles are optimal. An outer introducer sheath is affixed in the lesion to minimize repeated imaging and localization, followed by the use of cutting needles and devices. The commonly used biopsy devices offer adjustable throw lengths and are lightweight, thus allowing single-handed operation.

An important consideration when choosing appropriate needle systems is the amount of tissue expected to be required for accurate pathologic diagnosis. A 25- or 22-gauge FNA needle will inevitably yield a smaller amount of specimen for diagnosis than a 14-gauge Ackerman needle will. However, FNA is used for rapid on-site cytopathologic assessment of the adequacy and diagnostic nature of specimens to guide additional sampling with CNB, because CNB samples require 2 or more days for preparation before samples can be interpreted. Given the limitations of FNA

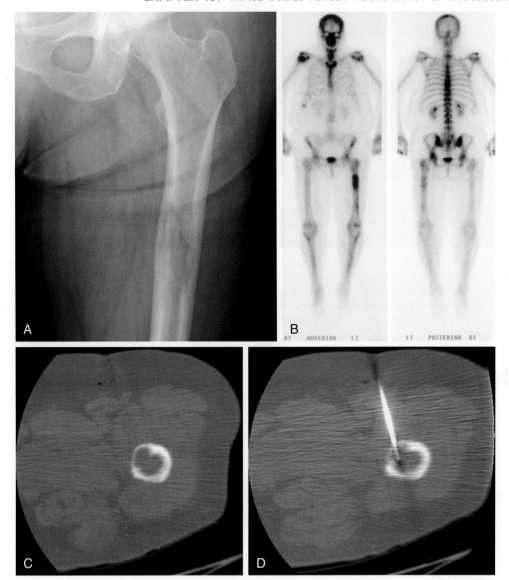

FIGURE 157-5. A, This 57-year-old woman complained of left groin and thigh pain and left leg weakness over past 3 weeks. Radiograph shows ill-defined lytic diaphyseal lesion. **B,** Bone scintigraphy shows increased metabolic activity over left proximal femoral diaphysis. **C,** Computed tomography shows endosteal erosion by lesion. **D,** Biopsy with 16-gauge needle reveals malignant lymphoma.

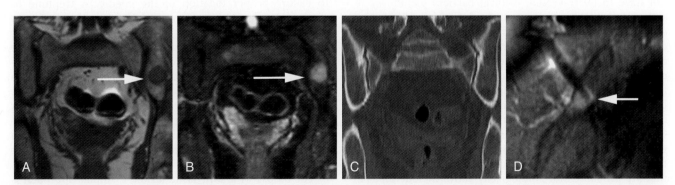

FIGURE 157-6. This 51-year-old woman with history of sarcoid and breast carcinoma was evaluated for pelvic pain. Preprocedure coronal T1-weighted **(A)** and short tau inversion recovery (STIR) **(B)** images show well-defined lesion in left ilium *(arrows)*, not demonstrated on computed tomography **(C)**. **D,** Intraprocedure axial STIR imaging with patient prone shows a susceptibility artifact represented by a 6-mm trephine needle with tip visualized in ilium lesion *(arrow)*. Biopsy revealed sarcoidosis. *(From Carrino JA, Blanco R. Magnetic resonance–guided musculoskeletal interventional radiology. Semin Musculoskelet Radiol 2006;10:159–74.)*

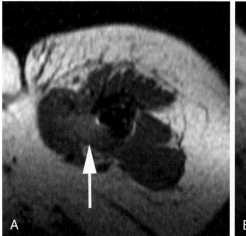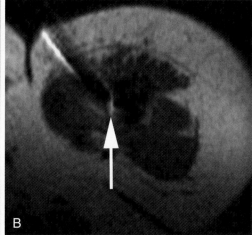

FIGURE 157-7. A, Biopsy around metal implant in 39-year-old woman after intramedullary rod placement and radiotherapy for uterine cancer metastatic to humerus. Intraprocedure contrast-enhanced T1-weighted image shows a peri-implant enhancing mass that was targeted for biopsy *(arrow).* Midfield magnetic resonance imaging reduces susceptibility artifact. Lesion was inconspicuous on computed tomography (not shown) because of metallic scatter artifact. **B,** Image taken during biopsy shows tip of coaxial introducer needle within lesion *(arrow).* Both fine-needle aspiration and core needle biopsy were diagnostic of recurrent metastatic uterine adenocarcinoma. *(From Carrino JA, Blanco R. Magnetic resonance–guided musculoskeletal interventional radiology. Semin Musculoskelet Radiol 2006;10:159–74.)*

and CNB, many interventionalists find that the two methods have complementary roles and perform both during each biopsy procedure. There are also instances in which the diagnosis will be made by one technique and not the other. Frequently, having both a cytopathologic and a histopathologic specimen increases diagnostic accuracy.[34]

TECHNIQUE

Anatomy and Approach

Knowledge of anatomic structures and relationships is fundamental for optimal performance of a percutaneous musculoskeletal biopsy. Compartmental anatomy greatly influences the needle approach, and such knowledge is critical for preventing unnecessary surgery and loss of limb function.

With regard to biopsy, the compartmental origin of the tumor must be taken into account so additional barriers do not have to be traversed. Natural barriers include bone, articular cartilage, fibrous septa, and origins and insertion of muscles. The underlying assumption is that malignant cells will seed the biopsy tract,[35-37] so any subsequent definitive surgery for control of local disease will require excision of the biopsy tract en bloc and irradiation of the field. The pathway for biopsy should avoid neurovascular bundles, pleural and peritoneal cavities, and the spinal canal. The cross-sectional anatomic imaging provided by CT or MRI is more ideal for biopsy of deep lesions. Optimally, the image-guided biopsy should be directed along the shortest path to the most biologically active area. Tissues that are probably more biologically active include areas of soft tissue ("solid") or the periphery of large cystic lesions, areas of enhancement, or positron emission tomography (PET)-avid regions[25]; for chondroid lesions it is critical to survey the lesion for atypical areas suspicious for dedifferentiation.[25,38]

Many studies have demonstrated that the best patient care is provided by a team approach that includes an orthopedic surgeon, radiologist, medical oncologist, and orthopedic pathologist, all of whom contribute to the accuracy and effectiveness of percutaneous biopsy.[4,20,22,39]

Technical Aspects

The patient is placed supine or prone depending on the location of the lesion and the trajectory route. When possible, a plane perpendicular to a flat surface of a bone is selected while avoiding neurovascular bundles, bowel, or large vessels. Using 5- or 3-mm-thick CT slices, images are taken through the lesion and localizing markers placed. Local anesthesia is given. Under sterile conditions, a small incision is made, and 0.5% to 2% lidocaine is administered subcutaneously. Conscious sedation is typically used for bone biopsy. A 22-gauge spinal needle is advanced to the bone cortex, with subsequent injection of lidocaine to permeate the periosteum. Reimaging of the lesion is performed to ensure proper location of the needle. A trephine or cutting needle is then burrowed through the cortex to create a tract through the periosteum. A coaxial outer sheath of the cannula is secured in the cortex for multiple passes. When on-site cytopathology is available, one strategy is to first acquire FNA samples for review and then proceed to CNB. Core specimens from a sclerotic bone lesion are most often placed in formalin and decalcified for later paraffin sections, whereas core specimens from a soft-tissue lesion do not require decalcification. When infection is suspected, fluid aspirates are placed in a culture tube for plating and analysis.

For biopsy of a soft-tissue lesion, a similar approach is taken to that for a bone lesion, but instead of the trephine needle, a soft-tissue biopsy gun device and an introducer sheath are used. For soft-tissue lesions, ultrasound may be used instead of CT or MRI (for superficial soft-tissue lesions).

CONTROVERSIES

When the diagnosis of malignancy, a benign tumor, or infection is established from a biopsy, a positive impact on management has been made; it is when the biopsy is "negative" or nondiagnostic that a management dilemma is created. Reports of normal, inconclusive, and nonspecific biopsy findings may arise from poor technique, missed lesions, inappropriate handling of specimens, or sampling of nonrepresentative portions of the lesion. From a pathology standpoint, a firm diagnosis can be made with a few abnormal cells for certain diagnoses such as metastatic carcinoma; however, a firm diagnosis of benignity is much harder and requires sufficient representative samples. The question often arises how to best handle "negative" biopsy results. Open biopsy and repeat percutaneous biopsy are valid choices, and the decision is often dictated by the clinical circumstances, suspicion for malignancy, and the need for treatment. Nevertheless, it should be emphasized that the effectiveness of the technique and the rate of nondiagnostic biopsy are related to the experience of the radiologists, cytopathologists, and histopathologists involved.[1,19,27]

In recent years, MRI guidance for biopsy has gained increasing recognition, and it has been used as an alternative to CT for lesions not visible on CT and other conventional modalities. However, its role vis-à-vis CT has yet to be ascertained.[29]

In the past, a soft-tissue mass was routinely subjected to biopsy under ultrasound guidance. More recently, ultrasound-guided attempts at biopsy of mixed osseous and soft-tissue lesions has been performed, with a reported accuracy of 97%.[39] Ultrasound can provide a quick alternative to conventional fluoroscopy- or CT-guided biopsy. However, for deep lesions, ultrasound should be used cautiously because there is a danger of violating critical soft-tissue compartments.

OUTCOMES

The spectrum of patients and radiologic lesions and the biopsy techniques and methods of analysis vary considerably in reported series. The reported accuracy of musculoskeletal biopsy under image guidance is in the range of 72% to 97%.[1-4,10,19,30-43] The reported accuracy of FNA has a wider range (23%-97%), with the lower accuracy attributed to benign lesions.[41] It should be noted that some 10% of aspirates produce inconclusive results, the majority (75%) being benign lesions.[2,41] Several studies have higher accuracy of CNB (89.7%-96%) to FNA (64%-88%),[14,44,45] whereas others have shown use of FNA and CNB are complementary and can increase diagnostic yield of biopsies.[41,46-48]

The diagnostic yield is higher for neoplastic than for non-neoplastic lesions. For neoplastic lesions, the accuracy for malignant neoplasms is higher than that for benign tumors in most series,[3,5,49-51] and the accuracy for metastatic disease is higher than that for primary disease.[4,5,42] However, studies have shown varied degrees of differentiation within a primary tumor volume, and even when confirmation is attempted with follow-up open biopsy, pathologic interpretation is still difficult.[1,3,52] Lesions that are particularly difficult to diagnose histologically are those with hemorrhage and fluid levels (e.g., aneurysmal bone cyst, telangiectatic osteosarcoma, giant cell tumor with an aneurysmal bone

cyst component), chondroid lesions (enchondroma and chondrosarcoma), fibrous tumors (differentiation of spindle fibrous tumor from fibrosarcoma and determination of low-grade malignant soft-tissue tumor (cellular intramuscular myxoma vs. low-grade myxoid sarcoma).[3,19,48] Some histologies that can be difficult to diagnose on initial CNB but successfully diagnosed with repeat sampling include lymphoma and histiocytosis, for which initial biopsy can be limited owing to crush artifacts.[19]

Biopsy of bone lesions with soft-tissue components (93%, 89%) has higher diagnostic accuracy than biopsy of lytic lesions (85%, 71%).[3,5] Moreover, it has been advocated that "cystic" bone lesions with areas containing substantial amounts of blood and necrotic material require biopsy of the wall for a higher yield, rather than biopsy of the fluid component.[3]

Some series have reported lower accuracy for biopsy of sclerotic lesions (69%).[5] It has been suggested that sclerotic lesions have low cellularity and often give a nondiagnostic result.[47,49,51] A recent study showed that CNB of such lesions is feasible, with a positive predictive value of 82% and a negative predictive value of 100%.[47] The less mineralized area is cited as being the less differentiated region and should be targeted for biopsy.

A series by Yang et al. reported an overall high accuracy of 89% in the interpretation of 453 of 508 needle biopsies, but a higher inaccuracy rate for malignant tumors (5%) compared with benign tumors (0%) in contrast to other studies.[19] In their series, the authors defined the nondiagnostic rate as meaning that the initial biopsy result had failed to define a clinical course for treatment. Hence, for malignant cases, the subsequent open biopsy or repeat needle biopsy was performed to establish the diagnosis, whereas for the benign cases, the initial biopsy results had led to either follow-up or an open biopsy to establish benign etiology. The malignant cohort showed higher statistical inaccuracy for certain histologies such as telangiectatic osteosarcoma and rare low-grade intraosseous osteosarcoma subtype (grade 1 fibroblastic osteosarcoma) as well as fibromyxoid sarcomas. The authors concluded that these histologic types were a potential pitfall for diagnosis by PNB and that for these particular subtypes, an open excisional biopsy could be considered for optimal management.[19] Ogilvie et al. also showed in their series that PNB has low diagnostic accuracy for myxoid histology.[48]

Infections have been reported to have a high diagnostic yield of 80% to 90% on aspiration, despite a low rate of positive culture.[5,53] In part, this may be due to antibiotic treatment before the time of biopsy, which will render culture of the biopsy sample negative despite histologic findings of inflammatory cell aggregates.

In some studies, biopsy location has been shown to be a factor in its accuracy. In a study of 359 patients, pelvic biopsy demonstrated the highest accuracy rate (81%), whereas spinal biopsy had the lowest rate (61%).[10] The difference in yield has been attributed to the difficulty in spinal access as opposed to pelvic access.[10] The series by Yang et al. demonstrated that lesions of the elbow and forearm had statistically higher nondiagnostic results compared to other locations.[19]

In other studies, diagnostic yield has been attributed to larger lesion size and larger specimen length.[54] In a series by Wu et al., CNB of 151 bone and soft-tissue lesions were evaluated prospectively and correlated to specimen and lesion size.[54] They found that diagnostic yield increased with size and specimen length, irrespective of the guidance modality used (CT vs. ultrasound), bone or soft-tissue lesions, or even needle gauge for CNB (14-18 gauge).[54] They also found cumulative diagnostic yield reached a plateau at either 3 or 4 specimens for all lesions and subtypes.[54] The only confounding variable encountered was that biopsy of lytic bone lesions had higher yield than sclerotic bone lesions (3.4 times).[54]

COMPLICATIONS

The range of reported image-guided percutaneous biopsy complications varies from 0.2% to 1.1% in the literature, but in practice it is probably less than 1%.[3,26] In contrast, in a study without image guidance, the complication rate was 15.9%.[8] Complications include pain, infection, spread of disease,[36,55,56] bone fracture, and hematoma. Site-specific complications are related to the surrounding anatomy. Pneumothorax, spinal cord damage, and vascular injury are rare events reported to be related to thoracic spine biopsy.[27,57] Local or even general anesthesia rarely produces any problem. Reportedly, prolonged paresis from an infiltrate or administration of local anesthetic close to nerves has been seen.[41,57] Mortality from a biopsy procedure is extremely low—0.02% in the largest review series of 9500 percutaneous skeletal biopsies by Murphy et al.—and is related to meningitis, which has led to death during spinal biopsy.[57]

POSTPROCEDURAL AND FOLLOW-UP CARE

Direct compression is applied for about 10 minutes to the site of the puncture, followed by a dressing covering the area around the skin puncture. Most wounds are small enough to not require sutures. Chest imaging, either radiography or CT, is obtained for thoracic spine lesions to rule out a possible pneumothorax. The patient should be observed during recovery to monitor analgesic control and check for dizziness, pain, weakness, ability to ambulate, bleeding, and general condition. The patient is released with instructions for medication and to contact the department or physician if any complications arise. Follow-up correlation of the imaging study with pathology results should be undertaken because aggressive-appearing lesions that produce a benign or low-grade histologic diagnosis may reflect a sampling error. For soft-tissue lesions, this can occur with a sarcoma when the less differentiated areas are not sampled. For chondroid bone lesions, a chondrosarcoma can be misdiagnosed as an enchondroma because of undersampling.

KEY POINTS

- Image-guided percutaneous needle biopsy has emerged as a safe, effective, and accurate tool for the diagnosis of musculoskeletal lesions. In many institutions, it has become the first test in assessing musculoskeletal lesions and has better patient tolerance, lower morbidity, and lower cost than conventional surgical biopsy.

- Indications for percutaneous biopsy vary widely, from assessment of whether a lesion is malignant or benign, to acquisition of a microbiological sample for suspected infection, evaluation of known systemic disease, and staging of a patient with a known primary. It has become a crucial part of the workup in patients with musculoskeletal lesions.

- As with any interventional procedure, image-guided percutaneous needle biopsy is not without its pearls and pitfalls. Knowledge of compartmental anatomy is crucial to success of the procedure in attaining a safe trajectory for biopsy and avoiding crucial organs and neurovascular bundles, as well as preventing violation of anatomic planes, with further spread of disease.

- Techniques of biopsy are based on the location of the lesion, its surrounding anatomy, and visibility of the lesion with each imaging modality. Selection of the proper imaging guidance system is often the key to obtaining adequate samples.

- Selection of image-guided biopsy based on diagnostic yield is important for patient outcome and expectations. Malignant lesions, metastatic lesions, and bone lesions with a large soft-tissue component have historically had higher diagnostic yield than benign lesions, primary lesions (especially for those with myxomatous or fibrous histology), and sclerotic bone lesions.

- Both core and fine-needle percutaneous biopsies are important and are complementary in increasing diagnostic yield of sampling. Repeat sampling may be warranted if there is high radiologic or clinical suspicion for a high-grade lesion or if there is suspected histology of lymphoma or histiocytosis.

- Integration of biopsy planning with an orthopedic oncologist is essential for planning the optimal approach, and collaboration with experienced musculoskeletal pathology staff is important for ensuring optimal patient care.

▶ **SUGGESTED READINGS**

Anderson MW, Temple HT, Dussault RG, Kaplan PA. Compartmental anatomy: relevance to staging and biopsy of musculoskeletal tumors. AJR Am J Roentgenol 1999;173:1663–71.

Bellaiche L, Hamze B, Parlier-Cuau, et al. Percutaneous biopsy of musculoskeletal lesions. Semin Musculoskelet Radiol 1997;1:177–87.

Bickels J, Jelinek JS, Shmookler BM, et al. Biopsy of musculoskeletal tumors: current concepts. Clin Orthop Relat Res 1999;368:212–9.

Choi JJ, Davis KW, Blankenbaker DG. Percutaneous musculoskeletal biopsy. Semin Roentgenol 2004;39:114–28.

Ghelman B. Biopsy of the musculoskeletal system. Radiol Clin North Am 1998;36:567–80.

Kattaparum SA, Rothensal DI. Percutaneous biopsy of skeletal lesions. AJR Am J Roentgenol 1991;157:935–42.

Ng CS, Gishen P. Bone biopsy. Imaging 2000;12:171–7.

Toomayan GA, Robertson F, Major NM. Lower extremity compartmental anatomy: clinical relevance to radiologists. Skeletal Radiol 2005;34:307–13.

Toomayan GA, Robertson F, Major NM, Brigman BE. Upper extremity compartmental anatomy: clinical relevance to radiologists. Skeletal Radiol 2006;35:195–201.

Weber KL. What's new in musculoskeletal oncology. J Bone Joint Surg Am 2005;87:1400–10.

Yang J, Frassica FJ, Fayad L, et al. Analysis of nondiagnostic results after image-guided needle biopsies of musculoskeletal lesion. Clin Orthop Relat Res 2010;468(11):3103–11.

Fichtinger G, Deguet A, Fischer G, et al. Image overlay for CT-guided needle insertions. Comput Aided Surg 2005;10(4):241–55.

Fritz J, U-Thainual P, Ungi T, et al. Augmented reality visualization with image overlay for MRI-guided intervention: accuracy for lumbar spinal procedures with a 1.5-T MRI system. AJR Am J Roentgenol 2012; 198(3):266–73.

Liu PT, Valadez SD, Chivers FS, et al. Anatomically based guidelines for core needle biopsy of bone tumors: implications for limb-sparing surgery. Radiographics 2007;27:189–206.

The complete reference list is available online at www.expertconsult.com.

CHAPTER 158

Ablation and Combination Treatments of Bony Lesions

Alexis D. Kelekis, Jean-Baptiste Martin, and Dimitrios Filippiadis

CLINICAL RELEVANCE

Primary or metastatic bone disease can become very painful, especially in cases of lytic lesions. Possible treatments include surgery, embolization, chemotherapy, radiotherapy, and palliative analgesics.[1]

Hypoxic cells with limited blood flow can be resistant to chemotherapy and external beam radiation therapy. These cells may be more sensitive to ablation because of increased cell sensitivity to heat in hypoxic state and decreased heat dissipation due to poor tumor perfusion.[2]

External beam radiation, although used frequently, provides pain relief in only 70% of patients treated.[3] Tumor destruction with ablation treatments, although fairly recent in its application within the musculoskeletal system, has evolved and seems effective for treatment of painful skeletal lesions. Such lesions can be treated by ablation, providing local tumor control either as a single-modality treatment or as an adjunct to surgical resection or other percutaneous techniques.[4,5]

Ablation can be curative for small lesions (up to 3-5 cm).[6] In bigger lesions, its main purpose is palliative treatment and to provide local control of the disease via a percutaneous approach. It can also help diminish local spread into muscle and can be used in conjunction with other techniques (vertebroplasty, surgery, radiotherapy), especially when the size of the lesion undermines bone stability.[6]

Ablation can be very effective for lesions spreading in soft tissues, diminishing tumor burden and mass effect on other organs.[7]

INDICATIONS

Ablation inside bone, especially when the cortex is intact, can have an oven effect and completely destroy small lesions. The most common benign lesion treated with radiofrequency ablation (RFA) is osteoid osteoma[5,8] (Fig. 158-1). Aneurysmal bone cysts can also be treated by RFA prior to filling, thus replacing the curettage technique (Fig. 158-2).

In the treatment of malignant painful lytic lesions spreading into bone and muscle, ablation can help provide local tumor control. When the lytic lesion is in a weight-bearing structure (involving > 40% of healthy bone), ablation must be accompanied by bone-supporting techniques (vertebroplasty, osteoplasty, intraosseous stent or surgery) to avoid the risk of bone collapse under the induced osteonecrosis.[6,7] Ablation can also help reduce the possible mass effect from the soft-tissue component of the lesion (Fig. 158-3).

Patients must be able to withstand the percutaneous approach as well as the ablation. When the lesion is deep in the bone structures, irritation of the periosteum is minimal and so is the pain sensation. On the contrary, when the lesion involves muscle structures or affects the periosteum, sedation is mandatory. Usually the treatment can be performed under monitored assisted conscious sedation[9,10] (Fig. 158-4).

CONTRAINDICATIONS

Absolute contraindications to ablation are the same as in any image-guided percutaneous procedure and include coagulopathy disorders, skin infection, immunosuppression, and absence of a safe path to the lesion without harming vital organs or structures.[8]

Relative contraindications depend on regional anatomy and the relationship of the lesion to the skin surface and vital structures. If the lesion is too close to the skin, adequate precautions to avoid skin burn should be observed, especially with monopolar electrodes.

As noted earlier, bone radiofrequency can be very effective when cortical bone is intact, producing an oven effect. When there is a severe lytic lesion of the cortex, electrical impulses can spread out easily, thus affecting surrounding vital structures. Especially in the spine, when the metastatic lesion is affecting the posterior wall, monopolar ablation can affect the nerves in the spinal canal.[7,11] In these cases, thermal monitoring of the epidural space can help prevent irreversible damage (Fig. 158-5). Injection of mediating solutions can help avoid damage of vital organs by either insulation or displacement of the structure one wishes to avoid.[7,11]

EQUIPMENT

There are multiple systems for RFA. Major categories include monopolar devices, bipolar devices, and coblation devices.

1. Monopolar systems require a grounding pad placed on the patient to "close" the electric circuit. Their main disadvantage is the formation of aberrant currents, which do not always allow for uniform energy deposition inside the lesion.[12] They can be divided into single electrode and multitined electrodes and are the most frequently used devices. Single electrodes have the advantage of small caliber but have smaller ablation radius. Different kinds of single monopolar devices exist to amplify treatment size. They can feature hot, cooled-tip, and water-perfused electrodes and work independently or in cluster mode. Depending on the type of electrode, the ablation shape changes. Multitined electrodes increase energy deposition by creating larger zones of coagulation and produce better lesion destruction.[2] There are three RFA systems available with expandable needle electrodes. The three

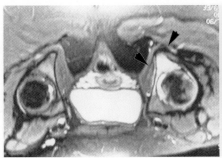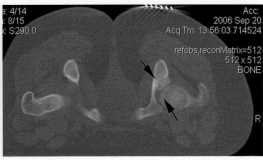

FIGURE 158-1. With patient in prone position, magnetic resonance imaging in short tau inversion recovery (STIR) sequence **(A)** shows bone edema of posterior column of right acetabulum *(arrowheads)*. **B,** Computed tomography image shows a hypodense lesion surrounded by sclerotic border. Lesion is characteristic of an osteoid osteoma.

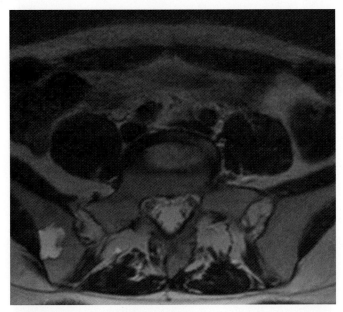

FIGURE 158-2. Aneurysmal bone cyst in right iliac wing. T2-weighted magnetic resonance imaging shows hyperintense signal of cyst, which reaches periosteum, making it a painful lesion.

systems differ in needle electrodes, generators, and the algorithms used to maximize coagulation volumes.

2. Bipolar devices do not require a grounding pad, because the current passes through the same or neighboring needles, thus diminishing the risk of aberrant currents. The distance between the electrodes can be variable depending on the type of needle used.[13,15]

3. Coblation is a controlled non–heat-driven process. It uses radiofrequency energy to excite the electrolytes in a conductive medium (e.g., saline solution), creating precisely focused plasma. The plasma's energized particles have sufficient energy to break molecular bonds within tissue, causing it to dissolve at relatively low temperatures (typically 40°C-70°C). The result is volumetric removal of target tissue.[14]

Microwave ablation (MWA) is a relatively recent ablation mode that delivers cytotoxic effects and cellular death by means of coagulation necrosis. Microwave antennae are inserted within the tumor and transmit high-frequency energy that facilitates molecular movement and frictional forces, resulting in temperature elevation and subsequent necrosis.[16] With MWA, a larger ablation zone is created within a shorter period of time. The applied energy extends approximately 2 cm around the antenna and not throughout the whole body as in RFA. The ablation zone is not governed by the heat sink effect produced by nearby vessels, and in contrast to RFA, no grounding pads are necessary. All the aforementioned factors make MWA the treatment of choice for large tumors in close proximity to a vessel.[17] Technical parameters of the ablation session are determined by the manufacturer of the antenna. In most protocols, 5 to 10 minutes of ablation is performed at 40 to 60 watts. When choosing appropriate therapeutic protocol, one must balance killing all malignant cells against minimizing surrounding tissue damage. A safety margin of 5 to 10 mm is mandatory for MWA. In selected cases, multiple antennae can be applied simultaneously, depositing energy in a synergistic fashion, which will result in even larger ablation zones.

Cryoablation is the application of extreme cold to destroy tumor cells by means of both direct cellular and vascular injury. In contrast to other ablation types, up to 25 probes can be used within the same lesion (depending on lesion size). In cases of multiple placements, probes should be more or less parallel and about 2 cm apart.[18] During the cryoablation session, two 10-minute cycles of freezing and one 8-minute intervening cycle of thawing are performed per position. As in all cases of ablation, a safety margin of roughly 5 mm is necessary to ensure complete tumor ablation. The size and shape of the iceball is governed by the expansion space at the tip of the probe. In cases where tumor location makes some kind of insulation necessary, fluid must be avoided (air via antimicrobial filter or CO_2 are more appropriate insulation agents). When the size of the lesion undermines bone stability and a combination of cryoablation and cement augmentation is necessary, one should wait until the tumor temperature rises back to normal levels to avoid cement leakages. In comparison to RFA, cryoablation seems to be less painful. Another advantage is the visibility of the iceball under computed tomography (CT) imaging during freezing, which allows visualizing the ablation margins.[18,19] The major factors governing a successful cryoablation session include rapid freezing to lethal temperature (around −40°C), slow thawing, and repetition of the same process. As in any image-guided percutaneous procedure, excellent monitoring is a requisite.

High-intensity focused ultrasound (HIFU) is application of locally concentrated acoustic waves (focused by an acoustic lens) that results in focal energy deposition. Tissue

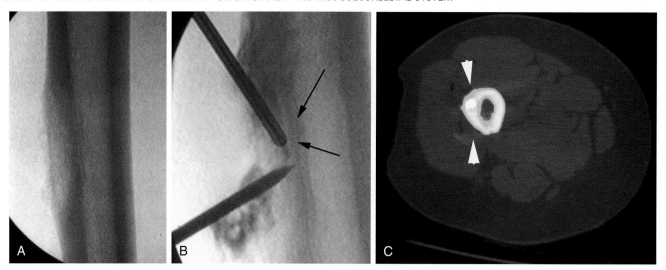

FIGURE 158-3. A, Painful lytic metastatic lesion from pulmonary cancer. **B,** Needle placement under fluoroscopy. Coblation radiofrequency ablation is seen inside puncture needle *(black arrows)*. **C,** Computed tomography scan post cement injection inside lytic lesion.

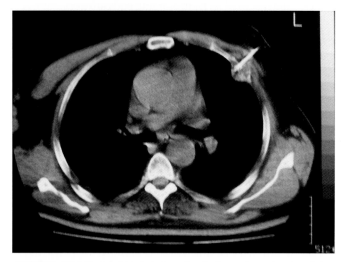

FIGURE 158-4. Painful lytic lesion of a rib from primary hepatocellular carcinoma, treated with monopolar radiofrequency ablation.

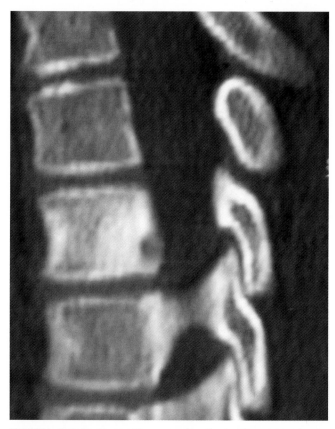

FIGURE 158-5. Computed tomography of osteoid osteoma of spine on posterior wall, making it a highly dangerous lesion to treat by radiofrequency.

absorption of this energy deposition results within seconds in frictional heating, causing focal temperature increase (sonication).[20] Since a single sonication's size is similar to a rice grain, multiple sonications arranged in such a way as to cover the whole tumor volume are necessary for ablation of a lesion. Bone readily absorbs this kind of acoustic energy, so in osseous lesions, application of lower energy levels results in higher temperature elevation. Since osseous lesions cause pain by means of their periosteal innervation, the heating of bone at temperatures above 60°C will effectively destroy the innervation of the periosteum, resulting in pain reduction. The typical sonication energy for osseous lesions is 1000 to 1500 joules, using a wide-beam approach and requiring shorter session duration (≈60 minutes). Treatment monitoring is performed by real-time ultrasound or magnetic resonance imaging (MRI). Because ultrasound cannot penetrate bone, intraosseous lesions are treated under MRI.[20-22] MRI-guided HIFU offers increased image quality with additional direct imaging of temperature changes (by means of thermal-sensitive sequences). The

technique totally lacks any invasive character (no needles are inserted inside the patient), but anesthesiologic control is required (ranging from conscious sedation to general anesthesia, with the decision varying among different centers). Owing to concerns for heat conduction through the bone to the spinal cord, HIFU is still not applied on vertebral bodies (an exception might include application of the technique on lesions of the spinous process). Similarly, care must be exercised when the target lesion is close to sensitive anatomic structures (e.g., blood vessels, nerves).

Since any kind of ablation apart from tumor necrosis results in bone weakening as well, combined therapies (ablation and cement augmentation) are necessary to achieve necrosis and at the same time support the bone to avoid postablation pathologic fractures (especially in the spine and other weight-bearing areas). To further enhance local tumor control, ablation can be combined with transarterial chemoembolization (especially for hypervascular lesions).[23]

Vertebral body support (VBS) is a recently developed percutaneous technique that in many ways resembles kyphoplasty. A significant difference is that in VBS, prior to cement injection, an endovertebral prosthesis (composed of polyetheretherketone [PEEK] polymer, nitinol, or titanium) is implanted inside the vertebral body, aiming at long-lasting height restoration. VBS technique includes the use of trocars through which the implant is inserted inside the vertebral body. Similar to bone augmentation, liquid polymer (polymethylmethacrylate [PMMA]) is then injected, creating a complex of implant and cement. The additional step in VBS is deployment of the implant to augment structural support.

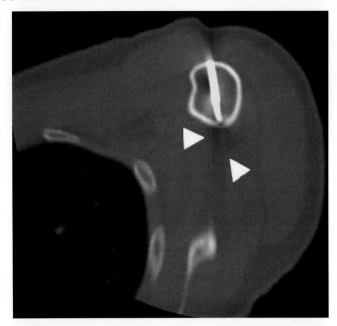

FIGURE 158-6. Puncture of an osteoid osteoma through normal bone, very proximal to neurovascular bundle *(white arrowheads)*.

TECHNIQUE

Anatomy and Approaches

The appropriate site for ablation should be evaluated for its proximity to neurovascular bundles, according to the anatomy of the location. If a neurovascular bundle is close or engulfed in the lesion, informed consent for possible neural deficit should be obtained.

In general, the approach should include a decent amount of subcutaneous fat (to avoid skin burns) and be as vertical as possible to the bone (to avoid skidding on the cortex). Puncture of the bone can be achieved with different tools to perform mechanical tapping, manual drilling, and electric drilling, depending on cortical thickness and distance of the lesion from the bone surface. An external trocar should be used to provide access, in which the radiofrequency probe is placed. The active tip of the probe should not be in contact with the needle and always extend forward, avoiding electrical discharge to the skin through the needle shaft.

If the lesion is too close to the skin and monopolar electrodes or microwave antennas are used, cooling down the skin might be necessary. The same applies for cryoablation, where warming of the skin is achieved with hot saline placed inside a sterile glove. One should choose the trajectory that achieves the shorter crossing of normal cortical bone. In some cases, however, crossing normal bone to reach the lesion cannot be avoided (Fig. 158-6).

If the location is intraarticular, a direct approach can be carried out provided the puncture needle is not bigger than 18 to 20 gauge. In such cases, the risk of cartilage or articular damage should be considered.

If the lesion will be excised, the approach should be discussed with the surgeon to include the tract in the operating field.

In cases of combined therapies (ablation and cement augmentation) at the same session, it is necessary to allow enough time between the two techniques for tumor temperature to decrease/increase (thermal/cryoablation, respectively) back to normal to avoid untimely cement polymerization due to the temperature. Whenever transarterial chemoembolization (TACE) or any other type of embolization is combined with the aforementioned techniques, it is better to perform the intravascular technique first and the ablation the morning after, with/without cement augmentation.

Technical Aspects

- Find the patient a comfortable position on the table.
- Inform the patient about the steps during the procedure.
- Obtain a direct trajectory to the lesion, trying not to cross neurovascular bundles.
- Minimize the crossing of normal bone.
- Discuss with the surgeon, if excision is to follow.
- Use ample local anesthetic and/or monitored sedation.
- Consider general anesthesia for prolonged procedures.
- Use sterile conditions.

CONTROVERSIES

RFA/MWA for bone is a new technique yet to be established. It is doubtful whether it can provide pain relief and secure bone strength, because the destruction and debulking of the mass can cause bone collapse. It is an adjunct tool to other bone-solidifying techniques (e.g., bone augmentation) in the effort to debulk tumor, especially when the lesion has extended into the soft tissues.[11]

The use of bone RFA has found its application mainly in osteoid osteomas, where it is considered reference treatment.[9] There are still authors, however, who consider conservative treatment[15] as primary treatment, arguing that these lesions might spontaneously regress.

It is still a fact that bone RFA/MWA has not found a primary independent role but still is an adjunct technique to our interventional armamentarium. Ablating the periphery of the lesion, such as the periosteum and soft-tissue ingredient of the tumor, should be part of the strategy when applying bone ablation techniques.[23,24]

Advantages of cryoablation include direct visualization of the ablation area (iceball in CT is seen as a hypodense ball with predictable geometry) and the fact that it is less painful than RFA, thus requiring lower levels of analgesia. Furthermore, with cryoablation, curative therapies of larger tumor volumes are achievable. However, in cases where large tumor volumes are ablated, precautions to preserve renal function (e.g., patient hydration), which might be endangered by the large amount of necrotic tumor tissue released into the systemic circulation. Disadvantages include the technique's duration, which is much longer (owing to cycle repetition); size of probes, which are bigger than RFA/MWA; the fact that gas tanks (with helium and argon) are necessary in the department; and the overall cost, which is higher.

An advantage of MWA is the fast and repeatable ablation zone, as well as the high-energy deposition, which is easily achievable on soft tissue. However, high and quick energy deposition can result in a disadvantage, since the exact form of the ablating zone cannot be visualized and in some cases even predicted. The energy deposition should be well monitored, especially where sensitive neural and vascular structures are adjacent.[23]

Advantages of HIFU include the fact that it does not require image-guided interventional skills and can be performed as an outpatient procedure. However, application of HIFU for curative therapies is still not possible. Advancements in technology are targeting high-density electronically steerable transducers with automatic tracking, water-permeable membranes for acoustic coupling, and built-in skin cooling systems. Possible use of ultrasound cavitation inside bone might help produce faster and bigger ablation zones.

Combined therapies (ablation, cement augmentation,[25] and embolization) result in significant pain reduction and mobility improvement, prevention of postablation pathologic fractures, and better local tumor control. However, more studies are necessary to evaluate the safety and efficacy of such combinations.

VBS with percutaneous implants is an alternative to vertebral augmentation, aiming at better mechanical properties. Inclusion of oncologic cases in the technique's indications remains controversial, compared to simple bone augmentation.

OUTCOMES

The purpose of RFA/MWA is to debulk tumor, especially in cases where it extends into soft tissue. It should be followed by solidifying techniques such as bone augmentation. Pain relief should occur 24 hours post ablation. Puncture sites might be painful for 5 to 7 days, but the pain should be superficial, heightened under local pressure. Deep throbbing pain should disappear by the next day. Analgesics should be administered to control local pain.

Cryoablation in cases of musculoskeletal lesions provides about 75% pain reduction (more or less the same success rate as thermal ablation). Initial reports of HIFU in cases of musculoskeletal lesions are that it provides about 85% pain reduction.

COMPLICATIONS

Complications can be due to the systematic primary disease, the anesthesia, or the procedure. Those involving the procedure include infection, needle placement, and current effect.

Infection of the skin or bone can be an issue requiring long-term antibiotic treatment, underscoring the necessity for strict aseptic conditions. Preoperative antibiotics are not mandatory but highly suggested by most interventional guidelines.[16] Preoperative antibiotic treatment should be adapted to hospital germ resistance.

Placement of the needle should be done under strict imaging conditions to avoid potential vital organs in the needle's path. Other structures to be avoided are nerves, vessels, and articulations. Puncture of these structures might cause nerve or vascular shearing, hydrarthrosis or hemarthrosis, and cartilage damage.

The RFA procedure can create aberrant currents, thus affecting neighboring structures. Specifically, neurovascular bundles are very sensitive to RFA energy deposition; permanent neurologic damage or vascular thrombosis are associated risks. Thermal damage can also affect normal bone, creating osteonecrosis in the periphery of the lesion; muscle, creating muscle atrophy and scaring; or skin burn, especially when the lesion is superficial.

Cryoshock phenomenon and iceball cracking resulting in hemorrhage have been described in 1% to 3.8% of liver and kidney cryoablation sessions. These are rarely encountered postablation syndromes, never described in bone treatments. As in the case of thermal ablation, temporary neuropraxia or permanent neural damage depend upon temperature and time.

POSTPROCEDURAL AND FOLLOW-UP CARE

Patients can be discharged on the same day, but usually 24 hours' supervision is advisable. Evaluation of the result should be performed 7 to 10 days post treatment and should include pain thresholds and entry site healing. Long-term follow up should include MRI and CT evaluation in 1, 3, and 6 months.

KEY POINTS

- Radiofrequency ablation is indicated for painful masses inside bone or soft tissue.
- Lesion size and the relationship of the lesion to neurovascular bundles are important considerations.
- Use of both the appropriate imaging modality to target the lesion and appropriate ablative technology to treat it are essential components of therapy.
- A temperature of 50°C to 100°C (or −20°C to −40°C for cryoablation) should be achieved and maintained throughout the entire target volume.

- In cases of weight-bearing locations, ablation should be accompanied with structural support (osteoplasty), in order to avoid the risk of bone collapse.
- Radiofrequency ablation can be combined with other therapeutic techniques such as vertebroplasty, kyphoplasty, and radiotherapy.
- Posttreatment neurologic and pain outcomes should be evaluated.

▸ SUGGESTED READINGS

Alda T, Kamran A. Palliative interventions for pain in cancer patients. Semin Intervent Radiol 2007;24(4):419–29.

Callstrom MR, York JD, Gaba RC, et al. Research reporting standards for image-guided ablation of bone and soft tissue tumors. J Vasc Interv Radiol 2009;20(12);1527–40.

Gangi A, Basile A, Buy X, et al. Radiofrequency and laser ablation of spinal lesions. Semin Ultrasound CT MR 2005;26:89–9.

Gangi A, Tsoumakidou G, Buy X, Quoix E. Quality improvement guidelines on bone tumor management. Cardiovasc Interv Radiol 2010; 33(4):706–13.

Goldberg SN, Gazelle GS, Mueller PR. Thermal ablation therapy for focal malignancy: a unified approach to underlying principles, techniques and diagnostic imaging guidance. AJR Am J Roentgenol 2000;174: 323–31.

Kelekis AD, Somon T, Yilmaz H, et al. Interventional spine procedures. Eur J Radiol 2005;55(3):362–83.

Sabharwal T, Salter R, Adam A, Gangi A. Image-guided therapies in orthopedic oncology. Orthop Clin North Am 2006;37:105–12.

The complete reference list is available online at www.expertconsult.com.

CHAPTER 159

Vertebroplasty and Kyphoplasty

David A. Pastel, Albert J. Yoo, Clifford J. Eskey, and Joshua A. Hirsch

Osteoporosis is a prevalent disease that affects 200 million people worldwide.[1] Fractures from osteoporosis have an incidence of roughly 150 per 100,000 in women (half this rate in men) and result in substantial pain, morbidity, and healthcare utilization.[2] In the United States alone, approximately 700,000 osteoporotic vertebral compression fractures occur each year.[3] Vertebroplasty and kyphoplasty are minimally invasive image-guided procedures that involve injection of bone cement into a fractured vertebral body, with the primary goal of pain relief and secondary goals of vertebral body stabilization and restoration of height. The primary difference is that with kyphoplasty, a cavity is created with a mechanical device before cement delivery.

Before the introduction of percutaneous vertebral augmentation, treatment of compression fractures consisted variably of bed rest, pain control (with nonsteroidal antiinflammatory drugs [NSAIDs], calcitonin, narcotics), and back bracing.[4] Percutaneous treatment of vertebral compression fractures was first performed in France in 1984 by Galibert and Daimond.[5] Vertebroplasty was first introduced in the United States in the early 1990s and rapidly gained widespread use based on observational data. In 2002, approximately 54,000 patients with vertebral compression fractures were treated with vertebroplasty or kyphoplasty. This number rose to 130,000 in 2007. Since that time, several landmark randomized prospective studies have been published. Two high-profile studies published in the *New England Journal of Medicine* in August 2009 that compared vertebroplasty to sham vertebroplasty for treating osteoporotic compression fractures found no statistically significant difference between the two groups.[6,7] These studies have been criticized for potential inclusion of patients with chronic fractures, absence of a control group without intervention, difficulty in recruitment, and inconsistent use of physical exam and bone marrow edema on magnetic resonance imaging (MRI) as inclusion criteria. These trials contrast with a more recent nonblinded randomized controlled trial where patients who underwent vertebroplasty for treatment of acute vertebral compression fractures experienced superior pain relief compared to a control group that was conservatively managed up to 1 year.[8] Another randomized controlled study comparing kyphoplasty to conservative management yielded similar results at 1 year.[9] The shortcomings of these trials underscore the difficulty in conducting adequately powered clinical trials. Despite the landmark work done to date, controversy still surrounds even the basic efficacy of vertebral augmentation procedures.

INDICATIONS

The primary indication for vertebroplasty and kyphoplasty is a painful unhealed compression fracture that has failed conventional medical therapy. This failure may represent inadequate pain relief from narcotic analgesia, undesirable side effects from narcotic analgesia, or hospitalization for pain. In the United States, the vast majority of fractures evaluated for treatment are related to primary osteoporosis. Other treatable fractures include those secondary to steroid-induced osteoporosis (e.g., transplant recipients, patients with chronic obstructive pulmonary disease or autoimmune disease),[10] metastatic disease, hematopoietic neoplasm (leukemia, multiple myeloma), or rarely trauma.[11] Vertebrae may also be treated if there is no fracture but a painful neoplasm or vascular tumor such as hemangioma. At this time, there is little justification for prophylactic treatment of unfractured vertebral levels because of the difficulty predicting which levels, if any, will sustain a fracture in the future.[12]

Pathologic fractures constitute an important subgroup of treatable fractures because of additional disease-specific issues that have to be addressed both before and during the procedure. One such issue includes the timing of vertebral augmentation in relation to tumoricidal treatment. Some practitioners advocate performing vertebral augmentation after radiation therapy to prevent the theoretic risk of tumor dissemination during pressurized cement injection.[10] However, others claim the procedure may be performed at any time—before, during, or after chemotherapy or radiation therapy.[13]

CONTRAINDICATIONS

The few absolute contraindications to vertebroplasty and kyphoplasty include current systemic or spinal infection, uncorrectable bleeding diathesis, insufficient cardiopulmonary health to tolerate sedation or general anesthesia, and myelopathy or radiculopathy secondary to fracture-related compromise of the spinal canal or neural foramina. In the case of infection, the patient must complete an adequate course of antibiotics and must be afebrile with resolution of leukocytosis before the procedure is performed. With regard to fracture-related neurologic dysfunction, some practitioners consider radiculopathy a relative contraindication.[10] The American College of Radiology practice guideline also lists allergy to cement or opacification agents as an absolute contraindication.

Relative contraindications substantially increase the risk or technical difficulty of the procedure. Patients with the following fracture features should be treated only by the most experienced practitioners:

- *Disruption of the posterior cortex* increases the risk for posterior cement leakage and therefore the risk for spinal cord or nerve root compression. Though rare in osteoporotic compression fractures, this feature is frequently seen in burst fractures and neoplasms. The integrity of the posterior cortex is best evaluated with computed tomography (CT).

• *Epidural extension of tumor* in the setting of pathologic fractures allows egress of cement into the spinal canal, because cement commonly fills the intraspinal soft-tissue mass.[14] Shimony et al. have demonstrated that vertebroplasty can be safely performed in this setting, even when epidural tumor is seen to contact the spinal cord or nerve roots.[15]

• *Substantial canal narrowing* (without neurologic dysfunction) increases the risk that even a small amount of cement leakage will produce neurologic compromise. However, even in the setting of spinal cord deformity and cord signal abnormality on preprocedural MRI, the procedure can be performed with a high rate of pain relief and without adverse neurologic sequelae.[16]

• *Marked loss of vertebral body height* (>70% loss of height) makes the procedure more difficult because there may be little space for placement of a cannula.

• *Poor visualization of osseous structures on fluoroscopy* increases the risk of improper needle placement and cement leakage but can be overcome with the use of CT.

PREPROCEDURAL WORKUP

Workup of patients for vertebral augmentation should (1) identify patients who will probably benefit from the procedure and (2) screen for the aforementioned contraindications. The decision to proceed with treatment must be based on a good history, physical examination, appropriate laboratory evaluation, and imaging.

History

• Vertebral compression fractures may occur with little or no trauma.

• Classic symptoms from an acute vertebral compression fracture include deep pain with sudden onset, midline location, and exacerbation by motion (especially flexion) and standing. Lateral radiation in a dermatomal pattern may be present.

• It is important to document failure of conventional medical therapy, which includes pain that is not adequately controlled by bed rest and analgesics, and intolerance to analgesics (e.g., adverse reaction, constipation). The trial of conservative therapy should not exceed 4 to 6 weeks, because pain from compression fractures usually resolves within this time.[12] There has been a growing trend toward earlier treatment with vertebral augmentation (within days), especially for patients who require hospitalization and parenteral narcotics.[10,12] However, vertebroplasty may be effective in an unhealed fracture even after more than 1 year has elapsed since the onset of pain.

• It is important to determine whether the patient is taking anticoagulant medication. Appropriate steps must be taken to ensure adequate coagulation at the time of the procedure.

Physical Examination

• The classic physical finding is point tenderness at the spinous process of the fractured vertebra, which may be the best predictor of clinical response.[10] Localization to a specific level, if possible, is important in targeting treatment in patients who have multiple compression fractures, some of which may be healed and do not require treatment. In difficult cases, examination can be performed with fluoroscopic assistance to localize the pain to a specific anatomic level.

• The absence of typical focal tenderness does not preclude the presence of unhealed fractures, and in one study did not result in difference in treatment outcome.[17] Atypical manifestations may be seen in Kümmell disease (see later), including radicular pain and pain remote from the fracture.[12]

• Assessment of lower extremity neurologic function is especially important in patients with symptoms suggestive of myelopathy, radiculopathy, or spinal stenosis.

Laboratory Evaluation

• Preprocedural laboratory screening for infection, coagulopathy, and metabolic abnormality is important. Every patient must have a complete blood cell count, routine coagulation study, and basic metabolic panel performed.

• Additional tests such as urinalysis, electrocardiography, chest radiography, or any combination of these tests are left to the discretion of the practitioner and local practice patterns.

Imaging

• Imaging of the spine is undertaken in all cases to confirm the clinical diagnosis, aid in identification of the acute painful fracture, identify potential difficulties, and plan the procedure.

• Radiographs can serve as the initial imaging evaluation; when recent previous radiographs are available for comparison, new compression fractures can be identified. In addition, identification of an *intraosseous vacuum phenomenon* (Kümmell disease) at a particular level points to that level as the probable source of pain and predicts a good response with regard to pain relief and restoration of height.[18]

• MRI is the test of choice for further evaluation and should be performed in all patients if not contraindicated. The single most useful sequence is a short tau inversion recovery (STIR) or T2-weighted sequence with fat saturation, on which unhealed fractures show hyperintense signal consistent with edema within the bone marrow (Fig. 159-1, *A*). In the case of retropulsion of fracture fragments, MRI is important in assessing the degree of spinal canal compromise and compression of the spinal cord or nerve roots. With regard to pathologic fractures, MRI is helpful in suggesting the diagnosis, which can be confirmed with intraprocedural bone biopsy, and allows evaluation of epidural extension of tumor.

• In patients who cannot undergo MRI (e.g., those with a pacemaker), bone scintigraphy is the test of choice. It allows differentiation of healed and unhealed fractures; unhealed fractures will take up the injected technetium-99m methylene diphosphonate tracer in much higher concentration. Bone scintigraphy highly predicts positive clinical response to vertebral augmentation.[19] The major

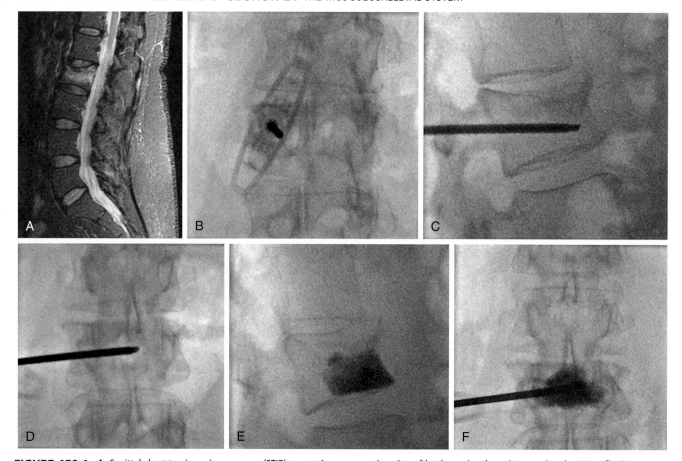

FIGURE 159-1. A, Sagittal short tau inversion recovery (STIR) magnetic resonance imaging of lumbar spine; hyperintense signal at L2, reflecting marrow edema, is consistent with an unhealed fracture. **B,** Needle placement with an "end-on" approach. Note parapedicular position of needle at lateral aspect of pedicle. **C,** Needle is advanced to anterior one third to one quarter of vertebral body. **D,** From parapedicular approach, needle tip achieves a midline position on anteroposterior view. **E,** Cement is injected until it reaches posterior one third to one quarter. **F,** Cement is deposited across midline.

disadvantage is poor spatial resolution, resulting in imprecise localization of the fracture, although single-photon emission computed tomography (SPECT) can be helpful in this regard. Bone scintigraphy with or without SPECT is limited in that it does not evaluate the spinal canal and its contents.

• CT is useful for preprocedural evaluation of the integrity of the posterior vertebral body cortex. This question is important in the setting of burst fracture or metastasis, where a fracture through the posterior cortex increases the risk of posterior leakage of cement or posterior displacement of bone or tumor during the procedure.[20]

TECHNIQUE

Anatomy

There are 7 cervical, 12 thoracic, and 5 lumbar vertebrae. Compression fractures most commonly occur in the lower thoracic and upper lumbar segments but may occur in any vertebra. The number of a particular vertebra (e.g., L5) is defined by counting down from the craniocervical junction. In practice, this information is not usually available, and it is common to count upward from the sacrum, a less

accurate method. However, in assigning the level of injury, the absolute number of a vertebra (e.g., L5) is less important than a careful match between the preprocedure imaging studies and the imaging used to guide the procedure.

Each vertebra consists of a vertebral body and a posterior vertebral arch. Of particular importance are the paired pedicles that form the bridge between the vertebral body and posterior arch and lie at the lateral aspect of the spinal canal. They also form the roof of the neural foramina. Orientation of the pedicles with respect to the vertebral body changes as one moves along the spinal axis. In general, the pedicles in the lumbar spine have a long axis parallel to the sagittal plane, whereas those of the thoracic spine angle anteromedially.

The marrow space of the cancellous bone communicates with a network of venous channels. Some of these channels coalesce to form the basivertebral plexus posteriorly in the midline, and others traverse small perforations in the cortex about the remainder of the vertebral body margin. These veins communicate with venous plexuses within the epidural space, neural foramina, and paraspinal tissue,[21] which in turn primarily drain into the lumbar and azygos veins. These venous channels are important because they represent possible pathways for extraosseous passage of polymethyl methacrylate (PMMA).

Technical Aspects

Sedation

Analgesia is necessary for vertebroplasty and kyphoplasty. In the majority of cases, it is achieved with a combination of local analgesics (e.g., lidocaine with bicarbonate, bupivacaine) and moderate sedation (intravenous midazolam and fentanyl). In some cases, general endotracheal anesthesia is required to provide adequate comfort and safety, but having the patient awake is desirable. A conscious patient can give feedback (e.g., increasing pain, neurologic dysfunction) that can alert the operator to potential complications, and neurologic examination during the procedure is possible. Kyphoplasty is performed with general anesthesia at most institutions but can be successfully undertaken with moderate sedation.[22,23] In all cases, continuous monitoring is performed with a minimum of electrocardiography, blood pressure measurement, and pulse oximetry. Drug delivery and monitoring are performed by anesthesiologists, nurse anesthetists, or certified nursing personnel. In patients with substantial preexisting respiratory or cardiac disease, an anesthesiologist can be asked to evaluate the patient and determine whether monitored anesthesia care is warranted. The patient should not eat or drink for at least 4 to 6 hours before the procedure.

Patient Positioning

Prone or oblique prone is the ideal patient position for thoracic and lumbar procedures. In addition to the clear advantage of easy access, with proper cushion support, this position maximizes extension of the fractured segments, thereby promoting reduction of kyphosis.[24] The patient's arms should be placed sufficiently toward the head to keep them out of the path of the fluoroscope. Analgesia should be considered before placement on the table, because this part of the procedure may be the most painful. Particular care must be taken when transferring aged or osteoporotic patients to avoid the potential development of new rib or vertebral fractures.

Antibiotic Prophylaxis and Skin Preparation

Infection risk is minimized with use of standard operating room guidelines for sterile preparation of the skin, draping, operator scrubbing, and use of sterile gowns, masks, and gloves. Antibiotic prophylaxis for these procedures comes in one of two forms. An intravenous antibiotic such as cefazolin (1 g) or clindamycin (600 mg in a patient allergic to penicillin) may be administered during the procedure. Alternatively, the PMMA may be mixed with an antibiotic (e.g., tobramycin 1.2 g) as the cement is being prepared, but many experienced practitioners have abandoned this once popular practice. There are few data to support or oppose antibiotic administration, but spine infections have been reported after these procedures[12,25] (see Complications section), and the presence of PMMA makes them difficult to treat successfully.

Needle Placement

The most important aspect of needle placement is to keep the needle trajectory lateral to the medial cortex and superior to the inferior cortex of the pedicle. This prevents entry of the needle into the spinal canal or neural foramen. The needle may be placed via a transpedicular or parapedicular approach. The *transpedicular approach* takes the needle from the posterior surface of the pedicle, through the length of the pedicle, and into the vertebral body. The long intraosseous path protects the postganglionic nerve roots and other soft tissues. However, the pedicle configuration can limit one's ability to achieve a final needle tip position near the midline. The *parapedicular approach* takes the needle along the lateral surface of the pedicle, and the vertebral body is penetrated at its junction with the pedicle. This approach permits more medial tip placement.

For either approach, there are two potential image guidance strategies: an end-on ("down the barrel") view and an anteroposterior view. The more straightforward approach uses the end-on view and is described here. This strategy involves an ipsilateral oblique view to place the fluoroscopy beam and needle tract perfectly parallel to each other:

- The image intensifier is first rotated to a true anteroposterior position, with the spinous process aligned midway between the pedicles.
- The craniocaudad angulation is changed to bring the pedicles to the midportion of the vertebral body. The image intensifier is then rotated approximately 20 degrees ipsilateral to the target pedicle so that the medial cortex of the pedicle is at the middle third of the vertebral body (Fig. 159-1, *B*). The vertebra adopts the "Scottie dog" configuration. This rotation can be continued only as long as the medial cortex of the pedicle remains clearly visible. The pedicle will have a round or ovoid shape. The pedicle should be centered in the field of view to avoid inaccuracies from parallax.
- The needle is placed so that it is "end on" to the image intensifier and appears as a dot. For the transpedicular approach, it is centered within the circle formed by the cortex of the pedicle. For the parapedicular approach, it is lateral to the lateral cortex of the pedicle (see Fig. 159-1, *B*).
- The skin and periosteum are anesthetized with subcutaneous lidocaine or bupivacaine via a 22-gauge needle along the planned trajectory. This smaller-gauge needle also provides an opportunity to assess and adjust the planned trajectory.
- A small nick is made in the skin, and an 11- or 13-gauge diamond-tipped needle stylet (sheathed in a cannula) is placed.
- Once the needle has been advanced to the bone surface, small corrections in the craniocaudad angulation can be made from a true lateral view (care is taken to angle the image intensifier so a true lateral view is obtained [Fig. 159-1, *C*]). For the parapedicular approach, the position at which bone is encountered (i.e., junction of pedicle and vertebral body) is more anterior on the lateral view.
- Once in the bone, the needle is advanced either with a drilling motion and controlled forward pressure or by carefully tapping the needle handle with an orthopedic hammer.
- The needle is then advanced through the pedicle while keeping the end-on appearance of the needle on the ipsilateral oblique view. The needle must be lateral to the medial cortex of the pedicle until it has traversed the entire pedicle on the lateral view.

• Once the needle has traversed the pedicle, the diamond-tipped needle may be replaced with a bevel-tipped needle for better maneuverability. The needle is advanced further using the lateral view to the anterior one third to one quarter of the vertebral body (see Fig. 159-1, *C*). For kyphoplasty, the cannula is pulled back to the posterior aspect of the vertebral body to allow insertion of the balloon tamp.

Additional Steps for Kyphoplasty

For vertebroplasty, PMMA is delivered through the cannula after needle placement, but kyphoplasty involves the additional steps of balloon insertion and inflation to create a cavity within the bone. After the needle stylet is removed, the balloon tamp is inserted through the cannula and slowly inflated with iodinated contrast material. The balloon is attached to a locking syringe with a digital manometer, and inflation is monitored with both the pressure transducer and intermittent fluoroscopy. Inflation continues until one of two conditions is met: the system reaches maximum pressure or maximum balloon volume, or the kyphotic deformity is corrected. This is typically done in a bipedicular fashion. The balloon is then deflated and removed.

Cement Placement

When ready for injection, cement consistency is similar to toothpaste. Wong and Mathis recommend a drip test in which the cement should ball up at the end of the needle and not drip downward, thus resulting in cement that is slightly more viscous than toothpaste.[26] Working time varies from 10 to 20 minutes, depending on temperature and the specific PMMA formulation being used. A variety of delivery systems are available for the cement, varying from a few 1-mL syringes with a spatula and mixing bowl to self-contained delivery devices (Fig. 159-1, *E*). A screw syringe injector with long flexible delivery tubing has the advantage of minimizing radiation exposure to the operator.[27]

Vertebroplasty

• The delivery system is connected to the cannula, and the cement is injected slowly.
• Careful fluoroscopic monitoring in the lateral plane is performed to ensure that the cement remains within the vertebra. Posterior or posterolateral leakage could result in irritation or damage to the spinal cord or nerve roots and should be avoided. Midline pain and pain related to the fracture are acceptable during cement injection. New pain with a different character should prompt oblique views.[13]
• The endpoints for cement injection include passage of cement beyond the marrow space and cement reaching the posterior quarter of the vertebral body on the lateral projection (see Fig. 159-1, *E*). In the case of cement leakage, one may wait 1 to 2 minutes to allow the cement to harden and then reinject to see whether the cement is redirected within the vertebral body.[28] Ideally, the cement will extend across the midline to the opposite pedicle by the end of the injection (Fig. 159-1, *F*). The optimal volume of cement is a matter of controversy (see later).
• The final portion of cement may be delivered by inserting the needle stylet. Alternatively, the cement may be

allowed to harden, and the needle removed with a gentle rocking motion to ensure that the cement within the cannula separates at the cannula tip. Manual compression is used to achieve hemostasis after the cannula is removed.

Kyphoplasty

• The cavity created by the balloon tamp allows injection of cement that is more viscous than that used for vertebroplasty. The cavity and more viscous cement theoretically minimize the risk of cement extravasation. Sufficient time is allowed for the cement to reach a doughy consistency with loss of the sheen of the initially mixed cement.
• Most practitioners use bone filler devices provided by Kyphon to inject KyphX cement. In our laboratory, we use a typical vertebroplasty injector system to inject PMMA for kyphoplasty. The delivery system is connected to the cannula, and the cement is injected slowly under fluoroscopic guidance. The cement fills the cavity in an anterior-to-posterior direction and should match or slightly exceed the volume of the inflated balloon tamp.

Vertebral Augmentation Device Updates

Since 2007, technology has advanced so extensively that the term *kyphoplasty* has expanded beyond its definition as the "balloon procedure" to include any device that creates a cavity before cement delivery. These devices have been developed in an effort to improve the safety and effectiveness of vertebral augmentation by allowing for improved targeting and control of cement delivery. The articulating VertecoR MidLine Navigational Osteotome needle (DFine Inc., San Jose, Calif.), for example, can be variably adjusted to 90 degrees, allowing for site and size-specific cavity creation. The ability to cross the midline with a single needle offers the additional benefit of a unilateral approach in most cases (Fig. 159-2).

Creating a cavity with a balloon or an osteotome needle displaces bone and, in the setting of malignant fractures, tumor. Thus, there are added risks when treating tumor-related compression fractures. There is the theoretical risk of causing the spread of tumor cells into the bloodstream and the risk of retropulsion of the tumor mass, especially when the posterior cortex is disrupted. These complications can occur during both cavity creation and cement delivery. Creating a cavity by removing, as opposed to displacing, pathologic tissue may mitigate these potential complications. The Cavity SpineWand (Arthro-Care Corp., Sunnyvale, Calif.) is a radiofrequency-based plasma ablation device placed through an 8-gauge working cannula. It uses a low-heat (40-70°C) plasma field to vaporize tumor, creating a cavity within the vertebral body. The result is tissue removal with minimal collateral tissue damage.

New, high-viscosity PMMA cements (VertaPlex HV [Stryker Instruments, Kalamazoo, Mich.] and KyphX HV-R [Medtronic Spine LLC, Sunnyvale, Calif.]) have the reported advantage of improved control of cement delivery without compromising working time. Viscous cement may be particularly useful in cases of lytic metastases and large cortical defects where there is a higher risk for cement extravasation. A recent modification heats bone cement with radiofrequency energy during delivery, thereby increasing

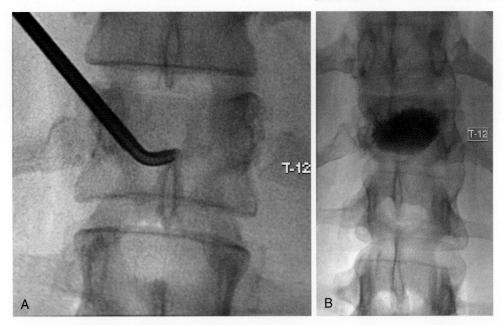

FIGURE 159-2. A, A 55-year-old female with T12 compression fracture. Unipedicular access to middle of vertebral body is achieved with articulating osteotome needle. **B,** Bone cement preferentially fills cavity.

viscosity without losing working time. With this device, a hydraulic device delivers the bone cement, allowing the operator to stand back from the radiation field.

A new bioactive alternative to PMMA is Cortoss Bone Augmentation Material (Orthovita Inc., Malvern, Pa.). It is an inherently radiopaque composite that has a faster in situ setting time than PMMA, reducing extravasation. It uses a mix-on-demand delivery system, allowing for very long working times.

These innovations appear to produce benefits in safety and perhaps efficacy, but there is little published evidence for such claims at this time.

SPECIAL TOPICS

Bipedicular versus Unipedicular Approach

Vertebroplasty and kyphoplasty can be performed with placement of bilateral needles or a single needle.[22] Most practitioners perform kyphoplasty with bilateral needle placement, although we reported a method of unilateral needle placement in these types of cases.[29] In either situation, the goal is to place cement across the midline within the vertebral body—we use placement of PMMA to the opposite pedicle as our general landmark. Therefore, use of a single needle with a relatively medial needle tip position is sufficient in many cases (see Fig. 159-1, *D*). If a unilateral approach is attempted but cement filling or balloon expansion does not cross the midline, a second system may then be placed on the other side. Kim et al. have demonstrated that there is no statistically significant difference in pain relief between the two approaches.[30] There are advantages to each approach. Advantages of a unipedicular approach include a decrease in procedure time and elimination of the risk associated with placement of a second needle. The major advantage of a bipedicular approach is facilitation of

PMMA injection, which is the most dangerous portion of the treatment.

Volume of Cement Injected

The optimal volume of cement is a matter of controversy, with some practitioners advocating the injection of maximum amounts of cement to completely fill the vertebral body and others advocating lower cement volumes with an emphasis on safety. The theoretical goal of more complete filling is to achieve restoration of biomechanical strength within the vertebral body to prevent refracture, without creating excess stiffness that may be transmitted to adjacent levels. Based on an in vitro biomechanical study, Mathis and Wong recommend cement filling to 50% to 70% of the residual volume of the vertebral body.[31] However, much smaller amounts of cement (<3 mL) appear to result in similar clinical outcomes as injection of larger volumes.[12] The decreased risk of cement extravasation with smaller volumes is an advantage of this approach, so long as one pays meticulous attention to the end of the injection criteria outlined earlier.

Vertebra Plana

When the vertebral body loses 70% of its original height, needle placement becomes a challenge. According to Stallmeyer et al., at least 8 mm of residual height is required for cannula placement.[10] The vertebra plana often adopts a bowtie configuration in which the center is compressed the most. It usually requires a lateral needle position and placement of bilateral needles.[32] Only a small amount of cement is needed to achieve pain relief.[13] If there is a cystic cleft within the fracture (i.e., Kümmell disease), the needle may be placed near the midline within the cleft in the hope of height expansion during needle placement and cement injection (see later).

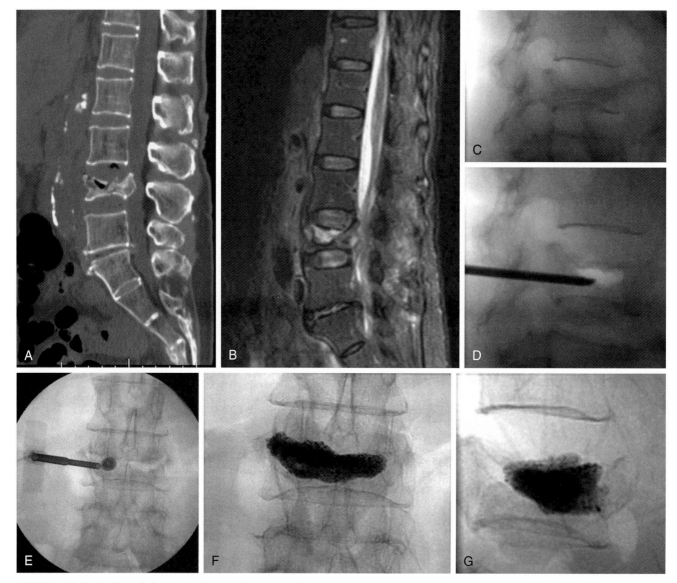

FIGURE 159-3. A, Kümmell disease in a 74-year-old woman with L4 compression fracture. Sagittal reformatted image from computed tomography scan of lumbar spine demonstrates retropulsion into spinal canal and intraosseous vacuum phenomenon. Also note fracture through posterior cortex. **B,** Sagittal short tau inversion recovery (STIR) image demonstrates fluid-filled cystic cleft where gas was previously seen. **C,** Lateral fluoroscopic image demonstrating severe height loss. **D,** During needle placement, there is expansion of cleft and increase in height of vertebral body, demonstrating dynamic nature of these lesions. **E,** Kyphoplasty balloon was inflated to maximum volume. Note further increase in cleft size, extending from right to left across entire vertebral body. **F-G,** Cement has filled cleft and further increased height of vertebral body. As demonstrated here, height increase is primarily a function of dynamic mobility of fracture fragments.

Fractures with Intraosseous Vacuum Phenomenon (Kümmell Disease)

The intraosseous vacuum phenomenon is thought to be related to osteonecrosis (Fig. 159-3). A fluid-filled cleft seen on MRI is an equivalent finding. Pain in this setting is believed to arise from motion between the unhealed fracture fragments. In some cases, this motion can even be seen under fluoroscopy as the height of the vertebral body changes with respiration. Prone positioning during the procedure promotes restoration of height because of the traction placed across the vertebral body. The needle should be placed into or as close to the cleft as possible so cement will fill the cleft. Vertebral augmentation yields significant rates of pain relief in the setting of an intraosseous vacuum phenomenon[33,34] and, in our experience, can provide considerable restoration of height. It is important to keep the patient prone for 10 to 15 minutes after injecting the cement to allow it to harden within the cleft before moving the patient off the fluoroscopy table. This is done to prevent cement from being squeezed out of the cleft when the patient moves.

Malignancy/Spinal Stenosis

Although vertebral augmentation may be performed in the setting of epidural tumor or spinal stenosis, there should be heightened awareness of the potential neurologic complications related to the presence of epidural or foraminal cement. Performing the procedure with the patient awake is an important safeguard because new pain, especially of a radicular quality, may be the first sign of dangerous cement leakage and should prompt a careful search for extraosseous cement. Cement injection volumes should be more modest than in routine cases. Limiting the cement to the anterior half of the vertebral body may be a good rule of thumb. Intrathecal contrast material may be instilled before the procedure to allow visualization of a mass effect on the thecal sac by tumor or bone displaced into the spinal canal during cement injection.

Safety of Multilevel Treatment

A patient who is to undergo vertebral augmentation may have multiple fractures that require treatment, and ideally, all the levels would be treated at one time. However, treating an excessive number of levels in a single session raises many concerns, including PMMA toxicity, difficulty for the elderly to lie prone and cooperate for the extended period that would be required, and extrusion of fat emboli from marrow during cement injection. There have been two reported deaths in patients who underwent vertebral augmentation at eight or more levels.[35] Although no guideline has been established, a good rule of thumb is to treat a maximum of three levels per session.[2,3]

Height Restoration

Studies have shown that the average increase in height is 2.2 mm for vertebroplasty and 4 mm for kyphoplasty.[36,37] For kyphoplasty, this translates to a mean decrease in kyphotic angle of approximately 6 degrees. It is unclear whether these results have any clinical significance. It appears that restoration of height is more a function of dynamic mobility of the fracture fragments (e.g., Kümmell disease) than the type of vertebral augmentation.[35] This has been confirmed in one study in which fractured levels containing gas achieved greater height restoration than those without gas.[24]

To date, there is no decided advantage of kyphoplasty over vertebroplasty with regard to pain relief, height restoration, or complications.

Cost-Effectiveness

Several studies evaluate the costs associated with vertebroplasty and kyphoplasty. Lad et al. (2009) assessed national trends by using data from the 2004 Nationwide Inpatient Sample.[38] In that year, approximately 23,000 vertebroplasties and kyphoplasties were performed at a cost of $672 million. Gray et al. (2008) reported that the nationwide inflation-adjusted charges for vertebroplasties increased from $76 million in 2001 to $152.3 million in 2005.[39] Although vertebroplasty is mostly performed in the outpatient setting, they found that the inpatient cases generated most of the costs. A retrospective chart review on 179 patients, comparing vertebroplasty to conservative management, found that vertebroplasty was more cost-effective at 1 week and 3 months.[40] At 12 months post procedure, no difference in costs between the two groups was found. A retrospective cohort study by Mehio et al. contrasted the hospital costs for vertebroplasty versus kyphoplasty in both the inpatient and outpatient population.[41] They found that vertebroplasty reduces hospital costs by nearly $5000 for inpatient procedures and by more than $4000 for outpatient procedures over kyphoplasty. These costs differences were observed despite older age and greater disease severity for the inpatient vertebroplasty group.

COMPLICATIONS

With adherence to careful technique and optimal visualization, the risk for morbidity or mortality is small. The risk is greater for malignancy-related fractures, with an overall complication rate of 5% to 10% versus 1% to 3% for osteoporotic fractures.[2,42] Potential complications that should be explained to the patient before consent include cement leakage, nerve or spinal cord damage resulting in paralysis or bowel/bladder dysfunction,[35,43] pulmonary embolism (secondary to cement or fat emboli[14,35,42]), infection (osteomyelitis, epidural abscess[25]), paraspinal hematoma, fracture (of a rib, pedicle, or vertebral body[12,14]), hypotension or depressed myocardial function (secondary to free methylmethacrylate monomer or fat emboli[14,35]), pneumothorax (for thoracic levels), and worsened pain or failure to treat.

Extraosseous passage of cement is a source of complications with both of these procedures. For vertebroplasty, small amounts of cement leakage are very common and occur in approximately two thirds of treated vertebra and slightly more frequently in pathologic fractures.[14,42,44] For kyphoplasty, a large low-resistance cavity is created and will fill first, thereby theoretically resulting in a lower rate of cement leakage.[23,36,45,46] For both procedures, most extraosseous cement produces no symptoms or long-term morbidity. However, even small amounts of PMMA adjacent to a nerve root, including cement within the foraminal veins, can produce radicular pain.[42] Experienced practitioners of vertebroplasty report a rate of symptomatic cement leakage that varies from 0% to 1% for treatment of osteoporotic fractures[44,47] and 4% to 8% for treatment of metastases.[20,48] Symptomatic leakage can also occur with kyphoplasty.[49] When radiculopathy is produced by cement leakage, the pain can be treated by nerve root block or systemic steroids. The need for surgical decompression is rare,[1] but it may be necessary when there is sufficient foraminal cement to cause frank nerve root compression or when sufficient cement has been placed in the spinal canal to cause cord compression or cauda equina syndrome.[48,50]

POSTPROCEDURAL AND FOLLOW-UP CARE

After the cement hardens, the cannulas are removed and manual compression is applied over the needle access to promote clotting and prevent bleeding complications. Transfer to the stretcher may be performed immediately after the procedure. The patient lies supine and flat in bed for 1 hour after the procedure and may be observed overnight in the hospital or discharged later the same day.[2,13,51] Assessment of the patient shortly after the procedure commonly reveals immediate relief or improvement of back pain. Frequently, the patient will be able to discriminate any new procedure-related pain, which is typically treated with NSAIDs and should resolve over a 24- to 72-hour period. In the setting of clinical deterioration indicative of cement leakage, cross-sectional imaging should be performed.

Postprocedural follow-up of patients is important. Up to a third of them will sustain a repeat fracture within 1 year, with the greatest risk in those with steroid-induced osteoporosis.[52,53] Patients should be seen for 3-week follow-up after the procedure and assessed with regard to pain, mobility, and need for pain medication. It is important to counsel them to report any sudden increase in back pain or new back pain, because it may indicate a new fracture. Imaging should be performed in this case to help elucidate the cause of new pain. Although the vast majority of recurrent fractures occur at new levels, a small percentage of patients suffer recurrent fractures at previously treated levels and may gain pain relief from repeat vertebral augmentation.[17] This being said, caution should be taken when interpreting marrow edema at a previously treated level, because according to one study, *normal* MRI findings after vertebroplasty include persistent or progressive marrow edema at the treated level in up to a third of patients and for up to 6 months after the procedure.[54]

- Since publication of two blinded randomized controlled trials in the *New England Journal of Medicine*, there has been controversy regarding the efficacy of vertebral augmentation, but two recent nonblinded randomized controlled trials show that vertebroplasty and kyphoplasty are highly effective.
- Complications are rare and generally result from unrecognized extraosseous leakage of the injected polymethyl methacrylate (PMMA). Complications include radiculopathy, paralysis, and pulmonary embolism. High-quality imaging, preferably in a biplane fluoroscopy suite, is necessary for safe performance of these procedures.

KEY POINTS

- Osteoporotic compression fractures are a common cause of pain and loss of independence in the middle-aged and elderly.
- Vertebroplasty and kyphoplasty are percutaneous procedures for the treatment of compression fractures that fail conventional medical therapy. The primary goal of these procedures is pain relief and associated improvement in mobility.

► SUGGESTED READINGS

Ortiz O, Mathis JM. Vertebral body reconstruction: techniques and tools. Neuroimaging Clin N Am 2010;20:145–58.

Jensen ME, Evans AJ, Mathis JM, et al. Percutaneous polymethylmethacrylate vertebroplasty in the treatment of osteoporotic vertebral body compression fractures: Technical aspects. AJNR Am J Neuroradiol 1997;18:1897–904.

Laredo JD, Hamze B. Complications of percutaneous vertebroplasty and their prevention. Skeletal Radiol 2004;33:493–505.

Mathis JM, Wong W. Percutaneous vertebroplasty: technical considerations. J Vasc Interv Radiol 2003;14:953–60.

The complete reference list is available online at www.expertconsult.com.

CHAPTER 160

New Directions in Bone Materials

Marc Bohner and Gamal Baroud

CLINICAL RELEVANCE

Osteoporosis has become a major health problem for most Western societies in recent decades. Strongly osteoporotic bone is so brittle, any move can result in bone fracture. In 1995, 1.5 million fractures in the United States were attributable to osteoporosis.[1] In 2000, 200,000 vertebral fractures were estimated to occur every year among the female U.S. population.[2] Even though these fractures are rather benign, they are associated with high morbidity and long hospital stays.[3] Repairing osteoporotic fractures with traditional osteosynthesis techniques is often very difficult owing to the inherent weakness of bone. The introduction of screw-locking osteosynthesis plates has improved therapy, but not for all indications. Therefore, new techniques should be proposed, investigated, and introduced.

One approach to heal or at least handle osteoporotic bone fractures is to inject a cementing bone substitute into bone. This technique, called *bone augmentation*, is particularly useful for vertebral fractures (the procedure is often called *vertebroplasty* [see Chapter 159]).[4] Unfortunately, dramatic negative outcomes of spine augmentation procedures have been reported in recent years.[5,6] Even though the cause of these negative results is in most cases associated with poor clinical practice, inadequate cement properties are also mentioned.[6] Therefore, the cement properties required by the given application should be well understood to design more adequate cements. The goal of this chapter is to review the present knowledge on cements designed for bone augmentation.

INDICATIONS

Exclusively bone cements developed for bone augmentation procedures should be used in vertebroplasty/kyphoplasty. Modifications of commercial cements that are often mentioned in leading publications[7,8] are prohibited, and hence the use of modified cements should be carefully weighed and discussed with the patient.[9]

CONTRAINDICATIONS

Bone cements developed for bone augmentation procedures should not be used for applications not mentioned by the manufacturer.

CEMENTS

In this section, the general properties of polymethyl methacrylate (PMMA) cements and calcium phosphate cements (CPCs) are described, and the two are compared. New cements and cement developments are also briefly reviewed.

POLYMETHYL METHACRYLATE CEMENTS

The first cement that was used for a bone augmentation procedure was a PMMA cement.[4] This cement consists of several ingredients that all have their importance[10]:

- A monomer called *methyl methacrylate* (MMA; transparent liquid; Mw = 100 g/mole) that will eventually react to form PMMA. The heat released by the latter reaction is very large (i.e., close to 57 kJ/mole), whereas the specific heat of PMMA is relatively low (i.e., close to 0.146 kJ/[mole·K]).[11] As a result, the heat released during the reaction is large enough to potentially heat up the cement by several hundred degrees during setting.
- A PMMA powder (or copolymers) used as a filler material, hence decreasing the total heat released per cement volume, as well as reducing shrinkage during setting (21% for pure MMA)
- A radiopacifier to ensure the cement can be seen radiographically (radiopacifier included in or added to PMMA powder). Typical powders are $BaSO_4$ and ZrO_2.
- Additives to initiate the polymerization reaction, commonly dibenzoyl peroxide (generally included in or added to PMMA powder) and N,N-dimethyl-p-toluidine (generally included in the liquid phase)
- Other additives such as stabilizers, inhibitors, radical catchers, coloring agents, antibiotics

In commercial formulations, the ratio between powder and liquid component is typically close to 2:3. Additionally, the radiopacifier content can easily reach 30%. For example, the powder component of Osteopal V (Heraeus Kulzer [see Table 160-1]) contains 14.16 g PMMA (40.0 w% of the total cement weight), 11.70 g ZrO_2 (33.1 w%), 0.14 g benzoyl peroxide (0.4 w%), and chlorophyll (coloring agent), and the liquid component contains 9.2 g MMA (26 w%), 0.19 g N,N-dimethyl-p-toluidine (0.5%), and chlorophyll. Since the MMA content is relatively small, shrinkage and volume heat release of commercial cement formulations are much lower than those of pure MMA cement.

Importantly, the curing (setting or hardening) reaction of PMMA cements is a polymerization reaction—that is, small monomers react together to form increasingly long polymer chains. Hardening occurs via entanglement of these polymer chains. Reaction stops when no more MMA monomers are present. The final porosity of the cement is very low.

In the early days of vertebroplasty, PMMA cements were modified to better fulfill the requirements of the application. In particular, the powder-to-liquid ratio was reduced to prolong the injection period, and more radiopacifier was added to increase radiologic contrast.[7,8] These changes considerably modified cement properties such as viscosity,

TABLE 160-1. List of PMMA Cements with 510(k) FDA Clearance for Vertebroplasty

Device Name	Applicant	Device Name	Applicant
BonOs Inject	AAP Biomaterials GmbH	Confidence Ex High Viscosity Bone Cement	DePuy Spine
Symphony VR Radiopaque Bone Cement	Advanced Biomaterial Systems	Confidence Fenestrated Introducer Needle*	DePuy Spine
Parallax Acrylic Resin with TRACERS	NeuroTherm	Mesh Fenestrated Introducer Needle*	DePuy Spine
Parallax Acrylic Resin with TRACERS-Ta	NeuroTherm	EBI Vertebroplasty Systems	EBI L.P.
Parallax Acrylic Resin cartridge with TRACERS	NeuroTherm	KyphX HV-R	Kyphon
Parallax Acrylic Resin cartridge with TRACERS-Ta	NeuroTherm	KyphX HV-R Bone Cement	Kyphon
		Kyphon XPEDE Bone Cement	Medtronic
Parallax contour vertebral augmentation device*	NeuroTherm	KyphX HV-R Bone Cement	Medtronic
ArthroCare Parallax contour vertebral augmentation device*	NeuroTherm	Arcuate Vertebral Augmentation System	Medtronic Sofamor Danek
Radiopaque Bone Cement	Cardinal Health	Cortoss Bone Augmentation Material	Orthovita Inc.
AVAflex vertebral augmentation needle*	Cardinal Health	Skeltex ISV	Skeltex Technologies Inc.
Inflatable bone tamp*	Cardinal Health	StaXx FX System	Spine Wave
AVAmax vertebral balloon model*	CareFusion	Stryker VertaPlex Radiopaque Bone Cement	Stryker Corp.
AVAmax vertebral balloon*	CareFusion	VertaPlex HV	Stryker Corp.
Vertefix Vertebroplasty Procedure Set	Cook Medical	IVAS 2-10 mm (10 gauge) Balloon Catheter*	Stryker Corp.
Modification to Vertebroplastic Radiopaque Bone Cement	DePuy Spine	Mendec Spine	Tecres Medical
Vertebroplastic Radiopaque Bone Cement	DePuy Spine	Kit Mendec Spine and Delivery System*	Tecres Medical
Space CPSXL Bone Cement	DFine Inc.	VSPSPN	Tecres Medical
Space 360 delivery system*	DFine Inc.	Spine-Fix Biomimetic Bone Cement	Teknimed
Modification to Space CPSXL Bone Cement	DFine Inc.	Opacity + Bone Cement	Teknimed
		Vertecem	Teknimed
Stabili ERX Bone Cement	DFine Inc.	F20	Teknimed
Confidence High Viscosity Bone Cement	DePuy Spine	Cohesion Bone Cement	Teknimed

*Device listed under the category "Polymethyl methacrylate (PMMA) bone cement" that does not appear to refer to a cement.
Listed in alphabetical order by company as of Aug 28, 2011; Classification Product Code: NDN—Cement, Bone, Vertebroplasty.
FDA, U.S. Food and Drug Administration; *PMMA,* polymethyl methacrylate.
(From Bohner M: Uebersicht über einspritzbare Zemente für die Vertebroplastie und die Kyphoplastie. IN Becker S, Ogon M (eds): Ballonkyphoplastie. Springer-Verlag: Wien, 2006. Used with kind permission from Springer Science+Business Media.)

setting time, monomer release, and mechanical properties. There was no cement accepted for vertebral bone augmentation procedures, so these changes were required, but at the clinician's and patient's risk. Nowadays there are cements designed specifically for the application (Table 160-1), and their use is recommended.

Calcium Phosphate Cements

CPCs were discovered in the early 1980s by LeGeros[12] and Brown and Chow.[13] Since then, CPCs have proved to be attractive bone-substitute materials.[14] The first in vitro attempt to use CPC for the augmentation of osteoporotic bone was performed in 1991.[15] A few years later, the first in vitro use for intravertebral reconstruction was proposed.[16]

To our knowledge, there is presently no CPC cleared by the U.S. Food and Drug Administration (FDA) for vertebroplasty applications, despite the fact that their clinical use has been described in the literature.[17-20]

CPCs generally consist of an aqueous solution and a powder that typically contains several calcium phosphate compounds. Upon mixing, the powder dissolves in the aqueous solution, and new crystals form (precipitate). The reaction proceeds until all reactive calcium phosphate compounds have reacted. Cement hardening occurs with the entanglement of calcium phosphate crystals (Fig. 160-1), leading to a highly porous structure. The final product has a porosity close to 40% to 60%, with pores ranging typically from 0.1 to 10 μm. It is worth noting that CPCs are mechanically much stronger in compression than in tension or shear because the entangled crystals are not well bonded.

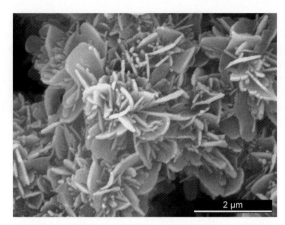

FIGURE 160-1. Typical structure of an apatite calcium phosphate cement showing entanglement of apatite crystals. *(From Bohner M: Uebersicht über einspritzbare Zemente für die Vertebroplastie und die Kyphoplastie. IN Becker S, Ogon M (eds): Ballonkyphoplastie. Springer-Verlag: Wien, 2006. Used with kind permission from Springer Science+Business Media.)*

Compressive strength is typically 5 to 10 times greater than tensile strength.

The two principal CPC types are apatite (e.g., hydroxyapatite, $Ca_5[PO_4]_3[OH]$) and brushite (also called *dicalcium phosphate dihydrate*, $CaHPO_4 \cdot 2H_2O$), depending on the end product of the setting reaction.[21,22] Most commercially available CPCs belong to the first category (e.g., α-BSM, Biopex, BoneSource, Calcibon, Cementek, Embarc, Kyphos, Mimix, Norian, Rebone (see list in Bohner[23]). In the past years, a few brushite CPCs have been used clinically: chronOS Inject, JectOS, Eurobone, and VitalOS.[23] The main difference between apatite and brushite CPCs lies in their solubility and hence resorption rate: brushite is much more soluble than apatite, so brushite CPC is in principle more rapidly resorbable than apatite CPC.

Difference Between PMMA and CPC

Because CPCs are the main candidates to replace PMMA in vertebroplasty, it is of interest to describe the primary differences between the two cements. Some very important differences are noteworthy (Table 160-2), and four of these will be described. First, PMMA cements are hydrophobic, whereas CPCs are hydrophilic, so the setting reaction of PMMA is barely affected by body fluids. This is in contrast to CPCs, where cement disintegration might occur, leading to the release of very large numbers of micro- and nanoparticles in the close environment of the cement and into blood. Second, the setting reaction occurs much faster in PMMA cements than in CPCs. As a result, reaction heat is released much faster from PMMA cements than from CPCs, leading to a much larger temperature increase in the former. So, even though CPCs are sometimes as exothermic as PMMA, they can be considered to set isothermally. Third, CPCs are very fragile materials. In particular, their shear and tensile properties are much lower than those of PMMA cements. As a result, clinicians are advised to use CPCs in simple/stable spinal fractures[17,24] or not to use them at all.[18] Fourth, CPCs are resorbable, contrary to PMMA cements, and should be replaced by bone and not simply resorbed. Presently, it is not clear how fast CPCs resorb and how much bone forms after CPC resorption in osteoporotic patients.

TABLE 160-2. Summary of Features of PMMA and Calcium Phosphate Cements

	PMMA Cement	CPC
Hydrophilicity	Hydrophobic	Hydrophilic
Injectability	Excellent	Critical
Setting time	<20 minutes	<20 minutes
Setting rate	Very high	Slow
Temperature change	Large	Negligible
Tensile strength	>50 MPa[10]	<15 MPa
Compressive strength	>70 MPa[10]	<100 MPa
Porosity	<40%*	40%-60%[†]
Pore diameter	—	0.1-10 μm
Resorption	No	Small to large
Bone–cement contact	Fair[55]	Excellent

*Porosity largely depends on preparation technique.[47] With vacuum mixing, values lower than 10% are typically obtained.
[†]Open porosity.
CPC, Calcium phosphate cement; *PMMA,* polymethyl methacrylate.
(From Bohner M: Uebersicht über einspritzbare Zemente für die Vertebroplastie und die Kyphoplastie. IN Becker S, Ogon M (eds): Ballonkyphoplastie. Springer-Verlag: Wien, 2006. Used with kind permission from Springer Science+Business Media.)

Other Cements

There are few new approaches in the field of polymeric and ceramic cements. One successful development in the field of methacrylate cements is represented by Cortoss (see Table 160-1), which has a more complex composition than traditional PMMA cements. The presence of three specific methacrylate components is meant to reduce toxic monomer release and improve the mechanical properties compared to PMMA cements. Additionally, a high ceramic fraction provides higher radiologic contrast and helps reduce the extent of the temperature increase during setting. However, this cement is stiffer, more hydrophilic, and tends to be less viscous than PMMA cements traditionally used in vertebroplasty. The high stiffness raises some concerns regarding the risk of fractures in vertebra adjacent to augmented vertebra. Another concern is the scattered vertebral fill that is attributed to the hydrophilic and liquid features of the cement. Such a fill appears mechanically sound because of the distributed stresses in the vertebra being augmented, yet might also be associated with a higher extravasation risk because of the dispersed filling. A less successful development is a nonresorbable cement based on a mixture of functional thiols, acrylic molecules, a reaction starter, a thixotropic agent, and barium sulfate (32 w%).[25] This cement has the unique feature of a compressive strength close to 30 to 40 MPa (cancellous bone has a value < 10 MPa), and an E-modulus lower than that of cancellous bone (close to 70 MPa compared to 100-500 MPa for cancellous bone and more than 1 GPa for PMMA cement). As a result, the augmentation of a vertebral body with this cement does not significantly affect the compliance of bone, which might reduce the risk of adjacent vertebral fractures.

In the field of ceramic cements, one of the most advanced projects presented in recent years was a nonresorbable cement based on calcium aluminate (Doxa AB, Sweden) that had a very low porosity and hence very great mechanical properties.[26] Indeed, flexural and compressive strengths close to 30 to 50 MPa and 150 to 180 MPa, respectively, were reported. The E-modulus was unfortunately very high, close to 10 to 12 GPa (cancellous bone: 0.1-0.5 GPa). Also there were concerns about the presence of aluminum in the cement. To our knowledge, development has been stopped recently. Another ceramic cement based on plaster of Paris (Cerament Bone Void Filler, Bone Support AB, Sweden) has been proposed as a bone void filler for spinal application. However, it is not meant to be used as stand-alone product, owing to its poor mechanical stability during resorption.

Technical Cement Requirements

In recent years, general understanding about the importance of cement properties and about what adequate cement properties are for vertebral bone augmentation procedures has been widely improved. As a result, new cements have been or are being designed that help enhance outcomes of the technique. Several important parameters are cement handling, viscosity, injection time, injectability, radiopacity, setting time, exothermic heat, mechanical properties, blood clotting properties, and monomer release. This section reviews these parameters.

Handling

Procedures such as cement mixing and filling syringes with cement should be easy and reliable. In that respect, most cements fulfill these requirements, even though improvements could be made. Efforts have lately provided two-liquid cements that are mixed during injection using a static mixer integrated in the cannula.[27-29] Cortoss is to our knowledge the only cement for vertebroplasty based on this principle.

Viscosity

Cement viscosity is a very important parameter for the application: it defines the injection pressure but more importantly the risk of extravasation.[30-34] In fact, the risk of extravasation decreases as cement viscosity increases, so it is important to find an adequate balance between a high cement viscosity that reduces extravasation risks and a low viscosity that enables low injection forces. Use of an adequate injection system is then required. A few years ago, a cement viscosity in the range of 100 to 1000 Pa·s appeared to be ideal. In recent years, the development of powerful cement injectors has triggered the development of more viscous cements, such as Confidence cement (see Table 160-1).

Injection/Working Time

Ideally, a cement should have a constant viscosity in the range noted earlier. Unfortunately, cement viscosity varies according to shear forces (generally shear-thinning) and as a function of time: after a decrease in the first seconds of mixing, viscosity increases considerably during curing, eventually leading to hardening. Since cement viscosity should be high to prevent extravasation, it is important to define an adequate injection window. In recent years, efforts have been made to provide cements that can be injected as

soon as they are mixed. Confidence cement belongs to this new generation (see Table 160-1). Another approach adopted by several companies has been to provide a tool or indications to determine at which time the cement can be injected. For example, Synthes developed a viscometer that is able to tell the surgeon when injection should be done. Unfortunately, the viscosity measurement is not performed on the cement present in the syringe. This problem was solved by Skeltex by offering a viscometer based on the measurement of the cement dielectric properties that can be mounted on the injection system and monitor cement viscosity during injection.

Injectability

Here, the *injectability* of a cement is defined as the ability of the cement to be injected without phase separation between fluid and powder. PMMA cements are very well injectable, contrary to CPCs, which tend to phase-separate or filter-press: above a certain injection pressure, the liquid phase is injected faster than the powder phase, eventually leading to plugging. When plugging occurs (e.g., in bone), cement injection is no longer possible. To improve CPC injectability, several approaches can be used—for example, increasing the liquid-to-powder ratio.[35] However, the most adequate approach appears to be the addition of a small amount of polymer gel into the mixing liquid (e.g., 0.5%-1.0% sodium hyaluronate gel) that lubricates the interparticle contacts without decreasing cement viscosity.[36]

Radiopacity

PMMA cements have hardly any radiologic contrast, contrary to CPC. However, both cement types require additional contrast. For PMMA cements, the choice is relatively easy because PMMA cements are not resorbable, so all radiopaque non- or poorly soluble powders, such as metal salts ($BaSO_4$, ZrO_2, $SrCO_3$) or metal powders (Ti, Ta, W), can be used. For CPC, the problem is more acute. CPCs are indeed slowly resorbable, so all added radiopacifying powders would be released over time. Most metallic salts (e.g. $BaSO_4$, ZrO_2) or metal powders (e.g., Ta) are insoluble, so use of radiopacifying powders represents a biocompatibility hazard. An alternative to this approach is to increase the powder-to-liquid ratio of the cement to increase its solid content. This strategy is possible but has limited efficacy and reduces cement injectability. It is also possible to add a liquid radiologic contrast agent such as iodine-based aqueous solutions. Unfortunately, a small fraction of the population is allergic to iodine. Interestingly, there is presently no guideline from the FDA concerning the minimum radiopacity required for the vertebroplasty application. At the moment, more is better.

Setting Time

The *setting time* of a cement is generally defined as the time required for the cement to reach a given mechanical strength. This property can be modulated quite easily, so most cements designed for vertebral bone augmentation have a setting time in the range of 5 to 20 minutes. Of note, the cement *setting rate* is more difficult to control; as soon as the setting reaction starts, the reaction cannot be slowed down or accelerated. Typically, PMMA cements harden very fast (20-30 minutes), whereas CPCs harden rather slowly (100% of mechanical strength is reached after 5-10 hours).

Exothermic Heat

The cause of pain relief following a vertebral bone augmentation procedure has been a topic of controversy. Two explanations have been proposed. First, pain relief results from mechanical stabilization of the vertebral body. This explanation is nowadays the most frequently mentioned. The second explanation is that pain relief results from nerve necrosis due to the considerable heat released from the cement. In that respect, it would be important to always use very exothermic and fast-setting cements such as PMMA cements.

Several studies have been published on the thermal effect of PMMA cements after vertebral bone augmentation (e.g., Belkoff and Molloy[37]). To better understand these studies, it is important to note that heat/exothermic release and temperature increase during setting are related topics, but not the same. Temperature increase not only depends on the rate of heat release but also on the rate of heat dispersion. In other words, very exothermic cement reactions do not necessarily lead to a temperature increase if heat release rate is very low (e.g., in CPC) or if heat dispersion is very good. Heat dispersion is favored when (1) the cement is in contact with a material with a high heat conductance (like a metallic implant), (2) the cement is in contact with a flowing liquid (e.g., blood), and (3) the cement piece has a high specific surface (ratio between cement surface and cement volume).

Mechanical Properties

The mechanical effect of vertebral bone augmentation has been investigated intensively. One particular point of interest is the potential negative effect of bone augmentation on fractures of adjacent vertebrae.[38] Even though finite element models suggest that vertebrae adjacent to a vertebra augmented with a stiff material such as PMMA or CPC are submitted to higher loads than normal,[39,40] it is not clear how important this effect is. Assuming that cement stiffness is a very important parameter and should be reduced, a problem occurs because it is difficult to reduce the stiffness of PMMA cements or CPC. In fact, the only possibility is to decrease cement porosity. This approach has been proposed by Bisig et al.,[41,42] who incorporated an aqueous phase into a PMMA cement paste based on the idea of DeWijn.[43] A report also exists on mixing blood and the cement.[44] Stiffness in the range of that of cancellous bone could be obtained with 40% aqueous fraction.[41] However, problems were encountered with particle release.[42] For CPC, this approach does not work because CPCs are already highly porous. Another approach could be to use new types of materials, such as the compliant cements mentioned herein. A second particular point of interest concerning the mechanical properties are the fatigue properties, particularly those of CPC, since CPCs are fragile materials and have much lower mechanical properties than PMMA cements. So far, there is very little information on the topic. In fact, to our knowledge only two studies on the fatigue properties of CPC have been published.[45,46] Here again, more work needs to be done, perhaps also in combination with in vivo studies.

Blood Clotting

This topic has received some attention after the death of a few patients following injection of a CPC (MAUDE Database; www.fda.gov/cdrh/maude.html) and presentation of the abstract of Bernards et al.,[47] who demonstrated that injection of CPC into the bloodstream of pigs provoked rapid embolization and death. Related and sometimes contradictory results by Axen et al.,[48] Takemoto et al.,[49] Aoki et al.,[50] and Krebs et al.[51] suggest that the most likely explanation for the negative outcome occurring sometimes after the use of CPC is blockage of blood capillaries with calcium phosphate particles released from the CPC. As a result, it appears essential to measure the cohesion of CPC—that is, the ability of the cement to harden in a liquid environment without releasing particles.[36] The fact that PMMA cements are hydrophobic (water repellent) and CPCs are hydrophilic could explain why PMMA does not trigger the same problems.[52]

Monomer Release

Release of MMA from PMMA cements during setting has been related to severe hypotension by an action on vascular smooth muscle.[53,54] Presently, a multitude of data are available in the field of hip arthroplasty, but little in the field of vertebral bone augmentation. Despite the fact that injected volumes of cements are lower in vertebral bone augmentation than in hip arthroplasty, it is of great importance to determine how much monomer is released from PMMA cements during setting. Four main reasons can be mentioned: (1) the liquid-to-powder ratio of cements used for vertebroplasty is generally lower than for hip arthroplasty, which should lead to more monomer release; (2) the setting time of cements used for vertebroplasty is generally longer than that for hip arthroplasty, which should lead to more monomer release; (3) vertebral bodies are very well irrigated bones; and (4) vertebral bodies are in very close proximity to the heart.

OUTCOMES

Vertebroplasty has been a very successful therapeutic approach, with complication rates close to 1%.[9] A lower rate is expected with the use of injection systems and cements specially designed for the application. Most of the know-how on the engineering side of vertebroplasty has been gained in the last decade, so more improvements are expected for the coming years. These improvements should lead to a decrease in complication rates.

COMPLICATIONS

As previously discussed, inadequate cement properties can lead to undesired events such as (1) poor injectability, preventing an adequate cement application[35] (for CPC); (2) low viscosity, leading to extravasation[30-34] (for all cements); (3) bad cohesion, leading to particle release into the bloodstream and resulting in capillary blockage[50] (for CPC); (4) too-early loading, leading to mechanical failure (for all cements); (5) low mechanical properties, leading to long-term cement failure and negative clinical outcome[17,18,24] (for CPC); or (6) too-high cement stiffness, leading to the failure of adjacent vertebra (for PMMA).[38,39]

POSTPROCEDURE AND FOLLOW-UP CARE

Once in place, the evolution of the cement should be assessed radiographically according to the normal surgical follow-up procedure to detect a cement failure or the occurrence of cement or bone resorption.

ACKNOWLEDGMENT

This contribution is a modified and translated version of a chapter by Marc Bohner entitled "Uebersicht über einspritzbare Zemente für die Vertebroplastie und die Kyphoplastie." and published in: "Ballonkyphoplastie"; Eds S. Becker, M. Ogon; Springer-Verlag/Wien, 2006. It is used here with kind permission from Springer Science+Business Media.

KEY POINTS

- The clinical outcome of bone augmentation such as vertebroplasty depends not only on the skills of the surgeon, but also on the properties of the injected material.

- A good knowledge of the cement properties required by the given application is a prerequisite for the design of adequate cement.

- Cements should have the following properties to provide a good short-term clinical outcome: easy handling, injectability, high radiopacity, adequate viscosity, rather long setting time (15 minutes), nontoxic, and non-clotting.

- Cements should have the following properties to provide a good long-term clinical outcome: isothermicity during setting, biocompatibility, adapted mechanical properties.

- Only commercial products sold for the given application should be used, or cement modifications should be discussed with the patient.

► **SUGGESTED READINGS**

Calcium phosphates and calcium phosphate cements:
Bohner M. Calcium orthophosphates in medicine: from ceramics to calcium phosphate cements. Injury 2000;31S(4):37–47.
Bohner M, Gbureck U, Barralet J. Technological issues for the development of more efficient calcium phosphate cements: a critical assessment. Biomaterials 2005;26:6423–9.

Polymethyl methacrylate cements:
Kühn KD. Bone cements: Up-to-date comparison of physical and chemical properties of commercial materials. Berlin Heidelberg: Springer-Verlag; 2000.

Cements for bone augmentation:
Heini PF, Berlemann U. Bone substitutes in vertebroplasty. Eur Spine J 2001;10:S205–13.
Lewis G. Injectable bone cements for use in vertebroplasty and kyphoplasty: state-of-the-art review. J Biomed Mater Res Part B: Appl Biomater 2006;76B:456–68.

Cement rheologic properties required for bone augmentation:
Baroud G, Bohner M, Heini P, Steffen T. Injection biomechanics of bone cements used in vertebroplasty. Biomed Mater Eng 2004;14(4):487–504.

General reviews on vertebroplasty:
Cotton A, Boutry N, Cortet B, et al. Percutaneous vertebroplasty: state of the art. Radiographics 1998;18:311–20.
Deramond H, Depriester C, Toussaint P, Galibert P. Percutaneous vertebroplasty. Semin Musculoskeletal Radiol 1997;1(2):285–95.
Mathis JM, Wong W. Percutaneous vertebroplasty: technical considerations. J Vasc Interv Radiol 2003;14:953–60.
Verlaan JJ, Oner FC, Dhert WJA. Anterior spinal column augmentation with injectable bone cements. Biomaterials 2006;27:290–301.

The complete reference list is available online at www.expertconsult.com.

CHAPTER 161

Minimally Invasive Disk Interventions

Gianluigi Guarnieri, Fabio Zeccolini, and Mario Muto

INTRODUCTION

When medical treatment has been unsuccessful for patients with low back pain (LBP) due to a small or contained herniated disk, minimally invasive techniques have recently been developed as "alternative" treatments to surgical intervention. Outcomes of these alternative treatments depend on the characteristics of the herniation itself and on the chosen technique.[1] Techniques include:

- Chemodiscolysis with chymopapain *(no longer used)*
- Automated percutaneous lumbar discectomy (APLD), developed by Onik
- Percutaneous laser disk decompression (PLDD)
- Intradiscal electrothermal therapy (IDET)
- Percutaneous coblation nucleoplasty
- Dekompressor percutaneous diskectomy
- Chemodiscolysis with O_2-O_3 mixture, with periradicular and periganglionic infiltration
- Jellified ethyl alcohol (DiscoGel)

All techniques can be performed under computed tomography (CT) or fluoroscopic guidance with the patient in prone position and under local anesthesia.[2] They offer good results, good patient compliance, low cost, and low complication rates. Patients need a short period of hospitalization, but most procedures can be performed in day surgery, and in cases of failed treatment, all techniques can be repeated once without interfering with surgery at a later date. All procedures can be performed at either cervical or lumbar levels. The rationale of all percutaneous treatments is to reduce the intradiscal pressure in different ways, creating the space required to decompress retropulsion or mass affect of the disk.

PATHOGENESIS OF LOW BACK PAIN

The pathogenesis of LBP is due to multifactorial mechanisms, but the two most common are mechanical causes that result in nerve root compression and acute inflammatory factors.

Mechanical Causes

Direct mechanical factors are direct compression of the herniated disk on the dorsal root ganglion (extraforaminal herniation) and mechanical deformation of the posterior longitudinal ligament and annulus, with nociceptor stimulation of the recurrent nerve of Luschka. *Indirect mechanical factors* are ischemia due to compression on afferent arterioles and nerve bundle microcirculation (with associated anoxic demyelination of nerve fibres) and venous stasis.

Inflammatory Factors

Cell-Mediated Inflammatory Reaction to Disk Protrusion

The nucleus pulposus is formed by proteoglycans immunologically segregated after birth. A herniated fragment may trigger an inflammatory process, with an autoimmune cell-mediated response led by macrophages, which results in a biohumoral immunologic response due to phospholipase A_2 (inflammatory inductor), which produces prostaglandin (PGE2) and leukotriene from arachidonic acid. In addition, disk degeneration is caused by matrix metalloproteinase (MMP)-1, MMP-2, MMP-3, and MMP-9, which degrade disk tissue and increase the inflammatory reaction.

INDICATIONS AND CONTRAINDICATIONS

General Exclusion Criteria

- Extruded herniated disk
- Free herniated fragment
- Recent disk or vertebral infection
- An upper arm deficit
- Sphincter dysfunction
- Extreme sciatica
- Progressive neurologic deficits of the involved body segment

The last three conditions are absolute indications for surgery. The best results are reported for small and medium-sized herniations within a normal spinal canal and without disk calcifications. Prognostic factors for an unsuccessful outcome are presence of a calcified herniated disk, high-grade spinal stenosis, a small descending herniated disk in the lateral spinal recess, failed back syndrome, and recurrent disk herniation.

General Inclusion Criteria

- *Clinical criteria:* LBP and sciatica resistant to conservative medical therapy, physiotherapy, and other interventions for a period not shorter than 2 to 3 months
- *Neurologic criteria:* paresthesia or altered sensitivity over the dermatome involved, mild muscle weakness, and signs of root ganglion irritation
- *Psychological criteria:* a firm resolve on the part of the patient to recover, with a commitment to cooperate and undergo subsequent physiotherapy with postural and motor rehabilitation

- *Neuroradiology (CT, MRI):*
  - Small and medium-sized herniated disks correlating with the patient's symptoms, with or without degenerative disk-vertebra disease complicated by intervertebral disk changes (protrusion, herniation)
  - Pain provoked by low-pressure contrast injection in the compromised disk during diskography for IDET, nucleoplasty, and APLD techniques
  - Residua of surgical (micro)-diskectomy, with herniation recurrence and/or hypertrophic fibrous scarring

CHOICE OF RADIOLOGIC GUIDANCE

All techniques require specific radiologic guidance with CT or fluoroscopy (DSA, C-arm). The choice among different techniques depends on personal preference and availability. Generally, all procedures can be performed under fluoroscopic guidance or CT without any significant difference. Use of CT helps identify the presence of bowel loops behind the psoas muscle, an absolute contraindication for any oblique approach to the disk.[2]

TECHNIQUE

The following are minimally invasive percutaneous techniques used in clinical practice to treat herniated lumbar disks.

Automated Percutaneous Lumbar Discectomy

APLD uses an instrument called a *nucleotome*, consisting of a compressed-air pneumatic pump connected to an "aspirating-cutting" probe with an external diameter of 2 mm. The probe is introduced into the disk through a 2.5-mm-diameter needle under fluoroscopic guidance. The nucleus pulposus is aspirated through a lateral window of the probe while a blade that moves coaxially within the probe destroys it and allows it to be drained.

This technique is indicated for all types and locations of disk protrusions or herniations without extrusion or free fragments. The success rate is about 70% to 80%. If the exclusion criteria are not considered, the success rate drops to 49.4%. When the procedure is not performed correctly, it may damage nerve roots or dural tissue. The most serious complication reported with this procedure is *cauda equina syndrome*, characterized by saddle anesthesia of the perineal region, retention or urine/fecal incontinence, and bilateral hyposthenia.[3-5]

Percutaneous Laser Disk Decompression

PLDD consists of introducing a soft flexible needle (0.8 mm) under fluoroscopic guidance into the nucleus pulposus of the herniated disk. Once the correct position of the needle is confirmed, a thin optical fiber connected to an Nd:YAG laser is introduced. The Nd:YAG is a special laser that works with a solid energy source, a yttrium aluminium garnet crystal doped with neodymium.

The action is based on the idea that the vertebral disk is a closed hydraulic system composed of the nucleus pulposus, made of water, surrounded by the fibrous annulus. An increasing water content of the nucleus pulposus causes a disproportionate increase of intradiscal pressure.

Vaporizing the nucleus pulposus leads to a reduction of intradiscal pressure and facilitates a relocation of the extruded nucleus pulposus into its original position. The laser vaporizes water in the nucleus pulposus, allowing decompression of disk pressure on the nerve root, with resolution of symptoms. It can be performed under CT or fluoroscopy guidance. If the hernia is contained, it is possible to perform PLDD under fluoroscopic guidance, releasing laser energy at the vertebral disk's center and posterior portion.

If the disk herniation is not contained but still connected to the intervertebral disk, it is better to perform the decompression procedure under CT guidance to better assess the connection of the disk and hernia portions. In this way, the laser energy can be released in multiple locations of the herniated disk, obtaining better vaporization and retraction of the hernia, with resultant root decompression and resolution of symptoms. The outcomes reported are success rates between 75% and 87% of cases, with an immediate reduction of back pain in 48% of cases. Septic and aseptic diskitis are the most common complications, with an average occurrence of 0% to 1.2% of cases. *Septic diskitis* is caused by introduction of microorganisms during positioning of the needle into the disk. Sterile technique is required. *Aseptic diskitis* is caused by the action of the laser itself on the disk and the adjacent vertebral plate.[6-12]

Uncommon complications such as intestinal perforation, cauda equina syndrome, and nerve root lesions with consequent impairments have been reported.

Intradiscal Electrothermal Therapy

IDET acts on the posterior aspect of the fibrous annulus, unlike other techniques where the action is on the nucleus pulposus. Under fluoroscopic guidance, a trocar is introduced into the intervertebral disk, then an electrothermal flexible catheter is introduced between the nucleus pulposus and annulus. The tip of the catheter has a resistor that, once placed near the posterior margin of the annulus, is warmed to 90°C for 16 to 17 minutes and then removed (Fig. 161-1). Warming the fibrous annulus reduces symptoms and stabilizes the disk lesion by reorganizing collagen fibers, strengthening the disk, cauterizing ring fissures, and ablating pain receptors.

IDET is indicated for treatment of a bulging disk or contained herniated disk without root compression symptoms and resistance to pharmacologic therapy and physiotherapy for more than 6 months. To obtain a better evaluation of a contained hernia, disk compression, or disk pressure, a previous diskography may be needed. The complication rate is 0.8%, with high frequency of osteonecrosis post IDET. The success rate is between 40% and 71% of cases.[12-17]

Percutaneous Coblation Nucleoplasty

In contrast to radiofrequency ablation, which uses high temperatures, coblation technology uses low temperatures (50°-70°C), obtaining the same results in a shorter time (2-3 inches vs. 15-17 inches). Under fluoroscopic guidance, a thermal coagulator (Perc-D coblation probe) is introduced into the nucleus pulposus, then a bipolar current is applied to the electrode tip, producing a radiofrequency field that

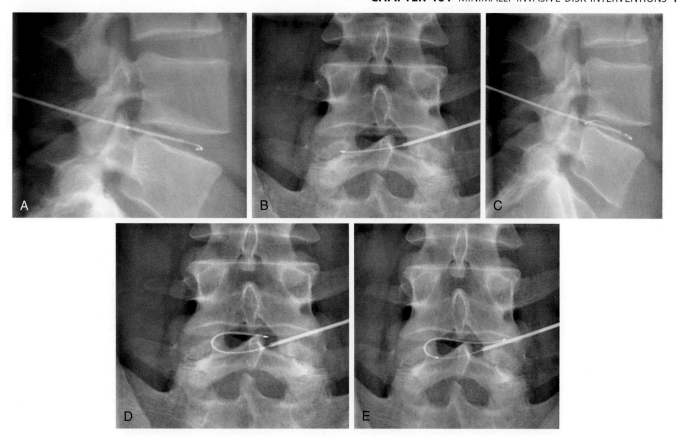

FIGURE 161-1. The LL **(A, C)** and AP **(B, D, E)** fluoroscopy controlo show the correct positioning of electrothermal catheter for intradiscal electrothermal therapy (IDET) in L4-L5 disk, using posterolateral approach and fluoroscopic guidance.

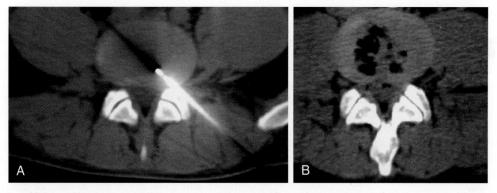

FIGURE 161-2. A, Coblation nucleoplasty at L4-L5, using computed tomography guidance and posterolateral approach in patient in prone position. **B,** Laterolateral and anteroposterior views of fluoroscopic guidance of correct positioning of needle at C5-C6 level.

breaks collagen bonds. Inside the nucleus, this creates "ionic plasma" containing simple molecules and ionized gases like O_2, H_2, and nitric oxide (NO) that will be removed through the needle used to introduce the electrode. The heat produced does not exceed 70°C and has a limited diffusion of 2 mm, creating a thermal lesion canal in the nucleus pulposus. Six manual 360-degree rotations of the probe without any other movements inside or outside the system creates six thermal lesion canals, with rapid dehydration of the nucleus and reduction of disk volume of about 10% to 20%. Subsequent contraction of the collagen

fibers reduces the protruded portion, with resultant decompression of the compressed root (Fig. 161-2). Integrity of the fibrous annulus is essential, otherwise the mechanism of retraction cannot happen. The best indication for this technique is symptomatic herniated (but *not* extruded) disk. Results obtained from controlled trials report resolution of pain symptoms in 70% to 80% of cases, with pain relief for at least 6 months. The risk of complications is very low. Principal complications are diskitis, anterior disk perforation caused by the probe, and cauda equina syndrome.[18-21]

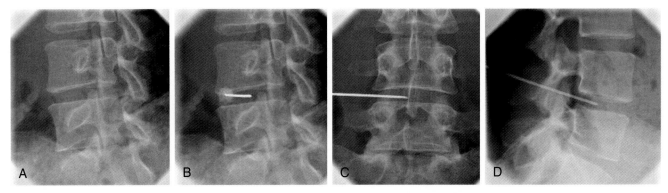

FIGURE 161-3. Dekompressor percutaneous discectomy at L4-L5 in patient in prone position and under fluoroscopy guidance, with oblique tube orientation by posterolateral approach.

Dekompressor Percutaneous Diskectomy

The aim of percutaneous diskectomy using the Dekompressor device is to remove the nucleus pulposus. A diskogram is suggested. The Dekompressor probe (Stryker, Kalamazoo, Mich.) is introduced through a coaxial 17-gauge trocar into the nucleus pulposus. The trocar can be curved manually if the access is difficult, especially when the herniated disk is at level L5-S1. After switching on the rotating engine, the probe is moved forward and backward, gradually removing tissue (Fig. 161-3). The procedure is complete when there is no more material to extract or when the radiologist feels satisfactory decompression has been obtained. The lumbar percutaneous diskectomy Dekompressor technique can be performed under CT or fluoroscopic guidance without technique limitations, but if it is performed with fluoroscopy guidance in patients in prone position, a posterolateral approach is needed to access the disk, using the lateral foramen as a landmark. The location of the hernia is the most important parameter for the efficacy of therapy. Indications are central or posterolateral and foraminal or extraforaminal herniated disk. Symptom reduction is better than 70% in 79% of foraminal posterolateral or extraforaminal hernia. This technique offers many advantages:

- The caliber of the probe is only 16 gauge (1.5 mm), reducing the risk of damage to the longitudinal posterior ligament and the annulus.
- The probe and trocar can be curved manually for difficult approaches.
- The probe rotation system allows nucleus aspiration not only in cases of central or paracentral herniation but also in cases of foraminal and extraforaminal herniated disk without root damage.
- Removing fewer than 3 cm of disk material results in a significant pressure decrease on the peripheral disk portion, resolving the disk-radicular conflict. Success is achieved in 70% to 79% of cases. Three cases of broken probes have been reported.[22-24]

Chemodiscolysis with O_2-O_3 Mixture with Periradicular and Periganglionic Infiltration

Ozone is an unstable, colorless, irritating gas with a sharp odor, oxidative power, and antiseptic, disinfectant, and antiviral properties. It is prepared and used in real time,

transforming a small percentage of O_2 to O_3 by special generators. The O_2-O_3 mixture is injected into the intradiscal space and foramen: 3 to 4 mL into the disk and 10 mL into the foramen. For treating the disk, 30 to 40 μm/mL is reported to be the best concentration to dehydrate the nucleus and reduce inflammation. The rationale is that the pain is due to mechanical compression on the root, with associated inflammatory changes in perigangliar and periradicular spaces. With the patient in prone position, the technique is usually performed under CT guidance for better evaluation of gas distribution into the disk or perigangliar space. The technique can also be performed under fluoroscopic guidance to control intradiscal or canal gas distribution. A needle is inserted into the nucleus pulposus (18-20 gauge, 7-10 cm length) by an oblique paravertebral approach, using the specific articular facet as a target (Fig. 161-4). Sometimes (especially at the L5-S1 level), when the "classic" oblique approach could be difficult for anatomic reasons, a further needle inclination of 30 degrees in the craniocaudal direction is necessary to reach the specific disk space, or a translaminar medial approach should be performed without fear of crossing the dural sac to reach the vertebral disk (Figs. 161-5 and 161-6). The needle is placed into the center of the disk, the gas mixture is slowly injected into the nucleus pulposus, then into the epidural and intraforaminal spaces, with a local antiinflammatory effect. Extruded herniated disk or free herniated fragments are contraindications. Diskography is not needed because it adds no diagnostic information necessary for the treatment and may affect the impact of the ozone gas. The oxygen-ozone mechanisms of action have been investigated and include:

- Antiinflammatory effect due to oxidative action on the chemical pain mediators
- Improvement of capillary blood perfusion and resolution of venous stasis, with better tissue oxygenation and reduction of root edema
- Direct action (through the oxygenation process) on the watery mucopolysaccharides of the nucleus pulposus, with secondary disk dehydration

No damage is reported if the O_2-O_3 goes into cerebrospinal fluid or the subarachnoid space. Success is reported in 70% to 80% of cases. No early or late neurologic or infectious complications have been reported following O_2-O_3 injection. A recent meta-analysis evaluating effectiveness and safety of ozone treatments for herniated lumbar disks

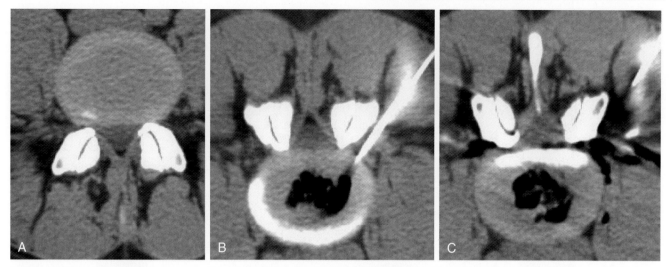

FIGURE 161-4. A, The Axial CT shows a mild protrusion at level L4-L5 in patien affected by right cruralgia. **B,** the Axial CT in patient in prone position shows a good distribution of O2-O3 gas in the centre of the disk and in right intraforaminal and perigangliar space **(C).**

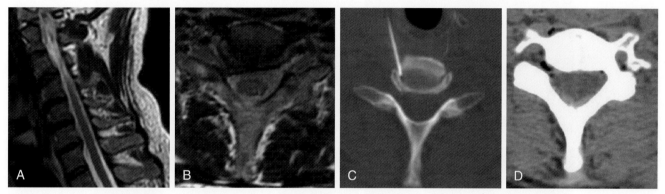

FIGURE 161-5. A, The Sagittal T2W MRI and the Axial **(B)** T1W MRI show a postero-lateral and right intraforaminal herniated disk at level C6-C7. **C,** The axial CT control shows the correct position of the needle into C6-C7 disk with right anterolateral approach. **D,** The axial CT post-treatment control shows the O2-O3 gas distribution into right foraminal space.

shows that pain and function outcomes are similar to the outcomes for lumbar disks treated with surgical diskectomy, but the complication rate is much lower (<0.1%), and recovery time is significantly shorter.[25-37]

Jellified Ethyl Alcohol (DiscoGel)

Jellified ethyl alcohol is a sterile viscous solution containing 96% pure ethyl alcohol, a cellulose derivative product, and an added radiopaque element, tungsten, that when injected into the vertebral disk at the cervical or lumbar level produces local necrosis of the nucleus pulposus. Its action is mechanical via dehydration of the turgescent protruding disk compressing the peripheral nerves of the cord and causing extreme pain. Using sterile technique and local anesthesia, the product is injected into the nucleus pulposus under CT or fluoroscopy guidance, with a posterolateral approach for the thoracic or lumbar level and an anterolateral approach for the cervical level. Preferably the disk is punctured using a small needle:

* 18 gauge for thoracic and lumbar disks, so as to reach the central region of the intraspinal space (Fig. 161-7)
* 20 gauge for cervical disks (Fig. 161-8)

The quantity of jellified ethyl alcohol injected varies between 0.2 and 0.8 mL, according to the dimension of the disk and extent of the hernia. Recommendations are:

* 0.2 mL of jellified ethyl alcohol for cervical disks
* 0.3 to 0.5 mL of jellified ethyl alcohol for thoracic disks
* 0.6 to 0.8 mL of jellified ethyl alcohol for lumbar disks

At the beginning of the injection, the patient may experience a transitional scalding sensation in the region of the injection, which disappears during the course of injection. To minimize this risk, the product must be injected very slowly. Once the product has been injected, the needle is left 2 minutes before being withdrawn. The viscosity of jellified ethyl alcohol depends on the temperature. If the product is warmed above room temperature, it becomes more liquid and is below optimum viscosity for injection. To increase its viscosity, jellified ethyl alcohol can be refrigerated just prior to injection. This agent is contraindicated in pregnant women, patients known to be allergic to one of its components, and patients in severe depression or any other condition making the interpretation of pain difficult. Experimental studies performed on pigs showed that injecting DiscoGel intradiscally, intraforaminally, epidurally, and intramuscularly produced no changes when the gel came in

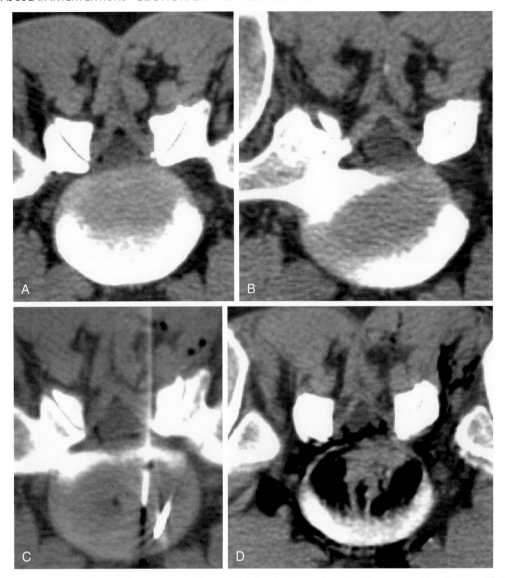

FIGURE 161-6. A-B, The axial CT show a right intraforaminal herniated disk at level L5-S1 in patient in prone position. **C,** The axial CT show one needle into L5-S1 disk by right translaminal approach and the another ones by right posterolateral approach. **D,** the post-treatment axial CT shows the O2-O3 gas distribution into disk and in the foraminal and gangliar spaces.

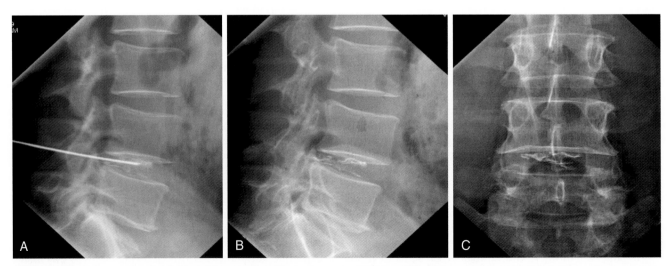

FIGURE 161-7. A, Laterolateral (LL) view of fluoroscopic guidance of correct positioning of DiscoGel needle into L4-L5 disk. **B-C,** LL and anteroposterior fluoroscopy after DiscoGel injection.

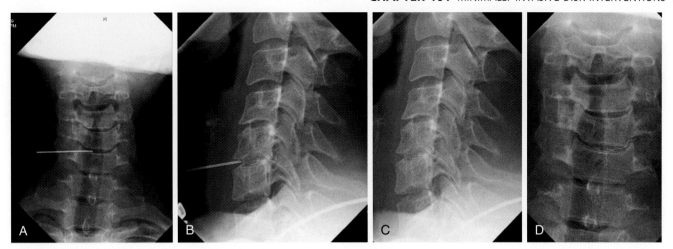

FIGURE 161-8. **A,** Anteroposterior (AP) view of fluoroscopic guidance of correct positioning of DiscoGel needle into C5-C6 disk. **B,** Laterolateral (LL) view of fluoroscopic guidance of correct positioning of DiscoGel needle into C5-C6 disk. **C,** LL fluoroscopy after DiscoGel injection. **D,** AP fluoroscopy after DiscoGel injection.

contact with nervous system structures or muscle tissue. In fact, no tissue alteration was found aside from inflammatory elements like lymphomonocyte cells and venous stasis, with same granular material staining black by the hematoxylin-eosin method (tungsten) in paravertebral tissue in muscular and connective tissue. The success rate is between 89% and 91% of cases, with no minor or major complications.[38-41]

Which Percutaneous Disk Treatment Do You Choose?

Clinical and diagnostic imaging selection criteria are very important to avoid overtreatment. Surgical indications have been previously discussed and should always be respected to exclude medicolegal problems. Our first choice is always intradiscal-intraforaminal CT-guided oxygen-ozone injection; this is related to its utility, reproducibility, rate of success, rate of complications, and lower cost. If this technique fails, we usually attempt a different technique. If LBP with radicular pain is prevalent, we suggest nucleo-plasty; if LBP with radiculopathy is prevalent, we suggest DiscoGel.

KEY POINTS

- Minimally invasive techniques can be a valuable alternative to traditional surgery, with low cost, low risk of complications, high utility, and high reproducibility, without preventing surgery at later date if they should fail.

- All techniques can be performed under computed tomography or fluoroscopic guidance with patients in prone position and under local anesthesia; a short period of hospitalization is necessary.
- All procedures can be performed at the cervical or lumbar level.
- The rationale for all percutaneous treatments is to reduce intradiscal pressure by creating the space required for retropulsion or digestion of the disk.
- Surgery remains indicated in emergency cases of neurologic deficit or severe low back pain.

▶ SUGGESTED READINGS

Gangi A, Dietemann JL, Mortazavi R, et al. CT-guided interventional procedures for pain management in the lumbosacral spine. Radiographics 1998;18(3):621–33.

Long DM. Decision making in lumbar disc disease. Clinical Neurosurg 1991;39:36–51.

Mathews RS. Automated percutaneous lumbar discectomy. In: Savitz MH, Chin JC, Yeung AT, editors. The practice of minimally invasive spinal technique. Richmond: AAMISMS Education LLC; 2000. p. 97–100.

Theron J, Cuellar H, Sola T, et al. Percutaneous treatment of cervical disk hernias using gelified ethanol. AJNR Am J Neuroradiol 2010;31: 1454–56.

Von Tulder MW, Koes BW, Bouter LM. Conservative treatment of acute and chronic non-specific low back pain. Spine 1997;22:2128–56.

The complete reference list is available online at www.expertconsult.com.

CHAPTER 162

Chemical and Thermal Ablation of Desmoid Tumors

David S. Pryluck, Joseph P. Erinjeri, and Timothy W.I. Clark

Desmoid tumors, or aggressive fibromatosis, are low-grade sarcomas composed of highly differentiated monoclonal fibroblasts with extensive collagen overgrowth. The incidence of sporadic desmoid tumors in the general population is estimated at two to five persons per million per year. Desmoids occur in 16% to 20% of patients with familial adenomatous polyposis (FAP) syndromes such as Gardner syndrome and produce significant morbidity. Desmoids are the second most common cause of death in patients with FAP, after colon cancer. Along with FAP, risk factors for desmoid tumors include surgical trauma, female gender, parity, bone malformations, and connective tissue disorders. Genetic risk has been associated with a mutation in the APC-β-catenin-Tcf pathway in both sporadic and FAP-associated desmoid tumors. Stabilization of β-catenin-Tcf in transgenic murine models has been shown to produce desmoids in 75% of unwounded animals after 3 months and excessive fibroblast proliferation in 100% of mice with cutaneous wounds after only 24 days.

Desmoid tumors are locally infiltrative, and although they rarely metastasize, extensive morbidity and even mortality can occur from compression of adjacent organs. Growth of desmoids is characterized by extension along fascial planes with invasion of neurovascular structures (Fig. 162-1, A). Primary surgical treatment consists of wide excision or limb amputation. Recurrence develops in 25% to 70% of cases despite tumor-free margins, often within several months after resection. In approximately 90% of patients with positive margins, disease rapidly recurs within several months after resection.

Therapy for desmoid tumors is extremely challenging and limited by the wide spectrum of the condition. The majority of the published literature is confined to single case reports, with a paucity of prospective studies.

Percutaneous image-guided techniques including chemical ablation, cryoablation, and radiofrequency ablation (RFA) are now being utilized as part of an interdisciplinary approach to treating desmoid tumors. These techniques, which have routinely been used in the treatment of hepatic, renal, and osseous neoplasms, may be uniquely suited for many of the challenges encountered in the treatment of desmoid tumors, and can be used as a primary treatment modality, an adjunct to chemotherapy or radiation, or as salvage therapy following postsurgical recurrence. The underlying goal should be improvement of pain and function in each patient. This chapter will discuss the mechanism of action, technical and clinical considerations, and a brief review of the existing medical literature for each technique as applied to the treatment of desmoid tumors.

CHEMICAL ABLATION

Percutaneous chemical ablation with 50% acetic acid or absolute ethanol has been used for in situ destruction of desmoid tumors (Fig. 162-2, B). The cytotoxic effects of acetic acid are derived from protein desiccation, lipid dissolution, and collagen extraction, whereas those of ethanol are attributed to cytoplasmic dehydration, denaturation of cellular proteins, and small vessel thrombosis. These effects culminate in coagulative necrosis indistinguishable from thermal ablation techniques. Instances of significant tumor reduction have been observed after even a single session of chemical ablation, suggesting that other mechanisms such as apoptosis or immune-modulated tumor destruction may also play a role in tumor regression.

Indications

Indications for percutaneous chemical ablation include:
- Biopsy-proven desmoid tumor
- Enlarging or symptomatic desmoid tumor (pain, limitation of limb motion), or recurrent tumor after previous surgical excision
- Percutaneously accessible without traversing lung, bowel, or other vital organs
- Lack of invasion of a major neurovascular structure or a vital organ within the intended treatment area
- Desmoid tumor 10 cm or less in maximum diameter by RECIST (Response Evaluation Criteria in Solid Tumors) criteria

Contraindications

- Neurovascular encasement within the intended treatment area
- Infiltration of vital structures, such as tumor encasement of bowel, ureter, aorta, and inferior vena cava. Desmoid tumors that abut but do not encase vital structures may be treated.
- Intercurrent infection
- Uncorrectable coagulopathy
- Pregnancy

Equipment

Devices needed for percutaneous chemical ablation of desmoid tumors are readily available in most interventional radiology practices and include:

Infusion Needle
Use of an infusion needle (e.g., Bernardino needle [Cook Inc., Bloomington, IN]) may have an advantage in that it has a conical tip with multiple side holes to permit diffusion and dispersal of the chemical agent. However, chemical ablation may also be performed with conventional 20- to 22-gauge Chiba-type needles. The extremely fibrous consistency of desmoid tumors makes needle insertion difficult, often producing bending or buckling of needles.

Injection System

The injection system consists of low-pressure connection tubing, a 1-mL calibrated polycarbonate Luer-Lok syringe, a 20-mL polycarbonate syringe as a reservoir for the chemical agent (i.e., 50% acetic acid), and a 3-way stopcock to enable refilling of the 1-mL syringe from the reservoir syringe during the treatment session.

Imaging

Real-time ultrasound with a high-resolution linear array transducer is optimal. This has the advantage of being able to monitor both real-time insertion of the infusion needle into the center of the tumor and chemical agent dispersal during injection to minimize the risk of nontarget tissue injury. If the tumor is not in an anatomic location accessible to ultrasound, percutaneous chemical ablation can also be performed with computed tomography (CT) or magnetic resonance imaging (MRI) guidance. In this imaging situation, the diffusion of acetic acid or ethanol will appear as a low-attenuation zone within the center of the lesion when CT is used or as a high–signal intensity zone within the center of the tumor on long TR (repetition time) sequences when MRI is used.

Technique

Anatomy and Approach

Chemical ablation of desmoid tumors involves targeting the center of the tumor through a percutaneous window that does not traverse collateral structures. Desmoid tumors may be oblong or irregular in shape and require insertion of more than one needle during the treatment session. Acetic acid is prepared in the hospital pharmacy by combining 10 mL of glacial acetic acid (U.S. Pharmacopeia) with 10 mL of sterile water. The resultant solution of 50% acetic acid is filtered through a Millex-GV 0.22-μm filter (Millipore, Bedford, MA) to ensure sterility. This solution is then delivered to the interventional radiology department in a stoppered sterile glass bottle. Patients must be informed

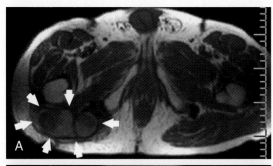
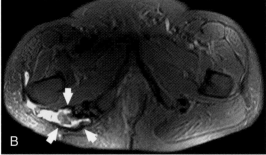

FIGURE 162-1. A, Axial magnetic resonance imaging (MRI) showing 9-cm gluteal desmoid tumor *(arrows)* that developed after wide excision. Tumor was producing a mass effect on sciatic nerve but was not encasing it. **B,** Axial T2-weighted MRI after three sessions of chemical ablation with acetic acid. Tumor was reduced to 2.5 cm *(arrows)* with some surrounding edema. Patient's pain and sciatica resolved.

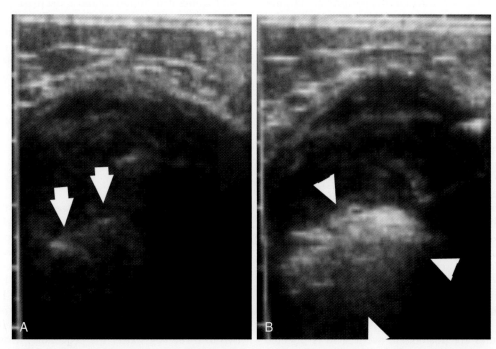

FIGURE 162-2. A, Ultrasound image of 8-cm upper extremity hypoechoic desmoid tumor after insertion of infusion needle *(arrows)* into center of tumor. **B,** Ultrasound image immediately after gradual injection of 2.5 mL of 50% acetic acid over a 5-minute period. Large hyperechoic area has formed around needle tip *(arrowheads)*.

that acetic acid is not approved for injection by the U.S. Food and Drug Administration (FDA), although it is used in various medical applications, including as a buffering agent for dialysate solutions and for diagnostic purposes during colposcopy to detect and characterize cervical lesions.

Infusion needles are positioned in the desmoid tumor under local anesthesia. Patients also receive conscious sedation (intravenous midazolam and fentanyl citrate) during the procedure for local pain during the injection. With ultrasound, the needles are positioned within the central core of the tumor before injection of the chemical agent.

After positioning of one to three needles within the center of the desmoid tumor, acetic acid is infused. Real-time ultrasound monitoring is preferable. *It is vital that an extremely slow rate of infusion be used.* For this reason, a calibrated 1-mL Luer-Lok syringe is helpful. This enables the operator to accurately monitor the rate and pressure of injection. Generally, acetic acid is injected at a rate of approximately 0.1 mL per 15 to 20 seconds. A rapid burst of the agent is undesirable; rather, the technique relies on steady and gradual dispersal of the agent. As acetic acid penetrates through the tumor, the baseline hypoechoic echotexture of the tumor will become immediately hyperechoic (see Fig. 162-2). Further injection is performed as the needle is slowly withdrawn away from the central core of the tumor in an attempt to render the inner aspect of the tumor as uniformly echogenic as possible. The volume of acetic acid during an individual treatment session is divided between the additional infusion needles. In total, no more than 10 mL of acetic acid is injected in a single treatment session. Even large tumors may require a much smaller volume than this to produce a large area of echogenicity in the tumor. Because desmoids are not encapsulated, great care must be taken to not allow extravasation of the agent through the interstices of the tumor. Care is also taken to ensure distribution of acetic acid in the peripheral margins. If the periphery of the tumor becomes hyperechoic during the injection, the infusion is stopped, and the needle is either repositioned or withdrawn.

All patients are given a dose of broad-spectrum parenteral antibiotic at the time of the procedure. Patients are discharged home after a period of 4 hours of observation and then seen back in the interventional radiology clinic the day after the procedure to assess overlying skin integrity and evaluate for local changes of tumor inflammation.

It is important to use a staged approach to therapy. Treatment sessions are spaced 4 to 5 weeks apart.

Technical Aspects
- Real-time ultrasound monitoring during chemical ablation is preferable.
- A single intravenous dose of a broad-spectrum antibiotic (e.g., cefazolin, vancomycin) is given.
- Conscious sedation is achieved with intravenous fentanyl citrate and midazolam.
- One to three needles (Bernardino, Chiba) are positioned within the center of the desmoid tumor under local anesthesia.
- Once the needles are positioned, acetic acid is injected through a single needle at a rate of approximately 0.1 mL per 15 to 20 seconds via a calibrated 1-mL Luer-Lok syringe.

- The desmoid tumor will change from a hypoechoic appearance to a bright echotexture during injection.
- The injection is performed to a sonographic endpoint to render the central two thirds of the tumor as uniformly echogenic as possible.
- Further injection is performed as the needle is slowly withdrawn away from the central core of the tumor in an attempt to render the inner aspect of the tumor as uniformly echogenic as possible.
- The needle is removed after aspiration to minimize seepage of acetic acid during tumor withdrawal.
- The same process is repeated with the remaining needle or needles.
- In total, no more than 10 mL of 50% acetic acid is injected during a single treatment session.
- When needles are reinserted during subsequent treatment sessions, brownish sterile fluid from necrotic tumor tissue as a result of previous treatment may be encountered. This fluid is aspirated before injection of additional acetic acid.

Outcomes

After our initial description of one partial response and a sustained complete response in two patients, we have performed approximately 60 additional treatment sessions of percutaneous chemical ablation in 20 cumulative patients. Our unpublished observations, including logistic regression of CT and MRI volumetric analysis of tumor regression patterns after chemical ablation, have shown that 60% of patients have a mean decrease in tumor volume of 30%. A subset of these patients will experience more dramatic responses, including those with complete resolution of enhancing tumor tissue on follow-up MRI. Parallel to a reduction in tumor size, these patients also experience improvement in function and a decrease in pain, many of whom required daily oral or transdermal narcotic analgesics (or both) before ablation. Moreover, these patients will no longer have central enhancement of their tumor on T1-weighted gadolinium-enhanced MRI. However, we currently limit treatment to patients with desmoid tumors that are 10 cm or less in maximum diameter and those who have a tumor located in an area that is percutaneously accessible without evidence of encasement of a major neurovascular structure or vital organ.

Complications

Complications relate to nontarget injury to skin, nerves, adjacent organs, and blood vessels. Infection can also develop within necrotic areas of the desmoid. Any patient in whom fever develops after percutaneous chemical ablation should be evaluated for an intratumoral abscess. Additional complications include transient hemoglobinuria from the effect of intravascular acetic acid, local erythema, and tenderness for several days after the chemical ablation session. The hemoglobinuria is mild and resolves within two to three voids after the procedure. Most patients also experience classic symptoms of postablation syndrome to a variable degree that are manifested as fever up to 101°F, local pain and tenderness, fatigue, and malaise. Patients in whom a skin burn develops require topical sulfonamide cream and plastic surgery consultation.

In our series, major complications occurred in three sessions (5%), including two patients in whom third-degree burns developed but resolved with wound care by a plastic surgeon; these patients did not require a skin graft, and their desmoid tumors decreased in size. An intratumoral abscess developed in another patient and required percutaneous drainage and several weeks of parenteral antibiotics.

THERMAL ABLATION

Thermal ablation, which includes percutaneous cryoablation and RFA, has also been used for in situ destruction of desmoid tumors. Cryoablation uses alternating cycles of rapid freezing and warming within a target tissue; rapid freezing induces formation of intracellular and extracellular ice crystals within the treated tissue, resulting in cellular injury. RFA uses high-frequency alternating current passed from an electrode into the surrounding tissue, which induces frictional heating, protein denaturation, and hydrolysis, resulting in cellular injury. For both cryoablation and RFA, thermal-induced cytotoxicity ultimately results in coagulative necrosis with eventual fibrosis and scarring.

Indications

Indications for percutaneous thermal ablation include:
• Biopsy-proven desmoid tumor
• Enlarging or symptomatic desmoid tumor (pain, limitation of limb motion) or recurrent tumor after previous surgical excision
• Percutaneously accessible without traversing lung, bowel, or other vital organs
• Lack of invasion of a major neurovascular structure or a vital organ within the intended treatment area

Contraindications

• Superficial tumors less than 1 cm subjacent to overlying skin
• Infiltration of vital structures, such as tumor encasement of bowel, ureters, aorta, and inferior vena cava
• RFA for desmoid tumors located within 1 cm of a vital structure (cryoablation may be possible in this situation)
• Neurovascular encasement within the intended treatment area
• Concurrent infection
• Uncorrectable coagulopathy
• Pregnancy

Equipment

Cryoprobes and Cryoablation Systems

Percutaneous cryoablation of desmoid tumors is performed using one or multiple cryoprobes inserted into the lesion under CT or ultrasound guidance. A cryoprobe is a modified hollow needle that functions as a high-pressure, closed-loop, gas expansion system. Rapid cooling and warming of the cryoprobe tip is achieved with the *Joule-Thompson effect*, by which rapid adiabatic expansion of a gas results in a change in temperature of the gas. When rapidly expanded at room temperature, gases such as argon and nitrogen exhibit Joule-Thompson cooling, while gases such as helium and hydrogen exhibit Joule-Thompson warming. These observations are the basis for current cryoablation techniques: rapid freezing of the cryoprobe tip using argon gas and rapid warming of the cryoprobe tip using helium gas.

Radiofrequency Ablation Electrodes and Systems

RFA systems include three basic elements: a power generator, one or multiple RF electrodes connected to the generator via a wire attachment, and grounding pads, which are attached to the patient's upper thighs and also connected to the generator via a wire attachment. Electrodes are modified needles, typically 14 to 17 gauge in diameter, that are inserted into the lesion under CT or ultrasound guidance. Electrodes function as the cathode in a closed electrical circuit; RF current travels from the generator to the electrode positioned within a tumor, through the patient toward the skin pads, and then back to the generator to complete the circuit. As RF current passes through the electrode, frictional energy is dissipated from the electrode tip into the surrounding tissues, resulting in local energy disposition and tissue burning.

Multiple RF systems and electrode configurations are commercially available in the United States. Currently available generators achieve outputs of up to 250 W. RF electrodes may be a single needle tip design or have multiple deployable prongs emanating from a central cannula at the electrode tip that create an umbrella-like configuration when deployed within a lesion. This multiprong configuration enables a larger, more reproducible ablation volume.

Imaging

Thermal ablation of desmoid tumors is typically performed using real-time CT or ultrasound guidance, both for probe placement and intraprocedural monitoring of the ablation zone. CT guidance for cryoablation has the advantage of guiding cryoprobe placement into the intended orientation and position within a lesion and direct visualization of iceball formation within the treatment zone. Using CT, the iceball will appear as a defined oblong or spherical low-attenuation region surrounding the cryoprobe active tip. If the lesion is not in an anatomic location accessible using CT guidance, real-time ultrasound can also be used. The iceball will appear as a brightly echogenic zone surrounding the cryoprobe active tip. As with cryoablation, CT has the advantage of guiding RFA probe placement into a lesion, as well as directly visualizing the position of ablation probe tines post deployment. Unlike with cryoablation, however, a clearly defined treatment zone cannot reliably be discerned using CT monitoring for RFA. Treated tissues may demonstrate a subtle decrease in attenuation following RFA, but this hypoattenuation, if present, is often too subtle to consistently determine the margins of a treatment zone. Real-time ultrasound monitoring during RFA is similarly limited because small foci of gas generated within treated tissues during burning can act as specular

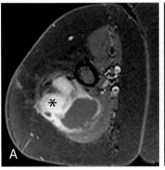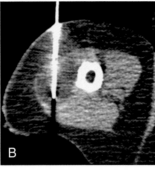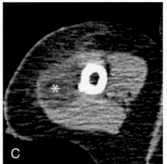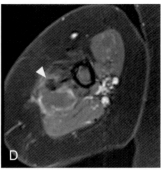

FIGURE 162-3. Percutaneous cryoablation of right upper extremity desmoid tumor in 44-year-old woman after prior percutaneous chemical ablation. **A,** Axial postcontrast T1-weighted magnetic resonance imaging (MRI) with fat suppression demonstrates right upper extremity desmoid tumor with lateral enhancing (*) and medial nonenhancing components, interposed between deltoid and triceps muscles. **B,** Under computed tomography guidance, two cryoprobes (Perc-17 [Endocare Inc., Irvine, Calif.]) were advanced into mass using posterolateral approach. A 10-minute freeze was performed, followed by an 8-minute active thaw, followed by a second 5-minute freeze. A single cryoprobe with real-time visualization of hypodense iceball formation is demonstrated in this image. **C,** Cryoprobes have been removed, and hypodense intratumoral iceball remains (*). **D,** Axial postcontrast T1-weighted spin echo with fat suppression MRI following three cryoablation treatment sessions over a 12-month time interval demonstrates marked decrease in tumor size and enhancement.

reflectors that scatter ultrasound beams, causing image distortion.

Technique

Anatomy and Approach

Cryoablation and RFA of desmoid tumors involve targeting the entirety of the lesion by creating ablation zones using one or multiple ablation probes inserted within the tumor. Ideally, the ablation zone will extend to at least 5 to 10 mm beyond the perceived border of the lesion to ensure an adequate kill zone and negative ablation margin. By using multiple ablation probes combined in series or in parallel, large lesions can be ablated in a single treatment session, as well as lesions that are oblong or irregular in shape that may extend beyond the ablation zone generated by a single probe. If using multipronged probes for RFA, particular care during prong deployment is necessary; the fibrous nature of the desmoid tumor can cause the prongs to bend or buckle. CT or ultrasound is used to confirm appropriate probe positioning prior to initiation of ablation.

Cryoprobes and RFA probes are inserted into the desmoid tumor under local anesthesia using CT or ultrasound guidance (Fig. 162-3). Although general anesthesia has been used in published reports of cryoablation and RFA, our patients typically receive conscious sedation (intravenous midazolam and fentanyl citrate) during the procedure for local pain during the ablation, with general anesthesia reserved for cases with extenuating circumstances. Such cases may include, for example, a pediatric patient who may experience difficulty remaining motionless during the ablation procedure. Interestingly, because of the inherent anesthetic effect of freezing, less sedation is typically required during cryoablation compared to either chemical ablation or RFA. Adequate sedation during RFA prior to commencement of burning is essential, because RFA can induce significant local pain for the patient, leading to increased anxiety, patient motion, and potential probe movement and dislodgement.

Cryoablation of desmoid tumors is typically performed with alternating cycles of an active freeze, followed by a passive thaw, followed by an additional active freeze (see Fig. 162-3). Endpoints of duration of each freeze/thaw cycle, as well as target temperature, are based upon previously determined treatment algorithms and may vary among device manufacturers. In published reports by Kujak et al., cryoablation was performed with a 10-minute initial freeze, followed by an 8-minute thaw, and then a second active freeze of 10 to 20 minutes. Current cryoablation systems use argon as the freezing agent, which can reach temperatures of as low as −186°C during active freezing. Intermittent monitoring of iceball formation during active freeze cycles is usually performed using noncontrast CT imaging.

RFA is performed as single or multiple sequential burns, depending upon the size and shape of the tumor being treated. Ablations are performed using predetermined endpoints of time, power, and temperature, which may vary among system manufacturers. In a published case report by Tsz-Kan et al. in which a desmoid tumor was treated with two sequential burns using four puncture sites (eight total ablations), primary ablations were performed with an initial RF power of 10 W, increased by 5 W every 2 minutes until a maximum power of 60 W, and the ablation was sustained until the maximum impedance was reached. Secondary ablations using the same puncture sites were performed with an initial power of 20 W, increased by 5 W every 1 minute until a maximum power of 60 W. In published reports by Ilaslan et al., ablations were performed for 10-minute intervals, with a target power of 50 W and temperature of 105°C.

All patients are given a dose of broad-spectrum parenteral antibiotic at the time of the procedure. Patients are discharged home after a period of 4 hours of observation and then seen back in the interventional radiology clinic the day after the procedure to assess overlying skin integrity and evaluate for local changes of tumor inflammation.

As with chemical ablation, it is important to use a staged approach to therapy. The need for additional treatment sessions will depend on an individual patient's response to initial ablation, and subsequent ablations should be spaced 4 to 8 weeks apart.

Technical Aspects

- One or multiple cryoprobes or RFA electrodes are positioned within the desmoid tumor under local anesthesia.
- CT is typically used to confirm appropriate cryoprobe or RFA electrode positioning prior to commencement of ablation.
- Conscious sedation is achieved with intravenous fentanyl citrate and midazolam.
- General anesthesia is reserved for selected cases (e.g., pediatric patients).
- Intermittent real-time CT monitoring during cryoablation is preferable; iceball formation can be used as an approximation of the effective kill zone.
- Real-time monitoring of RFA is limited with both CT and ultrasound.
- A single intravenous dose of a broad-spectrum antibiotic (e.g., cefazolin, vancomycin) is given.
- Cryoablation is performed in alternating cycles of initial active freezing, thawing, and refreezing, to endpoints of temperature and time based upon a predetermined treatment algorithm that may vary among cryoablation systems (10-minute initial freeze, 8-minute thaw, 10- to 20-minute refreeze in published reports).
- RFA is performed using predetermined endpoints of maximum power (50-60 W in published reports) to reach maximum impedance. Endpoints of time and temperature have also been used (10 minutes and 105°C in published reports).

Outcomes

The existing medical literature describing use of thermal ablation to treat desmoid tumors is limited to a single retrospective case series for cryoablation and a retrospective case report and case series for RFA. Kujak et al. described five patients with painful extraabdominal desmoid tumors treated with cryoablation, including a 9-year-old girl with a 3-cm lower back desmoid that recurred following prior surgery and chemotherapy; a 32-year-old woman with a 4.9-cm right scapular desmoid previously treated with chemotherapy; a 41-year-old woman with a 6.1-cm left scapular desmoid previously treated with chemotherapy; a 21-year-old man with a history of FAP and a 9.1-cm chest wall desmoid that invaded several thoracic neural foramina and encased several spinal nerve roots and recurred following prior surgery; and an 18-year-old young man with a history of FAP and a 10-cm desmoid tumor that involved the left posterior neck, supraclavicular, and axillary regions, including the brachial plexus and subclavian vessels, and had failed prior surgical resection, chemotherapy, and radiation therapy. The former three patients were referred for local tumor control, and complete tumor coverage by the cryoablation zones was achieved. The latter two patients were referred for palliation of pain symptoms caused by inoperable lesions that had encased major neural structures. Incomplete tumor coverage with the cryoablation zones

occurred in these two cases to protect involved nerves from thermal injury.

Positive long-term results were reported in the three patients in whom complete tumor ablation was achieved, including pain relief and diminution in tumor size; complete tumor regression was reported in two patients. For the remaining two patients with neural encasement by tumor, partial pain relief was initially observed 2 weeks following cryoablation. At long-term follow-up however, although one lesion had decreased in size from 9.1 cm to 4.9 cm at 58 months, the other lesion that initially measured 10 cm had enlarged at 36 months, with marked growth of the untreated portions. Also, local pain symptoms returned to pretreatment moderate levels for both patients. Additional ablations were not pursued in either case.

Tsz-Kan et al. described the use of RFA to treat a lower back desmoid tumor that recurred 4 months after surgery in a 47-year-old woman. Under CT guidance, eight ablations were performed via four puncture sites using a 15-gauge active expandable needle electrode. Serial follow-up MRI demonstrated progressive diminution in tumor size; no evidence of residual tumor was seen at 28 months' follow-up.

Ilaslan et al. reported using RFA to treat five desmoid tumors in four patients: a 59-year-old woman with recurrent desmoid tumors of the right calf and thigh following resection, re-resection, and radiation; a 5-year-old boy with Gardner syndrome and a recurrent left paraspinal desmoid following excisional biopsy; a 14-year-old girl with an enlarging left hip desmoid; and a 32-year-old man with a paraspinal desmoid. For the latter two patients, RFA was the initial therapy. In the case of the 14-year-old girl with the left hip desmoid, the mass was deeply embedded within the adjacent musculature. RFA was selected rather than surgery because of the lesion's location, size, and potential functional morbidity from surgical resection. Three lesions were less than 3 cm and required one ablation each; the two remaining lesions were larger than 3 cm, and required up to four ablations each, with intermittent electrode repositioning. Approximately 1 to 2 cm of normal adjacent tissue was included in the ablation zone. Clinical follow-up for all four patients and MRI follow-up for two patients demonstrated no evidence of desmoid tumor recurrence following RFA.

Complications

Similar to chemical ablation, potential complications of thermal ablation include nontarget injury to skin, nerves, adjacent organs, and blood vessels. Patients with superficial lesions located immediately subjacent to overlying skin are at particular risk for cutaneous thermal injury. In the case series presented by Ilaslan et al., one patient developed focal soft-tissue necrosis that required surgical débridement and skin grafting. Several techniques can be implemented during ablation to mitigate this risk, including thickening of the overlying skin with saline injections and cooling or warming of the skin overlying the ablation site. The risk of grounding pad burns is unique to RFA, and correct placement of these pads should be ensured prior to commencement of ablation. Patients in whom a skin burn develops require topical sulfonamide cream and plastic surgery consultation.

As with chemical ablation, infection can develop within necrotic areas of the desmoid following thermal ablation. If fever develops 4 days or more after percutaneous thermal ablation, the patient should be evaluated for an intratumoral abscess. In the case report presented by Tsz-Kan et al., the patient developed an abscess at the site of tumor necrosis during the first week after ablation that required catheter drainage and antibiotics. Some patients will experience classic symptoms of postablation syndrome to a variable degree within the first 48 hours following ablation, manifested as fever up to 101°F, local pain and tenderness, fatigue, and malaise. Other potential complications of thermal ablation include hemorrhage, tumor seeding from needle electrode placement and manipulation, and pneumothorax.

Postprocedural and Follow-up Care

Following percutaneous chemical and thermal ablation, all patients are discharged home with a prescription for oral narcotic analgesics. Postprocedural antibiotics are not routinely given. Patients will often supplement their oral narcotic analgesic with a nonsteroidal antiinflammatory agent. In general, following chemical ablation, patients are not reassessed with imaging until they have undergone a series of treatment sessions, typically 3 to 4 sessions 4 to 5 weeks apart. Patients are then re-imaged about 4 weeks after the final procedure, ideally with gadolinium-enhanced MRI. In general, following cryoablation or RFA, patients are re-imaged 4 weeks after each treatment session, also ideally with gadolinium-enhanced MRI. For chemical and thermal ablation, the imaging endpoint of treatment is conversion of the tumor to a low–signal intensity lesion on T1-weighted images, with lack of contrast enhancement after administration of gadolinium. Areas of edema and necrosis can form within a successfully treated desmoid tumor and produce areas of high signal intensity on long TR–weighted sequences.

A small subset of patients will require treatment again at some point in the future. Patients may remain at risk for developing desmoid tumors in new locations, particularly those with FAP and those who have previously undergone resection of desmoid tumors.

- Desmoid tumors (aggressive fibromatosis) are low-grade sarcomas.
- Sporadic desmoid tumors occur throughout the body, most commonly in the limbs, neck, trunk, or abdominal wall.
- In patients with familial adenomatous polyposis syndrome, the most common site is the abdominal mesentery or bowel wall.
- Treatment of desmoid tumors requires a multidisciplinary collaboration between the surgical oncologist, medical oncologist, interventional radiologist, and radiation oncologist.
- A staged approach is required for chemical and thermal ablation of desmoid tumors.
- Chemical ablation confines treatment to the center of the tumor.
- Cryoablation and radiofrequency ablation involve targeting the entirety of the tumor by creating ablation zones using one or multiple ablation probes.
- A decrease in desmoid size occurs gradually over a period of weeks to months.
- Gadolinium-enhanced magnetic resonance imaging is optimal for assessing tumor response to chemical and thermal ablation following treatment.
- Repeat treatment may be necessary months to years later if surveillance imaging shows a return of internal enhancement, clinical growth of the tumor, or both.

▶ SUGGESTED READINGS

Clark TW. Percutaneous chemical ablation of desmoid tumors. J Vasc Interv Radiol 2003;14:629–34.

Dahn I, Jonsson N, Lundh G. Desmoid tumors: a series of 33 cases. Acta Chir Scand 1963;126:305–14.

Hui GC, Tuncali K, Tatli S, et al. Comparison of percutaneous and surgical approaches to renal tumor ablation: metaanalysis of effectiveness and complication rates. J Vasc Interv Radiol 2008;19:1311–20.

Pignatti G, Barbanti-Brodano G, Ferrari D, et al. Extraabdominal desmoid tumor: a study of 83 cases. Clin Orthop Relat Res 2000;375:207–13.

The full list of Suggested Readings on this topic can be found at www.expertconsult.com.

CHAPTER **163**

Selective Nerve Root Block

L. Mark Dean

INTRODUCTION

Selective nerve root block (SNRB) is a fundamental technique used to perform regional anesthesia. This procedure is also used as a means for diagnosis and medical treatment. The physician attempts to prove that a particular nerve is the root source of the patient's symptoms by placing a needle adjacent to the nerve root sleeve as it emerges from the intervertebral foramen. The evaluation attempts to reproduce the patient's typical pain and then interrupt and alleviate the pain. This procedure is performed under the guidance of fluoroscopy, ultrasound, or computed tomography (CT) scan to confirm proper needle placement along the nerve root sleeve. This interventional procedure tests for the cause of pain that may be undiagnosed by magnetic resonance imaging (MRI), CT, discograms, and electromyograms.

The practice of recognizing and understanding dermatomal patterns has given practitioners the opportunity to better characterize pain and analyze the process of radicular pain. The understanding and application of techniques that interrupt pain from the neck, thorax, visceral organs, or lower extremities that can be adequately blocked at the spinal level continues to evolve.[1] As we better characterize pain patterns and as this process is readily adopted into clinical practice, the awareness of its efficacy will be more pervasive.[2]

This chapter attempts to place the practitioner within a standard, safe, and effective algorithm for the clinical evaluation of patients. Working through the patient's description of their symptoms, their behavior, and the pictures and pain diagrams they draw, the practitioner can determine the location and type of injection to be performed. This information will help practitioners who perform SNRB to determine the location or level for needle placement.

HISTORY

The creation and development of anesthetics has been an essential part of regional anesthetics. Since the proposition and theorization by Rene Descartes in the 17th century that physiologically there was a neural connection between the peripheral aspects of the body to the brain, doctrine has developed to confirm the transmission of nerve impulses.

ANATOMY

Tissues and Fascia

To perform SNRB, understanding the approach, location, and the layers of the tissue and fascia the needle must pass through gives the practitioner a higher level of safety and accuracy. The surrounding fascia, be it lipomatous or vascular, can affect selection of medication and determine whether adjuncts such as corticosteroids or vascular constrictors should be used. The location of the needle tip and selection of medications can greatly impact the efficacy of the injection and its perineural infiltration.

The brain continues as the spinal cord to T12 or L1 and is protected by the meninges and the bony vertebral column. The spinal meninges covering the cord is composed of the pia mater, arachnoid, and dura mater. Protection of the spinal cord is formed from 33 specialized vertebrae. The size of the central canal, the size of the alae, and curvature of the bones give the vertebrae functional ability and provide protection function to the cord and nerve roots (Fig. 163-1).

The neural foramen is the passageway for the spinal nerve as it exits the central canal. The anterior border of the foramen is framed by the uncovertebral joint and vertebral body. The pedicle of the vertebral body above supplies the roof, and the pedicle and lamina of the vertebrae below supplies the floor. The posterior aspect of the neural foramen is framed from the inferior and superior articular facets of the adjoining vertebrae (Fig. 163-2).

The spinal epidural space surrounds the cord and nerve roots and extends from the sacral hiatus inferiorly to the foramen magnum at the skull base. Between the epidural space and the spinal cord are the three layers of the meninges.

Nerves

There are 31 pairs of spinal nerves that extend from the cord. These nerve rootlets are covered by all layers of the meninges initially. The anterior and posterior rootlets coalesce to form the dorsal root ganglion, and the nerve root extends peripherally beyond the neural foramen. As the nerve roots approach the neural foramen, the dura thins.

The dorsal and ventral rootlets of the cord are covered by pia and arachnoid. Beyond the neural foramen, the pia and arachnoid form the perineural epithelium covering of the peripheral nerve. The dura extends primarily along the dorsal surface of the rootlets and extends lateral to the point where the anterior and posterior rootlets fuse to form the ganglia. This termination of dural tissue forms a small sleeve. The sleeve is of variable lengths.[3] The sleeve is pierced by arteries, veins, and lymphatics that communicate with the underlying subarachnoid space.

Also along this sleeve are permeations in the thinned dura where a layer of arachnoid mushrooms through and creates areas of granulation. The granulation is a permeable membrane for anesthetic to enter the subarachnoid space. These arachnoid granulations are continuous with the epineurium that surrounds the nerve beyond the neural foramen. This allows for a ready route for passage of local anesthetic onto the nerve root. The caudal nerve roots in the sacrum are more susceptible to neural blockade because they are only surrounded by epineurium.

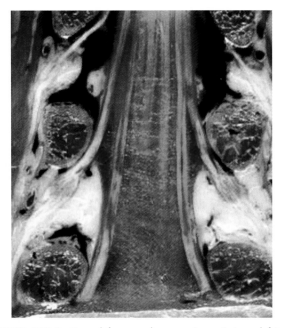

FIGURE 163-1. Coronal frozen cadaver specimen. Perineural fat and fascia surround nerve roots and ganglia. Nerve root ganglia lie below pedicle.

Nerve fibers carry afferent and efferent activity. Both motor activity and sensory perception travel along the peripheral nerve trunks. The dermatomal area a nerve innervates and its designated function differentiate the type of primary afferent fibers and the type of sensation that travels in the nerve root. The target or end muscle innervated is responsible for gross motor movement or fine motor activity. Information about proprioception and muscle spindle tone are transmitted to the brain along afferent tracts.

The anatomy of the nerve fiber, its diameter, and myelination can determine its physiologic response to anesthetics.[4] The myelination and diameter of the nerve are important in this process.

Nerve permeability regulates the readily available amount of anesthetic for blocking neural transmission. The amount of anesthetic, such as lidocaine, around the nerve root also affects its neural blockade activity. In addition, pH can enhance permeability of the perineural membrane. Local anesthetics are weakly acidic. These molecules are more stable at the acidic level, but the neutral anesthetic molecule passes across the membrane more readily.[5,6] Therefore, raising the pH with small aliquots of sterile sodium bicarbonate prevents significant dilution and is beneficial in creating the alkalized form of the anesthetic.[7]

Sources of Pain

There are potentially five perspective sources of back- or spine-mediated pain: the disc, facet joint complex, spinal cord and its extension as the nerve root, the bone or vertebral body, and the myofascia. Other than bone-mediated pain, which is transmitted by segmental nerves within the vertebral column, pain is transmitted via the nerve root. A

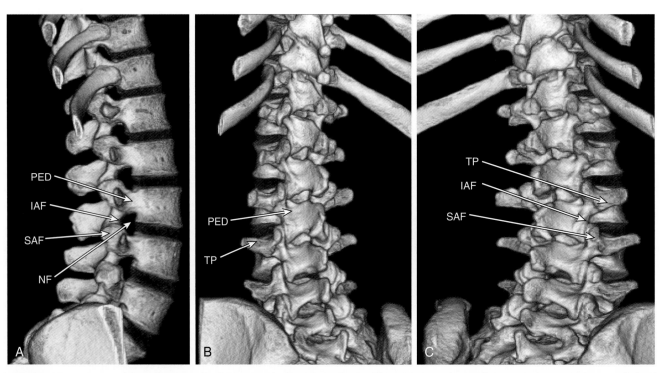

FIGURE 163-2. A, Lateral three-dimensional lumbar spine. Left oblique **(B)** and right oblique **(C)** views of neural foramen *(NF)* surrounded by pedicle *(PED)*, inferior articular facet *(IAF)*, superior articular facet *(SAF)*, and transverse process *(TP)*.

nerve root block is one of the dominant pathways for halting pain transmission. SNRB is designed to determine which level is producing provocative pain.

Pain from the zygapophyseal joint is referred to the adjacent paraspinal tissues. The pattern and potential distribution of perceptive pain in the cervical spine have been defined by Bogduk and Marsland, and in the thoracic spine by Fukui et al.[8,9] The lumbar spine and paraspinal and adjacent structures produce perceptive pain from the low back, buttock, and thigh areas. However, the lower lumbar medial branch nerves may convey pain that is perceived as low as the knee and occasionally the calf.

Disc-mediated pain is described as being mechanical if the disc is degenerating. Increased pressure and inflammation within the disc can create back, neck, or thoracic pain or paresthesias. Disc-mediated pain can arise in discs that are "normal appearing" and in discs that are degenerating. The input source of the innervated disc and the annulus is the sinuvertebral nerve. The sinuvertebral nerves are branches of the ventral rami, and the gray rami communicantes of the sympathetic chain.

Myofascial pain emanates from the superficial tissues that surround the vertebral column, such as the ligaments and muscle, and is conveyed through sensory fibers and relayed via the nerve root. SNRB can interrupt the specific pathway based on the dermatome being innervated.

Pain originating from within the cord or a primary nerve root can be due to several sources, including inflammation,

tumor, or defects such as a syrinx. Cord-mediated pain, however, is blocked more centrally.

INDICATIONS

SNRB serves to identify a specific a level where the pain generator arises. Pain relief after SNRB implicates a specific nerve as the source of pain. A selective block is therefore not only therapeutic in the alleviation of pain but diagnostic in determining the level at which therapy may be beneficial. Radicular pain creates sensory, motor, and reflex abnormalities in a clinical pattern manifested as pain, numbness, and weakness. Other dysesthesias can accompany the pain, such as tingling, itching, or hyperesthesia. Neck pain, headaches, and nuchal stiffness are not unusual from cervical nerves. Stiffness can be due to muscle spasms secondary to nerve irritation. Radicular pain is often described as shooting, stabbing, burning, or a dull ache. The patient's history, clinical findings, and physical examination are used to exclude causes such as tumor, infection, aneurysm, fracture, or cauda equina syndrome.

The location and distribution of pain can be diagrammed on a dermatomal map (Fig. 163-3). This valuable information can assist in determining whether single or multilevel disease is present. Recording factors such as time of day and response to aggravating or relieving factors helps characterize pain. An organic pain map has considerable diagnostic potential. It has a high degree of validity in the assessment

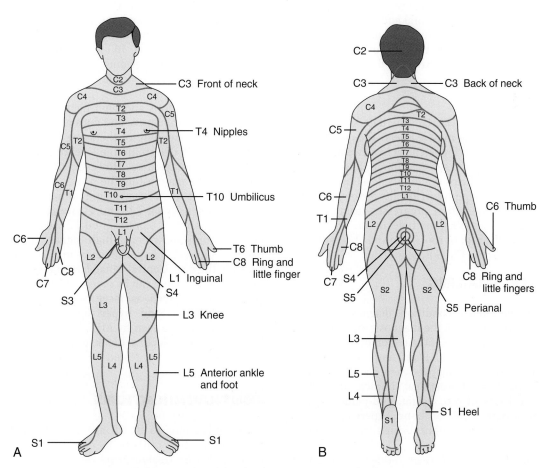

FIGURE 163-3. Anterior **(A)** and posterior **(B)** neuromuscular dermatome patterns.

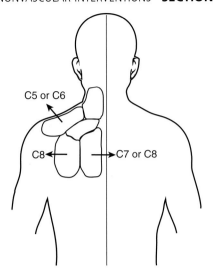

FIGURE 163-4. Dermatome pain pattern of cervical nerve roots.

of neurogenic pain and dysfunction and is reliable in showing concordance with the physical examination.[10] How pain is influenced by functional ability, mechanical loading, bending, sitting, standing, driving, or rest can further the evaluation.

Nerve roots cover a defined dermatome in most individuals, but the specific distribution or patterns are individualized. There is, however, considerable overlap in nerve root distribution. In the cervical region, the map is better defined (Fig. 163-4). In the thoracic region, the pattern of the thoracic nerve roots is segmental and covers a band or horizontal distribution. In the lumbar and sacral region, there is a more extensive distribution with overlap along the back and involvement of the buttocks and leg to the foot.

MAPPING

Needle electromyography (EMG) can detect waves and fibrillation potentials along muscle fibers. The motor nerve fibers innervating the muscles extend across two nerve root levels. EMG does not test sensory input. Based on the muscles involved, EMG helps predict the level of the radiculopathy. EMG detects signs of irritability as the process of denervation and reinnervation progresses from acute to chronic injury.[11,12] By sampling multiple muscles, it seeks to determine the specific root or roots involved. It is estimated that the specificity of the EMG is near 85%.[13]

DIAGNOSTIC IMAGING

Depending on the clinical condition, diagnostic imaging may provide the best clues to the diagnosis and level to be injected. Plain film evaluation of the region of concern provides a good diagnostic tool. Plain film radiography is readily available and cost-effective when diagnosing acute back pain.[14] Plain films of the cervical, thoracic, and lumbar spine may reveal loss of disc height, end-plate sclerosis, neural foramen narrowing, or bone hypertrophy. Plain films assist in ruling out other benign and malignant conditions.

Plain film images of the cervical, thoracic, and lumbar spine can be obtained without concern for an implant device, sedation, or claustrophobia. Spinal instruments such as screws and plates may limit evaluation of plain films but do not produce the multiple artifacts that would be seen with CT and MRI.[15] Plain film images are obtained in at least two planes, frontal and lateral. Special projections such as oblique views in the lumbar and thoracic region and pillars or odontoid views in the cervical spine are helpful in evaluating pathology and postoperative changes, including fusions.[16] In addition, congenital anomalies, fractures, osteoarthritic impingement, or bone erosion may be differentiated from tumor involvement with plain film radiography.

CT is the imaging tool that best visualizes the bones of the spine and is capable of determining the level of disc bulging or herniation in the spine. Gas within the disc, intraosseous herniation, and loss of disc height on sagittal reconstructions can all be seen with CT and can often predict a potential source of pain.

The discogram is a diagnostic tool for identifying discogenic back pain. Intradiscal injections create pressure, provide the opportunity to characterize spread of contrast material throughout the disc, and identify spillage into the epidural space. Concordant pain can be reproduced with injection of the offending disc. Correlation with a CT scan demonstrates the spread of contrast material through the nucleus pulposis and into the fissures of partially or completely torn annular fibers.

Myelograms are performed with the assistance of CT. This procedure allows access to the cerebrospinal fluid for diagnostic purposes. Intrathecal administration of iodinated contrast material allows detection of abnormalities encroaching on the spinal cord or nerve roots, including herniated disc, meningeal carcinomatosis, or spinal vascular malformation (Fig. 163-5). In patients with scoliosis, CT is the preferred imaging tool over MRI, which may have limitations with visualization of the sagittal plane (Fig. 163-6).

MRI uses protons and high-field-strength magnets for imaging. It is noninvasive and does not use x-rays. MRI has revolutionized imaging of the spine and surrounding soft tissues and can determine the level of a disc herniation or nerve root impingement. However, an abnormal disc may not indeed be manifesting the pain.

MRI shows loss of disc height, annular tears, and intradisc hypointensity on T1- and T2-weighted images. In the presence of annular tears, sagittal T2-weighted images with fat saturation show focal high signal, and subchondral marrow shows T2 hyperintensity in the vertebral bodies abutting the disc. Central canal, lateral recesses, and neural foraminal narrowing can be seen on MRI (Fig. 163-7). Associated changes such as facet hypertrophy, degenerative spondylolisthesis, and hypertrophy of the ligamentum flavum can also be seen by MRI. These findings are correlated with the selective block to determine which level or levels should be tested or should undergo neural blockade.

CONTRAINDICATIONS

Contraindications to SNRB are procedural or related to medications. If sensitivity to contrast media is present, patients can be treated prophylactically, or nonionated contrast media or gadolinium can be used.

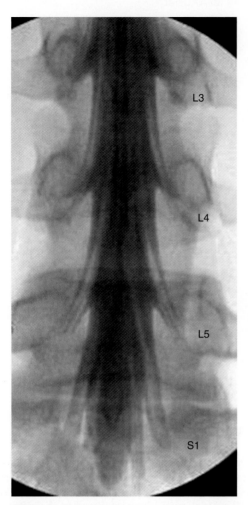

FIGURE 163-5. Normal posteroanterior lumbar myelogram. Nerve root sleeve terminates near neural foramen. An effective selective block is performed lateral to sleeve.

TABLE 163-1. Coagulopathy-Related Contraindications to Spinal Injection

Baseline laboratory data contraindicating injections include:
- International normalized ratio > 1
- Partial thromboplastin time > 50 seconds
- Prothrombin time > 15 seconds
- Platelets < 50,000/mm³

In patients with an uncorrectable coagulopathy, spinal injections are not recommended (Table 163-1). Spinal and paraspinal infection creates a risk of spread along the spinal canal.

A spinal injection or neural blockade of the nerves to the muscles used in respiration can create a thoracic block in a patient with a contralateral pneumothorax or severe chronic obstructive pulmonary disease (COPD). In the setting of a suspected tension pneumothorax, chest trauma or COPD pulmonary clearance is recommended to avoid an intraoperative crisis.[17]

DRUGS USED FOR SELECTIVE NERVE ROOT BLOCK

Anesthetics

Because local anesthetics are infiltrated as a fluid medium around the nerves, the fluid must diffuse through layers of fibrous tissue before it reaches the axons.[5] The rate of diffusion depends on adjacent scar tissue, and diffusion can be especially difficult in the setting of previous surgery. The rate of absorption by fat, uptake into the microvasculature, and local metabolism all determine the clinical potency of the injection. The final concentration that reaches the nerve is affected by these factors and by the length of nerve exposed to the drug solution. Injections in close proximity to the nerve reduces the need for diffusion and the volume of anesthetic required to achieve the desired block. Intimate proximity to the nerve root can be confirmed radiographically by CT scan or fluoroscopically.

Injection of water-soluble iodinated contrast or gadolinium in iodine-sensitive patients is beneficial to outline the nerve root and proximity to the ganglion and confirm the location of the needle. It also serves to exclude direct vascular uptake.

Blockade of the peripheral nerve can also be affected by drug absorption in surrounding tissues. This can be affected by use of a vasoconstrictor such as epinephrine. The rate of absorption in the vasculature is reduced, thereby leaving more anesthetic available for neural blockade and prolonging the anesthetic affect.[18]

Corticosteroids

Depot formulations of epidurally placed medications appear to prolong the local anesthetic effect. The slow release should also be accompanied by a decrease in the rate of systemic drug absorption and reduction of the potential for systemic toxicity.[19,20]

The analgesic effect of anesthetics is enhanced with corticosteroids. Steroids relieve pain by reducing nociceptive C-fiber transmission and by decreasing inflammation. Steroids inhibit the action of phospholipase A2, which releases arachidonic acid from cell membranes at the site of inflammation. Membrane injury causes accumulation of edema and release of unsaturated fatty acids. Altered membrane permeability in the setting of inflammation leads to intraneural edema and causes abnormal neural transmission.[21,22] Abnormal transmission along the nerve fiber results in creation of pain. Stabilization of the neural membrane by corticosteroids can inhibit sensitization of the nerve fiber and prevent the neural discharge that results in pain creation.

Corticosteroid medications have a therapeutic benefit. The recommended dose is not more than 50 mg triamcinolone or 80 mg methylprednisolone.[23] Corticosteroids have been used to prolong the therapeutic effect of the diagnostic test injection. The antiinflammatory effect decreases pressure along the nerve root as swelling subsides and autologous histamine substances such as substance P are diluted away. Symptom improvement can increase the time for the patient to confirm the injection is beneficial. An injection of 0.5 to 1.5 mL of contrast material is used to outline the nerve root. The volume of injected anesthetic should mirror the injected volume of contrast material. The goal of the contrast is to not only localize the nerve root but also demonstrate the extent of the spread of medication and perhaps avoid injection into the epidural space.

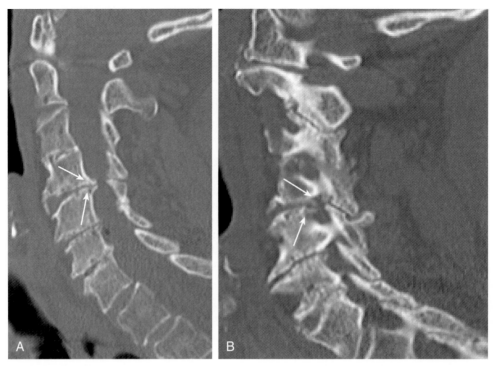

FIGURE 163-6. Near midline (**A**) and lateral (**B**) sagittal computed tomography scan of cervical spine in patient with scoliosis and radiating mid-neck and shoulder pain caused by bone and ligamentum flavum hypertrophy, narrowing C4 foramen.

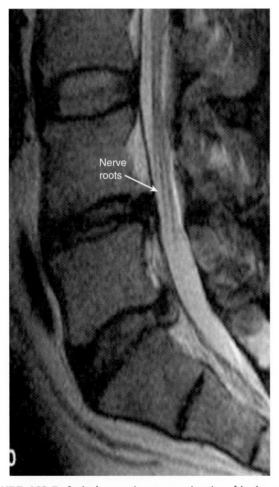

FIGURE 163-7. Sagittal magnetic resonance imaging of lumbar spine. Nerve roots (*arrow*) in narrowed spinal canal are adjacent to degenerating disc at L4-L5 and subligamentous herniation at L5-S1.

TECHNIQUE

SNRB can be performed in the cervical, thoracic, lumbar, and sacral spine. The procedure was initially performed without guidance and involved the use of a series of landmarks. The block could be performed in the sitting, lying, or oblique position. Most thoracic and lumbar injections are performed with the patient prone, whereas a cervical block can be performed from the decubitus or supine position. The chosen position should allow maximal exposure of the spine and neural foramen. A short roll can be place beneath the hips or chest in the prone position and under the neck in the supine position.

Most injections are performed using fluoroscopic guidance, but CT can also be used for needle guidance.[24] Its benefit is best seen in the cervical region where the avoidance of major blood vessels is critical (Fig. 163-8). The approach taken with the use of CT will be a direct axial one unless the CT scan gantry is angled. This approach allows the practitioner to avoid the primary vasculature of the vertebral and carotid arteries as well as the large branches of the subclavian artery, especially the superior thyroidal artery near the base of the neck. There are multiple small muscular branches of the vertebral artery that may not be avoidable, but recognition of their presence if bleeding develops as the vertebral artery is approached can be helpful. However, vigilance for the spinal artery during a cervical injection is important to avoid major complications. The precise location of a tortuous vertebral artery can be localized, especially near the skull base and at the base of the neck, before entering the foramen transversarium (Fig. 163-9). In the setting of a neck or shoulder mass, CT scan presents an excellent option to avoid direct transgression of the mass to gain access to the cervical nerve root.

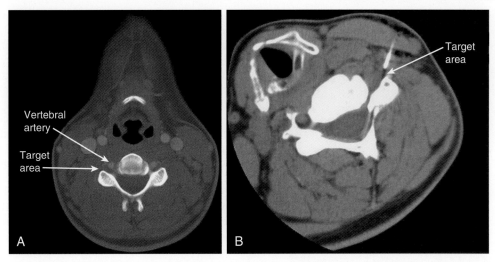

FIGURE 163-8. Axial computed tomography (CT) scan of cervical spine. **A,** Neural foramen and target for needle lie posterior to vertebral artery. **B,** Oblique projection shows needle at target site under CT guidance. *(Courtesy Dennis Griffin, MD.)*

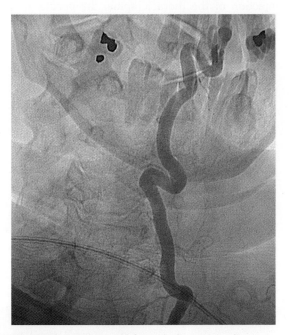

FIGURE 163-9. Unsubtracted left vertebral angiogram showing tortuous and unpredictable course of vertebral artery.

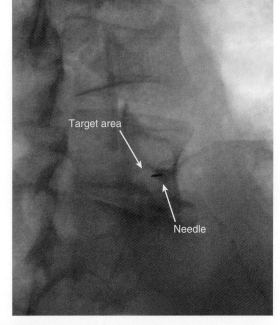

FIGURE 163-10. Oblique view of lumbar spine. A direct needle approach to target location was taken, below pedicle and lateral to inferior articular process of vertebrae.

The skin is prepped and draped using sterile technique. Local anesthetic is placed in the subcutaneous tissues. A 22- or 23-gauge spinal needle with a beveled tip is often used.

The basic technique is to stabilize the needle with the thumb and index finger or use a hemostat for measured advancement of the needle tip. The fluoroscope is positioned to optimize the position and alignment of the neural foramen. A gun-site or down-the-barrel projection is used when the target is the foramen. The goal is perineural placement of the needle (Fig. 163-10). To avoid puncture of the nerve root, the advancing needle tip is also visualized in the lateral and frontal projections. Ideal needle placement depends on the level of the spine being treated. In the cervical spine, the needle tip is placed posterior for the foramen

(Fig. 163-11). As the needle tip nears the neural foramen, care should be taken to avoid piercing the nerve root and vertebral artery. Success of the injection is not influenced by the length of the spinal needle bevel. In comparison with long-bevel needles, short-bevel needles do not reduce the rate of vascular injection.[25]

Cervical

For injection of the cervical spine, the needle end target is placed near the upper outer aspect of the foramen at the 10 o'clock position on the right and at the 2 o'clock position on the left of the patient. The patient can be placed in an oblique position, or the image intensifier is maneuvered to open the neural foramen and create the widest circle

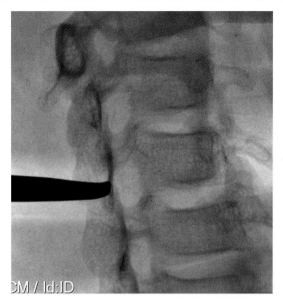

FIGURE 163-11. Oblique view of cervical spine. Target is located along posterior wall of foramen. Vertebral artery is anterior to neural foramen.

(Fig. 163-12). The nerve exits the foramen anterolaterally and inferiorly en route to form segments of the brachial plexus. The needle should be directed to engage the lip of the foramen posteriorly. The vertebral artery commonly lies anterior to the nerves and passes through a channel or foramen transversarium. Posterior to the needle are the articular facets (Fig. 163-13).

For the injection of the C2 nerve, a direct lateral or posterior approach is taken. The pathway is centered in a rectangle created between the spinal laminar line posteriorly and the odontoid anteriorly. The superior border is framed by the lamina of C1, and the floor is created by the lamina of C2. Using a posteroanterior projection, the needle tip is advanced until it passes the lateral third of the facet joint (Fig. 163-14). Oftentimes the patient's mouth has to be opened for adequate positioning and determination of landmarks.

Thoracic

For injection of the thoracic spine, the needle is angled along an inferolateral approach. The image intensifier is

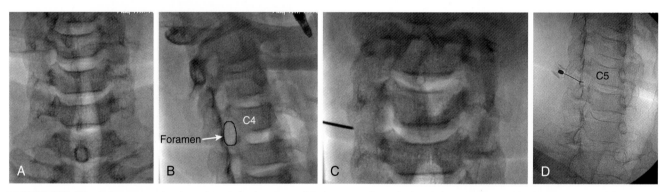

FIGURE 163-12. **A,** Posteroanterior view of cervical spine. **B,** Parallel alignment of vertebral end plates maximizes circular appearance of foramen for oblique projection. Frontal **(C)** and oblique **(D)** views of cervical spine show final location of needle for selective nerve root block.

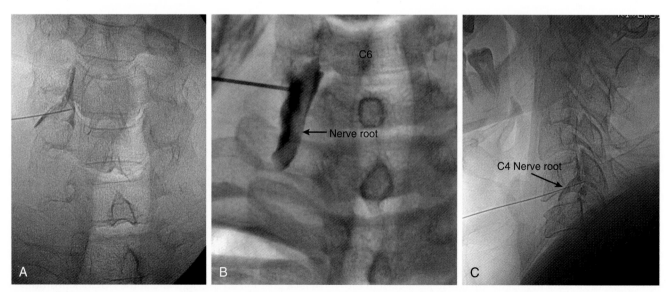

FIGURE 163-13. Frontal view of cervical spine for selective nerve root block at C5 **(A)** after injection of 0.5 mL of contrast material and **(B)** with C6 nerve root well surrounded by contrast material after injection of 1 mL. **C,** Lateral view shows final needle location and contrast material outlining nerve root origin. Note anterior-to-inferior projection of nerve root as it extends toward brachial plexus.

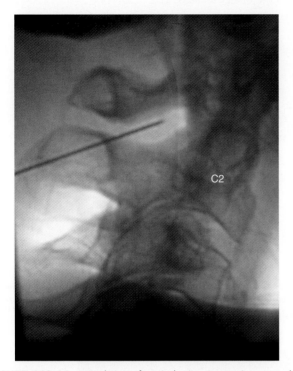

FIGURE 163-14. Lateral view of cervical spine. A posterior approach to C2 nerve root is taken for selective nerve root block. Needle tip is in center of a rectangle created by anterior adenoid, posterior aspect of spinal canal, upper rim of lamina of C1, and inferior rim of lamina of C2.

angled so it parallels the end plates of the vertebral bodies at the level that is being approached. the foramen is approached medially from the inferior aspect of the transverse process. A curved needle is used to touch the transverse process and then walked off its edge. Just deep to the anterior aspect of transverse process, the needle will give way beyond the bone contact with the bone. The needle is advanced in a lateral to medial direction (Fig. 163-15).

From an anteroposterior projection, the position of the needle is adequate when the lateral third of the pedicle is approached. From a lateral projection, the needle should not advance more anterior than the posterior wall of the vertebral body or anterior margin of the foramen. However, the anterior margin of the foramen can be difficult to see if the view is not a true lateral projection. Contrast material is injected to locate the nerve root and view it in the frontal and lateral projections (Fig. 163-16).

Lumbar

For injection of the lumbar spine, the vertebral bodies are squared and their end plates are paralleled by the image intensifier. The target is beneath the pedicle of the vertebrae or "eye of the Scotty dog" and is in the region of the safe triangle as described by Bogduk et al. (Figs. 163-17 and 163-18). This region is above the exiting nerve root.[26] A down-the-barrel approach is best; the needle is inserted

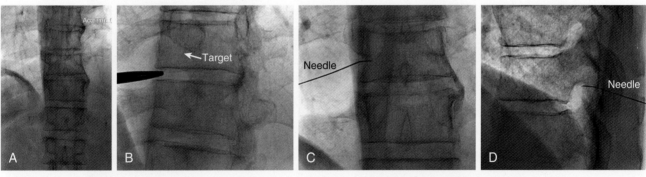

FIGURE 163-15. Posteroanterior view of thoracic spine for a selective nerve root block. **A,** End plates of vertebrae at selected level to be injected are parallel. Oblique view is used to select a site to project needle inferior and lateral to target. **B,** Inferior lateral angle of vertebrae can be used in a modestly built person, but a more lateral and inferior approach may be needed in an obese patient. Final location of the needle is shown in posteroanterior **(C)** and lateral **(D)** views.

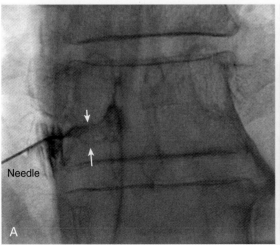

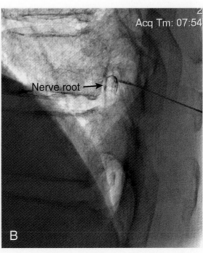

FIGURE 163-16. A, Posteroanterior view of contrast material outlining nerve root *(arrows)*. **B,** In lateral view of thoracic spine, contrast material surrounds nerve root as it exits foramen.

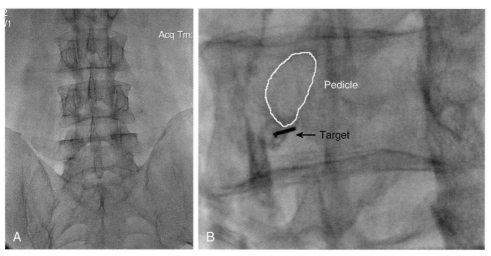

FIGURE 163-17. A, Posteroanterior view of lumbar spine with parallel end plates of vertebral body. **B,** Oblique view of lumbar spine that creates a safe projection to approach target in a down-the-barrel approach of needle to target. Pedicle size is maximized to create an ideal projection to approach target. Needle can approach nerve root because it is in "safe triangle." Base of triangle is formed by inferior aspect of pedicle; superior articular facet and lamina form medial wall. Outer wall is a direct vertical along posterior aspect of vertebral body.

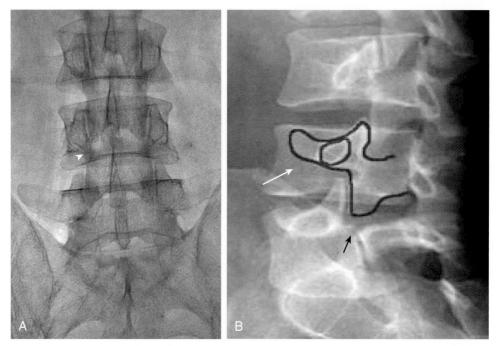

FIGURE 163-18. A, Posteroanterior view of lumbar spine showing safe triangle, with superior border created by pedicle and medial border by exiting nerve root. **B,** Target lies beneath the "eye" *(white arrow)* of the radiographic "Scotty dog" *(black arrow)*.

into the tissues in a paramedian direction through the muscle. This approach immediately below the pedicle and along the superior border of the foramen is chosen to avoid the exiting nerve root. From a posteroanterior approach, the needle is not advanced more medial than the lateral one fourth of the pedicle. The needle is aspirated to avoid blood or cerebral spinal fluid (Fig. 163-19).

Sacral

When injecting the sacral spine, the foramina are directly posterior nond are aligned so that the anterior and posterior foramina overlap. This approach creates a steep cephalocaudal view from the image intensifier. The image intensifier can also be made slightly laterally oblique to create a larger circle of the foramen. This places the image intensifier in a position perpendicular to the foramen, and the location of the individual sacral nerve roots can be predicted (Fig. 163-20).

The spinal needle is inserted into the foramen perpendicular to the dorsal surface of the sacrum (Fig. 163-21). The needle is advanced through the epidural space and is viewed from the lateral projection (Fig. 163-22). If the needle is seen approaching the anterior foramen and presacral space, the position of the needle is adequate. Contrast material can be injected to view the outline of the sacral nerve.

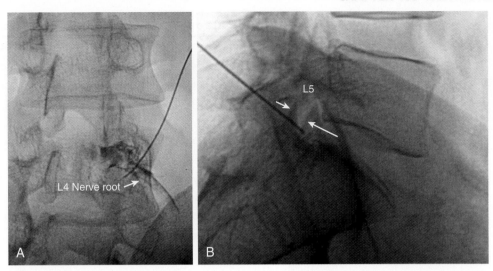

FIGURE 163-19. Oblique view of lumbar spine. **A,** Injection of 1 mL of contrast material shows outline of L4 nerve root. **B,** Lateral view of final needle position as L5 nerve root is targeted and opacified *(arrows)*.

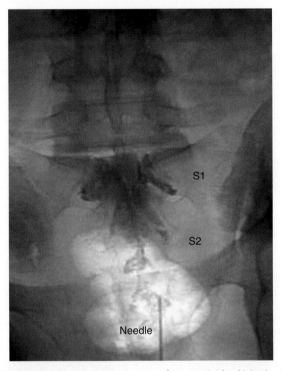

FIGURE 163-20. Posteroanterior view of sacrum. Epidural injection from caudal approach shows outline of sacral nerve roots.

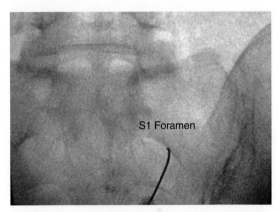

FIGURE 163-21. Posteroanterior view showing sacral foramen. Image intensifier is projected in a steep caudal approach to maximize circular orifice of neural foramen, and needle approaches along lateral margin of foramen.

At each level, a small quantity of contrast (1-2 mL) is injected to identify the nerve root. This also confirms the absence of epidural and vascular spread of contrast.[3] Anesthetic solution and corticosteroid medications are injected around the nerve root sleeve. The diagnostic value of the injection is maintained if epidural spread of contrast is avoided (Fig. 163-23). Using a 1-mL syringe, 1 mL of anesthetic solution is injected. The injected anesthetic may be lidocaine 1% in the cervical region or as strong as 4% in the lumbar region, or bupivacaine 0.5% can be used.

The injected contrast agent is viewed in two projections to confirm that vascular uptake is not occurring. The injection should be smooth, without great pressure. Small volumes are injected to exclude untoward respiratory or cardiac activity. The patient should be observed for changes in perception of pain.

OUTCOMES

SNRB is used primarily as a diagnostic tool, but it can have extended beneficial therapeutic effects as well. A paravertebral approach can create a zone of anesthesia to cover the ventral ramus, dorsal ramus, and the sinuvertebral nerve beyond the neural foramen. Larger volumes of injectate can extend to the medial branch nerve posteriorly or anteriorly, affect the sympathetic nerve, and cloud the diagnostic information. Awareness of where the contrast material is spreading is therefore essential.

Patients should be asked to draw and describe the location and type of pain they experience. This information is fed into the characterization of the pain and is useful to distinguish neuropathic from radicular from articular-based pain. Organic pain drawings are found to have a positive predictive value in outcome parameters[27] and have

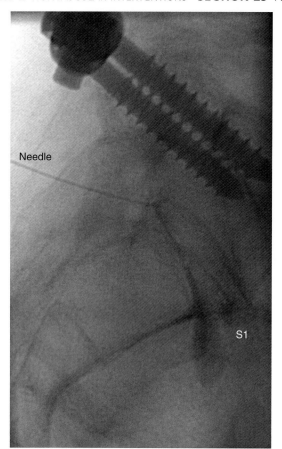

FIGURE 163-22. Lateral view of sacrum for selective S1 nerve root injection.

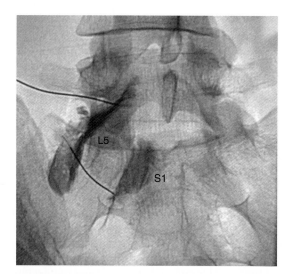

FIGURE 163-23. Posteroanterior view of sacrum for selective nerve root block of left L5 and S1 nerves.

been associated with positive radiologic and surgical findings of nerve root entrapment.[28,29]

Although patients often indicate that they hurt and describe a wide general area, they should be encouraged to define as specifically as possible where they perceive discomfort and where it travels to and draw it. This can be used

TABLE 163-2. Neurogenic versus Spondyloarthritic Pain	
Nerve	**Articular/Ligament**
Numbness	Popping
Sparking	Cracking
Shooting	Dull
Burning	Stiff
Crawling	Grating
Weakness	Sore
Atrophy	Achy
Temperature change	Sticking
Color change	Grinding
Stabbing	Catching
Tingling	

to determine where the initial injection is to be performed, but the diagram can also serve as a follow-up to assess regression of the symptoms.

In the lower part of the back, pain described as a focal dull ache, or shooting pain from the low back down the lateral thigh to the calf can have varied consequences. The patient's description of the pain can guide the clinician in differentiating nerve-mediated pain from spondyloarthropathy (Table 163-2). It is probable that some patients with nonradiating focal lumbosacral midline pain could have spondylolisthesis or facet-mediated arthrosis, and that others describing pain radiating down the leg may have a paracentral disc at the L4-L5 level. A good dermatomal map can be created by descriptions of the pain.

Concordant pain can be created along a nerve root by approaching it with the needle tip or by injecting contrast material nearby. Resolution of the primary pain by injection of the anesthetic confirms the appropriate level of injection. The efficacy of the selective block has been studied by Pang et al. and was used to predict which level was implicated in creating the radicular pain.[30] Nerve roots in the lumbar spine were infiltrated with anesthetic for diagnostic evaluation. This, however, can be challenging in the setting of multilevel disease or complex pain secondary to disc-mediated and facet spondylotic disease.

The difficulty associated with interpretation of pain in patients was studied by Wolfe et al.[31] They evaluated the perception of pain induced by the injection and mapped the creation of an anesthetic effect by SNRB to determine which levels matched which dermatomes. They also sought to determine what neighboring dermatomes created overlap on the pain map. The investigators found overlap by two to three dermatomal levels, both from the subjacent level below and also the supra-adjacent level above. The overlap created in the neural network is built-in redundancy that is a common theme seen at the level of the facet and medial branch nerves. Each rootlet provided sensory input from the level below, at the level of origin, and from the level above. Not uncommonly, however, some patients perceive pain not only from two levels above or below the primary root origin but also from the contralateral side. So the map is used as a template to predict where the initial injection should be placed.

TABLE 163-3. Thoracic Nerve Block

Spinal Level	Dermatomal Area
C7	Brachial plexus: index, third finger
T1	Brachial plexus: thumb
T2-T3	Intercostobrachial nerve: axilla
T4-T6	Anterior chest and cardiac area pain
T6-T9	Right upper quadrant, biliary area pain
T10-T12	Right lower quadrant, appendiceal pain
T12-L1	Right pelvic and ilioinguinal area, pain with hernia repair

The dermatomal map for the lower and upper extremities is well established. The thoracic region and the map for the visceral organs are less specific and less often used in clinical practice. The use of regional anesthesia can offer surgical colleagues a more specific and diagnostic clue to where and what is hurting the patient. Patients with chronic symptoms of right upper quadrant pain can respond to a positive block and help the practitioner distinguish acalculous biliary colic from renal or duodenal disease (Table 163-3).

Similarly, nonischemic angina or chronic anterior thoracic pain can be found to have a positive response to SNRB at the T5, T6, or T7 region. This can offer the cardiac patient an opportunity for long-term response to an injection for noncoronary pain. This information has been beneficial to spinal surgeons seeking a positive prediction for a good surgical outcome from decompression.

In patients with breast or head and neck cancer, the cancer can presumably affect the nerve, but chemotherapy or radiotherapy or concurrent therapies can create a disabling plexopathy. There is no specific study or clinical finding that can be used to distinguish which nerve roots are responsible for the pain. Patients with breast cancer can have an incidence of radiation-induced plexopathy as high as 9%.[32,33] A selective block of the lower trunks of the plexus at the C5, C6, or C7 roots tends to relieve this pain.

Not only has the map been shown to have diagnostic value, but Derby et al. also used the map and SNRB to predict surgical outcomes.[34] If perineural injection of steroid and anesthetic relieved the radicular pain by inhibiting release of arachidonic acid along the affected nerve root, it should predict a positive outcome from surgical decompression at that level.

North et al. used the diagnostic SNRB indirectly in the lumbosacral spine. Their study of a series of 33 patients led them to conclude that the selective block was not specific for a positive outcome, but that failure of the temporary block to relieve the pain would predict failure of a surgical procedure.[35]

Slipman et al. studied 20 patients retrospectively and reported a significant reduction in pain at an average of 5.8 months in 60% of them. This clinically effective intervention was used for cervical radiculopathy in treating atraumatic cervical spondylotic pain.[36]

Radicular pain creates a potentially dull, burning ache often associated with numbness, be it in the arm radiating from cervical nerve roots or in the thoracic or lumbar region. With radicular pain, pulsating or shooting discomfort can be perceived. This ache can be described as shocking or stabbing, but it is nonetheless annoying and not readily relieved. Patterns seen in the dermatomal map are typical for a radiculopathy across a single nerve root pathway (see Fig. 163-3).

SNRB can be difficult for the practitioner to master technically, but after a level of proficiency develops, diagnostic accuracy can be gained. Learning which level or levels produce the offending pain based on location and character can propel novice practitioners to an elevated status. The ability to determine the need for multiple injections or directly assess the neural pathway at the nascent levels is satisfying.

Postthoracotomy pain syndrome creates an interesting dilemma. It is probably due to intercostal nerve injury and can be predictive of which nerve roots are involved, based on the surgical site. The pain can be quite intense in the acute phase and distressing if it becomes chronic. However, for the practitioner, radiation of pain along nerves two or three levels above or below the surgical site can make controlling the pain difficult. Treatment of the acute postoperative pain and its underrecognized neuropathic pain by regional anesthetic nerve blocks can have a favorable impact on pain management.

The level of inflammation, patients' perception of how the pain is affecting their lives, and pain tolerance can determine how well they respond to an injection. It can be challenging to predict how patients will report their response to pain reduction, and this can be related to the presence of anxiety and depression.[37]

The objective of evaluating the diagnostic process in assessment of the patient's level of pain is to create a hypothesis about what is creating the pain and determine the level at which the pain is arising. The clinical information, imaging studies, physiologic analysis, and available assessments are evaluated to anticipate where the involved nerve roots are located. The experience of a seasoned practitioner, along with the use of a pain map for assessment, can create a high degree of reliability that the result of SNRB will be beneficial.

COMPLICATIONS

Possible complications of nerve root injection can result from procedure-related entities such as infection, bleeding, and allergic reactions to contrast media or anesthetic. Direct procedural complications may include leakage of cerebrospinal fluid from a tear along the nerve root sleeve, direct nerve puncture, and injection of material directly into the nerve root. Bowel or visceral perforation or injury can occur if the needle is advanced too far.

Vascular or ischemic injury, particularly on the left paravertebral region, can be created if the spinal arteries are lacerated or directly injected (Fig. 163-24). Direct injection can cause embolization of the spinal artery and devascularize the cord. Injection of the spinal artery can create inadvertent spread of anesthesia in another area of the spinal tract and produce unexpected results and nondiagnostic injections. In the cervical region, injection of the vertebral artery or its muscular branches (e.g., radiculomedullary artery or anterior spinal artery) places the patient at risk for particulate or air embolism, which can cause a stroke or

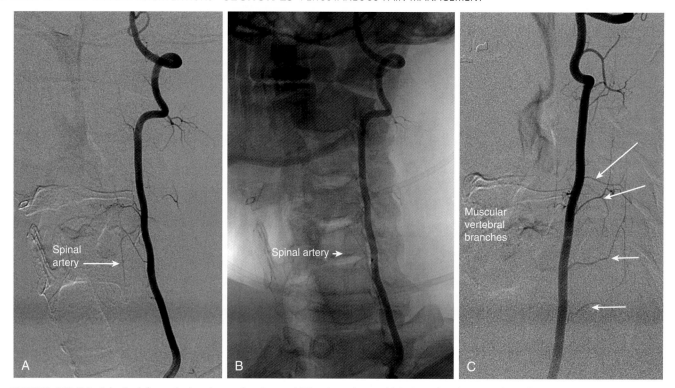

FIGURE 163-24. Selective left vertebral angiogram in subtracted **(A)** and unsubtracted **(B)** views show location of spinal artery. **C,** Subtracted angiogram of left vertebral artery showing many cervical muscular branches from vertebral artery *(arrows)*.

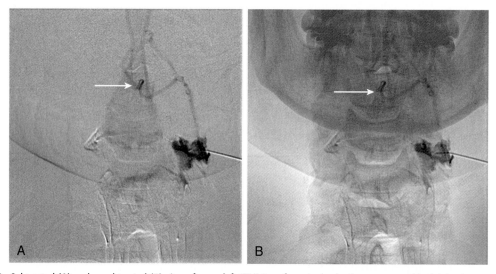

FIGURE 163-25. Subtracted **(A)** and unsubtracted **(B)** views from a left C5-6 transforaminal selective nerve root block injection revealed arterial uptake and opacification of spinal artery *(arrow)*.

paralysis (Fig. 163-25). In the lumbar and thoracic region, inadvertent injection or embolization of the artery of Adamkiewicz and the anterior spinal artery can result in spinal cord infarct and paralysis. The injectate itself can have untoward complications. Use of medications such as lidocaine with epinephrine can lead to tachycardia and arrhythmias.

The most common side effect of an injection is a back or neck ache from placement of the needle through the paravertebral muscles. Injecting large volumes of local anesthetic or inadvertent intravascular injections can produce a systemic toxic reaction. The reaction can manifest as perioral numbness, nausea, and dizziness. Intracerebral administration of anesthetics such as lidocaine can cause seizure activity.

These complications can best be avoided by test injections of contrast material or injections of small or test doses. Aspiration of the needle for blood or cerebrospinal fluid can determine whether the test should be discontinued or the needle adjusted. Injections should be performed under fluoroscopic or CT guidance and with cardiopulmonary assessment.

Long-duration or frequent injections of steroids can produce adrenal suppression or Cushing syndrome as a result of suppression of the hypothalamic-pituitary-adrenal axis. Suppression of endogenous corticosteroids causes a decrease in cortisol and adrenocorticotropic hormone (ACTH). Benzodiazepines are known to have a potentiating inhibitory effect on the hypothalamic-pituitary-adrenal axis, and patients given midazolam as conscious sedation have a more pronounced suppression of this pathway.[38]

Inadvertent subarachnoid injection of steroid can result in spinal analgesia. Preservatives or steroid medications can lead to arachnoiditis or meningitis.[39]

Avascular necrosis may occur as a complication of either intermittent or continuous corticosteroid treatment. It most commonly affects the femoral head, but the humeral head, elbow, or any bone in the body can be affected. It can create intense pain at a joint or in the limb around the joint, such as the hip, thigh, or knee, in the setting of hip involvement. Children treated for acute lymphoblastic leukemia from age 10 to 20 have a 14% increased risk for development of osteonecrosis following multiple prolonged courses of corticosteroids.[40]

PATIENT SELECTION

Pain that extends along a dermatomal pattern is considered radicular. Patients with radicular pain are considered to be better candidates for SNRB. Patients undergoing the injections are evaluated clinically and by imaging including routine x-rays, CT, and MRI to exclude other conditions that may imitate radicular symptoms. Patients for a diagnostic or therapeutic SNRB will often have:

- Known disc herniation or narrowed neural foramen
- Multilevel disc disease with unknown pain generator level
- Minimal or equivocal imaging findings
- Equivocal discogram
- Postoperative pain
- Equivocal neurologic or EMG analysis
- Atypical or complex radiating pain

MEDICATIONS

Diagnostic Injection

- Lidocaine hydrochloride 1%, methylparaben free (MPF), 0.5 mL (Xylocaine-MPF 1% [AstraZeneca Pharmaceuticals LP, Wilmington, Del.])
- Bupivacaine hydrochloride 0.25% MPF, 0.5 mL (Sensorcaine-MPF Injection 0.25% [AstraZeneca]) Or
- Lidocaine hydrochloride 4% MFP, 1 mL (Xylocaine-MPF 4% [AstraZeneca])

Therapeutic Injection

- Lidocaine hydrochloride 1% MPF, 0.5 mL (Xylocaine-MPF 1% [AstraZeneca])
- Bupivacaine hydrochloride 0.25% MPF, 0.5 mL (Sensorcaine-MPF Injection 0.25% [AstraZeneca])
- Triamcinolone acetonide injectable (40 mg/mL), 0.5 mL (Kenalog-40 [Apothecon, Princeton, N.J.])

Cervical

- Lidocaine hydrochloride 1% MPF, 0.5 mL (Xylocaine-MPF 1% [AstraZeneca])
- Bupivacaine hydrochloride 0.25% MPF, 0.5 mL (Sensorcaine-MPF Injection 0.25% [AstraZeneca])
- Betamethasone sodium phosphate and betamethasone acetate injectable suspension (6 mg/mL), 0.5 mL (Celestone Soluspan [Schering Corp., Kenilworth, N.J.])

PREPROCEDURE CARE

- Nothing by mouth (NPO) 2 hours prior to procedure or 6 hours if anxiolysis is to be provided.
- Stop anticoagulants per institution protocol.
- Stop antiinflammatory medications 4 days prior.
- Stop nutraceuticals 4 days prior.
- Provide list of medications.
- Provide lists of allergies.
- Provide medical historical data and imaging studies.
- Provide a copy of power of attorney, living will, and primary contact.

PROCEDURE CARE

- Pause and confirm prior to injection.
- Monitor blood pressure, pulse oximetry, heart rate.

POSTPROCEDURE CARE

- Observe patients for 30 minutes prior to discharge.
- Evaluate motor strength and coordination prior to discharge.
- Caution patients to avoid heavy lifting and strenuous activity.
- Instruct patients to avoid exposure of injection site to water for 24 hours or until healed.

POTENTIAL COMPLICATIONS

- Bleeding
- Thecal sac puncture and postural headaches
- Vasovagal reaction and ataxia
- Infection
- Allergic reaction to medication or contrast
- Pneumothorax in thoracic injections
- Paraplegia
- High spinal anesthesia

CASE STUDIES

Please visit www.expertconsult.com for seven clinical case studies involving SNRB techniques, along with additional downloadable illustrations.

KEY POINTS
• Selective nerve root block (SNRB) is an excellent tool for creating a zone of anesthesia over a specific area of the body, either for diagnostic or therapeutic purposes.
• The dermatomal map is the key to determining which nerve should be blocked, because most pain radiates well away from the root source.

- The distal aspect of where the symptoms lie on the dermatomal map should be determined, and that point identifies the level to be treated.
- Despite some general consistency from patient to patient in the area a nerve should cover, there can be variances due to redundancy in coverage from an adjacent nerve root, as well as variances in the area of the dermatomal map being covered.
- Correct setup and approach of the image intensifier before placing the needle are key to a successful injection.

▶ **SUGGESTED READINGS**

Bogduk N, April C, Derby R. Selective nerve root blocks. In: Wilson DJ, editor. Interventional Radiology of the Musculoskeletal System. London: Edward Arnold; 1995. p. 122–32.

Pang WW, Ho ST, Huang MH. Selective lumbar spinal nerve block, a review. Acta Anesthesiol Sin 1999;37(1):21–6.

Quinn SF, Murtagh FR, Chatfield R, Shashidhar HK. CT-Guided nerve root block and ablation. AJR Am J Roentgenol 1988;151:1213–16.

The complete reference list is available online at www.expertconsult.com.

CHAPTER 164

Stellate Ganglion Block

Brian M. Block

The stellate ganglion is the lowermost component of the three cervical sympathetic ganglia, which themselves are the extension of the sympathetic nervous system into the head and upper extremity. The stellate ganglion is composed of preganglionic fibers from the thoracic spinal cord traveling to one of the three ganglia and postganglionic cell bodies. Postganglionic fibers from all three ganglia join the brachial plexus and carotid and vertebral arteries. Stellate ganglion block (SGB) will cause a temporary block of sympathetic nervous function in the ipsilateral head, face, and upper extremity. The stellate ganglion is located in the anterior neck, anterior and adjacent to the longus colli muscle, just anterior to the C7 transverse process, lying between the carotid sheath and thyroid gland.

SGB is indicated for treatment of neuropathic pain in the upper extremity, head, and face. It has been used for over 100 years and is a relatively safe and effective adjunct to treatment of complex regional pain syndrome (also known as *reflex sympathetic dystrophy*), Raynaud vasospasm, postherpetic neuralgia, and iatrogenic vasospasm. Recent reports have suggested that SGB may also be useful for treatment of posttraumatic stress disorder and postmenopausal hot flashes. Historically, SGB was done blindly, using palpation of anatomic landmarks (C6 transverse process and cricoid cartilage), but imaging is now commonly used. SGB is done by placing a needle onto the transverse process of C6 or C7, withdrawing the needle 1 to 2 mm, and then injecting a solution of local anesthetic, typically using 12 to 15 mL. Complications to be avoided are intravascular injection, spinal or epidural injection, esophageal perforation, pneumothorax, and hematoma.

The full version of this chapter plus five figures and a table summary of features of sympathetic nervous system involvement are available at www.expertconsult.com.

CHAPTER 165

Facet Joint Injection

Theodore S. Grabow and Brian M. Block

CLINICAL RELEVANCE

Back and neck pain are among the most common medical complaints in developed countries. Prevalence of spinal pain is estimated at 66% in the general population, with 55% to 90% reported as low back pain, 44% cervical, and 15% thoracic.[1-3] Spinal pain is a significant burden on both the individual and society in terms of direct cost, economic loss, and suffering.[1-3] Spinal pain is most common in people 18 to 44 years of age and ranks second for chief complaints for outpatient visits, third for surgical procedures, and fifth for hospitalizations.[4] Most episodic symptoms resolve over days to weeks with only conservative therapy, but roughly a third of patients will progress to chronic pain, more commonly in smokers, women, and those with psychological distress, low physical activity, and other premorbid conditions.[3] Differential diagnosis of spinal pain includes vertebral body pathology, vertebral disc disease, spinal stenosis, nerve entrapment syndromes, paraspinal muscle pain, and facet joint disease, along with extraspinal ailments such as cancer, gastric/duodenal ulcer, pancreatitis, aortic aneurysm, nephrolithiasis, prostatitis/cystitis, and postherpetic neuralgia. Often the etiology of spinal pain is elusive, but facet syndrome is thought to be the cause of chronic spinal pain in approximately 30% of people with low back pain, 55% of those with cervical pain, and 40% of thoracic pain.[2,4-7] Diagnostic facet blocks should be part of an algorithmic approach to the clinical management of chronic spinal pain.[5,8] Recent trends in utilization have shown exponential growth in the number of patients receiving facet interventions,[9] as well as in the performance of facet interventions by non-physicians.[10]

INDICATIONS

The facet joint, also called the *zygapophyseal* or *Z-joint*, is a true synovial joint involved in the articulation of adjacent vertebral bodies.[6] The two facet joints and the intervertebral disc make a tripod support for each spinal level. Involvement of this joint in spinal pain is called *facet* or *zygapophyseal syndrome*. The association of facet joint pathology and pain was first described in 1911 by Goldthwait and termed *facet syndrome* by Ghormley in 1933.[6] Etiologies of facet syndrome include trauma, arthritis, inflammation, and degeneration.[6] Facet syndrome typically presents as axial low back pain, neck pain, or headaches.[11-15] Axial pain of thoracic facet origin has been described but is less common.[16] The thoracolumbar juncture is vulnerable to facet injury from the abrupt transition in facet joint orientation from the coronal to sagittal plane that occurs there anatomically.

The prevalence of lumbar facet arthrosis increases with advancing age.[17] Greater than 50% of adults over 30 years of age demonstrate arthritic changes of the facet joints.[18] The most commonly affected lumbar joint is the L4-5 facet joint, possibly owing to its sagittal orientation.[19] Comorbid vascular disease is also a risk factor for facet degeneration.[20]

The symptoms of facet syndrome are nonspecific and overlap with other diagnoses. The pain may be confined to the axial lumbar spine or referred to the buttock and thigh.[21] Pain may also have a pseudoradicular component but rarely radiates distal to the knee and is not exacerbated by the straight leg raise test.[4-6,21] In the cervical spine, pain is in the neck itself or may be referred to the head (cervicogenic headache), shoulders, or scapula.[11,12] Physical examination findings that suggest facet syndrome are pain aggravated by palpation of the paraspinal muscles, standing, spinal extension, and facet joint loading with rotation.[4-7,13] Pain is usually ameliorated by sitting and flexing the spine. Diagnostic scoring systems with signs and symptoms of facet syndrome have been developed, but results have not been consistent. Furthermore, some suggest that the physical exam is only sufficient to rule out major neurologic injury but insufficient to diagnose the source of the pain.[22]

Radiologic or scintigraphic (bone scan) studies are neither sensitive nor specific for diagnosing facet syndrome. Facet syndrome is suggested by findings of degeneration and hypertrophy of the facet joints (spondylosis), but these changes are ubiquitous with aging. Furthermore, many people with radiographic spondylosis have no pain.[4-6,17] Yet one study demonstrated that community hospital patients with spinal pain demonstrate an increased prevalence of increased uptake in the facet joint on single-photon emission computed tomography (SPECT).[23] Because of these ambiguities, facet syndrome often is considered a diagnosis of exclusion. Spondylolisthesis may be comorbid with facet syndrome because displacement of the vertebral bodies produces stress on the facet joints.[6] Similarly, prior spinal fusion can lead to adjacent segment degeneration (transition zone syndrome) and facet-mediated pain.[24]

In the acute and early chronic setting, conservative management should be considered. This may include physical therapy, analgesics, relative rest, acupuncture, or chiropractic manipulation.[5] If conservative therapy fails after 6 to 12 weeks and there is no evidence of neurologic impairment on physical exam or major radiologic abnormality, the diagnosis of facet syndrome can be considered. Because the physical exam and radiologic studies are inadequate to diagnose facet syndrome, current practice is to anesthetize the nerves to the facet joint to confirm the diagnosis. There is a 30% to 40% placebo response to most pain therapies, including facet block, so a double-block protocol (i.e., repeated injection) with different local anesthetics with different durations of action can be used to reduce the false-positive rate.[2,25] Placebo-controlled blocks could be done, but placebo studies are often unacceptable to the patient, physician, or payer. The facet joint may be anesthetized either by injecting local anesthetic directly into the joint capsule or by blocking the medial branch nerves that innervate the joint. Corticosteroid also can be injected into the joint to provide potentially longer-lasting analgesia through its antiinflammatory effect.

CONTRAINDICATIONS

Because of the proximity of the facet joint to the epidural and spinal spaces, contraindications to facet joint injection or medial branch block are identical to other neuraxial techniques. Absolute contraindications include patient refusal, systemic infection, skin infection overlying the injection site, coagulopathy, and thrombocytopenia. Relative contraindications include inability to lie prone or otherwise tolerate the procedure, pregnancy, allergy to contrast dye or local anesthetic, untreated psychological dysfunction, and baseline neurologic deficits that may be confused with or disguise procedural complications. Previous posterior spinal surgery is not a contraindication to facet injection but may increase the technical difficulty of the procedure.

EQUIPMENT

- Oxygen and monitors (e.g., blood pressure, pulse oximetry, electrocardiography)
- Sterile preparation and draping equipment
- 25-gauge needle for skin infiltration with 1% lidocaine
- 22-gauge spinal needles (3.5-inch length adequate for most blocks, but 5-inch needles may be needed for larger or obese patients)
- Local anesthetic for facet block (preservative free):
  - Diagnostic injectate:
    - 2% lidocaine (0.3-1 mL) or 0.25% to 0.5% bupivacaine (0.3-1 mL)
  - Therapeutic injectate:
    - 0.25% bupivacaine with corticosteroid, 2 to 3 mL total volume for extracapsular injection
    - 0.25% bupivacaine with corticosteroid, 1 mL total volume for intraarticular injection
- Corticosteroid for facet injection:
  - Triamcinolone acetonide (Kenalog) 10 mg per joint
  - Methylprednisolone acetate (Depo-Medrol) 10 mg per joint
  - Betamethasone acetate (Celestone) 3 to 6 mg per joint

TECHNIQUE

Anatomy

A *facet* is defined as a smooth, flat area of bone that is covered with cartilage and articulates with another bone. Each vertebra has four articular processes (facets), two superior and two inferior, that project from the lamina of the vertebra. Each facet articulates with the opposing facet of the adjacent vertebrae, sacrum, or skull to form a facet joint. Vertebral facet joints are true synovial joints with fibrous capsules that restrict range of motion of the spine and distribute axial weight, particularly with extension.[26] The joint is arranged sagittally in the lumbar region,

coronally in the thoracic region, and cephalocaudad oblique in the cervical spine. The joints are less defined in the cervical spine, allowing for a greater range of motion. The anterior portion of the joint is in close proximity to the ligamentum flavum and may actually fuse with the joint.

Innervation of the lumbar facet joint is from the medial branch nerve at the spinal level of the joint and also from one level above (Fig. 165-1).[26] The medial branch nerve is a derivative from the dorsal rami of the nerve root exiting the spinal cord and also innervates the interspinous ligament and the multifidus and rotatores muscles.[26] The nerve travels off the dorsal rami, around the inferior base of the superior articular process, then divides such that some fibers travel superiorly to innervate the superior facet joint of its respective vertebrae. Other fibers continue inferiorly to innervate the facet joint of the vertebra one level below. The L5 median branch travels inferiorly over the sacral ala before it travels around the base of the superior articular process of the sacrum.[26] Of all lumbar medial branch nerves, the L5 dorsal ramus has the most consistent location over the sacral ala. The remaining medial branches either lie at the junction of the transverse process and the corresponding articular pillar or slightly above or below this junctional location.

The thoracic dorsal medial branch nerves (T1-T4, T9-T10) cross the superolateral corners of the transverse processes then pass medially and inferiorly across the posterior surfaces of the transverse processes at each level.[27] Exceptions to this pattern occur at the midthoracic level (T5-T8), where the inflection point occurs more superiorly to the superolateral corner of the transverse process. The course of the midthoracic medial branches makes their routine blockade or radiofrequency denervation somewhat unpredictable. The T11 dorsal medial branch courses along the lateral margin of the superior articular process of T12, and the T12 dorsal medial branch assumes a course analogous to that of the lumbar medial branches.

The cervical medial branch nerves course along the lateral recesses of the articular pillars at the respective vertebral levels and divide superiorly and inferiorly to supply the C3-4 to C7-T1 facet joints. The C2-3 facet joint receives its major innervation from the third occipital nerve and a lesser contribution from the C3 dorsal rami. The C0-C1 and C1-C2 joints receive innervation from the C1 and C2 ventral rami and thus are amenable to intraarticular blockade only.

Approach

Although radiologic imaging cannot reliably diagnose facet syndrome, it is invaluable in performing facet injections and medial branch blocks. Traditional fluoroscopy (x-ray fluoroscopy) is typically used, but other modalities have been described, such as ultrasound[28] and computed tomography (CT).[29] Similarly, CT-fluoroscopy has been utilized for lumbar diagnostic facet injections[29] and facet rhizotomy[30] and may provide more accurate needle placement, more reliable blocks, and better pain control. However, a direct comparison between CT and fluoroscopy-guided lumbar facet rhizotomy demonstrated equal reduction in Visual Analog Scale (VAS) scores.[31] Recently, laser irradiation of the dorsal surface of the facet joint capsule has

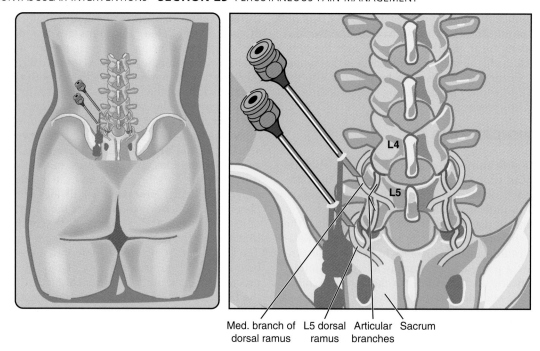

Med. branch of   L5 dorsal   Articular   Sacrum
dorsal ramus   ramus   branches

FIGURE 165-1. Lumbar zygapophyseal joint anatomy. *(Adapted from Waldman SD. Atlas of interventional pain management. 2nd ed. Philadelphia: Saunders; 2001.)*

been shown effective in reducing pain from lumbar facet syndrome.[32]

In preparation for lumbar facet block, the patient should be positioned prone. Pillows may be placed under the abdomen and ankles for comfort and to reduce lumbar lordosis. Monitors and supplemental oxygen should be used, and the patient may be sedated if necessary. For diagnostic blocks, sedation should be avoided if possible because it may be a confounding factor in determining the patient's response to the injection. After sterile preparation and draping, fluoroscopy is used to identify anatomic landmarks.

Diagnostic Lumbar Medial Branch Block

Use a radiopaque marker to identify the desired skin entry point. Anesthetize the skin with 1% lidocaine and a 25-gauge needle. With a posteroanterior (PA) view, insert the styleted 22-gauge needle and guide the tip to the superior, posterior, and medial border of the transverse process, (i.e., at the junction of the transverse process and superior articular process). This can be done by intentionally contacting the lamina overlying the pedicle and then walking off the bone superiorly (Fig. 165-2). It is not necessary to move completely off the transverse process, merely approaching the edge is sufficient. Needle tip position can be confirmed in an oblique view as well (Fig. 165-3). After negative aspiration for blood, diagnostic injection is performed with 0.3 to 1 mL of 1% lidocaine or 0.5% bupivacaine. The sacral ala must be identified for L5 medial branch blocks (Fig. 165-4; also see Fig. 165-3). As noted, blocks must be done at the level of and one level above the suspected facet joint. For example, to anesthetize the L4-5 facet joint, the median branch nerves of both L3 and L4 must be anesthetized. These nerves will lie along the transverse processes of L4 and L5, respectively, at the junction of the transverse process and superior articular pillar. However, successful

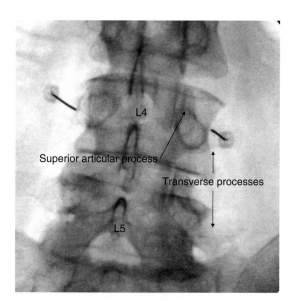

FIGURE 165-2. Posteroanterior fluoroscopy of L3 medial branch block showing needle placement at junction of transverse process and superior articular process of L4.

neurotomy of lumbar medial branch nerves may require multiple lesions within this target zone to ensure adequate destruction of the medial branches that may lie slightly above or below this location (see earlier).

Lumbar Facet Joint Injection: Diagnostic or Therapeutic

Rotate the fluoroscopic machine to an oblique position until it is in the plane of the posterior portion of the joint. The facet joint may not lie in a single plane but may be C-shaped. Therefore, the entire length of the joint may not be seen in one fluoroscopic view. In the appropriate angulation, the edges of the joint will be sharply and darkly defined (Fig. 165-5). Advance the spinal needle into the joint, and inject 0.1 to 0.3 mL of contrast to confirm joint entry. If correct placement is verified, deliver injectate with a total volume of no more than about 1 mL. The joints are very low volume, and capsular rupture has been described, which may cause future pain.[33] Injection should be done slowly, and if the patient reports pain, no further volume should be injected.

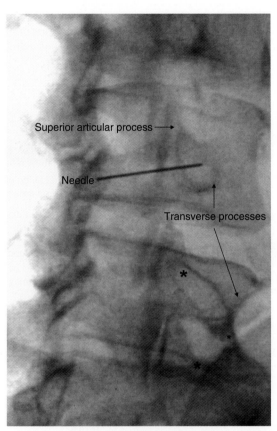

FIGURE 165-3. Right lateral oblique view of L3 medial branch block. Asterisks mark sites for blockade of right L4 and L5 medial branch nerves.

Diagnostic Cervical Medial Branch Block

The patient is positioned prone with the neck in a neutral position (i.e., looking straight down at the floor). A specialized positioner may be used, or pillows placed under the chest and forehead. Again, use a radiopaque marker to identify the desired skin entry point, and anesthetize the skin with 1% lidocaine. With a PA view, insert the styleted 22-gauge needle until it contacts the midpoint ("waist") of the articular pillar at its lateral border (Figs. 165-6 and 165-7). In the lateral view, the needle tip may be advanced off the pillar until it is just forward of the posterior border of the facet joints at the centroid of the articular pillar (see Fig 165-7, *B*). This forward advancement is unnecessary for diagnostic block but necessary for facet neurolysis.[11-14,34] Then 0.25 to 0.5 mL of 1% lidocaine or 0.25% bupivacaine is injected to anesthetize the medial branch nerve. CT guidance for facet medial branch block is shown in Figure 165-8. In general, the medial branches lie at the centroids of the articular pillars or slightly higher at C3 and C6. At C7, the medial branch has a variable location and may lie between the apex of the C7 superior articular process and the root of the C7 transverse process. As an example, since each cervical facet joint has dual nerve supply, the medial branches of C4 and C5 must be targeted to anesthetize the C4-5 facet joint. The C2-3 facet joint is innervated mainly by the third occipital nerve, which lies either transversely across the lateral axis of the C2-3 facet joint or a few millimeters above or below the joint line on lateral view. Successful block of the nerve supply to the C2-3 facet joint may require needle placement at any or all these locations.

Diagnostic Thoracic Medial Branch Block

The patient is positioned prone on the fluoroscopy table. Radiopaque markers can be used to identify proper needle entry points. The skin is anesthetized with 1% lidocaine. With PA view, insert the 22-gauge needle until it contacts the superolateral margin of the transverse process (see Anatomy for details). Then inject 0.5 mL of 1% lidocaine. Care must be exercised to avoid pneumothorax with thoracic medial branch block. Because of the variable anatomy of thoracic medial branch nerves in relation to their bony counterparts, there may not be a reliable technique that can

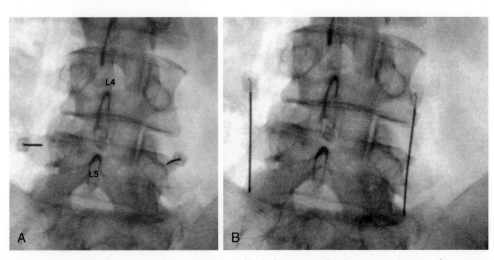

FIGURE 165-4. A, Posteroanterior (PA) fluoroscopy of L4 medial branch block showing needle placement at junction of transverse process and superior articular process on L5. **B,** PA fluoroscopy of L5 medial branch (dorsal rami at this level) block showing needle placement at junction of sacral ala and sacral superior articular process.

be used universally for local anesthetic blockade or denervation of all thoracic medial branch nerves.

OUTCOMES

A facet block is considered diagnostic of facet syndrome if
a patient reports a 50% reduction in pain score 30 minutes
after the procedure.[5] Since the false-positive rate may be as
high as 38%, a double-block paradigm has been recommended.[2,5] The blocks should be done with lidocaine and

bupivacaine on separate occasions a few weeks apart.
Patients should keep a pain diary for 8 hours after the block,
and the duration of analgesia should match the duration of
action of the anesthetic (60-90 minutes for lidocaine, 4-6
hours for bupivacaine).

Pain relief outcomes after corticosteroid facet injection
for therapy are mixed. Historical studies were small, nonrandomized, and retrospective.[1] Among the higher-quality
studies, results varied from positive to equivocal to
negative.[35-37] Confounding variables included nonuniform
methods and criteria for diagnosing facet syndrome,
varying techniques for performing joint injections and
medial branch blocks, and varying interpretations of similar
data.[1] Some authors describe successful block as being pain

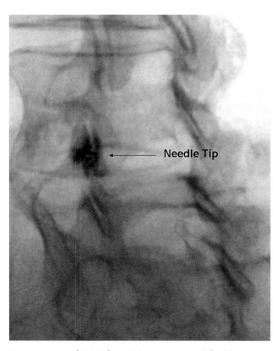

FIGURE 165-5. Left L4-5 facet joint injection in left oblique view. Note
contrast filling joint and nicely outlined walls of L5-S1 facet joint below.

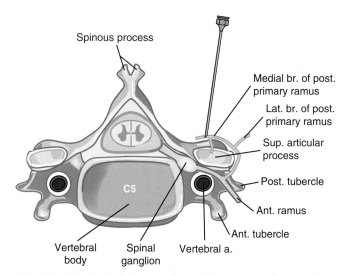

FIGURE 165-6. Cervical zygapophyseal joint anatomy. *(From Waldman
SD. Atlas of interventional pain management. 2nd ed. Philadelphia: Saunders;
2001.)*

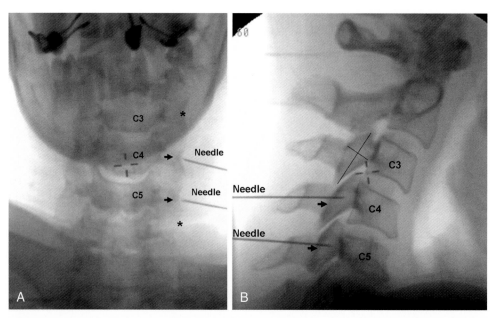

FIGURE 165-7. A, Posteroanterior view of left C4 and C5 medial branch block. Needle tips are in "waist" of lateral masses. *Asterisks* mark sites for C3
and C6 medial branch block. **B,** Lateral view of C4 and C5 medial branch blocks. Appropriate site for neurotomy is at midpoint of lateral masses. *Diagonal
lines* drawn on C3 show how to estimate best site for neurotomy.

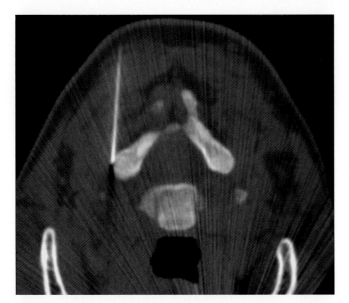

FIGURE 165-8. Computed tomography image of cervical facet block.

free for 3 months after injection. Other investigators consider this a failed block, since pain recurred. Interestingly, patients with positive facet joint findings on bone scan had a better response to facet joint steroid injection than those with no bone scan findings.[38] Similarly, patients who had positive SPECT findings of facet arthrosis, compared to those who did not, showed better response to medial branch blocks.[39] Accuracy in diagnosing lumbar facet joint pain can be increased and long-term outcomes can be improved by using the cutoff measure of 80% pain relief rather than 50% pain relief as the diagnostic criterion.[40] Serial facet joint injections using local anesthetic with or without steroid can provide long-term pain relief and functional improvement.[41-43]

Radiofrequency neurolysis can be considered if facet syndrome is diagnosed with medial branch block or joint injection.[34,44,45] Neurolysis may be more beneficial than intraarticular steroids, at least in the cervical spine.[46,47] For neurolysis, the cannulae are positioned in the same location as for medial branch block. Neurolysis can be done in the cervical, thoracic, and lumbar spine. Lesioning is usually done by radiofrequency at 80 to 85°C for 75 to 90 seconds. Multiple studies have demonstrated good pain relief after radiofrequency denervation. Success rates, defined as at least 50% pain relief, vary between 50% and 87%.[1,47-51] Positive results can be sustained over time by repeated rhizotomy.[52] Percutaneous lumbar cryorhizotomy, an alternative to radiofrequency rhizotomy, also has shown long-term benefit.[53] Meticulous patient screening using a combination of clinical history, physical examination findings, imaging tests, and response to diagnostic facet injections can improve outcomes in patients receiving radiofrequency lumbar facet denervation.[54] A recent 10-year prospective clinical study demonstrated that 68.4% of patients had better than 50% to 80% pain relief lasting from 6 to 24 months.[55] Unfortunately, much of the data supporting facet rhizotomy came from retrospective or uncontrolled studies.[47,50] Furthermore, some reviews have found no lasting benefit from rhizotomy.[1] Even reviews of randomized controlled trials have been critical of inadequate

screening criteria and inaccurate needle placement, and authors have proposed revised guidelines to improve results.[56,57] In studies demonstrating lasting benefit from rhizotomy, the diagnosis of facet syndrome was made by median branch block.[45,47,50,51,58] Studies that used intraarticular local anesthetic injection for diagnosis showed less benefit from rhizotomy.[49,59] A recent randomized controlled trial demonstrated three successful diagnostic facet blocks followed by multiple radiofrequency lesions at each site resulted in significant improvement in quality-of-life variables, global perception of improvement, and generalized pain scores.[60] Outcomes are worse when patients have comorbid depression,[61] advanced age,[62] and increased neuroforaminal stenosis.[62] In contrast, prominent local tenderness, percussion tenderness, pain on rising, extension and transitional movement, and good immediate response are associated with better outcome.[63]

COMPLICATIONS

Facet joint injection is safe, with about a 1% risk of minor complications, usually postprocedural pain.[64] Other complications include infection, facet capsular rupture, dural puncture with or without spinal anesthesia/total spinal, spinal headache, allergic reactions, vasovagal response, pneumothorax, and bleeding.[64] Significant bleeding from inadvertent puncture of the vertebral artery could occur as a complication of a cervical facet block. Case reports of complications include paraspinal abscess, meningitis, septic arthritis, and chemical meningitis.[65] Finally, there are reports of radiographic facet joint changes consistent with infection in noninfected patients after facet radiofrequency denervation.[66]

POSTPROCEDURE AND FOLLOW-UP CARE

After facet joint injection or medial branch block, the patient should be monitored for 15 to 30 minutes for improvement or worsening of back or neck pain. If sedation was used, postoperative monitoring should be instituted for at least 30 minutes or until the patient meets discharge criteria. Pain score at rest and with ambulation should be assessed before discharge. Discharge instructions and a pain diary should be provided. The patient should be instructed to call or seek immediate medical attention if signs or symptoms of complications arise. A phone call from a physician, nurse practitioner, or nurse is appropriate 24 to 48 hours after injection. Patients receiving diagnostic blocks should be scheduled for follow-up in 2 to 6 weeks. Patients receiving therapeutic blocks should be reevaluated in 2 to 4 months.

KEY POINTS

- Back and neck pain are some of the most frequent medical complaints and account for a significant amount of economic loss and suffering.
- The facet joint, also known as the *zygapophyseal* or *Z-joint*, is a true synovial joint that comprises two of the three articulating surfaces in the vertebral column. The facet joint receives its innervation from the medial branches of the dorsal primary rami.

- Facet joint pathology can lead to acute or chronic back, posterior thoracic, or neck pain, which is termed *facet syndrome*. Facet disease in the neck can produce cervicogenic headaches.
- Facet syndrome signs, symptoms, and radiologic findings are nonspecific and shared with other etiologies of back or neck pain.
- Facet joint injections and medial branch blocks are done for both diagnostic and therapeutic purposes. The gold standard for diagnosis is a positive response to facet block on more than one occasion. If facet syndrome is confirmed, treatment options include corticosteroid injection into the joint or neuroablation of the corresponding medial branch nerves.

▶ SUGGESTED READINGS

Berven S, Tay BB, Colman W, Hu SS. The lumbar zygapophyseal (facet) joints: a role in the pathogenesis of spinal pain syndromes and degenerative spondylolisthesis. Semin Neurol 2002;22(2):187–96.

Bogduk N, McGuirk B. An algorithm for precision diagnosis. In: Bogduk N, McGuirk B, editors. Medical management of acute and chronic low back pain An evidence-based approach: Pain Research and Clinical Management, vol. 13. Amsterdam: Elsevier Science BV; 2002. p. 177–86.

Bogduk N, McGuirk B. Causes and sources of chronic low back pain. In: Bogduk N, McGuirk B, editors. Medical management of acute and chronic low back pain An evidence-based approach: Pain Research and Clinical Management, vol. 13. Amsterdam: Elsevier Science BV; 2002. p. 115–26.

Curatolo M, Bogduk N. Diagnostic and therapeutic nerve blocks. In: Fishman S, Ballantyne J, Rathmell J, editors. Bonica's Management of Pain. 4th ed. Philadelphia: Lippincott; 2010. p. 1401–23.

Govind J, Bogduk N. Neurolytic blockade for non-cancer pain. In: Fishman S, Ballantyne J, Rathmell J, editors. Bonica's Management of Pain. 4th ed. Philadelphia: Lippincott; 2010. p. 1467–85.

Niemisto L, Kalso E, Malmivaara A, et al. Radiofrequency Denervation for Neck and Back Pain: A Systematic Review Within the Framework of the Cochrane Collaboration Back Review Group. Spine 2003;28(16):1877–88.

Slipman CW, Bhat AL, Gilchrist RV, et al. A critical review of the evidence for the use of zygapophysial injections and radiofrequency denervation in the treatment of low back pain. Spine J 2003;3(4):310–16.

The complete reference list is available online at www.expertconsult.com.

CHAPTER 166

Sacroiliac Joint Injections

Alexis D. Kelekis and Dimitris Filippiadis

CLINICAL RELEVANCE

At least once during their lifetime, the vast majority of the healthy population (70%-90%) will experience an episode of low back pain.[1] Degeneration or inflammation of the sacroiliac (SI) joint is a common cause (10%-27%).[2-5] However, defining the SI joint as the pain source can be quite difficult, mostly owing to overlapping of symptoms with those of facet or hip joint degeneration.[6,7] Therefore, infiltration as a diagnostic test can provide the foundation for establishing the SI joint as the pain source in these patients.

Symptoms of SI joint degeneration or inflammation can be persistent and refractory to conservative therapy (oral nonsteroidal antiinflammatory drugs [NSAIDs] and analgesics, bed rest, physiotherapy).[2-5] Steroid administration is believed to achieve a neural blockade that alters or interrupts the neural processes of encoding and processing noxious stimuli, the afferent fibers' reflex mechanisms, the neurons' self-sustaining activity, and central neuronal activity patterns.[8] In addition, corticosteroids inhibit synthesis and/or release of proinflammatory mediators, thus reducing inflammation. Local anesthetic interrupts the pain/spasm cycle and transmission of noxious stimuli.[8]

INDICATIONS[9-13]

- Patient with unilateral or bilateral low back or groin pain without neuralgia
- Patient with sitting intolerance
- Patient with low back or groin numbness or buttock tingling
- Symptomatic patient (any of the aforementioned symptoms) with positive imaging findings for SI joint degeneration

CONTRAINDICATIONS

Absolute[9-13]

- Local sepsis/skin infection at the puncture site
- Bacteremia or any active systemic infection (including tuberculosis)
- Allergy to any component of the injected mixture (local anesthetic, corticosteroid)
- Patient unwilling to consent to the procedure
- Pregnancy (due to teratogenic effects of ionizing radiation)
- Underlying clinical entity that contraindicates corticosteroid therapy (ulcer, severe hypertension, severe congestive heart failure with fluid retention, etc.)

Relative[9-13]

- Hemorrhagic diathesis (should be corrected before procedure)
- Anticoagulant therapy (should be interrupted before procedure)
- Immunodeficiency syndrome
- Allergy to contrast medium (in such cases, gadolinium can be used)
- Patient has already received maximum allowed dose of steroids for a given period (3-4 infiltrations within 6-12 month period)

EQUIPMENT[9-13]

- All necessary material for extensive local sterility (scrubs, sterile drapes and coverings, gloves, and gauzes)
- Nonionic contrast medium
- Spinal needle, 22 to 25 gauge, 90 or 110 mm length
- Syringe (n = 2), 3 to 5 mL (for contrast medium and injectate)
- Injectate containing local anesthetic (e.g., lidocaine hydrochloride or bupivacaine hydrochloride) and long-acting steroid (e.g., betamethasone, methylprednisolone, or cortivazol) at 1:1.5 ratio (total injectate volume ≈ 2.5 mL)
- For diagnostic purposes, a local intraarticular anesthetic alone is injected.

TECHNIQUE

Anatomy and Approaches

The SI joint is a diarthrosis between the sacral and iliac bones. The joint itself consists of two parts: inferiorly there is a synovial cartilaginous joint, and posterosuperiorly there is a fibrous part.[9] The sacral cartilage is 3 to 5 mm thick, and the iliac cartilage is only 1 mm thick.[9] The ventral rami of L4 and L5, the superior gluteal nerve, and the dorsal rami of S1, S2, S3, and S4 nerves innervate the SI joint.[1,2,10] In addition, the joint capsule and ligaments contain nerve fibers.[2,3,9]

SI joint infiltration is a minimally invasive image-guided technique that is performed on an outpatient basis. Fluoroscopy, computed tomography (CT), and magnetic resonance imaging (MRI) can be used for imaging guidance.[9-13] Although ionizing radiation is absent in MRI, the required cost and time are considered significant disadvantages. CT exposes the patient to ionizing radiation but can be reserved for cases with significant joint degeneration where intraarticular needle positioning is difficult.[14-16]

Fluoroscopy provides faster and dynamic needle placement with real-time evaluation of the contrast medium's spread inside the joint, which will verify both the desired and the extravascular needle position.[17-20] Cone beam CT (with pulsed fluoroscopy) may provide guidance (with fluoroscopic images, axial, and multiplanar reconstruction [MPR] CT-like images) at low radiation levels for both the patient and the medical staff.

Corticosteroids used in SI joint infiltrations can be particulate or non-particulate. The former may offer better and more lasting results, but for intravascular injection their crystals might act as emboli, occluding a vascular branch. The latter are free of such a complication (can be injected intravascularly without consequences), but success rates are lower and results are not long-lasting.[8]

Informed consent is necessary prior to the session.

TECHNICAL ASPECTS

The patient is placed in prone position on either the fluoroscopy or CT table.[9-13] In the absence of C-arm guidance, especially under fluoroscopy guidance, raising the contralateral hip by 20 to 30 degrees will place the lower joint space parallel to the x-ray beam, allowing direct entry to the synovial portion by means of a more or less vertical route. Alternatively, the patient is placed in a simple prone position, and the fluoroscopy beam is directed caudally and laterally, angulated about 25 degrees. Infiltration is performed under extensive local sterility. Local anesthesia is optional, and the decision varies among different centers throughout the globe. Under fluoroscopic guidance, a 22-gauge (90-110 cm) needle is advanced inside the SI joint, following a course parallel to the beam. The target point is located approximately 1 cm over the joint's inferior end[9-13] (Fig. 166-1). Once inside the joint, a minor resistance loss is felt. The desired intraarticular and extravascular needle placement is verified fluoroscopically after injection of a

small amount (0.1-0.5 mL) of nonionic contrast medium. The contrast medium will be seen lining the joint's margins or collecting at the joint's dependent portion (Fig. 166-2). Once in the desired position, the injectate is released within the joint. For difficult cases, alternative double needle techniques under fluoroscopic guidance have been described in the literature.[21] Beware of trespassing the articulation and ending in the anterior part of the sacrum, next to the iliac vessels.

In cases where CT is preferred as the guiding mode, scans with 5-mm axial images from the joint's middle portion to the distal end are performed.[9] Once again, the target point is located approximately 1 cm over the joint's inferior end[10-14] (Fig. 166-3). A 22-gauge (90-110 cm) needle

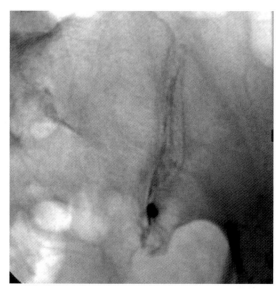

FIGURE 166-2. Anteroposterior projection of fluoroscopy-guided sacroiliac joint injection. Contrast medium is seen inside joint, verifying desired intraarticular position of needle.

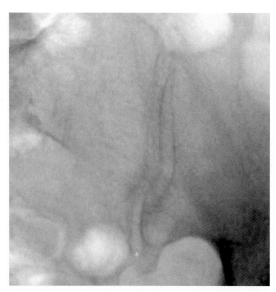

FIGURE 166-1. Anteroposterior projection of fluoroscopy-guided sacroiliac joint injection. Asterisk notes target point approximately 1 cm cephalad over end of joint.

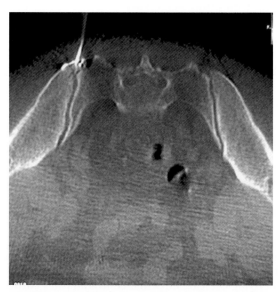

FIGURE 166-3. Cone beam computed tomography (axial image). Needle is seen within sacroiliac joint.

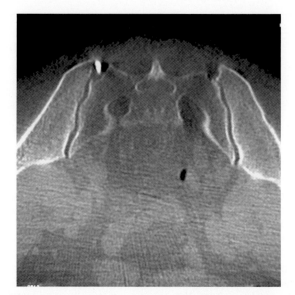

FIGURE 166-4. Cone beam computed tomography (axial image). Contrast medium is seen inside joint, verifying desired intraarticular position of needle.

is advanced directly into the SI joint following a route that is more or less parallel to the joint orientation. Once inside the joint, a minor resistance loss is felt. The desired intraarticular and extravascular needle placement is verified with a scan after injection of a small amount (0.1-0.5 mL) of nonionic contrast medium. The contrast medium will be seen lining the joint's margins or collecting at the joint's dependent portion (Fig. 166-4). Once in the desired position, the injectate is released within the joint.

CONTROVERSIES

- The SI joint acts as a source of pain, either due to synovial irritation or by means of joint fluid mediators that chemically irritate the innervating nerves.[9,22,23]
- Imaging guidance seems to be necessary for successful intraarticular needle placement. Prospective double-blind studies have shown that blind SI joint infiltrations succeed in intraarticular needle positioning in only 22%.[9]
- Duration of the pain reduction effect is questionable. In many cases, optimal results require a second infiltration session 7 to 10 days after the first one.[11] If the injections are short lived, one can opt for radiofrequency ablation.

OUTCOMES[9,11,14-16]

- Immediate pain relief in 50% to 80% of patients for a mean follow-up period of 10 ± 5 months
- Pain relief within 12 hours in 90% of patients for a mean follow-up period of 10 ± 5 months
- Pain relief less than 50% in patients with a history of spine surgery

COMPLICATIONS[9-13]

- Bleeding
- Infection
- Allergic reaction
- Transient lower extremity weakness or paresthesia (due to potential injectate spread along the nerve roots inside the epidural space or extravasation around the sciatic nerve)
- Transient pain exacerbation
- Contact of the needle with the sciatic nerve (in cases where needle is advanced too inferiorly)
- Intrapelvic puncture

POSTPROCEDURAL AND FOLLOW-UP CARE

SI joint infiltrations are performed as an outpatient procedure. Patients remain under observation for about 30 minutes after the session. Monitoring of vital signs is optional. Patient discharge is performed after motor strength and potential sensory deficit evaluation and always into the care of an accompanying person. Because initial pain relief is mainly due to the local anesthetic (steroids require 3 to 5 days to start acting), the patient is instructed to continue pain-relief medication. A follow-up appointment is scheduled 7 to 10 days after the infiltration session.

KEY POINTS

- Chronic low back pain may be caused by sacroiliac joint (SI joint) degeneration.
- Infiltration of the SI joint can be used for either diagnosis or treatment of chronic low back pain.
- Diagnostic tests verify the SI joint as the pain source in a patient with chronic low back pain.
- Therapeutic infiltrations decrease pain and improve mobility by reducing inflammation or treating degeneration of the SI joint.
- Imaging guidance ensures proper intraarticular needle positioning.
- Pain and mobility outcomes should be evaluated after the procedure.

▶ **SUGGESTED READINGS**

Forst SL, Wheeler MT, Fortin JD, Vilensky JA. The SI joint: anatomy, physiology and clinical significance. Pain Physician 2006;9(1):61–7.

Hansen HC, Mc Kenzie-Brown AM, Cohen SP, et al. SI joint interventions: a systematic review. Pain Physician 2007;10(1):165–84.

Kelekis AD, Somonb T, Yilmaz H, et al. Interventional spine procedures. Eur J Radiol 2005;55(3):362–83.

Rupert MP, Lee M, Manchikanti L, et al. Evaluation of SI joint interventions: a systematic appraisal of the literature. Pain Physician 2009;12(2):399–418.

The complete reference list is available online at www.expertconsult.com.

CHAPTER 167

Periradicular Therapy

Gianluigi Guarnieri, Roberto Izzo, and Mario Muto

INTRODUCTION

Low back pain (LBP) and neck pain (NP) are the most common spine diseases and the most common cause of absence from work in developed countries. Roughly 80% of adults suffer from back pain or LBP during a lifetime; 55% suffer from radicular pain, and of these, 44% experience pain in the cervical region, 15% in the thoracic, and 66% at the lumbar level.[1] Most symptoms revolve spontaneously within a few days or weeks with conservative medical therapy, but about a third of patients progress to chronic pain. The causes of chronic LBP or NP include vertebral body pathology, vertebral disk disease, spinal stenosis, nerve entrapment syndrome, and facet joint disease.

The diagnosis of LBP or NP is difficult and should be done by a multidisciplinary team. Clinical evaluation, imaging (computed tomography [CT], magnetic resonance imaging [MRI], electromyelography [EMG]), and a multi-specialist approach (radiologist, neuroradiologist, neurosurgeon, and neurologist) are essential. Many mini-invasive spinal procedures have been developed for managing these conditions, including percutaneous spinal analgesic injections into the epidural or foraminal space and facet joints, with good results and low rates of complications (1%).[2-4] Pathogenesis of LBP and NP are discussed in Chapter 161.

The full discussion of this topic is available at www.expertconsult.com.

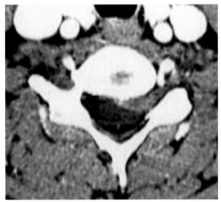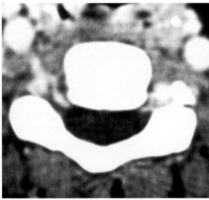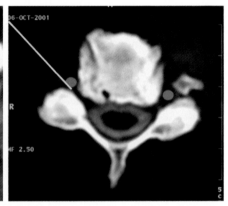

FIGURE 167-1. Patient affected by left posterolateral herniated disk at C5-C6 level. Illustration shows anterolateral approach to foraminal space.

CHAPTER 168

Epidural Steroid Injection

Brian M. Block and Theodore S. Grabow

CLINICAL RELEVANCE

Low back pain is a significant medical problem. It is widely prevalent, affecting patients of all ages, and greatly contributes to healthcare and disability costs. Bressler et al. estimated the frequency of back pain at 13% to 49% of patients over the age of 65.[1] Overall prevalence is 60% to 80%, moreso in industrialized countries, with peak prevalence between 45 and 60 years of age.[1-3] Low back pain disorders are expensive, accounting for one third of all disability costs in the United States. Of patients on disability, low back pain represents only 3% of subjects receiving compensation, but they receive 75% of payments. In 2006, the economic burden of back and neck pain on the United States was estimated at $85.9 billion and was increasing faster than the overall rate of medical inflation.[4] Patients with back pain had nearly twice the medical expenditures as patients without back pain.[4]

Lumbosacral radiculopathy, commonly known as *sciatica*, presents with a wide range of symptoms from mild intermittent low back and leg pain to severe neurologic compromise. Symptoms arise from mechanical compression of the lumbosacral nerve roots. Younger patients are more likely to suffer from intervertebral disc herniation, whereas older patients may have vertebral degeneration, facet joint hypertrophy, spondylosis, and osteophytes as the cause of their neuroforaminal stenosis, radiculopathy, and/or pain. Conservative treatment includes rest, oral antiinflammatory medications, oral corticosteroids, analgesics, and physical therapy.[5,6] The natural course of radicular pain is variable but typically resolves in a matter of weeks to months.[7] During this time, epidural steroid injection (ESI) can be helpful in alleviating symptoms and promoting a return to normal function. In complicated cases, surgery may be necessary to relieve nerve root compression. ESI can be an effective alternative to surgery in some patients and provide relief in cases where surgery has failed.[8]

INDICATIONS

- Radiculopathy/radiculitis: from herniated nucleus pulposus, degenerative stenosis
- Spinal stenosis: central or neuroforaminal
- Spondylosis causing axial pain

Radiculopathy is the best indication for ESI and has the best outcomes. A careful history and physical can optimize patient selection for ESI. Back pain or neck pain with radiation to the extremity, a dermatomal pattern of sensory loss, and presence of sciatic or brachial plexus stretch signs are symptoms of radiculitis and may predict better success with ESI.[9] In contrast, non-radiating axial pain, myofascial pain syndrome, facet and sacroiliac arthropathy, and neurogenic claudication respond less well to ESI.[10] However, there is a paucity of effective treatments for these pain syndromes

and a huge prevalence of them, so ESI is often done as a trial of therapy. Other axial pain treatments, such as sacroiliac joint steroid injections, zygapophyseal (facet) joint injection, and median branch denervation, can be effective if pain persists despite ESI.

Although there is a poor correlation between outcomes and imaging studies, computed tomography (CT) and magnetic resonance imaging (MRI) can be important tools for localizing the area of nerve root compression and ruling out other serious causes of back pain such as tumor.[2,9]

CONTRAINDICATIONS

- Coagulopathy, thrombocytopenia, or anticoagulant therapy
- Local or systemic infection
- Relative contraindications are uncontrolled diabetes, glaucoma, and immunocompromise.

Spinal/epidural hematoma and abscess are the major complications of epidural injection to be avoided. ESIs are never life saving, so any patient with overt risk for bleeding or infection should be postponed. Immunocompromised patients, such as those with HIV or cancer, may be at higher risk for infection, so extra care should be taken both in patient selection and technique for them. Injected steroids can worsen glaucoma and glucose control in diabetics.[9,11]

EQUIPMENT

- Sterile prep and drape
- Touhy needle for midline injection, 17 to 18 gauge for lumbar, 20 gauge for cervical injection
- Spinal needle (22 gauge) for transforaminal or caudal injection
- Extension tubing for transforaminal injection
- Injectable contrast solution such as Omnipaque or Isovue
- Steroid preparation (triamcinolone diacetate 40-80 mg, methylprednisolone acetate 40-80 mg, betamethasone 6-12 mg, or dexamethasone 8-16 mg)
- Preservative-free local anesthetic (lidocaine or bupivacaine) or saline for steroid diluent
- Intravenous access for cervical or thoracic injections
- Resuscitation and airway equipment
- Monitors, including pulse oximetry, blood pressure, and electrocardiography

TECHNIQUE

Anatomy

An understanding of the anatomy of the spinal column including the vertebrae, spinal cord and nerve roots, and ligamentous structures is necessary. The lumbar vertebra is

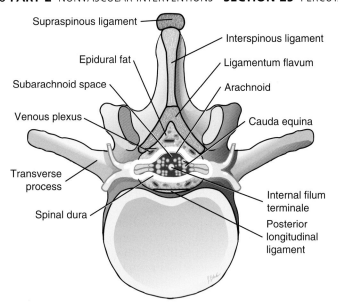

FIGURE 168-1. Lumbar epidural anatomy. *(From Waldman SD. Atlas of interventional pain management. 2nd ed. Philadelphia: Saunders; 2001.)*

comprised of a spinous process, two laminae, two transverse processes, two pedicles, and a vertebral body. Circumferentially, these structures make up the spinal canal, which contains the dural sac, spinal cord, cauda equina, and cerebrospinal fluid (CSF). Ligaments, from posterior to anterior, are the supraspinous, interspinous, and ligamentum flavum. The epidural space lies deep to the ligamentum flavum and is a potential space containing fat, blood vessels, nerve roots, and dural sac (Fig. 168-1). The epidural space extends laterally to the intervertebral foramen and anteriorly to the vertebral body. The inferior border of the epidural space is at the sacral hiatus, a U-shaped space between the inferior aspect of the sacrum and the coccyx. The hiatus is bounded laterally by the sacral cornua, with the sacrococcygeal ligament as the main structure between the skin and epidural space at this level.[12]

For the safe performance of transforaminal injections, knowledge of neuroforaminal anatomy is critical. The neuroforamen is bordered posteriorly by the zygapophyseal joints, superiorly and inferiorly by the pedicles, and anteriorly by the vertebral bodies and intervertebral disk. The neuroforamen contains the exiting nerve root in a dural sleeve and the radicular artery. At some levels, the radicular artery becomes the main blood supply to the anterior spinal cord and is then termed the *major anterior radicular artery* (artery of Adamkiewicz). The artery of Adamkiewicz usually arises from one of the left intercostal arteries, typically between T8 and L3,[13,14] but many different anatomic variations have been reported, including an origination from the lower lumbar segments.[15] The nerve root is thought to lie at the superior anterior aspect of the neuroforamen most (but not all) of the time, and the radicular artery is attached to the ventral surface of the nerve root. Previously, the superior and posterior aspect of the neuroforamen had been promoted as the "safe triangle" for transforaminal injection. However, a recent study of 113 subjects showed that the artery of Adamkiewicz lies in the superior half of the foramen 97% of the time. Thus placing the needle in the inferior half should reliably miss the artery.[14] The

intervertebral disk also lies in the inferior half of the foramen, so if this site is chosen for needle placement, care should be taken not to advance the needle too deeply and inject the disc annulus or nucleus. Intradiscal injection could be less effective, since the medications would not be applied to the inflamed nerve and may carry higher risks due to the potential for discitis or incitement of degenerative disk disease.

Approach

Interlaminar

This is the most common approach to the epidural space and is sometimes termed *translaminar*. Interlaminar epidural injection should not be done through an area of prior laminectomy, owing to the likelihood of dural puncture and headache.

The patient is positioned prone with a pillow under the lower abdomen to straighten the curve of the lumbar spine and open the interlaminar space. An anteroposterior (AP) fluoroscopic view is used to identify the targeted level in the midline. After sterile preparation and draping, the skin is infiltrated with lidocaine. A 17-, 18-, or 20-gauge Touhy needle with stylet is carefully inserted through the anesthetized area of skin and advanced to the supraspinous ligament. At this point, there will be greater resistance to needle advancement as the needle engages the dense fibers of the ligament. Fluoroscopy should be used to verify midline positioning of the needle. The stylet is removed, and a well-lubricated 5-mL syringe containing preservative-free saline or air is attached. A loss of resistance technique is used along with radiologic guidance. The needle is advanced slowly and incrementally through the ligaments. As the needle tip reaches the ligamentum flavum, even greater resistance will be encountered. Once the needle traverses the ligamentum flavum, there will be a loss of resistance to both needle advancement and syringe injection. Lateral fluoroscopy or CT guidance is very helpful in identifying the true epidural space (Fig. 168-2).

Once in the epidural space, the needle tip will be just anterior to the laminae and spinous processes. If aspiration is negative for blood and CSF, 0.5 to 3 mL of contrast is injected. Contrast solution should spread along the posterior epidural space and should be confirmed in the AP view (Fig. 168-3). Dural puncture, or "wet tap," is usually evident by the free flow of CSF and layering of contrast anteriorly along the vertebral body. Occasionally, dural puncture may occur unnoticed, or subdural extraarachnoid injection can occur.[16,17] In the first case, patients may report postdural puncture headache later (see later) or have immediate temporary weakness from spinal block from any injected local anesthetic. Subdural injection presents as a slow onset (10-15 minutes) of spinal block with weakness, sensory loss, and hypotension.[17]

ESI is also effective in the cervical spine, but with an increased risk of both minor and severe complications. In the cervical spine, meticulous care should be taken to avoid dural puncture. Cervical dural puncture can lead to persistent CSF leak and severe persistent headache.[18] Beyond dural puncture, direct and catastrophic spinal cord injury can also result from anterior needle positioning. Radiologic guidance should always be used for cervical injection. If the needle tip appears too anterior, without loss of resistance,

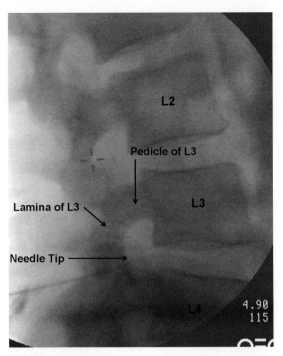

FIGURE 168-2. Lateral fluoroscopy showing needle placement just anterior to the facet line.

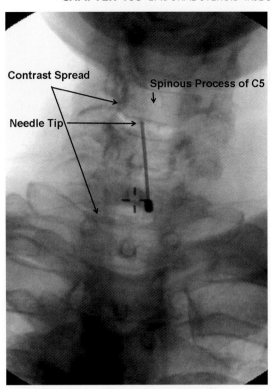

FIGURE 168-4. Cervical ESI at C5-6 in PA view. Note that needle placement is only slightly left of midline, yet the injectate spreads exclusively leftward in the tight cervical space.

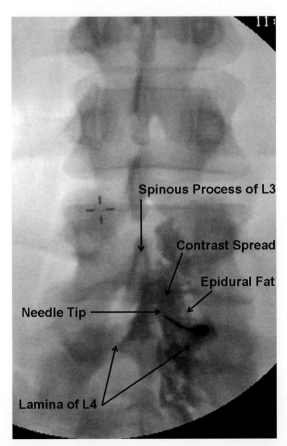

FIGURE 168-3. Posterior fluoroscopic image from L3-4 interlaminar epidural steroid injection. Needle tip and contrast spread is slightly to right. Epidural fat is seen as radiolucent globules within radiopaque contrast.

it may be lateral and should be repositioned. Also, the ligamentum flavum is much thinner in the cervical spine, so the tactile response during needle advancement will be less. In some cases, the ligamentum flavum fails to fuse and is completely absent.[19] Injecting a small amount (0.3 mL) of contrast can reveal whether the needle is in the epidural space or still too posterior (Figs. 168-4 through 168-6). Once epidural positioning is verified, the steroid mixture is slowly injected. There should be virtually no resistance to injection; any change in resistance warrants repeating the procedure at a different level. Patients often report pressure or mild discomfort during injection. However, complaints of pain should prompt the physician to stop injection and consider moving to a different level or using a smaller volume of injectate. Steroids should be diluted with *preservative-free saline.* Using local anesthetic as a diluent carries a risk of unrecognized subdural injection and late onset of cervical spinal or epidural block. In that event, the diaphragm and respiratory function could be compromised. In the cervical spine, total volume of injectate should be 3 to 6 mL, and in the lumbar spine, volume can be as little as 5 mL for an elderly patient with severe spinal stenosis or as much as 15 mL for a young patient with a herniated intervertebral disk.

Thoracic epidural steroid injection can also be done but is rarely needed.[20] In general, the approach is similar to that for lumbar injection. The major difference is that the spinous processes are angled from cephalad to caudad, which limits the needle trajectory along the midline. Paramedian trajectory is an alternative to midline placement. For a paramedian approach, the needle is inserted 1 to 2 cm off the midline and then slightly angled back to pierce the ligamentum flavum at the midline. As in the cervical spine, the spinal cord is vulnerable to direct injury, so lateral imaging is recommended.

Transforaminal

This approach is good for unilateral symptoms but has an increased risk of nerve and spinal cord injury. In fact, the risks of spinal cord injury appear to be so high in the cervical spine that some experts recommend avoiding cervical transforaminal injections entirely.[21] Thoracic transforaminal injections likely carry an increased risk of spinal cord injury similar to that of cervical injections, but no data are available for direct estimates. Transforaminal injections are

also appropriate for patients who have had spinal surgery at the level to be treated.

The patient is positioned prone, sterilely prepared, and draped. In the oblique view, the needle insertion site is just below the chin of the so-called Scotty dog (Fig. 168-7). The overlying skin is anesthetized, and a 22-gauge, 3.5- to 5-inch spinal needle is inserted. With intermittent fluoroscopic guidance, the needle is advanced to the neuroforamen. Bogduk et al. have described a fluoroscopically visualized

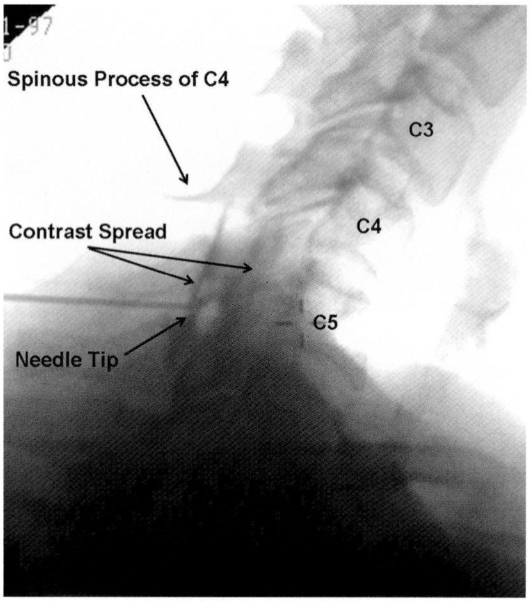

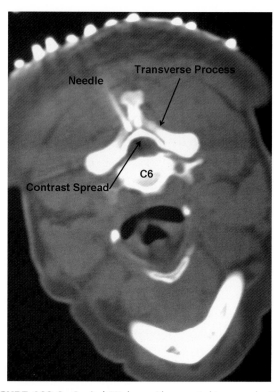

FIGURE 168-6. Cervical ESI done with computed tomography C6-7.

FIGURE 168-5. Lateral image from cervical ESI at C5-6. Note the contrast spread along the posterior dura and also down along the left nerve roots. The needle is just barely past the spinous processes.

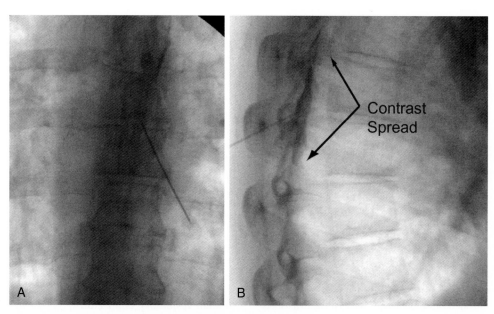

FIGURE 168-7. Thoracic ESI. **A,** The needle is placed from a right paramedian approach in the PA view. **B,** Lateral view shows contrast spread along the posterior epidural space.

safe triangle at the posterior superior end of the neuroforamen (Fig. 168-8).[20] Staying in this region will likely avoid contact or injury to the nerve root. As noted earlier, the safe triangle concept has been challenged recently.[14] In the lateral view, the tip will be in the posterior half of the neuroforamen just anterior to the facet line and just inferior to the pedicle (see Fig. 168-8). In the AP view, the needle tip should not be more medial than the midpoint of the superior pedicle (Fig. 168-9). Contrast should be injected with

live imaging to capture any vascular spread. Still images alone may miss the fact that the injectate is partially intravascular. Intravascular injectate may merely be less effective or may cause catastrophic spinal cord injury. Contrast should spread medially into the epidural space and distally down the nerve root. Low volumes (2-5 mL) of diluted corticosteroid are then injected after aspirating for blood or CSF. CT imaging has been safely used for transforaminal injection (Figs. 168-10 through 168-12). For cervical or thoracic injection, CT may even be superior for needle placement, given the complex anatomy in those regions. However, traditional CT does not allow "live" imaging during contrast injection and thus will not reliably detect intravascular injection. CT-fluoroscopy does allow live imaging, but in the case of intravascular injection, the contrast flow will be largely perpendicular to the plane of imaging, and this modality will not reliably detect intravascular injection.

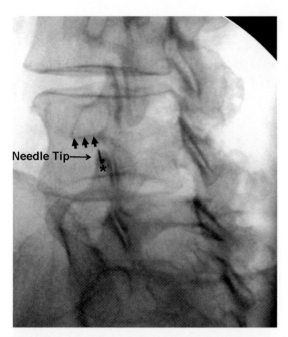

FIGURE 168-8. Left L4-5 transforaminal ESI. Needle placement is inferior to L4 pedicle, denoted by the arrowheads and just superior to the L5 superior aarticular process *(asterisk).*

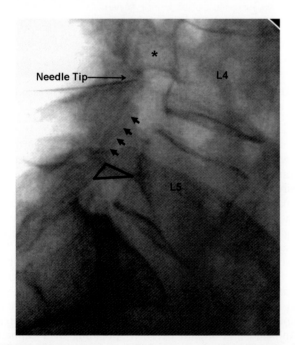

FIGURE 168-9. Lateral view of left L4-5 transforaminal ESI. Note that needle placement is only slightly anterior to the facet line *(arrowheads)* and just inferior to the pedicle of L4 *(asterisk).* The "safe triangle" for the L5-S1 neuroforamen is also marked.

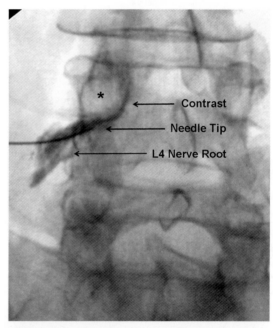

FIGURE 168-10. PA view of left L4-5 transforaminal ESI. Needle placement is abutting the L4 pedicle while contrast spreads both proximally into the epidural space and distally down the nerve root.

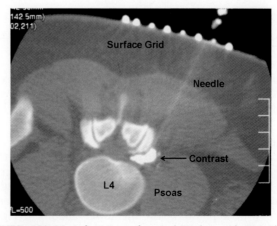

FIGURE 168-11. Left L4-5 transforaminal ESI done with CT guidance. Note contrast filling the neuroforamen.

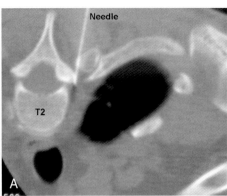
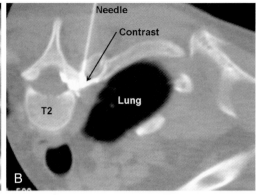

FIGURE 168-12. Left T2-3 transforaminal ESI done with CT guidance. **(A)** Needle placement before contrast injection. The overlying anatomy makes thoracic needle placement difficult with fluoroscopy. CT allows greater precision. **(B)** Contrast tracks along the nerve root and into the neuroforamen.

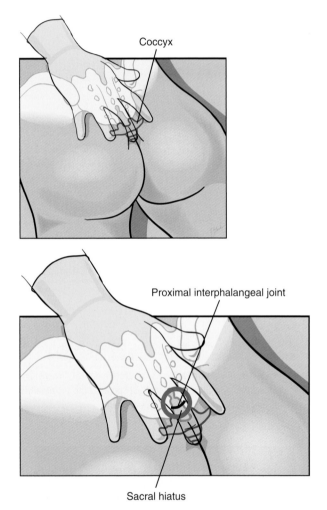

FIGURE 168-13. Anatomic cartoon depicting caudal epidural steroid injection. *(From Waldman SD. Atlas of interventional pain management. 2nd ed. Philadelphia: Saunders; 2001.)*

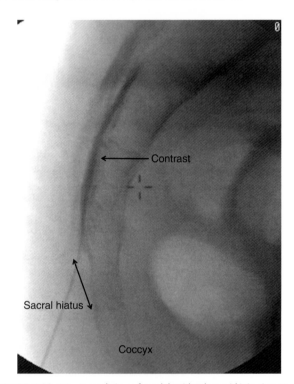

FIGURE 168-14. Lateral view of caudal epidural steroid injection. Needle trajectory is 45 degrees and clearly within spinal canal.

Caudal

This is the safest approach to the epidural space. The thecal sac ends at S1 in most patients, so the risk of dural puncture and headache is extremely low, and the risk of bleeding causing complication is neglible.[12] The patient is positioned prone with a pillow below the lower abdomen. Figure 168-13 shows the relevant anatomy and technique. The sacral cornua are palpated while AP fluoroscopy will reveal

the superior border of the sacral hiatus as an inverted U. Lateral fluoroscopy is generally used for needle insertion, because the sacral hiatus and caudal epidural space are easily visible (Fig. 168-14). A wide sterile preparation, particularly of the gluteal cleft, and draping is done, and the skin overlying the hiatus is infiltrated with lidocaine. A 22-gauge spinal needle is inserted at a 45-degree angle and advanced cephalad into the sacrococcygeal ligament. Traversing the ligament and entering the caudal epidural space will produce a noticeable loss of resistance to needle advancement. At this point, the needle angle is decreased and advanced 1 to 2 cm. Aspiration should be negative for blood and CSF. Using a lateral fluoroscopic view, contrast is injected and should be seen spreading in a cephalad direction. AP fluoroscopy is then used to verify bilateral spread of injectate (Fig. 168-15). Occasionally one-sided spread is desired for a patient with unilateral symptoms. In that case, the needle can be directed to one side after

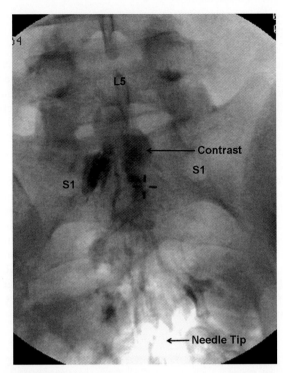

FIGURE 168-15. PA view of caudal ESI. Midline needle placement and bilateral contrast spread are observed.

piercing the sacrococcygeal ligament. Once needle position is confirmed, the steroid and anesthetic mixture is injected. Injectate volume should be 10 to 20 mL to ensure adequate cephalad spread to the lumbosacral nerve roots.

OUTCOMES

Onset of analgesia may be as soon as 10 minutes if local anesthetic is used, but this immediate analgesia is fleeting. The steroid component usually takes effect in 3 to 5 days to affect analgesia.[11] It is important to obtain preprocedural baseline measures of pain and functional limitations for comparison with postprocedure results.

Controlled studies attempting to evaluate long-term efficacy of ESI have had highly variable results. Hindrances in interpreting the many studies have been heterogeneous patient populations with poorly defined pain diagnoses, lack of appropriate controls, wide variability in treatment protocols, and poor outcome measures.[22] Systematic reviews of the literature reveal a full spectrum of conclusions with regard to efficacy. One early review concluded that 12% of patients had excellent results, 46% had fair results, and 25% failed treatment.[23] Other studies have concluded that ESI offers short-term benefit with unclear long-term efficacy.[24-26] A recent randomized controlled trial of 228 patients with sciatica found that ESI offered relief at 3 weeks, but without sustained improvement at 12 months.[27] Others have found efficacy of ESI up to 3 years in duration.[28] Transforaminal injections may be more effective than other approaches. In fact, transforaminal ESI may even reduce the need for surgery.[29] Overall, there is evidence for long-term benefit for both cervical and lumbar ESI.[30]

The nature of symptoms and the underlying diagnosis have been shown to make a difference in outcomes. Axial pain responds less well than radicular pain to cervical ESI.[31]

Patients with radicular symptoms from spinal stenosis respond less well than those with pain from disc herniation.[9,10] Recent randomized controlled trials have shown pain relief in 74% to 80% of patients and functional improvement in 69% to 71% of patients with chronic back pain from degenerative disc disease in the lumbar[32] and cervical spine.[33] Another study of ESI showed pain relief lasting 6 months for spinal stenosis, which was significantly better than controls.[34]

Several factors have been identified as decreasing the success rate of treatment for back pain. Imprecise medication delivery is an obvious cause of failed treatment that can be virtually eliminated with the use of radiologic guidance.[35] Patient factors also affect success. Patients with a greater number of previous treatments, greater dependence on pain medications, pain not increased with activity, and pain increased by cough all report less benefit from ESI.[36] Socioeconomic factors such as employment status and smoking also play a role.[37] In general, patients with secondary gains from remaining "ill" have lower success rates for all treatments.[36,37]

COMPLICATIONS

Overall, complications of epidural injections are quite low,[38-41] but catastrophic events including paralysis and death have been documented.[41,42] There are specific complications associated with these techniques. Awareness of the possible complications and vigilance for them can lead to early detection, hopefully before a serious adverse event occurs.

Postdural Puncture Headache

Headache is a common complication of any spinal or epidural procedure. Its prevalence has been reported as high as 30% following epidural anesthesia, lumbar puncture, and myelography. Symptoms typically arise within 48 hours of the procedure and usually resolve in about 3 to 7 days with minimal treatment. Postdural puncture headache (PDPH) is thought to arise from CSF leakage producing mild intracranial hypotension and traction on the meninges.[43] Use of needles smaller than 22 gauge has a decreased incidence of PDPH, because the potential dural tear is smaller. Conservative management consists of bed rest, hydration, and oral analgesics, including caffeine. In some cases, persistent PDPH necessitates use of an epidural blood patch, which is thought to work by increasing CSF pressure and sealing the dural tear, preventing further CSF leakage.[44] In the event of dural puncture, some patients are at higher risk for PDPH. Younger patients are much more prone to PDPH, but it is rarely seen in patients older than 60. Women are twice as likely as men to suffer PDPH, and patients with prior headaches are more prone. Lastly, thin patients (low body mass index) are at higher risk.[43]

Intrathecal Injection

Needle tip penetration of the dura can result in medication being introduced into the intrathecal space. Dural tear may be insidious and unnoticed during needle placement. Intrathecal local anesthetic can lead to spinal anesthesia with significant motor and sensory blockade, the duration of which depends on the local anesthetic agent used. Dense blockade of sympathetic fibers can cause significant hypotension, particularly with cervical injection but also with thoracic injection. For cervical injections, total spinal is also possible, causing immediate respiratory compromise. It is crucial to have emergency airway and resuscitation equipment at hand when performing these procedures. These risks stem from the local anesthetic component of the epidural injectate. Thus some clinicians elect to use only saline to dilute the steroid, especially in the cervical spine. Intrathecal Depo-Medrol injection has been suggested to cause arachnoiditis, but this may be related to the preservatives in the preparation.[45] Other steroid preparations, preservative-free solutions, or perhaps lower doses may not be harmful.[46]

Epidural Abscess and Meningitis

Although rare, infectious complications of epidural injections are potentially catastrophic. Overall mortality of purulent meningitis has been reported as 21%, and spinal procedures are a significant iatrogenic cause. The most common offending pathogens are *Staphylococcus* and other skin flora, reinforcing the importance of meticulous sterile technique. Management of infection consists of aggressive antibiotic therapy and possible surgical intervention for epidural abscess.[47]

Epidural Hematoma

As mentioned earlier, bleeding diatheses are an absolute contraindication to epidural injection. Epidural hematoma can happen acutely and result in significant spinal cord compression, paralysis, or cauda equina syndrome. Early recognition is crucial. Any suspicion of hematoma from worsened back pain, loss of extremity function, incontinence, and the like should warrant immediate neurosurgical consultation for possible evacuation.[48]

Paralysis/Anterior Spinal Artery Syndrome

There have been multiple case reports of permanent neurologic injury and spinal cord infarction following both midline ESI and transforaminal injections. The offending event has usually been a cervical transforaminal injection. Presumably there was injection into the vertebral artery or into a radicular artery feeding into the vertebral system, or direct injury to the artery.[49] Cervicomedullary ischemia resembling anterior spinal artery syndrome then resulted. Pathology studies have shown that the brain injury is likely due to hemorrhagic infarction induced by the depot carrier, and not necessary embolism from the particulate matter.[50] Embolic infarction can also occur with injection of air.[41] Paralytic complications are not limited to the cervical spine. Lumbar transforaminal injections have also caused paralysis from anterior spinal artery syndrome.[42]

Systemic Steroid Toxicity

As with any treatment involving steroids, systemic toxicity should be considered, and frequent use can result in adrenal suppression.[9,11] Commonly observed side effects include flushing, transient (weeks) elevations in blood pressure and blood glucose, and pedal edema.[11]

POSTPROCEDURE CARE AND FOLLOW-UP

Immediately following an ESI procedure with local anesthetic, a patient should be monitored in a recovery area for at least 15 minutes if lidocaine is used, 30 minutes for bupivacaine. During this time, the effectiveness of the injection can be assessed and compared to baseline findings, and any signs of complications can be detected. A neurologic exam should be performed, and patients should be asked to walk under observation before discharge.

Patients should be reassessed in 2 to 3 weeks. In some cases, a single injection will provide adequate relief indefinitely. In others where relief may be temporary, additional injections may be appropriate. Repeat injections should be based on patient response rather than a standardized treatment plan.[9] In general, practitioners recommend no more than three steroid injections within a 6-month period to limit systemic side effects.[11] Nonetheless, a wide range of practices with regard to dose, frequency, volume, and techniques for ESI exists.

KEY POINTS

- Epidural steroid injections are a widely used treatment for many painful lumbar spinal syndromes including radiculopathy, spinal stenosis, degenerative disk disease, postlaminectomy pain syndrome, spondylosis, and even undefined low back pain.

- Steroids can be injected into the cervical, thoracic, or lumbar epidural space. Anatomic location should match the pathology.

- There are three approaches to the epidural space: midline interlaminar, lateral transforaminal, and caudal. Selection of a particular technique should be based on the patient's symptoms, pathology, and anatomy.

- Radiologic guidance, fluoroscopy, or computed tomography greatly improve the success rate of any approach and reduce risk.

▶ **SUGGESTED READINGS**

Manchikanti L, Boswell MV, Singh V, et al. Comprehensive evidence-based guidelines for interventional techniques in the management of chronic spinal pain. Pain Phys 2009;12(4):699–802.

McLain RF, Kapural L, Mekhail NA. Epidural steroids for back and leg pain: mechanism of action and efficacy. Cleve Clin J Med 2004;71: 961–70.

Nelemans PJ, de Bie RA, de Vet HC, Sturmans F. Injection therapy for subacute and chronic benign low back pain. Cochrane Database Syst Rev 2000;CD001824.

Waldman S. Cervical epidural nerve block. In: Waldman SD, editor. Interventional Pain Management. 2nd ed. Philadelphia: W.B. Saunders Co; 2001. p. 373–81.

Waldman S. Lumbar epidural nerve block. In: Waldman SD, editor. Interventional Pain Management. 2nd ed. Philadelphia; W.B. Saunders Co; 2001. p. 415–22.

The complete reference list is available online at www.expertconsult.com.

CHAPTER 169

Image-Guided Intervention for Symptomatic Tarlov Cysts

Juan Carlos Baez, Gerald M. Wyse, and Kieran P.J. Murphy

Symptomatic Tarlov cysts cause chronic pelvic and lower extremity pain. These cysts may be large and can expand the spinal canal or cause erosion of overlying bone. Patel et al. describe a single-needle approach to Tarlov cysts in which they inject fibrin adhesive to treat the cyst.[1] This is a three-stage procedure: (1) cyst entry and aspiration, (2) injection of myelographic contrast material to ensure that a wide neck is not present, and (3) injection of tissue adhesive. Many of our initial patients were treated by this standard technique and experienced considerable pain that required significant sedation with fentanyl and midazolam. We believe this pain was caused by a flux in pressure in the cystic cavity during aspiration of the injected substances.

On reflection, it became apparent a two-needle technique was necessary. This method requires access with one needle placed superficially in the cyst and the other at the deepest point of the cyst. The superficial needle is placed to allow venting of any pressure or volume change within the system, and the deeper needle is used as the working lumen. Although the patient's pain once limited the volume we could aspirate or inject into a Tarlov cyst, we can now drain and fill it completely with minimal patient discomfort.

We have also been able to eliminate the need for myelographic contrast material. If the cyst is wide necked and communicates with the cerebrospinal fluid (CSF) space, it refills after drainage, and we do not inject tissue adhesive. This has allowed us to aspirate large (3- to 6-mL) Tarlov cysts, usually at the S2-S3 level, in a virtually pain-free fashion under computed tomography (CT) fluoroscopic guidance.

INDICATIONS

Patients with Tarlov cysts are complex to manage and have innumerable complaints. In our experience, narrow-necked Tarlov cysts may be symptomatic, whereas wide-necked Tarlov cysts are not. They can be differentiated by their T2 signal on magnetic resonance imaging (MRI). Wide-necked cysts have the same signal as the general CSF space around the cord, but narrow-necked cysts have higher signal than the adjacent CSF space. In 1993, Davis et al. published evidence of signal change within symptomatic cysts.[2] Their paper demonstrated that in 19 patients with 24 cysts, narrow-necked cysts were consistently more symptomatic than wide-necked cysts. The only patients we have treated with our CT-guided technique (now > 90 patients in the last 2 years) have been symptomatic with narrow-necked cysts. We have also treated patients with symptomatic wide-necked lesions who had previously undergone surgical repair and subsequently developed persistent CSF leaks.

It is not simple political correctness to state that careful patient selection, a multidisciplinary approach, and long-term follow-up and management are necessary in these patients. It is absolutely essential that scientific rigor be applied to this treatment paradigm. All patients are reviewed by both a professor of neurosurgery with an extensive career in spine pathology, and an associate professor of interventional neuroradiology. Patients are categorized into three types:

1. Good candidates with narrow-necked cysts go straight to fibrin injection under CT fluoroscopy.
2. Surgical candidates with wide-necked cysts proceed to surgical repair.
3. Candidates for whom a consensus cannot be reached undergo CT myelography with early and delayed imaging to examine the cyst neck. They are then treated appropriately according to the first two paradigms.

We switched to the two-needle technique when it became clear the pressure flux in the wall of the cyst induced severe pain in our patients. The two-needle technique not only markedly reduced patient discomfort and requirements for conscious sedation during the procedure, it also increased the amount of fibrin glue we could inject. We are conducting an ongoing study of this technique at our institution with institutional review board approval, and we will be publishing the results in future papers. The two-needle approach to aspiration and injection of any hollow viscus or joint space should be considered, whether it be a Tarlov cyst, a gallbladder, an abscess, an intracranial ventricle, or an arthrogram.

CONTRAINDICATIONS

Small Tarlov cysts (<1.5 cm) are rarely symptomatic. Surgical candidates with wide-necked cysts should undergo surgical repair.

EQUIPMENT

CT or CT fluoroscopy is necessary to identify the cyst and perform the two-needle technique safely. Fibrin glue is also needed and is available from the blood bank.

TECHNIQUE

We explain the technique by using a classic case we treated.

A 64-year-old woman had chronic pelvic and lower extremity pain, principally on the left side, that caused her to be bedridden for 20 hours a day for the previous 18 months. The patient, a highly functioning retired nurse with no psychological issues, required constant narcotic medication for severe pain. Informed consent was obtained, and we prepared and draped her back in the usual fashion. Local anesthesia was infiltrated into the skin, fat, and muscles underlying the left side of the sacrum. It is our habit to anesthetize the skin, fat, and periosteum overlying the cyst with an 18-gauge spinal needle. If the overlying bone is too thick to penetrate with an 18-gauge needle, we go coaxially through a 13-gauge spinal needle.

Diagnostic CT was performed to identify the lesion (Fig. 169-1). After the level of the lesion was determined, visualization was achieved with CT fluoroscopy at 13 frames a second and three levels with 4-mm slice thickness. Two 18-gauge needles were advanced in a parallel orientation into the cyst. The first was placed deep, and the second was placed superficially in the cyst. The patient experienced minimal pain at the point where the needles were passing through the dura and some minimal overlying residual thin lamina. The stylets were then removed from both needles. Through the deeper needle, we aspirated 5 mL of initially slightly blood-tinged and later clear fluid from the cyst (Figs. 169-2 and 169-3). During this aspiration, the more superficial needle acted as a vent tube, and air was seen to fill the cyst. The patient did not experience pain during this

procedure. We subsequently watched the cyst intermittently under CT fluoroscopy because we have found that wide-necked cysts will refill. If the cyst is narrow necked or has a ball valve, air persists in the cyst cavity, which allows us to fill it with fibrin glue with a greater degree of confidence. Since we have developed this technique, we have ceased injecting myelographic contrast material into the cyst and instead rely on the stability of the height of the air/fluid level in the cyst to indicate a narrow neck.

We then sequentially injected 4 mL of Tisseel VH fibrin glue (Baxter Healthcare Corp., Westlake Village, Calif.) into the cyst cavity (Fig. 169-4). Appropriate filling of the cyst is judged by development of symptoms or pain, thereby indicating that we are distending the cavity. This is usually synchronous with reflux of the fibrin glue back up the second needle. In this case, the patient experienced no pain, and we stopped the injection once we saw on CT fluoroscopy that the cavity was filled with fibrin material and some

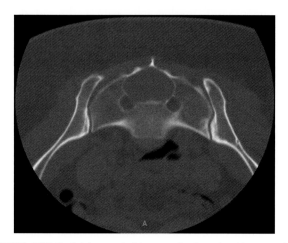

FIGURE 169-1. Axial computed tomography through mid-sacrum demonstrates a large cyst with extensive bony remodeling.

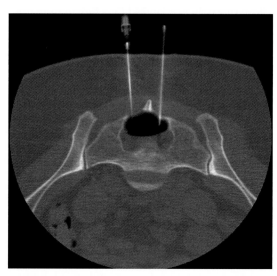

FIGURE 169-3. Axial computed tomography after aspiration of cyst demonstrates air/fluid level that remained stable for several minutes, indicative of a narrow-necked cyst.

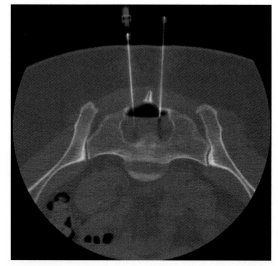

FIGURE 169-2. Axial computed tomography after placement of two 18-gauge spinal needles within cyst. One needle is placed deep for aspiration and the second superficially to act as a venting tube.

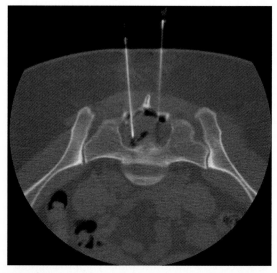

FIGURE 169-4. Axial computed tomography after fibrin glue injection.

material was coming back up the 18-gauge needle. We then removed both needles and dressed the puncture sites with bacitracin ointment and Opsite TM (Smith & Nephew, Inc., Largo, Fla.). The patient was subsequently placed on a gurney and returned to the holding area. She was observed for 1.5 hours as part of our conscious sedation protocol and then discharged home. On follow-up 8 days later, she was completely pain free and able to stop taking all her narcotics.

CONTROVERSIES

Although Tarlov cysts were first described in 1938, controversy still exists regarding whether aspiration or surgical intervention provides a therapeutic benefit for symptomatic patients.[3,4] Anecdotal evidence has suggested that recurrence of symptoms and surgical complications limit the benefits of surgery, but Voyadzis et al. showed statistically significant improvement with surgery in a series of 10 patients with Tarlov cysts.[4] Other studies have also supported the use of cyst fenestration.[5] The literature regarding the efficacy of aspiration and fibrin glue therapy remains mixed. We believe our method relieves symptoms in properly selected patients and is associated with minimal patient discomfort and morbidity. As noted earlier, results of our ongoing study of this technique at our institution will be published in future papers.

OUTCOMES

We report our experience with image-guided therapy for symptomatic Tarlov cysts in this section. Three- and 12-month follow-up of 30 patients treated by CT fluoroscopy-guided aspiration and fibrin glue injection was obtained. Thirty patients, 29 female and 1 male, were reviewed by an experienced neurosurgeon and interventional neuroradiologists.

We established three patient groups at initial screening: (1) candidates with imaging characteristics consistent with narrow-necked cysts on CT myelography or MRI were offered fibrin injection under CT fluoroscopy guidance, (2) candidates with imaging characteristics consistent with wide-necked cysts on CT myelography or MRI underwent surgical repair, and (3) those in whom we could not determine cyst neck diameter based on their imaging underwent CT myelography with early and delayed imaging to examine the cyst neck. They were then treated appropriately as described earlier.

A two-needle technique was used to overcome the weakness of the traditional single-needle approach. As already described, this method requires access with one needle placed superficially in the cyst and the other at the deepest point of the cyst, allowing pressure to remain nearly constant during the procedure and markedly reducing procedural pain.

Three-month follow-up was available on 30 patients: 63% were significantly better (19/30), 20% were the same (6/30), 13% were a little worse (4/30), and 3% were significantly worse (1/30). Twelve-month follow-up was available on 12 patients: 66% were significantly better, 16% were better, 8% were the same, and one patient was lost to follow-up. In none of our patients did aseptic meningitis develop after fibrin injection. We have now treated 88 Tarlov cysts in total and believe this is an interesting technique that delivers significant pain relief to an overlooked patient population.

COMPLICATIONS

No complications developed in any of our patients after fibrin injection to treat Tarlov cysts. The first paper by Patel et al. describing the single-needle technique, on the other hand, reported that aseptic meningitis developed in three of four patients.[1] We have published our results in the peer-reviewed literature.[6,7]

POSTPROCEDURAL AND FOLLOW-UP CARE

It is critical that these complex patients be monitored with serial office visits and telephone consultations.

KEY POINTS

- Tarlov cysts with narrow necks can be symptomatic.
- Narrow-necked cysts have higher signal than cerebrospinal fluid around the cord on T2-weighted magnetic resonance imaging.
- Fibrin glue placement is a successful therapy in appropriate patients.

▶ **SUGGESTED READINGS**

Acostav FL Jr, Quinones-Hinojosa A, Schmidt MH, Weinstein PR. Diagnosis and management of sacral Tarlov cysts. Case report and review of the literature. Neurosurg Focus 2003;15:E15.

Voyadzis JM, Bhargava P, Henderson FC. Tarlov cysts: a study of 10 cases with review of the literature. J Neurosurg 2001;95(Suppl 1):25–32.

The complete reference list is available online at www.expertconsult.com.

CHAPTER 170

Scalene Blocks and Their Role in Thoracic Outlet Syndrome

Juan Carlos Baez, Kieran P.J. Murphy, and Brian M. Block

Thoracic outlet syndrome (TOS) is a constellation of symptoms caused by compression of neurovascular structures as they traverse the superior thoracic outlet.[1] TOS can have neural components, vascular components, or both, and its causes include trauma, repetitive stress injury, congenital abnormalities, or combinations of these (e.g., congenital cervical rib combined with repetitive stress injury).[2,3] Vascular TOS is straightforward and can be documented by arteriography. Compression of the subclavian vessels leads to swelling, edema, and loss of blood flow to the upper extremity, particularly with exertion. Neurogenic TOS (nTOS) is more ambiguous. In nTOS the brachial plexus is presumably compressed, and such compression gives rise to pain, numbness, heaviness or other dysesthesia, and weakness in the upper extremity.[4] Electrodiagnostic studies may be abnormal in nTOS patients, but only in a minority, and results vary over time.[5] Given that many conditions (e.g., cervical radiculopathy, cervical spondylosis, shoulder joint and tendon pathology, myofascial pain syndrome, peripheral neuropathy, etc.) can lead to arm or neck pain, diagnosis of nTOS can prove difficult.

Treatment of nTOS is also controversial. The brachial plexus can be decompressed by either transaxillary or supraclavicular approaches. A recent case series of 170 patients showed that decompression was successful 65% of the time.[6] Interestingly, Landry et al.[7] monitored 79 patients with "disputed TOS" who had symptoms of nTOS but no electrodiagnostic confirmation. Fifteen of the patients underwent decompressive surgery at other centers, and the remaining 64 were managed nonoperatively. Outcome was no better or worse with surgery. Given these results, patient selection for surgery is crucial. Jordan and Machleder showed that temporary relaxation of the anterior scalene muscle (ASM) with an injection of local anesthetic can predict which patients will benefit from decompression.[8] The ASM lies directly anterior to the trunks of the brachial plexus (Fig. 170-1, A). Presumably, relaxation of the ASM temporarily "decompresses" the plexus, thereby predicting the results of surgical decompression. For the injection to be predictive, anesthesia of the adjacent plexus and sympathetic chain must be avoided. Jordan and Machleder used electromyography to position the needle directly in the ASM. The positive predictive value of their injections was excellent; 30 of 32 (94%) patients who received relief from the temporary block achieved a good outcome from surgical decompression. The negative predictive value was less impressive. Six patients underwent surgery despite a negative ASM block, and 3 (50%) had a good outcome from decompression.[8] They also found that chemodenervation with botulinum toxin leads to sustained relief with a duration of 88 days, consistent with the duration of chemodenervation.[9]

Because we have extensive experience using computed tomography (CT) and CT fluoroscopy for interventional procedures, we developed a CT-guided technique for ASM injection. All patients underwent a block as part of the workup for nTOS. These patients had a high pretest probability of TOS, given they had been referred for treatment of suspected nTOS.

A great advantage of CT-guided injection is that it facilitates fast, reliable, and accurate injection of local anesthetic into the ASM. The scans clearly show whether the local anesthetic is leaking out of the ASM and thus should be highly specific. As for safety, no complications occurred in the initial 14 patients. These numbers are small, but CT provides an excellent safety profile because nearby vital structures (internal jugular vein, carotid artery, cervical neuroforamina, vertebral artery, lung) can be seen and avoided.

These data are preliminary. Too few patients have proceeded to surgery on the basis of CT-guided ASM injections for sensitivity, specificity, and positive and negative predictive values to be calculated. However, these injections should be at least as good as electromyelography-guided injections.[8] To be clear, pain relief after ASM injection is not the gold standard for the diagnosis of TOS. Congenital abnormalities may compress the neurovascular bundle at the thoracic inlet, or the compression may be distal to the ASM.[10] However, pain relief after ASM injection does predict the outcome of surgical decompression.[8] A positive response to ASM injection will reassure patients and their surgeons that the operation is likely to be successful, whereas negative responses can spare other patients needless surgery.

CT-guided ASM injections are a novel approach to the diagnosis and treatment of nTOS. Further work must be done to determine the prognostic value of this technique and monitor for complications. The utility of chemodenervation with botulinum toxin via CT-guided injection also remains to be elucidated.

INDICATIONS

Neurogenic TOS is thought to be secondary to brachial plexus compression. In addition to pain, numbness, heaviness, and dysesthesia of the upper extremity, there can be atrophy of the thenar eminence, ulnar intrinsic hand musculature, and forearm muscles. Median sensory nerve function is intact, but the median nerve–mediated compound muscle action potential in the thenar eminence is reduced. Median antebrachial cutaneous nerve findings should be reduced or absent. Finally, the amplitude of the ulnar sensory nerve action potential is reduced. Unfortunately, although electrodiagnostic studies can indicate

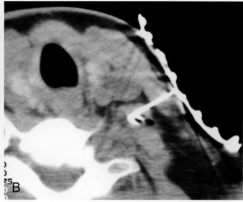

FIGURE 170-1. A, Computed tomography image at C6 level. A 22-gauge spinal needle has been in left anterior scalene muscle (ASM), and tomographic marker tape is visible on skin. **B,** ASM after injection of 0.25 mL iohexol (Omnipaque).

abnormalities, they are abnormal in only a minority of patients with symptoms of nTOS, and the results can change over time.[5] The lack of reliability of electrodiagnostic studies coupled with the multitude of pathologies resulting in arm and neck pain make the diagnosis of nTOS difficult.

CONTRAINDICATIONS

Contraindications to ASM injection include allergies to the local anesthetic or Botox. The patient must also be a reliable subject to determine the therapeutic efficacy of the injection.

EQUIPMENT

CT, CT fluoroscopy, or ultrasound can be used for the image-guided injections. The majority of these injections were performed with CT fluoroscopy, which has multiple advantages over conventional CT. More than 1 million CT-guided biopsy and drainage procedures are performed each year in the United States. However, unlike ultrasound and conventional x-ray fluoroscopy, conventional CT is unable to provide real-time guidance capability. In conventional CT-guided procedures, the operator positions the needle and steps out of the room to image the needle, thereby resulting in longer procedure times because multiple CT scans are needed to confirm appropriate needle or catheter position. CT fluoroscopy combines the benefits of conventional CT with the added value of real-time imaging capabilities. This imaging modality was first reported by Katada, Kato, et al. in the mid-1990s and has since developed into a powerful imaging tool with widespread application.[11-15] Recent advances in CT technology have led to development of new applications for CT fluoroscopy. In CT fluoroscopy, images are reconstructed and displayed every 0.17 second. Our CT scanner can be run by the operator from the tableside during a procedure, similar to an x-ray fluoroscopy suite. Three slices are acquired simultaneously: one centered and one each 4 mm cephalad and caudad to the central image. Each image is displayed simultaneously on a plasma screen monitor at the bedside at 13 frames per second. The physician operates the CT scanner from the tableside with a foot pedal to trigger imaging. We use intermittent imaging, but continuous imaging is also

possible. Continuous imaging offers optimal visualization during a procedure but results in greater radiation dosage to both the operator and patient.[16] We have used CT fluoroscopy for other interventional pain procedures as well, including sacroiliac joint injections and thoracic and lumbar nerve root blocks.[17] CT fluoroscopy is especially helpful for getting to "deep" structures such as the celiac plexus, splanchnic nerves, and superior hypogastric plexus.

TECHNIQUE

Anatomy and Approach

Patients were examined before the ASM block. Particular attention was paid to the neurologic and musculoskeletal examination. Data collected included strength, sensation, reflexes, radial pulses, provocative pain maneuvers including an elevated arm stress test, and the costoclavicular maneuver. Informed consent was obtained. Patients were placed supine on the CT gantry. In the first five patients, lateral tomograms were obtained and CT images were taken from the C4 to the T1 levels. In the remaining patients, a single scout CT image was taken at the level of the cricoid cartilage (C6). The ASM was identified as the muscle adjacent to the C6 articular pillar and anterior to the neuroforamen (see Fig. 170-1, A). Tomographic marker tape was placed on the neck. Extension tubing was connected to the needle before insertion to minimize needle movement after it was in the ASM. Under CT guidance, the needle was inserted through the skin and then into the ASM (see Fig. 170-1, A). Iohexol (Omnipaque 180) diluted 1:1 with preservative-free normal saline was injected once the needle was positioned in the ASM (Fig. 170-1, B). CT images showed the contrast agent within the ASM for 3 cm of cephalad-to-caudad imaging (Fig. 170-2). Finally, 2 mL of 0.25% bupivacaine with 16 mg of triamcinolone was injected.

OUTCOMES

Fourteen diagnostic injections have been performed in 14 patients thus far, along with one therapeutic injection of botulinum toxin (Botox) into one of the patients. Figures 170-1, 170-2, and 170-3 show representative CT images

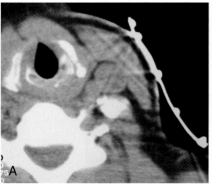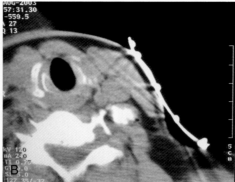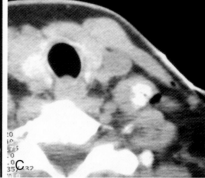

FIGURE 170-2. A, Same patient as in Figure 170-1 after injection of 2 mL bupivacaine and triamcinolone. Image was taken 10 mm cephalad of needle entry into anterior scalene muscle. **B,** Computed tomography (CT) image 15 mm caudad of image in **A. C,** CT image 15 mm more caudad than image in **B.**

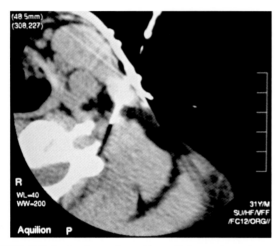

FIGURE 170-3. Another patient with needle in anterior scalene muscle for injection.

from the injections. Figure 170-2 clearly shows that the injectate is contained within the ASM along its length. Consistent with the usual demographics of nTOS patients, 93% were women. The average age was 39.7 ± 2.1 years (range, 25-52).

The blocks were easily accomplished in the CT suite, with the last five blocks taking roughly 15 minutes in the CT room. Needle placement appears to be no more painful than other injections for chronic pain. As seen in all populations of chronic pain patients, a minority report significant pain during the procedure, whereas others report none. No complications have occurred thus far, other than pain during needle placement. Two patients reported numbness in the hand appearing 15 minutes after the injection, probably caused by leakage of local anesthetic out of the muscle and onto the brachial plexus. The numbness was seen with the initial blocks in which we used 2.5 mL total volume of injectate. We have since reduced the total volume of local anesthetic to 2 mL and not had any patients report numbness.

COMPLICATIONS

Complications of ASM injections include potential phrenic nerve injury, dysphagia, pneumothorax, brachial plexus block or injury, and vertebral or carotid injection.

POSTPROCEDURAL AND FOLLOW-UP CARE

Close postprocedural follow-up is needed to ensure that the impact of the Botox injection and the implications of such injection on the risk/benefit ratio of surgical intervention are well understood. The great weakness of radiology is patient follow-up, and that will undermine and end any pain intervention program. Office staff must be available to ensure follow-up is performed.

KEY POINTS

- Thoracic outlet syndrome has both neural and vascular components.
- Image guidance is critical.
- Computed tomography (CT), CT fluoroscopy, or ultrasound can be used.
- Avoid the phrenic nerve, and know the anatomy.

▶ SUGGESTED READINGS

Braun RM, Sahadevan DC, Feinstein J. Confirmatory needle placement technique for scalene muscle block in the diagnosis of thoracic outlet syndrome. Tech Hand Up Extrem Surg 2006;10:173–6.

Demondion X, Herbinet P, Van Sint Jan S, et al. Imaging assessment of thoracic outlet syndrome. Radiographics 2006;26:1735–50.

Huang JH, Zager EL. Thoracic outlet syndrome. Neurosurgery 2004;55: 897–902.

The complete reference list is available online at www.expertconsult.com.

Index

Note: Page numbers followed by f indicate figures; those followed by t indicate tables.